	atropine	butorphanol (Stadol)	chlordiazepoxide (Librium)	chlorpromazine (Thorazine)	cimetidine (Tagamet)	codeine	dimenhydrinate (Dramamine)	diphenhydramine (Benadryl)	glycopyrrolate (Robinul)	heparin	hydromorphone (Dilaudid)	hydroxyzine (Vistaril)	meperidine (Demerol)	metoclopramide (Reglan)	morphine	nalbuphine (Nubain)	pentazocine (Talwin)	promethazine (Phenergan)	scopolamine	trimethobenzamide (Tigan)
atropine	—	C	I	C	C	U	C	C	C	U	C	C	C	C	C	C	C	C	C	U
butorphanol (Stadol)	C	—	I	C	U	U	I	C	U	U	U	C	C	U	C	U	U	C	C	U
chlordiazepoxide (Librium)	I	I	—	I	I	I	I	I	I	U	I	I	I	I	I	I	I	I	I	I
chlorpromazine (Thorazine)	C	C	I	—	U	U	I	C	C	U	C	C	C	C	C	U	C	C	C	U
cimetidine (Tagamet)	C	U	I	U	—	U	U	U	U	C	U	U	U	U	U	U	U	U	U	U
codeine	U	U	I	U	U	—	U	U	C	I	U	C	U	U	U	U	U	U	U	U
dimenhydrinate (Dramamine)	C	I	I	I	U	U	—	C	I	U	U	I	C	C	C	U	U	I	U	U
diphenhydramine (Benadryl)	C	C	I	C	U	U	C	—	C	U	C	C	C	C	C	U	C	C	C	U
glycopyrrolate (Robinul)	C	U	I	C	U	C	I	C	—	U	C	C	C	U	C	U	I	C	C	C
heparin	U	U	U	U	C	I	U	U	U	—	U	U	I	U	I	U	U	I	U	U
hydromorphone (Dilaudid)	C	U	I	C	U	U	U	C	C	U	—	C	U	U	U	U	U	C	C	U
hydroxyzine (Vistaril)	C	C	I	C	U	C	I	C	C	U	C	—	C	C	C	C	C	C	C	U
meperidine (Demerol)	C	C	I	C	U	U	C	C	C	I	U	C	—	C	I	U	C	C	C	U
metoclopramide (Reglan)	C	U	I	C	U	U	C	C	C	U	C	C	C	—	C	U	C	C	C	U
morphine	C	C	I	C	U	U	C	C	C	I	U	C	I	C	—	U	C	C	C	U
nalbuphine (Nubain)	C	U	I	U	U	U	U	U	U	U	C	U	U	U	U	—	U	C	C	C
pentazocine (Talwin)	C	U	I	C	U	U	U	C	I	U	U	C	C	C	C	U	—	C	C	U
promethazine (Phenergan)	C	C	I	C	U	U	I	C	C	I	C	C	C	C	C	C	C	—	C	U
scopolamine	C	C	I	C	U	U	C	C	C	U	C	C	C	C	C	C	C	C	—	U
trimethobenzamide (Tigan)	U	U	I	U	U	U	U	U	C	U	U	U	U	U	U	C	U	U	U	—

C, Compatible; **I**, incompatible; **U**, unknown or conflicting data.

MOSBY'S
Pharmacology
in
Nursing

MOSBY'S
Pharmacology in Nursing

LEDA M. McKENRY, R.N., M.S.N., M.B.A.

Associate Professor, University of Miami School of Nursing, Miami, Florida;
Director, University of Miami School of Nursing at Hextall Court, United Kingdom

EVELYN SALERNO, Pharm.D.

Associate Professor, Southeastern College of Pharmaceutical Sciences, North Miami Beach, Florida;
Associate Professor, Southeastern College of Osteopathic Medicine, North Miami Beach, Florida;
Director of Pharmacy Services, Hospice, Inc., Miami, Florida

With Contributions by

MARK C. HAMELINK, R.N., M.S.N., C.R.N.A., C.C.R.N.

Clinical Assistant Professor, The University of Texas Health Science Center, School of Nursing,
Houston, Texas

SEVENTEENTH EDITION

with **168** illustrations

The C. V. Mosby Company

ST. LOUIS • PHILADELPHIA • BALTIMORE • TORONTO   1989

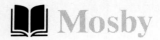

Acquiring editor: Don Ladig
Developmental editor: Robin Carter
Project manager: Mark Spann
Production editors: Stephen C. Hetager, Maureen Kenison, Barbara Terrell,
        Mary Wright, Suzanne Aboulfadl
Designer: John Rokusek

SEVENTEENTH EDITION

The C.V. Mosby Company
11830 Westline Industrial Drive, St. Louis, Missouri 63146

Library of Congress Cataloging–in–Publication Data

McKenry, Leda M.
    Mosby's pharmacology in nursing. — 17th ed./Leda M. McKenry,
Evelyn Salerno; with contributions by Mark C. Hamelink.
        p. cm.
    Rev. ed. of: Mosby's pharmacology in nursing/Anne Burgess Hahn,
Sandy Jeanne Klarman Oestreich, Robert L. Barkin. 16th ed. 1986.
    Includes bibliographies and index.
    ISBN 0-8016-3294-3
    1. Pharmacology. 2. Nursing. I. Salerno, Evelyn. II. Hamelink,
Mark C. III. Hahn, Anne Burgess. Mosby's pharmacology in nursing.
IV. Title. V. Title: Pharmacology in nursing.
    [DNLM: 1. Pharmacology — nurses' instruction. QV 4 M478m]
RM301.M39 1989
615'.1 — dc19
DNLM/DLC
for Library of Congress   89-2960
                                                                 CIP

TS/VH/VH   9   8   7   6   5   4   3   2

Nursing Consultants

Jean Krajicek Bartek, R.N., M.S.N.
University of Nebraska, Omaha, Nebraska

Ruth Bowen, R.N., M.S.
Texas Woman's University, Denton, Texas

Marilyn Edmunds, R.N., Ph.D.
The University of Maryland, Baltimore, Maryland

Mary Gardner, R.N., M.S.
The University of Lowell, Lowell, Massachusetts

Marion F. Hale, R.N., M.S.N.
Georgia State University, Atlanta, Georgia

Mark C. Hamelink, R.N., M.S.N., C.R.N.A., C.C.R.N.
The University of Texas Health Science Center, Houston,
Texas

Donna Ignatavicius, R.N., M.S.
DI Associates, Baltimore, Maryland

Marlene Lindeman, R.N., M.S.N.
University of Nebraska, Omaha, Nebraska

Barbara MacDermott, R.N., M.S.
Syracuse University, Syracuse, New York

Edwina McConnell, R.N., Ph.D.
Nurse Consultant, Madison, Wisconsin

Andrew McPhee, R.N.
Windham Regional Technical School, Willimantic, Connecticut

Susan Meeker, R.N., M.S.N.
St. Clair County Community College, Port Huron, Michigan

Michaelene Mirr, R.N., M.S.N., Ph.D. candidate
University of Wisconsin, Eau Claire, Wisconsin

Patricia Gonce Morton, R.N., M.S.
The University of Maryland, Baltimore, Maryland

Judith Myers, R.N., M.S.N.
St. Louis University, St. Louis, Missouri

Marian Newton, R.N., M.N.
Albany Veterans Administration Medical Center, Albany, New
York

Michelle Poradzisz, R.N., M.S.
DePaul University, Chicago, Illinois

Kathy Sindmack, R.N., M.S.
San Bernardino Valley College, San Bernardino, California

Yvonne Stock, R.N., M.N.
Iowa Western Community College, Council Bluffs, Iowa

Verlee Sutherlin, R.N., M.S.N., M.Ed.
Spokane Community College, Spokane, Washington

Mary Vande Berg, R.N., M.S.N.
Northern Michigan University, Marquette, Michigan

Richard E. Watters, R.N.
Grande Prairie Regional College, Grande Prairie, Alberta

Sheila Rankin Zerr, R.N., M.Ed.
University of Victoria, Victoria, British Columbia

Pharmacology Consultants

Carmen Aceves-Blumenthal, M.S.
Southeastern College of Pharmaceutical Sciences, North Miami Beach, Florida

Bruce Ackerman, Pharm.D.
University of Arkansas for Medical Sciences, Little Rock, Arkansas

James H. Culley, Pharm.D.
University of Arkansas for Medical Sciences, Little Rock, Arkansas

William Gerthoffer, Ph.D.
University of Nevada, School of Medicine, Reno, Nevada

Patricia Howard, R.Ph
University of Kansas Medical Center, Kansas City, Kansas

Keith Olsen, Pharm.D.
University of Arkansas for Medical Sciences, Little Rock, Arkansas

Harry E. Peery, R.N., Ph.D. candidate
University of Toronto, Toronto, Ontario

Alphonse Poklis, Ph.D.
Medical College of Virginia, Richmond, Virginia

Katherine Stefos, Ph.D., R.Ph.
M.D. Anderson Hospital and Tumor Institute, Houston, Texas

Scott Swigart, Pharm.D.
University of Nebraska Medical Center, Omaha, Nebraska

Cherie K. Whitmore, Pharm.D.
Hoechst-Roussel Pharmaceuticals, Inc., Somerville, New Jersey

Ronald A. Young, Pharm.D.
University of Arkansas for Medical Sciences, Little Rock, Arkansas

Preface

HISTORICAL PERSPECTIVE

Mosby's Pharmacology in Nursing has a long history of providing the nursing student, nurse educator, and practicing nurse with thorough and up-to-date pharmacology and nursing management. Currently in its seventeenth edition, *Pharmacology in Nursing* has its roots in *A Textbook of Materia Medica for Nurses* by A.L. Muirhead, published in 1919. In 1936 Hugh Alister McGuigan became the primary author, at which time the book was renamed *Materia Medica and Pharmacology.* In 1940 Elsie E. Krug joined McGuigan as coauthor, a role she was to hold until 1948 when she became the primary author. The book was renamed *Pharmacology in Nursing* in 1955, after ten successful editions. In all of its previous editions, *Pharmacology in Nursing* has sold nearly 2,000,000 copies, making it the most widely used and successful nursing pharmacology textbook book ever published.

THE REVISION

This edition of *Mosby's Pharmacology in Nursing* is intended for both the nursing student and the nurse practitioner. It is also useful to professionals in other health-related areas, as well as to readers wishing an in-depth consideration of the pharmacology of therapeutic drugs. We trust that this book's broad scientific approach to the subject will provide a basis for the understanding of drug therapy now and in the future.

This edition has been thoroughly revised and updated. The **focus** is on basic concepts of pharmacology, with special emphasis on the role of the nurse in developing a comprehensive approach to the clinical application of drug therapy through the use of the **nursing process.** With the increasing importance of pharmacology for the professional nurse, many nursing programs now offer specialized course work as a separate part of the curriculum. In this context, our goal has been to update and expand the scientific foundation that will provide the learner with rationales for clinical practice. This book is intended for use in conjunction with the most recent clinical recommendations.

Substantial portions of this edition have been reorganized and rewritten. The book is divided into two major parts. Part One, "Basic Concepts of Pharmacology," consists of three units. The first unit deals with the principles of pharmacology, and the second with the relationship of these principles to the nursing process. The third unit focuses on the biopsychosocial aspects of pharmacology, including psychologic and cultural aspects of drug therapy, drug therapy across the life span, and substance misuse and abuse. Part Two, "Clinical Aspects of Pharmacology," is composed of the broad pharmacologic units that have been retained and modified from the preceding edition. However, this section, which makes up the largest portion of the book, now consists of sixteen units, almost all of which focus on major drug categories. Finally, the sequence of the major drug classifications is based on organ systems, which facilitates ready retrieval of drug information.

We have maintained the **drug monograph format.** Each monograph includes the following topics: mechanism of action, pharmacokinetics, indications, side effects/

adverse reactions, significant drug interactions, dosage and administration (adults, children, and elderly, where appropriate), FDA pregnancy category, and nursing considerations. These topics, easily located by boldface type, provide a framework for integration of pharmacologic concepts, a prerequisite for effective drug therapy. The monographs appear in two formats: **group monographs,** which describe in a general manner the closely related pharmacologic properties of a group of drugs (e.g., major drug class, drug subclass) and **individual monographs,** which usually follow a group monograph and present specific information about individual drugs. In the process of revision, particular care has been taken to avoid overlap of material and to unify content through cross-references.

NURSING CONSIDERATIONS

Another major modification of *Mosby's Pharmacology in Nursing* involves the considerable expansion of nursing content. Each drug monograph ends with an instructive summary of **nursing considerations** using a modification of the nursing process. This modification has resulted in the use of the following headings within nursing considerations sections: **Assessment, Intervention, Education,** and **Evaluation.** The planning step has not been mentioned for individual drug monographs, and the implementation step has been divided into intervention and education for emphasis. This format has been used because the text deals with the generalities of various clients receiving specific agents, rather than with unique individual clients for whom specific goals could be established. For example, the assessment of any client receiving a particular drug should be much the same with respect to the agent that client is receiving. Planning and client outcomes, however, are quite specific for each individual client. Examples of sample **nursing care plans,** including **nursing diagnoses,** are given for major drug classifications to provide guidance for the reader. Nursing considerations for client education are discussed within each drug monograph to provide the nursing student and the practicing nurse with alternatives for assisting the client in attaining expected outcomes or goals. This organization reinforces the fact that effective and safe drug administration depends on firm scientific knowledge of clinical pharmacologic principles and on nursing professionalism. Thus, evaluation of responses to drug therapy requires attention to analysis of a variety of sophisticated data about the client and his or her condition. The nursing considerations sections also address drug therapy problems specific to the elderly, to children, and to other special client populations. Also included are explicit instructions to clients concerning **self-medication.** This approach adds to the nurse's expanding role in the administration of drugs. Much

more nursing care could have been included within the nursing considerations sections, but because of space limitations we have limited the discussions to nursing care specific to pharmacologic interventions and education. For more general nursing care related to nonpharmacologic interventions, the reader should supplement this book with an appropriate general nursing textbook.

NEW CONTENT

Despite the many pharmacologic advances and the large number of new drugs — more than **150 new drugs** have been added to this edition — an effort has been made to keep the book a manageable size. This was accomplished by condensing some material, deleting outdated information, and tailoring content to the knowledge base required of the nurse. We have also shortened many chapters and increased their number by dividing the material into more discrete units. As a result, we have been able to introduce new discussions involving **cultural aspects** of drug therapy and a new chapter on lifespan considerations. Chapter 8, "Drug Therapy Across the Life Span," focuses on the special requirements of pediatric, childbearing, and geriatric clients. Overview chapters have been added for the endocrine, reproductive, immunologic, and integumentary systems, as well as material on infections, inflammation, and fever. These chapters should provide the background to facilitate learning about drugs affecting these systems. Unit XIII, "Drugs Affecting the Reproductive System," has been expanded and includes not only drugs related to or prescribed for disorders of the reproductive system but also drugs prescribed for nonreproductive system conditions that might affect the client's sexuality. **Geriatric and pediatric considerations** and **patient and family education** have been expanded throughout. In addition, new illustrations serve as visual aids to reinforce learning, and the use of color throughout the book emphasizes important material. More than **75 new illustrations** have been added; color has been added to many of the existing illustrations. The bibliographic references have been expanded and updated. Finally, **new appendixes** include drug compatibility, drug interferences with laboratory tests, commonly used medications, food/drug interactions, medication administration information for home care, and an alphabetical listing of drugs by generic to trade name.

PEDAGOGY

Chapter objectives have been added at the beginning of each chapter to help students get an overview of material presented and to help them focus on important material. **Key terms** are set in color where defined in the text.

These terms are listed at the end of each chapter, with page number references to facilitate reviewing. Many **summary tables** and **boxes** providing material of further interest have been added throughout the book to supplement, reinforce, or help the student make comparisons among similar drugs.

ANCILLARIES

The **instructor's manual** that accompanies the textbook has been designed to aid the educator in presenting and preparing class lectures. It contains the following teaching tools: chapter overview, key terms, teaching strategies, and teaching objectives. Also included are 35 illustrations for conversion to transparency masters. More than 1000 **Testbank** questions are also included, available in hard copy or on software for Apple and IBM systems. A **rationale** accompanies each correct answer.

ACKNOWLEDGMENTS

The success of *Mosby's Pharmacology in Nursing* through sixteen editions reflects its high degree of scholarship and the contributions of many people. We have attempted to incorporate the many suggestions and constructive criticisms offered during the revision of this book. We invite today's readers to continue this sharing dialogue so that the book will continue to be current, informed, and accurate. We are grateful to students, colleagues, reviewers, and everyone who has helped this textbook to grow with the nursing profession.

Many people have been involved throughout the revision process. We wish to thank Don Ladig, our editor, and to acknowledge the highly skilled staff of The C. V. Mosby Company. We would like to extend special gratitude to Robin Carter for her patience and unusual ability to coordinate the innumerable problems and their solutions during the production of this book. We are grateful to Steve Hetager for his meticulous attention to detail throughout production and to John Rokusek for his design. We deeply appreciate the efforts of Mark Hamelink and Al Poklis, who generously shared their professional expertise. It is the loyal support, encouragement, and help of our colleagues, friends, and families for which we are most grateful and to whom we extend our love and appreciation.

Leda M. McKenry
Evelyn Salerno

Brief Contents

Detailed Contents

Note to the Reader

PART ONE

Basic Concepts of Pharmacology

UNITS

I
Principles of Pharmacology

II
The Nursing Process and Pharmacology

III
Biopsychosocial Aspects of Pharmacology

UNIT I

Principles of Pharmacology

CHAPTERS

Orientation to Pharmacology

Pharmacology is the study of the actions and effects of drugs within a living system. It deals with all drugs in society today—legal or illegal, prescription or nonprescription (over-the-counter), to prevent disease or to cure or treat illness—drugs in any context. The pharmacologic agents available today have controlled and, in some instances, cured cardiac disease, hypertension, cancer, psychiatric illness, polio, and hundreds of other illnesses. The result has been improved quality of life and, perhaps, extension of the life span. Medications also can potentially harm the client, which is reflected by the fact that the term "pharmaceutical" is actually derived from the Greek word for poison (Siler and others, 1982). Therefore, the nurse should understand thoroughly any medication before giving it to a client. The nurse must know the usual dose, route of administration, indication(s), significant side effects and adverse reactions, major drug interactions, and appropriate nursing assessment, planning, implementation, and evaluation techniques necessary to safely administer the drug.

A number of terms are fundamental to the knowledge base of nurses. The box on p. 6 lists some basic terms; more will be added as appropriate throughout the book.

HISTORICAL TRENDS

Primitive peoples believed that disease was caused by evil spirits inhabiting the body. This thought persisted

pharmacokinetics what the body does to a drug, that is, how a drug is altered as it travels through the body: its absorption, distribution, special tissue binding or affinity, metabolism, and excretion.

pharmacodynamics what drugs do to the body and how drugs interact with body tissue.

pharmacogenetics hereditary influences on an individual's response to a drug or drug category; possible basis for idiosyncratic (unexplainable) drug responses.

nonprescription or over-the-counter (OTC) drugs drugs that may be purchased without a prescription.

legend or prescription drugs drugs requiring a prescription to be dispensed.

indication an illness or disorder for the treatment of which a specific drug has a documented usefulness.

drug any substance used in diagnosis, cure, treatment, or prevention of a disease or condition. The United States Food and Drug Administration (FDA) definition of *drug* also includes any substance listed in *The United States Pharmacopeia* or *The British Pharmacopoeia* and all substances, other than foods or devices, capable of altering body structure or function. The terms *medication, medicine, medicinal,* and *medicament* are used more or less synonymously with the term *drug.*

action of a drug chemical changes or effects a drug has on body cells and tissues.

side effect an additional effect of a drug that is not necessarily the primary purpose of giving the drug. Side effects may be desirable or undesirable.

adverse reaction an unintended and undesirable response to a drug.

throughout the Egyptian period of medicine. Hippocrates advanced the idea that disease resulted from natural causes and could only be understood through study of natural laws. He believed the body had recuperative powers and saw the health care provider's role as assisting the recuperative process. Called the Father of Medicine, Hippocrates influenced the principles that control the practice of medicine today. Building on the teachings and practices of Hippocrates, Galen (131 to 201 AD) established a system of medicine and pharmacy that was recognized as the supreme authority for several hundred years.

The decline and fall of the Roman Empire marked the beginning of the medieval period (400 to 1580 AD). Germanic barbarians overran Western Europe and reverted to a medicine of folklore and tradition, similar to that of the Greeks before Hippocrates.

At the same time Christian religious orders built monasteries that became repositories for all learning, including pharmacy and medicine. They aided the sick and needy with good food, rest, and medicinals from their monastery gardens.

The Arabs' interest in medicine, pharmacy, and chemistry was reflected in the hospitals and schools they built, the many new drugs they contributed, and their formulation of the first set of drug standards.

In 1240 AD, Emperor Frederick II declared pharmacy to be separated from medicine. However, pharmacy was not truly established separately until the sixteenth century, when Valerius Cordus wrote the first pharmacopeia to be printed as an authoritative standard. Paracelsus, professor of physics and surgery at Basel, denounced "humoral pathology" and substituted the idea that diseases were actual entities to be combated with specific remedies. He improved pharmacy and therapeutics for succeeding centuries, introducing new remedies and reducing the overdosing so prevalent in that period.

In the seventeenth and eighteenth centuries great progress was made in pharmacy and chemistry. The first London pharmacopeia appeared in 1618. Many preparations that were introduced are still in use today, including tincture of opium, coca, and ipecac. In 1785, Englishman William Withering introduced infusion of digitalis for heart disease. Edward Jenner made his first public inoculation with smallpox vaccine in 1796.

During the nineteenth century, pharmaceutical chemistry emerged. Serturner's discovery of the alkaloid morphine in 1815 led to research on many vegetable drugs; quinine, strychnine, atropine, codeine, and others were found as a result. Ether and chloroform were first used as general anesthetics in the 1840s. The French *Codex* was issued in 1818 and was the first of the important national pharmacopeias. It was followed by the United States' *Pharmacopeia* in 1820, that of Great Britain in 1864, and Germany's in 1872.

Accurate study of dosage in the nineteenth century led to the establishment of large-scale manufacturing plants to produce drugs. Fewer drugs were prescribed, and knowledge of their expected action became more precise. Rational medicine had begun to replace empiricism.

In 1907 Ehrlich introduced salvarsan for syphilis; Banting followed in 1922 with the discovery of insulin for diabetes mellitus. The sulfonamides, penicillin, and other antibiotics revolutionized the treatment of infectious diseases. Cortisone was first used in 1949 and opened a new era in medical science. In 1955 and 1961, new poliomyelitis vaccines showed similar success.

In the late 1950s oral contraceptives were introduced and had widespread effects on the per capita birth rate and sexual mores.

More recently, research has discovered new classes of drugs that the body itself produces, for example, interferon, enkephalins, and endorphins.

Between now and the year 2000, the trends in health care and pharmaceutics will focus on the following:

1. Consumer health education expansion—consumers will probably be seeking information on preventive health care matters through computer software programs and other educational resources. People are motivated to take responsibility for health, disease prevention, and lowered costs for medical care.

2. Research—the thrust of research will be directed to finding new treatments, cures, or methods to prevent disease processes that limit the growth, everyday living, or average life span of the individual. Specific areas addressed will be preventing and treating heart attacks, stroke, and other devastating diseases of the cardiovascular system; reversing or curing viral diseases, with a primary focus on acquired immune deficiency syndrome (AIDS); dealing successfully with the muscular atrophic disease states; treating psychiatric illnesses; eliminating infectious disease; and, hopefully, making major in roads to combat the 100 or more diseases known as cancer.

3. Orphan drugs—research will be expanded to provide new incentives to develop drugs for the patients suffering from rare, chronic diseases, research that is usually unprofitable. In 1983 the FDA established an Orphan Drug Act that provides grants to encourage this research. Among the disorders benefiting from this research are hepatic porphyria, hemophilia, leprosy (Hansen's disease), Cushing's syndrome, and Tourette's disorder. Thirteen new drugs have already been approved to treat some of these disease states (Horowitz, 1987).

As a result of the current and projected trends the health care consumer will be asking for more information; one of the persons most often questioned is the nurse. The nurse will take on greater responsibility for professional judgment in the administration and supervision of drug therapy as new products—usually more potent, more complex, and, therefore, with greater potential for toxicity—appear on the market. Therefore, nurses must know about and use drug information resources to better care for their clients.

THE SCOPE OF NURSING RESPONSIBILITIES

Drugs can help or harm. Nurses, physicians, and clinical pharmacists are held legally responsible for safe and therapeutically effective drug administration. Specifically, nurses are liable for their actions and omissions and for those duties they delegate to others, who may include medication technicians, pharmacy technicians, practical nurses, or even physicians. They are personally responsible—legally, morally, and ethically—for every drug they administer or have administered, no matter who actually

prescribed it. Indeed, all members of a health team may be held liable for a single injury to a client. The increase in litigation against nurses and physicians indicates that society tolerates only a minimal margin of error in relation to human life. Claims have been brought against health professionals for drug errors that caused loss of life (*Norton v. Argonaut Insurance Co.,* the *Somera* case) and permanent injury (*Honeywell v. Rogers*). (*Murchison and Nichols, 1970*). When claims against health professionals are supported with evidence that the conduct of one or more health professionals helped to bring about the loss or injury, those parties may be held liable. The law, a legal and social norm, requires health professionals to be safe and competent practitioners and permits compensation to those harmed or injured.

However, the law is a protective force for the knowledgeable, competent, and responsible nurse. Nurses who are determined to safeguard patients from drug-induced harm will, for example:

• Use correct techniques and precautions
• Observe and chart drug effects explicitly
• Keep their knowledge base current
• Refer to authoritative sources in professional literature and to pharmacologists, pharmacists, and other respected colleagues
• Question a drug order that is unclear or that appears to contain an error
• Refuse to administer or refuse to allow others to order or administer a drug if there is reason to believe it will be harmful

The law, in turn, protects such nurses from unfair litigation.

Much remains to be learned about the actual mode of action as well as effects from prolonged use of many commonly prescribed drugs. Furthermore, there is increasing concern about drug-induced disease. Fortunately, drug therapy for most conditions or for illness prevention is temporary. However, some diseases require lifelong use of drugs to sustain life (such as insulin for diabetes mellitus) or prolonged use to maintain relatively normal physiologic or psychologic functioning (such as phenobarbital for seizure disorders).

Nurses are entrusted with potent and habit-forming drugs, and they must not abuse or misuse this trust. Used respectfully and intelligently, drugs are comforting and lifesaving. Used unwisely or with undue dependence, they can lead to tragedy. The nurse who combines diligent and intelligent observation with moral integrity and factual knowledge will be a safe and competent practitioner and a credit to the nursing profession.

In addition, the nurse must establish with the client a **"therapeutic alliance,"** a respectful and trusting relationship to facilitate the highest level of self-care attainable. The client is the most important participant in the team effort for safe and effective drug administration. Clients are not expected to be submissive, acquiescent, and nonquestioning followers of the health team's instructions, but must be motivated to assume responsibility for their own care; nurses must recognize that the power to comply is ultimately the client's. All the nurse's knowledge, skill, and ability are brought to bear on the establishment of a therapeutic alliance to facilitate the most appropriate level of self-care related to medications.

Pharmacology applies knowledge from many different disciplines, including anatomy and physiology, pathology, microbiology, organic chemistry and biochemistry, mathematics, psychology, and sociology. Thus, clinical drug therapy can be considered an applied science. The hundreds of drugs available present a formidable study if they had to be approached as individual agents. Fortunately drugs can be systematically classified into a reasonable number of drug groups based on chemical, pharmacologic, or therapeutic relatedness. Understanding the characteristic effects of a particular class of drugs at the subcellular, tissue, organ, or functional system level permits a student or practitioner to extrapolate information to a wide variety of drugs. A typical representative drug can be selected and studied and its specific characteristics compared to others in the same class. Gradually, the individual builds a knowledge base.

Lists of drugs, dosages, and their indications should not be regarded as dogma. New information is constantly being generated by laboratory research and by new scientific methods of evaluation. Occasionally there are reports that a drug, even an old and trusted one, is suspected of causing mutations, birth defects, cancer, or less serious secondary effects. Not only nursing students but also practicing nurses are challenged by the proliferation of drugs: most of the drugs on the market today were developed recently. Change is the only constant in pharmacology.

Pharmacology books must be kept up-to-date in the nurse's library. In addition, official current literature on drugs must be followed carefully, since new drugs only slowly make their way into more permanent literature. For the nurse working in a hospital or health service, physicians, instructors, in-service educators, and pharmacists will be on hand to help. In a more isolated practice, greater personal effort will be required to maintain currency. In any case, nurses must pay close attention to the drug therapy of their clients.

Learning is an active process. Therefore clinical experience with drugs is invaluable, for it enables the student to:

1. Note which drugs are most commonly used to treat certain diseases or specific signs and symptoms
2. Note the frequency with which certain drugs are administered
3. Observe which drugs are most effective in relieving particular signs and symptoms
4. Witness individual differences in clients' reactions to a specific drug
5. Relate knowledge obtained from authoritative sources to real-life situations

Regardless of what is to be learned, reasoning and the ability to analyze and synthesize information are prerequisites to understanding. These cognitive skills, along with perceptual skills, permit an individual to see meaningful relationships, make comparisons, and determine significance, all of which are essential for sound decision making.

THE NURSING PROCESS AND DRUG ADMINISTRATION

The *nursing process* is a systematic method for identifying actual or potential health care problems or impediments to the activities of daily living. It points the way to rational nursing actions and objective evaluation of care.

The direction of the nursing process is fairly universal in the field, although its structure may vary from the widely used pattern of four phases or steps: (1) assessment of data (this may culminate in a nursing diagnosis), (2) planning, (3) implementation, and (4) evaluation.

To apply the nursing process to drug therapy, nurses *assess* the medication needs of their patients partly in terms of how these needs are matched by the prescriber's orders. The result of this assessment by the nurse is the nursing diagnosis. Nurses make *plans,* which include goals that directly relate to their *nursing diagnoses.* The stage is then set for *implementing* the goals, using specific, rationale-based nursing actions. Such actions might simply be the preparation and administration of a medication as ordered, or they might include steps to withhold a dose and obtain a changed order. The final step is the *evaluation* of the outcome in terms of the original goals. Each time a nursing process is evaluated, nurses' knowledge bases increase and they become more valuable.

The nursing process is discussed in more detail in Unit Two: The Nursing Process and Pharmacology.

GOALS OF THIS TEXT

This text will orient the reader to nursing pharmacology and therapeutics by presenting a firm theoretic foundation and a practical approach to drug therapy applicable in many settings—the home, the clinic, the extended care facility, the office, the classroom, and the hospital.

Part One provides general principles, theories, and facts about all drugs and how they are given. Practical information is presented on how the nursing process is integrated with pharmacology, and general principles of action are given to facilitate a student nurse's learning in both academic and clinical environments. The rest of the book presents specific drug information about clinical applications and nursing considerations. Thus this book can be used both as a text and as a reference.

To find information about a particular drug in this book:

1. Look it up in the index
2. When you find the information about the drug, go to the beginning of the chapter or unit and read the material that precedes the specific discussion

Reading only the pages listed in the Index for the drug will illuminate only the drug's specifics, out of context and without necessary fundamental information about that class of drugs. Reading the background information offers an overall view and places the drug information into an understandable framework.

The specific drug information summarizes what is needed to administer drugs safely and competently. Each discussion is titled with some of the common names by which the particular drug is known. (Chapter 3 explains the various types of names and forms of drugs.) The names of drugs that are available in Canada but not in the United States are followed by a maple leaf symbol (♣).

The **mechanism of action** explains how the drug acts at the biochemical or cellular level to produce its therapeutic effects. The officially approved therapeutic purpose of the drug or the conditions for which it is used are detailed under **indications.** The **pharmacokinetics** section specifies how the drug is absorbed, distributed, associated with tissue, biotransformed or metabolized, and excreted. The section entitled **side effects/adverse reactions** details most of the common secondary effects that may be experienced when the drug is administered. The **significant drug interactions** section names drugs whose concurrent administration requires caution because the concomitant use may lead to an effect different from that of either drug when used alone. The **dosage and administration** section presents currently approved dosages as well as dosing intervals and frequency. It must be noted that not all drugs have been tested for safety and efficacy in administration to the elderly, pregnant women and those who are breastfeeding, or children; the **pregnancy safety** section in each monograph lists the FDA Pregnancy Safety Category. Routes and special techniques for drug preparation are also listed here in each monograph.

The nursing considerations section describes distinctive nursing measures:

Assessment: data gathering about an individual's experience with medications and/or identifying preexisting medical conditions that might influence the choice of dosage of drug

Intervention: special handling, timing of doses, and other significant aspects of the actual administration of a drug

Education: client teaching for the highest level of self-care related to medication administration

Evaluation: the ongoing monitoring of the client for safe and effective drug therapy

SUMMARY OF NURSING CONSIDERATIONS

Safe, therapeutically effective drug administration is a major responsibility of nurses. It depends on sound, current knowledge of medications and careful monitoring of their effects on patients. Ongoing laboratory and clinical research modifies and enlarges available drug information, necessitating continual effort to keep one's knowledge up-to-date. The mode of action of many commonly prescribed drugs, effects of their prolonged use, and the possibility of drug-induced disease are yet to be completely understood. There are many sources of current drug information, but even the most diligent student of these sources requires clinical experience to develop competence in drug administration. Few areas of nursing demand more intellectual curiosity, integrity, factual knowledge, and motivation to use reference sources.

KEY TERMS

action of a drug, page 6
administration, page 9
adverse reaction, page 6
dosage, page 9
drug, page 6
drug interactions, page 9
indication, page 6
legend drug, page 6
mechanism of action, page 9
nonprescription drug, page 6
over-the-counter (OTC) drug, page 6
pharmacodynamics, page 6
pharmacogenetics, page 6
pharmacokinetics, page 6
pregnancy safety, page 9
prescription drug, page 6
side effect, page 6
therapeutic alliance, page 7

BIBLIOGRAPHY

Atkinson, LD, and Murray, ME: Understanding the nursing process, ed 2, New York, 1983, Macmillan, Inc.

Carlson, JH, Craft, CA, and McQuire, AD: Nursing diagnosis, Philadelphia, 1982, WB Saunders Co.

Carpenito, LJ: Nursing diagnosis: application to clinical practice. Philadelphia, 1983, JB Lippincott Co.

Doenges, ME, Jeffries, MF, and Moorhouse, MF: Nursing care plans, Philadelphia, 1984, FA Davis Co.

Griffith-Kenny, JW, and Christenson, PJ: Nursing process: application of theories, frameworks, and models, ed 2, St Louis, 1986, The CV Mosby Co.

Horowitz, AM: On orphan drugs, Am Pharm NS27(4):33.

Ivey, M, and others: Pharmacotherapeutics in primary care, New York, 1984, Elsevier North Holland, Inc.

Krantz, JC: Historical medical classics involving new drugs, Baltimore, 1974, The Williams & Wilkins Co.

Lamonica, EL: The nursing process: a humanistic approach, Menlo Park, Calif, 1979, Addison-Wesley Publishing Co.

Leake, CD: An historical account of pharmacology to the twentieth century, Springfield, Ill, 1975, Charles C Thomas, Publisher.

Marriner, A: The nursing process: a scientific approach to nursing care, ed 3, St Louis, 1982, The CV Mosby Co.

Murchison, IA, and Nichols, TS: Legal foundations of nursing practice, New York, 1970, Macmillan, Inc.

Roger, FB: A syllabus of medical history, Boston, 1972, Little, Brown & Co.

Siler, WA, and others: Death by prescription, Tallahassee, Fla, 1982, Rose Printing Co, Inc.

Yura, H, and Walsh, MB: The nursing process: assessing, planning, implementing, evaluating, ed 4, East Norwalk, Conn, 1983, Appleton-Century-Crofts.

Legal Foundations of Pharmacology Practice

OBJECTIVES

After studying this chapter, the student will be able to:

1. Identify the process used in the development and evaluation of a new drug prior to marketing.
2. Differentiate between over-the-counter and prescription drugs.
3. Describe the United States procedure for evaluation of over-the-counter drugs for safety and effectiveness.
4. Describe the United States procedure for evaluation of prescription drugs for safety and effectiveness.
5. Identify legislative or authoritative source(s) for drug standards published in the United States and in Canada.
6. Describe the FDA pregnancy categories for drugs.
7. Discuss the nurse's role in drug research.
8. Discuss the changing nursing roles related to drug administration.

Since the beginning of time, people have searched for substances to treat illness and cure disease. The oldest prescriptions known were found on a clay tablet, written by a Sumerian physician about 3000 BC, or nearly 5000 years ago.

Many remedies of past civilizations lacked the information we take for granted today, such as the strength of the substances in a preparation or even the ingredients themselves. For example, an Egyptian doctor's cure for night blindness was the "liver of ox, roasted and crushed," or to cure blindness itself, one was instructed to mix a pig's eye with antimony, red ocher, and honey and pour the mixture into the blind person's ear (Modell and Lansing, 1967). These prescriptions were written about 1500 BC and clearly illustrate the knowledge gap that existed within even the basic sciences of anatomy and physiology. This type of medical practice, although perhaps not always as inappropriate, extended well into the nineteenth century. Standards for preparation, identification of ingredients, proof of effectiveness and safety, and government interventions are largely developments of the twentieth century.

UNITED STATES DRUG LEGISLATION

Before 1906, patent medicines and remedies were sold by medicine men in traveling wagon shows, drugstores, and mail order and by doctors, real or self-titled. Such products were not required to list ingredients on the label, so many contained drugs such as opium, morphine, heroin, chloral hydrate, and alcohol. Many persons (especially infants) were reportedly injured, became addicted, or died as a result of the dangerous ingredients or their quantities in these preparations.

In 1906 the first federal **Pure Food and Drug Act** was passed to protect the public from adulterated or mislabeled drugs. The law required the drug company to declare on the package label the presence of 11 identified (some of which were in the list just mentioned) dangerous and perhaps addicting drugs. This first law had limitations that were used by the patent medicine dealers for their own gain. For example:

1. False and misleading claims about the curative value of the product were not allowed *on the package,* which was described as a bottle, label, or wrapper that encircled the bottle. Claims made in advertisements, newspapers, or drug almanacs, by word of mouth, or on signs in store windows were not covered. Unscrupulous nostrum dealers took full advantage of this oversight.

2. Serial numbers were required for products containing any of the 11 dangerous drugs, and each label was to bear the words "Guaranteed Under the Food and Drugs Act." This meant that the dealer had registered his product and was legally responsible for it if it was improperly sold under this act. However, many patent medicine dealers implied that this was the government seal of approval. In response to this abuse, this clause was abolished in 1919.

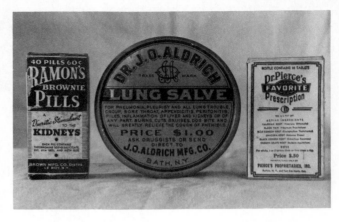

FIGURE 2-2 Patent medicines and remedies from the turn of the century.

3. Only drugs sold in interstate commerce (made in one state and sold to persons living in other states) were covered. Drugs made and sold within one state did not fall under the jurisdiction of this law.

The Food and Drug Act of 1906 designated *The United States Pharmacopeia* and *The National Formulary* as official standards and empowered the federal government to enforce them. Drugs were required to comply with the standards of strength and purity professed for them, and labels had to indicate the kind and amount of morphine or other narcotic ingredients present.

In 1912 Congress passed the Sherley Amendment, prohibiting use of fraudulent therapeutic claims.

A further update of the drug legislation occurred in 1938 with the passage of the federal Food, Drug, and Cosmetic Act. More than 100 deaths had occurred in 1937 as a result of ingestion of a diethylene glycol solution of sulfanilamide. This preparation had been marketed as an "elixir of sulfanilamide" without investigation of its toxicity. Under the 1906 law the only charge that could be made against the drug was that it was mislabeled, since it was labeled an "elixir" and the drug failed to meet the definition of an elixir as an alcoholic solution. The 1938 act prevented the marketing of new drugs before they had been properly tested for safety by requiring the manufacturer to submit an investigational new drug exemption to the government for review of safety studies before a product could be sold.

The Durham-Humphrey Amendment of 1952 further changed the 1938 drug act as it related to legend (prescription) drugs and refills, as follows:

1. Legend drugs could be dispensed by prescription only.
2. Legend drug prescriptions could not be refilled without physician authorization.
3. Some legend drugs could be prescribed by oral or telephone instructions.
4. With certain limitations, refills could also be authorized by oral or telephone means.

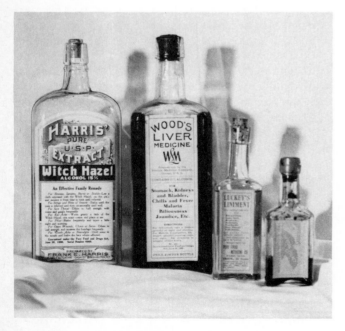

FIGURE 2-1 Patent medicines and remedies from the turn of the century.

LEGEND DRUGS

Legend drugs must bear the legend "Caution: Federal law prohibits dispensing without prescription." These include all drugs given by injection as well as the following:

1. Hypnotic, narcotic, or habit-forming drugs or derivatives thereof as specified in the law
2. Drugs that, because of their toxicity or method of use, are not safe unless they are administered under the supervision of a licensed practitioner (physician or dentist)
3. New drugs that are limited to investigational use or new drugs that are not considered safe for indiscriminate use by the public

---

This amendment also recognized a second class of drugs, over-the-counter drugs (OTCs), for which prescriptions are not required.

In 1958, Senator Estes Kefauver of Tennessee began a senate investigation into the drug industry when it became known that the drug companies were making huge profits and that some drug promotion was false or misleading. This investigation received little support until given impetus by the thalidomide tragedy, although for the United States it was more a might-have-been catastrophe than a real one. Thalidomide, a hypnotic marketed in Europe, was found to be responsible for severe deformities in babies whose mothers had taken the drug during the early stage of pregnancy. These events led to passage of the Kefauver-Harris Amendment in 1962.

The Kefauver-Harris Amendment required proof of both safety and efficacy before a new drug could be approved for use. This meant that all drugs introduced under the safety-only criterion in effect from 1938 to 1962 had to be evaluated. To do this the FDA signed a contract with the National Academy of Sciences and its research arm, the National Research Council (NAS/NRC), in 1966 to study all supporting data for all therapeutic claims. This program of study was called the Drug Efficacy Study Implementation (DESI). Early in the study it was agreed that each drug would be rated for effectiveness in each of its stated indications according to the following categories:

Effective: substantial evidence of effectiveness.
Probably effective: additional evidence required to rate the drug effective.
Possibly effective: eventual effectiveness possible, but little evidence of efficacy at the present time.
Ineffective: no substantial evidence of effectiveness.

Other rating categories have been formulated since that time:

Ineffective as a fixed combination: even though one or more components might be effective if used alone, the product is not acceptable in fixed dosage combination for reasons of safety or because there is no evidence of contribution of each component to claimed effect.
Effective but: although effective there is an appropriate qualification or restriction imposed on the drug, which is still under consideration by the NAS/NRC and the FDA; the drug is effective for some recommended uses but not for all, requiring labeling changes.
Exempt: less than effective, but a decision on whether to remove drug from the market is deferred pending completion of additional clinical studies.
Effectiveness to be determined: products not evaluated by NAS/NRC, which are undergoing FDA evaluation for effectiveness.
Effective/new safety issue: products never reviewed by the DESI process, which have now been discovered to have some harmful potential.

Thousands of drugs and therapeutic claims have been evaluated and "ineffective" drugs have been withdrawn from the market. Those rated as "possibly effective" or "probably effective" are being withdrawn or reformulated; however, a drug may remain on the market while claims are being modified and scientific data collected to substantiate the claims. Drugs in the "probably effective" and "possibly effective" categories must be upgraded to the "effective" category within time limits set by the FDA or the claims and drug withdrawn. On the other hand, the system allows the prescribing of an approved drug as therapy for a disorder for which the drug has not been FDA approved. The drug may be a fairly common one, and informed consent for this nonresearch application of the drug need not be obtained.

OVER-THE-COUNTER DRUG REVIEW

The over 300,000 over-the-counter drug products currently available contain approximately 700 active ingredients. In 1972, the FDA assembled an advisory review panel to perform an ingredient review, asking primarily the following:

1. Are the stated ingredients recognized as safe and effective for consumers to self-medicate?
2. Are the labeling, indications, dosage instructions and warnings sufficient? If they were found lacking, appropriate recommendations were to be developed.

This study, completed in 1983, found that approximately one third of the ingredients reviewed were safe and effective for labeled indications. Ingredients found particularly or potentially dangerous were either transferred to prescription status only (such as hexachlorophene, an antibacterial topical product with a potential for inducing neurologic toxicities) or removed entirely from the market. An example of the latter was camphorated oil or camphor liniment, which may be mistakenly taken orally for

SUMMARY OF IMPORTANT U.S. DRUG LEGISLATION

Food, Drug and Cosmetic Act of 1938	An act, implemented by the FDA, that mandates that drug manufacturers must test all drugs for harmful effects and that labels and other literature enclosed be accurate and complete. It also requires that medical devices be safe and effective and that cosmetics be safe. The FDA has the power to prevent the marketing of any drug it has adjudged to be incompletely tested or dangerous.
Wheeler-Lea Act of 1938	This act defines the criteria for nonfraudulent advertising of drugs, food, or cosmetics: no false claims, full disclosure of chemical formulas, including the amount of each ingredient. This act is implemented by the Federal Trade Commission.
Durkham-Humphrey Amendment of 1952	This amendment distinguishes more clearly between drugs that can be sold with or without prescription and those that should not be refilled without a new prescription and need to be so labeled. These latter are those drugs considered habit forming, narcotic, hypnotic, or potentially harmful.
Drug Amendment of 1962 (Kefauver-Harris Act)	This act is a result of the thalidomide tragedy, wherein severely deformed babies were born to European mothers who had taken the hypnotic thalidomide. It was only through the staunch efforts of a woman investigator working for the FDA that this drug was not officially approved in the United States. This drug is now barred from the United States and its possessions. This act gave the FDA increased power to (1) tighten controls over drug safety and over statements about adverse reactions and contraindications, (2) evaluate the actual drug testing methods used by manufacturers, and (3) determine drug effectiveness (of both prescription and nonprescription drugs), not just their relative lack of toxicity. As a result, many drugs have now been determined to be "ineffective," "possibly effective," and so on (about 50% of all prescription drugs). These drugs must be so designated and must eventually be improved to "effective" status or be removed from the market.
Controlled Substances Act of 1970 (Title II of the Comprehensive Drug Abuse Prevention Act of 1970)	The FDA and Drug Enforcement Agency of the Justice Department have jurisdiction to regulate and control the flow of drug traffic. This act categorizes controlled substances (drugs such as narcotics, amphetamines, barbiturates, sedatives and those that have potential for abuse) into five categories, called Schedules, based on their relative potential for abuse. Drugs in Schedule I offer the highest abuse potential. All controlled substances are limited in the number of times a prescription may be refilled.
Drug Regulation Reform Act of 1978	This act allows a shortened time period for new drug investigative efforts, thereby speeding new drug release to the public.

cod liver oil or castor oil and produce serious toxicity and even death. The benefits of this product did not outweigh the serious risks associated with its availability, so it was removed from the market.

PRESCRIPTION DRUGS SWITCHED TO OTC DRUG STATUS

The review panels and other interested parties suggested switching a number of prescription drugs to nonprescription drug categories, since such products were deemed to be safe for self-treatment by consumers without professional guidance. Examples of drugs that were changed from prescription to OTC status include diphenhydramine (Benadryl), which is now an active ingredient in OTC antihistamines and antitussive and hypnotic medications, and chlorpheniramine maleate (Chlor-Trimeton), which is now an OTC antihistamine. Topical hydrocortisone is now available as an antipruritic and sodium

fluoride rinse as an anticaries agent. A number of other products have been tentatively approved for OTC marketing. The reader is referred to Davidson (1986) for additional information.

CONTROL OF OPIOIDS (NARCOTICS) AND OTHER DANGEROUS DRUGS

Narcotic and drug abuse laws. The Harrison Narcotic Act, passed in 1914, was the first federal law aimed at curbing drug addiction or dependence. This was the first narcotic act passed by any nation. It established the word "narcotic" as a legal term. This act regulated the importation, manufacture, sale, and use of opium and cocaine and all their compounds and derivatives. Marijuana and its derivatives were also subject to this act, as were many synthetic analgesic drugs that proved to produce or sustain either physical or psychologic dependence.

This act and other drug abuse amendments now have

only historical import, since they have been superseded by the Comprehensive Drug Abuse Prevention and Control Act of 1970,* also called the **Controlled Substances Act** (CSA), which became effective May 1, 1971. This law was designed to provide "increased research into, and prevention of drug abuse and drug dependence; to provide for treatment and rehabilitation of drug abusers and drug dependent persons; and to strengthen existing law enforcement authority in the field of drug abuse." This law is also designed to improve the administration and regulation of the manufacturing, distributing, and dispensing of **controlled substances** by legitimate handlers of these drugs to help reduce their widespread dispersion into illicit markets.

The CSA classifies controlled substances solely according to their compared use and abuse potentials. Drugs are classified into numbered levels or schedules from Schedule I to Schedule V (Table 2-1). Drugs with the highest abuse potential are placed in Schedule I; those with the lowest potential for abuse are in Schedule V. These classifications are flexible. Drugs may occasionally be added or be changed from one schedule to another without new legislation. It might be anticipated, for example, that marijuana might be changed to another schedule if and when it is accepted for use in treating the nausea that may occur with cancer chemotherapy or for treatment of glaucoma. Some drugs with potential for dependence, such as ethanol and certain analgesics, are not listed as controlled substances. In practice, states may differ in their implementation of the Controlled Substances Act. Anyone handling controlled substances should follow the more inclusive or stringent requirements of the laws, federal or state.

In July 1973, the Drug Enforcement Administration (DEA) in the Department of Justice became the nation's sole legal drug enforcement agency; it replaced the Bureau of Narcotics and Dangerous Drugs.

Possession of controlled substances. It is, of course, unlawful for any person to possess a controlled substance unless it has been obtained by a valid prescription or order, or unless its possession is pursuant to actions in the course of professional practice. It is a federal offense to transfer a drug listed in Schedule II, III, or IV to any person other than the patient for whom the drug was ordered.

Drug suppliers and hospitals — as well as physicians, pharmacists, and nurses — are individually and collectively responsible for accounting for inventory and management of the flow and distribution of controlled substances. Institutional control of the flow of controlled substances is maintained by carefully recorded checks of the balance on hand, supplies added, and doses adminis-

---

*Current regulations can be obtained from the nearest Regional Director, Drug Enforcement Administration, or from the Drug Enforcement Administration, Department of Justice, Post Office Box 28083, Central Station, Washington, DC 20005.

tered. The nurse who is responsible for stock supplies of all drugs in each area of an agency usually orders the anticipated prescriptions each morning from the pharmacy. These drugs may be delivered periodically during the shift or workday. Control is maintained by actual counts of doses of each controlled substance by designated nurses at the beginning and end of each shift or workday. High accountability is demanded of the nurses who do this counting as well as all who handle controlled substances during the work period. Doses are recorded and tallied on a special form supplied by the pharmacy department (also on a client medication recording form). Thus, each dose is accounted for as it is administered, discarded, wasted, or withheld. All doses of controlled substances should be kept in double-locked cabinets or other secured areas, with the keys in the custody of a designated nurse. Although these protocols may seem to entail a needless waste of time, they are necessary to safeguard the control of drug flow. Routine delays caused by searching for the narcotics keys or by balky locks, key fumbling, and special recording forms should be counter-balanced by the efficient use of nursing time in client assessments and skilled administration techniques. Evaluation of the delays in the process and mechanisms to rectify them should be performed by nurses as part of their problem-identification and problem-management roles.

ADDITIONAL REGULATORY BODIES OR SERVICES

Food and Drug Administration. The Food and Drug Administration is charged with the enforcement of the federal Food, Drug, and Cosmetic Act. Seizure of offending goods and criminal prosecution of responsible persons or firms in federal courts are among the methods used to enforce the Act.

In addition, pharmaceutical firms must report at regular intervals to the FDA all adverse effects associated with their new drugs. The FDA also has an adverse-reaction reporting program with approximately 450 cooperating reporting sources. All health professionals are encouraged to relate an unusual occurrence or unusually high number of occurrences associated with a drug, its formulation, or packaging, and so forth. Communication may be made directly to the FDA by telephone and by completing a Drug Experience Report form. A response from the FDA will follow. The purpose of this program is to detect reactions that have not been revealed by previous clinical or pharmaceutical studies. Changes in the drug may be required, or it may be withdrawn from the market as was the drug benoxaprofen in 1982.

Public Health Service. The Public Health Service is an agency that is part of the U.S. Department of Health and Human Services. One of its many functions is the regulation of biologic products. This refers to "any virus, thera-

TABLE 2-1   Schedule of Controlled Substances

Schedule	Characteristics	Dispensing restrictions	Examples*
I	High abuse potential No accepted medical use—for research, analysis or instruction only May lead to severe dependence	Approved protocol necessary	Heroin, marijuana (cannabis), tetrahydrocannabinols, LSD, mescaline, peyote, psilocybin, methaqualone
II	High abuse potential Accepted medical uses May lead to severe physical and/or psychologic dependence	Written Rx necessary—only emergency dispensing permitted without written Rx (only required amount may be prescribed for emergency period) No Rx refills allowed Container must have warning label†	Opium, morphine, hydromorphone, meperidine, codeine, oxycodone, methadone, secobarbital, pentobarbital, amphetamine, methylphenidate, cocaine, and others
III	Less abuse potential than drugs in Schedules I and II Accepted medical uses May lead to moderate/low physical dependence or high psychologic dependence	Written or oral Rx required Rx expires in 6 months No more than 5 Rx refills allowed within a 6-month period Container must have warning label†	Preparations containing limited quantities of, or combined with, one or more active ingredients that are noncontrolled substances: codeine, hydrocodone, morphine, dihydrocodeine or ethylmorphine, and nonnarcotic drugs such as derivatives of barbituric acid except those that are listed in another schedule, glutethimide, methyprylon, chlorphentermine, mazindol, paregoric, and others
IV	Lower abuse potential compared to Schedule III Accepted medical uses May lead to limited physical or psychologic dependence	Written or oral Rx required Rx expires in 6 months with no more than 5 Rx refills allowed Container must have warning label†	Barbital, phenobarbital, chloral hydrate, meprobamate, fenfluramine, chlordiazepoxide, diazepam, oxazepam, clorazepate, flurazepam, lorazepam, dextropropoxyphene, pentazocine, and others
V	Low abuse potential compared to Schedule IV Accepted medical uses May lead to limited physical or psychologic dependence	May require written Rx or be sold without Rx (check state law)	Medications, generally for relief of coughs or diarrhea, containing limited quantities of certain opioid controlled substances

Courtesy Winthrop Laboratories, New York, N.Y. Modified from Ruggieri, N.L.: Drug Therapy 10(12):58-64, 1980, and the DEA pharmacist's manual—an informational outline of the Controlled Substances Act of 1970, U.S. Dept. of Justice, Washington, DC, June 1980. (Data apply to federal CSA and Uniform Controlled Substances Act; state laws may differ.)

*The examples cited constitute a partial listing. Individual hospital counsel should be consulted for a complete list for a particular state.

†Caution: Federal law prohibits the transfer of this drug to any person other than the patient for whom it was prescribed.

peutic serum, antitoxin, or analogous product applicable to the prevention, treatment, or cure of diseases or injuries of man." The Public Health Service exercises control over these products by inspecting and licensing the establishments that manufacture the products and by examining and licensing the products as well.

Product liability. In a majority of the states the rule of strict manufacturer's liability has been adopted. This doctrine holds manufacturers liable for injuries caused by defects in their products, drugs, or devices. **Product liability** exists (1) if a product is defective or not fit for its

reasonably foreseeable uses, (2) if the defect arose before the product left the control of the manufacturer, and (3) if the defect caused some person harm. If these three criteria are met, the manufacturer must pay money damages for the harm unless the liability can be shifted to some other party. Anyone harmed by a defective product has the right to sue the manufacturer for compensation.

Harm may be caused if the drug contains an ingredient whose danger is not commonly known, or if it contains an ingredient known to be harmful that one would not reasonably expect to find in such a product. Drugs containing potentially harmful ingredients must provide on the label warnings concerning its use; otherwise, the product will be considered defective and the manufacturer liable for resulting harm to unusually susceptible persons who unknowingly use it. Whether or not a product is defective depends on its compliance with current reasonable standards of safety. Manufacturers are legally responsible for knowing the effects of their products. If an unknown risk could have been discovered through a reasonable amount of research, the manufacturer will be held liable for any resulting harm.

Since nurses are accountable, they will want to stay alert to defects in the drugs they administer. Despite manufacturers' quality assurance programs, drug products are susceptible to errors in the manufacturing, packaging, and delivery processes. Although detection of chemical defects is usually outside the nurse's province, detection of observable physical defects is not. Nurses should learn to be keenly aware of physical characteristics of the drugs they administer and make comparisons before administering them. For example, unusual discoloration, other inconsistencies, precipitates, or foreign bodies in parenteral fluids should be considered suspect. Such observations warrant withholding the drug and contacting the pharmacy department or other authoritative source. It might mean that an entire stock supply or batch is defective. Recall of defective drugs is necessary to prevent patient harm.

Occasionally, human error can be expected to cause the wrong medication to be dispensed from the pharmacy. Again, the nurse is responsible for every medication administered. In this case the nurse who administers the wrong drug and the pharmacist who labeled it may both be held liable for any resulting patient harm. This liability has been sustained in the courts on several occasions. Helpful color photographs of many drug formulations can be found in a section of the *Physicians' Desk Reference* when such a question arises. Pharmacists may also provide verification.

CANADIAN DRUG LEGISLATION

In Canada, the Health Protection Branch (HPB) of the Department of National Health and Welfare is responsible for administration and enforcement of the Food and Drugs Act, as well as the Proprietary or Patent Medicine Act and the Narcotics Control Act. These acts are designed to protect the consumer from health hazards and fraud or deception in the sale and use of foods, drugs, cosmetics, and medical devices. Canadian drug legislation began in 1875 when the Parliament of Canada passed an act to prevent the sale of adulterated food, drink, and drugs. Since that time there has been food and drug control on a national basis.

Canadian Food and Drugs Act. In 1953 the present Canadian Food and Drugs Act was passed by the Senate and House of Commons of Canada. Since that time the law has been amended often. The Act stipulates that no food, drug, cosmetic, or device is to be advertised or sold to the general public as a treatment, preventive, or cure for certain diseases listed in Schedule A of the Act. Among the diseases included in the list are alcoholism, arteriosclerosis, and cancer. When it is necessary to provide adequate directions for the safe use of a drug used to treat or prevent diseases mentioned in Schedule A, that disease or disorder may be mentioned on the labels and inserts accompanying the drug. In addition, the Act prohibits the sale of drugs that are contaminated, adulterated, or unsafe for use and those whose labels are false, misleading, or deceptive. According to the Act, drugs must comply with prescribed standards as stated in recognized pharmacopeias and formularies listed in Schedule B of the Act, or according to the professed standards under which the drug is sold. Recognized pharmacopeias and formularies include the following:

Pharmacopoea Internationalis
British Pharmacopoeia
The United States Pharmacopeia/The National Formulary
Pharmacopée Française
The Canadian Formulary
British Pharmaceutical Codex

CSD means Canadian Standard Drug. This legend or the abbreviation must appear on the inner and outer labels of a drug to signify that it meets the standards prescribed for it.

Sale of certain drugs is prohibited unless the premises where the drug was manufactured and the process and conditions of manufacture have been approved by the Minister of National Health and Welfare. These drugs are listed in Schedules C and D and include injectable liver extracts, all insulin preparations, anterior pituitary extracts, radioactive isotopes, antibiotics for parenteral use, serums and drugs other than antibiotics prepared from microorganisms or viruses, and live vaccines. Distribution of samples of drugs is also prohibited, with the exception of distribution of samples of drugs to duly licensed individuals such as physicians, dentists, or pharmacists. Schedule F of the Act contains a list of drugs that can be sold and refilled only on prescription. Refills may be permitted at specified intervals but cannot exceed 6 months. Drugs listed in Schedule F include the antibiotics, hormones, and tranquilizers. They must always be properly and clearly labeled and include directions for use. Labels on containers of Schedule F drugs must be marked with the symbol Pr (prescription required). These drugs cannot be advertised to the general public other than giving of the name, price, and quantity of the drug.

Controlled drugs are those listed in Schedule G of the

Act and include amphetamines, barbituric acid and its derivatives (barbiturates), and phenmetrazine. Controlled drugs must be marked with the symbol ⟨C⟩ in a clear and conspicuous color and size on the upper left quarter of the label. The proper name of the drug must appear on the labels either immediately preceding or following the proprietary or trade name. Controlled drugs can be dispensed only on prescription.

When a controlled drug is dispensed by prescription, the labels must carry the following:
1. Name and address of the pharmacy or pharmacist
2. Date and number of the prescription
3. Name of the person for whom the controlled drug is dispensed
4. Name of the practitioner
5. Directions for use
6. Any other information that the prescription requires be shown on the label

Prescriptions for controlled drugs cannot be refilled unless at the time the prescription was issued, the practitioner so directed in writing and specified the number of times it could be refilled and the dates for, or intervals between, refilling. All information on the labels must be clearly and prominently displayed and readily discernible. Controlled drugs cannot be advertised to the general public.

Designated drugs are the following controlled drugs: (1) amphetamines, (2) methamphetamines, (3) phenmetrazine, and (4) phendimetrazine. Physicians may prescribe a designated drug for the following conditions: (1) narcolepsy, (2) hyperkinetic disorders in children, (3) mental retardation (minimal brain dysfunction), (4) epilepsy, (5) parkinsonism, and (6) hypotensive states associated with anesthesia. Permission can be obtained to prescribe amphetamines for patients with diagnoses other than those listed.

Restricted drugs are those listed in Schedule H of the Act and include the hallucinogenic drugs lysergic acid diethylamide (LSD), diethyltryptamine (DET), dimethyltryptamine (DMT), and dimethoxyamphetamine (STP; DOM). Sale of these drugs is prohibited. These drugs may be obtained for research by a qualified investigator if authorized by the Minister of National Health and Welfare. Precautions must be taken to ensure against loss or theft of a restricted drug.

The following are some of the additional requirements to be found in the Canadian Food and Drugs Act.

1. Labels of drugs must show:
   a. Proper name of the drug immediately preceding or following the proprietary or brand name
   b. Name and address of the manufacturer or distributor
   c. Lot number of the drug
   d. Adequate directions for use
   e. Quantitative list of medicinal ingredients and their proper or common names
   f. Net amount of drug
   g. Common or proper name and proportion of any preservatives used in parenteral drugs
   h. Expiration date if the drug does not maintain its potency, purity, and physical characteristics for at least 3 years from the date of manufacture
   i. Recommended single and daily adult dose; if the drug is for children the label must state: "Children: As directed by physician" or:

Age in Years	Proportion of Adult Dose
10-14	One-half
5-9	One-fourth
2-4	One-sixth
Under 2	As directed by physician

   j. A warning that the drug be kept out of the reach of children and any precautions to be taken (e.g., "*Caution:* May be injurious if taken in large doses for a long time. Do not exceed the recommended dose without consulting a physician." Warning is to be preceded by a symbol—octagonal in shape, red in color, and on a white background)
   k. Contraindications and side effects of nonprescription drugs
   l. On and after July 1, 1974, the drug identification number assigned to the drug, preceded by the words "Drug Identification Number" or the abbreviation "D.I.N."; to be shown on the main labels of a drug sold in dosage form (i.e., one ready for use by the consumer)
2. Other specific regulations, such as:
   a. Manufacturers must be able to demonstrate that a drug in oral dosage form represented as releasing the drug at time intervals actually is released and available as represented.
   b. Oral tablets must disintegrate within 45 minutes. Enteric-coated tablets must not disintegrate for 60 minutes when exposed to gastric juice but must disintegrate within an additional 60 minutes when exposed to intestinal juices.
   c. Drugs containing boric acid or sodium borate as a medicinal ingredient must carry a statement that the drug should not be administered to infants or children under 3 years of age.
   d. Safety factors such as sterility and absence of pyrogens must be assured in parenteral drugs.

The regulations allow the government to withdraw from the market drugs found to be unduly toxic. New drugs introduced to the market must have shown effectiveness and safety in human clinical studies to the satisfaction of the manufacturer and the government.

For more specific information, the nurse can obtain a copy of *Health Protection and Drug Laws* from Supply and Services Canada, Canadian Government Publishing Centre, Hull, Quebec KIA 059.

Canadian Narcotic Control Act. The regulations of the Canadian Narcotic Control Act govern the possession, sale, manufacture, production, and distribution of narcotics. The Canadian Narcotic Control Act was passed in

1961. This act revoked the Canadian Opium and Narcotic Act of 1952. The 1961 act has been amended a number of times.

Only authorized persons can be in possession of a narcotic. Authorized persons include a licensed dealer, pharmacist, practitioner, person in charge of a hospital, or a person acting as an agent for a practitioner. A licensed dealer is one who has been given permission to manufacture, produce, import, export, or distribute a narcotic. Practitioners include persons registered under the laws of a province to practice the profession of medicine, dentistry, or veterinary medicine. However, persons other than these may be licensed by the Minister of National Health and Welfare to cultivate and produce opium poppy or marijuana or to purchase and possess a narcotic for scientific purposes. Members of the Royal Canadian Mounted Police and members of technical or scientific departments of the government of Canada or of a province or university may possess narcotics in connection with their employment. A person who is undergoing treatment by a medical practitioner and who requires a narcotic may possess a narcotic obtained on prescription. This person may not knowingly obtain a narcotic from any other medical practitioner without notifying that practitioner that he or she is already undergoing treatment and obtaining a narcotic on prescription.

All persons authorized to be in possession of narcotics must keep a record of the name and quantity of all narcotics received, from whom narcotics were obtained, and to whom narcotics were supplied (including quantity, form, and dates of all transactions). In addition, they must ensure the safekeeping of all narcotics, keep full and complete records on all narcotics for at least 2 years, and report any loss or theft within 10 days of discovery.

The schedule of the Act lists those drugs, their preparations, derivatives, alkaloids, and salts that are subject to the Canadian Narcotic Control Act. Included in the schedule are opium, coca, and marijuana. Before a pharmacist legally may dispense a drug included in the schedule or medication containing such a drug, he or she must receive a prescription from a physician. A signed and dated prescription issued by a duly authorized physician is essential in the case of all narcotic medication prescribed as such or any preparation containing a narcotic in a form intended for parenteral administration. Medications containing a narcotic and two or more nonnarcotic ingredients may be dispensed by a pharmacist on the strength of a verbal prescription received from a physician who is known to the pharmacist or whose identity is established. Prescriptions of any narcotic may not be refilled.

There is one exception to the prescription requirement. Certain codeine compounds with a small codeine content may be sold to the public by a pharmacist without a prescription. In such instances the narcotic content can-

not exceed 8 mg per tablet or 20 mg/28 ml. In products of this kind, codeine must be in combination with two or more nonnarcotic substances and in recognized therapeutic doses.

Additionally, items of this nature are required to be labeled in such a fashion as to show the true formula of the medicinal ingredients and a caution to the following effect: "This preparation contains codeine and should not be administered to children except on the advice of a physician." These preparations cannot be advertised or displayed in a pharmacy. It is also unlawful to publish any narcotic advertisement for the general public.

Labels of containers of narcotics must legibly and conspicuously bear the proprietary and proper or common name of the narcotic, name of the manufacturer and distributor, the symbol *"N"* in the upper lefthand quarter, and net contents of the container and of each tablet, capsule, or ampule.

Although the administration of the Canadian Narcotic Control Act is legally the responsibility of the Department of National Health and Welfare, the enforcement of the law has been made largely the responsibility of the Royal Canadian Mounted Police. Prosecution of offenses under the Act is handled through the Department of National Health and Welfare by legal agents specially appointed by the Department of Justice.

The Narcotic Control Act defines a narcotic addict as "a person who through the use of narcotics has developed a desire or need to continue to take a narcotic, or has developed a psychological or physical dependence upon the effect of a narcotic." A person brought into court for a narcotic offense may be placed in custody by the court for observation and examination. If the person is convicted of the offense and found to be a narcotic addict, the court can sentence him or her to custody for treatment for an indefinite period.

Amendments to this Act place special restrictions on methadone. No practitioner can administer, prescribe, give, sell, or furnish methadone to any person unless the practitioner has been issued an authorization by the Minister of National Health and Welfare.

Application to nursing. A nurse may be in violation of the Canadian Narcotic Control Act if he or she is guilty of illegal possession of narcotics. Ignorance of the content of a drug in the nurse's possession is not considered a justifiable excuse. Proof of possession is sufficient to constitute an offense. Legal possession of narcotics by a nurse is limited to times when a drug is administered to a patient on the order of a physician, when the nurse is acting as the official custodian of narcotics in a department of the hospital or clinic, or when the nurse is a patient for whom a physician has prescribed narcotics. A nurse engaged in illegal distribution or transportation of narcotic drugs may be held liable, and heavy penalties are imposed for violation of the Canadian Narcotic Control Act.

DRUG STANDARDS

Drugs may vary considerably in strength and activity. Drugs obtained from plants, such as opium and digitalis, may fluctuate in strength from plant to plant and from year to year, depending on where the plants are grown, the age at which they are harvested, and how they are preserved. Since accurate dosage and reliability of a drug's effect depend on uniformity of strength and purity, standardization is necessary. The technique by which the strength and purity of a drug are measured is known as **assay.** The two general types of assay method used are chemical and biologic. Chemical assay is a chemical analysis to determine the ingredients present and their amounts. A simple example would be the determination of the concentration of hydrochloric acid in a solution to be used medically. Thus the acid content of a solution might be measured by titration. Then the acidity might be adjusted to the standard contained in a 0.1 normal solution.

Opium is known to contain certain alkaloids (*active principles* was the older term), and these may vary greatly in different preparations. The United States official standard demands that opium must contain not less than 9.5% and not more than 10.5% of anhydrous morphine. Opium of a higher morphine content may be reduced to the official standard by admixture with opium of a lower percentage or with certain other pharmacologically inactive diluents such as sucrose, lactose, glycyrrhiza, or magnesium carbonate.

In the case of some drugs, either the active ingredients are not known or there are no available methods of analyzing and standardizing them. These drugs may be standardized by biologic methods—**bioassay.** Bioassay is performed by determining the amount of a preparation required to produce a defined effect on a suitable laboratory animal under certain standard conditions. For example, the potency of a certain sample of insulin is measured by its ability to lower the blood sugar of rabbits. The strength of a drug that is assayed biologically is usually expressed in units. For example, insulin injection possesses a potency of not less than 95% and not more than 105% of the potency stated on the label, expressed in U.S.P. insulin units. Both the unit and the method of assay are defined, so that national and sometimes international standards exist.

Drug standards in the United States. Since 1980, the only official book of drug standards in the United States is *The United States Pharmacopeia* (USP). Any drug included in this book has met high standards of quality, purity, and strength. Drugs meeting these criteria can be identified by the letters U.S.P. following the official name. The U.S.P. is revised every 5 years by a group of elected scientific experts from a variety of fields, including nursing, pharmacy, pharmacology, and chemistry, to name a few, and by consumers.

The history of the standard reference books in the United States is interesting. The U.S.P., first published in 1820, has over the years been revised and published mainly by physicians. *The National Formulary* (N.F.) was established in 1888 by the American Pharmaceutical Association, and through the years it has been the project of pharmacists. In 1906, when the first Food and Drug Act was enacted, both of these privately issued compendia, the U.S.P. and the N.F., were established as the official standards by the United States government. In 1974, the United States Pharmacopeial Convention purchased *The National Formulary* from the American Pharmaceutical Association, and beginning in 1980, the only official book of drug standards in the United States was *The United States Pharmacopeia.*

Although there are numerous additional reference books and guides available on the market, two very valuable resources for drug information in a clinical setting are *U.S.P. Dispensing Information* and the *American Hospital Formulary Service* (AHFS) *Drug Information* book. The U.S.P.-DI is available in two volumes: Volume I (A and B), directed toward health care professionals, provides important information about a drug's indications, pharmacokinetics, precautions, dosing, warnings, and side effects. Volume II contains patient information on drugs, and many nurses, pharmacists, and physicians use this volume to teach patients about their medications. (The advantage of using this volume is that photocopies used in a health care setting do not require any prior permission to distribute. Automatic permission is granted to professionals who copy a limited quantity of monographs from this volume to distribute directly to their patients, free of charge.) The U.S.P-DI is issued annually, with regular supplement updates during the year. AHFS *Drug Information* is issued by the American Society of Hospital Pharmacists. It contains a comprehensive, evaluative approach to individual drugs. Not infrequently, it reviews some of the newer or investigational uses of medications. Both references are highly recommended as resources to the nurse, pharmacist, or physician.

Drug standards in Great Britain and Canada. The *British Pharmacopoeia* (B.P.) is similar to the U.S.P. in its scope and purpose. Drugs listed in the B.P. are considered official and subject to legal control in the United Kingdom and those parts of the British Commonwealth in which the *British Pharmacopoeia* has statutory force. It is published by the British Pharmacopoeia Commission under the direction of the General Medical Council. Dosage is expressed in metric system, although in some cases dosage is indicated in both metric and imperial systems.

The United States Pharmacopeia is used a great deal in Canada, and some preparations used in Canada conform to the U.S.P. instead of the B.P. because many of the drugs used in Canada are manufactured in the United States.

The *British Pharmaceutical Codex* (B.P.C.) is published by the Pharmaceutical Society of Great Britain. In general, it resembles *The National Formulary.*

The Canadian Formulary contains formulas for preparations used extensively in Canada. It also contains standards for new drugs prescribed in Canada but not included in the *British Pharmacopoeia.* The publication has been given official status by the Canadian Food and Drug Act.

The Physician's Formulary contains formulas for preparations that are representative of the needs of medical practice in Canada. It is published by the Canadian Medical Association.

INTERNATIONAL DRUG CONTROL

International control of drugs legally began in 1912 when the first "Opium Conference" was held at The Hague. International treaties were drawn up legally obligating governments to (1) limit to medical and scientific needs the manufacturing of and trade in medicinal opium, (2) control the production and distribution of raw opium, and (3) establish a system of governmental licensing to control the manufacture of and trade in drugs covered by the convention.

In 1961 government representatives formulated the "Single Convention on Narcotic Drugs," which became effective in 1964. This act consolidated all existing treaties into one document for the control of all narcotic substances by:

1. Outlawing their production, manufacture, trade, and use for nonmedicinal purposes
2. Limiting possession of all narcotic substances to authorized persons for medical and scientific purposes
3. Providing for international control of all opium transactions by the national monopolies (countries designated to produce opium, such as Turkey) and authorizing production only by licensed farmers in areas and on plots designated by these monopolies
4. Requiring import certificates and export authorizations

An **International Narcotics Control Board** was established to enforce this law. Since this is an immense task, it is impossible to prevent illicit trafficking in drugs. For example, during a 1-year period it was estimated that 1200 tons of opium were circulated in the illicit market when 800 tons were considered sufficient for world medical needs. Laws need to be frequently updated and strictly enforced, but the unfortunate fact is that financial support for regulation and enforcement is sometimes not equal to the task.

INVESTIGATIONAL DRUGS: RESEARCH TO MARKET

The multibillion dollar pharmaceutical industry is constantly screening substances with potential for marketability as new drugs. Prospective drugs may take years and huge amounts of capital to progress through the following FDA-required testing sequence:

A. Animal studies, to ascertain
   1. Toxicity
      a. Acute toxicity—as determined by the LD 50 (the dose that kills 50% of the animals). This is known as the median lethal dose
      b. Subacute toxicity
      c. Chronic toxicity
   2. Therapeutic index—the ratio of the median lethal dose to the median effective dose
   3. Modes of absorption, distribution, metabolism (biotransformation), and excretion of the substance
B. Human studies
   1. Phase I—initial pharmacologic evaluation
   2. Phase II—limited controlled evaluation
   3. Phase III—extended clinical evaluation

There is a noteworthy lack of correlation between levels of toxicity in animals and adverse effects in humans. In addition, many symptoms of adverse effects in animals simply cannot be determined in animals. A partial list of common human symptoms that are not measurably distinguishable in animals includes such effects as dizziness, nausea, drowsiness, nervousness, indigestion, headache, and weakness.

FDA approval process. The FDA approval process and specifications are as follows:

1. IND **(Investigational New Drug)**—if a pharmaceutical company or individual desires to investigate a new drug substance or an old drug for a new indication or at a different, unapproved dosage in humans, an IND application must be completed and submitted to the FDA. The IND will include evidence of drug safety by providing animal or clinical information, proof of the investigator's qualifications to perform this research, and evidence of the drug product's proven quality and strength. The investigation covered under the IND is divided into three phases:

   Phase I—initial pharmacologic evaluation. A small number of normal individuals (usually volunteers) will take the drug so that the investigators can determine the pharmacokinetics of the agent (absorption, distribution, metabolism, routes of elimination or excretion). Blood tests, urine analysis, vital signs, and specific monitoring tests are performed during this phase.

   Phase II—limited controlled evaluation. Now the drug will be administered at gradually increasing dosages to selected individuals with the targeted disease. For example, if the product is believed to have antihypertensive properties, individuals with documented hypertension would be chosen for this phase. During this phase, the individual will be closely monitored for drug effectiveness and for side effects. If no serious side or adverse effects occur, the study will progress to phase III.

Phase III — extended clinical evaluation. The drug is now tested in various centers in the United States, in larger numbers of individuals. Standards (protocols) have been developed and are to be followed at all investigative sites. The three objectives for this phase are: (1) clinical effectiveness, (2) drug safety determination, and (3) establishment of tolerated dosage or dosage range.

Several other factors are involved with this program. First, the investigator reports to the FDA after completion of each phase and needs approval from the FDA to progress to the following phases. Second, a double-blind study may be instituted, usually in phase II or phase III. A double-blind study involves the administration of the research drug or a placebo (such as milk sugar) and/or a marketed drug with the same pharmacologic effects as the drug being studied. All of the products are formulated to look the same and then packaged, usually by code numbers. Generally no one involved with the study will know which bottle of medicine the client is taking: the study drug (the active drug) or the placebo. Therefore bias will be eliminated and the evaluation will be done accurately, on the basis of therapeutic response. (The codes and content identification sheets are usually sealed and locked up by the Chief Investigator or Pharmacist, with instructions to break the code only in an emergency.)

2. NDA (New Drug Application) — following the completion of phase III of the IND and assuming the data collected indicate that the new drug is very promising, investigators will submit all the collected data to the FDA. After careful review of the information, the FDA may approve or reject the NDA. If the NDA is approved, the drug product can be marketed for the selected indication in the dosing schedules, as studied. If the NDA is rejected, the FDA may require additional studies or information before reconsideration.

3. ANDA (Abbreviated New Drug Application) (for generic drug approval) — generic formulations of currently marketed medications are not usually required to repeat all the previous steps before marketing. A company is required to prove that its product can produce the same therapeutic effects as the already marketed drug. Although nearly all generic drugs require the ANDA, the FDA may require different methods to prove generic equivalency, depending on the drug. For example, chlordiazepoxide (Librium) and amitriptyline (Elavil) require in vivo studies — that is, the generic drug must be given to humans and blood and urine studies data should be equivalent to data obtained when the name brand product is given, according to statistical analysis. Other drug products, such as chlorpheniramine (Chlor-Trimeton) and dexamethasone (Decadron) only need to prove that the manufacturing process is in compliance with Good Manufacturing Practice guidelines and that their quality control standards are equivalent. In other words, testing in humans is not required for the latter drugs. Thus the FDA establishes the criteria according to the drug product, the possibility of bioequivalency problems, or the lack of such problems. Drugs marketed before 1938, such as chloral hydrate and phenobarbital, do not require an approved ANDA before marketing.

The nurse should be aware of several of the limitations of the testing and marketing process. First, the number of persons studied is often limited; it usually averages between 500 and 3000. The studies are conducted for a limited time, and often certain types of individuals are excluded, including infants, children, pregnant women, persons with multiple disease states, and, frequently, geriatric individuals. If a drug is considered safe and effective during the time of study, with the previously mentioned limitations, it is marketed. Once marketed, the drug will be used in much greater numbers of clients, probably for longer periods, and it is inevitable that the drug will be reported to produce additional effects (possibly therapeutic but often adverse) that were not noted during the trial studies.

Therefore, a phase IV, or postmarketing surveillance period, has been advocated to monitor and tabulate information about new drugs in order to disseminate it to health care professionals and consumers. This is a more difficult phase to supervise, since it depends on the voluntary reports of persons in the medical field. The importance of this phase should not be underestimated, since it will affect many more people than the previous three phases combined.

Informed consent. All participants in experimental drug studies should be true volunteers and not subjected to any coercion. **Informed consent** should be obtained from them only after they have been given careful explanation of the purpose of the study, procedures to be used, and risks involved. New drug studies in children and psychiatric patients require special consideration. Beginning in 1983, new rules stipulated that both children's and parents' consent are required for research involving children if it is funded by the Department of Health and Human Services. In addition, these researchers must follow more rigorous guidelines to protect a child's rights. The rights of human participants in medical research have come to be protected under the umbrella of the **Nuremberg Code.** This code was developed under the aegis of American physicians as a result of the post–World War II trials at Nuremberg of Nazi physicians who had conducted experiments on political prisoners without their consent. The Code states essentially that:

1. Truly voluntary consent of the human subject is critical
2. The experiment must be proved to be valid or made possible only through the use of human subjects
3. The results and risks are justified by the study
4. Unnecessary suffering, death, or disability will be avoided
5. The experiment will be conducted in a careful and professional manner by scientifically qualified persons
6. The subject or investigator may terminate the experiment at any point that it is felt unendurable or impossible

Additionally, any experimental drug trials using humans, which are supported by the U.S. Department of Health and Human Services, must also meet federal guidelines for the protection of participants. Institutions supporting such investigational research have review boards that evaluate aspects of the research as it affects human subjects and that formally approve or disapprove research proposals accordingly.

NURSES AND DRUG RESEARCH

Nurses involved in research projects concerning human subjects, whether tangentially or directly, must be knowledgeable about the precepts of the Nuremberg Code and must protect clients by being ever alert to the possibility of subtle slip-ups in protocol or oversights in adherence to the tenets of the Code. The most important elements of the Code relate to subjects' rights to informed consent and to participation that is without coercion and fully voluntary. Although these rights would seem to be naturally assumed, they have occasionally been abrogated in the past (for example, instances of forced sterilization of retarded persons and of uninformed inoculations of military personnel with experimental drugs).

Informed consent refers to the written consent to an experimental procedure by individuals after they have received full and adequate explanation of the procedure itself, their full role in it, the expected effects, and the risks. This particular consent is heir to the flaws of other patient consents: the information conveyed may be incomplete or not delivered in nonmedical language or perhaps presented at a time when the individual is sleepy or sedated and not fully cognizant of the ramifications of what is being signed. It is the nurse's obligation to ensure that this does not happen and that it is the researcher or the physician, not the nurse, who gives full explanation and answers pertinent questions.

Expanding roles in nursing often include nurses on the team researching experimental drug development. Indeed, more nurses than ever before are conducting research of their own, much of it clinical even if not directly related to investigational drugs, using human subjects. Because of a healthy professional commitment to client well-being, nurses may find themselves caught in an ethical conflict. They likely may feel ambivalent about clients' right to know (vis-a-vis the Patients' Bill of Rights) and yet be uncomfortably aware that too much information may unduly influence a person's behavior or condition in some way and thereby adversely influence the variable under study. This is an area of ethics that awaits further study.

Nurses involved in clinical drug studies should be fully informed about the study and the drug under investigation. All information available to the physician, researcher, or pharmacist should also be available to the nurse.

Ethical and legal responsibilities mandate that a nurse's actions be based on adequate knowledge and skill and that clients be protected from foreseeable harm. This necessitates that the nurse know the recommended dosage range and route of administration, the desired therapeutic effect, and the undesired and toxic effects. Throughout the entire investigation the nurse must strictly adhere to the protocols of the study. Recordings of all observations should be as precise as possible, for they will have a direct influence on the study outcome.

NURSING LEGISLATION

Nursing practice is regulated not only by the previous drug standards and legislation but also by individual state nurse practice acts; joint policy statements among the state nursing associations, medical associations, and hospital associations; and institutional and agency policies. Institutions and agencies may set policies that interpret more specifically those actions allowable under state nursing practice acts, but they may not modify, expand, or restrict the intent of such acts. Personal and professional ethical standards further govern actual nursing decisions and judgments in practice.

FDA PREGNANCY CATEGORIES FOR DRUGS

The FDA has assigned pregnancy safety categories for drugs studied in humans and animals, based on documentation. The categories are as follows:

Category A: Studies indicate no risk to the fetus.

Category B: Animal reproductive studies indicate no risk to the fetus; adequate and well-controlled studies in pregnant women are unavailable.

Category C: Animal reproductive studies indicate an adverse effect on the fetus, but adequate and well-controlled studies in pregnant women are not available. Potential benefit versus risk must be evaluated, since use of the drug in selected pregnant women at risk may be warranted.

Category D: Human data or studies exhibit positive evidence of human fetal risk, but potential benefit versus risk may warrant the use of the drug in pregnant women.

Category X: Fetal abnormalities and positive evidence of fetal risk in humans are available from animal or human studies or from marketing reports. The risks of using this drug far outweigh the benefits; thus such drugs should not be used in pregnant women.

Modified from United States pharmacopeia dispensing information, 1987.

FDA CLASSIFICATIONS FOR NEWLY APPROVED DRUGS

To assist the professional in immediately classifying new drug entities, the FDA has developed the following method of drug classification. A number and a letter are assigned to each new drug at the IND phase or at the NDA review by the FDA. The manufacturer has a right to contest this classification and have it changed before the final classification is established.

NUMERICAL CLASSIFICATION:

1. A new molecular drug
2. A new salt of a marketed drug
3. A new formulation or dosage form not previously marketed
4. A new combination not previously marketed
5. A drug that is already on the market, a generic duplication
6. Product already marketed by the same company (This designation is used for new indications for a marketed drug.)

LETTER CLASSIFICATION:

A— Drug offers an important therapeutic gain.
B— Medication offers a modest therapeutic gain over drugs already on the market.
C— Drug offers little or no therapeutic gain over other marketed drugs.
M— Drug marketed in a foreign country.
R— Drug has individual unique conditions for approval that are outlined in NDA approval letter.
T— Drug has toxicity problem (such as carcinogenicity in animals).
U— Drug is apt to be used for treatment of children.
D— Drug has less safety or is less effective as compared with marketed drugs but has a compensating virtue (such as being available for persons who have not responded to or are unable to tolerate the alternative available drugs on the market).
P— The important feature of the product is the container or package, not the drug.

The above classification is available by request from the Freedom of Information Staff at the Bureau of Drugs (Food and Drug Administration, 5600 Fishers Lane, Rockville, MD 20857).

The nurse practice acts of individual states define conditions under which nurses may be licensed to practice professionally. One of their functions is to protect the public from unskilled, undereducated, and unlicensed nurses and to delineate clearly the scope of nursing as a health care profession. Another function is to protect nurses by defining clearly their responsibilities and freedoms. Every state nurse practice act includes laws and regulations on reciprocity and suspension or revocation of nurse licenses.

Changing nursing roles and nursing legislation. Clearly, the traditional roles of the nurse are changing and expanding along with newer techniques and approaches to drug therapy. These expanding roles often find the nurse in activities beyond traditionally accepted nursing practices, which challenge the judgment and accountability of the nurse legally. Two such areas are prescription writing and certain modes of drug administration.

Prescribing medications has been, in the past, a purely medical function as determined by state law, while medication administration has usually been delegated to nurses and occasionally to licensed pharmacists and other trained personnel. In reality, astute nurses have been indirectly prescribing for many years, using diplomatic ploys with physicians to attend to changing patient needs: "Will you write an order for Dulcolax for Mrs. Rommel? She hasn't had a bowel movement for 3 days." Now, certain expanding roles in nursing, along with increased education and expertise (e.g., certification as nurse practitioner by the American Nurses' Association), raise the issue of legalizing the prescribing function of nurse practitioners.

Two reports acknowledged this need, one from the American Medical Association in 1970 and the other from the Department of Health, Education and Welfare in 1971. Both clearly state that the prescribing of medications "may be the practice of medicine when carried out by a physician and the practice of nursing when carried out by the nurse." Several states as a result of this change have amended their nurse practice acts. These amendments have predominantly given authorization to the nurse practitioner to write prescriptions according to established protocols or under physician supervision or collaboration. Some states, such as Alaska, Idaho, Maine, New Hampshire, Nevada, New Mexico, North Carolina, Oregon, Tennessee, Vermont, Washington, Michigan, and Maryland have revised their nurse practice acts to encompass prescribing as a nursing function if the nurse meets special criteria (e.g., usually those certified in the nurse practitioner role).

A pilot program to assess the safety and cost effectiveness of prescribing by hundreds of California nurse practitioners has been reviewed and found by all accounts to have been highly successful. The study determined that $15 million a year could be saved in physicians' and pharmacists' salaries if this function were legally endorsed. However, the California Medical Association is not in accord.

Other states have nurse-prescribing bills pending. Many states and institutions therein have developed protocols for designating the types of clients to be treated by nurse practitioners. They have also developed formularies to aid in their selection of prescribed drugs and to provide reviews of their prescribing activities, usually by periodic chart audits. One evaluative study of 1000 nurse practitioner–generated prescriptions demonstrated high levels of accuracy, accountability, and legibility. Of these prescriptions 25% were for relief of discomfort, 25% were for contraceptive purposes (one fourth of these were for diaphragms), 40% were for antibiotics, 6% were written to treat chronic stabilized disorders, and a small number were prescribed by the physician consultant for controlled substances. Nonprescription preparations such as Pepto-Bismol, aspirin, and vitamin supplements were also recommended by nurse practitioners. Of the drugs ordered 99% were consistent with the related protocol. There was no evidence of any complications arising from the medication prescribed, and all were deemed appropriate in terms of safety and therapeutic usefulness. It is of interest to note that the ratio of drug prescriptions to clients was lower among the nurse practitioners than among the physicians.

The AMA Socioeconomic Monitoring System has ascertained that physicians who employ nurse practitioners or physicians' assistants are able to charge less for visits and to manage about 20% more client visits per week than those who do not. Physicians who employ nurse practitioners report that they are generally pleased. Those physicians who were polled stated that they fully expected that more nurse practitioners would be part of the health care delivery system in the future and that this would be for the better. The plethora of studies attesting to the nurse practitioner's functional effectiveness, safety, and acceptance by the client may offer one solution to the high costs, long waits, and depersonalization in health care today.

Drug administration was, for a very long period in health care history, a function of physicians only. In fact, nurses were kept ignorant of the medications the client might be receiving. Gradually, medication administration became an interdependent function. Now, nurses find that they are increasingly taking responsibility for suggesting and selecting drugs, their dosages, and regulation. For example, in specialty units of some acute care hospitals, nurses assume responsibility for titrating the infusion rate and the dosage of potent antihypertensive medications against blood pressure parameters. They frequently are responsible for titrating intravenous (IV) fluids to replace gastrointestinal drainage milliliter for milliliter. In the past, nurses were authorized to administer large-volume continuous IV infusions. Nurses now also administer medications by small-volume intermittent IV infusion (by "piggyback" or "rider"). Furthermore, although the procedure is not generally legitimized as a nursing function, some hospitals, particularly in their specialized care units, authorize nurses to give very small-volume, undiluted medications either directly into a vein by IV "push" or into IV tubing.

Generally, changing roles and functions and the laws that govern them are not enacted simultaneously. There is usually a time lag between the adoption of a new function and official approval. Thus nurses who prepare and inject admixtures intravenously, whatever the delivery system, are breaking new legal ground. Such procedures are potentially more risky than other medication procedures, and nurses who perform them are probably placing themselves in a tenuous legal position unless (1) they are qualified by virtue of adequate training, education, and experience and (2) there exists written sanction. Policies should be drawn up jointly by the administration of the hospital or agency and nursing representatives. These policy statements should carefully delineate the roles of nurses and physicians and present guidelines for these procedures. They should include a list of drugs and routes to be used only by physicians and a list of criteria for permitting nurses to give medications by an IV route or other system. Currently, there is a trend for pharmacy department personnel to draw up and mix admixtures in large-volume IV solutions before delivering the medication to the nursing area. This is done under controlled conditions in agency pharmacies, with the goal of reducing IV solution contamination.

Basically, at the implementation stage, three conditions should be met before a nurse may legally begin to administer a medication by any mode:

1. The medication order must be valid
2. The physician and nurse must be licensed
3. The nurse must know the purpose, actions, effects, and major side and toxic effects of the drug

A valid order is one that leaves no room for doubt as to the medication prescribed, its dose and route, dosing interval, and the prescriber's name/signature. Moreover, the drug must also be deemed appropriate for that specific client. Since nurses are legally, morally, and ethically responsible for their actions, they must assess the medication order for its preciseness, accuracy, and appropriateness.

The medication order must be written and worded in such a way that it is correct, complete, legible, and clearly understandable. If it is not, clarification must be sought from the prescriber. Creating a healthy, open, questioning atmosphere in the prescriber-nurse relationship avoids the very real hazard lurking behind "guessing," "assuming," and "not wanting to bother the doctor."

Although not every medication given in error results in actual client harm, the potential always exists. It is wise to avert such incidents by clarifying the prescribing situation in the following ways.

Verbal order. A physician's order is given verbally (often at a client's bedside), such as "Just give her a little Mylanta." It is then appropriate to remind the prescriber that nurses cannot give medication unless the order is in writing. If the order is not written at that time, it is often forgotten. If the medication has already been given and it has not been "signed for" by the prescriber, it is illegal until the order is written and signed. Managing this before the prescriber leaves the area is often not possible.

Telephone order. An order given over the telephone can easily be miscommunicated, misinterpreted, or not clearly heard, and such an order often remains too long unsigned by the prescriber. Many institutions have a specific policy that limits acceptance of verbal or telephone orders to emergency situations only. In any event, all orders should be signed by the prescriber as soon as possible. Nursing students should not be held responsible for following or transcribing *any* unsigned telephone or verbal orders.

Incomplete order. Orders that are not complete in medication name, dose, route, time, or signature must be clarified and completed before administration. Orders for medications to be given by the IV route are the ones most often found incomplete; frequently the rate of infusion is the part missing from the order.

Incorrect or inappropriate order. The order may be judged by the nurse to be incorrect or inappropriate for the client (for example, a dose too high for the client of low body weight or impaired renal function as evidenced by low creatinine clearance, or a medication ordered for a client with a recent myocardial infarction that is noted to have secondary effects of tachycardia or dysrhythmias). Here, the situation may be quite intimidating to the nurse, who is now in the position of challenging the judgment of the physician at the risk of incurring embarrassment, job threat, or both. Of course, such intimidation is not justifiable. It is the nurse's or nursing student's absolute right and responsibility to question *any* proposed action that is potentially harmful to a client. Often physicians and some nurses (and many consumers) are under the mistaken impression that nurses who merely act by following a physicians' order are absolved from any untoward results of that act. Actually, *no one can relieve a nurse of responsibility for actions;* to carry out an order than the nurse knows to be incorrect constitutes negligence. To change an order by modifying any part of it, if done without consultation with the prescriber, is similarly illegal.

If an order is believed to be in error, some suggested actions are as follows:

1. Validate the order by consulting an authoritative reference source (see Chapter 5 for suggested drug data references).

2. If the order is indeed apparently incorrect, objectively report the conflicting facts and discuss it with the prescriber in a factual, calm, nonblaming manner.

3. If the prescriber still wants the medication given as ordered after the nurse's objections have been raised, can the nurse give the medication if the prescriber takes full responsibility? Again, *no one* can

release nurses from full responsibility for every medication they give just because they are acting under a physician's order. To do so is to court a suit for negligence. This fact must be made clear to the prescriber as the rationale for the nurse's refusal to medicate.

If the prescriber chooses to administer the medication personally after the nurse refuses to do so in the belief that it could be potentially harmful to the client, the nurse should see that the facts of the situation are made known to the immediate supervisors, and consultation should be sought if necessary. If the drug is given, the medication record should reflect that it was the prescriber who gave it.

Invalid order. Orders signed by medical students, physicians' assistants, or nurse practitioners are not legally accepted as having been signed by a duly licensed physician (this is the wording of most nursing practice acts) and should not be implemented until actually signed by a physician (or the law is changed). Validity of orders written and signed by a nonlicensed intern or resident may be equivocal, depending on local law or policy.

Order for unfamiliar drug. Orders for a medication that is unfamiliar to the administering nurse must stimulate a nearly reflex reaction to "look it up or to ask the pharmacist." Administration of an unfamiliar drug while remaining in ignorance of its actions, its intended and side effects, and its adverse reactions (at the very minimum) is considered nursing negligence if it results in harm to the client. For instance, a nurse was found liable when a 3-month-old infant died after being given an injectable form of digoxin instead of the pediatric elixir. In another instance, a nurse was found negligent when prolonged infiltration of a levarterenol (Levophed) infusion went unobserved, causing permanent injury.

• • •

Astute nurses are not only alert to the set limits of functioning but also to the quality of functioning within those limits. Although legal suits can be initiated when a nurse exceeds the limits of accepted practice, few have actually been instituted. However, more can be anticipated in the near future as the public becomes more aware of nurses' liability. Most suits, however, are brought by clients or their families who feel they have been subjected to behavior or to a procedure that was not of the quality of practice reasonably expected of someone with a nurse's professional education and experience and under the particular circumstances. This is identified legally as malpractice. The nurse can take safeguards against malpractice resulting from errors of medication administration by observing the **Five Patient Rights:**

1. The *right medication* (the one that was prescribed and one that is not contraindicated)

2. The *right patient* (not someone else's medication by mistake, or one that is similar in appearance)
3. The *right dosage* as prescribed and appropriate (it may involve simple mathematical computations)
4. The *right form, route, and technique* as prescribed
5. The drug at the *right time* (usually within half an hour of the time indicated and at beneficial intervals as ordered)

The following are examples of nursing actions that support and facilitate the meeting of these expectations:

1. Refusing to allow administration of a drug against good nursing judgment
2. Preparing medications in a quiet, undisturbed environment conducive to thoughtfulness and accuracy
3. Comparing the information on the medication ticket or Kardex with the prescriber's order and medication chart to prevent wrong dosage, double-dosing, or the like
4. Looking up information about all new or unfamiliar drugs before administering them
5. Reading medication labels three times—when taking drug container from its storage place, when preparing the dose, and when returning the drug container to its storage place
6. Carefully calculating dosage as necessary, especially when working with decimals
7. Administering only drug doses that were self-prepared
8. Positively identifying the client by comparing the arm band and the name on the medication ticket or medication administration record.
9. Listening intently to clients when they question the administration of a particular drug, its color, size, dosage, or a possible allergy; clients frequently give nurses crucial data in this manner
10. Recording the administration of each dose as soon as possible
11. Observing carefully for side and toxic effects, reporting them, and documenting actions taken

Probably the most powerful fundamental force at work in the actual implementation of right and proper nursing practice is the nurse's own concept of ethical and moral correctness and responsibility. Both the American Nurses' Association (1968) and the International Council of Nurses (1973) have adopted similar codes of ethics for nurses, which can serve as a guide to standards of conduct, relationships, and practice. At the core of any such professional code is that its precepts spring from the reality that the client is a person with rights and dignity not to be subsumed under the needs or rights of any other person or the machinations of the institution or society at large. For example, clients have every right to know necessary information about a drug they are receiving and to refuse to take it after having given the courtesy of an explanation, no matter what the consequences.

For the nurse's part, accountability is a term that has gained increasing import, particularly as related to pharmacotherapeutics. Nurses are no longer considered to be merely "physicians' handmaidens" or to be accorded

"umbrella protection from litigation" by the physician and the institution. Nurses are increasingly expected to take the responsibility for and be answerable for the service they provide or make available.

In summary, basic guides to litigation-free, professional nursing practice and to medication administration in particular include:

1. Knowing the limitations of nursing practice in the community through awareness of the agency policies, joint medical and nursing practice statements, nursing practice acts, and state and federal laws; then abiding by them
2. Knowing the limitations of one's own skills, expertise, knowledge, and experience and never exceeding them
3. Informing involved personnel of and documenting thoroughly and carefully all happenings related to client care, especially those with potential legal implications
4. Maintaining a professional, caring, and collaborative relationship with clients and their families. Aside from this being a proper approach, it can act to dissolve potential dissatisfaction of clients with health care, with the institution, or with its policies.

SUMMARY OF NURSING CONSIDERATIONS

Early in a nursing career, the study of legal issues related to the administration of medications can seem a somewhat less than fascinating exercise. However, as the nurse builds practical experience, this study will prove its worth time and time again. Laws, acts, codes, and regulations shaping pharmacologic practice provide the boundaries for safe practice. Experience proves that knowing the accepted scope of nursing practice of one's nation, state, locale, and institutional community provides security and support for the nurse who aspires to provide harm-free care. Legal statutes only guide; nurses have to translate these guides into action. Often what guides best within legal constraints is the individual nurse's judgment based on his or her own code of ethics, professionalism, and sense of accountability. A fundamental precept is that what is best for the client usually turns out to be best for the nurse.

There are few hard and fast rules in nursing practice. Many specific questions about legalities in drug administration must be answered, and the answer is often, "It depends . . . ." This should not act to immobilize nurses and prevent them from acting in healthy, assertive ways. If they function within the accepted boundaries of practice, continue to stretch for new knowledge, and act accountably for the benefit of their clients, there is little that can harm their clients, themselves, their professional reputations, or their jobs. The sureness that comes with experience flourishes as they exercise these skills. And exercising these skills often demands that they stand up for what is right in client care despite pressures in the situation generated by time constraints or by others who want them to "just get on with it." Being human, nurses will occasionally fail to use the best judgment or to be perfect. This is reasonable, but it is also reasonable for nurses to aspire to structure their practice in ways that make it difficult to fail.

The neophyte nurse may be somewhat shaken by the wealth of background information necessary to safe practice. The more experienced nurse will probably grapple with the temptation to become complacent and to make dangerous assumptions about the limits of his or her practice. Both need equally to continue to read and question to improve the quality of their decisions, whether the issues stem from legal, ethical, or moral considerations.

The state of the art of drug development, evaluation, and prescribing, although sophisticated and well regulated in theory, may in practice be sometimes inadequate. Moreover, since all chemical substances such as drugs create side effects, adverse reactions, and interactions, and many have been identified as having questionable efficacy, it becomes increasingly compelling to avoid medicating, when feasible, and to substitute rational nursing measures. For example, nursing interventions to promote comfort, if instituted effectively and early in the pain cycle, can often substantially reduce pain so that "as necessary" medications become unnecessary.

KEY TERMS

BIBLIOGRAPHY

American Nurses' Association: Code for nurses with interpretive statements, Kansas City, Mo, 1976, The Association.

Bigbee, JL: Territoriality and prescriptive authority for nurse practitioners, Nurs Health Care 5(2):106.

Bigbee, JL, and others: Prescriptive authority for nurse practitioners: a comparative study of professional attitudes, Am J Public Health 74(2):162, 1984.

Black, JB, ed: Safeguarding the public: historical aspects of medical drug control, Baltimore, 1970, The Johns Hopkins University Press.

California RNs fight for the right to prescribe, Am J Nurs 83:700, 1983.

Corbett, KM, and Lynch, LC: Professional nursing issues in the administration of investigational antiarrhythmic medications, Heart Lung 13(4):395, 1984.

Creighton, H: Law every nurse should know, ed 4, Philadelphia, 1980, WB Saunders Co.

Davidson, DE, ed: Handbook of nonprescription drugs, ed 8, Washington, DC, 1986, American Pharmaceutical Association.

Department of National Health and Welfare: Patent medicines, no 14, Ottawa, 1971, Food and Drug Directorate, Educational Services.

Department of National Health and Welfare: Health protection and drug laws, Ottawa, 1980, Minister of National Health and Welfare, Educational Services, Health Protection Branch.

Department of National Health and Welfare: Food and drug act and regulations, 1972, with amendments to January, 1982, Ottawa, 1982, Queen's Printer and Controller of Stationery.

Department of National Health and Welfare: Narcotic control act and narcotic control regulations, Ottawa, 1982, Queen's Printer and Controller of Stationery.

Edmunds, MW: Evaluation of nurse practitioner effectiveness: an overview of the literature, Evaluation Health Professions 1 (1):11, 1978.

Gosselin, RA: Postmarketing surveillance, Apothecary 94(3):58, 1982.

Johnson, JB: Bioequivalence: a factor in product selection, Pearl River, NY, 1979, Lederle Publication, pp 667-669.

Johnson, JM: Clinical trials: new responsibilities and roles for nurses, Nurs Outlook 34(3):149, 1986.

Kallet, A, and Schlink, FJ: 100,000,000 guinea pigs: dangers in everyday foods, drugs, and cosmetics, New York, 1933, The Vanguard Press.

Marchette, L: Experimental drugs: where do you stand legally? RN 47(3):23, 1984.

Modell, W, and Lansing, A: Drugs, New York, 1967, Life Science Library, Time, Inc.

Munroe, D, and others: Prescribing patterns of nurse practitioners, Am J Nurs 82:1538, 1982.

Reidenberg, MM: The final report of the joint commission on prescription drugs, Hosp Pharmacy 15(8):4171, 1980.

Rosenaur, J, and others: Prescribing behaviors of primary care nurse practitioners, Am J Public Health 74(1):10, 1984.

Schneiweiss, F: Understanding the FDA's guarded system for classifying new drugs, Hosp Pharmacy 14(5):262, 1979.

S.C. nurses defend right to practice under MD protocols, Am J Nurs 83:851, 1983.

Sullivan, JA: Research on nurse practitioners: process behind the outcome, Am J Public Health 72:8, 1982.

Sultz, HA, and others: A decade of change for nurse practitioners, Nurs Outlook 31(3):137, 1983.

United States Pharmacopeia Dispensing Information. Easton, Pa, 1988, Mack Publishing Co.

Young, JH: The toadstool millionaires: a social history of patent medicines in America before federal regulation, Princeton, NJ, 1961, Princeton University Press.

CHAPTER
3

Drug Preparations and Formulations

OBJECTIVES

After studying this chapter, the student will be able to:

1. Describe the difference between chemical, generic, and trade names of drug products.

2. Differentiate between alkaloid, glycoside, gum, resin, and oil.

3. Describe the difference between permissive and mandatory drug substitution in the United States.

4. Name the four main sources of drug and biologic products.

5. Explain the importance of properly storing medication according to the manufacturer's specifications.

6. Identify nursing considerations for proper drug storage and distribution.

7. Identify common pharmaceutical preparations and dosage forms.

8. Discuss delivery systems available for the administration of medications.

NAMES OF DRUGS

As a drug passes through the investigational stage and the stages when it becomes accepted and marketed, it collects and keeps as many as three different types of names. The first is the chemical name, the second is the generic or nonproprietary name, and the third is the trade name.

The **chemical name** is a precise description of the drug's chemical composition and molecular structure. It is particularly meaningful to the chemist. For example, the chemical name of one of the commonly prescribed antibiotics is 4-dimethylamino-1,4,4a,5,5a,6,11,12a-octahydro-3,6,10,12,12a-pentahydroxy-6-methyl-1,11-dioxo-2-napthacenecarboxamide. Its generic name is tetracycline and it is also sold under a number of trade names—Achromycin, Mysteclin, and Panmycin, among others.

The **generic** or **nonproprietary name** is often assigned by the manufacturer with USAN (the United States Adopted Name Council of the U.S.P.) approval to denote a general class of pharmacologically similar drugs as designated by the U.S.P. The generic name is often derived from the chemical name and a simpler form. The generic name is not as easily remembered as the trade name, and thus is not as frequently selected by prescribers. However, the use of generic names is widely advocated to avoid confusion between trade names that are similar. The drug that is packaged under the generic name usually has the same therapeutic efficacy. In addition, it is much less expensive than the trade name drug, often costing only one-half to one-half as much. The **trade name, brand name,** or **proprietary name** is designated by the drug company selling it and is copyrighted; it is a proper noun and the first letter is capitalized. Trade names of drugs discussed in this book will be found enclosed in parentheses following the generic name.

Skilled marketing specialists work to give each of their company's drugs an easily spelled, short trade name that in some way communicates its major action or ingredient. To promote sales of the trade name drug extensive advertising is usually necessary, involving considerable expense, which is borne mainly by the consumer. However, much of the research in new drugs is done in laboratories of reputable drug firms, and, to realize a legitimate return for the cost of research, drug companies need to patent their products and have exclusive rights to their manufacture and sale.

Health care–related organizations have recognized the growing confusion among the public, health care providers, and prescribers resulting from the proliferation of "new" drugs and multiple names for each. Many of these "new" drugs are reformulations of established drugs (some whose patents may have expired after 17 years) designed to capitalize on an existing market. The United States Adopted Name Council of the U.S. Pharmacopeia Committee and the World Health Organization are working to facilitate world-wide standardization of drug names, and the AMA-USP Nomenclature Committee and the American Pharmaceutical Association are working to create simpler, more useful generic names through the use of more logical syllables. It is anticipated that these approved names will eventually be adopted as the official drug nomenclature.

DRUG SUBSTITUTION IN THE UNITED STATES

Nearly every state has a drug substitution law that either permits or mandates substitution on the part of the pharmacist, although the physician retains the prerogative to require the dispensing of a particular brand drug. In permissive states the physician must give express permission for substitution by either signing a special section on the prescription form or by checking the correct phrase on the prescription. If substitution is not wanted, the physician may note this by writing "Dispense as written," "Brand necessary," or "Medically necessary."

In states with a mandatory law, the pharmacist is required to dispense approved, less expensive, generic drugs to the patient. Several exceptions apply in such situations; for example, the consent of the client may be required before substitution, or the physician may mark the individual prescription with a term that prohibits substitution, such as "Medically necessary." Some states, such as Florida, have enacted a **negative drug formulary,** a

list of drugs that have a proven potential for different bioavailabilities or therapeutic problems and that may not be substituted for trade name drugs. If the physician orders a brand name for these products (see box for current Florida listing), then only that specific brand may be dispensed. If the physician orders any of these products by a generic name, which incidentally, is not recommended, then the pharmacist must select a product that is FDA approved and that has an NDA or an abbreviated new drug application number.

SOURCES OF DRUGS

Drugs and biologic products have been identified or derived from four main sources: (1) plants, examples of which are digitalis, vincristine, and colchicine; (2) animals and humans, from which drugs such as epinephrine, insulin, and ACTH are obtained; (3) minerals or mineral products, such as iron, iodine, and Epsom salts; and (4) chemical substances made in the laboratory. The drugs made of chemical substances are pure drugs, and some of them are simple substances, such as sodium bicarbonate and magnesium hydroxide. Others are products of complex synthesis, such as the sulfonamides and the adrenocorticosteroids.

Active constituents of plant drugs. The leaves, roots, seeds, and other parts of plants may be dried or otherwise processed for use as medicine and, as such, are known as crude drugs. Their therapeutic effect is caused by the chemical substances they contain. When the pharmacologically active constituents are separated from the crude preparation, the resulting substances are more potent and usually produce effects more reliably than does the crude drug. Some of the types of pharmacologically active com-

---

FLORIDA NEGATIVE DRUG FORMULARY LIST*

1. Digoxin
2. Digitoxin
3. Quinidine
4. Nitroglycerin
5. Warfarin sodium
6. Conjugated estrogens
7. Erythromycin
8. Chloramphenicol
9. Dicumarol
10. Phenytoin
11. Nitrofurantoin
12. Liotrix
13. Prednisone
14. Gamma benzene hexachloride

*List revised as of March 17, 1977 and is current as of June 2, 1987.

pounds found in plants, grouped according to their physical and chemical properties, are alkaloids, glycosides, gums, resins (balsams), and oils.

1. **Alkaloids** are organic compounds composed of carbon, hydrogen, nitrogen, and oxygen. They are alkaline in nature and are chemically combined with acids in the laboratory to form water-soluble salts, such as morphine sulfate and atropine sulfate. Synthetic alkaloids formulated in the laboratory have activity similar to plant alkaloids.

2. **Glycosides** are active plant substances that, on hydrolysis, yield a sugar plus one or more additional active substances. The presence of the sugar is not necessary for the action of the glycosides, but it is believed to increase the solubility, absorption, permeability, and cellular distribution. An important cardiac glycoside used in medicine is digoxin.

3. **Gums** are plant exudates. When water is added, some of them will swell and form gelatinous masses. Others remain unchanged in the gastrointestinal tract, where they act as hydrophilic (water-loving) colloids; that is, they absorb water, form watery bulk, and exert a laxative effect. Agar and psyllium seeds are examples of natural laxative gums, while methylcellulose and sodium carboxymethylcellulose are synthetic colloids. Gums are also used to soothe irritated skin and mucous membranes.

4. **Resins** are semisolid or solid plant exudates. The sap of certain trees also contains resin. Resins are not used as commonly today in medicine as they were in the past.

5. **Oils** are highly viscous liquids and are generally of two kinds, volatile or fixed. A **volatile** oil imparts an aroma to a plant, and because of their pleasant odor and taste, these oils were frequently used as flavoring agents. Peppermint oil and clove oil are examples of volatile oils occasionally used in medicine. **Fixed oils** are generally greasy and do not evaporate easily unlike volatile oils. Olive oil is a fixed oil used in cooking, while castor oil is an example of a fixed oil used in medicine.

DRUG CLASSIFICATION

Drug classification can be approached from two perspectives, by clinical indication or by body system. This book uses both approaches where appropriate. Examples of drugs classified by clinical indication include:

Chapter 15 — Central nervous system stimulants
Chapter 21 — Skeletal muscle relaxants
Chapter 61 — Antimicrobial and antiparasitic drugs

An example of drugs classified by body system is:

Unit Four — Drugs affecting the central nervous system

These drug groupings can assist the nurse to understand and memorize many of the individual agents avail-able for drug therapy. Learning pharmacology becomes easier when one understands the common characteristics of each drug classification and when a prototype drug within each group is studied thoroughly. When a new drug becomes available, the nurse will then be able to associate it with its drug classification and make inferences about many of its basic qualities before reading about its specific properties. Learning which of its qualities are different from the prototype drug and its dosage is extremely helpful.

Nurses need not be overwhelmed by long, involved drug names. Certain syllables can suggest information, such as the suffix "-caine" and its association with anesthetics; the syllable in cortisone derivatives "-cort-"; "ceph-," relating to cephalosporin-type antibiotics; and so on. The basic information to be learned about each major drug includes its generic name and one trade name, the category to which it belongs, its clinical uses, its mechanism of action, side effects and toxic effects, and other specifics associated with the nurse's role in administration of, evaluation of, and client teaching about that drug. "Looking it up" should become second nature to the nursing student as well as the practicing nurse, who should also encourage or initiate the development of a nurses' library shelf and a file of informative inserts about drugs frequently used in the clinical area. Nurses are professionally, morally, legally, and personally responsible for every dose of medication they administer.

PHARMACEUTICAL PREPARATIONS

Pharmaceutical preparations are the formulations that make a drug suited to various methods of administration. They may be made up by the pharmacist but more often are prepared by the pharmaceutical company from which they are purchased. The nurse who is informed about various preparations can make more astute judgments about their individual applications and appropriate recommendations to the prescriber when necessary.

Table 3-1 details common preparations and their various applications.

ALTERNATE DRUG DELIVERY SYSTEMS

Innovative advances in scientific technology and computerization provide impetus for the development of increasingly sophisticated drug delivery systems, particularly in the treatment of diabetes mellitus and cancer. However, medical devices are not subject to the same rigorous evaluation or regulation as are drugs. Some examples of these technologies include implanted drug deposits, membrane drug delivery systems, and needle-syringe pump assemblies.

Implanted capsules of a progestin hormone, called the norplant method, are being tested for contraceptive efficacy. Implantation takes 15 minutes and is immediately

TABLE 3-1   Various Forms of Drug Preparations*

Form	Examples/Remarks
PREPARATIONS FOR ORAL USE	
Liquid	
Aqueous solutions	Substances dissolved in water and syrups
Aqueous suspensions (shake well before administering)	Mixtures (solid particles suspended in liquid), emulsions (fats or oils suspended in a liquid with an emulsifier), magmas (milky suspensions), gels (suspensions of insoluble substances)
Spirits (alcohol solutions), e.g., whiskey, wine	
Elixirs (aromatic, sweetened alcohol and water solution containing a dissolved substance or medication)	
Tinctures (alcohol extract of animal or vegetable substances)	
Fluidextracts (concentrated alcoholic liquid extracts of vegetables)	
Extracts (e.g., syrup or dried extract of the active drug ingredients)	
Solid	
Capsules (gelatin-covered dry drug, used to avoid the problems of disintegration, instability, or taste; or in tiny beads for continuous release)	Tetracycline (Achromycin)
Tablets (powdered drug that is compressed and molded into small disks); may be scored to allow for half doses; may be coated for palatability, for ease in swallowing, to make identifiable or layered for sustained release or enteric coated (to protect drug from gastric secretions or to protect gastric mucosa from effects of the drug); enteric coated tablets are not to be broken or crushed for administration	Aspirin (acetylsalicylic acid) Enteric tablets/capsules have been found undigested in patients' stool and may cause local mucosal irritation; both capsules and tablets may "case harden" or deteriorate with age
Troches (lozenges that dissolve in the mouth)	Cēpacol throat lozenges
Powders and granules (loose or molded); for use with or without mixing in liquid	Potassium chloride for oral solution (K-Lor); psyllium hydrophilic mucilloid (Metamucil)
PREPARATIONS FOR PARENTERAL USE	
Ampules (sealed all-glass containers for liquid injectable medication; must be broken open for use); needle filters or IV in-line filters recommended	Diazepam (Valium)
Vials (glass containers with rubber stoppers for liquid or powdered medication — diluent must be added); before medication is withdrawn, air equivalent to the dosage volume must be added	Mix-O-Vial
Cartridges (usually a single-dose unit of parenteral medication that comes with or without needle attached to the glass cylinder); to be used with a specific injecting assembly mechanism	Tubex and Carpuject sterile needle units Bristoject units for injection
Large-volume intravenous infusions (suspended on hanger at bedside)	
Glass bottles, various sizes containing from 150 to 1000 ml for continuous infusion of fluid replacement with or without medications added via medication port; rubber stoppers with an air vent, either a long plastic tube through the solution and opening into air at top of inverted bottle (without air filter) *or* air inlet on administration set at juncture with bottle (with air filter); rigid, easy to handle, and biologically inert glass, but heavy and breakable	D$_5$W, normal saline; large-volume infusions are used for drugs that must be highly diluted (KCl) or that require steady blood levels (e.g., nitroprusside, oxytocin), or for total parenteral nutrition; most commonly used to replace fluids or electrolytes (see Chapter 70)
Flexible, collapsible plastic bags of polyvinyl chloride containing 150 to 1000 ml for continuous infusion of fluid replacement with or without medications added via small auxiliary tube port; needs no air vent; unbreakable, lightweight, but not biologically inert (may absorb some medication to inside of container, and some constituents of the plastic [plasticizers] may leach out into solution; this creates no currently known hazard to patient)	
Semirigid plastic container made of polyolefin in a (currently) limited variety of volume sizes for continuous fluid replacement with or without added medication via port; needs no air vent; biologically inert, impermeable to moisture, lightweight, unbreakable	

*See also text.

Continued.

TABLE 3-1 Various Forms of Drug Preparations*—cont'd

Form	Examples/Remarks

Ampules and vials as discussed previously

Pump-action vials with a plastic spike on top for inverting and injecting into a large-volume infusion

Special double-ended needles inserted into both the medication vial and the bottle for mixing and injecting into the large-volume intravenous infusion

Intermittent intravenous infusions (usually secondary IV setup)

Small plastic or glass bottles (volume: 50 to 250 ml solution) to which medication is added; to run as "piggyback," hung separately from primary (main) IV infusion, and run via a secondary administration tubing set for a period of 20 minutes to 2 hours; usually primary IV solution is run during the time between medication doses, but some institutions may infuse IV medication intermittently through an infusion lock or "heparin lock" without recourse to a primary IV solution at all. Volume-control sets are small-volume (100 to 250 ml) solutions; semirigid, calibrated plastic chambers or flexible plastic bags to which medication is added; the volume-control set is hung below an IV solution, which acts as diluent-reservoir for intermittent medication administration or as the primary infusion between doses of medication
    (right column) Medication: antibiotics — Soluset (Abbott Laboratories), Volu-Trole-A (Cutter Laboratories), Pedatrol (Travenol Laboratories)

Direct intravenous rapid injection

Intermittent infusion device consisting of a winged infusion needle with a short length of narrow tubing for intermittent injection of small doses of medication by needle and syringe; device stays in place between doses without any solution infusion (although to keep vein open, a diluted heparin solution is added to lock after each dose of medication); needle and syringe injection of very small volume of a drug directly into IV tubing via a port or the rubber bulb or directly injected into a vein itself; no solution infuses between doses
    (right column) Heparin lock, infusion lock; Emergency drugs; Cancer chemotherapy

PREPARATIONS FOR TOPICAL USE

Liniments (liquid suspension for lubrication; apply by rubbing)

Lotions (liquid suspensions; apply by patting on); can be protective, emollient, cooling, astringent, antipruritic, cleansing, etc.

Ointment (semisolid medicine in a greasy base) for local protective, soothing, astringent, bacteriostatic effects, or transdermal application for systemic effects (nitroglycerin, scopolamine)

Pastes (thick ointments) primarily for skin protection

Plasters (solid preparations that are adhesive, protective, or soothing)

Creams (emulsions containing an aqueous and an oily base)

Aerosols (fine powders or solutions in volatile liquids with a propellant)

PREPARATIONS FOR USE ON MUCOUS MEMBRANES

Drops (aqueous saline solutions with or without gelling agent to increase retention time in the eye); dropper tip should not touch anything except the solution itself, to retain sterility
    (right column) For eyes, ears, or nose

Instillation (aqueous solution of medications for topical action or occasionally for systemic action)
    (right column) Enemas, douches, mouthwashes, throat sprays, gargles

Aerosol sprays, nebulizers, inhalers (aqueous solutions of medication delivered by container designed to make droplets of a size appropriate to the location of the target membrane; i.e., the smaller the droplet, the farther it will travel down the bronchial tree); with or without a propellant, for bronchodilation or topical anesthesia
    (right column) Bronchodilators: metaproterenol sulfate (Alupent); teach patients to exhale fully before inhaling medication and to hold breath momentarily after deep inhalation; tolerance may build—do not overuse

Foams (powders or solutions of medication in volatile liquids with a propellant)
    (right column) Vaginal foams: for contraception

Powders, tablets, creams
    (right column) Vaginally, for contraception or vaginitis, etc.

Suppositories (medicinal substances mixed with a firm but malleable base, e.g., glycol, to facilitate insertion into a body cavity); generally should be refrigerated; may be used with an applicator
    (right column) Laxatives, vaginal suppositories

Continued.

TABLE 3-1   Various Forms of Drug Preparations — cont'd

Form	Examples/Remarks
MISCELLANEOUS DRUG DELIVERY SYSTEMS (EXAMPLES)	
Intradermal implants	
Pellets containing a small deposit of medication inserted in a dermal pocket; designed to allow medication to leach slowly into tissue	Testosterone Estradiol
Micropump system	
Small external pump, attached by belt or implanted, that delivers medication by needle in a continuous steady dose	Insulin Anticancer chemotherapy Narcotics
Membrane delivery systems	
Drug-laden polymer membrane instilled in the conjunctival fornix of the eye to deliver a steady flow of medication	Pilocarpine Corticosteroids
Pessaries and IUDs	
Drug enveloped or impregnated within the device for slow release of medication (e.g., hormones, copper, or other substance) to prevent contraception, etc.	
COMMON ACCESSORY ADDITIVES TO DRUG AND BIOLOGIC PREPARATIONS (INACTIVE INGREDIENTS; EXCIPIENTS)	
Preservatives (none in some medications because they inactivate the drug) pH stabilizers	
Bacteriostatic agents	Phenol, benzoic acid, thimerosal
Diluents as "fillers" when the drug dose is too small to work with	Sterile water, normal saline, bacteriostatic water, dextrose, lactose, starch, bentonite, kaolin, Fuller's Earth
Binding agents provide adhesion to a powdered drug to form a tablet	Acacia gum, methylcellulose, sugars
Lubricants prevent the drug product from sticking to the machinery during manufacture of tablets, etc.	Starch, lactose
Disintegrators to facilitate dissolution of product when appropriate	Starch (expands when exposed to water), sodium bicarbonate
Coatings	Gels, gums, waxes
Flavoring	Sugar or chocolate
Coloring	Dyes

effective. Contraceptive effects are said to last 5 to 7 years.

Small pumps weighing about half a pound are now available as portable infusion systems for continuous drug treatment of certain type I diabetic or cancer clients. The systems currently approved and in use generally consist of a battery, a programmable electronic "brain," an electric motor and pump, and a syringe, all of which are detachable as a unit from the small needle kept in place either in subcutaneous abdominal or thigh tissue (for diabetes) or by Silastic catheter inserted into an artery supplying the malignant tumor. These programmable pumps allow for various flow rates and an on-off feature. For clients with varying clinical needs, such a device appears to be quite efficient (Paice, 1984). Some systems are designed to be worn externally over clothing, stored in a pocket, or suspended from a belt or a neck chain (Figures 3-2 and 3-3). Others are implanted within a subcutaneous pocket in the lower abdomen and elsewhere. Epidural

morphine and intrathecal morphine have been successfully administered via implantable continuous drug delivery systems such as the Infusaid pump (Figure 3-4).

Topical ointment applications of nitroglycerin have been used to treat anginal pain for some time, and now microquantitative assay capabilities make possible precise unit dosages using transdermal modes. These products contain topical nitroglycerin in small unit-dose adhesive bandages that slowly release the medication over a 24-hour period. Some of them employ a semipermeable, rate-controlling membrane placed next to the skin (on the upper body, usually a hair-free area of the chest); others disperse the nitroglycerin evenly throughout a gel matrix. Nitrodisc, Nitro-Dur, and Transderm-Nitro are some trade name products. Similarly, motion sickness is treated with scopolamine (Transerm-V); duration of effects of one application behind the ear is about 3 days.

The student should be aware that new systems are similar to new drugs on the market — that is, widespread use

Directions for use of
Carpuject®
Sterile Cartridge-Needle Units

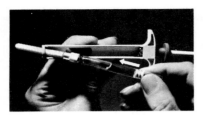

1 Insert CARPUJECT Sterile Cartridge-Needle Unit, needle end first, into open side of holder.

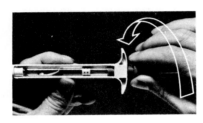

2 Advance and engage blue locking screw and turn *clockwise* beyond initial resistance until it will no longer rotate.

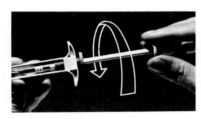

3 Advance plunger rod and screw *clockwise* onto threaded insert in rubber plunger.
To maintain sterility, leave needle guard in place until just before use.

Prepare CARPUJECT unit for administration in a normal manner, ie, remove needle guard, dispel air from cartridge, and proceed with injection.

FIGURE 3-1 Directions for use of Carpuject sterile cartridge-needle units with self-contained medication.

(Courtesy Winthrop-Breon Laboratories, New York, NY.)

often uncovers information or problems that were not previously documented. For example, reports have indicated that tolerance develops rapidly to the nitroglycerin patches, which can result in decreased effectiveness in as little as a 2-week time period (Abramowicz, 1984; Parker, 1985). Other studies report conflicting data in this area (Abramowicz, 1984). Therefore more research is necessary not only to document a problem but also to develop new ways to offset or reduce clinical setbacks.

DRUG STABILITY AND STORAGE

The potency and efficacy of drugs are affected by the way they are handled and stored. **Potency** is the strength per milligram of drug. **Efficacy** is the drug's maximum therapeutic ability. Deterioration, decomposition, or alteration of any drug or chemical compound begins as soon as it has been produced and proceeds gradually. Eventually this may result in altered effectiveness or toxicity of the drug, and this fact must be considered in the ordering, storing, dispensing, and administering of drugs.

Most drugs can be stored on the stock supply shelves or in the medication cart, but some must be stored according to specific manufacturer's directions (on the label or package insert) in order to retard deterioration (e.g., live vaccines, most reconstituted drugs, and most suppositories). Many drugs change composition or potency when

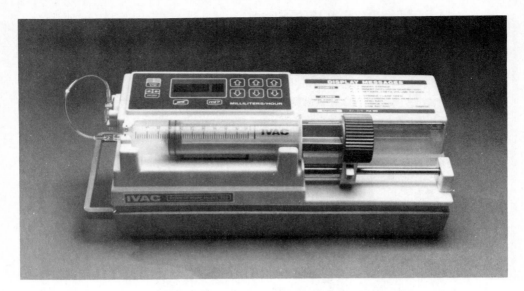

FIGURE 3-2   Microcomputer-controlled larger-volume syringe pump for use when there is a need for medication or fluids of up to 50 ml to be administered with accuracy and at a constant rate.

(Courtesy IVAC Corp., San Diego, Calif.)

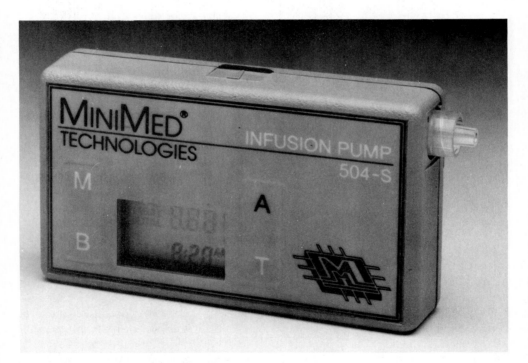

FIGURE 3-3   MiniMed Insulin Syringe. This pump (Infusion Pump 504-S) is one of the smallest and lightest available — it weighs only 3.1 ounces. The pump is easy to wear under clothing, carry in pockets, or attach to belts. Its features include a water-resistant package, long battery life (monthly change of batteries), and an alarm system to warn the user of an occlusion, an empty syringe, a runaway infusion, or a low or depleted battery. The unit can be preprogrammed for four basal variation rates in 24 hours, thus providing flexibility for the user. A 24-hour hotline is available to answer any questions on diabetes and the pump therapy.

(Courtesy MiniMed Technologies, Sylmar, Calif.)

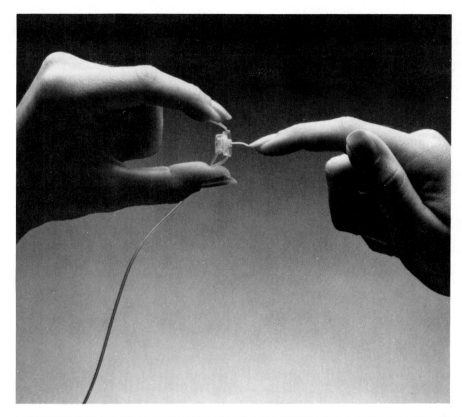

FIGURE 3-4 Sof-set, a soft teflon cannula and tubing that is inserted by needle, which is then withdrawn so the pump can operate without one. This product has a special adhesive dressing that inhibits bacterial growth.
(Courtesy MiniMed Technologies, Sylmar, Calif.)

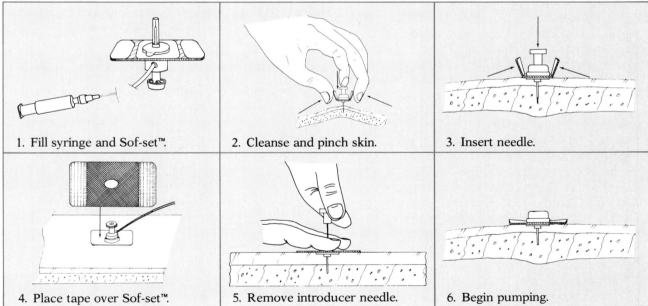

1. Fill syringe and Sof-set™. 2. Cleanse and pinch skin. 3. Insert needle.

4. Place tape over Sof-set™. 5. Remove introducer needle. 6. Begin pumping.

exposed to light, heat, moisture, or gases in the environment. The U.S.P. has defined the nomenclature used in instructions for prevention of changes resulting from heat:

Freeze—store below 0° C (32° F)

Store in a cold place—temperature no higher than 15° C (59° F)

Refrigerate—2° to 15° C (36° to 59° F)

Avoid excessive heat—temperature no higher than 40° C (104° F)

Medication refrigerators should be used solely for the storage of drugs and related necessities and should be cleaned out regularly, with expired drugs being returned to the pharmacy. At least one thermometer should be inside to monitor temperature maintenance.

The appropriate storage of drugs on the nursing unit is a nursing responsibility.

Amber-colored containers protect some medications (such as furosemide and nitroglycerin) against deterioration by light. This fact and its significance should be pointed out to clients who are self-medicating and who might otherwise transfer medications to a different container (to take to work, on vacation, and the like). Storage in a closed cabinet or other dark place should also be advised. If it is feasible, clients should be given information about how to tell if their medication has deteriorated (nitroglycerin no longer tingles under the tongue), and they should be told that the medication may need replacement if storage requirements have been abridged or if the medication's appearance or effects have changed.

Certain drugs given intravenously are significantly light-sensitive: amphotericin B; B complex vitamins; cisplatin; daunorubicin; doxorubicin; the essential amino acid for injection, NephrAmine; and nitroprusside. These should be checked for visible signs of deterioration, such as color change, precipitation, or gas formation. Deterioration may neutralize the drugs, make them toxic, or occur without these signs. Thus nitroprusside and amphotericin solutions for infusions should be kept covered with foil or an amber plastic bag (not a brown paper bag). Unless freshly prepared, all the other solutions should also be kept covered.

Tight lids can prevent degradation or change of the drug form or its active constituents by preventing exchange of moisture or gases within the container.

Clients who store drugs at home should be reminded that they *must* be stored out of reach of children — particularly those under 5, who are insatiably curious and may mimic adults' drug-taking behavior. The drug's childproof cap may serve only to slow the child down.

The expiration dates printed on drug labels mean simply that the drug contained is probably at its peak effectiveness until some point in time around that date. Since quality controls in drug production are subject to error rates similar to all other control programs, pharmaceutical companies tend to estimate these expiration dates somewhat conservatively. Thus, the drug is not instantly rendered useless or harmful by that date, but the effectiveness of the therapy may be gradually diminished and the drug may produce inadequate or occasionally toxic results some time after the printed date. The nurse should not administer doses from an outdated lot of drug or container; a fresh supply must be obtained.

Certain precepts should guide the way clients' drugs are stored, distributed, and accounted for. Health care agencies have developed policies that with variation, support these precepts as rules for client protection and prevent nurses from making errors. In addition, rational nursing judgments must enter into decision making,

allowing departure from these rules as a wise and necessary choice, but this should never be undertaken lightly. It should also be a practice to consult other expert personnel or authorities.

The following guidelines are not necessarily listed in order of importance.

1. All medicines should be kept in a special place, which may be a cupboard, closet, or room. The area should not be freely accessible to the public.
2. Narcotic drugs and those dispensed under special legal regulations must be kept in a locked box or compartment and accounted for at the end of each shift. Any dose that is wasted or discarded must be attested to by another nurse by initialing of such a notation.
3. In some hospitals each client's medicines are kept in a designated place on a shelf or compartment of the medicine cupboard or room or in a drawer of the medication cart. Such an arrangement means that the nurse must be careful to keep the client's medicines in the right area and to make certain that, when the client leaves the hospital, the medicines are returned to the pharmacy.
4. If stock supplies are maintained, they should be arranged in an orderly manner. Preparations for internal use should be kept separate from those used externally.
5. Some preparations, such as serums, vaccines, certain suppositories, certain antibiotics, and insulin, need to be kept on a refrigerator shelf, not on the door, to maintain a more constant cool temperature.
6. Labels of all medicines should be clean and legible. If they are not, they should be sent to the pharmacist for relabeling. *Nurses should not label or relabel medicines.*
7. Bottles of medicines should always be stoppered and protected from light, heat, and high humidity as necessary.

Intravenous drugs. Many intravenous drugs require a diluent to dissolve the medication, which then can be added to a larger-volume solution for administration. The storage times for such medications can vary, depending on the following:

1. The expiration date on the package for the fresh package of medication stored under the specific instructions of the manufacturer
2. The expiration time period allotted for the dissolved medication
3. The expiration time period allotted for the dissolved medication added to a larger volume of solution

To obtain accurate information for an individual drug, the reader is referred to the drug's package insert or the U.S.P.-DI, volume I. Table 3-2 illustrates the range of expiration times and storage requirements, even within the same drug classification (cephalosporin antibiotics).

SUMMARY OF NURSING CONSIDERATIONS

Close attention to all drugs the nurse administers helps the nurse learn to identify them, tailor their application, and spot errors before they occur. Expertise is built in just

TABLE 3-2 Expiration Times and Storage Requirements of Selected Intravenous Drugs

Drug	Stability after reconstitution at		
	Room temperature*	Refrigeration†	If frozen‡
cefamandole (Mandol)	24 hr	96 hr	6 mo
cefazolin sodium (Ancef, Kefzol)	24 hr	96 hr	3 mo
cefoperazone sodium (Cefobid, Cefobine)	24 hr	120 hr	3 to 5 wk, depending on concentration and parenteral solution used
cefoxitin sodium (Mefoxin)	24 hr	48 hr	Cannot be refrozen
cephalothin sodium (Keflin, Ceporacin)	12 hr (IM use)	96 hr	3 mo
cephradine (Velosef)	2 hr	24 hr	6 wk

Data from U.S.P.-DI, volume I, 1988.
*Room temperature: 15° to 25° C (59° to 77° F).
†Refrigeration temperature: 2° to 8° C (36° to 46° F).
‡Frozen: 20° C (−4° F).

this fashion. Learning names of drugs, their formulations, and their pharmacologic actions is best done in small increments and in a systematic way by making associations between information about a known drug in a classification, its close analogues, and clients cared for. The learning value of analysis and synthesis of these data in actual practice far outweighs that of memorizing long lists of unrelated drugs and their properties. Nurses in emergency departments and in community health are frequently challenged to identify medications from clients' personal unlabeled pill boxes or containers. Often many varieties of drugs and pieces of tablets are mixed together. Clients are often unable to assist in identification of their drugs, having never been properly educated by the health care system. The *Physicians' Desk Reference* for prescribed drugs and the *Physicians' Desk Reference for Nonprescription Drugs* provide actual photographs of drugs, which will assist the nurse in making visual identification. In addition, several states have passed legislation requiring identification codes or symbols on solid drug dosage forms. Although these markings may not be meaningful to the practicing nurse, pharmacists and local drug information centers can provide assistance in the identification of generic and trade products from them. Difficult identification problems may be referred to the FDA Drug Listing Branch or the FDA Division of Poison Control, both in Rockville, Maryland. Refer to Table 3-1 for descriptions and examples of some various drug forms now on the market. Various common routes of drug administration are discussed in Chapter 6.

In relation to drug preparation and formulation, the nurse can tailor the nursing intervention to individual client needs. For example, if a topical foam application is seen to be ineffective when it "runs" off the site, an avail-able ointment, cream, or film form may be recommended as more adherent. If a small child or an elderly client has difficulty swallowing pills, the drug form can be changed in collaboration with the prescriber to an equivalent dosage in elixir form. Such suggestions fall well within the province of nursing care.

If there is no elixir form of a drug available and another route is not feasible, some capsules or tablets may be physically altered to facilitate swallowing. Some capsules may be opened and some tablets crushed to a fine powder and mixed with a small amount of food, such as applesauce, pudding, or custard. Crushing can be done in several ways (it is not necessarily a sterile procedure): by placing the tablet in the bowl of one spoon and crushing with another spoon or by using a paper-lined mortar and a pestle or a special crushing device. A cold food such as ice cream or applesauce will tend to subdue a medication's bitter or oily taste. If the medication is added to a small amount of food, the client should be informed so that it may be entirely consumed on the first mouthful and none of the medication wasted or left unconsumed should the client refuse the rest. Liquid or powdered medication in water may be instilled after flushing of the client's nasogastric tube with a small amount of water, followed by additional water (total: approximately 60 ml). It is wise to medicate via nasogastric tube between tube feedings, if possible, so that drug-food interactions may be avoided and absorption improved. Sustained-release tablets often have layered coatings to delay dissolution and absorption of the drug over time (e.g., Theo-Dur); sustained-release capsules often contain similarly coated beads of the drug (Ornade Spansules). No sustained-release drug form should be crushed, chewed, or vigorously mixed with food for administration, because of the risk of overdosage when all of the drug is released for absorption at one time. Enteric-coated tablets (such as Dulcolax) contain drugs that could be neutralized or irritating if dissolved in stomach acids; they are intended to dissolve in the small intestine. Enteric-coated medication should be taken whole, on an empty stomach, with a full glass of water to ensure rapid passage to the small intestine. These, as well as certain other drug forms, because of their special construction, should not be crushed for administration.

Therapeutic effects of drugs also depend on their potency. Thus their freshness at the time of administration may depend on awareness of the expiration dates and the ways the drugs are stored, capped, and used. Gross deterioration and manufacturing defects may manifest themselves in unusual consistency (such as viscosity of liquids and crumbling of tablets) and in changes in color, odor, or sediment. Any deviation from the expected appearance of a drug should be discussed with the pharmacy department and possibly reported to the manufacturer and the FDA. In any event the suspected drug should not be administered or ignored. Childproof caps, although they deter curious investigation and emergency poisonings, do prevent easy opening, especially by arthritic hands. Clients can request regular caps from the pharmacist.

The growing wealth of drugs from which to prescribe challenges physicians in the field as much as it does nurses and nurse practitioners. Nurses find themselves increasingly in the position of making suggestions and actually prescribing. Recommendations may relate to the medication itself, the dose, the route, or the scheduled timing of doses. This is a highly professional interdisciplinary obligation with which the practicing nurse and the physician should become comfortable.

KEY TERMS

alkaloid, page 31
brand name, page 30
chemical name, page 29
efficacy, page 35
generic name, page 29
glycoside, page 31
gum, page 31
negative drug formulary, page 30
nonproprietary name, page 29
oil, page 31

potency, page 35
proprietary name, page 30
resin, page 31
trade name, page 30

BIBLIOGRAPHY

Abramowicz, M: Nitroglycerin patches, Med Letter 26(664):59, 1984.

Bergman, HD: Medical abbreviations, US Pharmacist 5(10):57, 1980.

Birdsall, C, and Uretsky, S: How do I administer medication by NG? Am J Nurs 84(10):1259, 1984.

British Pharmacopoeia, ed 10, London, 1980, The Pharmaceutical Press.

Drug substitution: where does your state stand? NARD J Oct 1980, p 44.

Florida Board of Pharmacy: Negative drug formulary, amended March 17, 1977, Chapter 21S-5.

Fredholm, N, Vignati, L, and Brown, S: Insulin pumps: the patients' verdict, Am J Nurs 84(1):36, 1984.

Goodman, L, Gilman, A, and Gilman, AG, eds: Goodman and Gilman's The pharmacological basis of therapeutics, ed 7, New York, 1985, Macmillan, Inc.

Nitroglycerin patch long-term use should include treatment-free interval, The Pink Sheet, FDC Rep 47(46):3, 1985.

Pageau, MG, Mroz, WT, and Coombs, DW: New analgesic therapy, Nursing '85 15(4):47, 1985.

Paice, JA: Intrathecal morphine sulfate for intractable cancer pain, J Neurosurg Nurs 16(5):237, 1984.

Parker, J: Cited in Nitroglycerin patches don't prevent nitrate tolerance in angina patients, Am Pharm NS25(7):20, 1985.

Pepper, GA: Revolution in dosage forms, Nurse Pract 11(5):76, 1986.

Ryan, JME: Troubleshooting the venous access system, Am J Nurs 85(7):795, 1985.

Speciale, JL and Kaalaas, J: Infuse-a-port: new path for I.V. chemotherapy, Nursing '85 15(10):40, 1985.

Strauss, S, and Sherman, M: Regulations pertaining to expiration dating of drug products, US Pharmacist 10(4):40, 1985.

United States Pharmacopeial Convention: Drug information for the health care provider, vol 1, Rockville, Md, 1987, United States Pharmacopeial Convention.

United States Pharmacopeia (Ed 21) and the National Formulary (ed 26), Rockville, Md, 1985, The United States Pharmacopeial Convention, Inc.

Waldman, SD, Feldstein, GS, and Allan, ML: Troubleshooting intraspinal narcotic delivery systems, Am J Nurs 87(1):63, 1987.

Wilkes, G, Vannicola, P, and Starck, P: Long-term venous access, Am J Nurs 85(7):793, 1985.

General Principles of Drug Action

OBJECTIVES

After studying this chapter, the student will be able to:

1. Discuss the three general properties of drugs.

2. Explain current theories of drug action: drug-receptor interaction, drug-enzyme interaction, and nonspecific drug interaction.

3. Describe the physiologic processes mediating drug action.

4. Cite examples of drug properties that influence pharmacokinetics.

5. Describe the three phases of drug activity: pharmaceutical, pharmacokinetic, and pharmacodynamic.

6. Describe nursing considerations related to patient variables altering drug responses.

7. List unusual and adverse responses to drug therapy.

8. Identify nursing assessments that can be used to detect actual or potential adverse drug reactions.

The number of drugs used in medical therapy has increased dramatically and continues to grow. Thousands of drugs exist. At the same time, the nurse's responsibilities concerning pharmaceutical agents have expanded. To approach the level of knowledge needed to meet these increased responsibilities, all health professionals must develop a fundamental theoretical framework within which to study and apply an understanding of drug therapy.

Nurses have traditionally administered drugs to clients. Today, in many health care delivery settings, the nurse's responsibility has shifted to ensuring safe administration of drugs by a variety of specially educated health workers and to observing and interpreting the client's response to drug therapy. However, the moral, ethical, and legal responsibility for drug administration remains the nurse's.

This chapter will present theories of drug action, physiologic processes mediating drug action, variables affecting drug action, and unusual and adverse responses to drug therapy. This knowledge the nurse can transfer to care of the unique problems of individual patients.

GENERAL PROPERTIES OF DRUGS

As stated earlier, a drug is a chemical that interacts with a living organism to produce a biologic response. This text deals with drugs administered in doses that obtain therapeutic, prophylactic, or diagnostic effects. These effects are achieved by some underlying biochemical and/or physiologic interaction between the drug and a functionally important tissue component (usually a receptor) in the body. Thus it is important to recognize the following general properties of drugs.

1. *Drugs do not confer any new functions on a tissue or organ in the body; they only modify existing functions.* Therefore the effects of drugs can be recognized only by alterations of a known physiologic function or process. Alteration in function is achieved by drugs that can replace, interrupt, or potentiate a physiologic process in specialized tissues. The following are examples: drugs used to treat anemia can replace iron to restore the adequate production of red blood cells. Atropine, on the other hand, can interrupt the rate of salivation in preoperative patients, which is an essentially abnormal state but a necessary one to decrease the surgical risk of aspiration. Finally, the administration of a cathartic can potentiate the rate of evacuation of the large intestine.

2. *Drugs in general exert multiple actions rather than a single effect.* Consequently, drugs may, in varying degrees, produce undesirable responses because of their potential to modify more than one function of the body. These unwanted effects may be avoided somewhat by administering more specific or more selective drugs. For example, metaproterenol is a selective beta$_2$ adrenergic agent used to produce bronchodilation. Yet a common side effect is beta$_2$ mediated muscle tremors.

3. *Drug action results from a physicochemical interaction between the drug and a functionally important molecule in the body.* Some drugs act by combining with a small molecule (e.g., antacids neutralize gastric acid) or producing alteration of cell membrane activity (e.g., local anesthetics). However, the major mechanism by which drugs interact is by combining with macromolecular components of tissues, such as receptors.

MECHANISMS OF DRUG ACTION

To produce its optimal desired or therapeutic effects, a drug must reach appropriate concentrations at its site of action. This means that the molecules of the chemical compound must proceed from their point of entry into the body to the tissues with which they react. In addition, the magnitude of the response depends on the dosage and the time course of the drug in the body. Therefore the concentration of the drug at its site of action is influenced by various processes, which may be divided into three phases of drug activity: pharmaceutical, pharmacokinetic, and pharmacodynamic. The sequential order of these phases is depicted in Figure 4-1.

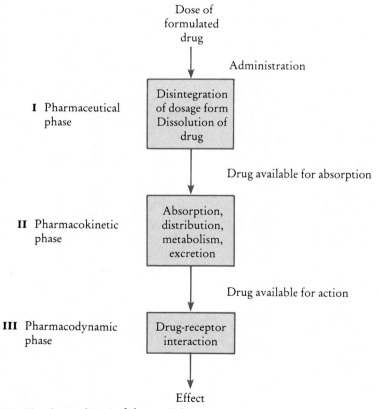

FIGURE 4-1   The three phases of drug activity.

(Modified from Ariens, EJ, and Simonis, AM: Molecular pharmacology, Orlando, Fla, 1964, Academic Press, Inc; from Bowman, WC, and Rand, MJ: Textbook of pharmacology, ed 2, London, 1980, Blackwell Scientific Publications.)

PHARMACEUTICAL PHASE

Pharmaceutics is the study of the ways in which various drug *forms* influence pharmacokinetic and pharmacodynamic activities. The drug may appear in solid form (tablet, capsule, or powder) or in liquid form (solution, suspension).

Dissolution refers to the rate at which a drug goes into solution. After ingestion, a solid drug (tablet or capsule) must first disintegrate before it becomes readily soluble in the body fluids. Following this process, the active drug ingredient is then *free* to enter solution. Thus the drug form is important, for the more rapid the rate of dissolution, the more readily the compound will cross the biologic membrane to achieve absorption. Obviously, oral drugs in liquid form are more rapidly available for gastrointestinal absorption than those in solid form (see Figures 4-2 and 4-3).

PHARMACOKINETIC PHASE

Pharmacokinetics is the study of the concentration of a drug during the processes of absorption, distribution, biotransformation, and excretion. The concentration that a drug attains at its site of action is influenced by four primary factors: the rate and extent to which a drug is (1) absorbed into body fluids, (2) distributed to sites of action or storage areas, (3) biotransformed or metabolized to breakdown products (metabolites), and (4) excreted from the body by various routes (see Figures 4-1 and 4-4).

Properties That Influence Pharmacokinetic Activity

Physicochemical Properties of Drugs

In general, drugs exist as weak acids or weak bases. Moreover, in body fluids they appear in either ionized or nonionized forms. The ionized (polar) form is usually water soluble (lipid insoluble) and does not diffuse readily through the cell membranes of the body. By contrast, the nonionized (nonpolar) form is more lipid soluble (less water soluble) and is more apt to cross the cell membranes. The influence of pH on these compounds is discussed under Absorption in this chapter.

Physicochemical Properties of Cell Membranes

The extent to which a drug attains pharmacokinetic activity (absorption, distribution, biotransformation, and excretion) depends on the rate at which drugs cross the cell membrane. The membrane consists of a bimolecular layer of lipids that contain protein molecules, which are irregularly dispersed throughout the lipid bilayer. The protein molecule itself may act as a carrier, an enzyme, a receptor, or an antigenic site. The drugs that are **lipid** (fat) **soluble** can pass through the lipid membrane, but those that are **water soluble** cannot. In this instance, the membrane, which appears to contain pores, permits the passage of small water-soluble substances such as urea, alcohol, electrolytes, and water itself.

Drug molecules, when free to move to sites of action, are transported from one body compartment to another by way of the plasma. However, free movement can be somewhat limited because these various sites are enclosed by membranes. Barriers to drug transport may consist of a single layer of cells, such as the villus in intestinal epithelium, or several layers of cells, such as skin. Nevertheless, in order for the drug to gain access to the interior of a cell or a body compartment, it has to penetrate cell membranes. All the physiologic processes mediating drug action—absorption, distribution, metabolism, and excretion—are predicated on two physicochemical properties: passive transport and active transport.

Passive transport. Passive transport of drugs occurs when the membrane is not required to generate energy to carry out the process.

Passive transport, or **passive diffusion,** is the random movement of a substance from a region of higher concentration to a region of lower concentration until equilibrium is established at the membrane. With this method of transport, the membrane does not actively take part in the transport. The vast majority of drugs are transported via this mechanism.

Carrier or active transport. Moderate-sized water-soluble molecules as well as moderate-sized ions, including the ionic form of most drugs, do not readily enter cells but require some means of transport. **Carrier transport,** or **active transport,** is believed to be conducted by "carriers" that form complexes with drug molecules on one

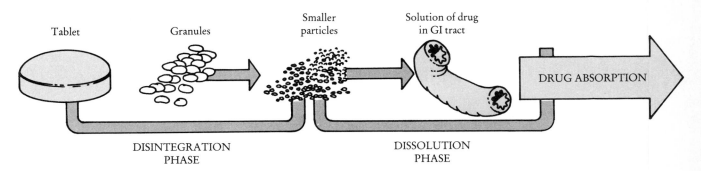

FIGURE 4-2 Phases of solid drug absorption.

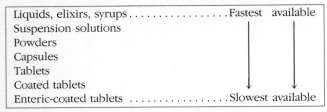

Liquids, elixirs, syrups . . . . .Fastest available
Suspension solutions
Powders
Capsules
Tablets
Coated tablets
Enteric-coated tablets . . . . .Slowest available

FIGURE 4-3   Availability or oral dosage forms.

surface of the membrane, carry them through the membrane, and then dissociate from them. The dynamics of active transport are similar to that of facilitated diffusion except that in this type of transfer an energy source is required. It involves the movement of drug molecules against the concentration gradient (from areas of low concentration to areas of high concentration) or, in the case of ions, against the electrochemical potential gradient such as occurs with the "sodium pump." Active transport is usually more rapid than passive diffusion.

Absorption

Absorption is a process that involves the movement of drug molecules from the site of entry into the body to the circulating fluids. Absorption begins at the site of administration and is essential to the three subsequent processes — distribution, metabolism, and excretion. The rate of drug absorption is significant because it determines when a drug becomes pharmacologically available in exerting its action. Of importance is that both the duration and the intensity of drug action are greatly influenced by the rate of this process. Accordingly, this type of response depends on the selection of the *route* of administration, the

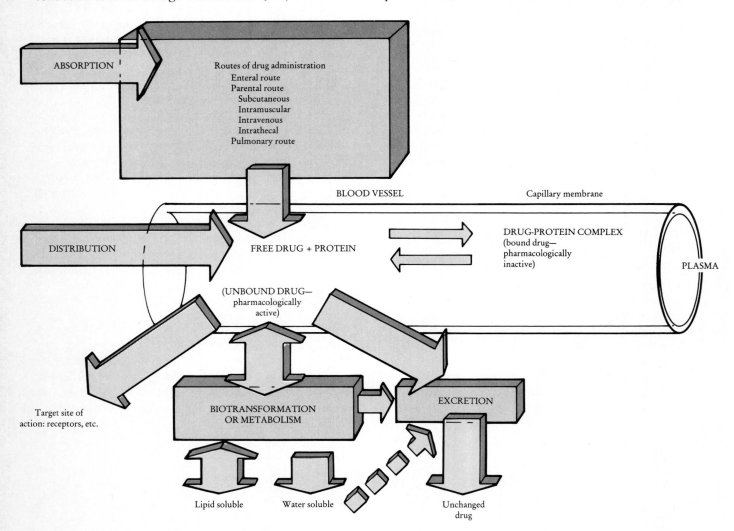

FIGURE 4-4   Schema of pharmacokinetic phase of drug action, showing absorption, distribution, biotransformation, and excretion of drugs. Note that only free drug is capable of movement for absorption, distribution to the target site of action, biotransformation, and excretion; the drug-protein complex represents bound drug, and because the molecule is large, it is trapped in the blood vessel and serves as a storage site for the drug.

dose of the drug, and the *dosage form* (tablet, capsule, liquid) of the agent administered.

Variables that Affect Drug Absorption

The rate and extent to which a drug is absorbed are influenced by the following:

1. Nature of the absorbing surface (cell membrane) through which the drug must traverse. The drug molecule may pass through a single layer of cells (intestinal epithelium), in which case transport is faster than when it traverses several layers of cells (skin). In addition, the size of the surface area of the absorbing site is another important determinant of drug absorption. Generally, the more extensive the absorbing surface, the greater the absorption of the drug and the more rapid its effects. Anesthetics are absorbed immediately from the pulmonary epithelium because of the vast surface area. Absorption from the small intestine, which offers a massive absorbing area, is more rapid than from a smaller absorbing surface, such as the stomach.

2. Blood flow to the site of administration. Circulation to the site of administration is a significant factor in the absorption of drugs. A rich blood supply (sublingual route) enhances absorption, whereas a poorly vascular site (subcutaneous route) delays it. A patient in shock, for example, may not respond to intramuscularly administered drugs because of poor peripheral circulation. Drugs injected intravenously, on the other hand, are placed directly into the circulatory system and are totally absorbed. This route of administration is desirable when speedy drug effects are necessary, but it carries the potential danger of achieving temporarily toxic responses in vital organs such as the heart or the brain. Therefore, to prevent deleterious effects, some drugs must be injected slowly. In addition, the decreased peripheral blood flow in patients with congestive heart failure or circulatory shock may cause a significant reduction in rate of transport of injected drugs to the target tissues, thereby considerably altering their efficacy.

3. Solubility of the drug. Again, to be absorbed, a drug must be in solution. The more soluble the drug, the more rapidly it will be absorbed. Moreover, because cell membranes contain a fatty acid layer, lipid solubility is a valuable attribute of drugs to be absorbed from certain areas — for example, the alimentary tract and the placental barrier. Chemicals and minerals that form insoluble precipitates in the gastrointestinal tract, such as barium salts, or drugs that are not soluble in water or lipids cannot be absorbed. Parenterally administered drugs prepared in oily vehicles, such as streptomycin, will be absorbed more slowly than drugs dissolved in water or isotonic sodium chloride.

4. pH. When in solution, drugs are a mixture of ionized and unionized forms. The unionized drug is lipid soluble and readily diffuses across the cell membrane: the ionized drug is lipid insoluble and nondiffusible. A drug that is acidic (e.g., aspirin) becomes relatively undissociated in an acid environment such as the stomach and therefore can readily diffuse across the membranes into the circulation. In contrast, a basic drug tends to ionize in the same acid environment and is not absorbed through the gastric membrane. The reverse occurs when a drug is in an alkaline medium. (see Figure 4-5.)

5. Drug concentration. Drugs administered in high concentrations tend to be more rapidly absorbed than drugs administered in low concentrations. In certain situations, a drug may be initially administered in large doses that temporarily exceed the body's capacity for excretion of the drug. In this way, active drug levels are rapidly reached at the receptor site. Once an active drug level is established, smaller daily doses of the drug can be administered to replace only the amount of the drug excreted since the previous dose. The initial and temporary overloading doses of the drug are **priming** or **loading doses,** while the smaller daily doses are **maintenance doses.** Such manipulation of drug dosage is frequently used, for example, with digitalis and steroid preparations in acute situations.

6. Dosage form. Drug concentration can be manipulated by pharmaceutical processing. It is possible to combine an active drug with a resin or another substance from which it is only slowly released or to prepare a drug in a vehicle that offers relative resistance to the digestive action of stomach contents (enteric coating). **Enteric coatings** on drugs are used for the following reasons: (1) to prevent decomposition of chemically sensitive drugs by gastric secretions (penicillin G and erythromycin are unstable in an acid pH), (2) to prevent dilution of the drug before it reaches the intestine, (3) to prevent nausea and vomiting, and (4) to provide delayed action of the drug.

Routes of Drug Administration

The mode of drug administration affects both the rate at which onset of action occurs and the magnitude of the therapeutic response that results. Therefore the choice of the route of administration is crucial in determining the suitability of a drug for an individual patient. For example, a patient who is vomiting will experience little or no appreciable gastrointestinal absorption of a drug when it is administered orally. Obviously, parenteral administration would be more beneficial in obtaining a therapeutic drug response.

Drugs are given for either their local or systemic effects. The *local* effect of a drug usually occurs at the immediate site of application, in which case absorption is a disadvantage. By contrast, when a drug is given for a *systemic* effect, *absorption is an essential first step* before the agent appears in the circulation and is distributed to a location distant from the site of administration.

A drug may enter the circulation either by being injected there directly — intravenously — or by absorption from depots in which it has been placed. The routes of drug administration can be classified into the following categories: (1) enteral (drugs administered along any portion of the gastrointestinal tract), (2) parenteral — subcutaneous, intramuscular, intravenous, intrathecal, (3) pulmonary, and (4) topical (see Figure 4-4.)

Enteral route. Generally, oral ingestion, or the **enteral** route, is the most commonly used method of giving drugs. It is also the safest (drug may be retrieved), most convenient, and economical route of administration. However, the frequent changes of the gastrointestinal environment produced by food, emotion, and physical activity make it the most *unreliable* and *slowest* of the commonly used routes.

Drugs are absorbed from several sites along the gastrointestinal tract.

Oral absorption. The oral cavity is lined with mucous membranes that consist of epithelial cells. These cells secrete saliva to begin digestion of food. Although the oral cavity possesses a thin lining, a rich blood supply, and a slightly acidic pH, little absorption occurs in the mouth. On the other hand, despite its small surface area, the oral mucosa is capable of absorbing certain drugs as long as they dissolve rapidly in the salivary secretions. The oral mucosa absorbs drugs by the **sublingual** and **buccal** routes. In sublingual administration the drug is placed under the tongue to permit tablet dissolution in salivary secretions. Nitroglycerin is administered in this manner, and the patient is advised to refrain as long as possible from swallowing the saliva containing the tablet form of

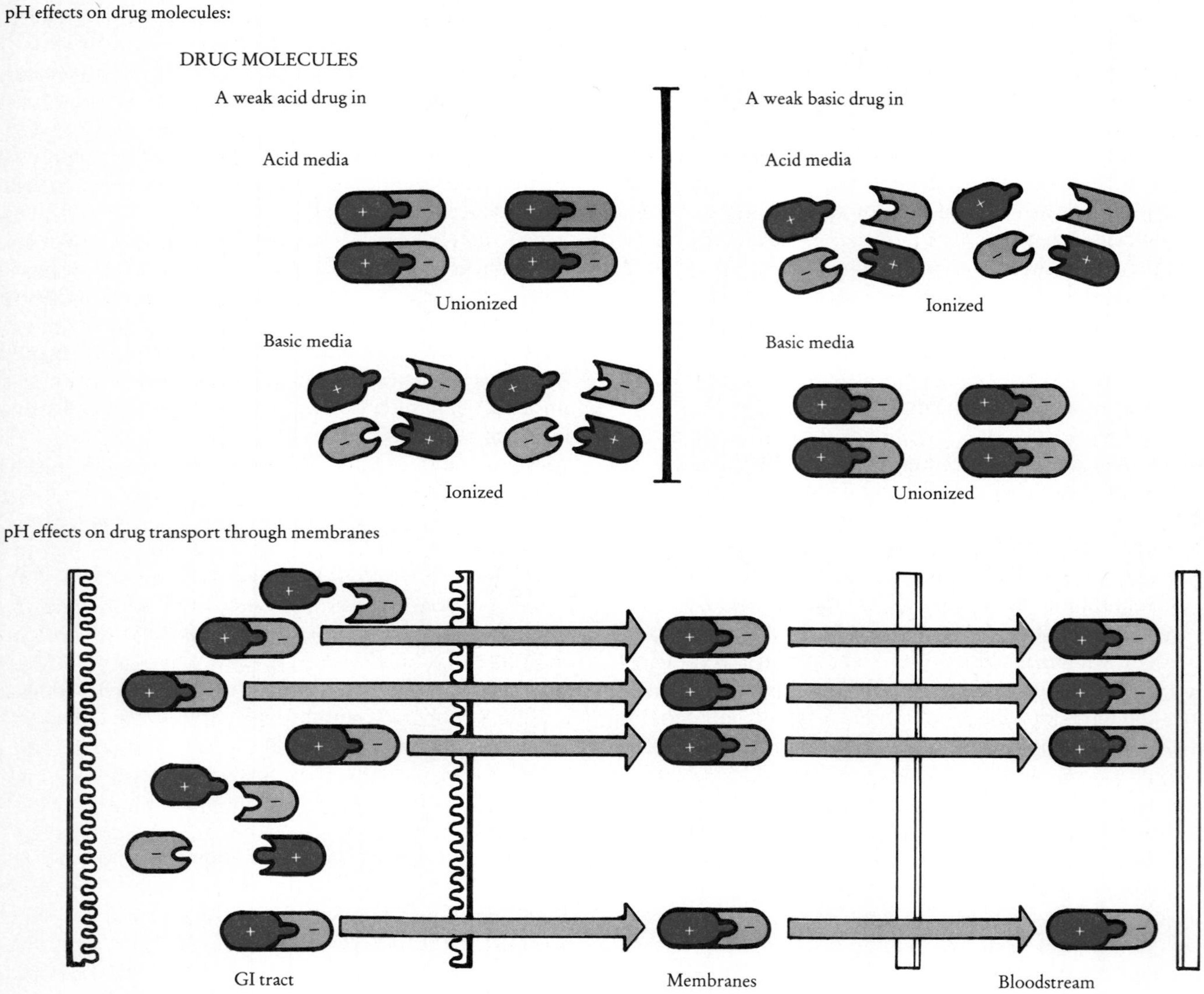

pH effects on drug molecules:

DRUG MOLECULES

FIGURE 4-5   Effect of pH on drug ionization and transport.

the drug. Because nitroglycerin is nonionic with a high lipid solubility, the drug readily diffuses through the lipid mucosal membranes. Following absorption, it enters the systemic circulation without preliminary passage through the liver. Accordingly, absorption is rapid, and the effects of the drug may become apparent within 2 minutes. In buccal administration the drug (tablet) is placed between the teeth and the mucous membrane of the cheek. Some hormones and enzyme preparations are administered by this route. The drug is absorbed rapidly and enters the general circulation directly without passing through the portal circulation. Both sublingual and buccal routes avert drug destruction by gastrointestinal fluids and the liver.

Gastric absorption. Although the stomach has a rich blood supply and large surface area, which provide excellent potential for drug absorption, it is not an important site for this process. The length of time a substance remains in the stomach is a significant variable in determining the extent of gastric absorption. This is governed by the pH of the drug and gastric motility.

In the stomach the pH is low (about 1.4), and drugs such as the barbiturates, which are slightly acidic, tend to remain nonionized and thus are readily absorbed into the circulation. Morphine and quinine are slightly basic; they ionize in the stomach and thus are poorly absorbed. A large majority of drugs are weak bases and on entry into the small intestine are absorbed because of the alkaline pH of the environment.

Generally, slowing the gastric emptying rate decreases drug absorption and vice versa. This is why so many drugs are administered on an empty stomach with sufficient water (8 ounces) to ensure their rapid passage into the small intestine, where drug absorption is increased because of the larger surface area available to the dissolving drug. Since some drugs cause gastric irritation, they are usually given with food. In addition, after drug administration, the patient should be encouraged to lie on the right side to hasten *gastric emptying time* (time required for the drug to reach the small intestine). Prolongation of emptying time increases the risk of destruction of unstable drugs (acetaminophen [Tylenol]) by gastric juices.

Small intestinal absorption. The small intestine with its many villi has a larger absorption area than the stomach. Also, it is highly vascularized. Drugs that are poorly soluble in the stomach pass into this region. Drug absorption occurs mostly in the upper part of the small intestine. The pH of the intestinal fluid is alkaline (7 to 8) and strongly influences the rate of absorption of the nonionized basic drugs. Increased intestinal motility caused, for example, by diarrhea or cathartics may decrease exposure to the intestinal membrane and thereby diminish absorption. Prolonged exposure, on the other hand, allows more time for absorption.

Rectal absorption. The surface area of the rectum is not very large, but drug absorption does occur because of extensive vascularity. In addition, drugs administered rectally are not subjected to hepatic alteration, since the blood that perfuses this region bypasses the liver. Some disadvantages to rectal administration of drugs include erratic absorption because of rectal contents, local drug irritation, and uncertainty of drug retention.

Parenteral route. The **parenteral** route refers to the administration of drugs by injection. It is the most rapid form of systemic therapy.

Subcutaneous. A **subcutaneous** injection means that a drug is given beneath the skin into the connective tissue or fat immediately underlying the dermis. This site can be used only for drugs that are not irritating to the tissue; otherwise severe pain, necrosis, and sloughing may occur. The rate of absorption is slow and can provide a sustained effect.

Intramuscular. **Intramuscular** administration means that a drug is injected into the skeletal muscle. Absorption occurs more rapidly than with subcutaneous injection, because of greater tissue blood flow.

Intravenous. The **intravenous** route produces an immediate pharmacologic response because the desired concentration of drug is injected directly into the bloodstream, thereby circumventing the absorption process. Drugs should be administered slowly to prevent adverse effects.

Intrathecal. **Intrathecal** administration means that a drug is injected directly into the spinal subarachnoid space, bypassing the blood-brain barrier. Many compounds cannot enter the cerebrospinal fluid or are absorbed in this region very slowly. When rapid effects of drugs are desired, as in spinal anesthesia or in treatment of acute infection of the central nervous system, this route may be used.

Pulmonary route. To ensure that normal gas exchange of oxygen and carbon dioxide is continuous in the lungs, drugs must be in the form of gases or fine mists (aerosols) when they are administered by inhalation. The lungs provide a large surface area for absorption, and the rich capillary network adjacent to the alveolar membrane may tend to promote ready entry of medication into the bloodstream. Drugs such as bronchodilators, mucolytics, and antibiotics are administered by various inhalation devices (nebulizers, pressure tanks) that propel the agents into the alveolar sacs and produce primarily local effects and at times unwanted systemic effects.

Topical route. Absorption of drugs applied topically to the skin and mucous membranes of various structures in the body is generally rapid.

Skin. Usually, drugs applied to the skin are employed as topical remedies to produce a local effect. Only lipid-soluble compounds are absorbed through the skin, which acts as a lipid barrier. To prevent adverse effects from systemic absorption of toxic chemicals, only an intact skin surface should be used. Massaging the skin enhances absorption of the drug because capillaries become dilated and local blood flow is increased as a result of the warmth created by the friction of rubbing.

Eyes. Administration of drugs in the eye produces a local effect on the conjunctiva or anterior chamber. Eyeball movements promote the distribution of drug over the surface of the eye.

Ears. Administration of drops into the auditory canal may be chosen to treat local infection or inflammatory conditions of the external ear.

Bioavailability

Bioavailability refers to the percentage of active substances in a drug that is absorbed and becomes available to the target tissue following administration. Thus drugs are **biologically equivalent** if they attain similar *concentrations* in blood and tissues at similar times; they are **therapeutically equivalent** if they provide equal *therapeutic effectiveness* in clinical trials. Of importance is the similarity of the absorption and therapeutic performances of drugs, which can be altered markedly by the ingredients and method of manufacture of an agent. Furthermore, different brands of the same drug can vary, and even different lots from a single manufacturer may show different levels of effectiveness. Thus the FDA is paying more attention to drug preparation and trying to ensure that the bioavailability of a drug conforms to uniform standards. Both the proportion of active drug and the percentage of its absorption are essential to attain therapeutic equivalence among all chemically similar drugs.

Distribution

Once a drug is absorbed into the bloodstream, it is immediately distributed throughout the body by the circulation of the blood. **Distribution** is defined as the transport of a drug in body fluids from the bloodstream to various tissues of the body and ultimately to its site of action (see Figure 4-6). The rate at which a drug enters the different areas of the body depends on the permeability of capillaries for the drug's molecules. As already discussed, lipid-soluble drugs can readily cross capillary membranes to enter most tissues and fluid compartments, whereas lipid-insoluble drugs require more time to arrive at their point of action. However, cardiac functions also affect the rate and extent of distribution of a drug; specifically, cardiac output (amount of blood pumped by the heart each minute) and regional blood flow (amount of blood supplied to a specific organ or

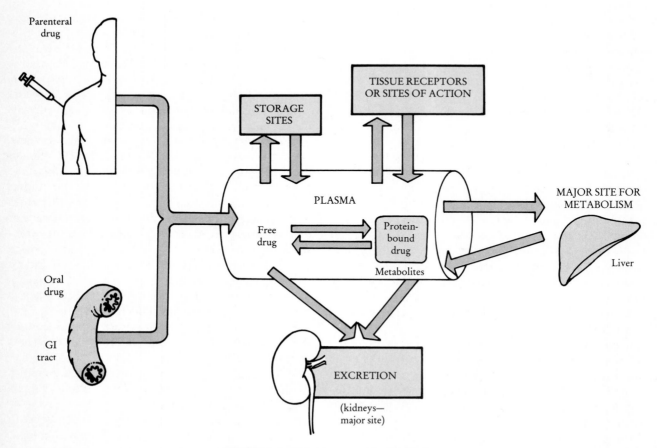

FIGURE 4-6 Drug transport in the body.

tissue) determine how much time is required. Most of the drug is first distributed to organs that have a rich blood supply: heart, liver, kidney, and brain. Afterward, the drug enters organs with a poor blood supply, which include muscles and fat.

Drug Reservoirs

Storage reservoirs allow a drug to accumulate by binding to specific tissues in the body. This sustains the pharmacologic effect of a drug at its point of action. The body's storage reservoirs involve two general types of drug pooling: **plasma protein binding** and **tissue binding**

Plasma protein binding. On entry into the circulatory system, drugs may come attached to proteins, mainly albumin contained in the blood. Thus, as free drug enters the plasma, it binds to the protein to form a drug-protein complex. This combination can also be reversed:

Free drug + Protein ⇄ Drug-protein complex

The formula indicates that equilibrium is established between the amount of free drug and the amount of drug that is bound to protein (drug-protein complex). Protein binding decreases the concentration of free drug in the circulation, thereby limiting the amount that travels to the site of action. The protein albumin molecule is too large to diffuse through the membrane of the blood vessel, so the bound molecule is trapped in the bloodstream and pharmacologically inactive. It becomes a circulating drug reservoir or storage depot (see Figure 4-4).

The equilibrium process is dynamic. As free drug is eliminated from the body, the drug-protein complex begins to dissociate so that more free drug is released to replace what is lost. As a result, the fact that the body temporarily stores the drug molecules in the drug-protein complex allows the drug to be available for a longer period of time. For example, a sulfonamide is highly bound to protein, and because free drug molecules are released slowly from the bound form, the antiinfective action of the antibiotic is long-lasting.

Degree of drug binding. Plasma protein binding is expressed as a percentage, which refers to the percent of total drug that is bound. Among the *highly protein-bound* drugs are bishydroxycoumarin (Dicumarol), which is 98% bound, and propranolol, which is 90% bound. Accordingly, a ratio exists between free and bound drug. In the case of propranolol this means that in a given period of time, 90% is bound to plasma proteins and only 10% of free drug is available for therapeutic use, eventual biotransformation, and excretion. Therefore if more than 10% of the drug is free to act within this same period of time, toxicity is likely to occur. Pentobarbital is 40% protein bound and represents a *moderately bound* drug, whereas guanethidine is only 1% to 8% protein bound and is a *low-bound* drug.

Competition for binding sites. Since albumin and other plasma proteins provide a number of binding sites, two drugs can compete with one another for the same site and displace each other. This competition may have dangerous consequences if particular combinations of drugs are administered. For example, serious problems can arise when a client who is satisfactorily stabilized on maintenance doses of warfarin, an anticoagulant, is *simultaneously* given aspirin, an analgesic. The aspirin may displace some of the protein-bound warfarin, thereby increasing the free drug level and causing severe hemorrhage. Because warfarin is normally highly protein bound, its continued administration may raise the concentration of free drug, causing further severe adverse reactions. Therefore the nurse must be alert to the potential dangers of drug interactions occurring when multiple agents are prescribed concurrently.

Hypoalbuminemia. **Hypoalbuminemia** is characterized by low levels of albumin in the blood. Either hepatic damage, such as cirrhosis of the liver, or some type of body cavity drainage may cause hypoalbuminemia. Furthermore, failure of the liver to synthesize enough of the plasma proteins needed to bind drugs means that more free drug is available for distribution to tissue sites. Therefore when a client is given the normal dosage of a drug that depends on plasma binding, more of the free form of drug is allowed into the circulation, resulting in possible overdosage and toxicity. Clients who require drugs that depend on protein binding for distribution generally receive albumin replacement. Meanwhile, the drug dosage is adjusted until the normal level of the plasma protein is reported.

Tissue binding

Fat tissue. Lipid-soluble drugs have a high *affinity* for adipose tissue, which is where these drugs are stored. Moreover, the relatively low blood flow in fat tissue makes it a stable reservoir for drugs. As an example, a lipid-soluble drug such as thiopental may stay in low concentrations in body fat for as long as 3 hours following administration. If this drug is given again before it is all excreted, it can produce a cumulative effect, since an additional amount of the agent will be stored in the fat tissue.

Bone. Some drugs have an unusual affinity for bone. For example, the antibiotic tetracycline accumulates in bone after being absorbed onto the bone-crystal surface. The drug is stored in the crystal lattice of bone. Tetracycline can interfere with the growth of bones when it accumulates in skeletal tissues of the fetus (by crossing the placenta from the mother) or young children. When the drug is distributed to unerupted teeth in a fetus or young child, discoloration of teeth results. Brownish pigmentation of permanent teeth also may result if this drug is given during the prenatal period or early childhood. See the box on p. 50 for specific actions of drugs in fetal tissues.

FETAL DRUG EFFECTS

Two major types of drug effects occur in the fetus. When given during the first trimester of pregnancy, some drugs induce aberrant development of organs and systems during the formation of these structures. This is known as a **teratogenic drug,** which is defined as an agent that causes physical defects in a developing embryo. Many drugs that cause anomalies are known to cross the placenta and exhibit teratogenicity.

The second type of drug affects the second half of pregnancy as well as delivery, causing respiratory depression in the newborn because of the under developed capacity of the infant to biotransform the drug and excrete it.

The rate of maternal blood flow to the placenta limits the availability of the drug to the fetus. Because passage of drugs is delayed, drugs take action in the mother more rapidly than in the fetus. This explains why an alert infant can be delivered to an anesthetized mother, provided that delivery occurs within 10 to 15 minutes of the time the drug is administered to the mother. Long-term administration of drugs to the mother, however, may produce adverse effects on the fetus. For example, infants born to mothers dependent on narcotics manifest withdrawal symptoms after delivery and removal from the flow of the products through the mother.

Unfortunately, the teratogenic effects of many drugs have not been adequately studied. Also, a potentially dangerous drug may be administered to a woman who is not aware of her pregnancy. It should be assumed that any drug will be able to pass the placental barrier, and the nurse must advise pregnant women not to take any drug without consulting the physician. Drugs should be administered during pregnancy only when the advantages greatly outweigh the potential risks to the fetus.

Barriers to Drug Distribution

Specialized structures, which are made up of biologic membranes, can serve as barriers to the passage of drugs at certain sites in the body. These include the blood-brain barrier and the placental barrier.

Blood-brain barrier. The blood-brain barrier is a special anatomic arrangement that allows distribution of only lipid-soluble drugs (e.g., general anesthetics, barbiturates) into the brain and cerebrospinal fluid. Actually, the barrier is made up of a row of capillary endothelial cells joined by continuous tight intercellular junctions. The capillaries are covered by a fatty sheath of glial cells. Consequently, compounds that are strongly ionized and poorly soluble in fat cannot enter the brain. Thus antibiotics that cross the blood-brain barrier with difficulty cannot be used to treat infections of the central nervous system. However, if a drug is instilled intrathecally, it bypasses the blood-brain barrier and directly treats the bacterial infection.

Placental barrier. The membrane layers that separate the blood vessels of the mother and fetus constitute the placental barrier. In addition, tissue enzymes in the placenta can metabolize some agents (e.g., catecholamines) by inactivating them as they travel from the maternal circulation to the embryo. Despite the thickness of the structure, it does not afford complete protection to the fetus. Unlike the blood-brain barrier, the nonselective passage of drugs across the placenta to the fetus is a well-established fact. Although lipid-soluble substances preferentially diffuse across the placenta, the barrier is also permeable to a great number of lipid-insoluble drugs. Consequently, many agents intended to produce a therapeutic response in the mother also may cross the placental barrier and exert harmful effects on the developing embryo. Among the drugs easily transported across the placenta are steroids, narcotics, anesthetics, and some antibiotics.

Biotransformation or Metabolism

Following absorption and distribution of a drug, the body eliminates the drug, first by biotransformation and then by excretion. **Biotransformation** (metabolism) chemically inactivates a drug by converting (transforming) it in to a more water-soluble compound, or metabolite, that can be excreted from the body (see Figure 4-5). The liver is the primary site of metabolism of drugs, but other tissues also may be involved in this process, namely the plasma, kidneys, lungs, and the intestinal mucosa.

Hepatic Biotransformation

After distribution to their sites of action, most drugs undergo metabolic changes or biotransformation. The chemical alterations are produced by microsomal enzyme systems, located largely in the liver, which consist of endoplasmic reticula, a series of membranes that appear as a network of canals within the cells. The microsomal enzymes usually affect biotransformation of lipid-soluble, nonpolar drugs. To increase polarity, they undergo one or both of two general types of chemical reactions. One type of transformation consists of oxidation, hydrolysis, or reduction. These chemical reactions result in increased polarity and water solubility of drug molecules. The second type, called conjugation, involves the union of the polar group of a drug with another substance in the body — glucuronide, glycine, methyl, or other alkyl groups. The conjugated molecule also becomes more polar, more water soluble, and therefore more excretable. These responses generally produce a loss in pharmacologic activity and occasionally are referred to as detoxication reactions.

Individuals vary considerably in the rates at which they metabolize drugs. The microsomal enzyme system can be depressed by conditions that affect hepatic function, such as starvation and obstructive jaundice. Individuals with liver disease, severe cardiovascular dysfunction, or renal problems may be expected to suffer from prolonged drug metabolism. Infants with immature metabolizing enzyme systems and the aged with degenerative enzyme function are major groups that experience depressed biotransformation. Genetically determined differences also affect metabolism. Some drugs (e.g., procainamide, hydralazine, and isoniazid) are metabolized by the acetyltransferase system. This system divides the population into "rapid acetylators" and "slow acetylators." The rapid acetylators metabolize a greater proportion of a drug dose than do the slow acetylators. The rapid acetylators may develop reactions caused by the metabolic products of a drug, whereas the slow acetylators may appear more sensitive to a drug by experiencing severe toxic effects. For example, an individual who is a slow acetylator and who is receiving procainamide is apt to develop a lupus-like syndrome, which is a serious adverse response.

If drug metabolism is delayed, cumulative drug effects may be expected and may be manifested as excessive or prolonged responses to ordinary doses of drugs. If drug metabolism is stimulated, a state of apparent drug tolerance is produced. A number of substances cause increased activity by hepatic microsomal enzymes, including CNS depressants, xanthines, pesticides, food preservatives, and dyes. Repeated administration of some drugs may stimulate the formation of new microsomal enzymes. This is thought to be the case with some hypnotic drugs, whose effect diminishes with prolonged administration.

Hepatic first-pass effect. Orally administered drugs absorbed from the gastrointestinal tract normally travel first to the portal system and then to the liver before entering the general circulation. However, some drugs may first be taken up by the hepatic microsomal enzyme system, so that a significant amount is metabolized before the drug ever reaches the systemic circulation. Consequently, only a small fraction of the dose is available for distribution to produce a pharmacologic effect. Thus the **hepatic first-pass effect** is defined as an initial biotransformation of drug (on passage through the liver from the portal vein) that produces a loss of pharmacologically active molecules. In some cases, the hepatic first-pass effect may result in complete elimination of the drug without the production of any pharmacologic activity. Hence a drug with an extensive hepatic first-pass effect is administered parenterally to bypass the liver, thereby preventing initial biotransformation.

Excretion

A drug continues to act in the body until it is biotransformed or excreted. Drug molecules — intact, changed, or inactivated — ultimately must be removed from their sites of action by physiologic channels involving mechanisms of excretion. **Excretion** is a process whereby drugs and pharmacologically active or inactive metabolites are eliminated from the body, primarily through the kidneys.

Organs of Excretion

Kidneys. Excretion via the kidneys remains by far the most important route of drug elimination. Some drugs are excreted almost unchanged in the urine, while other drugs are so extensively metabolized that only a small fraction of the original chemical substance is excreted intact.

Excretion is accomplished through passive glomerular filtration, active tubular secretion, and partial reabsorption (see Figure 4-7). The availability of a drug for glomerular filtration depends on its concentration in unbound form in plasma. Free, unbound drugs and water-soluble metabolites are filtered by the glomeruli, whereas protein-bound substances do not pass through this structure. After filtration, lipid-soluble compounds are not excreted; instead, they are reabsorbed by the tubular nephron and reenter the systemic circulation. The water-soluble compounds, on the other hand, fail to be reabsorbed and therefore are eliminated from the body.

Urinary pH varies between 4.6 and 8.2 and affects the amount of drug reabsorbed in the renal tubule by passive diffusion. Weak acids are excreted more readily in alkaline urine and more slowly in acidic urine; the reverse is true for weak bases. In cases of poisoning by weak organic acids such as aspirin or phenobarbital, alkalinizing the urine can result in increased urinary drug excretion. Raising the pH of the urine causes weak acids to become ionized, and subsequently these agents are excreted.

Urine may be alkalinized by administering sodium bicarbonate or tromethamine (Tham-E). By contrast, high doses of vitamin C or ammonium chloride acidify the urine and promote the excretion of basic drugs. By altering the pH of urine, increased elimination of certain drugs can be facilitated, thus preventing prolonged action or overdosage of a toxic compound. (See Table 4-1.)

Another technique to alter the rate of excretion of a drug is to produce a competitively blocking effect. As an example, probenecid may be used to block the renal excretion of penicillin; this prolongs the effect of the antibiotic by maintaining a higher therapeutic plasma level.

Drugs may also be eliminated through the use of extracorporeal dialysis, which was originally designed to substitute for renal function in cases of severe but temporary renal shutdown. Overdosage of drugs may lead to just

TABLE 4-1 Effect of Urinary pH on Drug Excretion

Weak acids	Weak bases
Phenobarbital	Amphetamines
Salicylates	Meperidine
Streptomycin	Quinidine
RATE OF EXCRETION IS:	**RATE OF EXCRETION IS:**
Increased in alkaline urine	Increased in acid urine
Decreased in acid urine	Decreased in alkaline urine

such a situation. By an artificial process resembling glomerular filtration, dialysis can achieve rapid reduction of high plasma levels of a drug. As a general rule, substances that are completely or almost completely excreted by the normal kidney can be removed by hemodialysis. Such substances include some CNS stimulants and depressants, some nonnarcotic analgesics, and metals.

Intestine. Although the major route of excretion of drugs is the kidney, many agents are eliminated through the intestine by biliary excretion. After metabolism by the liver, the metabolite is secreted into the bile and passed into the duodenum. It is then eliminated with the feces. Certain drugs such as fat-soluble agents many be reabsorbed by the bloodstream and returned to the liver. This is the **enterohepatic cycle.** These compounds are later excreted by the kidney.

Lungs. Most of the drugs removed by the pulmonary route generally are intact and not metabolites. Agents such as gases and volatile liquids (general anesthetics) that are administered through the respiratory system usually are eliminated by the same route. On inspiration, these agents enter the bloodstream and, after crossing the alveolar membrane, are distributed by the general circulation. The rate of gas loss depends on the rate of respiration. Therefore exercise or deep breathing, which causes a rise in cardiac output and a subsequent increase in pulmonary blood flow, promotes excretion. By contrast, decreased cardiac output, such as that occurring in shock, prolongs the period of time for drug elimination. Other volatile substances such as ethyl alcohol and paraldehyde, which are highly soluble in blood, are excreted in limited amounts by the lungs. The remaining amounts are largely metabolized in the liver and excreted in urine. However, these compounds can be easily detected because the individual expires the gases in to the atmosphere.

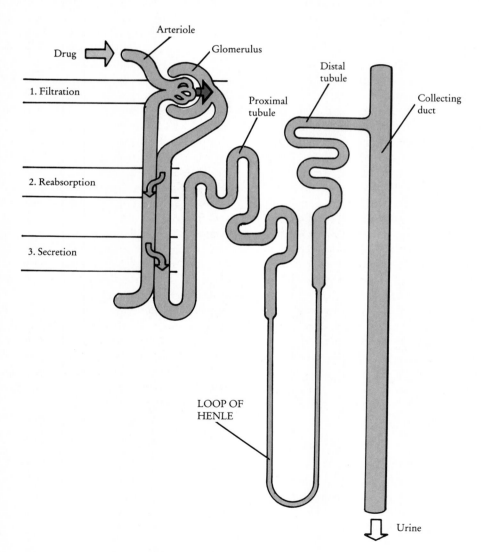

FIGURE 4-7 The drug excretion process.

Sweat and salivary glands. The excretion of drugs through sweat and saliva is relatively unimportant. This process depends on diffusion of lipid-soluble drugs through the epithelial cells of the glands. The elimination of drugs and their metabolites into sweat may be responsible for causing side effects such as dermatitis and several other skin reactions. Drugs excreted in the saliva are usually swallowed and undergo the same fate as other orally administered agents. Furthermore, certain compounds that are given intravenously also may be excreted into saliva and cause the individual to complain of the "taste of drug."

Mammary glands. Many drugs or their metabolites cross the epithelium of the mammary glands and are excreted in breast milk. Breast milk is acidic (pH 6.5), and therefore basic compounds such as narcotics (e.g., morphine and codeine) achieve high concentrations in this fluid. On the other hand, diuretics, barbiturates, sulfonamides, and other weak acids will be less concentrated in breast milk. A major concern arises over the transfer of drugs from mother to their breastfed babies. Although small quantities of any drug may be obtained in this manner, a cumulative effect can occur because of the undeveloped metabolizing system of the infant. Thus the nursing mother should be warned against taking any drug, because of its potential for reaching her infant. If medication is essential for the mother's health, the risk to the neonate can be diminished if the drug is given immediately after breast-feeding.

PHARMACODYNAMIC PHASE

Pharmacodynamics is the study of the mechanism of drug action on living tissue. It is concerned with the response of tissues to specific chemical agents at various sites in the body. The effects of drugs can be recognized only by alterations of a known physiologic function. That is, drugs *modify* physiologic activity but do not confer any new function on a tissue or organ in the body. The goal of drug therapy is to attain a therapeutic effect in a patient. Therefore, in this context, drugs are used for cure of disease, symptomatic relief of symptoms, diagnosis, and also prevention of disease or undesirable conditions.

Theories of Drug Action

The means by which drugs produce an alteration in function at their action is known as the *mechanism of action.* The mechanism of action of most compounds is believed to involve a chemical interaction between the drug and a functionally important component of the living system. Most drugs produce their effects by one of the following ways:

1. Drug-receptor interaction
2. Drug-enzyme interaction
3. Nonspecific drug interaction

Drug-receptor interaction. Structural specificity is an essential postulate of the receptor theory of drug action. This theory hypothesizes that drugs are selectively active substances that have a high affinity for a specific chemical group or a particular constituent of a cell. In essence the drug-receptor interaction theory states that a certain portion (active site) of the drug molecule selectively combines or interacts with some molecular structure (reactive site on the cell surface or within the cell) to produce a biologic effect. Thus a **receptor** is a reactive cellular site with which a drug can interact to produce a pharmacologic response. The relationship of a drug to its receptor has often been likened to that of the fit of a key into its lock. The drug represents the key that fits into the lock or receptor. Thus some sort of reciprocal or complementary relationship exists between a certain portion of the drug molecule and the receptor site of the cell.

It has been postulated that the drug molecule with the best fit to the receptor will produce the greatest response from the cell. It has been suggested that there must be some force that attracts a receptor and holds it in combination with a specific drug long enough to produce a pharmacologic response. It is believed that drug receptor binding may result from the formation of chemical bonds — hydrogen, covalent, ionic, or van der Waals forces — between the receptors on the cell and the active site of the drug. Following absorption, a drug gains access to the receptor after it leaves the bloodstream and is distributed to tissues that contain receptor sites. See the box on p. 54 for terms used in this theory of drug action.

The rate theory of drug action assumes that the most important factor determining drug activity is the rate at which drug-receptor combinations take place. It is concerned with an intensity of effect. It postulates that if a drug-receptor complex dissociates rapidly, it has high efficacy. Conversely, if there is slow dissociation, there is firm binding, prolonged occupancy, and low efficacy. Thus, drug antagonism is associated with slow kinetics and drug agonism with fast kinetics.

Drug-enzyme interaction. An interaction between drug and cellular enzyme is the second way by which drugs produce their effects. Enzymes are indispensable biologic catalysts that control all biochemical reactions of the cell. Drugs can inhibit the action of a specific enzyme and alter a physiologic response. For example, neostigmine, an agent used to manage the muscle weakness in myasthenia gravis, acts chemically by combining with acetyl cholinesterase to prevent this enzyme from inactivating acetylcholine at the neuromuscular junction.

Drugs that combine with enzymes are thought to do so by virtue of their structural resemblance to an enzyme's substrate molecule (the substance acted on by an enzyme). A drug may resemble an enzyme's substrate so closely that it can combine with the enzyme instead of with the normal substrate. Drugs resembling enzyme substrates are termed "antimetabolites" and can either block normal enzymatic action or result in the production of other substances with unique biochemical properties. The antimetabolites, then, become the receptor for the drug. However, although enzymes may be receptors, not all receptors are enzymes. An example of an antimetabolite is the anticancer drug methotrexate.

Nonspecific drug interaction. Some drugs demonstrate no structural specificity and presumably act by more general effects on cell membranes and cellular processes. These drugs may penetrate into cells or accumulate in cellular membranes, where they interfere, by physical or chemical means, with some cell function or some fundamental metabolic processes.

Cell membranes are complex lipoprotein structures that regulate the flow of ions and metabolites in a highly selective manner, thereby maintaining an electrochemical gradient between the interior and exterior surfaces of the cell. Structurally nonspecific drugs are exemplified by the general anesthetics, which are lipid-soluble compounds of unrelated chemical structure but with similar properties. It is believed that general anesthetics alter the properties of lipids in cell membranes of nerves rather than act on specific receptors.

DRUG-RECEPTOR INTERACTION TERMS

affinity the propensity of a drug to bind or attach itself to a given receptor site.

efficacy (intrinsic activity). The drug's ability to initiate biologic activity as a result of such binding.

agonist a drug that combines with receptors and initiates a sequence of biochemical and physiologic changes; possesses both affinity and efficacy.

antagonist an agent designed to inhibit or counteract effects produced by other drugs or undesired effects caused by cellular components during illness.

competitive antagonist an agent with an affinity for the same receptor site as an agonist; the competition with the agonist for the site inhibits the action of the agonist; increasing the concentration of the agonist tends to overcome the inhibition. Competitive inhibition responses are usually reversible.

noncompetitive antagonist an agent that combines with different parts of the receptor mechanism and inactivates the receptor so that the agonist cannot be effective regardless of its concentration. Noncompetitive antagonist effects are considered to be irreversible or nearly so.

partial agonist an agent that has affinity and some efficacy but that may antagonize the action of other drugs that have greater efficacy. Not infrequently, antagonists share some structural similarities with their agonists.

Other structurally nonspecific drugs may act by biophysical means that do not affect cellular or enzymatic functions. Drugs acting as a result of their obvious physical properties include the ointments and emollients. Hydrophilic indigestible substances exert a cathartic effect because of their physical action on the bowel. Examples of true chemical reactions that produce biologic effects are the interaction of a molecule such as lead with an antidotal drug and the neutralization by antacid drugs of hydrochloric acid present in gastric juice. Neither is considered a receptor interaction because there are no macromolecular tissue elements involved. Detergents, alcohol, oxidizing agents such as hydrogen peroxide, and phenol derivatives such as Lysol are also structurally nonspecific and act by irreversibly destroying the functional integrity of the living cell.

DRUG-RESPONSE RELATIONSHIP

After it is administered, each drug has its own characteristic rate of absorption, distribution, biotransformation, and excretion. These can be analyzed by performing a plasma level profile. In many instances nurses are required to monitor serum drug levels to help the physician determine the dosage, scheduling, and route of administration for an individual patient. These data also provide information concerning the degree of therapeutic effectiveness so that potential adverse reactions can be predicted, thereby preventing serious clinical problems.

Plasma Level Profile of a Drug

The plasma or serum level profile graphically demonstrates the relationship between the plasma concentration of a drug and the level of the therapeutic effectiveness over a course of time. After one dose is administered, the time course of the amount of drug in the body depends on the rates of absorption, distribution, metabolism, and elimination. By monitoring the plasma level of a compound, the efficacy and safety of drug therapy can be more closely controlled. The box on p. 55 lists important terms used in plasma level profiles and explains their interrelationships.

Biologic Half-Life

The rate of biotransformation and excretion of a drug determines its biologic **half-life** ($t\frac{1}{2}$). Moreover, the duration of a dosage can be demonstrated by the biologic half-life, which is defined as the time required to reduce to one half that amount of unchanged drug that is in the body at the time equilibrium is established. The half-life of each drug is different. One with a short $t\frac{1}{2}$, such as 2 or 3 hours, will need to be administered more often than one with a long $t\frac{1}{2}$, such as 12 hours.

The half-life does not change with the drug dose; it always takes the same amount of time to eliminate one half of the drug present in the body. If, for example,

10,000 units of a drug are administered and that drug has a half-life of 4 hours, then 5000 units of the drug will be excreted in 4 hours. In the next 4 hours, 2500 units will be excreted, with 1250 units more being excreted in the third 4-hour period. In hepatic dysfunction, in which drug metabolism is impaired, or in renal disorders, in which elimination may be prolonged, the half-life of a drug is lengthened. This usually necessitates reduction of drug dosage.

Therapeutic Index

The **therapeutic index** (TI) provides a quantitative measure of the relative safety of a drug. It represents a ratio between two factors: (1) **lethal dose** (LD 50), which is the dose of a drug that is lethal in 50% of laboratory animals tested, and (2) **effective dose** (ED 50), which is the dose required to produce a therapeutic effect in 50% of a similar population. The therapeutic index is calculated as follows:

$$TI = \frac{LD\ 50}{ED\ 50}$$

The closer the ratio is to 1, the greater the danger involved in administration of that drug to human beings. Obviously, in the human the dose that promotes a side

---

PLASMA LEVEL PROFILE TERMS

onset of action or latent period   interval between the time a drug is administered and the first sign of its effect

termination of action   point at which a drug effect is no longer seen

duration of action   period from onset of drug action to the time when response is no longer perceptible

minimal effective concentration   lowest plasma concentration that produces the desired drug effect

peak plasma level   highest plasma concentration attained from a dose

toxic level   plasma concentration at which a drug produces serious adverse effects

therapeutic range   range of plasma concentrations that produce the desired drug effect without toxicity (the range between minimal effective concentration and toxic level)

loading dose   bolus of drug given initially to attain rapidly a therapeutic plasma concentration

maintenance dose   the amount of drug necessary to maintain a steady therapeutic plasma concentration

---

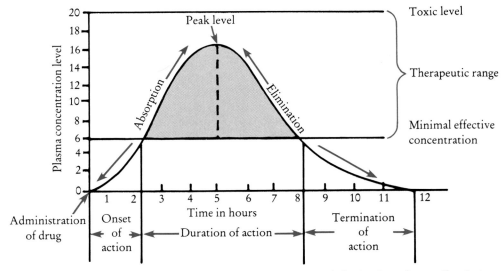

FIGURE 4-8   Plasma level profile of a drug. The absorption and elimination of an orally administered drug are depicted. *Onset of action:* after a dose of the drug is administered, there is a delay or a latent period required for absorption and distribution of the drug. In this case, it takes 2 hours. *Minimal effective concentration:* signifies the first sign of a drug effect. *Duration of action:* extends from the time of onset of action to the time when the response is no longer perceptible. With this drug it lasts 6 hours. *Peak level:* represents the maximal drug response — takes 5 hours. *Toxic level:* occurs when a higher dose is given and it exceeds the peak level. *Therapeutic range:* extends from some point below the toxic level to minimal effective concentration. The shaded area represents the therapeutic effectiveness of the drug where plasma levels are raised from the minimal effective concentration to the peak level (during absorption and elimination). *Termination of action:* when the plasma level falls below the minimal effective concentration, the action of the drug is ended — takes 4 hours. Time of complete absorption and elimination of drug varies with each compound.

effect or the first sign of a toxic response is of greater importance than the therapeutic index of the drug, since the physician's major concern is avoiding even an isolated fatality caused by drug toxicity.

ADVERSE RESPONSES TO DRUGS

Drugs can react in the body to produce unpredictable, harmful, and sometimes unexplainable responses. No drug is totally safe and absolutely free of toxic effects. Sometimes these effects are immediately apparent. At other times they may take weeks or months to develop. Some adverse reactions are relatively mild; others can be fatal. With the increasing numbers of drugs being used, the incidence of adverse reactions has increased and is presently a significant problem in medical therapeutics.

PREDICTABLE ADVERSE RESPONSES

Some factors alter the response to drug therapy. Deviant drug reactions can frequently be traced to the predictable influence of such variables. The nurse must be cognizant of characteristics that modify cell conditions and, therefore, the activity of a drug. These characteristics include age, body mass, sex, environmental milieu, time of administration, pathologic state, genetic factors, and psychologic factors (see Table 4-2).

Age. It is generally recognized that children and elderly persons are highly responsive to drugs. Infants often have immature hepatic and renal systems and, therefore, incomplete excretory and metabolic mechanisms. Aged individuals may demonstrate different responses to drug therapy because of deterioration of hepatic and renal function, which is often accompanied by concurrent disease processes, such as cardiovascular disease. Modifications of dosage for children may be calculated on the basis of body weight or surface area.

Body mass. The relationship between body mass and amount of drug administered influences the distribution and concentration of a drug. In order to maintain a desired drug concentration in individuals of various sizes, drug dosage must be adjusted in proportion to body mass. For a given dose of drug, the greater the volume of distribution, the lower the concentration of drug reached in various body compartments. Since the volume of interstitial and intracellular water is related to body mass, weight has a marked influence on the quantitative effects produced by drugs. The average adult drug dose is calculated on the basis of the drug quantity that will produce a particular effect in 50% of persons who are between the ages of 18 and 65 and weigh about 150 pounds (70 kg). Therefore, particularly for children and for very lean and for very obese individuals, drug dosage is frequently determined on the basis of amount of drug per kilogram of body weight or body surface area.

TABLE 4-2 Factors Altering Drug Responses and Summary of Nursing Considerations

Factor and pertinent description	Nursing considerations
Age Infants—immature body systems Children—dosage adjustment usually necessary Elderly—depressed hepatic and renal systems	Modify dosages. Children have a different physiologic profile and body mass distribution. Thus, dose per kilogram is individualized. It could be more or less than in an adult. Elderly clients may also have concomitant physical conditions that alter drug effects; altered excretion mechanism, too may require less drug or different scheduling of medication.
Body mass The greater the volume of distribution, the lower the concentration of drug in the body compartments Calculation: average adult dose based on drug quantity that will produce a particular effect in 50% of population between the ages of 18 and 65 and weighing about 150 pounds (70 kg)	Adjust dosage in proportion to body mass. For children, dosage frequently is determined on the basis of amount of drug per kilogram of body weight or body surface area
Sex Women--smaller than men; definite differences during pregnancy and in relative proportions of fat and water; drugs vary by water or fat solubility	Allow for size differential and whether a drug is water or lipid soluble. Avoid drugs during pregnancy unless an absolute necessity exists.
Environmental milieu Mood and behavior modified by (1) drug itself, (2) personality of the user, (3) environment of the user, and (4) interaction of these three factors; other factors: sensory—deprivation or overload; physical environment—cold vs heat, oxygen deprivation (altitude)	Be aware of the physical situation of the client with regard to heat and cold, interactions with other individuals, drug effects, and how the client generally reacts to situations.

TABLE 4-2 Factors Altering Drug Responses and Summary of Nursing Considerations—cont'd.

Factor and pertinent description	Nursing considerations
Time of administration Food—presence or absence Biologic rhythms—sleep-wake cycle, drug-metabolizing enzyme rhythms, corticosteroid secretion rhythm, blood pressure rhythms, circadian (24-hour) cycle in absorption and urinary excretion; also rhythm of drug receptor susceptibility	Give irritating drugs when there is food in the client's stomach. Follow manufacturer's recommendations. Make every effort to understand the client's normal and abnormal rhythms and seek possible relationships between the client's biologic rhythms and reactions to drug therapy. Administer drugs at same time of day. Altered body cycles (shift workers) may result in altered response to a drug.
Pathologic state Presence and severity of pathologic state—pain intensifies need for opiates; anxiety may produce resistance to large doses of tranquilizing drugs; presence of circulatory, hepatic, and/or renal dysfunctions interferes with physiologic processes of drug action	Take into account any pain, disease, or altered metabolic state of the client and adjust dosage accordingly.
Genetic factors Genetically determined abnormal/susceptability to a chemical, or "idiosyncratic response"	Be aware that any client may show an idiosyncratic response. Always monitor closely, especially when beginning therapy, for abnormal susceptibility. Be aware of common drug idiosyncrasies.
Psychologic factors Symbolic investment in drugs and faith in their efficacy Placebo effect Hostility toward or mistrust of medicine or health personnel	Be aware of the attitude and the impression the nurse creates at the time of drug administration, and use them to enhance the drug's effects.

Sex. Differences in drug effects related to the variable of sex result, in part, from size differences between men and women. Women are usually smaller than men, which will lead to high drug concentrations if dosage is prescribed indifferently. There are also demonstrable differences in relative proportions of fat and water in the bodies of men and women, and some drugs may be more soluble in one or the other. Some authorities also indicate that subjective factors regarding drug effects may vary with sexual differences, stating that women are more suggestible to drug effects than men. This, however, is a controversial hypothesis.

Since drugs taken by a pregnant woman might affect the uterus and/or the fetus as a result of placental transfer, the use of drugs is best avoided during pregnancy unless an absolute necessity exists.

Environmental milieu. Drugs affecting mood and behavior are particularly susceptible to the influence of the individual's environment. With such drugs one has to consider effects in light of four factors: (1) the drug itself, (2) the personality of the user, (3) the environment of the user, and (4) the interaction of these three components. Sensory deprivation and sensory overload may also affect responses to drugs. Physical environment can modify drug effects. For example, temperature affects drug activity: heat relaxes peripheral vessels and thus intensifies the actions of vasodilators, while cold has the opposite effect. The relative oxygen deprivation at high altitudes may increase sensitivity to some drugs.

Time of administration. It is well known that drugs are absorbed more rapidly if the gastrointestinal tract is free of food and that irritating drugs are more readily tolerated if there is food in the stomach.

Although the theory is highly speculative, if findings from drug research on animals are applicable to humans, the time of drug administration in relation to human biologic rhythms can significantly affect the response to various drugs. It seems quite plausible that in humans the sleep-wake rhythm, deep sleep and dreaming sleep cycle, drug-metabolizing enzyme rhythms, corticosteroid secretion rhythm, blood pressure rhythms, and circadian (24-hour) variation in absorption and urinary excretion contribute to the effective, ineffective, adverse, or toxic response to particular drugs. There may also be a circadian rhythm in drug receptor susceptibility. Chronopharmacology and chronotoxicology are new areas of interest, and the frequency with which drug rhythm reports are appearing in the literature is increasing. The nurse should make every effort to understand the client's normal and abnormal rhythms and seek to determine possible relationships between the client's biologic rhythms and reactions to drug therapy.

Pathologic state. The presence of a pathologic condition and the severity of symptoms may call for careful consideration of the type of drug administered and for adjustment in dosage. For example, the presence of severe pain tends to increase a client's requirement for opiates, and an extremely anxious individual can prove resistant to very large doses of tranquilizing and sedating drugs. Aspirin administered to a client with a fever will produce a decrease in temperature, whereas a client taking the drug for its analgesic effects will show no temperature change at all. Larger doses of insulin may be required for the client with diabetes whose condition is complicated by fever or infection. In addition, it bears repeating that the presence of circulatory, hepatic, and/or renal dysfunctions will interfere with the physiologic processes of drug action.

Genetic factors. Genetic differences may alter greatly the response of individuals to a number of drugs. Such differences may arise from genetically conditioned deficiencies in drug metabolism or in receptor sensitivity. These pharmacogenetic abnormalities often manifest themselves as "idiosyncrasies" and may be mistakenly diagnosed as drug allergies. For example, some individuals may lack pseudocholinesterase activity in their plasma. If they receive an injection of succinylcholine, which is normally hydrolyzed by plasma cholinesterase, they may become paralyzed and remain that way for a long time. The field of pharmacogenetics is of great interest, since it may provide a rational explanation for many so-called drug idiosyncrasies.

Psychologic factors. The client's symbolic investment in drugs and faith in their effects strongly influence and usually potentiate drug effects. The placebo effect is an outstanding example of how strong motivation can influence the emergence of desired drug effects. Conversely, hostility and mistrust of medicine and health personnel can diminish drug effects. It is important for nurses to realize that their attitudes and the impressions created at the time of drug administration may influence the therapeutic result.

IATROGENIC RESPONSES

Generally, the term **iatrogenic** diseases refers to adverse effects produced unintentionally in the treatment of a client. Iatrogenic diseases induced by drugs manifest themselves in five major groups: (1) blood dyscrasias, such as agranulocytosis, thrombocytopenia, aplastic anemia, and bone marrow depression; (2) hepatic toxicity, which is common and may take the form of biliary obstruction, hepatitis-like syndromes, and hepatic necrosis; (3) renal damage, particularly glomerular damage, which is a significant toxic effect of a number of drugs, including some antibiotics; (4) teratogenic effects, or drug effects causing malformations in the fetus as a result of placental transfer of drugs taken by a pregnant woman; and (5) dermatologic effects, such as acne, psoriasis, eczema, maculopapular rashes, and, rarely, erythema multi-

forme. By carefully monitoring a client's response to a drug, the nurse in some instances may be able to avert an iatrogenic disease.

In addition to these common and well-known drug-induced diseases, numerous other iatrogenic syndromes are specific to certain drugs. Ulceration of the gastrointestinal tract, for example, is a common result of long-term therapy with drugs such as aspirin, steroids, and potassium chloride. The relationship between oral contraceptive agents and thromboembolic phenomena is another untoward effect that may eventually be defined as an iatrogenic disease.

UNPREDICTABLE ADVERSE RESPONSES

Adverse drug reactions are one way of characterizing unpredictable and sometimes unexplainable drug responses that have not been optimally, clearly, and distinctly defined. The most common and best defined adverse drug reactions are the following. (See also the accompanying box.)

Drug allergy is an altered state of reaction to a drug, resulting from previous sensitizing exposure and the development of an immunologic mechanism. Substances foreign to the body act as antigens to stimulate the production of antibodies or immunoglobulins. Later, when a previously sensitized individual is again exposed to the foreign substance, the antigen reacts with the antibodies in ways that are damaging to body tissues. The antigen-antibody complex is not directly responsible for the manifestations of allergy. Rather, the complex reacts with various tissues and cells of the body by processes not clearly understood and causes them to release certain substances (for example, histamine), which then provoke the symptoms of allergy.

Allergic reactions may manifest themselves as a variety of symptoms, ranging from minor skin rashes to fatal hypotension. Reactions may be localized or widespread, and the symptoms can appear immediately or within hours to days after drug administration.

Immediate reactions occur within minutes of exposure to the chemical to which the person has been previously sensitized. Immediate and severe reactions are called anaphylactic reactions and are frequently fatal if not recognized and treated quickly. Signs and symptoms are severe, occur suddenly, and produce shock. The most dramatic form of *anaphylaxis* is sudden, severe bronchospasm, vasospasm, severe hypotension, and rapid death. Signs are largely caused by contraction of smooth muscles and may begin with irritability, extreme weakness, nausea, and vomiting and may proceed to dyspnea, cyanosis, convulsions, and cardiac arrest. Antihistamine drugs, epinephrine, and bronchodilators are indispensable in the treatment of anaphylactic shock.

DRUG RESPONSES

Drug allergy	Altered state of reaction resulting from previous sensitization and development of immunologic mechanism
	Body treats the drug as an antigen and produces antibodies that react in ways harmful to body tissues
	Manifestations range from minor skin rashes to fatal anaphylaxis are local or widespread, occur immediately or within hours to days following administration
	Life-threatening reactions: called anaphylactic reactions and are frequently fatal; signs and symptoms severe, occur suddenly, and produce shock; symptoms include sudden severe bronchospasm, vasospasm, severe hypotension, and death in the most severe form of anaphylaxis; signs are caused by contraction of smooth muscle and may begin with irritability, extreme weakness, nausea, and vomiting; may proceed to dyspnea, cyanosis, convulsions, and cardiac arrest; *Treatment:* antihistamine drugs, epinephrine, bronchodilators
	Mild reactions: rash, angioedema, rhinitis, fever, asthma, pruritus; may be immediate or appear 7 to 14 days after first administration of drug; delay reminiscent of "serum sickness" and characterized by angioedema, arthralgia, fever, lymphadenopathy, splenomegaly; also includes contact dermatitis; *Treatment:* avoid reexposure to that drug; skin tests may be performed to definitely diagnose response; do no reinstitute the therapy, since an anaphylactic response may then occur
Idiosyncrasy	Abnormal or peculiar response to drug; may be (1) overresponse or abnormal susceptibility, (2) underresponse that shows abnormal tolerance, (3) qualitatively different response than that expected, (4) unpredictable or unexplainable response
	Thought to result from genetic enzymatic deficiencies that lead to abnormal mechanism of metabolizing drug
Hypersensitivity	An exaggerated response to a drug; often incorrectly used as synonymous with allergy; usually idiosyncratic' not a true antigen-antibody reaction as seen with allergies
Tolerance	Decreased physiologic response to the repeated administration of a drug or chemically related substance
	Excessive increase in dosage required in order to maintain the required therapeutic effect
	Tolerance mechanism unknown; sometimes an effect resulting when prolonged administration of some drugs induces the synthesis of extra drug-metabolizing enzymes in the liver
	Cross-tolerance occurs between related chemicals
Tachyphylaxis	Quickly developing tolerance to the rapid, repeated administration of drug
Cumulation	Results when the body cannot metabolize one dose of drug before another dose is administered; that is, drug is excreted more slowly than it is absorbed and the concentration of drug within the body rises
	Requires adjustment of the dosage to avoid toxic effects brought on by the accumulation of drug in the body
	Reaction can occur rapidly or insidiously; for example, ethyl alcohol intoxication occurs rapidly, but poisoning with heavy metals occurs over a prolonged period of time as these substances are stored in various body tissues
Drug dependence	A state in which intense physical or emotional distrubance is produced if a drug is withdrawn; previously termed habituation or addiction; can be physical or psychic (for further details, see Chater 9.)
Drug interaction	Effects of one drug are modified by the prior or concurrent administration of another drug, thereby increasing or decreasing the pharmacologic action of one or both drugs; may be beneficial or detrimental
Drug antagonism	Conjoint effect of two drugs is less than the sum of the drugs acting separately
Summation (addition)	Combined effect of two drugs produces a result that equals the sum of the individual effects of each agent, 1 + 1 = 2
	Combination allows the administration of a lower dose of each drug, with a resultant decrease in adverse reactions
Synergism	Combined effect of drugs is greater than the sum of each individual agent acting independently; 1 + 1 = 3 or more
Potentiation	Concurrent administration of two drugs in which one drug increases the effect of the other drug

Mild allergic reactions may be characterized by the development of a rash, angioedema, rhinitis, fever, asthma, and pruritus. Some allergic reactions are delayed and may appear anywhere from 7 to 14 days after initial administration of the drug. *Delayed reactions* are frequently analogous to *"serum sickness"* and are characterized by angioedema, arthralgia, fever, lymph-adenopathy, and splenomegaly. Contact dermatitis, which results from direct skin contact with the eliciting drug, is also a delayed allergic response.

An individual who has had a mild allergic response to a particular drug should avoid reexposure to that drug and, optimally, should have skin tests performed in order to more definitely diagnose the response. Reinstitution of therapy with the same drug in a client who manifests allergic reactions is always dangerous, since an anaphylactic reaction may occur.

The term *"hypersensitivity"* is frequently used synonymously with allergy, but it is inappropriate because it is frequently confused with other kinds of adverse drug reactions. Since there is a lack of precision to defining hypersensitivity, it may be wise to avoid use of the term.

Idiosyncrasy is any abnormal or peculiar response to a drug that may manifest itself by (1) overresponse or abnormal susceptibility to a drug; (2) underresponse, demonstrating abnormal tolerance; (3) a qualitatively different effect from the one expected, such as excitation after the administration of a sedative; or (4) unpredictable and unexplainable symptoms. Idiosyncratic reactions are generally thought to result from genetic enzymatic deficiencies that lead to an abnormal mechanism of metabolizing drugs. This term has been used rather vaguely to describe drug reactions that are qualitatively different from the usual effects obtained in the majority of patients and that cannot be attributed to drug allergy.

Tolerance is said to exist when there is a decreased physiologic response to the repeated administration of a drug or a chemically related substance. It is a reaction that necessitates an excessive increase in dosage to maintain a given therapeutic effect. Drugs well known for their propensity to produce tolerance are tobacco, opium alkaloids, nitrites, barbiturates, and ethyl alcohol. The actual mechanism of tolerance is unknown. In some instances, prolonged administration of some drugs somehow induces the synthesis of extra drug-metabolizing enzymes in the liver, which may account for the patient's increased ability to tolerate larger drug doses than previously. *Cross tolerance* between related chemicals (such as between alcohol and some anesthetics) is a well-documented phenomenon. It is quite clear, however, that not all cases of tolerance are attributable to a drug's increased rate of metabolism. For example, the remarkable tolerance to morphine cannot be caused by its more rapid metabolic degradation.

Tachyphylaxis refers to a quickly developing tolerance to the rapid, repeated administration of a drug. It is quick in onset, and the client's initial response to the drug cannot be reproduced, even with larger doses of the drug.

Cumulation occurs when the body cannot metabolize one dose of a drug before another dose is administered. In other words, when drugs are excreted more slowly than they are absorbed, each new dose adds more to the total quantity in the blood and organs than is lost in the same amount of time by excretion. Unless drug administration is adjusted, sufficiently high concentrations can be reached to produce toxic effects. Cumulative toxicity can occur rapidly, as dramatically illustrated in ethyl alcohol intoxication, or it can occur insidiously, as is the case in poisoning with heavy metals, such as lead. The latter is stored in many body tissues and deposited in bones, therefore having prolonged effects on the body while accumulation continues.

Drug dependence is the term preferred over the previous terminology of "habituation" and "addiction." The World Health Organization has suggested the use of the term dependence in conjunction with the drug being described (e.g., barbiturate dependence or opiate dependence). Dependence can be physical or psychic. Physical dependence refers to a state of physiologic adaptation to a drug that manifests itself by intense physical disturbance when the drug is withdrawn. Psychic dependence is a state of emotional reliance on a drug in order to maintain a sense of well-being. Its manifestations may range from a mild desire for a drug, to craving, to compulsive use of the drug. Drug dependence will be explored in greater breadth and depth in Chapter 9.

Drug interaction occurs when the effects of one drug are modified by the prior or concurrent administration of another drug, thereby increasing or decreasing the pharmacologic action of each. Drug interactions may be either beneficial (e.g., probenecid prolongs the action of penicillins) or detrimental (e.g., aspirin increases the action of anticoagulants, causing hemorrhage).

Drug antagonism occurs when the conjoint effect of two drugs is less than the sum of the drugs acting separately.

Summation (addition) occurs when the combined effect of two drugs produces a result that equals the sum of the individual effects of each agent. The mathematical response is $1 + 1 = 2$. For example, codeine and aspirin both act as analgesics and when given together provide greater relief of pain than when eigher one is used alone. This combination allows the administration of a lower dosage of each drug, with a resultant decrease in adverse reactions.

Synergism describes a drug interaction in which the combined effect of drugs is greater than the sum of each individual agent acting independents. Mathematically the response is $1 + 1 = 3$. This can be exemplified by the use of a combination of drugs in treating hypertension. Each of the drugs lowers blood pressure, but in different ways; however, the combined effect produces a greater decrease in hypertension than if either drug were given alone.

Potentiation refers to the concurrent administration of two drugs in which one drug increases the effect of the other drug.

SUMMARY OF NURSING CONSIDERATIONS

The nurse's responsibilities in the administration of drugs require more than memorization of specific drugs, their actions, and their dosages. Rather, effective implementation depends on a sound comprehension of the theories of drug action, constituting knowledge that the nurse can transfer to the individual client, each with a specific diagnosis and definable individual needs. Such a background necessitates the understanding of theories of drug action, physiologic processes mediating drug action, variables affecting drug action, and unusual and adverse responses to drug therapy.

On entry into the body, a drug initiates a series of physiologic events before it reaches its site of action. The extent of drug absorption depends on the form in which the drug appears. Tablets or capsules must first disintegrate and then be dissolved in solution before absorption through the intestinal membrane can occur. However, the nurse should never crush an enteric-coated tablet, because the coating protects it from destruction by the acid pH of the stomach. To maintain its effectiveness, the drug appears in this form so it can disintegrate and dissolve in the alkaline pH of the intestine. Drugs that irritate the gastric mucosa must also be coated.

To obtain the maximal pharmacokinetic benefit of a drug, the time of administration is another important concern of the nurse. Oral drugs should be given ½ hour before meals with a glass of water (8 ounces). It is important to remember that the presence of food, which delays stomach emptying, tends to diminish the therapeutic effect of the drug. Occasionally, an agent must be administered with meals to prevent gastrointestinal irritation. The nurse should anticipate a rapid response when a drug is given intravenously, because the full dosage is placed directly into the bloodstream, thus bypassing the need for absorption.

Individuals with hepatic dysfunction are susceptible to drug overdosage, especially if the drug is highly bound to plasma proteins. Adverse responses can be prevented by the administration of albumin. In addition, the nurse should be alert to the client's response to a drug if there is a renal disorder. Since most agents are excreted by the kidneys, the client should be observed for a cumulative effect that may result from the continued administration of the drug. Usually, drug dosage is adjusted in individuals with hepatic or renal disorders so that adverse effects will be prevented.

In instances when the nurse is required to monitor serum drug levels, careful observations of the client's response to the drug provide information that aids the physician in determining the dosage of a drug, the frequency of administration, and the route of administration. The data are essential for promoting the optimal therapeutic benefit to the client and at the same time preventing potential adverse reactions.

Finally, the nurse should alert a pregnant woman about the danger of taking medications and, to prevent teratogenic effects, advise her to check with a physician before taking any drug. In addition, if a medication is required, the lowest possible dose of the prescribed drug should be administered.

KEY TERMS

absorption, page 44
active transport, page 43
bioavailability, page 48
biologically equivalent, page 48
biotransformation, page 50
buccal, page 46
carrier transport, page 43
dissolution, page 43
distribution, page 48
effective dose, page 55
enteral, page 46
enteric coating, page 45
enterohepatic cycle, page 52
excretion, page 51
half-life, page 54
hepatic first-pass effect, page 51
hypoalbuminemia, page 49
iatrogenic, page 58
intramuscular, page 47
intrathecal, page 47
intravenous, page 47
lethal dose, page 55
lipid soluble, page 43
loading dose, page 45
maintenance dose, page 45
parenteral, page 47
passive diffusion, page 43
passive transport, page 43
pharmaceutics, page 43
pharmacodynamics, page 53
pharmacokinetics, page 43
priming dose, page 45
plasma protein binding, page 49
receptor, page 53
subcutaneous, page 47
sublingual, page 46

BIBLIOGRAPHY

Clark, JB, Queener, SF, and Karb, VB: Pharmacological basis of nursing practice, ed 2, St Louis, 1986, The CV Mosby Co.

Clarke, G: Pharmacokinetics, Nurs Times 79(48):58, 1983.

Gilman, AG, and others, eds: Goodman and Gilman's the pharmacological basis of therapeutics, ed 7, 1985, New York, Macmillan, Inc.

Goth, A, and Vesell, ES: Medical pharmacology: principles and concepts, ed 11, St Louis, 1984, The CV Mosby Co.

Jones, B: How drugs act, Nurs Mirror 158(19):17.

Koch-Weser, J: Drug administration in hepatic disease, N Engl J Med 309:1616, 1983.

Lamy, PP: Prescribing for the elderly. Littleton, Mass, 1980, PSG Publishing Co, Inc.

Lamy, PP, and Breardsley, RS: The older adult and the pharmacist educator, Am Pharm NS22(5):40.

Levinson, RS, and Allen, LV: Physiological and pharmaceutical factors that affect the bioavailability of drugs, Cont Edu Guide Pharm 1(3):1, 1976.

Martin, RB: Drug interactions, Cont Educ Guide Pharm 1(1):1, 1976.

Schwartz, RH, and Yaffe, SJ, eds: Drug and chemical risks to the fetus and newborn, New York, 1980, Alan R Liss, Inc.

Smith, S: How drugs act: intolerance, idiosyncrasy and hypersensitivity, Nurs Times 80(51):34, 1984.

Smith, S: How drugs act: how drugs are absorbed and reach their destination, Nurs Times 80(48):24, 1984.

Smith, S: How drugs act: elimination and cumulation, Nurs Times 80(49):44, 1984.

Stockley, L: Drug interactions, London, 1981, Blackwell Scientific Publications.

UNIT II

The Nursing Process and Pharmacology

CHAPTER 5

Assessment, Nursing Diagnosis, and Planning

OVERVIEW OF THE NURSING PROCESS

The **nursing process** is applied to drug therapy to develop a systematic, organized approach to handling the wealth of data about clients and their drugs. It provides direction for rational nursing actions to manage problems related to drug therapies. Conceptually, the nursing process itself continues to be in a healthy state of evolution as nurse researchers and practitioners develop and test nomenclature and theories. Although current literature may not be in absolute agreement about all of the terminology or the distinctive phases in the nursing process, its concepts become more completely defined and more widely accepted with each passing year. The nursing process, however, is certainly a viable and practical organizing tool to apply to patient care.

The nursing process was the foundation of high-quality clinical practice long before it had been conceptualized and given a name. Its process and phases are analogous to scientific and problem-solving methods. Although other variations exist, in this book, it will be described here in four phases: (1) assessment, culminating in nursing diagnoses, (2) planning, (3) implementation, and (4) evaluation. Figure 5-1 diagrams these phases or steps, which are discussed in this chapter and in Chapter 6. It should be kept in mind that the steps of the nursing process have an ongoing, cyclic nature—no step should be considered completed or static.

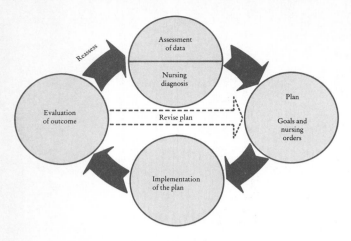

FIGURE 5-1 Nursing process.

ASSESSMENT OF DATA

The assessment phase of the nursing process is both the first phase and a continuous phase that ends only on discharge of the client. During assessment of data, all the facts relating to clients and their drug therapy, relationships with others, the health history, and the environment are collected and organized so that the nurse can begin to make inferences about any problems in drug therapy. The data that are collected and analyzed form the basis for development of a nursing diagnosis.

The client's status and the assessment data derived from these indicated sources are constantly changing. Nursing diagnostic statements will change as well. In collaboration with the physician, these changes may result in revision of the medical plan, such as drug deletions, additions, or dosage changes.

Nurses must have a sound base of knowledge about a client's disorder and drugs being administered, as well as the skill to use references to answer questions that arise. The ability to ask questions and seek answers about the data collected will form a solid foundation for the planning, implementation, and evaluation phases of the nursing process.

DRUG HISTORY GUIDELINES

Taking a **drug history** can be extremely useful for gathering data about an individual's experience with medications. Obtaining a comprehensive drug history requires a combination of nursing knowledge, interviewing skills, and a review of specific drug reference resources, whenever necessary. A drug history should explore the client's usage of prescription medications, usage of over-the-counter (OTC) drugs, self-treatment with herbal or home remedies, general and specific health history, and when possible, specific cultural factors that influence individual drug therapies. Figure 5-2 shows a sample drug history form.

A thorough drug history can provide extremely useful information for the entire health care team. For example, it can:

1. Explain a mysterious new symptom reported in the patient.
2. Provide clues about unreported chronic disorders.
3. Reveal learning needs or concerns regarding patient compliance with therapy.
4. Provide information crucial to prevent drug interactions, allergies, or side or toxic effects.
5. Help interpret laboratory tests reliably.
6. Identify the potential for drug-drug and drug-food interactions.

When a nurse is taking a drug history, it is important to communicate at the level of understanding appropriate for the client. Medical terminology may be confusing to the non–medically trained person; therefore the nurse should be familiar with local observances and, when applicable, ethnic or cultural expressions for specific diseases, illnesses, symptoms, and/or other information.

Open-ended questioning is preferred to direct "yes" or "no" questions during an interview. For example, to obtain information about a client's use of analgesics, a "yes" or "no" question would be: "Do you take analgesics? If 'yes,' name them." If the person is unsure of the meaning of the term *analgesia,* a "no" answer might be the natural response. The question can be reworded to ask, "What do you take when you have pain, such as a headache, backache, muscle sprain, or other type of ache or pain?" and the more descriptive information the nurse is seeking may then be forthcoming. Questions concerning over-the-counter drugs must often be accompanied by reminders from the interviewer. Commonly used product names or currently advertised brands may be suggested to jog the memory of the client. For example, aspirin is an ingredient in hundreds of OTC preparations; therefore simply asking the client if he or she consumes aspirin may limit the answer to only products labeled as aspirin. Suggesting trade name products, such as Anacin, Bufferin, or Alka Seltzer, would expand the possibility of obtaining a more thorough drug history.

If the interview is performed in the client's living quarters, the nurse should ask to see medications. Many individuals, especially the elderly, forget to report all the medications they have on hand for self-medicating purposes. Also the storage place for medications should be noted, since this may be important information if a potentially hazardous site is used. Storage in a bathroom cabinet or over a kitchen sink or stove may adversely affect many medications. Areas of heat and moisture are not recommended as proper storage areas for most drugs.

Evaluating the client's knowledge about proper dispos-

DRUG HISTORY

Patient's name _____ Sex _____ Age _____ Date of interview _____
Occupation   Physician

Diagnosis and past history (if relevant)
    Frequency of meals?   Special diet, prescribed
                                             or self-imposed:
Allergies/drug reactions (food and/or drugs; describe reaction, approximate date, and action taken or outcome):

Close family members with drug allergies (relationship, drug, and reaction):

Type/daily consumption   Smoking (type and amount):
    of alcohol:

Over-the-counter medications:
(List medications, dose, frequency, and when last dose was taken for following:)
Constipation (laxatives):
Diarrhea (antidiarrheal):
Gastric upset (antacids):
Pain, headache (analgesics):
Cold medication (antihistamine, decongestants):
Cough medicine (syrups/other forms):
Drugs for sleep:
Drugs to stay awake:
Drugs for menstrual conditions in premenopausal women:
Drugs for nerves:
Drugs for fluid retention:
Do you use any salt substitutes (obtain brand name; Morton Lite Salt, CoSalt, etc.)
Do you use any food supplements? Name and quantity per day:
Do you buy health food store products? Obtain complete listing and daily consumption.

Do you take vitamins? Note type, strength, and amount per day:

Current prescribed medications; include name, strength, and daily dosage:

Prescription medications taken during the previous three months:

Nurse _____

FIGURE 5-2 Sample drug history.

al of drugs (via the sink or toilet), ability to read and understand the labels on medication, and ability to locate expiration dates is part of assessing the individual's ability to safely store and consume medications. Studies have indicated that many persons (from one third to one half of various elderly populations) cannot read or do not understand drug package labels. This high incidence clearly indicates an area of concern that requires nursing assessment.

Information should also be obtained on the individual's general life-style, consumption of alcohol, use of caffeine-containing products, and smoking habits. All these factors may affect or modify a typical drug response. (See the section on drug interactions in this chapter for further information.)

CLIENT AND ENVIRONMENTAL DATA

Client and environmental data are collected from clients, their friends, or their relatives by subjective and objective observations. In addition to observation of clients and their environment, interactions of clients with others and notes from the history and physical examination sections of the chart are used as sources. At the initial interview the practitioner notes a client's past health history and does a physical examination to assess the client's current status. The resulting prioritized problem list directs the therapeutic approach.

Before compiling the nursing data base, rapport must be established if transfer of relevant information is to be made freely. Information obtained in the client's history and physical examination should be reviewed to select pertinent data. The nurse needs to gather data in certain areas to assess appropriateness of the planned drug therapy. If drug dosage and route of administration are not carefully selected, alterations in the various systems may result in either an increased or exaggerated drug effect or a decrease in drug response.

Table 5-1 lists the major factors to be evaluated and pertinent data to be obtained.

CURRENT CLIENT DRUG DATA

Drug data include information derived from the prescriber's orders or prescription and that gained from assessment of the drugs' effects on the patient, based on observation, vital signs, and laboratory reports. The characteristics of the drugs administered and the way they are ordered by the prescriber have an impact on the patient's nursing care.

Drug Orders and Prescriptions

"Medicating" a patient begins when the medication is suggested and authorized by a legally sanctioned prescriber, usually a licensed physician or dentist. These two professionals are currently the only ones legally allowed to initiate medication plans in all states. In several states, nurse practitioners or physicians' assistants have also been given that function legally; in other states this is under consideration. The practicing nurse should be aware of and follow the limitations outlined in the state nurse practice act.

The prescriber's orders are meant for the one who dispenses the medication. There are two different formats, the prescription blank and the order sheet. The prescription blank is given to the outpatient and is to be filled by a community pharmacist; it may look similar to Figure 5-3. For clients in an institutional setting, the order is written on an order sheet found in the client's chart (Figure 5-4). It is filled by the pharmacy within the institution or contracted for by the institution and sent to the medication area on the client's floor for access by the client's medication nurse.

The prescriber's order has seven elements that should be present and identifiable:

1. Patient's name and other identifying data
2. Date that the order was written
3. Medication name and strength
4. Dosage to be administered each time
5. Route of administration
6. Frequency of administration and any special instructions (e.g., "Give with orange juice" if the medication's taste is strong or unpleasant and the medication would not interact with the acidic solution)
7. Prescriber's signature

The "Five Rights" of medication administration referred to in many basic nursing texts are derived from these seven elements (omitting numbers 2 and 7). All parts of the order should be legible and clearly expressed. If there is any doubt, the prescriber must be contacted to validate or clarify. Obviously, to administer a drug under questionable instructions is to risk harm to the patient in an area with a high potential for error (see Chapter 6).

Safe nursing practice is to follow approved procedures in the particular work environment and to administer only drugs that are ordered in writing. Nursing *students* should be aware of special limitations imposed on their actions by the educational and/or clinical institution. In particular, they should be advised to follow only written orders. However, sometimes a verbal or telephoned order from a physician, often in response to the nurse's telephoned request, is unavoidable. When this occurs, it is best to copy the order as it is being given, then verify it by repeating it back to the. sender. Verbal or telephoned orders should be rare, involving circumstances of some urgency rather than convenience. Such an order must be clearly communicated and noted on the patient's chart by the nurse. It must be countersigned by the physician, usually within 24 hours in most institutions, *to be legal.* It is careless and negligent to allow the order to remain unsigned, because it violates both the law and institutional policy. This allows a precarious period of nursing vulnerability to malpractice charges. (See Chapter 2.)

Types of Drug Orders

It is probably obvious by now that, although outpatients are free to medicate themselves with any medication accessible, once an individual is admitted to a clinical institution, usually neither the client nor the nurse may legally administer any medication without a written order.

Contents of the prescriber's orders dictate the conditions under which the ordered drug may be administered. Several types of orders follow.

Routine order. The most common type is the **routine order,** which means that the drug as ordered is to be regularly administered until a formal discontinuation order is written or until a specified termination date is reached. Automatic termination or "automatic stops" may be explicit in agency policy. Automatic stop policies may be mandated for institutional accreditation or licensure requirements, or they may be applied variously by institutions. Such policies act as a stimulus to the prescriber to

TABLE 5-1   Client and Environmental Data

Factor	Questions for evaluation	Rationale
Medical diagnosis	Are the drugs ordered clinically indicated and corroborated by the best judgments according to authoritative literature?	The patient must be protected from wrongful harm; the administering nurse may be held legally accountable.
Age	Has the patient's age been considered? Have drug reactions occurred in the past?	The very young and the elderly are subject to a wide range and great intensity of side and adverse effects because of reduced functioning of body systems that absorb, transport, affect the metabolism of, and excrete drugs (see also Chapter 8).
Body mass	Was the dosage assessed in relation to total body weight, body surface area (weight-to-height ratio), and lean body mass?	For prescribing purposes, the person up to 12 years old is usually considered a child and given a pediatric dosage. The dose is based on the different physiologic and pharmacokinetic factors in the neonate, infant, or older child. The average weight of a 12-year-old child is about 90 pounds; an "average" adult weighs 150 pounds. An adult at or near the weight of 90 pounds who receives the "average adult dose" may exhibit signs of overdosage.
Inherited factors	Have genetic differences (pharmacogenetic variations) in enzyme production or destruction, which may cause apparent therapeutic failure or secondary effects when a drug is metabolized too rapidly, too slowly, or incompletely, been considered?	Many aberrant reactions (termed idiosyncrasy) are often acutely caused by genetic abnormalities. An example is the lack of the enzyme glucose-6-phosphate dehydrogenase, found in a small percentage of people of Mediterranean descent (Italians Greeks, Arabs, and Sephardic Jews) and in about 10% of American black males, less often in black females. Fava beans and medications such as aspirin, antimalarials, and sulfonamides, if taken by these susceptible people, may cause hemolytic anemia. Also, hypersensitivity (allergy) to specific medications often correlates with a tendency to other common allergies to certain foods, grasses, trees, molds, or animal dander.
Coexisting conditions	Are there disorders that affect any of the major body systems, especially those of the gastrointestinal tract or the circulatory, hepatic, or renal system, that will interfere with normal digestion, absorption, transport, metabolism, degradation, and detoxification or excretion of the drugs prescribed?	Impaired capacity for biotransformation may alter drug action and increase the possibility of toxic effects or therapeutic failure. Pregnancy or breast feeding precludes administration of all but essential medications (see Chapter 8).
Compliance	Is there a past history or other factors indicating that the patient, if self-medicating, will not follow medication instructions? (See Chapter 7 for full discussion of patient compliance.)	Attitudes and behavior conducive to positive health behavior depend on psychosocial, cultural, economic, cognitive, and physical factors—how the client views and values health and illness; how the client understands or accepts illness; what he or she knows about the drug in question; how he or she relates to the health care surroundings, system, and practitioners; how the client assigns control and decision making; whether the client communicates and thinks logically; how he or she has been educated; and whether he or she has manipulative skills, among others. Studies show that having faith in a therapy has a decidedly favorable effect on its outcome. A subtle approach is needed to evaluate these parameters.

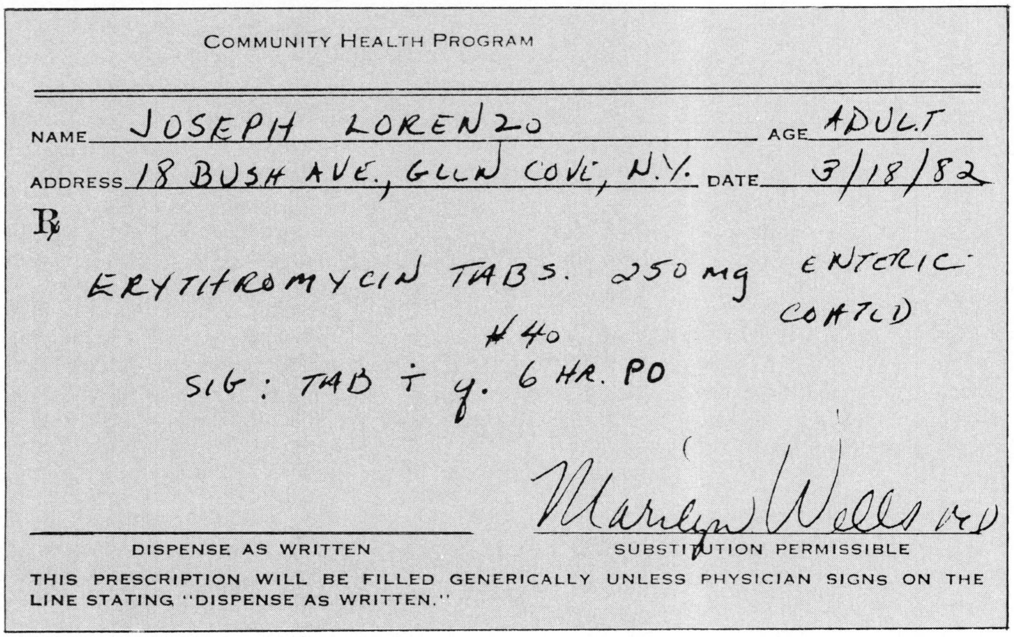

COMMUNITY HEALTH PROGRAM

NAME JOSEPH LORENZO AGE ADULT

ADDRESS 18 BUSH AVE., GLEN COVE, N.Y. DATE 3/18/82

℞

ERYTHROMYCIN TABS. 250 mg ENTERIC COATED

#40

SIG: TAB i q. 6 HR. PO

Marilyn Wells M.D.

DISPENSE AS WRITTEN SUBSTITUTION PERMISSIBLE

THIS PRESCRIPTION WILL BE FILLED GENERICALLY UNLESS PHYSICIAN SIGNS ON THE LINE STATING "DISPENSE AS WRITTEN."

FIGURE 5-3 Prescription blank.

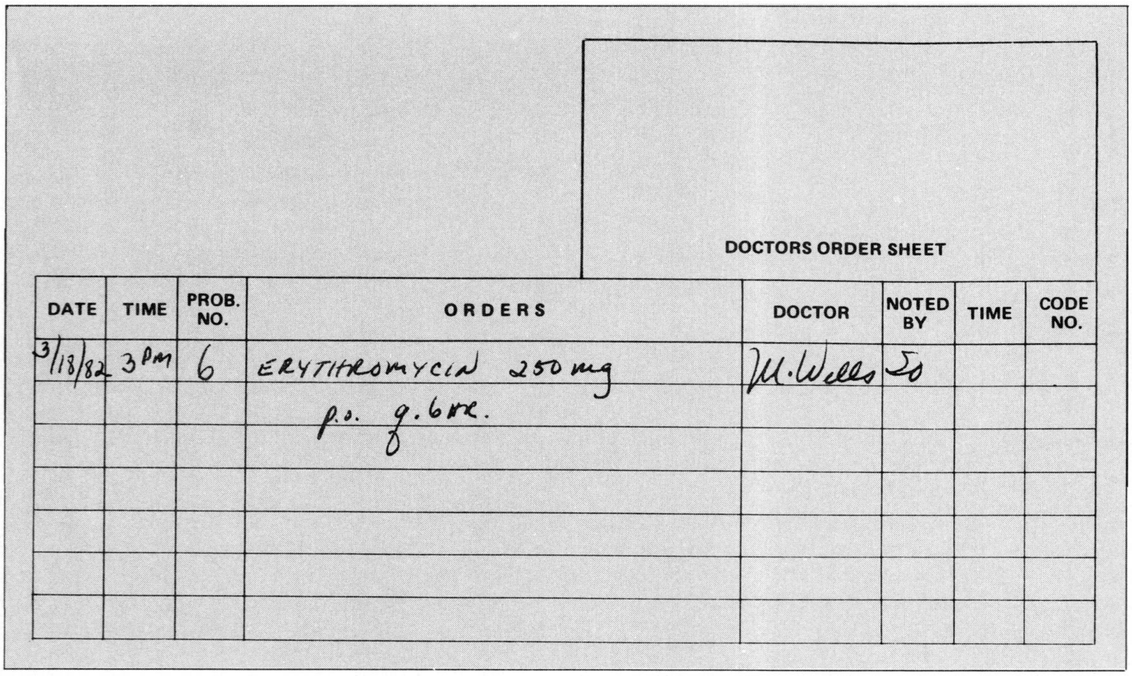

DOCTORS ORDER SHEET

DATE	TIME	PROB. NO.	ORDERS	DOCTOR	NOTED BY	TIME	CODE NO.
3/18/82	3 PM	6	ERYTHROMYCIN 250 mg p.o. q. 6 hr.	M. Wells	Jo		

FIGURE 5-4 Order sheet.

evaluate continued need for those drugs that require especially close attention.

Prn order. Prn drugs are to be administered by the nurse only "as necessary." Within the other criteria specified by the order, the decision of when to medicate is left to the nurse's judgment. This has implications for nursing autonomy similar to protocol orders.

Medications to reduce the perception of pain make up the bulk of **prn orders.** Keen nursing assessments of pain are required in order to carry out these prn orders appropriately. (See Chapter 11 for specifics for the evaluation of pain.) It is sufficient to note that pain is a very complex phenomenon, influenced by factors of subjectivity, emotions, and age, among others. The most dependable guide is that the pain is what and when the client says it is; assumptions by the nurse are not as reliable.

Research has demonstrated that patients are frequently undermedicated for pain. Children especially are frequently left to suffer, undermedicated for pain, under the assumption that their pain is less severe than it seems.

Single order. A **single order** is to be administered only once, at the time indicated. An example is a preoperative medication.

Stat order. A **stat order** is a single order that is to be administered immediately.

Protocol. A **protocol** is a set of criteria that serves as a directive under which medication may be given. Protocols may typically be one of two types: *standing orders* or *flow diagram protocols.* Standing orders are officially accepted sets of orders (not only for medications) to be applied routinely by nurses to the care of clients with certain conditions or under certain circumstances (e.g., as part of admission orders in some critical care units). Flow diagram protocols are criteria that give nurse practitioners guidelines for administration of certain treatments and medications on the basis of patient variables. These protocols provide the widest scope for application of nursing judgment and decision making of all the types of orders. Criteria and direction may be either very specific, for those with limited expertise or responsibility, or less specific and allow for greater latitude, self-reliance, and sophistication in decision making.

Assessment of Medication Orders

Patient. Every possible effort should be made to ensure that the patient receives the intended medication in the manner planned by the prescriber. Toward this end, patients with similar names should be widely separated in the health care setting, and all their paperwork must be clearly distinguishable. An identifying arm band must be kept on every patient and compared to identifying information that accompanies each dose of medication.

Date. The date that a medication order was written must be checked against other information for accuracy or for confirmation of when the last dose is to be given.

Medication. The medication's name may be written either in generic or trade name form. The patient should know the name of the medication if it is agency policy. If it is not, then nurses in the agency should be actively working with administrative leaders to reverse the policy. Patients should be told the names of their drugs while hospitalized so they can reasonably be expected to follow self-administration orders successfully at home! It is dangerous to keep patients ignorant of their medications. Exact names and dosages are crucial information for attending physicians to know if, for example, emergency treatment is needed.

Dosage and frequency. Drug dosages should be given as prescribed in the medication order unless nursing judgment detects, for example, that the size of the dose ordered falls outside the range of usual limits or that there are intervening factors in the patient-dosage, its frequency, or the route of administration. The drug would then not be administered or would be held until the nurse consults the prescriber on the question.

During the development of a drug the manufacturer makes determinations in regard to optimal range of dosage, frequency, and effective route for administration for most people. These are based on the known pharmacokinetics of the drug. For example, a drug that routinely undergoes biotransformation slowly may remain in the body system longer and produce more prolonged effects than another drug. Therefore it may effectively be given on a once-a-day basis, but a drug that is excreted rapidly may need to be given every 4 hours around the clock if effective tissue levels of the drug are to be maintained. Nursing judgments must be made in order to align an individual client's medication schedule with agency policy at appropriate intervals or to keep to a single schedule to meet a specific drug requirement (before or after meals) or a special need of the client. Some reasons to individualize administration time include client convenience and avoiding disturbing the client's rest, sleep, meals, visiting hours, other activities, or treatments. Rationales for other modifications in the medical plan should be discussed with the prescriber.

Route. Every medication order should include a specified route for administration. Making assumptions in this area is negligent. However, choice of the actual *site* of administration of injectables is a nursing or nurse-patient decision. For example, subcutaneous, intramuscular, and intravenous sites to avoid include any areas of obvious injury, disease, or lesions, even if minor; any that are noticeably erythematous (reddened), vesicular (blistered), open and weeping or pustular, ecchymotic (bruised), or scarred; and those previously overused for injection. Such areas may have impaired circulation or may be adversely affected by the injection itself or by the material injected. (Details may be found in Chapter 6.)

The ordered route of administration should routinely be assessed as to its efficacy, feasibility, or practicality. The oral route would naturally be precluded for the client who is nauseated or vomiting, for example. Prior consultation with the prescriber must be made before administering a drug by a different route, because dosage or other factors may have to be readjusted if bioavailability is affected by such changes.

EVALUATION OF PRIMARY AND SECONDARY EFFECTS

The ultimate effects of drugs on the body can be divided into two types. The main purpose of administering a medication is to utilize its **primary,** or therapeutic **effect.** All other consequences can be considered **secondary effects,** largely unintended and often nontherapeutic. Figure 5-5 illustrates the association between common terms that are used to describe the relative severity of secondary effects.

Drugs are developed and formulated to promote special effects; therefore the appearance of secondary effects demonstrates a continuing challenge to drug manufacturers. The crux of this problem is that most drugs cannot be made selective enough to be targeted at only one body system, organ, tissue, or cell. When the drug is circulated or distributed to other areas, reactions may range in severity from merely inconvenient or annoying side effects to very serious adverse effects. On the other hand, a side effect may actually be the sought-after primary effect under certain circumstances or may be exploited by the prescriber as a therapeutic effect along with the primary effects. For example, diphenhydramine (Benadryl) is an antihistamine that produces a high incidence of drowsiness or sedation-type side effects. If this antihistamine is prescribed for an irritable child afflicted with an itching, poison ivy rash, the effect of sedation becomes a desired secondary effect. But if diphenhydramine is prescribed for an allergic reaction in a person who handles dangerous machinery or drives a commercial vehicle for a living, this side effect is undesired. In such instances, the physician should probably select an antihistamine with a sedative side effect that is considerably reduced.

Primary and secondary effects are often dose related—that is, directly related to increases in dosage—or they may be related to the duration of that specific therapy.

In the assessment phase of the nursing process, it is essential to discover any **contraindications** to a drug's administration. A contraindication to administration of a drug has potential to be more harmful than do side effects and adverse reactions, which may be discerned only in the evaluation phase (see Chapter 6), after the administration of the drug. It is essential that the medicating process be assessed with regard to each medication's clinical indications and potential efficacy and any contraindications, especially any hypersensitivity (allergy) to the drug or any pathologic condition, etc., that would preclude its administration (see boxed material).

An allergic history **(hypersensitivity)** of any sort, even if unrelated to the medication, must be explored to

---

MEDICATIONS FREQUENTLY IMPLICATED IN HYPERSENSITIVITY (ALLERGIC) REACTIONS

Antibiotics: penicillin (the most common cause of drug-induced anaphylaxis), cephalosporins, tetracyclines, streptomycin, erythromycin, neomycin, nitrofurantoin, and sulfa drugs (very frequently)

Aspirin, hydantoins, acetaminophen, tolbutamide, gold salts, phenylbutazone, phenothiazines, histamines, aminopyrine, iodides, iron dextran, methylergonovine, quinidine, dipyrone, aminosalicylic acid, thiouracil, tranquilizers, anesthetics such as benzocaine (particularly troublesome because they are frequently used for application topically to irritated or delicate mucous membranes), tetracaine, procaine, lidocaine, and cocaine

Diagnostic agents such as iodinated contrast media (e.g., dye for IVP), iopanoic acid (Telepaque), sulfobromophthalein (BSP), dehydrocholic acid (Decholin), Congo red dye

Biologicals such as antitoxins, vaccines, gamma globulin, insulin, ACTH, enzymes, and their preservatives such as thimerosal, parabens, and antibiotics

---

rule out and prevent any possible allergic reaction. The occurrence of drug hypersensitivity reactions is extremely individualized, unpredictable except for history, and not usually closely dose related. The reaction may result in a very serious and life-threatening situation. Consequently the drug must not be given. Reactions may vary from mild rash to severe exfoliative dermatitis and from asthma to anaphylactic shock. They may include urticaria, angioneurotic edema, and drug fever.

An allergic drug response is caused by a specific reaction between a drug and the immune system. Most drugs are organic molecules with molecular weights of less than 1000 daltons. Such small molecules act as haptens; that is, they take on the ability to act as an allergen (to cause hypersensitivity or allergic reactions) only if they become bound to a carrier protein. This happens when the drug or its metabolite combines with tissue or plasma proteins

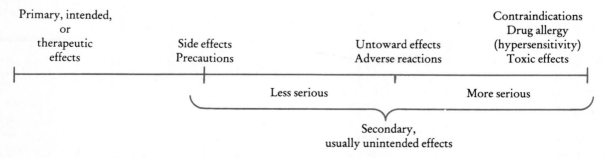

FIGURE 5-5 Terms indicating relative severity of medication effects—a continuum.

to form the drug-protein complex, the complete allergen, necessary to stimulate the immune response and provoke an allergic response. At initial exposure to the drug, allergic persons may exhibit a latent period of 10 to 20 days before the hypersensitivity reaction occurs. Reactions to reexposure to the drug may occur sooner, even immediately.

It is essential to place alerting stickers or notations as to patient's allergic history in the chart, Kardex, or other places according to agency policy. These locations need to be checked before any medications are given. Records may denote "no known allergy" (NKA), but usually this refers to drugs. Since there is often a correlation between one allergic response and the development of another, the patient's description of *any* past allergic manifestations—to drugs, inhalants, contactants, foods (typically: eggs, orange juice, chocolate, shellfish, strawberries), or whatever—must be clarified and evaluated. Often the patient erroneously defines an unexpected response as an allergic one. For example, the nausea following a meperidine (Demerol) injection may be labeled an allergic reaction by the patient, when in actuality it is likely to be only a normal, if exaggerated, side effect. Correcting such misinformation with the patient and in the records may become important because it makes that drug available for therapy when necessary. Before any questionable medications are administered, nurses should specifically inquire about previous experiences with these agents and, if necessary for a patient who has many allergies, discuss with the prescriber the need for a test dose. Special methods for those who must take medication to which they are allergic (e.g., aspirin, local anesthetics, or contrast media in diagnostic agents) include pretreatment medication in the form of antihistamines, prednisone, and ephedrine or cautiously increasing dosages of the allergy-provoking drug under supervision.

Other contraindications to drug therapy must be assessed before administration; evidence of other secondary effects usually appears only after the fact.

Drug Interactions

The complexity of modern pharmacotherapy is nowhere more obvious than in the ever-growing list of drugs that interact nontherapeutically with one another, with foods, and with fluids and that distort laboratory test results. That these chemical substances will interact with or potentiate one another is not surprising; this fact should always be kept in mind when medications appear either ineffective or harmful or when the accuracy of laboratory tests is crucial.

Variables influencing drug interaction include (1) intestinal absorption, (2) competition for plasma binding, (3) drug metabolism or biotransformation, (4) action at the receptor site, (5) renal excretion, and (6) alteration of electrolyte balance. The following are examples of these variables' effects that interact nontherapeutically with other drugs, food, juices, and other liquids and distort many laboratory test results:

1. Intestinal absorption: foods or antacids that contain calcium, magnesium, or aluminum may complex or bind tetracycline, resulting in reduced absorption of the antibiotic.
2. Competition for plasma protein binding: tolbutamide can be displaced from its binding on plasma proteins by bishydroxycoumarin, resulting in severe hypoglycemia. Many drugs are weak acids that are bound largely to plasma proteins. These weak acids may compete for binding sites on plasma proteins, thus increasing the free, active drug, which may have potent effects.
3. Drug metabolism or biotransformation: the monoamine oxidase inhibitors prevent the biotransformation of tyramine, which is present in aged cheese, liver, overripe fruit, and fermented meat (sausage, bologna, pepperonia, salami).
4. Action at the receptor site: there are numerous examples of one drug intensifying or antagonizing the action of another drug at the receptor site. For example, the antihistaminics decrease many effects of histamine, while cocaine increases the actions of epinephrine.
5. Renal excretion: probenecid inhibits the renal clearance of penicillin.
6. Alteration of electrolyte balance: the thiazide diuretics may cause hypokalemia, which predisposes to digitalis toxicity.

Not all drug interactions are dangerous; some are relatively insignificant or even beneficial. Tables listing known drug interactions should be posted in the medication area as references for nurses.

Drug-Drug Interactions

Some drugs commonly involved in clinically significant drug-drug interactions include coumadin, tricyclic antidepressants (MAO inhibitors), aminoglycosides, amphetamines, corticosteroids, digitalis glycosides, diuretics, sulfonamides, alcohol, antihypertensives, beta blockers, and theophylline. Before any such medication is given, an appropriate-source should be consulted to assess the drug, its mechanism, and any other medications given concurrently to determine the probability of interactions developing. This text gives this information in the context of specific drug monographs.

Other Drug Interactions

Drug-induced malabsorption of foods and nutrients. Drugs that change gastric or intestinal motility can alter the digestion or absorption of certain nutrients. Important drugs that affect these changes are stimulant cathartics and mineral oil and, at the other extreme, anticholinergics and narcotics. Long-term use of diuretics to treat such conditions as congestive heart failure can lead to serious potassium depletion. If the potassium loss is not corrected in patients taking digitalis, the heart may over-respond to the usual dose of digitalis. Some oral contraceptives impair folic acid absorption in undernourished patients.

Food-induced malabsorption of drugs. Fatty foods or foods low in fiber will delay stomach emptying by up to 2 hours, which may result in delayed and/or reduced drug absorption. Several medications, though, such as griseofulvin and possibly spironolactone, exhibit enhanced bioavailability (absorption) following a high-fat meal. Many tetracyclines can form insoluble complexes in the gastrointestinal tract if given at the same time as foods or drugs containing ions of calcium, aluminum, magnesium, or iron. Thus, administering tetracycline medication along with milk-based tube feedings or common antacids should be avoided. Ascorbic acid from citrus fruits or juices enhances absorption of iron, but carbonated soft drinks or acid juices (fruit or vegetable) can cause drugs to dissolve more quickly in the stomach than in the intestine or can neutralize them, thereby changing the intended rate or completeness of absorption.

Milk, coffee, eggs, tea, whole-grain breads and cereals, dietary fiber, and foods containing bicarbonates, carbonates, phosphates, or oxalates may all reduce iron absorption if given concurrently. Iron products should be spaced at least 1 hour before or 2 hours after the mentioned food substances are given.

Alteration of enzymes. Enzyme alterations, either induction or inhibition, may affect the metabolism of a food or drug. The natural extract of licorice is chemically similar to that of steroids, and therefore if taken in excess licorice can cause hypokalemia, retention of sodium and water with resultant hypertension, and alkalosis. Ingestion of large amounts would be contraindicated for patients who are concurrently taking potassium-losing diuretics or who have cardiovascular disease.

Likewise, consumption of large amounts of foods high in vitamin K (such as liver and green leafy vegetables) may reduce or antagonize the effectiveness of oral anticoagulants. Difficulty in maintaining the desired anticoagulant response with appropriately prescribed dosages indicates the need for an assessment of food and drug consumption.

Monoamine oxidase inhibitors (tricyclic antidepressants) act by inhibiting the breakdown of norepinephrine, a vasopressor substance. This excess norepinephrine is then stored in the neurons. The ingestion of certain tyramine-containing foods (aged cheeses, beef and chicken liver, pickled herring, broad beans, canned figs, bananas, avocados, soy sauce, active yeast preparations, beer, sherry in large quantities, Chianti wine, chocolate, anchovies, caffeine, mushrooms, raisins, sausages, dried fish, tuna fish, cola drinks, and many fermented foods) may elevate the quantity of norepinephrine to toxic levels, thereby precipitating hypertensive crises. OTC cold remedies containing ephedrine, phenylephrine, and phenylpropanolamine and amphetamines in general can act similarly, releasing stored quantities of norepinephrine. The net effect can be a headache, sudden climb in blood pressure to dangerous levels, cardiac arrhythmias, or intracranial bleeding.

Alcohol consumption. Of the more than 100 most frequently prescribed drugs, more than half contain at least one ingredient known to interact adversely with imbibed alcohol. An interaction is probable if the drug is known to affect the central nervous system or is metabolized by the liver. The effects are dose-related, and whether quantities of alcohol are used habitually, chronically, or only occasionally often makes a distinct difference in the direction of interactive effects. Patterns of alcohol consumption will likely have a bearing on the patient's concurrence with drug treatment and follow-through as well. Alcohol consumption should be limited or totally avoided if a client is taking narcotics, tranquilizers, sedatives, and other CNS depressant–type drugs, which may cause additive or synergistic respiratory and CNS depression. Thus it is obvious that patterns of alcohol consumption are important when a history is being taken.

The fact that many elixirs and tinctures are liquid formulations of drugs dissolved in alcohol is significant, especially in the assessment of pharmacotherapy for children. These preparations must be reassessed and cannot be assumed to have the same rates and degrees of absorption as the same drugs in aqueous solution, since bioavailability may be altered.

Cigarette smoking. The main pharmacokinetic effect of heavy cigarette smoking is the lowering of drug plasma levels by induction of microsomal enzyme systems responsible for increased drug metabolism or excretion. The rate of theophylline breakdown is increased, necessitating an increase in dosage of from $1\frac{1}{2}$ to 2 times the average dose. The usual doses of other drugs have diminished effectiveness in the heavy cigarette smoker—for example, the antidepressant imipramine; analgesics such as pentazocine, antipyyrene, phenacetin, and proproxyphene; vitamins C, B_{12}, and B_6; and the influenza vaccine. The absorption rate of insulin by the subcutaneous route is twice as slow as usual. Smoking also interacts with glutethimide, furosemide and propranolol. CNS depression and drowsiness are less frequent with diazepam (Valium), and drowsiness is reduced with chlorpromazine (Thorazine). When smoking is combined with use of estrogens, the risk of heart attack, stroke, and other circulatory disorders increases. Laboratory test results may also be somewhat outside the range of normal, depending on the duration of smoking history and inhalation practices. The white cell count is increased (in the absence of clinical infection); hemoglobin concentration, hematocrit, and red blood cell size are increased; and clotting time is reduced. Some investigators of cigarette smoking have found an abnormal increase in cholesterol, and others have found carcinoembryonic antigen levels as high as for persons with colon cancer, yet without other evidence of it. Therefore smokers can be expected sometimes to exhibit more numerous drug therapy "failures" or adverse effects, or they may even have fewer or different reactions to drugs than do nonsmoking patients. Certain laboratory test results must be interpreted in light of cigarette smoking history.

Food-initiated alteration of drug excretion. Changes in the pH of urine caused by food (making the urine overly acidic or alkaline) can have a significant effect on the excretion rates of some drugs, since pH influences the ionization of weak acids and bases. A drug will diffuse more easily from the urine back into the blood in its non-dissociated state, thereby prolonging drug action. Thus action of acidic drugs is prolonged when urine is acidic. Although it is quite difficult to override the kidneys' ability to regulate urine pH, an alkaline ash or acid ash diet, whether by purpose or not, can drive urinary pH above 8 or below 5, creating a medium for potential drug reactions. Continued taking of many antacid tablets each day in concert with quinidine administration was seen in one instance to create quinidine intoxication by shifting urinary pH toward the base and causing a serious arrhythmia necessitating hospitalization.

Drug Incompatibilities

Interactions occurring when drugs are mixed before administration, as in a single syringe or in intravenous fluids, are termed **drug incompatibilities.** Drugs that are physically incompatible may produce unwanted changes through processes such as liquefaction, deliquescence, or precipitation. Chemical incompatibilities may result when ingredients interact to form new compounds or are neutralized. If drug incompatibilities are anticipated, separate administration routes should be sought. Some drugs are highly incompatible in solution with many other drugs. Since solution incompatibilities are frequently time dependent, there may be fewer difficulties associated with mixing drugs in one syringe than in IV solutions; both drugs should be administered as soon after mixing as possible. Examples of drugs that are noted for interacting incompatibly with many other drugs in a *syringe* and that therefore should be administered alone include chloridiazepoxide, diazepam, pentobarbital, phenobarbital, phenytoin, secobarbital, and sodium bicarbonate.

Many drugs have explicit manufacturer's instructions for preparation (dilution and method of adding to selected IV parenteral solutions, which should be closely followed. A check for drug compatibility is indicated before two or more drugs are added to the same IV solution. Standard IV parenteral drug charts and guides are available for reference use (see appendix). Many hospital pharmacies are providing an IV preparation service that screens for incompatibilities before preparation and delivery to the nursing area.

With the increase in the number of potent drugs and the variety of combinations, use of the pharmacist's expertise in a controlled environment is probably a wise policy. If the nurse is required to prepare IV solutions on the nursing unit, then adequate references, including a list of incompatibilities, should be posted in the area where the nurses perform this duty. Open communication on a regular basis with the pharmacy department is necessary in order to obtain new or additional information and/or assistance, whenever necessary.

EXPLORING DRUG DATA

Any nursing process will be only as effective as the knowledge base and the analytic thought that go into it. Logic and judgment improve as the nurse's information base is perfected, partly as experience is tested against knowledge. Nowhere is ongoing self-learning more essential than in nursing pharmacotherapeutics. The "need to know" escalates, for example, when a nurse who is responsible for administering medications is confronted with an order for an unfamiliar drug or by an unexpected client symptom not usually associated with the diagnosis.

Realistically, it is not possible to know everything about all medications on the market, even the ones nurses use frequently. It is important to know where to get essential information as it becomes required. Various reference sources exist, each with its own emphasis, yet most are not completely adequate to meet the specialized needs of nursing pharmacotherapeutics.

Drug Information References

The following are references frequently used as drug information sources by nurses.

Physicians' Desk Reference (P.D.R.) (Oradell, N.J.: Medical Economics Co., Inc.) is the most commonly consulted reference in clinical settings. It is a concise compilation of specific information similar to that found enclosed with medication as it comes from the pharmaceutical distributor (package inserts). As such, it is of limited value for the nursing process, since it is written in "medicalese," lacks any nursing methodology, and lists long strings of secondary effects without regard to relative frequency or severity. It is probably best used as a quick reference with another source handy to fill in information gaps. However, both the P.D.R. and package inserts can be considered to give an FDA-approved and reliable discourse on drugs' clinical indications and safe ranges of dosages. The P.D.R. also lists the telephone numbers of pharmaceutical manufactures to consult for specific questions or emergencies and to report adverse reactions.

Users of this information for the purpose of prescribing should be aware that individual cases may allow for variation in use and dosage of a drug, even to exceed suggested dosage range, but that such individual variation should have a valid rationale. When this source is being used, it should be borne in mind that the material it contains is submitted by the pharmaceutical company producing the drug. Other references provide unbiased drug information, including expanded areas of clinical drug use and application, which is preferable to the utilization of a pharmaceutical industry–supported reference.

American Hospital Formulary Service (Bethesda, Md.: American Society of Hospital Pharmacists) is an objective overview in monograph form of nearly every available drug in the United States. It is kept current by periodically released supplements, and it includes extensive drug information. It is highly recommended as a source of drug information.

A.M.A. Drug Evaluations (Chicago: American Medical Association) is a source of information about specific drugs, even those that are being used for valid clinical applications different from those that have been approved thus far.

Nursing journals such as *American Journal of Nursing, Nursing '89* (etc.), and *R.N.* offer both general and specific drug information in nursing terms and with a nursing perspective.

Many *nursing pharmacology texts* such as this one follow the same approach as the nursing journals but also include a greater depth of information about physiology and pathology of specific medication uses. Some offer only drug highlights for quick reference use.

FDA Drug Bulletin (Rockville, Md.: Department of Health and Human Services, Public Health Service) is a free six-page newsletter published several times a year to inform health professionals about the results of recent FDA reviews of various drugs (usually common ones) and their new clinical findings. Each issue also includes a form for reporting unusual clinical experiences with drugs.

Physicians' Desk Reference for Nonprescription Drugs (Oradell, N.J.: Medical Economics Co., Inc.) was first published in 1980 in recognition of the proliferation of over-the-counter drugs and the public's growing health awareness and interest in participating in self-care management. The format is similar to that of the P.D.R., with identifying photographs of the drugs, pharmaceutical company addresses, and descriptions of individual drugs and compounds. It also includes a section on the self-care of minor health problems.

Handbook of Nonprescription Drugs (Washington, D.C.: American Pharmaceutical Association) deals with OTC drug information in general categories. Each chapter presents the relevant physiologic background first and concludes with a table comparing specific drugs.

The *National Formulary* (N.F.) (Rockville, Md.) is now combined with the *United States Pharmacopeia* (U.S.P.). The U.S.P. was the official reference recognized by the Federal Pure Food and Drug Act of 1906 and is still a required reference book for pharmacies in the United States. Its primary focus is drug sources, chemistry, physical properties, tests for identity, purity, assay, and official storage requirements. Hence its usefulness is directed more toward the pharmaceutical industry and pharmacists than toward the nursing profession.

United States Pharmacopeia Dispensing Information (Easton, Pa.: U.S. Pharmacopeial Convention, Inc.) is a reference first published in 1980 to meet the needs of those involved in dispensing and administration, to themselves or others, *after* the prescription has been written and filled. The information on each drug includes its category, precautions to consider, side effects, what to tell the client, dosage forms, and labeling. A section entitled "Advice for the Patient" gives the reader in nontechnical language pertinent essentials about the drug, describes its ramifications, and tells how to tailor its administration to life-style. A major advantage of this reference is the manner in which it presents side effects — that is, the incidence potential (rare to common) — and it clearly states which ones should be reported to the physician. It is a highly valuable source for nurses.

The Pharmacological Basis of Therapeutics (A.G. Gilman, L.S. Goodman, and A. Gilman, editors; New York: MacMillan, Inc.) is a thorough and respected reference text that is considered an authoritative source for those learning or working with pharmacology. It is not geared especially for nurses, nor does it contain specifics related to nursing pharmacotherapeutics, but it is an excellent reference work.

Other Drug Information Sources

Drug information centers are located throughout the United States to disseminate information about the clinical uses of drugs and related equipment. Both general and specific information can be obtained, with advice based on scientific literature. A team of specially trained pharmacists is available, and these centers are often located within a large medical center setting. Many difficult pharmacologic questions related to patient care can be

---

Allergic reactions have been reported following ingestion of food additives, such as monosodium glutamate (MSG), tartrazine, and sulfites. Tartrazine and sulfites are also used as additives, preservatives, and/or antioxidants in various medications. The most serious adverse reaction, resulting in some reported deaths, occurred most often in asthmatic patients. Current lists of foods and drug products containing tartrazine and sulfites should be reviewed in assessing reported allergic reactions. (See appendix.)

dealt with quickly by contacting the nearest Drug Information Center.

Drug manufacturers, package inserts, and pharmacists located in hospitals, skilled care facilities, and other agencies also provide similar information.

Agencies frequently furnish similar sources of information. The area or floor where a nurse works often has a card file of package inserts; ideally, a nursing library shelf on each floor contains pharmacology information and other material of interest. Any nurse can initiate the development of such material and request funds or supplies. The agency nursing inservice or education department is responsible for promoting ongoing and updated learning and can facilitate audiovisual aids, references, or a seminar program. Building a personal library and maintaining its currency are also important professional activities.

No text is a complete source of all the pharmacology information necessary for nursing practice. The nurse must gather reliable information from various sources to meet clinical needs.

ANALYSIS OF DATA

When data from the nursing assessment have been collected, the next phase is analysis — the critical evaluation of information to determine its meaning and importance. As with all phases of the nursing process, analysis is continuous. It is the *process* of interpreting data based on sound pharmacologic and nursing principles.

To facilitate analysis, the nurse may follow several steps. Initially, data are organized into categories. Categorization is accomplished by use of a planned systematic assessment, and gaps in data are noted. Once identified, missing information can then be obtained to complete the assessment. Accepted standards and norms are then applied to determine discrepancies between what is and what should be or could be, and conclusions are drawn regarding what actual, possible, or potential problems may be present. The culmination of analysis is the identification of specific areas toward which nursing help may be directed and may include a nursing diagnosis.

NURSING DIAGNOSIS

The American Nurses' Association has defined **a nursing diagnosis** as a description of an actual or potential health problem that nurses are capable of treating and licensed to treat. One criterion is that it features a problem for which nursing care provides the most appropriate treatment. Basically, a nursing diagnosis should be a summary statement to "engineer the uncertainty out of a patient care situation and thus minimize the number of incorrect inferences."[*]

[*]Shamsky, S.L., and Yanni, C.: In opposition to nursing diagnosis a minority opinion, Image: J. Nurs. Scholarship. 15(2):47, 1983.

The nursing profession is actively working toward standardization of nursing process terminology to facilitate communication among practitioners. A current aim is to classify groups of nursing diagnoses so that patterns will emerge, leading to categories of diagnoses. The North American Nursing Diagnosis Association (NANDA) has endorsed a classification of nursing diagnoses by human response patterns with approved terminology (Kim and others, 1987). Whenever possible, diagnostic statements used in this book are drawn from the list of NANDA-approved nursing diagnoses. The NANDA list and other widely circulated lists are not considered complete, but, rather, nurses are encouraged to test them and develop new ones.

Several examples of nursing diagnoses follow. Note that there could be countless ways to convey the same thoughts, all equally correct, and variations can arise from differences among individuals constructing the diagnoses and from the wording chosen. A nursing diagnosis includes two main components: a description of altered health status and an inferred reason for it. The main presenting symptom may also be included in the statement. The following list presents some sample nursing diagnoses:

Possible alteration in urinary elimination: urinary retention related to antihistamine therapy

Altered comfort: nausea/vomiting related to chemotherapy

Potential alteration in bowel elimination: diarrhea related to antibiotic administration

Fluid volume excess: edema related to steroid therapy

Noncompliance: failure to refill prescriptions related to inadequate financial resources to buy drugs

A nursing diagnosis forms the basis for the design of the subsequent phases of the nursing process: planning, implementation, and evaluation. The diagnosis differentiates between actual, potential, and possible problems. Table 5-2 defines each type and the corresponding focus of interventions.

NATURE OF NURSING ACTIONS

Nursing interventions may be categorized into three domains: **dependent** (or delegated), **collaborative,** and **independent.** Medicine diagnoses and treats pathologic or cellular responses, while nursing diagnoses and treats the *human response* (Sanford, 1987). Those activities legally requiring a physician directive, or dependent interventions, may constitute a significant portion of nursing practice related to pharmacology. A significant number of interventions require collaboration between nurses and other health care providers. Client conditions require differing ratios of medical (or other health care provider) and nursing input (Figure 5-6). Neither nurses nor other health-care providers possess exclusive respon-

TABLE 5-2   Nursing Diagnoses and Their Related Interventions

Type	Definition	Focus of nursing interventions
Actual (is present)	Validated major s/s*	To reduce or eliminate or promote positive diagnoses
Potential (may happen)	Presence of high-risk factors	To prevent onset
Possible (may be present)	Suspected to be present	To obtain additional data to rule out or confirm

From Carpenito, LJ: Nursing diagnoses in critical care: impact on practice and outcomes, Heart Lung 16(6, part 1):596, 1987.
*s/s, Signs and symptoms.

sibility for diagnosis and treatment of collaborative problems. Each group maintains its own responsibility throughout its involvement with the client. The independent domain involves the diagnosis and treatment of problems that are primarily nursing in nature. The nurse identifies these problems and assumes primary responsibility for ordering needed interventions.

UTILITY OF NURSING DIAGNOSIS

By describing human responses, nursing diagnosis distinguishes nursing from other health care disciplines. Nursing diagnoses are most useful in the independent domain. Their use provides a focus for goals and interventions: a *nursing diagnosis* is a clear, concise description of a problem that is uniquely addressed by nurses. The development of nursing diagnoses has added much to the refinement and description of nursing care by providing structure, focus, and language for clear communication.

Because of the early stage of development of nursing diagnosis, implementation of nursing diagnoses is hampered by divergent views, conceptual controversies, and confusing terminology. The nursing profession's health-related, strength-oriented emphases are not easily addressed by currently accepted nursing diagnoses, and it may be unrealistic to expect nursing diagnoses to describe all of nursing practice. Much of the nurse's role in pharmacotherapeutics encompasses the dependent and collaborative domains, areas not thoroughly addressed by nursing diagnoses. Throughout this textbook, the use of nursing diagnosis is encouraged but not forced upon situations in which it is inappropriate. As the evolution of nursing diagnosis continues, application to pharmacotherapeutics will become increasingly appropriate and useful.

PLANNING FOR DRUG THERAPY

The planning phase of the nursing process has two parts, setting goals (or **outcome criteria**) and specific plans for interventions that will implement the goals. The planning to meet the pharmacotherapeutic nursing needs of clients should be characterized by an orientation to (1) the client, (2) resources in the environment, and (3) the future. These in turn should be characterized by a balance between the real and the ideal.

Goals associated with medication needs of patients may be stated in many ways to encompass these three orientations. They must actually be stated (e.g., in the nursing care plan) to provide communication with the rest of the staff and to give clear direction for the subsequent implementation and evaluation phases. Otherwise, implementation and evaluation of the nursing care will be based on vague events and partially remembered and incomplete actions.

Goals are objectives to be met sometime in the future. Therefore the use of the words "will be" in the goal statement is appropriate. An approximation of time limits for the goal to be accomplished should be included in the statement to provide a way of measuring progress toward the goal, whether short term, intermediate, or long term: "by date of discharge," "in 3 days," "by 2 PM today," and so forth. The time limit should be the best estimate, not an edict carved in stone. The goal should be client oriented in that it *should describe what the client's condition or behavior will be at the outcome of nursing care,* not what the nurse intends to *do* for the client. For example, a goal is best stated as "Client will demonstrate understanding of drug regimen before discharge from the hospital," rather than "To promote understanding of the drug regimen by

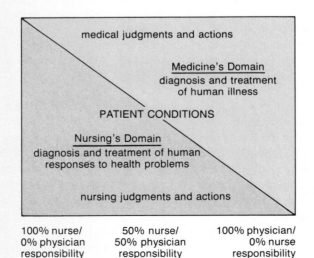

FIGURE 5-6   Professional interface model (PIM).

(From McLane, AM, ed: Classification of nursing diagnoses: proceedings of the Seventh Conference, St Louis, 1987, The CV Mosby Co.)

the time of discharge from the hospital." If the goal describes only what nurses do, they could work diligently to promote a client's understanding of a drug regimen, and success would merely be measured in the evaluation of what procedures were performed; yet the client may never have actually learned, which is the intent of the goal.

The nurse can prevent the blurring of the distinction between goals and interventions — two entirely different phases of the nursing process — by stating outcome criteria in terms of behavioral objectives for the client. If criteria are stated in words that depict nursing interventions or actions, such as "prevent," "provide," "promote," or "maintain," then evaluation of care becomes more an appraisal of what the nurse did by intervening than of the *client's condition.*

Finally, outcome criteria related to each nursing problem or diagnosis identified earlier may be ranked in priority to meet the client's needs.

The rest of the planning phase lays the ground work for carrying out specific actions in the implementation phase. Such plans for nursing actions should be supportable by applicable principles from the arts, sciences, and humanities, which are the foundations of nursing.

Development of a positive, accountable attitude through goal setting and planning for each nursing action strengthens what nurses do for clients and why. Outcome criteria and specific planning provide documentation for peers and preclude legal challenge, while first and foremost guiding the selection of appropriate caring actions. The completed abbreviated nursing care plan, as a blueprint for action, can be entered in writing in the Kardex or on the patient's chart and makes up the plan for nursing management.

SUMMARY OF NURSING CONSIDERATIONS

Although its structure and terminology may change, the nursing process remains an extremely useful clinical tool. It should be approached as framework for organizing patient care in creative and satisfying ways.

Professional nurses enhance their decision-making skills by carefully critiquing their clients' medication plans and maintaining a strong knowledge base about medications, including their indications, mechanisms, pharmacokinetics, and dosages.

The quality of nursing assessment relies on the nurse's ability to observe significant cues, to make sound inferences, and to recognize the client's individuality and establish rapport. Thus a nurse can develop a valid diagnosis, establish realistic goals with the client, and shape an effective nursing plan.

Medication administration is a highly visible, legal function of nurses. Since it depends heavily on the structure and content of prescriber's orders, conscientious assess-

ment of the drug order becomes a very healthy habit. Professional accountability for all disciplines demands open collaboration on questions about clients' medication orders and plans.

Underlying the routine of assessing medication therapy is the major goal of preventing harm. Assessment should emphasize preventing the client from receiving drugs that will interact, be incompatible, or evoke an allergic response; drugs that will not be degraded or excreted adequately; or drugs that will be transferred to a nursing infant or fetus. Creative nursing consists of finding ways to reschedule or space intervals between dosages of interactive drugs. If there is any question about pregnancy or breast feeding, administration of drugs should be suspended and the prescriber contacted for consultation. Unfortunately, the early part of pregnancy, when it may still be unsuspected, is one of the most potentially dangerous periods for teratogenesis (birth defects, miscarriage). If the mother's disorder is serious enough, drug therapy may have to be maintained nonetheless. This may occasionally also be true for a client with a contraindicating concomitant disorder or organ system impairment. Reactions caused by incompatibilities in solution may be avoided or minimized if drugs are administered as soon as possible after mixing. Allergic reactions, if anticipated, are usually grounds for a prescriber's decision to change drugs. However, a nurse is often the one who notes the offending allergenic substance via a client's history and other data. Again, effective nursing assessment can improve compliance, enhance therapeutic outcomes, and avoid negative secondary effects.

The nursing assessment culminates in the identification of specific problems (actual, possible, or potential). Interventions by the nurse to address identified problems may involve physician-directed (or dependent) interventions, collaborative interventions with other health care providers, or interventions that are solely the domain of nurses. Those problems falling within the independent nursing domain are best described by the nursing diagnosis, a concise statement of a problem that is uniquely addressed by nurses.

After the identification of problems and the formulation of a nursing diagnosis, goals in the form of outcome criteria are established. A specific plan is developed to direct nursing care toward meeting the goals. The development of goals and clear planning forms the basis for implementing and evaluating nursing care.

KEY TERMS

BIBLIOGRAPHY

American Hospital Formulary Service: AHFS drug information 88, Bethesda, Md, 1988, American Society of Hospital Pharmacists, Inc.

Asnes, R: Pain in childhood, Pediatr Consultant, 4(2), 1985.

Atkinson, LD, and Murray, ME: Understanding the nursing process, ed 3, New York, 1986, Macmillan, Inc.

Bell, SK: Guidelines for taking a complete drug history, Nursing '80, 10(3):10, 1980.

Breu, C, and others: Integration of nursing diagnoses in the critical care nursing literature, Heart Lung 16(6, part 1):600, 1987.

Burokas, L: Factors affecting nurse's decisions to medicate pediatric patients after surgery, Heart Lung 14(4): 373, 1985.

Campbell, C: Nursing diagnosis and intervention in nursing practice, ed 2, New York, 1984, John Wiley & Sons, Inc.

Carey, KW, ed: Nursing now: drug interactions, Springhouse, Pa, 1984, Springhouse, Corp.

Carlson, JH, and others: Nursing diagnosis, Philadelphia, 1982, WB Saunders Co.

Carnevali, DL: Nursing care planning: diagnosis and management, Philadelphia, 1983, JB Lippincott Co.

Carpenito, LJ: Nursing diagnosis: application to clinical practice, Philadelphia, 1983, JB Lippincott Co.

Carpenito, LJ: Actual, potential, or possible, Am J Nurs 85:458, 1985.

Carpenito, LJ: Nursing diagnosis: selected dilemmas in practice, Occup Health Nurs, 33(8): 397, 1985.

Carpenito, LJ: Nursing diagnosis in critical care: impact on practice and outcomes, Heart Lung 16(6, part 1):595, 1987.

Clark, JB, Queener, SF, and Karb, VB: Pharmacological basis of nursing practice, ed 2, St Louis, 1986, The CV Mosby Co.

Cohen, FL: Postsurgical pain relief: patient's status and nurse's medication choices, Pain 9:265, 1980.

Dudley, SR and Holm, K: Assessment of the pain experience in relation to selected nurse characteristics, Pain 18:179, 1984.

Edel, MK: Noncompliance: an appropriate nursing diagnosis? Nurs Outlook, 33(4):183, 1985.

Fadden, TC, and Seiser, GK: Nursing diagnosis: a matter of form, Am J Nurs 84(4):470, 1984.

Fehring, RJ: Methods to validate nursing diagnoses, Heart Lung, 16(6, part 1):625, 1987.

Gilman, AG, and others, eds: Goodman and Gilman's the pharmacological basis of therapeutics, ed 7, New York, 1985, Macmillan, Inc.

Griffith, JW, and Christensen, PJ: Nursing process: application of theories, frameworks, and models, ed 2, St Louis, 1986, The CV Mosby Co.

Hagey, RS, and McDonough, P: The problem of professional labeling, Nurs Outlook, 32(3):151, 1984.

Hansten, PD: Drug interactions, ed 5, Philadelphia, 1985, Lea & Febiger.

Hussar, DA: Geriatric drug interactions, East Hanover, NJ, Feb 1986, American Society of Consultant Pharmacists and Sandoz Pharmaceuticals.

Jacoby, MK: The dilemma of physiological problems: eliminating the double standard, Am J Nurs, 85:281, 1985.

Kim, MJ, and others: Pocket guide to nursing diagnoses, ed 2, St Louis, 1987, The CV Mosby Co.

Kritek, PB: Nursing diagnosis: theoretical foundations, Occup Health Nurs 33(8):393, 1985.

Lee, M, and others: Tartrazine-containing drugs, Drug Intell and Clin Pharm 15(10):782, 1981.

Loebl, S, and Spratto, G: The nurse's drug handbook, ed 4, New York, 1986, John Wiley & Sons, Inc.

Marks, RM, and Sachar, EJ: Undertreatment of medical inpatients with narcotic analgesics, Ann Intern Med 78:173, 1973.

Mather, L, and Mackie, J: The incidence of postoperative pain in children, Pain 15:277, 1983.

McLane, AM: Measurement and validation of diagnostic concepts: a decade of progress, Heart Lung, 16(6, part 1):616, 1987.

Miaskowski, CA: Nursing diagnosis within the context of the nursing process, Occup Health Nurs 33(8):401, 1985.

Mosby's Medical & Nursing Dictionary, ed 2 , St Louis, 1986, The CV Mosby Co.

North American Nursing Diagnosis Association: Classification of nursing diagnoses: proceedings of the Seventh Conference, St Louis, 1987, The CV Mosby Co.

Saint Margaret Hospital of Hammond: Pharmacy Drug Information Bulletin 11(8), 1985.

Sanford, S: Administrative applications of nursing diagnosis, Heart Lung, 16(6):600, 1987.

Shoemaker, JK: Characteristics of a nursing diagnosis, Occup Health Nurs 33(8):387, 1985.

Tartaglia, MJ: Nursing diagnosis: keystone of your careplan, Nursing '85, 15(3): 34, 1985.

Taylor, AG, and others: Duration of pain condition and physical pathology as determinants of nurses' assessments of patients in pain, Nurs Res 33:4, 1984.

Ted Tse, CS, and Bernstein, IL: Adverse reactions to tartrazine, Hosp Form 17(12):1625, 1982.

Truitt, CA and others: An evaluation of a medication history method, Drug Intell Clin Pharm 16:592, 1982.

United States Pharmacopeial Convention: Drug information for the health care provider, ed 6, vol 1, Rockville, Md. 1986, United States Pharmacopeial Convention.

Vandenbosch, TM, and others: tailoring care plans to nursing diagnoses, Am J Nurs 86:313, 1986.

Warren, JJ: Accountability and nursing diagnosis, J Nurs Adm 13(10):34, 1983.

Yura, H, and Walsh, MB: The nursing process: assessing, planning, implementing, evaluating, ed 4, Norwalk, Conn, 1983, Appleton-Century-Crofts.

Implementation and Evaluation

OBJECTIVES

After studying this chapter, the student will be able to:

1. Relate the implementation stage of the nursing process to the pharmacologic aspects of client care.

2. Identify the essential components of a written medication order.

3. Describe the factors considered in establishing the dosage, dosing intervals, and scheduling of medication.

4. Cite methods used to accurately measure the correct dosage or rate of administration of a medication.

5. Identify specific procedures used to maintain client safety during the preparation and administration of medications.

6. Differentiate between systemic effects and local effects of medications.

7. Cite the advantages and disadvantages of the various routes of medication administration.

8. Identify the landmarks for the administration of medications via the intramuscular route.

9. Cite the reasons for modifying administration methods for psychiatric clients and other clients with special needs.

10. Discuss the rationale for teaching clients about their prescribed medication regimens.

11. Discuss the importance of evaluation in the nursing process.

IMPLEMENTATION

The implementation phase of the nursing process consists of putting the goals into action. It is the actual giving of care as prescribed by the nursing care plan or nursing orders. The nurse, guided by the nursing care plan (formal or informal), with goals clearly in focus, can initiate proposed actions in an orderly way. The best chance for success lies in clear, frequent communication and collaboration with the client since any goal or action not viewed by clients as conguent with their own goals will decrease participation.

The implementation phase in drug therapy comprises all the steps of the administration of medications. It includes collaborating with the prescriber and medicating clients according to prescribers' orders, preparing drugs (including any necessary arithmetic calculations), techniques and procedures (with modifications for individual client situations), alertness to errors, recording medications given, and teaching clients about their drugs. Evaluation of goals follows and, depending on the specific goal, most often relates to some aspect of drug effects. Outcomes are measured and compared with the criteria established in the goals during the planning phase. Broader evaluation is done by nursing audit committees that critique the quality of nursing care administered to groups of clients, as well as individuals.

To perform all the functions of the nursing process, nurses must have strong interpersonal, cognitive, and psychomotor skills. Nursing actions are the product of foundational work in the psychosocial as well as the biologic and physical sciences.

DRUG ADMINISTRATION

The nursing function that is most closely identified with nursing by the public, and the one carrying the most legal vulnerability, is that of administering medications. It requires much preparation, a solid knowledge base, skilled decision-making abilities, and close attention to the "Five Rights" (see Chapter 5).

Technically, written medical orders are the only legal means for the administration of medications by nurses. Written orders constitute permanent legal records of the prescriber's plans and can be submitted as evidence in case of litigation. Thus, nurses must routinely ensure that (1) each order is appropriate, accurate, and complete and (2) the order is followed unerringly to completion, for nurses are held legally accountable for every dose of medication they administer. Free flow of communication between prescriber and nurse is crucial to fulfillment of this responsibility. Nurses must be ready to consult with the prescriber as necessary to clarify, understand, or suggest medication therapy as needed. Assertiveness is a quality that must be developed by professional nurses if they are to deal from an appropriate position of strength within the health care system to promote their clients' best interests while achieving equity for their own contributions.

What is the process by which a prescriber's order is translated into the administration of a medication? It is first transcribed by a ward clerk, head nurse (or nursing care coordinator), or primary nurse from an order sheet onto the Kardex, medication administration record (MAR) (Figure 6-1), or medication ticket or card (Figure 6-2). Accuracy in transcription of the medication order to the medication administration record is essential. If the order has been transcribed by a ward secretary, it should be verified by a nurse, who can then better relate the medication to the client and the diagnosis. The nurse must check the dosage of the medication and the age of the client, check for drug interaction possibilities and for allergies, and ensure the completeness of the order to prevent error (see box). Whatever the question concerning the physician's order, legally it can only be clarified with the physician who has written the order. Verifying an order with another physician who happens to be present or with a nursing colleague does not suffice.

The drug is requested in a daily supply from the institution's pharmacy department. When the supply arrives, it is stored in the medication room either as stock supply to meet general needs of clients on the floor or in an individual client's own medication box or drawer of a medication cart.

The nurse administers a drug by following the order as

written on the medication card, ticket, or MAR. Because of space limitation, physicians, pharmacists, and nurses rely on pharmacologic abbreviations or symbols for communication. These are often from the Latin and are universally used. Table 6-1 includes the most commonly used abbreviations, along with some symbols common to clinical practice. Although apothecary symbols are sometimes used, they are frequently misinterpreted and may be used incorrectly. The nurse should convert the apothecary measure to a metric measure when transcribing the medication order. In addition, prescribers should be encouraged to use the metric system to avoid errors. Abbreviations are a key to communication in the busy health field and should be learned. In addition, a number of physicians also use abbreviations for ordering specific medications. (See Table 6-2.) Because of the danger of misinterpretation, the use of variant or nonstandard abbreviations should be avoided. The nurse should review the approved abbreviation listing for the health agency.

When transcribed, the physician's order must contain all the elements described in Chapter 5. It must contain the *full name* of the patient (and bed location — for example, room 212, bed 2); the *date* the order was written; the *medication name, dosage, route,* and *frequency;* and, according to agency policy, the *name* or *initial* of the nurse responsible for the transcription. (See Figure 6-2.)

Types of Drug Delivery Systems

There are several pharmacy-nursing approaches to distributing and dispensing drugs to patients in an institutional setting: the floor stock system, individual client pre-

---

CHECKING TRANSCRIPTION

WHICH MEDICATION?

Is it quinine sulfate (a medication for leg cramps) or quinidine sulfate (a cardiac depressant)? Pentobarbital or phenobarbital? Digoxin or digitoxin? Ornade or ornase?

WHICH DOSE?

Is it a loop of an *f, g,* or *q,* or another zero?

Vital signs q 4h
Gentamycin 60 mg IV q 6h

ANYTHING MISSING?

Does Halcion i HS mean 0.125 mg or 0.25 mg?

scription orders, unit dose drug distribution, and a combination of these. In the floor stock system, all medications except those infrequently used are stored in bulk on the nursing unit in the medication room. The disadvantages of this system are the increased potential for medication errors because of the large array of stock medications to choose from, the economic loss caused by misplaced or forgotten charges and expired drugs to be returned, the need for frequent total drug inventorying, and the storage problems inherent in crowded medica-

PATIENT'S STAMP

MEDICATION RECORD

INIT	DO / SD	RD / NSD	MEDICATION DOSE, ROUTE, FREQUENCY	TOUR	TIME INTERVAL	DATE	DATE	DATE	DATE	DATE	DATE	DATE
				N								
				D								
				E								
				N								
				D								
				E								
				N								
				D								
				E								
				N								
				D								
				E								
				N								
				D								
				E								
				N								
				D								
				E								
				N								
				D								
				E								
				N								
				D								
				E								
				N								
				D								
				E								
				N								
				D								
				E								

RECOPIED BY: _____ DATE: _____

ALLERGIES:

—Medication given
O—Medication Omitted—
   Explanation on Nurses'
   Notes.
D/C—Medication Discontinued. In addition to this record, anticoagulant and Diabetic records are also maintained
D.O.—Date ordered
S.D.—Stop date
N.S.D.—New stop date

SIGNATURES

N	D	E	N	D	E	N	D	E	N	D	E	N	D	E	N	D	E	N	D	E

FIGURE 6-1 Sample MAR.

TABLE 6-1   Common Abbreviations and Symbols Related to Medication Administration*

Abbreviation	Unabbreviated form	Meaning	Abbreviation	Unabbreviated form	Meaning
a	ante	before	OU	oculus uterque	each eye
ac	ante cibum	before meals	pc	post cibum	after meals
ad lib	ad libitum	freely	PM	post meridiem	after noon
AM	ante meridiem	morning	PO	per os	by mouth, orally
bid	bis in die	twice each day	prn	pro re nata	according to necessity
c̄	cum	with	pt	patient	patient
cap	capsule	capsule	q	quaque	every
cc, cm³	cubic centimeter	cubic centimeter (ml)	qd	quaque die	every day
clt	client	client	qh	quaque hora	every hour
D/C or DC	discontinue	terminate	q4h, q4°	every 4 hours	every 4 hours around the clock
elix	elixir	elixir			
g, gm	gram	1000 milligrams	qid	quater in die	four times each day
gr	grain	60 milligrams	qod	quaque aliem die	every other day
gtt	gutta	drop	qs	quantum satis	sufficient quantity
h, hr	hora	hour	®	right	right
hs	hora somni	at bedtime	℞	receipt	take
IM	intramuscular	into a muscle	s̄	sine	without
IV	intravenous	into a vein	SL	sub linguam	under the tongue
IVPB	IV piggyback	secondary IV line	SOS	si opus sit	if necessary
kg	kilogram	2.2 lb	ss	semis	a half
KVO	keep vein open	very slow infusion rate	stat	statim	at once
Ⓛ	left	left	SC, SQ	subcutaneous	into subcutaneous tissue
L	liter	liter	tbsp	tablespoon	tablespoon (15 ml)
μg, mcg	microgram	one millionth of a gram	tid	ter in die	three times a day
			TO	telephone order	order received over the telephone
mg	milligram	one thousandth of a gram	tsp	teaspoon	teaspoon (4 or 5 ml)
mEq	milliequivalent	the number of grams of solute dissolved in one milliliter of a *normal* solution	U	unit	a dosage measure for insulin, penicillin, heparin
			VO	verbal order	order received verbally
min or m	minim	minim (⅟₁₅ or ⅟₁₆ ml)	ī, īī	one, two	one, two (as in "gr ī," "gr īī")
ml, mL	milliliter	one thousandth of a liter	ʒ	dram	4 or 5 ml
ng	nanogram	one billionth of a gram	℥	ounce or fluid-ounce	ounce (30 milliliters)
			×	times	as in two times a week
ō	no or none	no or none	>	greater than	greater than
OD	oculus dexter	right eye	<	less than	less than
OS	oculus sinister	left eye	=	equal to	equal to
os	os	mouth	↑, ↗	increase or increasing	increase or increasing
OTC	over-the-counter	nonprescription drug	↓, ↙	decrease or decreasing	decrease or decreasing

*It is recommended that certain abbreviations be abandoned if they can confuse.

tion rooms. In addition, because of fear of contamination, the bottles of unused drugs must often be discarded, not allowing the client for whom the drug was originally ordered to receive financial credit for drugs not administered. The individual order method of dispensing each type of medication daily to individual patients is an improvement, but it is rather unwieldy and time consuming. A combination of floor stock and individual orders is generally superior but has the disadvantages of both systems.

Single-dose packages of drugs are dispensed in the unit dose drug distribution method. Each oral dose, for example, may be a tablet encased in a blister pack or a paper tear-off strip of tablets. This packaging is said to be the safest and most economical method of drug distribution.

The advantages of using the unit dose system far outweigh the disadvantages. The most important advantages are increased medication safety and decreased errors, since drug computations are largely eliminated. The drug is already properly labeled and does not have to be prepared. All the nurse needs to do is deliver the package to the client, where it is opened at the bedside and administered. This may permit clients to check on their own drugs and be assured of proper medication and dosage. Unit dose packaging also decreases chances of deterioration and permits giving financial credit to the client for drugs not used. Disadvantages include increased cost to

TABLE 6-2 Drug Abbreviations

ACTH	adrenocorticotropic hormone
ASA	acetylsalicylic acid (aspirin)
CPZ	chlorpromazine
DES	diethylstilbestrol
DM	dextromethorphan
D$_5$W	5% dextrose in water
D$_5$S	5% dextrose in normal saline
DSS or DOSS	dioctyl sodium sulfosuccinate
DPH	phenytoin
DW	distilled water
EC	enteric coated
ETH & C	elixir terpin hydrate with codeine
Fe	iron
5-FU	5-fluorouracil
FUD	floxuridine
HC	hydrocortisone
K	potassium
KCl	potassium chloride
LOC	laxative of choice
MOM	milk of magnesia
6-MP	6-mercaptopurine
MS	morphine sulfate
MTX	methotrexate
Na	sodium
NS	normal saline
NTG	nitroglycerin
PAS	para-aminosalicylic acid
PB	phenobarbital
PCN	penicillin

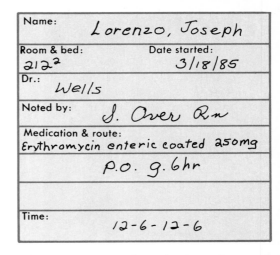

FIGURE 6-2 Transcription of a medication order onto the Kardex or a medication card or ticket.

set up the system and the need for additional pharmacy personnel to fill new orders and resupply the client's units each 24 hours. The administration of new and stat medication orders may be delayed while the medication order is sent to the pharmacy, filled, and then delivered back to the nurse rather than being immediately available on the unit. To avoid delays, emergency medications are often kept on each client unit for immediate access.

Strip packages make narcotic counting easier for nurses, since all packages in the strip are numbered. This also prevents contamination caused by pouring narcotic tablets into the hands for counting, which is a grossly improper technique. Prefilled unit dose disposable syringes are also available. Their advantages are:

1. Accuracy of dosage
2. Sterile product
3. Sharp needle
4. Elimination of suspected source of serum hepatitis (needle)
5. Less danger of drug absorption by personnel handling the drugs
6. Immediate availability of drug for use
7. Only medicine used is charged to client
8. Reduced likelihood of pilferage of narcotics
9. Less waste by breakage or incomplete use

Unit dose dispensing systems in hospitals may be centralized, decentralized, or a combination of both. In the centralized system the pharmacist and the pharmacy are located in a central area from which drugs are distributed to patient care areas. In the decentralized system, clinical pharmacists and satellite pharmacies are located in patient care areas and drugs are prepared and distributed to clients from those particular areas. In the combined system, medications are prepared in a central area, with clinical pharmacists assigned to various patient care areas to oversee drug therapy, thus providing safer and more controlled drug ordering and drug distribution.

Medication carts are used in some hospitals for distributing unit doses to the nursing unit and to the client's bedside. Each client has a drawer or tray for medications, which is restocked by the pharmacy staff.

Role of the Clinical Pharmacist

A present trend is toward more extensive use of clinical pharmacists stationed in nursing areas to work closely with physicians, nurses, and dietitians. Since pharmacists are educated in the compounding, dispensing, and control of drugs, they can be an invaluable resource for assistance in solving pharmacologic problems. Nurses frequently consult them about medication administration methods, dosages, drug identification, and secondary effects. Statistically, they are consulted by all health care disciplines most often about antiinfectives, analgesics, and cardiovascular drugs. The health care system today demands more of this kind of interdisciplinary collaboration and shared expertise for the benefit of all, especially the client.

Hospital pharmacies can have special "clean rooms" and specially filtered air for compounding various parenteral solutions. The pharmacist may be responsible for putting all additives into intravenous solutions and checking all such solutions for compatibility reactions.

Role of the Nurse

Regardless of changes in ordering, distributing, or administering drugs, nurses are still responsible for their clients' care 24 hours a day. Technology, clinical pharmacists, and unit package doses make it increasingly crucial to be well informed about drugs and their actions. Nurses must make observations of clients and their response to drug therapy, determine whether prn orders are to be given, and consult with prescribers about withholding, discontinuing, or changing drugs. They continue to take histories, to teach clients about drugs and their effects, to work collaboratively with pharmacists, and to help clients plan drug therapy after returning home.

PREPARING TO ADMINISTER DRUGS
Dosages, Dosing Intervals, and Scheduling

Understanding the medical rationale for selection of a particular dosage and frequency of administration requires a basic understanding of the drug in question. Within limits, increasing a drug's dose or frequency of administration increases pharmacologic effect but can also increase the risk of side and adverse effects. The various relationships involved can be represented as follows:

Optimal dosages → dose-response relationship

Optimal frequencies → time-response relationship

The variables to deal with in **dose-response relationships** are defined as follows:

Drug potency: absolute amount of drug required to produce a desired effect

Therapeutic index: relative margin of safety; the ratio of lethal dose to effective dose

Maximum effect: greatest response possible regardless of dose given

Time-response relationships deal with these variables:

Latency: time necessary for peak effect

Time for maximum effect: time after administration for the drug's effect to peak

Duration of action: length of times effect

These last variables are affected by route used, pharmacokinetics involved, and individual client **biorhythms.**

To avoid wide fluctuations in the serum concentration of a drug, doses are given at intervals to approximate a steady state without accumulation of the drug above plateau level. If the dosage interval is too short, drug accumulation with potential for toxicity will occur. If it is too long, serum concentration will drop because the drug will continue to be excreted and not replaced. Drugs with very short half-lives (see Chapter 4 for a discussion of drug half-life) will not accumulate if they are given orally and frequently, since very frequent doses are needed to achieve a steady state. Drugs with very long half-lives are often given once a day.

EXAMPLES OF CLINICAL APPLICATIONS OF DRUG DOSING

Blood levels of steroids administered between 7:30 AM and 8:30 AM may most closely match levels as they would occur normally.

Most antibiotics and antihypertensives should be administered around the clock to achieve a steady state in the bloodstream.

Anticoagulant dosages should be titrated with tests of the patient's own partial thromboplastin time or a similar determination.

Diuretics should not be administered late in the day or before appointments, when urinary urgency would be inconvenient for the client.

In drug studies, dosing relationships are interpreted on the basis of a normal curve, and dosages and dosing intervals are derived for treating the ideal "average" person in a population. This explains why certain medications with relatively long half-lives can usually be given once a day. Likewise, it explains why a drug scheduled to be given every 6 hours should not be expected to be as effective for most people if it is given arbitrarily four times a day during daylight hours. It is less likely that optimal serum levels or tissue levels will be maintained by the latter schedule. It also explains why, although dosage and dosing intervals have been studied statistically, drug therapy regimens must continually be reassessed for individual needs. Some people will always fall outside the "average" range in responding to a drug. In addition, dosing intervals may be modified in consideration of patient convenience and the effect on compliance.

Times to administer routine medications may be determined by agency policy. For example, qid drugs may be routinely given at 10 AM, 2 PM, 6 PM, and 10 PM, or at 9 AM, 1 PM, 5 PM, and 9 PM, and so forth. Special units, such as pediatrics, have other medication hours to coincide with the special needs of their clients. Based on client convenience and the need to avoid mealtimes or other activities that might interfere with either drug administration or its pharmacokinetics, nurses may choose autonomously to vary the times (but not the intervals) if the decision is based on solid rationale. For example, calcium supplements might be given at bedtime rather than 9 AM on a daily schedule because calcium is better absorbed at night. Drugs administered once daily, can usually be given according to a flexible schedule, perhaps just before or after a treatment that would interfere with a dosing time, such as a client's trip off the nursing unit to the physical therapy department or x-ray department. Drugs should be administered to clients as close to the time indicated as possible, but obviously a nurse cannot medicate each of a group of assigned patients at exactly the same time. Agency policies may vary, but usually they stipulate administration within ½ hour before or after the indicated time. Exempt from this flexibility are stat or one-time-only drug orders, such as those given before diagnostic procedures or surgery, and those medications administered at the most frequent intervals, such as q2h or q4h.

Drug effects are monitored by the prescriber and the nurse according to either *direct assessment* (by observation for clinical responses) or *indirect assessment* (by laboratory values or serum concentrations of the drug). Nurses, because of their unique presence and expertise, are most capable in assisting the prescriber to make keen assessments of clients' responses.

Dosage Measurement

When the specified amount of a drug is not prepackaged in single unit doses, the nurse must be able to choose from among the sometimes numerous drugs for the patient the right drug and the right dose. If the drug is formulated in units that are multiples of the dosage ordered, whether tablet or liquid, the computation to determine the correct dose is simple. If, however, the drug does not come in units that are multiples of the dose prescribed, if the drug must be dissolved in water, or if the order is written in the apothecary system and the drug is available only in metric units, dosage calculations will be necessary.

Flow rate calculations are necessary for certain therapies in order to set the proper amount for the desired dose effect. Intravenous infusions and oxygen therapies necessitate careful flow rate calculation. These therapies should be ordered by the prescriber in definitive amounts and rates. (See Chapter 70.)

The rate of replacement fluids with or without other additives by IV infusion may be regulated in one of two basic ways. One is by a simple *roller clamp* on the tubing, which can be manually adjusted to deliver the number of drops per minute that will provide the prescribed total amount over the prescribed time. Given the total volume of solution to be infused, the total number of minutes the solution is to be infused, and the drop factor (number of drops per milliliter that the tubing delivers—a small number that varies among tubing manufacturers and is found on the back of the tubing box), the prescribed drops per minute can be calculated and the set regulated by counting drops in the drip chamber of the tubing. A simple formula for IV flow rate calculation can be found in Exercise 12 later in this chapter. Details of regulating by manual clamps, the most common mode, may be found in a basic nursing text such as Potter and Perry (1988). (See Bibliography.)

Another way that infusions can be made to run more precisely is by the use of instrumentation such as IV controllers and pumps. These can be used in situations that require more accurate titration of infusion fluids or nutri-

ents than is provided by hand-adjusted roller clamps, which can allow up to a 5% error in flow rate within the first 15 minutes of flow and other variations thereafter. One study in a Boston hospital revealed that 37% of the hospitalized patients who died from drug-related causes did so from fluid overload or potassium excess (potassium is a frequent additive to intravenous infusions). Increased use of instrumentation for regulating IV flow rates can be predicted in the future.

Most of the instrumentation to regulate infusions consists of various applications of either **infusion controllers** or **infusions pumps.** These small boxlike devices are attached to IV poles. The infusion tubing is strung for regulation of rate to ensure automatic delivery of solutions at preselected rates or volumes. CAUTION: For instruments that can accommodate either macrodrip or microdrip tubing, the tubing must be appropriate for the drop factor used to calculate drop rate. A rate calculated on the basis of microdrip tubing but accidentally administered by macrodrip could seriously overdose or overhydrate a patient.

Infusion controllers (Figure 6-3) work simply by utilizing the force of gravity. Controllers are not capable of

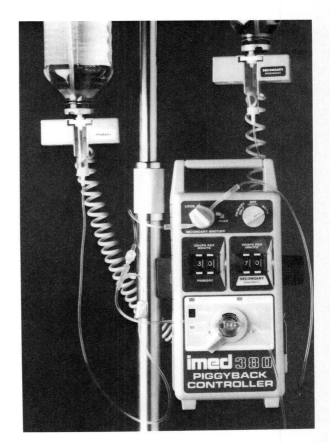

FIGURE 6-3 Intravenous controller for the simultaneous regulation of a primary or main intravenous infusion and a secondary, intermittent medication infusion.

(Courtesy IMED Corp. Warner-Lambert Co., Morris Plains, N.J.)

delivering rates with the accuracy of infusion pumps (which may be more useful in special situations in which there will be rises in back pressure that are transmitted to the fluid in the tubing; such is the situation in arterial infusions or when the patient is a restless child or a woman in labor.) However, unlike infusion pumps, IV controllers will not pump fluid into interstitial tissue if the infusion needle infiltrates. Controllers are useful in 80% to 85% of cases calling for intravenous therapy.

Infusion pumps are of at least two kinds, both delivering infusion fluids under positive pressure: (1) nonvolumetric ("infusion pumps"; Figure 6-4), which measures fluid volume delivery by drop rate (not as accurate since drop volume may vary), and (2) volumetric ("volume pumps"; Figure 6-5), which can measure very precisely even smaller volumes of infusion solution by milliliter per hour. This latter pump is especially useful for small children, total parenteral nutrition, and the administration of potent drugs by continuous IV infusion (such as streptokinase, dopamine, or nitroglycerin). Alarm readout messages (e.g., "Fix Me") may be displayed on the front panel of the instrument.

Similar instrumentation is made by several different manufacturers, which utilize various physical principles to sense pressures and pump fluid and read out the flow-rate settings and the like. Their capabilities include great-

er accuracy than other modes of infusion delivery systems and alarms to warn of blocked tubing, air in the tubing, or empty solution containers. All this capability sounds ideal, but like all mechanical devices, infusion pumps are subject to malfunction and therefore require continued watchfulness by nurses to ensure reliability and to maintain personal contact with the purpose of it all—the client. There is currently a growing body of literature on this type of equipment. Its intricacy presents nurses with still another challenge, although not an insurmountable one. The reader is referred to the excellent references at the end of this chapter to learn more.

Oxygen therapy is also ordered in units of flow rate. Oxygen is a medication that should be administered with care, especially to a client with a chronic obstructive pulmonary disorder or one who requires longer-than-usual continuous oxygen supportive therapy. Regardless of the delivery equipment (nasal cannula or "prongs," nasal catheter, mask, or tent), the oxygen order should specifically state the desired flow, usually in liters per minute

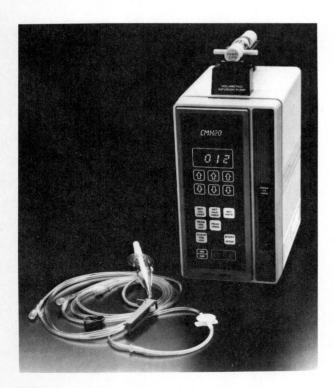

FIGURE 6-4 Infusion pump used when positive pressure provided by peristaltic action on the tubing produces the preset drop rate.

(IVAC 530 type; courtesy IVAC Corp., San Diego, Calif.)

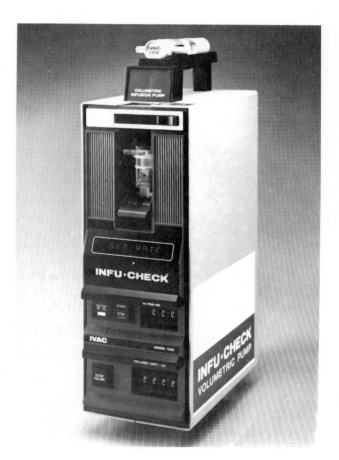

FIGURE 6-5 A positive pressure volumetric infusion pump, which ensures closer accuracy of the infusion in volumes of milliliters per hour than the slightly less accurate drops per minutes of other types of pumps.

(IVAC 630 type; courtesy IVAC Corp., San Diego, Calif.)

(e.g., 2 to 4 L/min) and, if necessary, by concentration desired. Regulation is usually by a flow meter calibrated in liters per minute, which is attached to a jar of oxygen-humidifying sterile distilled water to alleviate the drying effect of oxygen on respiratory mucosa.

Frequently, oxygen is ordered to be given "prn" or "on standby" for the client who can be anticipated to have occasional bouts of dyspnea or chest pain caused by coronary insufficiency. Full, continuous oxygen therapy for more than 24 hours can have serious consequences, since oxygen works to fuel oxidative body processes; certain tissues (especially lung and retinal tissues in the newborn) may literally burn themselves out. Clients with a history of chronic obstructive pulmonary disorders may also be at risk if the rate of flow routinely exceeds about 2 L/min. The bodily oxygen sensors in these clients have become accustomed to lower-than-normal blood oxygen levels accompanied by higher carbon dioxide levels. Their sensors have adapted to regulating respiratory excursions via higher-than-normal carbon dioxide levels. If these sensors are suddenly flooded with normal or high oxygen levels and correspondingly reduced carbon dioxide levels, the drive to initiate respiration is reduced or eliminated. Thus clients with chronic obstructive pulmonary disease may stop breathing if oxygen is delivered at or above the usual flow rates.

Most dosage calculations, however, deal with numbers of tablets to give or with changing from one unit of measurement to another. A dosage problem may be as simple as giving 10 grains of acetylsalicylic acid from a container of 5-grain tablets. It is almost as easy to figure out how many milliliters of morphine sulfate one must give if the container is labeled "15 mg = 1 ml" and the order reads "10 mg morphine sulfate SC." Complexity builds when the units of measurement in the medication order must be converted to a different type of unit in which the drug is available.

Currently three systems of measurements are in use for administering medications: the **metric system** (the most widely adopted and the most convenient), the **apothecary system** (which is being phased out), and the **household system** (the least accurate and not widely used except in home settings).

Metric system. The metric system of weights and measures was invented by the French at the end of the eighteenth century, and toward the end of the nineteenth century the Bureau of Weights and Measures was formed and given the challenge to develop metric standards for international use. The United States finally joined the worldwide trend toward adoption of the metric system with the enactment of the Metric Conversion Act of 1975.

The basic metric units of measurement are the meter, the liter, and the gram. The *meter* is the unit for linear measurement, the *liter* for capacity or volume, and the *gram* for weight. A meter is a little longer than a yard; a

liter is a little more than a quart; and a gram is a little more than the weight of a steel paper clip.

The metric system is a decimal system; the basic units can be divided into 10, 100, or 1000 parts; or the basic units can be multiplied by 10, 100, or 1000 to form secondary units that differ from each other by 10 or some multiple of 10. The names of the secondary units are formed by joining Greek or Latin prefixes to the names of the primary units (Table 6-3). Subdivisions of the basic units are made by moving the decimal point to the left, and multiples of the basic units are indicated by moving the decimal point to the right.

The meter is the unit from which the other metric units are derived. Centimeters and millimeters are the chief linear measures used in hospital work. Measurement of the size of body organs is made in centimeters and millimeters, and the sphygmomanometer used to measure blood pressure is calibrated in millimeters of mercury. There are approximately 2.5 cm (25 mm) in 1 inch.

The liter is the unit of capacity or volume and is equal to approximately 1000 cc or 1000 ml. The weight of a liter of water at 4° C is 1 kg. Because of the way it was originally defined, a liter is actually 1000.028 cc. However, *in practice the cubic centimeter and the milliliter are considered equal.* The difference is so small that it is of no importance except in determinations of extreme precision.

Fractional parts of a liter are usually expressed in milliliters or cubic centimeters. For example, 0.6 liter would be expressed as 600 ml or 600 cc. Multiples of a liter are similarly expressed: 2.4 liters would be 2400 ml or cc. The abbreviation cc is in the process of being dropped and is considered obsolete; either ml or mL may be used, according to the National Bureau of Standards.

The gram is the metric unit of weight that is used in weighing drugs and various pharmaceutical preparations. Originally, the unit of measurement for weight was the kilogram, but this proved too large to meet the practical

TABLE 6-3 Metric Prefixes, Meanings, and Relationships

Prefix	Meaning
Giga*	Billions
Kilo†	Thousands
Hecto	Hundreds
Deka	Tens
Base units of meter, liter, gram	One unit
Deci	Tenths
Centi†	Hundredths
Milli†	Thousandths
Micro†	Millionths
Nano	Billionths

Data from The International System of Units, National Bureau of Standards Publications No. 330, August 1977, U.S. Department of Commerce.
*Abbreviated G, as opposed to g for gram.
†Prefixes most commonly encountered in nursing.

needs of the pharmacist. The gram equals the weight of 1 ml of distilled water at 4° C.

The approved abbreviation for gram is g; G as the abbreviation for gram is no longer approved, since it conflicts with the abbreviation for the prefix *giga*. Gm is also not approved by the National Bureau of Standards.

As a review of Table 6-3 indicates, a decigram is 10 times greater than a centigram and 100 times greater than a milligram. To change decigrams to centigrams, one multiplies by 10; to change decigrams to milligrams, one multiplies by 100. To change milligrams to centigrams, one divides by 10; to change milligrams to decigrams, one divides by 100; to change milligrams to grams, one divides by 1000; and so forth. To figure out how many micrograms (μg) of medication there are in 1 milliliter, one determines how many milligrams are in a liter (or 1000 ml). The resulting number is the same as the number of micrograms in 1 milliliter.

The style of notation proposed by the International System of Units (referred to as SI) from the National Bureau of Standards is recommended except when it conflicts with proper English language norms:

Units are not capitalized (gram, not Gram).

No period should be used with abbreviations of units (ml, not m.l. or ml.).

A single space should be left between the quantity and the symbol (24 kg, not 25kg).

Large numbers may be separated into groups of three numbers, without comma (25 000, not 25,000).

Except in the apothecary system, only decimal notation should be used, not fractions (0.25 kg, not ¼ kg).

Numerical quantities less than 1 should have a zero placed to the left of the decimal point (0.75 mg, not .75 mg).

Abbreviations should not be pluralized (kg, not kgs).

Nurses need the foregoing as part of their knowledge base not only to use in preparing medications but also to interpret laboratory data (some are reported in milliliters, others in deciliters or nanograms, and so forth), to weigh patients (kilograms instead of pounds), and to figure flow rates of IV infusions. (Refer to the table of abbreviations and symbols, Table 6-1, as necessary.)

Until the metric system is fully accepted in clinical practice, nurses will deal with all three systems of measurement: metric, apothecary, and household. This chapter presents the basic logic of each system and the interrelationships among the systems (Table 6-4). The nurse can extract a few crucial relationships to memorize. These data can then be readily inserted where applicable as part of a formula or as half of a ratio-and-proportion equation often used for dosage calculation. A suggested practical list of equivalents that nurses should know is presented in Table 6-4.

Apothecary system. Only a few medications are now available in units of the apothecary system. It is less convenient and less precise than the metric system. The basic unit of weight is the *grain,* which is derived from the age-old standard of the weight of a single grain of wheat, a weight now variously accepted as approximately equivalent to 60 or 65 mg (60 mg is the more widely accepted of the two). Other units of weight commonly used in the apothecary system are the dram, the ounce, and the pound.

The basic unit of fluid volume is the *minim,* approximately equal to the volume of water that would weigh a grain, a very small amount, about 0.005 or 0.006 ml. Other volume measures, which may also be considered household measures, are the pint and the quart.

In written prescriptions, the placement of abbreviations and the type of numerals used in the apothecary system follow a more complex arrangement than in the metric system. In the apothecary system, the abbreviation is placed before the numeral. Whole numerical quantities usually are expressed in roman numerals (e.g., gr x for 10 grains.) Fractional quantities are usually expressed by arabic numerals rather than by decimals (e.g., gr ¼, not gr 0.25, for one-quarter grain). When comparing fractional amounts, remember that the larger the bottom number (the denominator), the smaller the quantity involved, given the same numerator. In other words, gr ¹⁄₂₀₀ is a smaller quantity than gr ¹⁄₁₅₀.

Household systems. Household measures include the glass, cup, tablespoon, teaspoon, and drops; pints and quarts are often included in this system as well as in the apothecary system. Recent changes in hospital reimbursement policies (e.g., DRGs [Diagnosis-Related Groups]), which have shortened hospital stays and correspondingly lengthened convalescence at home, and the increasing geriatric population have expanded the numbers of people under care at home. Because standardized measurements of household equipment usually do not exist in the home, the community health nurse may not have access to accurately calibrated measuring devices in the home. For example, the average teacup or coffee cup can hold from 5 to 9 ounces or more, not the accepted 8 ounces or half pint. The average household teaspoon can hold 4 to 5 ml or more of liquid medication rather than the standard 5 ml. A drop and a minim *cannot* be considered equivalents, since drop size will vary with the viscosity of the medication even when measured by an approved dropper. Therefore any listing of household measurements on a table of equivalent measures must be considered only approximations. Depending on the situation (e.g., medicating infants) and the need for precise dosage, such measures may or may not be adequate. Clients may need to obtain precise measuring instruments from the local pharmacy or the visiting nurse for medication administration at home.

Dosage Calculation

Challenges to the mathematical skills of nurses occur infrequently in the administration of medications. An

TABLE 6-4 Common Approximate Equivalents of Weights and Measures

Metric	Apothecary	Household
WEIGHT		
1 kg*	2.2 pounds	
1000 mg = 1 gram*	gr xv	
60 mg* (occasionally seen as 65 mg)	gr i̇	
30 mg	gr ss (one half)	
1 μg (mcg) = 0.001 mg		
VOLUME		
	4 quarts	1 gallon
1000 ml* = approx 1 liter = 1000 cc	Approx 1 qt	1 quart
500 ml	Approx 1 pint (½ qt)	16 ounces
240 or 250 ml	℥ viii (8 fluidounces)† = approx ½ pint	1 cup or 1 glass
30 ml* = approx 30 cc	℥ i̇ (1 fluidounce)	2 tbsp
Approx 16 ml = approx 16 cc	ʒ iv (4 fluidrams)	1 tbsp
8 ml	ʒ ii̇ (2 fluidrams)	2 tsp
4 to 5 ml	ʒ i̇ (1 fluidram)	1 tsp
1 ml* = approx 1 cc	Minims xv or xvi	Minims cannot be compared with drops

*These equivalents may be committed to memory for ready application to dosage problems.
†Note the small difference in the symbols for fluidounce and fluidram.

equation can be set up to apply what the nurse has learned about a few crucial equivalents and how that relates to what needs to be solved—all in a logical sequence or relationship. Calculators may not be appropriate in the nursing unit, for they tend to have exasperating battery failures or to "disappear" from busy hospital units and nursing homes. It is more reliable to develop and maintain a basic competence in mathematical calculations.

Following are some typical exercises to do, accompanied by explanations and answers. These exercises assume a working knowledge of decimals, fractions, and a ratio-and-proportion approach to problem solving. Again, if you are used to working with another method that works as well, use it instead—just check your answers and rationale with the following.

Exercises

1. If a drug is ordered in units different from the units on hand, the order must be mathematically translated into the units available. Thus if the medication order is written in terms of milligrams, yet the client's drug is supplied in grams, you must translate the needed dose into grams.

Question: A drug is ordered to be given in the amount of 1500 mg. How many grams would you give?
Answer: Knowing that there are 1000 mg in a gram, set up the ratio in logical sequence. The logic of the relationships ("this is to this as that is to that") remains constant in a ratio-and-proportion approach, but which of the relationships is set down first in the equation does not matter. Some people set down first, on the left side of the equation, the relationship between what has been ordered or what information is wanted in the problem and the unknown quantity, or x. Then on the right side of the equation they set down the known equivalents, the conversion factors, or the "givens." Once set up, the equation is solved by multiplying the means (middle adjacent numbers) by the extremes (numbers on each end):

$$1500 \text{ mg}:x = 1000 \text{ mg}:1 \text{ g}$$
$$1000x = 1500$$
$$x = 1.5 \text{ g}$$

Question: A dosage of 30 ml of cough syrup is ordered to be given qid. The label on the bottle of medication states that it contains a total of 240 cc. How many cubic centimeters would you give?
Answer: You need to know that 30 ml is roughly equivalent to 30 cc.

Question: 10 mEq of potassium chloride (KC1) is to be added to an IV infusion solution. KC1 is available for this application in vials of 40 mEq/20 ml. How many milliliters would you give?
Answer: Again set up the equation in logical sequence, possibly starting with the desired ingredient and the unknown quantity.

$$10 \text{ mEq}:x = 40 \text{ mEq}:20 \text{ ml}$$
$$40x = 200$$
$$x = \frac{200}{40} = 5 \text{ ml}$$

2. Sometimes medicaton for injection comes in powdered or concentrated liquid form and must be dissolved (reconstituted) or diluted before it can be injected. Most often directions as to how much diluent (dissolving or diluting solution) and what kind should be added by needle and syringe to the powder or liquid are on the label of the container of the drug. All that the nurse needs to know in order to determine the amount to give is on the label.

Question: A certain antibiotic has been ordered "750 mg IV." The drug comes in a 10-g multiple-dose vial (there is more than enough of the drug in the vial for one dose) in powdered form. The label reads, "Add 7.2 ml sterile water or sodium chloride solution for injection to yield 10 ml of reconstituted drug." After the diluent has been added, how many milliliters would you give?

Answer: 10 ml now contains 10 g; thus 1 ml equals 1 g. You should already know or be able to refer to a listing of standard equivalents to find out that 1 g equals 1000 mg. You may then start the equation by setting down the relationship between what you want to give and the volume that contains it. Then follow the same sequence of relationship on the other side of the equation which denotes what is available in which volume.

$$750 \text{ mg}:x = 1000 \text{ mg}:1 \text{ ml}$$
$$1000x = 750$$
$$x = \frac{750}{1000} = 0.75 \text{ ml}$$

Whenever a drug appears in concentrated form (powder or liquid), after the appropriate diluent has been added and well dispersed or dissolved, the same mathematical approach can be used, no matter what the size of the finished solution. NB: Do not fall into the trap of including the amount of *diluent* anywhere in your equation.

3. *Question:* The quantity of a certain medication is ordered as "gr xv," and the tablets on hand are in gr v dosage. How many tablets should be given?
Answer:

$$\text{gr } 15:x = \text{gr } 5:1 \text{ tablet}$$
$$5x = 15$$
$$x = \frac{15}{5} = 3 \text{ tablets}$$

4. *Question:* One quart bottle of potassium permanganate has been sent up from the pharmacy. The treatment order reads that a pint of potassium permanganate is used in each treatment of the client's skin condition. How much solution will be left after the first treatment?
Answer: One pint. You should know that 2 pints make 1 quart.

5. *Question:* How many pints should be requested from the pharmacy if a medication is to be given in 4-ounce doses three times a day for 2 days?
Answer: You need to know that 16 ounces are in 1 pint. Total number of ounces for the course of therapy = 4 × 3 × 2 = 24 oz, or 1½ pints.

6. *Question:* A client's medication has been ordered based on body weight. If the client weighs 150 pounds, how many kilograms is that?
Answer: You need to know that 1 kg is equal to 2.2 pounds.

$$150 \text{ lb}:x = 2.2 \text{ lb}:1 \text{ kg}$$
$$2.2x = 150$$
$$x = \frac{150}{2.2} = 68.2 \text{ kg}$$

7. *Question:* A medication order calls for 0.5 ml of a drug. If available syringes are calibrated only in minims, how many minims will you give?
Answer: You need to know that there are between 15 and 16 minims in 1 ml. Choose either figure to use.

$$0.5 \text{ ml}:x = 1 \text{ ml}:16 \text{ minims}$$
$$x = 0.5 \times 16$$
$$x = 8 \text{ minims}$$

8. *Question:* Atropine sulfate gr ¹⁄₁₅₀ is ordered. How many tablets would you give if the available supply is in tablets of 0.2 mg?
Answer: First you need to know that 1 grain is equivalent to 60 mg; then you can find how many milligrams are equivalent to gr ¹⁄₁₅₀. Second, you need to find out how many tablets will provide the milligram equivalent of gr ¹⁄₁₅₀.

$$\text{gr } ^1/_{150}:x \text{ (mg)} = \text{gr } 1:60 \text{ mg}$$
$$x = 60 \left(\frac{1}{150}\right)$$
$$x = \frac{60}{150} = 0.4 \text{ mg}$$

The second step may certainly be done without pencil and paper, but it is more likely to be accurate if not calculated in the head.

$$0.4 \text{ mg}:x = 0.2 \text{ mg}:1$$
$$0.2x = 0.4$$
$$x = \frac{0.4}{0.2} = 2 \text{ tablets}$$

9. *Question:* You may also be confronted with the reverse of the preceding question. How many grains would you give if 0.6 mg scopolamine has been ordered?
Answer:

$$0.6 \text{ mg}:x \text{ (gr)} = 60 \text{ mg}:\text{gr } 1$$
$$60x = \frac{0.6}{60}$$
$$x = \text{gr } 0.01 = \text{gr } ^1/_{100}$$

10. *Question:* Codeine gr ss is ordered; how many milligrams would you give?
Answer: You need to know that the symbol "ss" indicates the quantity one half.

$$\text{gr } ^1/_2:x \text{ (mg)} = \text{gr } 1:60 \text{ mg}$$
$$x = 60 \left(\frac{1}{2}\right)$$
$$x = \frac{60}{2} = 30 \text{ mg}$$

11. *Question:* The client is to take 6 ounces of magnesium sulfate solution, and the calibrations on the available measuring device are in milliliters. How many milliliters would you give?
    Answer: You need to know that 1 ounce is equivalent to 30 ml.

    $$6 \text{ oz}:x \text{ (ml)} = 1 \text{ oz}:30 \text{ ml}$$
    $$x = 6 \times 30$$
    $$x = 180 \text{ ml}$$

12. Although some practitioners may not technically consider IV infusions to be medications, we will practice figuring IV infusion rates here.

    The amount of IV solution to be infused during a given length of time is the IV flow rate. It is dictated by the prescriber's order, which should give the total amount of fluid and the number of milliliters that should be infused over each 1-hour period or less *or* the number of drops per minute that should be infused. Some prescribers are still writing IV orders that give only the total volume of solution to be infused (e.g., 1000 ml) over a longer period (e.g., 8 hours). Technically, such information is inadequate and the order should be clarified.

    If the order does not spell out the rate of flow in drops per minute, the following formula may be used to figure this out:

    $$\frac{\text{Total number of milliliters to be infused}}{\text{Total number of minutes infusion is to run}} \times \text{Drop factor}$$

    $$= \text{Rate in drops per minute}$$

    Question: If an order is given for 1000 ml D$_5$W to run for 8 hours and the drop factor is 10 drops per milliliter for the particular tubing used (other types deliver 15 drops or 60 drops — often used to infuse children), how fast should the IV infusion be set to run?
    Answer:

    $$\frac{1000 \text{ ml}}{480 \text{ min}} \times 10 = x$$

    $$\frac{100}{48} \times 10 = 20.8 \text{ drops (gtt)/min} = 21 \text{ gtt/min}$$

    A bit more challenging are some of the mathematics involved with IV rates for infusion pumps. These pumps are often used for giving drugs whose dosages must be calculated more closely.

    Question: Dopamine 400 mg is ordered to be added to 250 cc D$_5$W to be infused at a rate of 350 μg/min. It is to be regulated by a volumetric infusion pump that is calibrated to deliver the fluid in units of cubic centimeters per hour. At how many cubic centimeters per hour should the pump be set?
    Answer: Here you are asked to convert the "language" of one flow rate to the language of another. First you need to know that 1 μg is equal to 0.001 mg, so:

    $$350 \text{ μg}:x \text{ (mg)} = 1 \text{ μg}:0.001 \text{ mg}$$
    $$x = 0.350 \text{ mg or } 0.35 \text{ mg}$$

    Thus 0.350 mg is being infused every minute. Now you need to calculate the rate per hour. That is, if 0.35 mg is infused every minute, how many milligrams will be infused per hour?

    $$x:60 \text{ min} = 0.35 \text{ mg}:1 \text{ min}$$
    $$x = 60 \times 0.35$$
    $$x = (350)0.01$$
    $$x = 21 \text{ mg}$$

    Now convert to cubic centimeters per hour:

    $$21 \text{ mg}:x(\text{cc}) = 400 \text{ mg}:250 \text{ cc}$$
    $$400x = 21 \times 250 = 5250$$
    $$x = 13.125 \text{ or } 13 \text{ cc/hr}$$

13. *Question:* 30 mg of a drug for three times a day dosing has been ordered for a child who weighs 15 kg and is 90 cm tall. The recommended 24-hour total pediatric dosage is 90 to 150 mg/m^2. Is the ordered dose safe or unsafe for this child? Refer to the West nomogram (see Figure 9-2).
    Answer: According to the nomogram, a line drawn from points indicating 90 cm and 15 kg crosses the body surface area (BSA) column at the 0.62 point. This means that the child's body surface area is about 0.62 m^2. Multiply 0.62 by each of the numbers indicating the drug's range of safety to see if the ordered 24-hour dosage is within that range.

Some rules of thumb will become more important as the metric system predominates.

Place a zero to the left of the decimal point when there is no integer in the decimal.

Carry out problems to the hundredths place, and then round off only in the final answer.

Use judgment in rounding off numbers. The smaller the answer (the lower the number), the more significant the relative change in the answer made by rounding off.

Many excellent nursing texts are available that one can use to develop and practice arithmetic skills necessary in the administration of medications. (See the references at the end of this chapter.) Much more practice is necessary than is presented here for introductory purposes.

PROCEDURES AND TECHNIQUES OF ADMINISTRATION

Accurate and full identification of the client before each dose of medication is given ensures that the right person gets the right medication. Using the client's full name on all paperwork and in all references helps prevent mixups, as does being alert to similarities in names and geographically separating people with similar names. Nurses should not rely on memory to identify clients. *Checking the client's name on the arm band or name tag* against the name on the accompanying medication ticket is the *most reliable* mode of identification. Asking the client his or her name and comparing it with the name on the medication ticket, Kardex, or MAR is not foolproof. For example, a client may give his name as "William" (first name), and then be given medication intended for "Mr. Williams" (last name). Checking the client's name by calling it out and waiting for a corroborating answer is particularly risky; in a sleepy state, clients have been known to answer to almost any name. Reliance on names on bed tags or labels is dangerous because clients are often away from their beds; a bed can be inadvertently occupied by another client who is in a groggy state after returning, for example, from a laboratory test. Asking a family member is not foolproof either; a distraught family member may respond inappropriately. Again, the *surest* way to identify a patient before giving medication is to *check the arm band* or *identifying tag.* In an institutional setting, medications should not be administered to any client not wearing an identification band or tag. Each institution has a policy for the replacement of identification bands or tags inadvertently removed or lost, and this policy should be complied with and the band or tag restored before any medications are administered. One exception might be in the case of an emergency, in which a delay might be detrimental. Even in an emergency the client's identity should be verified by some method before drug administration.

Before administering medications, the nurse must also make sure that the drug order has not been changed in any way (e.g., discontinued or dosage changed) from what appears on the medications ticket or MAR. It is also wise to check the medication administration record to see that the dose about to be given has not already been given by someone else caring for the client (such as the private duty nurse or nursing student). Individual agency policies spell out the checking procedure to be used; these policies should be followed routinely to avoid error.

The following are recommended guidelines for distributing or administering drugs to patients.

1. When preparing or giving medicines, concentrate your whole attention on what you are doing. Do not permit yourself to be distracted while working with medicines.
2. Make certain that you have a written order for every medication for which you assume the responsibility of administration. (Verbal and telephone orders should be written out and signed by the prescriber as soon as possible. These orders should be used only in limited circumstances and not for the convenience of the prescriber.)
3. Make a habit of reading the label of the medicine and comparing it to the MAR carefully at least three times: first, when removing the drug from the supply drawer or medication cart; second, when placing the medication in a souffle cup, ounce cup, or syringe; and third, just before administering it to the client, before the container is discarded.
4. Make certain that the data on the medicine card or MAR corresponds exactly with the prescriber's written order and with the label on the client's medicine. If the card system is used, a card should accompany each dose. Sometimes skipping a dose of medicine may be as dangerous as an overdose.
5. Never give a medicine from an unlabeled container or from one on which the label is not legible.

6. If you must in some way calculate the dosage for a client from the preparation on hand and you are uncertain of your calculation, verify your work on paper by having some other responsible person—an instructor, nurse in charge, or pharmacist—check it. In some hospitals certain drug dosages, (e.g., insulin) are routinely verified by another nurse. Whenever the result of a calculation calls for more than two units of a drug to make a dose, double check the calculation. It is highly unusual for more than two units of a single drug to be administered in a single dose.
7. Measure quantities as ordered, using the proper equipment: graduated containers for milliliters, fluidounces, or fluidrams, minim glasses or calibrated syringes for minims, and droppers for drops. When measuring liquids, hold the container so that the line indicating the desired quantity is on a level with the eye. The quantity is read when the lowest part of the concave surface of the fluid (meniscus) is on this line.
8. Dosage forms such as tablets, capsules, and pills should be handled so that the fingers do not come into contact with the medicine. Use the cap of the container to guide or lift the medicine into the medicine glass or container you will be taking to the bedside of the client.
9. Avoid waste of medicines. Medicines tend to be expensive; in some instances a single capsule may cost the patient several dollars. Dropping medicine on the floor is one way of being wasteful.
10. When pouring liquid medicines, hold the bottle so that the liquid does not run over the side and obscure the label. This is known as "palming the label." Wipe the rim of the bottle with a clean piece of paper tissue before replacing the stopper or cover.
11. Always prepare an IV admixture before you label the container, and verify the dosage on the emptied additive container when labeling the IV container.
12. When preparing an injection, always label the syringe immediately. Keep the vial with the syringe, and do not rely on memory to determine what solution is in which syringe.
13. Never administer medication prepared by another person. In doing so, you accept the responsibility for accuracy, dose, correct medication, and so forth. If the person who prepared the medication has made an error, you are accountable for any harm done to the client.
14. If a client expresses doubt or concern about a medication or the dosage of a medication, reassure the client as well as yourself by rechecking to make certain that there is no error, before the medication is administered. You may need to recheck the order, the label on the medicine container, or the client's chart. The astute and caring nurse also recognizes that a client who refuses medication has the right to do so and that this behavior is giving a message about expressed or unexpressed feelings. The understanding nurse is not content to simply chart that the patient refused 10:00 AM medication. The client should be able to talk about whatever feelings caused the behavior, and this will help the client feel that his or her reaction, whatever it may be, is accepted. You thus provide the client opportunities to exercise some control over the environment.
15. Assist weak or helpless clients to take their medications. Do so as patiently and unhurriedly as possible.

16. Many liquid medicines should be diluted with water or other liquid. This is especially desirable when medicines have a bad taste. Exceptions to this rule include cough medicines that are given for a local effect in the throat. The client (in the sitting position) should be supplied with *at least 100 ml of water* for swallowing solid forms such as tablets or capsules, unless the individual is allowed only limited amounts of fluid. This will facilitate dissolution and reduce gastric irritation, if any. Esophageal erosion caused by an adherent tablet or pill has been reported when inadequate amounts of water were given.

17. *Remain with the client until the medicine has been taken.* Most clients are very cooperative about taking medicines at the time that the nurse brings them. However, sometimes clients are more ill than they appear and have been known to hoard medicines until they have accumulated a lethal amount and then take the entire amount, with fatal results. In some instances, however, clients may be permitted to keep medicines at their bedsides and take them as necessary, such as nitroglycerin and antacids. In fact, in some controlled situations in which clients self-administered medications, client satisfaction improved and nursing staff members felt that they had more time to instruct clients about their medications and not just distribute them (Anderson and Poole, 1983).

18. Stay, for at least 5 minutes, with the client receiving the first dose of an IV medication, especially antibiotics, and monitor closely for adverse effects.

19. Do not leave a tray or cart of medicines unattended. If you are in a client's room and must leave, take the tray of medicines with you. Similarly, do not leave the medication cart unattended in the hall; take it into the client's room with you.

20. Never chart a medicine as having been given until it has been administered. Nursing students should check the chart before giving a medication. MARs should document all medications, including prn's, one-time-only medications, and special drugs (e.g., heparin), in one place to allow the nurse to consider incompatibilities and/or duplications of similar drugs. The name of the drug, the dosage, the time of administration, and the route of administration should be noted on the medication record in the chart. In the recording of parenteral medications, the site of injection is always included. The patient's response, adverse as well as intended, to the medication should be recorded in the progress notes or nursing notes.

21. Always verify a drug's route of administration. Sometimes preparations for a specific route of administration may be used for another route. For example, Mycostatin suppositories developed for vaginal use may be used as an oral troche for an oral yeast infection, or some parenteral preparations may be diluted for oral use, such as vancomycin when indicated for pseudomembranous colitis. In this latter example and with other drugs, do not put oral drugs in syringes used for injection. Oral syringes that cannot accommodate a needle should be used to prevent accidental parenteral injection of an oral preparation.

22. Within an institutional setting, any unused medication should be returned to the pharmacy. According to institutional policy, the unused portion may be credited to the client's account. If it can be used for another client, the pharmacy will verify that it has been stored correctly and relabel it.

23. Borrowing medications from one client's supply for another client is not appropriate and leads to dosing errors. Only medications issued by the pharmacy and labeled for a specific client should be used for that client, except in the case of a stock medication kept on the nursing unit. Medications brought into the hospital by a client should be returned home with a family member or, if they are to be utilized in the institutional setting, sent to the hospital pharmacy to be verified and relabeled.

All medicine containers and trays should be scrupulously clean, and water supplied immediately after the medicine should be fresh. Carelessly prepared medicines and lack of consideration in the way a medicine is handed to a client can convey a demeaning or insulting message, whether intended or not.

When a medicine with an unpleasant taste is given, it is better to admit that it may be unpleasant than to make a client feel that his or her reaction is grossly exaggerated or silly. The nurse can attempt to improve the taste by diluting the medicine (if possible) or by offering chewing gum or hard candy immediately after the medicine.

If an injection is likely to sting or hurt, it is honest to tell the client beforehand. The client who is told is also more likely to deal with the pain more effectively than one who is not told. It is better to tell a child just before the injection rather than much beforehand, so that there is little time for the child to anticipate and grow anxious, thereby actually increasing the pain.

The route of administration of a drug is determined by its physical and chemical properties, the condition or status of the client, the desired action of the drug, its speed of absorption, and the rapidity of response desired. As a rule, drugs are administered for either local or systemic effects (see Chapter 5). Some drugs given locally may produce both local and systemic effects if the are partly or entirely absorbed; some drugs are applied for local absorption yet are targeted solely for systemic effect, such as nitroglycerin, ointment hormones, and scopolamine. There has been an increasing awareness that many more substances are absorbed through the skin than was previously believed. Toxic incidents in infants exposed to topically applied dermal medication are increasing. Some of these drugs are boric acid, iodides, hexachlorophene, corticosteroids, and rubbing alcohol. Care is advised in use of any topically applied drug on infants' skin. Yet a drug may be injected into a joint cavity and have little or no effect beyond the tissues of that structure.

Administration for Local Effects

Application to skin. Medications are applied to the skin primarily for the following effects:

1. *Astringent:* resulting in vasoconstriction, tissue contraction, and decreased secretions and sensitivity, thereby counteracting inflammatory effects

2. *Antiseptic* or *bacteriostatic:* to inhibit growth and development of microorganisms
3. *Emollient:* for a soothing and softening effect to overcome dryness and hardness
4. *Cleansing:* for the removal of dirt, debris, secretions, or crusts

These medications may be applied in the form of a lotion, tincture, ointment or cream, foam, wet dressing, tampon, bath, or soak. The effectiveness of medicinals applied to the skin for local effect is limited by the fact that highly specialized layers of skin resist penetration of many (but not all) foreign substances to protect the internal body environment. Topical absorption is increased when the skin is thin or macerated, when there is increased drug concentration, when there is prolonged contact of the drug with the skin, or when the drug is combined with a solvent-penetrant (e.g., dimethyl sulfoxide [DMSO] and acyclovir are under study for topical use in this way). See information, presented in Chapter 8, on topical drugs and the instillation of eyedrops and eardrops.

Application to mucous membranes. Drugs are well absorbed across mucosal surfaces, and therapeutic effects are easily obtained. However, mucous membranes are highly selective in their absorptive capacity and vary in sensitivity. To produce the same effects, a drug applied to oral (buccal or sublingual) mucosa may be twice as concentrated as that applied to nasal mucosa, while its concentration may be reduced one fourth to one half for application to delicate membranes of the eye or urethra. Aqueous solutions are quickly absorbed from mucous membranes, whereas oily liquids are not. Oily preparations should not be applied to nasal or respiratory mucosa by sprays or nebulae, since the droplets of oil may be carried to terminal portions of the respiratory tract and retained there, causing lipoid pneumonia.

Respiratory mucosa may be medicated by means of inhalation or insufflation. The **inhalation** method utilizes sprays or nebulae, whereby the drug is sprayed into the throat by a nebulizer; aerosols are delivered by a flow of air or oxygen under pressure to disperse the drug throughout the lower respiratory tract. In the **insufflation** method a fine powder is blown or sprayed onto nasal mucosa. Drugs so administered tend to have both a local respiratory and a systemic effect. The respiratory mucosa offers an enormous surface of absorbing epithelium. If the drug is volatile and chemically absorbable, and if there is more in the inspired air than in the blood, the drug is instantaneously absorbed. This fact is of significance in emergencies. Amyl nitrite, oxygen, and carbon dioxide are examples of volatile and gaseous agents that are given by inhalation.

Drugs in suppository form can be used for their local effects on the mucous membranes of the vagina, urethra, or rectum. Packs and tampons may be impregnated with a drug and placed in a body cavity; these are used particularly in the nose, ears, and vagina. Drugs may also be painted or swabbed on a mucosal surface, instilled (e.g., a vaginal douche), or administered via irrigation or injection (such as intralesional injection for psoriasis or local intraarterial injection for cancer).

Administration for Systemic Effects

Drugs that produce a systemic effect must be absorbed into the bloodstream and carried to the cells or tissues capable of responding to them. The route of administration used depends on the nature and amount of drug to be given, the desired rapidity of effect, and the general condition of the patient. Routes selected for systemic effect include the following: skin, oral, sublingual, rectal, and parenteral (injection). Routes of parenteral administration include the intradermal (or intracutaneous), subcutaneous, intramuscular, intravenous, intraspinal (or intrathecal), and sometimes intracardiac, intrapericardial, intraosseous, and intraperitoneal.

Oral administration. Oral administration is the safest, most economical, and most convenient way of giving medicines. Therefore it is the preferred route unless some distinct advantage is to be gained by using another way. Most drugs are absorbed from the small intestine; only a few are absorbed from the stomach and colon. This explains the ineffectiveness of cathartics and enemas in the attempt to remove most toxins and overdoses in cases of poisoning.

Following oral administration, drug effects are *slower* in onset and *more prolonged* but *less potent* than when drugs are given parenterally. Thus when a steady-state in pharmacokinetics is desired it is often more closely approached with oral than with parenteral administration. When rapid, high dosages are needed as loading doses or in emergencies, the parenteral route may be used. Strategies for wise pain care, if carefully tailored to individual needs, can exploit these characteristics of oral and parenteral routes for analgesics. For the client in low-level or chronic pain, the oral route for analgesics can be more successful than other routes in promoting a steady state (fewer oscillations) in pain relief. Acute pain may submit to an initial dose of analgesic by the parenteral route, followed by oral doses. Altered effects from oral administration may result from (1) variation in absorption as a result of drug composition, gastric or intestinal pH and motility, food content, or a pathologic condition within the gastrointestinal tract or (2) alteration of the drug resulting from its retention, inactivation, or partial destruction by the liver if the drug traverses the hepatic circulation before entering the general circulation.

Disadvantages of oral administration of certain drugs are that (1) they may have an objectionable odor or taste or be bulky to swallow, (2) they may harm or discolor the teeth, (3) they may irritate the gastric mucosa, causing nausea and vomiting, (4) they may be aspirated by a seriously ill or uncooperative individual, (5) they may be destroyed by digestive enzymes, and (6) they may be inappropriate for some patients, such as those who must be given nothing by mouth.

Sublingual administration. Drugs given sublingually are placed under the tongue, where they should be retained until dissolved and absorbed. The thin epithelium and rich network of capillaries on the underside of the tongue permit both rapid absorption and rapid drug action. In addition, there is greater potency than with oral administration, since the drug gains access to the general circulation without traversing the liver or being affected by gastric and intestinal enzymes. Many of the same effects apply also to *buccal* administration, whereby a tablet is held in the mouth in the pocket between gums and cheek for local dissolution and absorption.

The number of drugs that can be given sublingually is limited (e.g., nitroglycerin tablets). The drug must dissolve readily, and the client must be able to cooperate; the client must understand that the drug is not to be swallowed and that taking a drink must be avoided until the drug has been absorbed. However, usually little harm is done if a sublingual drug is inadvertently swallowed; effects may be neutralized or delayed slightly.

Rectal administration. Rectal administration of certain preparations can be used advantageously when the stomach is nonretentive or traumatized, when the medicine has an objectionable taste or odor, or when it can be changed by digestive enzymes. It is also a reasonably convenient and safe method of giving drugs when the oral method is unsuitable, as when the individual is either a small child (or infant) or is unconscious.

Use of the rectal route avoids irritation of the upper gastrointestinal tract (however, aminophylline suppositories often irritate the rectal mucosa) and may promote higher bloodstream drug titers because venous blood from the lower part of the rectum does not traverse the liver. The suppository as a drug vehicle is often superior to the retention enema because the drug is released at a slow but steady rate to ensure a protracted effect. One disadvantage of the retention enema is unpredictable retention of the drug; another is that some of the fluid may pass above the lower rectum and be absorbed into the portal circulation. An evacuant enema before administration of rectal medication is usually advisable. The amount of solution that can be given rectally is usually small.

Parenteral administration. Strictly speaking, parenteral administration means administration by any route other than oral; thus technically it could be defined to include topical or inhalation administration. In practical usage, however, parenteral usually means administration by the use of a needle (see Table 6-5).

Parenteral administration of drugs includes all forms of drug injection into body tissues or fluids using a syringe and needle or catheter and container (Figures 6-6 and 6-7). Drugs given parenterally must be sterile, readily soluble and absorbable, and relatively nonirritating. Since parenteral administration of drugs can be hazardous, precautions are required: (1) aseptic technique must be used to avoid infection and (2) accurate drug dosage, proper rate of injection, and proper site of injection are essential to avoid harm such as **lipodystrophy** (atrophy or hypertrophy of subcutaneous fat tissue), abscesses, necrosis, skin slough, nerve injuries, prolonged pain, or periostitis. *An injected drug is irretrievable,* and an error in dosage or method or site of injection is not easily corrected.

With drugs given parenterally (as compared with orally), (1) the onset of drug action is more rapid (except as noted previously), (2) the dosage is often similar, since drug potency remains unaltered, and (3) the cost of drug therapy may be greater. Parenteral administration of drugs requires specialized knowledge, aseptic technique, and manual skill to ensure safety and therapeutic effectiveness. Most methods of parenteral administration may be performed by the nurse, but some are usually done only by a physician. The nurse should know and adhere to agency policy. Clients and family members may also learn to administer injections.

Intradermal. Intradermal or intracutaneous injection means that the injection is made into the upper layers of the skin almost parallel to the skin surface (Figure 6-8). The amount of drug given is small, and absorption is slow. This method is used to advantage in testing for allergic reactions and for giving small amounts of a local anesthetic. In a test for allergic reactions, minute amounts of the solution to be tested are injected just under the outer layers of the skin. The medial surface of the forearm and the skin of the back are the sites frequently used. These injections are best made with a fine, short needle (26 or 27 gauge) and a small-barrel syringe (such as a tuberculin syringe) (Figure 6-9).

Subcutaneous (SC). Small amounts of drug in solution are given subcutaneously usually by means of a 25-gauge (or thinner) needle and syringe. The needle is inserted through the skin with a quick movement, but the injection is made slowly and steadily (Figure 6-10). The nurse should slightly withdraw the plunger of the syringe before injecting the drug, to make sure that a blood vessel has not been entered. The angle of insertion should usually be 45 to 60 degrees (but can be any angle from 30 to 90 degrees, depending on needle length and depth of fat pads), and insertion should be made on the fat pads of the abdomen, the outer surface of the upper arm, or the anterior surface of the thigh, or occasionally the lower abdominal surface (heparin). In these locations there are fewer large blood vessels, and sensation is less keen than on the medial surfaces of the extremities. Massage of the part after injection tends to increase the rate of absorption but should be avoided after injection of some drugs, such as heparin, to minimize bruising as the drug spreads through the tissues. Disposable syringes and needles contribute to aseptic safety of the procedure but also to cost and problems of storage and disposal. Subcutaneously injected medicines are limited to drugs that are highly soluble and nonirritating and to solutions of limited volume (ideally no more than 1 ml).

Irritating drugs given subcutaneously can result in the formation of sterile abscesses and necrotic tissue, espe-cially if injections are made repeatedly in the same site. Care should be exercised to avoid contamination and to rotate sites. Subcutaneous injections are not effective in individuals with sluggish peripheral circulation (i.e., the client in shock).

The introduction of large amounts of solution (500 to 1000 ml in adults) into subcutaneous tissues is known as **hypodermoclysis.** Isotonic solutions of sodium chloride or glucose are administered this way. The needle is

TABLE 6-5　Suggested Injection Guides

Route	Common areas	Region	Needle sizes*	Volume injected (ml)		Examples of medications by this route
				Average	Range†	
Intradermal (intracutaneous)	Skin (corium)	Inner aspect of mid forearm or scapula	26 or 27 gauge × ³⁄₈ in	0.1	0.01 to 1.0	Tuberculin, allergens, local anesthetics
Subcutaneous	Beneath the skin	Lateral upper arms; thighs; abdominal fat pads except the 1-in area around umbilicus and tissue over bone; upper back; upper hips	25 to 27 gauge × ½ to ⅝ in‡	0.5	0.5 to 1.5	Epinephrine (non-oily), insulin, some narcotics, tetanus toxoid, vaccines, vitamin B_{12}, heparin
Intramuscular	Gluteus medius	Dorsogluteal	20 to 23 gauge × 1½ to 3 in‡	2 to 4	1 to 5	Most intramuscular and Z-track injections
	Gluteus minimus	Ventrogluteal	20 to 23 gauge × 1½ to 3 in‡	1 to 4	1 to 5	All intramuscular medications
	Vastus lateralis	Anterolateral midthigh	22 to 25 gauge × ⅝ to 1 in‡	1 to 4	1 to 5	Almost all intramuscular medications
	Deltoid	Upper arm below shoulder	23 to 25 gauge × ⅝ to 1 in‡	0.5	0.5 to 2	Vaccines, absorbed tetanus toxoid, most narcotics, epinephrine, sedatives, vitamin B_{12}, lidocaine
Intravenous bolus	Cephalic and basilic veins	Dorsum of hand and forearm; antecubital fossa	18 to 23 gauge × 1 to 1½ in	1 to 10	0.5 to 50 (or more by continuous infusion)	Antibiotics, vitamins, fluids and electrolytes, antineoplastics, vasopressors, corticosteroids, aminophylline, blood products

Modified from Newton, M., and D.W.: Guidelines for handling drug errors, Nursing '79 9(7):18, 1979.

*Needles used for withdrawing medication from a container should be changed before injecting medication drawn (1) from ampules, because irritating medication may cling to needle (filter-needles should be used to withdraw medication from ampules) and (2) from vials, because needles are dulled after insertion through rubber tops; disposable needles are thus labeled "for one-time use only."

†Administration of the largest volumes listed here should be avoided if possible by dividing the dose and using different sites or by using another route in consultation with prescriber.

‡See text for discussion of factors influencing choice of needle length.

longer than that used for a regular subcutaneous injection, and it is inserted into areas of loose connective tissue such as that under the breasts, in the upper surfaces of the thighs, and in the subscapular region of the back. Fluids must be given slowly to avoid overdistention of the tissues. Hyaluronidase is sometimes added to the solution to facilitate the spread and absorption of fluid by decreasing the viscosity of the ground substance in connective tissues. Most prescribers prefer IV infusion of fluids to hypodermoclysis because the amount of absorption is more readily determined.

Intramuscular (IM). Deeper injections are made into muscular tissue, through the skin and subcutaneous tissue, when a drug is too irritating to be given subcutaneously. Irritation may also occur with some drugs given intramuscularly, however. Larger doses can be given by intramuscular injection — up to 5 ml — than by subcutaneous injection. SC or IM absorption is delayed in circulatory collapse (i.e., shock states); the IV route is then chosen.

A drug may be given intramuscularly in an aqueous solution, an aqueous suspension, or a solution or suspension of oil. Suspensions form a depot of drug in the tissue, and slow, gradual absorption usually results. Two disadvantages are sometimes encountered when preparations in oil are used: the patient may be sensitive to the oil, or the oil may not be absorbed. In the latter case, incision and drainage of the oil may be necessary. Few drugs are formulated in oil.

Criteria for selection of a safe intramuscular injection site include distance from large, vulnerable nerves, bones, and blood vessels and from bruised, scarred, or swollen previous injection or infusion sites. The type of needle used for IM injection depends on the site of the injection, the condition of the tissues, the size of the client, and the nature of the drug to be injected. Needles from 1 to 1½ inches in length are common. The usual gauge is 21 to 23 *(the larger the number, the finer the*

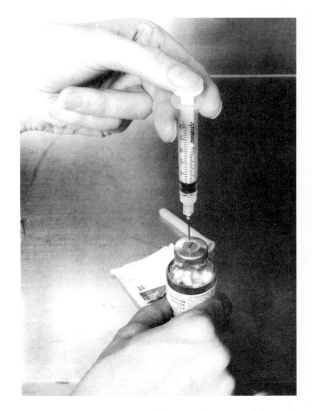

FIGURE 6-7 Withdrawing medication from a rubber-topped vial. To prevent a vacuum the vial is inverted to inject a volume of air equivalent to the volume of medication to be withdrawn. If a large amount is to be withdrawn, it may be necessary (in order to be able to continue to withdraw the liquid) to alternate actions (while the needle remains inserted) of instilling air and withdrawing medication. Another method is to use a second needle as an airway in the vial top, maintaining the tip of the medication needle within the liquid; otherwise, only air will be drawn up. Current literature is equivocal about the procedure of drawing an additional 0.1 to 0.3 ml bubble of air into the syringe after the precise medication dosage has been drawn up. This bubble will rise to the top of the medication dose in the syringe when injected to form an absorbable plug so that irritating medication will not back up the skin track made by the needle.

(From Potter, P., and Perry, A.: Fundamentals of nursing: concepts, theory, and practice, St. Louis, 1985, The C.V. Mosby Co.)

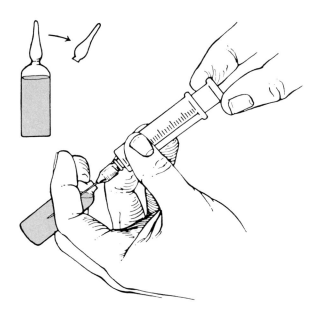

FIGURE 6-6 Withdrawing medication from an ampule. The ampule on the left will break easily when pressure is exerted at the constricted portion. An ampule may be made so that a metal file must be used at the neck to secure a clean break. A filter needle should be used to withdraw medication; glass particles might otherwise be drawn up. An in-line tubing filter may also be used for intravenous infusions.

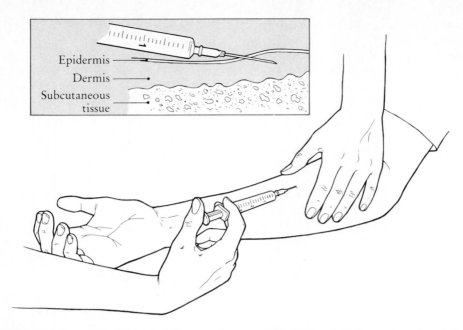

FIGURE 6-8　Intradermal injection. The needle penetrates epidermis and goes into dermis but not subcutaneous tissue. (Note that the skin is not pinched up.)

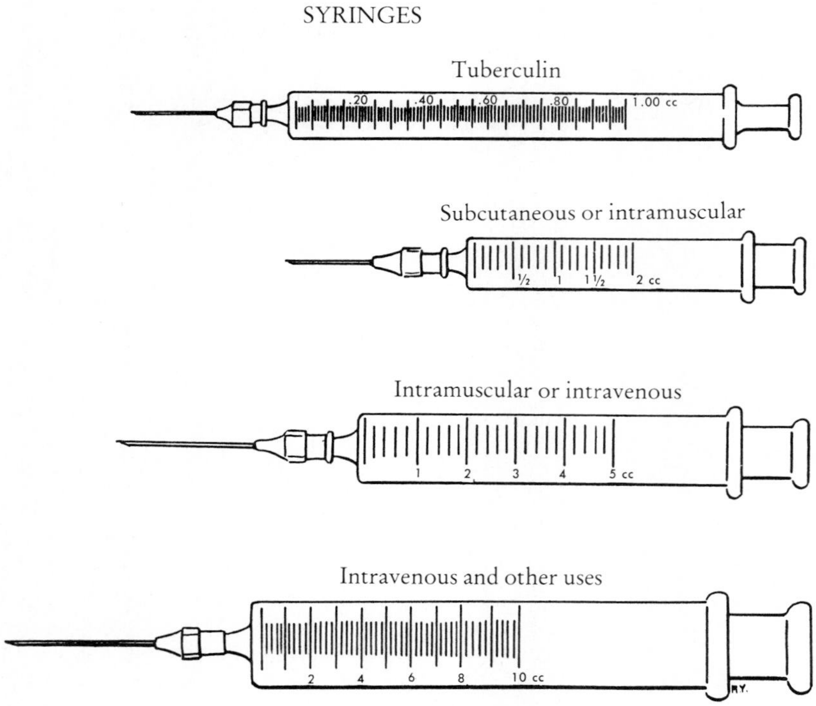

SYRINGES

Tuberculin

Subcutaneous or intramuscular

Intramuscular or intravenous

Intravenous and other uses

FIGURE 6-9　These syringes are used to accurately measure varying amounts of liquids and liquid medications. The uppermost syringe is known as a tuberculin syringe and is graduated in 0.01 cc (ml). It is a syringe of choice for administration of very small amounts. The 2 cc syringe is the one commonly used to give a drug subcutaneously or intramuscularly. It is graduated in 0.1 cc. The larger syringes are used when a larger volume of drug is to be administered intramuscularly or intravenously; for withdrawing blood for laboratory testing; or for obtaining urine specimens from urinary catheters (20 cc syringes may be preferred for the last two uses). These syringes and needles are not drawn to scale (e.g., the tuberculin syringe is much thinner and shorter than the others).

needle). Fine needles can be used for thin solutions and heavier needles for suspensions and oils. Needles for injection into the deltoid area should be ⅝ to 1 inch in length, the gauge again depending on the material to be injected. The deltoid can readily absorb up to 2 ml of

drug. For many IM injections the gluteals are preferred because of fewer nerve endings and less discomfort at this site. The needle must be long enough to avoid depositing the solution of drug into the subcutaneous or fatty tissue. The depth of insertion depends on the amount of subcu-

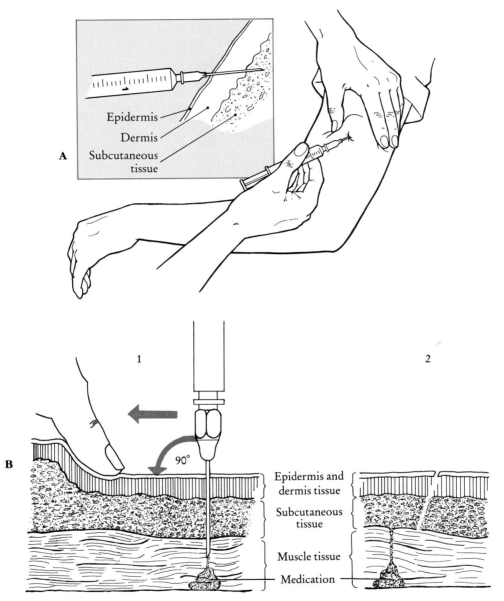

FIGURE 6-10   A, Subcutaneous injection. The skin surface has been cleansed, and the syringe is held at the angle at which the needle will penetrate subcutaneous tissue. The left hand is used to pinch the arm gently but firmly. When the needle has been inserted into the subcutaneous tissue, the tissue of the arm is released and the solution is steadily injected. Based on the patient's condition or the medication to be injected, nursing judgment may dictate a different angle or an approach different from pinching up the skin. **B,** Z-track intramuscular injection method, which is useful for administration of medication known to cause pain or permanent staining of superficial tissues. *1,* The skin is stretched to one side and medication injected as usual, perpendicular to the skin surface. *2,* Needle is then removed and the skin allowed to return to resting position, sealing off the deposited medication from the track made by the needle. The site is not massaged in this method.

taneous tissue and will vary with the weight of the patient. (See Nursing Considerations for discussion of needle and syringe selection.)

It is essential to locate the appropriate landmarks to delimit the areas safe for injections (Table 6-4 and Figure 6-11). IM injections may be given into such clearly defined areas of musculature as the gluteal region of the lower back (provides slowest absorption), the deltoid area, and the anterolateral thigh. At first it seems to most nursing students that the fleshy part of the buttock is a logical intramuscular site. It is not, since underneath, centrally, and running diagonally is the sciatic nerve, which if damaged can result in permanent leg paralysis. Every attempt must be made to avoid this area.

There are now two acceptable ways to map appropriate IM sites in the gluteal region. The formerly used method of dividing the gluteus medius into imaginary quadrants and injecting into the upper outer quadrant is out of favor because it does not necessarily prevent an injection into the sciatic nerve, especially if its course runs abnormally in an individual.

The nurse can best locate the *dorsogluteal site* (the muscle underneath is the gluteus medius) by asking the client to lie face down and exposing the entire area so that the landmarks and injection site can be clearly located. The proper site for this injection is outlined by an imaginary diagonal line drawn from the area of the greater trochanter of the femur to the posterior iliac spine. The injection should be given at any point between that imaginary straight line and below the curve of the iliac crest (hipbone) (see Figure 6-11, *A*).

The *ventrogluteal site* can be made accessible with the patient in a supine, prone (which is awkward), or side-lying position. This site is used for IM injections in either children or adults and could be used more often than it is. To locate it on the left side, the nurse should palpate for the left greater trochanter with the right palm, point the right index finger to the anterior superior iliac spine, and extend the middle finger toward the iliac crest. The injection should be made into the center of the V formed between the index and middle fingers (see Figure 6-11 *B*). The left hand is likewise used to detect landmarks in the right hip.

Either of the two gluteal sites is preferred for the Z-track method.

The *mid-deltoid area* is the muscular area in the arm formed by the rectangle bounded on the top by the edge of the shoulder and on the bottom by the beginning of the axilla (see Figure 6-11, *D*). The deltoid muscle has a considerably higher blood flow than the other IM injection sites and, for rapid onset, is the area of choice for many small-volume (2 ml or less) medications.

The *vastus lateralis* is a muscular area in the upper outer leg. The potential area for injection is a long rectangular area just lateral to the frontal plane of the thigh. Its top boundary is found about one handsbreadth below the greater trochanter, and the bottom boundary is about one handsbreadth above the knee (see Figure 6-11, *C*). This area can accommodate volumes of medication the same size as the gluteus medius and is distant from any major blood vessels or nerves, but injection here may be more painful than in the buttocks.

Relaxation and comfort may be enhanced during an IM injection into the gluteal muscles if the client lies in a prone position with a pillow under the legs just below the knees, and in a toes-in position (to relax the buttocks). The side-lying position is an alternative. To prevent local postinjection complications (such as discomfort, scars, abscesses), no two injections should be made in the same spot during a course of treatment.

For the IM injection, the needle and syringe assembly is held as if it were a dart while the other hand stretches taut the skin of the injection site. The nurse can test sensitivity of the area by tapping it with the fingers. If the muscle mass underlying the injection site is inadequate to accommodate the length of the needle, the flesh may instead be pinched up before needle insertion. The injection should be made *perpendicular to the skin surface,* from a distance of about 2 inches, in one quick motion. If possible, the needle should not be inserted to its full depth and a small portion of needle should be left accessible above the skin so that the needle might be retrieved should it break, a very rare event. It is necessary to make certain that the needle is not in a blood vessel, thus causing the unintended deposit of medication into the bloodstream instead of muscle tissue (also very unusual). This is ascertained by pulling out the plunger *slightly* after the needle is in place in tissue (termed "aspiration"). A slight pinkish tinge to the medication may be seen close to the needle hub, or a small amount of blood may enter the barrel of the syringe, if the needle is in a blood vessel rather than in tissue. If this is the case, needle and medication-filled syringe should be withdrawn and discarded before continuing. In certain instances injection of oily or particulate medicines or killed bacteria by such an inadvertent IV administration could result in a serious emergency.

Contrary to popular belief, needle puncture of the skin is not always the prime source of discomfort associated with injections, although a dull needle such as one inserted through a vial's rubber stopper will certainly contribute to pain. Also, it is not the length of the needle that causes pain, but the diameter; a 3-inch needle will hurt no more than a ⅝-inch one if the diameter is similar. Except for the psychologic aspect of anxiety about needles, most injection pain is thought to occur from stretching of tissue (pain receptors in the skin) as it accommodates the volume of the drug; from irritation from the drug itself; from unsteadiness in the injector's technique, which results in jiggling of the needle during overly slow insertions; during aspiration; while the injector is reaching for the antiseptic swab at completion; or from wet antiseptic on the skin during insertion. Firm pressure applied to the needle-tissue juncture with an antiseptic swab will prevent discomfort as the needle is withdrawn. Massaging the site (except after heparin, iron dextran products, and others) acts to disperse the medication and may also reduce any discomfort.

Intravenous (IV). When an immediate effect is desired, when for any reason a drug cannot be injected into other tissues, or when absorption may be inhibited by poor circulation, the drug may be given directly into a vein as an *injection* or as an *infusion.* The technique of this method requires skill and asepsis, and the drug must

be highly soluble and capable of withstanding sterilization. This method is of great value in emergencies. The dose and amount of absorption can be determined with accuracy. However, the rapidity of absorption and the fact that there is no recall once the drug has been given constitute dangers worthy of consideration. From this standpoint it is one of the least safe methods of administration. Precautions must be taken to prevent extravasation of drug or fluids into surrounding tissue **(infiltration).**

In IV **injection** ("IV push") a comparatively small amount of solution (also referred to as a bolus) is given by means of a syringe into IV tubing, into a heparin lock, or directly into a vein over a 1- to 7-minute period. The drug

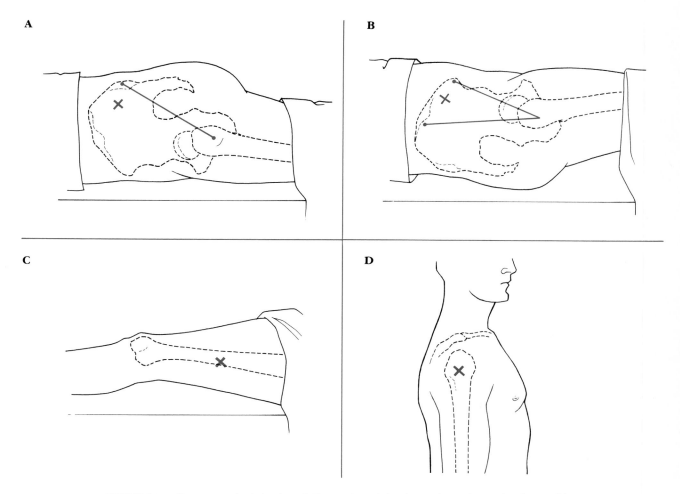

FIGURE 6-11 Intramuscular injection. **A,** Dorsogluteal site, located anterior to the diagonal line from the trochanter to the posterior iliac spine. An injection near the middle of the buttocks may result in an injury to the sciatic nerve. The needle is inserted in with a quick firm movement, entering perpendicular to the skin. After aspiration to make certain the needle is not in a blood vessel, the solution is injected slowly and steadily. **B,** Ventrogluteal intramuscular injection site. The **V** fans out from the greater trochanter between the anterior iliac spine and iliac crest. The injection site (**X**) is centered at the base of the triangle. **C,** Vastus lateralis (midlateral thigh) intramuscular injection site — a handsbreadth below the greater trochanter and a handsbreadth above the knee and halfway between the front and side of the thigh. **D,** Mid-deltoid intramuscular injection site — below the acromion and lateral to the axilla.

is dissolved in a suitable amount of normal (physiologic) saline solution or some other isotonic solution. The injection is usually made into the median basilic or median cephalic vein at the bend of the elbow (Figure 6-12). However, another large accessible vein may be used. Factors that determine the choice of a vein for IV therapy are related to the thickness of the skin over the vein, the closeness of the vein to the surface, the presence of a firm support (bone) under the vein, and the need to use a larger vein for concentrated or irritating substances. The veins in the antecubital fossa are readily accessible, although the veins of the back of the hand are also sometimes used for infusions. Leg veins are avoided because of their potential for phlebitis.

A vein that is normally distended with blood is much easier to enter than a partially collapsed one. A tourniquet is drawn tightly around the extremity proximal to the IV site to distend the vein, the air is expelled from the syringe, and the needle is introduced pointing proximally, bevel up. A few drops of blood aspirated into the syringe indicate that the needle is in the vein; the tourniquet is then removed and the solution injected slowly. As in all types of injections, the needle, syringe, and solution must be sterile; hands must be scrupulously washed, and antiseptic must be applied to the insertion site and allowed to dry. An IV bolus dose is the method of choice for rapidly administering drugs in an emergency because it is a reliable way to achieve optimal drug blood levels rapidly. It is also the way to administer certain IV medications that may be incompatible in solution: digoxin, diazepam, furosemide, diazoxide, certain anticancer drugs, and diagnostic agents in dye form. A 20-gauge needle is commonly used for IV push or bolus doses.

Many drugs given intravenously must be given slowly to avoid cardiac, neurologic, or respiratory changes. Only drugs for which the nurse knows the dosage rate should be given IV, to avoid a potentially fatal problem.

In IV **infusion,** a larger amount of fluid is given, usually starting with 1 L. The solution flows by gravity from a graduated glass bottle or plastic bag through tubing, connecting tip, and needle or catheter into a vein. Or it may be infused with an IV controller or pump.

Infusions are most commonly given to relieve tissue dehydration, to restore depleted blood volume, to dilute toxic substances in the blood and tissue fluids, to supply electrolytes or drugs, to provide an IV line if an emergency is anticipated, or to provide a fluid challenge to evaluate kidney function.

The fluid is usually given slowly to prevent reaction or fluid overload, which may impair cardiac or pulmonary function, especially in elderly clients or those with cardiac disease. Ordinarily 8 hours are required for every 1000 ml of fluid, depending on the condition of the client and the nature of and reason for the solution. For children the rate will be slower and is determined by age, weight, and urinary output.

See Unit 18 for discussion of various IV infusion solutions and parenteral nutrition, and Chapter 29 for discussion of blood products.

A number of commercial solutions are used in IV replacement therapy. Some solutions contain not only salts of sodium and potassium but also salts of calcium

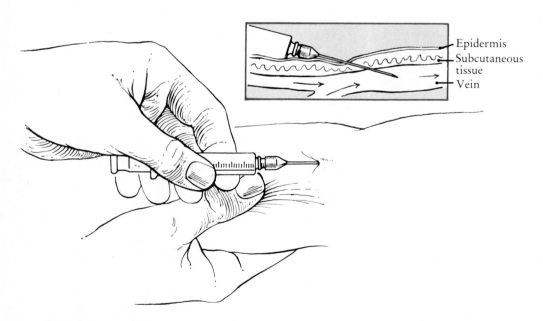

Epidermis
Subcutaneous tissue
Vein

FIGURE 6-12 Intravenous injection. The skin has been cleansed with a solution of alcohol. Thumb of right hand holds the skin taut. Withdrawal of blood indicates needle is in the vein. Solution is injected slowly and steadily.

and magnesium. Vitamins are also added to IV fluids when necessary.

Total parenteral nutrition (TPN) or hyperalimentation is the infusion of an individual's total basic nutritional needs via an infusion catheter into a large central vein and/or into a peripheral one. The choice of site depends partly on the phlebitis-causing potential of the medium. Fat emulsions have a much lower potential for causing phlebitis than hypertonic dextrose solutions used for TPN.

Whole blood and blood products are likewise given intravenously to restore depleted blood volume as well as constituents of the blood. Blood products should be introduced through IV tubing that has been primed with a normal saline infusion solution rather than dextrose solution, which would cause "stickiness" of red blood cells, causing them to clump artificially, possibly clogging the needle or causing hemolysis. Insertion of an 18-gauge or larger needle when blood products are expected to be infused will help minimize trauma to cells. Tubing should also be of the sort that incorporates a filter to trap cell particles and clumped cells to prevent them from circulating or clogging the needle.

Some drugs, such as antibiotics, are administered by **intermittent infusion** (known as "IV piggyback" [IVPB] or "IV rider" in some parts of the United States). They are given via a setup that is secondary to the primary IV infusion and that is hung in tandem and connected to the primary setup.

Most intermittent diluted drug infusions are meant to have a total infusion time of 20 or 30 minutes to 1 hour, depending on factors such as package insert instructions related to the amount of diluent required and the potential for vein wall irritation by the drug. Again, references for more detailed information can be found at the end of this chapter.

Particulate matter (which can consist of tiny chunks of rubber stoppers or glass slivers from ampules) in IV infusion solutions is disturbingly common. It can be introduced during manufacture, during changing of the solution bottle, or during administration of a medication. One study showed that all twelve antibiotic injectables tested contained extraneous particles. The resulting potential for phlebitis is high. It is recommended that in-line filtering devices be used for all IV therapy. Optimal filtration is provided by 0.22-μm filters; most organisms, except certain strains of *Pseudomonas* and the viruses, are filterd out by 0.45-μm in-line filters. To prevent injection of larger particles, disposable needles with 5-μm filters can be used to draw medication up.

Stainless steel scalp-vein needles ("butterfly needles") (Figure 6-13, *A*) produce lower rates of infection and phlebitis, but plastic catheters (over-needle catheters; Figure 6-13, *B*) or cannulaes (through-the-needle catheters; Figure 6-13, *C*) tend to decrease the incidence of infiltra-

tion and work best when an infusion needle will be in place for a long period. Advantages and disadvantages must be weighed at the time of insertion. (See Table 6-6.)

IV devices that are inserted only by a physician are the subclavian through-the-needle catheter and the Hickman catheter. The subclavian through-the-needle catheter (12 inches or 30 cm) is used when poor venous access prohibits the use of peripheral veins or when irritating solutions must be infused directly into a large central vein to avoid phlebitis. The Hickman catheter is implanted surgically and is utilized for long-term IV therapy.

Although starting infusions and drawing blood were traditionally the duty of physicians, many nurses today perform these functions, especially in critical care areas. Probably one of the most effective approaches is the preparation of IV teams whose sole job is to maintain, remove, and replace IV needles, catheters, and so forth. However, such teams may prove to be a mixed blessing; even though they become very proficient at their job, they also may serve to further fragment a client's care.

Table 6-7 lists data to assess for IV needle site complications and suggests concomitant nursing interventions.

Intrathecal. Intrathecal (into a sheath) injection is also known as intraspinal, subdural, subarachnoid, or lumbar injection. The technique is the same as that required for a lumbar puncture. Nurses do not usually directly administer drugs intraspinally. However, the filling of a drug reservoir of an implanted intraspinal delivery system may be required. Special preparation of the nurse is needed, and the manufacturer's instructions should be followed closely.

• • •

In addition, drugs are occasionally administered by intracardiac, intrapericardial, intraperitoneal, and intraosseous injections; however, policy does not usually cover nurses to administer drugs by these routes.

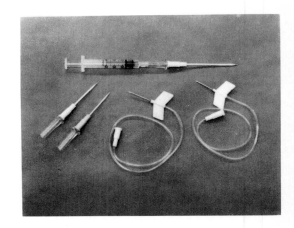

FIGURE 6-13 IV needles.

Psychiatric Clients and Special Situations

Psychiatric clients. Giving medicines to a psychiatric client may assume pronounced symbolic meanings. Meaningful interpersonal relationships are generally found outside medical situations. Psychiatric clients, however, frequently are unable to develop such relationships and look to health care providers for security and affection. Even then, their emotional deprivation may be concealed by an appearance of hostility or disdain.

In addition, immediate personal needs of the client and the current symptoms that the client is experiencing will influence the situation. Overwhelming anxiety, depression to the point of suicide, pain of an uncanny nature, or distortions of thought that constantly separate the client from others demand of the nurse much care in any contact. To the individual in a state of psychologic disequilibrium, that which is taken by mouth or given by injection may hold threats and symbolic meanings rarely noted by other clients. The fear of poisons or supernatural effects of capsules or the suggestions of witchcraft ascribed to a needle often reach a high degree unless the nurse is able to understand the client's concerns and respond appropriately. The psychiatric clients tendency toward impulsiveness and increased emotional sensitivity must constantly be kept in mind. The complexity and subtle implications inherent in administering medications to psychiatric clients make strong and persistent demands on professional nursing awareness, wisdom, and judgment. Although very successfully employed otherwise, nursing aides or mental health aides unlicensed as registered nurses are in a perilously unsafe position if they administer medications to psychiatric clients.

No practical suggestions can take the place of the techniques practiced by the psychiatric nurse, but the following factors should be considered in the general handling of medications for the psychiatric client:

1. Drugs for use in emergencies must be anticipated and readily available.
2. Medicines should be given in paper, not glass, containers. The psychiatric client is often so impulsive that all possible precautions must be taken to avoid accidents, and glass is always a potential suicide weapon.
3. Precautions should be used whenever drugs are administered or stored.
4. *The nurse must remain with the client until oral medications have been swallowed.* This principle is basic in the giving of all medications but of particular importance to the depressed and suicidal client; such individuals may conceal capsules in the mouth for long periods, only to hoard them until a lethal supply has been accumulated. Frequently, measures such as piercing the capsule case and staying with the client until the drug is dissolved or using liquid preparations will ensure the actual ingestion of the drug.
5. It is often necessary not only to urge psychiatric clients to take medication but also to insist on its acceptance. The psychiatric client is frequently an indecisive, emotionally confused individual who tends to doubt everything. These clients often press the nurse for detailed information about a drug prescribed and frequently rebel because of minor discrepancies in information. Paradoxically, however, they comply quickly if a positive yet interested attitude is demonstrated without undue explanation.
6. It is of utmost importance to report all drug refusals to the prescriber in charge. In the meantime it is frequently also important to persuade the client to take the medicine. Omission of doses may cause the blood level of psychotropic drugs to be lowered so that larger doses than usual may eventually be needed. IM administration of psychotropic

TABLE 6-6 Intravenous Needles in Common Use by Nurses

IV needle	Length of needle	Length of tubing	Indication
Wing-tip or scalp-vein needle (E-Z Set or Butterfly)	½ to 1¼ in (1.3 to 3.1 cm)	3 to 12 in (7.5 to 30 cm)	Client in stable condition; IV fluids or medications of short duration; intermittent IV push injections, indefinite period of time
Over-the-needle catheter (Abbocath, Jelco, or Angiocath)	Varies	1¼ to 5½ in (3.1 to 13.8 cm); 1¼ to 2 in (3.1 to 5 cm) most commonly used	Client in unstable condition (needs large volume replacement); only available veins are poor; caustic medications to be administered
Through-the-needle catheter (Intracath)	1½ to 2 in (3.8 to 5 cm)	8 to 36 in (20 to 90 cm)	Client has poor venous access; long-term IV therapy; extremely caustic medications (continous chemotherapy, total parenteral nutrition)

drugs assists in calming the client within a relatively short period of time, so that oral preparations may then be given. The oral route of administration is preferred and should be reinstituted as soon as possible.

Special situations

Swallowing difficulty. The following suggestions are for clients who have difficulty swallowing oral medications. If the cause is a diminished swallow reflex, however, the drug should be given by another route after consultation with the prescriber.

1. Have the client drink some water *just before* taking the medication and drink only a small amount *with* the medication. *Following* the drug, at least 100 ml of liquid should be taken. Clients are capable of taking fluids more easily if they are in Fowler's position (upright sitting position).
2. Instruct the client to place the tablet at the midpoint of the tongue and toss it back to the throat with the water. For the hemiplegic client, place the tablet on the unaffected side of the tongue for swallowing.

If the head is tipped slightly forward, the act of swallowing follows more naturally; choking is more likely when the head is tilted back. Initiation of the mechanical act of swallowing may be facilitated by massaging the laryngeal prominence (Adam's apple) or the area just under the chin.

Medications may be crushed (except enteric-coated or sustained-action forms), or capsules may be opened and contents sprinkled on a small portion of easy-to-swallow food such as applesauce or gelatin desserts. The client should be told about this procedure and instructed to eat the medicated contents first so that very little remains unadministered if the rest is refused. This approach for children should be used cautiously, since the particular food may be rendered distasteful and be rejected by the child in the future.

Medications may be liquefied for drinking by the addition of water, or they may be administered by instillation into the mouth next to the cheek by a large syringe with or without a short tubing attached.

Suggestions for clients with a tracheostomy tube in place. The tube should have a cuff, and it should be inflated whenever any substance is taken by mouth, in order to prevent it from accidentally entering the lungs. If there is an external attachment in place to allow the patient to talk, a T-piece should be substituted. After the medication has been swallowed, the cuff is deflated after suctioning is performed.

Suggestions for administering medications to clients with a nasogastric (NG) or gastrostomy tube

1. Follow the procedure for administering tube feedings, with these additional precautions.
2. Check placement of the tube before giving medications or tube feedings.
3. Give medications and tube feedings at separate intervals in case the stomach contents must be aspirated or the tube irrigated later.
4. Assess for potential drug-food interactions (penicillin G and most tetracyclines) if you must administer drugs with a feeding, just as you would with any oral drugs. See Chapter 3 for cautions about tablet crushing. If appropriate, a paste made with a few drops of mineral oil added to the crushed tablets,

TABLE 6-7   Common Intravenous Needle Site Complications

Needle site data	Infiltration	Clot over needle opening or obstruction	Phlebitis	Infection at site of needle insertion
Color	Pale	No change	Red	Red over site
Temperature	Cool to cold	No change	Warm to hot	Warm at site
Swelling	Rounded	None	Cordlike vein path	Small amount at site
Pain	Yes, usually	None	Yes	None usually
Flow	Slowed or stopped	Slowed or stopped	No change or may be slowed	No change
Nursing actions	Tourniquet proximally (flow continues—infiltration) Lower bottle (blood in tubing—no infiltration) Discontinue IV Call IV team Get order for warm compresses and elevate part	Check for infiltration Resposition arm Raise IV container, close clamp, coil tubing, release quickly Call IV team	Discontinue IV *usually* Call IV team Note irritating solution (Valium, Keflin, KC1 running too fast) Warm compresses; elevate and immobilize part	Do not discontinue IV until IV team advice has been sought or physician has been notified (it may be the only vein available for essential infusion)

then mixed with water and instilled down the tube, is thought to keep the drug from sticking to the tube.

5. Crush and administer the medication first, before the feeding; flush the tubing before and after the medication to prevent the drug from sticking to the inside of the tube.

6. Afterward, position the client upright and turned slightly to the left side if the medication is for local effect in the stomach (e.g., antacids) and should remain there for a time.

Suggestions for rectal administration

1. If the anal area is irritated, or if diarrhea, rectal bleeding, or hemorrhoids are present, request an order for medication by a different route.

2. Make certain that there is no fecal bulk in the rectum to obstruct free flow of the medicated enema or the action of a suppository.

3. Do not divide a dose of a suppository drug form by cutting it (the active drug constituent may not be evenly distributed in the suppository.)

Refrigerated suppositories will soften and cannot be inserted if they are handled or carried in the pocket for even a brief period. Cold running water will restore rigitidy to suppositories. To be retained for effective therapy, suppositories and enema tubing must be inserted beyond the internal anal sphincter (2 to 3 inches).

PREVENTING AND REPORTING ERRORS

It may help to be aware of some of the pitfalls with regard to medication administration. The accompanying box recounts actual errors related to medication administration to call attention to some common but careless nursing acts.

To prevent medication administration errors, the following guidelines should be observed:

1. Question the calculations or order if it appears that multiple tablets or several vials are necessary to prepare a single dose.

2. Carefully read all labels for *all* the "Five Rights," including the drug's name—the pharmacist can make a mistake, too, by sending the wrong medication.

3. Be wary about ambiguous orders or drug names, or drug names that include numerals. Consult with the prescriber if in doubt.

4. Be alert to unusually large dosages or excessive increases in dosages ordered.

5. When in doubt, check the order out with the prescriber, a pharmacist, and the literature. Check even simple calculations with a peer.

6. Double-check with an allergic client about all new drugs as they are added to the treatment plan.

7. Routinely refer to drug interaction charts. Commit common interactive drugs to memory.

8. Question the use of nonstandard abbreviations and symbols; do not use them yourself.

9. Read the package insert carefully for specific instructions when giving a drug for the first time.

10. Do not use slang names or colloquialisms that may be unfamiliar to others.

ERRORS IN MEDICATION ADMINISTRATION

1. Not knowing why a medication was to be administered caused one nurse to irrigate a client's bladder with a topical antiinflammatant, Burow's solution, instead of the genitourinary antibiotic irrigant distributed by a manufacturer of a similar name. This caused another nurse to delay giving a dose of medication essential to recuperation after cancer chemotherapy because she believed it to be "just a vitamin" instead of folinic acid.

2. Not identifying clients by their arm bands caused several nurses to give medication to the wrong individuals in the right beds. One of the nurses even asked a client his name, which turned out to be similar to another client's. One nurse called out her client's name, and the wrong person responded. The result was the same—they all got the wrong medication.

3. Not checking with the prescribing physician caused one nurse to give her patient 30 ml of milk of magnesia every hour rather than every night because she misinterpreted the "qn" (an unacceptable abbreviation) order for "qh". Another nurse gave 2.5 mg of digoxin instead of 0.25 mg; although the order was wrong, the nurse did not recognize that it was excessive. The result was that the client received a toxic dose of medication.

---

11. Do not decipher illegible orders or make assumptions. Do not accept incomplete orders. Obtain a clear copy from the prescriber.

12. Do not accept verbal or telephone orders except in an emergency. Nursing students should refer such requests to other practicing staff nurses.

13. Question a drug form used in an unfamiliar way (e.g., suspensions are usually given orally; an IV drug form ordered to be administered by feeding tube).

14. Question an unusual single order containing more than one drug.

15. Mistakes seem to breed other errors. It is axiomatic that when one thing goes wrong in a client's care, other mishaps follow inexorably. No one knows why.

16. Stay alert! Question! Learn!

In a large Michigan hospital, medication errors accounted for almost 41% of the incidents with potential for a lawsuit. Nursing errors accounted for 65% of these medication errors. Wrong dosage headed the list. Many computer programs for updating dosage calculation skills now exist, and more are on the way. Innumerable helpful instructional materials, including programmed learning texts, are available; some are listed at the end of the chapter. All personnel who, as part of their jobs, must calculate dosages should be alert for gaps in their mathematical competence. To double-check calculations with others when uncertain and to maintain proficiency by practice are practical, professionally necessary actions. This assumes another essential step: that all calculations are *written down* on paper to be checked.

To err is human. However, to admit its possibility and one's susceptibility is essential. To safeguard one's client as well as one's reputation and psyche, the first step in a suspected medication error is to backtrack to double-check one's actions or computations to see if an error occurred. Next is the step requiring the most accountability: to consult one's instructor or superior to inform him or her and to gain perspective and objective support. The client's prescriber should also be informed. Actions to correct drug effects and to normalize the client's condition follow. Precise, objective documentation of the event and the circumstances is made both on the chart and on a special form, the incident report. This report is an intra-agency communication that is analyzed by the agency's risk management personnel to develop procedures for preventing the same or similar incidents.

CLIENT TEACHING

Updating clients and keeping them informed about their treatment and other necessary information should be an ongoing activity that occurs naturally during any interaction with clients. Teaching should be a part of the plan in any nursing process. It may be a formal plan (e.g., a diabetic teaching program), or it may be a simple impromptu discussion based on a question the client raises.

Although teaching-learning interactions between client and nurse are among the most necessary and professionally demanding, teaching clients is not as visible as bathing them, taking their vital signs, or giving them injections. When it is done, it may not be seen as important enough to be noted in nursing progress notes. However, success in client learning has a direct bearing on success in convalescence at home. Strong rationales for teaching clients come from the many state nurse practice acts that define teaching as a necessary part of nursing, thereby giving it the power of a state mandate: one could be sued for not teaching clients. Accreditation committees recognize the importance of client teaching and look for documentation when they visit. Thus the resistance of other disciplines to client teaching by nurses is becoming less of an issue than it was in the past. Studies show that nurses actively engage in discussions about medications: 66% discuss them with physicians at least once a week, and 85% discuss them with clients monthly; 95% of the clients followed nurses' recommendations and passed them along to others.*

Basic to any learning are the following tenets:

1. Clients must be ready to learn. If they are in pain, about to be

*Nursing '84 14(4):17, 1984.

discharged, or emotionally upset, they will be too distracted to assimilate information.
2. The atmosphere must be conducive to learning. Privacy, some quiet, and a rapport between the nurse and the client that is facilitated by understanding of cultural or personal differences all aid the dynamics of learning.
3. Information must be presented at the level of clients' understanding. The nurse should find out what they already know and start from there.
4. Information should be presented beginning with the simple and building to the complex. Too much too fast will overwhelm clients. A good starting place is responding to a client's questions. The goal is to meet the client's learning needs, *not* the nurse's need to teach.
5. Learning and motivation will be enhanced by rewarding positive behavior. For example, relief of pain after clients put into use new learning will be its own reward; sometimes verbal rewards, such as a compliment on performing a procedure well, can be effective motivation.
6. Active participation should be encouraged at each step.
7. Specific feedback from clients is necessary in order to evaluate if learning has taken place. It is not enough just to "tell" clients over and over again. Return demonstration is perhaps the best way to evaluate the degree of success achieved in teaching.

Clients need to learn the following about their medications: the names of the medications (write them down), what they are for and how to recognize the proper effects (in very specific ways), some of the major secondary effects (expected and tolerable, and those representing toxicity), what to do if they miss a dose, how to store the medication, how to take it (e.g., with meals), and whom to call if there is a problem. It can be expected that clients will forget many of the instructions; a printed fact sheet or checklist to take home will be helpful to many clients and should augment the verbal explanation. Chapter 7 discusses essential information the client should know, from a client perspective.

RECORDING DRUG ADMINISTRATION

Recording the administration of each dose of medication as soon as possible after it is given leaves a documented record if there is any question as to whether the client received the dose. Otherwise, the client may inadvertently receive a second dose from another nurse or nursing student. The busy nurse who "double-pours" (prepares two doses at one time—an illegal practice) may also be tempted to record the second dose at the same time the first dose is recorded. Medications should not be recorded (charted) before they are actually given, because something may come up to prevent that dose from being administered. Then the medication record, which is a legal document, will have to be corrected carefully and perhaps an incident report filed.

Several different forms are used to record medications

for each client. These forms usually include areas to note each medication name, date, dose, route, and time, and the administering nurse's initials (see Figure 6-1). Extra notations may be added in certain instances. For example, when digitalis is given, the apical and radial pulses taken just before administration may be noted ("AP, 78; RP, 76"). If the pulses are found to be outside the normal limits established by that agency, the medication should not be given, the record should be marked "held" and initialed, and the prescriber should be consulted. Clients also have the right to refuse treatment, including medications, and sometimes do, despite explanations. "Refused" is then noted in the appropriate spot on the medication record, with the reason for the client's refusal. Medication may also be recorded as "discarded" or "wasted" if only part of it was administered and the rest had to be discarded (as in a prefilled syringe), or if the medication was dropped or contaminated. If the medication is a controlled substance, its disposal must be witnessed and initialed in the special record for this drug.

Routine (or continuous) daily medications usually are recorded on one type of form. Once-only, loading dosages, prn medications, and stat medications should be recorded on the same MAR. Administration of a controlled substance is recorded both on the prn medication sheet and on that particular drug's sheet (which includes a running tally of the balance of the controlled substance). A notation should usually be made, in the progress notes on the clients chart, relating to the assessment of the need for the administration of any prn medication and the client's response to its effects.

Potential for error in drug administration is almost limitless. Some mistakes of significance can be rectified if discovered and acted on quickly. Also, if an error was properly reported and appropriate actions were taken, courts tend to look more kindly on the nurse than if these were not done. Courts generally recognize the humanness of people, including nurses, and recognize the potential for error in clinical practice.

EVALUATION

Evaluation is the completing step in the nursing process, which facilitates the delivery of high-quality nursing care in regard to pharmacotherapeutics. While planning nursing care and establishing goals, the nurse determines what kind of evaluation will take place and when and how it will be done. Clear and specifically stated goals make it easy to determine whether the intended outcomes have been achieved, or the degree of achievement. Evaluation includes both subjective and objective data. When evaluating the nursing care for a patient undergoing drug therapy, the nurse looks at several areas:

1. Therapeutic response to the drug
2. Secondary or unwanted effects

3. Compliance
4. Learning

In evaluating therapeutic response, the nurse must have a clear understanding of the therapeutic goals. Evaluation may center on a reduction of symptoms, decreased frequency of attacks, enhanced organ function, elimination of infection, or a multitude of other goals. Evaluation looks for a drug's therapeutic response, but it is also directed toward detection of *any* response that may be attributed to the drug. An awareness of the pharmacology of the drug used and potential effects guides this evaluation. **Compliance** refers to following the prescribed regimen correctly. In the hospital setting, evaluation may look at nursing care (was the drug administered in the correct dose and at the right time, with appropriate precautions?), while evaluation of outpatients is directed toward the patient. Research indictes that at least one fourth of all outpatients fail to follow prescribed drug therapy correctly. Finally, the nurse will have to determine if educational goals are being met. Often, clients can report back what they have been told, yet be unable to apply this knowledge. Asking hypothetical questions and observing return demonstrations are helpful techniques for evaluation of learning.

SUMMARY OF NURSING CONSIDERATIONS

The implementation phase of the nursing process with regard to drug therapy begins when the nurse takes action to attain the goals established as described in Chapter 5. Nursing interventions are directed at the actual administration of drugs, which includes the preparatory steps as well as the subsequent recording of drug administration.

The traditional Five Rights—to ensure the right client, the right medication, the right route, the right dose, and the right time—are still reliable criteria for competent, safe, and individualized medication administration. So that nurses who are eager to provide high-quality care might have some of their penetrating questions answered, some of the theoretical bases for selection of drug dosages and dosing intervals have been included in this chapter. Examples have been presented of typical kinds of dosage calculations that sometimes challenge nurses, even those who have been practicing for a long time. Answers and explanations have also been included. Common drug routes and sites and some of the newer transdermal and syringe-pump modes have been detailed and illustrated. Specialized and personalized nursing care of the psychiatric client, incorporating basic tenets of comfort, dignity, honesty, and patience when medications are given, has been discussed. Special helps have been presented for medication administration to those with a tracheostomy or nasogastric tube.

Evaluation of nursing functions in medication administration includes a critique of one's own techniques, but it is not limited to that. The environment should be made conducive to high-quality care by the nurse's efforts toward thoughtful and safe medication administration. Enough time must be set aside, and double-checking of calculations should be routine. Careful identification of clients is essential to ensure that the right person receives the medication as intended. Since nurses are in the position of being on the client care scene and taking care of clients as no one else does, they are uniquely placed to detect even subtle secondary drug effects, interactions, or incompatibilities.

Prevention of errors in medication administration is crucially important to nurses, since it is an area fraught with much potential for irreversible harm to patients. Alert attention to all of the details of medication administration, including client comments, must be maintained so that safety is not abridged and clients obtain the most beneficial effects of the drugs they take. Recording a drug dose is the final act of communication; it signifies that the drug was given and assures accountability by the nurse who "signs for it."

In short, the actual act of administering medications—the implementation or intervention phase of the nursing process—demands a solid knowledge base, well-practiced skills, commitment to continuous learning, and intense, unremitting concentration in order to sustain the best interests of the client. Potential for error is rife; medication administration cannot be a casual act or the risk will escalate.

Evaluation of therapeutic effects, secondary effects, compliance with the prescribed regimen, and patient learning follows the implementation phase of the nursing process. It allows the nurse to determine if goals were met and measures the effectiveness of nursing care.

KEY TERMS

apothecary system, page 89
biorhythms, page 86
compliance, page 110
dose-response relationship, page 86
drug potency, page 86
duration of action, page 86
household system, page 89
hypodermoclysis, page 98
infiltration, page 103
infusion, page 104
injection, page 103
infusion controllers, page 87
infusion pumps, page 87
inhalation, page 96
insufflation, page 96
intermittent infusion, page 105
latency, page 86
lipodystrophy, page 97

maximum effect, page 86
metric system, page 89
therapeutic index, page 86
time for maximum effects, page 86
time-response relationship, page 86

BIBLIOGRAPHY

Anderson, K, and Poole, C: Self-administered medication on a postpartum unit, Am J Nurs 83(8):1178, 1983.

Bing, CM, and O'Donnell, J: Check this chart. . . . before infusing two critical care drugs through the same I.V. line, Nursing '84 14(11):50, 1984.

Birdsall, C, and Uretsky, S: How do I administer medication by NG? Am J Nurs 84(10):1259, 1984.

Brown, CS, Wright, RG, and Christinsen, DB: Association between type of medication instruction and patients' knowledge, side effects, and compliance. Hosp Community Psychiatry 38(1):55, 1987.

Chaplin, G, Shull, H, and Welk, PC, III: How safe is the air-bubble technique for I.M. injections? Nursing '85 15(9):59, 1985.

Cheung, P: Learning your tables, Nurs Times 82(42):40, 1986.

Clayton, M: A simple way to calculate IV and IM doses, RN 48(12):41, 1985.

Cluff, LE: Patient compliance: changing patterns of disease and health care costs, Hosp Formul 20:503, 1985.

Cohen, MR: Medication error columns, Nursing '83 to Nursing '87 vols 13-17, 1983-1987.

Cohen, MR: Drug-induced anaphylaxis, Nursing '85 15(2):45, 1985.

Curren, AM: Math for meds: a programmed text, ed 3, 1979, Seal Beach, Calif, Wallcur.

Cushing, M: Drug errors can be bitter pills, Am J Nurs 86(8):895, 1986.

Goodman, LS, and Gilman, A, eds: The pharmacological basis of therapeutics, ed 6, New York, 1986, MacMillan, Inc.

Hansen, MS, and Woods, SL: Nitroglycerin ointment: where and how to apply it, Am J Nurs 80(12):1122, 1980.

Hill, MN: Drug compliance, Nursing '86 16(10):50, 1986.

Hussar, DA: Drug interactions, Nursing '86 16(8):34, 1986.

Keane, CB, and Fletcher, SM: Drugs and solutions, ed 4, Philadelphia, 1980, WB Saunders Co.

McGovern, K: 10 steps for preventing medication errors, Nursing '86 16(12):36, 1986.

Miyares, MU: Medication aids your elderly patients will love, RN 48(11):44, 1985.

Morce, NA: On patients and drug regimes, Am J Nurs 85(1):51, 1985.

Motz-Harding, E and Good, F: The right solution: mixing I.V. drugs thoroughly, Nursing '85 15(2):62, 1985.

National Bureau of Standards, US Department of Commerce: The International System of Units (SI), special pub. no. 330, 1977.

Northrop, CE: Don't overlook discharge teaching about drugs, Nursing '86 16(11):43, 1986.

Pierce, ME: Reporting and following up on medication errors, Nursing '84 14(1):77, 1984.

Potter, PA, and Perry, AG: Fundamentals of nursing, ed 2, St Louis, 1988, The CV Mosby Co.

Wyeth Laboratories: Intramuscular injections.

UNIT III

Biopsychosocial Aspects of Pharmacology

CHAPTER 7

Psychologic and Cultural Aspects of Drug Therapy and Self-Medication

OBJECTIVES

After studying this chapter, the student will be able to:

1. Discuss the influence of culture and psychological beliefs on drug therapy.

2. Discuss on a symbolic level what drugs mean to clients.

3. Identify factors that affect client compliance.

4. Differentiate between the advantages and disadvantages of self-treatment using nonprescription medication.

5. Identify principles used in client education concerning self-administration of nonprescription medications.

Cultural background, ethnic practices, psychological beliefs, and tradition influence both health beliefs and treatment results. Effectively caring for clients from different cultural groups requires an understanding of the predominant ethnic-specific influences and an assessment of the individual client to determine how those cultural influences affect health needs. Since nearly 2,000 cultures and subcultures exist, it is impossible for the nurse to have a working knowledge of all of them. Instead, nurses and other health care professionals should study the predominant cultural groups in their communities. The literature from transcultural nursing and anthropology (see bibliography listing) provides valuable insights into various health care beliefs and practices.

Health beliefs and practices related to pharmacology are evident in all cultures. Some similarities exist in the way the use of drugs is perceived, most often regarding the value that the appropriate use of medications is to reach optimal health. Although most individuals share common views regarding life patterns, significant differences occur in values, beliefs, and attitudes. Clients bring to health settings psychological and cultural differences in perceptions of masculine and feminine roles, in rural and urban backgrounds, in ethnic groups, and in social classes that influence drug usage. To administer medications effectively and to teach clients self-administration requires an understanding of the predominant cultural influences within the community, a knowledge base of the psychologic aspects, and an assessment of the individual client to determine how these influence health needs.

PSYCHOLOGIC ASPECTS OF DRUG THERAPY

Every drug administered to a client has a symbolic meaning and a potential psychologic effect in addition to its pharmacodynamic action. A drug not only alters the function or structure of some part of the body, but it may also influence the behavior, sense of well-being, and mental state of the client. Psychologic responses of clients to symbolism may mimic pharmacologic reactions, adverse effects, or even allergic reactions to drugs. A profound reaction may be observed in clients receiving placebos.

Medications tend to be more effective when individuals believe in their capacity to get well, when they have a strong desire to get well, and when they believe that the health personnel expect the medication to be effective and say so. Clients' past and present conditioning to drugs, illness, hospitals, nurses, and other health personnel as well as their health goals are determinant factors in the response to drugs. Nurses must remember that among the major deterrents to successful drug therapy are divergent goals of the client and the health personnel. An accurate appraisal of the client's goal in seeking health advice and therapy is important to planning and implementing an effective plan of care.

SYMBOLIC MEANING OF DRUGS TO CLIENTS

Medications may be a symbol of *help* to the client. This meaning is strengthened and drug effectiveness enhanced when physicians or nurses suggest to a client that a particular drug will be of benefit or help. Repeated suggestions to the client that the drug is beneficial further reinforce its therapeutic value. This is similar to the relief a mother's kiss gives to her child's pain; the assurance it gives makes the child feel better. Investigation of the effects of drugs on the mind has resulted in the conclusion that some drugs are effective only in the presence of an appropriate mental state.

Drugs may also be viewed as symbols of *danger*. Clients may interpret *cure* as a serious threat to their emotional security if illness is being used to meet a need for dependence. Taking medication may also be objectionable if there is a strong need to exhibit an image of independence; adverse reactions may even result. The client may complain of dry mouth, nausea, vomiting, palpitation, fatigue, and other vague feelings of discomfort. The individual may resist taking the medication, refuse to have the prescription refilled, or even throw the drug away.

Many people have ambivalent feelings about taking medications. An expressed desire to regain health may coexist with an unconscious reluctance to give up the *secondary gains* of the sick role. These gains can include freedom from responsibilities and extra attention. Individuals may report secondary drug effects or find reasons why they cannot take the medication to retain these benefits.

Clients may harbor unsubstantiated notions about medications. Some patients believe a medication is too strong or not needed any longer, and therefore may refuse to take the drug, decrease the amount of drug taken at any one time, or decrease the number of times the drug is taken. This behavior may be suspected when a drug known to be effective for a specific condition is ineffective in a particular client with that condition.

A client who believes the drug is too weak may take the drug too often, request the drug more often than prescribed, increase the amount of drug taken, or continue drug therapy for longer than prescribed. Symptoms of overdosage may then develop.

Some fantasies concerning resistance evolve from fears. Individuals tend to fear radioactive drugs such as ^{32}P or ^{131}I and to fear dependence on drugs that have antidepressant, analgesic, or sedative effects. Although few people today believe in cure-all remedies, some have blind faith in a certain medication and insist on taking it habitually.

Clients who believe they are allergic to a certain drug, for real or imagined reasons, are likely to react with fear or panic when administration of that drug is contemplated. A detailed personal history and (if possible) tests for drug allergy should be used to corroborate or refute the client's belief. Rejection of a client's claim of allergic response without evidence is an unwise assessment of data and negligent, to say the least.

The route of administration of a drug and the financial cost of treatment as well as a client's conscious and unconscious attitudes toward drugs, physicians, nurses, illness, and so on influence the extent, duration, and intensity of the client's response to medication. Studies indicate that when a client is angry, resentful, or hostile, certain medications used in usual doses may not be effective.

A client's illness may affect the emotional response to a drug. When the illness is short, recovery complete, and medical and drug expense not too great, the client tends to have a positive reaction to drugs, hospitals, and health and nursing personnel. Strong negative reactions toward drugs or health personnel result when clients are falsely reassured that they will make a quick and complete recovery, and when drugs are both ineffective and expensive, or symptoms of allergy, side or toxic effects, or overdosage occur. Preparing clients for the realistic limitations of drugs, for side and adverse effects, and for drug expense tends to create reasonable expectations.

In any chronic illness a client may suddenly rebel against ill health and resist therapy with life-sustaining medications. When this occurs, clients may be testing to see if they are really dependent on the drugs, or they may be attempting a real or symbolic act of self-destruction. A stressful event or decision may be the root cause. Support, caring, or objective assistance in coping will be necessary.

To avoid causing the client unnecessary concern or to deflect time-consuming questions, many health care providers are reluctant to present any negative aspects when teaching client's about drugs. A clear, nonthreatening explanation about the purpose of the medication and how it may affect them is the least clients deserve. On the whole, most clients prefer knowing the potential risks of drug therapy; this also tends to increase their participation and to engender trust. Litigation could also ensue if clients suffer harm from unrecognized secondary effects of a drug because they were not informed. The nurse should be aware that some people do not want to know details of their treatment, and some are very suggestible.

It is just as important to *listen intently to what the patient says* about the medication, the feelings associated with it, and the condition for which it has been prescribed. Then the health care provider can begin to see the situation from the client's point of view and develop an understanding of the client's motivation to seek health care. Does the individual see the treated condition as a physical threat? How much of a threat; how susceptible? How much control does the client want to exert over the condition; how probable is it that such control will reduce the threat adequately? Until these concerns and other personal factors are at least briefly explored, the success of treatment is uncertain.

EFFECTS OF DRUGS ON THE MIND

Many common drugs have a secondary effect on the client's mind. Drugs may interfere with judgment, mood, sense of values, motor ability, and coordination. Certain antihistaminics used to treat allergies may decrease alertness and cause drowsiness, depression, and predisposition to accidents. Antihypertensive agents may cause depression. Barbiturates and tranquilizers may induce inattentiveness and confusion and reduce initiative. Drug-induced depression calls for discontinuance or a decreasing dosage of the offending drug. Clients should be watched for self-destructive tendencies, since pharmacologic literature has abundant examples of those with drug-induced depressions who have attempted suicide.

CULTURAL INFLUENCES ON HEALTH CARE

Published anthropologic and transcultural studies have offered nurses extensive information on how to assess cultural factors in their clients. Creative cultural measures for improved therapeutics and comfort are available in numerous books and research articles (Henderson, 1981; Bullough, 1982; Shubin, 1980).

Dr. M.L. Leininger (1978), a nurse-educator credited as the major voice of the transcultural strand in nursing, has suggested asking questions such as the following to assess client's cultural influences: "Could you tell me about yourself and your family?" "How do you keep well?" "What made you become ill?" If the nurse has gained the confidence of the client and family, feelings and beliefs will be more openly discussed. If the nurse treats this information with respect and incorporates some of the important aspects in the nursing care plan, then the client is apt to respond more readily to therapy.

Many cultural groups avoid standard American medicine until either their herbal or home remedies are totally ineffective or they have become acutely ill. Haitian, Hispanic, Cuban, Vietnamese, Samoan, Jamaican, Chinese, American Indian, and other clients generally follow this practice. Nurses should be aware of this reluctance to seek standard medical care. When the need arises, such individuals should be counseled on appropriate methods to use in seeking health care.

In an institutionalized setting, diets palatable and/or acceptable to the individual can be problematic. Many private and some public hospitals have recognized this problem and offer ethnic meals as alternatives to the standard fare. Dietary concerns are also intertwined with cultural beliefs. For example, many ethnic groups (Italian, Mexican, Cuban, and others) believe they need their own cultural foods to help hasten the recovery process. Discussing food preferences and preferred methods of preparation with clients is often very important for the well-being of the client.

The common process of leaving ice water at bedside for the administration of medications is a procedure we take for granted today. Some cultures though, such as the Chinese, Chinese-Americans, and Israelis, believe cold drinks are unhealthy for the sick person and may therefore avoid this fluid intake. This should be discussed with the individual and, if medically acceptable, hot tea or an alternate substitute should be provided.

PLACEBO THERAPY

In the past when a physician had no medicine to offer a client who expected treatment, a "sugar pill," or **placebo**, was given to placate the sick individual. A placebo is any treatment—medication, surgical or diagnostic procedure, or nursing action—that elicits a client's response simply because of its intent rather than its known active properties. A placebo is most often a formulation of a pharmacodynamically inert substance such as lactose or sugar, distilled water, normal saline, or a small dose of an innocuous substance such as a vitamin. In medicine, placebos are employed in one of two ways: in experimental drug studies (e.g., before the drug's approval by the FDA) or, much more rarely, to satisfy a client's unwarranted demand for a particular medication when in the considered judgment of the prescriber withholding a dose will impede psychologic or physical health.

Some documented facts about placebos follow.

- In one large study of placebo effects, 36% of the individuals with 1-day postoperative pain reported satisfactory relief. In another study, half the clients who had had wisdom teeth extracted were given morphine, the other half a saline injection. One third of this placebo group also reported significant pain relief. Thus placebos can work against severe pain in some instances. Furthermore, pain relief with administration of a placebo does not mean the client did not have real pain.

- Placebos may work in some physiologic way even though the ingredients may not be pharmcodynamically active. Objective measures show that placebos can alter gastric peristalsis, cause eosinophilia, increase serum hydrocortisone, decrease serum lipids, and cause anaphylactic reactions and that placebo-induced pain relief can be negated by a narcotic antagonist. Ten percent of clients even report side effects of nausea and vomiting.

- People who have positive responses to placebos are not especially anxious, gullible, or neurotic. They are people who are able to use their mental and physiologic capacity to obtain pain relief from a placebo. Statistically, they are likely to be college graduates with independent, responsible life-styles.

- Of 15 individuals 13 obtained pain relief despite being told outright that they were getting a placebo that had helped other clients. Given the right supportive environment, honesty may still be the best policy.

- A nurse cannot legally administer any drug, even a placebo, without a prescriber's order.

Although giving a placebo can, on occasion, be amazingly effective, it should never be administered lightly. Placebos are usually prescribed for extremely unusual situations where no other course of action seems viable. Because most people respond to honest, straightforward rationales, prescribers who value an open relationship with their clients will not write an order or prescription when it is not warranted, and they will explain the rationale behind their decision. Philosophically, most nurses seem to agree and, if given a choice, choose to administer the ordered placebo only after all other alternatives have been thoroughly explored.

SELF-MEDICATION

Public interest in self-care management is at an all-time high, as exemplified by the numerous self-care books and clinics that now abound. One of the most effective and inexpensive ways to counteract rising health care costs may be through expanded, educated self-care management. Studies show that half the people visiting a general practitioner have already started a self-treatment plan that helps more than 60% of the time. If these people were also helped to learn when to seek medical supervision and how to follow treatment advice wisely, they would have a still better potential for health.

Nurses, with their commitment to collaboration with the client to further health, can educate clients, as can pharmacists, physicians, and many other health care professionals. Consumer information pamphlets abound, even printed by the FDA in large type for the visually impaired, offer valuable advice about drug interactions, health foods, and nonprescription pain relievers.

Development of the science of public health has led to the realization that the state of a nation's health does not depend exclusively on the interplay between professional medical practice on the one hand and bacteria, malignancy, and other causes of disease on the other. The influence on community health of the individual's personal attempts at self-medication or at life-style alterations has frequently been ignored or underestimated.

Drugs sold without prescription can induce sleep or wakefulness, relieve pain or tension, or supply the body with vitamins and minerals. Remedies can be purchased for any part of the body. Sales of prescription and non-prescription (or over-the-counter [OTC]) drugs have established the pharmaceutical industry as a continually growing multi-billion dollar industry. Concern over the use of home remedies and self-medication is not new, but rather continues to be a controversial subject.

The practice of self-medication is based on the tradition of folk remedies. Before medicine became as sophisticated as it is today, home remedies were as successful as the contents of the doctor's little black bag.

SELF-ADMINISTRATION OF PRESCRIPTION DRUGS

Purchasing drugs. People who are 65 years and older have the highest per capita expenditures for prescription drugs. These elderly and the poor are the most likely to need prescription drugs and the least able to pay for them. Nurses are responsible for assessing the client's ability to obtain prescription medications, and, if necessary, referring them to an appropriate community agency whose resources will meet their needs.

Practical information about some prescription drugs is available to consumers via package inserts produced by the pharmaceutical industry or by the American Medical Association. Information includes the drug's purpose, possible side and adverse effects, and the best way to take the drug. Some pharmaceutical industry claims state that this service may add up to 18¢ to the consumer's cost of each prescription.

More than 1000 common drugs are listed annually in the *U.S. Pharmacopeia Dispensing Information (U.S.P.D.I.)*, which is geared partly to inform those who dispense or administer prescription drugs and partly for those who take them. Section II, entitled "Advice to the Patient" offers jargon-free guidelines for safe and informed self-administration of prescription drugs by generic name. The U.S.P.D.I. may be available to the consumer by health practitioners or pharmacists who can reproduce for distribution a limited number of pages from the Advice section.*

Compliance. The word "compliance" means the degree to which clients take medication instructions seriously, concur with them, and follow through. It is a term that can have an offensively controlling ring to it, implying that the prescriber directs the client who must follow those directions. Since compliance is the standard accepted term, it is used here; but "concurrence with therapy" and "adherence to instructions" are synonyms.

Why do clients seek medical care and then not follow through on the suggested medication plan at home? There are many reasons, some personal, some social, some psychological, some cultural. Everyone is a potential "noncomplier," whether intentionally or not. Studies show that 33% to 60% of prescription drugs purchased are never taken completely as directed. In addition, some clients never fill the prescription, most take them at unscheduled times, and many stop taking the medication early.

The consequences include inexplicable medication failures with continuing symptoms or overdoses. Medication not used may be kept and taken inappropriately later when its potency and chemical activities may have changed. Prescribers tend simply to increase the drug dosage or change medications when confronted with apparent medication failures instead of investigating for noncompliance with the therapeutic plan.

The following are examples of situations known to foster **noncompliance.**

1. The client is chronically ill or on prolonged therapy. The symptoms in chronic illness tend to grow worse, then improve in a cyclic fashion. Clients do not often get to see any clear causal relationship

between taking or not taking the prescribed medication methodically and the waxing and waning of symptoms. It has been shown that the routine action of reviewing medications with clients and inquiring how they are taken at home dramatically increases compliance. It should be stressed that medication will have to be taken for the rest of the individual's life and should not be precipitously discontinued.

2. The client is relatively asymptomatic or feels better. Reasons for needing to take the drug completely should be explained. Many people are not aware that organisms mutate, for example; and that to ensure their eradication in the first place, antibiotic medications should be completed as prescribed.

3. The medication is expensive or inconvenient to obtain. Prescription by generic name and explanations may be effective in remotivating the client if this is the problem.

4. The medication instructions are complex and not easily understood. "Take with meals" means twice a day to the person who always skips breakfast, for example. Or it may mean before or after meals for some people. Written instructions with a sample of the drug taped to them help as a reminder when the client is home and has forgotten what was heard in the office or in the hospital when being discharged.

5. The medication is unwieldy to take because the bottle cap is difficult for arthritic hands or there are complicated mixing or measuring directions. Measuring cups or droppers can be offered, and the client can be told that easy-to-remove caps can be requested when the medicine is purchased.

6. The medication tastes unpleasant or must be taken at inconvenient times (during sleep hours, at work) or too many times a day to be feasible. Medication can be mixed with or taken with various liquids that are both pleasant and compatible. Medication prescriptions can often be changed after consultation with the prescriber to higher doses given less frequently or to a sustained-action form if available and if feasible.

7. The therapeutic plan contains many different medications, so the drug-taking schedule is complicated. Occasional systematic review of the medications by the prescriber or the nurse is necessary to see if the client still needs all of them and simplify the care plan. Confrontation of the client's habits is necessary when medication containers remain full when they should be empty. Written schedules with sample drugs attached are helpful. Also small medication boxes with separate compartments for

*The U.S.P.D.I. is available for purchase from: Secretary of the USPC Board of Trustees, 12601 Twinbrook Parkway, Rockville, MD 20852.

each dosing time are available at pharmacies. The nurse may suggest that the client keep the medication near equipment used at a specific time each day (such as a coffee cup or toothbrush).

8. Most people wait more than an hour in the physician's office. Waiting longer than this has been correlated with a distinct drop in following the prescriber's medication instructions. Often the wait is unavoidable, but the situation can be improved if the practitioner is empathic.

9. The client does not understand or accept the illness or disorder, or the explanation of the illness or treatment plan does not fit the client's concepts of illness, health care, or health. Typical of the factors that influence attitudes toward treatment are the extent to which clients believe (a) themselves to be susceptible to the illness, (b) the illness to be serious, and (c) that they will benefit from taking action. *Giving information, therefore, is not the entire answer.* It helps to seek active participation of the client in the health and nursing process and to show interest in and respect for client ideas, feelings, and beliefs.

10. The client and health care practitioners perceive the clients problems or goals in divergent ways, yet do not effectively communicate this.

11. The medication is seen as an artificial additive or contaminant to the body or as a crutch on which dependence should be limited.

12. Side effects are severe or interfere with functioning in daily activities.

13. The client has problems of memory or confusion.

SELF-TREATMENT USING NONPRESCRIPTION DRUGS

Advantages. The individual has a right to practice self-medication. Throughout history the public has searched for medicines to relieve ailments and has tried almost every natural material known in the battle against pain, discomfort, and disease.

That the public is health conscious is evident by the number of OTC and nonprescription drugs available. Many ailments are minor and temporary, and the client wants to eliminate discomfort as quickly as possible. Minor ailments do not always require the expertise of a physician; but because many nonprescription drugs can interact with prescription drugs, it is best to check with a member of the health care team. Minor complaints can be successfully treated by nonphysicians. Indeed, if individuals sought medical advice for every minor ailment (colds, headaches, minor wounds, temporary gastrointestinal upsets, or minor burns), health care providers would be unable to attend to individuals who need professional medical care. However, self-medication, if misused or abused, can be harmful. Risks can be reduced by professionally implemented client teaching.

Disadvantages. Most preparations available before the twentieth century were fairly harmless vegetable concoctions. Modern chemistry and pharmacology produced literally thousands of preparations for self-medication. Some are quite effective for certain minor ailments, some are potentially dangerous, and some are worthless. Americans are generally overmedicated. They have developed a casual attitude toward drug use and believe every discomfort or disorder requires chemical treatment.

Today, OTC drugs can be bought in drugstores, supermarkets, restaurants, and vending machines. Annually, this is a $5 to $6 billion industry. Widespread sales promotion via the media encourages self-medication. Since the hazards are generally insufficiently detailed in advertisements and commercials, persistent abuse of medications and resultant toxic effects are fairly common. Many drugs tested as being harmless can actually cause serious secondary effects. Aspirin may upset the gastrointestinal tract or cause bleeding; one 5-grain aspirin impairs platelet aggregation to some extent for up to 1 week. Serious, complex problems can develop from vitamin and mineral overuse (with vitamin A or D overdosage, for example). Habitual use of certain laxatives may prevent absorption of fat-soluble vitamins or cause colon atony so that the treatment perpetuates constipation. Few established dosage limits exist for the use of OTCs by the pregnant or breast-feeding woman, and effects on the fetus and neonate may be extremely harmful. Therefore *no drug of any sort should be taken by a pregnant or breast-feeding woman until a health care provider is consulted.* Many OTC drugs are intended only for adults, not for children; the dosage should not simply be altered for administration to children. Additionally, *the prescriber should be consulted before the patient takes any drug that may have caused a previous allergic reaction.*

Often, a surprising lack of critical judgment is employed when evaluating a newly marketed drug. Typically there is an initial overreaction, especially to new OTC or well-marketed prescription drug: a "honeymoon phase" occurs when the agent is introduced with fanfare and used and prescribed somewhat casually for a time. Then when longer-term results are apparent and new secondary reactions are discovered, its reputation suffers for a while, and its use may be overcautiously controlled. After another time period, use again builds to a more moderate level as the prescribers and the public recognize that judicious use under specified circumstances is the rational approach.

Habitual self-medication with nonprescription drugs may mask a serious condition, prevent diagnosis, endanger the individual's life, or create long-term, expensive medical problems. Health care providers have an obligation to understand how taking medication "fits" with clients' understandings, attitude, and life-styles. The accompanying box outlines how to understand and explore the risk-benefit ratio when consumers are contemplating the use of nonprescription drugs. An additional factor for consideration is cultural influences on self-medicating behaviors.

CULTURAL INFLUENCES ON SELF-MEDICATING BEHAVIORS

While research on the elderly and on their consumption of nonprescribed medications is limited and in some instances conflicting, a study conducted on the four predominant cultural groups in Miami reported important implications for the nurse and other members of the health care team (Salerno, 1985). The cultural groups studied via a descriptive survey design were Hispanics, Haitians, American blacks, and Caucasian Americans.

This study reviewed the factors influencing the elderly of these groups to choose and use OTC substances. An added feature was the development of a Self-Medicating Behavior Safety Scale (SMBS). This scale was applied to all persons interviewed (110 subjects), and a numerical value for safety was calculated for each client. The pharmacist-investigator reviewed all questionnaires and extracted data to answer the question: "Was there any difference between the cultures for potential for misuse or abuse of OTC medications?"

The following data were extracted from this study:

1. The Haitian elderly reported the highest number of health problems, but the greatest usage of OTC products was reported by the Caucasian subjects. The mean usage per group was Caucasian, 7.4; Black American, 4.4; Haitian, 5.8; and Hispanic, 2.4.

One should be cautious in applying self-reported health information, however. The nurse should be aware of the "yea-saying" tendencies of minority groups when the are asked about their health or health care attitudes, meaning the answer is often an effort to please a member of the dominant group and/or health care provider. This behavior is much greater for minorities of Spanish heritage than for others (Aday, 1980). Scott (1978) reported that the Cuban population seems to be more highly motivated toward preventive medicine and tends to report fewer illnesses than do other minority groups. Lopez-Aquires (1984) advises caution with the use of the traditional measure of self-reported health perception among Hispanics, since their findings indicate that Hispanics significantly underestimate their objective health problems and conditions.

GENERAL BENEFITS AND RISKS OF OVER-THE-COUNTER MEDICATIONS

BENEFITS

Occasional use of certain simple preparations can be highly effective for specified minor, usually self-limiting conditions (Table 7-1).

Cost is low in relation to prescription drugs, and the cost of a physician's visit is eliminated.

The client regains some control over personal health care.

Directions and some possible secondary effects are listed on the label.

Condition is immediately treatable. OTC medications are as accessible as the nearest store supply, and a wait for a physician's appointment is eliminated.

RISKS

Treatment depends on patient judgment in differentiating a minor condition from a major, more complex one and in selecting appropriate medication.

Signs and symptoms of a serious condition may be masked by the medication.

Costs in the long run may be higher if a serious condition progresses while improperly treated.

Substances taken as OTC drugs are not always viewed as "drugs" with potential for harm, and dosing may be exceedingly casual.

RISKS — cont'd

Available combination preparations very often contain useless or harmful stimulants or depressants (caffeine or alcohol) and allergy-producing preservatives in addition to the active ingredient.

Professional advice to integrate the drug into an overall plan (e.g. to prevent interactions) is absent unless all drugs are obtained from one source that keeps a drug profile on clients.

Dosage may be too low to be effective, risking decisions by the client to overdose or delay needed professional treatment.

Many do not read labels, and most label print is too small for easy reading, even with glasses, by those with failing eyesight.

Professional follow-up for other conditions may be avoided unknowingly.

OTC drug self-treatment promotes the idea that there is a "magic bullet" for every ailment, major or minor, and that no discomfort should be tolerated.

OTC drug containers are especially vulnerable to criminal package tampering if they are kept accessible on shelves or are not in tamper-proof containers.

2. The ability to read and understand the label of a typical OTC (generic) cold medicine was tested on all individuals. The findings here were particularly alarming. Over 50% of the subjects could not read or comprehend the package label. Other studies (Knapp and Knapp, 1980; Robinson and Stewart, 1981) reported 33 percent of their subjects also had this problem. This high incidence has explicit implications for all health care personnel working with the elderly. Many geriatric clients may need help in choosing an appropriate OTC medication and with specific instructions concerning the proper way to take the medication.

3. The influencing factors reported to affect their choice of OTC products were significantly different with the four groups. While all relied highly on the suggestions of others, professionals included, the Caucasians reported a high reliance on reading materials, television, radio, and self-knowledge influencing their choice of OTC products. This has been supported by other researchers (Knapp, 1980). American blacks indicated that availability of OTC medications was very important, while the Haitians reported self-knowledge as the most important factor. Nearly all cultural groups utilized drugstores or pharmacies as their primary site to purchase OTC preparations.

4. The most common types of OTC products used by all groups were gastrointestinal (antacids, antidiarrheals and laxatives) and analgesics (aspirin and acetaminophen products). Interestingly, the Caucasian subjects reported a high usage of vitamins while the Haitians reported a high usage of herbals and teas. The latter was not a major report of the other groups. But this finding is not surprising, as Scott (1978) reported that many Haitians self-treat with herbs and home remedies before orthodox health care is sought.

5. Statistics concerning forgetfulness in taking medications was also significant between all four groups. Each group used memory as the most common system used to remember to take medication. The Caucasian group reported they tended to use memory less and relied on special devices or systems to help them remember, yet they had the greatest incidence of forgetting to take their medications.

6. The evaluation of abuse and misuse of nonprescribed medications was largely dependent on the items listed in the Self-Medicating Behavior Safety Scale. While the researchers reported no differences between the four groups studied, the group mean was only 8.4. (The scale ranged from 1 to 15 with 15 (100%) being the highest and safest score possible.) The lowest score for safety, 7.6 (51%) was recorded by the Haitian group, 8.03 by Caucasians, 8.63 by Hispanics, and 10.9 (73%) by black Americans. The overall findings were in the low to low-average range for safety for all four groups.

A review of items #4 and #5 of the SMBS indicated that 56% of all subjects in the study used OTC medications inappropriately. The Caucasian group, at 81% inappropriate usage, was the highest. The latter was mainly demonstrated in inappropriate use of vitamins and health food products, with dosages in excess of U.S. RDAs,* and in some instances, approaching megadosages. Examples quoted from the article (Salerno, 1985) include:

One individual believed all OTC substances were "foods" and she not only consumed large amounts of such products, but also advised all her friends to do the same. Another interviewee reported taking vitamin K tablets to treat "blood spots" or "skin bruises." Many unapproved indications were offered as reasons for consuming nonprescribed substances by all four groups interviewed. Examples included taking vitamin C "to help the eyes" or "whenever it rains"; Milk of Magnesia tablets "whenever dizzy"; Pepto Bismol for "hard stools"; Alka-Seltzer for "throat allergies"; Bufferin for "indigestion or greasy food"; and aspirin "to clean out stomach" or "for heat in the stomach." While some expressions were endemic to a specific culture, the basic need for guidance and valid professional advice was evident.

7. Other potentially dangerous situations noted included a number of drug-drug interactions, such as the frequent use of antacids by clients taking digoxin, cimetidine, tetracycline, or others; the use of OTC sympathomimetics in hypertensive patients; and the use of alcohol by clients taking aspirin, nitrates, antihypertensives, and CNS depressants. Many clients were not aware of the possible interactions or the alternate methods (spacing drugs apart with antacids) employed when using such medications. Foreign drugs were being taken along with American medications, and in several instances, duplicate consumption of the same medications under different names was identified.

Another study performed in California concerned Chinese and Hispanic elders and OTC drug usage. Race was determined to be the important variable in the use of OTC preparations in this project. The Chinese elderly who were interviewed preferred topical preparations to treat pain, while the Hispanic group used mostly internal analgesics. Hispanics used more OTC products than the Chinese, an average of 3.8 to 2, respectively. One reason cited was, perhaps, their broad definition of the term "nerves." Hispanics tend to define nerves as nervousness, anxiety, restlessness, palpitations, high blood pressure and insomnia (Hess, 1986, p. 317). With such a wide variety of illnesses defined as "nerves," the preparations used

*U.S. Recommended Daily Allowances published by FDA (Davidson, 1986).

may also be varied, depending on the person's symptoms and his or her perception of etiology.

Because in China many folk remedies usually consist of a single dose of a liquid preparation, taking tablets or capsules on a regular schedule would perhaps be confusing to the older Chinese client. This may be why this group prefers teas and topical remedies.

The nurse should be aware of possible cultural influences on medicating behaviors of their clients. Such information may be used to guide the nurse to ask the right questions during the initial history, to be aware of possible reasons for noncompliance or lack of adherence to a therapeutic drug regimen, and to help identify specific areas needing additional client teaching.

LEGAL CONTROLS OVER NONPRESCRIPTION DRUGS

Self-treatment with drugs and home remedies has always existed, but legislative controls are relatively recent. Control over nonprescription drugs has steadily increased in Canada, most European countries, and the United States. Drug laws are not intended to restrict arbitrarily the availability of drugs for self-medication but to make drug consumption safer and more effective, reserving legend drugs (those for prescription) for the more sophisticated and more potent formulations or for those with complex instructions. During very recent years there has been a change. The U.S. FDA has approved the change of several prescription drugs (e.g., some low-dose tablet-form bronchodilators and certain topical cortisone preparations) to nonprescription status (Table 7-2).

Many nonprescription drugs have limited potency, whereas prescription agents are considerably stronger. Thus analgesics such as aspirin are available for the relief of minor aches and pains, but agents such as morphine that relieve visceral pain are not available without a prescription. A nonprescription drug, like a prescription drug, must be proved safe and effective in the conditions for which it is recommended. This rule has resulted in the withdrawal of many harmful and ineffective agents from the market. Nonprescription medicines must be safe and effective within a wide range of dosage. This provides wide protection against misuse. Most drugs capable of causing dependence, addiction, or abuse are no longer available across the counter. Many nonprescription drugs

---

CONSUMER EDUCATION TOPICS

1. Awareness that OTC medications are truly drugs, just as are prescription drugs, and deserve the same care in use.
2. Identification of some types of medications that are considered useful for home treatment (see Table 7-1).
3. Advising patient about safety precautions
   a. Choose OTCs that have clear and understandable labels.
   b. Heed instructions and explain warnings on labels—for example, "Do not drive or operate machinery while taking this medication" or "Discontinue use if rapid pulse, dizziness, or blurring of vision occurs" (see Figure 7-1).
   c. Check all medications periodically for expiration dates and for deterioration. Discard outdated or deteriorated medications.
   d. Discard unused portions of drugs and do not share these with friends or family even if they appear to have symptoms like your own. Do not even save them for yourself without asking a prescriber.
   e. Keep all medications out of children's reach, and never refer to medications as "candy" to induce children to take the medication.
   f. Do not take any medication in the dark.
   g. Do not mix medications in one container. Store drugs in the original container with the original label. Keep tightly capped.

   h. If you suspect a mistake or overdose, call your local Poison Control Center, prescriber, or pharmacist. Have the medication container at hand.
   i. Learn both the generic and brand or trade names of prescribed drugs. Learn the appearances of your drugs.
   j. Tell the prescriber and pharmacist about any allergies or other conditions you have as well as any previous unusual reactions, current pregnancy, or if you are breast-feeding.
   k. Take the medication precisely as directed and for the length of time prescribed. Ask the health practitioner or consult the U.S.P.D.I. about what to do if one dose of the medication is omitted. Do not just stop the medication on your own.
4. Instruction that nonprescription drugs do not usually cure a condition but rather just make the symptoms bearable. Treated conditions that persist, recur, or produce unusual reactions should be seen by a health care provider.
5. Counseling and instruction, when appropriate, about alternate nursing therapies or therapies that accompany drug taking (e.g., instruct about increasing fluids, activity, and roughage to reduce a laxative habit).
6. Warnings about certain drugs that can produce physical and psychological dependence (e.g., analgesics, stimulants, and laxatives).

TABLE 7-1 Common Useful Over-the-Counter Preparations*

Medication	Use
Analgesic balm or ointment	Muscular aches
Analgesic tablets, nonnarcotic	Headaches, minor aches, pains, fever
Antacids	Indigestion or upset stomach
Antidiarrheal compounds	Mild, uncomplicated diarrhea
Antihistamines	Allergies
Antiseptics	
Liquid, cream, spray	Minor cuts and scrapes
Mouthwash	Mild sore throat
Throat lozenges	Mild sore throat
Calamine cream or lotion	Insect bites, minor itching, poison ivy
Contraceptives	Prevention of unwanted pregnancy or sexually transmitted diseases
Cough syrup	Excessive coughing caused by colds
Ipecac syrup	Accidental poisoning emergency
Laxatives, mild	Constipation
Motion or travel sickness remedies	Dizziness, nausea, vomiting
Nasal decongestants	Nasal stuffiness resulting from colds or allergies
Skin creams or lotions	Chapped skin, diaper rash
Sunburn and other burn treatments	Sunburn, other minor burns
Vitamin preparations	Dietary supplement

*Container label should be read carefully and the health care provider contacted if there are questions.

are of low toxicity and pose little threat to the average consumer when directions are followed, but many others do, especially if the consumer is allergic, pregnant, or breast-feeding or has disorders other than the one being treated.

According to law, all nonprescription drugs must show this information on their labels:

1. Name of the product
2. Name and address of the manufacturer, packer, or distributor
3. Net contents of the package
4. Active ingredients and the quantity of certain ingredients
5. Name of any habit-forming drug contained in the prescription
6. Cautions and warnings needed for the protection of the user
7. Adequate directions for safe and effective use

Drugs purchased in a grocery store or supermarket or from mail-order houses or vending machines do not always allow access to professional advice as needed from a pharmacist, who is usually on the premises when purchases are made from drug stores or pharmacies. Pharmacists are able to observe the drug-buying habits of their customers, keep a drug profile or drug history on each customer, and explain and advise consumers when a visit to the physician or prescriber is necessary. A well-run pharmacy can make a valuable contribution to the health of a community.

SUMMARY OF NURSING CONSIDERATIONS

Medications tend to be more effective when clients believe in their capacity to get well and in the drug itself. An accurate assessment of clients' past and present conditioning to drugs, illness, hospitals, nurses, and other health care personnel as well as their own health beliefs and practices all influence their response to drug therapy. This assessment is most important in planning and implementing an effective care plan.

From the onset of drug therapy the client should be advised in a nonthreatening manner of the purpose of the medication and any possible side or adverse effects. All questions should be answered in a straightforward manner. It is important to listen to what the client has to say about the medication, the feelings associated with the drug and whether they are based on fear or anxiety, and the perception of the condition for which it has been prescribed.

Client education plays an important role when, at discharge, the individual needs to follow a prescribed medication plan. Routinely reviewing medications with clients and inquiring about how medications are taken at home have been shown to increase compliance in following a medication plan. The client should be told if a medication must be taken for life and should understand that the decision to discontinue medication should be made in consultation with the prescriber.

The nurse should make sure the client thoroughly understands the medication instructions. Written schedules and instructions for taking medications, with a sample of the drug taped to them, will remind clients when they are at home and have forgotten what they heard in the office or on discharge from the hospital.

Clients should be told of the potential serious side effects of mixing OTC drugs with prescription drugs and mixing different types of prescription drugs. The prescriber and pharmacist should always be told about any allergies or other conditions as well as current pregnancy or if the client is breast-feeding. The pharmacist can check for any type of severe drug interaction and can possibly substitute an equivalent drug after discussion with the prescriber.

MEDICATION WARNINGS

□ **1** Avoid alcoholic beverages while taking this medication.

□ **2** Swallow these tablets. Do not chew them. **Do not take if coating is cracked.**

□ **3** Do not drive a car or operate machinery if this medication makes you drowsy. If you have to drive home, wait until you get home to take your first dose.

□ **4** Do not allow this medication to contact the skin, eyes, or clothing.

□ **5** Take this medication on an empty stomach either 1 hour before meals or **2 hours after meals. You may drink water.**

□ **6** Do not take this medication with fruit juice.

□ **7** Take this medication _____ hour(s) before meals.

□ **8** Do not take this medication with milk or milk products. You may drink water or juice.

□ **9** Take this medication with at least 8 ounces of water.

□ **10** Take this medication immediately after meals.

□ **11** This medication may discolor the urine or stools.

□ **12** Do not take this medication with antacids.

□ **13** Do not take aspirin with this medication.

□ **14** Do not take mineral oil with this medication.

□ **15** Take orange juice, bananas, and other foods high in potassium while taking this medication.

□ **16** Avoid tyramine-rich foods such as cheese, pickled herring, and wine while taking this medication.

□ **17** Count your pulse (by feeling at the wrist) each time before taking this medication. If it is less than 60 beats a minute, do not take the dose. Contact the prescriber.

□ **18** Do not take this medication if pregnant or breast-feeding or if you have ever had an allergic reaction to it. Instead, contact prescriber for instructions.

□ **19** Do not take this medication if you have the following medical problems or symptoms:

FIGURE 7-1 Instruction sheet for the patient: medication warnings. Nurses and doctors in clinics or offices may want to reproduce this instruction sheet for use with clients.
(Modified from Martin, E.W.: Hazards of medication, Philadelphia, J.B. Lippincott Co.; from Nursing Update, Sept. 1972.)

The client should learn to check all medications for expiration dates and deterioration and to discard those that are outdated and deteriorated. Clients should be instructed *never* to share medications with friends or family because of the potential unknown effects.

Clients should be reminded that nonprescription drugs are not curative but offer only symptomatic relief and that they should see a health care provider when treated conditions are persistent or recurrent or when unusual reactions occur.

KEY TERMS

cultural background, page 115
health beliefs, page 115
noncompliance, page 119
placebo, page 117

BIBLIOGRAPHY

Anderson, K, and Poole, C: Self-administered medication on a postpartum unit, Amer J Nurs 83(8):1178, 1983.

Brown, CS, Wright, RG, and Christensen, DB: Association between type of medication instruction and patients' knowledge, side effects, and compliance, Hosp & Comm Psychiatry 38(1):55, 1987.

Bullough, VL, and Bullough, B: Health care for the other Americans. New York: Appleton-Century-Crofts, 1982.

Cluff, LE: Patient compliance: changing patterns of disease and health care costs, Hosp Formul 20:503, 1985.

TABLE 7-2   Prescription Drugs Now Marketable as Over-the-Counter Drugs

Drug/trade name	Dosage	Indication	Drug/trade name	Dosage	Indication
acidulated phosphate fluoride rinse	0.02% fluoride; 10 ml twice daily	Anticaries	hydrocortisone acetate (topical)/Many	0.25%-0.5%; not more than 3-4 times daily	Antipruritic
brompheniramine maleate/Dimetane	4mg/4-6 hr (Adult)	Antihistamine	ibuprofen/Advil	200 mg/4-6 hr	Analgesic (antiinflammatory agent)
chlorpheniramine maleate/ Chlortrimeton	4 mg/4-6 hr (Adult)	Antihistamine	miconazole nitrate/Micatin	2%; morning and night	Antifungal (except *Candida*)
diphenhydramine hydrochloride/ Benadryl	25-50 mg/4-6 hrs (Adult)	Antiemetic, antihistaminic	phenylephrine hydrochloride/ Various	0.5 mg aqueous sol. up to 4 times daily and not to exceed 2mg/24 hr	Anorectal vasoconstrictor
dyclonine hydrochloride/ Dyclone	0.05% to 0.10% as rinse, mouthwash, gargle or spray no more than 3-4 times daily 0.05% to 0.10% concentrate in lozenge (equal to 1-3 mg per lozenge) every 2 hr if necessary	Anesthetic/analgesic	pseudoephedrine hydrochloride (oral)/Sudafed	30-60 mg/4 hr (Adult)	Nasal decongestant
			pyrantel pamoate (Antiminth)	11 mg/kg in a single dose orally	Pinworms
			oxymetazoline hydrochloride (topical)/Afrin	0.05% aqueous sol. 2 times daily (in the morning and evening)	Nasal decongestant
ephedrine sulfate/Various	2-25 mg aqueous sol. up to 4 times daily and not to exceed 100 mg/24 hr	Anorectal vasoconstrictor	sodium fluoride rinse/ Fluorigard	0.05%; 10 ml once daily	Anticaries
			Stannous fluoride gel	0.4%; once daily	Anticaries
epinephrine hydrochloride/ Various	100-200 μg aqueous sol. up to 4 times daily and not to exceed 800 μg/24 hr	Anorectal vasoconstrictor	stannous fluoride rinse	0.1%; 10 ml once daily	Anticaries
haloprogin/Malotex	1%; morning and night	Antifungal (except *Candida*)	xylometazoline hydrochloride (topical)/ Otrivin	0.1% aqueous sol. every 8-10 hr	Nasal decongestant
hydrocortisone (topical)/Many various	0.25%-0.5%; not more than 3-4 times daily	Antipruritic			

Modified from FDA Drug Bulletin 13(3):29, Nov. 1983, and Davidson, 1981.

Davidson, DE, ed: Handbook of nonprescription drugs, ed 8, Washington, DC: American Pharmaceutical Association, 1986.

Department of Health and Human Services: Rx drugs switches to OTC, FDA Drug Bull 13(11):29, 1983.

Gilman, A, and others, eds: Goodman and Gilman's The Pharmacological Basis of Therapeutics, ed 7. New York: MacMillan Publishing Co, 1985.

Gossel, TA: The changing nature of OTCs: why—and how—to keep up to date, RN 46(9):73, 1983.

Henderson, G, and Primeaux, M: Transcultural Health Care. Menlo Park: Addison-Wesley Publishing Co, 1981.

Hess, P: Chinese and Hispanic elderly and OTC drugs, Geriatric Nursing 7(6):314, 1986.

Hill, MN: Drug compliance, Nursing '86 16(10):50, 1986.

Knapp, D, and Knapp, D: The elderly and nonprescribed medication, Contemp Pharm Practice 3(2):85, 1980.

Leininger, M: Transcultural nursing: concepts, theories, and practices. New York: John Wiley & Sons, 1978.

Leininger, M: Transcultural nursing '79. New York: Masson Publishing USA, Inc, 1979.

Lopez/Aquires, W, and others: Health needs of the Hispanic elderly, J Amer Geriatric Soc, 191-198, 1984.

Martinez, RA: Hispanic culture and health care: fact, fiction, folklore. St Louis: The CV Mosby Co, 1978.

McCaffery, M: Would you administer placebos for pain? Nursing '82 12(2):80, 1982.

Miyares, MU: Medication aids your elderly patients will love, RN 48(11):44, 1985.

Northrop, CE: Don't overlook discharge teaching about drugs, Nursing '86 16(11):43, 1986.

Orque, MS, Block, B and Monrroy, L: Ethnic nursing care, a multicultural approach. St Louis: The CV Mosby Co, 1983.

Robinson, JD, and Stewart, RB: Elderly: understanding their non-prescription needs, Am Pharm NS21(11):48.

Salerno, E, and others: Self-medicating behaviors, Fla J Hosp Pharm 5(3):13, 1985.

Scott, CS: Health and healing practices among five ethnic groups in Miami, Florida. In Bauwens, E: The anthropology of health. St Louis: The CV Mosby Co, 1978.

Shubin, S: Nursing patients from different cultures, Nursing 80 10(6):78, 1980.

U.S. Pharmacopeia Convention: Advice for the patient, Vol II, USPDI, ed 8. Rockville: Mack Printing Co, 1988.

Wood, CS: Human sickness and health: a biocultural view. Palo Alto, Calif: Mayfield Publishing Co, 1979.

CHAPTER 8

Drug Therapy Across the Life Span

The effects of pharmaceutical agents vary in clients of different ages. The reasons for these differences are complex. Understanding the rationale behind these effects will assist the nurse to administer medications safely and evaluate their responses appropriately, regardless of the client's age. In addition, the client's age might also determine special techniques of administering medication to provide greater safety for the client. In this chapter special factors related to neonates, infants and children, and the elderly will be discussed. These are, of course, artificial categories because life is a continuum in which development, maturity, and then degeneration occur without any distinct demarcation. Individuals mature and decline and/or have special needs at different ages, at different rates, and under different circumstances, that affect drug response in characteristic ways.

CHILD-BEARING CLIENTS

Any substance ingested or absorbed by a woman is likely to reach the fetus by way of maternal circulation or to be transferred to the breast-fed neonate by way of breast milk if the substance is in sufficient concentration and is well distributed. Thus drugs taken by the mother potentially can cause serious harm to the fetus or neonate. No drug is known to be *absolutely* safe for the developing embryo, but some oral medications that are inactivated in the mother's stomach or not absorbed by the maternal gastrointestinal tract are assumed to be relatively safe. However, many drugs and other substances have yet to be identified as harmful to the fetus.

Considerations for drug therapy in the child-bearing client center on the effects of drugs administered to the mother on the developing fetus or nursing infant. The **neonate** (birth to about one month of age), **infant** (one month to two years), older child, and geriatric client all have unique needs and nursing considerations based on both physiologic and psychosocial developmental levels.

The child-bearing client takes, on average, four or more drugs (other than vitamins) during pregnancy, and the fetal effects of these drugs are unknown. Shepard (1982) has indicated that there are more than 600 substances with some degree of "teratogenicity," or ability to cause developmental abnormalities of offspring when taken by a parent, based on experiments in animals. Only about 25 are known to cause human malformations.

Parents now ask health professionals more questions than in the past. Nurses are called on to supply accurate information, provide rationales, discuss the options available, and support parents' decisions. Prescribers and parents may have to make difficult choices between the benefits to the mother and the risks to the fetus or neonate. A judgment may need to be made between the risks to both if the mother's illness is not treated by a certain drug and the risks to the fetus if the drug is administered. This dilemma illustrates the absolute necessity for nurses to keep up to date in their drug knowledge and highly skilled at information retrieval from reliable sources. Parents should make the ultimate decision, with informed, sensitive input from all appropriate health professionals.

DRUG TRANSFER TO THE FETUS: PHARMACOKINETICS AND THE PLACENTA

Pregnancy does not seem to have much effect on drug absorption from the gastrointestinal tract, but protein binding is decreased, freeing more drug for placental transfer. Biotransformation of drugs in the liver is probably delayed in pregnancy, but renal excretion may be more rapid because renal blood flow increases dramatically as a result of increased cardiac output and glomerular filtration rate. (See Chapter 4.)

At the placental interface, transfer of drugs and other substances is affected primarily by simple diffusion and partly by active transport. Transfer across the placenta depends on the chemical properties of the drug: its molecular weight, spatial configuration, protein binding capabilities, pKa, and lipid solubility, as well as its distribution and concentration gradient. The potential for transfer is proportional to the period of time the drug

remains in the maternal bloodstream. Transfer is greater during late gestation because of enhanced uteroplacental blood flow, increased placental surface at the interface, thinner membranes separating maternal blood flow and placental capillaries, lowered pH of fetal circulation (and thus more receptivity to ionized basic drugs), more physical interruption in membranes, and an increased proportion of free drug available to the circulation. Pathologic processes in the placenta, such as inflammation, degeneration, or partial separation, can increase blood flow and thus drug transfer. Not much is known about drug metabolism in the placenta itself, but it is thought to be a less active process. Certain drugs can alter placental enzyme activity necessary for degradation of substances and for energy-dependent transport mechanisms.

Many drugs are carried across the placenta within minutes, especially if administered intravenously (see box below). Thus the historical concept of the placenta as a completely protective barrier to circulating substances must be discarded. Most drugs that cross the placenta stabilize in the fetus at a level between 50% to 100% of the maternal level. Some (such as diazepam and local anesthetics) stabilize at levels even higher than the mother's blood levels. However, continued exposure of the fetus to a drug is more important than the rate of placental transport.

Within the fetus, drug effects may be more significant and prolonged than in the mother because of (1) probable lower enzyme concentrations and enzymatic reaction rates of drug metabolism and (2) slower excretion rates. Fetal excretion of drugs takes place via maternal resorption and excretion by the fetal kidneys into amniotic fluid, which, under ordinary circumstances, the fetus often swallows.

On occasion, various fetal complications such as anemia and syphilis exposure have been actively treated by drugs in utero. The drug delivery routes chosen have been either the passive, transplacental approach or direct

---

DRUGS THAT CROSS THE PLACENTA RAPIDLY*

ampicillin	meperidine
barbiturates	penicillin G
cephalothin	phenytoin
diazepam	propranolol
ethanol	salicylates
kanamycin	streptomycin
lidocaine and other local anesthetics	sulfonamides
	tetracycline

*Especially if administered intravenously.

instillations into the amniotic fluid. These modes are still controversial.

It is, however, well documented that many unintended fetal drug doses via maternal circulation produce harmful fetal effects. The embryo or fetus runs the risk of developing the usual side or toxic effects, just as the mother does. Also, doses can be lethal or **teratogenic** (causing fetal organ defects); **mutagenic** (causing genetic mutations); or **carcinogenic** (causing or accelerating the development of cancer, sometimes much later). An example of the last is the precancerous or cancerous cell changes discovered in youths whose mothers took the hormone diethylstilbestrol (DES) during pregnancy.

Every embryo undergoes a series of precisely programmed steps from cell proliferation, differentiation, and migration to organogenesis. The critical periods for drug effects on the fetus are the first 2 weeks of rapid *cell proliferation,* when drug exposures can be lethal to the embryo, and the *third through the tenth weeks of pregnancy,* when the axial skeleton, muscles, limbs, and organs are developing most rapidly.

An unfortunate example is the hypnotic drug thalidomide, which caused abnormal limb development (phocomelia) in many children whose mothers were administered the drug during pregnancy. Beyond the tenth week of pregnancy, the results are more likely to be physiologic or behavioral alterations and delays in growth.

Advice that all drugs be avoided during pregnancy and while breast-feeding cannot always be followed. Some maternal conditions (e.g., hypertension, epilepsy, diabetes, and infection) place both mother and fetus in serious jeopardy if left untreated. Although authoritative literature and drug package inserts routinely warn that drugs have not been tested for use in pregnancy, breast-feeding, or for infants, much empiric data and some research are accumulating. The FDA now rates drugs as to their safety for use during pregnancy. This rating is discussed in Chapter 2.

Obvious legal and ethical problems associated with research experiments on such vulnerable subjects and with obtaining consent have delayed the generation of necessary data. Well-controlled research, although fraught with ethical dilemmas in research design, is undeniably needed. Nurses are well-positioned to participate in this important research, and they should do so.

Some drugs considered relatively safe during pregnancy, depending on the situation, are listed in Table 8-1. Certain categories of drugs are expressly contraindicated during pregnancy, or are used only when the risk-benefit situation has been carefully considered and thoroughly discussed with the client. These are listed in the box. Although some of these are mentioned in Table 8-1, their use should be severely curtailed, with only those pregnant women whose life and that of the fetus would be in jeopardy without drug treatment receiving them. One variable to be considered is the dose that reaches the embryo or fetus. This depends on the maternal dosage, the maternal volume of distribution, and the metabolic clearance rate of the mother. The fetal gestational age at time of exposure, duration of therapy planned, fetal and maternal genotypes, and any other drugs administered concurrently are also factors in prescribing decisions. Dosages, dosing intervals, and duration of treatment may be manipulated carefully to avoid harmful effects. Ethyl alcohol, especially at or near time of conception, is associated with the fetal alcohol syndrome, which produces both growth and mental retardation (see box on p. 131). Other very common substances such as aspirin, vitamin supplements, caffeine, and nicotine are suspected to cause adverse reactions in the fetus.

One difficulty with these and other substances is that effects on the embryo may occur before the woman is aware that she is pregnant. Women of child-bearing age who are not using contraceptives and who are sexually active should be prescribed for carefully and should be instructed to use OTC medications cautiously. Education and prevention are considered the best therapy.

ROLE OF THE NURSE

Most nursing goals related to these topics should be aimed at ensuring that parents know that any foreign substance absorbed by the mother may have lifelong effects on the child. A balance must be maintained between protecting the child and dealing constructively with the family; creating *unnecessary* family concern is not appropriate. Essential to these aims is cooperating with the prescribing clinician, providing an environment for free ex-

---

DRUGS CONSIDERED RELATIVELY UNSAFE DURING PREGNANCY

alcohol	methyltestosterone
aminopterin	methylthiouracil
chlorpropamide	norethindrone
cocaine	paramethadione
diazepam	phenothiazines
diethylstilbestrol	phenytoin
estrogens	propranolol
heroin	propylthiouracil
iodide	secobarbital
lithium	tetracycline
mepivacaine	thalidomide
mercury	trimethadione
methadone	warfarin*
methotrexate	

*Considered unsafe during first trimester and last month of pregnancy.

ALCOHOL AND THE CHILD-BEARING CLIENT: FETAL ALCOHOL SYNDROME

Although the public is becoming aware of the hazards of using drugs during pregnancy, many people do not include alcohol in the category of drugs. The teratogenic effects of intrauterine alcohol exposure on the fetus are well documented. Heavy use of alcohol by the child-bearing client has been associated with retarded growth, a pattern of congenital anomalies, and neurologic dysfunction of the infant. These effects seem to be dose related, so that the greater the maternal alcohol consumption during pregnancy, the more severe the infant's symptoms. Although the exact mechanism of **fetal alcohol syndrome** (FAS) has not yet been specified, studies have demonstrated that counseling to decrease maternal alcohol intake has a beneficial effect on the health of the mother and infant. The nurse must be aware of clients who are at risk of FAS and be prepared to provide client education, counseling, and referral.

change of information, and, if possible, forestalling parental feelings of guilt or fear associated with drug administration, whether planned or inadvertent. The following information should be conveyed.

1. Potential harm to the child resulting directly from substances the mother is exposed to and potential danger to both mother and child if treatment is not begun must both be weighed. These decisions must be made with the prescriber whenever exposure to an unfamiliar substance or drug is contemplated. Not everything is known at this time about effects on the child; and as more information becomes available, accepted guidelines may change.

2. Over-the-counter medications and other common substances such as aspirins, vitamin supplements, alcohol, caffeine, and nicotine are drugs and thus can cause detrimental effects.

3. Any prescription written by a professional who is not a specialist in the care of pregnancies or nursing mothers should be evaluated by an obstetrician or pediatrician. The prescription may need to be changed by the specialist to a safer drug or dosage.

4. If a questionable substance is absorbed by the mother, close health care supervision is essential. If real potential for fetal or infant injury results, the parents need ongoing support as they endure the sometimes long wait for effects to be manifested. If birth defects or toxic effects are present, or if invasive diagnostic tests or a therapeutic abortion is to be performed, objective psychologic intervention may help the parents endure this critical period.

PEDIATRIC CLIENTS
NEONATES

Since newborns are small and immature, lacking many of the protective mechanisms that allow older children and adults to be relatively resistant to stressors of all kinds, they require special considerations. Their skin is thin and permeable, their stomachs lack acid, and their lungs lack much of the mucous barrier. Neonates regulate body temperature poorly and become dehydrated easily. Their liver and kidneys are immature and cannot manage foreign substances as well as older children and adults. Specific factors affecting medication use in neonates are listed in the box on p. 132.

BREAST-FED INFANTS

Almost *all* forms of drugs in maternal circulation can be readily transferred to the colostrum and breast milk. Since drugs or their biotransformed products are handled by different pathways in the infant and the fetus, the impact of maternal medications on the infant probably differs (is probably less) from that on the fetus. This difference can serve as a guide in prescribing for the breast-feeding mother. Typical nontherapeutic outcomes in the breast-fed infant are signs of the drug's usual side or toxic effects. Adverse effects may occur, such as gray-brown stains of the later-erupting teeth as a result of tetracycline therapy over 10 days in length or allergic sensitization to penicillin. Most drug products that reach the neonate via breast milk have undergone maternal biotransformation and are probably less than the original dose. However, immaturity of the neonate's liver and kidney systems limits the capacity for further metabolism and excretion.

Data about infant's capabilities for drug absorption, digestion, distribution, metabolism, and excretion are scant and conflicting. In general, the proved benefits of continuing breast-feeding must be weighed on an individual basis against the risks of maternal medication to the infant. Although the mammary glands are a relatively insignificant route for maternal drug excretion and the drug level in breast milk is usually less than the actual maternal dose, the infant's actual dose depends largely on the volume of milk consumed. Thus a single measurement of a drug in human milk will not accurately reflect the total dose the infant receives.

The concentration of the drug in maternal circulation depends on the relationship among several factors: dosing and route of administration, the drug's distribution, its protein binding, and maternal metabolism and excretion. The mammary alveolar epithelium presents to any potentially transferable substance a lipid barrier with water-filled pores. It is most permeable to drugs during the collostrum stage of milk production—during the first

SUMMARY OF SOME PEDIATRIC PHARMACOKINETICS INFLUENCING DOSING PRINCIPLES

AGE

Effects of drugs are the most unpredictable among neonates because of the varying rates of system development.

FORM OF DRUG

Liquids and suspensions disperse quickly in gastrointestinal fluids and are therefore more readily absorbed. For example, absorption of digoxin tablets may be up to 85% complete; in elixir form it may be 100% complete. Percutaneous absorption of *topical preparations* is readily achieved in the neonate through the preadolescent; therefore inadvertent systemic circulation can result in toxicity (e.g., boric acid or steroids applied to inflamed, broken, or eczematous skin).

DISTRIBUTION

Since most drugs are distributed in body water, increases in total body water and extracellular volume may also increase the volume of drug distribution. Compared with adults, neonates have proportionately higher volumes of total body water and a higher ratio of extracellular to intracellular fluid; therefore, higher dosages of aqueous-soluble drugs may be needed to achieve effective blood levels in the newborn. The blood-brain barrier in the newborn is also fairly ineffective against drugs.

BIOTRANSFORMATION

Various liver enzyme systems for metabolism generally mature unevenly. For example, acetylation is deficient in the newborn; yet sulfation is enhanced.

ELIMINATION

Renal excretory mechanisms progress to maturity after 1 year of age. Excretion of some substances (e.g., aminoglycosides) through the renal system may be delayed because of immaturity before that age, resulting in higher circulation levels and longer duration of action than desirable.

BREAST FEEDING AND MARIJUANA

Clinical studies have demonstrated hazardous effects, impaired DNA and RNA formation, and structural changes in the brain cells of nursing laboratory animals whose mothers were given marijuana. Anecdotal reports of drowsiness in breast-fed infants after the mother smoked marijuana have been documented. A study (Perez-Reyes, 1982) indicates that marijuana's active substance (tetrahydrocannabinol) is concentrated and secreted in human breast milk and thereby ingested by the infant.

How should nurses respond to the dilemma of a breast-feeding mother who refuses to stop using marijuana? If recreational use is limited to only once or twice a month, it may be better for the mother to continue to breast-feed rather than wean and institute bottle-feeding. If use of marijuana is more than just once or twice a month, bottle feeding of formula should be urged as an alternative to breast feeding, to protect the nursing infant from the hazards of marijuana use.

week of life. Drug factors that enhance drug excretion into milk are nonionization, low molecular weight, solubility in fat and water, plasma binding versus milk-protein binding, and the relationship of plasma pH and milk pH (7.4 and 7.1, respectively). Transfer of an active or passive form of a drug's metabolites into maternal plasma and then to milk depends mainly on passive diffusion. The absorptive processes of the infant's gastrointestinal tract and drug distribution are estimated to be similar to those in the adult, which means that lipid-soluble substances are well absorbed. The infant's age (thus the amount of drug-containing milk consumed) and the relative immaturity of the infant's important organs bear greatly on the outcome. If the drug is fat-soluble, it may be more highly concentrated in breast milk at the end of feedings and at midday. Since the infant's total serum protein is lower in comparison to the adult's, more free drug is available to the circulation. Metabolic reactions in the infant's liver are slower than the older child's; consequently, drug biotransformation may likewise be delayed. Other factors in the neonatal period may present risks: inadequate body temperature control, hypoxemia, or inadequate nutrition, for example. Drug excretion is delayed in the neonate because it is largely via the kidneys, where immature glomerular filtration rates and tubular functioning are maintained for several months. The extreme variability among drug effects and infants' capabilities makes it difficult to decide whether the mother should take a drug and whether or not she should breast-feed.

Human milk contains small, fixed amounts of many substances absorbed by the mother. Considerable evidence shows that certain other substances are incontrovertibly contraindicated unless necessary for survival and unless their effects are closely monitored. The usual recommendation is that breast-feeding be temporarily interrupted (usually for 24 to 72 hours) and the breasts pumped to remove drug-containing milk. Less often, it is advisable to cease breast-feeding altogether. Dosages and routes may also be changed. It is recommended that the following drugs be avoided while breast-feeding unless absolutely necessary: marijuana (inhibits lactation and

TABLE 8-1   Some Drugs Considered Relatively Safe for Use in Pregnancy

Agent	Recommendations and cautions*	Agent	Recommendations and cautions*
ANALGESICS		**ANTIHYPERTENSIVES**	
acetaminophen	Considered safest analgesic during pregnancy	methyldopa	Safest of antihypertensives during pregnancy (especially as substitute for diuretics in pregnancy for diastolic blood pressure > 110 mm Hg in the 3rd trimester)
ANTIASTHMATICS			
cromolyn sodium	Relatively safe	hydralazine	Safest for hypertensive crises in pregnancy
metaproterenol (aerosol)	Relatively safe for mild, intermittent episodes. Avoid oral form		
theophylline	Relatively safe if blood levels are closely monitored	**ANTIINFECTIVES**	
		erythromycin	For use as substitute for penicillin hypersensitivity
ANTICOAGULANTS		metronidazole	Not to be used during the 1st trimester
heparin	For use during 1st trimester; use caution if given during last trimester	miconazole	Relatively safe during pregnancy
		penicillin and derivatives	Relatively safe during pregnancy
ANTICONVULSANTS			
phenobarbital	For use only if necessary to maintain seizure control; if given during pregnancy, monitor neonate during first 24 hours for neonatal coagulation defect (bleeding)	**ANTITHYROID DRUGS**	
		propylthiouracil	For use only if absolutely necessary (e.g., for hyperthyroidism); use lowest dose possible
ANTIDIABETICS		**ANTITUBERCULOSIS DRUGS**	
insulin	Relatively safe as drug of choice	isoniazid	Relatively safe during pregnancy
		rifampin	
ANTIEMETICS		ethambutol	
pyridoxine	Relatively safe for morning sickness	**CARDIAC GLYCOSIDES**	
doxylamine	For use as necessary for severe nausea or vomiting	digoxin	Relatively safe. Maternal plasma levels should be closely monitored. Dosages may be increased toward the end of gestation and decreased for 6 weeks after delivery
prochlorperazine			
promethazine			
trimethobenzamide			

*Recommendations are likely to change; therefore manufacturers' package inserts should always be consulted. No drugs are known to be *absolutely* safe during pregnancy. The use of many substances, including most drugs not on this list, should be carefully considered by the obstetrician as to risks and benefits. See drug monographs for specific drug information; see also bibliography. Consult references for sources of information about drugs in this table.

passes into breast milk causing possible impairment of DNA and RNA formation and structural brain cell damage), sulfa (in G-6-PD deficiency), metronidazole, atropine, quinidine, reserpine, hydralazine, benzodiazepines, meprobamate, MAO inhibitors, lithium, acetohexamide, chlorpropamide, tolazamide, tolbutamide, sex hormones, cascara, danthron, pyridoxine (which, in large doses, inhibits lactation), more than 2 ounces of alcohol per day, caffeine, nicotine, iodides, radioactive iodine, and technetium-99.

Drug effects may be minimized by substituting formula for the midday breast-feeding, since that is the feeding highest in fat content and thus more likely to contain higher amounts of fat-soluble drug products. In addition, breast-feeding mothers who must be treated with medications can time their doses to be taken right *after* breast-feeding so as much time as possible elapses and the drug can reach a relatively low concentration before the next feeding (see Table 8-2).

With radioactive substances, therapy is of short dura-

tion or if merely a diagnostic radioisotope test is to be done, breast-feeding must be interrupted until all radiation is absent from milk samples. Breast-feeding will probably be terminated when the drug is so potent that minute amounts may profoundly affect the infant, when the drug has high allergenic potential, when the mother exhibits evidence of decreased renal function (which augments drug excretion into breast milk), or when there are serious pathologic conditions requiring prolonged drug administration of high dosages.

Changes in the activity levels of the fetus or nursing infant signal dangerous effects resulting from drug administration; parents should be taught how to assess and report unusual fetal inactivity or infant apathy.

Alternatives to drug therapy. Both health professionals and clients place high value on pharmaceutical solutions to health concerns. However, many illnesses are self-limited or cause only minor discomforts that end or decrease without medication or with non-drug alternatives, such as relaxation techniques rather than tranquil-

TABLE 8-2   Some Drugs Considered Relatively Safe While Breast-Feeding

Agents	Recommendations and precautions*	Agents	Recommendations and precautions*
ANALGESICS		**BRONCHODILATORS**	
acetaminophen aspirin mefenamic acid propoxyphene	Relatively safe in breast-feeding	ephedrine cromolyn sodium theophylline	Safe; destroyed in infant's GI tract Observe for infant irritability or insomnia
ANTIINFECTIVES		**PSYCHOTROPIC DRUGS**	
cephalexin cephalothin oxacillin penicillin erythromycin sulfonamides	Safe during breast-feeding; not found in breast milk Relatively safe after 1 mo, but may sensitize the infant Safe after 1 mo Safe; but last-month drug administration may cause neonatal jaundice	chlorpromazine phenothiazine tricyclic antidepressants **ANTIDIABETICS** insulin **THYROID DRUGS**	Appear safe, although found in milk; may cause drowsiness in baby Safe; destroyed in the GI tract
CARDIOVASCULAR DRUGS		thyroid hormones	Relatively safe if monitored for thyroid function and response
digoxin guanethidine methyldopa propranolol	Safe if maternal serum levels are closely monitored Safe in recommended dosages Assumed to be safe; no adverse reports Relatively safe at lowered maternal dosages (higher drug levels in breast milk than in maternal bloodstream because of high lipid solubility of drug)	**GASTROINTESTINAL DRUGS** antacids metoclopramide laxatives (except cascara & danthron) **PESTICIDES**	Safe; electrolytes should be monitored Under usual conditions found less in human milk than in cow's milk
DIURETICS		**AIR POLLUTANTS**	
chlorothiazide hydrochlorothiazide furosemide	Excreted in breast milk; no problems documented in humans Fluids and electrolytes must be closely monitored		Have not been found in human milk
ANTICONVULSANTS		**VACCINES**	
primidone phenytoin	Relatively safe with close observation	RhoGAM	Considered safe

*Over time, recommendations may change; therefore manufacturer's package inserts should always be consulted by pediatricians and nurses. Many substances should be avoided during the period of breast-feeding. (Details about specific drugs are located under relevant chapter headings in this text.) Consult bibliography for sources of information.

izers. The effect of any medication should be weighed against the mother and child's physical and psychologic stress of abrupt weaning.

Other considerations might be to delay the mother's pharmacologic therapy until the infant is weaned on his or her own or to select another drug to meet the therapeutic goal without interfering with breast-feeding. The age and maturity of the child must be considered also; as the infant develops physiologically the drug's ability to cause harmful effects will diminish. The frequency of feedings should also be considered. An infant dependent on breast milk for total nutrition will receive higher doses of drugs than an infant breast-feeding only once or twice a day and taking other forms of nourishment.

OTHER PEDIATRIC CLIENTS

Drug administration to pediatric clients requires special knowledge and approaches. Physicians may prescribe the dosage of medication, but it is the nurse's responsibility to know the safe dosage range of any medication administered to children. A standard dosage of medication is nonexistent in pediatrics; medications are usually ordered according to the weight or body surface area of the child. Some pharmaceutical companies continue to supply medications in a standard adult dosage strength, and the nurse must be able to evaluate the correct dosage before administering the medication.

Weight as a basis. Following is a formula for calculating estimated safe dosages based on weight alone (Clark's rule). Because this is based on weight alone, it is somewhat imprecise for children under 3 years old.

$$\frac{\text{Average adult dose} \times \text{Weight of child in pounds}}{150} = \text{Estimated safe dose}$$

Example: How much acetaminophen (Tylenol) should a 1-year-old child weighing 21 pounds receive if the average adult dose is 10 grains?

$$\text{Answer:} \frac{10 \text{ (grains)} \times 21 \text{ (weight in pounds)}}{150} = \text{gr } 1\frac{2}{5}$$
$$= \text{gr } 1\frac{1}{2}$$

A nurse preparing calculated dosages of digitalis, insulin, barbiturates, and narcotics should have the calculations as well as the prepared medication dosage checked by another nurse before the drug is administered. Pediatric dosages are often minute, and a slight mistake in calculating the amount of medication to be administered results in greater proportional error.

Pediatric dose calculation based on weight alone implies that the pediatric client is a small adult, which is not true. Physiologic differences in the infant when compared to an adult may definitely affect the amount of drug needed to produce a therapeutic effect. For example, infants have a body composition that is approximately 75% water (adults have 50% to 60%) and less fat content than the adult. (See box on p. 136.) Therefore, water-soluble drugs are generally administered in larger doses to infants/children per body weight than to an adult. A good example of this is the water soluble drug gentamicin, an intravenous antibiotic. Recommended dosages from U.S.P.D.I., Volume I, 1988 are: older neonates and infants, 2.5 mg/kg every 8 hours; children, 2.0-2.5 mg/kg every 8 hours; and adults, 1.0-1.7 mg/kg every 8 hours.

Rules based on weight, such as Clark's rule, are generally taught and used by students in clinical areas to assess pediatric dosages. While useful as a guide, their accuracy for a number of drugs is questionable. If the student is uncertain regarding dosage, the following sources are recommended: the drug monograph in a package insert; U.S.P.D.I., Volume I; AHFS; or a pharmacist.

Body surface area as a basis. More than 100 years ago, Hufeland suggested that drug doses should be calculated on size or proportional amount of body surface area (BSA) to weight. Many physicians continue to use weight as the basis for calculating drug doses and body surface area for calculating fluid requirements. Most clinicians advocate using body surface area for determining drug dosage for adults as well as children. Physicians usually carry a simple slide rule or nomogram, such as the West nomogram (Figure 8-1) to make rapid BSA conversions from weight and height. It is believed that the larger amount of total body water (TBW) in children, as well as the percentage of water in body weight and the part of

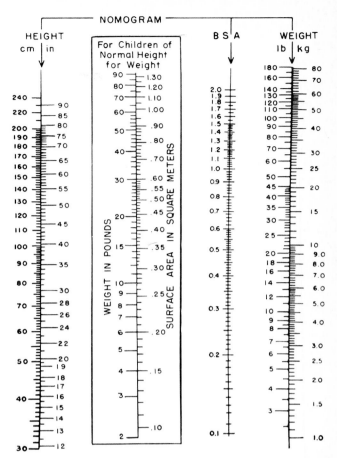

FIGURE 8-1 BSA is indicated where straight line that connects height and weight levels intersects BSA column or, if patient is about average size, from weight alone (enclosed area).

(Modified from data of E. Boyd by C.D. West.)

that percentage formed by extracellular water, accounts for the fact that children tolerate or require larger doses of some drugs on an mg/m² basis.

For the 75% of drugs that have no established pediatric dosage, calculating the child's dosage as a fraction of the average adult dose using Clark's rule is really too imprecise for most applications, yet it may be used (mg per kg) where the dosage according to body surface area has not been established. *The surface area rule is the most accurate.* As a relationship between height and weight, it can provide a more precise guide to the maturity of the child's organs and metabolic rate of functioning for effective pharmacokinetics. The dosage should be tailored to the individual child according to the amount of medication per square meter of body surface area. *The BSA rule for children's dosages* follows:

Child's approximate dose =

$$\frac{\text{Child's BSA in square meters} \times \text{Adult dose (from nomogram)}}{1.73}$$

ROLE OF THE NURSE

Although these rules have been devised for relating adult doses to infants and children, it must be emphasized that *no rules or charts are adequate to guarantee safety of dosage at any age,* particularly in the neonate. No method takes into account all variables, particularly individual tolerance differences. Astute, accurate nursing observations of how individual children react to drugs can assist in choosing drugs and dosages.

The administration of medications to infants and children is both challenging and frustrating. Giving injections skillfully will enhance security and help to gain a child's cooperation. A sound knowledge of growth and development also provides the nurse with information about how a child might be approached, whether reasoning will help or hinder the process, and whether assistance will be needed. The principles of safe administration of medication apply to all age groups, but children differ from adults, and the nurse has added responsibilities.

Ideally, a child will cooperate more readily with a nurse who has established a positive relationship. The child may also find it easier to accept the discomforts accompanying injections and some oral medications from the nurse who

is associated with daily hygiene, feeding, holding, play, and happy times. In addition, the nurse will feel less guilty when the child associates the nurse with pleasure and comfort most of the time, and discomfort only when necessary to get well.

When a child is afraid or anxious, the natural response is to strike out at the frustration or avoid it. By accepting this behavior as a natural response, the nurse will be able to deal with it and be honest when a medication or procedure will be unpleasant or painful.

Truthful explanations to children are essential. Children have a right to some explanation of any procedure that concerns them. The timing and type of explanation should be geared to the child's ability to perceive and understand. For the child 2 years of age or younger very simple explanations such as "I have some medicine for you to drink" or "I have an injection to give you, and it will hurt a little" are sufficient. Long explanations to children through 5 years of age do little more than prolong the anticipation and increase anxiety or fear. Telling 4-year-olds to stop kicking, hitting, or other avoidance behavior only conveys to them that they are not understood and they will receive little or no help with their feelings of frustration about being medicated.

Many children are courageous, or like to be considered so, and appealing to their courage is sometimes effective. Children 4 years old or over may choose to hold their own medicine cup, or drink unassisted, and to take pills from the container without any assistance from the nurse. Because of the sense of achievement that follows, they may want to save the medicine cups to show their parents.

Oral medications. Success in administering oral medications usually requires a kind but firm approach with a positive attitude. No doubt that the child will take the medicine should be reflected in choice of words or tone of voice. The nurse might say, "Jimmy, it's time to take your yellow medicine" or "Do you want to take your pill now or with your Jell-O?" This indicates that Jimmy is expected to cooperate and to do it willingly. It also allows the child some control over the situation. An unwise approach that reveals doubt on the nurse's part might be: "I have your yellow pill Jimmy. Will you take it for me, please?"

Nurses should try to be aware of how a medicine tastes so that they can answer such questions as, "Does it taste bad? Will it burn my mouth?" A helpful reply would be, "It tastes like cherry to me. Tell me what it tastes like to you." Often the child will accept the suggestion to taste and find out. However, if the medication is bad tasting, attempting deceit or lying to the child is as futile and destructive as it is to an adult.

Disagreeable-tasting medications should be disguised if at all possible. Small amounts of honey, syrup, jam, fruit, and some fruit juices are suitable sweet vehicles for less

---

PHYSIOLOGICAL DIFFERENCES, INFANT TO ADULT

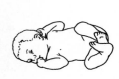
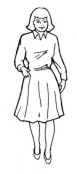

BODY WATER CONTENT

Age	Total body water (%)
Premature	86
Full-term	70
Adult	55

OTHER VARIABLES

Body fat: less in infants
Liver metabolism
Kidney function: less in infants; reaches adult values between 6 and 12 mos.
Selected drugs in neonate*: prolonged effect

Data from Katcher, 1983.

*Drug half-life (hr) in neonate (and adult): indomethacin 20 (6-7), diazepam 25-100 (15-25), theophylline 18-26 (3-9), and phenytoin 15-105 (10-20).

palatable drugs. Some pills can be crushed and suspended in small amounts of these substances as long as the two are compatible. Infants and children swallow many liquid medications more readily if mixed with a sweet substance or diluted with a small amount of water. (If large amounts of water or other substances are used and the child refuses to take all of the mixture, estimating the amount of medication the child received is difficult.) Fortunately, many drugs are available in palatable syrups or suspension form well suited for administration to infants and children. The box below offers further guidelines.

Caution must be exercised to prevent aspiration when giving oral medications to children. (See Special Situations later in this section for modifications as necessary.) Medications must be given to infants slowly and in small amounts to avoid choking. Liquid medications may be administered by nipple, plastic medicine cup, plastic dropper, or a plastic syringe without the needle. Water

should be swished through the inside of these *first* to prevent medication from sticking, thereby undermedicating. Glass cups, droppers, or syringes should be avoided because of the obvious danger of breakage in the child's mouth. A dropper or syringe is best suited for placing a liquid medication along one side of the infant's tongue. Older infants and toddlers seem to prefer to take their medications from a plastic medicine cup. If children are held or placed in a sitting position, they are less likely to aspirate the medication than if lying on their backs. When administering a medication with a dropper or syringe, the nurse may purse the infant's lips with one hand to keep the medicine from running out of the mouth. Droppers and syringes used for medication should be kept clean, reserved for only one client's use, and rinsed or washed before returning them to the medication bottle.

If the child refuses to cooperate even after explanations and encouragement, the nurse may have to ask whether the child will take the medication alone or will need the nurse to give it. Physical coercion is seldom necessary, but if used, it should be mild and used with dispatch and firmness, since aspiration is a danger. The nurse must not combine force with anger or resort to force when one nurse has been unable to administer the medication. Careful consideration should be given to such factors as: Why does the child resist? Does the child disapprove only of one nurse? Have past experiences with medications given at home or in the hospital frightened the child? Will forcing a medication cause a struggle that will negate the effects of a drug given for sedation? If mild restraint is necessary, the nurse should explain to the child that this form of treatment is necessary. The child will not cooperate if force is seen as a punishment for inability to cooperate; often the child loses confidence in all personnel.

Topical medications. Children have a large skin surface area in proportion to total body weight. Their skin, especially neonates', is particularly thin, permeable, and without much protective oil. Although adults absorb much more medication through intact skin than was previously believed, the child is at increased risk for systemic medication administration. The discovery that hexachlorophene can cause encephalopathy in newborns and that topically applied boric acid can cause systemic poisoning testifies to the hazard of applying drugs to children's skin, especially for prolonged contact or over broken skin areas. Plain soap and water may be preferred for abrasions or open lesions, replacing medicated dressings.

Subcutaneous injections. There are wide swings in the amounts of subcutaneous fat during the childhood years. Neonates have proportionately smaller amounts; these increase slightly to 23% by 1 year of age. From 1 to 5 years of age they drop to between 8% to 12%. Then the amounts of bodily fat climb to about 20% when the child reaches the age of 10. Lipid-soluble drugs have an affinity for fat tissue; less subcutaneous fat means that lower dos-

---

GUIDELINES FOR DRUG ADMINISTRATION

1. Parents are frequently good sources of information about successful methods or vehicles of giving medications to their children.
2. Try to avoid using essential foods such as milk, cereal, or orange juice, since the child may refuse to accept that food in the future.
3. Never underestimate children's reactions. They may not require that the taste of medication be disguised.
4. A sip of cold fruit juice, ice chips, a frozen fruit-bar, or a mint-flavored substance before and after the administration of an unpalatable medicine may effectively dull its taste.
5. Sugarless vehicles such as those sweetened by saccharin should be used to disguise the taste of medications given to diabetic children or those on a ketogenic diet.
6. Honey and syrup are ideal for suspending drugs that do not dissolve easily in water.
7. Since fruit syrups are usually acid, they should not be used for medicines that react in an acid medium (e.g., sodium bicarbonate, soluble barbiturates and penicillin).
8. Elixirs have an alcohol base that, when undiluted, may cause the child to either refuse them or to cough and choke; they may also cause a drug-drug interaction. Small amounts of water added to elixirs of phenobarbital or chloral hydrate occasionally help.
9. Nursing time can be saved by recording the most successful method of administering medications and pertinent nursing orders on the child's care plan. This also saves the child frustration, fear, and anxiety.

ages of drugs such as diazepam and barbiturates are necessary to maintain blood levels. In addition, less subcutaneous tissue for injections may be available. An alternate route may need to be selected—oral, intramuscular, or intravenous.

Intramuscular injections. The principles and techniques of the administration of injections are similar to those for adults.

Most authorities believe that the risk of sciatic nerve injury is too great to warrant the use of the gluteal site of administration. The sciatic nerve is the largest nerve in the body; its normal pathway is the hollow midway between the ischial tuberosity and the greater trochanter, covered by the gluteus maximus muscle. This pathway, however, varies a great deal from individual to individual. In addition, the small size of the gluteal mass in the infant or neonate and the potential neurotoxicity of many drugs enhance the possibility of iatrogenic trauma secondary to IM injections. Trauma of this kind is the leading cause of sciatic neuropathy in infancy. A lesion at this height of the sciatic nerve is usually tragically associated with marked permanent disability.

The younger the child, the less muscle tissue may be available for IM injections anywhere on the body. If repeated injections are necessary, the available sites may become overused, inflamed, or dystrophic, requiring concerted efforts by the nurse to develop systematic plans for rotating sites and *communicating them* to the rest of the staff. The vastus lateralis muscle is the site of choice for IM injections in children under 3 (Figure 8-2). The ventrogluteal site is preferred for the child over 3 years old who has been walking for a year or two (Figure 8-3). The dorsogluteal muscles should not be used for injections in the child under 4 to 6 years old if other IM sites are available. These muscles should not be used for injections at all until the younger child has been walking for at least 1 year.

For injection into the left gluteals, the thumb is placed on the trochanter and the middle finger on the iliac crest. The index finger placed midway between the thumb and middle finger will indicate a safe injection area. Infants should receive no more than 0.5 ml in each injection site. Small children can tolerate a volume of up to 1 ml at each site. The deltoid muscle is likewise not used for children under 5 years of age because of its underdevelopment. Rather than the skin being held taut, as for adults, the muscle mass may instead be pinched up. The needle will thus avoid striking deeper-lying structures such as nerves, bones, or blood vessels. The IM injection is still made at a 90-degree angle to the top of the massed flesh. Preferred needle sizes for pediatric IM injections are 25- to 27-gauge and ½ to 1 inch in length. A 21- or 22-gauge needle may be preferred if a viscous medication such as procaine penicillin is to be given. In the interest of safety, the child should usually be restrained for an injection and the injec-

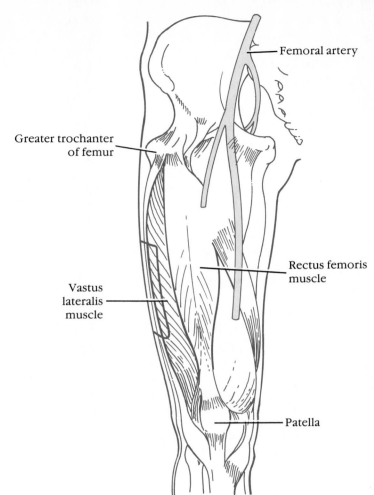

FIGURE 8-2 Vastus lateralis site for intramuscular injection. The vastus lateralis site is located on the medial outer aspect in the center third portion of the thigh in children. The belly of the muscle is one-third the distance between the greater trochanter and the knee. It is the preferred site in children, since it is well developed at birth. It is also recommended for adults because the muscle is large and can take up to 5 ml of medication per single injection. In the adult the site for injection is from one hand's breadth below the greater trochanter to a hand's breath above the knee. The injection should be given at the right angle to the muscle or on an angle slightly toward the knee.

tion given rapidly. Two or more persons should be available for children over 4 years of age despite promises that they will "hold still." An extra sterile needle may be carried in a pocket in case a needle becomes contaminated when a child moves unexpectedly. A child's attention may be distracted from the injection by asking the youngster to wiggle the toes. Since children enjoy trying out each other's beds, the identifying armband must be checked before giving each medication.

Rectal administration. When oral administration is difficult or contraindicated, the rectal route is often

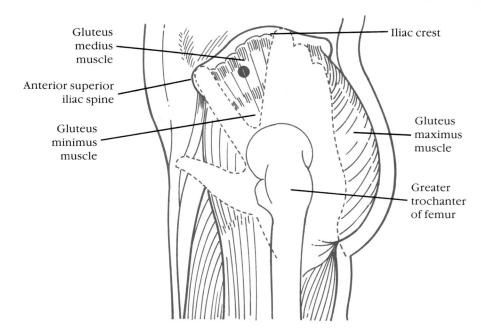

FIGURE 8-3   Ventrogluteal site for intramuscular injection. To locate this site, the nurse palpates the greater trochanter of the femur with the heel of the hand. The index and middle fingers are spread to form a **V** from the anterior superior iliac spine to just below the iliac crest. The triangle formed between the index finger, the middle finger, and the crest of the ilium is the injection site. The injection is made in the center area of the triangle with the needle directed slightly toward the iliac crest or at a right angle to the muscle. This site is relatively free from major nerves and vessels and has a larger muscle mass and less subcutaneous tissue than the dorsogluteal site. It is recommended for adults and children over 3 years of age who have been walking.

advised. Many children perceive use of the rectal route as an extreme invasion of their bodies or anticipate pain as a result. It may help to let them insert the suppository. Several drugs, such as sedatives, aspirin, and antiemetics, are available in suppository form. Suppositories made with a cocoa butter base will melt rapidly at normal body temperature, releasing the drug for absorption. After a suppository is inserted in an infant, the buttocks should be held or taped together for 5 to 10 minutes to relieve pressure on the anal sphincter and thereby help to ensure retention and absorption of the medication. Infants and children with diarrhea, however, may easily expel suppositories with explosive stools. Likewise, a suppository inserted into a child with a constipation problem or a rectum full of stool will be surrounded with stool and will have little chance for absorption of its contents.

Pharmacists and nurses often divide suppository doses by cutting them to obtain correct doses. This is a dangerous practice, since all the medication might be contained in one area of the suppository. If divided doses must be administered, the pharmacist should be the one to divide the suppository; it should be cut lengthwise and weighed to ensure as accurate a dosage as possible.

Nose drops, eardrops, and eyedrops. Aqueous prepa-

rations of nose drops are the only safe preparations to use, if it is deemed necessary to use them at all, because of the danger of aspiration. Many nose drop preparations contain vasoconstrictors, and prolonged or excessive use may be harmful. Infants are nose breathers, and nasal congestion will inhibit their sucking. For this reason, nose drops, if necessary, should be instilled 20 minutes to ½ hour before feedings.

To instill *nose drops* (Figure 8-4):
1. Hold the infant in your arm, allowing the head to fall back over the edge of your arm, or place a small pillow under the shoulders and allow the head to fall back over the edge of the pillow.
2. Place your free arm so that the forearm is around the far side of the child's head, stabilizing the head between your forearm and your body. Use your hand to stabilize the arms and hands.
3. With your free hand you can then instill the prescribed drops with minimum struggle and maximum accuracy.

The instillation of *eardrops* requires a knowledge of anatomic structure, since the shape of the auditory canal of a young child is different from that of an adult. Gentle massage of the area immediately anterior to the ear will

standardized—all droppers are not manufactured to deliver drops of the same volume. Viscosity of drugs also varies, affecting the drop size.

Eyedrops and eardrops are more comfortably tolerated if they are warmed (if not contraindicated) before instillation. This can be achieved by running warm water over the side of the bottle without the label or immersing the bottle in some warm water in a medicine cup. Even carrying the bottle in a pocket for half an hour or so will take the chill off the drops.

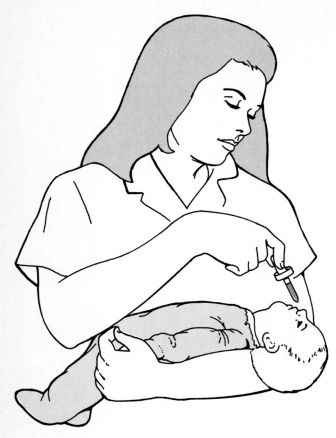

FIGURE 8-4   Administration of nose drops.

facilitate the entry of the drops into the ear canal (Figure 8-5).

Eyedrop instillation is done in the same way with children as with adults except that the head may be stabilized by an assistant. Many eyedrops cause a burning sensation for a few seconds, so if both eyes are to be medicated it is wise to do the second instillation quickly before the patient begins to blink and tear as a reaction to the burning sensation occurring in the first eye medicated. Mild pressure for 30 seconds over the inner canthus next to the nose will prevent premature drainage of the medication away from the eye. (See Figure 8-6.)

Aqueous preparations of nose, ear, and eye drops may support the growth of bacteria and fungi. For this reason small volumes of such medications are ordered and should be used for only *one* individual (not shared by family members). The dropper (especially eye droppers) should not be permitted to become contaminated by touching anything but medication or rinsing water from the tap at any time. It should never be inverted so that medication or water runs into the rubber bulb to form a medium for microbiologic growth or to flavor the medication with a rubber taste. A dropper from one medication should usually not be used to measure and administer another type of medication because droppers are not

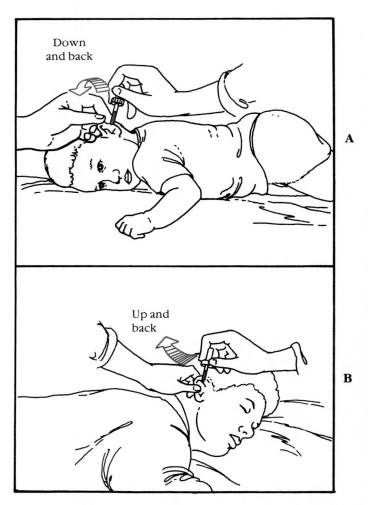

FIGURE 8-5   Administration of eardrops. The infant or child is positioned on the unaffected ear. **A,** The nurse pulls the pinna down and back to administer eardrops to infants and children under 3 years of age. **B,** When administering eardrops to children older than 3 years and adults, the nurse gently pulls the pinna up and back. The nurse should stabilize his or her hand on the patient's head for safety and instill the prescribed number of drops. The drops are directed toward the ear canal to avoid hitting the tympanic membrane, which can cause pain. The patient should remain in the position for 5 to 10 minutes. Otic drops should be warmed before they are instilled, to prevent nausea or vertigo.

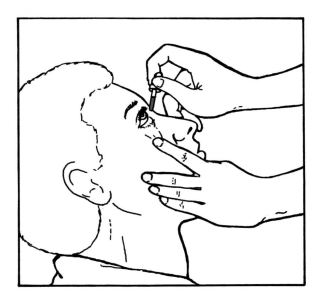

FIGURE 8-6 Administration of eyedrops. The client should be asked to look up so that the cornea reflex is diminished, and the dropper should be introduced from the side. The lower lid is gently retracted, and the drops are instilled into the conjunctival sac. Drops should not be placed directly onto the cornea. After the drops are instilled, the lid is gently released.

Intravenous medications. The use of IV drug therapy is widespread on most pediatric services for several reasons. In children with vomiting and diarrhea, medications given by mouth may be vomited, losing precious time in drug management. These same children may have poor absorption of drugs and fluids as a result of dehydration or peripheral vascular collapse, so that drugs administered via the IM route may be equally ineffective. For premature or physiologically distressed neonates, it may be preferable to give certain high-osmolality drugs by IV rather than give the syrup or elixir forms by the oral route. These infants are prone to necrotizing entercolitis (NEC) and death when administered feedings or oral drugs that have an osmolality greater than that of body fluids. Although elixirs of theophylline, phenobarbital, calcium, digoxin, and dexamethasone all have osmolalities 10 times greater than body fluids and have been implicated in causing NEC, analysis shows that the contained additives actually raise the medication's osmolality. Related studies continue.

The pediatric nurse responsible for the administration of IV drugs may find the suggestions in the box above helpful (see also Chapter 6).

Most older children may be given fluids or drugs intravenously following the same principles and techniques used for adults. The younger and smaller the child, the narrower the margin for error.

Neonates, infants, and children must be adequately restrained so as not to dislodge or pull out an infusion

GUIDELINES FOR IV DRUG ADMINISTRATION

1. IV drug therapy should be used only if other channels of drug administration are impracticable. Pediatric nurses skilled in giving medications to children via other routes may be able to influence prescribers' decisions regarding successful routes of drug administration.
2. For small infants a scalp vein or a superficial vein of the wrist, hand, foot, or arm may be most convenient and most easily stabilized. Scalp veins have no valves, and thus infusions may be in either direction. They are the most frequent sites for infant infusions. Older children may receive infusions through any accessible vein.
3. A too-rapid IV infusion or injection may cause "speed shock": rapid fall in blood pressure, respiratory irregularity, blood incoagulability, and even death. Preventive measures include use of the minidropper (note that the milliliter per hour in the order translates to the drops per minute with this tubing), calibrated volume control chambers, and infusion pumps.
4. Total parenteral nutrition (TPN) solutions are usually infused into the vena cava or innominate or subclavian veins approached via the external or internal jugular veins. Occasionally, the inferior vena cava is entered via the femoral vein.
5. Once a drug is injected intravenously, the drug's action is relatively irreversible.
6. Drugs must be properly diluted. Too much emphasis cannot be placed on the caution: GIVE THE SMALLEST POSSIBLE DOSE AT THE SLOWEST POSSIBLE RATE.

needle or catheter once it is in place. Some of the following may be helpful hints to the nurse caring for a client receiving IV therapy (see also Figure 8-7).

1. The needle or catheter should be fixed with plastic tape.
2. When a loop of tubing directly above the needle is secured to the tape, tension is relieved from the needle should it be pulled by sudden movement.
3. Since most children move about or are restless, it is necessary to support the limb with a padded arm board and immobilize the site of IV therapy. Support should extend to the joints above and below the site (with arm boards or IV boards).
4. If the infusion bottle is too high, the pressure in the vein will increase, causing fluid seepage into the surrounding tissues.

Other factors influencing drug dosages. Again, the dosage of most agents is related to the child's age, weight, and height. A child's bodily systems grow and develop at varying rates. This makes for unpredictable primary and secondary effects in pediatric medication administration.

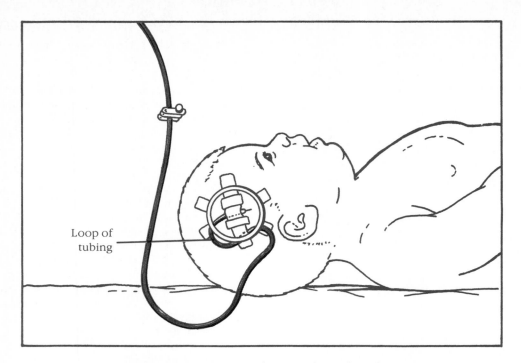

FIGURE 8-7   Securing a scalp vein infusion for infants.

One example of secondary effects specific to children is discoloration of teeth and depression of enamel growth in the child under 8 years of age with administration of tetracycline liquid medications. (This adverse reaction is well-documented, but many prescriptions for this drug are still being written for this age group, according to the FDA.) Skeletal growth of children receiving long-term adrenocortical steroids is similarly impaired.

Individual variations are noted in children's response to digitalis, insulin, opiates, and oral enzyme products; dosages require careful titration. Paradoxical responses are noted with a few drugs; responses may be directly opposite that which could be expected in the adult. Excessive reactivity to atropine by infants may be related to immaturity of the central nervous system. In addition, many drugs that are safe and effective for adults have not been tested for use with children, nor have dosages been established, because of the complex medicolegal issues involved in experimentation on children.

GERIATRIC CLIENTS

Although individuals who are over 65 represent 11.2% of the total population of the United States today, they use about 25% of the prescribed drugs. Over-the-counter drugs are also consumed in great numbers. The elderly tend to have more diseases and are given various medications. The elderly's use and abuse of drugs, especially laxatives and analgesics, seem to be widespread. It is not surprising, then, that many hospital admissions of the elderly are related to drug side effects or adverse effects.

PHYSIOLOGIC CHANGES

As people age they undergo a variety of physiologic changes that increase their sensitivity to drugs and drug-induced disease. General loss in body weight of many elderly clients may require reevaluation of dosages used for them; the criterion for dosage should be shifted from age to weight. Some older clients weigh no more than the average large child, and some weigh a lot less; yet they are prescribed the larger "adult" doses. In another case, stimulants are generally less effective in elderly individuals, and large doses are often necessary. However, CNS depressants produce intensified effects in the elderly. Sedatives and hypnotics tend to produce paradoxical side effects of irritability, incontinence, confusion, and disorientation.

Pharmacokinetics are altered in the aging client because of reduced gastric acid and slowed gastric motility, resulting in unpredictable rates of dissolution and absorption of drugs. Changes in absorption may occur when acid production decreases, altering the absorption of weakly acidic drugs such as barbiturates. However, few studies of drug absorption have shown clinically significant changes occurring with advanced age.

Changes in body composition, such as increased proportion of body fat and decreased total body water, plasma volume, and extracellular fluid, have been noted in the elderly. The increased proportion of body fat increases the body's ability to store fat-soluble compounds such as phenothiazines and barbiturates, and thus increases the accumulation of those drugs. The reduced lean body mass affects drug distribution by decreasing the volume in which the drug circulates, thereby causing higher peak levels. The risk of toxicity with water-soluble drugs increases as total body water decreases. Decreased serum albumin for binding drugs leads to increased amounts of free drug in the circulation. Disorders common to the aging person such as congestive heart failure (CHF), which may impair liver function, influence biotransformation by decreasing the metabolism of drugs and increasing the risk of drug accumulation and toxicity. Renal function may be impaired because of loss of nephrons, decreased blood flow, and glomerular filtration rate. A reduction in renal function is also secondary to CHF. Decreased renal clearance may cause increased plasma drug concentrations and longer half-lives of drugs and active metabolites that the kidney usually excretes. Special precautions include careful monitoring of the elderly client for a safe drug regime.

THE ROLE OF THE NURSE

In view of the effects just outlined and the multiplicity of drugs prescribed for elderly clients, their occasionally unreliable memories, senses, and inadequate financial status, and propensity for adverse secondary effects, nurses must make every attempt to simplify the geriatric drug therapy plan. Often what passes for senility is drug-induced lethargy or confusion.

In the administration of medications, the geriatric client may have special needs. They may have slowed reflexes and reduced understanding of treatment. It helps to organize the dispensing of medication so that enough time is allowed for clients who require a great deal of attention, possibly by medicating them last, and yet all clients will receive their medication on time. A nurse has roughly an hour's range in which to distribute all the medications during one administration period.

Diminished taste sensation usually keeps unpalatable drugs from being much of a problem, but many older individuals may have difficulty swallowing, especially if they have sustained a cerebrovascular accident (stroke). (See the discussion of special situations in Chapter 6.)

Selection of sites for injectable medications in elderly clients may present the nurse with a challenge. Since muscle mass declines with age, suitable sites for intramuscular injection may be fewer than in younger individuals and will require more skill and effort in palpating to detect muscles of adequate body and size. On the other hand, decreased sensory perception, including perception of pain, may make injections less painful.

Physical problems often interfere with the ability of the older client to comply with prescribed drug regimens. Some older clients may be unable to read labels or locate drugs because of failing eyesight; others, such as arthritic clients, may have difficulty opening bottles or handling small pills, (particularly child-proof containers) while the hard-of-hearing client may not hear all of the instructions. The logistics of obtaining drugs and the economic cost may be a deterrent to complying with therapy. Multiple drug therapy may simply be too complex for the client to manage without assistance. The nurse can simplify drug administration and scheduling as much as possible. Dosage schedules and calendars often help the forgetful client. Drug packaging that is easy to use and clearly labeled, as well as printed directions and drug information, help to ensure compliance in the older client.

Probably the most important part of the nursing process for aging clients is the nurse's ability to communicate patience, warmth, and understanding and to treat the elderly as persons with dignity and with the ability to reason, to feel, and to contribute.

KEY TERMS

carcinogenic, page 130
fetal alcohol syndrome, page 131
infant, page 129
mutagenic, page 130
neonate, page 129
teratogenic, page 130

BIBLIOGRAPHY

American Society of Hospital Pharmacists: AHFS Drug Information Service. Bethesda: American Hospital Formulary Service, 1988.

Chasnoff, and others: Cocaine use in pregnancy, New Engl J Med 311:127, 1985.

DeMino, J: The emergence of synthetic opioids—a summary, PharmAlert 14(4):1, 1984.

Erbe, RW: Drugs and pregnancy: what are the dangers? Consultant 23(11):185, 1983.

Fanaroff, AA, and Martin, RJ, eds: Behrman's neonatal-perinatal medicine: diseases of fetus and infant. St Louis: The CV Mosby Co, 1984.

Fielo, S, and Rizzolo, MA: The effects of age on pharmacokinetics, Geriatric Nurs 6(11/12):328, 1985.

Hurd, PD, and Butkovich, SL: Compliance problems and the older patient: assessing functional limitations, Drug Intell & Clin Pharm 20(3):228, 1986.

Katcher, BS, and others: Applied therapeutics, ed 3, San Francisco, Applied therapeutics.

Lamy, PP: New dimensions and opportunities, Drug Intell & Clin Pharm 19(5):399, 1985.

Linn, S, Schoenbaum, SC, and others: The association of marijuana use with the outcome of pregnancy, Am J Public Health 73(10):1161, 1983.

Mathieson, A: Old people and drugs, Nursing Times 82(2):22, 1986.

Nahas, G and Panon, W, eds: Marihuana: chemistry, biochemistry, and cellular effects. New York: Springer-Verlag, 1976.

Office of Research, Demonstrations, and Statistics; Health Care Financing Administration: Medicare-use of prescription drugs by aged persons enrolled for supplementary medical insurance, 1967-1977. Baltimore: Department of Health and Human Services, 1981.

Oppeneer, JE and Vervoren, TM: Gerontological pharmacology: a resource for health practitioners. St Louis: The CV Mosby Co, 1983.

Perez-Reyes, M, and Wall, ME: Presence of 9-tetrahydrocannabind in human milk (Correspondence), New Engl J Med 307:819, 1982.

Riordan, J, and Riordan, M: Drugs in breast milk, Amer J Nurs 84(3):328, 1984.

Rossett, HL and Weiner, L: Identifying and treating pregnant patients at risk from alcohol, CMA Journal 125:149, 1981.

Rossett, HL, Weiner, L, and Edelin, KC: Treatment experience with pregnant problem drinkers, JAMA 249:2029, 1983.

Shepard, TH: Detection of human teratogenic agents, J Pediatr 101(5):810, 1982.

Smith, S: How drugs act: drugs at different ages, Nursing Times 81(2):37, 1985.

Todd, B: When the risks outweigh the benefits, Geriatric Nurs 7(7/8):212, 1986.

United States Pharmacopeial Convention. Drug information for the health care provider, ed 7. Rockville: US Pharmacopeial Convention, Inc, 1987.

Wade, B, and Bowling, A: Appropriate use of drugs by elderly people, J Adv Nurs 11:47, 1986.

Zarlengo, DG and Uhl, HSM: Drug therapy: the geriatric patient, Hosp Formul 18(2):196, 1983.

CHAPTER 9

Substance Misuse and Abuse

Although most drugs are prescribed and administered carefully, all drugs have the potential to be misused or abused. The prescribing of drugs without adequate exploration of the client's presenting complaint, for example, represents drug misuse by a physician. Prolonged and unsupervised administration of drugs for symptomatic relief is another example. In general, **drug misuse** refers to nonspecific or indiscriminate use of drugs, including alcohol. **Drug abuse** refers to self-medication or self-administration of a drug in chronically excessive quantities, resulting in psychic and/or physical dependence, functional impairment, and deviation from approved social norms.

Drug abuse is neither a new nor a recent phenomenon. It has been known throughout history as one expression of an individual's search for relief of physical, psychologic, social, and economic problems. Indeed, investigators suggest that epidemics of drug abuse have occurred throughout human history (Brecher, 1972). Contemporary drug abuse has attained prominence as an issue with moral, legal, religious, social, intrapsychic, and medical implications.

Drug abuse is not a problem confined to any particular socioeconomic, cultural, or ethnic group. It is a major medical, social, and interpersonal problem affecting individuals from all economic backgrounds and across the life span.

Bissell and Haberman (1984) studied alcoholism and the use of other drugs with alcohol in U.S. professionals, including doctors, nurses, dentists, attorneys, social work-

TOP TEN DRUGS ABUSED IN THE UNITED STATES*

EMERGENCY ROOM

1. alcohol in combination
2. heroin
3. cocaine
4. diazepam
5. phencyclidine
6. aspirin
7. acetaminophen
8. marijuana
9. flurazepam
10. amitriptyline

MEDICAL EXAMINERS

1. alcohol in combination
2. heroin
3. cocaine
4. codeine
5. amitriptyline
6. diazepam
7. phencyclidine
8. D-propoxyphene
9. quinine
10. phenobarbital

*As reported by emergency rooms (from January to June, 1984) and Medical Examiners' offices (from July to December, 1983) from 26 metropolitan areas in the United States. Data from National Institute on Drug Abuse 1985. Statistical Series: Data from the Drug Abuse Warning Network (DAWN): Semiannual Report, Trend Data through January to June, 1984. Rockville, MD: U. S. Department of Health and Human Services.

ers, and college women. They followed a group of approximately 400 professionals for 5 to 7 years after locating the individuals from Alcoholics Anonymous programs. Nearly two thirds of the sample were graduated in the top third of their class.

Alcoholism or alcohol abuse with other drugs usually affected a professional in his or her first 15 years of practice. Drinking interfered with individual life-style at a median age of 28 for women and 30 for men. When asked reasons for seeking help from Alcoholics Anonymous, males reported family and economic pressures or difficulty with their profession, while women cited health problems, shame, or guilt as their primary reasons.

The combination of alcohol and other drugs was quite prevalent, especially with physicians and nurses. This group reported the greatest addiction to hard narcotics. Meperidine (Demerol) was their narcotic of choice because it was readily available in their settings and because it produced less pupillary constriction than the other opioids. Most physicians and nurses stated that they received their drugs through professional channels. Oth-

er professionals with combination drug abuse obtained their drugs from street sources.

When asked why they combined alcohol with other drugs, many professionals answered that they were not taught that alcohol can cause insomnia and aggravate agitation and depression. Therefore when such symptoms occurred, they had a tendency to blame other problems, such as stress, financial difficulties, marital problems, and fatigue for the symptoms. Medication was often prescribed for relief of these symptoms by attending physicians, while questioning regarding the use of alcohol was frequently overlooked.

Career pressures and accessibility of a supply of drugs place health care professionals at greater risk for drug abuse. Unfortunately, some impaired health professionals are in practice. They constitute a hazard to client well-being and to themselves, so they cannot be ignored, overlooked, or left unreported. It is vital that health agencies be alert to suspected drug abusers on its staff. Many agencies and most states have active rehabilitation programs for impaired health professionals.

Drug and alcohol abuse in the workplace costs businesses an estimated $43 billion to $85 billion a year in the United States. (Lawrence, 1983). Absenteeism, stealing, embezzlement, tardiness, and health care costs, which nationally are over $50 billion annually for the treatment of alcohol- and drug-related problems, are just a few of the cost factors related to substance abuse. Persons abusing alcohol and/or other substances will usually demonstrate a reduction in their job efficiency over time that is reflected by their attendance record, general behavior on the job, and job performance. (See Fig. 9-1.)

In an effort to identify persons with alcohol- and drug-related problems, many businesses, government agencies, and health-related facilities are performing drug analysis or urine drug tests under specified conditions on their employees. Drug screens may also be part of a pre-employment physical examination. While a number of testing procedures are available, it is important to know the analytic techniques used and the purpose and the limitation of any tests performed. Such testing often affects the individual's reputation and employment, so knowing the sensitivity of the test is very important. Is the test being given to screen a population for drug use or is it specific for a particular drug substance? Generally, the screening method tests are very sensitive, although not always as specific as the confirming tests. Therefore, false-positive and false-negative results may occur. To ensure accuracy, a second test specific for the agent reported in the screening test is necessary. Physicians interpreting the tests should be familiar with drugs known to cross react or give a false-positive result with the test in use. If the individual reports taking such a medication, an alternate, more specific drug test could then be ordered. (See boxed material on page 148.)

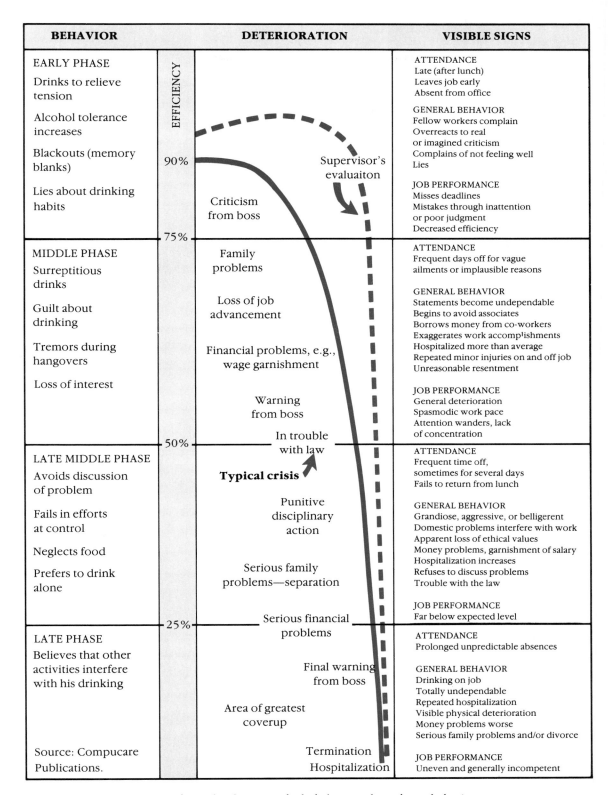

BEHAVIOR	DETERIORATION	VISIBLE SIGNS
EARLY PHASE Drinks to relieve tension Alcohol tolerance increases Blackouts (memory blanks) Lies about drinking habits	EFFICIENCY 90% 75% Criticism from boss Supervisor's evaluaiton	**ATTENDANCE** Late (after lunch) Leaves job early Absent from office **GENERAL BEHAVIOR** Fellow workers complain Overreacts to real or imagined criticism Complains of not feeling well Lies **JOB PERFORMANCE** Misses deadlines Mistakes through inattention or poor judgment Decreased efficiency
MIDDLE PHASE Surreptitious drinks Guilt about drinking Tremors during hangovers Loss of interest	Family problems Loss of job advancement Financial problems, e.g., wage garnishment Warning from boss In trouble with law 50%	**ATTENDANCE** Frequent days off for vague ailments or implausible reasons **GENERAL BEHAVIOR** Statements become undependable Begins to avoid associates Borrows money from co-workers Exaggerates work accompl¹ishments Hospitalized more than average Repeated minor injuries on and off job Unreasonable resentment **JOB PERFORMANCE** General deterioration Spasmodic work pace Attention wanders, lack of concentration
LATE MIDDLE PHASE Avoids discussion of problem Fails in efforts at control Neglects food Prefers to drink alone	**Typical crisis** Punitive disciplinary action Serious family problems—separation Serious financial problems 25%	**ATTENDANCE** Frequent time off, sometimes for several days Fails to return from lunch **GENERAL BEHAVIOR** Grandiose, aggressive, or belligerent Domestic problems interfere with work Apparent loss of ethical values Money problems, garnishment of salary Hospitalization increases Refuses to discuss problems Trouble with the law **JOB PERFORMANCE** Far below expected level
LATE PHASE Believes that other activities interfere with his drinking Source: Compucare Publications.	Final warning from boss Area of greatest coverup Termination Hospitalization	**ATTENDANCE** Prolonged unpredictable absences **GENERAL BEHAVIOR** Drinking on job Totally undependable Repeated hospitalization Visible physical deterioration Money problems worse Serious family problems and/or divorce **JOB PERFORMANCE** Uneven and generally incompetent

FIGURE 9-1   Relationship between alcohol abuse and employee behaviors.

(Redrawn from Lawrence, C, Jr: As workers get high, so do prices, The Miami Herald, Oct 24, 1983, p C-1.)

DRUGS THAT MAY RESULT IN FALSE-POSITIVE RESULTS IN RADIOIMMUNOASSAY OR ENZYME-MULTIPLIED IMMUNOASSAY TESTS

TESTING FOR	FALSE-POSITIVES REPORTED IN PRESENCE OF
amphet-amines	diethylpropion (Tenuate) ephedrine (in Tedral, Quadrinal, Primatene) nylidrin (Arlidin) phenylpropanolamine (in Alka-Selter Plus Cold Medicine, Dexatrim)
barbiturates	phenytoin (Dilantin)
opiates	chlorpromazine (Thorazine) D-propoxyphene (Darvon) dextromethorphan (the DM in many cough-cold preparations)
phencyclidine (PCP)	chlorpromazine (Thorazine) dextromethorphan (see above) diphenhydramine (Benadryl) meperidine (Demerol) thioridazine (Mellaril)

Data from Council on Scientific Affairs, 1987.

TIME VERSUS DRUG DETECTION IN URINE

DRUG	DETECTION IN URINE (HOURS)
amphetamines	48
barbiturates	
Short-acting	24
Long acting	168
cocaine	48 to 72
marijuana	
One-time use	72
Daily use	240

Data from Council on Scientific Affairs, 1987.

thing that provides relief from problems, and the drug generally is used as an adjustive, coping mechanism. Since very few drugs or substances without CNS effects are abused, one of the predominant factors contributing to drug abuse appears to be intrapsychic—a desire to alter one's state of mind. This desire may arise from a number of factors, such as curiosity, boredom, peer pressure, multiple and diverse alienation, hedonism, affluence, and the attention paid to drug abuse by the mass media. All or any combination may lead to misuse of drugs and substances. More individual or subjective reasons are personal inadequacy or failure, conflicts terminating in tension, feelings of shame, and a predisposition to depression, which may lead to emotional and behavioral problems (see boxed material on p. 149).

Pleasure-seeking behavior (hedonism) often seems to be a factor in drug abuse. Among other goals, it may represent escape from inner tensions, a search for euphoria, an attempt to explore unknown aspects of cognitive function, or an attempt to discover one's self. More specifically, some psychologic hypotheses have been advanced in relation to persons prone to use drugs as escape mechanisms. Persons with potentially drug-dependent predispositions are described as having strong psychologic dependence, low threshold of frustration, fear of failure, and feelings of inadequacy. Other authorities dispute the "addiction-prone" personality hypothesis, maintaining that everyone has the potential to become dependent on something.

Types of Drugs and Substances Abused

All drugs have some abuse potential, and some sources indicate that drug abuse may be related to the personality characteristics of the user. Perhaps among the more frequently abused chemically active substances are the xanthines, found in coffee, tea, chocolate, and colas. Although these substances rarely are perceived as drugs by the lay public, they produce mild stimulant and euphoric effects,

Urine testing for specific drugs may detect substances used days or even a week before testing. (See boxed material.) Such tests give evidence of use or prior exposure to a drug only; they do not indicate the individual's pattern of drug abuse or degree of drug dependency (Council on Scientific Affairs, 1987).

It is beyond the scope of this chapter to explore all aspects of drug abuse in depth, rather the focus is on drug actions and the treatment of drug abuse. However, the nurse is urged to investigate independently other aspects of the complex phenomenon of drug abuse to achieve a more holistic frame of reference.

ETIOLOGIC FACTORS OF DRUG ABUSE

A characteristic common to most drugs that cause dependence is that they are initially taken because the individual believes that a desirable pharmacologic effect will result. To cause dependence, then, a drug must produce favorable, pleasant, unusual, or desirable effects. The person who is dependent on a drug has found some-

DRUG ABUSE CONSIDERATIONS

FACTORS

Abuse of drugs or substances that are dependence producing is a multifaceted complex including the influence of the following factors:
1. Social
2. Cultural
3. Economic
4. Political
5. Religious
6. Personal
7. Personality
8. Initial disease state
9. Pharmacologic profile of the drug or substance
10. Change in vogue, popularity, or access

CHARACTERISTICS

The four characteristics of drugs of abuse are
1. Altered state of consciousness
2. Development of tolerance
3. Rapid onset of action of desired effects
4. Abstinence syndrome *may* appear if drug is discontinued abruptly after extended period of use

STAGES

The four states of the seduction process in the drug experience are
1. Experimentation (social recreational use)
2. Occasional use
3. Regular use
4. Dependence

*This seduction process ceases with dependence, when individual control is lost and the drugs themselves become the central theme in negotiating life.

DRUG ABUSE TERMINOLOGY

Drug abuse self-medication or self-administration of a drug in chronically excessive quantities, resulting in psychic and/or physical dependence, functional impairment, and deviation from approved social norms

Drug misuse nonspecific or indiscriminate use of drugs, including alcohol, caffeine, and nicotine

Drug Abuse Warning Network (DAWN) federal agency that monitors data on medical and psychologic problems associated with drug abuse; it identifies currently abused drugs and patterns of drug abuse and monitors changing trends or new abuse substances; such data may be used to develop new drug controls or to reschedule drugs already on the market

Hallucinogenic tendency of a drug to produce auditory and /or visual hallucinations; hallucinogenic effects are not uniform, nor are they a primary property of all consciousness-altering drugs

Psychotomimetic ability of a drug to chemically induce symptoms of psychosis

Psychedelic mind-altering drug self-administered for its subjective effects of altering perception, thought, and feeling and for social-recreational purposes

Psychic (psychologic) dependence emotional reliance on a drug; manifestations range from a mild desire for a drug to a craving to repeated compulsive use for subjectively satisfying or pleasurable effects

Physical (physiologic) dependence adaptive physiologic state occurring after prolonged use of a drug; discontinuation causes intense physical disturbances (objective withdrawal symptoms) that are relieved by readministering the same drug or a pharmacologically related drug

Tolerance tendency to increase drug dosage to experience same effect formerly produced by a smaller dose

Cross-dependent drugs drugs capable of relieving withdrawal symptoms that result from withdrawal of another drug

and their use may lead to psychic and physical dependence. Nicotine and ethyl alcohol (ethanol) are the most frequently misused and abused drugs, with consequent physical and **psychic dependence.** Reserpine, anticholinergics, steroids, phencyclidine (PCP, angel dust), phenethylamines (e. g. , amphetamines, epinephrine), pentazocine, cardiac glycosides, and L-dopa are examples of other drugs that may induce altered states of perception, thought, and feelings and drug-induced psychoses as a result of prolonged and concentrated therapeutic use or abuse.

However, as previously indicated, few drugs without CNS effects are misused or abused. (See boxed material.)

The major categories of commonly abused drugs are opioids and related compounds, barbiturates and other sedative-hypnotics: antianxiety and antipsychotic agents; amphetamines, cocaine, and other CNS stimulants; cannabis drugs; other mind-altering drugs that have been vari-

ably classified as mood modifiers and include the psychotomimetic agents (hallucinogens); inhalants; and anabolic steroids. When used for prolonged periods, depressant drugs such as the opiates, cannabis drugs, barbiturates, and alcohol generally produce both physical and psychic dependence. Stimulant drugs such as the amphetamines and cocaine appear to produce psychic dependence and tolerance and may be associated with some physical dependence in increased dosages. The other mind-altering drugs have variable and, at this time, questionable dependence-producing qualities, but it seems generally agreed upon that they all produce psychic dependence and have a rapid onset of action.

Drug abuse may take several forms. (1) *Experimental*

abuse occurs when individuals use drugs in an exploratory way and after which they accept or reject continuing use of the drugs. (2) *Social-recreational drug abuse* may occur only in social contexts; drugs that are frequently abused in social situations are alcohol, marijuana, cocaine, nicotine, and caffeine. (3) *Episodic drug abuse* refers to the periodic abuse of excessive amounts of a drug. (4) *Compulsive drug abuse* is characterized by irrational, irresistible, or compelling abuse of a drug. (5) *Ritualistic drug abuse* may be related to religious practices.

Polydrug or multiple drug abuse is common. Marijuana, alcohol, and other depressants frequently are used together and in conjunction with CNS stimulants. Heroin may be used with cocaine, pentazocine and tripelennamine, alcohol, or other depressants.

Patterns in use also develop regionally. The common use of LSD in the 1960s led to the use of speed (amphetamines) in the middle to late 1960s; in the early 1970s downers (CNS depressants) were used heavily. About the same time PCP use became common and remained so into the late 1970s. In the 1980s cocaine became popular again, and its abuse is seen more frequently but initially was somewhat curtailed by its high cost. Since 1985 cocaine use has become extremely popular throughout the United States.

The 1980s have also documented the development of synthetic "designer drugs" produced by illegal laboratories or chemists. The molecular structure of a controlled substance is modified to produce a new variant that mimics the effects of the original drug. The types of drugs most commonly modified and sold are analogs of meperidine (Demerol), fentanyl (Sublimaze), and MDMA (3, 4-methylenedioxymethamphetamine) from the illicit psychedelic agent MDA (methylenedioxyphenylethylamine). When "designer drugs" are identified, the Drug Enforcement Agency enacts regulations to ban them. Until it is banned, such a substance is legal to make, sell, or use. Once a substance is outlawed, underground chemists will make a new, legal variation of the product; and it will be sold until a ban against it is established. Thus "designer drugs" are constantly changing and should be considered to be potentially dangerous substances. Contaminants have been identified in these products, and overdoses and deaths have been reported with their use (National Institute on Drug Abuse 1985).

PHARMACOLOGIC BASIS OF PHYSICAL DRUG DEPENDENCE AND TOLERANCE

Psychic and physical dependence on a drug can exist independently or simultaneously. Both types of dependence can potentially lead to compulsive patterns of drug use in which the user's life-style is focused on procurement and administration of the drug.

Several hypotheses attempt to explain the pharmaco-logic basis of the physiologic adaptation that occurs in tolerance and physical drug dependence.

Tolerance may exist with either psychologic or physical dependence and may be viewed in two ways. **Receptor site (tissue) tolerance** is a form of adaptation in which the effect produced depends both on the concentration of the drug and on the duration of the exposure. In this type of tolerance the clinical effect of the drug is reduced as the duration of exposure continues.

The second type of tolerance is **metabolic (pharmacologic) tolerance,** which refers to an aspect of drug disposition. Prolonged exposure to a drug can change the body's metabolic response to that drug, increasing drug clearance with repeated ingestion. For example, with prolonged exposure to barbiturates, the steady state blood concentrations will fall progressively with continued administration of the same dose. This may be an attribute of the barbiturate's effect on hepatic microsomal enzymes to stimulate their own metabolism.

PATHOPHYSIOLOGIC CHANGES CHARACTERISTIC OF CHRONIC DRUG ABUSE

Physical and psychic dependence on drugs is frequently associated with debilitated physical states caused by the user's extensive involvement in procuring and using the drug. Malnutrition, dehydration, and hypovitaminosis often are evident. Respiratory complications such as pneumonia, pulmonary emboli, and abscesses frequently are associated with neglect, debilitation, and the respiratory depression produced by CNS depressants. The intravenous administration of illicit drugs often leads to a high incidence of sepsis, hepatitis, and AIDS as a result of the use of contaminated equipment. In addition, cellulitis, sclerosis of the veins, phlebitis, and skin abscesses may occur. Death from accidental overdose is common. Overdosage is a particularly significant potential danger because illegal drugs are notoriously unreliable in regard to the potency of their active ingredient. The drugs are frequently well adulterated with various substances by the time they reach the user (Table 9-1). If an individual who has been using cut drugs unknowingly receives pure or stronger drugs, the risk of toxicity and death exists. Overdosage also may occur when an individual who has been withdrawn from drugs for some time (thereby having lost accumulated tolerance) injects the previous usual dose, which now is in excess of the tolerance level.

As a consequence of all these factors, the life expectancy of persons who are physically dependent on drugs is generally lower than that of nondependent individuals.

Table 9-2 presents common drug groups that are abused, along with signs and symptoms of acute intoxication. (The box on pp. 152 to 153 lists clinical signs and symptoms that may be found in a substance abuser and may be used as an aid to diagnosis of drug abuse.)

TABLE 9-1 Illicit Drug Adulterants

Illicit drug(s)	Adulterants	Diluents
cocaine	lidocaine, procaine, antipyrine, boric acid, ethyl aminobenzoate (Benzocaine), ephedrine, tetracine, phenylpropanolamine, barbiturates, amphetamines, CNS stimulants, caffeine, A.S.A., methapyrilene, PCP	Dextrose, quinine, inositol, mannitol, lactose, talcum powder
heroin	strychnine, tripelennamine, procaine, caffeine, barbiturates, PCP, methapyrlline, cocaine, scopolamine, pentazocine, propoxyphene, antihistamines, quinine, dyes, amphetamines, phenylpropanolamine, hashish, those adulterants listed under cocaine	Similar to those of cocaine
marijuana	PCP, hashish oil, organic solvents	
LSD	PCP, MDA, ethyl aminobenzoate, benzodiazepines, antihistamines	
amphetamines and their derivatives	Caffeine, phenylpropanolamine	

TABLE 9-2 Signs and Symptoms of Acute Drug Intoxication

Drug(s) abused	Signs and symptoms
cannabis drugs	Tachycardia and postural hypotension, conjunctival vascular congestion, clear sensorium, distortions of perception, dryness of mouth and throat, possible panic
opiates	Depressed blood pressure and respiration; fixed, pinpoint pupils; depressed sensorium; coma; pulmonary edema
barbiturates and other general CNS depressants	Depressed blood pressure and respirations, ataxia, slurred speech, confusion, depressed tendon reflexes, coma, shock
amphetamines	Elevated blood pressure, tachycardia, other cardiac dysrhythmias, hyperactive tendon reflexes, pupils dilated and reactive to light, hyperpyrexia, perspiration, shallow respirations, circulatory collapse, clear or confused sensorium, possible hallucinations, paranoid feelings
hallucinogenic agents	Elevated blood pressure, hyperactive tendon reflexes, pilorection, perspiration, pupils dilated and reactive to light, anxiety, distortion of body image and perception, delusions, hallucinations

OPIOIDS AND RELATED COMPOUNDS
OPIATES AND OPIATE DERIVATIVES

The opium derivatives are one of the most abused categories of drugs, although some other narcotics also are abused. The pharmacologic types of drugs that cause opiate-like dependence include the opium alkaloids (heroin, morphine), the semisynthetic group (hydromorphone, oxymorphone), and the synthetic group (meperidine, levorphanol, methadone). Of the opiates, heroin, D. propoxyphene (Darvon), methadone, oxycodone (Percodan) and morphine are the most often abused; heroin (diacetylmorphine) is the most potent of the five.

Mode of administration. The opium derivatives generally can be administered percutaneously (absorbed through the mucous membranes) by sniffing, by subcutaneous injection (known as *skin popping*), or by direct IV injection (*mainlining*). The rate of absorption is correspondingly increased, with mainlining producing almost immediate drug effects.

Mechanism of action and effects. The opium deriva-

tives, being narcotics, act as CNS depressants, probably acting on the sensory cortex, psychic or higher centers, and thalami. Because these drugs elevate mood; relieve tension, fear, and anxiety, and produce feelings of peace, euphoria, and tranquility, they are particularly likely to lead to physical and psychic dependence. Rapid intravenous injection of these drugs produces warm, flushing sensations described as being similar to sexual orgasm. This is followed by a soothing state that seems to be best characterized as a state of complete drive satiation. The individual "high" on opiates feels no need to satisfy drives for basic biologic needs and is often described as being "on the nod"—drowsy, content, and euphoric. The drugs do not produce hallucinogenic or psychotomimetic effects.

Acute overdosage. Acute overdosage of opiate-type substances may result in coma, pulmonary edema, and cessation of respiration. These outcomes are dose dependent and are related to the degree of individual tolerance. Symptoms occur rapidly in most clients. What constitutes

CLINICAL SIGNS AND SYMPTOMS OF DRUG ABUSE*

CENTRAL NERVOUS SYSTEM

Coma: amphetamines, antihistamines, atropine, barbiturates, chloral hydrate, diazepam, ethanol, glutethimide, meprobamate, methaqualone, narcotics, PCP, pentazocine, propoxyphene, quinine, scopolamine, sedative-hypnotics, toluene, tricyclic antidepressants

Ataxia (incoordination): atropine, barbiturates, cocaine, ethanol, glutethimide, hallucinogens, opiates, PCP, phenothiazines, propoxyphene, toluene, tricyclic antidepressants

Tetanic rigidity: caffeine, methaqualone, morphine, PCP, phenothiazines, scopolamine

Convulsions: amphetamines, antihistamines, atropine, barbiturates, benzodiazepines, caffeine, cocaine, ethanol, ethchlorvynol, glutethimide, meprobamate, methaqualone, methyprylone, opiates, PCP, propoxyphene, tricyclic antidepressants

Muscle weakness or paralysis: alcohol, hallucinogens, morphine, PCP, quinine

Muscle spasm: atropine, cocaine, methaqualone, phenothiazines

Anesthesia: barbiturates, benzene, cocaine, ethanol, ketamine, PCP

Paresthesia: barbiturates, benzene, cocaine, hallucinogens, morphine, psilocybin, quinine

Muscle fasciculations (twitchings): atropine, ethanol

Hallucinations: amphetamines, atropine, barbiturates, caffeine, cocaine, ethanol, ketamine, LSD, morphine, PCP, psilocybin

Headaches: atropine, barbiturates, benzene, caffeine, cocaine, ephedrine, ethanol, morphine, scopolamine, toluene, tricyclic antidepressants

CARDIOVASCULAR SYSTEM

Circulatory collapse or shock: amphetamines, antihistamines, barbiturates, benzodiazepines, boric acid, caffeine, chloral hydrate, cocaine, ephedrine, ethanol, methaqualone, opiate withdrawal, procainamide, procaine, propoxyphene, quinine

Bradycardia: codeine, ethchlorvynol, lidocaine, narcotics, quinine, sedative-hypnotics

Tachycardia: amphetamines, antihistamines, atropine, caffeine, cocaine, codeine, ephedrine, ethanol, glutethimide, methaqualone, methyprylon, PCP, quinine

Hypertension: amphetamines, ephedrine, glutethimide, methaqualone, PCP

Hypotension: barbiturates, benzodiazepines, caffeine, chloral hydrate, glutethimide, lidocaine, LSD, meprobamate, methyprylon, narcotics, propoxyphene, quinine

Dysrhythmias: amphetamines, meprobamate, propoxyphene, quinine, toluene, tricyclic antidepressants

Vasoconstriction: amphetamines, cocaine, ephedrine

Hemorrhage, petechiae, purpura: barbiturates, benzene, quinine

RESPIRATORY SYSTEM

Rapid or deep breathing: amphetamines, atropine, barbiturates, boric acid, caffeine, chloral hydrate, cocaine, ethanol, LSD, quinine

Slow or labored breathing: atropine, barbiturates, benzene, benzodiazepines, chloral hydrate, cocaine, ethanol, ethchlorvynol, glutethimide, heroin, methaqualone, methyprylon, morphine, narcotics, propoxyphene, quinine, tricyclic antidepressants

Breath odor: ethanol, fetid or pearlike with chloral hydrate, pungent with ethchlorvynol

Respiratory paralysis: barbiturates, ethanol, hypnotics, lidocaine, opiates, PCP, procaine, toluene

Cough: benzene, ethanol

DIGESTIVE SYSTEM

Anorexia: amphetamines, cocaine, codeine, ethanol, morphine

Dysphagia: atropine, cocaine, ephedrine, tricyclic antidepressants

Thirst: atropine, chloral hydrate, morphine

Salivation: cocaine, morphine, quinine

Dry oral mucosa: amphetamines, antihistamines, atropine, benzene, glutethimide, morphine, scopolamine, tricyclic antidepressants

Nausea and vomiting: antihistamines, atropine, benzene, benzodiazepines, boric acid, caffeine, cocaine, codeine, ephedrine, ethanol, lidocaine, LSD, marijuana, opiates, propoxyphene, quinine, toluene

Colic: morphine

Diarrhea: boric acid, chloral hydrate, cocaine, quinine

Bloody stools: morphine

Constipation: anticholinergics, barbiturates, codeine, ephedrine, glutethimide, morphine, tricyclic antidepressants

Abdominal pain: benzene, chloral hydrate, cocaine, codeine, morphine, procaine, quinine, tricyclic antidepressants

Gastroenteritis: atropine, benzene, chloral hydrate, codeine, ethanol, nonbarbiturates, sedative-hypnotics

SKIN AND MUCOUS MEMBRANES

Pruritus: atropine, boric acid, opiates, scopolamine

Rash, urticaria: barbiturates, gluthethimide, halogens, LSD, meprobamate, methaqualone, nonbarbiturates, procaine, quinine, sedative-hypnotics

Dryness: atropine, benzene, boric acid, ephedrine, ethanol, heroin, morphine, scopolamine

Perspiration: ethanol, tricyclic antidepressants

Flush: amphetamines, antihistamines, atropine, codeine, ephedrine, ethanol, morphine, scopolamine

Pallor: barbiturates, benzene, cocaine, ephedrine, heroin

---

*From the Bio-Science Handbook of Clinical and Industrial Toxicology, ed 1, Van Nuys, Calif, Bio-Science Laboratories Main Laboratory, 1979.

CLINICAL SIGNS AND SYMPTOMS OF DRUG ABUSE—cont'd

Discoloration of skin
   Cyanosis: barbiturates, ethanol
   Jaundice yellow: benzene, chloral hydrate, nitrobenzene
   Red: atropine, boric acid, scopolamine
Bullae: barbiturates, glutethimide
Burns, irritation, corrosion, ulcers: boric acid, cocaine, glutethimide, pentazocine
Dermatitis inflammation: amphetamines, atropine, barbiturates, benzene, boric acid, chloral hydrate, cocaine, codeine, ephedrine, morphine, quinine, toluene
Alopecia: boric acid, chloral hydrate, morphine
Hirsutism: antidepressants, barbiturates
Exfoliation or desquamation: boric acid
Needle marks (referred to as *tracks*): amphetamines, barbiturates, cocaine, narcotics, pentazocine, propoxyphene

UROLOGIC DISORDERS

Glycosuria: atropine, caffeine, morphine
Hematuria: benzene
Oliguria: atropine, morphine, quinine
Polyuria: atropine, benzene, caffeine, cocaine, ethanol, scopolamine
Porphyrinuria: benzene
Proteinuria: benzene, caffeine, ethanol, methaqualone, morphine, quinine, toluene
Urobilinogenuria: benzene, chloral hydrate, cocaine, quinine

HEMATOLOGIC DISORDERS

Anemia: barbiturates, benzene, ethanol, meprobamate, morphine, quinine

Hemolysis: benzene, quinine
Leukopenia: benzene, meprobamate
Polycythemia: benzene

AUDITORY, PERSONALITY, AND VISUAL DISTURBANCES

Auditory disturbances
   Hearing impairment: atropine, benzene, cocaine, quinine
   Tinnitus: benzene, codeine, morphine, quinine
Personality alteration (such as irritability, confusion, delirium, psychosis): amphetamines (psychosis), antihistamines, atropine, barbiturates, benzene, benzodiazepines, caffeine, cocaine, codeine, ephedrine, ethanol, ethchlorvynol, hallucinogens, LSD, marijuana, morphine, pentazocine, PCP, procaine, scopolamine, toluene
Visual disturbances
   Blindness (partial or complete): ethanol, phenothiazines, quinine
   Blurred vision: alcohol, atropine, barbiturates, benzodiazepines, CNS depressants, ephedrine, hallucinogens, lidocaine, morphine, quinine, scopolamine
   Color distortions: ethanol, hallucinogens, LSD, quinine
   Miosis (pinpoint pupil): benzodiazepines, caffeine, chloral hydrate, codeine, heroin, morphine, pentazocine, propoxyphene
   Blank stare: PCP
   Mydriasis: amphetamines, cocaine, glutethimide, hallucinogens, belladonna alkaloids (atropine)

---

a lethal dose depends on the individual's tolerance for the drug.

Opiate toxicity is manifested in various ways. Pupils are generally found to be pinpoint (miotic), but they may be dilated in mixed overdose conditions or severe acidosis. Thrombophlebitis, scarred veins, puckered scars from subcutaneous injections, severe acidosis, bradycardia, itching caused by histamine release, hypotension, hypoxia, muscle spasm, respiratory depression, and urinary retention also occur. There is rapid absorption of the opiates following either oral or intravenous administration. These drugs tend to delay motility and gastric emptying time, so that the revival of the client may increase peristalsis and thus further increase absorption of the drug, producing a coma cycle. Chronic abuse may result in abscesses, myelitis, anaphylaxis, dysrhythmias, cellulitis, endocarditis, fecal impaction, glomerulonephritis, hyperglycemia or hypoglycemia, myoglobinuria, osteomyelitis, encephalopathy, tetanus, and thrombophlebitis. These

are caused by a spectrum of factors ranging from injection technique to adulterants in the substance of abuse. An overdose with methadone may produce prolonged toxicity of 24 to 48 hours, including respiratory depression.

The treatment of choice for acute overdosage is administration of an antagonist and respiratory support. Attention is focused on reversal of shock and treatment of apnea. The opiates depress brainstem sensitivity to carbon dioxide, and heavy dependence on a hypoxic respiratory drive device is paramount. When the triad of miotic pupils, coma or stupor, and bradypnea (respirations slowed to a rate of four to six per minute) appears, the administration of naloxone (Narcan) may differentiate narcotic poisoning from other conditions.

Naloxone is a pure narcotic antagonist and reverses the toxic effects of opiates and derivatives such as heroin, morphine, methadone, pentazocine, and propoxyphene. The usual adult dose is 0.4 to 0.8 mg intravenously. If a site for intravenous injection is not found because of abuse

ANTICIPATED DESIRED CNS EFFECTS FROM ABUSED NARCOTIC-LIKE DRUGS

Euphoria
Alteration to pleasurable mood changes
Drowsiness
Floating sensation
Transient hallucinations
Disorientation
Unusual dreams
Unreality
Delusions
Depersonalization
Apathy
Mental clouding
Lethargy
Visual disturbances

injection sites, the intramuscular (producing a longer lasting effect) or subcutaneous route may be used. Larger doses may be required to treat acute overdoses of codeine, propoxyphene, and pentazocine. If a single dose fails, a dose of 2 mg or more may be used intravenously. Failure to respond to high doses of a narcotic antagonism may indicate a mixed substance overdose or involvement of a nonopiate substance.

Blood and urine samples should be examined with a multiple drug screen to aid in diagnosis. Heroin itself may not be detected in the urine because it appears as a derivative of morphine and may be detected from 12 to 24 hours after administration. It is necessary to provide support of blood pressure and maintenance of respiration following response to naloxone. Pupils may be dilated if hypoxemia is severe or if the overdose is from meperidine; miosis is observed in barbiturate, ethanol, and phenothiazine overdoses.

Children with a known or suspected narcotic overdose may receive 0.01 mg/kg as the first dose. Naloxone may be diluted with Sterile Water for Injection. If the child is not responsive to the first dose, one or two additional intravenous doses may be given at 2- to 3-minute intervals.

Naloxone reverses apnea and coma within minutes. The naloxone must be titrated to the client's arousal with a respiratory rate in a range of 10 to 20 breaths per minute. Intravenous administration may be repeated to reverse narcotic respiratory depression in 2- to 3-minute intervals. Repeated doses may be required at 1- to 2- hour intervals, depending on the amount and type of drugs (short- or long-acting) and the interval since the last administration of the narcotic. A positive response to naloxone is characterized by dilation of the pupils and an increase in respiratory function, blood pressure, and cardiac rate.

After satisfactory response is attained, the client is kept under observation, and naloxone doses are repeated as necessary, since the duration of action of some narcotics (morphine, heroin, methadone) exceeds that of naloxone (1½ to 2 hours).

Physical dependence and acute abstinence syndrome. In a patient physically dependent on opiates an abrupt and complete reversal of narcotic effects with naxolone may precipitate an acute abstinence syndrome. Although the opiate abstinence syndrome may be reversible by administration of opiates, the administration of narcotics to maintain a drug-dependent client is prohibited by law except if the person is an inpatient who was admitted for an emergency procedure or is being detoxified or maintained in an approved federal drug-treatment program. Methadone usually is considered the drug of choice in the treatment of this clinical condition.

Physical dependence on opiates usually is described in terms of the opium derivative heroin, since the other derivatives manifest similar symptoms. Physical dependence on heroin is evident in the withdrawal syndrome that develops if the drug is withheld and in the marked tolerance that develops with continued use of the drug. Also, because persons dependent on heroin so frequently feel satiated, physical, emotional, and social deterioration often occurs. The individuals may feel little need for food and become grossly malnourished and weak. Preoccupation with obtaining the drug makes participation in the usual social and vocational aspects of life difficult, if not impossible. As the drug craving grows, tolerance to the drug also increases, and eventually the motivation for using the drug becomes oriented more to the avoidance of withdrawal symptoms and less to the achievement of euphoria.

Withdrawal symptoms. The initial withdrawal symptoms are related to the half-life of the narcotic being used. Symptoms of withdrawal from heroin are autonomic in origin and appear within 8 hours after the last dose in individuals who are physically dependent. These symptoms are less life-threatening than with other substances of abuse. They may originally be manifested as restlessness, chills and hot flashes, piloerection on the skin (which gives rise to the term "cold turkey"), rhinorrhea, drowsiness, lacrimation, mydriasis, sneezing, yawning, generalized anxiety, abdominal cramps, lower back pain, lower extremity cramps (which probably resulted in the phrase "kick the habit"), vomiting and diarrhea, anorexia, diaphoresis, muscular twitching, elevated pulse rate, blood pressure, and temperature, and a craving for the drug. Such symptoms usually are followed by a restless sleep known as *yen* from which the client may awaken irritable, weak, and depressed. Depending on the drug used, the abstinence syndrome develops within 2 to 48 hours and peaks at 72 hours.

Occasionally withdrawal symptoms are severe enough

to result in cardiovascular collapse. If withdrawal is untreated, it may continue for up to 7 to 10 days, after which the physical dependence of the body on the presence of opiates is eventually lost. Psychic dependence continues for a longer period; some authorities claim it continues forever.

Treatment of opiate dependence

Withdrawal programs. Generally, opiate withdrawal is difficult, and repeated relapses to drug abuse can be expected. Abrupt and complete withdrawal (*cold turkey*) can be accomplished but is generally avoided as a dangerous and inhumane approach. Therapeutic withdrawal from an opiate may be somewhat more comfortably achieved by successively tapering the drug's dosage over a period of several days.

The choice of withdrawal program is partly influenced by the following factors: the client's physical condition, the duration of drug dependence, the type and amount of drug being taken, motivations for drug abuse and withdrawal, and whether the individual is also dependent on other drugs. In some instances, depending on these factors, opiate withdrawal may need to be accomplished within a hospital and with close medical supervision.

In identifying criteria for evaluating opiate withdrawal, one should note that recovery from morphine-type dependence is not equated with cure. Regardless of repeated relapses to drug abuse, therapeutic programs should continue. Progress in withdrawal may be indicated by progressively longer periods of abstinence from opiates without resort to the use of other psychoactive drugs and by the client's growing confidence in the ability to function effectively without drugs.

Therapeutic community programs. The ultimate goal of using any substance to treat dependency is to provide relief from the compulsive craving for the drug of abuse. To achieve rehabilitation, the abuser needs to turn to more than another substance. The individual also needs human dignity, sincerity, compassion, warmth, self-respect, and hope with positive reinforcement. To achieve independence and become a self-sustaining, productive member of the community, the abuser must be provided with emotional and social support. These human resources have not been effectively addressed by many treatment programs, and failures have resulted.

Because persons withdrawing from drugs frequently cannot make the transition easily, groups of persons who have decided to abstain from drug use can meet or live together in an attempt to support and guide one another. Such therapeutic community programs as Phoenix House and halfway houses have been established that include group psychotherapy and self-help approaches. Ultimately an individual should emerge from such a program with sufficient personal growth and appropriate support systems to be able to manage life satisfactorily without resorting to drug abuse.

Methadone detoxification and withdrawal. A currently preferred method of withdrawal is substitution of methadone hydrochloride, a program pioneered by Drs. Vincent Dole and Marie Nyswander. Methadone hydrochloride is a synthetic opiate analgesic that, by virtue of cross-tolerance, permits effective substitution of methadone dependence for heroin dependence. Its effectiveness against heroin dependence results from its ability to forestall the euphoriant effects of heroin and the craving for the drug without producing heroin's deleterious physical and mental effects. When properly administered, methadone allows the individual to function adequately, without intellectual or emotional impairment.

Methadone is taken orally, generally in daily doses of 15 to 20 mg and ranging up to 120 mg. Methadone is usually initiated in a 20 mg dose and titrated in 5 to 10 mg increments until symptoms are suppressed. Detoxification may be accomplished by 5 mg/day (to 25 mg), and then decreasing it by 2.5 mg/day. Methadone therapy is initiated empirically based on client symptoms. As a general guide, 1 mg methadone is substituted for 20 mg meperidine, 4 mg morphine, and 2 mg heroin.

For a review of recommended dosages and dosage adjustments, the reader is referred to current drug abuse references or the most recent edition of the American Hospital Formulary Service (McEvoy, 1988).

Regular administration results in the development of tolerance to methadone and cross-tolerance to heroin. The client will not experience the opiate-induced "rush" and euphoria unless higher doses than usual are used. When the abuser is being treated with methadone, supportive psychologic or psychiatric counseling may relieve some of the burdens that led to drug dependence. During this phase the methadone may be gradually withdrawn, usually at a rate of 20% reduction in daily dosage. However, this is controversial, since this program is not always successful. Previous opiate abusers who are unable to negotiate life in a drug-free state may revert to their former dependence or alternative substance abuse or may return to the methadone therapy detoxification. (For a discussion of methadone maintenance, see boxed material on p. 156.)

Methadone maintenance. In the United States, methadone may be administered to opioid dependent individuals for detoxification purposes. The drug is given in decreasing dosages over 3 weeks, the time allotted for complete drug withdrawal. Maintenance programs are defined as administration of regular or consistent dosages of methadone for longer than 3 weeks. Admittance to a methadone maintenance program usually requires a minimum of a 2-year history of opioid dependence with demonstration of a current physiologic dependence on an opioid-type substance. Maintenance methadone treatment programs require both FDA and state licensing and/or approval. The ultimate goal of these programs is

METHADONE TREATMENT PROGRAMS

Methadone, if used as an analgesic, may be stocked and dispensed from any licensed pharmacy. But methadone for use in the treatment and/or maintenance of opioid abstinence syndrome must follow the guidelines of the U.S. FDA.

1. Methadone products may only be stocked and dispensed by hospital or community pharmacies or facilities that are approved by the FDA and appropriate state regulatory boards.
2. Only oral dosage forms may be dispensed in accordance with the Federal Methadone Regulations (21CFR 291.505)
   a. Detoxification programs may not extend beyond 21 days and may not be repeated until 1 month following the previous course.
   b. Although the oral dosage form is preferred, if the client cannot swallow oral medications, parenteral methadone may be used initially.
   c. If methadone is given beyond 3 weeks, a detoxification program has progressed to a maintenance-treatment program.
3. The goal of a program is eventual withdrawal of the drug. The success of a program depends on the client being goal-oriented, along with the use of supportive services (medical, social, psychologic, and vocational).
4. Although maintenance programs are limited to government-approved agencies only, if addicted clients are hospitalized for medical reasons and are officially enrolled in an approved, documented program, they may receive temporary maintenance therapy during their critical hospitalization period.
5. For additional and specific guidelines, check both state and federal regulatory bodies.

complete withdrawal from drug dependency for the participant.

Nurses should be aware that addicts hospitalized with medical conditions other than addiction may require pharmacologic support with methadone or opioids during their stay. Such individuals should be referred to an approved methadone maintenance program for follow-up care.

Methadone dependence does occur, but it is less serious than heroin dependence. Withdrawal symptoms are less severe but last for a longer period. Methadone withdrawal programs generally include supplemental rehabilitation techniques such as vocational and social rehabilitation. After individuals have functioned free from heroin for a sufficient period, secured steady employment, and readjusted their life-style, theoretically they can be withdrawn from methadone maintenance. Some treatment centers report having accomplished withdrawal from methadone through the use of chlorpromazine, whereas others maintain that methadone may need to be taken indefinitely. Whether the latter can be avoided still is being researched.

Heroin maintenance. In a number of countries, notably Great Britain, physicians are permitted to prescribe heroin and other opioids for persons who have a history of intractable dependence, thereby maintaining them and preventing withdrawal symptoms. Prescriptions currently are issued only through designated hospitals and the National Health Service. When such a system is implemented appropriately, it appears that the drug user can function normally and will seldom seek supplemental or illicit sources of drugs. There are, however, several reasons why such programs sometimes do not operate effectively and may be abused. Allowing clients to determine their own dose of the drug and supplying the drug in a form and quantity such that it can be easily resold or misused are examples of the ways in which such systems can be abused.

Clonidine treatment. Clonidine (Catapres), a sympatholytic antihypertensive (central alpha adrenergic stimulator) drug approved for treatment of hypertension, is being investigated for relieving symptoms of acute withdrawal in dependence on to opioids, such as heroin and methadone. Opioid withdrawal symptoms theoretically are thought to be a function of the hyperactivity of the locus ceruleus, a major noradrenergic nucleus of the brain. Inhibitory receptors in the locus ceruleus are thought to be stimulated by opioids and by stimulation with clonidine through the alpha-2 adrenergic receptors.

A dosage of 5 μg/kg/day of clonidine to start increasing up to 17 μg/kg/day has been used to prevent the withdrawal syndrome. The dose is dependent on the individual's tolerance and quantity and type of narcotic agonist used. The daily dosage is administered in equally divided doses over a 24-hour period and individually titrated to the client's response. The dosage is gradually tapered by 0.1 or 0.2/mg daily at the end of the treatment to avoid emergence of the withdrawal syndrome and headaches. The clinical usefulness of clonidine is limited by the drug's sedative and hypotensive effects, and extremely close supervision of the client is necessary to monitor side effects, adverse effects, and any manipulation of the dose by the client. Physical dependence on opioids is eliminated by this detoxification process, and nonpharmacologic intervention can be used to address the remaining psychic dependence.

ANALGESICS

pentazocine (Talwin)

Pentazocine HCl (Talwin) 50 mg orally is considered approximately equivalent as an analgesic to 60 mg (1 grain) of codeine. Sharp increases in the incidence of drug abuse involving pentazocine have led the Drug Enforcement Administration to place this drug in the controlled status (Class IV) under the Controlled Substances Act.

Pentazocine's potential for producing psychic and physical dependence is significant even in low doses, and infants born to pentazocine-dependent women experience withdrawal immediately postpartum. Pentazocine can cause psychotomimetic reactions such as visual hallucinations, feelings of depersonalization, and nightmares.

The CNS effects of pentazocine are similar to those of the opioids, including analgesia, sedation, and respiratory depression (reversed by naloxone). In high doses pentazocine causes increases in blood pressure and heart rate. Lung problems may be caused by the talc binders and other particulate matter from crushed tablets accumulating in the lungs. Other clinical effects include seizures and ulceration and severe sclerosis of the skin and subcutaneous tissue and muscles, caused by subcutaneous or intramuscular injections. These ulcerated areas may measure 8 × 5 cm, and extensive cellulitis is observable. Such areas often require debridement and grafting. The combination of pentazocine with other CNS depressants such as barbiturates and alcohol may be lethal.

Pentazocine and PBZ (tripelennamine) abuse first appeared in the late 1960s to the 1970s. Shortages or high cost of heroin in large metropolitan areas contributed to the substitution of pentazocine and tripelennamine, known as *T's and blues* (*T* for Talwin and *blue* for the color of the generic tablet of tripelennamine). T's and blues are oral tablets that are mixed together in solution and injected either through a cotton filter intravenously, like heroin, or subcutaneously, possibly resulting in abscess and necrotic tissues (many users require hospitalization and grafting). Drug abusers have indicated that tripelennamine is used to increase the onset of action and prolong the duration of the euphoria produced by pentazocine. Abusers report that when injected intravenously, T's and blues produce a rush "indistinguishable from a heroin rush" (Seabolt, 1984).

To discourage abuse, the manufacturer sought alternate formulations of pentazocine to market. Other companies have had to take similar steps because of street abuse of their products (e.g., Darvon Compound to Darvocet-N). Eventually the manufacturer released a combination of pentazocine and naloxone (Talwin-Nx). The addition of naloxone nullifies or cancels the rush effect of the pentazocine-tripelennamine combination. Hopefully, this will reduce the abuse potential of pentazocine.

The treatment of pentazocine dependence is gradual reduction of the drug itself in a controlled environment. The psychotomimetic effects should be observed closely in a controlled environment and may persist for 5 to 7 days.

propoxyphene (Darvon, Novopropoxyn✳)

Use of propoxyphene products in excessive doses, either alone or in combination with other CNS depressants including alcohol, is a significant cause of drug-related deaths. Fatalities within the first hour of overdose are not uncommon. In a survey of deaths from overdosage conducted in 1975, in approximately 20% of the fatal cases death occurred within the first hour (5% occurred within 15 minutes). Propoxyphene should not be taken in doses higher than those recommended by the physician, and clients should be so warned. The judicious prescribing of propoxyphene is essential for safe use of this drug. With clients who are depressed or suicidal, consideration should be given to the use of nonnarcotic analgesics.

Because of its added depressant effects, propoxyphene should be prescribed with caution for those individuals whose medical condition requires the concomitant administration of sedatives, tranquilizers, muscle relaxants, antidepressants, or other CNS depressant drugs. Clients should be cautioned against the concomitant use of propoxyphene products and alcohol because of potentially serious CNS additive effects of these agents. Many of the propoxyphene-related deaths have occurred in individuals with previous histories of emotional disturbances or suicidal ideation or attempts as well as histories of misuse of tranquilizers, alcohol, and other CNS active drugs. Some deaths have occurred as a consequence of the accidental ingestion of excessive quantities of propoxyphene alone or in combination with other drugs.

The clinical effects of overdose occur within ½ hour and include nausea, vomiting, and drowsiness followed by stupor and coma. Within ½ to 1 hour of an oral overdose, respiratory arrest, hypotension, and grand mal seizures often occur. Miotic pupils are frequently seen, and the individual may experience diabetes insipidus, pulmonary edema, cardiac dysrhythmias requiring cardiopulmonary resuscitation, bundle branch block, nonspecific ST and T wave alterations, prolongation of the QRS complexes, and hypoglycemia.

There is a high incidence of toxic psychosis, convulsions, and coma. The peak plasma level occurs 2 to 3 hours after a therapeutic dose, with a therapeutic half-life of 6 to 12 hours. However, the active metabolite, norpropoxyphene, attains peak plasma concentration in 4 hours and has a half-life of 30 to 36 hours.

The drug also may be abused by parenteral administration of the oral form. The tablet or contents of the capsule is dissolved in ethyl alcohol (vodka), placed in a syringe with a cotton filter or cigarette filter, and injected intravenously.

The severe and sometimes unpredictable course of propoxyphene intoxication has stimulated an interest in its clinical kinetics. It is primarily metabolized in the hepatic microsomal enzyme system through the major metabolic pathway of demethylation to norpropoxyphene and is primarily eliminated by renal excretion. The most severely intoxicated individuals with the highest plasma levels also have metabolites with the longest half-life, which may indicate dose-dependent kinetics. Total urinary excretion of all metabolites is about 7 days. The systemic availability is reduced corresponding to extensive first pass metabolism of 30% to 70%, and the half-life is 8 to 24 hours for propoxyphene and 18 to 29 hours for the metabolite norpropoxyphene. The ranges indicate pronounced intraindividual dose-independent variations in oral clearance. Transient changes in hepatic blood flow at the time the drug passes through the liver may influence kinetics of high-clearance drugs such as propoxyphene. This is further influenced by a high-affinity binding site in some tissues, which also occurs with tricyclic antidepressants.

Norpropoxyphene has less CNS depressant effect than propoxyphene but a greater anesthetic effect on the myocardium, similar to that of amitriptyline and antidysrhythmic drugs such as lidocaine and quinidine. Electrocardiographic monitoring is essential in management of overdosage.

Propoxyphene is pharmacologically related to the opioids; however, it may not elicit the narcotic response when naloxone is administered, and the client will need more protracted respiratory support measures. Overdose may be accompanied by seizures requiring anticonvulsants, and emergence from a coma may require restraints before administration of naloxone because of the client's disorientation, agitation, and confusion.

Clients need psychologic and emotional support during this time. A quiet, calm environment with reduced sensory stimulation may reduce the incidence of disorientation and agitation. The nurse should use a simple, direct approach when communicating with reality orientation and reassurance.

The FDA Drug Bulletin has carried the warning that propoxyphene should not be taken during pregnancy. The warning against use during pregnancy is based on demonstrations of withdrawal symptoms in newborn infants from mothers taking the drug during pregnancy. The symptoms include tremors, irritability, high-pitched cry, diarrhea and weight loss with ravenous appetite, and infrequently, seizures.

SEDATIVE-HYPNOTICS
BARBITURATES

It is generally known by the lay public that the barbiturates and some nonbarbiturate sedative-hypnotics can cause physical as well as psychic dependence. It appears that short-acting barbiturates, in addition to drugs such as glutethimide (Doriden), methaqualone, chloral hydrate, methyprylon (Noludar), and ethchlorvynol (Placidyl), are most likely to produce physical dependence, possibly

because they produce sudden and forceful desired effects (rapid onset of action). The lipid solubility enables the drug to enter the central nervous system rapidly, with immediate appearance of effects.

Because these drugs are more extensively described in other chapters, mechanisms of action and effects are not explored here. Rather, this section focuses on acute intoxication and withdrawal syndromes resulting from dependence on these drugs. Table 9-3 presents the therapeutic and toxic serum reference values for some of these agents.

Intoxication from barbiturates must be differentiated from other causes of intoxication. The client's breath odor is an indicator with alcohol, inhalants, and chloral hydrate but not with the barbiturates. The effects of barbiturate intoxication resemble those of alcohol intoxication and include emotional lability, muscular incoordination, difficulty in cognitive processes, and sedation. Toxic doses lead to stupor and respiratory depression. The reasons for barbiturate abuse are similar to those for ethyl alcohol abuse: both drugs produce disinhibition and mild euphoria.

Specific and efficient antidotes to offset barbiturate/depressant drug overdoses are not available. Individuals dependent on the sedative-hypnotics should never be abruptly withdrawn because the withdrawal syndrome accompanying cessation of barbiturate administration is one of the most dangerous in the field of drug abuse. The withdrawal syndrome may begin with weakness, tremulousness, restlessness, anxiety, insomnia, gastrointestinal disturbances, and orthostatic hypotension that may last 3 to 14 days. The syndrome starts in the first 24 hours, possibly leaving the patient too weak to get out of bed. Symptoms of psychoses may progress to confusion, delirium, and hallucinations. Major convulsive seizures are more common in barbiturate withdrawal than in alcohol withdrawal. Agitation and hyperthermia may lead to exhaustion, cardiovascular collapse, and death.

Coma and apnea from single high doses of mixed depressants may lead to high morbidity and mortality. If the withdrawal syndrome is untreated, it usually ends by the fourteenth day of drug abstinence, and its end generally is preceded by prolonged sleep. Clients experiencing barbiturate withdrawal must be hospitalized because even though the syndrome appears mild 24 hours after the last dose, convulsions and cardiovascular collapse may occur on the second or third day and last up to 2 weeks.

Treatment of barbiturate withdrawal generally consists of substitution of the drug with a longer-acting barbiturate such as phenobarbital. Dosage of the substitute is slowly tapered over a period of several weeks until it is completely withdrawn.

Some investigators prefer pentobarbital to phenobarbital as a withdrawal agent, and there is some controversy

TABLE 9-3 Therapeutic and Toxic Reference Values for Some Sedative-Hypnotics

Substance of abuse	Therapeutic levels (μg/ml)	Toxic levels (μg/ml)
BARBITURATES		
short-acting (blood, serum, plasma)	1-5	>5
intermediate-acting (blood, serum, plasma)	5-14	>30
long-acting (blood, serum, plasma)	15-35	>40
amobarbital (blood)	5-8	>30
secobarbital (blood)	3-5	>5
pentobarbital (blood)	1-4	>5
NONBARBITURATES		
methyprylon (blood)	<10	>30
chloral hydrate (trichloriethanol—TCE— and trichloroacetic acid)	2-6 (urine), 2-3 hr after ingestion 0.8-1.2 mg TCE/100 ml blood, 30-60 min after 1 g chloral hydrate	
ethchlorvynol (blood)	0.5-6.5	>20
glutethimide (blood, serum)	2-6	>10

concerning the dose equivalents. Some clinicians use 30 mg phenobarbital for 100 mg pentobarbital, and others use a milligram-per-milligram equivalency. Phenobarbital detoxication may produce disinhibition and euphoria and may result in fewer client management problems than pentobarbital substitution. Phenobarbital permits safer withdrawal with fewer blood level fluctuations and less risk of overdose fatality in the sedative-hypnotic-dependent individual.

Some abusers inject the tablet or capsule oral forms of the barbiturates and sedative-hypnotics intravenously, which can result in serum hepatitis, septicemia, pulmonary emboli, papilloma, bacterial endocarditis, abscesses, tetanus, and various skin rashes. Because of the highly alkaline sclerosing of veins, phlebitis and extravascular abscesses occur with intravenous-injection abuse of barbiturates.

Long-acting barbiturates (phenobarbital, mephobarbital, metharbital, primidone [15% converted to phenobarbital]) are not generally the substances of abuse. Doses over 8 mg/kg have produced some toxic manifestations depending on the individual's exposure or dependence on the drug. Because of enzyme induction, long-term barbiturate use increases the metabolism of the barbiturate. Hepatic enzymes degrading barbiturates increase rapidly, metabolize the barbiturates, and reduce the barbiturate effect. Drug-dependent individuals have been known to take up to 1 g of barbiturate daily. Doses in therapeutic ranges may achieve levels as high as 5 mg/100 ml; however, clients on long-term therapy or those who abuse the drug may sustain higher levels. In individuals who have not developed tolerance to barbiturates, a blood level of 3.5 mg/ml for the short-acting barbiturates or 8 mg/ml or more for the long-acting barbiturates can be fatal.

Some clinical effects observed following acute overdosage are depression, coma, hypotension, hypoxia, hypothermia, depressed kidney function caused by cardiovascular depression, respiratory or cardiac arrest, and aspiration pneumonia. Physical dependence has been observed with chronic ingestion of 300 to 700 mg daily for about 2 months. Withdrawal (lasting up to 14 days) causes tremors, anorexia, insomnia, nausea, vomiting, muscular weakness, and hypotension. Convulsions (clonic-tonic, isolated, or status epilepticus) may ensue 16 to 24 hours after the last dose of the drug. Withdrawal may occur in neonates of mothers who abuse phenobarbital and may be seen soon after delivery or delayed up to 2 weeks. Hyperirritability and seizures may occur in neonates for several months following withdrawal.

Treatment of the adult with phenobarbital poisoning should include forced alkaline diuresis. Withdrawal may be treated with phenobarbital by a gradual reduction regimen over a 3-week period.

Short-acting barbiturates possess clinical effects similar to those of the longer-acting derivatives. In this case, forced diuresis is of no value. Hemodialysis is also ineffective; however, it may be used in clients with severe acid-base or fluid and electrolyte problems even though the drug is not dialyzable. The seizure from barbiturate withdrawal may be treated with diazepam given intravenously. Withdrawal after the last dose may be treated with phenobarbital in a dosage of 30 mg for each 100 mg short-acting barbiturate used, administered in divided doses three or four times daily for a gradual decrease. If withdrawal symptoms continue, the dosage should be increased until the client is comfortable; then once the client's condition is stabilized, the drug is gradually withdrawn over a period of 3 weeks.

NONBARBITURATES

ethchlorvynol (Placidyl)

Prolonged use of ethchlorvynol may result in tolerance, physical dependence, and psychic dependence. Dependence has been observed in individuals taking 1 g dosages over prolonged periods (4 to 5 months).

Some signs and symptoms of chronic intoxication are incoordination, tremors, ataxia, confusion, slurred speech, hyperreflexia, diplopia, and generalized muscle weakness. Some reversible symptoms are toxic amblyopia, nystagmus, and peripheral neuropathy. If the liquid in the capsule form is injected intravenously, pulmonary edema can result.

Severe withdrawal symptoms similar to those of barbiturate and alcohol withdrawal may occur as late as 9 days following abrupt cessation after prolonged use of this drug. Signs and symptoms of ethchlorvynol withdrawal are convulsions, delirium, schizoid reactions, perceptual distortions, retrograde amnesia, ataxia, insomnia, slurred speech, anxiety, irritability, agitation, tremors, anorexia, dizziness, nausea, vomiting, weakness, sweating, muscle twitching, and weight loss. Coma has been reported to last 12 days before recovery; a flat electroencephalogram may be seen during coma, but supportive care must be continued. Overdose-induced hypotension responds to fluids and vasopressor agents. A neonatal withdrawal syndrome has also been observed.

Respiratory depression necessitates artificial ventilation. Close nursing monitoring should include observations for bradycardia, pulmonary edema, peripheral neuropathy, cardiac arrest, respiratory arrest, and hypothermia. The half-life of the drug in an overdose may be more than four times that of the therapeutic half-life (25 hours).

The nurse should be alert for mixed ingestion, as in other cases of substance abuse. Alcohol potentiates this drug result so that lower levels of ethchlorvynol lead to a coma.

The client who manifests withdrawal symptoms is given either ethchlorvynol or phenobarbital (30 mg phenobarbital for each 350 mg ethchlorvynol abused) and the dosage tapered gradually over a period of days or weeks. The addition of a phenothiazine may be necessary for the client exhibiting psychotic withdrawal symptoms. Hospitalization in the withdrawal stage is absolutely necessary. There is a narrow margin between the toxic and therapeutic dose ranges for this drug, and dependency is produced even with lower doses. Overdose symptoms usually disappear in 1 to 2 weeks.

Since ethchlorvynol is very lipid soluble, a period as long as 9 days may elapse between the last dose and the appearance of withdrawal symptoms. Since this is a tertiary alcohol, a characteristic pungent odor of the breath is frequently noted.

glutethimide (Doriden)

Glutethimide is widely abused. Signs and symptoms of chronic intoxication include impairment of memory and ability to concentrate, impaired gait, ataxia, tremors, hyporeflexia, and slurring of speech. Withdrawal reactions ranging from nervousness and anxiety to grand mal seizures are seen upon abrupt cessation of the drug after prolonged use. Abdominal cramps, chills, numbness of extremities, and dysphagia are also found.

Acute overdosage is a life-threatening situation. Signs and symptoms of acute intoxication vary in severity with the ingested dose and are difficult to distinguish from barbiturate intoxication. Mild intoxication produces drowsiness and lethargy; and moderate to severe intoxication produces different degrees of coma, which may last as long as 4 or more days. The nurse should be alert for mixed drug ingestion (such as hypnotics, sedatives, alcohol, and illicit drugs) and suicide attempts.

Glutethimide produces significant anticholinergic effects, including adynamic ileus (diminished or absent peristalsis), urinary retention (atonic urinary bladder), dryness of the mouth, mydriasis, irritability, and convulsions. These effects are potentiated by a mixed drug ingestion involving, among other substances, alcohol. There is also depressed or absent response to painful stimuli, hypotension, and inadequate ventilation, sometimes with cyanosis. Sudden apnea may occur with manipulation such as gastric lavage or endotracheal intubation.

Cyclic coma (coma to wakefulness to coma) occurs because of the continued periodic absorption of the glutethimide from the gastrointestinal tract. The anticholinergic effects (cholinergic blockade) of glutethimide lower the motility of the gastrointestinal tract until the drug is metabolized, after which motility is resumed; following this, more glutethimide is absorbed, and the coma begins again. This pattern may be interrupted by increasing the emptying time of the gastrointestinal tract with a cathartic and charcoal to absorb the drug and lavage or emesis. Prolonged coma may be caused by the accumulation in brain and plasma of the toxic active liver metabolite 4HG (4 hydroxy-2-ethyl-2-phenylglutarimide).

The anticholinergic effect and cyclic coma necessitate a period of observation to determine the toxicity of the ingestion. Death has occurred following ingestion of 5 g (10 tablets of 500 mg), and survival has been reported with ingestion of 35 g. The lethal dose is in a range of 10 to 20 g.

A phenobarbital equivalent dose of 30 mg is recommended for each 250 mg glutethimide abused in cases of withdrawal. Overdose is a potential problem, since there is a narrow therapeutic-lethal range and active metabolites are present.

One gram of glutethimide combined with 240 mg of

codeine is used as a substitute for heroin to produce heroin-like effects. This combination is called a "load." The codeine is obtained either from the Class V antitussives that contain 240 mg codeine in 120 ml of the product or from acetaminophen or aspirin products containing codeine. The Class V cough-suppressant product is referred to as "syrup." The nurse should be aware of the possibility of an overdose of both codeine and glutethimide in a client who admits to "loading."

methaqualone (Tualone-300♣, Hyptor♣, Quaalude♣)

Methaqualone, a well-documented drug of abuse, was officially withdrawn from the U.S. market in 1984. While no longer legally available, methaqualone is still sold illegally (Dominquez, 1987). Analyzed samples of street "ludes" (methaqualone) have been found to contain methaqualone or diazepam.

Methaqualone, a hypnotic agent, was first released in 1965. Abuse of methaqualone can cause severe psychic and physical dependence. Abusers describe the effects produced by the drugs as sensual, euphoric, and similar to those of opiate drugs. Multiple drug abuse often occurs with methaqualone, and the concomitant abuse of alcohol may worsen the prognosis.

Acute overdose may result in delirium and coma, with restlessness, irritability, and hypertonia, progressing to convulsions. Spontaneous vomiting and increased secretions frequently occur and may lead to aspiration pneumonitis or respiratory obstruction. Large overdosages may result in cutaneous and pulmonary edema, hepatic damage, renal insufficiency, bleeding, shock, and respiratory arrest. Coma has been reported with doses of 2.4 g and death with a dose of 8 g, although individuals have survived doses of 22 g. Hyperexcitability and hyperreflexia are seen frequently in addition to myoclonic jerking, tetany, and tachycardia. Myocardial damage may result from use of this drug.

Withdrawal symptoms are familiar to those of barbiturate withdrawal, and there may be hallucinations, jitteriness, irritability, agitation, depression, and abdominal pain within 16 to 24 hours. Convulsions are experienced by 20% to 40% of individuals and can be controlled with intravenous administration of diazepam. The convulsions produced with this drug make overdose more dangerous than with other sedative-hypnotics that have a potential for causing dependence.

Because the drug is rapidly absorbed from the gastrointestinal tract, emesis or lavage is necessary in addition to cathartics and charcoal. Pulmonary edema is a contraindication to the use of forced diuresis. Hemodialysis is reserved for the person who is severely intoxicated with levels over 11 mg/100 ml.

Withdrawal is initiated either with methaqualone or phenobarbital (30 mg phenobarbital for each 250 to 300 mg methaqualone abused). Methaqualone is used in decreasing dosages, and phenobarbital is usually initiated with a dose not exceeding 180 mg daily in the adult, titrated to client comfort when symptoms of withdrawal subside for 1 or 2 days, and then gradually reduced. Continued absorption of the drug remaining in the gastrointestinal tract produces erratic peak plasma levels. Further, in abuse the continued exposure may be accounted for by differential metabolism of the drug. It is estimated that levels exceeding 2.5 mg/100 ml are intoxicating in most individuals.

methyprylon (Noludar)

Methyprylon can cause dependence similar to that of barbiturates and alcohol in high dosages over extended periods. Symptoms reported in methyprylon intoxication are coma (lasting up to 30 hours), hypotension, respiratory depression, tachycardia, hypothermia, hyperthermia, somnolence, confusion, constricted pupils, and paradoxic excitability. The most dangerous complication is the hypotension.

The symptoms of withdrawal are restlessness, auditory and visual hallucinations, diaphoresis, polyuria, excitement, confusion, and convulsions on the abrupt cessation of the drug.

Methyprylon is water and lipid soluble, and most of the dose is excreted as a metabolite in the urine with a therapeutic half-life of up to 6 hours. Toxic blood levels are 3 to 5 mg/100 ml and 10 mg/100 ml is potentially lethal: therapeutic blood levels are less than 10 μg/ml (1 mg/100 ml).

Withdrawal syndrome is treated with phenobarbital. The dose used is 30 mg, equivalent to 300 mg methyprylon. The nurse should be alert for mixed substance abuse.

ALCOHOLS

Although there are many different kinds of alcohols, the term "alcohol" usually refers to ethyl alcohol. Methyl alcohol, propyl alcohol, butyl alcohol, and amyl alcohol are examples of other alcohols.

ethyl alcohol

Ethyl alcohol has been known in an impure form since earliest times, and it is the only alcohol used extensively in medicine. Many of the OTC "nighttime" cough and cold remedies are abused because of their considerable sedative potential, since they contain 25% alcohol (50-proof) with antihistamines. Ethyl alcohol was formerly thought to be a remedy for almost any disease or disorder. It is a colorless liquid and lighter than water, with which it mixes readily. It lowers surface tension and acts as a good solvent for a number of substances. Ethyl alcohol, also referred to as ethanol or grain alcohol, is the product of the fermentation of a sugar by yeast.

Mechanism of action. Ethyl alcohol may have either a local or a systemic action.

Local. Ethyl alcohol denatures proteins by precipitation and dehydration. This is said to be the basis for its germicidal, irritant, and astringent effects. It irritates denuded skin, mucous membranes, and subcutaneous tissue. Subcutaneous injection of alcohol may cause considerable pain and sloughing of the tissues. When it is injected into or near a nerve alcohol may cause nerve degeneration and anesthesia. Alcohol evaporates readily from the skin, producing a cooling effect and reducing the temperature of the skin. When rubbed on the surface of the body it acts as a mild counterirritant. It dries and hardens the epithelial layer of the skin and helps to prevent bed sores when used externally. However, its use on dry and irritated skin is usually contraindicated.

Solutions of ethyl alcohol that measure 70% by weight seem to exert the best bactericidal effects. High concentrations have a marked dehydrating effect but do not necessarily kill bacteria. Ethyl alcohol in proper concentration is considered an effective germicide for a number of uses, but it does not kill spores.

Systemic. Modern scientific authorities do not consider alcohol to be a stimulant, popular ideas to the contrary. What sometimes appears to be stimulation results from the depression of the higher faculties of the brain and represents the loss of inhibitions acquired by socialization. Alcohol is thought to interfere with the transmission of nerve impulses at synaptic connections, but how this is accomplished is not known. It causes progressive and continuous depression of the central nervous system (cerebrum, cerebellum, spinal cord, and medulla). Its action is comparable to that of the general anesthetics. The excitement stage, however, is longer; and when the anesthetic stage is reached, definite toxic symptoms are present. The margin between the anesthetic and the fatal dose is a narrow one.

The action of alcohol varies with the individual, one's tolerance, the presence or absence of extraneous stimuli, the rate of ingestion, and gastric contents. Small or moderate quantities produce a feeling of well-being, talkativeness, greater vivacity, and increased confidence in one's mental and physical power. The personality becomes expansive, and there is a general loss of inhibitions. The finer powers of discrimination, concentration, insight, judgment, and memory are gradually dulled and lost. Large quantities may cause excitement, impulsive speech and behavior, laughter, hilarity, and, in some cases, pugnaciousness in some persons, while others may become melancholy or unduly sentimental. The intoxicated individual usually becomes ataxic, mutters incoherently, has disturbance of the special senses, is often nauseated, may vomit, and eventually lapses into stupor or coma.

The respiratory center is not depressed except by large doses.

Cardiovascular. Alcohol depresses the vasomotor center in the medulla and causes dilation of the peripheral blood vessels, especially those of the skin. This causes a feeling of warmth. Heat is also lost from the interior, which accounts for the fact that an intoxicated person may freeze to death more quickly than a nonintoxicated person. Alcohol also depresses the heat-regulating mechanism; and before the advent of the modern antipyretics, it was used to reduce fever.

Small doses (10 to 25 ml) produce an insignificant increase in the pulse rate, caused mainly by the excitement and the reflex effect on the gastrointestinal tract. Larger doses (over 25 ml) produce the same effect but may be followed by lowered blood pressure caused by the effect on the vasoconstrictor center. Only high concentrations of alcohol depress the heart.

Gastrointestinal. The effect of alcohol on the function of the digestive organs depends on the presence or absence of gastrointestinal disease, the degree of alcohol tolerance, the concentration of the alcohol, and the type and amount of food present. Small doses of alcohol will stimulate the secretion of gastric juice rich in acid. Salivary secretion is also reflexly stimulated. Large and concentrated doses of alcohol tend to inhibit secretion and enzyme activity in the stomach, although the effect in the intestine seems to be negligible. However, when large quantities of alcohol are taken over prolonged time periods, gastritis, nutritional deficiencies, and other untoward results have been observed.

Pharmacokinetics. Alcohol does not require digestion before absorption. A small amount is absorbed in the stomach while most is absorbed in the small intestine. Approximately 90% of the alcohol is metabolized by alcohol dehydrogenase in the liver. In the presence of alcohol dehydrogenase, alcohol is oxidized to acetaldehyde; acetaldehyde oxidizes to acetic acid, which is buffered to an acetate that eventually oxidizes to carbon dioxide and water. The process of alcohol metabolism occurs at a fairly constant rate; a person weighing 70 kg usually metabolizes 20 to 30 ml of 90 proof spirits (45% alcohol) or 8 to 12 ounces of beer (4% alcohol) or 3 ounces of wine or champagne (12% alcohol) per hour.

Alcohol that escapes oxidation is excreted by way of the lungs and kidneys, and some is found in a number of excretions such as sweat.

Alcohol produces an increased flow of urine because of the increase in fluid intake. It has been suggested that alcohol may also act as a diuretic through CNS depression and inhibition of antidiuretic hormone (ADH) release. If the individual has preexisting renal disease, the kidney may be further damaged. Large and concentrated doses of alcohol are thought to injure the renal epithelium.

After absorption, alcohol is distributed in the tissues of the body in approximately the same ratio as their water content. Therefore a rough estimate of the quantity consumed may be obtained from an analysis of the blood and urine (Table 9-4).

At times alcohol is injected into a nerve to destory sensory nerve fibers and relieve pain associated with a severe and protracted neuralgia, such as trifacial neuralgia (tic douloureux), or inoperable cancer. An injection of 80% ethyl alcohol is used. Effects may persist for 1 to 3 years, until regeneration of the peripheral nerve fibers takes place, or be permanent.

Alcohol is used to produce vasodilation in peripheral vascular disease. Concentrated solutions often produce greater peripheral vasodilation than any other drug. The pain of Buerger's disease may be relieved by oral ethyl alcohol. Alcohol may be prescribed to decrease the frequency of anginal attacks but effects are said to be unreliable. Benefits to the person with a cardiac condition, if they occur, are believed to result from the rest and relaxation that the alcohol produces.

Alcohol has been used as an appetite stimulant for patients with poor appetite during periods of convalescence and debility. Alcohol may be used as a hypnotic for older persons who do not tolerate other hypnotics.

Dosage and administration. See box for various preparations of ethyl alcohol. Dosage varies with the purpose for which the alcohol is administered. When whiskey is prescribed as a vasodilator, 30 ml may be ordered to be given two or three times a day.

Drug interactions. The most commonly used and abused drug in America is alcohol. It interacts with many prescription and OTC drugs, resulting in serious adverse effects leading to emergency room admissions or even death. The magnitude of this potential interaction is enormous. Most people, professionals and lay persons alike, are not fully cognizant of some of the most significant alcohol-drug interactions. (See Table 9-5.)

The National Safety Council regards concentration of alcohol in the blood up to 0.05% as evidence of unquestioned sobriety. Concentrations between 0.051% and 0.149% are regarded as grounds for suspicion and for use of performance tests, and anything more than 0.15% is evidence of unquestioned intoxication. The states differ as to what is accepted as a legal limit.

The effects of alcohol may become apparent when the individual attempts to operate machinery such as an automobile. Visual acuity (especially peripheral vision) is diminished, reaction time is slowed, judgment and self-control are impaired, and the individual tends to be complacent and pleased with himself. Many drivers will take

CONTENT OF ETHANOL IN VARIOUS SOLUTIONS

BEVERAGES	Alcohol content (%)	Alcohol proof
Beer	4	8
Wine (red/white)	12	24
Brandy	30-45	60-90
Whiskey, vodka	45	90
Martini, Manhattan	30	60
Daiquiri, Alexander	15	30
OTC MEDICINALS		
Actol Expectorant	12.5	25
Formula 44-D	20	40
Prunicodeine	25	50
Nyquil	25	50
Elixir terpin hydrate with codeine (various)	39-44	78-88

Data from Osol, 1980; Davidson, 1986; Hinds, 1985.

TABLE 9-4 Relation Between Clinical Indications of Alcohol Intoxication and Concentration of Alcohol of the Blood and Urine

Stage	Blood alcohol (%)	Urine alcohol (%)	Clinical observations
Subclinical	up to 0.11	up to 0.15	Slight evidence of performance deterioration possible, such as motor function; coordination; personality or mood and mental acuity.
Emotional instability	0.09-0.21	0.13-0.29	Decreased inhibitions; emotional instability; slight muscular incoordination; slowing of responses to stimuli
Confusion	0.18-0.33	0.26-0.45	Disturbance of sensation; decreased pain sense; staggering gait; slurred speech
Stupor	0.27-0.43	0.36-0.58	Marked decrease in response to stimuli; muscular incoordination approaching paralysis
Coma	0.36-0.56	0.48-0.72	Complete unconsciousness; depressed reflexes, subnormal temperature; anesthesia; impairment of circulation; possible death
Death (uncomplicated)	Over 0.44	Over 0.60	

TABLE 9-5   Selected Significant Alcohol-Drug Interactions

Substances interacting with alcohol	Mechanism	Possible effect(s)
I. antihistamines antidepressants opioid analgesics sedative-hypnotics antianxiety agents antipsychotic drugs	Additive	Enhanced CNS depressant effects
II. disulfiram (Antabuse) chlorpropamide (Diabinese) other oral antidiabetic agents (to varying degrees) metronidazole (Flagyl)	Inhibition of dehydrogenase in metabolism of alcohol, leading to acetaldehyde accumulation (disulfiram or a "disulfiram-type reaction")	Most severe effects seen with disulfiram and alcohol: flushing, stomach pain, head throbbing, increased heart rate, hypotension, sweating, nausea and vomiting. With antidiabetic agents: mild to severe hypoglycemia
III. phenytoin (Dilantin)	Increase or decrease in liver metabolism	In chronic alcohol abuse: possible decrease in anticonvulsant effect, due to increased metabolism. In acute alcohol use: a possible decrease in metabolism, causing increased serum level of phenytoin and toxicity
IV. salicylates	Additive	Increased gastrointestinal irritability and bleeding
V. nitrates nitroglycerin	Additive	Vasodilation leading to hypotension, syncope

chances when under the influence of alcohol that they would never take ordinarily. This leads to disaster, as accident statistics reveal.

Indications. Ethyl alcohol is used topically as an astringent and antiseptic. It is a popular disinfectant for the skin. Alcohol rubs are given to prevent decubiti on the back and buttocks. It is an excellent solvent and preservative for many medicines and medicinal mixtures (spirits, elixirs, fluidextracts).

At times 80% ethyl alcohol is injected into a nerve to destroy sensory nerve fibers and relieve pain associated with a severe and protracted neuralgia, such as trifacial neuralgia (tic douloureux) or inoperable cancer.

Toxic Alcohols

Isopropyl alcohol and methyl or wood alcohol are very toxic when taken internally. When some alcoholic individuals are unable to purchase ethanol (ethyl alcohol), they substitute agents such as isopropyl (rubbing) alcohol, methyl alcohol (antifreeze), or any available substance that might prevent alcohol withdrawal. This is a dangerous practice with serious systemic effects.

isopropyl alcohol

Isopropyl alcohol is a clear, colorless liquid with a characteristic odor. It compares favorably with ethyl alcohol in its antiseptic action. It has been recommended for disinfection of the skin and for rubbing compounds and lotions to be used on the skin. Its bactericidal effects are said to increase as its concentration approaches 100%.

Isopropyl alcohol is occasionally misused as a beverage. It can cause severe poisoning and death. The first symptoms are similar to intoxication from ethyl alcohol, but the symptoms progress to coma from which the patient may not recover.

methyl alcohol (wood alcohol, methanol)

Methyl alcohol is prepared on a large scale by the destructive distillation of wood. It is also prepared synthetically. It is important in medicine chiefly because of the cases of poisoning caused by its ingestion.

The main effects are on the central nervous system. However, intoxication does not occur as readily as with ethyl alcohol unless large amounts are consumed. Methyl alcohol is oxidized in the tissues to formic acid, which is poorly metabolized. This is the basis for the development of a severe acidosis.

Symptoms of poisoning include nausea and vomiting, abdominal pain, headache, dyspnea, blurred vision, and cold clammy skin. Symptoms may progress to delirium, convulsions, coma, and death. In nonfatal cases the individual may become blind or suffer from impaired vision. Treatment is directed toward the relief of acidosis since this seems to be related to the severity of the visual symptoms. Large amounts of sodium bicarbonate may be needed to treat acidosis successfully. Obviously, methyl alcohol is much more toxic than ethyl alcohol. One dose of 60 ml has been known to cause permanent blindness. Fluids containing methyl alcohol usually bear a "Poison" label.

Drugs Used in Treatment of Chronic Alcoholism (Alcoholism Deterrent)
disulfiram (Antabuse)

Disulfiram is used to sensitize an individual to alcohol by bringing about an unpleasant alcohol-disulfiram reaction. This disulfiram reaction begins with flushing in the face and develops into intense vasodilation of the face, neck, and upper part of the body. Hyperventilation and increased pulse rate may occur. Nausea occurs in 30 to 60 minutes along with facial pallor, hypotension, and copious vomiting. There is usually an intense feeling of discomfort, pulsating headache, palpitations, dyspnea, syncope, and a constrictive feeling in the neck. The reaction lasts from 30 minutes to several hours, as long as alcohol is being metabolized; it is then followed by drowsiness and sleep. This experience is so unpleasant that use of alcohol tends to repel the individual.

Mechanism of action. In the body alcohol is oxidized to acetaldehyde. Disulfiram inhibits the enzyme aldehyde dehydrogenase, which converts acetaldehyde to acetate. This permits acetaldehyde to accumulate and cause unpleasant toxic effects. Disulfiram has few effects unless the person ingests alcohol.

Indication. Alcohol deterrent.

Pharmacokinetics. Metabolism is hepatic and initial effect may be delayed up to 12 hours because of localization in adipose tissue; twenty percent of a dose remains in the body for 1 week or more. Renal excretion of metabolites occurs in addition to excretion of carbon disulfide via the lungs. Five to twenty percent of each dose is eliminated unchanged in the feces. Because of slow and incomplete absorption and eliminations, effects persist for up to 2 weeks after therapy is stopped. Clients should be warned not to ingest any alcohol-containing substance during this time.

Alcohol is available in prescription drugs, OTC drugs, liquid cough-cold analgesic products, foods, flavoring, mouthwashes, salad dressings, and the like, and the individual should be warned of possible interaction and the need to check all liquids for alcohol. Psychotherapy aimed at mental and social rehabilitation should accompany disulfiram therapy, and all clients should carry disulfiram treatment identification. Disulfiram is available in 250 and 500 mg tablets.

Side effects/adverse reactions. The most frequent side effect is sleepiness. Less frequent are headache, rash, stomach upset, increased tiredness, metallic taste, and decrease in sexual potency in males. If side effects continue, increase, or disturb the client, the physician must be informed. Adverse reactions are less frequent but include ocular pain or visual changes, psychosis, weakness, tingling sensation, pain or numbness in hands or feet, and jaundice. If adverse reactions occur, medical intervention may be necessary.

Significant drug interactions. When disulfiram is given with:

Drug	Possible Effect and Management
anticoagulants	Increased anticoagulant effects; dosage adjustments may be necessary; monitor closely
phenytoin (hydantoins)	Increased serum levels of hydantoins; monitor serum levels before and during anticoagulant therapy; dosage adjustments may be necessary
isoniazid (INH)	Increased CNS side effects (ataxia, inability to sleep, dizziness, increased irritability); disulfiram dosage may need to be reduced or stopped; monitor closely
metronidazole	Confusion and psychotic episodes; avoid this combination
paraldehyde	Increased serum levels of paraldehyde and acetaldehyde resulting from inhibition of acetaldehyde dehydrogenase; concurrent use not recommended

Dosage and administration

Adults. Initial, 0.5 g orally daily for 7 to 14 days; maintenance, 250 mg orally daily

Pregnancy safety. FDA category undetermined

ANTIANXIETY AND ANTIPSYCHOTIC AGENTS

In the late 1970s to 1980s, the number of prescriptions for antianxiety agents soared. Psychoactive agents were freely prescribed and taken. Women in particular were overmedicated, for reasons such as the following:

1. Women see physicians more often than men do. The National Center for Health statistics reports that approximately 60% of physician visits are with women. It has been said that men generally seek physicians advice when they are ill, while women seek medical help when they are healthy (e.g., advice on birth control, prenatal care, birth of a child, routine Pap smears, and breast examinations).
2. Females are more vocal in reporting emotional problems or feelings than males. Physicians may not know how to appropriately respond to these "nonmedical" complaints, so they prescribe deazepam (Valium) or a similar benzodiazepine (Hughes and Brewin, 1979). The physician's prescriptions also meet the expectation of the client, that is, they are a confirmation of an ailment. In many instances, nonchemical approaches are not even considered.
3. Sexual bias among physicians has been asserted (Cooperstock in Hughes, 1979). When males and females visited the physician with the same complaints of emotional unhappiness (depression, crying periods, tension, worry, and anxiety), physicians prescribed tranquilizers for the females while ordering tests and therapies for male clients (Hughes & Brewin, 1979; Nellis, 1980). This resulted in more prescriptions for psychoactive drugs for the women as compared to men.

The problem of overprescription of psychoactive drugs also affects elderly clients. In the United States, Canada, and the United Kingdom, prescriptions for psychotropic drugs increase proportionately with age (Hyams, 1984). A study of the Department of Health, Welfare and Education reviewed the records of over 250,000 individuals living in nursing homes and discovered that nearly 47% of them were receiving psychotropic drugs. In Canada, a review of 1431 chronically ill elderly revealed that about 25% of them were receiving psychotropic medications. A different Canadian study of outpatient elderly reported similar percentages (26%) taking psychotropic drugs. This study also reported that in nearly 10% of these elderly the drugs were the cause of their symptoms (Hyams, 1984).

A study of the association between the risk of hip fractures in the elderly and the use of psychoactive drugs illustrates the potential dangers with these agents (Ray & others, 1987). A total of 1021 cases and 5606 controls were evaluated in this study. Forty-two percent of the studied population was over 85 years old, and 77% were women. Four categories of psychotropic medications were reviewed: (1) antianxiety or hypnotic drugs with short half-lives (less than 24 hours), (2) antianxiety or hypnotic agents with long half-lives (longer than 24 hours), (3) tricyclic antidepressants, and (4) antipsychotic agents. Categories 2, 3, and 4 were associated with increased risk and incidence of hip fractures.

Both the antianxiety and antipsychotic agents can lead to psychic and physical dependence. Abrupt withdrawal of phenothiazine-type drugs may result in anxiety, insomnia, gastrointestinal disturbances, and muscular discomfort. Abrupt discontinuance of benzodiazepines such as chlordiazepoxide (Librium), diazepam (Valium), and clorazepate (Tranxene) may produce withdrawal symptoms such as insomnia, increased irritability and nervousness, stomach pain, muscle cramping, nausea and vomiting, fear, tremors, sweating, headaches, decreased ability to concentrate, and increased tiredness. Such reactions have been reported even in clients abruptly stopping dosages of benzodiazepines within the usually recommended therapeutic range. The symptoms described occur more frequently and are more severe in individuals who suddenly withdraw from the short-acting benzodiazepines. (See boxed material.)

Overdosage

Benzodiazepines. Benzodiazepine overdosage may cause sleepiness and minor extrapyramidal signs with some excitement. Because of the high probability of a mixed ingestion, one must watch for possible deep coma, marked hypotension, and respiratory depression. Other effects include dry mouth, tachycardia, dilated pupils, and absent bowel sounds. Abrupt cessation of a benzodiazepine may result in withdrawal symptoms if the drug has been taken daily for several months or years. Hallucinations, confusion, and seizures often are reported. These effects may be overcome by gradually withdrawing the drug. Flumazepil (Ro 15-1788) is a product marketed in

---

BENZODIAZEPINE CLASSIFICATIONS

SHORT-ACTING (Half-life less than 24 hours)

alprazolam (Xanax)
lorazepam (Ativan, Apo-lorazepam♣, Novolorazem♣)
oxazepam (Serax, Ox-Pam♣, Zapex♣)
temazepam (Restoril)
triazolam (Halcion)

LONG-ACTING (Half-life longer than 24 hours)

chloriazepoxide (Librium, Apo-Chlorax♣, Medilium♣)
clorazepate (Tranexe)
diazepam (Valium, Apo-Diazepam♣, E-Pam♣)
flurazepam (Delmane, Novoflupam♣)
halazepam (Paxipam)
prazepam (Centrax)

Europe as a benzodiazepine receptor antagonist. While human studies are limited, the reports of the antagonist effects of this drug on benzodiazepine are quite impressive. Flumazepil can be given orally or intravenously and appears to have no pharmacologic effects of its own. This product has been given in both known and suspected cases of benzodiazepine toxicity and is a potentially promising investigational drug (Drake, 1986).

Phenothiazines. Phenothiazine overdosage most often produces stiff neck, ataxia, protruding tongue, reduced activity and attentiveness, and psychomotor slowing. Initial symptoms may include agitation, hyperactivity, and seizures. Disturbance of the temperature-regulating processes by phenothiazines creates hyperthermia or hypothermia. The alpha-blocking and anticholinergic effects of phenothiazines frequently produce tachycardia, lethargy, and somnolence. The quinidine-like effect of the phenothiazines may produce a widening of the QRS complexes and ventricular tachycardia. The nurse should remember not to administer other sedatives, barbiturates, narcotics, or anesthetics concurrently with phenothiazines, since the potentiation of these depressant drugs may create respiratory depression and increased CNS effects.

CNS STIMULANTS

Amphetamines and cocaine are the most commonly abused CNS stimulants.

AMPHETAMINES

Amphetamine was first synthesized in Germany during the 1930s. This stimulant soon became very popular worldwide. Some governments, including the Soviet Union, gave amphetamines to factory workers to increase their output. Although initially considered successful, in time these experiments were deemed to be unsuccessful. During World War II amphetamines were given to U.S. soldiers to help them improve their strength and reduce fatigue during battle.

In the 1950s and 1960s, tremendous amounts of amphetamines were produced and available both legally and illegally. Drug manufacturers were advising physicians to prescribe these products for the depressed housewife, for overweight persons, or to make someone happy and energetic (Weil and Rosen, 1983). Although Sweden classified amphetamines as "prescription only" in 1939, the United States did not institute this control until 1954. But even the prescription requirement did not curtail the abuse of amphetamines seen in many countries, including the United States, Sweden, and Japan (Brecher, 1972).

Abuse of oral amphetamines was reported as early as 1940. Intravenous use of amphetamines began in the 1950s and increased in popularity in the 1960s, when physicians in the San Francisco Bay area prescribed it for pain and as a treatment for heroin addiction.

In the 1960s new federal drug amendments were passed to control the manufacture and distribution of amphetamines, and physicians, pharmacists, and others involved in illegal uses were arrested.

Amphetamine abuse is still reported in the Drug Abuse Warning Network, but cocaine is clearly the leading CNS stimulant abused.

Mechanism of action. The amphetamines are synthetic indirect sympathomimetic amines that are chemically and pharmacologically related to epinephrine and norepinephrine. The exact mechanism by which amphetamines act is unknown, but they cause CNS stimulation probably by releasing catecholamines (norepinephrine and dopamine) from sympathetic nerve terminals. Oral doses are absorbed from the GI tract and concentrated in the kidneys, lungs, and brain. Peak effects occur 15 minutes after intravenous administration. Approximately half the administered does is excreted unchanged, with the balance being metabolized as deaminated metabolites. The half-life of the metabolites in the urine varies with changes in urine pH. Amphetamine is a basic drug with a **pK$_a$** level of 9.9 (pK$_a$ is the point at which half the amount in the body is ionized and half is nonionized). Its half-life in recipients with an acidic urine (pH less than 6.6) ranges from 7 to 14 hours. In recipients with alkaline urine (pH over 6.7, as from use of sodium bicarbonate), the half-life range is prolonged to 18 to 34 hours.

Deaths have occurred with doses of 5 mg/kg or more. Tolerance develops, and response is variable, since chronic abusers use from 5 to 8000 mg/day. The desired effects occur within 1 hour after ingestion. Because amphetamines and related derivatives possess a high pK$_a$, acid diuresis will enhance amphetamine excretion. The goal of acidification is to achieve a urine pH between 4.5 and 5.5.

Effects. The amphetamines usually are abused because they produce an elevation of mood, a reduction of fatigue, a sense of increased alertness, and "invigorating aggressiveness." Amphetamines do not create extra physical or mental energy; rather, they promote expenditure of present resources, sometimes to the point of hazardous fatigue, which is often unrecognized. Intravenous injection results in marked euphoria, an orgasmic feeling known as the **flash** or **rush,** a sense of great physical strength and capacity, and a sense of crystal-clear thinking. The user feels little or no need for rest, sleep, or food and may continually engage in vigorous activity that may be perceived as exhilarating and creative. To an objective observer, however, inefficient, stereotyped, and repetitious behavior is common during an amphetamine high.

Depending on the dosage of the drug taken, the individual may experience a "run" of variable length, perhaps several days. Some amphetamine users force themselves to lie down and close their eyes for a few hours during such a run and also will force-feed themselves in an attempt to prolong the run. Termination of the drug's use may result from a variety of factors, such as exhaustion, fright, or inability to obtain more of the drug. Withdrawal of the drug is followed by long periods of sleep. On awakening, the individual often feels hungry, extremely lethargic, and profoundly depressed, a phenomenon known as **crashing.** The risk of suicide during this period must be considered.

The stimulant properties of amphetamines can cause dramatic cardiorespiratory effects, such as tachycardia, dyspnea, chest pain, and hypertension. Users of amphetamines may panic because these signs and symptoms are those of a myocardial infarction. To deal with these disturbing symptoms, amphetamine users often use depressants, or **downers.** Some drugs (such as dextroamphetamine sulfate and amobarbital) combine a CNS stimulant with CNS depressant in an attempt to minimize the overstimulation produced by the amphetamine ingredient.

Amphetamines are also said to be psychotomimetic. Although there is some conflicting evidence regarding the cause of amphetamine psychosis, it is claimed that heavy users may develop psychosis characterized by aggression, delusions of persecution, depression, paranoia, euphoria, and fully formed visual and auditory hallucinations. Some authorities suggest that these symptoms may be related to the insomnia produced by prolonged amphetamine abuse because sleep deprivation, in and of itself, leads to psychologic disturbance. Marked tolerance to amphetamines occurs.

Oral tablets are sometimes crushed for use in an intravenous solution. Although intravenous administration of amphetamine alone is not associated with pulmonary microemboli, tablet fillers such as magnesium silicate (talc) and cornstarch may produce pulmonary emboli, resulting in granuloma formation within the lung. Pulmonary emboli have also been observed following injection of methylphenidate tablets. Talc may also appear in the cornea of the eye after chronic parenteral administration of solutions made from oral tablets of methylphenidate. Because the lungs act as filters for these large talc particles intravenous abusers who complain of nonspecific pulmonary symptoms should be examined for talc-containing microemboli; an eye examination may reveal the same source of talc.

Withdrawal symptoms. Although amphetamines do not appear to lead to physical dependence, as identified by the criterion of a characteristic and reproductible withdrawal syndrome, most authorities maintain that the signs and symptoms characteristic of crashing constitute just such a syndrome.

Preparations. Chemically, there are three types of amphetamines: salts of racemic amphetamines, dextroamphetamines, and methamphetamines, all of which vary in degree of potency and peripheral effects. Dextroamphetamine is said to have fewest peripheral effects, such as hypertension and tachycardia.

Treatment of amphetamine toxicity. Diazepam is the drug of choice for the treatment of hyperactivity caused by amphetamines. The nurse must question the client about concurrent use of other drugs such as barbiturates. Chlorpromazine may be used only if the ingested substance is a pure amphetamine or an amphetamine combined with a barbiturate. However, if the ingested drug is said to be MDA, DMT, DOM, or similar designer agents, chlorpromazine is contraindicated because synergistic hypotension results. It is also contraindicated in persons with seizure disorders because chlorpromazine increases the possibility of seizures. If hypertension does not respond to chlorpromazine, or in an emergency in which the individual is refractory to chlorpromazine, the choice is phenoxybenzamine, phentolamine, diazoxide, or sodium nitroprusside. The intravenous route of chlorpromazine is effective with a slow infusion.

Marked suicidal depression often follows an amphetamine overdose and chronic abuse by 24 to 72 hours; withdrawal results in sleepiness and apathy.

COCAINE

Cocaine is classified as a narcotic but is a tropine, related to the belladonna alkaloids. A potent CNS stimulant, cocaine is used therapeutically mostly as a local anesthetic, since it is likely to cause toxic side effects when administered by other routes. Cocaine as a social-recreational drug of abuse is popular for its effects: elation and euphoria. It also produces increased energy, like the amphet-

amines, and may lead to a similar psychotic state with strong elements of paranoia.

The purity of the illicitly produced drug varies greatly (generally 5% to 10%). This short-lived CNS stimulant is often diluted or cut with agents such as amphetamines, boric acid, quinine, mannitol, procaine, and lidocaine. The vasoconstricting effect of cocaine may be responsible for limiting its own absorption. Abusers of this drug may mix it with alcohol, a concoction known as a "liquid lady."

Cocaine may be administered by sniffing (snorting) the white, fluffy crystalline powder (which resembles snow, hence the name), by direct intravenous injection, or by smoking (transalveolar route) the converted base form ("free base"). It may be inhaled from a small spoon, rolled dollar bills, lengthened finger nail, or an inhalation device designed for cromolyn sodium. Sniffing causes vasoconstriction, which limits the amount of cocaine absorbed from the nasal mucosa into systemic circulation. Sometimes cocaine is mixed with heroin for heightened effects and to diminish dysphoria, a combination known as a **speedball.**

The cocaine hydrochloride salt is converted to the free-base form by the use of a solvent such as diethyl ether. The freebase form is heat resistant, lending itself to smoking in any form including "coke pipes." Smoking freebase cocaine produces a more intense effect and is dangerous because of the possibility of an excessive dose being administered. The free base solvents are inflammable and may explode during the process, causing further harm to the user.

Free base cocaine has largely been replaced by crack. Crack cocaine is also a free base but it is made without any volative chemicals. It became popular because of its availability in smaller amounts at a much lower cost then free base cocaine and because its use does not require any elaborate paraphernalia. The cocaine market has thus become affordable to all economic groups. (See boxed material for cocaine names and description.)

Cocaine is rapidly metabolized, and the abuser of cocaine may use the drug every half hour or less to maintain the high. Cocaine is metabolized in the liver by hepatic esterases, and plasma hydrolysis is the result of serum cholinesterase. It is absorbed from all mucous membranes. The serum levels are not proportional to the toxicity, and the elimination half-lives by oral, intranasal, and intravenous routes are similar (50, 80, and 60 minutes, respectively). Cocaine stimulation of the CNS initially affects the intellect (cognition) and behavior (affective domain).

At this time there is no absolute level known to be lethal. Toxic effects have been reported with a 20 mg dose and fatal outcomes with 1200 mg. The rapidity of the increase in blood level may be as important in determin-

---

COCAINE NAMES AND DESCRIPTION

	STREET NAMES	SOURCE/COMMENTS
Freebase cocaine	Base, baseball, white tornado, snow toke	Purified base made by using volatile chemicals
Basuco cocaine	Coca paste, pasta	Crude form of cocaine; derived from coca leaves; mixed with tobacco or marijuana smoked; cheapest form of cocaine and usually the most contaminated form
Crack cocaine	Rock, gravel	Base product; up to the early 1980s rock cocaine usually referred to chunks of pure cocaine hydrochloride; today the term usually refers to crack

---

ing fatal reactions as the peak blood concentration. Factors other than blood concentration of cocaine must be examined. These factors include tolerance, reverse tolerance, previous history of cocaine abuse, individual susceptibility, and presence of other drugs.

Initial symptoms of cocaine use are restlessness, mydriasis, hyperreflexia, vasoconstriction, tachycardia, hypertension, hallucinations, nausea, vomiting, and muscle spasms, which may be followed by respiratory failure, convulsions, coma, and circulatory collapse. In chronic abusers a toxic cocaine psychosis (similar to paranoid schizophrenia) is often found, characterized by hallucinations and paranoid delusions. Skin eruptions (with itching and compulsive scratching) caused by self-inflicted skin irritation are also frequently observed. The energetic client may be prone to outbursts of violent behavior. Blood in the nose and a perforated nasal septum are frequently seen in those who chronically snort cocaine. A large dose of cocaine has direct cardiotoxicity, but death from overdose may result from respiratory failure.

Physical dependence now appears to be an emerging characteristic of cocaine abuse. Strong psychologic dependence is also evident. (For discussion of drugs used to lessen the symptoms of cocaine withdrawal, see boxed material.)

CANNABIS DRUGS (MARIJUANA)

The cannabis drugs are derived from the leaves, stems, fruiting tops, and resin of both female and male hemp plants, *Cannabis sativa.* The potency of the active ingredient, tetrahydrocannabinol (δ^9-THC), is greatest in the flowering tops of the plant and seems to vary according to the climatic conditions under which the plant is grown. In the U.S. the plants grow wild or are illegally cultivated and thus potency varies. The only legal cultivation is that by the federal government for research purposes.

The availability of more potent species and varieties of

DRUGS TO REDUCE SYMPTOMS OF COCAINE WITHDRAWAL

Initial clinical studies with amantadine (Symmetrel) and bromocriptine (Parlodel) have reported promising results in reducing the craving for cocaine during cocaine abstinence. Additional studies on a longer term basis are currently being performed (El-Mourad, 1986; Bohach, 1987). Cocaine acts to stimulate the release of dopamine in the brain initially, which provides the user with a feeling of pleasure. The crash period, or low period, with dopamine may result from a drop of dopamine level in the brain. This drop is believed to induce the craving for more cocaine and perhaps is responsible for the depression seen during this period. Because both amantadine and bromocriptine produce elevated levels of dopamine in the brain, their use may lessen the symptoms associated with cocaine withdrawal.

---

marijuana and the alarming increase in use among young teenagers (12 to 14 years of age) require a new attitude of concern toward the substance. Imported marijuana and that grown under scientifically controlled conditions is often 10 times as potent as the domestic variety smoked in the past. Some of the marijuana from Central and South America has 4% to 6% THC compared with 0.2% to 4% in that grown in the U.S.

Preparations. Marijuana (average grown in the U.S. 0.2% to 4% THC) and hashish (5% to 12% THC) are the most common forms of cannabis drugs used in the U.S. Hashish refers to the powdered form of the plant's resin, which is five to ten times as potent as some varieties of marijuana. Other forms of cannabis drugs, used in such countries as Jamaica, Mexico, Africa, India, and in the Middle East, include *bhang, ganja,* and *charas,* which correspond, respectively, to American marijuana, hashish, and unadultered resin. In Morocco *kif* is used, whereas in South America a cannabis drug often used is called *dagga*.

Mode of administration. Cannabis drugs may be absorbed when administered by oral, subcutaneous, or pulmonary routes, but they are most potent when inhaled. Either the pure resin or the dried leaves of the cannabis plant may be smoked in pipes or cigarettes. Because the smoke is acrid and irritating, some users prefer to smoke marijuana through a water pipe. The smoke is inhaled deeply and retained in the lungs as long as possible to achieve maximal saturation of the absorbing surface. Powdered hashish and marijuana may also be mixed with foods, a mode of administration that delays the drug's absorption. The sedative-hypnotic effects of smoking are rapid and generally last 2 to 3 hours, while the effects of the orally ingested drugs may not begin for several hours. Hashish oil injected intravenously has a high incidence of mortality.

THC is the major active constituent of marijuana, and biologic activity may be caused by the 11-hydroxy metabolite. Marijuana cigarettes (joints) illicitly used in the U.S. generally have 1% to 2% THC and weigh approximately 500 mg, yielding from 5 to 10 mg THC. The effective dose may be reduced by half when the dose is smoked, yielding from 2.5 to 5 mg THC per 500 mg weight.

Potency varies with plant strain and cultivation. Marijuana cigarettes usually produce moderate to intense psychopharmacologic effects, reaching a peak in 15 minutes and lasting 1 to 4 hours.

Marijuana cigarettes may be *dusted* (treated) or saturated with PCP (known as *super grass*), which may cause PCP overdosage. Hashish oil is also used on marijuana cigarettes.

Marketed products. Dronabinol (Marinol, THC or delta-9-THC) capsules are available for the treatment of nausea and vomiting induced by cancer chemotherapy that is not responsive to standard therapies. A synthetic product that closely resembles THC, nabilone (Cesamet), is also available in the United States. Both products have a high potential for abuse, so they are closely regulated under the Federal Controlled Substances Act.

Mechanism of action. All the cannabis drugs seem to act as CNS depressants. They depress higher brain centers and consequently release lower centers from inhibitory influences. Although some controversy exists regarding their classification, the cannabis drugs are not narcotic derivatives but are legally classified as controlled substances. They are more frequently classified as sedative-hypnotic-anesthetics or psychedelic drugs. Like the sedative-hypnotics, they appear to depress the ascending reticular activating system. As their dosage increases, their effects proceed from relief of anxiety, disinhibition, and excitement to anesthesia. If dosage is high enough, respiratory and vasomotor depression and collapse may occur.

Research has yielded some marijuana homologs and analogs (such as synhexyl, which is one third as potent as marijuana). These should permit standardization of dosage and provide more information regarding structure-activity relationships of the cannabis drugs.

Pharmacokinetics. Peak plasma levels of THC after smoking one marijuana cigarette are reported to be from 0.020 to 0.050 µg/ml. Within a few hours these values decrease to between 0.005 and 0.010 µg/ml. Only trace amounts of the unmetabolized THC are detected in the urine.

The liver is the primary site of metabolism, and the major route of elimination of THC is bile and feces. Prolonged enterohepatic circulation is reported with this lipophilic drug, and it is highly protein bound in the serum. Reports of death or overdose are rare. Both THC and its metabolites may be detected in plasma and urine for several days. Marijuana may alter barbiturate and ethyl alcohol metabolism.

Effects. The drug has intoxicating, mind-altering properties. It induces an anxiety-free state of relaxation characterized by a feeling of extreme well-being. Perceptions of time and space are distorted. Ideas flow freely and disconnectedly; interruptions in thought that are blanks or gaps similar to **epileptic absence** may occur. There may be states of inwardness and/or occasional excitement in the form of hilarity. Hallucinations can occur with high doses of the drug but are generally reported to be pleasant. Dissociative phenomena also are reported. There has been some controlled research with this drug, and some experiments suggest that impaired decision making and psychometric performance are related to the use of marijuana. The drug experience is highly subjective; the presence of an altered state of consciousness may not be perceived by the novice until he or she is sensitized to it by colleagues. Some factors that influence the psychologic and behavioral effects of marijuana are drug dose, user's personality, user's drug expectations, environment, social influences, and life experiences.

The incidence of adverse reactions to marijuana appears to be low. Minor side effects include immediate tachycardia and delayed bradycardia, delayed hypotension, conjunctival vascular congestion (red eyes), dryness of the mouth and throat, hyperphagia, delayed gastrointestinal disturbances, possible vasovagal syncope, and enhanced appetite and flavor appreciation. More serious side effects are psychologic and include fear, panic (especially among first-time or naive users), feelings of paranoia, disorientation, memory loss, confusion, and a variety of perceptual alterations. Marijuana has been known to percipitate acute psychotic reactions and toxic psychoses in poorly organized personalities. The incidence of adverse effects appears to be highest in novice users of the drug. However, these adverse effects generally appear to be short lived and self-limiting.

Apparently psychic and physiologic dependence and tolerance to marijuana develops with long-term, regular use. The effects of prolonged abuse of marijuana have not yet been scientifically proved. However, there seems to be some indication that amotivational states, apathy, memory problems, and some loss of mental acuity may occur. Physiologically, the possibility of chronic, long-term use of marijuana cigarettes leading to chronic bronchitis and emphysema cannot be discounted.

There has also been some question regarding the use of marijuana leading to the use of opiates. This "stepping-stone" use is somewhat controversial, and some authorities state that any progression in drug use stems from personality and environmental factors rather than from the pharmacologic properties of marijuana. The multiple drug use theory lends support to this hypothesis, stating that a person predisposed to abuse one drug is also likely to abuse other, and perhaps stronger, drugs.

Treatment of the rare acute overdose is directed at the symptoms. If depressive, hallucinatory, or psychotic reactions occur, the client is taken to a quiet, nonthreatening area and given positive verbal reassurance. The psychologic effects are short lived, ranging from a few minutes to about 4 hours. If the patient shows signs of excessive agitation, panic, or disorientation, an oral dose of 5 to 10 mg diazepam may be useful.

Withdrawal symptoms. Physiologic withdrawal symptoms after discontinuation of marijuana use have been reported. Some restlessness, anxiety, irritability, and insomnia may be associated with withdrawal, but these symptoms are generally mild and of short duration.

PSYCHEDELIC DRUGS (HALLUCINOGENS, PSYCHOTOMIMETICS, AND PSYCHOTOGENS)
LSD AND RELATED COMPOUNDS

Classifications of the most common hallucinogenic agents include (1) lysergic acid diethylamide (LSD) and its variants, dimethyltryptamine (DMT) and its analogs, and psilocybin, and (2) mescaline, DOM, and the anticholinergic hallucinogens. The phenylethylamine derivatives, such as mescaline, are structurally related to catecholamine, whereas LSD and DMT have structural relationships to serotonin that may involve the action of these agents as hallucinogens.

LSD

LSD is a colorless, odorless, and tasteless substance that is a synthetic derivative of lysergic acid, a compound that naturally occurs in ergot and some varieties of morning glory seeds. It is structurally related to ergonovine, an ergot alkaloid.

Users of LSD today are better informed about the effects than they were in the 1960s, when there was a high incidence of bizarre or adverse effects to the substance such as loss of control and intense hallucinations. The strengths used today are approximately 85 μg compared to levels of 150 μg used in the 1960s, which may be the reason for the lesser degree of adverse effects. The doses used today produce effects such as visual trails of color or light, laughing, facial grimacing, and bruxism. Forms of street LSD are microdots (tablets 2.5 × 5 mm or smaller) and blotter acid (a 6 × 6 cm square blotter paper either plain or with figures drawn on it).

Therapeutic uses. A number of potentially therapeutic uses of LSD have been proposed, all of which merit more investigation. These include the drug's use in the treatment of chronic alcoholism and in the reduction of intractable pain as occurs in malignant disease and in phantom limb sensations. For a time some psychiatrists used the drug to induce psychosis, thereby helping the client revive repressed memories, the influence of which could then be dealt with by the client and therapist. The psychotomimetic effects of the drug have also generated the theory that some chemical imbalance may cause schizophrenia. However, such preliminary data regarding the therapeutic uses of LSD require much more research.

Dosage and administration. Pharmacologically, on a weight-for-weight basis, LSD is more active than almost any other drug. It can be detected in the body at concentrations of 1 part per billion. The human body reacts to relatively minute doses of the drug; 100 to 250 μg administered orally can produce intense depersonalization for up to 12 hours in the majority of subjects.

LSD is usually distributed as a soluble powder and can be ingested in capsule, liquid, or tablet form. An obsolete mode of ingestion is from an aqueous solution on sugar, although the drug can be licked off any object impregnated with it, such as a cookie, a stamp, or blotting paper. The drug may also be administered subcutaneously, intramuscularly, or intravenously. It is readily absorbed from the intestinal tract and mucous membranes as well as from body fluids.

Mechanism of action. LSD acts pharmacologically as a sympathomimetic agent. These effects, however, are secondary to the profound psychologic changes it also produces. The drug is believed to be a serotonin antagonist and inactivates monoamine oxidase and acetylcholinesterase. Cross-tolerance to mescaline and psilocybin has been demonstrated. The exact biochemical mechanism of action, however, is not currently known.

Pharmacokinetics. After oral ingestion LSD is absorbed rapidly, strongly bound to plasma protein, with high concentrations found in the liver, kidneys, and lungs. Less than 1% of the orally administered dose will penetrate the central nervous system, but intense psychic alterations occur at levels of less than 3 μg LSD per gram of brain tissue. The concentrations of LSD in the brain are thought to be in the pituitary and pineal glands, the hypothalamus and limbic system, and the auditory and visual reflex areas. In humans the half-life of LSD is almost 3½ hours. This is close to the duration of the peak psychosensory effect, which decreases over an 8- to 12-hour period. The substance is metabolized to inactive metabolites in the liver and excreted in the urine.

Effects. The effects of LSD usually begin within 20 to 50 minutes after administration. Like effects of other mind-altering drugs, they cannot be reliably predicted. Autonomic nervous system changes are relatively mild and may include tachycardia, hypertension, nausea, vertigo, and diaphoresis. Effects vary widely among individuals and are in part related to the dosage, the mental state of the individual, and the environment. The drug experience may also vary for the same individual from time to time ("good trip" vs. "bad trip").

The initial reaction to the drug may be one of vague anxiety and sometimes nausea. Later there are general changes of perception involving sound, sight, touch, body image, and time. Brightness of colors may be intensified, for example, and there is generally heightened awareness of the environment, creating a flood of sensations and impressions. There may be synesthesia, that is, the translation of one type of sensory experience into another sensory modality, such as "hearing a color." Every perception assumes an increased sense of significance and meaning. Changes in cognitive functioning and value judgment formation may occur (good and bad may become equal). Blurring of boundaries may occur between the self and the environment, and an ineffable state of transcendence may be achieved.

However, unpleasant experiences with LSD are also rather frequent. Clinically, evidence of impaired judgment in the toxic state is frequent, and examples of such behavior are well known, as demonstrated, for example, by LSD users attempting to stop traffic with their bodies. Altered states of consciousness may cause psychosis to develop or trigger a latent psychosis into activity. The release of repressed material may cause an acute panic psychosis. Feelings of acute panic and paranoia during a toxic LSD psychosis can result in homicidal thoughts and actions. Toxic delirium, with altering and alternating levels of consciousness, follows toxic psychosis, and the experience generally resolves in a stage of exhaustion in which the user feels "empty," unable to coordinate thoughts, and depressed. During this time suicide is a definite risk.

Significant unfavorable reactions induced by LSD include prolonged, delayed, and recurrent reactions such as depression and long-term schizophrenic or psychotic reactions. The recurrent reactions have been described as **flashback phenomena,** referring to the transient, spontaneous repetition of a previous LSD-induced experience that is unrelated to renewed administration of the drug. Moreover, a bad trip (anxiety or panic reaction) on LSD is likely to be a paranoid experience, and tendencies toward violence can be characteristic of LSD intoxication.

Research reports of chromosomal damage related to LSD ingestion are increasing, although there appears to be some variation in susceptibility to chromosomal breaks that is of unknown origin. The drug does not seem to cause physical dependence, but tolerance occurs rapidly, and psychic dependence is frequent.

The chemical effects of LSD might be negated by administration of a tranquilizer, a barbiturate, or nicotinic acid. It is specifically recommended that chlorpromazine *not* be administered in LSD toxicity because chlorpromazine may accentuate anticholinergic-like drug effects and may, in high doses, lead to severe hypotension or confusion, further compounding the situation. In any case, the administration of medication is recommended only as an adjunct to crisis intervention psychotherapy. A "talk-down" approach in a quiet environment is often used. It consists of directing the person's attention away from perceptions that produce panic and providing reassurance that the experience will dissipate and that no permanent harm has been done. Hospital practices of administering massive doses of tranquilizers, applying restraints, and isolating such individuals are to be avoided. The client's dramatically heightened awareness of the environment and distorted perceptions may render these measures traumatic rather than therapeutic.

Pregnant women should be especially cautioned against taking LSD. Because lysergic acid is the base of all ergot alkaloids, it has uterine stimulant properties that can adversely affect a pregnancy. It may also have adverse cytogenetic effects.

Withdrawal symptoms. Insofar as is known, no withdrawal symptoms follow discontinuation of long-term use. Tolerance develops in 3 to 7 days but disappears within 7 days of abstinence.

mescaline

Mescaline is the chief alkaloid extracted from mescal buttons (flowering heads) of the peyote cactus, and it produces subjective hallucinogenic effects similar to those produced by LSD. Like the amphetamines, mescaline belongs to the phenylethylamine group, and its chemical structure distantly resembles that of norepinephrine. It is usually ingested in the form of a soluble crystalline powder that is either dissolved into teas or capsulated. The usual dose of mescaline is about 500 mg. Each button contains about 45 mg mescaline.

The effects of mescaline from a dose of 5 mg/kg (6 to 12 buttons) appear within 2 or 3 hours and may last 4 to 12 hours or longer. Doses of up to 500 mg are characterized by prodromal abdominal pain, nausea, vomiting, and diarrhea, which are followed by vivid and colorful visual hallucinations.

Mescaline is not a very potent psychotomimetic, and the oral dose of 5 mg/kg in adults is 4000 times larger than the equivalent milligram dose of LSD. After oral ingestion a syndrome of sympathomimetic effects of anxiety, hyperreflexia, static tremors, and psychic perturbations with vivid visual hallucinations is encountered. The half-life of mescaline is about 6 hours, and it is excreted in the urine.

Peyote cactus is used internally by Southwestern Plains Indians in religious practices.

psilocybin

Psilocybin is a drug derived from Mexican mushrooms *(Psilocye mexicana)*. It produces subjective hallucinogenic effects similar to those produced by mescaline but of shorter duration.

A phosphate ester of DMT, psilocybin is found in the Mexican mushroom at a concentration of about 0.3%. In vivo dephosphorylation by alkaline, phosphatase converts psilocybin to psilocin, the most active psychotogen of the N-alkylated tryptamines. Since the molecule is less polar because of the loss of the phosphoric acid radical, psilocin is able to penetrate the blood-brain barrier more efficiently and therefore produce relatively greater hallucinogenic potency compared with psilocybin. Psilocin is not as potent as LSD (about 0.01% as active on a milligram-for-milligram basis) and creates a lesser psychedelic state, but when equivalent doses are used, the individual may be unable to differentiate between the two drugs.

The 5 hydroxy-DMT (bufotenine from the skin and parotid glands of the toad *Bufo marinus* and the cahobe bean) has less psychotomimetic activity than psilocin.

Within $\frac{1}{2}$ to 1 hour after ingestion of 5 to 15 mg psilocybin a hallucinogenic dysphoric state begins. A dose of 20 to 60 mg may produce effects lasting 5 or 6 hours. The mood is pleasant to some users, and others experience apprehension. The user has poor critical judgment capacities and impaired performance ability. Also seen are hyperkinetic compulsive movements, laughter, mydriasis, vertigo, ataxia, paresthesias, muscle weakness, drowsiness, and sleep.

phencyclidine (PCP)

Phencyclidine was developed in the late 1950s as an anesthetic for dissociative anesthesia, a cataleptic state in which the person appears to be awake but is detached from the surroundings and unresponsive to pain. The drug is related chemically to ketamine (Ketaject, Ketalar), an anesthetic used primarily for children, and the analgesic meperidine (Demerol).

An increased frequency of emergency room visits for PCP-induced problems of intoxication, psychosis, and overdosage has been recorded. Its illicit manufacture for less than $100 can bring thousands of dollars in sales. The piperidines necessary to manufacture PCP are now under government regulation, which has prompted clandestine laboratories to seek new chemical derivations for their sale of PCP analogs. PCP is frequently misrepresented and distributed as THC, mescaline, or LSD to the naive user or buyer of abuse substances. The most current application of the drug is soaking a dark wrapper cigarette in PCP, referred to as "Shermans" or "longs." In addition, marijuana is frequently soaked with PCP. Smoking is the preferred route, since it permits the user to regulate the amount ingested.

Pharmacokinetics. PCP is rapidly metabolized in the liver to inactive metabolites, and ingestion of large amounts results in high concentrations of the unmetabolized drug in urine. PCP is lipophilic and has a half-life of $\frac{1}{2}$ to 1 hour in small doses and from 1 to 4 days in larger doses. The pK_a of the drug is 8.5. The "ion trapping" of the drug into extravascular areas, which are more acidic than the serum, is thought to be a major cause of prolonged toxicity. The recirculation of the drug secretion to the acidic gastric fluid and reabsorption in the small intestine may also account for the prolonged toxicity and offer a key to the management of the toxicity of overdosage. These observations have led to treatment using urine acidification with diuresis and continuous gastric drainage in severe intoxication to enhance elimination. Urinary excretion is enhanced when the urine is acidified to 5.5 pH or less with ascorbic acid. The fact that PCP may be found in adipose tissue may indicate that the long-term effects are related to its lipophilic nature. Possibly during a nutritional fast PCP is released and resulting symptoms are interpreted as a flashback.

Effects. In humans common peripheral signs include flushing, profuse sweating, nystagmus, diplopia, ptosis, analgesia, and sedation. Other effects of PCP are as follows:

1. A state similar to alcohol intoxication with ataxia and generalized numbness of extremities
2. Psychologic effects that usually proceed in three stages:
   a. Change in body image and feelings of depersonalization
   b. Perceptual distortions (visual or auditory)
   c. Discomforting feelings of apathy, estrangement, or alienation
3. Disorganization of thought and derealization that is greater than with LSD
4. Impairment of attention span, motor skills, and sense of body boundaries, movement, and position
5. Hallucinations that can recur unpredictably for days, weeks, or months

PCP is similar to ketamine in producing stages of anesthesia. In addition, excitation, paranoid behavior, self-destructive acts (because sensation or feeling of pain is absent), horizontal and vertical nystagmus, tachycardia, hypertension, seizures, increased reflexes, muscle rigidity, respiratory depression, and coma with open eyes may ensue. PCP is a strong sympathomimetic and hallucinogenic dissociative anesthetic agent. Since the drug is now classified as a controlled substance (Class II), penalties for illegal manufacture have been enacted and enforced.

Effects of PCP are claimed by some investigators to mimic schizophrenia more accurately than those of other psychotomimetics or hallucinogenics. Like the symptoms of schizophrenia, the effects of PCP are reduced by sensory deprivation. Currently no chemical antidote exists for inhibiting the effects of PCP. Keeping the user quiet and away from sensory stimuli may decrease the intensity of some of the effects.

Toxic effects. The pressor effects of PCP may cause hypertensive crisis, intracerebral hemorrhage, convulsions, coma and death.

Intoxication and treatment. The clinical symptoms and signs of PCP intoxication are dose related. The waxing and waning of the intoxicative signs may be related to the pharmacokinetics of enteric reabsorption for the alkalized (nonionized) PCP with the recirculation and redistribution of the agent, as described earlier.

Low overdosage. A low dose is considered to be 2 to 5 mg. This may be achieved by smoking or by intranasal use. Serum level ranges from 25 to 90 μg/ml. With low overdosage the individual is conscious but disoriented and may exhibit self-destructive acts of violence. The client often has a characteristic blank, open-eyed stare.

Treatment includes rest, minimal sensory stimulation in a quiet, lowly lit room, positive verbal reassurance, and psychologic support. The client is oblivious to the environment, which should be nonthreatening. The client should be protected from self-inflicted injury. The nurse should not "talk down" the anxious individual to the extent that anxiety is intensified or agitation produced. If treatment with an antipsychotic drug is necessary, the butyrophenone haloperidol is preferred. Use of phenothiazine has resulted in hypotension, and other drugs with anticholinergic properties should also be avoided.

Intravenous diazepam may be used for myoclonic convulsions and seizures and to calm the person. The dosage is usually 2.5 mg at 1- to 15-minute intervals for adults. Oral administration is used for cooperative individuals. Diazepam will also relieve muscle spasm, diminish somatosensory dissociation, and make the client more open to treatment.

Moderate overdosage. A moderate dose is 5 to 25 mg with a serum level of 90 to 300 μg/ml. The individual is unconscious, in no immediate danger of dying, responsive to noxious or painful stimuli, and unable to respond to verbal command.

Treatment is initially begun with a diuretic along with urinary acidification by administration of ascorbic acid until the urinary pH is 4.5 to 5.5. Ammonium chloride should not be given since ammonia-breakdown products place a burden on the damaged hepatocellular complex.

Deep oropharyngeal suctioning or intubation is used only when absolutely imperative. The somatosensory sys-

tem is deadened, so pain and stimulation of the autonomic reflex system of the airway should be avoided.

High overdosage. A high overdosage is generally 25 mg or more, with a serum level of 300 μg/ml or more. Individuals taking such large doses may have underlying suicidal tendencies. This dose produces an adrenergic crisis and status epilepticus, possibly with fatal results. Respiratory failure is very late and occurs frequently. The person is comatose and unresponsive to deep pain stimuli. This client must be hospitalized and vital life processes maintained.

Management of clients with a high overdose is the same as for those with a moderate overdose. Periodic respiration occurs; apnea is a terminal sign, and protective airway reflexes are lost. The increased respiration with orotracheal secretions and sustained vomiting often initiates aspiration pneumonitis. At this stage, if the tachycardia and hypertension continue, congestive heart failure and a cerebrovascular accident may result. Boardlike stiffness and myoclonus increase with opisthotonos and tonic-clonic seizure activity to status epilepticus, and the airway is lost.

All medical efforts are directed to management of the airway and control of status epilepticus. Fixed dilated pupils are a sign of deep intoxication. An expert should perform orotracheal intubation. A large-bore nasogastric tube is used for flushing gastric contents, since it is suggested that ion trapping of PCP occurs in an acid gastric content. Periodic lavage with a solution of 0.1 N hydrochloric acid to maintain a gastric pH of 2 is recommended. Since PCP has a high pK_a level and is ionized in an acid medium, PCP is not absorbed as long as it remains in the highly acidic gastric juice. When PCP passes to the small intestine where the pH is alkaline, it becomes nonionized and unable to pass through the semipermeable membrane of the intestine to be absorbed into the blood. This is the key to the ion trapping and the reason for maintaining a highly acid pH in the stomach and urine.

The treatment of overdosage with high amounts of PCP should also include keeping the person cool with sponging or use of a hypothermia blanket. Propranolol (1 mg) may be given intravenously over 1 to 5 minutes to a maximum of 10 mg to titrate the hypertensive spikes and dysrhythmia. There should be a standing order for diazoxide for hypertensive crisis (150 to 300 mg over ½ minute by intravenous push). The pulmonary system must be protected from edema (aspiration pneumonitis). Symptomatic control of status epilepticus is achieved by intravenous anticonvulsant therapy, as indicated.

When the clients are recovering from moderate to high overdosages, a severe, life-threatening dopaminergic storm may occur in addition to anxiety or depression and confusion. The anxiety/depression state is different in each user, but the use of diazepam or haloperidol may control such reactions. The dopaminergic storm may be controlled with propranolol, since it crosses the blood-brain barrier and acts on the dopaminergic receptor sites of the limbic system to calm the client.

The use of PCP causes a wide range of subjective effects requiring careful observations of the overdosed client. The prolonged and severe behavioral disturbances may progress to respiratory and cardiovascular emergencies as serum levels of the drug change.

INHALANTS

Volatile hydrocarbons and aerosols are other substances of abuse. Representatives of this group are toluene, xylene, benzene, gasoline, paint thinner, typewriter correction fluid, lighter fluid, and airplane glue.

Volatile hydrocarbons are often used as propellants in aerosol products. When sniffed (inhaled), these agents may produce a rapid general CNS depression with marked inebriation, dizziness, floating sensations, exhilaration, and intense feelings of well-being that are at times seen as reckless abandonment, disinhibition, and feelings of increased power and aggressiveness similar to those seen with alcohol intoxication. Inhalation may result in bronchial and laryngeal irritation, transient euphoria, headache, giddiness, vertigo, ataxia, and renal tubular acidosis, especially with glue sniffing. At high doses confusion and coma occur with blood dyscrasia. Depression may follow these early excitatory effects. Chronic toluene abuse will lead to hepatic and renal toxicity, and death from cardiac dysrhythmia and respiratory failure has been reported. Recovery from lower doses may be seen in 15 minutes to a few hours. Inhalants are used mainly by young children and preteens (6- to 15-year-olds).

Butyl nitrite is a clear, yellow liquid sold as a room deodorizer under trade names such as Rush, Bolt, and Bullet. The substance is sold in drug paraphernalia shops, and adult book stores and by mail order. The opened container is placed under the nose, and the individual inhales in deep, nasal breaths and becomes dizzy, feels faint, and possibly loses consciousness. This rush lasts less than 1 minute and may include a headache, perspiration, and flushing, all caused by rapid vasodilation. It strongly resembles the effects achieved from amyl nitrite (a prescription smooth muscle relaxant and vasodilator). The FDA may change the status of butyl nitrite from a room odorizer or deodorizer because of its potential for abuse and for harmful effects. Amyl nitrite is sometimes abused to heighten a sexual orgasm in both partners. Both butyl nitrite and amyl nitrite lower blood pressure and reduce the heart's oxygen consumption.

ANABOLIC STEROIDS

Anabolic steroids are synthetic formulations produced from testosterone, the male hormone. Young people are taking these agents to look good and to improve their chances of winning in sports and in athletic competitions.

(See boxed material.) Lamb (1984) estimated that 80% to 100% of participants in weight lifting, discus throwing, and javelin throwing use anabolic steroid products. The abuse of these drugs is widespread and has been documented in young school-age students as well as in older persons and in both male and females.

Since 1984, many organizations have denounced or publicly banned the use of anabolic steroids, including the American College of Sports Medicine, the American Medical Association, the National Collegiate Athletic Association, the International Olympic Committee, and the U.S. Powerlifting Federation. Many states have also passed laws to ban or limit the selling of such products (Duncan and Shaw, 1985; Duda, 1986).

Nevertheless, the debate continues over the use of steroids. Many physicians have prescribed anabolic steroids, especially for underweight persons and/or for athletes seeking an edge in the competitive field. Many steroidal preparations are available and are used orally and parenterally. Table 9-6 lists some of the commonly used steroids by generic and trade names and the recommended therapeutic dose. Many athletes do not follow these recommendations and use dosages far in excess of the stated dosages. While the dosage of methandrostenolone (Dianabol) was recommended at 5 mg/day, some athletes were taking 1000 to 1500 mg daily for extended periods. This misuse led to the withdrawal of this product from the market in 1982. "Stacking" of drugs or taking multiple anabolic steroids at one time is a practice employed by a number of athletes. This usually includes taking very large

---

MAJOR EFFECTS ASSOCIATED WITH ANABOLIC STEROIDS

ANDROGEN-TYPE EFFECTS

Increased growth and development of the seminal vesicles and prostate gland
Increased body and facial hair
Increased production of oil from the sebaceous glands
Deepening of the voice
Increased sexual interest and desire
Enhancement of abstract and spatial dimension thinking ability
Increase in different aspects of male behavior (e.g., aggressive behavior)

ANABOLIC-TYPE EFFECTS

Increased organ and skeletal muscle mass
Increased calcium in bones
Increased retention of total body nitrogen
Increased hemoglobin concentration
Increased protein synthesis

Data from Duncan and Shaw, 1985.

TABLE 9-6   Selected Listing of Commonly Used Anabolic Steroids

Generic and trade name(s)	Recommended adult dosage
dromostanolone (Drol-ban*)	Antineoplastic dosage: 100 mg IM three times a week
ethylestrenol (Maxibolin)	4 mg orally daily
nandrolone (Anabolin IM, Durabolin, Androlone)	Females: 50-100 mg weekly IM Males: 100-200 mg IM weekly
oxandrolone (Anavar)	2.5 mg orally two to four times daily
oxymetholone (Anadrol, Anapolon♣)	1-5 mg orally/kg daily
stanozolol (Winstrol)	2 mg orally three times daily

*Dromostanolone's primary indication is for the treatment of women with inoperable breast cancer. The other products listed have other indications alone or in addition to the antineoplastic use; such as anabolic, antianemic, and antiosteoporotic agents and as a preventative against angioedema (hereditary). Many of these substances plus various testosterone preparations are or have been used, abused, or misused by athletes (U.S.P.D.I., 1988; Duncan and Shaw, 1985).

dosages of the steroids on an 8-week cycle schedule while following a regular strenuous exercise program (perhaps on isolated muscle groups) and consuming a high-protein diet. The long-term effects of such a schedule have not been studied, but documented short-term effects include increased aggressive behavior and some masculinization in the female.

The American College of Sports Medicine has released a position paper (Duncan and Shaw, 1985) that briefly states:

1. The use of anabolic steroids in individuals under 50 years old does not usually result in improved endurance, strength, lean body mass, or body weight.
2. Scientific documentation does not indicate that excessive doses of these drugs positively or negatively affect the performance of an athlete.
3. Continued use has resulted in reports of liver disease in some individuals; the disease process was reversible in some persons but irreversible in others.
4. Males taking anabolic steroids have had a decrease in testicular size and function and in sperm production. Whether these effects are reversible or irreversible is unknown.
5. Education is necessary to curb the misuse and abuse of these drugs.

This statement is directed to athletes, coaches, doctors, trainers, and physical education instructors. The general public should also be informed of the potential risks associated with short-term and long-term consumption of anabolic steroids.

MAJOR ADVERSE EFFECTS OF ANABOLIC STEROIDS

FEMALES

Oily skin; acne
Decrease in breast size, ovulation, lactation, or menstruation
Hoarse and deep voice tone (usually irreversible)
Clitoral enlargement
Unusual hair growth and/or male type baldness (usually irreversible)

MALES

Prepuberty
Increased size of penis, number of erections, and secondary male characteristics
Postpuberty
Priapism (continuing erections), difficult/increased urination
Increase in breast size (gynecomastia)
Testicular atrophy, oligospermia, impotence

BOTH SEXES

Hypercalcemia
Edema of feet or legs
Jaundice, liver impairment
Liver carcinoma (rare)
Urinary calculi
Hypersensitivity
Insomnia
Iron deficiency anemia
Nausea, vomiting, anorexia, stomach pains

THE NURSE'S ROLE IN SUBSTANCE AND DRUG ABUSE

Great diversity exists both among substances that may be abused and the manner of the abuse. The role of the nurse may involve prevention, detection, treatment, and rehabilitation. Preventive nursing roles both inside and outside the hospital environment include education regarding drugs of all types, particularly those prone to producing dependence. Promoting useful coping mechanisms and acceptable alternatives to drugs may prove beneficial.

Health care providers, including nurses, have a high rate of substance abuse and related problems. Nurses must be aware of the potential for drug or substance abuse among themselves and other health care providers and be alert to recognize and deal with this problem should it arise.

Each nurse must evaluate his or her own feelings and responses to drug abuse. Some nurses tend to react with disgust or disdain, behavior which often increases a client's low self-esteem and results in ineffective lectures and scare tactics. Another common response of the nurse is that of "enabler": someone who shields the client from the consequences of substance abuse or unintentionally encourages continued substance abuse. The most effective response is to recognize and confront the problem directly. Nurses must acknowledge that if left untreated, substance abuse often results in death. However, appropriate treatment can often help these individuals overcome their problems and restore them to productive lives without dependence on harmful substances or drugs.

Since substance abuse transcends the boundaries of economics, social class, race, and ethnic background, all clients have the potential to abuse substances or be affected by someone who does. The following discussion is focused on the client who is suspected or known to abuse substances or drugs.

ASSESSMENT

Assessment includes both physical and psychologic signs and symptoms of substance abuse. The nurse should closely observe both verbal and nonverbal responses to questions since an element of denial may often be ascertained in clients who abuse substances. The nonverbal response may provide additional information, contradict, or reinforce what is verbally stated.

Physical assessment includes vital signs, pupillary signs, and skin (especially for needle marks or "tracts" and abcesses that are often seen with injected drug abuse) and, collecting data on nutrition, elimination, and sleep patterns. For specific findings related to the substances used, see the box on pp. 152 to 153. Diagnostic tests may be used to detect drugs or their metabolites in the blood or urine. The nurse should be aware of the possibility of falsely positive results (see box, p. 148).

Past medical history of the client may include prior treatment of drug abuse or history of drug-related illness such as hepatitis, abcesses, or bacterial endocarditis. A thorough drug history for current or past use of OTC, prescribed, or social/recreational drugs should be taken and should include the frequency, magnitude, and circumstances of drug use and abuse as well as the development of withdrawal symptoms if the drug was stopped.

INTERVENTION

Interventions include monitoring of vital signs and administering medications (if prescribed for treatment of withdrawal). Clients abusing substances often have nutrition deficiencies as well as other health problems, which should be corrected.

The nurse should use a straightforward and receptive approach with clients abusing substances. Therapeutic communication should be focused on increasing self-esteem and confronting manipulative behavior while teaching effective coping mechanisms and problem solving. A client cannot restructure a manner of thinking, feeling, and acting until he or she achieves a new image. Many abusers suffer from deprivation of basic needs such as physical closeness and emotional openness, which may in part be caused by the dissolution of basic family relationships. Such deprivation affects individual needs and the expectations of what one is entitled to in these meaningful relationships. Lack of fulfillment of these needs leads to a pronounced disequilibrium.

A multidisciplinary approach often serves these clients best since they frequently have many health, personal, and social problems that must be addressed. Referral to appropriate agencies (i.e., Alcoholics Anonymous, Narcotics Anonymous, and Alanon) will assist in the follow-up care of these individuals and provide much needed support and encouragement.

EDUCATION

The nurse should assist the client to develop effective coping mechanisms and "non-drug strategies" to deal with stress. Education of the client and family should include drugs and abused substances, particularly those prone to producing dependence.

EVALUATION

Evaluation is focused on how the client has tolerated the withdrawal period and developed new coping strategies. After the withdrawal period, the client must decide to remain drug free. Relapses may occur and should not be viewed as the nurse's failure. Ultimately the decision to use and abuse drugs remains with the client.

Referral to appropriate agencies (see Interventions) is beneficial. The long-term support is essential in helping these clients remain drug free.

ACUTE DRUG INTOXICATION AND WITHDRAWAL

Signs of acute intoxication differ according to the drug abused and may manifest themselves variably, as indicated in Table 9-3. Drug overdose and intoxication may be life threatening. Immediate goals are to stabilize and maintain vital functions and minimize damage. Supportive treatment is combined with specific treatment once the drug has been identified. This is a time of acute psychologic stress for the client, and the nurse must remember to treat the whole patient, not just a physiologic system.

Physical and/or psychologic withdrawal symptoms may follow abrupt cessation of drug or substances use. Promotion of adequate nutrition, safety, rest, and orientation are areas of general nursing interventions during this time. Medications may be administered to reduce the withdrawal symptoms. Rehabilitation begins during the withdrawal period and is continued in an attempt to avoid relapse.

KEY TERMS

crashing, page 167
DAWN, page 149
downers, page 167
drug abuse, page 145
drug misuse, page 145
epileptic absence, page 170
flash, page 167
flashback phenomena, page 172
hallucinogenic, page 149
metabolic tolerance, page 150
pK$_a$, page 167
pharmacologic tolerance, page 150
physiologic dependence, page 149
psychedelic, page 149
psychic dependence, page 149
receptor site tolerance, page 150
rush, page 167
speedball, page 168
tissue tolerance, page 150

BIBLIOGRAPHY

Abramowcz, M: Adverse effects of cocaine abuse, Med Lett Drugs Ther 26:662, May 25, 1984.

American Hospital Formulary Service: AHFS drug information '87, Bethesda Md, 1988, American Society of Hospital Pharmacists.

Aranow, R, and others. Phenycyclidine overdose: an emerging concept of management, J. Am Coll Emerg Physicians 7:56, 1978.

Avery, GS: Drug treatment. ed 2, New York, 1980, Adis Press.

Benzodiazepine abuse: what are the data? Psychopharmacol Bull 18(3):87, 1982.

Berdmann, E, and others: Stopping valium, New York, 1982, Warner Books.

Berkow, R, ed: The Merck manual of diagnosis and therapy, vol. 1, ed 14, Rahway, NJ, 1987, Merck, Sharp & Dohme Research Lab oratory.

Bernstein, JG: Kids and drugs: recreational use, Drug Ther. 14(3):193, 1984.

Bissell, C, and Haberman, PW: Alcoholism in the Professions, Oxford, 1984, Oxford University Press.

Blum, K: Handbook of abusable drugs, New York, 1984, Gardner Press, Inc.

Bohach, C: Combating cocaine dependence, amantadine tested as withdrawal aid, Street Pharmacologist 2(1):1, 1987.

Brecher, EM: Licit and illicit drugs, Boston, 1972, Little, Brown, & Co.

Brewer, C: Controlling the demon, Nurs Times, 1986, p. 46.

Burt, MR: Prevalence and consequences of drug abuse among U.S. military personnel, 1981-1982, Am J Drug Alcohol Abuse 8(4):419, 1980.

Cherry, N, and others: Solvent sniffing in industry, Hum Toxicol 1(3):289, 1982.

Council on Scientific Affairs: Scientific issues in drug testing: council report, JAMA 127(22):3110, 1987.

Davidson, DE, ed: Handbook of nonprescription drugs, ed 8, Washington, DC, 1986, American Pharmaceutical Association.

Dietch, J: The nature and extent of benzodiazepine abuse: an overview of recent literature, Hosp Community Psychiatry 34(12):1139, 1983.

Dominquez, R: SP lab: 1986 analysis summary, Street Pharmacologist 11(3):1, 1987.

Dominquez, RA, and Goldstein, BJ: 25 years of benzodiazepine experience: clinical commentary on use, abuse, and withdrawal, Hosp Formul 20(9):1000, 1985.

Drake WC: Ro-1788 (flumazepil): an antidote for benzodiazepine intoxication? Pharm Alert 16(3):1, 1986.

Drew, LP: Drug dependence: an appraisal of the disease concept, Aust NZ J Psychiatry 16(2):55, 1982.

Drug abuse related to prescribing practices, JAMA 247(6):864, 1982.

Duda, M: California proposes tougher steroid law, The Physician and Sports Medicine 14(2):40, 1986.

Duda, M: Do anabolic steroids pose an ethical dilemma for U.S. physicians? The Physician and Sports Medicine 14(11):173, 1986.

Duncan, DJ, and Shaw, EB: Anabolic steroids: implications for the nurse practitioner, Nurse Pract 10(12):8, 1985.

El-Mourad, R: Bromocriptine in the treatment of cocaine craving, Street Pharmacologist 10(12):4, 1986.

Evens, RP, and others: Alcohol: vehicle and active drug, US Pharmacist 6(3):33, 1981.

Fredrick, DS: Alcoholism: medical consequences and therapy, US Pharmacist 5(6):47, 1980.

Gaskin, J: Nurses in trouble, Can Nurse 82(4):31, 1986.

Gonzales, ER: Methaqualone abuse indicated in injuries, deaths nationwide, JAMA 246(8):813, 1981.

Goodman, AG, and others, eds: Goodman and Gilman's the pharmacological basis of therapeutics, ed 7, New York, 1985, Macmillan, Inc.

Goyan, JE: Prescribing of minor tranquilizers, FDA Drug Bull 10(1):2, 1980.

Grabowski, J, ed: Cocaine: pharmacolgy, effects, and treatment of abuse, NIDA research mongraph 50, Washington, DC, 1984, National Institute of Drug Addiction.

Gram, L, and others: D-propoxyphene kinetics after single oral dose and intravenous doses in men, Clin Pharmacol Ther 26(4):463, 1979.

Green, PL: The impaired nurse: chemical dependency, J Emerg Nursing 10(1):23, 1984.

Greenblatt, DJ, and others: Current status of benzodiazepines, part 2, N Engl J Med 309(7):410, 1983.

Hall, J: Counting heads: how do you measure abuse? Street Pharmacologist 10(10):1, 1986.

Hall, JN: Cocaine smoking ignites America, Street Pharmacologist 9(1):1, 1986.

Halpern, JS, and Davis, JW: "T's" and blues, J Emerg Nursing 8(3)150, 1982.

Hanenson, IB: Quick reference to clinical toxicology, Philadelphia, JB, Lippincott Co.

Hansten, PD: Drug interactions, ed 5, Philadelphia, 1985, Lea & Febiger.

Herfindal, ET, and Hirschman, JL: Clinical pharmacy and therapeutics, ed 3, Baltimore, 1984, The Williams & Wilkins Co.

Hershey, CO, and Miller, S: Solvent abuse: a shift to adults, Int J Addict 17(6):1085, 1982.

Hinds, M, ed: How much blood alcohol content per drink, Informed Families of Dade County 2(6):1, 1985.

Holland, DJ: Cocaine use and toxicity, J Emerg Nursing 8(4):166, 1982.

Hopkins, DR, and others: Benzodiazepine withdrawal in general practice, J R Coll Gen Pract 32(245):758, 1982.

Hughes, R, and Brewin, G: The tranquilizing of America, New York, 1979, Warner Books.

Hutchinson, S: Chemically dependent nurses: the trajectory toward self-annihilation, Nurs Research 35(4):196, 1986.

Hyams, DE: Central nervous system anxiolytics and hypnotics. In Brocklehut, JC, ed: Geriatric pharmacology and therapeutics, Oxford, 1984, Blackwell Scientific Publications.

Johnson, R, and Connelly, JC: Addicted physicians: a closer look, JAMA 245(3):253, 1981.

Kandel, DB, and Logan, JA: Patterns of drug use from adolescence to young adulthood. I. Periods of risk for initiation, continued use, and discontinuation, Am J Public Health 74(7):660, 1984.

Katcher, BS, and others: Applied therapeutics: the clinical use of drugs, ed 3, San Francisco, 1983, Applied Therapeutics, Inc.

Kelly, L: Are nurses dipping in Demerol? NJ Nurse 12(4):18, 1982.

Khantzian, EJ, and McKenna, GJ: Acute toxic and withdrawal reaction associated with drug use and abuse, Ann Intern Med 90(3):361, 1979.

Krough, CME, ed: Compendium of pharmaceuticals and specialties, ed 21, Toronto, 1986, Southern Murray.

Lachman, VD: Why we must take care of our own, Nursing '86 4:41, 1986.

Lamb, D: Anabolic steriods in athletics: how well do they work and how dangerous are they? Am J Sports Med 12(1):31, 1984.

Lamy, PP: Drug abuse by older adults: who is responsible? Am Pharm NS22(10):5, 1982.

Lawrence, C, Jr: As workers get high, so do prices, The Miami Herald, Oct. 24, 1983, p Cl.

McEvoy, GK, ed: AHFS drug information '87, Betheseda, Md, 1988, American Society of Hospital Pharmacists.

McKenna, GJ: Methadone and opiate drugs: psychotropic effect and self-medication, Ann NY Acad Sci 398:44, 1982.

Mclellan, AT, and others: Is treatment for substance abuse effective? JAMA 247(10):1423, 1982.

Morgan, DA, and Johnson, VE: Intervention: a process for helping impaired physician, J Fla Med Assoc 69(11):937, 1982.

Morse, RM, and others: Prognosis of physicians treated for alcoholism and drug dependence, JAMA 251(6):743, 1984.

Morton, A. The nurse addict: a state of emotional bankruptcy? Nurs. Mirror 159(6):16, 1984.

National Institute on Drug Abuse: Patterns and trends of drug abuse: a national and international perspective, Rockville, Md, US Department of Health and Human Services.

National Institute on Drug Abuse: Statistical series: data from the Drug Abuse Warning Network (DAWN)—semiannual report, trend data through January-June 1984, Rockville, Md, 1985, US Department of Health and Human Services.

Nellis, M: Too many overuse drugs pharmacists hear, Drug Topics, Aug 15, 1980.

Niven, RG: Adolescent drug abuse, Hosp Community Psychiatry 37(6):596, 1986.

Novak, A: The deliberate inhalation of volatile substances, J Psychedelic Drugs 12(2):105, 1980.

O'Connor, D: The use of suggestion techniques with adolescents in the treatment of glue sniffing and solvent abuse, Hum Toxicol 1(3):313, 1982.

O'Malley, PN, and others: Period, age, and cohort effects on substance use among American youth, 1976-82, Am J Public Health 74(7):682, 1984.

Osol, A, ed: Remington's pharmaceutical sciences. Easton, Pa, 1980, Mack Publishing Co.

Pallikkathayil, L, and Tweed, S: Substance abuse: alcohol and drugs during adolescence, Nurs Clin North Am 18(2):313, 1983.

Peden, NR, Pringle, SD, and Crooks, J: The problem of psilocybin mushroom abuse, Hum. Toxicol 1(4):417, 1982.

Penny, JT: Spotlight on support for impaired nurses, Am J Nurs 86(6):689, 1986.

Perry, PJ, and Alexander, B: Sedative hypnotic dependence: patient stabilization, testing, and withdrawal, Drug Intell Clin Pharm 20(7):532, 1986.

Platt, D: Alcohol-drug interactions, The Apothecary 94(6):35, 1982.

Pointer, J: Typewriter correction fluid inhalation: a new substance of abuse, J Toxicol Clin Toxicol 19(5):493, 1982.

Rappolt, RT, and others: Emergency management of acute phenycyclidine intoxication, J Am Coll Emerg Physicians 8:68, 1979.

Ray, OS: Drugs, society, and human behavior, ed 3, St Louis, 1983, The CV Mosby Co.

Ray, WA, and others: Psychotropic drug use and the risk of hip fracture, N Eng J Med 316:363. 1987.

Reed, MT: The dependent nurse, Nurs Times 79(3):12, 1983.

Rice, MA, and Kibbee, PE: Review: identifying the adolescent substance abuser, MCN 8:139, 1983.

Richards, ML, and others: Phenycylidine psychosis, Drug Intell Clin Pharm 13:336, 1979.

Rickels, K: Benzodiazepines in the treatment of anxiety, Am J Psychother 36(3):358, 1982.

Riordan, CE, and Kleber, HD: Rapid opiate detoxification with clonidine and naloxone, Lancet 1:1079, 1980.

Robert, DJ: Abuse of aerosol products by inhalation, Hum Toxicol 1(3):249, 1982.

Ross, CA: Gasoline sniffing and lead encephalopathy, Can Med Assoc J 127(12):1195, 1982.

Rosser, WW: Benzodiazepine prescription to middle-aged women: is it done indiscriminately by family physicians? Postgrad Med 71(4):115, 1982.

Ryan, CV: Drug diversion: the legal aspect, Okla Nurse 26(1):6, 1981.

Schnoll, SH: Street PCP scene: issues on synthesis and contamination, J Psychodelic Drugs 12(3-4):229, 1980.

Schnoll, SH: Aiding the drug abuser, Hosp Med 19(9):116, 1983.

Schnoll, SH, and others: Cocaine dependence, Med Times 113(4):46, 1985.

Seabolt, J: Drug information request: Talwin-Nx, PharmAlert: Student Committee on Drug Abuse Education, University of Maryland School of Pharmacy 15(1):3, 1984.

Segal, M, and others: The 1980 prevention objectives for alcohol and drug misuse: progress report, Public Health Rep 98(5):426, 1983.

Shinn, AF, ed: Evaluation of drug interactions, St Louis, 1985, The CV Mosby Co.

Showalter, CV: T's and blues: abuse of pentazocine and tripelennamine, JAMA 244(11):1224, 1980.

Solvent abuse (editorial), Lancet 2(8308):1139, 1982.

Stahl, SM, and Kasser, IS: Pentazocine overdose, Ann Emerg Med 12(1):28, 1983.

Stewart, DC: The use of clinical laboratory in the diagnosis and treatment of substance abuse, Pediatr Ann 11(8):669, 1982.

Surgeon General's warning on marijuana, Morbid Mortal Week Rep 31(31):428, 1982.

Tommasello, T: Cocaine dependence and treatment: the pharmacological aspects, PharmAlert 15(1):1, 1984.

United States Pharmacopeial Convention: USPDI-88: drug information for the health care provider, ed 7, Rockville, Md, 1988, United States Pharmacopeial Convention.

Volans, G, and others: Solvent abuse: current findings and research needs, Hum Toxicol 1(3):201, 1982.

Walsh, JM and Hawks, RL: Drug screening: is it reliable? US Pharmacist 12(3):107, 1987.

Washington, AM and Resnick, RB: Clonidine in opiate withdrawal: review and appraisal of clinical findings, Pharmacotherapy 1:140, 1981.

Washington, AM, and others: Opiate and cocaine dependencies, Postgrad Med 77(5):293, 1985.

Watson, JM: Solvent abuse: presentation and clinical diagnosis, Hum Toxicol 1(3):231, 1982.

Weil, A, and Rosen, W: Chocolate to morphine: understanding mind-active drugs, Boston, 1983, Houghton Mifflin Co.

Wetli, CV: Changing patterns of methaqualone abuse: a survey of 246 fatalities, JAMA 249(5):621, 1983.

Woolf, DS, and others: Guidelines for management of acute phencyclidine intoxication, Crit Care Update 7(6):16.

Yamaguchi, K, and Kandel, DB: Patterns of drug use from adolescence to young adulthood: II. Sequences of progression, Am J Public Health 74(7):668, 1984.

PART TWO

Clinical Aspects of Pharmacology

UNITS

IV
Drugs Affecting the Central Nervous System

V
Drugs Affecting the Autonomic Nervous System

VI
Drugs Affecting the Cardiovascular System

VII
Drugs Affecting the Blood

VIII
Drugs Affecting the Urinary System

IX
Drugs Affecting the Respiratory System

X
Drugs Affecting the Gastrointestinal System

XI
Drugs Affecting the Visual and Auditory Systems

XII
Drugs Affecting the Endocrine System

XIII
Drugs Affecting the Reproductive System

XIV
Drugs Used in Neoplastic Diseases

XV
Drugs Used in Infectious Diseases and Inflammation

XVI
Drugs Affecting the Immunologic System

XVII
Drugs Affecting the Integumentary System

XVIII
Intravenous and Nutritional Therapy

XIX
Miscellaneous Agents

UNIT IV

Drugs Affecting the Central Nervous System

15

Central Nervous System Stimulants

16

Psychotherapeutic Drugs

17

Drugs for Specific CNS-Peripheral Dysfunctions

Overview of the Central Nervous System

The nervous system consists of the **central nervous system (CNS)** and the **peripheral nervous system (PNS)** (Figure 10-1). The PNS will be discussed in Chapter 18. This chapter will review the primary areas of the CNS, with focus on the specific areas affected by drug therapy.

The CNS, composed of the brain and spinal cord, essentially controls all functions in the body. The PNS is the network that transmits information to and from the CNS, thus alerting the CNS of internal and external changes, such as muscle tension, blood vessel alterations, pain, fever, sound, smell, taste, touch, and sight. This information is integrated, and instructions are then relayed to appropriate cells or tissues to produce the necessary actions and environmental adjustments. Information concerning these actions and adjustments is again fed back into the CNS. The constant feeding of information into the CNS permits continuous adjustment to be made in the instructions sent to various tissues to ensure effective control of body functions.

BRAIN

The **brain** can be physically divided in various ways. A simplified developmental or embryonic approach is to divide it into the forebrain, brainstem, and cerebellum. The forebrain is made up of the **telencephalon** (which

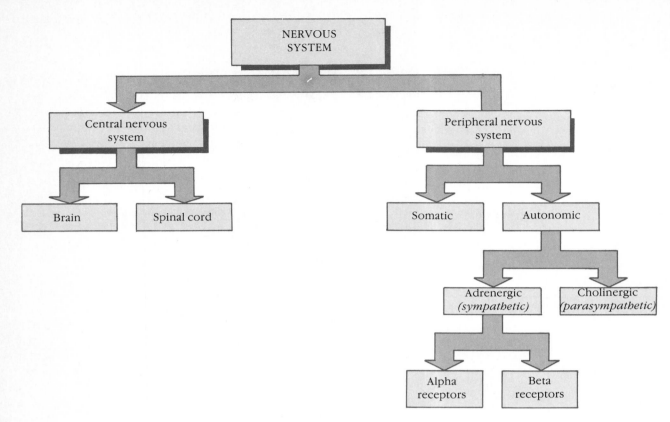

FIGURE 10-1   Overview of the nervous system.

is located anterolaterally and includes the cerebrum) and the diencephalon (which arises from the midbrain but is considered part of the forebrain; it is located posteriorly and includes the thalamus and hypothalamus). The brainstem includes the midbrain, pons, and medulla oblongata. The cerebellum is attached to the cerebrum and brainstem in the occipital region of the head (Figure 10-2).

Telencephalon

Cerebrum. The **cerebrum** is the highest functional area of the brain, where memory storage, sensory, integrative, emotional, language, and motor functions are controlled. The cerebrum consists of two hemispheres (right and left) connected by fibrous tracts. The outer surface of the cerebrum is called the **cerebral cortex** or gray matter of the brain, and it covers the four lobes into which each hemisphere is divided. These lobes are named for the bones of the skull under which they lie—frontal, parietal, occipital, and temporal. The frontal lobe contains the motor and speech areas. The sensory cortex is located in the parietal lobe, the visual cortex in the occipital lobe, and the auditory cortex in the temporal lobe. Association areas lie near these areas and act in conjunction with them. In addition, large parts of the cortex are concerned with higher mental activity—reasoning, creative thought, judgment, memory—those attributes that are unique to humans and separate them from other animals.

Drugs that depress cortical activity may decrease acuity of sensation and perception, inhibit motor activity, decrease alertness and concentration, and even promote drowsiness and sleep. Drugs that stimulate the cortical areas may cause more vivid impulses to be received and greater awareness of the surrounding environment. In addition, increased muscle activity and restlessness may occur. The specific response brought forth by a drug depends to a large extent on the personality of the individual, the emotional and physiologic state, the specific attributes of the drug, and a host of other factors.

Diencephalon. The **diencephalon** (between-brain) is composed of the thalamus, hypothalamus, and part of the third ventricle.

Thalamus. The **thalamus** is composed of sensory nuclei and serves as the major relay center for impulses to and from the cerebral cortex. It also registers such sensations as pain, temperature, touch, and many types of sensory impulses and relays this information to the cerebrum.

The thalamus enables the individual to have impressions of pleasantness or unpleasantness, and it also appears to play a part (with the reticular activating system) in arousal or alerting signals in the individual. (See Reticular Activating System later in this chapter for a further description.) Drugs that depress cells in the various portions of the thalamus may interrrupt the free flow of

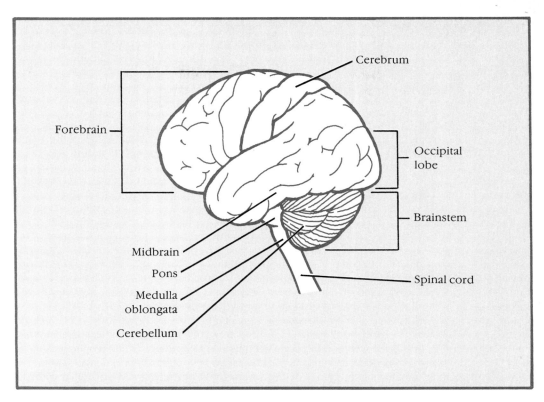

FIGURE 10-2   Surface of human brain.

impulses to the cerebral cortex. This is one way in which pain may be relieved.

Hypothalamus The **hypothalamus** lies below the thalamus and is vital for maintaining vital functions and for the well-being of the individual. It is a major link between the mind and body, and it connects the nervous system to the endocrine gland mechanism. Functions of the hypothalamus include regulating body temperature, carbohydrate and fat metabolism, and water balance; the appetite center and pleasure or reward centers are also believed to be located here. There is evidence that a center for sleep and wakefulness also exists within the hypothalamus. Some of the sleep-producing drugs are thought to depress hypothalamic centers.

Neurons in the hypothalamus release hormones that affect the anterior pituitary gland. Growth hormone, hormones that affect sexual glands or functions, and thyroid and the adrenal cortex hormones are under the control of the hypothalamus. The hypothalamus is also involved with the control of emotions along with other specific areas in the brain. These functions of the hypothalamus may be affected by drugs. An example is the use of antidepressants to treat the symptoms of depression. The action of tricyclic antidepressants on the hypothalamus often reverses the symptoms of weight loss, anorexia, decreased libido, and insomnia associated with depression. Other psychotherapeutic agents may cause a number of hypothalamic side effects, including breast en-

gorgement, lactation, amenorrhea, appetite stimulation, and alterations in temperature regulation.

Brainstem. The **brainstem** is composed of the midbrain, pons, and medulla ablongata and is the source of 10 of the 12 cranial nerves (see box on p. 188); the exceptions are the olfactory and optic nerves that originate in the diencephalon. The **midbrain** contains nerve tracts to and from the cerebrum. It is also the source of the third (oculomotor) and fourth (trochlear) cranial nerves; some optic fibers are also located here. The midbrain serves as a relay station from higher areas of the brain to lower centers. The source of the fifth, sixth, seventh, and eighth cranial nerves is the **pons.** It also contains a center that controls involuntary respiratory regulation. The midbrain and pons are affected by drugs as they stimulate or depress the reticular activating system. The **medulla oblongata** contains the vital centers: the respiratory, vasomotor, and cardiac centers. Such centers are referred to as vital because they are necessary for survival. Other essential functions also originate here, such as vomiting, hiccuping, sneezing, coughing, and swallowing reflexes.

If the respiratory center is stimulated by drugs, it will discharge an increased number of nerve impulses over nerve pathways to the muscles of respiration. If it is depressed, it will discharge fewer impulses, and respiration will be correspondingly affected. Other centers in the medulla that respond to certain drugs are the cough center and the vomiting center. The medulla, pons, and mid-

CRANIAL NERVES

CRANIAL NERVE	TYPE OF NERVE	FUNCTION
I Olfactory	Sensory	Smell
II Optic	Sensory	Sight
III Oculomotor	Motor	Movement of eye and eyelid muscles, pupillary constriction
IV Trochlear	Motor	Eye muscle for downward and inward motion of eye
V Trigeminal	Motor	Chewing, lateral jaw movement
	Sensory	Sensations of the face, scalp, oral cavity, teeth, and tongue
VI Abducens	Motor	Eye movements
VII Facial	Motor	Facial expressions
	Sensory	Taste
VIII Acoustic	Sensory	Hearing, equilibrium
IX Glossopharyngeal	Motor	Swallowing, salivation
	Sensory	Taste, throat sensations
X Vagus	Motor	Voice production, decrease in heartbeat, swallowing, increased peristalsis
	Sensory	Gag reflex; sensations of throat, larynx, and abdominal viscera
XI Spinal accessory	Motor	Head and shoulder movements
XII Hypoglossal	Motor	Tongue movements

Drug effects, toxicity, or both have been reported to affect various cranial nerve functions. For example, ototoxicity or eighth cranial nerve damage has been reported with aminoglycoside antibiotics. Vincristine, an antineoplastic agent, may produce ptosis (cranial nerve III), trigeminal neuralgia (cranial nerve VII), facial palsy (cranial nerve V) and jaw pain. Since various medications have the potential for affecting the cranial nerves adversely, the student should be familiar with the functions of the cranial nerves.

brain constitute the brainstem and contain many important correlation centers (gray matter) as well as ascending and descending pathways (white matter).

Cerebellum. The **cerebellum** contains centers for muscle coordination, equilibrium, and muscle tone. It receives afferent impulses from the vestibular nuclei, as well as the cerebrum, and plays an important role in the maintenance of posture. Drugs that disturb the cerebellum or vestibular branch of the eighth cranial nerve cause dizziness and loss of equilibrium.

SPINAL CORD

The **spinal cord,** a center for reflex activity, also functions in the transmission of impulses to and from the higher centers in the brain and may be affected by the action of drugs. Ascending sensory tracts conduct up to the brain from peripheral nerves and descending motor tracts conduct down from the brain to peripheral nerves.

A cross section of the spinal cord reveals an internal mass of gray matter enclosed by white matter (Figure 10-3). The butterfly-shaped gray matter is divided into horns; the **afferent** (sensory) **nerve fibers** are located in the dorsal or posterior section, whereas the **efferent** (motor) **nerve fibers** exit from the ventral or anterior horns. For example, when a pain impulse reaches the dorsal

horn, the impulse will be transmitted along special tracts (lateral spinothalamic tract) to the thalamus, which then distributes the message to other areas of the brain. The brain responds by means of the descending efferent fiber pathways to inhibit or modify other incoming pain stimuli. (See the discussion of gate theory in Chapter 11.) Large doses of spinal stimulants may cause convulsions; smaller doses may increase reflex excitability.

When a drug is described as having a central action, it means that it has an action on the brain or the spinal cord.

BLOOD-BRAIN BARRIER

The **blood-brain barrier** is actually a covering of nerve cells (astrocytes) that encircle the brain's capillary walls. This covering prevents the passage of many drugs or large molecules into the brain, but it will allow small molecules (such as water, alcohol, oxygen, and carbon dioxide), glucose, gases, and lipid-soluble substances to penetrate this barrier. Such selective processing allows the brain a degree of security against the toxic effects of some drugs on the CNS, but in large doses or in instances of meningeal inflammation the permeation of such substances across the blood-brain barrier would increase. Current research is studying methods to increase the permeability of the blood-brain barrier to specific therapeu-

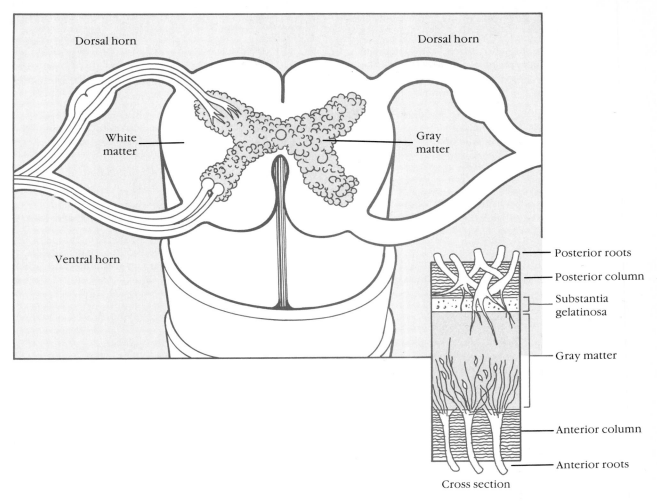

FIGURE 10-3 Cross section of spinal cord.

tic agents, such as antibiotics or antineoplastic agents, needed to treat a localized brain infection or brain tumors.

CNS FUNCTIONAL SYSTEMS

The three major CNS functional systems affected by selected drug or chemical administration include (1) the reticular activating system, (2) the limbic system, and (3) the extrapyramidal system.

Reticular Activating System. The **reticular activating system** (RAS) is a diffuse system of nuclei in the brainstem that permits a two-way communication between the RAS and the cerebral cortex. The primary functions of the RAS are as follows:

1. Consciousness and arousal effect
2. An alerting mechanism
3. A filter process that allows for concentration

The gray matter of the pons and the midbrain, when stimulated, transmits impulses to the thalamus, which fur-

ther transmits the impulse to various areas of the cerebral cortex. This results in consciousness or awakening and, possibly, an arousal effect. Arousal reactions require an external signal, such as a pain stimulus, an alarm clock, or bright lights. The cerebral cortex may signal the RAS or vice versa, but the end result is activation of both areas that may lead to additional transmission of impulses throughout the body (e.g., skeletal muscle activation). Inactivation of the RAS results in sleep, whereas injury or disease may produce a lack of consciousness or comatose state.

The alerting mechanism's primary function is self-preservation, for example, waking up at night because of a chilly sensation. Once awakened, the individual can assess the situation and discover the reason for awakening, perhaps the blanket on the bed had fallen to the floor. The sensation of feeling chilly activated the RAS and caused the awakening, but the situation had to be assessed to determine why the chilliness had occurred.

The filter mechanism allows the individual to decrease

the perception of monotonous stimuli that usually surround us. It permits us to concentrate on a specific at a given time. For example, imagine attending a large birthday party where nearly everyone is talking to someone at the same time. A functioning RAS will allow us to focus on the conversation or person we are interested in by filtering out all the other conversations. In other words, it permits us to have selective concentration.

Many drugs act on the RAS. Anesthetics dampen its activity and induce sleep, whereas amphetamines stimulate or activate the system. LSD and some of the other hallucinogenic agents may act on the RAS by interfering with its ability to filter out stimuli; therefore, the person taking this substance is bombarded by all kinds of wanted and sometimes unwanted stimuli. In contrast, it is a proposed theory that chlorpromazine stimulates the activity of the RAS and reinstitutes the activity of the filtering process, thus making it useful in reducing hallucinations in the psychotic patient and in patients experiencing an untoward reaction to LSD.

Limbic system. The **limbic system** is a border of subcortical structures that surround the corpus callosum (Figure 10-4). This system forms a ring around the top of the brainstem that consists of the portions of the brain remaining after the cerebral hemispheres and cerebellum have been removed.

The emotions of anger, fear, anxiety, sexual feelings, pleasure, and sorrow are related to this system. Learning and memory have been associated with the hippocampus.

The limbic system is extremely complex in its functioning. It may work with or inhibit other parts of the brain such as the cerebral cortex, brainstem, or hypothalamus to normalize expressions of emotions, influence their ultimate expression to other than normal, or affect the biologic rhythms, sexual behavior, and motivation of an individual.

Drugs that affect the limbic system are the benzodiazepines, meprobamate, and morphine. The benzodiazepines and meprobamate are believed to suppress the limbic system, preventing it from activating the reticular formation, thus resulting in drowsiness and sleep, especially in patients with anxiety. Morphine is thought to alter the subjective reactions of the patient to pain in addition to abolishing pain stimuli received by special areas within the limbic system.

Extrapyramidal system. The **extrapyramidal system** is a somatic motor pathway located in the CNS that affects skeletal muscles. This system is associated with coordination of muscle group movements and posture. Antipsychotic agents that block dopamine receptors may produce side effects or adverse effects related to this system. For further discussion of these effects see Chapter 16.

SYNAPTIC TRANSMISSION IN THE CNS

The **synapse** is the junction point from one neuron to the next. There is evidence that transmission of impulses at synapses in the CNS is humoral (through a secretion). Many neurotransmitters are still to be identified. When released, they affect the postsynaptic neurons to stimulate or inhibit their activity.

Inhibition of motor neuron activity may be presynaptic or postsynaptic. Studies indicate that **presynaptic inhibition** occurs in the brain and is widespread at the spinal

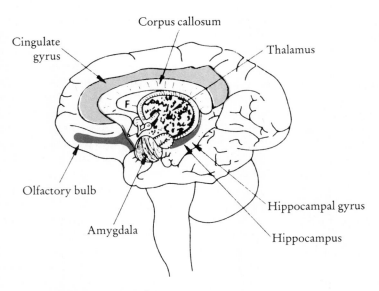

FIGURE 10-4 Limbic system.

(From Bowman, WC, and Rand, MJ: Textbook of pharmacology, ed 2, London, 1980, Blackwell Scientific Publications.)

level, affecting transmission in afferent fibers from skin and muscle. The function of presynaptic inhibition is probably to suppress weak inputs that would otherwise cause unnecessary responses. This modulation of nerve impulses results in less transmitter substance being liberated. The net effect is a limiting or "inhibiting" of impulses to postsynaptic nerve fibers. Inhibition is important for orderly function.

Postsynaptic inhibition may be the result of changes in the membrane permeability of the postsynaptic cells caused by release of chemical transmitters from presynaptic nerve endings.

Upper motor neurons are scattered throughout the cerebral cortex; a number of them are located in the motor cortex. About three fourths of the nerve fibers from these motor neurons cross to the opposite side at the level of the medulla, descend to the spinal cord, and synapse with interneurons, which in turn synapse with the lower motor neurons. Almost all motor neurons of one side are controlled by the motor cortex of the other side. Therefore injury to the motor cortex of the right side causes paralysis on the left side of the body (hemiplegia). Systems other than the upper and lower motor neuron systems are concerned with voluntary movement, but lower motor neurons form the common final pathway for stimuli for voluntary movement.

Some of the **neurotransmitters** that will be discussed are acetylcholine, the catecholamines (dopamine, norepinephrine, and epinephrine), serotonin, and neuroactive peptides (enkephalins, endorphins, and dynorphins).

Acetylcholine. **Acetylcholine** is the best known chemical transmitter of nerve impulses. Not all parts of the CNS contain acetylcholine. Those areas that have high concentrations are the motor cortex, thalamus, hypothalamus, geniculate bodies, and anterior spinal roots; very low concentrations are found in the cerebellum, optic nerves, and dorsal roots of the spine. Acetylcholine can cause cardiac inhibition, vasodilation, gastrointestinal peristalsis, and other parasympathetic effects.

Lower motor neurons release acetylcholine at the neuromuscular junction, causing contraction in striated (voluntary) muscle. The concentration of acetylcholine must be high, since a large number of muscle fibers must respond synchronously for striated muscle contraction to occur and also because acetylcholine is very rapidly destroyed by the enzyme cholinesterase.

Catecholamines and related substances. **Catecholamines** (dopamine, norepinephrine, and epinephrine) and the amine serotonin (5-hydroxytryptamine) are synthesized, stored, and metabolized in the brain. These substances do not easily penetrate the blood-brain barrier, but their precursors do. The effect of injected catecholamines on the CNS is slight in comparison with the effect on the autonomic nervous system. However, an increase in catecholamines and serotonin causes cerebral stimula-

tion. Drugs, such as reserpine, that release catecholamines and reduce amine concentration in the brain have a depressing or sedative action. Methyldopa lowers the serotonin and norepinephrine levels and this, too, has a cerebral depressing effect.

Special staining techniques indicate that there are adrenergic (sympathomimetic) and serotoninergic tracts within the CNS. Dopamine, a catecholamine, is especially concentrated in the basal ganglia. The low level of dopamine at this site in individuals suffering from Parkinson's disease led to the therapeutic approach of using its precursor L-dopa with good results in many cases.

Neuroactive peptides. Neuroactive peptides may be considered neuromodulators, neurohormones, or neurotransmitters. Studies indicate that a peptide may affect neuronal activity by increasing or decreasing the synthesis, release, or breakdown of neurotransmittes, neurohormones, or neuromodulators. Basically, little is known of the catabolism, conservation, storage, or synthesis of the neuroactive peptides. Our knowledge is only beginning to uncover the neuroreceptor mechanisms of these substances.

The parenteral or intracerebral injection of these components causes potent behavioral effects. A number of these peptides exist in tissues other than the CNS, primarily in the gastrointestinal tract cells (myenteric plexus). Studies are being done to provide more information about the functions, sites of activity, and mechanisms of action of these peptides. A continual search to find additional neuroactive peptides and other substances having a role in neurotransmission is in progress.

Enkephalins, endophorins, and dynorphins are three major polypeptides found in the brain that have opioid activity. **Enkephalins** may block opiate receptors in the dorsal horn of the spinal cord by blocking the release of substance P. **Substance P,** a transmitter of pain impulses in the nerve fibers, has been proposed to be transmitter for the primary afferent sensory fibers. Enkephalins behave as inhibitory neurotransmitters, decreasing the perception and emotional aspect of pain. Studies indicated that enkephalins may bind to the same neuroreceptor membranes as morphine, and the concept of internal opiates or natural pain killers developed. The enkephalins allow modification and control of the perception of pain.

Endorphins (from "endogenous morphine") is a general term that includes many peptides in the brain that suppress pain. These peptides are also found in the pituitary gland, intermediate lobe, and the corticotroph cells of the adenohypophysis. Subgroups of endorphins have been isolated and identified, including beta-endorphin, an analgesic substance that is much more potent than enkephalin.

Technology has shown that the brain, pituitary gland, and gastrointestinal tract each have enkephalins and beta-

> Jogging and other strenuous types of prolonged sports or exercises reportedly increase the release of endogenous polypeptides. Whereas acute pain may also stimulate the release of endorphins (and possibly other polypeptides), chronic pain usually results in a reduction of endorphin levels. Endorphin levels are decreased in depressed persons but are said to be elevated in happy, cheerful persons (Dolphin, 1983).

endorphins. These peptides are not found in the same cells. Further, the brain cells containing beta-endorphin are different from those that contain enkephalins.

Dynorphin is an endorphin found in the pituitary gland, hypothalamus, and spinal cord. This is the most potent pain-relieving substance discovered; dynorphin is 50 times more potent than beta-endorphin and 200 times more potent than morphine.

Naloxone, a potent opiate antagonist, reverses the analgesic effect of narcotics. Animal studies demonstrate that if naloxone is administered after enkephalins or endorphins are given, it will reverse the analgesic effect produced by the polypeptides. Endorphin release in the body is higher following acupuncture and transcutaneous electrical nerve stimulation, and both effects may be reversed by the use of naloxone. It has been proposed that the analgesic response associated with the use of a placebo may be due to an increased release of endorphins in the body.

From peptide research may come pain relievers with fewer side effects and minimal to no addiction potential, and we may also gain increased understanding of mental disorders and addiction mechanisms.

Neurobiologists are only now beginning to understand what these and other yet to be discovered peptides are doing in the brain and spinal cord. Only basic research will provide the answers to the peptide cascade and an understanding of the functions in the nervous system.

KEY WORDS

acetylcholine, page 191
afferent nerve fibers, page 188
blood-brain barrier, page 188
brain, page 185
brainstem, page 187
catecholamines, page 191
central nervous system, page 185
cerebellum, page 188
cerebral cortex, page 186
cerebrum, page 186
diencephalon, page 186
dynorphins, page 192
efferent nerve fibers, page 188
endorphins, page 191
enkephalins, page 191
extrapyramidal system, page 190
hypothalamus, page 187
limbic system, page 190
medulla oblongata, page 187
midbrain, page 187
neurotransmitter, page 191
peripheral nervous system, page 185
pons, page 187
postsynaptic inhibition, page 191
presynaptic inhibition, page 190
reticular activating system (RAS), page 189
spinal cord, page 188
substance P, page 191
synapse, page 190
telencephalon, page 185
thalamus, page 186

BIBLIOGRAPHY

Anthony, CP, and Thibodeau, GA: Textbook of anatomy and physiology, ed 11, St Louis, 1983, The CV Mosby Co.

Beck, EW, and others: Mosby's atlas of functional human anatomy, St Louis, 1982, The CV Mosby Co.

Boss, BJ, and Stowe, AC: Neuroanatomy, J Neurosurg Nurs 18(4):214, 1986.

Bullock, BL, and Rosendahl, PP: Pathophysiology, Boston, 1984, Little, Brown & Co.

Carey, KW: Pain (Nursing now series), Springhouse, Pa, 1985, Springhouse Corp.

Conway-Rutkowski, BL: Carini and Owens' neurological and neurosurgical nursing, ed 8, St Louis, 1982, The CV Mosby Co.

Dolphin, NW: Neuroanatomy and neurophysiology of pain: nursing implications, Int J Nurs Stud 20(4):255, 1983.

Goth, A, and Vesell, ES: Medical pharmacology principles and concepts, ed 11, St Louis, 1984, The CV Mosby Co.

Katcher, BS, and others: Applied therapeutics: the clinical use of drugs, ed 3, San Francisco, 1983, Applied Therapeutics, Inc.

Kerr, FWL: The pain book, Englewood Cliffs, NJ, 1981, Prentice-Hall, Inc.

McClintic, JR: Human anatomy, St Louis, 1983, The CV Mosby Co.

Mountcastle, VB: Medical physiology, vol 1 and 2, ed 14, St Louis, 1979, The CV Mosby Co.

Price, SA, and Wilson, LM: Pathophysiology: Clinical concepts of disease processes, New York, 1982, McGraw-Hill Book Co.

Stewart, D: Turning on the endorphins, Amer Pharm NS20(10):50, 1980.

West, BA: Understanding endorphins: our natural pain relief system, Nursing '81 11(2):50, 1981.

CHAPTER 11

Analgesics and Antagonists

OBJECTIVES

After studying this chapter, the student will be able to:

1. Describe the physiology, characteristics, and types of pain.

2. Explain the effect of opioid binding with the four major opioid receptors.

3. Discuss special considerations for use of CNS analgesics and antagonists in the very young or old client.

4. Describe the nurse's role in opioid therapy.

5. Differentiate among the opioid analgesics, opioid antagonist, and opioid agonist-antagonist agents.

6. Formulate an appropriate plan of care for individual clients who require the administration of CNS analgesics or antagonists..

Pain, an unpleasant sensation of physical discomfort, is one of the most common problems afflicting humans. It is the most distressing symptom of illness or trauma reported by clients. This is unfortunate since the potent analgesics currently available are both safe and effective when health care providers properly select the **analgesic,** or pain-killing medication, and apply pain management techniques based on the pharmacokinetics of the drug and the individual client's response. The greatest abuse with narcotic analgesics is not inducing addiction, rather it is using too little medication too infrequently to control pain.

Why do clients experience pain?

1. Is it fear of tolerance or addiction on the part of the health care provider or client? Study results indicate that health care providers are overly concerned about the danger of inducing **addiction,** or physiologic dependence on a drug (Marks and Sachar, 1973; Cohen, 1980). Porter and Jick (1980) reviewed nearly 40,000 hospital charts and reported that nearly 12,000 of them had received narcotic analgesics. Of this group only four cases of addiction were documented in clients with no previous history of drug abuse. Study results have indicated that the risk of addiction for hospitalized clients receiving narcotics at regular intervals, even for prolonged periods, is minimal.

Tolerance, or the need to increase the dose of an analgesic to maintain the desired effect, is another concern in practice. Tolerance is not usually seen in clients who have severe acute or chronic pain for which there is a physical cause, such as trauma, tumor growth and invasion, and postsurgical pain. Clients in pain respond differently to an analgesic than individuals seeking euphoric effects from the drug. One must not confuse physical dependence with tolerance. **Physical dependence** is an altered physiologic condition in a long-term drug abuser who requires consistent use of the drug to avoid withdrawal symptoms.

Clients with cancer may receive large amounts of narcotics to control the pain without the adverse effects of respiratory depression or excessive sedation. Pain specialists believe this is the result of **selective tolerance,** that is, tolerance to some of the effects of the drug without interfering with the drug's analgesic effect.

2. Is it ignorance of basic pain management principles by the physician? Bonica (1980) reviewed medical school curricula in the U.S. and found that very few schools include pain management techniques or even the basic pharmacology of narcotic drugs. Such information may or may not be acquired in the clinical setting of internship and residency, depending on the training the senior physicians in the facility had. Often, misconceptions or dealing with the problem of pain in an empirical manner takes precedence over basic pain management techniques.

Bonica examined textbooks on oncology and reported that seven leading oncology texts contained nearly 5500 pages but devoted less than 20 pages to pain management: Thus he concluded that pain is not an important topic to academicians and oncology clinicians.

3. Is it failure on the part of the health care provider to listen to the client? Published studies have indicated that approximately 75% of clients interviewed in hospital settings had moderate to severe pain even though analgesics were available and ordered for them. Chart reviews substantiated the lack of administering prescribed analgesics by health care providers (Marks and Sachar, 1973; Cohen, 1980). A physician survey indicated that physicians tended to underestimate the effective dosage range of a drug and overestimate its length of action. Therefore many orders were insufficient for effective pain management, leading to undertreatment (Marks and Sachar, 1973).

PAIN COMPONENTS AND CONCEPTS

Because of its highly subjective nature, pain is difficult to define. Pain can be viewed as having two components: the physical component, the *sensation of pain,* which involves the nerve pathways and the brain, and the psychologic component, the *emotional response to pain,* which is the product of such factors as the individual's anxiety level, previous pain experience, age, sex, and culture.

Research has shown that a relatively constant pain threshold exists in all persons under normal circumstances. For example, heat applied to the skin at an intensity of 45° to 48° C will initiate the sensation of pain in almost all individuals. However, pain tolerance—the point beyond which pain becomes unbearable—varies widely among individuals and in one individual under different circumstances. Figure 11-1 shows factors affecting the pain threshold.

Pain can be classified in various ways. It may be acute or chronic. **Acute pain** has a sudden onset and usually subsides with treatment. Examples of acute pain include the pain of acute myocardial infarction, acute appendicitis, and kidney stones. **Chronic pain,** such as accompanies cancer and rheumatoid arthritis, is a persistent or recurring pain that is difficult to treat (Table 11-1).

Pain may also be classified by its source as superficial, visceral, or somatic. **Superficial pain** arises from skin or mucous membranes. **Visceral or deep pain** has its origin in the smooth musculature or organ systems. This pain is often difficult to localize since it is dull and aching. Visceral pain may also be referred, that is, felt at a site distant from its origin, such as the pain of a myocardial infarction that is experienced initially in the arm. **Somatic pain** arises from the skeletal muscles, facies, ligaments, vessels, or joints. Superficial and visceral pain may be relieved by narcotic analgesics; somatic pain may respond better to nonnarcotic analgesics.

Pain may also originate from psychogenic causes. Psychiatric illness, including anxiety and depression, has been known to cause severe pain. Obviously, in such a case drug therapy will not bring relief; rather, psychotherapy is indicated.

The great variation in the pain experience has prompted much research and led to the proposal of several theories of pain transmission and pain relief. The **gate control theory,** proposed by Melzack and Wall in 1965, attempts to explain the modulations in the pain experience (Figure 11-2). This theory proposes that a mechanism in the dorsal horn of the spinal cord (the "spinal gate") can alter the transmission of painful sensations from the peripheral nerve fibers to the brain. The "spinal gate" is closed by large-diameter afferent fibers (the fast-acting A-delta fibers) and opened by small-diameter afferent fibers (the slower-acting C-delta fibers). The "gate" is further influenced by descending control inhibition from the brain. Thus gentle stimulation of large-diameter fibers will "close the gate" to stop perception of slower-acting painful stimuli. It is on this theory that many nondrug regimens for pain relief are based, including massages or use of counterirritants. It is also a foundation of the Lamaze theory of "natural childbirth."

Anxiety
Sleeplessness
Tiredness
Anger
Fear, fright
Depression
Discomfort
Pain
Isolation

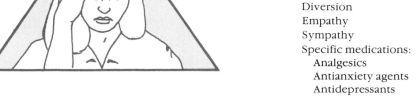

Lower

PAIN THRESHOLD

Raise

Symptom relief, such as in:
Sleep
Rest
Diversion
Empathy
Sympathy
Specific medications:
  Analgesics
  Antianxiety agents
  Antidepressants

FIGURE 11-1   Factors affecting pain threshold.

TABLE 11-1   Acute and Chronic Pain

Onset	Usually sudden	Usually of long duration
Characteristics	Generally sharp, localized, may radiate	Dull, aching, persistent, diffuse
Signs and symptoms	Physiologic response: increased blood pressure and heart rate, sweating, pallor	Physiologic response: often absent
	Emotional response: increased anxiety and restlessness	Emotional response: client may be depressed, withdrawn, expressionless, and exhausted
Therapeutic goals	Relief of pain Sedation often desirable	Relief of pain Sedation *not* desirable
Drug administration		
Timing	As needed or upon request often adequate	Regular preventive schedule
Dose	Standard dosages often adequate	Individualized according to client response
Route	Parenteral	Oral

The Nurse's Role in Pain Therapy

Nurses must use all of their skills to successfully manage clients who are experiencing pain. The nurse often instigates or coordinates the implementation of pain management.

Assessment. Accurate assessment of pain relies on both subjective and objective information. While "pain" cannot be observed (pain is a perception, not an object), the physical and psychologic signs and symptoms of pain can be assessed. Each client perceives and reacts to pain differently based on physical, emotional, and/or cultural influences. Assessment of pain includes both the quantity of pain (the duration and intensity [severity] of pain) and the quality of pain (sharp, dull, burning, radiating, stab-

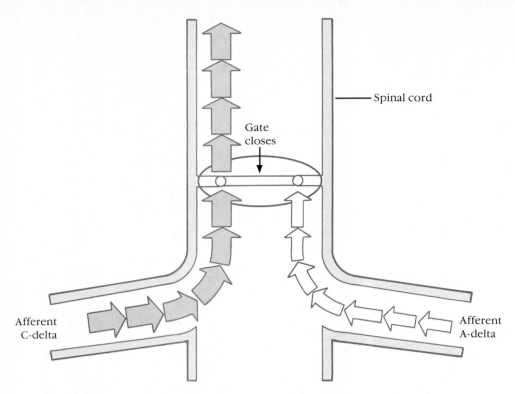

FIGURE 11-2 Gate control theory. Activity from A-delta (large afferent) fibers excites activity in the substantia gelatinosa, thus closing the gate to C-delta, pain-stimulating carrying fibers.

bing, or cramping). The nurse should allow the clients, in their own words, to describe their pain and what seems to intensify or relieve it. Pain may bring forth many emotions from the client, such as fear, anger, or impatience. There are a number of physiologic responses, usually sympathetic in nature, to pain that include increased blood pressure, pulse, and/or respirations; sweating; pallor; restlessness and/or agitation.

Intervention. All clients in pain should receive nursing care directed toward reducing the perception of, and reaction to, pain and to enhance the analgesic effect of medications. The nurse often has significant influence over pain medication through p.r.n. (when needed) prescribing of analgesic medications. As previously mentioned, the greatest abuse of analgesics is in the under-utilization, which results in failure to adequately relieve or control pain. Analgesics should be used *before* the pain reaches peak intensity and painful events occur.

It is well known that anxiety exacerbates pain and causes muscle tension. Relaxation techniques can be effective in reducing the amount of pain experienced. Simple methods that promote comfort, a quiet, pleasant environment, or proper body position may prove very effective. Rhythmic breathing, counting, and purposeful relaxation of muscle groups are among the techniques nurses can teach clients. More advanced methods include biofeedback and hypnosis. An example of a highly suc-

cessful relaxation technique for pain control is the psychoprophalactic or "Lamaze" method of rhythmical breathing and focusing to blunt the perception of pain during labor and delivery. The same techniques also are useful for the management of many other types of acute pain.

Transferring the client's focus of attention away from the painful stimulus is known as distraction. This technique greatly improves the client's ability to cope with chronic pain. Clients may even find that they have developed the ability to distract themselves without realizing it. Watching television, visiting with friends, walking or working on a project can be effective distractions.

Stimulating the client's skin to relieve pain, or cutaneous stimulation, has been found to be very effective in pain management. Transcutaneous electrical nerve stimulation (TENS) is a method of applying a small electrical current to skin areas over nerves or around surgical incisions; it works very well in selected situations. TENS has been shown to cause both the release of natural analgesic substances (endorphins) and interference with pain impulse conduction (see gate control theory, p. 194). Nurses have used cutaneous stimulation for years in the form of massage, stroking, and application of heat and cold.

The nurse should always remember to question the clients about pain relief methods they have used in the past. Reinforcing methods used in the past and supplementing these methods with new techniques often lower the need for pain-relieving medications.

Education. Instructing the clients in various self pain-relief techniques is an important part of pain therapy, especially in chronic pain. The nurse can provide the client with a method of dealing with pain. The nurse may know many techniques for dealing with painful situations that can be taught to the client, such as the technique of applying firm pressure to an abdominal incision with a pillow (*splinting* an incision) to reduce the discomfort of coughing.

Clients given drugs for relief of pain should be informed of the medicaiton's purpose. Analgesic effects may be enhanced by positive suggestion. Clients who self-administer pain-relieving medications should be taught adverse effects, proper dosage, drug or food interactions, correct administration, and safe storage of medications.

Evaluation. Following the implementation of pain relief therapy, an evaluation of effectiveness must be made. Assessment once again evaluates the physiologic responses and the client's perception of pain. One common method of quantifying pain is to have the client rate the pain on a scale of 0 to 10 with 0 representing the absence of pain and 10 representing intolerable pain. Rating the pain before and after treatment serves to document the response to treatment.

In evaluation of pain relief drug therapy, the nurse also looks at several parameters. These areas include compliance with therapy and the development of addiction, dependence, tolerance, or adverse effects.

OPIOID RECEPTORS

Research concerning the binding of opioid medications in the brain and other body organs has identified at least eight different **opioid receptors.** In the CNS, four major receptors have been identified; mu, kappa, delta, and sigma. Analgesia has been associated with the mu and kappa receptors, whereas the sigma receptors demonstrate dysphoric and **psychotomimetic** (inducing psychotic behavior) drug effects. Delta receptors appear to be involved with affective behavioral responses. (See Table 11-2 for receptor effects.)

Naloxone, the narcotic antagonist, has an affinity for all the opioid receptors, but its affinity for the mu receptors is 10 times greater than for the other receptors sites. Morphine has an affinity for the mu and kappa receptors, whereas pentazocine and nalbuphine antagonize mu receptors but have a greater attraction for kappa and delta receptors (Gilman and others, 1985).

OPIOID ANALGESICS-AGONISTS

Opium in the crude form was used until well into the nineteenth century, before the chief alkaloid, morphine,

TABLE 11-2 Opioid Receptor Responses

Receptors	Response
Mu	Supraspinal analgesia, respiratory depression, euphoria, and drug dependence
Kappa	Spinal analgesia, sedation, and pupillary constriction
Sigma	Anxiety, dysphoria, hallucinations, nightmares
Delta	Not identified

NARCOTIC TERMINOLOGY

For years morphine and similar opioid drugs were referred to as narcotics. The term **narcotics** is now considered obsolete and rarely is used to describe the effects of a potent analgesic. Narcotic is derived from a Greek word meaning the induction of stupor or sleep; therefore it could have been referring to sleep-inducing medications. It has also been used to described a CNS depressant, a dependence-producing medication, and a drug that may have neither effect but is still listed under the restrictions of the federal narcotic law, now known as the Controlled Substances Act. Since many drugs fit this description (see Chapter 2) (barbiturates, benzodiazepines, alcohol, and hypnotics, etc.), the term *narcotic* lacks specificity and is no longer acceptable to use interchangeably with opioid analgesics.

was isolated. The discovery of other alkaloids soon followed, and their use came to be preferred to that of the crude preparations.

Opiate refers to drugs that contain or are extracted from opium, whereas **opioid** designates synthetic drugs that have pharmacologic properties similar to opium or morphine. Today opioid is a term used for both natural and synthetic products that have morphine-like effects. In a generic sense, the terms are considered interchangeable.

Morphine is still obtained from opium because of the difficulty encountered in synthesizing it in the laboratory. Many analgesics are available now, but none has been proved to be clinically superior to morphine. All new analgesics are compared to morphine, which is the standard, in potency and in side or adverse effects. Over-the-counter (OTC) analgesics, are effective in mild-to-moderate pain situations and are included in the **step approach system** of pain management (see box on p. 198).

morphine

Mechanism of action. The active principles of opium are alkaloids, of which there are some 20 in number,

STEP SYSTEM APPROACH TO PAIN MANAGEMENT IN CANCER (WHO*)

A three-step approach to pain management involves using the mild analgesics (nonopioid) first and progressing to stronger analgesics in the second and third steps.

Step 1: Mild pain

Aspirin or acetaminophen, 650 mg every 4-6 hr.

Step 2: Moderate pain

Aspirin or acetaminophen with codeine, 60 mg every 4-6 hr.

Step 3: Severe pain

Morphine preparations (oral or rectal), individually dosed according to client response

In addition to the above progression, the following is recommended:

1. Administer medications on a *scheduled* basis to prevent pain.
2. Administer analgesics in adequate doses at appropriate intervals based on the drug's pharmacokinetics.
3. Evaluate frequently and add additional adjuvant medications as necessary (i.e., anticonvulsants, antianxiety agents, antidepressants, or steroids).

*World Health Organization guidelines for the use of oral agents to control cancer pain.

although only three are used widely in the practice of medicine—morphine, codeine, and papaverine. Morphine and codeine act mainly on the CNS, where they produce a combination of depressing and stimulating effects. Both increase smooth muscle tone and promote contraction of smooth muscle; whereas papaverine has little effect on the nervous system but produces relaxation of certain smooth muscles in the body.

As previously mentioned; morphine produces its potent analgesic effects by combining with receptor sites in the brain called opioid receptors. This interaction alters the client's pain perception and emotional response to the pain-provoking stimulus. Two receptors (mu and kappa) are involved with analgesia, and they are located in various areas of the CNS. Kappa receptors are mainly distributed in the cerebral cortex and spinal cord, whereas mu receptors are widely distributed in the CNS but are especially noted in the limbic system, thalamus, hypothalamus, and midbrain. Thus morphine's action on the limbic system reduces the unpleasant emotional response to pain that is typically evoked by a pain stimulus. Pain signals to the brain may be hindered or stopped by inhibitory impulses received at the dorsal horn neurons by descending neural-inhibiting responses. Therefore the perception of pain will also be reduced.

Indications

1. Pain treatment. The analgesic effect of morphine is indicated for the treatment of severe pain. Morphine may be administered by numerous routes, depending on the client's diagnosis, physical condition, and individual response. Generally, the oral step system is the preferred approach for terminally ill clients experiencing pain (see boxed material).
2. Diarrhea treatment. The gastrointestinal effects produced by morphine include a decrease in peristalsis and glandular secretions. Although this usually results in the side effect of constipation, this effect has been used therapeutically to treat diarrhea. Usually the less potent opioids such as codeine and opium tincture are used for this purpose. They are considered safer than morphine and are effective in the treatment of diarrhea.

TABLE 11-3   Pharmacokinetic Overview of Morphine Dosage Forms

Dosage form	Onset of action (min)	Peak effect (min)	Duration of action (hr)
Oral			
Solution*, syrup†, tablets	10-30	60	4-5
Extended release tablets‡	—	—	8-12
IM	10-30	30-60	4-5
IV		20	4-5
SC	10-30	50-90	4-5
Epidural§	15-60	—	Up to 24
Intrathecal§	15-60	—	Up to 24
Rectal‖	20-60	—	4-5

*Roxanol, M.O.S., and Morphitec (not commercially available in U.S.), MSIR.
†Morphite, and Morphitex-1, Morphitec-5 (not commercially available in U.S.).
‡M S Contin, Roxanol SR.
§Duramorph (preservative-free).
‖R.M.S. suppositories.

3. Treatment of clients with lung cancer, pain aggravated by coughing, or an unproductive nagging cough. Small doses may cause depression of the cough center, and this secondary effect may be useful. However, in clients with a cough caused by a cold, less potent and potentially safer medications are usually preferred, such as codeine or the nonnarcotic antitussive, dextromethorphan.

4. Treatment of congestive heart failure and myocardial infarctions. In clients with congestive heart failure and pulmonary edema, morphine's peripheral vasodilation effect on veins and arteries can be very useful in aiding cardiac function and reducing the seepage of fluid into the lungs. Morphine is also used to treat clients with myocardial infarctions because (1) it does not produce significant changes in heart rate and blood pressure at the usual dosages ordered and (2) the calming effect it induces along with the peripheral vasodilation effect may result in a decreased work load on the heart that would be beneficial during an acute myocardial infarction.

Pharmacokinetics

Absorption. May be administered orally, intramuscularly, intravenously, subcutaneously, epidurally, intrathecally, and rectally. For onset, peak, and duration of action see Table 11-3

Distribution. Widely distributed in all body tissues

Metabolism. Liver

Excretion. Mainly excreted in urine with approximately 7% to 10% excreted in the bile and feces

Side effects/adverse reactions. See Table 11-4.

Significant drug interactions. When morphine is given with:

Drug	Possible Effect and Management
alcohol or other CNS depressants	May result in enhanced CNS depression, respiratory depression, and hypotension. Reduce dosage of one or both drugs and monitor closely.
monamine oxidase (MAO) inhibitors	Test dose with ¼ of the dose of morphine (or any prescribed opioid analgesics) to ascertain compatibility of the medications. The possibility of inducing excitability, hypertension, or hypotension; increased sweating; convulsions; respiratory depression; fever; and cardiac dysfunctions exists. Therefore it is usually recommended that caution be taken and reduced dosages of opioids be prescribed for clients receiving MAO inhibitors.
naltrexone	Will produce withdrawal symptoms in clients dependent on opioid medications. Avoid concurrent administration in clients receiving opioids therapeutically.

Dosage and administration. See Table 11-5.

Pregnancy safety. FDA Category C. See also Table 11-6.

Opioid Use in Children

Children are often untreated or inadequately treated for pain. The following are misconceptions that, unfortunately, persist in clinical areas today. The reasons given by health care providers for undertreatment are numerous and include the following: infants lack the ability to communicate the site and intensity of pain, therefore they do not feel pain; children do not experience pain or interpret pain the way adults do; children will not remember pain; pain is a learned response; it is unsafe to give potent analgesics to young children because of the increased potential for inducing respiratory depression or addiction.

The pain for an injection is often believed to cause more pain for children than the underlying pain necessitating its administration. Young children are unable to make the connection between an immediate pain from the injection and the pain relief experienced later. Their reaction to the injection may interfere with nursing judgment, resulting in nonmedication and unnecessary pain for the child.

The health care provider should consider medicating the pediatric client for pain in the same circumstances as the adult client would be given medication. In children under 2 years of age with observably increased irritability, anorexia, loss of interest in play, and in whom the assessment of whether the problem is "merely" irritability or pain is inclear, the decision to medicate appropriately is justified. Medicating in this instance should lead to a more comfortable, less anxiety-ridden child. In the child over 2, the health care provider should know how the child's age and stage of development will influence his or her ability to perceive and communicate the experience. The approach to the child should be individualized, using the child's words and gestures for communication. Figure drawings may be helpful for the child to point out "where it hurts." Other signs of discomfort, such as restlessness, decreased activity, anorexia, whining, and crying should be assessed. The child's parents are to be consulted regarding the child's pain status; since they are most familiar with the child.

As with adults, pain is best managed if the client is medicated early rather than when the pain becomes severe. To decrease the possibility of the child denying pain to avoid an injection, the nurse may administer analgesics by an alternative route. Children find suppositories, elixirs, and tablets crushed in applesauce more acceptable than injections. The nurse can assist the child in associating the medication with the relief from pain by indicating that it will make him or her "feel better." The nurse must check to see if the medication has been effective and remind the child that he or she probably "feels better" because of the medication.

Guidelines for administration of injections to the child are found in Chapter 8.

TABLE 11-4 Side Effects/Adverse Reactions to Opioid Analgesics

Drug(s)	Side effects*	Adverse reactions†
Opioid analgesics Prototype: morphine	More frequent: Vertigo, faintness, light-headedness that occurs most often in ambulatory clients. Fatigue, sleepiness, nausea and/or vomiting, increased sweating, and constipation Less frequent: Dry mouth, headache, anorexia, abdominal cramping, nervousness, increased anxiety, mental confusion, visual hallucinations, and nightmares	Seizures, tinnitus, jaundice (hepatic toxicity), pruritus, skin rash or facial edema (allergic reaction), breathing difficulties, respiratory depression, excitability (paradoxic reaction seen mainly in children), and tachycardia

*If side effects continue, increase, or disturb the client, inform the physician.
†If adverse reactions occur, contact physician since medical intervention may be necessary.

TABLE 11-5 Morphine Analgesic Dosage and Administration

Route	Adults	Children	Elderly
IV	4-10 mg diluted in 4-5 ml water administered slowly	0.05-0.1 mg (50-100 μg)/kg body weight administered slowly	Geriatric clients more susceptible to opioid drugs, especially respiratory depression effects; lower dosages than usually prescribed adult dose recommended
IM	5-20 mg every 4 hr		
SC	5-20 mg every 4 hr.	0.1-0.2 mg (100-200 μg)/kg body weight every 4 hr; do not exceed 15 mg/ dose	
Epidural (lumbar region)	1-5 mg initially; assess in 1 hr; if adequate for pain relief, 1-2 mg increments may be administered; 10 mg in 24 hr maximum		
Intrathecal	0.2-1 mg as single dose only; repeated dosage by this route not recommended		
Oral (individualized)	Initially 10-30 mg every 4 hr for morphine sulfate syrup, oral solution, and tablets; may be increased according to pain severity, client's weight, and client's response	Not established; must be individualized	
Preoperative		0.5-0.1 mg (50-100 μg)/kg body weight, IM; do not exceed 10 mg/dose.	

For pediatric dosing of mild to moderate pain, acetaminophen tablets, liquid, or suppositories are usually the analgesic prescribed. The health care provider should see package insert or consult a physician or selected references for recommended pediatric dosages (Korberly, 1985).

Aspirin containing products carry the warning of a possible association between their use and Reye's syndrome

Text continued on p. 201.

TABLE 11-6 FDA Pregnancy Safety Classification of Common Opioid Agonists, Antagonists, and Agonist-Antagonists

Category*	Drug
C	morphine
	codeine
	hydromorphone
	alphaprodine
	naltrexone
	pentazocine
B	nalaxone
Pregnancy safety not currently established by the FDA	meperidine
	methadone
	levorphanol
	oxycodone
	oxymorphone
	propoxyphene HCI
	butorphanol tartrate
	nalbuphine HCI

*See FDA pregnancy categories for drugs in Chapter 2.

CONTINUOUS INFUSION OF OPIOIDS

Continuous infusions of opioids are used when traditional routes of administration are inappropriate or have failed to provide satisfactory pain relief, as with the client with intractable vomiting or severe local bruising following IM or SC injection, and/or the client with severe pain unrelieved by oral, rectal, or intermittent parenteral opioid dosing.

Before starting the infusion, the nurse should obtain a baseline blood pressure and respiratory rate and rhythm. All previous medication orders for pain are discontinued. The solution is administered using a microdrip infusion set and infusion control pump with an alarm. The client's current pain treatment requirements and degree of pain control will determine the initial infusion rate. Infusion rate adjustments thereafter are based on objective and subjective evidence of pain relief and side effects. The client should be monitored for potential respiratory depression every hour for the first 4 hours and routinely thereafter. If the client's respiratory rate falls below the established limit, the nurse should reduce the rate of flow, notify the physician, and have naloxone ready to administer. Mechanical ventilation may be preferred to naloxone to relieve the respiratory depression, since naloxone will also diminish the client's pain relief.

---

in both children and teenagers. It is recommended that the use of aspirin be avoided with influenza, varicella, and acute febrile conditions. Pediatric clients also appear to be more susceptible to the toxic side effects of aspirin, especially children with elevated temperatures and dehydration.

When stronger analgesics are necessary, acetaminophen with codeine or, if necessary, morphine or opioid derivatives may be indicated. The health care provider should monitor closely for respiratory depression, especially in the very young, elderly, or very ill client (see box). In such clients lower analgesic dosages or alternate opioids may be necessary.

Pregnancy, Labor, and Delivery

Teratogenic (tending to cause fetal malformation) or birth defects have not been documented in humans with

---

TIME REQUIRED TO PRODUCE MAXIMAL RESPIRATORY DEPRESSION EFFECTS WITH OPIOID ANALGESICS

APPROXIMATE TIMES	ROUTE OF ADMINISTRATION
Within 7 minutes	IV
Within 30 minutes	IM
Within 90 minutes	SC

From Pain, nursing now, Nursing '85 Books, Springhouse, Pa, 1985, Srpinghouse Corp.

ANALGESIC EQUIVALENCY CHART

All analgesics are compared to 10 mg (IM) morphine to determine an analgesic dosage equivalent. Such information is very useful for healthcare professionals assessing potency and considering drug alternatives.

ANALGESIC	IM DOSE (mg)	ORAL DOSE (mg)
morphine	10	20–60
hydromorphone	1.5	7.5
oxycodone	N/A*	30
levorphanol	2	4
methadone	10	20
meperidine	75	300

SUPPOSITORY DOSAGE FORM

Hydromorphone, 3 mg, is approximately equivalent to 7.5 mg oral dosage and 1.5 mg IM dosage.

Morphine, 10-30 mg, is considered nearly equivalent to the recommended oral dosage (10-30 mg or more as necessary). Individualize dosage according to client response.

Oxymorphone, 5-10 mg, is approximately equivalent to 1 mg of IM oxymorphone. (1 mg IM oxymorphone is equivalent to 10 mg IM morphine.)

*N/A, Not available.

the use of morphine, codeine, hydrocodone, hydromorphone, or opium. However, animal studies report that very high doses of morphine, hydrocodone, and hydromorphone may produce teratogenic effects. Therefore the use of such potent analgesics during pregnancy should be carefully assessed (risk vs potential benefit) before use.

Opioid analgesics also cross the placenta, so that routine use of such drugs in the mother may lead to physical drug dependence in the fetus. After birth, severe withdrawal reactions may occur in the neonate. Pregnant women in methadone maintenance programs may demonstrate a fetal distress syndrome in utero and usually deliver an underweight baby at birth.

Since the opioid analgesics cross the placenta to enter fetal circulation, the potential for inducing respiratory depression in the fetus must be considered. If at all possible, such drugs should be avoided in the delivery of a premature infant because the respiratory depressant effect is enhanced. Because of its extended duration of action, methadone should not be used in obstetrics. Morphine, codeine, and, perhaps, other opioids reportedly prolong labor.

Several analgesics used when labor pain and contractions are regular include meperidine (intramuscularly or subcutaneously) 50 to 100 mg every 1 to 3 hours; or pentazocine lactate injection intramuscularly (30 mg) or intravenously (20 mg) on a 2- to 3-hour schedule when necessary for pain.

Opioid Use in The Elderly

Analgesic dosing in the elderly usually requires dosage and dosing interval adjustments according to the client's therapeutic response and/or the development of undesirable side effects (confusion, excessive untoward CNS effects, respiratory depression). The height, weight, and body surface area are not accurate measures for dosing analgesics in the elderly.

Studies have reported that analgesia lasts longer in the geriatric client because of a decrease in drug clearance from the body (McCafferty, 1986). Although lower dosages of analgesics are often recommended for the aged, this approach should generally not be the rule. Kaiko's study (1980) indicated age was not a significant factor in determining analgesic dosage, but it was important in establishing the frequency of drug dosing. Both dosage and drug frequency should be titrated to the individual's response to the analgesic medication. The presence of unwanted adverse effects would influence drug dosage and drug frequency.

The intramuscular and subcutaneous routes of analgesic administration may also be influenced by the aging process. The elderly may have a diminished circulatory process, which would result in slower absorption of drugs administered by these routes. Administering additional dosages in such a situation may result in unpredictable or increased drug absorption, which increases the potential for adverse side effects.

The elderly client may be less likely to ask for pain medication because of an acceptance of pain as a part of old age, not wanting to be a "bother," or denying discomfort as a cultural and ethnic issue. Nonverbal communication, such as irritability, anorexia, decreased activity, or gripping an object, should be carefully assessed. The decreased activity resulting from pain increases the risk of immobility complications, especially in the elderly client. The stress of the pain experience leads to fatigue and anxiety, reducing the elderly client's diminished physical and psychologic resources.

Because the elderly client may be taking many drugs concurrently, health care providers should be aware of specific drug interactions with analgesic therapy.

Careful nursing care should be used in working with the elderly client experiencing pain.

Adjuvant Medications

Adjuvant medications are commonly added to opioid analgesics to enhance pain control or relief in specific conditions. The nonsteroidal antiinflammatory agents (NSAIAs) have been found to be effective for the treatment of bone pain. Cancer metastasis to the bone results in increased production of prostaglandins, which in turn causes osteolysis and a lowered peripheral pain threshold. The NSAIAs include aspirin, diflunisal, ibuprofen, indomethacin, fenoprofen calcium, naproxen, piroxicam, and sulindac. They have antiinflammatory and analgesic properties that are associated with inhibition of prostaglandin synthesis. Such agents are also indicated for the treatment of pain and inflammation caused by rheumatoid arthritis, osteoarthritis, and various other acute and chronic musculoskeletal and soft tissue inflammations (see Chapter 61).

Psychotropic (acting on the mind) agents and corticosteroids have also been prescribed with systemic analgesics. Although selected phenothiazines are useful in treating nausea and vomiting induced by opioid analgesics, the routine use of antidepressants in clients with chronic intractable pain to potentiate analgesia is a debatable issue. Twycross and Lack (1984) have advocated the use of coanalgesia in clients exhibiting inadequate pain relief from opioids following large increases in dosage. Coanalgesia may include corticosteroids, NSAIAs, antianxiety and antidepressant medications, or nondrug measures such as nerve blocks or radiation therapy.

Treating intractable pain with antidepressants does not always produce uniform results. Pilowsky et al. (1982) studied the effect of amitriptyline on pain in a pain clinic population and reported subjective pain improvement at weeks 2 and 4 but no difference when amitriptyline was compared with placebo at week 6. Therefore, the efficacy of antidepressant therapy on pain needs additional research.

Corticosteroids are beneficial in cancer pain that originates in a fairly restricted area, such as intracranially; alongside a nerve root; or in pelvic, neck, or hepatic areas. Dexamethasone is prescribed for an increase in intracranial pressure and for relief of pain caused by pressure on a nerve. Corticosteroids may also relieve pain by inhibiting the release of prostaglandins and thus improving the inflammatory process. Hypercalcemia tends to reduce the pain threshold, whereas this effect may be reversed by the increased excretion of calcium induced by corticosteroids. Additional effects of appetite stimulation and elevation of mood have also been useful in selected cases.

Treatment of Opioid Overdose

Naloxone hydrochloride (Narcan) should be available on every nursing unit where opioid medications are used. Naloxone is an opioid antagonist; that is, it can reverse opioid-induced respiratory depression and sedation by displacing the opioids at the receptor site. In opioid-dependent individuals, it can also induce acute drug withdrawal.

The intravenous route of administration is the preferred method of administering naloxone. Its effects are seen within 2 minutes. It can also be given intramuscularly or subcutaneously but the onset of action is then seen within 2 to 5 minutes. Naloxone is shorter acting than most opioids; therefore, to prevent the recurrence of respiratory depression, it must be administered by a continuous infusion or by repeated injections (intramuscularly or subcutaneously). See drug monograph for additional information about naloxone.

The Nurse's Role in Opioid Therapy

Assessment. A thorough assessment of the client's pain as to location, severity, quality, and intensity needs to be accomplished to establish a baseline for management of the client's condition. It is necessary to individualize the drug dose and its frequency based on the potency and duration of action of the specific drug used, severity of pain, condition of the client, other medications that the client is receiving concurrently, and the client's response to the analgesic regimen. The nurse should observe the client's response to the analgesic and record the degree and duration of pain relief and any adverse effects that may occur.

Vital signs should be taken and recorded before morphine sulfate is given. Morphine can cause respiratory depression; if client's respiratory rate is less than 12/min, the dose may need to be withheld or decreased. The nurse's assessment is important information required by the physician to determine the possibility of adverse drug effects on the client. Other signs of opioid overdose are cold and clammy skin, drowsiness, dizziness, restlessness and mental confusion, pinpoint pupils, and decreasing pulse rate and blood pressure.

Oral and injectable opioid analgesics produce unacceptable or undesirable effects such as nausea and vomiting, constipation, urinary retention, cough reflex sup-

ndx Selected Nursing Diagnoses Relating to Opioid Therapy

Nursing diagnosis	Outcome criteria	Nursing interventions
Ineffective airway clearance (potential) related to cough reflex suppression	Evidence of good pulmonary ventilation	Reposition the immobile client frequently. Teach turning, coughing, and deep breathing.
Altered comfort related to nausea and/or vomiting	Absence of and/or decrease in nausea and/or vomiting	Administer prescribed antiemetics. Administer oral analgesics with food. Reduce noxious environmental stimuli. Apply cool cloth to the face.
Constipation	Evidence of client's normal bowel patterns	Assess client's bowel status. Increase fluid consumption. Instruct in high-fiber diet. Encourage ambulation. Obtain an order for a stool softener and/or a bulk-forming laxative. Provide relaxed environment for elimination.
Alteration in patterns of urinary elimination related to urinary retention	Evidence of urinary status with urgency and/or retention	Increase fluid intake to about 3000 ml daily, unless contraindicated. Administer sitz bath. Provide relaxed environment for elimination. Suggest a dose reduction or switch to alternative therapy.
Sensory/perceptual alterations	Evidence of alertness and orientation to environment	Assist to ambulate. Safeguard with side rails. Caution against driving and other hazardous activities. Caution against taking alcohol and other CNS depressants concurrently.

pression, and CNS effects. In many instances, these effects may be overcome by appropriate nursing care (see nursing diagnosis table).

Tolerance is another undesirable effect of narcotic analgesics. An increase in analgesic dosage may be needed to provide the same degree of analgesic effectiveness. Lack of reliable data has led to many misconceptions about tolerance. Tolerance, for example, does not always occur. It is sporadic and unpredictable. One client may take the same dosage of the same opioid for years and never need an increase, whereas other clients with similar pain problems may require periodic increases. In the majority of clients with genuine pain, who are receiving opioids in therapeutic doses, the dependence liability is relatively uncommon; and most do not report euphoria or psychologic dependence. Tolerance in clients needing pain relief (not tolerance in clients who take drugs for pleasure) is managed by gradually decreasing the dose when analgesic effect is achieved. Once pain is controlled (e.g., removal of a tumor that is causing the pain), a lower dose will maintain analgesic effects. The need for an increase in the analgesic dosage will usually be a result of the disease process or progression. The nurse should assess for pupillary constriction. As the drug is eliminated from the body, the pupils return to normal. Continued constriction of the pupils with early return of the symptoms for which the medication was administered may indicate a developing tolerance because the drug has not yet been eliminated from the body but has diminished effectiveness.

Abstinence syndrome may occur after prolonged use of opioid analgesics. Gradually decreasing the dosage of the medication as the severity of the pain decreases may diminish the development of withdrawal symptoms.

Intervention. Preventive pain treatment with analgesics involves the frequent administration of analgesics on a regular fixed-time interval in anticipation of pain. Analgesics are to be given before the client's anticipation of the recurrence of pain or before it reaches an intensity that makes the client feel a loss of control. The client should actively participate in the pain treatment process with trust and confidence and be able to assist in planning a schedule of pain medication based on life-style. This fixed-schedule method of administration decreases suffering until the next scheduled dose because a blood level of the analgesic has been reached that controls the client's pain. If an order for the fixed-time schedule is unavailable, it is the nurse's responsibility to teach the client to request medication before the pain becomes severe. Oftentimes clients are unaware that they need to ask for pain medication, since none of their own medications is on a demand schedule.

The nurse should encourage client and family willingness and belief to participate in the reinforcement of the pain-treatment process. Combinations of optimal doses of NSAIAs and narcotic agonists indicated for pain may permit lower doses of the opioid agonist.

A stepped-care approach (see boxed material earlier in chapter) is the optimal plan to follow because it uses nonopioid analgesics progressing to other stronger analgesics to manage the client's pain with the most effective dosage.

After administering the medication, the nurse should provide comfort measures to allow the best effect: reduction of environmental stimuli, placing the client on bedrest, and back massage. Nonpharmacologic measures for pain such as these and others (relaxation techniques and cutaneous stimulation) may be used concurrently, as well as considered as substitutes for pharmacologic interventions with some clients.

Injection sites should be rotated to prevent induration and abscess. If analgesic medication is required for more than 2 weeks, oral, intravenous, or other routes of administration should be considered. For prolonged pain relief, epidural or intrathecal administration may be considered (see box on p. 212 for additional information).

When a narcotic is administered intravenously, naloxone must be on hand because the risk of respiratory distress is markedly increased with this route of administration.

Repeated intramuscular or subcutaneous administration of opioids to clients in shock, who may have impaired perfusion, may cause an overdose when the client's circulation is restored.

Morphine sulfate intensified oral solution (Roxanol) (20 mg/ml) comes with a specific calibrated dropper; no other dropper should be used for the medication, which is diluted in 30 ml or more of fluid or semisolid food. The nurse or client should make sure the entire dose is removed from the dropper.

When changing the client's medication from one route of administration to another in collaboration with the physician, the nurse must check the dosage against the "Analgesic Equivalency Chart."

Education. Since **orthostatic hypotension** (a form of low blood pressure that occurs when a person stands) can occur in ambulatory clients, caution the client about rising quickly from a supine position.

Roxanol is the most convenient method for receiving oral morphine but requires careful instruction of the client. Because it is a controlled substance, the client should be instructed to prevent theft by drug-dependent individuals.

Opioids can impair the client's mental and/or physical abilities, so caution should be exercised when the drug is prescribed for ambulatory clients or for anyone who will be driving a car or operating any type of machinery. Clients should be instructed to call for assistance if they wish to smoke or to ambulate.

The dose may be altered by a physician if a client is

receiving other opioid analgesics. CNS depressants, cyclic antidepressants, neuroleptics, anxiolytics, ethanol, or sed-ative-hypnotics. Since the combination of any of these can produce CNS depression, the client needs to be reminded that the combination of ethanol and their normal dosage of hydromorphone can render them incapable of normal functioning.

Evaluation. Because opioid analgesics are frequently used inappropriately, the nurse should be aware and report any instances of suspected abuse.

Since some health professionals are not well versed in pain control, nurses should take the initiative in reversing the undertreatment of clients in pain. Educating others within the clinical setting is important to promote comfort for the client.

opium preparations

Opium contains several alkaloids that include mor-phine and small amounts of codeine and papaverine. The effects of opium result from the presence of morphine in the preparations. The mechanism of action and pharmaco kinetics and the same as or similar to morphine.

1. Opium tincture. Contains 10 mg morphine/ml and is used as an antidiarrheal agent and, when diluted, for the treatment of neonatal opioid dependence.
2. Camphorated tincture of opium (paregoric). Con-tains 2 mg morphine/5 ml. It is an **antidiarrheal** agent (an agent inhibiting diarrhea). In some in-stances, it has been used to treat neonatal opioid dependence, but the latter use is controversial. Par-egoric contains camphor, which can cause serious toxicity including seizures and respiratory depres-sion, and benzoic acid, which can displace bilirubin from albumin. Both substances may enhance the typical problems seen in such infants (such as con-vulsions and hyperbilirubinemia); therefore, many physicians seem to prefer the use of diluted opium tincture to paregoric.
3. Opium alkaloid hydrochloride injection (Panto-pon). Contains 10 mg morphine/ml. It is used as an analgesic for the relief of severe pain.
4. Opium and belladonna suppositories, No. 15A (B & O Supprettes). Contain 30 mg powdered opium (10% morphine and other alkaloids) and 16.2 mg powdered belladonna alkaloid (the principle alka-loids of belladonna are atropine and scopolamine). No. 16A contains 60 mg powdered opium and 16.2 mg belladonna extract. The preparations are used to relieve moderate to severe pain reported with ure-teral spasms and have also been prescribed for breakthrough pain between injections of opioids.

Side effects/adverse reactions. See Table 11-4.
Significant drug interactions. See morphine.
Dosage and administration. See Table 11-7.

NURSING CONSIDERATIONS

Opium tincture may be diluted with water for admin-istration; the solution will beome milky. Other liquid forms of opioids may be given with fruit juice to increase their palatability.

If rectal suppositories are being used to administer opioids, the rectum should be emptied first to enhance absorption of the drug.

codeine (methylmorphine)

Codeine is available in sulfate and phosphate salts and marketed as oral tablets, oral solution, and injectable dos-age forms. Codeine is absorbed well after either oral or parenteral administration and is excreted by means of the kidney, mainly as norcodeine and free and conjugated morphine. Oral administration is used for analgesic, **anti-tussive** (cough suppressant) and antidiarrheal effects. Codeine may also be injected for treatment of mild to moderate pain. See Tables 11-8 and 11-9 for dosage forms and adult and pediatric dosages.

Pregnancy safety. FDA category C.

TABLE 11-7   Dosage and Administration for Opium Preparations

	Adults	Children
opium tincture	0.3-1 ml (usually 0.6 ml) four times daily orally; maxi-mum 6 ml in 24 hr	Not established
camphorated tincture of opium (paregoric)	5-10 ml orally one to four times a day; maximum 10 ml four times daily	0.25-0.5 mg/kg body weight one to four times a day orally
opium alkaloid hydrochloride injection (Pantopaon)	5-20 mg every 4 or 5 hr when needed IM or SC	Not established
B & O Supprettes	One suppository rectally once or twice a day or as ordered by physician	Not established

TABLE 11-8 Pharmacokinetic Overview of Selected Opioid Dosage Forms

Drug/dosage form	Onset of action (min)	Peak effect (min)	Duration of action (hr)
codeine			
Oral	30-45	60-120	4
IM	10-30	30-60	4
SC	10-30		4
hydrocodone bitartrate			
Oral	10-30	30-60	4-6
hydromorphone hydrochloride			
Oral	30	30-90	4
IM	15	30-90	4
IV	10-15	15-30	2-3
SC	15	30-90	4
Rectal	N/A*	N/A*	6-8
meperidine			
Oral	15	60-90	2-4 (usually 3)
IM	10-15	30-50	2-4 (usually 3)
IV	1	5-7	2-4 (usually 3)
SC	10-15	30-50	2-4 (usually 3)
methadone			
Oral	30-60	90-120	4-6†
IM	10-20	60-120	4-5†
IV		15-30	3-4
alphaprodine			
IV	1-2	N/A*	½-1½
SC	Within 10 (range, 2-30)	N/A*	1-2 or greater
levorphanol			
Oral	10-60	90-120	4-5
IM	N/A*	60	4-5
IV	N/A*	Within 20	4-5
SC	N/A*	60-90	4-5
oxycodone			
Oral	N/A*	60	3-4
oxymorphone			
IM	10-15	30-90	3-6
IV	5-10	15-30	3-4
SC	10-20	N/A*	3-6
Rectal	15-30	2	3-6
propoxyphene			
Oral	15-60	120	4-6

*N/A, Not available.
†With active metabolites and continuous dosing, half-life and duration of action may increase to 22 to 48 hours.

TABLE 11-9 Dosage and Administration for Codeine (Methylmorphine)

	Adults	Children
Tablets/solution		
Analgesic	15-60 mg (most commonly 30 mg) orally every 3-6 hr as needed	Not recommended for premature infants; not established for newborns; 0.5 mg/kg body weight or 15 mg/m² body surface orally every 4-6 hr as needed
Antidiarrheal	30 mg orally one to four times a day	0.5 mg/kg body weight up to four times a day
Antitussive	10-20 mg orally every 4-6 hr; maximum 120 mg in 24 hr	Not established for children less than 2 yr old; 2-6 yr, 2.5-5 mg orally every 4-6 hr—maximum 30 mg/day; 6-12 yr, 5-10 mg orally every 4-6 hr—maximum 60 mg/day
Injection	15-60 mg (most commonly 30 mg) IM, IV, or SC every 4-6 hr as needed	Not recommended for premature infants; not established for newborns; 0.5 mg/kg body weight or 15 mg/m² body surface IM or SC every 4-6 hr as needed

NURSING CONSIDERATIONS

Oral codeine should be administered with milk or food to reduce any gastrointestinal distress. Codeine has been added to cough elixirs because it acts as a cough suppressant. The nurse should encourage fluid hydration, which will help to liquify sputum.

hydrocodone bitartrate (Dicodid, Vicodin, Hycodan, Robidone✦)

In the U.S. Hycodan is marketed as a combination including homatropine; in Canada Hycodan is hydrocodone bitartrate only. Although the product name is similar in both countries, the formulation is not identical. Hydrocodone bitartrate is used an an analgesic and autitussive. See Table 11-10 for dosage and administration.

hydromorphone hydrochloride (Dilaudid, Dilaudid HP)

Hydromorphone is a semisynthetic opioid, used for its analgesic and antitussive effects, that has a faster onset of action but a shorter duration of action than morphine. See Table 11-11 for dosages.
Pregnancy safety. FDA Category C.

NURSING CONSIDERATIONS

Hydromorphone can produce a dose-related respiratory depression if the dosage exceeds what is normal for the client; signs of respiratory depression should be observed for. This may not be a drug of choice for clients with chronic obstructive pulmonary disease because they have decreased respiratory rate and poor respiratory drive. In addition to its respiratory depressive capabilities, hydromorphone can exaggerate an already increased intracranial pressure. This drug may not be one of choice for clients with head injuries or increased intracranial pressure.

meperidine (Demerol, Pethidine hydrochloride✦)

Meperidine is one of the most commonly prescribed opioids in a hospital setting (McCafferty, 1986). Its pharmacologic profile is similar to morphine with several noted differences.
1. It is believed to interact more strongly with kappa receptors than morphine (Gilman and others, 1985).
2. Its duration of action is shorter than morphine. See Table 11-7 for onset, peak, and duration of effect.
3. Most equivalency charts (see box on page 201) note oral meperidine as a 300 mg dosage equivalent to 10 mg intramuscular morphine. The manufacturers for meperidine market the oral preparation in 50 and 100 mg tablets. Therefore oral dosages of meperidine frequently prescribed are considered to be much less effective than the injectable form.
4. A major metabolite of meperidine produced in the liver is normeperidine. Normeperidine is further metabolized (partially) to the conjugated form and then excreted from the body. Prolonged administration and/or increasing the daily dosages of meperidine has produced significant mood changes (sadness, anger, restlessness, apprehension) and stimulation of the CNS

TABLE 11-10 Dosage and Administration for Hydrocodone Bitartrate

	Adults	Children
Antitussive	5 ml syrup orally every 4-6 hr as needed 5 mg tablet orally every 4-6 hr as needed	0.15 mg/kg body weight orally every 6 hr as needed
Analgesic	5-10 mg tablet orally every 4-6 hr as needed	

TABLE 11-11 Dosage and Administration for Hydromorphone Hydrochloride

	Adults	Children
Analgesic tablets	2 mg tablet orally every 3-6 hr as needed; may increase to 4 mg or more if necessary every 4-6 hr; dosage should be individualized according to client's pain, response to medication, and appearance of adverse effects	Individualize according to age, size, and individual's response
Suppositories	3 mg rectally every 4-8 hr as needed for pain	Not established
Injectable	2 mg every 3-6 hr IM, IV, or SC; increase to 3 or 4 mg every 6 hr if necessary to control pain	Individualize according to age, size, and individual's response

(McCafferty, 1986; Gorman and Warfield, 1986). Increased serum levels of normeperidine are responsible for the excitatory effects (i.e., quivering, tremors, and multifocal myoclonus [grand mal] seizures).

Although the use of meperidine for only a few days may generally result in mild and tolerable problems, meperidine should probably be avoided in clients requiring prolonged usage or high-dose continuous therapy and when renal or liver dysfunction are present. The nurse should be aware that naloxone (opioid antagonist) will antagonize meperidine but not normeperidine and may in some instances cause further CNS excitation and seizures.

Management for normeperidine toxicity includes stopping the meperidine and substituting an alternate opioid, such as morphine. If seizures occur, an anticonvulsant (diazepam or others) may be used.

Meperidine produces a vagolytic effect on the heart; therefore its use should probably be avoided or closely monitored in clients with dysrhythmias and/or myocardial infarction. In addition to drug interactions common to opioids, meperidine is contraindicated for clients receiving MAO-inhibiting agents currently or within the previous 2 weeks. Very severe, unpredictable reactions (severe respiratory depression, hypotension, hypertension, seizures, **hyperpyrexia,** or exceptionally high fever, increased excitablity) and at times, death have resulted. This is a serious and avoidable drug interaction.

Dosage and administration. See Table 11-12 for dosages.

Pregnancy safety. Not established.

NURSING CONSIDERATIONS

Assessment. Vital signs should be monitored and recorded before and after administration of meperidine. It can cause tachycardia and hypotension. Practice nursing measures to avoid postural hypotension and syncope. The nurse should raise side rails for clients on bedrest.

Meperidine is contraindicated in severe dysfunction of the liver (since the drug is inactivated in the liver), in certain conditions involving the gallbladder and the bile ducts (since meperidine causes contraction of these structures), and in clients with head injury, increased intracranial pressure, increased CSF, respiratory depression, or shock. Respiratory depression occurs as with morphine but is of shorter duration.

Meperidine causes CNS excitation ranging from irritability to seizures. When administered with a phenothiazine such as promethazine, which also lowers the seizure threshold, the client is at higher risk for seizures.

Meperidine should be used with caution in clients who have artrial flutter and other supraventricular tachycardias, since meperidine may increase ventricular response through vagolytic action.

Meperidine is not administered for chronic pain, because of its short duration of action. It may be given orally but is more effective intramuscularly.

Tissue irritation is common with the administration of intramuscular meperidine. Clients frequently experience muscle damage, poor absorption, and pain during injection.

Common side effects with meperidine are dizziness, drowsiness, nausea and vomiting, constipation, increasd sweating, and hypotension.

Meperidine is contraindicated in clients receiving MAO inhibitor therapy or in those who have received it during the previous 14 days, since concurrent administration may produce coma, severe respiratory depression, and hypotension. In addition, meperidine potentiates CNS depressants.

Intervention. Before mixing meperidine in solution with another medication, consult a specific reference,

TABLE 11-12   Dosage and Administration for meperidine

	Adults*	Children*
Analgesic	50-150 mg every 3-4 hr as needed IM or SC; 15-35 mg hourly by IV infusion as needed using an infusion pump; dosage should be individualized according to client's age, weight, and severity of pain	1.1-1.76 mg/kg body weight IM or SC; do not exceed 100 mg every 3-4 hr as needed
Preoperatively	50-100 mg IM or SC 30-90 min before anesthesia	1-2.2 mg/kg body weight IM or SC; do not exceed 100 mg 30-90 min before anesthesia
Obstetric analgesia	50-100 mg IM or SC when regular contractions occur; may be repeated every 1-3 hr as needed	
Intravenous infusion	Dilute meperidine to 1 mg/ml and titrate according to client's needs, anesthesia used, and type and length of operation.	

*IM preferred route of administration for both adults and children.

because it tends to be physically and chemically incompatible with a wide range of substances.

Meperidine is diluted for IV administration; however, it is not the recommended route of administration. It needs to be titrated for the client's response because of its respiratory depressant effects.

Meperidine dosage should be gradually tapered because abstinence symptoms, such as nausea, vomiting, and diarrhea, can occur. Such symptoms should be reported to the physician so that the dosage may be adjusted.

Education. The nurse should caution the client about rising too quickly because of the drug's hypotensive effects.

methadone (Dolophine, Methadose)

Methadone was discovered by German chemists during World War II. It is an effective analgesic with properties similar to morphine with the exception of its extended half-life. The duration of action for methadone is usually listed at 4 to 6 hours, but with repeated oral dosing, the half-life may extend from 22 to 48 hours (perhaps even longer in the elderly and clients with renal dysfunction, etc.). This extended half-life is not related to its analgesic effect. To control pain methadone is administered every 3 to 4 hours or, with repeated dosing and dosing adjustments based on the individual's response, every 6 to 8 hours. See Table 11-13 for dosages.

Because of its extended half-life, methadone is approved by the FDA for use in detoxification and maintenance treatment programs. Methadone dependence is substituted in individuals who are physiologically dependent on heroin, opium, or other opioids. See Chapter 9 for methadone treatment program.

Mechanism of action. See morphine.

Indications. Analgesic or treatment of opioid abstinence syndrome.

Pharmacokinetics. Similar to morphine. See Table 11-8.

Side effects/adverse reactions. See Table 11-4. With methadone, the miotic and respiratory depressant effects may be present more than 24 hours. Excessive sedation is also reported in some clients following a regular dosing schedule.

Significant drug interactions. See morphine.

Dosage and administration. See Table 11-13.

Pregnancy safety. Not established.

NURSING CONSIDERATIONS

Assessment. When the client is receiving methadone for treatment of heroin abuse, the nurse should be aware of possible outside sources of OTC drugs and alcohol, such as liquid cough preparations with alcohol and alcohol beverages brought in by friends and family.

Although most adverse effects dissipate in the initial 3 weeks of therapy, constipation and diaphoresis may persist.

Intervention. Overdosage of this drug can cause extreme respiratory depression. Naloxone should be readily available for intravenous administration. The antagonist action is only 1 to 3 hours, and the action of methadone is 36 to 48 hours or more; thus repeated doses of nalozone for up to 8 to 24 hours may be required to treat respiratory depression.

When methadone is used for detoxification and maintenance therapy, it is administered as an oral liquid. If dispersable tablets are used, they are dissolved in 120 ml of water or citrus flavored solution, such as Tang, Kool-Aid, or fruit juice. Dissolution takes a minute or so and may be enhanced by using cold and/or acidic solvents. If

---

TABLE 11-13   Dosage and Administration for Methadone

	Adults	Children
Analgesic		
Oral solution	5-20 mg every 4-8 hr; adjust dosage or dosing interval according to client's response	Individualize according to client's age, size, and response to medication
Oral tablet	2.5-10 mg every 3-4 hr initially. In chronic dosing, adjust dosage and interval according to client's response	
Treatment of opioid abstinence syndrome		
Detoxification	15-40 mg orally or as solution (10 mg/ml) once daily or as necessary to control documented withdrawal symptoms. Reduce dosage at 1-2 day intervals based on client's response. Parenteral dosage form only indicated if client is unable to take oral medication.	
Maintenance	Individualize according to client's response	

the concentrated oral solution is used, it should be diluted in at least 90 ml of solution to enable the complete dosage to be received.

It has been used for the terminally ill, and each hospital may have a different formula for the pain cocktails, which may contain different quantities and different ingredients, such as hydromorphone, cocaine, morphine, or methadone and hydroxyzine.

Education. Since methadone is commonly given on an outpatient basis for withdrawal from heroin or morphine-like drugs, the client should be cautioned about operating a car or other potentially dangerous equipment because mental and physical abilities may be impaired.

Orthostatic hypotension is a common side effect, which can last for several weeks. Clients should be instructed to rise slowly from a recumbent position and to sit or lie down in the event of dizziness or faintness.

alphaprodine (Nisentil)

Alphaprodine is a synthetic opioid agonist-analgesic similar pharmacologically to morphine and meperidine. It has a more rapid onset of action and a shorter duration of action than meperidine. Alphaprodine is metabolized and excreted in the urine as either the free drug or the glucuronide metabolite.

Alphaprodin is used in the treatment of presurgical or obstetric pain as an adjunct to anesthesia in surgical procedures or urologic examinations and as an analgesic for pediatric dentistry. (The last use is controversial and, if used, trained personnel must closely monitor the client,

and resuscitative equipment and naloxone should be available for emergency use.)

If used with other CNS depressants (such as alcohol, other opioids, general anesthetics, psychotropic agents, hypnotics, barbiturates, sedatives, and antidepressants [tricyclic and MAO inhibitors]), the dosage of alphaprodine should be reduced and the client closely monitored. Severe respiratory depression, hypotension, coma, cerebral injuries, and death have been reported as a result of potentiation of CNS-depressant effects.

Pediatric and geriatric clients are more susceptible to the adverse effects of alphaprodine, especially the respiratory depressant action. Usually lower dosages than adult dosages should be considered for the elderly client. This medication should only be administered by health care professionals trained in its use. See Table 11-14 for dosages.

Pregnancy safety. FDA Category C.

NURSING CONSIDERATIONS

Alphaprodine should be used with caution in clients with head injury, increased intracranial pressure, CNS depression, respiratory depression, chronic obstructive pulmonary disease (COPD), and liver or renal disease. If it is used for a client with any of these disorders, vital signs should be taken before and frequently after administration of the drug. Nursing considerations for alphaprodine are essentially the same as with meperidine, except alpha-

TABLE 11-14   Dosage and Administration for Alphaprodine

	Adults	Children
Obstetric analgesia	40-60 mg SC given after cervical dilation has begun and repeated at 2-hr intervals if needed	Should not be used for children 12 yr or less because safety and effectiveness not determined except for dental procedures.
Presurgical use Major surgery Minor surgery	10-20 mg IV; 20-40 mg SC 20 mg IV; 40 mg SC	For dentistry, dose is usually 0.3-0.6 mg/kg body weight submucosally—should not be administered by any other route to children
Cystoscopy (urologic procedure)	20-30 mg IV or an alternate dosage schedule for adults: 0.4-0.6 mg/kg body weight IV not exceeding a 30 mg initial dose. If necessary, an additional 0.1-0.15 mg/kg body weight may be given 15 min later. 0.4-1.2 mg/kg body weight SC; do not exceed 60 mg as initial dose. If necessary, 0.1-0.3 mg/kg body weight may be given 15 min later. Maximum dose IV or SC is 240 mg in 24 hr. Use lower dosage ranges until individual's response to drug can be determined	

NOTE: Do not administer IM: erratic and severe adverse effects including death have been associated with IM administration.

prodine does not have a vagolytic effect. It has a more rapid onset and shorter duration than meperidine.

When administered intravenously or submucosally (as by a dentist), a narcotic antagonist (naloxone), oxygen, and artificial ventilation equipment should be available to counteract any respiratory depression.

Alphaprodine is not administered intramuscularly, because its absorption is erratic by this route and severe adverse reactions have occurred.

Intravenous doses of alphaprodine should be administered in a dilute solution slowly over several minutes, since too rapid administration may cause severe respiratory depression, hypotension, and cardiac arrest.

levorphanol (Levo-Dromoran)

Levorphanol is an opioid analgesic used for moderate to severe pain, such as visceral pain associated with terminal cancer, renal and biliary colic, myocardial infarction, and trauma. It is also used as a preanesthetic narcotic as well as for the relief of postoperative pain.

Adult dosages are 2 to 3 mg orally or subcutaneously, every 6 to 8 hours for analgesia. Dosage and time interval should be individualized according to severity of pain and the client's response to the medication. Levorphanol has also been given intravenously, as an adjunct to anesthesia, but optimal adult dosages are not established.

Pediatric doses are individualized by physician according to the client's age, weight, and therapeutic response to the medication.

Pregnancy safety. Not established.

NURSING CONSIDERATIONS

The actions of levorphanol are identical to morphine, but the effective dose is one fourth that of morphine.

Levorphanol should not be confused with levallorphan tartrate (Lorfan), which is used as a narcotic antagonist and sometimes as an antidote for levorphanol. If levallorphan is mistakenly given to a person who is chemically dependent on narcotics, it can cause an **abstinence syndrome** (a collection of symptoms that occur on withdrawal from a drug on which one is physically dependent). Although levallorphan tartrate has been discontinued by the U.S. manufacturer, it may continue to be available until existing supplies are depleted.

oxycodone hydrochloride (Percodan, Tylox, Percocet, Supeudol✽)

Oxycodone HC1 is approximately 10 times more potent than codeine and nearly equivalent in potency to morphine. It is available alone and in combination prep-

arations, that is, with aspirin (Percodan) or acetaminophen (Tylox, Percocet).

Adult doses are 5 mg orally 3 to 6 hours or, if combined with acetaminophen, every 4 to 6 hours as necessary for pain. Increase if required according to pain severity and the individual's response to medication. (Suppositories are not currently available in the United States, but they are available in Canada. Adult dosage is 10 to 40 mg rectally, 3 or 4 times daily.)

Pediatric doses are individualized according to age and size.

Pregnancy safety. Not established.

oxymorphone hydrochloride (Numorphan)

Oxymorphone is pharmacologically similar to morphine with the following exceptions. In equivanalgesic dosages, oxymorphone usually causes more nausea, vomiting, and psychic effects (euphoria) than morphine. It may also be less constipating and causes less suppression of the cough reflex than morphine. Oxymorphone is a potent analgesic used for moderate to severe pain; preoperatively used; for obstetric analgesia or as adjunct therapy for the treatment of anxiety caused by dyspnea resulting from pulmonary edema associated with left ventricular failure.

Adult doses are 1 to 1.5 mg IM or SC every 3 to 6 hours as needed for pain. IV dose is 0.5 mg. Dosages may be adjusted according to pain severity and client's response to the medication. Rectally: 5 mg every 4 to 6 hours as needed.

Pediatric dosage has not been established.

Pregnancy safety. Not established.

NURSING CONSIDERATIONS

Oxymorphone should be given with milk or meals to decrease the incidence of gastrointestinal distress. It tends to cause more nausea and vomiting than **equivanalgesic** (equal pain killing) doses of morphine sulfate.

propoxyphene hydrochloride (dextropropoxphene, Darvon, Dolene, Novopropoxyn✽)
propoxyphene napsylate combinations
propoxyphene combinations

Propoxyphene hydrochloride is a synthetic analgesic that is structurally related to methadone. Although indicated for the treatment of mild to perhaps moderate pain, it is generally considered to be a mild analgesic. Controlled studies have reported that propoxyphene HC1, 65 mg, is equivalent or less effective than acetaminophen, 650 mg; aspirin, 650 mg; or codeine, 65 mg. When combined with aspirin or acetaminophen, propoxphene combinations are generally as effective as codeine and aspirin.

Propoxyphene binds to opioid receptors and produces an analgesic effect similar to codeine and the opioids. The hydrochloride dosage form is more rapidly absorbed than the water-insoluble napsylate formulation, although peak serum levels are approximately equivalent. The bioavailability of propoxyphene hydrochloride, 65 mg, is equivalent to that of propoxyphene napsylate, 100 mg. The half-life of propoxyphene is 6 to 12 hours.

Propoxyphene crosses into the CSF and is believed to cross the placenta.

Metabolism occurs mainly in the liver where approximately ¼ of the dose is metabolized to norpropoxyphene. Norproxyphene has less CNS-depressant effects than propoxyphene, but it has greater local anesthetic activity. Its half-life is 30 to 36 hours.

Both propoxyphene and norpropoxyphene are excreted in the urine.

Adult doses are propoxyphene HC1, 65 mg, or propoxyphene napsylate, 100 mg, every 4 hours as needed, but no more than 390 mg/day propoxyphene HC1 or 600 mg/day of propoxyphene napsylate.

Pregnancy safety. Not established.

NURSING CONSIDERATIONS

Propoxyphene should be used with caution with clients who have a history of excessive alcohol intake and is contraindicated in those who are suicidal or addiction prone. Preparations containing propoxyphene taken in excessive doses, or in combination with alcohol or other CNS depressants, are a major cause of drug-related deaths.

INTRASPINAL ANALGESIC INFUSION

An experimental type of analgesic therapy—continuous intraspinal morphine infusion—reduces the client's pain without diminishing CNS functioning. An implantable infusion device is connected to an implantable catheter placed in the epidural or intrathecal space. The system, which is refilled by injection through a septum into a central chamber of the device, administers the medication continously. The client and family are taught how to care for the device and how to evaluate the response to the therapy. The device is usually refilled every 2 weeks by a home health care provider. Study is continuing with this unique method of pain control, which promises relief for clients with intractable pain while increasing the quality of life.

Ambulatory clients should be cautioned about driving a car or operating dangerous machinery, since their mental and physical judgment may be impaired.

OPIOID ANTAGONISTS

The term "agonist" means "to do" and the term "antagonist" means "to block." Opiates or drugs that act to relieve pain are agonists, and opiates that block the effect of an agonist are the antagonists. In an opiate possessing both agonist and antagonist components, the antagonist portion acts to abate addiction and the agonist portion acts to relieve pain. Continuous contact with the receptor site is essential for addiction.

It has been theorized that a variety of subtypes of opioid receptors are located in the CNS. Each may represent a different therapeutic effect and/or side or adverse reaction relating to the opioid medication. Two receptors (mu and kappa) have been associated with analgesic effects and several specific side effects/adverse reactions. (See box on Opioid Receptor Response) Sigma receptors mediate both the subjective and psychotomimetic effects of the opioids with a mixed activity, that is agonist and antagonist properties (pentazocine and others). Naloxone and naltrexone are opiate antagonists; that is, they competitively displace the opioid analgesics from their receptor sites, thus reversing their effects. The major difference is naloxone must be administered parenterally, whereas naltrexone is available as an oral dosage formulation.

Antagonists block the subjective and objective effects of the opiates and will precipitate withdrawal symptoms in patients physically dependant on opioids. Naloxone and naltrexone are opioid antagonists; therefore they have been used to reverse the adverse or overdose effects of opioids (alphaprodine, codeine, diphenoxylate, fentanyl, heroin, hydromorphone, levorphanol, meperidine, methadone, morphone, oxymorphone, opium derivatives, and propoxyphene) and of the partial agonists (agonist-antagonist drugs such as butorphanol, nalbuphine, and pentazocine). Respiratory depression induced by nonopioids (barbiturates, etc.), CNS depression, or a disease progression will not usually respond to antagonist drug therapy.

In an opioid analgesic overdosage, naloxone and naltrexone will reverse the respiratory depression, sedation, pupillary **miosis** (contraction), and euphoric effects; they may also reverse the psychotomimetic effects of the agonist-antagonists analgesics (pentazocine and others). Both drugs are believed to work at all three receptor sites, but their greatest activity is for the mu receptors.

Naltrexone, 50 mg orally, will block the effects of 25 mg of intravenous heroin for approximately 24 hours; if the dose is doubled to 50 mg, the blockage is extended an additional 24 hours. This is why naltrexone is used for the maintenance of an opioid-free state in detoxified, formerly addicted opioid individuals. Other uses for naltrexone are under investigation and include sudden infant death syndrome, other pulmonary diseases, and the treatment of various forms of addiction including bulimia and compulsive gambling. Proven safety and effectiveness for such uses are necessary before naltrexone can receive government approval for these indications (Weintraub & Evans, 1984).

The Nurse's Role in Opioid Antagonist Therapy

Nurses will administer opioid antagonists in the emergency treatment of opioid overdose as well as in maintenance therapy of former opioid addicted individuals. The nurse must have an understanding of opioid analgesics as well as opioid antagonists to provide nursing care to these clients.

Assessment. Clients should be observed carefully; opioid antagonists should either not be administered or administered with extreme caution if the client is known or suspected to be physically dependent on opioids (including newborns of dependent mothers) because abrupt and complete reversal of opioid effects will produce an acute abstinence syndrome in the physically dependent client.

PATIENT-CONTROLLED ANALGESIA

Patient-controlled analgesia (PCA) is a new drug delivery system that allows the client to assist in the regulation of his or her own pain medication. By providing small doses at short intervals, it allows the client to maintain therapeutic levels. Relief comes more quickly than with intramuscular injections. And because clients control this pain, they experience less fear and anxiety and do not depend on the health care provider's availability for pain control.

A PCA unit has an infusion pump, a timing device, and a computer. To administer a dose, the client presses a button on a cord, similar to a call light, and the infusion pump delivers a single dose of intravenous analgesic. To prevent drug overdosing, the timing device permits the delivery of no more than a specific number of doses per hour. The computer records the doses used. The role of the health care provider in client and family teaching with PCA must begin before surgery. Explanation and demonstration of the system stress that the client need only push the button to maintain control of the pain. Although it may not completely eliminate pain, clients have obtained better pain relief without repeated injections. Portable units are available for home use, which allows for greater client independence.

Intervention. To verify abstinence from opioids, as is frequently done before naltrexone therapy, a naloxone challenge test may be done. This test should not be done in the presence of withdrawal symptoms (body aches, diarrhea, gooseflesh, sneezing and runny nose, irritability, diaphoresis, trembling and weakness, abdominal cramping, tachycardia, nausea and vomiting) or opioids in the urine. If administered intravenously, an initial dose of 0.2 mg is given and the client is observed for 30 seconds for symptoms of withdrawal. If no symptoms occur, an additional 0.6 mg may be administered and the client is observed for 20 minutes. If administered subcutaneously, 0.8 mg is given, and the client is observed for 45 minutes. If withdrawal symptoms occur, the test should be repeated at an appropriate interval.

Continued nursing observation is necessary for the client who has responded to naloxone, and doses should be repeated as necessary, since the duration of action of some opioids exceeds the duration of action of naloxone. The intravenous infusion rate of administration should be titrated according to the client's response. An intensive care unit is probably the most appropriate place for this client until the effects of the drug have completely abated. Clients should be observed for a day or longer regardless of the apparent recovery.

It should be remembered that naloxone has no effect on respiratory depression caused by nonopiate drugs. If the client has taken multiple drugs, the naloxone will reverse only the opioids. In the reversal of opioid toxicity, the respiratory rate and volume will increase and the blood pressure will return to normal if it has been depressed.

Nalaxone should be used with caution in clients with preexisting ventricular irritability because ventricular tachycardia and fibrillation may occur. It is recommended that naloxone not be mixed with other agents because it becomes unstable. After dilution, any unusual solution should be discarded after 24 hours. Additional resuscitive measures, such as oxygen and/or mechanical ventilation, should be available when necessary to counteract opioid overdosage.

The major indication for naltrexone is the treatment of opioid dependency and addiction, and it should be used as an adjunctive measure to a comprehensive drug rehabilitation program involving counseling and psychotherapy.

Naltrexone therapy should not be instituted until the client has been completely detoxified as evidenced by being opioid free for 7 to 10 days, absence of withdrawal symptoms, and abstinence verification by a negative urinalysis for opioids and/or naloxone challenge test.

If, in an emergency situation, an opioid analgesic is required for a client receiving naltrexone therapy, its administration should be accomplished in a hospital setting where careful monitoring is available. Because high doses of the analgesic will be required to overcome the effects of naltrexone, the client will be at high risk for prolonged respiratory depression and circulatory collapse.

Education. When opioid antagonists are used in emergency treatment, client education should be focused on assisting the client to cope with the immediate situation. Instructions should be given to keep the client informed of what is to occur and to help the client cooperate with treatment procedures, even when the client appears unresponsive.

Discussion of the dangers of drug abuse or dependence may be appropriate at some time after emergency treatment. Compliance with naltrexone therapy is improved if someone other than the client (health care provider or family member) administers the naltrexone.

Evaluation. When opioid antagonists are used to counteract opioid overdose, close monitoring is essential. The danger exists that the duration of the antagonist action will be less than the duration of the opioid. In this case the symptoms of overdose may again manifest themselves. The nurse's close evaluation of therapy will identify the recurrence of opioid overdose and allow instigation of appropriate supportive therapy or repeat administration of antagonists, before the situation becomes life threatening.

After administration of antagonists, evaluation takes place to help identify the development of opioid withdrawal syndrome in the possible opioid dependent patient. When naltrexone is used for maintenance of the opioid-free state in former opioid addicted individuals, follow-up evaluations are needed to reinforce and ensure compliance.

naloxone hydrochloride (Narcan)

Mechanism of action. See general discussion of opioid antagonists

Indications
1. Indicated for complete or partial reversal of opioid depression and respiratory depression induced by opioids, propoxyphene, and the partial agonists.

2. May be used as a diagnostic agent in cases of suspected opioid overdosage (see nursing considerations).

Pharmacokinetics

Absorption. Inactivated orally, in doses effective parenterally.

Onset of action. 1 to 2 minutes (intravenous); 2 to 5 minutes (intramuscular or subcutaneous)

Peak. 5 to 15 minutes

Duration of action. Depends on administered dose and route of administration. Generally, intramuscular dose results in a prolonged effect.

Distribution. Rapidly throughout the body; it crosses the placenta.

Metabolism. Liver

Excretion. Kidneys

Side effects/adverse reactions. See Table 11-15.

Significant drug interactions. None significant

Dosage and administration. See Table 11-16.

Pregnancy safety. FDA category B

naltrexone (Trexan)

Mechanism of action. See general discussion of opioid antagonists.

Indications. See naloxone (No. 1 under indications).

Pharmacokinetics

Absorption. Rapidly, following oral administration. Undergoes extensive first-pass metabolism because only 5% to 20% of a dose reaches systemic circulation.

Onset of action. 15 to 30 minutes

Peak. Usually within 2 hours

Duration of action. Dose dependent; generally a single 50 mg oral dose of naltrexone blocks the effects of 25 mg intravenous heroin for up to 24 hours; if naltrexone is increased to 100 or 150 mg, the antagonizing heroin (25 mg) effects will be prolonged to 48 or 72 hours, respectively.

Distribution. Widely and variable. In humans, naltrexone and its metabolites have been distributed in saliva and erythrocytes. It is unknown whether naltrexone crosses the placenta or passes through breast milk.

Metabolism. Primarily in the liver. The major metabo-

TABLE 11-15   Naloxone and Naltrexone: Side Effects/Adverse Reactions

Drug(s)	Side effects*	Adverse reactions†
naloxone	Nausea, vomiting, tremors, increased sweating, nervousness	Tachycardia, hypertension
naltrexone	Insomnia, nervousness, nausea, vomiting, abdominal distress, headaches, tiredness, generalized joint and muscle pain	Respiratory distress, hypertension, tachycardia, hallucinations, paranoia, confusion, severe depression

*If side effects continue, increase, or disturb the client, inform the physician.
†If adverse reactions occur, contact physician because medical intervention may be necessary.

TABLE 11-16 Dosage and Administration for Naloxone Hydrochloride

	Adults	Children
Opioid antagonist	In emergencies, IV route preferred, although IM or SC may be used; 0.01 mg/kg body weight or 0.4 mg administered in single dose. If necessary, IV dose may be repeated at 2-3 min intervals. Dosage must be individualized according to response. Some clients may require higher initial dosages (e.g., 0.8-1.2 mg), others, if physically addicted and not in danger, may receive lower doses initially (0.1-0.2 mg). Dosages may be repeated at 2-3 min intervals, if necessary. For longer-acting effect, additional naloxone may be given by continous IV infusion or by IM route	
Verification of abstinence from opioids	See "Nursing Considerations"	
Depression induced by opioids postoperatively	0.1-0.2 mg IV every 2-3 min until adequate ventilation achieved and client recovery observed without presence of significant pain. Dosage may be repeated at 1-2 hr intervals. Carefully titrate dosage to avoid breakthrough of severe postoperative pain	
Depression induced by opioid analgesics		Neonates: 0.01 mg/kg body weight IM or SC through umbilical vein. Dose may be repeated every 2-3 min until desired effect observed
Opioid overdose		Children: substitute IV route for umbilical vein and proceed as above for neonate.

lite of naltrexone is 6-β-naltrexol, which also possesses opiate antagonist activity. Several other metabolites have also been identified.

Excretion. Kidneys
Side effects/adverse reactions. See Table 11-15.
Significant drug interactions. None significant
Dosage and administration

Adults. Treatment with naltrexone is started cautiously, generally 25 mg orally with close monitoring for withdrawal signs and symptoms for approximately 1 hour. If no withdrawal effects occur, give the balance of the daily dosage. See Table 11-16. Maintenance: Usually 50 mg orally every 24 hours. A variety of other dosage schedules have been advocated depending on the individual and client compliance. For example, 100 mg every other day or 150 mg every third day.

Children. Not established
Pregnancy safety. FDA category C

OPIOID AGONIST-ANTAGONIST AGENTS

Although the exact mechanism of action of the **opioid agonist-antagonist agents** is unknown, these agents have both analgesic and opiate antagonist effects. It has been proposed that drugs such as nalbuphine competitively antagonize mu receptors, but they are partial agonists at the kappa and sigma receptors. Whereas pentazocine has a weaker mu receptor antagonistic action, it has a stronger agonist effect at the kappa receptors. Buprenorphine has some agonist effect at the mu receptor sites (see box "Opioid Receptor Responses"). Generally, these drugs have a lower dependency potential than opioids, and withdrawal symptoms are not as severe as those reported with the opioid agonist medications. The opioid agonist-antagonist agents have pharmacokinetics, adverse effects, and significant drug interactions similar to morphine.

butorphanol tartrate (Stadol)

Butorphanol tartrate is indicated for treatment of moderate to severe pain. It has been used preoperatively and for the treatment of postpartum discomfort and pain. The adult dosage is 1 to 4 mg (usually 2 mg) intramuscularly every 3 to 4 hours as necessary or 0.5 to 2 mg (usually 1 mg) intravenously every 3 to 4 hours if needed. Pediatric dosage has not been established.

NURSING CONSIDERATIONS

Assessment. Use with caution as a preoperative medication with hypertensive clients because butorphanol may increase the blood pressure. It should not be administered to clients with coronary insufficiency, myocardial infarction, or ventricular dysfunction because its use has not been evaluated in these cases.

If there is some suspicion that the client is physically dependent on narcotics, butorphanol should not be given until the person is detoxified. Since butorphanol is a narcotic agonist-antagonist, it would only counteract the effects of the original narcotic, set up a need for an increase in the dosage, and precipitate an abstinence syndrome.

Butorphanol may elevate CSF pressure; therefore it should be used with caution in clients with head injuries or preexisting increased CSF pressure.

Because butorphanol is metabolized in the liver, it should be given with caution to clients with comprised or impaired renal or hepatic function. Because of decreased metabolism of the drug in the liver, side effects and greater activity may result.

The safety of the use of butorphanol in pregnancy before the labor period has not been established, but the safety to the mother and fetus following the administration of butorphanol during labor has been established. Clients receiving butorphanol during labor have experienced no adverse effects other than those observed with commonly employed analgesics; however, this drug should be used with caution in women delivering premature infants.

Butorphanol tartrate can cause respiratory depression if the dose exceeds 4 mg as a single dose. If the usual intramuscular dose of 2 mg is insufficient to relieve the client's pain, the dose can be increased by 1 to 4 mg every 3 to 4 hours. It is important for the nurse to assess the client's response to this medication and to be aware of any signs of respiratory depression. These could be changes to rate, depth, or regularity of respiratory rate.

pentazocine (Talwin)

Pentazocine is indicated for the treatment of moderate pain. Pentazocine HCl tablets (Talwin) are no longer available in the U.S. because of the incidence of pentazocine abuse; it has been reformulated to include naloxone in the oral preparation. Orally naloxone is not pharmacologically active, but if this formulation is injected, naloxone will block the effects of pentazocine. (See Table 11-17 for pentazocine HCl and naloxone HCl dosage.)

NURSING CONSIDERATIONS

Tissue irritation as evidenced by pain on injection, induration, and nodules may occur at injection sites.

nalbuphine hydrochloride (Nubain)

Nalbuphine HCl is an analgesic for moderate to severe pain, used preoperatively as an adjunct to anesthesia and for obstetric analgesia. The adult dosage is 10 mg (intramuscular, intravenous, or subcutaneous) every 3 to 6 hours as necessary. For a single dose the maximum is 20 mg; the maximum total daily dosage is 160 mg. The pediatric dosage has not been established.

buprenorphine (Buprenex)

One of the newest agents to be released in this category is buprenorphine hydrochloride (Buprenex). It is said to be 30 times as potent as morphine sulfate and also has an extended duration of action. The latter effect is attributed to buprenorphine's strong affinity for the mu receptor sites and its very slow release from these receptors. See Table 11-18 for the pharmacokinetics of agonist-antagonist medication.

TABLE 11-17   Dosage and Administration for Pentazocine

	Adults	Children
analgesic (pentazocine HCl and naloxone HCl)	50 mg pentazocine orally every 3-4 hr as necessary. If needed, single dose may be increased to 100 mg; maximum daily dosage is 600 mg	Not established
pentazocine lactate injection		
Analgesia	30 mg IM, IV, or SC every 3-4 hr as necessary	
Obstetric analgesia	30 mg IM or 20 mg IV when contractions are regular. May be repeated two or three times at 2-3 hr intervals.	
Maximum	Equivalent of 360 mg/day. Single dose 30 mg IV or 60 mg IM pentazocine	

TABLE 11-18   Pharmacokinetic Overview of Agonist-Antagonist Medications

Drug/dosage form	Onset of action (min)	Peak effect (min)	Duration of action (hr)
buprenorphine HCl			
IM	15	60	Up to 6 hr (some clients 10 hr or longer)
IV	More rapidly	Less than 60	Up to 6
butorphanol tartrate			
IM	10-30	30-60	3-4
IV	2-3	30	2-4
nalbuphine HCl			
IM	Within 5	60	3-6
IV	2-3	30	3-4
SC	Within 15	NA*	3-6
pentazocine			
Oral	15-30	60-90	3
IM	15-20	30-60	2-3
IV	2-3	15-30	2-3
SC	15-20	30-60	2-3

NA, Not available.

Although overdosage of the opioid agonist and agonist-antagonist drugs usually responds to naloxone, buprenorphine overdosage has at times required the use of doxapram, a respiratory stimulant. Therefore both naloxone and doxapram should be available in facilities using buprenorphine.

Buprenorphine HCl is used for treatment of moderate to severe pain. The adult dosage (13 years of age and older) is 0.3 mg (1 ml) intramuscular or slow intravenous administration. For severe pain, dosages up to 0.6 mg have been given.

Pregnancy safety. FDA category C.

KEY TERMS

BIBLIOGRAPHY

American Hospital Formulary Service: AHFS Drug Information 88, Bethesda, Md, 1988, American Society of Hospital Pharmacists, Inc.

Alberico, JG: Breaking the chronic pain cycle, Am J Nurs 84: 1222, 1984.

Anthony, CP, and Thibodeau, GA: Textbook of anatomy and physiology, ed 11, St Louis, 1983, the CV Mosby Co.

Bast, C, and Hayes, P.: Patient-controlled analgesia, Nursing '86 16:25, 1986.

Bast, C, and Hayes, P.: PCA: a new way to spell pain relief, RN 49(8):18, 1986.

Baumann, TJ, et al: Patient controlled analgesia in the terminally ill cancer patient, Drug Intell Clin Pharm 20:297, 1986.

Beauclair, TR, and Stoner, CP: Adherence to guidelines for continuous morphine sulfate solutions, Am J Hosp Pharm 43:671, March, 1986.

Bonica, JJ: Cancer pain. In Bonica, JJ, ed: Pain, New York, 1980, Raven Press.

Burgess, KE: Cerebral depressants: their effects and safe administration, Nursing 85 15(8):47, 1985.

Burokas, L.: Factors affecting nurses' decisions to medicate pediatric patients after surgery, Heart Lung 14(4):373, 1984.

Cleeland, CS: The impact of pain on the patient with cancer, Cancer 54(11):2635, 1984.

Cohen, FL: Postsurgical pain relief: patients' status and nurses' medication choices, Pain 9:265, 1980.

Comparative effects of common analgesic orders, RN 46(5):45, 1983.

Cundy, JM: Postoperative analgesia, Nurs Times 19(11):59, 1983.

Cushing, M: Cause of death: drug or disease? Am J Nurs 86:943, 1986.

D'Apolito, K: The neonate's response to pain, MCN 9(4):256, 1984.

Dennis, EMP: An ambulatory infusion pump for pain control: a nursing approach for home care, Cancer Nurs 7(4):309, 1984.

Faherty, BS, and Grier, MR: Analgesic medications for elderly people postsurgery. Nurs Res 33(6):369, 1984.

Foley, KM: The practical use of narcotic analgesics, Med Clin North Am 66(5):1091, 1982.

Foley, KM, and Sundarescan, N: Management in cancer pain. In DeVita, VT, Jr, Hellman, S, and Rosenberg, SA: Cancer principles and practice of oncology, ed 2, vol 2, Philadelphia, 1985, JB Lippincott Co, p 1940.

Fraulini, KE, and Gorski, DW: Don't let perioperative medications put you in a spin, Nursing '83 13(12):26, 1983.

Friedman, FB: PRN analgesics: controlling the pain or controlling the patient? RN 46(3):67, 1983.

Gever, LN: Infusing morphine safely, Nursing '83 13(2):32, 1983.

Gilman, AG, and others, eds: Goodman and Gilman's the pharmacological basis of therapeutics, ed 7, New York, 1985, Macmillan, Inc.

Gorman, ES, and Warfield, CA: The use of opioids in the management of pain, Hosp Pract, vol 21, no 7, 1986.

Grey, D: Intrathecal morphine: relief from intractable pain, Can Nurse 79(1):50, 1983.

Grinde, JW, and others: Pain management by epidural analgesia: the challenge for nursing, Heart Lung 13(2):105, 1984.

Hannan, D, and others: Pain: portable relief for terminal patients, RN 48(1):37, 1986.

James, EC, and Gellathy, TA: Pain management by epidural analgesia, Heart Lung 13(2):103, 1984.

Kaiko, RF: Age and morphine analgesia in cancer patients with postoperative pain, Clin Pharmacol Ther 28:823, Dec, 1980.

Kanner, RM, and Portenoy, RK: Are the people who need analgesics getting them? Am J Nurs 86:589, 1986.

Katcher, BS, and others: Applied therapeutics: the clinical use of drugs, ed 3, Spokane, Wash, 1983, Applied Therapeutics.

Kline, S: Recovery room care for the child in pain, MCN 9(4):261, 1984.

Korberly, BH: Pharmacologic treatment of children's pain, Pediatr Nurs 11(4):292, 1985.

Larrat, EP, and Mattea, E.J.: Pain cocktails: survey of formulations used in US hospitals, Hosp Formul 21:497, 1986.

Lipman, AG: Reassessment of pain management (editorial), Clin Pharm 5(10):825, 1986.

Marks, RM, and Sachar, EJ: Undertreatment of medical inpatients with narcotic analgesics, Ann Intern Med 78(2):173, 1973.

McCafferty, M: IV morphine for children, Am J Nurs 84:1153, 1984.

McCafferty, M: Problems with meperidine, Am J Nurs 84, 525, 1984.

McCafferty, M: Narcotic analgesia for the elderly, Am J Nurs 85:296, 1986.

McGivney, WT, and Crooks, GM, (eds): The care of patients with severe chronic pain in terminal illness, JAMA 251(9):1182, 1984.

McGuire, L: 7 myths about pain relief, RN 46(12):30, 1983.

McGuire, L, and Dizard, S: Managing pain in the young patient, Nursing '82 12(8):52, 1982.

McGuire, L, and Wright, A: Continuous narcotic infusion: it's not just for cancer patients, Nursing '84 14(12):50, 1984.

Narcotic and opioid analgesics, Nursing '83 13(10):64, 1983.

Oles, KS: Pharmacokinetics in the aged. II. Commonly used drugs in the elderly, Hosp Formul 19:53, 1984.

Pageau, MG, and others: New analgesic therapy: relieves cancer pain without oversedation, Nursing '85 15(4):47, 1985.

Paice, JA: Intrathecal morphine sulfate for intractable cancer pain, J Neurosurg Nursing 16(5):237, 1984.

Pain, nursing now, Nursing '85 Books, Springhouse, Pa, 1985, Springhouse Corp.

Panyotoff, K: Managing pain in the elderly patient, Nursing '82 12(8):52, 1982.

Paris, PM: Narcotics, Emerg Med 18(7):66, 1986.

Physicians Desk Reference (PDR), ed 40, Oradell, NJ, 1986, Medical Economics Co.

Pilowsky, J, and others: A controlled study of amitriptyline in the treatment of chronic pain, Pain 14:169, 1982.

Portenoy, RK: Continuous infusion of opioids, Am J Nurs 86:318, 1986.

Porter, J and Jick, H: Addiction rare in patients treated with narcotics, N Engl J Med 302:123, 1980.

Regnard, C, and Newburg, A: Pain and the portable syringe pump, Nurs. Times 79(26):25, 1983.

Rimar, JM: Alphaprodine hydrochloride for obstetrics, MCN 10(2):187, 1985.

Saunders, DC: Principles of symptom control in terminal care, Med Clin North Am 66(5):1169, 1982.

Schaffner, AT, and Dieterich, D: Streetwise narcotic safety: precautions in home care, Am J Nurs 86:707, 1986.

Scott, JG, and Rigney-Radford, K: Factors affecting the management of pain, MCN 9(4):253, 1984.

Sheredy, C: Factors to consider when assessing responses to pain, MCN 9(4):250, 1984.

Traub, S: Clonidine for opiate withdrawal, Hosp Formul 20:77, Jan 1985.

Twycross, R, and Lack, S: Oral morphine in advanced cancer, Beaconsfield, England, 1984, Beaconsfield Publishers, Ltd.

United States Pharmacopeial Convention: Drug Information for the health care provider, ed 6, Rockville, Md, 1986, United States Pharmacopeial Convention, Inc., Mack Printing Co.

Warbinek, E, and others: Managing intractable pain, Nursing '85 15(5):33, 1985.

Warfield, CA: Patient-controlled analgesia, Hosp Pract 20(7):32L, 1985.

Warfield, CA: Treating traumatic pain, Hosp Pract 21(3):48M, 1986.

Warfield, CA: The use of opioids in the management of pain, Hosp Pract 21(6):48A, 1986.

Warfield, CA, and Dahlman, LE: Intraspinal narcotics for pain control, Hosp Pract 19(2):148B, 1984.

Warfield, CA, and Warfield, R: Postoperative analgesia, Hosp Pract 19(6):85, 1984.

Weintraub, M, and Evans, P: Naltrexone: a potent oral narcotic antagonist for opiate addiction, Hosp Formul 19:449, 1984.

White, JP: Meeting pain head on, Drug Topics 53 1:144, Feb 7, 1983.

Whitman, HH: Sublingual morphine: a novel route of narcotic administration, Am J Nurs 84:939, 1984.

WHO proposes cancer pain guidelines, Consultant pharmacists' Washington report 2(10):1, 1986.

Zollo, M: Management of pain in critically ill children, MCN 9(4):258, 1984.

CHAPTER
12

Anesthetics

OBJECTIVES

After studying this chapter, the student will be able to:

1. Describe common general anesthetic agents.

2. Identify the significant physiologic changes observable in the client at each stage of anesthesia.

3. List common drugs that interact with anesthetic agents and the possible result of concomitant use.

4. Identify disease and risk factors that can alter response to anesthesia.

5. Discuss nursing measures to prevent or treat common postoperative complications.

6. Discuss the use and side effects of local anesthetics.

7. Apply nursing process to the client receiving general or local anesthetic agents.

Anesthetic drugs are CNS depressants that possess two characteristics: they have an affinity for nervous tissue and their action is reversible, with nerve cells returning to normal on elimination of the drug from the cells. There are three major categories of anesthesia: general, regional, and local. General anesthesia may be administered by intravenous or inhalation routes of drug administration; whereas regional anesthesia is achieved by injecting a local anesthetic drug near a nerve trunk or into specific sites (spinal, caudal). Local anesthesia may be applied topically or by setting up a field block in an area that encircles the operative field (infiltration anesthesia). Spinal, epidural, caudal, and nerve block anesthesia have been referred to as both regional and local anesthesia. The effect of application of regional anesthesia is related to the target nerve and its distribution in the body, whereas local anesthesia is generally a blockade of the nerves in the infiltrated tissues.

To simplify the anesthetic categories, this chapter will present two broad major classifications: general anesthetic agents and local anesthetic agents.

General Anesthesia

General anesthesia is a drug-induced state in which the CNS is altered to produce varying degrees of analgesia, depression of consciousness, skeletal muscle relaxation, and reflex reduction in the body. It is an important mode of therapy, especially for surgical procedures.

ACTION OF GENERAL ANESTHETICS

General anesthetics affect all excitable tissues of the body at concentrations that produce anesthesia. They vary widely in chemical structure, and the concentrations required of different anesthetics to produce a given state of anesthesia also differ greatly.

Although many theories of anesthesia have been proposed, none satisfactorily explains the basic mechanisms of action. Indeed, different anesthetics may have different modes of action, and no single theory may suffice.

The **Overton-Meyer theory** stresses the relationship between the lipid solubility of an anesthetic agent and its potency; the greater the solubility in fat, the greater the effect. Since the nerve cell membrane has a high lipid content, the Overton-Meyer theory explains why anesthetics are preferentially taken up by the brain. However, not all lipid-soluble substances possess anesthetic activity.

When an anesthetic gas is first administered, the **concentration gradient** from alveolar air to blood is steep, and therefore absorption of the gas into the blood is rapid. With time the concentration of gas in alveolar air, blood, and tissues approaches equilibrium, and absorption of the gas slows. When the anesthetic is stopped, the reverse process occurs. Elimination is very rapid at first and then slower. Equilibrium of anesthetics in the fat depots of the body is more slowly reached than in other tissues and is more slowly eliminated. This effect probably is caused by the relatively small blood supply to the fat depots. Alveolar walls are highly permeable to anesthetics, and free diffusion occurs between the alveoli and capillary membranes. Much investigational work is being done in this area, but regardless of the ultimate explanation, anesthesia is produced by progressively increasing the amount of the anesthetic agent, first in the blood and subsequently in the nervous system.

Unlike many other drugs, the anesthetics that can be given by inhalation were thought to be absorbed, transported, and excreted by the body without undergoing significant chemical change. There is evidence, however, for some quantitative hepatic metabolism of many anesthetics. They primarily are exhaled and excreted by the lungs, except for small amounts metabolized by the liver and excreted by kidneys and skin. Associations have been made between biotransformation of inhalation anesthetics and toxicity. The metabolic rate of inhaled anesthetics may be modified by the concentration being inhaled; for example, halothane metabolism is modified in a dose-dependent manner. An inhaled anesthetic may inhibit metabolism of other drugs. Anesthetics are relatively safe agents when used with skilled supervision, since their anesthetic effect can be rapidly reversed by elimination from the lungs, if respiration is maintained satisfactorily. This possibility of rapid removal by breathing permits the safe use of drugs when a surprisingly small difference exists between an anesthetic dose and a fatal dose.

The pattern of depression is similar for all anesthetics—irregular and descending. The medullary centers are depressed last. Fortunately, the medulla is spared temporarily, since it contains the vital centers concerned with heart action, blood pressure, and respiration.

Initially, anesthesia produces a loss of the perception of sight, touch, taste, smell, awareness, and hearing. Usually unconsciousness is produced. The two classes of general anesthetics are inhalation anesthetics (gases or volatile liquids) and intravenous agents.

BALANCED ANESTHESIA

A combination of drugs is necessary to produce all the desired effects sought with anesthesia. Analgesia, muscle relaxation, unconsciousness, and amnesic effects cannot be produced by a single anesthetic. The induction of anesthesia using a combination of drugs, each for its specific effect, rather than using a single drug with multiple effects, is termed **balanced anesthesia.** For example, anesthesia may be induced with a short-acting barbiturate or a benzodiazepine then an opioid analgesic, a skeletal muscle relaxant; and an anesthetic gas will be administered by the anesthetist. The specific drugs and dosages will depend on the procedure to be performed, the physical condition of the client, and the client's response to the medications. The advantage of balanced anesthesia is a lower reported incidence of postoperative nausea, vomiting, and pain.

STAGES OF GENERAL ANESTHESIA

Anesthesia generally consists of four stages (Table 12-1). The stages of anesthesia vary with the choice of anesthetic, speed of induction, and skill of the anesthetist. Current practice of inducing anesthesia with an intravenously administered anesthetic before inhalation anesthesia promotes rapid transition from consciousness to surgical anesthesia, and the early stages of anesthesia are not seen. If the drug is given slowly enough, however, usually all stages can be observed. They are most easily seen when an anesthetic gas is used as the only anesthetic. Not all stages may be seen with all anesthetics.

Stage 1: analgesia. This stage begins with onset of anesthetic administration and lasts until loss of consciousness. Smell and pain are abolished before consciousness is lost. Vivid dreams and auditory or visual hallucinations may be experienced. Speech becomes difficult and indistinct. Numbness spreads gradually over the body. The body feels stiff and unmanageable. Hearing is the last sense lost.

Nursing considerations. The nurse should maintain a quiet and tranquil environment for the client because even low voices and equipment sounds may be inter-

TABLE 12-1 Stages of Anesthesia

CNS effects	Stage 1	Stage 2	Stage 3 planes				Stage 4
			1	2	3	4	
Consciousness	Maintained Analgesia Euphoria Some distortion of perceptions Variable amnesia	Lost	Absent	Absent	Absent	Absent	Absent
Respiration	No alteration, or increased rate with some irregularity	Rapid, irregular	Regular	Regular, but expirations longer than inspirations	Diaphragmatic	Thoracic ceased Diaphragmatic depressed	No respiratory movement Respiratory paralysis
Skeletal muscles	Normal tone	Tone increased	Small muscles relaxed	Large muscles relaxed	Complete relaxation	Complete relaxation	Diaphragm paralyzed
Eyes							
Pupils	Reaction to light	Dilated	Constricted	Mid-dilation	Increasing dilatation	Dilated	Dilated
Movements	Unchanged	Increased	Increased	None	None	None	None
Tear secretion				Decreased	Decreased	Absent	
Reflexes							
Lid	Present	Present	Absent	Absent	Absent	Absent	Absent
Corneal	Present	Present	Present	Absent	Absent	Absent	Absent
Pharyngeal or "gag"			Absent				
Laryngeal				Absent			
Cough					Absent in large bronchi	Absent in small bronchi	
Heart rate		Increased	Decreased				
Blood pressure	Unchanged	Increased	Normal	Normal	Decreased	Decreased	Decreased
Venous pressure	Unchanged	Increased	Unchanged				Increased

preted as excessively loud and may be counterproductive to the anesthetic.

Before anesthesia is begun, restraining straps are placed on the client; and he or she is covered for warmth and modesty.

Stage 2: excitement. This stage varies greatly with individuals but begins with loss of consciousness. Reflexes are still present and may be exaggerated, particularly with sensory stimulation such as noise. The client may struggle, shout, laugh, swear, or sing. Autonomic activity, muscle tone, eye movement, and rapid and irregular breathing increase. Irregular respiration may cause uneven absorption of anesthetic; a period of apnea followed by a few deep breaths may produce a high concentration of anesthetic in the blood.

The variability in this stage results from (1) the amount and type of premedication, (2) the anesthetic agent used,

and (3) the degree of external sensory stimuli. Since the advent of balanced anesthesia, excitement during induction is rare. However, this stage is important for classifying and analyzing drug effects in investigational studies.

Nursing considerations. Except to restrain for safety reasons, the client should not be touched during this stage.

Stages 1 and 2 constitute the *stage of induction.*

Stage 3: surgical anesthesia. The third stage is divided into four planes of increasing depth of anesthesia. Which plane a client is in is determined by the character of the respirations, eyeball movement, pupil size, and degree to which reflexes are present. Most operations are done in plane 2 or in the upper part of plane 3 (see Table 12-1). As the client moves into plane 1, the respiratory irregularities of the second stage usually have disappeared and respiration becomes full and regular. As anesthesia deepens, respiration becomes more shallow and also more rapid. Paralysis of the intercostal muscles is followed by increased abdominal breathing; finally, only the diaphragm is active. The eyelid reflex is lost and the eyeballs, which exhibit a rolling movement at first, gradually move less and then cease to move. Normally, if the pupils were reflexly dilated in the second stage, they now constrict to about their size in natural sleep. The reaction to light becomes sluggish. The pupils dilate as plane 4 is approached.

The client's face is calm and expressionless and may be flushed or even cyanotic. The musculature becomes increasingly relaxed as reflexes are progressively abolished. Most abdominal surgery cannot be performed until the abdominal reflexes are absent and the abdominal wall is soft. The body temperature is lowered as the anesthetic state continues. The pulse remains full and strong. Blood pressure may be elevated slightly, but in plane 4 the blood pressure drops and the pulse becomes weak. The skin, which was warm, now becomes cold, wet, and pale.

Nursing considerations. The approval of the anesthetist should be obtained before preparing the skin and surgically draping the client.

Stage 4: medullary paralysis (toxic stage). The fourth stage is characterized by respiratory arrest and vasomotor collapse. Respiration ceases before the heart action, so artificial respiration may lighten the anesthetic state (if a gaseous agent has been used) and save the client's life.

Nursing considerations. The nurse is part of the surgical team in providing resuscitative measures; the necessary drugs, equipment, supplies; and other assistance as necessary.

SIGNIFICANT DRUG INTERACTIONS INVOLVING GENERAL ANESTHETICS

Among the dangers facing a surgical client is an unexpected drug interaction occurring in preparation for or during anesthesia. Anesthetists must always be cognizant of the interactions between anesthetics and the maintenance drug therapies used in a wide range of illnesses. A serious drug interaction may be underway before surgery, and the surgical anesthesia may complicate the interaction. A critical analysis of the surgical candidate's drug regimen (prescribed and OTC) should be evaluated in relation to the anesthetic drugs and preanesthetic drugs to be used.

In obtaining a drug history, the nurse should ask the client to list all medications consumed in the 2- to 3-week preoperative period. Various pharmacologic classes of medication may result in adverse reactions in clients anesthetized for surgery (see box on p. 224).

Many other drugs have the potential for inducing an unwanted effect intraoperatively or postoperatively. Concurrent administration of various drugs with anesthetic agents requires close supervision and monitoring of the surgical client. As a general guideline, if a drug is needed for treatment preoperatively, it should be continued through surgery. Unnecessary drugs should be discontinued, for a period at least five times the half-life of the drug, prior to surgery. Drugs having significant interactions with anesthetic agents should be replaced, when possible, with an alternative medication prior to surgery. Notable exceptions are MAO inhibitors; anticoagulants, if surgical hemostasis is needed; and dosage adjustments for insulin and corticosteroids.

SPECIAL ANESTHESIA CONSIDERATIONS

Many disease states and risk factors can alter the individual's response to anesthesia (see box on p. 224).

THE NURSE'S ROLE IN THE USE OF GENERAL ANESTHETICS

Nursing during the perioperative period encompasses three distinct phases: preoperative, intraoperative, and postoperative. While these phases are connected, nursing care during each phase differs in its approach to the client and nursing care goals.

Preoperative preparation. The night before surgery, sedatives or hypnotics may be administered to ensure a sound and restful sleep. The time of the administration of this medication provides an opportunity to assess the client's anxiety regarding the anticipated operative procedure. The mental state of the client should be noted, and any undue anxiety or expressions of fear of death should be reported at once. Appropriate intervention should take place before surgery. Severe anxiety or fear, unless allayed, affects both the autonomic and central nervous systems and may cause reactions that are detrimental physiologically and psychologically. Anxious clients may resist relaxation and fight the anesthetic. A greater amount of anesthetic therefore is required, and toxic levels of drugs may be administered inadvertently. Preoperative teaching and counseling by the nurse assists in allaying the client's anxiety.

In addition to the preanesthetic medications, all of the preparation for surgical procedures should be carefully explained to clients. The necessity for postoperative coughing, deep breathing, frequent turning, and use of spirometers should be taught to the client preoperatively. These activities help to prevent the postoperative complications of general anesthetics such as hypostatic pneumonia and atelectasis. The preoperative teaching promotes cooperation when the client is asked to perform these activities that often cause discomfort after a surgical procedure.

Food is usually withheld after the evening meal, and

ADVERSE REACTIONS IN ANESTHETIZED CLIENTS RESULTING FROM VARIOUS PHARMACOLOGIC CLASSES OF MEDICATION

Anticoagulants (heparin, coumidin): Usually discontinued 48 hours before surgery to reduce the increased risk of hemorrhage.

Antidysrhythmics: May induce a decreased cardiac output, decreased heart rate, and bronchospasms; for example, propranolol HCl (beta-adrenergic blocking agent). Quinidine, procainamide, and lidocaine may reduce cardiac conduction, increase peripheral vasodilation, and potentiate neuromuscular blocking agents, such as tubocurare.

CNS depressants (opioids, hypnotics, etc.): May increase the risk of enhanced CNS depressant effects.

Sympathomimetic or vasoconstrictive agents (epinephrine, phenylephrine, or methoxamine): If combined with local anesthetic agents should be carefully dosed and closely monitored. Ischemia leading to sloughing of tissue or gangrene may occur in fingers, toes, or areas that have end arteries.

Antihypertensive agents (such as guanethidine [Ismelin], methyldopa [Aldomet], and reserpine): Combined deplete the synthesis or storage of norepinephrine in the sympathetic (adrenergic) nerve endings and may result in severe hypotension when combined with anesthetics and analgesics. Physicians may consider reducing or stopping such medications before surgery.

Corticosteroids: When used as long-term chronic therapy, usually produce adrenal gland suppression, which may result in hypotension during surgery. Since the stress of anesthesia and surgery usually increases the need for and release of endogenous corticosteroids, it is recommended that corticosteroid dosages be increased in the perioperative period.

Cholinesterase inhibitors (such as echothiophate iodide [Phospholine Iodide] and demecarium bromide [Humorsol], and exposure to organophosphate insecticides): May prolong succinylcholine blockade. Extended apnea and death have been reported with this combination. It is generally recommended that the eyedrops be stopped approximately 2 weeks before elective surgery.

Antibiotics: Particularly aminoglycoside antibiotics (e.g., amikacin, gentamicin, kanamycin, neomycin, netilmicin, streptomycin, tobramycin), clindamycin, tetracyclines, and polymixin antibiotics may potentiate the neuromuscular blocking agent or cause neuromuscular blockade. A reduction in the dose of the neuromuscular blocking agent may be necessary, along with careful **titration** or careful dosing of the drug for the client, to response. Clients with myasthenia gravis, Parkinson's disease, and other neuromuscular disorders must be monitored carefully.

DISEASE AND RISK FACTORS THAT CAN ALTER RESPONSE TO ANESTHESIA

Alcoholism: The alcoholic client may have a variety of associated disease states, including liver dysfunction, pancreatitis, gastritis, and esophageal varices. The anesthetic requirements for such a client may be increased owing to the increase in liver-metabolizing enzymes and the development of cross-tolerance. The alcoholic client should be monitored closely during the postanesthetic period for alcohol withdrawal syndrome, since diazepam or other pharmacologic agents may be required.

Obesity: Overweight or obese clients may have cardiac insufficiency, respiratory problems, atherosclerosis, hypertension, and an increased incidence of diabetes, liver disease, and thrombophlebitis. In such clients obtaining the desired depth of anesthesia and muscle relaxation may be a problem. Generally, fat-soluble anesthetics, especially those with toxic metabolites such as methoxyflurane (Penthrane), should be avoided.

Smoking: Individuals who smoke usually have an increasingly rigid arterial vascular system, adrenal gland stimulation, and perhaps lung disease (bronchitis, emphysema, carcinoma, etc.) Therefore postoperative complications are six times more common in smokers than in nonsmokers. Smoking also increases the client's sensitivity to muscle relaxants.

Young age: The physical characteristics of a neonate may predispose the infant to upper airway obstruction or laryngospasms during resuscitation or anesthesia. A small mandible and neck, a narrow cricoid ring, and a large body water compartment with a high extracellular water turnover rate, immaturely functioning liver and kidneys, and a rapid metabolic rate all contribute to the need for careful considerations of the infant/pediatric client. Drug dosages and administered fluids must be carefully calculated using the body weight or the surface area of the child. Generally halothane and nitrous oxide are commonly used in pediatrics because the incidence of hepatitis (pg. 228) in children is considered rare after halothane usage. Neonates are usually more sensitive to the nondepolarizing muscle relaxing agents (See Unit 5, Chapter 24)

Advanced age: The effect of aging is determined by a generalized decline in organ function (approximately 1% per year after age 30), the existence of chronic disease processes, or both. As the number and complexity of illnesses increase with age, the complexity of drug treatment also increases, which results in greater potential for drug interactions and side effects. Generally, an increased and prolonged drug effect is seen in the elderly. Mortality rates for the aged patient undergoing major surgery may be 4 to 8 times higher than for younger patients.

standard procedure is to give the client nothing to eat or drink after midnight. This procedure helps prevent aspiration if vomiting occurs as a response to anesthesia.

Attention should be given to the client's drug history in preoperative preparation. Withholding maintenance medications while the client is NPO for surgery will have the physiologic impact of abrupt withdrawal. Specific orders should be obtained from the primary physician regarding rescheduling the time of administration, a change in the route of administration of the client's standing medications, or both. When a parenteral form of medication is not available, permission may sometimes be given for the client to take oral medications with a small amount of water (30 to 60 ml) while the client is held NPO before surgery.

In addition, some medications may remain in the client's system and interact to cause serious problems such as arterial hypotension and circulatory collapse or respiratory depression. See the box regarding these drugs and their interactions.

Premedication is used less commonly now than in the past. Drug choice takes into account the client's age, weight, physical condition, level of anxiety, anesthetic method selected, as well as duration and type of surgery. Not including drugs in the preoperative preparation of some clients may be appropriate, while others may need aggressive pharmacologic intervention to produce the desired preoperative state. When prescribed, a combination of drugs, such as morphine or meperidine, hydroxyzine, and atropine, is generally used for the immediate preoperative preparation of the client for surgery. In this instance, atropine is used to block the action of acetylcholine at parasympathetic nerve endings, to overcome vagal effects of anesthesia, and to dry secretions. (It may cause tachycardia in addition to the mild cerebral stimulation.) A dose of 0.4 or 0.6 mg is most useful in adults, but as high as 2 mg is needed to produce palpitations and cardiac effects such as a rapid heart rate.

Narcotics, barbiturates, or anxiolytics administered before the client is taken to surgery promote serenity, amnesia, and smooth induction. It is important that the nurse administer the medications at the exact time as ordered, since a narcotic given too close to the time of administration of the general anesthetic may achieve its full effect during anesthesia and cause severe respiratory depression.

The time it takes to complete specific surgical procedures is variable, and it becomes impossible for many preoperative medications, other than for the first cases of the day, to be ordered for a specific time. In these instances, the preoperative medication is ordered "on call" from the operating room.

All the physical tasks involved with the client's preparation for surgery (i.e., signing surgical permits, final voiding before surgery, taking vital signs) should be accomplished before the preoperative medication is administered. Once the medication is administered, the client should be placed on bed rest with the side rails up and the call light within reach. This decreases stimulation and favors the action of the medication. In addition, the consent for anesthesia, surgery, or both is not considered valid if the client has received sedation before signing.

Intraoperative considerations. The nurse has a highly specialized role within the operating room. The nursing responsibilities entail the maintenance of safety, physiologic monitoring, and psychologic support for the client, but the nurse's role in relation to the administration of anesthetic agents is that of a supportive one to the physician administering the anesthetic. The clinical role of the nurse anesthetist, who assumes a more direct responsibility for the administration of anesthetics, requires a formal certification program for advanced practice of that speciality.

Postoperative considerations. The major objective of the immediate postoperative period is to assist the client in recovering from the effects of the anesthesia and the surgery safely, comfortably, and as quickly as possible. With general anesthesia, careful monitoring is required until the client is alert and oriented to time and place, with vital signs stabilized for at least 30 minutes. Regional anesthesia requires that reflexes and sensation have returned to the affected area and the vital signs have returned to the client's preoperative norms before intensive monitoring ceases.

In addition, a variety of signs and symptoms may be observed in the postoperative client. Nurses should be aware of the more common postoperative complications and the possible causative factors to enable them to determine effective modes of intervention (see box).

With increasing numbers of surgeries being done at ambulatory surgical centers, the nurse should be concerned with client-family teaching for the client who is returning home to recover more fully from the anesthesia and the surgery. In addition to specifics regarding the client's operative procedure and its relevant postoperative care, the nurse should prepare the client for some psychomotor impairment during the first 24 hours following anesthesia and caution against attempting tasks that require alertness and coordination, such as driving. The client should be instructed to avoid using alcohol or other CNS depressants within the first 24 hours unless prescribed by the physician.

TYPES OF GENERAL ANESTHETICS

General anesthetics are usually divided into two groups: (1) the inhalation anesthetics, which include gases and volatile liquids, and (2) intravenous anesthetics, which include barbiturates and nonbarbiturates.

COMMON POSTOPERATIVE COMPLICATIONS AND POSSIBLE CAUSATIVE FACTORS

Hypotension: May result from an excess of nonvolatile drugs that depress the vasomotor center. When narcotics are given, the client's pain must be assessed thoroughly and vital signs recorded. Narcotics should be avoided because they may increase hypotension. However, severe pain can also cause hypotension. In these cases a narcotic may both alleviate pain and increase blood pressure.

Nausea and vomiting: May be caused by stimulation of the vomiting center or by anoxia during anesthesia. Postoperatively the nurse can administer antiemetics and position the client on his or her side to prevent aspiration.

Hypoventilation: May result from excess or cumulative effects of drugs administered during anesthesia. Neuromuscular blocking agents such as curare, anectine, and *d*-tubocurare can cause hypoventilation. Maintaining a patent airway until the client has fully responded is important in the postoperative period.

Oliguria (scanty urination): **Oliguria** is very common after anesthesia as are bladder *atony and urinary retention* after perineal and genital operations.

Nerve injury: May follow spinal anesthesia or malpositioning during general anesthesia. Brachial, radial, ulnar, and perineal nerves are most likely to be injured. The operating room nurse is responsible for taking appropriate measures to protect the client from nerve damage; knowledge of proper positioning for the particular surgical procedure is essential.

Intestinal distention and at times *paralytic ileus:* May occur from the anesthetic agent, postoperative sedation, or a combination of both. Nursing measures to assess for distention include auscultation of the abdominal area for bowel sounds and frequent assessment of the client's nasogastric tube.

Thrombosis: May result from the stasis of blood in the lower extremities. Nursing measures to prevent this include application of an elastic stocking or Ace bandage, early ambulation, and frequent change of position for the client on bed rest.

Shock: Clients should be closely observed for signs and symptoms of shock, a not uncommon postoperative complication. Early detection of impending shock and institution of proper therapy may prevent or at least modify its severity. Rate, volume, and rhythm of the pulse should be noted, as well as the client's color and skin temperature. A rapid, thready, weak pulse; cyanosis or extreme pallor; cold, clammy skin; and low blood pressure are characteristic signs of shock. Checking for bleeding at the operative site is important; if the client continues to lose blood postoperatively, hemorrhagic shock may occur. Postoperative shock also may result from extensive surgical trauma, prolonged operating time, prolonged deep anesthesia, or even inadequate anesthesia.

Atelectasis: Clients should be adequately ventilated postoperatively to prevent **atelectasis** (collapse of the lung). Nursing measures include encouraging clients to take deep breaths and cough every hour. Change of position to prevent pooling of pulmonary secretions also can help to improve ventilation.

Hypothermia/hyperthermia: Since inhalation agents depress the hypothalamus and therefore can elevate or reduce body temperature, clients should be monitored for **hypothermia or hyperthermia** (subnormal temperature or high fever) during the recovery phase. If clients were febrile before surgery, their temperature should be monitored postoperatively.

Malignant hyperthermia: **Malignant hyperthermia** rarely may occur during the administration of many anesthetic agents. With concurrent use of succinylcholine, the onset may be more abrupt. The body temperature may increase as much as $1°$ C ($1.8°$ F) every 5 minutes, reaching reported highs of $43°$ C ($109.4°$ F). The operating room personnel should have a preplanned course of action, including the availability of dantrolene sodium, a complete change of anesthesia circuit, hyperventilation with 100% oxygen, methods to lower body temperature rapidly, and other symptomatic treatment.

INHALATION ANESTHETICS

Inhalation or *volatile* anesthetics are gases or liquids that can be administered by inhalation when mixed with oxygen. These can effect a concentration in the blood and brain to depress the CNS and cause anesthesia. They have the following characteristics:

1. They are complete anesthetics and thus can abolish superficial and deep reflexes.
2. They provide for controllable anesthesia, since depth of anesthesia is easily varied by changing the inhaled concentration.

3. Allergic reactions to these agents are uncommon.
4. Rapid recovery can occur as soon as administration ceases, since the anesthetic is excreted in expired air.

Conversely, a rare but very dangerous adverse effect of inhaled, fat-soluble anesthetics is malignant hyperthermia. This is an emergency situation, whereby the client's temperature suddenly escalates and if not treated appropriately and promptly the client may die. The use of neuromuscular blocking agents has also been associated with this adverse effect, especially when they are used in conjunction with the inhalation anesthetics. For treatment of malignant hyperthermia see nursing considerations for dantrolene in Chapter 21.

Nitrous oxide, ether, and chloroform are three of the earliest used anesthetics (over 100 years). Ether and chloroform are generally considered obsolete anesthetic agents today. Ether has a wide safety margin and is an excellent muscle relaxant, but it is also inflammable and explosive; has a slow, unpleasant induction; and the recovery phase is marked with nausea and vomiting. It also irritates the mucous membranes with resulting increased mucus production, laryngeal spasms, and coughing episodes. Thus ether is rarely used today except in developing countries where resources are limited.

Chloroform, a volatile liquid, is hepatotoxic and nephrotoxic so its usage is also obsolete.

The Nurse's Role in the Use of Inhalation Anesthetic Agents

The actual administration of general anesthesia is conducted by a physician or nurse who has specialized training in anesthetic management, which is beyond the scope of this text. General nursing measures discussed herein are focused on the care of the client after surgery is completed.

Assessment. The vasodilating effect on smooth muscle may cause a drop in temperature and blood pressure; shivering and tremors may be observed postoperatively. Monitor the client's temperature and blood pressure closely during the immediate postoperative period. The recovery phase of volatile anesthetic agents is generally short and they leave no analgesia residue; thus the postoperative analgesia phase will be short. Thoroughly assess the client for postoperative pain.

Intervention. Use caution when changing the client's position during the recovery phase. In addition to the vasodilation, compensatory vasoconstriction mechanisms are depressed, which may result in a significant drop in blood pressure with position changes (orthostatic hypotension). Oxygen is administered during the immediate recovery period to compensate for the respiratory depression from the anesthetic agents as well as the increased oxygen needs of the body from shivering. Pain relief medications will provide relief of immediate postoperative pain. The nurse should remember that any sedative or analgesic probably will need to be decreased one half to one fourth for the first dose after surgery. Measures to avoid heat loss from vasodilation include using warm blankets, covering the head with a blanket, and using a hyperthermic automatic blanket.

Education. To allay fears, explain preoperatively to these clients that they will receive oxygen during the recovery period and be closely monitored until the anesthetic effects are completely worn off.

Gases

Two gases available for general inhalation anesthesia are cyclopropane and nitrous oxide. Cyclopropane is a flammable agent that is also explosive when combined with oxygen, whereas nitrous oxide is nonflammable. Therefore the most commonly used agent is nitrous oxide for dental surgery, minor surgery, and during labor. It is often combined with other anesthetics to enhance its effects so it is used extensively in major surgery.

cyclopropane

Mechanism of action. See Action of General Anesthetics.

Indications. Anesthesia and obstetric analgesic.

Pharmacokinetics. Gas administration.

Metabolism and excretion. Mainly by the lungs

Side effects/adverse reactions. Postanesthesia nausea, vomiting, headache, and slowing of heart rate. Adverse effects include respiratory depression, hypotension, cardiac dysrhythmias, and postoperative delirium.

Significant drug interactions. Primarily with aminoglycosides and sympathomimetics. See previous drug interaction section. Also cyclopropane is explosive and flammable so adequate antistatic safeguards should be implemented.

Dosage and administration. Gas administered in a closed system with oxygen. Analgesia, 3% to 5% continuous inhalation. Anesthesia, 25% to 50% for induction, lowered to 10% to 20% for maintenance.

nitrous oxide

Mechanism of action. See Action of General Anesthetics.

Indications. Anesthesia and obstetric analgesia.

Pharmacokinetics. Gas administration.

Excretion. 100% unchanged through the lungs.

Side effects/adverse reactions. Postoperative nausea, vomiting, or delirium.

Significant drug interactions. None significant.

Dosage and administration. General anesthesia: 70% with 30% oxygen inhalation for induction; 30% to 70% with oxygen for maintenance; analgesia: 20% to 40% with oxygen.

NURSING CONSIDERATIONS

At the termination of nitrous oxide anesthesia, the rapid movement of large amounts of nitrous oxide from the circulation into the lungs may dilute the oxygen in the lungs leading to a phenomenon known as **diffusion hypoxia**. To prevent this the anesthesiologist/anesthetist usually administers 100% oxygen to clear the nitrous oxide from the lungs. During recovery the client should be administered humidified oxygen by mask, and encouraged to breathe deeply to promote ventilation.

Volatile Liquid Anesthetics

The volatile, nonflammable liquid anesthetics are commonly used anesthetic agents. The liquid is vaporized and usually combined with oxygen or nitrous oxide and administered to the client by inhalation. The anesthetic is rapidly distributed by way of the blood flow to body tissues including the brain, liver, and kidneys. Excretion of inhaled volatile liquid anesthetics is mainly by the lungs. (For a discussion of anesthetic gases as an occupational health hazard, see the boxed material.)

halothane (Fluothane, Somnothane)

Mechanism of action. See Action of General Anesthetics.
Indications. General anesthesia.
Pharmacokinetics. See Table 12-2.
Side effects/adverse reactions. See Table 12-2.
Significant drug interactions. Halothane sensitizes the myocardium to the effects of catecholamines (epinephrine, norepinephrine, or dopamine) or sympathomimetic agents (e.g., ephedrine, metaraminol). These agents may produce serious cardiac dysrhythmias in the presence of halothane. Levodopa, which pharmacologically increases the quantity of dopamine in the CNS, should be discontinued at least 6 to 8 hours before halothane is administered. Halothane is the only volatile anesthetic agent that sensitizes the myocardium.

Systemic aminoglycosides, lincomycins, polymyxins, and capreomycin when given concurrently with any of the volatile anesthetics may result in skeletal muscle weakness, respiratory depression, or **apnea** (absence of respiration). Patients usually require mechanical ventilation. If these medications are used, the dosage of the nondepolarizing neuromuscular blocking drugs should be decreased to one third or one half of the usually prescribed dosage.

Dosage and administration. See Table 12-2.
Pregnancy safety. Not established.

methoxyflurane (Penthrane)

Methoxyflurane is the only volatile anesthetic agent, which is used for obstetric analgesia at concentrations of 0.3%-0.8%. It is highly metabolized; and a by-product of this metabolism is free fluoride, which is toxic to the kidney (nephrotoxic). Because of the potential for nephrotoxicity, it is rarely used except for obstetric analgesia. Its clinical effects, although similar to halothane, are more potent.

enflurane (Ethrane)

Enflurane is only slightly metabolized in the body. Its clinical effects are similar to halothane, only it is less potent. Enflurane may cause seizures when given at high concentrations; therefore, it is not recommended for use in seizure-prone patients (epileptics, head injuries).

isoforane (Forane)

Isoforane is the newest of the volatile anesthetic agents. It undergoes an extremely low degree of metabolism. Isoforane has a more rapid action than the other inhalation agents and causes less cardiovascular depression. It has not been associated with toxicity.

WASTE ANESTHETIC GASES AS OCCUPATIONAL HEALTH HAZARD

Chronic exposure of health care providers in the operating room to waste anesthetic gases may present a significant occupational health hazard. Studies have demonstrated an increased incidence of spontaneous abortions among women exposed to nitrous oxide, as well as among wives of men who are exposed. In addition, neurologic, hepatic, and renal disorders have been seen in the chronically exposed. Health care providers should protect themselves by avoiding the area within a foot of the client's mouth and nose where the breath contains exhaled anesthetic agents. Healthcare providers should be active in establishing exposure monitoring programs to detect unsafe levels caused by faulty equipment and unsafe practices.

HALOTHANE HEPATITIS

Although controversial, halothane has been implicated as possibly causing liver damage, or *halothane hepatitis*. While the mechanism is not known, some experts believe it to be caused by a hypersensitive-type reaction to a metabolite of halothane. The diagnosis is made on the clinical findings of unexplained fever, eosinophilia, rashes, and abnormal liver function tests within 2 weeks of exposure, especially after a repeat exposure. The syndrome is more common in older and obese clients and is not seen in children. The National Halothane Study by the Committee on Anesthesia, National Academy of Sciences, National Research Council (1966) concluded that the occurrence of halothane-induced hepatic damage could not be ruled out, but was rare. Even though halothane is considered safe, its use is generally avoided in the presence of liver disease as are repeat exposures within a short time interval.

TABLE 12-2 Volatile Liquid Anesthetic Agents

| Agent | Pharmacokinetics | | | Anesthetic dose (volume %) | | Toxicity | Side effects/adverse reactions |
	Absorption	Metabolism	Excretion	Induction	Maintenance		
halothane (Fluothane, Somnothane)	by lungs	20%-25% by liver	Over 80% unchanged by the lungs; remainder excreted or metabolized through kidneys	up to 4	0.5-2.5	May cause "halothane hepatitis" (see box)	Hypotension, cardiovascular depression, lowered body temperature, respiratory depression, malignant hyperthermia Emergency—shivering and trembling, confusion, hallucinations, nervousness, increased excitability
methoxyflurane (Penthrane)	by lungs	about 50% by liver	50% unchanged by lungs; remainder excreted as metbolites through kidneys	1-3 (0.3-0.8 obstetric analgesia)	0.25-1.0	Dose-related nephrotoxicity (renal tube damage) from fluoride metabolite	see halothane
enflurane (Ethrane)	by lungs	about 2.5% by liver	Over 87% unchanged by lungs; remainder excreted as metabolites through kidneys	2-5	1.5-3.0	—	see halothane
isofane (Forane)	by lungs	less than 1%	Almost all through lungs: less than 1% as metabolites through kidneys	1.5-3.0	1-3	Nephrotoxic from fluoride metabolites (unlikely [except in cases of renal insufficiency] due to small degree of metabolism)	see halothane

INTRAVENOUS ANESTHETICS

Intravenous anesthetic agents are used for induction or maintenance of general anesthesia, to induce amnesia, and as an adjunct to inhalation-type anesthetics. The major groups include ultrashort-acting barbiturates, nonbarbiturates, dissociative anesthetics, and neuroleptanesthesia. Intravenous anesthetics are valuable to allay emotional distress, since many clients dread having a tight mask placed over their face while they are fully conscious. These anesthetics reduce the amount of an inhalation anesthetic required. The principal drug used for this purpose is thiopental sodium.

The intravenous anesthetics most commonly used are the ultrashort-acting barbiturates. These drugs are rapidly taken up by brain tissue because of their high oil-water solubility. For example, equilibrium between brain and blood occurs within 1 minute after injection of thiopental. Shortness of action results from the drug being quickly redistributed into the fat depots of the body. Amount of body fat affects drug action; the greater the amount of body fat, the briefer the effect of a single intravenous dose. With prolonged administration or large doses, however, prolonged drug action results in delayed recovery; this is caused by saturation of fat depots and the slow rate of drug release (10% to 15% per hour).

The Nurse's Role in the Use of Intravenous Anesthetic Agents

Within this text, the nurse's role in intravenous general anesthetics does not include administration of the anes-

---

PHARMACOKINETICS OF INTRAVENOUS ANESTHETIC BARBITURATES

Onset of action: 20 to 60 seconds
Dosage for induction of general anesthesia:
  Methohexital: 1 mg/kg body weight
  Thiamylal: 2 to 3 mg/kg body weight
  Thiopental: 3-4 mg/kg body weight
  Adjustments are made, based on concomitant disease state or physical impairment.
Duration of action:
  Methohexital: 5 to 7 minutes
  Thiamylal: 10 to 30 minutes
  Thiopental: 10 to 30 minutes
Absorption: Rapid onset and extremely short duration
Distribution: Throughout body; accumulation in fatty tissues, followed by redistribution from brain to lean body mass in emergence
Metabolism: Hepatic
Excretion: Kidneys

---

thetic. The focus of the role does include, however, client care during the recovery period that follows the anesthetic.

Assessment. The nurse should remember that the dose of any sedative or analgesic probably will need to be decreased by 1/3 to 1/4 for the first dose after surgery; thereafter the dose of the analgesic will be titrated according to the client's needs. Titration is not a nursing measure, but the nurse must assess the client's response to the analgesic and relay the information to ensure adequate medication dosage. Assessment of the client's cardiovascular and respiratory status should be done at frequent intervals.

Intervention. The nurse should note that intravenous anesthetics are seldom used alone for anesthesia, except for short procedures such as electroconvulsive therapy, cast application or removal, and hypnosis. When they are used, resuscitative equipment should be close to the client.

Education. Generally there is some impairment of psychomotor skills for 24 hours following the administration of these drugs. The client should be instructed not to engage in any activities requiring alertness and coordination, such as driving.

Caution the client to avoid alcohol and CNS depressants for the first 24 hours after taking these drugs except as prescribed by the physician.

Ultrashort-Acting Barbiturates

Ultrashort-acting barbiturates include thiopental sodium (Pentothal), thiamylal sodium (Surital), and methohexital sodium (Brevital sodium).

Mechanism of action. These ultrashort-acting barbiturates are CNS depressants that produce hypnosis and anesthesia without analgesia. They frequently are combined with other drugs for muscle relaxation and analgesia in balanced anesthesia.

Their exact mechanism of action for anesthesia, anticonvulsant effects, or the reduction of intracranial pressure (indication for thiopental) is unknown although a variety of theories have been proposed. General anesthesia with ultrashort-acting barbiturates is believed to result from suppression of the reticular activating system.

Indications. See previous section.

Pharmacokinetics. See box.

Side effects/adverse reactions. Most commonly during recovery period shivering and trembling are noted. Less frequently reported are nausea, vomiting, prolonged somnolence, and headache. Serious adverse effects include emergence delirium (increased excitability, confusion, and hallucinations, cardiac dysrhythmias (tachycardia, bradycardia, myocardial depression, or dysrhythmias), hypersensitivity reaction (bronchospasm; rash; hives; edema of eyelids, lips, or face; and hypotension), respiratory depression, and thrombophlebitis.

ADVANTAGES AND DISADVANTAGES OF INTRAVENOUS ANESTHETICS

Disadvantages. Swelling, pain, ulceration, tissue sloughing, and necrosis if drug infiltrates into tissue; thrombosis and gangrene if arterial injection occurs; and hypotension, laryngospasm, and respiratory failure from overdosage or prolonged administration. Muscle relaxation and analgesic effects are minimal.

Advantages. Rapidity with which unconsciousness is induced, amnesic effects, prompt recovery with minimal doses, and simplicity of administration. Intravenous anesthetics are nonirritating to mucous membranes, and use is not accompanied by the hazard of fire or explosion.

Significant drug interactions. Careful assessment and close monitoring are required when the intravenous barbiturates are used in combination with other CNS depressants (enhanced depression effects), diuretics, antihypertensive agents, and calcium-blocking drugs (hypotension may occur).

Dosage and administration. See box.

Pregnancy safety. Thiopental, FDA Category C. Other barbiturates, not established.

NURSING CONSIDERATIONS

Intravenous barbiturates must be administered by personnel trained in their use and in management of possible complications. Continuous monitoring is essential while these barbiturates are being administered. Barbiturates cause depression of respiratory and cardiovascular functions. Resuscitation equipment, an endotracheal tube, suction, and oxygen must be on hand when ultrashort-acting barbiturates are administered for anesthesia.

Ultrashort-acting barbiturates are very alkaline and therefore irritating to the tissues. Care should be taken to avoid extravasation of the drug into the tissues during intravenous injection; pain, swelling, ulceration, and necrosis may occur. Intraarterial injection may result in tissue necrosis and gangrene.

Intravenous barbiturates are incompatible with a wide range of solutions, including bacteriostatic diluents and lactated Ringer's solution. The nurse should consult the drug insert or specialized reference before mixing substances and should not administer them if they are cloudy or there is a precipitate. Thiamylal and thiopental solutions should be freshly prepared and used within 24 hours.

Nonbarbiturates

Nonbarbiturate intravenous anesthetic agents include etomidate, a short-acting hypnotic; opioids fentanyl, sufentanil, and alfentanil; and ketamine, which produces a dissociative anesthetic. Several drugs also may be combined to produce neuroleptanesthesia.

etomidate (Amidate, Hypnomidate)

Etomidate is a short-acting, nonbarbiturate hypnotic used for the induction of general anesthesia.

Mechanism of action. Etomidate is reported to decrease the activity of the reticular formation in the brainstem (in animals). Its cardiac and respiratory effects are minimal, so this product may be advantageous for the client with impaired cardiac functions, respiratory functions, or both.

Indications

1. Used intravenously in induction of general anesthesia and in concomitant anesthesia for supplementation of a subpotent anesthetic agent (nitrous oxide in oxygen).
2. Maintenance of anesthesia for short procedures (dilation and curettage or cervical conization).

Dosage and administration. See Table 12-6.

Pregnancy safety. FDA Category C.

NURSING CONSIDERATIONS

Since the recovery time for etomidate is short, the nurse should observe for any respiratory depression or hyperventilation. Blood pressure should be monitored for possible hypertension and hypotension. The nurse should monitor cardiac status for any dysrhythmias.

fentanyl, sufentanil, and alfentanil

Adjunct medications for anesthesia include fentanyl (Sublimaze), sufentanil (Sufenta), and alfentanil (Alfenta). All three are opioid analgesics used for balanced anesthesia (see earlier section) and in combination with oxygen, nitrous oxide, or both for the induction and maintenance of anesthesia. When combined with a neuroleptic agent, such as droperidol, fentanyl, sufentanil and alfentanil may be used for neuroleptanalgesia or neuroleptanesthesia (see p. 235).

Mechanism of action. See opioid receptors in analgesics chapter. These agents have been theorized to produce their effects at the mu receptor.

Indications. See introductory paragraph, this section.

Pharmacokinetics. See Table 12-3.

Side effects/adverse reactions. See Table 12-4.

Significant drug interactions. See Table 12-5.

TABLE 12-3   Pharmacokinetics of Nonbarbiturates

Agent	Distribution	Onset of action	Peak effect and duration of action	Metabolism	Excretion
etomidate (Amidate, Hypnomidate)		Hypnosis occurs within 1 min and duration is 3-5 min. Recovery time is shortened in adults by use of 0.1 mg IV fentanyl 1 or 2 min before induction of anesthesia, since less etomidate is then necessary		Rapid hepatic; plasma levels of present or free drug rapidly decrease within 30 min after injection and then more slowly, producing half-life of 1.25 hr (75 min)	75% excreted by kidneys in urine during first day of administration
fentanyl (sublimaze), sufentanil (Sufenta), and alfentanil (Alfenta)	All cross blood-brain barrier and are rapidly distributed to various tissues. Protein binding high; half-life triphasic—distributive phase, redistributive phase, elimination	Fentanyl, analgesic: 7-15 min IM or 1-2 min IV. Loss of consciousness depends on high doses and rate of administration (usually 4-5 min, rate of 0.4 mg/min IV). Sufentanil, analgesic: immediate. Loss of consciousness depends on high doses and rate of administration (usually 1-1.6 min, rate of 0.3 mg/min). Alfentanil, analgesic: immediate	Dose dependent. Fentanyl peak analgesic effect 20-30 min IM, 3-5 min IV; duration, 1-2 hr IM, 0.5-1 hr IV. Sufentanil peak analgesic effect almost immediate; duration of action less than 1 hour. Alfentanil, peak analgesic effect almost immediate; duration of action is dose dependent but generally less than 30 min	Liver; sufentanil may also have intestinal metabolism.	Kidneys

Dosage and administration. See Table 12-6.
Pregnancy safety. FDA Category C.

See also nursing considerations for opioid analgesics, Chapter 11.

Nurses should carefully monitor all clients receiving fentanyl during surgery, since respiratory depression is a side effect and all precautions need to be taken; an oral airway and oxygen should be readily available. CNS depressants can potentiate the respiratory and sedative effects of fentanyl, so the dosage of any sedative or analgesic should be reduced by one third to one fourth.

The client should be made to lie down if experiencing nausea, vomiting, dizziness, or syncope.

Dissociative Anesthetic
ketamine hydrochloride (Ketalar)

Mechanism of action. Ketamine is a rapid-acting, nonbarbiturate, intravenous anesthetic. It is a derivative of the psychotomimetic drug of abuse phencyclidine. Ketamine acts on the midbrain within the reticular formation, as do the barbiturates. It produces analgesia and amnesia but not muscular relaxation. The mechanism of action is not fully known. It blocks afferent transmission of impulses associated with the affective-emotional aspect of pain perception. It may also suppress spinal cord activity. Ketam-

TABLE 12-4 Side Effects/Adverse Reactions of Nonbarbiturates

Agent	Side effects/adverse reactions
etomidate (Amidate, Hypnomidate)	Most commonly reported during recovery period are nausea and vomiting; less often reported are hypotension, hypertension, dysrhythmias, and breathing difficulties. Involuntary muscle movements reported especially when fentanyl not given before induction with etomidate. Pain at injection site also reported.
fentanyl (sublimaze), sufentanil (sufenta), and alfentanil (Alfenta)	Most common are drowsiness, hypotension, bradycardia, and respiratory problems (allergic reaction). Less frequent are chills, nausea, vomiting, increased weakness, dizziness, constipation, depression, pruritus, muscle spasms, and increased excitability (paradoxical reaction). Convulsions reported with fentanyl; dysrhythmias reported with sufentanil.

TABLE 12-5 Significant Drug Interactions with Nonbarbiturates

Agent	Drug interactions
etomidate (Amidate, Hypnomidate)	With other CNS depressants, client should be monitored for enhanced CNS depression. For less significant but potential drug interactions, see listing under IV barbiturates.
fentanyl (Sublimaze), sufentanil (Sufenta), and alfentanil (Alfenta)	Concurrent usage with CNS depressants may result in enhanced CNS depressant effect, hypotension, and respiratory depression. Dosage adjustment and careful monitoring are required. When other opioid agonist analgesics are used during recovery phase, dosage should be ¼ to ⅓ the usually recommended dosage. Naltrexone blocks effects of opioid analgesics. If opioid is necessary for elective surgery, naltrexone should be stopped for several days before scheduled operation.

ine has been called a *dissociative anesthetic*; that is, it produces a **cataleptic state** in which the client appears to be awake but detached from his or her environment and unresponsive to pain. The client's eyelids usually do not close, **nystagmus** (rapid, involuntary oscillation of the eyeballs) is common, and slight involuntary and purposeless movements may occur.

Ketamine increases secretions of salivary and bronchial glands; therefore the administration of an anticholinergic agent (such as atropine) may be necessary. Ketamine may increase blood pressure, muscle tone, and heart rate. Respiration is usually not depressed. After recovery, the client has no recall of events while under the influence of ketamine.

Indications
1. Ketamine has its greatest usefulness for diagnostic studies in infants and children and for repeated anesthesia in burned children.
2. It is best suited for short diagnostic or surgical procedures not requiring skeletal muscle relaxation.
3. It is recommended for induction of anesthesia when a barbiturate is contraindicated.

Pharmacokinetics

Onset of anesthesia. Within 30 sec IV, 3-4 min IM if dose is 5-10 mg/kg body weight

Duration of action. 5-10 min IV for dose 2 mg/kg body weight or 12-25 min IM for dose 10 mg/kg body weight

Metabolism. Liver. Termination of anesthetic action occurs with redistribution from the CNS and liver biotransformation

Excretion. Kidneys (90%)

Side effects/adverse reactions. See box.

Significant drug interactions. None reported.

Dosage and administration. See Table 12-7.

Pregnancy safety. Not established.

TABLE 12-6 Dosage and Administration for Nonbarbiturates

Agent	Adults	Children
etomidate (Amidate, Hypnomidate) Anesthesia induction	0.2-0.6 mg/kg body weight	Children over 10 yr, 0.2-0.6 mg/kg body weight
fentanyl (Sublimaze) Adjunct to general anesthesia		Children 2-12 yr, 2-3 μg (0.002-0.003 mg)/kg body weight IV
Minor surgery	2 μg (0.002 mg)/kg body weight IV	Children less than 2 yr, no established dosage
Major surgery	2-20 μg (0.002-0.02 mg)/kg body weight IV. High doses are used for open-heart surgery, complicated neurosurgery, or orthopedic procedures, i.e, 20-50 μg (0.02-0.05 mg)/kg body weight IV	
Primary agent in major surgery	50-100 μg (0.05-0.1 mg)/kg body weight IV given with oxygen, nitrous oxide, or both and neuromuscular blocking agent	
Presurgical or postoperative use	0.07-1.4 μg (0.0007-0.0014 mg)/kg body weight IM	
sufentanil (Sufenta) Adjunct to general anesthesia	Low dosages, 0.5-1 μg (0.0005-0.001 mg)/kg body weight IV initially. Additional dosages of 10-25 μg may be given as needed. Moderate dosages, 2-8 μg/kg body weight IV initially. Additional dosages of 25-30 μg may be given as needed	
Primary agent in major surgery	8-30 μg/kg body weight IV initially with oxygen. Additional dosages of 25-50 μg may be given as needed	Initially, 20-25 μg/kg body weight IV given with 100% oxygen. Maintenance, up to 25-50 μg IV
alfentanil (Alfenta) Adjunct to general anesthesia	8-20 μg (0.008-0.002 mg)/kg body weight IV initially. Additional dosages of 3-5 μg/kg as needed for short duration (<1 hr). Longer anesthetics may use initial dose of 130-245 μg (0.130-0.345 mg)/kg body weight. May also be administered as continuous infusion 50-75 μg (0.05-0.075 mg)/kg initially; with 0.5-3 μg (0.0005-0.003 mg)/kg/min	Use in children under age 12 not recommended

NURSING CONSIDERATIONS

Observe ketamine-anesthesized clients for blood pressure elevation, tachycardia, bradycardia, dreaming, delirium, hallucinations, euphoria, and increased muscle tone. Ketamine is contraindicated in clients with hypertension, increased intracranial pressure, intracranial lesions, intracranial surgery, or a history of psychiatric problems or alcoholism.

Monitor cardiac status and observe for respiratory depression. Do not arouse these clients until they awake on their own, and warn these clients not to drive or engage in hazardous activities for 24 hours or more after recovery from ketamine.

When clients are given ketamine, protect them from visual, tactile, and auditory stimuli during emergence to decrease the possibility of psychic effects. Up to 50% of unpremedicated clients report dreams and hallucinations as the medication wears off. These dreams and hallucina-

---

SIDE EFFECTS/ADVERSE REACTIONS OF KETAMINE

MOST COMMONLY REPORTED

Hypertension and increased pulse rate; an emergence reaction, such as distortion in body image, delirium, explicit dreams, illusions, and dissociative-type experiences. In some clients, flashback of vivid dreams with or without illusions may occur weeks later

LESS COMMONLY REPORTED

Hypotension, bradycardia, respiratory depression, vomiting

TABLE 12-7   Dosage and Administration for Ketamine

	Adults	Children
Anesthesia induction	1-2 mg/kg body weight IV or 5-10 mg/kg body weight IM. Maintenance, 10-30 μg/kg body weight by infusion at rate of 1-2 mg/min. Dosage needs to be carefully assessed and individualized	See adult dosage recommendations
Sedation and analgesia	0.2-0.75 mg/kg body weight IV over 2-3 min initially, followed by 0.005-0.02 mg/kg body weight/min as continuous infusion; IM, 2-4 mg/kg body weight initially, followed by 0.005-0.02 mg/kg body weight/min as continuous IV infusion	

tions can occur up to 24 hours after administration of ketamine. Administer ketamine on an empty stomach, since it has a tendency to cause vomiting.

Ketamine produces a dissociative state; the client may not appear to be asleep but is dissociated from the environment.

Neuroleptanesthesia

Neuroleptanesthesia is a general anesthesia produced by a combination of a neuroleptic (antipsychotic) such as droperidol, diazepam (Valium), or ketamine (Ketalar) and a narcotic analgesic, most commonly fentanyl but sometimes meperidine (Demerol), morphine, or pentazocine (Talwin). It is used primarily for procedures that require the client's cooperation.

An example of this classification is droperidol and fentanyl (Innovar injection). Innovar consists of 1 part fentanyl to 50 parts droperidol.

droperidol and fentanyl (Innovar injection)

Mechanism of action. See above and Indications.

Indications

1. Innovar is used to produce neuroleptic anesthesia. Droperidol is a neuroleptic drug with prolonged action. This combination produces a state in which clients are neither asleep nor awake but in a state of profound analgesia and psychomotor sedation. This state permits the client to undergo short procedures requiring consciousness cooperation, such as bronchoscopy and cystoscopy without pain.

2. Innovar is also used as a premedication for anesthesia and as an adjunct for induction and maintenance of anesthesia.

3. Innovar has lost some of its earlier popularity, since clinical investigation has demonstrated that the depression of respiratory rate and alveolar ventilation may persist longer than the analgesic effect.

Pharmacokinetics. Fentanyl characteristics: See previous section. Droperidol: Onset of action, 30 minutes. Duration of action 2 to 4 hours; alteration of consciousness may persist up to 12 hours.

Metabolism. Liver.

Excretion. Kidneys.

Side effects/adverse reactions. See box on p. 236.

Significant drug interactions. Innovar when given concurrently with opioid analgesics may lead to respiratory arrest. Other CNS depressants may result in enhanced CNS depressant effects.

Dosage and administration. See Table 12-8.

Pregnancy safety. Not established.

SIDE EFFECTS/ADVERSE REACTIONS OF INNOVAR

MOST COMMONLY REPORTED

Hypotension, hypertension, dystonia, increased hyperexcitability, anxiety, sweating

LESS FREQUENTLY REPORTED

Bronchospasm, emergence delirium (hallucinations), chills, shivering, depression, nightmares. Respiratory depression reported when opioid analgesic used in combination; this can lead to respiratory arrest. Concurrent usage should be avoided, but if necessary, reduce dosage of opioid 1/4 to 1/3 usual dosage

---

TABLE 12-8   Dosage and Administration for Innovar

	Adults	Children
Premedication for general anesthesia	0.5-2.0 ml given ¾-1 hr before surgery IM	0.25 ml/20 lb body weight IM
General anesthesia adjunct		Combined dosages for induction and maintenance average 0.5 ml/20 lb body weight
Induction	1 ml/20-25 lb body weight administered slowly IV. Individualize dosage, since smaller dosages have been found adequate depending on client's response.	
IV infusion	Add 10 ml innovar to 250 mg D5W, administer slowly until desired effect is obtained	
Maintenance	Used in combination with other anesthetics	
Without general anesthesia for diagnostic procedures	0.5-2.0 ml IM approximately ¾-1 hr before procedure	

NURSING CONSIDERATIONS

Innovar produces neuroleptic analgesia; the client is usually free of pain, not necessarily asleep, easily aroused, able to cooperate, but psychologically indifferent to the environment, which is beneficial when the client must participate in breathing. Assess the client frequently for any signs of respiratory depression, because increased rigidity of the respiratory muscles may result in insufficient breathing. Innovar should be used with caution in clients with renal, respiratory, cardiovascular, or hepatic impairment.

Postoperatively, the client may not complain of pain because droperidol alters *perception* of pain. In these clients pain may manifest itself as restlessness, agitation, or any number of other nonspecific complaints. If the client does experience pain, the normal dosage of analgesic may be decreased by one third to one fourth. Droperidol potentiates the actions of barbiturates and narcotics, so the analgesic dosage will be decreased until all the droperidol is eliminated. Some alteration of consciousness may last for 12 hours after the last dose.

Since droperidol has hypotensive effects, monitor blood pressure until the drug effects have dissipated completely. Orthostatic hypotension is possible. If given droperidol preoperatively, the client should be assisted if ambulation is necessary. If the hypotension is caused by hypovolemia, several approaches may need to be taken. Fluids may be ordered to treat hypotension, the client may be repositioned to improve venous return (supine with feet elevated) and a vasopressor may be given.

PREANESTHETIC AGENTS

Various medications are used as preanesthetic agents to reduce undesirable effects produced by apprehension or induction and maintenance of anesthesia. See Table 12-9 for a review of some of the common agents.

Local Anesthesia

Local anesthesia refers to the rendering of a portion of the body insensitive to pain. Unlike general anesthesia, consciousness is not depressed with local anesthesia. Local anesthetic agents may be applied to an area or injected into tissues where they produce their effect in the immediate area only; hence the term local anesthesia. Local anesthetic drugs may also be injected around a nerve or nerve trunk (spinal, epidural) to produce anesthesia in a large region of the body. This is referred to as **regional anesthesia.**

SURFACE OR TOPICAL ANESTHESIA

The use of surface, or topical, anesthesia is restricted to mucous membranes, damaged skin surfaces, wounds, and burns. The local anesthetic is applied in the form of a solution, ointment, gel, cream, or powder to produce loss of sensation by paralyzing afferent nerve endings. Local anesthetics do not penetrate unbroken skin. Topical anesthesia is used to relieve pain and itching and to anesthe-tize mucous membranes of the eye, nose, throat, or urethra for minor surgical procedures. Cocaine in a 4% to 10% solution continues to be one of the most widely used agents for topical anesthesia.

Local anesthesia may also be achieved by freezing. Low temperatures in living tissues produce diminished sensation. This form of anesthesia is sometimes employed for minor operative procedures. Packing an extremity in ice may be used for the major operative procedure of amputation of part of an extremity, particularly in elderly and debilitated persons or in clients considered to be at high risk if given a general anesthetic. Tissues that are frozen too intensely for too long may be destroyed.

Ethyl chloride is a local anesthetic that can be used to produce this effect, although it is not employed extensively.

LOCAL ANESTHETICS

Local anesthetics are drugs used to abolish pain sensation in a particular part of the body (Tables 12-10 and 12-11). The *basic mechanism of action* of these drugs is unknown, but most act by stabilizing or elevating the threshold of excitation of the nerve cell membrane without affecting resting potential. This action is a result of reduction of membrane permeability to all ions; thus depolarization and transmission of nerve impulses are prevented.

TABLE 12-9 Preanesthetic Agents

Drug classification	Agent most frequently used		Desired effect
	Generic name	Trade name	
Narcotic analgesics	morphine		Sedation to decrease tension and anxiety, provide analgesia, and decrease amount of anesthetic used
	meperidine	Demerol	
Barbiturates	pentobarbital	Nembutal	Decreased apprehension
	secobarbital	Seconal	Sedation
			Rapid induction
Phenothiazines	promethazine	Phenergan	Sedation
			Antihistaminic
			Antiemetic
			Decreased motor activity
Anticholinergics	glycopyrolate	Robinol	Inhibition of secretions, vomiting, and laryngospasms
	atropine	—	
	scopolamine	—	Sedation (with scopolamine)
Skeletal muscle relaxants	succinylcholine (depolarizing)	Anectine	Promotion of muscular relaxation
		Quelicin	
		Sucostrin	
	d-tubocurarine (nondepolarizing)	Sux-cert	
Intravenous barbiturate	thiopental	Pentothal	Rapid induction

TABLE 12-10   Local Anesthetics—Administration and Use

Method	Tissue affected	Preparation used	Examples of drugs used	Therapeutic use
Topical	Sensory nerve mucous membranes and dermis	Solution Ointment Cream Powder	cocaine benzocaine ethyl aminobenzoate lidocaine tetracaine bupivacaine	Relief of pain or itching Examination of conjunctiva
Infiltration	Sensory nerve endings in subcutaneous tissues or dermis	Injection	etidocaine procaine prilocaine lidocaine chloroprocaine mepivacaine	Minor surgery
Block	Nerve trunk	Injection	etidocaine procaine prilocaine lidocaine chloroprocaine mepivacaine	Dental and limb surgery Sympathetic block
Spinal (subarachnoid block)	Spinal roots	Injection	dibucaine procaine tetracaine lidocaine	Abdominal surgery Muscle relaxation

TABLE 12-11   Properties of Commonly Used Local Anesthetics

	cocaine	procaine	benzocaine
Trade names	—	Novocain	Americaine Hurricaine
Potency	2-3 times that of procaine		Very low
Onset of action	1 min	2-5 min	Immediate
Duration	½-1 hr	½-1 hr	During contact only
Dose	1%-4% topically 5%-10% for anesthesia of nose and throat	0.25%-2%, depending on method of administration 10% for spinal anesthesia Not used topically	Variable 5%-20% ointment topically
Toxicity	4 times more toxic than procaine when injected subcutaneously	Least toxic of all local anesthetics	Relatively nontoxic
Precautions	Not recommended for infiltration, nerve block, or spinal anesthesia Repeated use causes psychic dependence Repeated use in eye may cause clouding, pitting, ulceration of cornea, and mydriasis	Overdose or rapid injection may cause stimulation	Suitable for topical use only Sensitization may develop

Table 12-11 presents some commonly used local anesthetics and their properties. The alcohols (phenol, cresol, menthol, and benzyl alcohol) are seldom employed today. Benzyl alcohol, an aromatic alcohol of low potency, is used topically with procaine to extend procaine's duration of action. Examples of benzoic acid esters are cocaine, hexylcaine, and piperocaine. Examples of PABA esters are procaine, chloroprocaine, and tetracaine, which are all metabolized by plasma cholinesterase. Examples of the amides are dibucaine, etidocaine, lidocaine, prilocaine, mepivacaine, and bupivacaine, which are not metabolized by plasma cholinesterase but are excreted in the urine and metabolized in the liver (see Table 12-11).

Vasoconstrictors (epinephrine) are used with the local anesthetic to decrease the systemic absorption and prolong the anesthetic's duration of action. They are not used for nerve blocks in areas where there are end arteries (fingers, toes, ears, nose, penis) because ischemia may develop, resulting in gangrene.

Mechanism of action. The mechanism of action of local anesthetics is inhibition of the depolarization phase of the nerve cell membrane by means of diminishing sodium ion permeability. This leads to a failure in propagated action potential, causing blockade of conduction.

A number of local anesthetic agents cannot be injected.

However, because they are absorbed slowly, they can be used safely on open wounds, ulcers, and mucous surfaces. They occasionally cause dermatitis and allergic sensitization, which necessitate their discontinuance.

Topical anesthetics for skin disorders, shown in Table 12-12, are used primarily to relieve pruritus, discomfort, pain, and soreness; indications for mucous membranes are similar. The anesthetics are poorly absorbed through the intact skin, but from mucous membranes and skin breaks and sores (abrasions, trauma, ulcers, and so on) absorption is increased, involving the possibility of systemic involvement. When employed in the oral cavity (mouth and pharynx), interference with swallowing may occur. The nurse should be aware of this, since aspiration may occur if food is ingested within 1 hour after use of an oral topical anesthetic, particularly in children.

Indications. Local anesthetics are capable of abolishing all sensation, but pain fibers are affected first, probably since they are thinner, unmyelinated, and more easily penetrated by these drugs. Loss of pain is followed in sequence by loss of response to cold, warmth, touch, and pressure. Most motor fibers also can be anesthetized when an adequate concentration of the drug is present over sufficient time.

Pharmacokinetics. The parenteral local anesthetics have complete systemic absorption, which is decreased

lidocaine	tetracaine	mepivacaine	dibucaine
Xylocaine Lignocaine	Pontocaine	Carbocaine	Nupercainal
2 times that of procaine	10 times that of procaine	2 times that of procaine	10-20 times that of procaine
Immediate	5-10 min	Less rapid than procaine	10 min
1-1½ hr	1½-2 hr	More prolonged than procaine or lidocaine (2-2.5 hours)	3-4 hr
0.5%-4% for injection 2% and 5% topically	0.5%-2% topically 0.15%-0.25% for injection	1%-2% solution	0.25%-2% for injection or topical application
See procaine	More toxic than procaine, but toxic effects rare because of low dosage used	2 times that of procaine; less than lidocaine	10 or 20 times that of procaine
When administered rapidly or in large doses, may cause convulsions and hypotension	May cause vasodepressor effects	Has vasoconstrictor action	Tissue sloughs when injected subcutaneously

TABLE 12-12 Topical Local Anesthetics

Amides
  lidocaine (Xylocaine, Anestacon, Xylocard)
  dibucaine (Nupercaine, Nupercanal)
Esters
  Benzoic acid type
    cocaine
    hexylcaine (Cyclaine)
    piperocaine (Metycaine)
    proparacaine (Ophthaine, Alcaine, Ophthetic)
  p-aminobenzoic acid type
    benzocaine (Americaine, Hurricaine)
    butamben picrate (Butesin Picrate)
    tetracaine (Pontocaine)
Miscellaneous
  Cyclomethycaine (Surfacaine)
  dimethisoquin (Quotane)
  diperodon (Diothane)
  dyclonine (Dyclone)
  pramoxine (Tronothane)
Pregnancy safety: tetracaine and dyclonine, FDA category
C; other anesthetics, not established

by the addition of a vasoconstrictor such as epinephrine. The amide type varies in protein-binding capacity. Bupivacaine and etidocaine are highly protein bound, whereas lidocaine and mepivacaine are moderately bound to protein. The amide type is hepatic, with only minor renal involvement, but the esters (PABA derivatives) are hydrolyzed primarily by plasma cholinesterases to PABA. The half-life of the ester types is as follows: bupivacaine, $3\frac{1}{2}$ hours; etidocaine, $2\frac{3}{4}$ hours; lidocaine, $1\frac{1}{2}$ hours; and mepivacaine, 2 hours. Onset of action is a function of the anesthetic technique employed, the type of block desired, dosage, and the pK_a (negative logarithm of ionization constant) of each anesthetic. The time it takes for a drug to reach a peak concentration depends on the block type but ranges from 10 to 30 minutes.

REACTIONS TO LOCAL ANESTHETICS

Local anesthetics produce vasodilation by direct action on blood vessels and by anesthetizing sympathetic vasoconstrictor fibers. This action can cause rapid absorption of the drug; when rate of absorption exceeds rate of elimination, toxic effects can occur. To decrease rate of absorption and incidence of toxic effects by allowing more time for metabolic degradation and to prolong local anesthetic effects, epinephrine or other vasoconstrictor drugs are used. Dosage of vasoconstrictors must be carefully determined to prevent ischemic necrosis at the injection site. Since local anesthetics are potentially toxic drugs, a client's age, weight, physical condition, and liver function must be taken into account in determining drug dosage. Caution is advised, with the use of amide anesthetics in clients with compromised livers, since the liver is the site of their metabolism.

Most reactions to local anesthetics result from overdosage, rapid absorption into systemic circulation, and individual hypersensitivity or allergic response.

Central nervous system. At first the CNS may be stimulated and cause anxiety, restlessness, confusion, dizziness, tremors, and even convulsions. Then depression may occur, and unconsciousness and death may ensue.

Cardiovascular system. Myocardial depression, bradycardia and hypotension can occur because of smooth muscle relaxation and inhibition of neuromuscular conduction. The client suddenly becomes pale, feels faint, and has a drop in blood pressure. Cardiac arrest can be the result of a cardiovascular reaction.

Anesthetics containing a vasoconstrictor are employed with caution in clients receiving drugs that may change blood pressure, such as monoamine oxidase inhibitors, phenothiazines, and tricyclic antidepressants. The combination may produce severe hypotension or hypertension. Cardiac dysrhythmias occur when catecholamine vasoconstrictors (e.g., epinephrine) are used with clients receiving cyclopropane, halothane, or trichloroethylene.

Allergic reaction. True allergic reactions are said to be uncommon. Sometimes a reaction is thought to be allergic when it is really caused by overdosage. However, allergic reactions can occur. They may be relatively mild (hives, itching, skin rash), or they may be acutely anaphylactic.

The allergic reactions are characteristically manifested by cutaneous lesions, urticaria, or edema. They may result from various factors, such as hypersensitivity, idiosyncrasy, or diminished tolerance. These rare hypersensitivity reactions are usually limited to the ester type of anesthetics. The most important risk of local anesthetics is a dose-related CNS toxicity, which may progress from sleepiness to convulsion. Clients from families that exhibit malignant hyperthermia (hyperpyrexia) should be administered only ester-type local anesthetics, since amide-type anesthetics are known for this reaction. Skin testing for sensitivity is of doubtful value. Allergy to PABA derivatives has not demonstrated a cross-sensitivity to the amide type (lidocaine).

Small test doses are frequently given by the physician to gauge the extent of the client's sensitivity to the anesthetic agent. The anesthetic agent chosen, its concentration, the rate of injection, and physical and emotional factors in the client all influence reactions to local anesthetics.

THE NURSE'S ROLE IN THE USE OF LOCAL ANESTHETICS

Unlike general anesthetics, nurses often administer topical local anesthetic agents. Therefore, the nurse has a much broader role in relating to these agents.

Assessment. Assess the client for previous response to local anesthetics and the existence of preexisting diseases or drug allergies. During and after administration of a local anesthetic, monitor the client for signs of toxicity, allergy, or other adverse reactions. It is especially important to monitor cardiac status for dysrhythmias and hypertension when a local anesthetic containing a vasoconstrictor such as epinephrine is administered.

Intervention. Do not use the local anesthetic solution if it is cloudy, discolored, or contains crystals. Solutions that do not contain preservatives should be discarded after the vial has been opened. Resuscitative equipment must be available in case the client has an anaphylactic reaction.

If local anesthetics are used as ointments or creams, thoroughly cleanse and dry the area before applying. When the suppository form of the agent is used, chill in the refrigerator 30 minutes, remove wrapper, and moisten with water or lubricant to insert. Note that when local anesthetics are used topically in the nose or throat, they may cause paralysis of the upper respiratory tract, leading to possible aspiration. Measure the preparation accurately. Apply with a cotton swab; swishing should be used for mouth and gums and gargling for application to the throat. Do not allow the local anesthetic to be swallowed unless specifically cleared with the physician.

Education (for local anesthetics that may be self-administered by the client). Instruct the client to use the preparation exactly as prescribed; not to use more, or more often, or for a longer period of time.

Caution the client not to inhale while using the topical aerosol or spray dosage forms.

Instruct the client in the use of the provided applicator for rectal aerosol foam preparation. Avoid using if bleeding hemorrhoids are present.

If local anesthetic preparations are used topically in the nose or throat, instruct the client not to eat for 1 hour after administration, since this may lead to aspiration. Because of the variability in response, each client must be able to swallow before food is offered. Advise the client not to chew gum while the anesthetic is in effect, since there is the risk of biting the tongue or buccal mucosa.

ANESTHESIA BY INJECTION

Anesthesia by injection is accomplished by infiltration, conduction, spinal, caudal, and saddle block.

Infiltration anesthesia is produced by injecting dilute solutions (0.1%) of the agent into the skin and then subcutaneously into the region to be anesthetized. Epinephrine often is added to the solution to intensify the anesthesia in a limited region and to prevent excessive bleeding and systemic effects. Repeated injection will prolong the anesthesia as long as needed. The sensory nerve endings are anesthetized. This method of administration is used for minor surgery such as incision and drainage or excision of a cyst (see Table 12-13).

Conduction, or **block, anesthesia** means that the anesthetic is injected into the vicinity of a nerve trunk that supplies the region of the operative site. The injection may be made at some distance from the surgical site. A single nerve may be blocked, or the anesthetic may be injected where several nerve trunks emerge from the spinal cord (paravertebral block). A more concentrated solution is required because of the thickness of nerve trunk fibers. This method of anesthetics is often used for foot and hand surgery.

Spinal anesthesia is a type of extensive nerve block sometimes called a *subarachnoid block.* The anesthetic solution is injected into the subarachnoid space and affects the lower part of the spinal cord and nerve roots (see next section).

For *low spinal anesthesia* the client is placed in a flat or Fowler's position. A solution with a specific gravity greater than that of spinal fluid is used, since it tends to diffuse downward. For *high spinal anesthesia* Trendelenberg's position with the head sharply flexed is used, along with an anesthetic solution of lower specific gravity than that of spinal fluid (which tends to diffuse upward) or a solution with the same specific gravity as spinal fluid (which may diffuse upward or downward, depending on position used). Solutions with the same specific gravity as spinal fluid act primarily at the site of injection.

Onset of anesthesia usually occurs within 1 to 2 minutes after injection. Duration of anesthesia is 1 to 3 hours, depending on the anesthetic used. Spinal anesthesia is used for surgical procedures on the lower abdomen, inguinal area, or lower extremities; it may be the method of choice for clients with severe respiratory problems or with liver, kidney, or metabolic disease. Marked hypotension, decreased cardiac output, and respiratory inadequacy tend to occur during anesthesia and are considered to be disadvantages of this method of anethesia.

Postoperatively, headache is the most common complaint; this may be accompanied by difficulty in hearing or seeing. Headache may be postural and occur only in the head-up or sitting or standing position. This symptom is the result of the opening in the dura made by the large spinal needle, which may persist for days or weeks, permitting loss of cerebrospinal fluid. Headache and auditory and visual problems following lumbar puncture result from decreased intracranial pressure. These symptoms usually are alleviated when spinal fluid pressure returns to normal. Paresthesias such as numbness and tingling may occur after spinal anesthesia; they are usually locally in the lumbar or sacral areas and disappear within a relatively short time. The success and safety of spinal anesthesia depend primarily on the anesthetist's skill and knowledge.

Caudal anesthesia is produced by injecting an anesthetic solution into the caudal canal, the sacral part of the vertebral canal containing the cauda equina, or the bundle of spinal nerves that innervates the pelvic viscera. It is

TABLE 12-13   Pharmacokinetic Overview of Selected Injected Local Anesthetic Drugs

Generic name	Trade name	Metabolism	Use	Dosage and administration
SHORT-ACTING (½-1 HR)				
chloroprocaine	Nesacaine Nescaine-CE	Ester compound- metabolized by cholinesterases in plasma and liver to a PABA compound. Excretion: kidneys	Nesacaine—infiltration and regional anesthesia Nesacaine—CE for caudal and epidural anesthesia	Usual adult dosage for infiltration nerve blocks: 30-800 mg as 1% or 2% solutions, depending on site and length of surgical procedure Caudal and epidural: 40-500 mg as 2% or 3% solution. (Without epinephrine) Usual pediatric dosage for infiltration nerve blocks: up to 20 mg/kg body weight
procaine HCl	Novocain	Ester compound— same as above	Infiltration, nerve block, spinal anesthesia, epidural block	Usual adult dosage for infiltration: 0.25% - 0.5% solution, 350-600 mg, up to 1 g Peripheral nerve block: 500 mg as 0.5%, 1%, or 2% solution Spinal and epidural dosage vary with individual client, procedure, and degree of anesthesia desired Pediatric dosage: not available
INTERMEDIATE DURATION (1-3 HR)				
lidocaine	Xylocaine, Xylocard♣	Amide compound Metabolism: liver to active and toxic metabolites Excretion: kidneys	Infiltration, nerve block, spinal, epidural	Usual adult dosage depends on site and length of surgical procedure Pediatric dosage: same as adult Lidocaine is available with and without epinephrine
mepivacaine HCl	Carbocaine HCl	Amide compound—see above	Infiltration, nerve blocks, caudal, epidural	Available alone and with levonordefrin (vasoconstrictor). Dosage depends on site and length of surgical procedure. Adult maximum dosage: Dental, up to 6.6 mg/kg body weight (300 mg maximum per appointment). Other usages, up to 7 mg/kg body weight. Pediatric, up to 5 or 6 mg/kg body weight

used in obstetrics and for pelvic or genital surgery. Its advantage over spinal anesthesia is that the anesthetic does not have direct access to the spinal cord and medullary centers. Thus the respiratory muscles and blood pressure are not directly affected, and undesirable effects are less likely to occur.

Saddle block is sometimes used in obstetrics and for surgery involving the perineum, rectum, genitalia, and upper parts of the thighs. The client sits upright while the anesthetic is injected, following a lumbar puncture. The client remains upright for a short time, until the anesthetic has taken effect. The body parts that contact a saddle when riding become anesthetized, hence the name.

INJECTABLE LOCAL ANESTHETICS

The short-, intermediate-, and long-acting local anesthetics for injection are listed in Table 12-13. Generally the onset of action for an anesthetic is the result of drug concentration and the targeted nerve-tissue area. Potency and duration of anesthetic action increase with drug lipid solubility.

The adverse reactions of injected local anesthetics generally require medical intervention (see Table 12-14). The significant drug interactions are limited (see box), but this does not preclude a variety of unexpected responses, thus indicating the need for close observation.

Pregnancy safety. Bupivacaine, chloroprocaine, dibu-

TABLE 12-13   Pharmacokinetic Overview of Selected Injected Local Anesthetic Drugs—cont'd

Generic name	Trade name	Metabolism	Use	Dosage and administration
INTERMEDIATE DURATION (1-3 HR)—cont'd				
prilocaine HCl	Citanest Citanest Forte Xylonest✤	Amide compound—see above	Infiltration, peripheral nerve blocks, caudal, epidural	Available alone or with epinephrine (vasoconstrictor). Although dosages vary with site and length of procedure, the adult maximum dosages are as follows: Dental, up to 400 mg as a 4% solution in 2-hr period. Other usages, 400 mg maximum in debilitated clients and clients with liver impairment Healthy adults, 600 mg maximum Pediatric maximum: Dental, children up to 10 yr, 40 mg (4% solution) maximum. Other procedures, individualize dosage; 1% solution recommended
LONG DURATION (3-10 HR)				
bupivacaine	Marcaine Sensorcaine Carbostesin✤	Amide type—see above	Infiltration, caudal, epidural, peripheral nerve blocks	Available alone or with dextrose (Marcaine spinal) or with epinephrine. Dosages vary with site, additional drugs, and length of procedure.
dibucaine HCl	Nupercaine	Amide type—see above	Caudal, spinal	Available alone and with dextrose (heavy solution Nupercaine). Dosage varies with site of injection, additional drugs if ordered, and length of procedure.
etidocaine	Duranest	Amide type—see above	Infiltration; peripheral nerve blocks, caudal and epidural nerve blocks	Available alone and with epinephrine. Dosages vary with site and length of procedure.
tetracaine HC1	Prontocaine HCl Amethocaine HCl✤ Minims✤	Ester compound—see above	Saddle block (low spinal), up to costal margin, spinal anesthesia	Available alone and with dextrose. Dosages vary with site and length of procedure.

caine, mepivacaine, procaine, and tetracaine—FDA Category C. Etidocaine, lidocaine, and prilocaine—FDA Category B.

KEY TERMS

apnea, page 228
atelectasis, page 226
balanced anesthesia, page 221
cataleptic state, page 233
caudal anesthesia, page 241
concentration gradient, page 221
conduction anesthetic, page 241
diffusion hypoxia, page 227

general anesthesia, page 220
hyperthermia, page 226
hypothermia, page 226
infiltration anesthetic, page 241
local anesthesia, page 237
malignant hyperthermia, page 226
neuroleptanesthesia, page 235
nystagmus, page 233
oliguria, page 226
Overton-Meyer theory, page 221
regional anesthesia, page 237
saddle block, page 242
spinal anesthetic, page 241
titration, page 224

TABLE 12-14 Injected Local Anesthetic Drugs: Adverse Reactions

Drug(s) or method of administration	Adverse reactions*
Epidural block or high spinal	Cyanosis caused by methemoglobinemia (reported with all local anesthetics but most prevalent with prilocaine). Symptoms may include weakness, breathing difficulties, increased heart rate, dizziness, or collapse Diplopia, seizures, tinnitus, increased excitability, shivering, involuntary shaking (stimulation of CNS) Skin rash; edema of face, lips, mouth, throat (allergic reaction; these effects are most often reported with ester compounds); anaphylaxis and severe hypotension rarely reported Diaphoresis, hypotension, bradycardia or irregular heart rate, pale skin color (cardiovascular depression) Nausea, vomiting
Central Nerve Blocks	Neuropathies or neurologic effects, including headaches; paresthesia or paralysis of lower legs; breathing difficulties; severe hypotension; bradycardia; backache; reduction or loss of sexual functions, bladder control, or bowel movements
Spinal anesthesia	Meningitis-type effects: headaches, nausea, vomiting, and stiff/sore neck
Dental anesthesia	Numbed or tingling feeling of lips and mouth, edema of lips or mouth (allergic effect)
Epinephrine or other vasoconstrictors	Hypertension, shaking, increased anxiety or nervousness, tachycardia, headache, chest pain (sympathomimetic or adrenergic effects)

*If adverse reactions occur, contact physician because medical intervention may be necessary.

SIGNIFICANT DRUG INTERACTIONS OF INJECTED LOCAL ANESTHETIC MEDICATIONS

Although the potential of an adverse drug interaction is present with many drugs, the most significant are as follows:

Prior or concurrent administration of CNS depressant drugs may result in additive CNS depression effects. Adjust dosages and monitor closely.

Vasoconstrictor agents, such as epinephrine, norepinephrine, or phenylephrine, in combination with local anesthetics may result in impaired circulation of the area resulting in sloughing of tissue. If used for end arteries, such as toes or fingers, ischemia resulting in gangrene may result. Extreme caution is advised.

BIBLIOGRAPHY

Ackerman, J: Monitoring waste nitrous oxide: one medical center's experience, AORN J 41(5):895, 1985.

American Hospital Formulary Service: AHFS Drug Information 88, Bethesda, Md, 1988, American Society of Hospital Pharmacists, Inc.

Biddle, CJ: Operating room workers: between Scylla and Charybdis, Occup Health Nurs 32(6):320, 1984.

Boucher, BA Witth, WO, and Foster TS: The postoperative adverse effects of inhalational anesthetics, Heart Lung 15(1):63, 1986.

Brown, DG Wetterstroem, N, and Finch, J: Anesthetic gas exposure: protecting the OR environment, AORN J 41(3):590, 1985.

Carey, KW ed: Nursing photobook: caring for surgical patients, Springhouse, Pa, 1982, Nursing 82, Books.

Catron, D: The anesthesiologist's handbook, ed 2, Baltimore, 1978, University Park Press.

French, MM and Phillips, KF: When seconds count: treating malignant hyperthermia, RN 47(11):26, 1984.

Gilman, AG, and others, eds: Goodman and Gilman's the pharmacological basis of therapeutics, ed 7, New York, 1985, Macmillan, Inc.

Hansten, PD: Drug Interactions, ed 5, Philadelphia, 1985, Lea & Febiger.

Hemminki, K, Kyyronen, P, and Lindbohm, M: Spontaneous abortions and malformations in the offspring of nurses exposed to anaesthetic gases, cytostatic drugs, and other potential hazards in hospitals, based on registered information of outcome. J Epidemiol Community Health 39(2):141, 1985.

Numphrey, MJ, and Blanch, TJJ: Malignant hyperthermia: rapid treatment and problematic prevention, Consultant 24(6):61, 1984.

Paris, PM: No more pain: ketamine, J Emerg Med 18(7):155, 1986.

Pories, WJ: Anesthesia, J Emerg Med 18(5):201, 1986.

Rogers, AL, and Sturgeon, LC, Jr: Malignant hyperthermia, AORN J 41(2):369, 1985.

Spencer, RT Nichols, LW, Lipkin, GB, Waterhouse, HP, West, FM, and Bankest, EG: Clinical pharmacology and nursing management, ed 2, Philadelphia, 1986, JB Lippincott Co.

Stehling, L and Brown, D: Malignant hyperthermia: more than a rising temperature, Diagn Med 6(3):58, 1983.

United States Pharmacopeia Convention: Drug information for the health care provider, ed 8, Rockville, Md, 1988, US Pharmacopeia Convention, Inc.

Van Den Eeden, SK, and Wilkinson, WE: Health screening for hospital personnel exposed to waste anesthetic gases, Occup Health Nurs 33(2):73, 1985.

CHAPTER

13

Antianxiety, Sedative, and Hypnotic Drugs

OBJECTIVES

After studying this chapter, the student will be able to:

1. Describe the physiology and stages of sleep.

2. Differentiate between antianxiety, sedative, and hypnotic drug effects.

3. Discuss the nurse's role in sedative-hypnotic therapy.

4. Discuss the special considerations for use of antianxiety, sedative, and hypnotic agents in the pediatric and geriatric clients.

5. Identify the characteristics of commonly used benzodiazepines and barbiturates.

6. Formulate an appropriate plan of care for individual clients who require the administration of antianxiety, sedative, or hypnotic agents.

Antianxiety or **anxiolytic** agents are used to reduce feelings of anxiety, that is, apprehension, nervousness, worry, or fearfulness. Anxiety is usually a normal response of the individual psychologically and physiologically to a personally threatening situation. A threat to one's health, body, loved ones, job, or life-style may result in anxiety. Generally this anxiety stimulates the person to take a purposeful or deliberate action to counteract or offset the anxiety-producing state. When a person is unable to cope with a persistently stressful situation because the excessive anxiety interferes with daily functioning, help is necessary. Although many nonpharmacologic modalities are available, the antianxiety agents are most commonly prescribed for the treatment of anxiety. For proposed site of action for the benzodiazepines, see "Limbic System" in Chapter 10, "Overview of the Central Nervous System."

Sedatives and **hypnotics** are CNS depressant drugs. Although sedatives were commonly prescribed before the advent of the benzodiazepine family, their general use today has declined. Sedatives are chemical substances that reduce nervousness, excitability, or irritability by producing a calming or soothing effect. Hypnotics are used to induce sleep. The major difference between a sedative and a hypnotic is the degree of CNS depression induced. Small doses of a CNS-depressing agent may be used for a sedative effect, whereas larger dosages may be used for hypnotic effects. Barbiturates have been used extensively as sedative-hypnotic agents, but because of their low degree of selectivity and safety, they have been largely replaced by the safer benzodiazepines.

MECHANISMS OF ACTION OF BENZODIAZEPINES

Benzodiazepines do not exert a general CNS depressant effect; instead there is a wide range of selectivity seen with the various members of this class. Some of the general pharmacologic properties of this class include muscle relaxant, and antianxiety, anticonvulsant, and hypnotic effects. Although their exact mechanism of action is unknown, they appear to act at the limbic, thalamic, and hypothalamic areas of the CNS. Stimulation of the gamma-aminobutyric acid (GABA) receptors in the reticular activating system will block stimulation and arousal of the limbic and cortical areas, especially after stimulation of the brain stem reticular activating system. Presynaptic inhibition is enhanced, which may result in reduction of the spread of seizure activity, especially in the thalamus, cortex, and limbic areas of the CNS. The skeletal muscle relaxant effects are believed to be caused by blockade of the **monosynaptic** and **polysynaptic reflexes**, and they also may directly decrease the motor nerve and muscle activity.

MECHANISMS OF ACTION OF BARBITURATES

Important actions of the barbiturates are those of sedation and hypnotic effect. Barbiturates have been shown to depress the neurons and synapses of the ascending reticular formation of the brain stem, and this effect may be responsible for the reduction in electric activity of the cortex. Since the ascending reticular formation receives stimuli from all parts of the body and relays impulses to the cortex (thus promoting wakefulness and alertness), depression of the ascending reticular formation decreases cortical stimuli, reducing the need for wakefulness and alertness.

There is evidence that the barbiturates act at all levels of the CNS. The extent of effect varies from mild sedation to deep anesthesia, depending on the drug selected, method of administration, dosage, and the reaction of the individual's nervous system. The barbiturates are not usually regarded as analgesics and cannot be depended on to produce restful sleep when insomnia is caused by pain. However, when combined with an analgesic the sedative action seems to reinforce the action of the analgesic and to alter the client's emotional reaction to pain.

All of the barbiturates used clinically depress the motor cortex of the brain in large doses, but phenobarbital, mephobarbital, and metharbital exert a selective action on the motor cortex, even in small doses. This explains their use as anticonvulsants.

Ordinary therapeutic doses have little or no effect on medullary centers, but large doses, especially when administered intravenously, depress the respiratory and vasomotor centers.

Smooth muscles of blood vessels and of the gastrointestinal organs are depressed after large amounts of barbiturates, but clinical doses do not usually produce untoward effects. Motility of the gastrointestinal organs may be reduced and emptying of the stomach delayed slightly, but there is apparently little interference with the ability to respond to normal stimuli. Uterine muscle is affected little by the hypnotic doses of barbiturates, and the force of uterine contractions at the time of childbirth is not diminished unless anesthesia has been produced by one of these drugs.

The effect of barbiturates (and also benzodiazepines) may result from their action on the inhibitory neurotransmitter, GABA. Research indicates their activity on a cellular level is different.

PHYSIOLOGY OF SLEEP

Sleep can be defined as a recurrent, normal condition of inertia and unresponsiveness during which an individual's overt and covert responses to stimuli are markedly reduced. During sleep a person is no longer in sensory contact with the immediate environment, and stimuli that have bombarded the senses of sight, hearing, touch, smell, and taste during waking hours no longer attract attention or exert a controlling influence over the individual's voluntary and involuntary movements or functions. It certainly is not difficult to understand that everyone needs to escape from constant stimuli.

Sleep research has shown that sleep is not one level of unconsciousness; it actually consists of two basic stages occurring cyclically:

1. Rapid eye movement (REM)
2. Non–rapid eye movement (non-REM)

During sleep, the individual moves through **REM sleep,** then through the four stages of **non-REM sleep,** with 4 considered the deepest level of non-REM sleep. The stages of sleep are based on electrical activity that can be observed in the brain by means of an electroencephalogram (EEG). The EEG provides graphic illustrations of brain waves, which are an indication of the electrical activity occurring in the brain. See box for a description of the stages of sleep.

From the standpoint of dreaming, sleep consists of two main functional states. One is called "slow wave," nondreaming, or nonrapid eye movement (non-REM) sleep. The other is referred to a "paradoxical," dreaming, or rapid eye movement (REM) sleep. It should be kept in mind that REM sleep is not synonymous with light sleep, since it takes a more powerful stimulus to arouse an animal or person from REM sleep than from synchronous slow wave sleep.

STAGES OF SLEEP*

STAGE	CHARACTERISTICS	AVERAGE TIME (%) SPENT IN STAGES IN YOUNG ADULTS
Non-REM Sleep		
Stage 1	Dozing or feelings of drifting off to sleep. Person can be easily awakened. Insomniacs have longer stage 1 periods than normal.	3%-6%
Stage 2	Person is relaxed but can be easily awakened. Has occasional REM and also some slight eyeball movements.	40%-52%
Stage 3	Deep sleep, difficult to wake person up. Respirations, pulse, and blood pressure may decrease.	5%-8%
Stage 4	Sleepwalking or bedwetting may occur. Person very hard to wake up. If awakened, may be very groggy. Dreaming especially about daily events.	10%-19%
REM Sleep	Rapid eye movements occur here. Vivid dreams occur during REM sleep. Respirations may be irregular.	23%-34%

*A complete cycle takes approximately 90 minutes.

Sleep research indicates that there is psychologic and physiologic needs for the body to maintain an equilibrium between the various stages of sleep. Physiologic functions of the body tend to be depressed during nondreaming sleep. For example, it is known that:

1. Blood pressure falls (10 to 30 mm Hg)
2. Pulse rate is slowed
3. Metabolic rate is decreased
4. Gastrointestinal tract activity is slowed
5. Urine formation slows
6. Oxygen consumption and carbon dioxide production are lowered
7. Body temperature slightly decreases
8. Respirations are slower and more shallow
9. Body movement is minimal.

Dreaming sleep tends to increase most of these parameters, and body movements are more noticeable—turning, jerking, arms and legs moving, talking, crying, or laughing—and, of course, eye movements can be seen under the closed lids. The dynamic physiologic equilibrium of the body continues to be maintained even during sleep. Depression of physiologic functions occur during deep sleep, and an increase in functions occurs during dreaming. Repeated studies have shown that when individuals are deprived of deep sleep, they become physically uncomfortable, tend to withdraw from society and their friends, are less aggressive and outgoing, and manifest concern over vague physical complaints and changes in bodily feelings. The overall impression made by persons deprived of deep sleep is that of a depressive and hypochondriac reaction.

However, dreaming sleep is also important. From studies in which individuals were deprived of dreaming sleep (every time the subjects attempted to dream, as evidenced by rapid eye movements, they were awakened and not permitted to dream), the following results were observed. During their waking hours the individuals became less well integrated and less effective. They showed signs of confusion, suspicion, and withdrawal. They appeared anxious, insecure, and irritable; they had greater difficulty concentrating; they had a marked increase in appetite with a definite weight gain; and they were introspective and unable to derive support from other people.

Many psychologists and psychiatrists believe that wish fulfillment finds expression in dreams, and potentially harmful thoughts, feelings, and impulses are released through the dream so that there is no interference of the functioning of the personality during waking hours.

It is also known that in dream deprivation studies, the longer dream deprivation continues, the greater the increase in attempts to dream, until the individual begins to dream almost on falling asleep. When subjects are finally permitted to dream, a marked increase of dreaming is noted for the entire night, and as much as 75% of the night may be spent in dreaming. This amount diminishes for each suceeding recovery night until the individual has once again established his or her normal sleep pattern.

Research has shown that deep sleep takes priority over dreaming sleep when there has been prolonged sleep deprivation. In other words, deep sleep needs will be met first, after which dreaming sleep needs will be met. The body attempts to reestablish the normal equilibrium between the sleep stages.

Each individual establishes his or her own normal sleep pattern, which will vary somewhat from night to night and which is influenced by the individuals's emotional and physical state. For most individuals, any alteration in sleeping habits will cause problems in falling asleep, staying asleep, or both. Since drugs affect an individual's physical or emotional state, they also influence his or her sleep pattern.

PEDIATRIC DRUG USE

The use of antianxiety, sedative, or hypnotic agents in children is limited in practice. Childhood anxiety disorders usually respond better to counseling and psychotherapy than to medications (Anxiety, 1980). Also, young children are much more sensitive to the CNS-depressant effects of this classification of drugs. **Paradoxical reactions,** or reactions contrary to the expected reaction, have been reported with the use of barbiturates in both children and geriatric clients. These include increased excitability, hostility, confusion, hallucinations, and, perhaps, an acute elevation of body temperature.

Sedation though may be indicated for particular situations if carefully selected (drug and dosage) for the individual child (e.g., the treatment of severe anxiety associated with an acute attack of asthma, as an adjunct preanesthetic agent, or in the treatment of convulsive disorders). But the use of such medications in children requires careful drug selection and dosage and close monitoring and assessment by the health care providers.

GERIATRIC DRUG USE

Careful drug selection and dosage are necessary to avoid producing excessive CNS depression in the elderly. The aging process is usually associated with physiologic alterations including a decline in metabolism and in many organ functions, especially liver and kidney functions. Since drug half-lives may be extended, selecting agents with shorter half-lives and no active metabolites may be safer for the geriatric client. The elderly client should also be monitored for paradoxical reactions (i.e., increased excitability, rage, hostility, confusion, and hallucinations, which have been reported with both the benzodiazepines and barbiturates). The appearance of such adverse effects indicates immediate discontinuance of the medication and consultation with the prescribing physician.

The short-acting benzodiazepines are much safer than the barbiturates and are effective anxiolytic and hypnotic agents. Oxazepam, lorazepam, temazepam, alprazolam, and triazolam have short to intermediate half-lives, and they are usually recommended for the elderly client requiring a benzodiazepine. Barbiturates should be avoided in the elderly because enhanced CNS depression, confusion, ataxia, and paradoxical reactions are commonly reported.

One of the most frequent complaints of the elderly is **insomnia** (difficulty falling asleep, staying asleep, or waking up early in the morning). Age-related physiologic changes may also contribute to the changes in sleep patterns reported. A recent study indicated that sleep problem complaints were more common with women and generally were most common with elderly subjects 80 years of age and older (Cornoni-Huntley and others, 1986). Chloral hydrate and benzodiazepines are usually the agents of choice in treating insomnia in the elderly. When possible, physicians often suggest the elderly limit their hypnotic dosages to three or four times a week, allowing client selection of the nights they need to take their medication. This schedule usually results in enhanced effectiveness, less daytime drowsiness or sedation, and a decreased potential for inducing tolerance to the medication. Careful assessment, monitoring, and re-evaluation for the need of hypnotics on a regular basis is highly recommended.

THE NURSE'S ROLE IN SEDATIVE-HYPNOTIC THERAPY

Assessment. The nurse should find out what a client's sleep habits are and how he or she ensures good sleep at home. A thorough sleep history is required before a regimen of medications is instituted. Such a history includes the following information:

- What does the client do about environmental control, which includes ventilation, lighting, and noise?
- What does the client do about physical care? Does he or she shower before retiring or go for a walk?
- What does the client do about food? Does he or she snack before retiring?
- What does the client do about quiet recreation, such as reading, before sleep?

Various problems may cause the client to have insomnia. These include circadian rhythm irregularities, sleep apnea, restless leg syndrome, intake of alcohol or caffeine, and poor sleep hygiene, which is characterized by irregular bedtimes, daytime napping, and strenuous exercise or heavy eating just before bedtime.

When a client is admitted, a thorough drug history should be taken and all medication brought from home removed for the client's safety.

Intervention. Since nurses are in a strategic position to influence the client's sleep, it cannot be stressed enough that caution must be exercised when making decisions about giving or repeating an hs or a prn order for a sleeping medication. Immediately resorting to administering a sleeping medication when a client complains of being unable to sleep may be doing the client more harm than good. An assessment of the client and alternate methods of relaxing the client must be considered.

The nurse should try using supportive nursing measures (e.g., a back rub, reduction of environmental stimuli, or a warm drink) either alone, before barbiturates are given, or in conjunction with the drug.

The nurse should prepare the client for sleep, raise the side rails on the bed, and caution the client to ambulate only with assistance. The normal adult dose may cause excitement, depression, or confusion.

Every effort should be made not to disrupt the sleeping client, if at all possible, medications are scheduled before sedatives or hypnotics are given. Vital signs are taken before the client falls asleep. Numerous interruptions for various aspects of care can do nothing but further alter the client's sleep pattern.

Since clients can become physically and psychologically dependent on these drugs, gradually taper off the medications to avoid an abstinence syndrome reaction.

Education. The client should be cautioned against driving a car, operating machinery, or participating in any activity that may be dangerous while the he or she is taking these drugs. Although the client may deny feeling sleepy the next day, his or her performance may show definable impairment because therapeutic levels of some of these drugs are retained.

Clients and their families need to be taught ways to promote good sleep without resorting to drugs, which includes OTC drugs (Sominex, NyTol, Sleep-eze, Unisom).

Stress to the client that sedative or hypnotic drugs should never be taken in combination with alcohol, antihistamines, antianxiety agents, antidepressants, or antipsychotic agents because they will produce an enhanced CNS-depressant effect.

Evaluation. Evaluation of compliance and effectiveness may be facilitated by use of a written "sleep diary." Among the information recorded in the diary are activities and eating before sleep, bedtimes, waking times, naps, and medication administration. Review of the diary will help identify success of therapy or areas of poor sleep hygiene. Indicators of effectiveness also include patient reports of feelings of rest and wakefulness without residual drowsiness or "drug hangover" during the daytime.

BENZODIAZEPINES

Benzodiazepines are among the most widely prescribed drugs in clinical medicine. Their popularity probably results from their anxiolytic effects occurring at nontoxic doses. Drowsiness and undesirable CNS depression occur less frequently with benzodiazepine agents than with comparable doses of meprobamate or barbiturates.

Mechanism of action. See "Mechanisms of Action of Benzodiazepines" on p. 246. Also, the limbic system, associated with the regulation of emotional behavior, contains a highly dense area of benzodiazepine receptors

in the amygdala that may correspond to specific antianxiety action of certain drugs. These proposed benzodiazepine receptors may share some sites of action with other drugs (alcohol, meprobamate, barbiturates) and may further explain cross-tolerance to these drugs. The benzodiazepines' receptor concentration in the dorsal spinal cord may account for their muscle relaxant effect; an endogenous benzodiazepine-like substance also may exist. GABA, an inhibitory neurotransmitter, affects benzodiazepine receptors, and a benzodiazepine receptor may be a portion of a GABA receptor. Benzodiazepines enhance the action of GABA at its receptors. The identification of psychotropic drug receptors is leading to the discovery and understanding of the time and course of receptor site occupancy. This knowledge will allow more effective therapeutic use of the agents affecting mood and behavior and will further explain how the drugs exert their action in the neurotransmitter interaction within the CNS.

Indications

1. *Anxiety disorders.* Benzodiazepines, with the exception of clonazepam, flurazepam, temazepam, triazolam, and midazolam, are indicated for the treatment of anxiety. Several benzodiazepines (alprazolam, oral lorazepam, and oxazepam) are used as adjunct medications to treat anxiety associated with depression.
2. *Alcohol withdrawal.* Chlordiazepoxide, clorazepate, diazepam, and oxazepam are often used for treatment of alcohol withdrawal syndrome.
3. *Preoperative medication.* Parenteral chlordiazepoxide, diazepam, lorazepam, and midazolam are used preoperatively to reduce anxiety and to help induce general anesthesia; the latter three drugs decrease the client's memory of the procedure. These three drugs are also used for endoscopic procedures to decrease anxiety and tension and to produce an anterograde **amnesic effect.**
4. *Sleep disorders.* Flurazepam, temazepam, and triazolam are usually prescribed for sleep disorders, such as insomnia, demonstrated by difficulty falling asleep, staying asleep, or early morning awakenings. Flurazepam is reported to be effective for up to 28 days, whereas temazepam's effectiveness may be demonstrated up to 35 days of daily administration.
5. *Seizure disorders.* Clonazepam is available orally as an anticonvulsant. See Chapter 17 Anticonvulsants. Also, parenteral diazepam is indicated for intractable, repetitive seizures, such as status epilepticus. Oral diazepam may be used for short-term adjunct therapy (1 to 2 weeks) with other anticonvulsants for the treatment of convulsions.
6. *Cardioversion.* Diazepam can be given intravenously before **cardioversion** (restoration of the heart's

rhythm by electrical countershock) to reduce anxiety and decrease the client's recall of the procedure.

7. *Neuromuscular disease.* Benzodiazepines, especially diazepam, may be useful as an adjunct medication for the treatment of skeletal muscle spasms caused by muscle or joint inflammation or spasticity resulting from upper motor neuron dysfunction, such as cerebral palsy and paraplegia.

Pharmacokinetics. Benzodiazepines are readily absorbed from the GI tract. Clorazepate dipotassium and diazepam are the most rapidly absorbed drugs in this class, whereas oxazepam, prazepam, and temazepam are absorbed more slowly. The more rapidly absorbed benzodiazepines produce a more prompt and intense onset of action.

After one dose, the benzodiazepines are dispersed rapidly to the body's fluids and tissues. This produces a rapid decrease in circulating drug, and the effects of a single dose end quickly. Lorazepam is not as extensively distributed and may have a longer duration of action, since effective blood concentrations may be more prolonged. After multiple doses, these drugs accumulate in the body's fluids and tissues. This saturation of storage sites allows for greater blood concentration and longer action. Accumulation in storage sites also accounts for the prolonged action of benzodiazepines after they have been discontinued.

The GI tract and the liver are the sites of metabolism either for the active drug forms or inactive metabolites. The acid pH of the stomach is the site of conversion of clorazepate to its active form, desmethyldiazepam. Prazepam is transformed in the wall of the GI tract or during the first pass through the liver to desmethyldiazepam, but this process is not as rapid as clorazepate conversion.

These drugs are highly protein bound and lipid soluble and are excreted by the kidney. Protein binding is reduced in newborns, alcoholic clients, and those with cirrhosis or renal insufficiency. Because oxazepam and lorazepam are inactivated in one step by the liver, they may be preferred agents in elderly clients and those with liver disease.

The injectable benzodiazepines include chlordiazepoxide, diazepam, and lorazepam. The onset of action of these agents after intravenous administration is approximately 1 to 5 minutes. After intramuscular injection, the onset of action is approximately 15 to 30 minutes.

See Table 13-1 for a pharmacokinetic overview of selected benzodiazepam drugs.

Side effects/adverse reactions. See Table 13-2.

Significant drug interactions. The following effects may occur when benzodiazepines are given with the drugs listed below:

Drug	Possible Effect and Management
CNS depressants, such as alcohol, opioid analgesics, anesthetics; MAO and tricyclic antidepressants	Enhanced CNS depressant effects reported. Monitor closely as the dosage of one or both drugs may need to be adjusted. Opioid analgesics should generally be reduced by one-third the dose when used in combination with benzodiazepines.

Dosage and administration. See Table 13-3.

Pregnancy safety. Alprazolam, halazepam, lorazepam, midazolam, (parenteral)—FDA Category D; temazepam, triazolam—FDA Category X; other benzodiazepines—not established.

THE NURSE'S ROLE IN BENZODIAZEPINE THERAPY

Assessment. Reassessment of the medication's efficacy as an antianxiety agent or as a sedative-hypnotic should be done periodically over the course of therapy.

Pregnant clients usually should avoid using benzodiazepines, since their use is associated with increased risk of congenital anomalies. Female clients of childbearing age should be advised that if they should become pregnant or intend to become pregnant during anxiolytic therapy, they should immediately notify the physician who prescribed these drugs about the advisability of conception. At that time a decision about discontinuing the drug must be made.

Nursing mothers should not be given benzodiazepines. Because of their molecular size, the benzodiazepines and their metabolites probably are excreted in breast milk.

For elderly or debilitated clients, the initial dose should be small and increments added gradually, based on the response of each client, to preclude ataxia or excessive sedation. Doses of benzodiazepines sufficient to control anxiety cause unwanted drowsiness less frequently than equivalent doses of barbiturates or meprobamate. The benzodiazepines have high therapeutic effectiveness and low addiction potential and lethality; they are generally desirable agents for anxious elderly clients. These drugs occasionally cause paradoxical reactions such as agitation and confusion, but these occur to a lesser degree than with barbiturates.

The nurse should remember that elderly clients are more vulnerable to the adverse effects of these drugs. Excretion is delayed in this population, and thus the half-life increases. They may allow the client to attain therapeutic blood levels with a single dose rather than two or three doses per day. Daytime sedation can be reduced if the single daily dose is administered at bedtime. If the elderly client is continent, ambulatory, and alert, excessive doses of the benzodiazepines may produce an incontinent, nonambulatory, or confused client. Careful titration to individual needs is essential in elderly clients.

Text continued on p. 255.

TABLE 13-1 Pharmacokinetic Overview of Selected Benzodiazepine Drugs

Generic name	Trade name	Onset of action (min)*	Peak plasma concentration (hr)	Half-life (hr)	Active metabolites (half-life in hr)
alprazolam	Xanax	Oral 15-45	1-2	12-15	alpha-hydroxy-alprazolam (12-15)
chlordiazepoxide	Librium Libritab Apo-Chlorax♣ Medilium♣	Oral 15-45 IM 15-30 IV 1-5	0.5-2 N/A† N/A	5-30	desmethylchloridazepoxide (18) demoxepam (14-95) desmethyldiazepam (30-200) oxazepam (5-15)
clonazepam	Clonopin Rivotril♣	Oral 30-60	1-2 (some patients from 4-8 hr)	18-50	none
clorazepate	Tranxene Tranxene-SD Novoclopate♣	Oral 30-60	1-2	Parent drug not active	desmethyldiazepam (30-200) oxazepam (5-15)
diazepam	Valium Apo-Diazepam♣ E-Pam♣	Oral 15-45 IM within 20 IV 1-3	0.5-1.5 0.5-1.5 N/A	20-70	desmethyldiazepam (30-200) temazepam (9.5-12.4) oxazepam (5-15)
flurazepam	Dalmane Apo-Flurazepam♣	Oral 15-45	0.5-1	2.3	desalkylflurazepam (30-200) N-1-hydroxyethylflurazepam (2-4)
halazepam	Paxipam	Oral N/A	1-3	14	desmethyldiazepam (30-200)
prazepam	Centrax	Oral N/A	6 hr for metabolite desmethyldiaze-pam (single dose)	Parent drug not active	desmethyldiazepam (30-200) oxazepam (5-15)
lorazepam	Ativan Apo-Lorazepam♣	Oral 15-45 IM 15-30 IV 5-15	2-5 1-1.5 N/A	10-20	None
oxazepam	Serax Ox-pam♣ Zapex♣	Oral 45-90	2-4	5-15	None
midazolam HCl	Versed	IM 15 IV 3-5	½-1	1-5	1-hydroxymethyl and 4-hydroxy midazolam
temazepam	Restoril	Oral 25-27	2-3	9.5-12.4	None
triazolam	Halcion	Oral 15-30	1.3	1.6-5.4	None

*Onset of action of various dosage formulations; not all trade names are available in multiple dosage forms. Usually the first named trade name is available in various dosage forms.

†N/A, Information not available.

TABLE 13-2 Benzodiazepines—Side Effects/Adverse Reactions

Drug(s)	Side effects*	Adverse reactions†
benzodiazepines	More frequent: drowsiness, hiccups (especially with midazolam), lassitude, loss of dexterity	Increased behavioral problems seen mostly with children (anger, decreased ability to concentrate)
	Less frequent: dry mouth, nausea, vomiting, headaches, constipation, abdominal cramping, unsteadiness, dizziness, blurred vision	Insomnia, increased excitability, hallucinations, apprehension (paradoxical reaction)
		Pruritus, skin rash, sore throat, elevated temperature, increased bruising or bleeding episodes, mental depression, hepatitis, confusion, mouth or throat sores, muscle weakness
		Muscle tremors, tachycardia, shortness of breath or breathing difficulties have been reported with midazolam

*If side effects continue, increase, or disturb the client, inform the physician.

†If adverse reactions occur, contact the physician because medical intervention may be necessary.

TABLE 13-3 Dosage and Administration of Selected Benzodiazepines

Adults	Elderly	Children
ALPRAZOLAM		
Antianxiety, 0.25-0.5 mg orally 3 times daily. Dosage may be titrated if needed, up to a maximum of 4 mg/day.	0.25 mg orally 2-3 times daily. Increase dosage if necessary, according to client's requirements and individual response.	Not established for children less than 18 yr.
CHLORAZEPATE		
Antianxiety: 7.5-15 mg orally, 2-4 times daily, or 15 mg at bedtime initially, then adjust dosage according to client's requirements and individual response.	7.5-15 mg orally initially, increase dosage gradually according to client's response and drug tolerance.	
Sedative-hypnotic: for acute alcohol withdrawal syndrome, 30 mg orally initially, then 15 mg orally 2-4 times a day for the first 24 hr; 15 mg 3-6 times daily for the second day; 7.5-15 mg 3 times a day the third day; 7.5 mg 2-4 times daily the fourth day; and 3.75 mg 2-4 times a day thereafter.		
Anticonvulsant: up to 7.5 mg 3 times daily initially then increase dose as necessary with the following limitations: limit increase to 7.5 mg/wk and daily dosage should not be more than 90 mg/day.		For children 9-12 yr, 7.5 mg orally initially, twice daily. Dosage may be increased by 7.5 mg increments weekly but should not exceed 60 mg daily. Dosage not established for children less than 9 yr.
CHLORDIAZEPOXIDE		
Antianxiety: 5-25 mg orally 3-4 times daily or 50-100 mg IM or IV initially, then 25-50 mg 3-4 times a day as needed. Sedative-hypnotic: 50-100 mg orally initially for acute withdrawal syndrome. Repeat when needed up to 300 mg/day. Maintenance therapy usually requires a reduced dosage. Parenterally, 50-100 mg IM or IV initially; if necessary, dosage may be repeated in 2-4 hr.	Antianxiety: 5 mg orally 2-4 times daily. If necessary, increase dose gradually according to client's requirements and individual response.	Antianxiety: for children 6 yr and older, 5 mg orally 2-4 times daily, increased gradually according to child's requirements and response. Dosage not established for younger children. Parenterally, children 12 yr and older, 25-50 mg IM or IV. Dosage not established for younger children.
DIAZEPAM		
Antianxiety: 2-10 mg orally in tablet form 2-4 times daily. Extended release capsules, 15-30 mg orally daily. Parenterally, preoperatively, individualize dosage. Generally, 10 mg IM or IV given before surgery. For treatment of psychoneurosis, 2-10 mg IM or IV; may repeat in 3 or 4 hr if needed.	2-2.5 mg orally once or twice a day or titrated to the individual's requirements and tolerance. Use of the extended release capsules is only recommended for persons maintained on a 5-mg tablet 3 times a day, then a 15-mg capsule daily may be substituted. Parenterally, 2-5 mg IM or IV initially. Titrate further dosage according to client's requirements and tolerance.	Children 6 mo and older, 1-2.5 mg or 0.04-0.2 mg/kg body weight or 1.17-6 mg/m^2 body surface area given orally 3 or 4 times daily. Not recommended for infants less than 6 mo of age. Dosage increases should be gradual and carefully monitored. Parenterally, no established dosage for neonate less than 30 days old.
Sedative-hypnotic: for acute alcohol withdrawal syndrome, 10 mg orally 3-4 times daily for the first 24 hr, then 5 mg 3-4 times daily therafter as needed. Extended release capsules, 30 mg orally for the first 24 hr, then 15 mg daily if needed. Parenterally, 10 mg IM or IV initially, then 5-10 mg in 3 or 4 hr when necessary.		

TABLE 13-3   Dosage and Administration of Selected Benzodiazepines—cont'd

Adults	Elderly	Children
Anticonvulsant: 2-10 mg orally 2-4 times daily. Extended release capsules, 15-30 mg daily. Parenterally, status epilepticus or severe convulsive episodes (recurrent) 5-10 mg IM or IV initially; repeat dosage if needed at 10-15 min intervals. Maximum dosage 30 mg. If required, the therapy may be repeated in 2-4 hr.		For infants more than 30 days old and less than 5 yr old, 0.2-0.5 mg IV (preferred) or IM, every 2-5 min up to maximum dosage of 5 mg. If repeated therapy is necessary, repeat in 2-4 hr. Children 5 yr and older, 1 mg every 2-5 min up to maximum dosage of 10 mg (IM or IV, latter is preferred). If necessary, dosage may be repeated in 2-4 hr.
Skeletal muscle relaxant: 2-10 mg 3 or 4 times daily. Extended release capsule, 15-30 mg daily. Parenterally, for muscle spasms, 5-10 mg IM or IV initially, repeat in 3-4 hr if needed. Tetanus requires larger dosages.		Tetanus—infants more than 30 days old and less than 5 yr, 1-2 mg IM or IV. May repeat every 3-4 hr if necessary. Children 5 yr and older, 5-10 mg IM or IV, repeat in 3-4 hr if necessary. NOTE: For IV dosages in infants and children, medication should be given over a 3-min period in a dose that does not surpass 0.25 mg/kg body weight. Wait 15-30 min before repeating dosage.
Amnesic effect: for cardioversion, 5-10 mg IV, 5-10 min before performing procedure. Endoscopic, dosages up to 20 mg IV (which is the preferred route of administration), titrate dosage according to client's response. Administer just before performing this procedure. IM doses (5-10 mg) may be given half hour before procedure.		
FLURAZEPAM		
Sedative-hypnotic, 15 or 30 mg orally.	15 mg orally to start. Increase dose if necessary and tolerated by client.	Dosage not established in children less than 15 yr old.
HALAZEPAM		
Antianxiety, 20-40 mg orally, 3-4 times daily.	20 mg orally once or twice a day. Titrate dosage according to client's response and tolerance.	Dosage not established for children less than 18 yr old.
LORAZEPAM		
Antianxiety, 1-3 mg orally 2-3 times daily. Sedative-hypnotic, 2-4 mg orally at bedtime. Parenterally, antianxiety, sedative hypnotic, amnnesic: 0.05 mg/kg body weight IM up to 4 mg maximum administered 2 hr before surgery to obtain greatest amnesic effect. IV, 0.044 mg/kg body weight or 2 mg dose, whichever is less. To produce amnesic action, doses up to 0.05 mg/kg body weight may be given (do not exceed 4 mg). This dose is given 15-20 min before surgery to obtain the greatest amnesic effect.	1-2 mg orally daily in divided dosages. Titrate dosage according to client's response and tolerance.	Dosage not established for children less than 12 yr old for oral dosage forms. For injectable, dosage not available for children less than 18 yr old.

Continued

Adults	Elderly	Children
MIDAZOLAM		Dosages not available for children up to 18 yr.
Sedation for presurgical and amnesic effects: 70-80 µg (or 0.07-0.08 mg of base)/kg body weight, usually administered IM 30-60 min before operation. It may be given with atropine and decreased dosages of narcotics. Sedation for endoscopic or cardiovascular scheduled procedures: if clients have been medicated with opioids, the dosage of midazolam should be reduced by 25%-30%. If not premedicated, IV dose is 35 µg base/kg body weight given before the procedure. Dosages up to 0.1 mg/kg body weight may be given if necessary. If additional dosages are needed, 25% of the initial dose (or increments of 25%) may be administered. Adjunct to general anesthesia: if not premedicated with opioids or other sedatives, for clients up to 55 yr old, 0.2-0.4 mg base/kg body weight IV given in 5-30 sec. For full effect to occur, wait at least 2 min. For clients more than 55 yr old, for healthy or good-risk clients, an initial 0.3 mg base/kg body weight IV given over 20-30 sec. For clients more than 55 yr old who have multiple or severe disease states, 0.2-0.25 mg base/kg body weight IV over 20-30 sec. Doses of 0.15 mg/kg body weight have been effective for some clients. If induction is not completed, increments of 25% of the initial dose or inhalation-type general anesthesia may be added. If clients are premedicated with sedatives or opioids and are 55 yr old or less, administer 0.15-0.25 mg base/kg body weight IV over 20-30 sec. If more than 55 yr old, give 0.2 mg (to healthy good-risk surgical clients) or 0.15 mg (to clients with severe disease states)/kg body weight.		
OXAZEPAM		
Antianxiety, 10-30 mg orally, 3-4 times daily. Sedative-hypnotic, for acute alcohol withdrawal syndrome, 15 or 30 mg orally 3-4 times daily.	10 mg orally initially, 3 times daily. Titrate dosage to 15 mg orally 3 or 4 times daily, according to client's response and tolerance.	Not recommended for children less than 6 yr. Dosages not available for children 6-12 yr old.
PRAZEPAM		
Antianxiety, 10 mg orally 3 times daily (20-60 mg/day as a range). Or an alternate dose is 20-40 mg at bedtime.	10-15 mg orally daily (in divided doses), titrate according to client's requirements and tolerance.	Dosages not available for children 18 yr and less.
TEMAZEPAM		
Sedative-hypnotic, 15 or 30 mg.	15 mg orally, titrate dosages according to client's requirements and tolerance.	Not available for children up to 18 yr.
TRIAZOLAM		
Sedative-hypnotic, 0.25-0.5 mg orally.	0.125 initially, then titrate dosage according to client's requirements and tolerance.	Not available for children up to 18 yr.

BENZODIAZEPINE TOLERANCE AND DEPENDENCY

Concern about overuse or overprescribing of benzodiazepines leading to tolerance, dependency, and withdrawal problems was discussed in Chapter 9. Several general guidelines are offered to reduce the potential for drug abuse with this drug classification.

1. Benzodiazepines are antianxiety agents (i.e., they are used to control the symptoms of anxiety but are not curative agents).
2. Benzodiazepines are indicated for short-term therapy or on an as needed only basis. The dosage would be the minimum necessary to produce the desired effect. The client should be re-evaluated every 2 weeks to ascertain the effectiveness of the medication, the need for continued therapy, or both.
3. When a benzodiazepine is being discontinued, the dosage should be tapered over 2 weeks. In clients receiving the short-acting benzodiazepines (lorazepam, alprazolam), severe withdrawal symptoms have been reported if the medications were abruptly stopped. Switching to a longer half-life benzodiazepine for a few weeks before instituting the tapering procedure has resulted in a reduction of the more serious withdrawal symptoms, such as tonic-clonic seizures.
4. Concurrent consumption of two or more benzodiazepine agents even for daytime anxiety and bedtime insomnia is considered inappropriate therapy. Using one benzodiazepine to accomplish both purposes would be preferred, because (a) effectiveness is usually equivalent, (b) the drug will be better tolerated and controlled by the client, and (c) the therapy will be less expensive.

From Dommisse, CF, and Hayes, PE: Current concepts in clinical therapeutics: Anxiety disorders. Clin pharm 6(3):196, 1987.

When depression accompanies the client's anxiety, the incidence of suicidal tendencies is significant. This may necessitate further protective measures to avoid self-destructive acts such as multidrug overdosage. As small an amount of the drug as possible should be available to such a client at any one time. This requires accurate medical office data about prescriptions and their refill dates and ensures greater control by the prescriber.

Take periodic blood counts (neutropenia) and liver function tests (jaundice) on clients receiving benzodiazepines for prolonged periods. Also, the usual precautions in treating clients with impaired renal or hepatic function should be observed. In animal studies hepatomegaly and cholestasis were observed.

Dosages should be carefully determined for clients with renal impairment, especially when administering chlordiazepoxide and diazepam, since active metabolites may accumulate and produce toxicity. Flurazepam hydrochloride should be avoided, whereas other agents, such as clonazepam, lorazepam, oxazepam, and temazepam, seem to pose no risk of toxicity in renal impairment.

Multiple physical and psychiatric problems frequently occur together and may require treatment with several drugs. Multiple drug therapy is sometimes referred to as "polypharmacy." A client may benefit diagnostically and therapeutically from an evaluation made on the basis of a drug-free baseline.

Some clients abruptly withdrawn from high doses or therapeutic doses of benzodiazepines taken over prolonged periods exhibit symptoms of withdrawal. These may resemble the symptoms of anxiety for which the drug was originally prescribed. A mild withdrawal syndrome is characterized by feelings of tension or anxiety, anorexia, GI symptoms such as diarrhea, weakness, and lethargy, light-headedness, tremor, and mild numbness. Other clients who exhibit moderately severe symptoms report anxiety, apprehension, restlessness, insomnia, increased frequency of dreaming, anorexia-induced weight loss, dysphoric moods, and palpitations. Rarely clients exhibit seizures and delirium. These symptoms usually begin 24 to 72 hours after withdrawal. When the client is withdrawn from a short-acting benzodiazepine, symptoms peak in about 5 to 7 days and subside after 7 to 10 days. The withdrawal syndrome of the long-acting benzodiazepines peaks at about 5 days but may last 2 to 4 weeks. Withdrawal symptoms can be relieved by administering a dose of the anxiolytic agent. The withdrawal syndrome can be avoided by gradually tapering the dose of the anxiolytic agent and supporting the client during this period with other anxiety-relieving techniques.

Intervention. The nurse should avoid intramuscular administration because the preparations are highly alkaline and irritating to tissues. Absorption is also erratic by this route of administration.

Administer intravenous preparations slowly because apnea, hypotension, bradycardia, and cardiac arrest have been known to occur with rapid administration. Arteriospasm, with resultant gangrene, will be caused by accidental intraarterial, rather than intravenous, administration.

Education. The client should be instructed to avoid alcohol and other CNS depressants while taking benzodiazepines.

The client should be cautioned not to take more than the prescribed dosage if the medication seems less effective, but to consult the prescriber.

If on a scheduled dosing regimen (such as use as an anticonvulsant), take the dose right away if dose missed but remembered within 1 to 2 hours. If remembered much later, do not double next dose, skip the missed dose and continue regimen.

SELECTED BENZODIAZEPINES

alprazolam (Xanax)

Alprazolam is used only as an antianxiety agent. Accumulation is minimal after multiple doses and elimination rapidly follows termination of therapy.

chlordiazepoxide (Librium, Libritab, Apo-Chlorax✤, Medilium✤)

In addition to its use as an antianxiety agent and a sedative-hypnotic, chlordiazepoxide is used as an antitremor agent and for relief of acute alcohol withdrawal symptoms.

Intravenous administration is preferred because intramuscular absorption is slow and erratic. Intravenous administration should be slow over a period of at least 1 minute. The nurse should be careful *not* to use the intramuscular diluent when preparing solution for intravenous administration since it has a tendency to form air bubbles.

When preparing a chlordiazepoxide solution for intramuscular administration, use only the manufacturer's diluent and administer the drug deeply into the muscle. Mixing the drug with sodium cloride or sterile water for injection will cause pain on injection.

Solutions should be used immediately after reconstitution, and any unused solution should be discarded.

After receiving the drug parenterally, the client should be kept resting in bed and monitored carefully for up to 3 hours for decreases in respiratory rate, heart rate, and blood pressure.

Because of the long-acting metabolites that remain in the blood stream for several days, the client should be monitored for accumulative effects of the drug.

clonazepam (Clonopin)

Clonazepem is used as an anticonvulsant and in treatment of panic disorders.

When used as an anticonvulsant, clients receiving long-term therapy should avoid abrupt withdrawal since this may precipitate seizures.

chlorazepate (Tranxene, Tranxene-SD, Novoclopate✤)

Chlorazepate is used as an antianxiety agent, sedative-hypnotic, anticonvulsant, and for relief of acute alcohol withdrawal symptoms.

When given orally, it is one of the most rapidly absorbed benzodiazepines.

Accumulation of active metabolites may be significant with long-term therapy.

diazepam (Valium, Valrelease, Apo-Diazepam✤, E-Pam✤, Meval✤, Neo-Calme✤, Novadipam✤)

Diazepam is used as an antianxiety agent, sedative-hypnotic, anticonvulsant, and skeletal muscle relaxer. Parenteral diazepam is an amnesic and is used orally as an antitremor agent.

Intravenous administration should be accomplished slowly, at least 1 minute for each 5 mg of the drug to prevent apnea, hypotension, bradycardia, or cardiac arrest. The client should be observed at bedrest for at least 3 hours after parenteral administration.

To minimize the occurrence of thrombophlebitis following intravenous administration of diazepam, the vein can be flushed with at least 1 mg of saline per milligram of diazepam. Injection should be made into a large vein, not small veins, such as found on the back of the hand, wrist.

Diazepam is not compatible with aqueous solutions. If direct intravenous injection is not possible, the drug should be slowly injected through an infusion tube as close to the point of insertion in the patient as possible.

Continuous intravenous infusion is *not* recommended since diazepam may precipitate in the infusion bag and the medication may be absorbed by the plastic infusion bags and tubing.

When used parenterally for perioral endoscopy, the use of a topical anesthetic is recommended. Increased coughing, decreased respirations, dyspnea, hyperventilation, and laryngospasm have been known to occur; measures to assist with respirations should be available.

See Chapter 14 for nursing considerations of diazepam in its use as an anticonvulsant.

flurazepam (Dalmane, Apo-Flurazepam✤, Somnol✤)

Flurazepam is indicated only for use as a sedative hypnotic.

The client should be instructed that 2 to 3 nights may be required before flurazepam becomes effective.

Elimination is slow since metabolites remain in the body several days. This may produce unwanted daytime carryover effects that result in poor coordination and drowsiness. Overcome carryover effects by using lower doses and administering medication every other evening. The client must be warned of the sustained effect of the active metabolites.

halazepam (Paxipam)

Halazepam is indicated for use only as an antianxiety agent. It has a long half-life and active metabolites, which may be significant when multiple doses are administered. Elimination may take several days or even weeks.

lorazepam (Ativan, Alzapam, Loraz, Novolorazem✤)

Lorazepam is indicated for use as an antianxiety agent and sedative hypnotic. Parenteral lorazepam is also indicated as an annesic, anticonvulsant, antitremor agent, and skeletal muscle relaxant.

Lorazepam must be diluted with a compatible diluent

immediately before intravenous use. It may be infused directly into a vein or through intravenous tubing. Infusion rates should not exceed 2 mg/min.

Intraarterial injection may cause arteriospasm and possibly gangrene.

Intramuscular lorazepam is injected, undiluted, into deep muscle mass.

After receiving a parenteral dosage of lorazepam, the client should be observed at bed rest for at least 1 hour for decreases in respiratory rate, heart rate, and blood pressure.

midazolam (Versed)

Midazolam, the newest of the commonly used benzodiazipines, is used for its antianxiety, sedative-hypnotic and amnesic effects, as well as an adjunct to general anesthesia. Midazolam is only used in parenteral form. Unlike diazepam, it does not cause thrombophlebitis and irritation on injection.

Dosages should be individualized according to the health status of the client. The range between therapeutic dosage and unconsciousness or disorientation appears to be narrow, necessitating close monitoring of the client.

The client should be instructed not to engage in tasks requiring alertness, such as driving, until the effects of midazolam have abated or until the day after administration, whichever is longer.

As with diazepam, when used for perioral endoscopic procedures, a topical anesthetic agent should also be used and measures to support respiration (O_2, suction airway) should be available.

oxazepam (Serax, Zapex❋)

Oxazepam is indicated as an antianxiety agent and sedative-hypnotic. Accumulation is minimal during multiple-dose therapy with rapid elimination following termination of therapy.

prazepam (Centrax)

Prazepam is indicated only as an antianxiety agent. It is one of the least rapidly absorbed benzodiazepines after oral administration, and accumulation of active metabolites may be significant in long-term therapy.

temazepam (Restoril, Razepam)

Temazepam is indicated as a sedative-hypnotic. Only minimal accumulation occurs during multiple doses and elimination is rapid.

triazolam (Halcion)

Triazolam is indicated only as a sedative-hypnotic. Since overdosage may occur at only 2 mg, which is only 4 times the maximum recommended dose, the nurse should be especially alert for the signs and symptoms of overdosage of this drug.

BARBITURATES

The barbiturates were once the most commonly prescribed class of medications for hypnotic and sedative effects. With only a few exceptions, they have been largely replaced by the benzodiazepines.

Classification. The barbiturates are classified according to the duration of their action as long-, intermediate-, short-, and ultrashort-acting drugs. This means that the short-acting drugs produce an effect or onset in a relatively short time (10 to 15 minutes) and peak over a relatively short period (3 to 4 hours). Short-acting barbiturates are used for treating insomnia, for preanesthetic sedation, and in combination with other drugs for psychosomatic disorders. Long-acting barbiturates require over 60 minutes for onset and peak over a period of 10 to 12 hours. Long-acting barbiturates are used for treating epilepsy and other chronic neurologic disorders and for sedation in clients with high anxiety. Ultrashort-acting barbiturates are used as IV anesthetics. Thiopental sodium, which belongs to the ultrashort-acting group of barbiturates, acts rapidly and can produce a state of anesthesia in a few seconds. Intermediate-acting barbiturates have an onset of 45 to 60 minutes and a peak in 6 to 8 hours.

Mechanism of action. See "Mechanisms of Action of Barbiturates" on p. 246.

Indications

Hypnotic. Although barbiturates are indicated for the treatment of insomnia, they have generally been replaced by the benzodiazepine family of drugs. If barbiturates are used, they are only indicated for short-term use, since they tend to loose their effectiveness in 14 days or less.

Antianxiety. Barbiturates have been used for sedative effects in treating anxiety and nervousness. But for daytime use the benzodiazepines have largely replaced the barbiturates primarily because they produce less drowsiness or ataxia.

Anesthetic. Short-acting barbiturate anesthetics, such as thiopental and methohexital, are used for selected surgical procedures, especially for surgery of short duration. These barbiturates were discussed more fully in Chapter 12.

Preanesthetic. The short-acting barbiturates, such as pentobarbital sodium, are selected for their preanesthetic effect. They are often ordered to be given the night before surgery to enable the client to sleep and may be ordered to be given the morning of the operation. Diazepam and other benzodiazepines are often used today for this purpose, that is as a preanesthetic agent to help with anesthesia induction, to reduce anxiety, and to induce an amnesic effect.

Anticonvulsant. Barbiturates are used to prevent or control convulsive seizures associated with tetanus, strychnine poisoning, meningitis, eclampsia, and epilepsy. They may be prescribed alone or in conjunction with other anticonvulsant drugs. Phenobarbital has been used for epilepsy (generalized tonic-clonic) and for seizures induced by fever, whereas mephobarbital and metharbital, also long-acting barbiturates, are also useful for the symptomatic treatment of certain types of epilepsy.

Hyperbilirubinemia. Although not an approved indication, phenobarbital (oral and injectable) is often used to prevent or treat hyperblirubinemia in neonates and in clients with congenital nonhemolytic unconjugated hyperbilirubinemia.

Pharmacokinetics. Barbiturates are readily absorbed after oral, rectal, and parenteral administration. The most soluble sodium salts are absorbed faster than the free acids. Most of the barbiturates, with the exception of barbital, undergo change in the liver before they are excreted by the kidney. They are excreted either in a partly altered form, a partly unchanged form, or a completely altered form. The longer-acting barbiturates are said to be metabolized or chemically altered more slowly than the rapidly acting members. The slower a barbiturate is altered or excreted, the more prolonged is its action. If excretion is slow and administration prolonged, cumulative effects will result.

Side effects/adverse reactions. See Table 13-4.

Significant drug interactions. The following effects may occur when barbiturates are given with the drugs listed below:

Drug	Possible Effect and Management
corticosteroids (adrenocorticoids, glucocorticoid, mineralocorticoid, corticotropin)	When given with barbiturates (especially phenobarbital), corticosteroids may have enhanced metabolism and a decrease in therapeutic effects. Dosage adjustments may be necessary. Monitor closely.
alcohol and CNS depressants	Enhanced CNS depressant effects may result. Monitor closely and perhaps decrease the dosage of one or both drugs to reduce the possibility of inducing this effect.
anticoagulants (coumarin or indanedione types)	Decrease in anticoagulant effects caused by enhanced metabolism. Monitor closely; prothrombin time tests may be necessary to determine dosage changes of the anticoagulant.
anticonvulsants (hydantoin)	Hydantoin metabolism may be affected by the addition of barbiturates. The effect on hydantoin is undependable and unpredictable; therefore serum levels of hydantoin should be closely monitored when combination therapy is used.
divalproex sodium or valproic acid	Monitor barbiturate serum levels closely, since the metabolism of barbiturates may decrease, leading to elevated levels and an increase in CNS depression and neurologic dysfunction. The half-life of valproic acid may also be reduced, which would also require monitoring of blood levels and dosage adjustments.

TABLE 13-4 Barbiturate Side Effects/Adverse Reactions

Drug(s)	Side effects*	Adverse reactions†
barbiturates	More frequent: ataxia, drowsiness, dizziness, hungover effect Less frequent: nausea, vomiting, insomnia, constipation, restlessness, faintness, headache, night terrors	Hypersensitivity reaction such as skin rash, exfoliative dermatitis, Stevens-Johnson syndrome, sore throat, fever, edema, serum sickness, apnea, bronchospasms, urticaria. Any age client but especially elderly or debilitated clients may exhibit confusion, disorientation, and mental depression. In children, elderly, and debilitated clients, a paradoxical reaction (increased excitability) may occur. Rarely but reported effects include hallucinations and increased bleeding tendencies. Chronic use may result in osteomalacia and rickets (bone pain or aching, anorexia, myalgia, loss of weight). Toxic signs include very severe confusion and persistent irritability. Acute toxic effects may include bradycardia, confusion, respiratory problems (apnea, laryngospasm), ataxia, extreme weakness, and visual disturbances.

*If side effects continue, increase, or disturb the client, inform the physician.
†If adverse reactions occur, contact physician as medical intervention may be necessary.

Dosage and administration. For pharmacokinetic information and dosage of selected barbiturates, see Table 13-5.

Pregnancy safety. FDA Category D.

THE NURSE'S ROLE IN BARBITURATE THERAPY

Barbiturates have proved to be useful drugs when used appropriately. Because of their potential for dependence, tolerance, abuse, or misuse, the role of the nurse is essential in providing safe and effective drug therapy.

Assessment. The nurse should assess and note the sleeping pattern of the client. This observation can influence the physician's decision on the type of barbiturate to prescribe. Clients who become disoriented or confused by the barbiturate should not be restrained. Rather, the client should be reoriented and a calm environment promoted.

Porphyria is a hereditary disease that involves errors in the formation or excretion of porphyrins (molecular components of hemoglobin, myoglobin, and various enzymes). Acute intermittent porphyria is characterized by irregular and unpredictable attacks, which may include abdominal distress, elevated blood pressure, psychotic episodes, and neuropathy. Acute intermittent porphyria may be aggravated through barbiturate inducement of the enzyme necessary for porphyrin synthesis.

The nurse should avoid giving barbiturates to clients with hypersensitivity to them, respiratory conditions (with dyspnea or obstruction), previous dependency on barbiturates, and porphyria, and elderly persons and children with paradoxical reactions.

If a client tells the nurse that he or she is hypersensitive to this group of drugs, the nurse should withhold the medication and then record the statement and inform the physician. Seriously impaired hepatic or renal function may also constitute a contraindication for the use of these drugs, although only the physician can decide whether the degree of damage warrants the use of a different type of drug.

See general nursing considerations regarding sedatives and hypnotics.

Intervention. The nurse should be aware that barbiturates may be combined in the same capsule so that a long-acting and a short-acting or moderately long-acting preparation can be used to advantage for the client who has difficulty in both getting to sleep and remaining asleep for the desired number of hours.

To hasten the onset of sleep with oral administration, the rate of absorption may be increased by administering barbiturates well diluted or on an empty stomach.

When administering barbiturates intramuscularly, the nurse should not give more than 5 ml at any one site because the preparations are irritating to the tissues.

With the exception of anesthesia and control of status epilepticus, barbiturates are infrequently prescribed to be administered by the intravenous route. If the intravenous route has been prescribed, medication should be administered slowly and in diluted form, according to the directions. If the barbiturate is to be infused in an intravenous solution, monitor the infusion rate closely, since rapid injection can be dangerous. The airway should be patent and emergency resuscitative equipment should be available when the medication is given intravenously.

For intravenous injection, the nurse should use the larger veins to decrease the risk of irritation. The intravenous site should be assumed for any signs of thrombophlebitis or extravasation.

Barbiturates may be administered rectally if the oral or parenteral route is undesirable. A retention enema may be prepared from the soluble salt of the barbiturate if a rectal dosage form is not available.

Education. Instruct the client to use the barbiturate only as directed. The client should not alter the dosage or take the drug more often or for a longer period than ordered.

Barbiturates may impair mental and physical functioning. Caution must be exercised to avoid dangerous activities if affected by barbiturates in this manner.

Barbiturates may affect the developing fetus. If a client is pregnant or may become pregnant during therapy, the client should discuss it with her doctor. Barbiturates will also pass into breast milk and may affect the nursing baby.

Barbiturates may cause mental or physical dependence or tolerance. The clients should consult their physicians if they experience the signs or symptoms of dependence or no longer receive the full effect of the drug.

If a scheduled dosing regimen (as when used as an anticonvulsant) and a dose is missed, take the dose immediately if remembered within 1 to 2 hours of the scheduled time; otherwise, skip the dose and continue with the regimen.

Abrupt withdrawal may precipitate seizures in the epileptic patient. Abstinence syndromes (see Chapter 9) may be seen after abrupt withdrawal in any patient after long-term therapy.

Barbiturates interact with many other drugs and alcohol. Inform the client not to take any additional medications while taking a barbiturate unless it has been approved by the prescriber or pharmacist. Dangerous interactions may occur.

Evaluation. Evaluation is focused on detection of adverse or side effects, monitoring compliance, and effectiveness of the therapy. Indicators of effectiveness include sleep time, daytime wakefulness, and client reports on feelings of rest and wakefulness. Tolerance develops to all barbiturates during long-term therapy, but it develops at unpredictable rates. The development of tolerance, as well as possible dependence, is closely evaluated. Monitoring for paradoxical reactions, allergic reactions, or drug interactions is also essential. The nurse should func-

TABLE 13-5 Pharmacokinetic Overview of Selected Barbiturate Drugs

Generic name	Trade name	Half-life (hr) Mean	Half-life (hr) Range	Indications/dosage
SHORT-ACTING				
pentobarbital	Nembutal Novopentobarb🍁 Pentogen🍁	*	15-50	*Oral dosage forms* Adult: sedation, 20 mg 3-4 times daily; hypnotic, 100 mg orally at bedtime. Elderly and debilitated clients: lower doses usually required. Children: sedative, 2-6 mg/kg body weight daily; preoperative, 2-6 mg/kg body weight, maximum 100 mg/dose; hypnotic, dosage not established. *Parenteral dosage form* Adult: sedative-hypnotic, 150-200 mg IM for preoperative sedative and hypnotic dosage; IV, 100 mg initially, if necessary give additional small doses at 1 min intervals up to a maximum of 500 mg for hypnotic effect; anticonvulsant, IV, 100 mg initially, if necessary give additional small doses at 1 min intervals up to a maximum of 500 mg. Elderly and debilitated clients: lower dosages are usually necessary. Pediatric: hypnotic, 2-6 mg/kg body weight, maximum dose of 100 mg, administered IM; IV, 50 mg initially, if necessary give additional small doses at 1 min intervals until desired goal is reached. Sedative: preoperative, 2-6 mg/kg body weight to a maximum of 100 mg/dose, IV. Anticonvulsive: IM, or IV, 50 mg initially; if necessary, give additional small doses at 1-min intervals. *Rectal dosage form* Adult: sedative, 30 mg 2-4 times daily; hypnotic, 120-200 mg at bedtime; for elderly and debilitated clients, give lower doses and monitor closely. Pediatric: hypnotic, dosage not available for children less than 2 mo old; children 2-12 mos, 30 mg; children 1-4 yr old, 30 or 60 mg; children 5-12 yr old, 60 mg; children 12-14 yr old, 60 or 120 mg. Sedative: 2 mg/kg body weight or 60 mg/m^2 body surface 3 times a day. Preoperative: children less than 2 mo old, dosage not available; children 2-12 mo old, 30 mg; children 1-4 yr old, 30-60 mg; children 5-12 yr old, 60 mg; children 12-14 yr old, 60-120 mg.
secobarbital	Seconal Novosecobarb🍁	28	15-40	*Oral dosage forms* Adult: hypnotic, 100 mg bedtime; sedative, 30-50 mg 3-4 times daily for daytime usage; preoperative, 200-300 mg, 1-2 hr before surgery. Elderly or debilitated clients: use lower doses. Pediatric: hypnotic, 50-100 mg; sedative, 2 mg/kg body weight or 60 mg/m^2 body surface, 3 times daily; preoperative, 2-6 mg/kg body weight to a 100 mg dose maximum, 1-2 hr before surgery.

*The mean half-life is dependent on the dose.

TABLE 13-5 Pharmacokinetic Overview of Selected Barbiturate Drugs—cont'd

Generic name	Trade name	Half-life (hr)		Indications/dosage
		Mean	Range	
				Parenteral dosage form
				Adult: hypnotic, 100-200 mg IM or 50-250 mg IV; sedative, 1.1-2.2 mg/kg body weight IV from 10-15 min before dental procedure; nerve block, 100-150 mg IV, anticonvulsant, tetany, 5.5 mg/kg body weight IM or IV, every 3-4 hr if needed.
				Elderly or debilitated clients: lower doses may be necessary.
				Pediatric: hypnotic, 3-5 mg/kg body weight or 125 mg/m² body surface to a maximum of 100 mg IM; rectally, 1%-1.5% solution—administer 5 mg/kg body weight to children weighing up to 40 kg; children weighing 40 kg and over, give 4 mg/kg body weight; preoperative sedative, 4-5 mg/kg body weight; anticonvulsant (tetany), 3-5 mg/kg body weight or 125 mg/m² body surface per dose IM or IV.
INTERMEDIATE-ACTING				
amobarbital	Amytal Isobec♣ Novamobarb♣	25	16-40	*Oral dosage forms*
				Adult: hypnotic, 65-200 mg at bedtime; sedative, 50-300 mg daily in divided doses; preoperative, 200 mg oral capsules, 1-2 hr before surgery; during labor, 200-400 mg oral capsules, may repeat in 1-3 hr if necessary to a 1 g maximum.
				Elderly or debilitated clients: lower doses may be necessary.
				Pediatric: hypnotic dosage not available; sedative, 2 mg/kg body weight or 60 gm/m² body surface 3 times daily; preoperative, 2-6 mg/kg body weight up 100 mg maximum dose.
				Parenteral dosage forms
				Adult: hypnotic, 65-200 mg IM or IV; sedative, 30-50 mg IM or IV, 2 or 3 times a day; anticonvulsant, 65-500 mg IV.
				Elderly or debilitated clients: lower doses may be necessary.
				Pediatric: hypnotic, children up to 6 yr old, 2-3 mg/kg body weight per IM dose; children 6 yr old and older, 2-3 mg/kg body weight per IM dose; IV dose is 65-500 mg per dose; sedative, preoperative, 65-500 mg IV or 3-5 mg/kg body weight per dose; anticonvulsant, children up to 6 yr old, 3-5 mg/kg body weight or 125 mg/m² body surface per IM or IV dose; children 6 yr old and older, 65-500 mg/IV dose.
aprobarbital	Alurate	24	14-34	
butabarbital	Butisol Buticaps Day-Barb♣ Neo-Barb♣	100	66-140	
talbutal	Lotusate	15	N/A	

Continued.

TABLE 13-5 Pharmacokinetic Overview of Selected Barbiturate Drugs—cont'd

Generic name	Trade name	Half-life (hr) Mean	Range	Indications/dosage
LONG-ACTING				
mephobarbital	Gemonil	34	11-67	
metharbital	Mebaral	N/A	N/A	
phenobarbital	Luminal Gardenal✽	79	53-118	*Oral dosage form* Adult: elixir, capsule, oral solution, and tablets; hypnotic, 100-320 mg at bedtime; sedative, 30-120 mg in 2 or 3 divided doses; anticonvulsant, 60-250 mg daily in divided or single dose; antihyperbilirubinemic, 30-60 mg 3 times daily. Elderly or debilitated clients: lower doses may be necessary. Pediatric: hypnotic, dosage not established; sedative, 2 mg/kg body weight or 60 mg/m² body surface 3 times daily; preoperative, 1-3 mg/kg body weight; anticonvulsant, 1-6 mg/kg body weight in divided or single dosages; antihyperbilirubinemic, neonates, 5-10 mg/kg body weight for a few days after birth; for children up to 12 yr old, 1-4 mg/kg body weight 3 times daily. *Parenteral dosage forms* Adult: hypnotic, 100-325 mg IM or IV; sedative, 30-120 mg daily in 2 or 3 divided doses; preoperative, 130-200 mg 1 to 1½ hr before surgery; postoperative, 32-100 mg IM; anticonvulsant, 100-320 mg IV, repeat if needed to a maximum of 600 mg in 24 hr; status epilepticus, 10-20 mg/kg body weight by slow IV; may repeat if needed. Elderly or debilitated clients: lower doses may be necessary. Pediatric: hypnotic, individualized; sedative, 1-3 mg/kg body weight IM or IV; postoperative, 8-30 mg IM; anticonvulsant, 10-20 mg/kg body weight IV initially as a loading dose; then maintenance dosage is 1-6 mg/kg body weight daily; status epilepticus, 15-20 mg/kg body weight given IV-over 10-15 min; antihyperbilirubinemic, 5-10 mg/kg body weight daily IM for a few days following birth.

tion as a client-advocate when evaluation suggests that a change in drug therapy is needed.

MISCELLANEOUS SEDATIVES AND HYPNOTICS

A number of sedatives and hypnotics do not fall into the previously discussed drug classes, but they will be discussed here because they are available for client use with prescription.

chloral hydrate (Noctec, Novochlorhydrate✽)

Mechanism of action. The CNS depressant effects produced are believed to be caused by its active metabolite, trichloroethanol. Its exact mechanism of action though is unknown.

Indications. Sedative, hypnotic.

Pharmacokinetics

Absorption. Oral and rectal dosage forms are rapidly absorbed

Metabolism. In liver and erythrocytes to active metabolite, trichloroethanol; further liver metabolism is to inactive metabolites

Onset of action. Hypnotic dose (500-100/mg) within 30 minutes

Half-life. Approximately 7 to 10 hours

Excretion. Kidneys

Side effects/adverse reactions. See Table 13-6.

TABLE 13-6   Miscellaneous Sedative-Hypnotic Side Effects/Adverse Reactions

Drug	Side effects*	Adverse reactions†
chloral hydrate	More frequent: nausea, abdominal distress, vomiting Less frequent: ataxia, dizziness, drowsiness	Skin rash or urticaria, confusion, increased excitability (paradoxical reaction), hallucinations
ethchlorvynol	More frequent: visual disturbances, nausea, vomiting, abdominal distress, increased weakness, facial numbness, dizziness Less frequent: ataxia, confusion, daytime sedation or drowsiness	Skin rash or urticaria, increased excitability or nervousness (paradoxical reaction), jaundice, diplopia, trembling, slurred speech, weakness, or numbness in the hands or feet
glutethimide	More frequent: daytime sedation or drowsiness Less frequent: visual disturbances, ataxia, confusion, headaches, nausea, vomiting, dizziness	Skin rash, sore throat, fever increased bleeding tendencies, severe weakness, confusion, trembling, CNS disturbances (memory recall problems, lack of concentrating ability)
meprobamate	More frequent: drowsiness or increased clumsiness Less frequent: visual disturbances (blurred or changes in distant or near sight), diarrhea, dizziness, euphoria, headache, nausea or vomiting, increased weakness	Skin rash, urticaria, pruritus, slurred speech, increased confusion or persistent dizziness, ataxia, increased bleeding tendencies, sore throat, elevated temperature, increased excitability (paradoxical reaction), tachycardia, respiratory difficulties (wheezing, shortness of breath).
methyprylon	More frequent: daytime sedation, headache, dizziness Less frequent: nausea, vomiting, diarrhea	Skin rash, increased excitability (paradoxical reaction), mouth sores or increased bleeding tendencies, respiratory difficulties, confusion, increased weakness.
paraldehyde	More frequent: unpleasant mouth odor, drowsiness; nausea, vomiting, and abdominal distress reported with oral preparations Less frequent: ataxia, dizziness, hangover-type effects	Skin rash, coughing (reported with IV use only), hepatitis, thrombophlebitis at injection site, tremors, confusion, increased nervousness or irritability (caused by metabolic acidosis from overdose), respiratory difficulties, increased weakness.
propiomazine HCl	Most frequent: dry mouth, increase in daytime sedation, dizziness Less frequent: confusion, diarrhea, nausea, vomiting, respiratory difficulties, skin rash, abdominal distress, tachycardia, increased restlessness	Thrombophlebitis or pain and swelling at injection site.

*If side effects continue, increase, or disturb the client, inform the physician.
†If adverse reactions occur, contact physician because medical intervention may be necessary.

Significant drug interactions. The following effects may occur when chloral hydrate is given with the drugs listed below:

Drug	Possible Effect and Management
alcohol or other CNS depressants	Enhanced CNS depression effects may result. Monitor closely and perhaps reduce the dosage of one or both drugs.
anticoagulants (coumarin or indandione)	Within the first few weeks especially, the anticoagulant may be displaced from its protein binding, leading to an enhanced hypoprothrombinemic effect. Monitor closely.

Dosage and administration. See Table 13-7.
Pregnancy safety. FDA Category C.

NURSING CONSIDERATIONS

Since the elixir has an unpleasant taste and odor, it may be difficult for clients, particularly children, to take. To make the elixir more palatable, the nurse should mix it with fruit juice or some type of chilled fluid (such as ginger ale).

If the client is getting this as a preoperative medication, flavored extract (e.g., peppermint extract, banana extract) should be added to make it more palatable.

Since the drug can cause gastric irritation, the nurse should administer it after meals with an 8-ounce glass of fluid. Its use should be avoided in clients with esophagitis, gastritis, or gastric or duodenal ulcers.

TABLE 13-7   Chloral Hydrate Dosage and Administration

	Adults	Children
Oral		
Hypnotic	500-1000 mg orally 15-30 min before bedtime.	50 mg/kg body weight or 1.5 g/m² body surface orally at bedtime. Maximum single dose is 1 g.
Sedative	250 mg orally 3 times/day after meals.	8.3 mg/kg body weight or 250 mg/m² body surface to a maximum of 500 mg 3 times daily after meals.
Preoperative	500-1000 mg orally ½ hr before surgery.	
Premedication (before electroencephalographic examination)		20-25 mg/kg body weight orally.
Withdrawal from alcohol	500-1000 mg orally, may repeat at 6-hr intervals. Maximum adult dosage is 6 g daily.	
Suppositories		
Hypnotic	500-1000 mg rectally at bedtime.	50 mg/kg body weight or 1.5 g/m² body surface area at bedtime, up to maximum of 1 g/single dose.
Sedative	325 mg 3 times a day. Maximum adult dosage is 2 g daily.	8.3 mg/kg body weight or 250 mg/m² body surface rectally 3 times daily.

Clients taking chloral hydrate concomitantly with oral anticoagulants should be monitored for hypoprothrombinemic effects, since chloral hydrate potentiates oral anticoagulants.

The nurse should instruct clients with diabetes to use Tes-Tape or Clinitest tables for urine testing or blood glucose testing, because chloral hydrate can cause a false-positive reaction with Benedict's or Fehling's solution.

ethchlorvynol (Placidyl)

Mechanism of action. CNS depressant effects are similar to chloral hydrate and barbiturates. Exact mechanism of action is unknown.

Indications. Sedative-hypnotic.

Pharmacokinetics

Absorption. Good from GI tract

Distribution. Highly localized in lipid or fat tissues; has been located in the CSF, brain, bile, liver, kidneys, and spleen

Metabolism. 90% metabolized in the liver; some metabolism also occurs in the kidneys

Half-life. Approximately 10 to 20 hours

Onset of action. Within 15 to 60 minutes

Duration of action. Approximately 5 hours

Excretion. Kidneys

Side effects/adverse reactions. See Table 13-6.

Significant drug interactions. See information for chloral hydrate on p. 263.

Dosage and administration. See Table 13-8.

Pregnancy safety. FDA Category C.

TABLE 13-8   Ethclorovynol Dosage and Administration

Adults	Elderly	Children
Sedative-hypnotic, 500-1000 mg orally at bedtime.	May require decreased dosage because this group may be more sensitive to this drug.	Not available.

NURSING CONSIDERATIONS

The drug may produce transient giddiness and ataxia in some clients because it is absorbed rapidly. The symptoms should be lessened by administering the drug with milk or food.

If the client awakens in the early morning hours after a bedtime dose of ethchlorvynol, a single additional dose of 100 to 200 mg may be administered.

The nurse should check to see that the dosage for elderly, debilitated clients is reduced to the smallest effective amount.

As with similar drugs, the nurse should inform the client that driving or operating any machinery that requires alertness should be avoided. The effects of the drug could last at least 5 hours.

See the general nursing considerations for sedatives and hypnotics.

glutethimide (Doriden)

Mechanism of action. CNS depressant similar to barbiturates. The mechanism of action is unknown.
Indications. Sedative-hypnotic.
Pharmacokinetics
Absorption. Irregular from the GI tract
Distribution. Mostly in lipid or fat tissues, has also been detected in the brain, liver, bile, and kidneys
Metabolism. Liver
Half-life. Approximately 10 to 12 hours
Onset of action. Within ½ hour
Duration of action. 4 to 8 hours
Excretion. Kidneys
Side effects/adverse reactions. See Table 13-6.
Significant drug interactions. See information for chloral hydrate on p. 263.
Dosage and administration. See Table 13-9.
Pregnancy safety. FDA Category C.

NURSING CONSIDERATIONS

Glutethimide can decrease bowel activity, so the nurse should take actions to help prevent constipation. Dependence on a laxative can lead to lazy bowel. Therefore the nurse should encourage fluids, fruits, roughage, and exercise.

See general nursing considerations for sedative-hypnotic drugs.

meprobamate (Equanil, Miltown, Meditran✹, Neo-Tran✹)

Mechanism of action. CNS depressant similar to barbiturates. Exact mechanism of action is unknown. It appears to act at the hypothalamus, thalamus, limbic system, and spinal cord.
Indications. Antianxiety.

Pharmacokinetics
Absorption. Good
Distribution. Throughout the body
Metabolism. Liver
Half-life. Approximately 10 hours
Excretion. Kidneys
Side effects/adverse reactions. See Table 13-6.
Significant drug interactions. Alcohol and CNS depressant effects; see data for chloral hydrate.
Dosage and administration. See Table 13-10.
Pregnancy safety. Not established.

NURSING CONSIDERATIONS

See general nursing considerations under antianxiety, sedative, and hypnotic agents.

methyprylon (Noludar)

Mechanism of action. Similar to barbiturates. Exact mechanism of action is unknown, but in animals an elevated threshold of arousal centers in the brain stem has been demonstrated.
Indications. Sedative-hypnotic.
Pharmacokinetics
Absorption. Good
Distribution. Little information available
Metabolism. Liver
Half-life. 3 to 6 hours
Onset of action. Within 45 minutes
Duration of action. 5 to 8 hours
Excretion. Kidneys
Side effects/adverse reactions. See Table 13-6.
Significant drug interactions. Alcohol and CNS depressants, see comments on chloral hydrate.
Dosage and administration. See Table 13-11.
Pregnancy safety. FDA Category B.

TABLE 13-9   Glutethimide Dosage and Administration

Adults	Elderly	Children
250-500 mg orally at bedtime to induce hypnotic effect. If necessary, dose may be repeated but only if it is 4 hr or more until arising.	Usually more sensitive to this drug, therefore smaller dosages initially (not exceeding 500 mg) at bedtime are usually prescribed.	Not available for children up to 12 yr.

TABLE 13-10   Meprobamate Dosage and Administration

Adults	Elderly	Children
400 mg orally 3 or 4 times daily or 600 mg twice daily, up to a maximum of 2.4 g.	May be more sensitive to this drug. Lower dosage and/or monitor closely.	Not recommended in children up to 6 yr.

TABLE 13-11   Methyprylon Dosage and Administration

Adults	Elderly	Children
200-400 mg orally at bedtime	May have increased sensitivity to this drug. Monitor closely or use lower dosages.	Not recommended for children less than 12 yr old. Children 12 and older, 50 mg orally at bedtime. Increase dosage if necessary up to 200 mg, according to client's requirements and tolerance of drug.

NURSING CONSIDERATIONS

See general discussion under sedatives and hypnotics.

paraldelhyde (Paral)

Mechanism of action. CNS depressant effects are similar to alcohol, barbiturates, and chloral hydrate. Exact mechanism of action is unknown. Also depresses ascending reticular activating system.

Indications. Sedative-hypnotic, anticonvulsant.

Pharmacokinetics

Absorption. Good from GI tract and IM sites

Distribution. Appears in CSF about ½ to 1 hour after administration, but levels are approximately 25% less than blood serum levels; other tissue distribution not available

Metabolism. Liver

Onset of action. Hypnotic, within 15 minutes

Duration of action. Approximately 8 hours

Excretion. By the lungs; only trace amounts excreted in urine.

Side effects/adverse reactions. See Table 13-6.

Significant drug interactions. Alcohol and CNS depressants, see data on chloral hydrate. Also interacts with disulfiram; that is, disulfiram decreases paraldehyde metabolism, which may lead to increased blood levels of paraldehyde and acetaldehyde. Do not give disulfiram to clients receiving paraldehyde.

Dosage and administration. Anticonvulsant:

Adults: 10-20 ml rectally or up to 12 ml (diluted to a 10% solution) orally via gastric tube, as needed every 4 hours. IM dose is 5 to 10 ml. IV infusion: add 5 ml to 100 ml of sodium chloride (0.9%) solution; administer slowly, not faster than 1 ml/min.

Children: Orally or rectally: 0.3 ml/kg or 12 ml/m² body surface. IM: 0.15 ml/kg or 6 ml/m² body surface. IV: 0.1-0.15 ml/kg diluted in sodium chloride injection (0.9%); administer slowly.

Pregnancy safety. Not established.

NURSING CONSIDERATIONS

Intervention. To give this drug orally, the nurse should dilute it well in a suitable medium such as flavored syrup, iced fruit juice, or milk; fluid should be chilled to minimize the odor and taste. Dilution also decreases gastric irritation.

When given by intramuscular or intravenous route, a glass syringe should be used. Paraldehyde will react with plastic syringes and cause a decomposition to toxic compounds.

For emergencies only (e.g., convulsions) paraldehyde should be administered by intravenous route. Two ml of the drug should be diluted with 4 ml of saline solution and 1 ml of the diluted solution (0.5 ml of active drug); it should be given cautiously over 1 minute.

When giving this drug by the parenteral route (rarely done), the nurse should have available resuscitative equipment in the event of a cardiorespiratory arrest. The client should be kept in the side-lying position to prevent aspiration of bronchial secretions, which are increased after administration of the drug.

Because it cannot be used after the container has been opened for longer than 24 hours, the container should be marked with the date and time it was opened.

The nurse should not use the drug if it is colored or smells like acetic acid.

When giving this drug by the intramuscular route, the nurse should give no more than 5 ml per injection site and rotate the sites. Subcutaneous administration should be avoided because paraldehyde is irritating to the tissues.

The nurse should keep the client in a well-ventilated room, since the exhaled drug can be very pungent.

For rectal doses, paraldehyde should be diluted with 1 to 2 parts of olive oil, cottonseed oil, or normal saline solution to prevent rectal tissue irritation.

Because the solution is extremely volatile, the nurse should avoid contact with eyes, skin, and clothing. The solution and its fumes should be kept away from a heat source, open flame, or spark.

Education. The nurse should prepare the client for the strong unpleasant breath odor that results from administration of the drug and should instruct the client in oral hygiene.

See additional nursing considerations related to use in alcohol withdrawal syndrome, Chapter 9.

propiomazine hydrochloride (Largon)

Mechanism of action. Although the exact mechanism of action is unknown, propiomazine is a phenothiazine with sedative properties at therapeutic dosages.

Indications. Sedative-hypnotic.
Pharmacokinetics
Absorption. Good
Distribution. Probably widely throughout the body, similar to other phenothiazines
Metabolism. Unknown but suspected to be in liver
Time to peak effect. 40 to 60 minutes by way or IM route; 15 to 30 minutes by way of IV route
Duration of action. Approximately 3 to 6 hours
Excretion. Unknown but may be kidneys and biliary tract as occurs with other phenothiazines
Side effects/adverse reactions. See Table 13-6.
Significant drug interactions. Alcohol and CNS depressants, see comments on chloral hydrate. Also, with epinephrine, concurrent use may lead to severe hypotension. Monitor closely.
Dosage and administration. See Table 13-12.
Pregnancy safety. Not established.

NURSING CONSIDERATIONS

The nurse should inject only a clear solution into undamaged veins because this drug causes severe chemical irritation and thrombophlebitis. Intravenous injections are given slowly to prevent transient hypotension. Perivascular extravasation should be avoided because of chemical irritation.

When other sedatives are administered with this drug, dosage should be reduced by one fourth to one half.

The nurse should relieve the side effect of xerostomia by providing mouth care, unless the client has received the medication preoperatively.

The nurse should monitor the client's vital signs, particularly blood pressure, for 5 hours after intramuscular or intravenous administration because of the drug's hypotensive effect. If hypotension occurs, administration of the drug should be discontinued and the physician notified. If vasopressors are required, norepinephrine should be used rather than epinephrine. When epinephrine is used in combination with propiomazine, the vasopressor effect may be reduced or possibly reversed.

TABLE 13-12 propiomazine hydrochloride Dosage and Administration

Adults	Children
Preoperative, 20-40 mg IM or IV; local nerve block or spinal anesthesia adjunct, 10-20 mg IM or IV; obstetrics, 20-40 mg IM or IV, may repeat in 3 hr if needed	For sedation before surgery, before anesthesia, or postoperatively: children up to 27 kg, 0.55-1.1 mg/kg body weight IM or IV; children 2-4 yr, 10 mg IM or IV; children 4-6 yr, 15 mg IM or IV; children 6-12 yr, 25 mg IM or IV

KEY TERMS

amnesic effect, page 249
antianxiety, page 245
anxiolytic, page 245
cardioversion, page 249
hypnotic, page 245
insomnia, page 248
monosynaptic reflex, page 246
non-REM sleep, page 246
paradoxical reaction, page 248
polysynaptic reflex, page 246
REM sleep, page 246
sedative, page 245

BIBLIOGRAPHY

American Hospital Formulary Service: AHFS drug information 88, Bethesda, 1988, American Society of Hospital Pharmacists Inc.

Ameer B and Greenblatt DJ: Lorazepam: a review of its clinical pharmacological properties and therapeutic uses, Drugs 21:161, 1981.

Anxiety, Fla Pharm J, March 1980, p. 22.

Betts TA and Birtle J: Effect of two hypnotic drugs on actual driving performance next morning, Br Med J 285:852, 1982.

Brocklehurst, JC: Geriatric pharmacology and therapeutics, Oxford, 1984, Blackwell Scientific Publications.

Burgess KE: Cerebral depressants: their effects and safe administration, Nursing '85 15:47, 1985.

Cornoni-Huntley J and others: Established population for epidemiologic studies of the elderly. Pub No 86-2443, Silver Springs, Md, 1986, National Institute on Aging, US Department of Health and Human Services.

Csernansky JG and Hollister LE: Withdrawal reaction following therapeutic doses of benzodiazepines, Hosp Formul 18:900, 1983.

Dolly FR and Block AJ: Effect of flurazepam on sleep-disordered breathing and nocturnal oxygen desaturation in asymptomatic subjects, Am J Med 73:239, 1982.

Dominquez RA and Goldstein BJ: 25 years of benzodiazepine experience: clinical commentary on use, abuse, and withdrawal, Hosp Formul 20:1000, 1985.

Dommisse CF and Hayes PE: Current concepts in clinical therapeutics: anxiety disorders. Part 2, Clin Pharm, 6(3):196, 1987.

Fagan DR and Illsley SS: Benzodiazepine hypnotics: a comparative review of recently approved agents, Hosp Formul 20:491, 1985.

Filligim JM: Double-blind evaluation of temazepam, flurazepam, and placebo in geriatric insomniacs, Clin Ther 4(5):369, 1982.

Finley R, editor: Insomnia in the elderly: principles in management, Drug Ther Elderly 1(1):1, 1986.

Gilman AG and others, editors: Goodman and Gilman's the pharmacological basis of therapeutics, ed 7, New York, 1985, Macmillan Publishing Co.

Hicks R and others: The pharmacokinetics of psychotropic medication in the elderly: a review, J Clin Psychiatry 42:374, 1981.

Lader MH: Short-acting benzodiazepines in insomnia, J Clin Psychiatry 44:47, 1983.

Methaqualone abuse implicated in injuries and death nationwide: medical news, JAMA 246:813, 1981.

Muzet, A, Johnson, LC, and Spinweber, CL: Benzodiazepine hypnotics increase heart rate during sleep, Sleep 5(3):256, 1982.

Owen JA: Alprazolam: a new benzodiazepine approved for anxiety disorders, Hosp Formul 18:950, 1983.

Pakes GE and others: Triazolam: a review of its pharmacological properties and therapeutics efficacy in patients with insomnia, Drugs 22:81, 1981.

Ramsey R: The aging kidney: impact on drug therapy, Drug Ther Elderly 1(6):23, 1986.

Reynolds, R, Lloyd, DA, and Slinger, RP: Cholestatic jaundice induced by flurazepam hydrochloride, Can Med Assoc J 124(7):893, 1981.

Scharf MB and others: Lorezepam: efficacy, side effects, and rebound phenomena, Clin Pharmacol Ther 31(2):175, 1982.

Solomon F and others: Sleeping pills, insomnia and medical practice, N Eng J Med 300(14):803, 1979.

Sussman N: The benzodiazepines: selection and use in treating anxiety, insomnia, and other disorders, Hosp Formul 20:298, 1985.

Tilley S and Weighill VE: How nurse therapists assess and contribute to the management of alcohol and sedative drug use among anxious patients, J Advanced Nurs 11:499, 1986.

Triazolam: a new benzodiazepine for insomnia, Med Lett Drugs Ther 25(631):137, 1983.

Triazolam: the latest FDA approved hypnotic, Int Drug Ther Newsletter 18:1, 1983.

United States Pharmacopeia Convention: Drug information for the health care provider, ed 8, Rockville, Md, The Convention, 1988.

Vacik JP and Palmer GC: The pharmacological basis for rational clinical application of benzodiazepines, Prim Care Dec 1980.

Whaley LF and Wong DL: Nursing care of infants and children, ed 2, St Louis, 1983, The CV Mosby Co.

Wincor MZ: Insomnia and the new benzodiazepines, Clin Pharm 1:425, 1982.

Anticonvulsants

OBJECTIVES

After studying this chapter, the student will be able to:

1. Describe the international classification description of epileptic seizures.

2. Identify observations to be made about a client having a seizure.

3. Discuss the nurse's role in anticonvulsant drug therapy.

4. Identify the major anticonvulsant drug classifications including examples of drugs and their primary method of seizure control activity.

5. List the common side effects/adverse reactions of anticonvulsants.

6. Formulate an appropriate plan of care for the individual client receiving an anticonvulsant drug or drugs.

CLASSIFICATION OF EPILEPSY

Epilepsy occurs in approximately 0.5% to 1% of the population. In 50% of the cases, the cause of epilepsy is unknown; in this instance it is called **primary** or **idiopathic epilepsy. Secondary epilepsy** may be traced to trauma, infections, cerebrovascular disorder, or other illnesses that contribute to epilepsy. Detection of contributing factors has been advanced by computed tomography (CT scans) and nuclear brain scans.

Epilepsy is regarded as a symptom of disease or disorder of the brain rather than a disease in itself. It is associated with marked changes in the electric activity of the cerebral cortex, and these alterations are often detected in the electroencephalogram. Therefore the EEG is often a valuable aid to the physician in making a diagnosis. In addition to the EEG, other laboratory tests such as routine blood and urine series, calcium, blood sugar, electrolytes, phosphorus, and sometimes renal and hepatic function tests are done to assist in the determination of the diagnosis.

Epileptic seizures vary and have been traditionally classified according to grand mal seizures, petit mal seizures, jacksonian epilepsy, and psychomotor attacks. A new classification of seizures, however, has been implemented and is being more extensively used because it more adequately describes the seizure of the client. It is called the International Classification of Seizures. Table 14-1 presents it with the traditional terms and characteristics. For

TABLE 14-1   International Classification of Seizures

Type	Characteristics
Partial seizures	
Simple	1. No impairment of consciousness
	2. Motor symptoms (formerly called jacksonian)
	3. Sensory (hallucinations of sight, hearing, or taste); somatosensory (tingling)
	4. Autonomic—autonomic nervous system responses
	5. Psychic (personality changes)
Complex	1. Impaired consciousness
	2. Cognitive (memory impairment, confusion)
	3. Affective (bizzare behavioral effects)
	4. Psychosensory (automatisms—repetition, purposeless behaviors)
	5. Psychomotor (complex symptoms that may include an aura, automatism [i.e., chewing, swallowing movements], unreal feelings, bizzare behaviors, and motor seizures)
	6. Compound (tonic, clonic, or tonic-clonic seizures)
Secondarily generalized	
Generalized seizures	1. Widespread involvement of both cerebral hemispheres
	2. Tonic-clonic seizures (formerly called grand mal)
	3. Tonic (sustained contractions of large muscle groups)
	4. Clonic (various dysrhythmic contractions in the body)
	5. Myoclonic (unaltered consciousness, isolated clonic contractions)
	6. Absence (formerly called petit mal—brief loss of consciousness for a few seconds, no confusion, EEG demonstrates 3/second spike wave patterns.
	7. Atonic (head drop or falling down symptoms)
Unclassified	1. Available data incomplete, inadequate, or lacks classification status (such as neonatal seizures)

the purpose of this text, both seizure classifications will be used.

Partial simple motor (jacksonian) epilepsy is described by some as a type of **focal seizure;** it is associated with irritation of a specific part of the brain. A single part, such as a finger or an extremity, may jerk and such movements may end spontaneously or spread over the whole muscu-lature. Consciousness may not be lost unless the seizure develops into a generalized convulsion.

Partial complex (psychomotor) seizures are characterized by brief alterations in consciousness, unusual stereotyped movements (such as chewing or swallowing movements) repeated over and over, temperamental changes, confusion, and feelings of unreality. These seizures are often associated with grand mal seizures and are likely to be resistant to therapy with drugs.

Generalized absence, simple or complex (petit mal) seizures are most often seen in childhood and consist of temporary lapses in consciousness that last for a few seconds. Clients appear to stare into space or daydream, are inattentive, and may exhibit a few rhythmic movements of the eyes (slight blinking), head, or hands. They do not convulse. They may have many attacks in a single day. EEG records a 3/second spike wave pattern. Sometimes an attack of generalized absence seizures is followed by a generalized tonic-clonic–type seizure; when the child reaches adulthood, other types of seizures may occur. Research is exploring the possibility of using drug combination therapies for childhood seizures as a prophylactic measure to avoid the development of other seizure patterns in adulthood.

Tonic-clonic generalized (grand mal) epilepsy is the type most commonly seen. Such attacks may be characterized by an aura and the sudden loss of consciousness. The aura is specific to the individual; that is, it may consist of numbness, visual disturbance, or a particular form of dizziness that warns the client of an approaching seizure. The client falls forcefully and has a series of **tonic** (stiffening) and **clonic** (rapid, synchronous jerking) muscular contractions. The eyes roll upward, the arms flex, and the legs extend. The force of the muscular contractions causes air to be forced out of the lungs, which accounts for the cry that the client may make on falling. Respiration is suspended temporarily, the skin becomes diaphoretic and cyanotic, perspiration and saliva flow, and the client may froth at the mouth and bite the tongue if it gets caught between the teeth. Incontinence may occur. When the seizure subsides, the client regains partial consciousness, may complain of aching, and then tends to fall into a deep sleep.

Status epilepticus is a recurrent seizure generally lasting 30 minutes or more without an intervening stay of consciousness. A 10% or 20% mortality rate results from anoxia in this medical emergency. *The major cause of status epilepticus is noncompliance with the drug regimen;* other causes include cerebral infarction, cerebral infection, or low blood concentration of calcium or glucose. The treatment of status epilepticus is discussed later in this chapter.

Mixed seizures are seen in some clients who have more than one type of seizure disorder. This is significant because different types of seizures respond specifically to certain anticonvulsant drugs. The aim of therapy is to find the drug or drugs that will effectively control the seizures with a minimum of undesirable side effects and restore physiologic homeostasis to arrest convulsive activity.

RELATIONSHIP OF AGE TO SEIZURES

A relationship of age to onset of an epileptic seizure state exists. Most clients diagnosed as having epilepsy have their initial seizure before the age of 20; however, seizures may have an onset at any age in life. Idiopathic (undefined, unascertainable, or genetic in origin or cause) seizures are often diagnosed between the ages of 5 and 20. Onset before or after this age period is often from nonidiopathic (identifiable, ascertainable) causes and is termed symptomatic (acquired, organic) epilepsy.

Neonatal seizures occur in newborn children less than 1 month old. Among the more common causes of neonatal seizures in this age-group are the following: congenital defects or malformation of the brain, abnormality or infections (meningitis, encephalitis, abscess) within the CNS, hypoxia (in utero or during delivery), premature birth, and defects in metabolism. These epileptic seizures are also referred to as **organic, symptomatic,** or **acquired** because they may be caused by an identifiable preceding condition or cause.

In infants less than 2 years of age the seizure types most frequently diagnosed include generalized tonic-clonic seizures and partial seizures. The atonic epileptic seizure seen in later development (ages 2 to 5 years) may be preceded by infantile spasms in those less than 2 years. The infantile spasm is not classified as a type of epileptic seizure itself. Among the more common causes of infant seizures are those causes as seen in the neonatal stage and additionally injury in the perinatal period, infection, exposure to toxins (in utero caused by maternal exposure or drug use, misuse, or abuse), maternal exposure to x-rays, and postnatal trauma.

In children 2 to 5 years old the seizure types that are frequently diagnosed include generalized tonic-clonic seizures and atonic seizures. The causes are similar to those mentioned in newborns and infants with the addition of chronic diseases involving the CNS. The parents of the child may wrongly believe the child has a behavioral disorder rather than a treatable seizure disorder.

In the age group 6 years and older, brain tumors and vascular disease may cause seizures. Sometimes the convulsive seizure is associated with a brain infection, head trauma, fever, growth of scar tissue, cerebrovascular disease, the presence of a toxin or a poison, or drug withdrawal.

In children 5 to 16 years old the seizure types that emerge in diagnosis are absence seizures and generalized tonic-clonic seizures, which may be idiopathic in origin. Seizure types such as partial, myoclonic, and less commonly generalized tonic-clonic seizures may be caused by neurologic diseases, infection, postnatal trauma, or head trauma (accident or sport).

Within the age group 16 to 25 years, the generalized seizures may be idiopathic in origin. The partial seizure and less commonly seen generalized seizures may result from the use of alcohol, social recreational drug use, drug abuse or misuse, or head injury.

In clients over 20 years of age, the seizures emerging often are of the generalized type, which may be idiopathic. Also seen are partial seizure and less commonly generalized seizures, which may have been precipitated by trauma to the head or a tumor of the brain, or, in middle aged and elderly clients, a cerebrovascular disease.

DRUG THERAPY

The effectiveness of anticonvulsant drugs is often measured by the amount of increased voltage necessary to provoke an electroconvulsion in an animal who has previously received the anticonvulsant to be tested or by the degree of their antagonism to chemical substances capable of producing convulsions. Pentylenetetrazol is a drug against which anticonvulsants are measured for effectiveness.

The anticonvulsants may be classified into the following groups:

Barbiturates—phenobarbital, mephobarbital, metharbital; amobarbital, pentobarbital, and secobarbital are for parenteral use only

Hydantoins—phenytoin, mephenytoin, ethotoin

Succinimides—ethosuximide, methsuximide, phensuximide

Oxazolidinediones—paramethadione, trimethadione

Benzodiazepines—clonazepam, diazepam, clorazepate, lorazepam

Miscellaneous—valproic acid, carbamazepine, divalproex, primidone, phenacemide, acetazolamide, magnesium sulfate

The exact mode and site of action of these drugs are still unknown at the molecular level. Stabilization of the cell membrane by altering cation transport (sodium, potassium, calcium) either by increasing sodium efflux or decreasing sodium influx is a proposed mechanism (AHFS, 1988). The main pharmacologic effects are (1) to increase motor cortex threshold to reduce its response to incoming electric or chemical stimulation, or (2) to depress or reduce the spread of a seizure discharge from its focus (origin) by depressing synaptic transport or decreasing nerve conduction. For example, hydantoins suppress the seizure by stabilizing cell membrane excitability, thus reducing the spread of seizure discharge, whereas barbiturates reduce neuron excitability and increase the motor cortex threshold to electric stimulation.

Although there is no ideal anticonvulsant drug, if there were, a number of characteristics would be considered highly desirable:

1. The drug should be highly effective but exhibit a low incidence of toxicity.
2. The drug should be effective against more than one type of seizure and for mixed seizures.
3. The drug should be long acting and nonsedative so that the client is not incapacitated with sleep or excessive drowsiness.
4. The drug should be well tolerated by the client and inexpensive, since the client may have to take it for years or for the rest of his or her life.
5. Tolerance to the therapeutic effects of the drug should not develop.
6. The drug should control seizures and permit a client to function effectively in any environment.

The present-day drugs that are considered especially satisfactory and safe are phenobarbital and phenytoin sodium. The barbiturates have been discussed (see Chapter 13), but their use as anticonvulsants is emphasized again. They are an important group of drugs for this purpose, especially the longer-acting agents. Phenobarbital is effective against most types of epileptic seizures except certain absence types. It is considered one of the safest anticonvulsants. Its chief disadvantage is that it must often be given in doses that produce apathy and sleepiness.

PHARMACOKINETICS

See Table 14-2. Although anticonvulsant agents are usually given orally, there are a few parenteral forms. These are reserved for occasions when the parenteral form is the best choice of therapy. Table 14-3 lists these condi-

TABLE 14-2 Pharmacokinetic Overview of Selected Anticonvulsant Drugs

Generic name	Trade name	Fate	Therapeutic plasma levels in adults (μg/ml)	Serum half-life (hr)	Time to reach steady-state
carbamaze-pine	Tegretol Apo-Carbamaze-pine♣ Mazepine♣	Absorption: slow and variable Metabolism: liver Excretion: urine, feces	4-12 (in adults)	1 dose: 25-65 Multidose: Adults: 12-17	40 hr (range 8-55 hr)
clonazepam	Clonopin Rivotril♣	Absorption: good Metabolism: liver Excretion: urine	0.020-0.080	20-44	4-8 days
divalproex	Depakote Epival♣	Absorption: 1-3 hr Metabolism: liver Excretion: urine, small amount from feces and lungs	50-100	6-16	30-85 hr
ethosuxim-ide	Zarontin Petinimid♣ Suxinutin♣	Absorption: good Metabolism: liver Excretion: urine, bile, feces	40-100	Adults: 56-60 Children: 30-36	Adults: 12 days Children: 6 days
methsuxim-ide	Celontin Petinutin♣	Absorption: good Metabolism: liver Excretion: urine	10-40	1-3 Active metabolite: 36-45	5-15 hr
phenobarbi-tal	Luminal and various other manufacturers	Absorption: good Metabolism: liver Excretion: urine	10-40	Adults: 53-118 Children: 40-70	Adults: 10-25 days Children: 8-15 days
phenytoin	Dilantin Epanutin♣ Eptoin♣	Absorption: orally, slow; poor in neonates Metabolism: liver Excretion: urine and feces	10-20	Adults: 14-22 (range 7-42)	7-10 days
primidone	Mysoline Sertan♣ Mylepsine♣	Absorption: good Metabolism: liver Excretion: urine	5-12	primidone: 3-24 phenobarbital: 72-144 PEMA: 24-48	
valproic acid	Depakene Epilim♣ Ergenyl♣ Urekene♣	Absorption: complete and rapid Metabolism: kidney Excretion: urine; small amount from lungs and feces	50-100	Adults: 6-16 Children: 4-14	Adults: 30-85 hr Children: 20-70 hr

TABLE 14-3 Parenteral Use of Anticonvulsant Agents

Parenteral drug	Use
barbiturates, especially phenobarbital, also amobarbital, pentobarbital sodium, and secobarbital sodium	Eclampsia, status epilepticus, severe recurrent seizures, tetanus, convulsant drug toxicity, other convulsive states
phenytoin	Status epilepticus, seizure during neurosurgery
magnesium sulfate	Severe toxemias of pregnancy (pre-eclampsia and eclampsia)
paraldehyde injection	Status epilepticus, tetanus, eclampsia, convulsant drug toxicity
benzodiazepines: diazepam, lorazepam	Status epilepticus; severe, recurrent seizures

tions or situations and the parenteral drugs indicated for the treatment of each.

DOSAGE ADJUSTMENTS

Anticonvulsant drugs may exhibit varying blood levels in different clients after each client has received the same dose. This variation results from a complex of interrelated factors including individual client compliance; individual absorption, metabolism, distribution, and excretion, which may be caused by genetic and/or environmental factors; concomitant ailments, such as renal or hepatic dysfunctions; concurrent medication; diet; and physical status. Certain drugs require an adjusted dosage to obtain optimal therapeutic effects, and this dosage may have wide client variation.

Therapeutic dosage ranges are intended to serve merely as rough guides to therapy; they are not firm limits. The ranges provide a point from which the dosage of a drug may be individualized to account for the extremes in variation to response and adverse effects. The client beginning anticonvulsant therapy should have serum levels measured to establish his or her individual level/dose ratio. This level tends to be a constant measure for an individual, although it varies considerably among clients. The time required to reach a steady serum level is generally about four to five times the elimination half-life of a drug. A convenient time for serum level measurement is 1 month after initiating therapy, since levels measured much earlier may be lower than the steady-state level finally achieved.

The **serum half-life** of a drug (the time required for the serum level to drop 50% when no additional drug is administered) is a measure of its rate of excretion and depends on the client's age. As discussed in Chapter 4, the pharmacokinetics of a drug are affected by age. For exam-

ple, drug metabolism is relatively slow in the neonate, but in infants and young children it is higher on a milligram per kilogram of body weight basis than it is for an adult. Usually the elderly, with a decrease in their metabolism, require a lower dosage schedule. (See Chapter 8)

One of the characteristics of the anticonvulsant drugs is that either the parent drug or the active metabolite has a long serum half-life, so the exact daily medication schedule is seldom critical. Administration of these drugs may be one to three times daily.

The first serum concentration after the first intravenous dose is half the peak value attained during long-term administration. Therefore the client can attain steady-state serum concentration quickly if the first intravenous dose is twice the maintenance dose. In adults, for example, a loading (intravenous) dose of phenytoin (1000 mg or 13 to 14 mg/kg, which is twice the usual maintenance dose of 300 to 400 mg/ half-life of about 24 hours) will produce a therapeutic serum concentration of 10 to 20 μg/ml. The intravenous route is necessary because phenytoin is absorbed very slowly and erratically by the intramuscular route because the water solubility of the drug decreases and phenytoin crystals precipitate in the muscle. A high degree of local irritation has also been reported with intramuscular injection.

THE NURSE'S ROLE IN ANTICONVULSANT DRUG THERAPY

A client for whom anticonvulsants have been prescribed is treated most effectively with a holistic approach. This client has many special problems, including the fear of sudden loss of physical and emotional control and the stigma concerning seizures. In recent years, emphasis has been placed on public education regarding epilepsy to dispel the myths associated with it. This individual needs information about the seizure condition and its management, along with psychosocial support from the nurse. The client should understand that the condition can be controlled or modified with medication. The goal is to attain maximum seizure control with minimal medication side effects. The anticonvulsant or combination of such drugs prescribed depends on the *type* of seizure, whether the client is having *more than one type of*

RESOURCE FOR BOTH THE CLIENT AND THE NURSE

Epilepsy Foundation of America
4351 Garden City Drive
Landover, Maryland 20785
(301) 459-3700

seizure, or whether the seizures are *difficult to control.* Finding the appropriate regimen for each client takes time.

Check the chart of major side effects and adverse reactions (Table 14-4); it is divided according to frequency, importance, and recommendations regarding when to report such effects to the prescribing physician.

Assessment. Alone with a general assessment and drug history, assessment of the client with a convulsive disorder includes data specific to the seizures. These data include the number of seizures within a specific time; precipitating events or activities; presence of sensations or perceptions that the client experiences before a seizure, called an aura; and the character of seizures (see box below). Often the nurse will not be present when a seizure has occurred. In this situation family, friends, or other witnesses may provide valuable information about the seizure. The most common medical test to evaluate seizure activity is the electroencephalogram (EEG), a recording of electrical activity generated by the brain made by placing electrodes on the scalp. Subjective data to be obtained include the client's understanding and reaction to the convulsive disorder and drug therapy.

Intervention. Anticonvulsant drugs should be administered intravenously in emergency situations (such as status epilepticus) because of the slow absorption from the intramuscular injection site and the low peak serum levels achieved. The anticonvulsant drugs should be administered using as long an interval between doses as possible, depending on their half-life. The anticonvulsant drugs that have an elimination half-life of 24 hours or more gen-erally need to be administered only once a day to maintain a therapeutic serum concentration. The daily dose may be administered at bedtime to overcome the sedation seen with peak levels of anticonvulsant drugs. In a non-emergency situation it is best to make changes in drug therapy with one drug at a time. The nurse and the client must be aware that each time a new anticonvulsant drug is started or the dose of a drug is increased or decreased, it takes four to five elimination half-life intervals (so the concentration of the drug has dropped by 95%) to reach the new steady-state serum concentration and to achieve the total therapeutic effect of the new drug regimen.

Many of the anticonvulsants have known blood levels of an optimal therapeutic range, that is, the level of medication needed to control seizures (see Table 14-2). When serum levels of anticonvulsants are ordered, they should be scheduled for a time greater than 8 hours since the last dose of medication was given.

Education. The client should understand that anticonvulsants take days or weeks to reach an effective level in the body. A missed dose may result in a seizure in a few days, and taking a dose will not prevent an impending seizure.

Although the client may be seizure free for some time and may perceive that a "cure" has occurred, the medication dose should not be decreased or stopped without consultation with the physician.

During initiation or change of therapy, the client should avoid activities that require coordination and alertness until response to the drug therapy has been determined.

OBSERVATIONS TO BE MADE ABOUT A PERSON HAVING A SEIZURE

Aura	Presence or absence, nature if present; ability of patient to describe it (somatic, visceral, psychic)	Relaxation (sleep)	Duration and behavior
Cry	Presence or absence	Postictal phase	Duration; general behavior; ability to remember anything about the seizure; orientation; pupillary changes; headache; injuries present
Onset	Site of initial body movements; deviation of head and eyes; chewing and salivation; posture of body; sensory changes	Duration of entire seizure	
Tonic and clonic phases	Movements of body as to progression; skin color and airway; pupillary changes; incontinence; duration of each phase	Level of consciousness	Length of unconsciousness if present

From Phipps, WJ, Long, BC, and Woods, NF: Medical-surgical nursing: concepts and clinical practice, ed 3, St. Louis, 1987, The CV Mosby Co.

TABLE 14-4 Anticonvulsants: Side Effects/Adverse Reactions

Drug(s)	Side effects*	Adverse reactions†
barbiturates (phenobarbital, mephobarbital, metharbital)	More frequent: drowsiness, dizziness, tiredness, hangover-type effects Less common: nausea, vomiting, constipation, headaches, insomnia, increased irritability, nervousness	Rashes; hives; fever; sore throat; sores on lips or in mouth; pain in chest, muscles, bones, or joints; confusion; depression or paradoxical excitement in children or elderly clients (exfoliative dermatitis; Stevens-Johnson syndrome; osteomalacia or rickets with chronic dosing)
hydantoins (phenytoin, ethotoin, mephenytoin)	More frequent: hirsutism (excessive hair growth seen primarily with phenytoin), constipation, nausea, vomiting, drowsiness, dizziness Less common: headaches, insomnia, distortion of facial features (thick lips, broadening of nasal tip, jaw protuberance), diarrhea (mostly with ethotoin)	Gingival hyperplasia (bleeding, sensitive or overgrow on gum tissue); rarely seen with ethotoin Slurred speech, nystagmus, hand trembling, increased irritability or nervousness, skin rash, behavioral changes, ataxia, blood dyscrasias (thrombocytopenia), and skin rashes reported more often with mephenytoin
succinimides (ethosuximide, methsuximide, phensuximide)	More frequent: headaches, epigastric pain, anorexia, hiccups, nausea, vomiting Less common: drowsiness, lethargy, irritability, dizziness	Rash, pruritus (possibly Stevens-Johnson syndrome), mood changes, sore throat and fever (agranulocytosis), increase in bleeding or bruising (thrombocytopenia)
oxazolidinediones (paramethadione, trimethadione)	More frequent: headache, drowsiness, dizziness, photophobia Less frequent: loss of appetite, weight loss, alopecia, pruritus, lethargy, nausea, vomiting	Visual changes, edema, rash, sore throat and fever, enlarged lymph glands, increased bleeding and bruising, and hepatitis
benzodiazepines (clonazepam, diazepam, clorazepate)	More frequent: drowsiness, ataxia, lethargy Less frequent: blurred vision, diplopia, constipation, headache, nausea, vomiting, incontinence, slurred speech, dry mouth	Insomnia, hallucinations, confusion, exictability, paradoxical rage, depression, muscle weakness, vivid dreams, muscle weakness, sore throat, fever, increased bleeding or bruising, hepatic dysfunction
miscellaneous valproic acid divalproex	More frequent: tremors, mild gastric distress, diarrhea, weight gain, irregular menses Less frequent: dizziness, drowsiness, alopecia (transient), headache, depression, constipation, hyperactivity, increased irritability	Hepatotoxicity (usually during first 6 months of therapy), abdominal cramps, nausea and vomiting, anorexia, ataxia, rash, increased bleeding or bruising, hepatitis, loss of seizure control
carbamazepine	More frequent: vertigo, drowsiness, nausea or vomiting, dizziness Less frequent: Dry mouth, headache, diarrhea, myalgia, arthralgia, leg cramps, photosensitivity, altered skin pigmentation, alopecia, anorexia, increased sweating	Increased release of antiduretic hormone resulting in hyponatremia, activation of latent psychosis, blurred vision, diplopia, confusion, hives, pruritus, rash, oculomotor disturbances, nystagmus, visual hallucinations, lethargy, weakness, hostility, stupor, edema
primidone	More frequent: drowsiness, ataxia, dizziness Less frequent: anorexia, headaches, impotence, nausea, or vomiting that usually decreases with continued drug usage	Rash, edema, swelling of eyelids, hives, unusual fatigue, confusion, restlessness, increased excitability (paradoxical reaction in children and elderly), difficult breathing
phenacemide	Anorexia, weight loss, drowsiness, tiredness, dizziness, insomnia, headache, muscle pain	An extremely toxic drug; has produced hepatitis, jaundice, fatal liver necrosis, severe bone marrow depression (aplastic anemia, agranulocytosis), acute psychoses, increase in suicide potential, nephritis

*If side effects continue, increase, or disturb the client, inform the physician.
†If adverse reactions occur, contact the physician, since medical intervention may be necessary.

Continued

TABLE 14-4 Anticonvulsants: Side Effects/Adverse Reactions—cont'd

Drug(s)	Side effects*	Adverse reactions†
acetazolamide	More frequent: diarrhea, increased frequency of urination, anorexia, metallic taste, nausea, vomiting, weight loss, paresthesias Less frequent: Drowsiness, nervousness, fatigue	Fever, sore throat, increased bleeding or bruising, rash, hives, confusion, depression, tinnitus, transient myopia, trembling, severe muscle weakness, shortness of breath, malaise
magnesium sulfate		Reduced respiratory rate, depression of reflexes, flushing, hypotension, hypothermia, ECG changes (adverse effects require *immediate* notification of physician and treatment)

ndx Selected Nursing Diagnosis for the Client on Anticonvulsive Medications

Nursing diagnosis	Outcome criteria	Nursing interventions
Knowledge deficit related to newly prescribed or altered anticonvulsant drug therapy	The client will describe: the seizure condition; how the drug therapy relates to the condition; how and when to take the medications; common drug interactions; safety precautions; common side effects and which of these warrant reporting; storage requirements of the drugs; demonstrate less anxiety related to fear of the unknown, loss of control, and misconceptions	Assess learning needs and learning readiness Plan with the client and family for the achievement of realistic goals Provide information to meet outcome criteria
Noncompliance related to medication regimen	The client will: self-administer medications safely and accurately	Determine the client's reasons for noncompliance and take appropriate teaching/counseling interventions Provide needed drug information concerning rationales for the specific client's seizure status Discuss the increased possibility of seizures with noncompliance
Potential for injury related to effects of anticonvulsant drug therapy	The client will: maintain anticonvulsant drug therapy without untoward side effects, adverse reactions, and toxicity	Administer drug safely and accurately Observe client for drowsiness, ataxia, behavioral changes, slurred speech, mental confusion, vertigo, and excessive sedation (see drug monographs for drug specific side effects/adverse reactions) Instruct client about symptoms to be reported Explain the importance of Medic Alert card/tag Discourage self-altering of medication regimen Caution against activities requiring coordination and alertness until responses to drugs are known

The client should be encouraged to use moderation in his or her life-style, follow an appropriate diet, and get sufficient rest and exercise. Stressful situations should be avoided; if this is not possible, the physician should be notified for dosage adjustment in ongoing stressful conditions. Drinking alcohol and taking OTC medications should be cautioned against (see specific drug for interactions or effects).

The client and family should be taught seizure precautions, and the importance of wearing a Medic Alert tag/card (obtainable at local pharmacy) should be explained.

Medications should be stored at home away from light and heat and out of the reach of children, since overdosage is especially dangerous in children. Outdated and discontinued medications should be flushed down the toilet.

The nurse should suggest that the family keep a daily record of the number and type of seizures that occur during drug therapy. This is one measure of the efficacy of the medication(s) and will help the physician determine if an increased dosage or an additional agent is needed.

Evaluation. Therapeutic alternatives are selected (monotherapy or polytherapy) that best control the client's seizure. Therapeutic drug monitoring includes interpreting results of serum concentrations with the client's clinical response. This monitoring has reduced the need of polydrug anticonvulsant therapy and added greater efficiency in drug selection for each client. A significant number of clients have seizure recurrences after treatment withdrawal. The withdrawal procedure should be initiated with close medical supervision (within a hospital), especially when polydrug anticonvulsant therapy is being adjusted or when inadequate seizure control is recognized. Seizures may occur even after long periods that were seizure free. Fewer seizures occur when the withdrawal is planned or gradual or when the dose is reduced to minimal maintenance therapy.

Increased anticonvulsant serum levels may signal impending toxic effects. Generally, adverse effects are more serious at higher serum levels. Maintaining a serum level within the therapeutic range is a challenge for some clients. The challenge surfaces when other drugs are added or deleted from the client's regimen, a client is noncompliant, there is an organ system dysfunction as seen in the hepatorenal systems, or undesirable drug effects cause the client to withdraw from drug therapy. When the client becomes fully informed about the drug therapy and need for serum concentrations within the therapeutic range, this may reduce therapeutic failures caused by noncompliance or adverse effects. Epilepsy may worsen during pregnancy, and status epilepticus increases in frequency during gestation and labor. Some of the anticonvulsants appear in breast milk. Emotional stress (psychologic, occupational, physiologic, marital, economic) may influence seizure frequency.

BARBITURATES

Barbiturates, especially phenobarbital, have been used for many years for the treatment of generalized tonic-clonic and partial seizures. This class of medications is relatively inexpensive, efficacious, and has a low incidence of side effects. Phenobarbital is one of two anticonvulsants most commonly prescribed in the United States; the other is phenytoin.

Mephobarbital (Mebaral) is converted by the liver-metabolizing enzymes to phenobarbital, whereas metharbital (Gemonil) is metabolized to barbital in the liver. All three barbiturates are long-acting compounds, but there is little or no advantage in using the latter two instead of phenobarbital, the most commonly prescribed barbiturate.

The parenteral dosage forms of amobarbital, pentobarbital, and secobarbital have been used in emergency treatment of seizures (Table 14-3). The oral dosage forms are generally not indicated for the treatment of seizure disorders because of their potent sedative-hypnotic effects.

Mechanism of action. Sedative, hypnotic, and anticonvulsant effects may be the result of nonselective CNS depression or of the ability of barbiturates to increase and/or mimic GABA-inhibiting action at the synapses. Barbiturates also increase the threshold of the motor cortex to electric activation.

Indications. Treatment of anxiety (although generally barbiturates have been replaced by the benzodiazepines), insomnia, epilepsy, acute convulsive states, and febrile convulsions and as an adjunct to anesthesia (preoperative use)

Pharmacokinetics. See Table 14-2. (See also Table 13-5.)

Side effects/adverse reactions. See Table 14-4. Also, apnea, bronchospasm, and respiratory depression may occur following rapidly administered, intravenous injections of barbiturates. Severe symptoms of withdrawal may occur in individuals who have a barbiturate dependency from prolonged use at high dosages. Anxiety, trembling, nausea, vomiting, insomnia, orthostatic hypotension, seizures, hallucinations, and even death may result if the drug is withdrawn abruptly. Gradual withdrawal in a controlled setting is usually recommended for the treatment of dependence.

Significant drug interactions. The following effects may occur when barbiturates, especially phenobarbital, is given with the drugs listed below:

Drug	Possible Effect and Management
adrenocorticoids or corticosteroids (prednisone, etc.)	Effects may be decreased because of enhanced metabolism produced by barbiturates. Dosage adjustment may be necessary.
alcohol, anesthetics, CNS depressants (sedatives, hypnotics, narcotics)	Enhanced CNS depressant effects, respiratory depression; use extreme caution in combining such medications. Usually the dosage of one or both drugs should be reduced.
anticoagulants (coumarin or indandione types)	Effects may be decreased because of enhanced metabolism produced by barbiturates. Closely monitor prothrombin time. Dosage adjustment of anticoagulants may be necessary.
hydantoin anticonvulsants	Unpredictable effects on hydantoin metabolism may occur. Serum levels should be closely monitored when drugs are given concurrently.

Drug	Possible Effect and Management
divalproex sodium or valproic acid	Two effects may result from this combination: (1) valproic acid half-life may be decreased, which would require a dosage adjustment to maintain control; or (2) metabolism of barbiturates may be decreased, which can result in elevated barbiturate serum levels and toxicity. Monitor barbiturate levels, since a dosage adjustment may be necessary.
ascorbic acid, vitamin D	An increase in urinary excretion of ascorbic acid is reported. The increased metabolism of vitamin D may lead to a vitamin D deficiency in clients on long-term barbiturate therapy. Supplementation with vitamin D (to prevent osteomalacia) and ascorbic acid may be necessary.

Dosage and administration. See Table 14-5.

Pregnancy safety. Barbiturates have been rated as category D by the FDA. Use during pregnancy has resulted in an increase in fetal abnormalities. Coagulation defects have also been reported (see "Nursing Considerations").

The Nurse's Role in Barbiturate Therapy

Assessment. Combination of these drugs with alcohol, antihistamines, antianxiety agents, antidepressants, or antipsychotic agents should be avoided because they may result in an enhanced CNS-depressant effect.

Pediatric and geriatric clients may be more sensitive to barbiturates and may respond to lower doses or may react with depression, confusion, or even excitement to the drug.

For clients receiving concurrent anticoagulant therapy, prothrombin times should be monitored carefully. Anticoagulant dose may need adjustment.

These drugs should be used very cautiously in pregnant women because they can cause neonatal hemorrhage and an increased incidence of teratogenic effects. If given throughout the third trimester, physical drug dependence and withdrawal reactions have been reported in the neonate from birth to approximately 2 weeks.

Intervention. If barbiturates are administered intravenously, the nurse should ensure that the airway is patent and resuscitative equipment is readily available.

When drug therapy is initiated, the client may have some drowsiness and dizziness. Safety precautions should be taken when the client is ambulatory until the response to the medication has been ascertained.

Since the drug dosage schedule initially will be different until the correct dosage maintenance level is achieved, it is important that the nurse follow the dosage schedule accurately.

The appearance of side effects or adverse reactions may require basic nursing measures such as reassurance, safety, or comfort, or it may indicate the need for further consultation (see Table 14-4).

If barbiturates are used during pregnancy, the nurse should consult with the client's physician to see if the client is to receive vitamin K in the last month of pregnancy to prevent hemorrhagic complications of delivery and in the newborn.

Education. Clients should be instructed to return to their physician routinely for CBC, blood chemistry studies, and drug blood level tests.

The client should be cautioned to avoid driving a car or operating potentially hazardous machinery until the response to drug therapy has been determined.

Self-alteration of prescribed medications or consumption of over-the-counter drugs should be discouraged without consultation with the physician. Over-the-counter drugs may interfere with or enhance the drug's effectiveness. If used in combination with alcohol, CNS depression may occur. Abrupt withdrawal of the drug is contraindicated and could result in severe abstinence syndrome. Dosage should be tapered under a physician's supervision.

Clients taking oral estrogen-containing contraceptives should be aware that concurrent use of barbiturates may result in decreased contraceptive reliability, and they may wish to use a nonhormonal method of birth control or consult with their prescriber about a progestin-only oral contraceptive.

Women using this drug therapy should be instructed to report to their physician if they become pregnant. Barbi-

TABLE 14-5 Phenobarbital Dosage and Administration

	Adults	Children
Anticonvulsant Oral	60-250 mg daily in single or divided doses	1-6 mg/kg body weight daily in single or divided doses
Injectable	100-320 mg, repeated if necessary to maximum of 600 mg in 24 hr	10-20 mg/kg body weight as single loading dose; maintenance dose is 1-6 mg/kg/day IV.
Status epilepticus	10-20 mg/kg by slow IV injection; repeat if necessary	15-20 mg/kg IV over 10-15 min

turates have been shown to cause an increase in fetal abnormalities. Barbiturates are excreted in the breast milk and can cause CNS depression in the nursing infant.

Evaluation. During prolonged barbiturate therapy, liver and renal function will be monitored (usually through blood and urine testing) at periodic intervals determined by the client's physician.

Determination of serum drug levels may be performed to monitor drug levels. The optimal blood levels are determined by response to seizure control and appearance of toxic effects.

amobarbital

Amobarbital is indicated for use as a sedative-hypnotic and anticonvulsant. Only the parenteral form is used as an anticonvulsant. Amobarbital should be administered deep intramuscularly to reduce the possibility of sterile abcesses and sloughing of tissue. When administered intravenously to an adult, the rate of injection should not exceed 100 mg/min. Parenteral solutions should be clear and without precipitate when reconstituted. The solution should be used within 30 minutes of reconstitution, since it hydrolyzes easily.

phenobarbital

Phenobarbital is the most common barbiturate used to treat epilepsy. There are many dosage forms (tablets, elixers, solutions, and parenteral forms) and strengths available. The nurse must exercise special caution to ensure the proper dose is given as prescribed.

Several weeks of phenobarbital therapy may be necessary to achieve the maximum anticonvulsant effects. When administered intravenously, 15 to 30 minutes is required to reach the maximum anticonvulsant effect. It is important to wait for the anticonvulsant effect to develop before administering additional doses to avoid excessive barbiturate-induced depression. When administered intravenously, phenobarbital should be administered slowly to avoid respiratory depression; a rate of 60 mg/min should not be exceeded. Resuscitative equipment should be readily available.

The optimal blood concentration of phenobarbital should be determined by seizure control and appearance of toxic effects. A serum concentration of 10 to 40 μg/ml is usually desired.

mephobarbital

Mephobarbital is a barbiturate indicated for use only as an anticonvulsant. Therapy is usually begun with small doses and increased over a period of 4 to 5 days until the optimal dosage has been established. Since mephobarbital is metabolized to phenobarbital, serum levels of phenobarbital may be monitored. Mephobarbital is available in oral dosage forms only.

metharbital

Metharbital is used only as an anticonvulsant. It is metabolized to barbital, and serum barbital concentrations may be monitored. Metharbital is available in oral dosage forms only.

HYDANTOINS

The prototype hydantoin is phenytoin (Dilantin, Diphenylan), which was developed from a search for an anticonvulsant that would cause less sedation than the barbiturates. Phenytoin is a drug for primary treatment of all types of epilepsy except absence seizures. Two other hydantoin drugs are used for their anticonvulsant effects, ethotoin (Pegonone) and mephenytoin (Mesantoin). The use of ethotoin and mephenytoin is usually reserved for those clients whose symptoms could not be controlled with other drugs or those who had significant adverse effects from other anticonvulsants. In addition, both drugs are only available in the oral form, which limits their usefulness when a rapid response or parenteral route is needed.

Phenytoin and some other hydantoins appear to inhibit the spread of seizure activity by possibly promoting sodium efflux from neurons, and they tend to stabilize the threshold against hyperexcitability caused by excess stimulation or environmental changes capable of reducing membrane sodium gradient. This includes the reduction of post-tetanic potentiation at synapses. The loss of post-tetanic potentiation prevents cortical seizure foci from detonating adjacent cortical areas. The hydantoins as a group act to reduce the maximal activity of brain stem centers responsible for the tonic phase of grand mal seizures.

The Nurse's Role in Hydantoin Therapy

Intervention. When using the suspension dosage form, the nurse must shake the container vigorously before measuring out the dose in a graduated or exact measuring device (oral syringe). Clients with enteral tube feedings and pediatric clients have been undermedicated and, later, overmedicated because of improper shaking of the container.

Oral preparations should be given with meals to decrease gastric distress. The appearance of side effects or adverse reactions may require nursing intervention ranging from basic nursing skills to urgent consultation with the physician (see Table 14-4).

Nasogastric tube administration of phenytoin. Studies have reported that administration of phenytoin suspension without dilution or follow-up irrigation of the nasogastric tube after the phenytoin was given led to a significant decrease in plasma phenytoin concentrations (Cacek and others, 1986). When phenytoin was administered to clients receiving enteral feedings, a significant decrease in absorption of oral phenytoin may occur. Until further research is performed, it is recommended that phenytoin suspension be diluted before administration and that the nasogastric tube be irrigated with 20 ml of fluid (D5W, normal saline). If the client is receiving an enteral feeding, the phenytoin should be administered intravenously; if this is not feasible, the serum concentrations of phenytoin should be monitored frequently (Yuen, 1984).

Education. One of the side effects of these drugs is gum hyperplasia; it is therefore important that oral hygiene be emphasized. Clients should be encouraged to brush frequently, floss, and massage their gums. As the tissue overgrowth is usually greater and more apparent anteriorly than posteriorly, the client, particularly the adolescent, may have body image concerns. A program of professional dental prophylaxis and an aggressive program of plaque control by the client will minimize hyperplasia. Clients should be instructed to inform their dentists that they are taking hydantoins, so the dentist can observe and monitor for periodental problems.

Clients who have diabetes should be instructed to report any changes in blood or urine sugar concentrations. Hydantoins may affect blood sugar levels.

The client should be advised of possible skin changes. An erythematous-type rash with or without fever should be reported immediately to the physician. Hirsutism or excessive body and facial hair growth is reported in some clients. This side effect is particularly troublesome in young women. This alteration in body image will require supportive nursing care.

Evaluation. When clients are taking hydantoins, serum levels should be monitored. It takes approximately 7 to 10 days before recommended serum levels are achieved. It is particularly important that serum levels be monitored closely in clients with renal and hepatic impairment. The client with impaired liver function, the elderly, or those who are very ill may demonstrate early toxic signs. A small percentage of persons metabolize the drug slowly because of limited enzyme availability that may be genetically determined. The metabolism of hydantoins is dose dependent at therapeutic doses.

The nurse should monitor closely for documented drug interactions that may alter the client's response to medications. (See drug-interaction section.) Because some drugs can impair or enhance the effects of phenytoin, monitoring of drug serum levels will be important for accurate dosage administration and as a mechanism of determining compliance.

The hydantoins are contraindicated in hypersensitivity, hepatic dysfunction, and hematologic disorders. Abrupt withdrawal may precipitate status epilepticus. There is an elevated incidence of birth defects in children born to mothers using anticonvulsants, although most deliver normal infants. Cautious administration is needed in clients with acute intermittent porphyria.

phenytoin sodium extended (Dilantin)
phenytoin (Dilantin, various)

Mechanism of action. See general discussion of anticonvulsants.

Indications
1. Used in the treatment of epilepsy. It is more effective for grand mal than petit mal seizures.
2. It is frequently prescribed in combination with phenobarbital.
3. It may be prescribed for clients following surgical operations on the brain, after head trauma, and for status epilepticus to prevent seizures.

Pharmacokinetics. See Table 14-2.

Side effects/adverse reactions. See Table 14-4. Signs of hydration overdose or toxicity include blurred or double vision, nausea, vomiting, slurred speech, clumsiness, unsteadiness or staggering walk, dizziness, fatigue, confusion, and hallucinations. In addition, the diverse signs of toxicity seen with intravenous phenytoin are cardiovascular collapse, CNS depression, and hypotension (seen with rapid intravenous administration resulting from propylene glycol solvent). The rate of administration (not to exceed 50 mg over 1 minute) is important, since severe cardiotoxic reactions and fatal outcomes are reported in elderly or gravely ill patients.

Significant drug interactions. A serious interaction between phenytoin and alcohol is the development of cross-tolerance to phenytoin in clients with epilepsy who are also heavy drinkers. Chronic alcohol use speeds up the metabolism of the drug apparently by enzyme induction and makes normal doses inadequate.

The following effects may occur when hydantoin are given with the drugs listed below:

Drug	Possible Effect and Management
anticoagulants (coumarin or indandione type)	A decrease in metabolism may cause an increased serum level and/or toxicity of hydantoins. Anticoagulant effect may be initially increased but will decrease with continuous combined usage. Monitor closely.
adrenocorticoids, corticosteroids, estrogens, or oral contraceptives	An increase in metabolism may decrease the therapeutic effects of these medications—monitor closely because a dosage adjustment may be necessary.
carbamazepine	A decrease in therapeutic effect may occur with one or both drugs. Serum drug levels should be closely monitored.
chloramphenicol, cimetidine, disulfiram, isoniazid, oxyphenbutazone, phenylbutazone, or sulfonamides	A decrease in metabolism may cause an increased serum level and/or toxicity of hydantoins.

Drug	Possible Effect and Management
diazoxide, oral	May decrease phenytoin effects and decrease the hyperglycemic action of diazoxide. This combination should be avoided.
folic acid	Hydantoins deplete folate from the body. Folic acid consumption may lower the serum hydantoin levels, leading to a possible loss of seizure control.
lidocaine, propranolol, and possible other beta-blocking agents	If given with IV phenytoin, additive cardiac depressant effects may occur. Hydantoins may also increase the metabolism of lidocaine.
methadone	Methadone metabolism may be increased by chronic dosing of phenytoin, which may precipitate an acute withdrawal reaction in clients being treated for narcotic dependence. Be aware that methadone dosages may need to be adjusted whenever phenytoin is started or discontinued.
trimethadione	Avoid concurrent use with mephenytoin because the risk for aplastic anemia increases.
valproic acid	Monitor serum levels of phenytoin (preferably unbound phenytoin) closely, since variable responses have been reported. Adjustments of dosage may be necessary according to the client's clinical response.
xanthines	Monitor serum concentrations of both drugs. If phenytoin plasma levels are in the therapeutic range, an increase in metabolism of xanthines (except for dyphylline) will occur. Also, if given with xanthines, a decrease in phenytoin absorption may result; monitor closely.

Dosage and administration. See Table 14-6.
Pregnancy safety. Not established

NURSING CONSIDERATIONS

Intervention. If the state of the client is such that immobilization of an extremity is impossible because of convulsions or inaccessible veins, then the intramuscular route may be useful. If the administration does not terminate the seizure, the nurse must consult with the prescriber to consider other anticonvulsants, intravenous barbiturates, general anesthesia, or other measures. The intramuscular route is not recommended for the treatment of status epilepticus, since the plasma levels of phenytoin in the therapeutic range cannot be readily achieved. Absorption is slow and erratic, and pain and necrosis may occur at the injection site.

The manufacturer supplies a special diluent for parenteral use. Because the preparation dissolves slowly, warming the vial in warm water after the diluent has been added is recommended to hasten dissolution. Only a clear solution is to be administered.

Because intravenous phenytoin is an irritant to the veins (and is incompatible with many solutions and medications), it is recommended that the intravenous line be flushed with normal saline (0.9% sodium chloride injection) before and after administration of this drug.

Some clients complain of burning and pain at the intravenous injection site. Because phenytoin is a highly alkaline solution, burning and pain raise suspicion that there may be a poorly seated needle, extravasation, or a fluid load that is being infused too quickly into a small vein. The nurse should restart the infusion into a large vein, using a larger gauge needle. Subcutaneous injection may cause inflammation and necrosis and should not be done.

The addition of phenytoin solution to an intravenous infusion is not recommended because of the lack of its solubility (the solution is made with propylene glycol 40%, alcohol 10%, water 50%, and pH adjusted with sodium hydroxide to 12) and the resultant precipitation.

The manufacturer does not recommend adding parenteral phenytoin sodium to intravenous solutions or mixing it with any other medications, since precipitation (even microcrystals) may occur. Since a number of physicians prescribe intermittent infusions of phenytoin, the USP DI (1988) has stated that all the following criteria must be met in such situations:

1. Parenteral phenytoin sodium is mixed with sodium chloride 0.9% injection (normal saline) only. The mixture is made immediately before administration of the infusion. The concentration of phenytoin in solution is between 1 and 10 mg/ml.
2. A 0.22 μ filter must be used in the administration of this solution and the infusion should be finished within 4 hours.
3. The administration rate for the infusion should be a maximum of 50 mg/min. Reduce to 25 mg/min in clients that might develop hypotension, have cardiovascular disease, or are receiving sympathomimetic adjuvant medications. Elderly, seriously ill, or debilitated clients or clients with liver function impairment should generally receive a lower dose at a much slower rate of administration.
4. Monitor blood pressure and cardiac function closely.
5. Carefully observe the admixture for crystals, cloudiness, or precipitation.

In the same manner that digitalization is accomplished, the nurse may encounter dilatinization in a manner that may place the client within the therapeutic range within 20 to 30 min to as long as 15 days.

The following are examples of methods used to accomplish reaching a therapeutic serum range of 5 to 20 μg/ml after the initial dose.

TABLE 14-6　Phenytoin Dosage and Administration

	Adults	Children
Oral	Anticonvulsant, 100 mg 3 times a day; dosage adjustments made at 1-3 wk intervals as necessary (up to 600 mg/day maximum). Loading dose method: 12-15 mg/kg body weight divided into 2 or 3 doses over 6 hr, then 1.5-2 mg/kg administered on subsequent days.	Initially, 5 mg/kg body weight divided in 2 or 3 doses/day (maximum 300 mg/day). Maintenance, 4-8 mg/kg or 250 mg/m² body surface area daily (divided doses, 2 or 3 per day).
IV injection	Status epilepticus, 10-20 mg/kg IV at rate of up to 50 mg/min (maximum, 1.5 g in 24 hr). Elderly, seriously ill, or debilitated clients or clients with liver dysfunction should receive smaller total dose given at slower IV rate (e.g., 50 mg over 2-3 min).	Status epilepticus, 15-20 mg/kg IV at a rate of 1-3 mg/kg/min.
IM injection	Not recommended if oral or IV routes are available; causes tissue irritation and delayed and erratic absorption. Should only be used as last choice for maximum of 1 wk. If IM administration required for client formerly stabilized on oral drug, compensating dosage adjustment needed to maintain therapeutic plasma levels. IM dose is 50% greater than oral dose to maintain these levels. When client returned to oral route, dose reduced by 50% of original oral dose for 7 days to compensate for excessive plasma levels resulting from sustained release from IM site of injection.	

1. The administration of 1000 mg of phenytoin by the IV route at less than 50 mg/min in adults (or 10 to 15 mg/kg in children at 25 mg/min) will achieve therapeutic range in 20 to 25 min. Monitor pulse, blood pressure, and respirations.
2. The administration of 1000 mg orally in adults (about 1 mg/kg in children) usually administered in divided doses followed by the usual maintenance dose starting 24 hours after the loading dose. Dividing the dosages (such as 400/mg, 300/mg, and 300/mg, at 2-hr intervals) will help reduce the adverse effects of epigastric pain and GI distress.
3. The administration of oral phenytoin (dilantin delayed action) to adults at 300/mg every 8 hours for 3 doses, followed thereafter by 300 mg daily achieves therapeutic range within 24-30 hr. This method is frequently used but is initially associated with mild ataxia in most clients.
4. An outpatient method is oral administration of 300 mg/day in adults (or 5 mg/kg/day in children) given daily without a loading dose. This method will achieve a therapeutic range in 5-15 days with minimal side effects.

The nurse can readily determine that the rate and time for dilantinization is a function of the client's clinical situation. The dose-related side effects increase with the rapidity at which the client is dilantinized to the therapeutic range. Proceeding cautiously and slowly is clinically prudent. Nystagamus (bilateral and vertical) develops at levels of 10 to 20 μg/ml; ataxia, drowsiness, and diplopia are seen at levels about 30 μg/ml; and lethargy is seen at 40 μg/ml.

Parenteral phenytoin should be used with caution in clients with hypotension and severe myocardial insufficiency.

The effects of phenytoin on ventricular automaticity (fibrillation) prohibit its use in sinus bradycardia, sinoatrial block and second- and third-degree atrioventricular block and in clients with Adams-Stokes syndrome.

Education. The client should be cautioned against exchanging brands since the bioavailability of phenytoin may vary. Generic phenytoin and Dilantin from Parke-Davis are not the same. Dilantin capsules are the only form of extended phenytoin sodium available; all the rest are prompt acting. The generic phenytoin capsules are a prompt-acting form of the drug. The chewable tablets are from Parke-Davis and are a prompt-acting form. The extended form can be used for once-a-day dosing and for those clients who are stabilized on a 300-mg divided dosage. It is important that the client and family have this information explained clearly.

When discussing the appropriate means of administration of the suspension dosage form, the nurse should stress that very vigorous shaking of the container is mandatory before measuring out the dose in a graduated or exact measuring device (oral syringe). Clients should be cautioned against unsupervised self-administration of other drugs while taking any of the hydantoins, since they interact with a variety of drugs.

Any patient with epilepsy should carry an identification card that indicates the medication he or she is taking.

mephenytoin (Mesantoin)

Mephenytoin is chemically similar in structure, activity, and pharmacokinetics to phenytoin, but it is less potent as an anticonvulsant. It produces more sedation than phenytoin, but this side effect is dose related. It also has a greater potential for producing blood dyscrasias and dermatologic effects than the other hydantoins. This product is usually reserved for clients whose seizures are not controlled with safer anticonvulsants.

Mephenytoin is only available for oral administration with the dose individualized according to age and response. The usual adult dose is 200 to 600 mg daily in three divided doses and for children, 100 to 400 mg daily in three divided doses. Administration of mephenytoin with oxazolidinedione anticonvulsants is not recommended because of the increased potential of producing blood dyscrasias such as leukopenia, neutropenia, agranulocytosis, thrombocytopenia, and pancytopenia.

ethotoin (Peganone)

Ethotoin is similar to phenytoin but less effective and offers little advantage over phenytoin. Side effects of ataxia, hirsutism, and gum hyperplasia are rare and ethotoin may be substituted for phenytoin to reduce these side effects. Ethotoin is available only for oral administration with dosage individualized according to response. Maintenance dosage (usually divided into four to six doses) of less than 2 g is usually not effective and the maximum daily adult dose is 5 g.

SUCCINIMIDES

The succinimides include ethosuximide (Zarontin), methsuximide (Celontin), and phensuximide (Milontin).

Mechanism of action. The succinimides produce a variety of effects, such as increasing the seizure threshold and reducing the spike and wave pattern of absence seizures by decreasing nerve impulses and transmission in the motor cortex.

Indications. Ethosuximide and phensuximide are indicated for the treatment of absence seizures, whereas methsuximide is reserved for absence seizures that are nonresponsive to other medication.

Pharmacokinetics. See Table 14-2.

Side effects/adverse reactions. See Table 14-4.

Significant drug interactions. The following effects may occur when succinimides are given in combination with the drugs listed below:

Drug	Possible Effect and Management
carbamazepine	Results in increased metabolism of succinimide anticonvulsants and decreased serum levels. Monitor serum levels especially when either drug is added, increased, decreased, or deleted from the drug regimen.
haloperidol	May change the pattern or frequency of seizures. Dosage adjustment of the anticonvulsant may be required. Also serum levels of haloperidol may be reduced, which may result in decreased effectiveness.
phenothiazines, thioxanthenes, antidepressants, loxapine, or maprotiline	May result in a decrease in the effectiveness of the anticonvulsant, enhance CNS depression, and also may lower the seizure threshold. Monitor closely because dosage modifications may be necessary.

Dosage and administration. See Table 14-7.
Pregnancy safety. Not established

NURSING CONSIDERATIONS

To decrease stomach distress, the succinimides may be taken with milk, food, or antacids.

Liver, renal, and hematologic studies should be evaluated periodically because of the drug's possible effects on these systems. Report any signs of liver, kidney, or hematologic disorders to the physician. The succinimides side effects and adverse reactions are listed in Table 14-4. The nurse should caution the client about drowsiness and other possible CNS disturbances. When dosage adjustments are made or medications added, serum drug levels may be ordered. The nurse should explain the importance of serum blood levels to the client who needs to have serum levels drawn frequently. The client should be cautioned that withdrawal of the succinimides may precipitate absence seizures. Adverse personality changes can occur while the client is taking this medication; the nurse should stress the importance of reporting any behavioral changes to the physician.

If the client is taking phensuximide, the nurse should caution him or her that the drug may change the color of the urine to pink, red, or red-brown; this is harmless.

TABLE 14-7   Succinimide Dosage and Administration

Drug	Adults	Children
ethosuximide (Zarontin)	Orally, initially 250 mg twice a day, increased as necessary at 4-7 day intervals; maximum total daily dose is 1.5 g.	Orally, for children 6 yr old and older, follow adult schedule. For children up to 6 yr, initial dose is 250 mg/day, increased by 250 mg at 4-7 day intervals. Maximum total daily dose is 1 g.
methsuximide (Celontin)	Orally, initial dose is 300 mg daily, increased as necessary by 300 mg increments at 1-wk intervals until seizures controlled or maximum daily dose of 1.2 g reached.	Dosage is individualized. 150 mg capsules available for pediatric dosage adjustments.
phensuximide (Milontin)	Orally, initial dose is 500 mg twice a day, increase by 500 mg increments at 1-wk intervals until seizures controlled or maximum daily dose of 3 g reached.	Pediatric dose similar to adult schedule.

OXAZOLIDINEDIONES

The oxazolidinediones include paramethadione (Paradione) and trimethadione (Tridione).

Mechanism of action. They appear to elevate the threshold for cortical seizures, decrease extension of focal discharges, and decrease the spike and wave patterns seen with absence seizures during an electroencephalogram.

Indications. They are indicated for treatment of absence seizures that are nonresponsive to other medications.

Pharmacokinetics

Absorption. Rapidly orally

Metabolism. To active metabolites in liver

Half-life. Paramethadione, biphasic 1.2-24 hr; trimethadione, 12-24 hr; active metabolite has 16-13 day half-life

Excretion. Kidneys

Side effects/adverse reactions. See Table 14-4.

Significant drug interactions. The following effects may occur when oxazolidinediones are given in combination with the drugs listed below:

Drug	Possible Effect and Management
haloperidol, phenothiazines, antidepressants, thioxanthenes, loxapine, or maprotiline	May result in a decrease in the effectiveness of the anticonvulsant and enhance CNS depression. Seizure threshold may also be lowered. Monitor closely since dosage modifications may be necessary.
mephenytoin	Increased risk of aplastic anemia when given concurrently with trimethadione. Monitor closely.

Dosage and administration. See Table 14-8.

Pregnancy safety. Paramethadione has been rated as FDA Category D. Coagulation defects have been reported with both paramethadione and trimethadione resulting in bleeding in the neonate during the first 24 hours after birth.

NURSING CONSIDERATIONS

Paramethadione should be administered with food or milk to decrease gastric irritation. The tablets (trimethadione chewable tablets) may be crushed with a small amount of water for ease of administration, if necessary. Paramethadione capsules should not be chewed or crushed since they contain an oily liquid. A solution is available for clients unable to swallow tablets. Paramethadione oral solution has a high alcohol content (65%); therefore it is recommended the dose be diluted in 4 ounces of water or juice before administration, especially to little children.

The drugs are not recommended for clients with hepatic or renal disease, disease of the optic nerve, or blood dyscrasias. Their use in pregnant women may cause malformation of the fetus (FDA category D).

Careful medical supervision of the client receiving the medication is essential. It is advisable for the client to have periodic examinations of the blood to detect early signs of toxic effects, since rare instances of aplastic anemia have been reported. Serum blood levels will be drawn frequently to control the level of the drug in relation to the seizure status of the client.

It may take from 1 to 4 weeks before the drug reaches

TABLE 14-8   Paramethadione and Trimethadione: Dosage and Administration

Drug	Adults	Children
paramethadione	Oral, 300 mg 3 or 4 times daily, increased at 1-wk intervals (300 mg/day increment) until seizures are controlled, toxic symptoms appear, or maximum limit of 2.4 g/day is reached.	Oral solution available. Children up to 2 yr, 100 mg 3 times a day; children 2-6 yr, 200 mg 3 times a day; children more than 6 yr, 300 mg 3 times a day.
trimethadione	Oral, 300 mg 3 or 4 times daily, increase 300 mg/day at weekly intervals until seizures are controlled, toxic symptoms appear, or maximum limit of 2.4 g/day is reached.	Oral solution, 13 mg/kg body weight or 335 mg/m² body surface 3 times a day.

its therapeutic levels, so clients may continue to experience seizures. It is important that the client recorded the time, type, and length of seizure and report this to the physician.

One of the adverse reactions of the drugs is ophthalmic damage. The nurse should caution the client to report any visual disturbances, particularly day blindness. If vision blurs in the sunlight, the client should be advised to wear sunglasses and report the problem to the physician.

Since renal damage is a possibility, the client should be instructed to report edema, urinary frequency, burning on urination, and cloudy urine. Periodic urinalysis should be done.

These drugs tend to have more toxic effects than other drugs used to treat seizure activity. The client should be instructed to be observant for the toxic effects and report them to the physician.

BENZODIAZEPINES

The benzodiazepines include clonazepam (Clonopin), diazepam (Valium), clorazepate (Tranxene), and lorazepam (Ativan).

Mechanism of action. The benzodiazepines appear to suppress the propagation of seizure activity produced by foci in the cortex, thalamus, and limbic areas.

Indications. Clonazepam may be useful in tonic-clonic, simple partial, complex partial, absence, and various generalized seizures. It has been used alone but more often, it is prescribed as an adjunct to other anticonvulsants to establish seizure control.

Diazepam is used parenterally in status epilepticus or in severe recurrent convulsive seizures, but the oral dosage form is not an effective preventive for maintenance control. The oral diazepam dosage form has been used as an adjunctive medication for short-term treatment in convulsive disorders (such as 1 to 2 weeks therapy.)

Clorazepate has been prescribed as an adjunct medication for the treatment of simple partial seizures.

Lorazepam parenteral is used for the treatment of status epilepticus.

Pharmacokinetics. See Table 14-2 and Chapter 13.

Side effects/adverse reactions. See Table 14-4 and Chapter 13.

Significant drug interactions. CNS depressants, such as narcotic analgesics, alcohol, antidepressants, hypnotics, sedatives, general anesthetics, may result in additive or synergistic CNS-depressant effects. Generally, the dosage of one or both drugs should be reduced. Monitor closely.

Dosage and administration. Dosages are usually individualized for each patient and are increased with caution to avoid adverse effects. Some patients may require higher doses than indicated. In elderly or debilitated persons and those taking other CNS-depressant–type medications, a lower dose with a slow increase is prudent.

clonazepam (Clonopin): anticonvulsant adult dosage, oral, initially 0.5 mg three times daily with increases of 0.5-1 mg every third day until seizures are controlled, side effects occur, or the maximum of 20 mg/day is reached. Pediatric anticonvulsant oral dose (less that 10 years old or 30 kg body weight), initial 0.01-0.03/kg body weight in divided doses (three times a day); if necessary, increase by 0.25-0.5 mg every three days until seizures are controlled, side effects occur, or the maximum maintenance dose of 0.1-0.2 mg/kg body weight is reached.

diazepam (Valium): adult status epilepticus or severe recurrent convulsive seizure dosage is 5-10 mg IM or IV (preferred method) initially; repeat at 10-15 min intervals if necessary to a maximum of 30 mg; inject slowly—at least 1 minute for each 5-mg dose administered intravenously. Pediatric anticonvulsant dose (from 1-5 yr of age), 0.2-0.5 mg IM or IV (preferred method) every 2-5 min to a maximum of 5 mg; this regimen may be repeated if necessary, in 2-4 hr. Children 5 years or older, 1 mg every 2-5 min IM or IV (preferred method) to a maximum of 10 mg; this regimen may be repeated if necessary, in 2-4 hr. Adult oral anticonvulsant dose, 2-10 mg two to four times daily.

clorazepate (Tranxene): adult oral dose, initial, up to 7.5 mg three times daily; increase if necessary by 7.5 mg/wk to a maximum of 90 mg/day. Pediatric anticonvulsant dose, for children 9-12 years old, orally, up to 7.5 mg twice daily; increase if necessary by 7.5 mg/wk to a maximum of 60 mg daily.

Pregnancy safety. See Chapter 13.

NURSING CONSIDERATIONS

Assessment. Clients undergoing long-term benzodiazepine therapy can become physically dependent on the drug and show signs and symptoms of withdrawal when the drug is discontinued.

Baseline vital signs should be taken before diazepam or lorazepam is given and then observed at bed rest for at least 1 hour for decreases in respiratory rate, heart rate, and blood pressure.

Intervention. Diazepam is insoluble in water; therefore each milliliter of the parenteral form contains 40% propylene glycol, 10% ethyl alcohol, 5% sodium benzoate and benzoic acid as buffers, and 1.5% benzyl alcohol as a preservative. If this ratio is altered, the diazepam is insoluble.

Lorazepam must be diluted with a compatible diluent immediately before intravenous use. It may be infused directly into a vein or through intravenous tubing. Infusion rates should not exceed 2 mg/min.

Because of the short-lived effect of intravenous benzodiazepine administration, seizures, although brought under prompt control, may recur. The nurse should be ready to readminister the drug. Benzodiazepines are not for maintenance; once seizure control is achieved, agents useful in long-term seizure control should be considered. Tonic status epilepticus has been precipitated in some clients treated with intravenous diazepam for petit mal status or petit mal variant status. The nurse must exercise extreme care (monitor respirations every 5 to 15 minutes and before each intravenous dose) in administering parenteral benzodiazepines (especially by the intravenous route) to elderly or very ill clients or those with compromised pulmonary reserve because of the possibility of apnea and/or cardiac arrest.

Resuscitative equipment should be available because of the possible occurrence of hypotension, tachycardia, and respiratory depression.

In the neonate (age 30 days or less) the efficacy and safety of parenteral diazepam are not established. Prolonged CNS depression has been reported in the neonate, probably resulting from the inability to biotransform diazepam into the inactive metabolites. The benzoate in the injectable form has been reported to displace other drugs and bilirubin from the plasma protein binding sites, causing jaundice.

The combination of diazepam and cimetidine may cause drug accumulation and drug toxicity, since both of these drugs are metabolized by hepatic microsomal oxidases. It is therefore necessary to observe for adverse reactions elicited by either drug or a combination of the drugs. Adverse reactions from the combination may necessitate a reduction in dosage of either drug or both drugs.

To minimize the occurrence of thrombophlebitis following intravenous injection of diazepam, the vein can be flushed with 1 ml of saline per milligram of diazepam.

If benzodiazepines are intended to be given along with a narcotic, the dose of the narcotic should be reduced.

Diazepam is a drug that may be subject to abuse by medical and nursing professionals and clients. This is a controlled drug; therefore the nurse is responsible for proper documentation of the drug's distribution and use.

Education. When benzodiazepines are given for treating convulsive disorders, an abrupt withdrawal of the medication can cause an increase in frequency or severity of seizures. Clients should be instructed to take their medication as directed.

Diazepam does cross the placental barrier and has been associated with causing cleft lip in the infant.

Risk/benefit ratio should be carefully considered in the client during pregnancy.

It is not advisable that alcohol or other CNS depressants be combined with benzodiazepines. Severe drowsiness, respiratory depression, and apnea may occur.

MISCELLANEOUS ANTICONVULSANTS

valproic acid (Depakene) and divalproex sodium (Depakote)

Mechanism of action. The mechanism by which valproic acid exerts its anticonvulsant effects has not been fully established. It has been proposed that its activity is related to increased brain levels of the inhibitory neurotrasmitter GABA. By competitive inhibition it prevents the reuptake of GABA by glial cells and axonal terminals. The drug has a marked effect on the generalized spike wave discharges (3/sec) in the EEG.

Indications. For use as sole and adjunctive therapy in the treatment of simple and complex absence seizures, including petit mal, and as adjunctive therapy in clients with multiple seizure types including absence seizures.

Pharmacokinetics. See Table 14-2. Chemically, valproate sodium is converted in the stomach to valproic acid, which is rapidly absorbed from the gastrointestinal tract. Divalproex sodium is a **prodrug,** a combination of valproic acid and valproate sodium, in an enteric coated tablet. Divalproex dissociates into valproate, which is then absorbed in the small intestine.

Side effects/adverse reactions. See Table 14-4.

Significant drug interactions. The following effects may occur when valproic acid and divalproex sodium (a drug that contains 50% valproic acid and sodium valproate) are given with the drugs listed below:

Drug	Possible Effect and Management
alcohol, anesthetics (general), CNS-depressant–type drugs	May result in potentiated CNS-depressant effects.
anticoagulants, coumarin, indan-dione types, heparin, or thrombolytic agents	Increased risk of bleeding and hemorrhage; monitor closely for early signs if given in combination.
aspirin, dipyridamole, or sulfin-pyrazone	Increased risk of bleeding and hemorrhage; monitor closely or the physician might consider alternative therapeutic agents.
barbiturates or primidone	Phenobarbital and primidone serum levels may increase, resulting in increased depression and toxicity. Monitor since dosage adjustment by the physician may be necessary.
carbamazepine and phenytoin	Breakthrough seizures may occur because of decreased serum levels of carbamazepine or valproic acid. Phenytoin protein binding may be affected when combined with valproic acid. Therefore monitor closely using serum levels as a guide for physician dosing adjustments.

Dosage and administration. Adults and children, range of 15 to 60 mg/kg/day, starting at the lowest dose and increasing by 5 to 10 mg/kg at weekly intervals as needed. The dose may be given with or immediately after meals to decrease gastrointestinal upset. The dose should be the lowest consistent with seizure control.

Pregnancy safety. FDA category D.

NURSING CONSIDERATIONS

Intervention. The drug should be administered with or after meals to avoid gastric irritation. The client should avoid chewing or crushing the tablets and capsules; the nurse should avoid giving the tablet form with milk because of possible early dissolution and local irritation to the mouth and throat. Syrup is available for clients unable to swallow tablets or capsules. Divalproex sodium is prescribed for clients unable to tolerate the gastrointestinal irritation produced by valproic acid.

When other anticonvulsant drugs are used in combination, the dosage of valproic acid and/or the other anticonvulsants may need to be adjusted to maintain serum levels and seizure control.

Education. The client should be instructed not to chew the tablet/or capsule, since it will irritate the mouth and throat. Combining this drug with alcohol or other CNS depressants can cause a potentiation of sedation. This drug can cause a false-positive ketone test in diabetic clients; these clients should be instructed to consult their physicians about using some other form of diagnostic tool for ketones. The client should be instructed to be aware of signs of decreasing mental alertness, which can occur when valproic acid is given alone or in combination with other anticonvulsants.

The drug is excreted in breast milk and can cause CNS depression in the nursing infant. Birth defects (spina bifida) have occurred when this drug was taken during the first trimester of pregnancy. Clients taking this drug who are considering pregnancy may need to be given another anticonvulsant that has no documented risk of causing birth defects.

The client should be told to report to the physician if any of the following side effects occur: visual disturbances, rash, diarrhea, light-colored stools, jaundice, and protracted vomiting.

Evaluation. Valproic acid has been shown to cause liver dysfunction; therefore the client should be instructed to report signs of liver dysfunction, such as spontaneous bleeding and/or bruising, immediately to the physician. The client should have liver function studies done at least every month during the first 6 months of therapy when heptotoxicity is most likely to occur.

carbamazepine (Tegretol)

Mechanism of action. The exact mechanism of action is unknown, although this drug's effects are somewhat similar to those of phenytoin.

Indications. Carbamazepine is indicated in the treatment of epilepsy for clients who are refractory or have not responded to phenytoin, phenobarbital, or primidone, for partial seizures with complex symptomatology, for generalized tonic-clonic seizures, for psychomotor seizures, and for mixed seizure patterns.

This drug is also indicated in the treatment of pain associated with true trigeminal neuralgia.

Pharmacokinetics. See Table 14-2. Autoinduction of metabolism occurs, and half-life decreases with repeated doses.

Side effects/adverse reactions. See Table 14-4.

Significant drug interactions. The following effects may occur when carbamazepine is given with the following drugs:

Drug	Possible Effect and Management
anticoagulants, oral (coumarin or indandiones)	Monitor for a decreased anticoagulant effect. Increased hepatic microsomal enzyme activity increases anticoagulant metabolism, resulting in a decreased half-life and effect. Dosage adjustments of anticoagulant may be necessary during and after treatment with carbamazepine.
estrogen-containing contraceptives	Decrease in contraceptive reliability; clients should be advised to use a nonhormonal birth control method or to discuss the possibility of an oral progestin product with their physician.
loxapine, maprotiline, thioxanthenes or tricyclic antidepressants	May reduce the convulsive threshold and/or enhance CNS depressant effects; dosage adjustment may be necessary to control seizures and reduce side effects. Monitor closely.
monoamine ozidase (MAO) inhibitors	Hypertensive crisis, elevated temperatures, severe convulsions, and even death have been reported with this combination. When switching from one therapy to another (MAO to carbamazepine or vice versa), at least a 14-day, drug-free interval is recommended.

Dosage and administration. See Table 14-9.
Pregnancy safety. FDA category C

NURSING CONSIDERATIONS

Intervention. Carbamazepine should be administered with meals to reduce gastrointestinal irritation.

Education. The importance of compliance with drug therapy should be stressed with all clients taking this drug.

Clients should report to the physician if they have any signs of hematologic dysfunction such as easy bruising, bleeding, sore throat or mouth, or malaise.

It is not uncommon for the client to be drowsy during the initial therapy; clients should be cautioned about this so that they can avoid driving a car or operating hazardous equipment.

This drug is used specifically for the pain of trigeminal neuralgia. It should not be used as a routine analgesic.

Carbamazepine can cause breakthrough bleeding in women taking oral contraceptives. Women should be told that it may interfere with the effectiveness of the contraceptive, so other forms of birth control measures may need to be used.

Carbamazepine is excreted in breast milk, so it may not be recommended in nursing mothers. Abrupt withdrawal of the drug (in clients with epilepsy) can precipitate a seizure.

In middle-aged or elderly clients, carbamazepine may decrease salivary flow and contribute to the development of caries, periodontal disease, or discomfort. Chewing gum may ease discomfort from the dry mouth.

Evaluation. Blood studies (CBC, liver function studies, BUN), urinalysis, physical examinations, ophthalmic examinations, and ECG should be done before beginning carbamazepine therapy. Then the blood studies should be done every 2 weeks during the second and third months and then every month while the patient is taking this medication.

primidone (Mysoline)

Mechanism of action. Primidone and its metabolites, phenobarbital and phenylethylmalonamide (PEMA), contribute to anticonvulsant activity. The mechanism of action is unknown, but primidone and its metabolites all appear to have active anticonvulsant effects.

Indications. Primidone is used for control of generalized and complex seizures.

Pharmacokinetics. See Table 14-2.

Side effects/adverse reactions. See Table 14-4.

TABLE 14-9 Carbamazepine Dosage and Administration

	Adults	Children
Oral anticonvulsant	Initial, 200 mg twice daily, increased by 200 mg/day in divided doses until response noted; maximum 1200 mg/day; maintenance, range 800-1200 mg/day in divided doses.	Children up to 6 yr, initially 5 mg/kg/day in divided doses; increase weekly if necessary to 10 mg/kg/day, then to 20 mg/kg/day. Maintenance, usually requires between 10 and 20 mg/kg/day to maintain therapeutic serum level. Children 6-12 yr, initially 100 mg twice a day; increase by 100 mg/day until desired response is obtained. Maintenance, usually between 400 and 800 mg/day in divided dosages.

Significant drug interactions. The following effects may occur when primidone is given with the drugs listed below:

Drugs	Possible Effect and Management
adrenocorticoids, glucocorticoid, or corticotropin (ACTH)	Decreased therapeutic effects of these medications when used concurrently with primidone; monitor closely since physician may need to increase dosage during and after primidone.
CNS depressants	Enhanced CNS and respiratory depression reported. Monitor since physician may need to adjust dosages.
tricyclic antidepressants	May see enhanced CNS depression, decrease in convulsive threshold, and decrease in primidone effects. Physician may need to increase primidone to control seizures.
monoamine oxidase (MAO) inhibitors	May prolong the effects of primidone; dosage adjustments may be necessary. Monitor closely.

Dosage and administration. See Table 14-10.
Pregnancy safety. Not established

NURSING CONSIDERATIONS

See barbiturate discussion in this chapter. Clients with reported reactions to barbiturates may be intolerant of primidone. The nurse should shake oral suspension well for consistent dosing.

phenacemide (Phenurone)

Phenacemide is used for clients with severe epilepsy,

TABLE 14-10 Primidone Dosage and Administration

Adults	Children
Oral, initially 100-125 mg at bedtime for 3 days, increase by 100 or 125 mg twice a day for the fourth through the sixth day, then increase by 100-125 mg 3 times a day until the ninth day. On day 10 dosage of 250 mg 3 times a day is established and may be altered according to needs of client up to 2 g/day.	Children up to 8 yr. initially 50 mg orally at bedtime for 3 days, increase to 50 mg twice a day through day 6, then increase to 100 mg twice daily through day 9. On day 10 maintenance dose of 125 or 250 mg 3 times a day may be given and adjusted according to client response.

especially partial seizures with complex symptoms that are refractory to other medications. This drug is extremely toxic and should be reserved for use *after* all available anticonvulsants were proven ineffective. It may cause liver, blood, and psychologic problems, such as personality changes, bone marrow depression, and hepatitis. Deaths have been reported with its use so some physicians believe it is too toxic for routine use.

acetazolamide (Diamox)

Acetazolamide is a carbonic anhydrase inhibitor usually prescribed for the treatment of open-angle glaucoma. It is used in combination with other anticonvulsant agents for the treatment of absence seizures, generalized tonic-clonic seizures, mixed seizures, and myoclonic seizure patterns.

Mechanism of action. Acetazolamide's mechanism of action is unknown. It has been theorized that inhibiting carbonic anhydrase in the CNS may result in an increase in carbon dioxide that retards neuronal activity. Systemic metabolic acidosis may also play a part in its action.

Pharmacokinetics. See Chapter 43.
Side effects/adverse reactions. See Chapter 43.
Significant drug interactions. The following effects may occur when acetazolamide is used with the drugs listed below:

Drugs	Possible Effect and Management
amphetamines, mecamylamine, or quinidine	Alkalinization of the urine may increase or prolong the effects and side effects of these drugs. Dosage alterations may be required, especially when a drug is added, increased, decreased, or deleted. Monitor closely. Mecamylamine should not be used in clients receiving acetazolamide because of the altered excretion.
methenamine	Effectiveness may be reduced because of the alkaline urine produced by acetazolamide. Do not use concurrently.

Dosage and administration. Adult, anticonvulsant, oral 8 to 30 mg (initial dose is usually 10/mg)/kg/day in four divided doses (usually 375 to 1,000 mg/day). Pediatric dosage, see adult recommendations.
Pregnancy safety. Not established

NURSING CONSIDERATIONS

The nurse should administer acetazolamide with food to decrease gastric irritation. Since bioequivalence problems have been reported, it is recommended that different generic brands not be used interchangeably for this product. Maintenance of an increased fluid intake is recommended, especially in clients with a history of gout or hypercalciuria. The nurse should closely monitor serum electrolytes and inform the physician if fever, sore throat, bleeding, hives, skin rash, difficult breathing, confusion, depression or difficulty or pain on urination occurs.

The nurse should caution the client that drowsiness and dizziness may occur, therefore the client should avoid driving a car or operating potentially hazardous machinery until the response to this drug has been determined. Diabetic clients should be informed that an increase in blood or urine glucose is usually reported with this medication. The nurse should advise the client on the signs of hypokalemia (dry mouth, muscle cramps, nausea, vomiting, tiredness, mood changes,); if they occur, the client must be urged to report them to the physician. Discontinuance of acetazolamide should be under the physician's guidance.

magnesium sulfate

Mechanism of action. Magnesium sulfate has a depressant effect on the CNS, which reduces striated muscle contractions. In addition, magnesium sulfate blocks peripheral neuromuscular transmission by reducing acetylcholine release at the myoneural junction, reducing the sensitivity of the motor endplate and lowering the excitability of the motor membrane.

Indications

1. Anticonvulsant: prevention and control of seizures related to toxemias of pregnancy (see box) and control seizures related to acute nephritis in children
2. Uterine relaxant: treatment of uterine tetany and inhibit contractions of premature labor
3. Replacement therapy: for magnesium deficiency

Pharmacokinetics. About one third of dietary ingested magnesium is absorbed from the GI tract. With intravenous administration, onset of action is immediate with approximately 30 minutes duration of action: with intramuscular, onset is about 1 hour with a 3 to 4 hour duration of action. Magnesium undergoes no metabolism and is excreted by the kidneys.

Side effects/adverse reactions. Sweating, flushing, depressed reflexes, hypotension, hypothermia, reduced heart rate, circulatory collapse, respiratory depression.

Significant drug interactions

CNS depressants: When barbiturates, opiates, general anesthetics or other CNS depressants are used, dosage of these agents should be adjusted to avoid additive CNS depressant effects.

Neuromuscular blocking agents: Excessive neuromuscular blockade has occurred when these drugs are administered with magnesium sulfate.

Cardiac glycosides: Serious changes in cardiac function, including heart block may occur if calcium is administered to counteract magnesium overdose.

Dosage and administration. See Table 14-11.

TOXEMIA OF PREGNANCY (PREECLAMPSIA AND ECLAMPSIA)

Toxemia of pregnancy is a syndrome of elevated blood pressure, edema, and proteinurea, which occurs in about 5% of all pregnancies in North America. The syndrome is described in clinical terms because its cause is unknown. Preeclampsia is another term for the syndrome. Depending on the severity of symptoms, preeclampsia may be classified as mild, which may be treated at home or severe, which requires hospitalization for monitoring and treatment. If the disease progresses, convulsions will occur and the syndrome is classified as eclampsia, which is derived from a Greek word used to describe convulsions. Sensory changes that occur in severe preeclampsia and eclampsia include headache, epigastric pain, blurred vision, and hyperreflexia. Therapeutic goals for the treatment of toxemia of pregnancy are control of blood pressure, prevention of convulsions, maintenance of renal function and provision of optimal conditions for the fetus. Treatment is symptomatic since the only "cure" for toxemia is delivery of the baby. Convulsions may still occur up to 48 hours after delivery, necessitating continued therapy in the immediate postpartum period.

TABLE 14-11 Magnesium Sulfate Dosage and Administration for Seizure Control

Adults	Elderly	Children
IM: 1 to 5 g (8-40 mEq) as a 25%-50% solution up to 6 times/day in alternate buttocks.	Often lower dosage is required because of reduced renal function	IM, 20 to 40 mg (0.16-0.32 mEq) kg of body weight as a 20% solution
IV: 1-4 g (8-32 mEq) as a 10%-20% solution, rate not to exceed 1.5 ml of 10% solution/min.		
IV infusion: 4 g (32 mEq) in 250 ml of D$_5$W or 0.9% NaCl. Administration rate not to exceed 4 ml/min		

Pregnancy safety. Magnesium sulfate is administered in the treatment of toxemias of pregnancy. The drug crosses the placenta, with fetal blood levels approximately equal to maternal blood levels, and produces similar effects in the neonate as in the mother. Decreased reflexes, muscle tone, blood pressure, and respiratory depression may be seen if the mother received magnesium shortly before delivery. It is recommended that magnesium sulfate *not* be administered during the 2 hours before delivery, if possible.

NURSING CONSIDERATIONS

Magnesium sulfate should not be used in the presence of heart block, significant heart damage, or renal failure. Caution must be exercised in the presence of renal function impairment or respiratory disease.

Extreme care must be taken to avoid overdosage and toxic serum concentrations. Intravenous infusions should be administered with a regulating or controlling device.

The client must be closely monitored for the possible development of magnesium toxicity. ECG should be monitored continuously during intravenous administration. Serum magnesium determinations may be obtained as clinically indicated. The patellar reflex or knee jerk is an indication of CNS depression from magnesium. The petellar reflex should be checked before beginning therapy and before each dose. The disappearance of the reflex indicates excessive serum levels of magnesium. The respiratory rate should be at least 16/minute before administration of a parenteral dose.

An intravenous calcium salt (calcium gluconate, calcium gluceptate, or calcium chloride) should be available when parenteral magnesium is administered.

KEY TERMS

acquired seizures, page 271
clonic, page 270
epilepsy, page 269
focal seizures, page 270
idiopathic epilepsy, page 269
organic seizures, page 271
primary epilepsy, page 269
prodrug, page 286
secondary epilepsy, page 269
serum half-life, page 273
status epilepticus, page 270
symptomatic seizures, page 271
tonic, page 270
tonic-clonic generalized epilepsy, page 270
toxemia of pregnancy, page 290

BIBLIOGRAPHY

AHFS Drug Information 88, 1988, American Hospital Formulary Service, Bethesda, American Society of Hospital Pharmacists, Inc

Beniak, J: Patient education in epilepsy, J Neurosurg Nurs 14(1):19, 1982

Breland, BD, and Barnes, WP: Pharmacokinetic principles in relation to serum drug sample collection, South Med J 74(12):1439, 1981

Burgess, KE: Cerebral depressants: their effects and safe administration, Nursing '85 15(8):46, 1985

Cacek, TT, and others: In vitro evaluation of nasogastric administration methods for phenytoin, Am J Hosp Pharm 43:689, 1986

Campbell, C: Nursing diagnosis and intervention in nursing practice, ed 2, New York, 1984, John Wiley & Sons

Carpenito, LJ Nursing diagnosis: application to clinical practice, Philadelphia, 1983, JB Lippincott

Cohen, MR: Medication errors: don't mix Dilantin with dextrose solutions, Nursing '83 13(6):19, 1983

Commission on Classification and Terminology of the International League Against Epilepsy: Proposal for revised clinical and electroencephalographic classification of epileptic seizures, Epilepsia 22:489, 1981

Gever, LN: Anticonvulsants, Nursing '84 14(4):41, 1984

Gever, LN: Your role in valproic acid therapy, Nursing '82 12:104, 1982

Gilman, AG, and others, eds: Goodman and Gilman's The pharmacological basis of therapeutics, ed 7, New York, 1985, Macmillan Publishing Co

---

SIGNS OF HYPERMAGNESEMIA

Approximate serum concentration (mEq/L):
  4-6: therapeutic range, mild depression of deep tendon reflexes
  5-10: depression of deep tendon reflexes; prolonged PQ interval or widened QRS inverval on ECG
  10: loss of deep tendon reflexes
  12-15: respiratory paralysis; complete heart block
  25: cardiac arrest

Signs of hypermagnesemia, which may begin at a serum concentration at or above 4 mEq/L, include flushing, hypotension, sweating, depressed reflexes, reduced respiratory rate, hypothermia, flaccid paralysis, circulatory collapse, slowed heart rate, and CNS depression. Treatment of overdose:
  Discontinue drug administration
  Artificial respiration if necessary
  Intravenous administration of 5-10 mEq of calcium (10-20 ml of 10% calcium gluconate) to reverse respiratory depression or heart block
  Peritoneal or hemodialysis may be required if renal function is reduced

Keys, PA: Valproic acid: interactions with phenytoin and pheno-barbital, Drug Intell Clin Pharm 16(10):737, 1982

Lesser, RP, and Pippenger, CE: Choosing an antiepileptic drug; the care for individualized treatment, Postgrad Med 77(4):225, 1985

Lindsay, ML: Living with epilepsy, Nurs Times 78:1115, 1982

Mancall, EL, and others: Pharmacologic therapy of seizures in the elderly, Hosp Pract, Nov 1984, p 223

Naylor, P: The positive approach, Nurs Mirror 153: 1981

Ozuna, J, and Friel, P: Effect of enteral tube feeding on serum phenytoin levels, J Neurosurg Nurs 16(6):289, 1984

Parrish, MA: A comparison of behavioral side effects related to commonly used anticonvulsants, Pediatric Nurs, 10(2):149, 1984

Rosenberg, JM, and others: Finding the therapeutic window, RN, July 1980, p 46

Sasso, SC: Phenobarbital for neonatal seizures, MCN 9(5):347, 1984

Sasso, SC: Phenytoin for seizure disorders, MCN 9(4):279, 1984

Steinkruger, M: Photosensitive epilepsy, J Neurosurg Nurs 17(6):355, 1985

Trekas, J: Managing epilepsy: don't forget the patient, Nursing '82 12(10):62, 1982

United States Pharmacopeial Convention: Drug information for the health care provider, ed 6, Rockville, Md, 1986, United States Pharmacopeial Convention, Inc

Wilder, BJ, and Schmidt, RP: Current classifications of epilepsies: guide to seizure control and characteristics, Postgrad Med 77(4):188, 1985

Yuen, GJ: Agents affecting phenytoin bioavailability, Drug inter-actions Newsletter 4(10):37, 1984

Central Nervous System Stimulants

The CNS stimulants may produce dramatic effects, but their therapeutic usefulness is limited because of the multiplicity of their actions and side effects. Also, repeated administration and large doses tend to precipitate convulsive seizures, coma, and exhaustion. The number of drugs that stimulate the CNS is large, but the number actually used for this purpose is limited.

Stimulants are classified on the basis of where they exert their major effects in the nervous system—on the cerebrum, the medulla and brainstem, or the hypothalamic limbic regions. **Amphetamines** are mainly stimulants of the cerebral cortex; **analeptics** act mainly on the centers in the medulla and the brainstem; and **anorexiants** suppress the appetite, perhaps by a direct stimulant effect on the satiety center in the hypothalamic and limbic regions. These drugs may also affect other parts of the nervous system. The drugs that act primarily on the medullary centers are said to be the best analeptics.

Cerebral stimulants were commonly prescribed in the past for obesity and to counteract CNS-depressant overdosage, but such use today is considered obsolete. Although the CNS stimulants suppress appetite, tolerance develops to the anorexic effect usually before the weight reduction goal is reached. Treatment of severe CNS depression with stimulants is also discouraged, since close monitoring and supportive measures have been found to be quite successful without the production of

PHARMACOLOGIC MANAGEMENT OF ADD

Studies indicate that about 80% of children with ADD no longer have problems after puberty. However, 20% continue to have ADD and need medication through adolescence. In either case, medication schedules are a challenge for the provider.

Although stimulant medications are available in short-acting (4-hour) and long-acting (8-10 hour) forms, it is general practice to establish a daily schedule using the short-acting form. The dosage required will be learned from empiric experience. For this reason, the prescriber needs to work closely with the client, the parents, and school personnel in evaluating results and planning dosages.

During school hours, management of the distractibility and hyperactivity is necessary. But it may be equally important to contain these symptoms at other times of the day to promote the child's psychosocial development by participating in club membership, religious activities, or social events. Rather than use a continuous approach to dosing, it is more helpful to consider the client's life in 4-hour units and provide a dosage appropriate to the needs of that time block. For example, the client might take 10 mg of a short-acting stimulant at 8 AM and again at noon on a school day but add another dose at 4 PM if a music lesson is planned for that evening.

undesirable adverse effects. CNS stimulants, with their narrow therapeutic index between effectiveness and toxicity, may induce cardiac dysrhythmias, hypertension, convulsions, and/or violent behavior. Thus the CNS stimulants have limited use in practice today; that is, they are primarily used for the treatment of **attention deficit disorder (ADD)** with hyperactivity and narcolepsy.

ADD with hyperactivity is a syndrome characterized by distractibility, a short attention span, impulsive behavior, and hyperactivity. Stimulant medications tend to decrease the distractibility and hyperactivity, resulting in an increased attention span.

Narcolepsy is characterized by excessive drowsiness and uncontrollable sleep attacks during the daytime. In addition, the client may exhibit a sleep paralysis (inability to move that occurs immediately on falling asleep or on awakening), **cataplexy** (stress-induced generalized muscle weakness), and **hypnagogic** illusions or hallucinations (vivid auditory or visual dreams occurring at onset of sleep). CNS stimulants are useful in controlling the daytime drowsiness and excessive sleep patterns, whereas tricyclic antidepressants are being tested in conjunction with the stimulants for cataplexy and sleep paralysis.

Cerebral stimulants can increase excitability by (1) blocking the activity of the inhibitory neurons or their respective neurotransmitters, or (2) enhancing the production or release of the excitatory neurotransmitters (see Figure 15-1). Neurons transmit messages by means of axons to neighboring neurons. When stimulatory neurons are activated (depolarized), a chemical neurotransmitter is released into the synaptic cleft located between neurons. The neurotransmitter may bind on the receptors and when sufficient quantities are attached, the postsynaptic neuron will be activated (depolarized). The two general groups of neurotransmitters are excitatory and inhibitory. Excitatory neurons may release either acetylcholine, norepinephrine, or dopamine (only one type of neurotransmitter per neuron), whereas inhibitory neurons release GABA and glycine, substances that stabilize the neuron to reduce its response to incoming stimuli. GABA is stored in the presynaptic inhibitory neuron, whereas glycine is located in the postsynaptic inhibitory neuron.

Strychnine, a toxic alkaloid used in pesticides, was previously a commonly used circulatory and respiratory stimulant. It was also available in many over-the-counter preparations such as tonics, laxatives, and analgesics up to approximately 1970. It has no legitimate use in medicine today, but it is an important research product because it selectively blocks the postsynaptic inhibitory transmitter glycine. Picrotoxin, another powerful stimulant with limited use in therapeutics, blocks the presynaptic inhibitory transmitter GABA. Both block the receptors on their respective sites, thus reducing or antagonizing the inhibitory effects, which results in excessive muscle activity such a muscle spasms of the face and neck, lockjaw, nystagmus and generalized, violent spasms and convulsive episodes. Since the majority of CNS stimulants do not affect the inhibitory neurons, they are classified as analeptics, that is, drugs that enhance the production or release of the excitatory neurotransmitters. Amphetamines, anorexiant drugs, caffeine, doxapram, methylphenidate, and pemoline all have CNS stimulatory effects.

anorexiant drugs

Anorexiant or appetite suppressant drugs include a variety of medications that are used to treat exogenous obesity (see Table 15-1). Amphetamines affect the neurotransmitter norepinephrine, producing marked euphoria, stimulation, and abuse potential. The anorexiant drugs are lipid soluble and cross the blood-brain barrier.

Phenmetrazine affects norepinephrine and, like amphetamine, produces marked euphoria, stimulation, and abuse potential. Phentermine and diethylpropion affect norepinephrine and produce mild euphoria and mild to moderate stimulation with minimal abuse potential.

Mazindol affects dopamine and adrenergic receptors and has the same CNS effects as diethylpropion, with minimal abuse potential. Fenfluramine increases serotonin, which depresses the CNS while producing appetite suppression. It also increases glucose use and has minimal

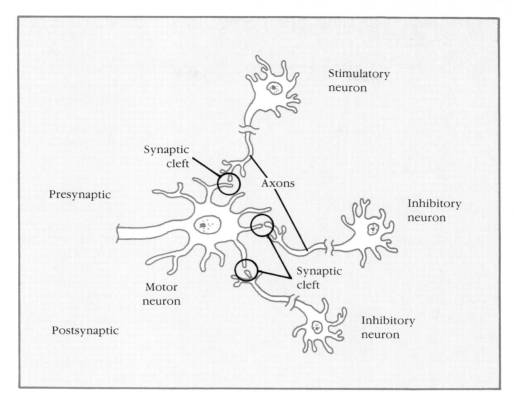

FIGURE 15-1 Neuron transmission.

abuse potential. Fenfluramine would be the drug of choice for anxious individuals or for clients who should avoid the use of CNS-stimulant drugs (such as those with hyperthyroidism, agitation, and advanced arteriosclerosis).

Since anorexiants have a number of limitations, careful selection of the clinical choices is necessary to minimize the unwanted effects. As appetite suppressants, they are recommended as an adjunct to other regimens, such as physical exercise, behavior modification, and restriction of caloric intake, for a short period, usually 6 to 12 weeks. Tolerance to the anorectic effect usually occurs within 6 to 12 weeks.

Side effects/adverse reactions. See Table 15-2.

Significant drug interactions. See box. Concurrent use or use within 14 days of monamine oxidase inhibitors (MAO) with anorexiants should be avoided, since potentiated sympathomimetic effects, including hypertensive crisis, may result. Avoid administration of concurrent CNS-depressant drugs with fenfluramine because enhanced CNS depression may result.

NURSING CONSIDERATIONS

Assessment. Adverse effects of anorexiant drugs, except for fenfluramine, usually relate to overstimulation, such as nervousness, restlessness, insomnia, and anxiety. Because of this effect the drugs are contraindicated for clients with hyperthyroidism, hypertension, advanced arteriosclerosis, glaucoma, and agitated states. Blood pressure and pulse should be monitored to assess whether response is adverse to the drug.

Tolerance is a frequent occurrence with anorexiants, and the client should be assessed for the possibility of habituation and addiction. These drugs are generally contraindicated in clients with a history of substance abuse.

Intervention. These drugs are to be used only as a short-term adjunct to a total weight reduction program than includes a suitable diet, appropriate exercise regimen, and behavior modification related to the cause of overeating.

Preparations that are administered on a daily basis should be administered in the morning to decrease insomnia. Avoid administering anorexiant drugs within 6 hours of sleep times.

These drugs should be administered with caution to clients with diabetes, since the need for insulin may be decreased as a result of the concomitant dietary regimen. Blood and urine glucose levels should be monitored closely.

General anesthesia should be administered with caution.

Do not administer anorexiants during or within 14 days

TABLE 15-1   Anorexiant Medications

Generic name	Trade name	Pregnancy safety FDA category	Recommended dosages
benzphetamine	Didrex	X	Adults, 25-50 mg orally, 1-3 times daily. Not recommended in children less than 12 yr old.
diethylpropion Tablets	Tenuate Tepanil Propion♣ Regibon♣	Unclassified	Adults, 25 mg 3 times daily, 1 hr before meals. Not recommended in children less than 12 yr old.
Extended-release capsules	Nobesine♣		Adults, 75 mg orally daily, at mid-morning. Not recommended in children less than 12 yr old.
Extended-release tablets	Tenuate Dospan Tepanil Ten-tab		Adults, 75 mg orally daily, at mid-morning. Not recommended in children less thatn 12 yr old.
fenfluramine Tablets	Pondimin Ponderal♣	C	Adults, 20 mg initially orally, 3 times daily, ½-1 hr before meals. May increase by 20 mg daily at weekly intervals up to 40 mg 3 times a day. No established pediatric dose (less than 12 yr).
Extended-release capsules	Ponderal Pacaps♣		Adults, 60 mg orally, initially, daily. May be increased to 120 mg daily if necessary. Not recommended in children less than 12 yr old.
mazindol	Mazanor Sanorex	C	Adults, 1 mg initially orally once a day before breakfast. Increase to 1 mg 3 times daily, an hour before meals or 2 mg daily, an hour before lunch. Not recommended in children less than 12 yr old.
phendimetrazine Tablets	Adphen Bontril PDM and others	Unclassified	Adults, 17.5-70 mg orally, 2 or 3 times daily, an hour before meals. Not recommended in children less than 12 yr old.
Capsules	Anorex Statobex		Capsules, same as tablet directions.
Extended-release capsules	Adipost Bontril Slow Release		Adults, 105 mg orally daily, ½-1 hour before breakfast. Not recommended in children less than 12 yr old.
phenmetrazine Tablets	Preludin	Unclassified	Adults, 25 mg orally, 2 or 3 times daily, an hour before meals. Not recommended in children less than 12 yr old.
Extended-release tablets	Preludin		Adults, 75 mg orally daily. Not recommended in children less than 12 yr old.
phentermine Tablets	Adipex-P Phentrol	Unclassified	Adults, 8 mg orally ½ hour before meals or 30-37.5 mg daily before breakfast. Not recommended in children less than 12 yr old.
Capsules	Dapex Fastin Obephen		Adults, capsules same as above.
Extended-release capsules	Parmine		Adults, 30 mg orally before breakfast. Not recommended in children less than 12 yr old.
Resin capsules	Ionamin		Adults, 15 or 30 mg orally daily before breakfast. Not recommended in children less than 12 yr old.

TABLE 15-2 Side Effects/Adverse Reactions of Anorexiant Medications

Side effects*	Adverse reactions†
Most frequent: insomnia reported with all except fenfluramine; euphoria reported with all except fenfluramine and mazindol	CNS depression and confusion reported with diethylpropion and fenfluramine
Increased nervousness and irritability with all except fenfluramine	Allergic rashes or hives reported with fenfluramine
Diarrhea and increased daytime sedation reported mostly with fenfluramine	
Dry mouth with fenfluramine and mazindol	

*If side effects continue, increase, or disturb the client, inform the physician.
†If adverse reactions occur, contact the physician, since medical intervention may be necessary.

of an MAO inhibitor regimen. The interaction with these drugs may result in profound potentiation of the anorexiant effect and a hypertensive crisis may develop.

The use of fenfluramine is contraindicated in clients with alcoholism because depression and psychosis have occurred. It is also contraindicated in clients with a history of depression, since they become depressed or more depressed following withdrawal of the drug.

Education. Clients should be cautioned not to self-regulate the dosage if the drug seems to be less effective but to consult the physician.

Clients should be cautioned that these drugs impair their ability to perform tasks requiring physical coordination and alertness.

Clients should be instructed in ways to minimize unpleasant taste and dryness of mouth with mouth rinses and sugarless candies.

Evaluation. Adverse effects of these drugs, except for fenfluramine, usually relate to overstimulation, such as nervousness, restlessness, insomnia, and anxiety. Fenfluramine is different from the other anorexiants because its adverse effects relate to drowsiness and depression. Diarrhea may be significant enough to decrease the dosage or end the course of fenfluramine.

amphetamines

Mechanism of action. Although their exact mechanism of action is unknown, amphetamines increase the release of catecholamines (norepinephrine from stored sites in nerve terminals), block reuptake of dopamine and norepinephrine following release into the synapse, and inhibit the action of monoamine oxidase (MAO). The result is an increased stimulating effect on the cerebral cortex and reticular activating system, thus increasing alertness and response to incoming stimuli. Increased wakefulness, euphoria, or elation may be noted. Long-term amphetamine abuse can lead to chorea, which is mediated by alterations in the physiology of the basal ganglia; chorea is also seen with cocaine, which reduces dopamine levels.

Amphetamines used over long periods can produce psychologic and physical dependence. Prolonged use of amphetamines leads to the development of tolerance.

Indications. Treatment of ADD with hyperactivity; narcolepsy.

Pharmacokinetics.

Absorption. Good

Distribution. Distributed to body tissues, with especially high concentrations in the brain and cerebrospinal fluid.

Half-life. The half-life depends on urinary pH. Generally amphetamine, 10-30 hr; dextroamphetamine, 10-12 hr for adults and 6-8 hr in children; methamphetamine, 4-5 hr.

Metabolism. Liver

Excretion. Kidneys. pH dependent. Excretion may be increased in an acidic urine and decreased in a more basic urine.

Side effects/adverse reactions. See Table 15-3.

Significant drug interactions. The following effects may occur when amphetamines are given with the drugs listed below:

Drug	Possible Effect and Management
beta-adrenergic blocking drugs (systemic and ophthalmic)	May result in increased alpha-adrenergic effects resulting in hypertension, bradycardia, and possible heart block. If necessary to use both classifications, labetalol, a beta-blocking agent that also has alpha-blocking effects, may reduce the risk of producing the above effects. Monitor closely.
digitalis glycosides	May result in an increase in cardiac dysrhythmias. Avoid usage or, if necessary, monitor very closely.
monoamine oxidase (MAO) inhibitors	Because of increased release of catecholamines, headaches; dysrhythmias; vomiting; sudden, severe hypertension; and possibly hyperthermia may result.

TABLE 15-3 Side Effects/Adverse Reactions of Amphetamines

Side effects*	Adverse reactions†
More frequent: euphoria, increased irritability, nervousness, insomnia, restlessness	More frequent: tachycardia or irregular heart rate
Less frequent: excessive sweating, dry mouth, abdominal cramps, impotency, alterations in sexual desire, diarrhea or constipation, dizziness, anorexia, nausea or vomiting, weight loss, blurred vision	Less frequent: allergic reaction including urticaria, hives, angina or chest pain, tremors, hyperreactive reflexes, dyskinesia
	High dosage or prolonged consumption: CNS mood changes including depression, increased agitation, psychosis; drug dependency and tolerance may also develop

*If side effects continue, increase, or disturb the client, inform the physician.
†If adverse reactions occur, contact the physician, since medical intervention may be necessary.

Drug	**Possible Effect and Management**
thyroid hormone	May result in increased effects and side effects of either medication. Also, thyroid hormone may increase the risk of coronary insufficiency in clients with coronary artery disease.

Dosage and administration. See Table 15-4.
Pregnancy safety. FDA Category C.

NURSING CONSIDERATIONS

Assessment. The nurse should be aware that amphetamines should be avoided by persons with hypertension and cardiovascular disease and by those who are unduly restless, anxious, agitated, and excited.

Nurses should assess pulse and blood pressure of clients receiving amphetamines to monitor for adverse cardiovascular effects of the drug.

Amphetamines should be used with caution in elderly and debilitated clients or those with a history of homicidal or suicidal tendencies.

Intervention. The last dose should be administered not later than 6 hours before the client's bedtime; if a sustained-release product is used, the last dose should be administered not less than 10 to 14 hours before bedtime to avoid insomnia.

The dose should be given 30 to 60 minutes before the client's meal. Dietary and behavior modification is essential if the drug is to be successful as an anorexiant. If weight loss is not desired, administer the drug with or after meals.

Help client overcome a dry mouth with sugarless candy, gum, or ice chips.

The dosage should be gradually reduced before discontinuing the drug following prolonged, high dosage to avoid withdrawal manifestations such as psychotic symptoms and lethargy.

Since fatigue occurs as the drug effects diminish, the nurse should be aware that the client will need more rest and sleep.

The nurse should know that some clients (e.g., those with bronchial asthma who are sensitive to tartrazine dye) should not use some of these dosage forms.

Education. The client should be instructed not to self-regulate the dose; the habit-forming potential should be stressed. If the effect of the drug seems to decrease, the nurse should caution the client not to increase the dosage but to consult the physician.

The nurse should inform the client of the CNS and cardiovascular side effects of the drug.

Clients should be cautioned that amphetamines may impair their functioning in the performance of tasks requiring mental alertness and physical coordination. These drugs are frequently abused by athletes, students, and drivers for the purpose of increasing alertness but may result in an impaired ability to function.

The client should be instructed to swallow the sustained-release tablet whole without breaking, chewing, or crushing.

The nurse should caution the client to keep the drug securely stored to avoid unintended use by another person.

Evaluation. Caution should be used and the possibility of psychologic dependence and addiction should be considered in clients with a history of addiction to alcohol or other drugs. The nurse should evaluate for potential dependence in all clients receiving the drug.

Children receiving amphetamines for a prolonged period should have their growth carefully monitored, since the drug is thought to inhibit growth. These children should also be reevaluated periodically for the need for amphetamines to treat disorders of attention deficit by the interruption of the course of therapy and monitoring for the return of behavioral symptoms.

doxapram (Dopram)

Mechanism of action. Stimulates respiration by acting on the peripheral carotid chemoreceptors at low doses. At

TABLE 15-4   Amphetamine Dosage and Administration

	Adults	Children
Amphetamine		
Narcolepsy	5-20 mg 1-3 times daily	Children to 6 yr, dosage not determined; 6-12 yr, 2.5 mg orally twice daily; increase by 5 mg/day at 1-wk intervals until therapeutic effect or adult dosage achieved. Children 12 yr and older, 5 mg orally, increasing dose by 10 mg/day at weekly intervals until therapeutic effect or adult dosage achieved.
Attention deficit disorder		Children up to 3 yr, not recommended. 3-6 yr, 2.5 mg orally; increase dosage by 2.5 mg/day at weekly intervals until desired therapeutic response achieved. 6 yr and older, 5 mg orally 1 or 2 times/day; increase by 5 mg/day at weekly intervals until desired therapeutic response achieved.
dextroamphetamine capsules, dextroamphetamine sulfate extended release capsules (Dexedrine, Spancap No. 1), dextroamphetamine sulfate elixir (Dexedrine), dextroamphetamine sulfate tablets (Dexampex, Dexedrine, Ferndex)—capsules, tablets, and elixirs:		
Narcolepsy	5-20 mg orally 1-3 times daily.	Children up to 6 yr, dosage not determined. 6-12 yr, 2.5 mg orally twice daily; increase by 5 mg/day at weekly intervals until therapeutic effect or adult dosage achieved. 12 yr and older, 5 mg orally twice daily; increase by 10 mg/day at weekly intervals until therapeutic effect or adult dosage achieved.
Attention deficit disorder		Children up to 3 yr, not recommended. 3-6 yr, 2.5 mg orally daily; increase dosage by 2.5 mg/day at weekly intervals until therapeutic response achieved. 6 yr and older, 5 mg orally once or twice/day; increase dosage by 5 mg daily at weekly intervals until therapeutic response achieved.
dextroamphetamine sulfate extended release capsules (use this dosage form after therapeutic dosage/day established:		
Narcolepsy	5-30 mg daily	Up to 6 yr, see above recommendations. 6-12 yr, 5-15 mg orally daily. 12 yr and older, 10 or 15 mg daily, orally.
Attention deficit disorder		Children up to 6 yr, see above recommendations. 6 yr and older, 5-15 mg orally daily.
methamphetamine hydrochloride tablets (Desoxym, Methapex), methamphetamine hydrochloride extended release tablets (Desoxyn):		
Attention deficit disorder		Children up to 6 yr, not recommended. 6 yr and older, 2.5-5 mg orally 1 or 2 times daily; increase dosage by 5 mg/day at weekly intervals until therapeutic effect achieved (usually 20-25 mg/day).

higher dosages, the medullary respiratory center is stimulated.

Indications. Treatment of respiratory depression induced by a drug overdose, chronic obstructive pulmonary disease, or postanesthetic effects.

Pharmacokinetics. Injectable: intravenous dosing
Onset of effect. 20-40 sec
Peak effect. 1-2 min
Duration of action. 5-12 min
Excretion. Kidneys
Side effects/adverse reactions. See Table 15-5.
Significant drug interactions. Administration of doxapram with monamine oxidase (MAO) inhibitors or vasopressors may result in increase in blood pressure or a hypertensive crisis. Monitor closely.
Dosage and administration. See Table 15-6.
Pregnancy safety. Not established

NURSING CONSIDERATIONS

A patent airway should be established and an adequate oxygen supply ensured before administering to clients with respiratory depression in an attempt to prevent aspiration.

Because intravenous administration tends to cause hemolysis, only dilute solutions should be administered at a slow rate of infusion. To decrease local tissue reaction and thrombophlebitis, various injection sites should be used to avoid extravasation.

Doxapram hydrochloride has a narrow margin of safety. The nurse should observe for early signs of toxicity, such as increased blood pressure and pulse rate, disrhythmias, dyspnea, and increased skeletal response with increased deep tendon reflexes and spasticity. The nurse should monitor pulse, blood pressure, and deep tendon reflexes frequently to avoid overdosage, and the rate of the infusion should be adjusted on the basis of these assessments.

Arterial blood gases should be analyzed before initiation of therapy as a baseline and every 30 minutes thereafter to avoid the possibility of respiratory acidosis.

Because narcosis may recur, close monitoring of the client is necessary until full alertness has been maintained for an hour. Doxapram is a *temporary* measure to correct acute respiratory insufficiency. Mechanical assistance with

TABLE 15-5   Side Effects/Adverse Reactions of Doxapram

Side effects*	Adverse reactions†
Less frequent: urination difficulties, headache, diarrhea, dizziness, cough, hiccups, confusion, warm or burning feeling, nausea or vomiting, sweating	Less frequent/rare: chest pains, tachycardia, extrasystoles, hemolysis, thrombophlebitis, dyspnea, tachypnea
	Overdosage: hypertension, convulsions, trembling, tachycardia, increased deep tendon reflexes

*If side effects continue, increase, or disturb the client, inform the physician.
†If adverse reactions occur, contact the physician, since medical intervention may be necessary.

TABLE 15-6   Doxapram Dosage and Administration

Indication	Adults	Children
Drug-induced CNS depression	1-2 mg/kg body weight IV; may repeat in 5 min. Maintenance, 1-2 mg/kg body weight every 1-2 hr until desired therapeutic response achieved. Maximum, 3g/day. If additional drug dosages necessary, schedule 24 hr from initial dose given in this treatment. Intermittent IV infusion, 1-3 mg/min until therapeutic response achieved or for 2-hr maximum time period. If needed, infusion can be repeated after ½-2 hr, with total dose maximum of 3 g.	Not recommended in children less than 12 yr old.
Chronic obstructive pulmonary disease with acute **hypercapnia** (excessive amounts of CO_2 in blood)	IV infusion, administer 1-2 mg/min; if necessary, administration rate may be increased to 3 mg/min. Maximum time for infusion with no additional infusions recommended, 2 hr.	
Postanesthesia respiratory depression	IV, 0.5-1 mg/kg body weight; do not exceed 1.5 mg/kg as single dose. If needed, dose may be repeated every 5 min up to maximum total dosage of 2 mg/kg body weight.	

ventilation is safer, more reliable, and effective for long-term (over 2 hours) therapy.

methylphenidate hydrochloride (Ritalin)

Mechanism of action. The mechanism of central action is unknown. Pharmacologic actions are similar to amphetamines, with CNS and respiratory stimulation; sympathomimetic activity is also reported. Sites of action are the cerebral cortex and subcortical areas. Methylphenidate also appears to block the reuptake of dopamine into the dopaminergic neurons. In ADD with hyperactivity, methylphenidate decreases motor activity and increases the attention span. In narcolepsy, it appears to stimulate the cortex and subcortex including the thalamic area to increase alertness, lift the spirits, and increase motor activity.

Indications. ADD and narcolepsy.

Pharmacokinetics

Absorption. Good

Peak serum concentration. Tablets in 1.9 hr in children; extended release tablets in 4.7 hr in children

Metabolism. Liver

Excretion. Kidneys

Side effects/adverse reactions. See Table 15-7.

Significant drug interactions. The following effects may occur when methylphenidate hydrochloride is given with the drugs listed below:

Drug	Possible effect and management
other CNS stimulants	May result in additive CNS stimulation effects causing increased nervousness, irritability, insomnia, dysrhythmias, and convulsions. Monitor closely.
monoamine oxidase (MAO) inhibitors	May result in hypertensive crisis. Do not give drugs concurrently or within 14 days of administration of an MAO inhibitor.
pimozide	Should not be administered together. Withdraw client from methylphenidate before starting pimozide therapy. Concurrent use may mask reason for tic development because methylphenidate may also induce tics. Pimozide is indicated for the treatment of tics in clients with Gilles de la Tourette's syndrome.

Dosage and administration. See Table 15-8.

Pregnancy safety. Not established

NURSING CONSIDERATIONS

Assessment. Methylphenidate must be used with caution in clients with epilepsy because the drug can lower

---

TABLE 15-7   Side Effects/Adverse Reactions of Methylphenidate Hydrochloride

Side effects*	Adverse reactions†
More frequent: anorexia, increased nervousness, insomnia (usually more frequent in children) Less frequent: headache, nausea, abdominal pain, drowsiness, dizziness	More frequent: hypertension, tachycardia Less frequent: chest pain, trembling or uncontrolled movements of body, rash, fever of unknown origin, increased bruising Overdosage: confusion, delirium, dry mouth, euphoria, increased fever and sweating, severe headaches, hypertension, tremors, muscle twitching, irregular heartbeats, vomiting, convulsions, and possibly coma

*If side effects continue, increase, or disturb the client, inform the physician.
†If adverse reactions occur, contact the physician, since medical intervention may be necessary.

TABLE 15-8   Methylphenidate Hydrochloride Dosage and Administration

Drug	Adults	Children
methylphenidate hydrochloride tablets (Ritalin)	5-20 mg orally 2 or 3 times daily, 30-45 min before meals	For ADD with hyperactivity: children up to 6 yr, dosage not established; 6 yr and older, 5 mg orally twice daily before breakfast and lunch. Increase dosage by 5-10 mg weekly to maximum of 60 mg daily. Generally, if improvement not seen after dosage adjustments over 30 days, stop medication.
methylphenidate hydrochloride extended-release tablets (Ritalin-SR)	20 mg orally 1-3 times daily every 8 hr on empty stomach	Children up to 6 yr, not established. 6 yr and older, 20 mg orally 1-3 times daily.

the convulsive threshold. It also should be used with caution in clients with hypertension. Long-term therapy should be accompanied by repeated medical examinations and tests for complete blood and platelet counts.

Use of methylphenidate in pregnant or lactating women is not recommended.

Use of methylphenidate is contraindicated in clients with glaucoma.

Intervention. Dosage should be calculated for each client based on the response to the drug. Extended-release forms of the drug should be used only after the initial therapy has established the appropriate dosage for the client.

The nurse should administer the last dose several hours before bedtime to avoid insomnia.

Sole dependence on methylphenidate for treatment of ADD is discouraged. Other therapies (psychologic,educational, social) should be used in conjunction with the drug therapy.

When symptoms of ADD are improved, interruption of drug therapy during times of low stress may be possible. The client may be given medication-free weekends, holidays, or vacations.

Education. The client should be instructed to administer the medication on an empty stomach 30 to 45 minutes before eating. Extended-release forms should be swallowed whole, not crushed, broken, or chewed.

Do not increase the dose if the medication seems less effective.

Regular visits with the client's physician are needed to monitor progress of the drug therapy.

If the client takes large doses over an extended period, withdrawal must be gradual. Caution the clients that they should *not* stop taking the medication without checking with the prescribing physician.

Evaluation. Tolerance and psychologic dependence have occurred with long-term use, and abnormal behavior and psychotic episodes have been observed. When the drug is withdrawn, careful supervision is required since severe depression may result.

Clients should be monitored for weight loss from appetite suppression. Children, in particular, should be assessed on a regular basis for physical growth, since there may be suppression of normal weight gain.

Methylphenidate must be used cautiously in emotionally unstable persons and in those with a history of drug dependence or alcoholism. Drug abusers have used it as a substitute for amphetamines.

The drug should be discontinued periodically to reassess the therapeutic need as indicated by the return of symptoms.

pemoline (Cylert)

Mechanism of action. The mechanism of central action is unknown. Pemoline may act by means of dopaminergic mechanisms.

Indications. ADD with hyperactivity.

Pharmacokinetics

Absorption. Good.

Half-life. 12 hours.

Peak serum concentration. In 2 to 4 hours with peak effect reached in 3 to 4 weeks.

Metabolism. Liver, partially.

Excretion. Kidneys.

Side effects/adverse reactions. See Table 15-9.

Significant drug interations. None have been reported.

Dosage and administration. See Table 15-10.

Pregnancy safety. FDA category B.

NURSING CONSIDERATIONS

Pemoline should be administered in the morning to avoid insomnia at night.

Pemoline must be used cautiously in emotionally labile clients and in clients with a history of drug dependence or alcoholism.

The drug should be discontinued periodically to reassess the need for its administration as indicated by a return of symptoms. The nurse should caution the client that the most common adverse effects are insomnia and anorexia. These are dose related and may be decreased by a dosage adjustment by the physician.

TABLE 15-9 Side Effects/Adverse Reactions of Pemoline

Side effects*	Adverse reactions†
More frequent: anorexia, insomnia, weight loss	Rare: jaundice
Less frequent: dizziness, daytime sedation, irritability, depression, nausea, rash, and abdominal pain	Overdosage: increased agitation, confusion, euphoria, hallucinations, severe headaches, hypertension, elevated temperatures, increased sweating, convulsions, fast heart rate, enlarged pupils, vomiting, uncontrollable muscle movements of eyes

*If side effects continue, increase, or disturb the client, inform the physician.
†If adverse reactions occur, contact the physician, since medical intervention may be necessary.

TABLE 15-10 Pemoline Dosage and Administration

pemoline tablets and pemoline chewable tablets (Cylert)	Children less than 6 yr, not established. 6 yr or older, 37.5 mg orally each morning. Dosage may be increased by 18.75 mg daily on weekly basis until therapeutic response noted or maximum of 112.5 mg per day is reached.

The client should be prepared for an initial weight loss with a return to the normal weight in 3 to 6 months.

Parents should be counseled that the beneficial effect of the medication may not be apparent for 3 to 4 weeks, but that it is important to the success of the regimen that the drug be administered as prescribed.

Also see the discussion of nursing considerations in methylphenidate therapy.

caffeine

Caffeine is a stimulant found in many beverages, foods, over-the-counter drugs, and prescription drugs (see box below). In the United States, it has been estimated that 7 million kg of caffeine are consumed annually. Caffeine has been implicated in many controversial adverse health

---

APPROXIMATE CAFFEINE CONTENT IN FOOD, DRINKS, AND DRUGS

SUBSTANCE/QUANTITY	CAFFEINE (mg)
Brewed coffee, 6 oz	100-150
Instant coffee, 6 oz	85-100
Decaffeinated coffee, 6 oz	2-5
Tea, 6 oz	60-72
Cocoa, 6 oz	50
Cola drink, 12 oz	40-72
Milk chocolate, 1 oz	3-6
Bittersweet chocolate, 1 oz	25-35

OVER-THE-COUNTER PRODUCTS	
Anacin	32
Ayds Extra Strength	200
Dexatrim Capsule	200
NoDoz	100

PRESCRIPTION PRODUCTS	
Fiorinal capsules plain or with codeine	40
Norgesic Forte	60
Darvon Compound	32

EFFECTS OF CAFFEINE

CNS. Although all levels of the CNS may be affected, regular doses of caffeine (100-150 mg) will stimulate the cortex to produce increased alertness and decreased motor reaction time to both visual and auditory events. Drowsiness and fatigue generally disappear. Larger dosages may affect the medullary, vagus, vasomotor, and respiratory centers, resulting in slowing of the heart rate, vasoconstriction, and increased respiratory rate. Studies attribute such effects to competitive blockade of adenosine receptors and accumulation of cyclic AMP. Thus caffeine is being investigated for the treatment of neonatal apnea, generally as an adjunct to nondrug measures and as an alternative to theophylline.

Cardiac. Caffeine stimulates the myocardium, bringing about both an increased heart rate and an increased cardiac output. This effect is antagonistic to that produced on the vagus center; consequently, a slight slowing of the heart may be observed in some individuals and an increased rate in others. The latter effect usually predominates after large doses. Overstimulation may cause tachycardia and cardiac irregularities.

Vascular. Caffeine constricts cerebral blood vessels, resulting in decreased cerebral blood flow and oxygen tension in the brain. Thus caffeine is used in analgesic products and in combination with ergotamine to enhance pain relief and, perhaps, to produce more rapid onset of action. When given with ergotamine, the enhanced effect is believed to be a result of better absorption of the ergotamine in the presence of caffeine.

Caffeine appears to dilate peripheral blood vessels, thereby decreasing peripheral vascular resistance. But this effect is usually offset by the increase in heart rate and cardiac output. Therefore the overall blood pressure response will largely depend on the dosage and the effects that predominate in the individual.

Skeletal muscles. Caffeine affects voluntary skeletal muscles to increase the contractual force and decrease muscle fatigue.

Gastrointestinal. Caffeine increases secretion of pepsin and hydrochloric acid from the parietal cells. This is the reason coffee is restricted in clients who have a gastric or duodenal ulcer.

Renal. Caffeine produces a mild diuretic effect by increasing renal blood flow and glomerular filtration rate and by decreasing the reabsorption of sodium and water in the proximal tubules.

Additional effects. Caffeine also increases metabolic activity, inhibits uterine contractions, increases glucose levels by stimulating glycolysis, and increases catecholamine levels in plasma and urine.

effects, such as cancer, fibrocystic breast disease, and birth defects. Because caffeine has an effect on many body functions, both its short-term and possible long-term effects are of concern (see box for description of effects of caffeine).

Mechanism of action. Multiple mechanisms of action for caffeine include an increase in calcium ion permeability within the sarcoplasmic reticulum; phosphodisterase competitive inhibition, creating cyclic AMP accumulation; and competitive blocking of adenosine receptors.

Indications. Treatment of tiredness or drowsiness; adjunct to analgesics to enhance relief of pain

Pharmacokinetics

Absorption. Good

Distribution. All body compartments; will cross and enter the CNS and readily crosses the placenta

Metabolism. Liver. In adults caffeine is metabolized to theophylline and theobromine, whereas in the neonate only a small portion is metabolized to theophylline.

Half-life. Plasma distribution half-life: 3.5 hr in adults, 70-100 hr in neonates. Elimination half-life: 6 hours in adults, 36 to 144 hours in the neonate; between 4 and 6 months of age, the adult value will be achieved

Peak plasma level. 50 to 75 minutes

Therapeutic plasma levels. 6 to 13 μg/ml; adverse effects reported in levels above 20 μg/ml

Excretion. Adults: kidneys, with only 1% to 2% excreted unchanged; neonates: kidneys, approximately 85% excreted unchanged

Side effects/adverse reactions. See Table 15-11.

Significant drug interactions. The following effects may occur when caffeine is given with the drugs listed below:

Drug	Possible effect and management
other CNS-stimulating drugs, other caffeine-containing medications or drinks	May result in increased CNS stimulation and undesirable side effects, such as increased nervousness, irritability, insomnia, dysrhythmias, and seizures. Monitor closely.
monoamine oxidase (MAO) inhibitors	With large doses of caffeine may produce hypertension or dangerous dysrhythmias. Monitor closely.

Dosage and administration. See Table 15-12.

Pregnancy safety. Not established (also see box on p. 305).

NURSING CONSIDERATIONS

Assessment. Assessment of caffeine intake should be a routine part of the nursing drug history. This includes caffeine intake from foods and beverages, as well as from medications.

Caffeine may exacerbate gastric ulceration in peptic ulcer disease and so should be used cautiously in clients with a history of peptic ulcer.

Because of its suspected potential for causing dysrhythmias, it is recommended that clients with symptomatic cardiac dysrhythmias or palpitations and clients in the recovery phase of acute myocardial infarctions avoid using caffeine.

TABLE 15-11   Side Effects/Adverse Reactions of Caffeine

Side effects*	Adverse reactions†
More frequent: irritation of GI tract resulting in nausea, increased nervousness, or jittery feelings	More frequent in neonates: abdominal swelling or distention, vomiting, body tremors, tachycardia, jitters, or nervousness
	Overdose: increased temperature, headache, increased irritability and sensitivity to pain or touch, increased urination, confusion, dehydration, abdominal pain, agitation, muscle twitching, nausea and vomiting, tinnitus, insomnia, and convulsions

*If side effects continue, increase, or disturb the client, inform the physician.
†If adverse reactions occur, contact the physician, since medical intervention may be necessary.

TABLE 15-12   Caffeine Dosage and Administration

	Adults	Children
caffeine tablets (NoDoz, Quick Pep, Vivarin)	100-200 mg orally, repeat in 3-4 hr if necessary. Maximum, 1000 mg in 24 hr.	Children less than 12 yr old, use not recommended.
caffeine extended-release capsules (Caffedrine, Dexitac)	200-250 mg orally, repeat in 3-4 hr if necessary. Maximum, 1 g/day.	Children less than 12 yr old, use not recommended.

CAFFEINE AND PREGNANCY

The FDA has warned women to avoid or to decrease caffeine consumption during pregnancy. Although there is no direct link between human malformation and caffeine intake, a daily consumption of caffeine (600 mg or more) has been associated with human fetal death and birth defects. Nurses in various settings should instruct pregnant and childbearing-age women to avoid drugs and sodas containing caffeine. Women who continue to drink coffee during their pregnancy should be encouraged to drink decaffeinated or instant coffee and to limit their coffee intake to 2-3 cups a day. Those who drink tea should decrease the brewing time or select a decaffeinated brand or herb tea. The best solution would be to substitute fruit and vegetable juices or water for beverages that contain caffeine.

Education. A client who is or may become pregnant should be advised to avoid or limit her consumption of caffeine-containing foods (e.g., coffee, tea, cola drinks, cocoa, and milk chocolate) and drugs (e.g., over-the-counter stimulants, analgesic combinations, and cold preparations), because there is evidence that caffeine may be an animal teratogen. Further studies are needed to establish a relationship between caffeine and human birth defects.

Caffeine passes into breast milk and may accumulate in nursing infants. Research suggests that when nursing mothers consume large amounts of caffeine, their babies may appear jittery and have trouble sleeping.

When taken close to bedtime, medications and beverages containing caffeine may interfere with sleep. Caffeine is not intended to replace sleep and should not be used for that purpose.

Clients with a hypersensitivity to caffeine should be alerted to its combination with analgesics (acetaminophen, aspirin, and phenacetin) for the treatment of headache. Because the adverse CNS effects for the drug are increased in children, these same combination preparations should be avoided for pediatric use.

Evaluation. The question is sometimes raised whether or not caffeine causes physical and psychologic dependence. Many persons note that if they do not have their usual cup or two of coffee in the morning, they feel irritable and nervous and develop a headache. This probably indicates psychologic and physical dependence. Such clients should be instructed to decrease their caffeine intake by gradually reducing the number of servings of coffee, cola, and tea or by mixing the amounts with decaffeinated preparations and gradually decreasing the proportion of the caffeinated form.

KEY TERMS

analeptics, page 293
anorexiants, page 293
amphetamines, page 293
attention deficit disorder (ADD), page 294
cataplexy, page 294
hypercapnia, page 300
hypnagogic, page 294
narcolepsy, page 294

BIBLIOGRAPHY

American Hospital Formulary Service: Drug information '88, Betheseda, Md, 1988, American Society of Hospital Pharmacists, Inc

Berkow, R, ed: The Merck manual of diagnosis and therapy, vol 1, General medicine, Rahway, NJ, 1982, Merck, Sharp & Dohme, Inc

Brooten, D, and Jordan, CH: Caffeine and pregnancy, J Obstet Gynecol Nurs 12(3):190, 1983

Brown, RT, Slimmer, LW, and Wynne, ME: How much stimulant medication is appropriate for hyperactive school children? J Sch Health 54(3):128, 1984

Brugess, KE: Nursing alert: understanding the spectrum of cerebral stimulants, Nursing '85 15(7):50, 1985

Freeman, DJ: The effectiveness of doxapram administration in hastening arousal following general anesthesia in outpatients J Assoc Nurs Anesthetists 54(1):16, 1986

Gilman, AG, and others, eds: Goodman and Gilman's the pharmacological basis of therapeutics, ed 7, New York, 1985, Macmillan Publishing Co

Hall, JN: Update on designer drugs, Street Pharmacologist 11 (3):3, 1987

Hallal, JC: Are coffee, cold tablets, and chocolate innocuous or is their caffeine hazardous to your patient's health? Am J Nurs 86(4):424, 1986

Handbook of nonprescription drugs, ed 8, Washington DC, American Pharmaceutical Association and The National Professional Society of Pharmacists, 1986

Kunkel, DB: The toxic emergency Top Emerg Med 17(21):81, 1985

Kurppa, K, and others: Coffee consumption during pregnancy and selected congenital malformations: a nationwide case-control study, Am J Public Health 73(12):1397, 1983

Pagliaro, AM, and Pagliaro, LA: Pharmacologic aspects of nursing, St Louis, 1986, The CV Mosby Co

Physicians' desk reference, ed 40, Oradell, NJ, 1986, Medical Economics

Raebel, MA, and Black, J: The caffeine controversy: what are the facts? Hosp Pharm 19(4):257, 1984

Rossignol, AM: Caffeine-containing beverages and premenstrual syndrome in young women, Am J Public Health 75(11):1335, 1985

Silver, LB, and Brunstetter, RW: Attention deficit disorder in adolescents, Hosp Community Psychiatry 37(6):608, 1986

United States Pharmacopeia Convention: Drug information for the health care provider, ed 8, Rockville, Md, 1988, United States Pharmacopeia Convention, Inc

Worthington-Roberts, B, and Weigle, A: Caffeine and pregnancy outcomes, J Obstet Gynecol Nurs 12(3):21, 1983

CHAPTER 16

Psychotherapeutic Drugs

OBJECTIVES

After studying this chapter, the student will be able to:

1. Discuss the use of drug therapy in psychiatry.

2. Identify the common psychotropic drugs.

3. Differentiate between phenothiazine derivatives, tricylclics, monoamine oxidase inhibitors, and lithium.

4. Discuss nursing measures to prevent or treat the common side effects/adverse reactions of psychotherapeutic agents.

5. Identify common tyramine-containing substances and their interaction with MAO inhibitor drugs.

6. Formulate an appropriate plan of care for individual clients who require the administration of psychotherapeutic agents.

Medications discussed in this chapter will include the **antipsychotic agents,** antidepressants, and lithium. Such drugs are used to treat psychoses and affective disorders, especially schizophrenia, depression, and mania. The student is referred to Chapter 10 for a review the physiology and functions of the various components of the central nervous system (CNS). It is necessary to review the CNS functional systems (i.e., reticular activating system, limbic and extrapyramidal systems, plus acetylcholine and catecholamines) to enhance understanding of this chapter.

ANATOMY AND PHYSIOLOGY OF EMOTIONS

To understand the action of drugs in alleviating the symptoms of mental illness, the health care provider must have knowledge of the functioning of the nervous system. The trend toward a holistic view of human beings and their phenomenologic experience no longer allows the practitioner to separate the functions of the mind from the body. Neurophysiologists traditionally have identified each part of the nervous system by a specific function or made tentative architectonic maps of the cerebral cortex, allocating specific functions to various areas of the brain. Research has indicated a change in this perspective. The brain is considered to be a single organ composed of various structures that produce a final, unified effect when they react on each other normally. The interrelationship of various structures is intricate, and allocating special functions to each structure is difficult.

Research has revealed methods for measuring certain types of brain activity, and such information has made it possible to speculate in some detail on the physiologic substrates of emotional activity. For purposes of clarity in the discussion of the neuroanatomic and neurophysiologic bases of emotions, the various aspects of the nervous system are discussed under the following headings:

1. Central nervous system
2. Autonomic regulation
3. Biochemical mechanisms

CENTRAL NERVOUS SYSTEM

The CNS functions in the coordination and direction of activities in the tissues and organs of the body. The various parts and levels of the CNS form a closely related and integrated series of mechanisms and systems through which the human being achieves adjustment and adaptation to the environment. The CNS is responsible for consciousness, behavior, memory, recognition, learning, and the more highly developed attributes such as imagination, abstract reasoning, and creative thought. In addition, it serves to coordinate such vital regulatory functions as blood pressure, heart rate, respiration, salivary and gastric secretions, muscular activity, and body temperature. Discussion is limited to consideration of CNS functions believed to affect the emotions and behavior.

The cerebrum, the largest part of the brain, is divided into two hemispheres. The outer surface of the cerebral hemispheres is composed of gray matter known as the cerebral cortex. It is believed to be the site of consciousness and is divided into sensory, motor, and association areas. These areas receive sensations from organs of special sense (sight, hearing, smell, taste), as well as from the skin, muscles, joints, and tendons (touch, pain, temperature). Large parts of the cortex now appear to function as a whole in providing the anatomic basis for such mental attributes as recognition, memory, intelligence, imagination, and creative thought.

Beneath the cortex are tracts of fibers comprising the white matter, which connect the lower centers of the brain, spinal cord, and associated areas of the cortex with each other. The basal ganglia (corpus striatum, claustrum, amygdaloid nucleus) are located near the lateral ventricle of the cerebrum. The hippocampus, a mass of gray matter lying close to the lateral ventricle, is connected by a tract of fibers (the fornix) to the mamillary bodies in the hypothalamus. The hippocampus, the fornix, the amygdaloid nucleus, the hippocampal gyrus, and the uncus are collectively referred to as the limbic system. This system is believed to be concerned with the conscious experience of emotion.

The midbrain, pons, and medulla form the part of the brain below the cerebrum. The midbrain contains the nuclei of cranial nerves III and IV. The pons is mainly a pathway for ascending and descending tracts of the fibers. The medulla oblongata is continuous with the spinal cord. It contains vital groups of synapses that are concerned with the reflex control of blood pressure (vasomotor center), heart rate and force (cardiac center), respiration (respiratory center), and vomiting (vomiting center). The reticular formation consists of a complex network of cell bodies and interlacing fibers in the medulla, pons, midbrain, and diencephalon. The reticular activating system (Figure 16-1) is believed to function in alerting the cortex to sensory stimuli and in originating the emotional reactions associated with somatic sensory experiences (pain, touch, hearing, sight). Experimental stimulation of this system produces alertness in behavior, whereas a decrease in its activity leads to relaxation and drowsiness. The reticular activating system has its upper end in the posterior hypothalamus and lower thalamus.

The cerebellum lies on the dorsal side of the pons and is attached to the brainstem. It functions as part of the feedback mechanisms concerned with subconscious control of equilibrium, posture, and movement.

The thalamus and hypothalamus are located in the region of the brain that is called the diencephalon (the "between-brain"). Most sensations are relayed through the thalamus to the cerebral cortex. The conscious appreciation of pain is said to be located in the thalamus. In recent years knowledge about the functions of the hypothalamus gradually has increased. Despite extensive research and experimentation, however, there still seems to be some question of its specific mode of function. It has been conjectured that the hypothalamus contains integrative mechanisms that, in addition to their effect on behavior patterns, also aid in regulating the basic human life functions (control of water excretion, appetite, sleep-wake mechanisms, temperature, blood pressure). The hypothalamus seems to function through its relationships with other parts of the nervous system and endocrine system. It is part of a system of complex circuits within the brain so strategically placed that its derangement may have profound effects.

These interrelationships among the various circuits in the brain produce patterns of behavior that can be modified by external situations or by internal autonomic adjustments. This allows the individual to adapt to changes in both external and internal environments.

AUTONOMIC REGULATION

The functions of the sympathetic and parasympathetic visceral nervous systems are discussed in Chapter 18. These systems play an important role in the production of behavior. An understanding of these mechanisms is the basis for learning the actions and side effects of the drugs

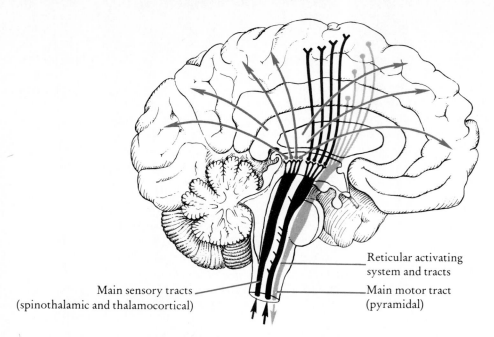

Reticular activating
system and tracts

Main motor tract
(pyramidal)

Main sensory tracts
(spinothalamic and thalamocortical)

FIGURE 16-1   Reticular activating system.

affecting mood and behavior. The importance of these systems' reactions in the production of behavior is paramount in gaining an understanding of drug action or the behavioral manifestations of side effects from the use of drugs.

BIOCHEMICAL MECHANISMS

The functions of the CNS depend on the actions of certain neurohormonal agents located in the brain and peripheral tissues. These neurohormones are stored in inactive forms, and at the right moment nerve impulses release their free forms, which then stimulate transmission of appropriate reactions.

Nerve impulses are conducted along the nerve cell by electric impulse and between nerve cells by chemical means. The **neurotransmitter** is the chemical substance that transmits an impulse or message from neuron to neuron; it is synthesized and stored in the presynaptic neuron. When the presynaptic neuron is stimulated by an electric impulse, it releases the neurotransmitter into the synapse, allowing it to cross the synapse and come into contact with the postsynaptic site. This in turn is the stimulus to which the postsynaptic site responds.

The postsynaptic cell may be another nerve cell that responds by releasing a neurotransmitter, or it may be a muscle cell that responds by contracting or relaxing, as discussed earlier. In either case the neurotransmitter exerts its action by interacting with the **receptor** (a specialized protein), located on the outermost part of the postsynaptic cell. This produces both electric and biochemical change within the postsynaptic cell.

The postsynaptic cell can be made more or less sensitive to the neurotransmitter by various processes or chemicals. **Desensitization,** or reduced sensitivity of the postsynaptic cell, can be caused by **tachyphylaxis, tolerance,** or **refractory responses,** which require more neurotransmitter to produce a response in the postsynaptic cell. **Supersensitivity,** or increased sensitivity of the postsynaptic cell, can be caused by prolonged blockade with drugs called **antagonists,** which bind to the postsynaptic cell without activating it. In these cases the postsynaptic cell responds to less neurotransmitter substance.

Evidence shows that acetylcholine is released from central neural tissue, such as the surface of the cerebral cortex, into the cerebrospinal fluid during activity. The rate of release is proportional to the level of activity. This is how it is known that some central synapses are cholinergic.

Norepinephrine also has been found in the CNS. Tyrosine and dopamine are normal constituents of the brain and known precursors of norepinephrine synthesis. High concentrations of norepinephrine are found in the hypothalamus, medulla, limbic system, and cranial nerve nuclei. Low concentrations are found in the striatum and caudate nucleus, where dopamine, the immediate precursor of norepinephrine, is found in high concentration (Figure 16-2). It is believed that both norepinephrine and dopamine function as transmitters. They have widespread inhibitory and excitatory effects on a wide variety of centrally mediated functions, such as sleep and arousal, affect, and memory. Thus some central synapses are **adrenergic.**

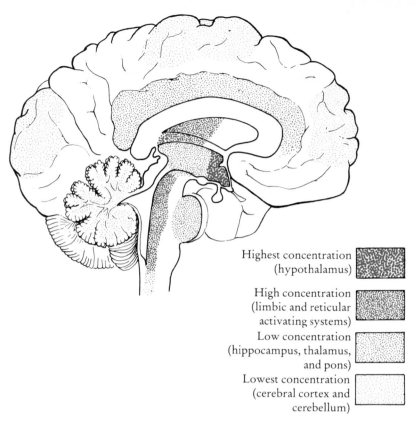

Highest concentration
(hypothalamus)

High concentration
(limbic and reticular
activating systems)

Low concentration
(hippocampus, thalamus,
and pons)

Lowest concentration
(cerebral cortex and
cerebellum)

FIGURE 16-2   Comparative concentrations of serotonin and norepinephrine in various parts of the brain.

Serotonin is another transmitter substance found in the CNS. Areas rich in serotonin include the hypothalamus, pineal gland, midbrain, and spinal cord (see Figure 16-2). Serotonin is synthesized in the brain and stored in the subcellular particles. Alteration of the level of serotonin in the nervous system is associated with changes in behavior. Many drugs mimic or block the action of serotonin on peripheral tissues and produce changes in mood and behavior, which suggests that they interfere with the action of serotonin and norepinephrine in the brain.

Other proposed central neurotransmitters include histamine, amino acids (i.e., glutamate, glycine, excitatory transmitters, aspartate, and GABA, substance P (a polypeptide composed of 13 different amino acids), prostaglandins, and the endorphins.

The relationship of dopamine to major psychoses is receiving much attention. Drugs such as the phenothiazines block the effects of dopamine and function as antipsychotic agents.

ROLE OF DRUG THERAPY IN PSYCHIATRY

Drugs play an important role in contemporary approaches of psychiatric care. The development of the tranquilizing drugs opened many avenues of treatment previously unavailable. Although many emphasize milieu factors in therapy, drug therapy is a valuable adjunct to providing comprehensive psychiatric care.

Drug therapy alleviates symptoms and allows the client an opportunity to participate more easily in other forms of treatment. Drugs temporarily modify behavior, whereas other therapies, such as psychotherapy, can shape behavior and produce a permanent change. Some drugs disrupt patterns of behavior or modify the electric patterns of fields within the brain that produce changes. However, any enduring effects on behavior are more likely to result from the individual's concurrent interaction with the environment. Since incoming information must be translated into biochemical changes before it can affect nervous system function, environmental transactions, as with drugs, may affect similar pathways before influencing behavior. Their effects can be additive, potentiating, or antagonistic, depending on their nature and direction. The milieu may potentiate the effectiveness of the drug or detract from it.

In the past, physicians selected psychotherapeutic agents on the basis of the diagnostic category—schizophrenia, manic-depressive syndrome, or psychoneurosis. More recent proposals, however, have indicated a radical change in the physician's approach.

The pharmacologic treatment of psychiatric disorders would appear to be similar to that of somatic disorders—modifying the most disabling components of the client's behavior so that the client may cope more effectively with the environment and take advantage of the therapeutic milieu available. The physician should try to match a particular drug's therapeutic advantages to the client's symptoms. This implies a thorough assessment of the individual before drug administration including the specific disabling features of the client's behavior, a decision about the goals of therapy, the dynamics involved, and the specific changes sought. Other factors helpful in making an accurate assessment of the client's need for drug therapy are:

1. Degree of agitation or behavioral arousal
2. Degree of overactivity or underactivity
3. Patterns of affective response to stress (avoidance or escape, aggression, fear, inhibited withdrawal)
4. Degree of social withdrawal
5. Nature and dynamics of depressive elements present
6. Sleep problems
7. Need for environmental control
8. Current health status
9. Possible drug dependence
10. Past drug history—effectiveness of response to drugs
11. Knowledge, thoughts, and feelings regarding medications

When the physician establishes the need for drug therapy, it must be decided what agent or combination of agents is best suited for the client's total health needs. This requires an intimate knowledge of the behavioral actions, pharmacologic effects, and potential adverse reactions of the agents used, as well as an awareness of the many individual and environmental factors present.

The additional effects or side effect profile of a drug is a useful tool in helping the physician select an appropriate antipsychotic agent (Table 16-1). If a drug with a strong sedation property is desired, chlorpromazine or thiridazine would probably be selected. If extrapyramidal side effects are particularly troublesome, the same two drugs have the least potential of inducing extrapyramidal side effects; thioridazine has the greatest anticholinergic effect, thus reducing its potential for this adverse effect.

If anticholinergic side effects such as dry mouth, blurred vision, constipation, and urinary retention continue and are disturbing to the client, the physician could select an agent with less potential of inducing such effects, such as fluphenazine (Prolixin, Permitil), thiothixene (Navane), or haloperidol (Haldol).

Continuous nursing and medical evaluation based on observation of the drug's effects is needed. An increase or reduction of dosage may be indicated to achieve the desired effects. Health care providers play an important role in the evaluation and assessment of a client's response to drug therapy. They should be aware of the criteria the physician uses in selecting psychotherapeutic

drugs and the expected effects so they can observe and report on the client's progress. This progress is evaluated by monitoring the client's behavioral and affective responses to the medications; the client's knowledge of the drug therapy; the presence and extent of expected side effects and adverse reactions and their response to dosage adjustment and supportive nursing interventions; and the potential for, or existence of, drug or food interactions. Knowledge of the action of drugs also assists health care providers in understanding the interpersonal responses that occur in the therapeutic client relationship with the client.

ANTIPSYCHOTIC OR NEUROLEPTIC AGENTS
HISTORICAL BACKGROUND

Between 1900 and 1950 the population of the United States doubled, and the population in public mental hospitals quadrupled. The increase was from 130,000 to over a half million clients. During this time, the average length of confinement was usually years, and the trend was definitely toward an increase in clients admitted to such institutions yearly. Also, client and employee injuries caused by combative or abusive clients led to the use of physical restraints and client isolation.

For hundreds of years the treatment of mentally disturbed clients consisted of isolation (i.e., hidden in cellars or attics in their homes); if they came to the attention of local authorities, they were transferred to jails or homes for the insane. Actual therapies before the antipsychotic agents were limited to water or ice pack therapies, straitjackets or the use of other physical restraints, shock therapy with insulin or electricity, lobotomy, and the use of a few drugs, such as paraldehyde, chloral hydrate, and the barbiturates.

Chlorpromazine (Thorazine) was the first **tranquilizer,** released in the early 1950s. However, the term "tranquilizer" had been used approximately 200 years ago by Dr. Benjamin Rush. Dr. Rush, an early pioneer in the mental health field and a signer of the Declaration of Independence, invented a restraining chair named the "tranquilizing chair" (Lyons and Petrucelli, 1978). This chair was modified by the addition of a pulley system, so that the extremely agitated client would be seated and restrained in the chair and the chair would be raised off the ground and rocked back and forth until the client was quieted (Figure 16-3). Thus the name tranquilizer chair. Neither the tranquilizer chair nor the tranquilizing agents cure mental illness. They have been and are used to control the symptoms associated with this disease state; the chair provides physical and eventually physiologic restraints, whereas the antipsychotic and tranquilizing agents constitute a chemical control of the symptoms.

The advent of antipsychotic drugs has proved to be a revolutionary force in the psychiatric field. Institutionalization time has decreased from years to months for many

TABLE 16-1 Classification of Selected Antipsychotic Agents and Potential Side Effects

Chemical class, generic name (trade name)	Potential frequency of side effects*				
	Sedation	Hypotension	Extrapyramidal	Anticholinergic	Antiemetic
PHENOTHIAZINE, ALIPHATIC					
chlorpromazine (Thorazine, Chlorpropamide♣, Largactil♣)	4	4	2	3	4
PHENOTHIAZINE, PIPERIDINE					
thioridazine (Mellaril, Novoridazine♣, Apothioridazine♣)	4	4	1	4	1
mesoridazine (Serentil)	4	2-3	1	2-3	1
PHENOTHIAZINE, PIPERAZINE					
trifluoperazine (Stelazine, Soloazine♣)	2	1	4	1	4
fluphenazine (Permitil, Prolixin, Apo-Fluphenazine♣)	1	1	4	1	1
perphenazine (Trilafon, Phenazine♣, Apo-Perphenazine♣)	1-2	1	4	2	4
prochlorperazine maleate (Compazine, Stemetil♣)	1-2	1	4	2-3	4
BUTYROPHENONE					
haloperidol (Haldol, Apo-Halperidol♣, Novoperidol♣)	1-2	1	4	2-3	1-2
THIOXANTHENE					
thiothixene (Navane)	1-2	1	2	1	†
DIHYDROINDOLONES					
molindone (Lidone, Moban)	3	1	3-4	3-4	†
DIBENZOXAZEPINES					
loxapine (Loxitane, Daxolin, Loxapac♣)	2-3	2-3	4	2-3	†

*Potential frequencies are ranked from the least (1) to most frequent occurence (4).
†Not documented or unknown.

clients, and others live at home and are treated at community mental health centers. The reported incidences of injuries have declined, along with the decrease in size or closing of many large public mental health facilities.

PHENOTHIAZINE DERIVATIVES

Discovery of the phenothiazine derivatives arose out of research in the area of the antihistamines. Chlorproma-zine hydrochloride was introduced in 1951 and has found wide acceptance in the treatment of mental illness. Additional investigation of the action of chlorpromazine in producing undesirable side effects led to the development of numerous derivatives, which now comprise the largest group of psychotropic agents.

About two thirds of all antipsychotic drugs are phenothiazine derivatives. They are commonly divided chemically into the following three subgroups: (1) the aliphatic

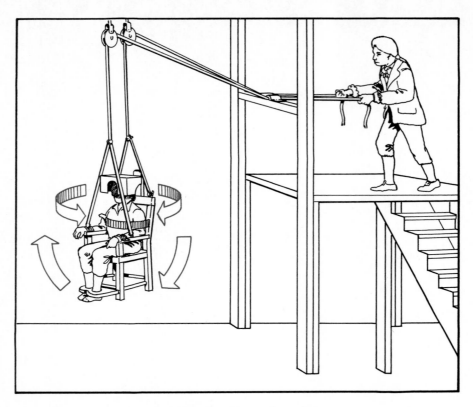

FIGURE 16-3 Tranquilizer chair.

compounds (chlorpormazine, triflupromazine), (2) the piperidine compounds (mesoridazine, piperacetazine, thioridazine), and (3) the piperazine compounds (acetophenazine, carphenazine, fluphenazine, perphenazine, prochlorperazine, trifluoperazine). Although a close structural similarity exists, thioxanthene derivatives (thiothixene, chlorprothixene) are not phenothiazine derivatives. The chemical structure of these compounds and specific information regarding their action, effects, and adverse reactions are presented separately after the general discussion of similarities. The type of action is essentially similar with all phenothiazine derivatives; individual compounds vary chiefly in their potency and in the nature and severity of their side effects.

Mechanism of action. Although the exact mechanism of action for the antipsychotic effects is unknown, a primary effect is the blockage of dopamine receptors in specific areas of the CNS. Dopamine is a major neurotransmitter in the subcortical and basal ganglia areas of the brain. These are the areas associated with emotions, cognitive functioning, and motor functions. Thus the major therapeutic effects and side affects are a result of the dopamine blockade in these areas.

In addition, phenothiazines may also produce an alphablocking effect (hypotension), depression of hormonal release from the hypothalamus and pituitary glands, blockade at the chemoreceptor trigger zone (antiemetic effect), and depression of activity of the reticular acting system (sedative effect). It has also been proposed that haloperidol decreases the release of growth hormone and increases the release of prolactin from the pituitary. Thiothixene also increases prolactin release in the body.

Indications
1. Treatment of psychosis
2. Treatment of nausea and vomiting (especially, chlorpromazine, perphenazine, prochlorperazine, triflupromazine)
3. Sedative
4. Treatment of Gilles de la Tourette's syndrome (haloperidol)

Pharmacokinetics
Absorption. Orally, usually good
Metabolism. Liver
Onset of action. Orally, between 30 minutes and 1 hour; IM, within 30 minutes with exception of fluphenazine enanthate and fluphonazine decoanoate
Duration of action. haloperidol, average 21 hours (range 13 to 35 hours)
loxapine, up to 12 hours
thiothexene, approximately 30 hrs
phenothiazines, 6 to 36 hours or more (this depends on the dosage and frequency of drug administration)
Excretion. Primarily kidneys

Side effects/adverse reactions. Table 16-2.

Significant drug interactions. The following effects may occur when antipsychotic agents are given with the drugs listed below:

Drug	Possible Effect and Management
alcohol, CNS depressants	May result in enhanced CNS depression, respiratory depression, and hypotensive effects. The excitatory CNS response to barbiturate anesthetics may also be increased, especially with phenothiazines. Reduce drug dosage to one-fourth to one-half usual dose.
antithyroid medications	Increases the risk for agranulocytosis when phenothiazines are given concurrently.
epinephrine	Antipsychotic agents may block alpha-adrenergic receptors, thus concurrent administration of epinephrine may result in severe lowering of the blood pressure (hypotension) and tachycardia.
extrapyramidal inducing medications (such as amoxapine, droperidol, metoclopramide, reserpine, metyrosine, papaverine)	May result in increased frequency and severe extrapyramidal effects.
levodopa	Concurrent use may render levodopa ineffective in controlling parkinson's disease.
lithium	Phenothiazines may (1) decrease GI absorption of chlorpromazine by as much as 40%, (2) increase the rate of lithium excretion in the kidneys, (3) increase extrapyramidal symptoms, and (4) induce nausea and vomiting which are signs to monitor for lithium toxicity; the antiemetic phenothiazines may mask these signs. With haloperidol, extrapyramidal side effects may be in-

Drug	Possible Effect and Management
	creased also. Although controversial, there are reports of irreversible neurologic and brain damage when both drugs are given for longer periods than the first couple weeks. If given concurrently, monitor clients closely since dosage reductions may be necessary.
guanadrel or guanethidine	Concurrent use with antipsychotic agents, especially loxapine and thiothixenes, may reverse the hypotensive drug effectiveness. Closely monitor all clients receiving this drug combination.
metrizamide	When given concurrently with phenothiazines, may lower the seizure threshold. Discontinue phenothiazines at least 2 days before and also for 1 day after a myelogram.

Dosage and administration. See Tables 16-3 to 16-5.
1. Before beginning antipsychotic therapy, the client (most especially the geriatric client) should have a drug-free period to rule out drug-induced psychiatric illness. Visual and auditory hallucinations have been reported with anticonvulsants, baclofen, cimetidine, and levodopa, whereas anticholinergic-induced psychosis has been seen with amitriptyline (especially in children and the elderly) and other tricyclic antidepressants (Salerno, 1986).
2. The dosage of the antipsychotic agents may vary according to the individual, the reason for treatment, and client's response to the medication. It is best to titrate from a low dose, increasing when necessary to produce a therapeutic response, which usually occurs within days to a couple of months. Continue at this dosage for 14 days and then gradually decrease dosage to lowest amount that produces a therapeutic response.
3. When stopping antipsychotic therapy, gradually reduce the dosage over 2 or 3 weeks. When antipsy-

TABLE 16-2 Side Effects/Adverse Reactions of Antipsychotic Medications

Side effects*	Adverse reactions†
More frequent: sleepiness, dizziness, dry mouth, constipation, and nasal congestion reported with aliphatic and piperidine phenothiazines and thioxanthenes. Incidence is less with the piperazine phenothiazines with the exception of perphenazine.	Visual changes, hypotensive episodes (more common with aliphatic and piperidine phenothiazines, thioxanthenes, and possibly, molindone.)
thioxanthenes, skin sensitivity to the sun.	Dystonia and/or parkinson-type side effects including shuffle in walk, arm or leg stiffness, tremors, masklike facial expression, dysphagia, imbalance, muscle spasms or unusual twisting effects of face, neck, or back (more common with aliphatic and piperazine phenothiazines, thioxanthines, loxapine, molindone, and haloperidol).
loxapine, most often seen are blurred vision, confusion, dizziness, dry mouth, and increase in body weight.	
haloperidol, usually blurred vision, constipation, dry mouth, and increase in body weight.	Akathisia, increased pacing, restlessness, and insomnia (more often reported with haloperidol, loxapine, thioxanthene).
molindone, usually sedation, blurred vision, dry mouth, and constipation.	Tardive dyskinesia, a very serious adverse reaction (see box).

*If side effects continue, increase, or disturb the client, inform the physician.
†If adverse reactions occur, contact the physician, since medical intervention may be necessary.

TABLE 16-3   Dosage and Administration of Aliphatic Phenothiazine

	Adults	Elderly	Children
chlorpromazine oral tablets/liquid	10-50 mg orally, 2-6 times daily as required. Usual maximum dosage is 1000 mg daily, although increases to 2000 mg daily for a short time have been used. Maintenance therapy, 1000 mg or less per day usually adequate.	Should receive lower than adult dosages, increasing as necessary according to response and/or development of side effects.	Infants less than 6 mo, not established. 6 mo old and older, 0.55 mg/kg orally or 15 mg/m² body surface area 4 times a day as necessary and tolerated.
chlorpromazine hydrochloride extended release capsules	30-300 mg orally 1-3 times daily. Adjust dosage as necessary.	Same as above.	Not recommended.
chlorpromazine hydrochloride injection	25-50 mg IM, repeat in 1 hr if necessary, then every 3-12 hr as necessary. 25-50 mg diluted to concentration of 1 mg/ml IV. Dilute with NaCl injection and administer at rate of 1 mg/min.	Same as above.	Infants less than 6 mo, not established. 6 mo or older, 0.55 mg/kg body weight or 15 mg/m² body surface area IM or IV every 6-8 hr as necessary. Maximum per day, 40 mg for children 6 mo-5yr, with up to 75 mg daily for 5-12 yr olds.
chlorpromazine suppositories	50-100 mg rectally 3 or 4 times daily as necessary.	Same as above.	Infants less than 6 mo, not established. 6 mo and older, 1 mg/kg body weight, rectally 3 or 4 times daily as necessary.
promazine tablets (Sparine)	10-200 mg every 4-6 hr; maximum of 1 g daily.	Lower initial dose, increase as needed and tolerated.	Children less than 12 yr, dosage has not been established. 12 yr and older, 10-25 mg every 4-6 hr with adjustments as needed.
promazine injection (Prozine, Sparine)	10-200 mg IM, repeat in 4-6 hr as needed and tolerated. IV, administered slowly after dilution to 25 mg or less/ml with NaCl injection	Same as above.	Children less than 12 yr, dosage has not been established.
triflupromazine injection (Vesprin)	Antiemetic IM 5-15 mg every 4 hr, up to 60 mg daily; IV 1 mg as needed (up to 3 mg daily). antipsychotic IM 60 mg as needed, up to 150 mg daily.	Lower initial dose, increase as needed and tolerated.	Less than 2½ yrs, dosage not established. Over 2½ yrs, IM 200-250 mcg (0.2-0.25 mg) per kg of body weight, not over 10 mg daily. IV, not recommended, may cause hypotension and rapid onset of severe extrapyramidal reactions.

TABLE 16-4 Piperidine Phenothiazine Dosage and Administration

	Adults	Elderly	Children
thioridazine oral tablets/liquid	25-100 mg orally 3 times daily as necessary. Maintenance, 10-200 mg orally 2-4 times daily. Maximum dosage is 800 mg daily.	Should receive lower than adult dosages, increasing as necessary according to response and/or development of side effects.	Children less than 2 yr, not established. Children 2-12 yr, 0.25-3 mg/kg body weight or 7.5 mg/m², orally 4 times daily or 10-25 mg 2 or 3 times daily.
mesoridazine besylate oral tablet/liquid	10-50 mg orally 2 or 3 times daily as necessary up to 400 mg/day maximum.	Same as above.	Children less than 12 yr, not established. Children 12 yr and older, same as adult dosage.
mesoridazine besylate injection	25 mg IM; may repeat in 30-60 min if necessary.	Same as above.	

TABLE 16-5 Piperazine Phenothiazine Dosage and Administration

	Adults	Elderly	Children
trifluoperazine hydrochloride tablet/liquid	1-5 mg twice daily initially, titrate dosage as necessary up to maximum of 40 mg daily.	Should receive lower than adult dosage, increasing as necessary according to response and/or development of side effects.	Children less than 6 yr, not established. 6 yr and older, 1 mg once or twice daily, titrate dosage as necessary.
trifluoperazine hydrochloride injection	1-2 mg IM every 4-6 hr as necessary. Maximum is 10 mg daily.	Same as above.	Children less than 6 yr, not established. 6 yr and older, 1 mg once or twice a day IM.
fluphenazine hydrochloride tablet/liquid	0.5-2.5 mg orally 1-4 times daily, adjust dosage as necessary.	Same as above.	0.25-0.75 mg orally 1-4 times daily.
fluphenazine decanoate injection (Prolixin decanoate, Modecate)	12.5-25 mg IM or SC; may repeat in 1-3 wk as necessary. Maximum, 100 mg/dose.		Children less than 12 yr, not established. 12 yr and older, see adult dosage.
fluphenazine Enanthate injection (prolixin enanthate, Moditen)	25 mg IM or SC; repeat in 1-3 wk as necessary. Maximum, 100 mg.		Same as decanoate.
fluphenazine hydrochloride injection	1.25-2.5 mg IM every 6-8 hr as necessary. Maximum 10 mg daily.	Same as above	Same as decanoate.
perphenazine tablet/liquid	2-16 mg orally, 2-4 times a day as necessary.	Same as above.	Same as decanoate.
perphenazine extended-release tablets	8-16 mg orally 1-4 times daily as necessary.	Same as above.	Not recommended for children.
perphenazine injection	5-10 mg IM every 6 hr as necessary. IV, dilute 5 mg with NaCl injection to 0.5 mg/ml and administer at rate of 1 mg/min. Maximum for ambulatory clients, 15 mg daily; for hospitalized clients, up to 30 mg daily.	Same as above.	Same as decanoate.

Continued.

TABLE 16-5 Piperazine Phenothiazine Dosage and Administration—cont'd

	Adults	Elderly	Children
prochlorperazine maleate tablets/ prochlorperazine edisylate liquid	5-10 mg orally 3-4 times daily as necessary up to 150 mg daily.	Same as above.	Children less than 2 yr or 9 kg, not established. 2 yr and older or more than 9 kg, 0.1 mg/kg body weight or 2.5 mg/m^2 body surface area 4 times daily orally.
			Antiemetic: children 9-13 kg, 2.5 mg once or twice a day; not to exceed 7.5 mg in 24 hr. Children 14-17 kg, 2.5 mg 2 or 3 times daily; not to exceed 10 mg in 24 hr. Children 18-39 kg, 2.5 mg 3 times daily or 5 mg twice a day; not to exceed 15 mg in 24 hr. Antipsychotic or sedative: children 2-12 yr, 2.5 mg orally 2 or 3 times daily. Check literature for further instructions.
prochlorperazine maleate extended-release capsule	10-75 mg orally every 12 hr as necessary. Maximum, 150 mg daily.	Same as above.	Not recommended.
prochlorperazine edisylate injection	Antiemetic or sedative: 5-10 mg IM every 3 to 4 hr as necessary. Maximum, 40 mg/day. Antipsychotic: 10-20 mg IM every 4-6 hr as necessary. Maximum, 200 mg/day.	Same as above.	Children less than 2 yr or 9 kg, not established. Children 2-12 yr, 0.132 mg/kg body weight IM.
prochlorperazine suppositories	25 mg rectally twice daily as needed.	Same as above.	Children less than 2 yr or 9 kg, not established. Children 9-13 kg, 2.5 mg rectally once or twice daily; not to exceed 7.5 mg/24 hr. Children 14-17 kg, 2.5 mg 2 or 3 times daily; not to exceed 10 mg/24 hr. Children 18-39 kg, 2.5 mg rectally 3 times daily or 5 mg twice daily; not to exceed 15 mg/24 hr. See directions for further instructions.

chotic agents have been given to clients in high doses or for a long time and are suddenly discontinued, nausea, vomiting, dizziness, tremors, and dyskinesia have been reported.

4. Antipsychotic agents may cause a number of cardiovascular effects, including hypotension (caused by alpha-adrenergic blockade), tachycardia (anticholinergic effect), myocardial depressant effects, and electrocardiographic alterations affecting ST, T wave, and widening of QRS interval. The most cardiotoxic agents are chlorpromazine and thrioidazine, and when possible they should be avoided in clients with cardiac disease. The high-potency antipsychotics, such as haloperidol, have fewer cardiotoxic effects so they may be the preferred agents in such clients.

5. In the past, many clients said to be resistant to drug therapy were found to be noncompliant with the prescribed therapy. Many psychotic clients deny their illness or may see the consumption of medications as being associated with dependence or weakness. Clients refractory to antipsychotic medications should be reviewed for:

a. Compliance. The physician may order a plasma serum level of the medication, if such a test is available, to determine the reliability of the client; or the drug order may be switched to a liquid formulation to be administered in a supervised setting.

b. The physician should adjust the dosage according to the individual needs of the client. Inadequate doses or the development of drug toler-

TARDIVE DYSKINESIA

Tardive dyskinesia (TD) is a potentially irreversible neurologic disorder that primarily involves the buccolingual and masticatory muscles. This adverse effect to the antipsychotic agents may occur within a few months or years of treatment or after these agents have been discontinued. The risk of inducing TD increases with total dosage of the drug given and the length of the treatment period.

Incidence: Although 0.5%-65% of the treated population may develop this syndrome, recent reports place the percentage of clients at risk as 10%-20%.

Presenting features:

Facial: grimacing or scowl expression, facial tics, arching of the eyebrows

Ocular: blinking, eyelid spasms (blepharospasm)

Oral/buccal: lip smacking, lower lip thrusting, sucking, puffing of cheeks, chewing of the cheeks (the inside of the mouth should be checked for this)

Lingual/masticatory: lateral jaw movements, tongue protrusion or thrusting such as "fly catching movements," tongue in lip or cheek resulting in an observable bulge in the specific area (Figure 16-4).

Systemic effects: foot tapping; rocking from side to side; arms, hands, and fingers may display a jerking motion and/or a writhing motion **(choreoathetoid)** (Figure 16-5); pelvic thrusting motions.

Treatment: Prevention only. Early assessment and diagnosis is crucial in preventing the development of an irreversible disorder. Decreasing or discontinuing the antipsychotic agent if possible is the recommended procedure (Kalachnik, 1983). At present, there is no known effective treatment for TD.

Data from Kalachnik, JE: Tardine dyskinesia, Minn Pharmacist 37(4):14, 1983.

ance may result in an inadequate response to the medication.

c. Questionable oral bioavailability. Although this is not considered a common possibility, it is a variable to be considered. The physician may switch from an oral solid dosage form to a liquid formulation and also adjust the dosage as necessary, based on the individual's response or development of side effects. Switching to another antipsychotic agent may also be considered.

6. Rapid neuroleptization or high dose. Aggressive treatment is used in clients with acute psychosis who may exhibit dangerous and/or destructive behaviors. Usually intramuscular therapy with a high-potency antipsychotic agent (such as haloperidol) is given, often on an hourly schedule, until the desired effects are achieved. If a client will take oral medication, then high-dose oral therapy may be substituted.

7. Once-a-day dosage schedule. Once a client is stabilized on antipsychotic medications, the entire daily dosage may be prescribed to be given at bedtime. The long duration of action of these drugs makes a single bedtime dosage feasible. This dosage schedule has increased client compliance, lowered medication costs, decreased side effects, and decreased or eliminated the need for simultaneous hypnotic medication.

This dosage schedule would require both careful drug and client selection before implementation. Using a drug with a high anticholinergic potential in an elderly client or an individual with cardiovascular disease may result in an increased potential for cardiotoxic effects. In such cases, multiple (two or three times daily) daily dosages are indicated.

8. Long-acting injections. Depot fluphenazine enanthate and fluphenazine decanoate are available for clients who are persistently noncompliant, do not understand the need for taking medications, or have a high frequency of relapses (psychotic episodes). Fluphenazine decanoate is often used in preference to the enanthate because the duration of action is approximately 2 weeks longer (an injection may last from 1 to 4 weeks). Clients receiving fluphenazine decanoate may exhibit a slight decrease in extrapyramidal side effects as compared with clients taking the enanthate formulation. Converting from an oral antipsychotic agent to fluphenazine decanoate requires various conversion considerations. The reader is referred to Katcher and others (1983) for this information.

9. Antipsychotic medications have been classified as low-potency, intermediate-potency, and high-potency drugs. The basis for the classification is the quantity of medication necessary to produce an equivalent effect when compared with other agents in the same category. For example, 50 mg of chlorpromazine is considered to be approximately equivalent to 25 mg of mesoridazine or 1 mg haloperidol. Thus chlorpromazine is a low-potency agent, mesoridazine an intermediate-potency agent, and haloperidol is a high-potency drug (see box on p. 318). The student is cautioned not to confuse potency with effectiveness, potency refers to the quantity of a drug necessary to produce an equivalent effect as compared with another drug in the same classification. Effectiveness measures the therapeutic response to various agents and this may range from less effective, equivalent in effectiveness, or greater in effectiveness, depending on the individual drugs being studied.

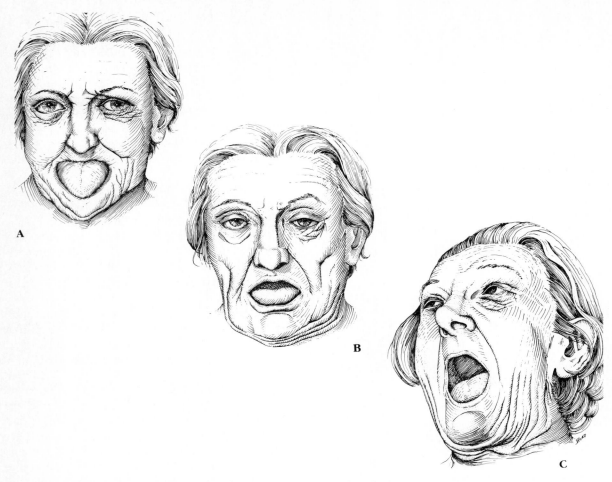

FIGURE 16-4 Persistent tardive dyskinesia. **A,** In-and-out movements of the tongue. **B,** Sucking and smacking of the lips. **C,** Lateral jaw movements. Lingual and facial hyperkinesias.

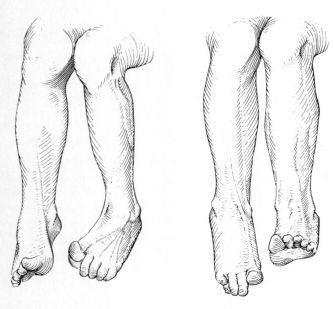

FIGURE 16-5 Abnormal (choreoathetoid) movements of extremities in persistent tardive dyskinesia. Complication of long-term therapy with antipsychotics (neuroleptics).

ANTIPSYCHOTIC DRUG EQUIVALENCY DOSAGES

DRUG	EQUIVALENT DOSE (mg)
Low potency	
chlorpromazine	100
thioridazine	100
Intermediate potency	
molindone	10
loxapine	15
High potency	
trifluoperazine	5
perphenazine	8
thiothixene	4
haloperidol	2
fluphenazine	2

Data from Knoben, JE, and Anderson, PO: Handbook of clinical drug data, ed 6, Hamilton, Ill, 1988, Drug Intelligence Publications, Inc.

10. Acetophenazine. (Tindal), promazine (Sparine), triflupromazine (Vesprin) are available on the market, but they are not commonly used today.

The Nurse's Role in Phenothiazine Therapy

Assessment. The nurse should assess the client for sensitivity to aspirin, since some individuals have a cross-sensitivity with the dye tartrazine (FD&C yellow No. 5) found in tablets of some phenothiazines.

These drugs should not be administered to clients with a history of narrow-angle glaucoma, urinary hesitancy or retention, prostatic hypertrophy, or acute or chronic respiratory problems, such as asthma or emphysema.

Phenothiazines should be used cautiously in clients with a history of convulsive disorders because of their action in reducing the convulsive threshold. Adequate anticonvulsant therapy needs to be maintained.

The nurse should be aware that phenothiazines are contraindicated in comatose clients because of the CNS depressive effect.

Intervention. Dosages of phenothiazines are individualized according to client response so that the lowest effective dose may be used. Dosages are increased more slowly and in smaller increments with elderly or debilitated clients.

Note that in institutional settings the severely agitated or combative client may be given larger intramuscular doses of the neuroleptics. Haloperidol and thiothixene have been given hourly to severely agitated clients to prevent them from hurting themselves or others. When symptoms are under control, the clients can be given the drug orally. Because of the half-life of the intramuscular doses, the first oral dose should be given 12 to 24 hours after the last intramuscular dose.

Note that in most cases concurrent treatment with more than one neuroleptic agent is not indicated. If the client does not respond to a particular drug, usually the dose of that drug should be increased or a different drug prescribed. Occasionally a client may respond best to a combination of two drugs from different classes. However, the potentiation and a lowered margin of safety of such combinations require greater precautions for client safety.

Since administration of large doses over a prolonged time may lead to anticholinergic psychoses or tardive dyskinesia, adverse reactions may be prevented by providing periodic "drug-free holidays" during which the client does not receive phenothiazines to prevent these adverse reactions. Because of the long elimination half-life of these drugs, "holidays" should last several weeks.

Maintenance dosage should be periodically evaluated for a possible reduction in the dosage or cessation of drug therapy. Clients with preexisting renal or hepatic disease may require reduced dosage.

When preparing phenothiazines, the nurse should be aware that the injectable forms tend to be physically and/or chemically incompatible with a wide range of solutions. The nurse should check the package insert for compatibility information about the specific drugs being prepared.

Avoid freezing phenothiazine solutions. Discolored solutions, slightly yellowed, may be used. However, if marked discoloration or a precipitate is apparent, the solution should not be used.

Skin and eye contact with phenothiazine solutions should be avoided because it may cause contact dermatitis and irritation. Exposed areas should be washed immediately to minimize the effect.

Oral forms of phenothiazines should be administered with food or a full glass of milk or water to decrease gastric irritation.

Phenothiazines should not be administered concurrently with antacids or antidiarrheals; hours of administration should be altered to allow 2 hours between doses of these medications.

Administration of the maintenance dosage at bedtime facilitates sleep and decreases drowsiness during the daytime.

Gradual reduction of the dosage over several weeks for clients on high or long-term dosages will help prevent withdrawal symptoms of nausea, vomiting, irritability, trembling, and transient dyskinetic signs. The only rationale for abrupt withdrawal is the occurrence of severe side effects/adverse reactions.

In pregnant women, the risk of administration of these drugs should be weighed against the expected therapeutic outcome.

Education. The nurse should caution clients against driving, operating dangerous machinery, or performing tasks that require absolute precision, motor coordination, and mental alertness.

The client should be instructed that the medication may take several weeks to effectively treat the disorder.

To prevent photosensitivity, the nurse should advise the client to stay out of the sun, use sunscreen lotion, or wear protective clothing to prevent solar erythema or the nurse should assist clients by providing the necessary protective measures. A dark, purplish brown skin pigmentation induced by light (photosensitivity) has been reported in hospitalized psychiatric clients who were given large dosages of phenothiazines for 3 to 10 years.

The nurse should caution the client that dry mouth can be a bothersome adverse effect and contribute to the development of caries, gum disease, and oral condidiasis. The client should be instructed in the use of proper oral hygiene. Xerostoma may affect the fitting of full dentures; referral should be made for dental care for this and other dental problems.

Phenothiazines also affect regulation of body temperature; clients should be cautioned to avoid extremes of environmental temperature (i.e., swimming in cold water or walking in hot, humid weather), which could lead to hypothermia and respiratory distress or hyperthermia and heat prostration, respectively.

The client should be instructed to avoid alcohol and other CNS depressants, since they increase the CNS depressant effects of the phenothiazines. Using these drugs concurrently with extrapyramidal reaction–causing medications will increase the frequency and severity of extrapyramidal effects.

Evaluation. If orthostatic (postural) hypotension occurs and causes severe difficulties or serious hazards, the nurse should alert the physician, who may institute one of the following remedial measures: (1) a change of medication to one of the phenothiazine derivatives that does not produce this side effect with such frequency, (2) reduction of dosage, or (3) discontinuation of medication for 24 hours with a gradual buildup of dosage as tolerated. The client who complains of dizziness, light-headedness, or palpitation may be experiencing orthostatic hypotension. This can easily be confirmed when the client's blood pressure is compared in the prone and standing positions. The client should be instructed to rise slowly from the recumbent position and to sit on the edge of the bed for a few minutes before attempting to stand. Support and reassurance may be necessary to allay the client's anxiety. Explaining orthostatic hypotension also may help him or her understand this experience and reduce anxiety. Clients should be encouraged to remain in a recumbent position for 1 hour after initial doses, parenterally administered doses, or large oral doses (rarely) of the phenothiazines to minimize hypotensive episodes.

The nurse should be alert to signs of agranulocytosis such as sore throat, fever, or weakness in clients taking these drugs; this usually occurs between weeks 4 and 10. When these symptoms appear, the drug is usually discontinued; the nurse should hold the dose and notify the physician as soon as possible. White blood cell and differential counts are required periodically.

Because of possible ocular changes, including particle deposition in the cornea and lens and pigmentary retinopathy (decreased vision, brownish coloring of vision, impaired night vision, and pigment deposits on the fundus), indicate on the client's record that the eye change may be related to dosage levels or therapy duration. The client on a long-term regimen or moderate to high dose therapy should have periodic ophthalmologic examinations. Exposure to light may increase the possibility of ocular changes; therefore the client should be instructed to wear sunglasses.

The nurse should monitor the client closely for early signs of tardive dyskinesia, usually small, wormlike motions of the tongue. Since there is no known effective treatment for tardive dyskinesia, phenothiazine should be discontinued immediately and the prescriber notified.

These drugs should be administered cautiously to clients with heart disease since they may precipitate hypotension. If hypotension necessitating drug interaction occurs, norepinephrine or phenylephrine may be administered. Since phenothiazines tend to reverse epinephrine's vasopressor effects, epinephrine may not be effective in reversing hypotension.

These drugs should not be administered to clients with a history of narrow-angle glaucoma, urinary hesitancy or retention, prostatic hypertrophy, or with acute or chronic respiratory problems, such as asthma or emphysema.

The client should be monitored for signs and symptoms of urinary hesitancy or retention, prostatic hypatrophy, narrow angle glaucoma, or respiratory problems (e.g., intake and output for urinary retention and/or constipation).

Hepatic function tests, urine bilirubin, and bile examinations should be done weekly during the first month of therapy to assist in the detection of cholestatic jaundice. Clinically, the client should be observed for yellow skin, nausea, flulike symptoms, and rash. Phenothiazines are to be discontinued immediately.

The nurse should monitor the client for **neuroleptic malignant syndrome** (hyperthermia, dehydration, cardiovascular instability, hypoxemia, and muscular rigidity). Therapy is essentially symptomatic and supportive with the phenothiazine being discontinued immediately.

Depression, especially if the client is not closely supervised, may account for the greater incidence of suicide in psychiatric clients undergoing drug therapy than in those receiving only institutional care.

Nursing considerations for selected phenothiazine derivatives. Each of the three subgroups of phenothiazine has unique considerations for the nurse.

Aliphatic phenothiazines. The aliphatic phenothiazine derivatives consist of chlorpromazine (Clorizine, Ormazine, Promaz, Thorazine), promazine (Prozine, Sparine), and triflupromazine (Vesprin) (see Table 16-3).

The oral route of administration is preferred unless the client is unable to take an oral dose. When given with at least 120 ml of fruit juice or other liquids or semi-soft foods, chlorpromazine becomes more palatable; however, the client should be informed that the medication is in the substance.

When given intramuscularly, it should be injected deeply and slowly in divided doses of not more than 1 ml per injection site. Irritation of the subcutaneous tissues can be reduced by diluting the drug with 0.9% sodium chloride injection and injecting the drug by the "Z tract" technique. Massaging the clients injection site helps reduce local irritation. Some clients have been known to develop abscesses at the injection site, which are believed to result from large doses of this substance being administered in one area. Use of the intramuscular route when administering chlorpromazine is usually indicated when the client refuses the tablet or concentrate form or when the most immediate effect of the drug is desired. If the client is severely agitated, combative, or struggling, the nurse should take care to follow safe administration technique. This technique usually requires enough well-trained personnel to restrain the client adequately while the medication is being given.

Intravenous administration of the undiluted drug should be avoided. If used for direct intravenous administration, chlorpromazine hydrochloride should be diluted to at least 1 mg/ml and administered at a rate of 1 mg/min for adults and 0.5 mg/min for children. For intravenous infusion, the drug should be added to 500 to 1000 ml of 0.9% sodium chloride solution and administered slowly. In both instances, the client should be kept recumbent to minimize hypotension.

Piperidine phenothiazines. The piperidine phenothiazine derivatives consist of mesoridazine (Serentil) and thioridazine (Mellaril-S, Apo-Thioridazine, Mellaril, Novoridazine, Thioridazine) (see Table 16-4).

The oral concentrate solution should be diluted with a half glass (120 ml) of water, orange juice, or grape juice just before administration, to make it more palatable.

Contact with liquid forms of the drug should be avoided because contact dermatitis may result.

Piperazine phenothiazines. The piperazine phenothiazine derivatives consist of fluphenazine (Moditen, Prolixin, Permitil), perphenazine (Trilafon, Phenazine, Apo-Perphenazine), prochlorperazine (Compazine, Chlorazine, Stemetil), and trifluoperazine (Stelazine, Suprazine, Terfluzive, Novoflurazine) (see Table 16-5).

The fluphenazine hydrochloride oral concentrate solution should not be mixed with fluids containing caffeine (coffee, tea, cola), tannic acid (tea), or pectinates (apple juice) because a physical incompatibility may occur. As with fluphenazine, perphenazine oral concentrate should not be mixed with the preceding solutions. Instead, dilute with at least 60 ml of lemon-lime carbonated beverage or pineapple, orange, tomato, or grapefruit juice for each 5 ml of concentrate.

Decanoate and ethanthate, the long-acting forms of fluphenazine, are oil preparations; they may be given subcutaneously using a 21-gauge or larger needle.

Intravenous administration of perphenazine is limited to recumbent hospitalized adult clients and requires the availability of resuscitative equipment and drugs for the treatment of severe hypotensive episodes or extrapyramidal responses in the client. If administered by fractional intravenous injection, the solution should be diluted to 0.5 mg/ml of 0.9% sodium chloride and administered slowly, 1 mg per injection at intervals of at least 1 to 2 minutes. Blood pressure and pulse should be assessed continuously during intravenous administration.

BUTYROPHENONE DERIVATIVES
haloperidol (Haldol)

The butyrophenones are structurally different from the phenothiazines and the thioxanthines but have similar properties in terms of antipsychotic efficacy. The receptor-blockade activity in the CNS may be at the level of the dopamine receptors. They have relatively less effect on the norepinephrine and epinephrine receptors and are probably more potent than most of the phenothiazine agents in their dopaminergic effects and possess a significant degree of extrapyramidal effects. The drug has both antiemetic and antipsychotic effects. Research conducted in Europe in the area of anesthesia brought this compound into view as a possible antipsychotic agent. Subsequent use indicated its effectiveness in the control of hyperactivity associated with the manic phase.

Dosage and administration. See Table 16-6.
Pregnancy safety. Not established

NURSING CONSIDERATIONS

In addition to the general nursing considerations for phenothiazines, the following points should be noted:
- A special dropper should be used for oral liquid administration; if diluted with tea or coffee, a precipitate will form. Butyrophenone may be administered from a premeasured oral syringe without diluting if desired.
- The emotional status should be assessed carefully since there may be a rapid mood swing from mania to depression when haloperidol is administered to the client with a bipolar disorder.

thiothixene hydrochloride (Navane)

Thiothixene, a thioxanthene derivative, resembles the piperazine phenothiazines in its tranquilizing and antiemetic actions and to a lesser degree in its spasmolytic and hypotensive effects. Its indications for use, side effects, precautions, and drug interactions are the same as those for the phenothiazines. Extrapyramidal symptoms and insomnia occur frequently with this drug.

Dosage and administration. See Table 16-7.
Pregnancy safety. Not established

NURSING CONSIDERATIONS

See the general nursing considerations for phenothiazines.

DIHYDROINDOLONE DERIVATIVE
molindone (Moban)

Mechanism of action. Molindone is an antipsychotic agent, chemically an oxygenated indole (dihydroindolone), that represents a new chemical class resembling reserpine. In theory molindone acts on the ascending

TABLE 16-6 Butyrophenone Dosage and Administration

	Adults	Elderly	Children
haloperidol tablet/liquid	0.5-5 mg orally 2 or 3 times daily, adjust dosage as necessary. Maximum, 100 mg/day.	0.5-2 mg orally 2 or 3 times daily; increase as necessary.	Children less than 3 yr, not established. Children 3-12 yr, 15-40 mg/kg body weight. Psychotic conditions, 0.05 mg/kg body weight orally, divided into 2 or 3 doses daily. Increase dose if necessary by 0.5 mg increments at 5-7 day intervals up to a total daily dose of 0.15 mg/kg body weight daily. Pediatric doses above 6 mg/day are usually unnecessary.
nonpsychotic conditions and Tourette's syndrome			0.05 mg/kg body weight orally divided into 2 or 3 doses daily. Increase dose if necessary by 0.5 mg increments at 5-7 day intervals up to a total daily dose of 0.075 mg/kg body weight daily.
haloperidol injection	Acute psychosis: 2-5 mg IM, may repeat at 1-hr intervals or every 4-8 hr if client's symptoms are under control. Maximum dosage, 100 mg/day.		Not established.

TABLE 16-7 Thioxanthene Dosage and Administration

	Adults	Elderly	Children
thiothixene capsules/ liquid	2 mg orally 3 times/day or 5 mg twice/day. Increase dosage as necessary to a maximum of 60 mg daily.	Lower than adult dose, increasing as necessary according to response and/or development of side effects.	Children less than 12 yr, not established.
thiothixene hydrochloride injection	4 mg IM 2-4 times daily. Adjust dosage as necessary to maximum of 30 mg daily.	Same as above.	Not established.

reticular activating system, with activity similar to major tranquilizers such as phenothiazines.

Dosage and administration.   Table 16-8.
Pregnancy safety. Not established

NURSING CONSIDERATIONS

In addition to the general nursing considerations for phenothiazines, the following point should be noted. The tablet form contains calcium sulfate which may impair the absorption of tetracycline and phenytoin. The client should be informed about this interaction.

DIBENZOXAPINE DERIVATIVE
loxapine succinate (Loxitane, Loxapac✽)

Loxapine has structural similarity to the phenothiazines but is a member of a distinct chemical class of antipsychotic drugs, the dibenzoxapines.

Dosage and administration. See Table 16-9.
Pregnancy safety. FDA category C

NURSING CONSIDERATIONS

In addition to the general nursing considerations for phenothiazines, the following points should be noted:

TABLE 16-8   Dihydroindolone Dosage and Administration

	Adults	Elderly	Children
molindone hydrochloride tablet/liquid	Initial dose, 50-75 mg daily in divided doses. May increase to 100 mg daily in 3 or 4 days. Dosage must be individualized. Maximum, usually 225 mg/day.	Lower than adult dose, increasing as necessary according to response and/or development of side effects.	Not recommended for children less than 12 yr.

TABLE 16-9   Dibenzoxapine Dosage and Administration

	Adults	Elderly	Children
loxapine hydrochloride liquid/loxapine succinate capsule	10 mg orally twice daily; increase slowly during first 7-10 days as necessary. Maintenance dose, 15-25 mg orally 2-4 times daily. Maximum, 250 mg/day.	3-5 mg twice daily initially.	Children less than 16 yr, not established.
loxapine hydrochloride injection	12.5-50 mg IM every 4-6 hr as necessary. Maximum, 250 mg/day.		Same as above.

- The nurse should administer the loxapine succinate oral concentrate with the calibrated dropper, which has 1 ml equal to 25 mg only. The drug should be mixed with orange or grapefruit juice shortly before administration.
- Loxapine hydrochloride is to be administered only intramuscularly. The nurse should caution the client that temporary drowsiness may occur when initial therapy starts and when dosage is increased. Tolerance develops as therapy continues. It may require several weeks of therapy to obtain optimal effects. An ECG should be performed periodically and with dose adjustment, since the drug may potentiate cardiac dysrhythymias.

ANTIDEPRESSANT THERAPY
CLASSIFICATIONS

Affective disorders, or mood disturbances, include depression, which is the most common affective disorder, and mania or elation. Mania will be discussed later in this chapter.

Over the years many classifications of depression have been used, such as the time during life that depression occurred (childhood, adolescent, or senile depressions), or the reason for the depression, such as reactive (exogenous) depression or endogenous depression. Reactive depressions are often a person's response to a loss (loss of pleasure or interest in activities and everyday living caused perhaps by the loss of a loved one or the presence of a debilitating illness) or disappointment (from not meeting one's expectations, loss of a job, pet, friend, or lover). This is usually referred to as "the blues" or normal depression (Berkow, 1982), which generally remits in several months without the use of antidepressant medications. The mobilization of support systems and, if necessary, psychotherapy are useful adjuncts in **exogenous depression.**

Endogenous depressions are characterized by the absence of external causes for depression. This type of depression may be due to genetic determination and biochemical alterations (Csernansky and Hollister, 1982). Antidepressant medications are very useful in the treatment of this type of depression.

The current classification for depressive disorders (Andreason and others, 1980) has eliminated the use of the above terminology. Instead, major affective disorders are defined as bipolar disorders (mixed type and manic) and major depression (single episode or recurrent episodes), along with atypical affective disorders, which include depression. Psychiatrists have debated over whether the new classification was an improvement over the previous (endogenous, exogenous, or manic depression) types of classification, since it is important for the clinician to have a diagnostic framework to work from.

The recognition of atypical depressions was considered a benefit (Csernansky and Hollister, 1982). Atypical depression usually does not meet the criteria for major depression or any other affective illness, thus it is characterized as atypical. Criteria for major depression include the presence of mood changes (sadness, despondency, anxiety, crying spells, guilt feelings, self-pity, pessimism, loss of interest in life and social activities), psychologic symptoms (low self-esteem, poor concentration, hopeless or helpless feelings, suicidal or increased focus on death), physiologic manifestations (sleep disturbances that may range from insomnia to hypersomnia, decreased interest in sex, complaints of fatigue, loss of energy, menstrual dysfunction, headaches, palpitations, constipation, loss of appetite, and weight loss or weight gain), and thinking alterations (a decrease in concentration or attention span, complaints of poor memory, confusion, delusions relating to health, persecution, or religion, and hallucinations if the client is also psychotic). Mood variations are usually diurnal and often worse in the morning.

Atypical depressions usually are of briefer duration and not as severe as a major depression. Often they are nonresponsive to the tricyclic antidepressants. Mood changes are usually worse in the evening; panic attacks, phobias such as agoraphobia, and physiologic complaints are often present. Csernansky and Hollister (1982) believe the MAO inhibitors are the drugs of choice for this type of depression.

Other measures to treat depression include electroshock therapy, psychotherapy, reduction of environmental stressors, and milieu therapy. In a number of cases, antidepressant drug therapy in combination with one or more adjunct measures is more effective than drug therapy alone.

ETIOLOGY OF AFFECTIVE DISORDERS

No single etiologic factor has been identified as the cause of affective disorders. Psychiatrists believing in psychosocial therapies will probe to identify stressful events or mental conflicts in one's life that preceded the onset of depression. Psychiatrists adhering to the biologic theory tend to explain affective disorders according to the monoamine theory (i.e., catecholamine [norepinephrine, dopamine, epinephrine] and indolamine [serotonin] levels in the CNS). Many practitioners today believe that both psychosocial and biologic factors lead to a common pathway that results in an affective disorder.

Many factors are involved with affective disorders, such as genetics, psychosocial events (divorce, death of a mate), physiologic stress (illness, infection, childbirth), and personality traits. Any combination of these factors may also affect the CNS's biochemical mechanisms leading again to the idea of the common pathway for affective disorders (Katcher and others, 1983).

Monoamine Theory in Affective Disorders

Centrally acting monoamines, especially norepinephrine and serotonin, have been theorized as the cause of depression and mania. A deficiency in central norepinephrine has been associated with depression, whereas an excess of norepinephrine is believed to be related to mania. Both norepinephrine and serotonin may be important substances in regulating affective behaviors, and the most important receptors for them appear to be in the limbic system (Bachmann and Sherman, 1983).

The tricyclic antidepressants may block the reuptake of one or both monoamines into the adrenergic neuron. This blockade will lead to elevated levels of norepinephrine and serotonin in the synapse areas. MAO, an enzyme found in the mitochrondia of nerve cells, is responsible for metabolizing norepinephrine within the nerve. MAO inhibitors block this enzyme, leading to increased levels of norepinephrine available for release to the synapse area. Although the mechanism of action of many antidepressants is inhibition of reuptake of norepinephrine or serotonin or inhibition of the MAO enzyme system, not all antidepressants have this effect. Therefore it is believed that the full range of antidepressant central activity of these medications is probably unknown (Figure 16-6).

SELECTION OF A TRICYCLIC ANTIDEPRESSANT

When drug therapy is indicated, the tricyclic antidepressants are usually the first drugs prescribed. No single agent is an ideal antidepressant because all of them may induce undesirable side or adverse effects; thus researchers are constantly searching for new antidepressant agents. See the box on page 325 for investigational antidepressant drugs according to chemical structures and comments.

Newer antidepressants include maprotiline, which is equivalent in effectiveness to the tricyclic antidepressants, but convulsions occur nearly three times more often with maprotiline than with the tricyclic agents. This high seizure potential has resulted in a decrease in the maximum recommended daily dose of this product. Amoxapine is also an effective antidepressant agent. But this product is the only antidepressant capable of causing extrapyramidal effects and tardive dyskinesia, which appears to be due to an amoxapine metabolite with dopamine-blocking effects. Amoxapine is also considered to be less potent than most of the tricyclic agents, thus requiring higher doses to produce an effect equivalent to the tricyclic agents. Trazodone, with the least anticholinergic effect, has the greatest margin for safety in overdose when compared with the other antidepressants. It also does not affect cardiac conduction, so it may be a safer product for the client with heart disease. Fluoxetine, while equivalent to the tricyclic agents in efficacy and onset of action, has a number of notable differences. It is usually given once daily (in the

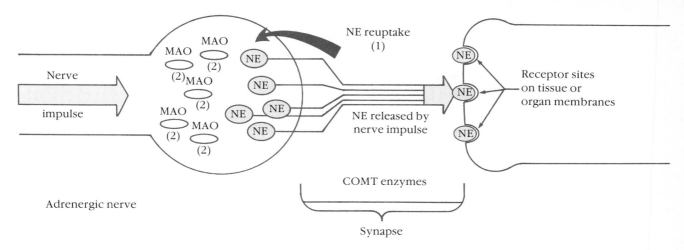

FIGURE 16-6 Proposed action of antidepressant drug therapy. Normally norepinephrine (NE) is released from storage sites within the adrenergic nerve by the arrival of a nerve impulse. The released NE may be metabolized within the nerve by MAO enzyme or following the activity of NE at the receptor sites, by catechol-O-methyltransferase (COMT) enzymes located in the synaptic cleft. Most NE is taken back into the nerve and stored by way of the reuptake mechanism. Antidepressant drug therapy: (1) tricyclic antidepressants block the reuptake of released NE and prevent it from re-entering the adrenergic nerve. (2) MAO inhibitors block MAO located on surface of the cell mitochrondia. The result is more NE available for release or present in the synapse area. See text.

INVESTIGATIONAL ANTIDEPRESSANTS

CHEMICAL STRUCTURE AND GENERIC NAME	COMMENTS
Unicyclic fluvoxamine	Potent serotonin inhibitor with no active metabolites; lacks anticholinergic activity
Bicyclic viloxazine	Norepinephrine reuptake inhibitor; appears to have amphetamine-type effects; lacks anticholinergic activity.
Tricyclic chlorimipramine	Marketed in Europe for the past decade; potent serotonin reuptake inhibitor with an active metabolite that inhibits norepinephrine reuptake; used to treat obsessive-compulsive behaviors
Tetracyclic oxaprotiline	Potent inhibitor of norepinephrine reuptake

morning); it has little or no anticholinergic or cardiovascular side effects, and it is capable of inducing weight loss.

Generally, physicians select sedating antidepressants (amitriptyline, doxepin) that are potent serotonin reup-

take blocking agents for the agitated depressive client. The potent blockers of norepinephrine reuptake (desipramine, nortriptyline) are reserved for the withdrawn depressive client. Selection of an antidepressant is empiric, taking into consideration the side effect potential of each antidepressant compared with the medical problems of the individual client.

For example, a client with a history of cardiac dysrhythmias may be considered a poor candidate for antidepressant drugs. Yet imipramine, nortriptyline, and maprotiline have documentation of reducing premature ventricular contractions by continuous ECG client monitoring (Veith, 1985). Thus judicious selection and careful client monitoring should reduce the risk of adverse effects in selected depressed individuals.

Hypotension, especially in the elderly, places some clients at risk for orthostatic hypotension with many of the antidepressant drugs. Trazodone (Desyrel) and the investigational drug bupropion appear to have a lower potential of inducing cardiovascular side effects (Edmond and Simpson, 1985). *Plasma levels* of the tricyclic antidepressants can vary widely between different individuals and often do not correlate with dose or therapeutic response. Physicians may order that serum levels be monitored to help identify the noncompliant client. A low plasma level should initially indicate the need to interview the client for adherence to the prescribed schedule. Seeking out reasons for noncompliance (side effects that are intolerable to client, misunderstanding of directions, lack of finances to purchase medications) can then be identified and perhaps resolved.

If compliance is verified and serum levels still remain low, dosage adjustments may be necessary, or the physician might consider switching to a different tricyclic agent. If the client is nonresponsive to a predominantly norepinephrine-potentiating medication, a serotonin-potentiating agent might be indicated (see Table 16-10). Biochemical differences may be present in the individual that would indicate a trial with the opposite reuptake blocking agent.

The elderly often have reduced liver drug metabolizing enzymes, thus higher serum drug levels and a greater potential for side effects exist. Many physicians start geriatric clients at one-third to one-half the usual adult dosage, adjusting as necessary according to therapeutic response or presence of undesirable side effects.

Mechanism of action. See Etiology of Affective Disorders.

Indications. Treatment of depression and enuresis (imipramine).

Pharmacokinetics

Absorption. Orally, very good

Metabolism. Primarily liver. Active metabolites produced in liver:

amitriptyline: nortriptyline
amoxapine: 7-hydroxyamoxapin, 8-hydroxyamoxapine
desipramine: 2 hydroxydesipramine
doxepine: desmethyldoxepin
imipramine: desipramine

Onset of antidepressant effect. Usually within 2 to 3 weeks. (For half-life, serotonin- or norepinephrine-blocking potential, and side effects, see Table 16-10.)

Excretion. Kidneys

TABLE 16-10 Pharmacokinetic and Blocking Potential of Selected Tricyclic and Tetracyclic Antidepressants

Generic name	Trade name	Serum half-life (hr)	Blockade of reuptake* of Norepinephrine	Serotonin	Sedative effects	Anticholinergic effects	Orthostatic hypotension
TRICYCLIC							
amitriptyline	Elavil Apo-amitriptyline♣ Levate♣	10-50	+	++++	++++	++++	++++
amoxapine	Asendin	8-30	†		Yes	Mild	Low
desipramine	Pertofrane Norpramin	12-54	++++		+	+	++
doxepin	Adapin Sinequan Triadapin♣	6-19	?/weak	?/weak	++++	++	+++
imipramine	Tofranil Tofranil PM Impril♣	13-28	++	++	+++	+++	++++
nortriptyline	Aventyl Pamelor	18-93	+++	++	++	++	++
protriptyline	Vivactil Triptil♣	54-198	Unknown	Unknown	+	+	++
trimipramine	Surmontil	9-11	Yes	Yes	Yes	Moderate	Low
TETRACYCLIC							
maprotiline	Ludiomil	27-58	Yes	No	Yes	Yes	Low
TRIAZOLOPYRIDINES							
trazodone	Desyrel	Unknown	No	Yes	Low	Lowest	Low
BICYCLICS							
fluoxetine	Prozac	Unknown	No	Yes	None	Very low	Low

Adapted from United States Pharmacopeial Convention: Drug information for the health care provider, ed 8, Rockville, Md, 1988, The Convention; Edmond, MPI, and Simpson, GM: New antidepressants: a review, Hosp Formul 20:580, 1985.
*Yes/no indicates activity but is not quantified. + = Low or slight activity; ++++ = high or greatest activity.
†Amoxapine blocks norepinephrine and dopamine reuptake but not serotonin.

Side effects/adverse reactions: See Table 16-11.

Significant drug interactions. The following effects may occur when tricyclic antidepressants are given with the drugs listed below:

Drug	Possible Effect and Management
alcohol or CNS depressants	May result in enhanced CNS depressant effects; avoid concurrent use.
antithyroid drugs	Increase risk of inducing agranulocytosis; avoid concurrent use if possible.
cimetidine	May inhibit metabolism of tricyclic agent leading to increase serum levels and toxicity; monitor closely.
clonidine, guanadrel, or guanethidine	May decrease the antihypertensive effects of these drugs; monitor closely since dosage changes or alternate antihypertensive agents may be necessary. Clonidine and tricyclic antidepressants may increase risk of CNS depression; monitor closely.
contraceptives, oral	May increase or decrease tricyclic serum levels; monitor closely for decreased therapeutic response or drug toxicity; dosage adjustments may be necessary.
extrapyramidal-inducing medications	Amoxapine and extrapyramidal-inducing drugs (phenothiazines, haloperidol, metoclopramide, reserpine, thioxanthenes) may increase risk and severity of extrapyramidal adverse effects; monitor closely.
metrizamide	Concurrent use of tricyclic antidepressants increases risk of inducing seizures because tricyclic antidepressants lower the seizure threshold. Discontinue tricyclic agents for at least 2 days before and 1 day after a myelogram.
MAO inhibitors	Contraindicated in outpatient settings; hypertensive crises, severely elevated temperatures, convulsions, and death have been reported with concurrent administration of MAO inhibitors and tricyclic antidepressants. Before switching from one classification to the other, at least a 2-week drug-free period from either category should be instituted. If concurrent use is prescribed in an inpatient setting, it would require strict supervision and close monitoring because of the potentially serious adverse effects.
sympathomimetics	Increase possibility of potentiating cardiovascular toxicities (severe hypertension, dysrhythmias, tachycardia) or severely elevated body temperatures. If this combination cannot be avoided, monitor very closely. If possible, avoid this combination.

Dosage and administration. See Table 16-12.

Pregnancy safety. Amitriptyline, amoxapine, trimipramine, FDA category C; desipramine, doxepin, imipramine, nortriplytine, protriptyline, FDA category unclassified; maprotiline and nomifensine, FDA category B

The Nurse's Role in Tricyclic Antidepressant Therapy

Assessment. Tricyclic antidepressants should not be administered to clients with increased intraocular pressure, history of urinary retention, or history of narrow-angle glaucoma, because these medications possess significant anticholinergic properties; hyperthyroid clients or those taking thyroid medication, because of the possibility of cardiovascular toxicity; or individuals with a past history of seizure disorders, because this class of drugs has been demonstrated to lower the seizure threshold; clients receiving guanethidine, methyldopa, clonidine, or similar agents, because the tricyclic antidepressants block the pharmacologic effects of these drugs. The following list summarizes the conditions that contraindicate administration of tricyclic antidepressants:

Glaucoma (narrow angle)	Angina pectoris
Kidney disease	Congestive heart failure
Pyloric stenosis	Paroxysmal tachycardia
Epilepsy	Benign prostatic hypertrophy
Overactivity, overstimulation, or agitation	Before surgery
	Pregnancy (risks to fetus)
Impaired liver function	Hyperthyroidism
Myocardial infarction (recent)	

Clients must be closely assessed for suicide potential at the start of therapy and monitored closely throughout therapy for suicide potential. The risk of suicide increases as therapy improves the client's depressed state and energy levels increase.

Intervention. Note that the possibility of suicide is inherent in any severely depressed client and persists until a significant remission occurs. The suicidal risks of tricyclic antidepressants are especially high, and suicide attempts with tricyclic antidepressants are frequently seen in many emergency departments. When a client has a serious overt suicidal potential and is not hospitalized, the quantity of the tricyclic antidepressant should not exceed 1 week's supply. In schizophrenic clients activation of the psychosis may occur, requiring reduction of the dosage or the addition of a major tranquilizer to the therapeutic regimen. Manic or hypomanic episodes may occur in individuals with the cyclic type of disorders. If this occurs, the tricyclic antidepressant should be discontinued until the episode is relieved and then may be reinstituted at a lowered dosage if still needed in the therapy.

Initial dosages in adolescent, elderly, and debilitated clients should be lower and increased gradually. The medication should not be withdrawn abruptly.

Education. During initiation or change of therapy, the client should avoid activities that require coordination and alertness until response to the tricyclic antidepressant therapy has been determined.

Self-alteration of the prescribed medications or consumption of other medication including over-the-counter medications should not be done without consultation with the prescriber. Clients should be specifically instructed to avoid alcoholic beverages during the tricyclic antidepressant regimen.

Orthostatic hypotension may occur. The nurse should

TABLE 16-11   Side Effects/Adverse Reactions of Tricyclic and Tetracyclic Antidepressants

Drugs(s)	Side effects*	Adverse reactions†
TRICYCLIC		
	Most frequent: dizziness, dry mouth, headache, increased consumption of sweets, nausea, weakness, weight gain, unpleasant taste Less frequent: sweating, diarrhea, gas, insomnia, vomiting	Most frequent: not reported Less frequent: confusion, constipation (especially in geriatric clients), hypotension, dysrhythmia, nervousness, tremors, insomnia, tachycardia or bradycardia, visual pain or blurred vision
amoxapine only		Less frequent: impairment of sexual functioning; extrapyramidal side effects (trouble speaking or swallowing, shuffle walk, slow movements, trembling, stiffness of arms and legs, loss of balance); tardive dyskinesia (abnormal chewing movements, lip smacking—see previous description under psychotropics)
TETRACYCLIC		
maprotiline	Most frequent: dizziness, blurred vision, dry mouth, pruritus, rash, insomnia, weakness, headache	Less frequent: severe constipation that may lead to impaction or paralytic ileus, nausea or vomiting, convulsions, tremors, increased excitement
TRIAZOLOPYRIDINE		
trazodone	Most frequent: sedation, dry mouth, nausea, vomiting, headache, dizziness, blurred vision Less frequent/rare: diarrhea, constipation, increased weakness, muscle pain or aches.	Less frequent: muscle tremors, confusion Rare: hypotension, bradycardia or tachycardia, painful delayed erection of the penis, rash, excitement
BICYCLIC		
fluoxetine	Most frequent: anorexia, weight loss, nausea, increased nervousness, anxiety, insomnia Less frequent: tremors, dry mouth, sweating, diarrhea	Rare: convulsions

*If side effects continue, increase, or disturb the client, inform the physician.
†If adverse reactions occur, contact physician, since medical intervention may be necessary.

instruct the client to come to a standing position slowly and carefully to avoid feeling faint.

Since dry mouth is a common side effect, the client should be taught appropriate oral hygiene to prevent caries and other dental problems. In addition, breath mints may be reassuring to the client in social situations.

The nurse should caution the client that therapeutic response to tricyclic antidepressants is not immediate. It may be 10 to 14 days before there is demonstrative effect and 30 days for full effect.

Note that an emerging public health problem is tricyclic antidepressant poisoning or overdosage in children. Doses in excess of 10 mg/kg body weight are potentially dangerous. The incidents are characterized as accidental, since most occur when the drug is given to a household member for depression or to an enuretic child. Alert the adult family member to the possibility of accidental overdosage and the need for security and administrative responsibility over the medication.

Evaluation. In resistant cases of depression in adults, a dose of 2.5 mg/kg body weight/day or higher may have to be exceeded in the hospital. If such a dose or higher is necessary, maintain ECG monitoring during the initiation of therapy and at appropriate intervals during stabilization of the dose.

When tricyclic antidepressants are administered to pregnant patients, the potential benefits should be weighed against the potential fetal risks.

Employ extreme caution (monitoring, nursing observations) when the tricyclic antidepressants are administered to clients with any evidence of cardiovascular disease because of the possibility of conduction defects, dysrhythmias, myocardial infarction, cerebrovascular accidents, and tachycardia. The quinidine-like cardiac effects are well documented in the literature.

Overdosage and treatment. Nearly a half million cases of tricyclic antidepressant drug overdoses occur yearly in the United States. In 1983 and 1984 the annual reports of

TABLE 16-12   Dosage and Administration of Tricyclic and Tetracyclic Antidepressants

	Adults	Elderly	Children
amitriptyline tablets	25 mg orally 2-4 times daily; adjust dosage as necessary. Maximum daily dose, up to 150 mg if outpatient; up to 300 mg daily for hospitalized clients.	10 mg orally 3 times daily and 20 mg at bedtime; adjust dosage as necessary.	Children less than 12 yr, not established. Adolescents, same as elderly dosage.
amitriptyline HCl injection	20-30 mg IM 4 times daily.		Children less than 12 yr, not established.
amoxapine tablet	50 mg orally 3 times daily. Adjust dosages on every third day basis if necessary; increase to 100 mg orally 3 times daily. Do not increase over 300 mg/day until this dosage is determined to be ineffective after minimum 2-wk trial. Maximum per day, institutionalized clients, up to 600 mg daily in divided dosages.	25 mg orally 3 times daily; if necessary, may increae to 50 mg 3 times a day after 3 days.	Children less than 16 yr, not established.
desipramine tablet/capsule	25-50 mg orally 3 times a day; increase dosage as necessary. Maximum daily dosage, adult up to 200 mg/day; elderly up to 100 mg/day.	25-50 mg daily in divided dosages; increase if necessary.	Children less than 12 yr, not established. Adolescent, same as elderly.
doxepin capsules/liquid	25 mg orally 3 times daily; increase as necessary. Maximum daily dosage, up to 150 mg daily for outpatients; up to 300 mg daily for institutionalized patients.		Children less than 12 yr, not established.
imipramine tablet	25-50 mg orally 3 or 4 times daily; adjust dosage as necessary. Maximum daily dosages, up to 200 mg daily for outpatients; up to 300 mg/day for institutionalized patients.	30-40 mg daily in divided doses; adjust dosage as necessary.	Antidepressant dosage: children less than 6 yr, not recommended; 6 yr and older, not recommended for anti-depressant use; may be used for antienuretic or attention deficit disorders with hyperactivity. Adolescents, same as elderly. Antienuretic: 25 mg orally daily 1 hr before sleep. If desired response is not achieved within 1 wk, increase to 50 mg at night for children under 12 and to 75 mg for children over 12. May give half dosage in midafternoon and one half at bedtime. This, at times, has proved more effective than single bedtime dosing.
imipramine pamoate capsule	75 mg orally at bedtime; increase dosage as necessary. Usually 150 mg at bedtime is optimum dosage. Maximum daily dosage, up to 200 mg daily for outpatients; up to 300 mg for institutionalized patients.		Children less than 12 yr, not established.
imipramine hydrochloride injection	25-50 mg IM 3 or 4 times daily. Maximum daily dosage, up to 300 mg/day.		Children less than 12 yr, not recommended
nortriptyline capsule/liquid	25 mg orally 3 or 4 times daily; adjust dosage as necessary.	30-50 mg in divided dosages daily; adjust dosage as needed. Maximum daily dosage, up to 100 mg/day.	Children less than 12 yr, not established. Adolescents, same as elderly.

Continued.

TABLE 16-12   Dosage and Administration of Tricyclic and Tetracyclic Antidepressants—cont'd

	Adults	Elderly	Children
protriptyline tablets	5-10 mg orally 3 or 4 times daily. Adjust dosage as necessary. Maximum daily dosage, up to 60 mg/day.	5 mg orally 3 times daily. Adjust dosage as necessary. If daily dosage is above 20 mg/day for an elderly person, closely monitor for cardiovascular responses.	Children less than 12 yr, not established. Adolescents, same as elderly.
trimipramine maleate capsule	25 mg orally 3 times daily; adjust dosage as needed. Maximum daily dosages, up to 200 mg/day for outpatients, up to 300 mg/day for institutionalized patients.	25 mg orally twice daily; adjust dosage as necessary. Maximum daily dosage, up to 100 mg/day.	Children less than 12 yr, not established. Adolescents, same as elderly.
tetracyclic antidepressants maprotiline tablets	75 mg orally in divided dosages daily for 2 wk; adjust dosage as necessary by 25 mg/day increments. Maintenance dose, usually 150 mg daily administered at bedtime. Hospitalized clients: 100-150 mg orally daily; increase dosage as necessary. Maximum dosage: up to 150 mg daily as outpatient; up to 225 mg daily for institutionalized clients	25 mg daily initially; gradually increase dose as necessary. Maintenance dosage, 50-75 mg daily.	Children less than 18 yr, not established.

TRIAZOLOPYRIDINE

trazodone	50 mg orally, 3 times a day. Dose may be increased by 50 mg/day, at 3-4 day intervals as necessary. Maximum for outpatients: 400 mg/day; for inpatients: 600 mg/day.	Usually require lower dosages.	Not recommended for children under 18 years old.

BICYCLIC

fluoxetine	20 mg orally in the morning for several weeks. If necessary, dose may be increased by 20 mg/day (morning and noon schedule). Maximum daily dose is 80 mg/day.	Usually require lower dosages.	Not available.

the American Association of Poison Control Centers reported the tricyclic drug classification was the number one cause of death from drug overdoses. Therefore it is important that health care professionals know how to deal with tricyclic overdose.

The signs and symptoms of overdosage may vary in severity, depending on many factors, including but not limited to the amount of the tricyclic antidepressants ingested and absorbed, age of the individual, and interval between ingestion and initiation of treatment modality. Any acute overdosage or unwarranted ingestion (even in children) of any amount must be considered as serious and potentially fatal.

The CNS abnormalities caused by overdosage may be agitation, ataxia, choreoathetoid movements, coma, convulsions, drowsiness, hyperactive reflexes, muscle rigidity, restlessness, and stupor. Cardiac abnormalities may include the following: dysrhythmia, ECG evidence of impaired conduction, signs of congestive heart failure, and tachycardia. Quinidine-like effects are common in poisonings with tricyclic antidepressants.

These additional conditions may also be present: cyanosis, diaphoresis, hyperpyrexia, hypotension, mydriasis, respiratory shock, and vomiting. Renal failure is seen with amoxapine overdose.

Since no specific antidote is known, the treatment for tricyclic antidepressant overdose is supportive and symptomatic. It necessitates hospitalization and close medical attention for the CNS involvement, respiratory depression, and cardiac dysrhythmias of sudden onset. This is suggested at all times, even when the quantity ingested is alleged to be small or the initial degree of intoxication apparently is minor or moderate. Each client having ECG abnormalities must have continuous cardiac monitoring for not less than 72 hours, coupled with close observations until well after the cardiac status has returned to normal, since after the apparent recovery period a relapse may occur. Cardiac dysrhythmias have occurred up to 6 days after massive doses of tricyclic antidepressants and may be treated with lidocaine (phenytoin for dysrhythmias retractory to lidocaine). The reported greater sensitivity of children to acute tricyclic antidepressant overdosage necessitates hospital cardiac monitoring for at least 4 days or more.

If the client is not comatose and is alert, the stomach should be promptly emptied by inducing emesis followed by lavage. If the client is obtunded, the airway should be protected with a cuffed endotracheal tube before beginning the lavage and emesis should be induced. The lavage in continued for at least 24 hours, based on the degree of intoxication. In children and adults the use of 0.9% or 0.45% saline solution avoids water intoxication. The use of activated charcoal instilled as a slurry may reduce absorption; however, this is done only after ipecac-induced emesis has occurred. If these two agents (activated charcoal, ipecac syrup) are used concurrently, the charcoal will absorb the ipecac and therefore reduce substantially its emetic effect.

The use of physostigmine salicylate is directed at clients with life-threatening signs (coma with respiratory depression, severe hypertension, uncontrollable seizures). There are reports of very slow (over 2 minutes) administration of physostigmine to reverse some of the CNS and cardiovascular effects of tricyclic antidepressants. The adult dose should start with 1 and 2 mg (slow intravenous injection at 1 mg over 1 minute). This initial dose may be repeated in 10 to 15 minutes, not exceeding a total of 4 mg. In children the initial dose is 0.5 mg slowly and intravenously and repeated at 10-minute intervals to arrive at the minimal effective dose, which should not exceed 2 mg. The minimal effective dose may be repeated as necessary every 30 to 60 minutes because the duration of action of physostigmine is short. Slow intravenous use of physostigmine is mandatory because rapid injections may possibly cause physostigmine-induced convulsions. Physostigmine can increase conduction blocks, causing cardiac arrest, and can aggravate tricyclic antidepressant- or phenothiazine-induced conduction abnormalities. It may also cause bronchospasm, muscle weakness, an increase in respiratory secretions, and bradycardia.

Adequate respiratory exchanges must be maintained without the use of respiratory stimulants. Shock may be treated with supportive measures, such as intravenous fluids, oxygen, and corticosteroids. The use of digitalis may induce further conduction abnormalities and thus aggra-

vate a previously sensitized myocardium. Extreme care must be exercised if rapid digitalization is required because of congestive heart failure.

The tendency to convulsions may be reduced by minimizing external stimulation. If anticonvulsants are necessary, diazepam, short-acting barbiturates, paraldehyde, or methocarbamol may be useful. Barbiturates should be avoided, since MAOIs may have been ingested recently. Hyperpyrexia may be controlled by ice packs, cooling sponge baths, and a cooling blanket.

Since the tricyclic antidepressants are rapidly fixed in the tissues, hemodialysis, peritoneal dialysis, exchange transfusions, and forced diuresis have been generally unsuccessful and ineffective. The level of tricyclic antidepressants in the blood and urine may not correlate with the degree of intoxication or reflect the severity of the poisoning and is thus an unreliable index in the clinical management of this tricyclic antidepressant–overdosage syndrome, but it does have diagnostic value.

MAO INHIBITOR ANTIDEPRESSANTS

The monoamines (norepinephrine, dopamine, serotonin) are CNS transmitters. Norepinephrine is also a peripheral transmitter at the sympathetic neuroeffector junction. MAO is widely distributed throughout the body, with the highest concentrations in the brain, liver, and kidneys. It is located on the surface of the mitochrondria of cells in the previously mentioned areas and also in the adrenergic nerve terminals. MAO regulates the metabolism of catecholamines and serotonin, and in the liver it is an important substance because it inactivates monoamines such as tyramine, that are absorbed from the gut into the portal circulation.

Two types of MAO enzymes have been identified and named MAO-A and MAO-B. MAO-A appears to have a preference for serotonin and is located throughout the body, with high concentrations located in the human placenta. MAO-B is mainly contained in human platelets, but approximately equal amounts of both types are found in the liver and brain. The MAO inhibitor drugs currently in use are nonselective.

The MAO inhibitors (MAOIs) are capable of blocking or diminishing the activity of MAO. The result is a net increase in brain amine levels. MAOIs also block amine uptake, and this may account for their clinical usefulness. During early clinical trials of MAOIs as antidepressants, orthostatic hypotension was encountered as a common but inconsistent side effect, and many MAOIs were then produced and studied specifically as antidepressant and antihypertensive agents.

MAOIs encompass a variety of activities: as an antidepressant, as an antineoplastic agent (procarbazine), as an antibiotic (furazolidone), and as an antihypertensive agent (pargyline hydrochloride). The MAOIs discussed in this section are the agents used as antidepressants: the hydrazines—isocarboxazid (Marplan) and phenelzine (Nardil), and the nonhydrazine, tranylcypromine sulfate (Parnate). Evidence shows that the primary properties seem to have special relevance to their psychiatric or mood alteration activity, reserpine reversal (reserpine decreases the concentration of norepinephrine in the central and peripheral nervous system), and potentiation of indirect-acting pressor amines. The MAOIs are indicated primarily in resistant depressions (to tricyclic and tetracyclic antidepressants) and anxious and hostile depressions, especially those also involving panic attacks and/or phobic symptoms.

MAOIs can increase the concentration of all central amines, although different effects on the individual amines are possible. For example, some of the MAOIs may increase dopamine or norepinephrine concentrations to a more extensive degree than serotonin concentrations, whereas other MAOIs may raise the level of serotonins to a greater degree than those of norepinephrine and dopamine. The increase in amine concentration is associated with behavioral hyperactivity (amphetamine-like psychomotor stimulation with large doses) produced by the MAOIs and, in some cases, with the exacerbation of psychotic symptoms. In lower doses the antiphobic and antidepressant activities are seen. In general these compounds are most effective in reversing the dysphoric state and its attendant vegetative disturbances in clients with depressive syndromes.

The therapeutic doses of the MAOIs require days to weeks to attain a maximal therapeutic effect. MAOIs produce an irreversible inactivation of MAO by forming a stable complex with the enzyme; thus degradation of biologic amines by this route is prevented and as such does not inhibit MAO production. Recovery from the effect of MAOIs thus depends on enzyme regeneration, which may occur over several weeks. MAOIs inhibit enzymes other than MAO; such as dopamine-β-oxidase, diamine oxidase, amino acid decarboxylases, and choline dehydrogenase. Inhibition occurs only in very high doses and may be responsible for some of the toxic effects of MAOIs.

Mechanism of action. See previous section.

Indications. Treatment of mental depression. See previous section.

Pharmacokinetics

Absorption. Very good from GI tract

Metabolism. Liver

Onset of action. In some individuals from 7 to 10 days; full effect usually takes from 4 to 8 weeks of therapy

Duration of action

Phenelzine and isocarboxazid—irreversibly binds MAO activity; may take up to 2 weeks for recovery.

Tranylcypromine—Produces reversible binding; thus recovery takes between 3 and 5 days for MAO activity

Excretion. In bile and kidneys

Side effects/adverse reactions. See Table 16-13.

Significant drug interactions. The following effects may occur when MAO inhibitors are given with the drugs listed below:

Drug	Possible Effect and Management
alcohol or CNS depressants	May enhance CNS depressive effects. If alcohol contains tyramine, may result in severe hypertensive reaction. Avoid concurrent use.
local anesthetics containing epinephrine or cocaine	May result in very severe hypertensive reaction. Avoid concurrent use.
anesthetics, spinal	Hypotensive response may be increased. If spinal anesthesia is planned, discontinue MAOIs at least 10 days before surgery.
antidepressants, tricyclic, carbamazepine, maprotiline, or other MAO inhibitors (furazolidone, pargyline or procarbazine)	May result in severely elevated temperatures, hypertensive crises, severe seizures, and death. Before switching from one of these medications to a MAO inhibitor or vice versa, a 2-week drug-free period should be instituted.
antidiabetic agents, oral, or insulin	Enhanced hypoglycemic effects reported. Reduction in oral hypoglycemic agent may be required during or even after concurrent drug therapy.
antihistamines or antimuscarinics (such as atropine, etc.)	May enhance CNS depressant effects of antihistamines. May increase anticholinergic effects that could lead to a paralytic ileus. Monitor clients closely receiving this combination.
caffeine (drug products, coffee, tea, chocolate, cola, etc.)	May result in severe cardiac dysrhythmias or hypertension. Avoid concurrent use.
dextroemthorphan	May result in increased excitability, hyperpyrexia and hypotension. Avoid concurrent use.
doxapram	Avoid concurrent use. Enhanced hypertensive effects may result.
guanadrel, guanethidine, or rauwolfia alkaloids	Severe hypertension may be produced. Withdraw MAOI at least 7 days before starting therapy with these agents. Rauwolfia alkaloid, if an MAOI is added to a medication schedule already containing a rauwolfia alkaloid, serious CNS depression may result. Or, if a rauwolfia alkaloid is added to a medication schedule already including an MAOI, hypertension and increased excitability may result. If at all possible, avoid concurrent use.

levodopa	*Avoid this combination.* Severe and sudden hypertensive crisis reported. Before starting levodopa therapy, the client should be withdrawn from MAOIs with at least a 2- to 4-week drug-free period.
meperidine and maybe other opioid narcotics	Severe hypertension, increased excitability, sweating, and rigidity reported with concurrent use. Also in some individuals, hypotension, seizures, elevated temperature, respiratory depression, cardiovascular collapse, coma, and death reported, which may be caused by serotonin accumulation from the MAOI. To avoid this reaction, avoid the use of meperidine for at least 14 to 21 days after a MAOI is stopped. Morphine and other narcotics are not reported as causing such a severe reaction, but it is recommended that the opioid dosage be reduced to one-fourth the usual dosage. Monitor closely whenever opioids or anesthesia adjuncts (fentanyl, alphaprodine, or sufentanil) are given to clients who has received MAOIs in the previous 2 or 3 weeks.
methyldopa	Severe headache, hypertension, hallucinations, and increased excitability have been reported. Avoid concurrent use.
methylphenidate	Concurrent use may result in a hypertensive crisis. At least a 2-week drug-free period should be allowed before instituting either therapy.
sympathomimetics, systemic	Direct acting (dopamine, mephentermine, metaraminol, dobutamine, methoxamine, and phenylephrine) or indirect acting (amphetamines, phenylpropanolamine, and psudoephedrine) or combination effects (ephedrine) should not be given during or within 2 weeks of an MAOI. Severe hypertensive crisis, elevated temperatures, cardiac dysrhythmias, headaches, vomiting have been reported.
tyramine or high pressor-containing foods and beverages (see box)	Sudden, severe hypertensive crisis has been reported. Client teaching is critical for individuals receiving MAOI drugs. Other drugs and tyramine or high pressor amine–containing foods or beverages must be avoided during therapy and for a minimum of 2 weeks after therapy is discontinued.

TABLE 16-13 Side Effects/Adverse Reactions of MAOIs

Side effects*	Adverse reactions†
More frequent: orthostatic hypotension, tremors, insomnia, headache, muscle twitching (during sleep), increased weakness, blurred vision, constipation, impaired sexual function, sleepiness, increased eating and weight gain, difficulty in urination	More frequent: orthostatic hypotension (dizziness when changing physical positions), falling down or fainting spells Less frequent: diarrhea, edema of feet and legs, increased nervousness, tachycardia Overdosage: increased anxiety, confusion, severe dizziness and drowsiness, elevated temperature, severe headache, hypotension or hypertension, irregular pulse, sweating, convulsions, severe insomnia, respiratory difficulties, hallucinations. Signs appear in 12 hr and reach maximum effect in 24-48 hr. Hospitalization and close monitoring are indicated

*If side effects continue, increase, or disturb the client, inform the physician.
†If adverse reactions occur, contact physician, since medical intervention may be necessary.

Dosage and administration. See Table 16-14.
Pregnancy safety. Not established

The Nurse's Role in MAO Inhibitor Therapy

Because of the possible food-drug interactions, the nurse should teach the client and family which foods may cause a severe reaction. (See box on p. 334.)

During hospitalization, the nurse should note that the depressed client's anorexia may prompt well-meaning family members or friends to bring supplementary foods to the client or a little wine to stimulate the appetite. Careful nursing observation during visiting hours and instruction of the family regarding these restrictions can avoid serious consequences. Communication with the hospital dietitian may also prevent these foods from appearing on the client's hospital menu. As the client's depression lifts or if electroshock therapy is used concomitantly with drug therapy, reinstruction of the client may be necessary. These foods and beverages should not be ingested for at least 2 to 3 weeks after discontinuance of drug therapy.

The nurse should teach the client and family to recognize the adverse effects of this drug, to know the dietary precautions, and to understand drug reactions that precipitate adverse reactions. This knowledge may avert the cardiovascular effects.

TABLE 16-14 MAOIs: Dosage and Administration

	Adults	Children
isocarboxazid tablet (Marplan)	30 mg orally in single dose or in divided doses daily until therapeutic response is noted. Then reduce dosage to maintenance level of 10-20 mg/day. Maximum, 30 mg/day.	Children less than 16 yr, not recommended.
phenelzine sulfate tablets (Nardil)	15 mg orally 3 times daily. Increase dosage if necessary up to 60 mg/day until desired effect (or side effects) is evident. Maximum dosage, 90 mg/day. Maintenance, 15 mg daily or every other day, or higher if necessary.	Children less than 16 yr, not recommended.
tranylcypromine sulfate tablet (Parnate)	30 mg orally daily; increase dosage at 1-3 wk intervals by 10 mg/day if necessary, up to 60 mg/day. Maintenance, 10-20 mg orally daily.	Children less than 16 yr, not recommended.

TYRAMINE-CONTAINING SUBSTANCES

Tyramine content of foods varies according to the references reviewed. This variation may result from different conditions or preparation of the foods, different food samples, or different producers or manufacturers. The major goal should be to advise the client to avoid foods and drinks with reported moderate to high tyramine content as follows:

  Cheese: aged (blue, boursault, natural brick, brie, camembert, cheddar, emmenthaller, gruyere, mozzarella, parmesan, romano, roquefort, stilton)

  Meat and fish: beef and chicken liver, unrefrigerated, fermented; caviar, fish, unrefrigerated, fermented; fish, dried; herring, dried salted; and spoiled pickled, fermented sausages (bologna, pepperoni, salami, summer sausage) and any other unrefrigerated, fermented meats

  Vegetables: overripe avocado and overripe fava beans

  Fruit: overripe figs, bananas, and raisins

  Alcoholic beverages: red wines, especially Chianti; sherry; beer; liquors

Other foods may contain tyramine or high-pressor amines but when eaten in moderation and only when fresh, they are said to be less apt to cause a serious reaction (USP DI, 1988). Such foods include yogurt, sour cream, cream cheese, cottage cheese, chocolate, avocado/guacamole, and soy sauce.

Since orthostatic hypotension is a common side effect, the nurse should instruct the client to come to a sitting or lying position slowly to avoid syncope.

Drowsiness occurs during initiation or change of therapy, so the client should be instructed to avoid activities requiring coordination and alertness until the response to therapy has been determined.

The client should be alerted to the signs and symptoms of hypertensive crisis: severe headache and/or chest pain, increased photosensitivity, nausea and vomiting, bradycardia or tachycardia, and diaphoresis. The client should check with the physician or hospital emergency department immediately.

The client should wear a medical identification band that indicates MAOI therapy and should be instructed to alert health care providers to the MAOI regimen if dental or emergency care is required.

The nurse should advise the client to observe all the rules of caution involved in MAOI therapy for at least 14 days after the medication is discontinued.

MAOIs should not be administered to clients with cerebrovascular defects, cardiovascular disease, hypertension, congestive heart failure, history of liver disease or abnormal liver function tests, and pheochromocytoma (since the tumors secrete pressor substances).

Periodic liver function tests (bilirubins, alkaline phosphatase, or transaminase) should be performed and darkened urine and jaundice as signs of drug-induced hepatitis should be monitored. Blood pressure should be regularly monitored to detect evidence of pressor amine response and orthostatic hypotension. In clients with impaired renal function, the MAOIs should be used with caution to prevent accumulation.

The drug should be discontinued immediately when any adverse signs and symptoms occur. Fever should be managed by external cooling. Either phentolamine mesylate (5 mg slowly intravenously to avoid hypotensive effect) or pentolinium tartrate (3 mg intravenously) is used to control severe hypertension reactions.

The nurse should be aware that overactive, overstimulated, or agitated clients usually do not respond well to MAOIs. These drugs are also contraindicated in many other conditions.

It should be noted that the suicidal tendencies present with the client's condition may compound the nursing care problem because of the delayed effect of these drugs in relieving suicidal tendencies. This effect presents an additional risk to the client during initial phases of drug therapy. The nurse should be alert to the possibility of any impulsive ingestion of these substances.

Since the risk of suicide is frequently higher near the end of the depressive cycle, attention should be given to the possibility of suicidal attempts during this period. Overt patient behavior may indicate a remission of depressive symptoms; however, this may be caused by drug action and not by alleviation of pathologic processes. Antidepressants should generally be continued for several months after the remission of symptoms and should never be discontinued abruptly, since a relapse may occur.

ANTIMANIC DRUGS

Mania is characterized by the presence of speech and motor hyperactivity, reduced sleep requirements, flight of ideas, grandiosity, elation, poor judgment, aggressiveness, and possibly hostility. The manic state is seen with recurrent manic symptoms with little or no depression, whereas bipolar affective disorders have both an acute manic phase and a hypomanic state or alternating periods of mania and depression. Lithium is considered the drug of choice for this disorder.

lithium carbonate capsules (Lithonate, Eskalith, Carbolith✲, Lithizine✲)
lithium carbonate tablets (Eskalith, Lithane, Lithotab)
lithium carbonate extended-release tablets (Eskalith CR, Lithobid, Duralith✲)
lithium citrate syrup (Cibalith-S)

Mechanism of action. Not established. It is theorized that lithium accelerates the presynaptic destruction of catecholamines, inhibits transmitter release at the synapse, and decreases postsynaptic receptor sensitivity, with the result that the presumed overactive catecholamine systems in mania are corrected. Other effects of lithium include interference with the formation of adenylcyclase, inhibition of serotonin turnover, increased synthesis of serotonin, and its intracellular affinity. Sodium in the cells has been reported to increase as much as 200% in manic patients. Lithium and sodium are both actively transported across cell membranes, but lithium cannot be as effectively pumped out of the cell as sodium. Thus lithium accumulates in the cells, which results in a decrease in intracellular sodium and perhaps an improvement in the manic state (Walker and Brodie, 1978).

Indications. Treatment of manic-depressive illness. Also see box.

Pharmacokinetics

Absorption. Completely absorbed in 6-8 hours.

INVESTIGATIONAL USES FOR LITHIUM

Depression: When tricyclic antidepressants are not effective, the addition of lithium to the therapy has reportedly improved the antidepressant effect
Headaches: May be useful in preventing cluster headaches
Neutropenia: Used in treatment of clients with chronic neutropenia; may reduce the incidence of infections in clients treated with antineoplastic-induced neutropenia

---

Metabolism. None
Half-life average
Adults: 24 hours
Adolescents: 18 hours
Geriatric: up to 36 hours
Time to peak serum levels
Syrup: 30 minutes
Extended release tablets: 4 hours
Therapeutic serum levels for treatment of manic depression
Acute: 1 to 1.5 mEq/L
Maintenance: 0.6 to 1.2 mEq/L
Clinical response. Usually reported in 1 to 3 weeks.
Excretion: Kidneys, unchanged (95%), sweat (4% to 5%).
Side effects/adverse reactions. See Table 16-15.

TABLE 16-15 Side Effects and Adverse Reactions of Lithium

Side effects*	Adverse reactions†
Most frequent: tremors of hands (slight), thirst, nausea, increased urination	Most frequent: tachycardia, increased weakness, weight gain, respiratory difficulties, (on exertion), fainting, and irregular pulse rate
	Early signs of toxicity: diarrhea, anorexia, muscle weakness, nausea, vomiting, tremors, slurred speech, drowsiness
	Later signs: blurred vision, convulsions, severe trembling, confusion, ataxia, increased production of urine

*If side effects continue, increase, or disturb the client, inform the physician.
†If adverse reactions occur, contact the physician, since medical intervention may be necessary.

Significant drug interactions. The following effects may occur when lithium is given with the drugs listed below:

Drug	Possible Effect and Management
antithyroid drugs, calcium iodide, potassium iodide, or iodinated glycerol	May enhance the hypothyroid and goitrogenic effects or either drug; monitor closely.
antiinflammatory analgesics, nonsteroidal	May decrease excretion of lithium leading to increased lithium levels and toxicity; monitor closely.
diuretics	Decreased lithium excretion resulting in an increased lithium level and toxicity. A reduction in lithium dosage may be indicated. Monitor closely. (See box below for other factors.)
molindone	Concurrent use may result in neurotoxicity, as evidenced by confusion, convulsions, delirium, or abnormal EEG changes. Avoid concurrent administration.

Dosage and administration. See Table 16-16.
Pregnancy safety. FDA category D

NURSING CONSIDERATIONS

Intervention. Lithium should not be administered to pregnant women during the first trimester unless the potential benefits outweigh the risks to the fetus. Lithium is excreted in breast milk of lactating mothers in quantities sufficient to affect the child with lithium toxicity, prohibiting its use in breast-feeding mothers.

Education. Client compliance, cooperation, and commitment to adhere strictly to all therapy is essential. The family should be advised in language they can understand of all ramifications of therapy, including effects related to serum level.

The nurse should discuss the overt clinical signs of lithium toxicity with the client, family, or closest companion. Some of these symptoms are diarrhea, vomiting, tremors, mild ataxia, lack of coordination, drowsiness, and muscular weakness. If any of these signs appear, the client is to discontinue therapy and promptly notify the physician.

Advise the client of facilities where prompt and accurate serum lithium determinations may be obtained.

Discuss with the client and family the importance of a normal diet, since lithium decreases sodium reabsorption by the renal tubules, which may produce sodium depletion. An intake of 2500 to 3000 ml of liquid daily during the initial stabilization period is essential. The client should be cautioned to avoid fluid depletion, such as limiting coffee, tea, and cola intake because of their diuretic effect and avoiding exercise, saunas, and exposure to hot weather. The client should be advised to seek the assistance of a health care provider for illnesses that cause diaphoresis, vomiting, and/or diarrhea.

The nurse should advise the client about the necessity of taking the medication consistently—initially because it takes 1 to 3 weeks for improvement of the condition and thereafter even though the symptoms may abate. The nurse should assess carefully for compliance to the regimen, particularly if the client has had an increase in weight. Weight gain is a major cause of noncompliance, especially in women clients.

The importance of regular visits to the physician for the monitoring of serum lithium levels should be stressed with the client.

FACTORS AFFECTING LITHIUM SERUM LEVELS

Increased by:
  Diarrhea
  Diuretics   } Retain
  Low-salt diets   } lithium
  High fevers or strenuous exercise
Decreased by:
  High salt intake   } Enhanced
  High intake of sodium bicarbonate } lithium
                  excretion
  Pregnancy

TABLE 16-16   Dosage and Administration of Lithium

	Adults	Elderly	Children
lithium carbonate tablets/capsules/syrup	Acute mania: 600 mg orally 3 times daily; adjust dosage as necessary according to client's response and development of side effects/adverse reactions. Maintenance: 300 mg 3 or 4 times daily, adjusted as necessary. Maximum, 2.4 g/day.	Usually require a lower dosage.	Children less than 12 yr, not established.
lithium carbonate extended-release tablets	900 mg orally twice a day or 600 mg orally 3 times a day; adjust dosage as necessary. Maintenance: 450 mg orally twice daily or 300 mg 3 times daily; adjust dosage as necessary. Maximum daily dose, 2.4 g/day.	Usually require a lower dosage.	Same as above.

Impairment of alertness may occur, so the client should be instructed to avoid activities requiring coordination and close attention until the response to therapy has been determined.

Evaluation. The nurse should assess the history of manic episodes, occurrence, and degree of severity, along with the cyclic appearance of pattern. Family intervention for treatment when manic-depressive symptoms appear is essential.

Since lithium also is secreted in the saliva and the plasma concentration/salivary concentration ratio is fairly constant, salivary lithium levels should be monitored.

KEY TERMS

adrenergic, page 308

affective disorders, page 323

antagonist, page 308

antipsychotic, page 306

choreoathetoid, page 317

desensitization, page 308

endogenous depression, page 323

exogenous depression, page 323

mania, page 335

neuroleptic malignant syndrome, page 320

neurotransmitter, page 308

receptor, page 308

refractory responses, page 308

supersensitivity, page 308

tachyphylaxis, page 308

tardive dyskinesia, page 317

tolerance, page 308

tranquilizer, page 310

BIBLIOGRAPHY

Abramowicz M, editor: Drugs that cause psychiatric symptoms, The Medical Letter 23(3):9, 1981.

Alverno L and Wang RIM: Tardive dyskinesia: implications for future psychochemotherapy, Hosp Formul 16:183,1981.

American Hospital Formulary Service: AHFS Drug Information '88, Bethesda, Md, 1988, American Society of Hospital Pharmacists, Inc.

Andreason N and others: Affective disorders and diagnostic and statistical manual of mental disorders, ed 3, Washington, DC, 1980, American Psychiatric Association.

Bachmann KA and Sherman GP: Pharmacotherapeutic management of psychiatric problems. In PRN: pharmacy review notes, ed 2, Toledo, 1983, Council of Ohio Colleges of Pharmacy.

Berkow R, editor: The Merck manual of diagnosis and therapy, ed 14, Rahway, NJ, 1982, Merck Sharp & Dohme Research Lab.

Biekhimer LJ and DeVane CL: The neuroleptic malignant syndrome: presentation and treatment, Drug Intell Clin Pharm 18:462, 1984.

Crismon ML: Drug induced extrapyramidal syndromes, US Pharmacist 7 (1):30, 1982.

Csernansky JG and Hollister LE: Pharmacologic guidelines in the management of atypical depression, Hosp Formul 17:711, 1982.

Csernansky JG and Hollister LE: The schizophrenic refractory to neuroleptic therapy, Hosp Formul 17:981, 1982.

Csernansky JG and Hollister LE: Psychotropic medications: the risk of teratogenesis, Hosp Formul 19:719, 1984.

DeVane CL and Ahsanuddin KM: Use of psychoactive drugs in children, Drug Intell Clin Pharm 17:562, 1983.

Dominquez RA: Evaluating the effectiveness of the new antidepressants, Hosp Community Psychiatry 34(5):405, 1983.

Doyal LE and Morton WA Jr: The clinical usefulness of lithium as an antidepressant, Hosp Community Psychiatry 35(7):685, 1984.

Edmond MPI and Simpson GM: New antidepressants: a review, Hosp Formul 20:580, 1985.

Feather RB: The institutionalized mental health patient's right to refuse psychotropic medication, Perspect Psychiatr Care 23(2):45.

Forgnone M: Tyramine in food and beverages, Drug Inform Pharm Resource Center Newslett 6(5):169, 1981.

Gelenberg AJ: Psychiatric emergencies: the psychotic patient, Drug Therapy (Hospital) 6:25, 1981.

Gold DD Jr: Pharmacotherapy of schizophrenia Hosp Formul 19:153, 1984.

Gilman AG and others: Goodman and Gilman's the pharmacological basis of therapeutics, ed 7, New York, 1985, Macmillan Publishing Co.

Grimm PM: Psychotropic medication: nursing implications, Nurs Clinics No Amer 21(3):397, 1986.

Groves JB and others: Psychoactive-drug use among adolescents with psychiatric disorders, Am J Hosp Pharm 43:1714, 1986.

Harris B: Drugs and depression, Am J Nurs 86(3):292, 1986.

Huston LD: Do psych patients really need those drugs? RN 50(2):90, 1987.

Ingalls K: Monitoring and testing lithium intoxication, US Pharmacist 8(9):M-1, 1983.

Jewwell JA and Chemij M: Tardive dyskinesia, the involuntary movement disorder that no one really understands, Can Nurse 79(6):20, 1983.

Kalachnik JE: Tardive dyskinesia, Minn Pharmacist 37(4):14, 1983.

Kane, JM: Neuroleptics in the treatment of schizophrenia, Hosp Therapy li(9):111, 1986.

Katcher BS and others: Applied therapeutics: the clinical use of drugs, ed 3, San Francisco, 1983, Applied Therapeutics, Inc.

Ketai R: Psychotropic drugs in the management of psychiatric emergencies, Postgrad Med 58:87, 1975.

Knober JE and Anderson PO: Handbook of clinical drug data, ed 6, Hamilton, Ill, 1988, Drug Intelligence Publications, Inc.

Labson LH, editor: How you can help the schizophrenic, Patient Care 18(1):99, 1984.

Lauler DP, editor: Schizophrenia: the role of allied health professionals, New York, 1971, Medcom.

Levenson AJ and others: Major tranquilizers and heart disease: to use or not to use, Geriatrics 35(10):55, 1980.

Levenson JL and Mishra A: Managing depression in the elderly cardiac patient, Geriatric Med Today 6(1):79, 1987.

Lithium for cluster headache, Med Lett 21(19):77, 1979.

Lyons AS and Petrucelli RJ: Medicine: an illustrated history, New York, 1978, Harry N. Abrams, Inc.

Moriarty RW: Tricyclic antidepressant poisoning, Drug Therapy 6:73, 1981.

Pagliaro AM and Pagliaro LA: Pharmacologic aspects of nursing, St Louis, 1986, The C.V. Mosby Co.

Physician's Desk Reference (PDR), ed 40, Oradell, NJ, 1986, Medical Economics Co.

Portnoi UA and Johnson JE: Tardive dyskinesia, Geriatric Nurs 3(1):39, 1982.

Responding to overdose with tricyclic antidepressants, Am Pharm NS27(5):17, 1987.

Rosenbaum JF: Psychotropic drugs and the cardiac patient, Drug Therapy (Hospital) 5(3):80, 1980.

Rubin EH: Psychotropic therapy: special concerns in the elderly, Hosp Pract 21(10):95, 1986.

Rubin J, editor: Drugs: nurse's reference library, Springhouse, Pa, 1982, Intermed Communication, Inc.

Salerno E: Psychopharmacology and the elderly, Topics Geriatric Rehab 1(2):35, 1986.

Salzman C and Hoffman SA: Clinical interaction between psychotropic and other drugs, Hosp Community Psychiatry 34(10):897, 1983.

Shillcut SD and Easterday JL: Geriatric therapeutics: safe and effective use of antipsychotic agents, Hosp Formul 21:462, 1986.

Silverman JJ and Bloom VL: Tricyclic antidepressant plasma levels and the diagnosis and treatment of depression, Hosp Formul 17:206, 1982.

Simpson, GM, Pi, EH, and Sramek, JJ: An update on tardive dyskinesia, Hosp Community Psychiatry 37(4):362, 1986.

Sriwatanakul K: Author's reply, low tyramine diet, Drug Therapy Hospital 7:11, 1982.

Stanaszek WF and Carlstedt, BC: Schizophrenia, US Pharmacist 11:33, 1986.

Turnquist AC: The issue of informed consent and the use of neuroleptic medications, Int J Nurs Stud 20(3):181, 1983.

United States Pharmacopeial Convention: Drug Information for the Health Care Provider, ed 8, Rockville, Md, 1988, The Convention.

van der Kolk BA: Psychopharmacological issues in posttraumatic stress disorder, Hosp Community Psychiatry 34(8):683, 1983.

Veith RC: Antidepressants and the depressed cardiac patient, Primary Cardiology, 11(6):97, 1985.

Walker JI and Brodie HK: Current concepts of lithium treatment and prophylaxis, J Cont Educ Psychiatry, 1978.

Weber SS and others: Diazepam in tardive dyskinesia, Drug Intell Clin Pharm 17:523, 1983.

Weiner RD and others: The price of psychotropic drugs: a neglected factor, Hosp Community Psychiatry 34(6):531, 1983.

Youssef FA: Adherence to therapy in psychiatric patients: an empirical investigation, Int J Nurs Stud 21(1):51, 1984.

CHAPTER
17

Drugs for Specific CNS-Peripheral Dysfunctions

OBJECTIVES

After studying this chapter, the student will be able to:

1. Explain the neurotransmitter balance theory in Parkinson's disease.

2. Name the two neurotransmitters that centrally affect motor function and balance.

3. Discuss medications used to treat Parkinson's disease.

4. Discuss medications used to treat myasthenia gravis.

5. Apply nursing considerations to the treatment of Parkinson's disease, myasthenia gravis, dementia, and Alzheimer's disease.

Parkinson's disease, myasthenia gravis, dementia, and Alzheimer's disease, are examples of the major CNS-neuromuscular disorders. Because each syndrome is essentially progressive and often incapacitating, appropriate assessment, intervention, and evaluation are important measures for nursing.

PARKINSON'S DISEASE

Parkinson's disease is a progressively debilitating disorder of the CNS. The cause is unknown; however, genetic and viral causes have been postulated. The disease is caused by a degeneration of the dopamine-producing neurons of the substantia nigra, which produces a dopamine/acetylcholine imbalance. The correct balance of dopamine and acetylcholine is important in regulating posture, muscle, tone, and voluntary movement (Figure 17-1). Drug therapy is aimed at correcting this imbalance by increasing dopamine levels and blocking acetylcholine levels. The classes of drugs used in treatment are (1) drugs with central anticholinergic activity (anticholinergics and antihistamines) and (2) drugs that affect brain dopamine levels to enhance dopaminergic mechanisms.

DRUGS WITH CENTRAL ANTICHOLINERGIC ACTIVITY

Symptoms of Parkinson's disease caused by an excess of cholinergic activity are muscle rigidity and muscle

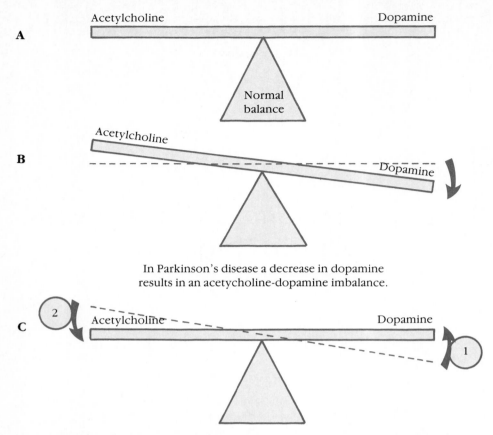

FIGURE 17-1   Central acetylcholine/dopamine balance. **A,** Normal "balance" of acetylcholine and dopamine. **B,** In Parkinson's disease, a *decrease* in dopamine results in an acetylcholine/dopamine imbalance. **C,** Drug therapy in Parkinson's disease aims at increasing the dopamine level, which restores the acetylcholine/dopamine balance toward normal by (1) increasing the supply of dopamine or (2) blocking or lowering acetylcholine levels.

tremor. The muscle rigidity or increased tone appears as **"ratchet resistance"** or **"cogwheel rigidity,"** wherein the affected muscle moves easily, then meets resistance or remains fixed in the new position. The muscle tremors appear to have a "to and fro" movement caused by the sequence of contractions of agonistic and antagonistic muscles involved. The tremors are usually worse at rest and are commonly manifested as "pill-rolling" motion of the hands and a bobbing of the head.

Three groups of drugs with central anticholinergic activity are used to treat Parkinson's disease: anticholinergic agents, antihistamines, and ethopropazine, a phenothiazine. These agents are used in the treatment of mild Parkinson's disease and as an adjunct to dopamine-replacement therapy.

Anticholinergic Agents

Drugs which inhibit or block the effects of acetylcholine are referred to as **anticholinergic** drugs (see Chapter 21 for a more complete discussion). The belladonna

---

PARKINSON'S DISEASE INDUCED BY DESIGNER DRUGS

Designer drugs, or chemical variations of illegal or controlled substances, are an ever-increasing problem in the United States. Such products are usually not illegal but generally are produced to induce the psychoactive effects of selected illegal products. Often the user consumes an unknown substance that may or may not be the desired product. Reports indicate that **MPTP,** a chemical produced as an analog of meperidine in the clandestine laboratories, has been sold on the streets as heroin, cocaine, or a contaminant of other products.

MPTP has reportedly induced a degenerative CNS disorder characterized by tremors and muscle paralysis similar to the symptoms of Parkinson's disease. In a number of cases the paralysis reported has been permanent.

alkaloids, atropine and scopolamine, were the first centrally active (i.e., crossing the blood-brain barrier) anticholinergic agents used to treat parkinsonism and for many years were the only drugs available for such treatment. These drugs have been supplanted by synthetic anticholinergics, which were developed in an effort to produce drugs as effective as the belladonna drugs but with fewer side effects.

The anticholinergics that readily cross the blood-brain barrier can produce slight to moderate improvement in functional capacity. The usefulness of these drugs is limited to their side effects and their tendency to be less effective with continued use. Some anticholinergics are also used to control the extrapyramidal reactions, such as rigidity, akinesia, tremor, and akathisia, caused by antipsychotic drugs such as the phenothiazines.

Mechanisms of action. Anticholinergic drugs block central cholinergic excitatory pathways, returning the dopamine/acetylcholine balance in the brain (especially, the basal ganglia) to normal. The effects of the anticholinergic agents include decreased salivation and relaxation of smooth muscle with a decrease in tremors. Decreased rigidity and akinesia (in nearly 50% of the clients) are also reported. Some agents, procyclidine and trihexyphenidyl, may have a direct relaxing effect on smooth muscle.

Indications. Treatment of Parkinson's disease; treatment of drug-induced extrapyramidal reactions

Pharmacokinetics

Absorption. Good

Onset of action

benztropine oral: 1 to 2 hours

benztropine IM/IV: within minutes

ethopropazine, oral: 0.5 to 1 hour

trihexyphenidyl oral: 1 hour

diphenhydramine: see antihistamines, Chapter 38

Duration of effect

benztropine (orally, IM, or IV): 24 hours

ethopropazine, oral: 4 hours

procycline, oral: 4 hours

trihexyphenidyl, oral: 6 to 12 hours

Metabolism. Undetermined

Excretion. Probably kidneys

Side effects/adverse reactions. See Table 17-1.

Significant drug interactions. The following effects may occur when anticholinergics are given with the drugs listed below:

Drug	Possible Effect and Management
alcohol and CNS depressant	May result in enhanced CNS depressant effects; monitor closely.
other antimuscarinic* or anticholinergic medications	May result in enhanced anticholinergic effects. Monitor for constipation because bowel impaction and/or paralytic ileus may be produced. Increased fluid intake, exercise, stool softeners, and/or laxatives may be necessary.
antacids	Concurrent administration may reduce absorption and therapeutic effects of anticholinergic agents. Separate antacids and anticholinergics by 1 to 2 hours.

*Drugs which block cholinergic receptors at postganglionic parasympathetic synapses and a small number of postganglionic sympathetic synapses (atropine, scopolamine). See Chapter 21.

Dosage and administration. See Table 17-2.

Pregnancy safety. Benztropine tablets, FDA category unclassified; biperiden lactate injection, FDA category C; ethopropazine hydrochloride tablet, FDA category unclassified; procyclidine hydrochloride tablet, FDA category unclassified; trihexyphenidyl hydrochloride extended-release capsule, FDA category unclassified

NURSING CONSIDERATIONS

Assessment. The nurse should note that anticholinergic drugs are contraindicated in children less than 3 years old and in clients with acute narrow-angle glaucoma or pyloric or duodenal obstruction.

Intervention. With beginning therapy, the dosages are low, increasing every 5 to 6 days until a therapeutic level can be obtained. In the same fashion, when the drug is to be withdrawn, it is done so gradually. Tolerance may develop if the therapy is prolonged, which may require an

---

TABLE 17-1 Side Effects/Adverse Reactions of Anticholinergic Drugs

Side effects*	Adverse reactions†
More frequent: blurred vision, mydriasis, constipation, dry skin, anhidrosis, urinary hesitancy, pain on urination, nausea, vomiting, photophobia, drowsiness, xerostomia, dysphagia	Less common: confusion seen mostly in elderly receiving high doses, pain in eyes (result of increased intraocular pressure), and skin rash (face, upper trunk, uticaria, dermatitis)
Less frequent: orthostatic hypotension, euphoria (reported most often in elderly receiving high doses), headaches, abdominal pain, sore mouth and tongue, increased numbness in hands or feet, muscle cramping, nervousness	Overdosage: ataxia; dry mouth, nose, throat; difficulty breathing; tachycardia; flushed, red, dry skin; seizures; hallucinations; insomnia or severe CNS depression; mood changes

*If side effects continue, increase, or disturb the client, the physician should be informed.
†If adverse reactions occur, the physician should be contacted because medical intervention may be necessary.

TABLE 17-2   Dosage and Administration of Anticholinergic Drugs

	Adults	Elderly	Children
benztropine tablets (Apo-benztropine♣, Cogentin)	Parkinson's disease: 1-2 mg orally daily. Dosage may be adjusted as necessary. Drug-induced extrapyramidal reactions: 1-4 mg once or twice daily or 1-2 mg 2 or 3 times a day. Maximum dosage, 6 mg/day.	Lower dosages may be necessary, since elderly are more sensitive to these medications.	Children less than 3 yr old, not recommended. 3 yr and older, individualized dosage.
benzotropine mesylate injection (Cogentin)	Parkinsonism: 1-2 mg IM or IV daily; adjust dosage according to individual's need and response. Drug-induced extrapyramidal reactions: 1-4 IM or IV once or twice daily. Maximum dosage, 6 mg/day.	See tablets.	See tablets.
biperiden tablet (Akineton)	Parkinson's disease: 2 mg orally 3-4 times daily. Adjust dose as necessary, according to individual's need and response. Drug-induced extrapyramidal reactions: 2 mg orally 1-3 times daily.	Lower dosages may be necessary, since elderly are more sensitive to these medications.	Not established.
biperiden lactate injection (Akineton)	Drug-induced extrapyramidal reactions: 2 mg IM or slow IV. If necessary, may repeat at 30-min intervals to maximum of 4 doses/day.	See above.	Drug-induced extrapyramidal reactions: 0.4 mg/kg body weight or 1.2 mg/m^2 body surface IM. If necessary, may repeat at 30-min intervals up to maximum of 4 doses/day.
ethopropazine hydrochloride tablet (Parsidal, Parsitan♣)	Parkinson's disease: 50 mg orally once or twice daily. Adjust dosage as necessary and tolerated up to maximum of 600 mg/day divided into 3 or 4 doses/day.	Same as above.	Not established.
procyclidine hydrochloride tablet (Kemadrin, PMS Procyclidine♣, Procyclid♣)	Parkinson's disease: 2.5 mg orally 3 times daily after meals initially. Increase to 5 mg 3 times daily, and if needed 5 mg at bedtime may be ordered according to client's response and need. Maximum in 24 hr, 20-30 mg divided into 3 or 4 doses. Drug-induced extrapyramidal reactions: 2.5 mg orally initially 3 times daily. Increase by 2.5 mg increments daily as needed and tolerated by client.	See above.	Not established.

Continued

TABLE 17-2 Dosage and Administration of Anticholinergic Drugs—cont'd

	Adults	Elderly	Children
trihexyphenidyl hydrochloride tablets or elixir (Artane, Aparkane tablet♣, Apo-Trihex tablet♣)	Parkinson's disease: 1-2 mg orally first day; increase by 2 mg at 3-5 day intervals until therapeutic response or maximum dose of 10-15 mg daily (divided in 3 or 4 doses) is reached. Drug-induced extrapyramidal reactions: 1 mg orally initially daily; increase dosage until therapeutic response or maximum dose of 5-15 mg/day is reached.	Same as above.	Not established.
trihexyphenidyl hydrochloride extended-release capsule (Artane Sequels)	Parkinson's disease: 5 mg orally after breakfast. If necessary, additional 5 mg capsule may be taken 12 hr later. Maximum daily dosage, 15 mg.	Same as above.	Not established.

increase in dosage. If another antiparkinsonism drug is to be substituted for the initial drug, the dosage of the first drug should be gradually decreased, while the substitute is gradually increased.

These drugs should be administered with meals, to decrease gastrointestinal distress.

Freezing of the injection solutions and elixir forms of these drugs should be avoided.

Adverse CNS effects of benzotropine are reduced by a single bedtime dose.

Intravenous injections of biperiden should be given slowly and the client monitored carefully, since hypotensive reactions occur more frequently with this route of administration.

Education. The nurse should arrange for the client to check with a pharmacist, physician, or other prescriber for drug interactions before taking any other drugs, including over-the-counter drugs.

The client should be cautioned that these drugs impair physical and mental functioning (i.e., drowsiness and blurred vision) and that care should be taken when driving or operating machinery.

The nurse should alert the client to the dangers of heat exhaustion during warm weather because of the decreased ability to perspire. This caution should also be of concern to clients with fever because hyperthermia may result.

The client should be instructed to avoid other CNS depressants such as alcohol, barbiturates, and narcotics while taking the drugs.

The client should be instructed to change position slowly if orthostatic hypotension is a problem.

The nurse should advise the client to use hard candy, gum, mouthwash, or bits of ice to relieve dryness of the mouth.

The client should be counseled to have yearly ophthalmic examinations. The intraocular pressure determinations are of particular importance because increased ocular tension may occur.

Evaluation. In clients with bladder neck obstruction, urinary retention may occur. In clients with hiatal hernias, esophageal reflux will be aggravated with these drugs because of gastric retention.

Dysrhythmias have been noted as a result of these drugs, but they are are dose-related. The vital signs should be monitored and changes in the cardiac status should be observed.

The nurse should not administer with other drugs that have anticholinergic properties, since they have an additive effect. They should not be administered with antacids because antacids interfere with their absorption; therefore the nurse should administer anticholinergic drugs at least an hour before administering antacids.

The nurse should observe the client for symptoms of paralytic ileus and report symptoms of abdominal pain, distention, and constipation to the physician.

Because of the decrease in peristalsis, gastrointestinal transit is prolonged and the absorption of other drugs may be impaired. For this reason, these drugs are also contraindicated in clients with diarrhea. If the cause is infectious, the diarrheal symptoms will be prolonged by retention of bowel contents.

Caution should be taken with clients with chronic pulmonary disease because the resultant decrease in bronchial secretions may lead to bronchial mucus plugs.

Elderly clients are more sensitive to these drugs and require less than the usual adult dose.

The nurse should observe the client for xerostomia, a reduction in the volume of saliva. This symptom is important and should be reported, not only because the extreme dryness of the mouth usually is a discomfort to the client but also because xerostomia limits the amount of drug that can be administered. From this symptom, the progression of adverse effects is interference with visual accommodation and difficulty in urination.

DRUGS AFFECTING BRAIN DOPAMINE

Three classifications of drugs affect brain dopamine: those that release dopamine, those that increase brain levels of dopamine, and dopaminergic agonists. The drugs of choice in the treatment of Parkinson's disease are those that increase the brain levels of dopamine. The other two classifications are used as adjuncts or when therapy normally used is contraindicated.

The drugs affecting brain dopamine have their major effect on the akinesia seen in Parkinson's disease. **Akinesia** is a difficulty in or a lack of ability to initiate muscle movement caused in Parkinson's disease by decreased levels of brain dopamine. The client with akinesia exhibits a masklike facial expression, impairment of postural reflexes, and eventually an inability for self-care.

Mechanisms of action. Drugs affecting brain dopamine increase the level of brain dopamine, thus creating a balance between dopamine and acetylcholine in the brain, especially in the basal ganglia area.

Drugs that Increase Brain Levels of Dopamine
levodopa (L-dopa, Dopar, Larodopa)

Mechanism of action. Levodopa crosses the blood-brain barrier intact. It is decarboxylated to dopamine, replacing the missing brain dopamine and balancing dopamine/acetylcholine concentrations.

Indications. Treatment of (idiopathic, postencephalitic, symptomatic, or parkinsonism associated with cerebral atherosclerosis.)

Pharmacokinetics

Absorption. By active transport; approximately 30% to 50% reaches systemic circulation

Distribution. To most body tissues; CNS receives less than 1% of the dose because of peripheral metabolism

Metabolism. The enzyme decarboxylase converts levodopa (95%) to dopamine in the stomach, intestines, and also the liver.

Half-life. 1 to 3 hours

Onset of action. Usually improvement is seen within 2 to 3 weeks (although other clients may require levodopa for up to 6 months to obtain a therapeutic effect)

Peak concentration. 1 to 3 hours

Duration of action. Up to 5 hours per dose

Excretion. Kidneys

Side effects/adverse reactions. See Table 17-3.

Significant drug interactions. The following effects may occur when levodopa is given with the drugs listed below:

Drug	Possible Effect and Management
anesthetics, hydrocarbon inhalation	May result in dysrhythmias. Discontinue levodopa 6 to 8 hours before hydrocarbon anesthetics, especially halothane.
anticonvulsants, haloperidol or phenothiazines	May result in decreased levodopa effects because hydantoin anticonvulsants increase levodopa metabolism and haloperidol and phenothiazines block dopamine receptors in the brain. When hydantoin and levodopa are given concurrently, monitor closely; increased doses of levodopa may be necessary. If at all possible, avoid the combination of haloperidol or phenothiazines with levodopa. If this combination must be used, monitor the client closely because therapeutic changes of dosages may be necessary.
monoamine oxidase (MAO) inhibitors	Not recommended. This combination may result in a hypertensive crisis. MAO inhibitors should be discontinued 2 to 4 weeks before starting levodopa therapy.

TABLE 17-3   Side Effects/Adverse Reactions of Levodopa

Side effects*	Adverse reactions†
More frequent: increased anxiety, nervousness, and confusion (especially in elderly); constipation; nightmares	More frequent: difficult urination, depression, orthostatic hypotension, mood changes, increased aggressiveness, irregular heart rate, severe nausea or vomiting, choreiform, involuntary movements of body (face, arms, hands, tongue, head and upper body)
Less frequent: diarrhea, headache, anorexia, tremors, insomnia, red flushing of skin, dry mouth, weakness; darkening of the urine or sweat reported (insignificant)	Less frequent: hypertension, abdominal pain (caused by development of duodenal ulcers), increased weakness caused by hemolytic anemia

*If side effects continue, increase, or disturb the client, the physician should be informed.

†If adverse reactions occur, the physician should be contacted because medical intervention may be necessary.

Drug	Possible Effect and Management
pyridoxine	Not recommended. Dosages of 10 mg or more may reverse the antiparkinsonian effect of levodopa.

Dosage and administration. See Table 17-4.
Pregnancy safety. Not established

NURSING CONSIDERATIONS

Assessment. Levodopa is not recommended for children less than 12 years old, pregnant women, nursing mothers, or clients with undiagnosed skin lesions or a history of melanoma because these lesions may be activated.

Intervention. Levodopa should be administered before meals since food impedes the drug's action.

Nausea and vomiting occur in 80% of the clients in early levodopa therapy. However, tolerance with regard to these symptoms develops with continued use of the drug.

Geriatric clients are more sensitive to levodopa and require smaller doses.

The nurse should monitor vital signs during periods of dosage regulation.

Education. The client should be cautioned to change position slowly if orthostatic hypotension is a problem.

The nurse should advise the client to be monitored periodically for increased intraocular pressure.

The client should be instructed to call the physician if symptoms of overdosage develop (involuntary muscle twitching and involuntary winking).

The nurse should caution the client receiving prolonged high-dosage therapy that the "on-off" syndrome may occur (see box above).

The client should be advised that involuntary movements of the face, mouth, tongue, and head often develop with prolonged therapy and that the physician should be notified of these symptoms so that drug dosage can be adjusted.

The nurse should inform the client that urine and perspiration may be darkened but that this has no significance.

ON-OFF SYNDROME OF PARKINSONISM

The on-off syndrome refers to a complication following prolonged levodopa therapy (2 years or more). The client will fluctuate from being symptom free ("on") to demonstrating full-blown Parkinson's symptoms ("off") any time during therapy. These effects may last for minutes to hours and are believed to be caused by altered sensitivity of the dopamine receptors or to serum level changes in levodopa.

Treatment may require more frequent administration of levodopa or levodopa-carbidopa and the addition of a direct-acting dopamine agonist, bromocriptine. Scheduling of meals and consumption of high-protein meals may also affect levodopa absorption. Perhaps taking levodopa 15 minutes before meals with a cracker (not milk since it may produce erratic drug absorption) and spacing protein equally over all meals may improve drug absorption and serum levels of levodopa.

Drug-free periods are also used to help reestablish receptor sensitivity to levodopa. Some medical centers advocate from 1 to 2 days to a 10- to 14-day "drug holiday" to permit resensitization of dopamine receptors. Following the latter regimen, most clients only need one-third to one-half their previous levodopa dosage. Such a program should be instituted under specific guidelines in a hospital setting so that close monitoring is available to reduce problems and avoid complications (Lannon and others, 1986).

The client should be cautioned to avoid foods high in vitamin B_6 and vitamins containing B_6 because B_6 decreases the effects of levodopa. See also general discussion of nursing considerations.

Evaluation. Levodopa should be administered with great caution to clients with severe cardiovascular, pulmonary, renal, hepatic, or endocrine disease; peptic ulcer; narrow-angle glaucoma; diabetes; psychiatric disturbances; or a history of cardiac dysrhythmias. Levodopa may increase dysrhythmias in predisposed clients. It may aggravate pulmonary conditions. Intraocular pressure may increase and precipitate an acute attack of glaucoma.

TABLE 17-4 Levodopa Dosage and Administration

	Adults	Elderly	Children
levodopa capsule (Dopar, Larodopa); levodopa tablet (Larodopa)	250 mg orally 2-4 times daily. Dosage may be increased by 100-750 mg/day at 3-7 day intervals until therapeutic response achieved. Maximum, 8 g/day.	Elderly and postencephalitic clients: may require lower dosage, since they are more sensitive to this medication.	Children less than 12 yr, not established. 12 yr and older, follow adult dosage.

There is increased risk of depression in clients with a psychiatric history. Upper gastrointestinal bleeding has been stimulated in clients with peptic ulcers.

Periodic evaluations need to be done for hepatic, cardiovascular, and renal functioning, including hemoglobin determinations and complete blood count.

levodopa-carbidopa (Sinemet)

Mechanism of action. Sinemet is the combination of levodopa with the dopa decarboxylase inhibitor, carbidopa. Carbidopa competes for the enzyme dopa decarboxylase, thus retarding the peripheral breakdown of levodopa. Carbidopa does not cross the blood-brain barrier as does levodopa and does not interfere with the intracerebral transformation of levodopa to dopamine. Because carbidopa prevents much of the peripheral conversion of levodopa to dopamine, the incidence of systemic side effects of levodopa, such as, nausea, vomiting, and cardiac dysrhythmias, is decreased. The CNS effects of levodopa are a greater risk with this combination because more levodopa is reaching the brain to be converted to dopamine.

The addition of carbidopa to levodopa reduces the required dose of levodopa to 25% of the original levodopa dosage. The available levodopa-carbidopa combination dosage forms include 10/100 (10 mg of carbidopa and 100 mg of levodopa), 25/100 (25 mg of carbidopa and 100 mg of levodopa), and 25/250 (25 mg of carbidopa and 250 mg of levodopa). To obtain the peripheral inhibitor effect of carbidopa, a minimum of 70 mg (range 70 to 100 mg) per day is necessary. Nausea and vomiting are reported in clients receiving dosages lower than 70 mg/day of carbidopa. Therefore three combination dosage forms are available to the physician to permit greater flexibility in prescribing sufficient amounts of both levodopa and carbidopa for the client. The manufacturer recommends that physicians not prescribe more than 200 mg of carbidopa per day. As with levodopa alone, the decarboxylation to dopamine replaces the missing brain dopamine and balances dopamine/acetylcholine concentrations.

Indications. Treatment of idiopathic, postencephalitic, and symptomatic Parkinson's disease.

Pharmacokinetics. For levodopa, see previous section; for carbidopa, see following data.

Absorption. Fairly good (40% to 70% of oral dose)

Distribution. Widely to many body tissues with exception of CNS

Metabolism. Insignificant

Excretion. Kidneys

Significant side effects/adverse reactions. See Table 17-5.

Significant drug interactions. See levodopa drug interactions—all noted with exception of pyridoxine. Interaction between levodopa and pyridoxine does not occur in the presence of carbidopa.

TABLE 17-5 Side Effects/Adverse Reactions of Levodopa-Carbidopa

Side effects*	Adverse reactions†
See Table 17-3.	More frequent: Choreiform and involuntary movements will be seen earlier in combination therapy than with levodopa alone. It is reported in 50%-80% of clients and is dose-related. Eyelid spasms or closing may be early sign of drug overdose. Mental or mood changes may also occur earlier and be dose-related.
	See also Table 17-3.

*If side effects continue, increase, or disturb the client, the physician should be informed.
†If adverse reactions occur, the physician should be contacted because medical intervention may be necessary.

Dosage and administration. See Table 17-6.
Pregnancy safety. Not established

NURSING CONSIDERATIONS

It is unnecessary to advise the client to avoid foods containing vitamin B_6.

See also nursing considerations for levodopa.

Dopamine-Releasing Drug
amantadine hydrochloride (Symmetrel)

Mechanism of action. A synthetic antiviral compound. The exact mechanism of action is not completely known. It is postulated that amantadine releases dopamine and other catecholamines from neuronal storage sites. It also blocks the uptake of dopamine into presynaptic neurons, thus permitting peripheral and central accumulation of dopamine. Amontadine may also give the client a sense of well-being and elevation of mood. It is less effective than levodopa but produces more rapid clinical improvement and causes fewer untoward reactions.

Indications. Antidyskinetic (treatment of parkinson's disease); antiviral (systemic agent).

Pharmacokinetics

Absorption. Very good

Metabolism. None

Half-life. 11 to 15 hours with normal renal function

Onset of antidyskinetic action. Usually within 48 hours

Peak serum levels. Reached within 2 to 4 hours; level 0.3 μg/ml. Steady-state reached within 2 to 3 days with daily drug administration. Steady-state level 0.2 to 0.9 μg/ml. Levels above 1.5 to 2 μg/ml are considered toxic.

Excretion. Kidneys

Side effects/adverse reactions. See Table 17-7.

TABLE 17-6 Carbidopa and Levodopa Dosage and Administration

	Adults	Elderly	Children
carbidopa and levodopa tablet (Sinemet)	Clients not previously on levodopa therapy: start oral dosage at 10/100 or 25/100 3 times daily. Increase dosage as needed every 1 or 2 days until desired response is obtained. Clients previously on levodopa therapy: discontinue levodopa at least 8 hr before instituting combination therapy then (1) if client was receiving less than 1.5 g levodopa daily, start with 10/100 or 25/100 of carbidopa/levodopa 3 or 4 times daily; increase at 1- or 2-day intervals until desired response obtained. (2) If client was receiving more than 1.5 g levodopa daily, then 25/250 carbidopa/levodopa orally 3 or 4 times daily, increasing if necessary at 1- or 2-day intervals until desired response obtained. Be aware that conversion from levodopa to combination levodopa-carbidopa requires only 25% of original dosage of levodopa initially. Maximum, up to 200 mg carbidopa and 2 g levodopa daily. If additional levodopa necessary, give as single agent.	Geriatric and postencephalitic clients may require a lower dose, since they are more sensitive to this combination.	Children less than 18 yr, not established.

TABLE 17-7 Side Effects and Adverse Reactions of Amantadine HCl

Side effects*	Adverse reactions†
More frequent: impaired concentration, dizziness, increased irritability, anorexia, nausea, nervousness, purple-red skin spots (livedo reticularis usually seen with chronic therapy) Less frequent: blurred vision; constipation; headache; vomiting; dryness of mouth, nose, and throat; and skin rashes	More frequent: confusion, hallucinations, mental or mood variations Less frequent: orthostatic hypotension, difficult urination Rarely reported: slurred speech, blurred vision, oculogyric crisis Overdose: severe confusion, insomnia, nightmares, seizures Chronic therapy: monitor for congestive heart failure: increased edema of feet and lower legs, difficulty breathing, rapid increase of body weight

*If side effects continue, increase, or disturb the client, the physician should be informed.
†If adverse reactions occur, the physician should be contacted because medical intervention may be necessary.

Significant drug interactions. The following effects may occur when amantadine is given with the drugs listed below.

Drug	Possible Effect and Management
alcohol	Not recommended. Increased CNS side effects, such as confusion, light-headedness, orthostatic hypotension, and fainting spells reported. Avoid concurrent use.
CNS stimulants	Additive CNS stimulation reported; side effects include increased nervousness, irritability, difficulty sleeping, and at times, seizures and cardiac dysrhythmias. Closely monitor clients receiving concurrent stimulant therapy.

Dosage and administration. See Table 17-8.
Pregnancy safety. FDA category C

NURSING CONSIDERATIONS

Assessment. Use is contraindicated in pregnant women and will cause vomiting, urinary retention, and skin rash in the infant of the nursing mother to whom it is administered.

Intervention. Therapy should be discontinued gradually. Abrupt cessation of the drug may cause exacerbations of parkinsonism symptoms within 24 hours and onset of parkinsonian crisis within 3 days.

Education. The client should be informed that a reduction in benefits occurs after 4 to 12 weeks of therapy. Compliance with a full course of therapy is necessary.

The nurse should instruct the client not to drink alco-

TABLE 17-8   Amantadine Hydrochloride Dosage and Administration

Adults	Elderly	Children
Antidyskinetic: 100 mg orally once or twice daily. Maximum dosage, 400 mg/day.	No specific recommendations.	No specific recommendations.

hol while taking this drug because it may result in dizziness, fainting, and confusion.

See also general discussion of nursing considerations.

Evaluation. Dopamine-releasing drugs should be administered cautiously in the presence of impaired renal function, since the drug will accumulate and increase the risk of CNS toxicity. They should be used cautiously in elderly clients and in those with epilepsy, psychoses, and liver, cardiac, or cerebrovascular disease. The administration of urine-acidifying agents will increase the rate of excretion from the body.

Dopaminergic agonist

bromocriptine (Parlodel)

Mechanism of action. An ergot alkaloid derivative marketed as the first agonist of dopamine receptor activity. Activates postsynaptic dopamine receptors, stimulating the production of dopamine and correcting the brain dopamine/acetylcholine imbalance.

Indications. Antidyskinetic, lactation inhibitor, growth hormone suppressant, antihyperprolactinemic

Pharmacokinetics

Absorption. Approximately 28% of a dose is absorbed, but only 6% reaches systemic circulation

Half-life. Biphasic: alpha, 4 to 4.5 hours; beta 45 to 50 hours

Onset of activity. From single dose: antiparkinsonism, 1/2 to 1 1/2 hour

Peak concentration. 1 to 3 hours

Peak effect. 2 hours

Metabolism. Liver

Excretion. Metabolites of bromocriptine in bile (approximately 95%) and kidneys (2.5% to 5%)

Side effects/adverse reactions. See Table 17-9.

Significant drug interactions. When bromocriptine is given with estrogens, progestins, or oral contraceptives, the hormones may cause amenorrhea and possibly galactorrhea, which counteracts the effects of bromocriptine. Do not give concurrently.

Dosage and administration. See Table 17-10.

Pregnancy safety. Not established

TABLE 17-9   Side Effects/Adverse Reactions of Bromocriptine

Side effects*	Adverse reactions†
More frequent: drowsiness, headaches, nausea	More frequent: light-headedness, hypotension
Less frequent: the following usually occur after high-dose therapy: diarrhea or constipation, dry mouth, nightime leg cramps, anorexia, depression, abdominal cramps, stuffy nose, vomiting, tingling or pain in fingers or toes on exposure to cold	Less frequent: confusion; hallucinations; uncontrolled movements of body, face, tongue, arms, hands, and head

*If side effects continue, increase, or disturb the client, the physician should be informed.
†If adverse reactions occur, the physician should be contacted because medical intervention may be necessary.

TABLE 17-10   Bromocriptine Dosage and Administration

	Adults	Children
bromocriptine mesylate capsules (Parlodel); bromocriptine mesylate tablet (Parlodel)	1.25-2.5 mg orally daily. Increase dosage as necessary. Maintenance dosage usually 10-20 mg in divided doses. Dosage increases should be made at 2-3 day intervals.	Children less than 15 yr, not established.

NURSING CONSIDERATIONS

Assessment. Bromocriptive should be used cautiously with clients receiving drugs known to have hypotensive action because there will be an additive effect. There is also an additive effect with other antiparkinsonism drugs.

Intervention. The nurse should administer with meals or milk to decrease the adverse effect of nausea.

The dosage is initiated at a low level and gradually increased to the minimum effective dosage.

Education. The nurse should caution clients to use a contraceptive measure, since this drug may result in a restoration of fertility. A mechanical barrier device, such as a diaphragm or condom, should be suggested rather than oral contraceptives, because oral estrogen contraceptives increase the risk of stimulating prolactin-secreting cells. Pregnancy tests should be performed not less than every 4 weeks during therapy along with the use of contraceptive measures. A positive result of a pregnancy test should be reported to the physician immediately.

The nurse should caution clients that drugs may impair physical and mental functioning and that they should take care when driving or operating machinery.

Evaluation. If used with clients with a psychiatric history, the medication may exacerbate the condition.

Blood pressure should be monitored; 1% to 5% of the clients have symptomatic hypotension.

Other common effects include constipation, nausea, nasal congestion, and tingling or pain in the fingers and toes when exposed to the cold. These effects occur in 30% to 60% of the clients being treated for Parkinson's disease with this medication.

This drug prevents lactation.

The client should be instructed to limit alcohol consumption, since it increases CNS side effects.

The client should be taught to prevent or minimize constipation by increasing dietary fiber, increasing fluid intake to 3000 ml daily, performing moderate exercise daily, and establishing a regular time of day for bowel elimination.

The nurse should advise the client to limit exposure to the cold or to wear protective clothing to prevent discomfort of the fingers and toes.

See also the general discussion of nursing considerations related to anticholinergic agents.

MYASTHENIA GRAVIS

Myasthenia gravis is a progressive and presently incurable disease characterized by the loss of, or decrease in, acetylcholine receptors caused by an autoimmune process resulting in skeletal muscle weakness and fatigue. Because of its involvement with the production of antibodies, the thymus gland is believed to have a role in the causation of myasthenia gravis. Nearly 15% of all myasthenia gravis clients have a thymoma, or tumor of the thymus gland.

Symptoms of myasthenia gravis usually become worse with exertion and are less noticeable with rest. Stress, infection, menses, surgery, and other factors may also increase the symptoms. The most common early reported symptoms are ptosis and diplopia. Dysarthria, dysphagia, and limb weakness, especially of the upper extremities, also occur in the advanced stages. The client may complain of shoulder fatigue after shaving or combing the hair or of hand weakness, that is, finding it difficult to open doors or kitchen jars or performing repetitive tasks, such as lawn work or playing the piano.

The most serious effects of myasthenia gravis are dysphagia and respiratory muscle weakness, since these may result in aspiration pneumonia or respiratory failure. Treatment of this disease state may include thymectomy,

cholinesterase inhibitors, plasmapheresis, and, at times, corticosteroids. The mainstay though is cholinesterase-inhibitor drugs, such as anticholinesterase drugs.

DRUGS USED IN MYASTHENIA GRAVIS

The **anticholinesterase** agents are drugs that enhance cholinergic action by blocking the effect of cholinesterase. These drugs act by inactivating or inhibiting cholinesterase at the sites of acetylcholine transmission, permitting the accumulation of acetycholine. Because of their ability to increase the amount of acetylcholine at the myoneural junction, the cholinesterase inhibitors are primarily used for the diagnosis and treatment of myasthenia gravis and for their local effects in the eye (see Chapter 43). These drugs are used also for urinary retention and paralytic ileus and as an antidote for the curariform effects of the nondepolarizing skeletal muscle relaxants.

ambenonium chloride (Myetelase✤)
edrophonium chloride injection (Tensilon)
neostigmine bromide tablet (Prostigmin)
neostigmine bromide injection (Prostigmin)
pyridostigmine bromide syrup and tablet (Mestinon)
pyridostigmine bromide extended-release tablets (Mestinon Time-spans)
pyridostigmine bromide injection (Mestinon, Regonol)

Mechanism of action. These drugs are cholinergic and act by inhibiting cholinesterase; acetylcholine released by the parasympathetic nerves accumulates in the synapse area to increase muscle strength duration of action at the motor end plate.

Indications. Treatment of myasthenia gravis, antidote for curariform (nondepolarizing neuromuscular blocking agents) blockade, diagnostic aid for myasthenia gravis, used postoperatively to prevent or relieve abdominal distention and urinary retention

Pharmacokinetics

Absorption. Orally, all are poorly absorbed from the gastrointestinal tract; IM, neostigmine is rapidly absorbed

Onset of action
ambenonium: within 30 minutes
edrophonium: IM within 2 to 10 minutes; IV within 30 to 60 seconds
neostigmine: orally within 45 to 75 minutes; IM within 20 minutes; IV within 4 to 8 minutes
pyridostigmine: oral tablet/syrup, within 30 to 45 minutes; extended-release tablet, 30 to 60 minutes; IM within 15 minutes; IV within 2 to 5 minutes

Duration of effect
ambenonium: 3 to 8 hours
edrophonium: IM within 5 to 30 minutes; IV, approximately 10 minutes

neostigmine: oral and parenteral, 2 to 4 hours

pyridostigmine: oral syrup, tablets, 3 to 6 hours; extend-ed release tablet, 6 to 12 hours; parenteral, 2 to 4 hours

Metabolism. Mainly liver (neostigmine, pyridostig-mine)

Excretion. Kidneys

Side effects/adverse reactions. See Table 17-11.

Significant drug interactions. The following effects may occur when cholinesterase inhibitors are given with the drugs listed below:

Drug	Possible Effect and Management
other cholinesterase inhibitors (such as demecarium, echothiophate, and isofluro-phate)	This combination of drugs is not recommend-ed and should definitely be avoided, since serious additive toxicity may result.
guanadrel, guaneth-idine, mecamyla-mine, or trimet-haphan	These are ganglionic blocking agents that may antagonize the action of the cholinesterase-inhibitor drugs, resulting in increased mus-cle weakness, respiratory muscle weakness, and difficulty in swallowing. Avoid concur-rent drug therapy.
procainamide	The neuromuscular blocking action and, pos-sibly, antimuscarinic effect of procainamide may antagonize the action of the cholines-terase inhibitor drugs. If used concurrently, monitor client closely.

Dosage and administration

ambenonium chloride (Mytelase). Ambenonium is a slowly reversible, cholinesterase inhibitor; therefore it may accumulate at cholinergic synapses and produce increased, prolonged effects. Because of the narrow mar-gin between first appearance of side effects and serious toxicity, ambenonium is usually reserved for clients not responding adequately to neostigmine or pyridostigmine or for clients who are hypersensitive to the bromide com-ponent in both drugs. See Table 17-12.

edrophonium chloride injection (Tensilon). Edro-phonium chloride injection is used to diagnose myasthe-nia gravis. Because of its short duration of action, it is not indicated for the treatment of myasthenia gravis. See Table 17-12.

neostigmine bromide tablets (Prostigmin). See Table 17-12.

neostigmine methylsulfate injection (Prostigmin). See Table 17-12.

pyridostigmine bromide syrup/tablet (Mestinon). See Table 17-12.

pyridostigmine bromide extended release tablet (Mestinon Timespans). See Table 17-12.

pyridostigmine bromide injection (Mestinon, Regon-ol). See Table 17-12.

TABLE 17-11   Side Effects/Adverse Reactions of Anticholinesterase Agents

Side effects*	Adverse reactions†
More frequent: nausea, vomiting, diarrhea, abdominal cramps, increased sweating, or drooling	Rare effect: red swelling at site of injection (pyridostigmine only), skin rash (caused by bromide ion of neostigmine or pyridostigmine)
Less frequent: increased urge to urinate, pinpoint pupils, eye watering, increased bronchial secretions	Overdose effects: blurred vision, severe diarrhea, increased salivation, increase in bronchial secretions, severe nausea or vomiting, respiratory difficulties, severe abdominal pain, bradycardia, increased weakness, ataxia, confusion, slurred speech, muscle weakness (especially in arms, neck, shoulders, and tongue)

*If side effects continue, increase, or disturb the client, the physician should be informed.

†If adverse reactions occur, the physician should be contacted because medical intervention may be necessary.

Pregnancy safety. Ambinonium chloride tablets, not established; idrophonium chloride injection, not estab-lished; neostigimin methylsulfate injection, FDA category C; pyridostigmine bromide injection, not established

NURSING CONSIDERATIONS

Assessment. Assess neuromuscular status (ptosis, diplo-pia, speed, ability to swallow, respiratory function, ex-tremity strength) before administration of the drug.

Caution should be used in clients with asthma, pneu-monia, or atelectasis. An increase in bronchial secretions may aggravate these conditions.

Antimyasthenics may cause an increase in dysryth-mias.

Intervention. These drugs are initiated at a dosage less than that required to produce the client's maximum strength, and the dosage is gradually increased at intervals of 48 hours or more. Oral dosage forms may take several days to produce any change. If the last dosage increment does not produce a corresponding increase in the client's muscle strength, the dose will need to be reduced to its previous level. Because it is essential that the smallest dose for maximum result by used, the nurse's assessment and documentation of the client's health status is criti-cal.

TABLE 17-12 Dosage and Administration of Cholinesterase Inhibitors

	Adults	Children
ambenonium chloride tablets (Myte-lase)	Antimyasthenic dosage: 2.5-5 mg orally 3 or 4 times a day. Adjust dosage every 24-48 hr as necessary.	0.3 mg/kg body weight or 10 mg/m^2 body surface divided in 3 or 4 doses/day orally. Increase dosage when necessary to 1.5 mg/kg body weight or 50 mg/m^2.
edrophonium chloride injection (Tensilon)	10 mg IM. If cholinergic reaction results, repeat test in ½ hr using 2 mg dose to rule out possibility of false-negative effect. IV, 2 mg given over 15-30 sec. If no response after 45 sec, give 8 mg. NOTE: if a cholinergic effect results after a 2-mg dose, discontinue test and give atropine IV at dose of 0.4 mg. If necessary to repeat test, it may be done after 30 min has elapsed.	
neostigmin bromide tablets (Prostigmin)	15 mg orally every 3-4 hr. Adjust dosage as necessary. Maintenance, 150 mg over 24 hr orally. Selection of dosage times should be determined by client's response and need.	2 mg/kg body weight or 60 mg/m^2 divided into 6 or 8 doses.
neostigmine methylsulfate injection (Prostigmin)	Antimyasthenic: 0.5 mg IM or SC. Base additional doses on client's response. Diagnostic aid for myasthenia gravis: 1.5 mg given with 0.6 mg atropine IM or SC. If significant improvement in muscle weakness appears within few minutes to 1 hr, it is an indication of myasthenia gravis.	Antimyasthenic: 0.01-0.04 mg/kg body weight IM or SC every 2-3 hr. (Dose of 0.01 mg/kg of atropine may be given with each dose or with alternate doses to offset muscarinic side effects.) Diagnostic aid for myasthenia gravis: 0.04 mg/kg body weight or 1 mg/m^2 body surface IM. IV, 0.02 mg/kg body weight or 0.5 mg/m^2 body surface.
pyridostigmine bromide syrup/tablet (Mestinon)	Antimyasthenic: 60-120 mg orally every 3 or 4 hr. Adjust dosage as needed. Maintenance usually ranges from 60 mg to 1.5 g/day orally.	7 mg/kg body weight or 200 mg/m^2 body surface area divided into 5 or 6 doses orally daily.
pyridostigmine bromide extended-release tablet (Mestinon Timespans)	Antimyasthenic: 180-540 mg once or twice daily; allow at least 6 hr between dosages	
pyridostigmine bromide injection (Mestinon, Regonol)	Antimyasthenic: 2 mg every 2-3 hr IM or IV.	Neonates of myasthenic mothers, 0.05-0.15 mg/kg body weight every 4-6 hr IM.

The drugs administered for myasthenia gravis are best given with food or milk to decrease adverse muscarinic effects, such as abdominal cramping, nausea, and vomiting. However, if dysphagia is a problem, the medication should be administered 30 to 45 minutes before meals and a rest period from the medication until meal time should be provided to allow for peak muscle strength for eating. This may be enhanced by serving frequent, regular, soft foods and encouraging the client to take small bites of food at a time with frequent rest intervals. The main meal should be served at the time of day when the client has the most strength.

The nurse should be prepared for crisis intervention with medications, (edrophonium and neostigmine) for myasthenic crisis and (atropine) for cholinergic crisis. Basic resuscitative equipment should be available suction catheters, AMBU bag, oxygen, and intubation tray.

The drugs should be administered on time since they are rapidly metabolized. A delay of 15 to 20 minutes in administration may cause beginning impairment of the muscles involved in swallowing and respiration.

The nurse must be especially alert to the route of administration because the oral dosage is 30 times greater than parenteral doses.

It should be noted that atropine sulfate, 0.06 to 1.2 mg, may be administered before or concurrently with these drugs to prevent adverse effects such as excessive secretions and bradycardia.

When using these agents to counteract curariform drugs, the nurse should administer them along with artificial ventilation and oxygen therapy. They should be used only when some definite sign of voluntary respiration can be observed.

The nurse should administer intravenous pyridostigmine bromide very slowly to prevent thrombophlebitis.

A client who has had prolonged drug therapy may become refractory to the drug. By decreasing the dosage or withdrawing the drug for a few days under medical supervision, responsiveness may be restored.

Education. The client with myasthenia gravis should be instructed to take the medication as ordered, using an alarm clock for precise timing of doses if necessary. An adequate supply of medications should be kept on hand. The family should also be instructed about timing of doses.

The client and family should maintain a log of symptoms. This will assist them to be aware of what events, such as emotional stress, menstruation, or infection, worsen the symptoms and how they respond to medication. The client should be taught to observe for therapeutic effects of the drug: a decrease or absence of ptosis; improved chewing, swallowing, and speech; increased skeletal muscle strength; and less fatigue. Activities should be planned to take advantage of the drug's peak effectiveness.

When stabilized, the client can be taught to recognize muscarinic effects (diaphoresis, salivation, slowed heart rate, and decreased blood pressure) and modify the medication dosage or take atropine if needed. The greater the control the client has over the therapeutic regimen, the less the feeling of powerlessness the client will have in the face of a devastating debilitating disease.

The client should be cautioned to avoid alcoholic beverages for 1 hour after medications, since they hasten drug absorption.

Tonic water should be avoided because it may contain quinine, which increases weakness.

Evaluation. When treatment is initiated, the client should be observed closely for signs of toxic effects. Atropine sulfate and equipment for respiratory support should be on hand. Observation for cholinergic effect should be ongoing when these drugs are used. The time of onset of weakness indicates whether the weakness is caused by overdosage or underdosage. If the weakness begins about 1 hour after administration of the drug, it would suggest overdosage. If it occurs after 3 or more hours, the weakness is usually caused by underdosage. The nurse should observe for subtle changes in the client's speech and facial expression. Ptosis increases and the ability to swallow decreases early as weakness increases.

Blood pressure, pulse, respirations, movement of the respiratory muscles, respiratory rate, tidal volume, and inspiratory force should be monitored. The nurse should check vital capacity by asking the client to take a deep breath and count as high as possible without taking another breath; most people can count as high as 40 or 50. All these observations are important because symptoms usually seen in respiratory distress, such as nasal flaring and intercostal or suprasternal retractions, may not occur because of muscle weakness. Arterial blood gases should also be monitored. Dosage, route of administration, and frequency of the medication depend on the client's clinical response, the remissions and exacerbations of the disease, and the stresses experienced by the client.

These drugs should be used with extreme caution in clients with bronchial asthma. Note that these drugs are contraindicated in clients with intestinal or urinary obstruction, peritonitis, recent ileorectal anastomoses, or acute peptic ulcer. They should be avoided in clients with decreased gastrointestinal motility because the drug may accumulate and cause toxicity when gastrointestinal motility is restored.

DEMENTIA

Dementia, or mental impairment, affects about 3 million elderly Americans. Although approximately 15% of the impaired may have an undetectable, reversible disorder; an additional 20% to 25% may have an undiagnosed contributing problem that is treatable by more than symptomatic treatments. Therefore, nearly 1 million Americans have an unrecognized but potentially treatable condition that may have directly, or perhaps, indirectly, caused dementia. See the boxed material on p. 353 for selected potentially reversible causes of dementia.

Generally, most irreversible dementias are caused by Alzheimer's disease (50% to 60%) and multi-infarct dementia (approximately 35%). **Multi-infarct dementia** was formerly known as cerebrovascular arteriosclerosis and is the result of localized infarcts of brain tissue. Other irreversible dementias include Huntington's chorea and Creutzfeldt-Jakob disease. Alzheimer's disease is discussed below.

The syndrome of dementia usually develops slowly. Early signs include depression; loss of ability to concentrate; and increased anxiety, irritability; and agitation. Intellectual ability is usually first to decline; then recent memory (such as names of acquaintances or recent events); followed by the loss of orientation as to time, place, and person. Personal habits will decline; the person may become loud or obscene, or some personality characteristics that were present might become magnified. Helplessness, total dependency, and loss of manual skills may occur next. In the final stages, the person may be bedridden with loss of sphincter control and eventually will die, usually of bronchopneumonia.

POTENTIALLY REVERSIBLE CAUSES OF DEMENTIA

*D*rugs, chemicals, or toxins
  a. Bromides
  b. Mercury
  c. Drugs such as butyrophenones, phenothiazines, diuretics, sedatives
*E*motional problems
  a. Depression
  b. Chronic alcoholism
*M*etabolic disorders
  a. Hyperglycemia
  b. Hypothyroidism
  c. Hypopituitarism
*E*ye/ear deprivation
  a. Blindness
  b. Deafness
*N*utritional deficits
  a. Vitamin B_{12} deficiency
  b. Folic acid deficiency
  c. Niacin deficiency
*T*umors/trauma, acute
  a. Subdural hematoma
  b. Brain metastasis
  b. Brain tumors
*I*nfections and/or fever
  a. Viral infections
  b. Bacterial (tuberculosis)
  b. Bacterial (endocarditis)
*A*rteriosclerotic events
  a. Vascular occlusion
  b. Stroke

Modified from Lamay, P. P.: Prescribing for the elderly, Littleton, Colo. 1980, PSG Publishing Co.

The physician should rule out all the possible reversible causes of dementia. Then treatment should be instituted to try to prevent or reduce the ongoing damage and to support the client and family in managing this disease process. Drug treatment is only indicated for symptom control, that is, the use of low dosage antipsychotic agents for treating severe agitation, delusions, and hallucinations, or antidepressants for severe depression. Supportive care should include proper nutrition, moderate exercise if permitted, vitamins if indicated, and the use of environmental aids in a consistent fashion, such as night lights, and daily calendar reminders.

ALZHEIMER'S DISEASE

Alzheimer's disease is a slowly progressive, irreversible disease that is tragically incurable. It affects more than 1.5 million Americans and is considered to be the major underlying reason for over 50% of all nursing home admissions. Other names for this disease include presenile dementia for disease occurrences before the age of 65 and senile dementia for occurrences after age 65.

The first three problems identified in clients with Alzheimer's disease are usually memory loss, loss of logical thinking or judgment, and an increased tendency to wander as a result of progressive disorientation. Later stages may include development of a seizure disorder and incontinence. Clients may be unable to feed or groom themselves, speak, or recognize simple objects or familiar persons.

In the terminal or last phase, the client wants to touch or examine all objects with their mouth **(hyperorality),** exhibits a decrease or loss in emotions, may be bulimic, and may also have a compulsion to touch everything in sight. Insomnia, night time wandering, and restlessness have also been reported. The progressive deterioration of brain cells may lead to increased dependency for all needs, decreased mobility to the point of being bedridden, and eventually death.

Researchers are still searching for the cause of Alzheimer's disease. Currently the theories under study include (1) a deficiency in acetylcholine, a major neurotransmitter in the brain; (2) the outcome of a slow virus or infection that attacks selected brain cells; (3) genetic predisposition; (4) autoimmune theory, that is, the body fails to recognize host tissue and attacks itself, and (5) aluminum theory; autopsy studies have reported finding 10 to 30 times the normal amount of aluminum in the brain. Is aluminum the cause for Alzheimer's disease? Many questions remain to be answered about this disease state.

Unfortunately, there is no pharmacologic method known to cure, treat, retard, or prevent Alzheimer's disease. Current prescribing is directed toward symptom control. Small dosages of antipsychotic agents, such as haloperidol, 0.5 to 5 mg/day, have been prescribed for delusions and hallucinations. Two precautions though: first, start with a low dosage and only gradually increase the dose, if necessary. Monitor closely for side effects. And second, be aware that antipsychotic agents, or any medications with a high anticholinergic potential, could worsen the cognitive functioning of the client.

To treat depression, antidepressants with a low anticholinergic profile, such as desipramine or trazodone, have been used. Start at one third to one half the usual adult dose for Alzheimer's disease clients and increase slowly as necessary. The antianxiety agents, especially those with a short to intermediate half-life, such as lorazepam, oxazepam, or alprazolam, are generally selected for clients exhibiting severe anxiety. Be aware though that if such agents are used to treat agitation in clients with dementia (or specifically Alzheimer's disease), the potential for inducing a paradoxical reaction is present. Such clients may respond with an increase in activity, restlessness, and agitation. So it is important for the physician to differentiate between agitation and anxiety. If the benzodiazepine antianxiety agents are used, they should be closely monitored because symptoms change with time. Short-term use or reevaluation at least every 3 to 6 months is necessary.

NURSING CONSIDERATIONS

In the pharmacologic management of clients with Alzheimer's disease, care needs to taken to provide for their safety and comfort. With most of the medications prescribed for the treatment of the symptoms of Alzheimer's disease, the nurse should understand that the elderly excrete and metabolize these drugs less efficiently. Smaller dosages are required to produce the desired effect. The nurse's assessment of subtle changes in the client's health status and the documentation of them will allow prescribers to more closely individualize medication dosages. Drugs should be avoided that have side effects of depression, confusion, alteration of sleep patterns, or those that compromise respiratory function.

Alzheimer's disease remains, in many ways, a perplexing illness. Besides providing appropriate care, the nurse should keep abreast of medical and nursing research findings, be committed to conducting nursing studies regarding the care of Alzheimer's disease, and share ideas about effective nursing interventions with colleagues.

KEY TERMS

akinesia, page 344
anticholinergic, page 340
anticholinesterase, page 349
Alzheimer's disease, page 353
cogwheel rigidity, page 340
dementia, page 352
designer drugs, page 340
hyperorality, page 353
MPTP, page 340
multi-infarct dementia, page 352
myasthenia gravis, page 349
Parkinson's disease, page 339
ratchet resistance, page 340

BIBLIOGRAPHY

American Hospital Formulary Service: Drug information '87, Betheseda, Md, 1987, American Society of Hospital Pharmacists, Inc.

Bergman HD: Therapy for parkinson's disease, Journal of Practical Nursing 36(2):18.

Berkow R, editor: The Merck manual of diagnosis and therapy, ed 14, Rahway, NJ, 1982, Merck, Sharp, and Dohme Research Lab, Inc.

Calne S: Parkinson's disease: helping the patient with a movement disorder, Can Nurse 80(11):35, 1984.

Charles, R, Truesdell, ML, and Wood, EL: Alzheimer's disease: pathology, progression, and nursing process, Geron Nurs 8(2):69, 1982.

Emmick MD: Alzheimer's disease: etiology, degenerative effect and the need for adaptive nutritional support, Today's Nurs Homes 7(5):33, 1986.

Feldman RG: Parkinson disease: individualizing therapy, Hosp Pract 20(1):80A, 1985.

Finley R, editor: Dementia in the elderly: focus on Alzheimer's disease, Drug Ther Elderly 1(3):9, 1986.

Glick A: Is an Alzheimer's unit appropriate for your facility? Today's Nurs Home 7(2):31, 1986.

Kess R: Suddenly in crisis: unpredictable myasthenia, Amer J Nurs 84(8):994, 1984.

Lamy PP: Prescribing for the elderly, Littleton, Colo: PSG Publishing Co.

Lannon MC and others: Comprehensive care of the patient with parkinson's disease, J Neurosci Nursing, 18(3):121, 1986.

LaPorte HJ: Reversible causes of dementia: a nursing challenge, J Geron Nurs 8(2):74, 1982.

Lindsay M: Myasthenia gravis, Nurs Times 80(4):38, 1984.

Maletta GJ and Hepburn K: Helping families cope with Alzheimer's: the physician's role, Geriatrics 41(11):81, 1986.

Mancoll EL: Therapy of neurologic disorders in the elderly, Hosp Pract 19(10):106E, 1984.

Mayer RF: Getting myasthenia patients through a crisis, Emer Med 98(5):110, 1986.

Noroian EL: Myasthenia gravis: a nursing perspective, J Neurosci Nurs 18(2):74, 1986.

Nutt JG: Turning off the "on-off" syndrome in parkinsonism, Emer Med 16(18):60, 1984.

Palmer MH: Alzheimer's disease and critical care: interactions, implications, interventions, J Geron Nurs 9(2):86, 1983.

Paulson GW and others: Avoiding mental changes and falls in older parkinson's patients, Geriatrics 41(8):59, 1986.

Pinizzotto AJ: Behavioral management issues in caring for persons with Alzheimer's disease, Today's Nurs Home 4(4):13, 1983.

Reisberg B: Dementia: a systematic approach to identifying reversible causes, Geriatrics 41(4):30, 1986.

Seybold ME: Myasthenia gravis, Hosp Med 22(5):139, 1986.

Shinn AF: Evaluation of drug interactions, St Louis, 1985, The CV Mosby Co.

Stokes L: Good days and bad days, Nurs Mirror 160(22):42, 1985.

Todd B: Therapy for parkinson's disease, Geriatric Nurs 6(2):117, 1985.

United States Pharmacopeia Convention: Drug information for the Health Care Provider, ed 6, Rockville, Md, 1986, The Convention.

UNIT V

Drugs Affecting the Autonomic Nervous System

CHAPTER

18

Overview of the Autonomic Nervous System

OBJECTIVES

After studying this chapter, the student will be able to:

1. Describe the reflex control system.

2. Explain the major differences between the parasympathetic and sympathetic divisions of the autonomic nervous system.

3. Name the primary neurotransmitters for each system.

4. Relate the primary disposition of the neurotransmitters following release from their respective nerves.

5. Name the three basic characteristics of the autonomic nervous system.

Autonomic means self-governing. The **autonomic nervous system (ANS)** functions primarily as a regulatory system for maintaining the internal environment of the body at an optimal level (homeostasis). This system automatically controls the function of smooth muscle, cardiac muscle, and glandular secretions, which interact in many vital physiologic tasks. Digestion of a meal, pressure of circulating blood, and many other processes are internally regulated by the ANS.

REFLEX CONTROL SYSTEM

The nervous system in general is the important control and communication system of the body. It collects information about conditions inside and outside of the body. The simplest means by which the nervous system responds to environmental change is through the action of the reflex arc. The term **reflex arc** is essentially anatomic; it is defined as the automatic motor response to sensory stimuli. The work it does is the **reflex act.** In any reflex a nerve fiber conducts a nerve impulse. These impulses are the basis of communication of information through the nervous system.

The reflex act consists of two major functional processes: the *sensory input* and the *motor output.* The first component of the reflex arc is the *receptor,* which detects environmental changes such as temperature, pressure in blood vessels, and distention in the viscera. These changes are responsible for producing a stimulus in the receptor. Information from the sensitized receptor is then transmitted as a nerve impulse along the *afferent neuron* to the *central nervous system,* the site of integration. The CNS then issues instructions as an altered motor nerve impulse along the *efferent neuron* to the *effector,* which produces the appropriate movements of muscles and glands (see *1* and *2* of Table 18-1).

The information carried *to* the central nervous system (sensory input) and instructions sent *from* the central nervous system (motor output) constitute a **feedback control mechanism.** That is, information fed back to the central nervous system from a receptor is modulated so that nerve impulses may vary in frequency and pattern according to the degree of activity required of the effector. The control of visceral function is involuntary, so the feedback mechanism must include all the components of a control system essential for performing the reflex act. Therefore reflex action functions as a feedback mechanism, operating from a receptor to an effector. Its purpose is to prevent extreme changes in function that may create a disturbance in the internal environment.

A good example of feedback control is the blood pressure–regulating reflex. Again, the sequence of events follows the pattern of the reflex arc. The carotid sinus in the carotid artery and the aortic sinus in the aortic arch serve as pressure receptors *(baroreceptors)* that are highly sen-

sitive to stretch and the degree of wall stretching is determined by the amount of pressure within these vessels. Thus any *increase in blood pressure* stimulates the baroreceptors, and this information is conveyed as nerve impulses along the *afferent neuron* to the *vasomotor center in the medulla.* The medulla is the central nervous system site for integration of blood pressure. After the appropriate neuronal connections, a *decrease in sympathetic discharge* is conducted along the *efferent neuron* to the *effectors* and produces relaxation of arteriolar smooth muscles. This relaxation causes dilation of the arteries and a reduction in blood pressure (see *3* of Table 18-1). This is only a partial explanation of blood pressure regulation, since a decrease in arterial pressure produces the opposite response in the same neuronal pathway. In addition, this control mechanism operates in coordination with cardiac function.

NERVOUS SYSTEM CLASSIFICATION

The nervous system is classified on the basis of the reflex arc (see *4* of Table 18-1). The two main divisions are (1) the central nervous system and (2) the peripheral nervous system. The central nervous system consists of the brain and spinal cord and performs the important integrative functions from the peripheral sources. The peripheral system has two divisions: the **somatic nervous system,** which innervates *voluntary* or skeletal

TABLE 18-1   Schema of Components of Feedback Control Mechanisms

	Sensory input			CNS connection	Motor output		
1. Reflex arc (anatomy)	Receptor	→	Afferent neuron	→ CNS†	→ Efferent neuron	→	Effector
2. Reflex act (physiology)	Stimulus	→	Sensory nerve impulse	→ Integration Motor → nerve impulse	Motor response (motion)		
3. Blood pressure regulation ↑ BP	Barorecptor (anatomy)	→	Afferent neuron	→ Medulla	→ Efferent neuron	→	Arteriolar smooth muscle
	Stimulus (physiology)	→	Afferent impulse	→ VSMC	→ Decrease in sympathetic nerve impulse	Vasodilation (↓ PR + CO → ↓ BP)	
4. Visceral nervous system	←	Visceral afferent system: sensory nerve impulse	→ CNS			Motor response	
				CNS	→ Visceral efferent system (ANS): motor nerve impulse		

†CNS, Central nervous system; BP, blood pressure; VSMC, vasomotor center; PR, peripheral resistance; CO, cardiac output; ANS autonomic nervous system; ↑, Increase; ↓, decrease.
*The *sensory input* carries sensory information such as pain, temperature, or pressure *to the central nervous system.* The *motor output* conducts the altered impulse *from the central nervous system* to the effector and produces motor activity or motion such as muscle contraction or glandular secretion. NOTE: The visceral efferent system or autonomic nervous system performs motor activity.

muscles, and the autonomic nervous system, which influences the *involuntary* activities of smooth muscles, cardiac muscles, and glands. The afferent fibers of both systems are the first link in the reflex arc by carrying sensory information to the central nervous system. Following integration at various levels in the brain, the motor outflow from the central nervous system is conducted along either the somatic efferent system or the visceral efferent system. Both of these systems constitute the final link in the reflex arc. (See Figure 18-1.)

Several centers in the central nervous system integrate all autonomic nervous system activities. There is evidence that the hypothalamus, in particular, performs such integrating activities. It contains centers that regulate body temperature, water balance, and carbohydrate and fat metabolism. It also integrates mechanisms concerned with emotional behavior, the waking state, and sleep. The medulla oblongata integrates the control of blood pressure, respiration, and cardiac function. A series of "vital

centers," including the vasomotor center, respiratory center, and cardiac center, respectively, coordinates these activities. The midbrain, limbic system, cerebellum, and cerebral cortex all are involved in the control of and in physiologic functions regulated by the autonomic nervous system. Remember, the autonomic nervous system is part of the central nervous system, not a distinct entity.

DIFFERENCES BETWEEN THE PARASYMPATHETIC AND SYMPATHETIC SYSTEMS

The autonomic nervous system is organized into two subdivisions: (1) the parasympathetic system and (2) the sympathetic system. The anatomic arrangement of each system consists of two motor nerves, a preganglionic nerve and a postganglionic nerve, with a ganglion (group of nerve cell bodies) connecting the two neurons (Figure 18-2).

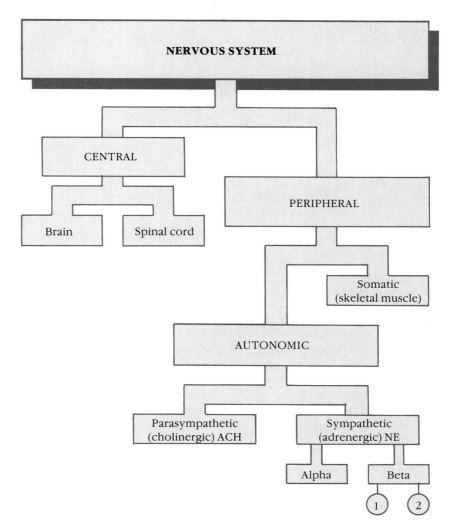

FIGURE 18-1 Divisions of the nervous system.

PARASYMPATHETIC SYSTEM

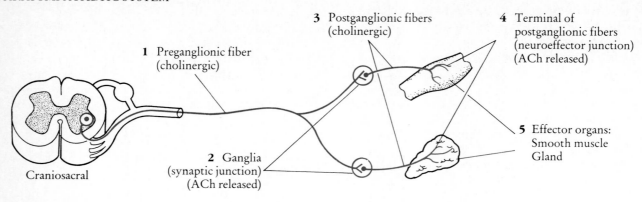

SYMPATHETIC SYSTEM

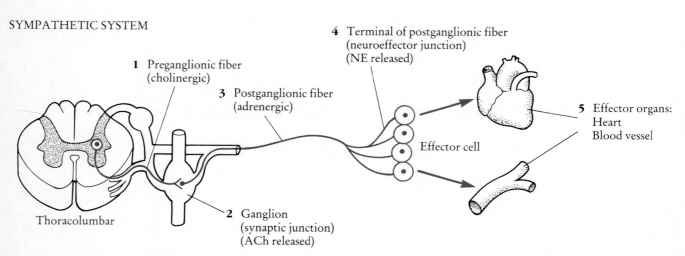

FIGURE 18-2 Preganglionic and postganglionic fibers and neurohormonal transmitters of the autonomic nervous system. The order in which the nerve impulse travels is numbered. Parasympathetic neuron releases acetylcholine (ACh) and acts on the ganglia and effector organs. Sympathetic neuron releases acetycholine (ACh), which acts on the ganglion, and norepinephrine (NE), which stimulates the effector organs.

Physiologic differences. Since the parasympathetic system and the sympathetic system simultaneously innervate many of the same organs, the opposing actions of the two systems balance one another. The parasympathetic system functions mainly conserve energy and restore body resources of the organism, otherwise known as the system of rest and digestion. These include cardiac deceleration, a rise in gastrointestinal activities associated with increased digestion and absorption, and an increase in excretion. In contrast, the sympathetic system mobilizes the organism during emergency and stress situations, and so it is called the "fight or flight" system. These functions involve expenditure of energy, such as emotional stress, and increases in the blood sugar concentration, heart

activity, and blood pressure (Table 18-2 presents effector organ responses).

Anatomic and pharmacologic differences. The parasympathetic system's preganglionic fibers emerge with the cranial nerves III, VII, IX, and X and at the sacral spinal levels from about S3 through S4. The tenth cranial nerve or vagus nerve has extensive branches that supply fibers to the heart, lungs, and almost all the abdominal organs. The parasympathetic system is also called the cholinergic system because the neurotransmitter released by its postganglionic fiber is acetylcholine (ACh).

The sympathetic system is also called the thoracolumbar system because its preganglionic fibers originate in the spinal cord from the thoracic segment T1 to the lum-

TABLE 18-2 Classification of the Effector Organ Responses to Autonomic Nerve Impulses

Effector organs	Response to parasympathetic (cholinergic) impulses	Response to sympathetic (adrenergic) impulses	
		Receptor	Response
Cardiovascular system			
Heart			
Sinoatrial node	Decreased heart rate	Beta$_1$	Increased heart rate
Atrioventricular node	Decreased conduction velocity	Beta$_1$	Increased automaticity and conduction velocity
Ventricles	No innervation	Beta$_1$	Increased force of contraction and conduction velocity
Arterioles (smooth muscle)			
Coronary	Dilation	Alpha, beta$_2$, dopaminergic	Constriction and dilation
Skin and mucosa	Dilation	Alpha	Constriction
Skeletal muscle	No innervation	Cholinergic	Dilation
Cerebral	Dilation	Alpha	Slight constriction
Mesenteric	None	Alpha, beta$_2$, dopaminergic	Constriction and dilation
Renal	None	Alpha, beta$_2$, dopaminergic	Constriction and dilation
Veins	None	Alpha, beta$_2$	Constriction and dilation
Lung			
Bronchial muscle	Bronchoconstriction	Beta$_2$	Relaxation (bronchodilation)
Bronchial glands	Stimulation		Inhibition
Gastrointestinal tract			
Motility	Increased motility	Alpha, beta$_2$	Relaxation (decreased motility)
Sphincters	Relaxation	Alpha	Contraction
Exocrine glands	Increased secretion	?	Decreased secretion
Salivary glands	Dilation: copious, watery secretion	Alpha	Constriction: thick, viscous secretion
Gallbladder and ducts	Contraction		Relaxation
Kidney	None	Beta$_2$	Renin secretion
Urinary bladder			
Detrusor muscle	Contraction	Beta$_2$	Relaxation
Sphincter	Relaxation	Alpha	Contraction
Eye			
Radial muscle	Contraction of sphincter	Alpha	Contraction (mydriasis)
Iris	Muscle (miosis, pupillary constriction)		
Ciliary muscle	Contraction		No innervation
Liver	Glycogen synthesis	Beta	Glycogenolysis, gluconeogenesis
Pancreas			
Acini	Secretion	Alpha	Decreased secretion
Islets (beta cells)	None	Alpha	Decreased secretion
Skin	None	Beta$_2$	Increased secretion
Sweat glands	No innervation	Cholinergic	Increased sweating
Pilomotor muscle	No innervation		Contraction (gooseflesh)
Lacrimal glands	Increased secretion		No innervation
Nasopharyngeal glands	Increased secretion		No innervation
Male sex glands	Erection		Ejaculation

TERMINOLOGY

Over the years, various terminology has been used to describe the divisions of the autonomic nervous system. The anatomic names are sympathetic and parasympathetic, and the corresponding functional terms, which relate to the primary neurotransmitters for each system, are adrenergic and cholinergic, respectively. Generally, the terms are used interchangeably—that is, sympathetic or adrenergic and parasympathetic or cholinergic nervous systems. It is important to understand the terms parasympatho*mimetic* and sympatho*mimetic*, which means to mimic or produce an effect similar to activation of either system. Parasympatho*lytic* or sympatho*lytic* implies blocking the normal effects seen with activation of either system. Anticholinergic is synonymous with parasympatholytic.

ANATOMIC	FUNCTIONAL	PRIMARY NEURO-TRANSMITTER
Sympathetic	Adrenergic	norepinephrine (NE)
Parasympathetic	Cholinergic	acetylcholine (ACH)

---

bar segment of L2 levels. Because the postganglionic fiber of this system releases the neurotransmitter norepinephrine or epinephrine from the adrenal medullary cells, the sympathetic system is also called the adrenergic system (Figure 18-2 and Table 18-3).

NEUROHUMORAL TRANSMISSION

There is general agreement that information in the nervous system is transmitted both electrically and chemically. This phenomenon occurs because nerve cells have two special characteristics: (1) They can conduct electrical signals. *The passage of a nerve impulse or an action potential along a nerve fiber or a muscle fiber is called* **conduction.** (2) They have intercellular connections with other nerve cells and with innervated tissues such as muscles and glands. The presence of a specific chemical at these connections determines the type of information a neuron can receive and the range of responses it can yield in return. *The passage of a nerve impulse across a synaptic or neuroeffector junction with the use of a chemical is called* **neurohumoral transmission**.

Although each nerve fiber may conduct an impulse along the neuron, it is solely the chemical substance called the *neurotransmitter* or **neurohormone** that permits the action potential of a neuron to cross (1) the **synaptic junction** from one neuron to another neuron or

---

TABLE 18-3   Differentiating Characteristics Between the Parasympathetic and Sympathetic Nervous Systems

Characteristic	Parasympathetic nervous system	Sympathetic nervous system
Origin	Craniosacral	Thoracolumbar
Structure innervation	Cardiac muscle	Cardiac muscle
	Smoothe muscle	Smooth muscle
	Glands	Glands
	Viscera	Viscera
Ganglia	Near the effector (vagus, atria of heart)	Near central nervous system
Length of fibers	Preganglionics (long)	Preganglionics (short)
	Postganglionics (short)	Postganglionics (long)
Ratio of preganglionics to postganglionics	Divergence in minimal (1:2), very discrete, fine responses	High degree of divergence (1:11, 1:17)
Response	Discrete	Diffuse
Ganglion transmitter	Acetylcholine	Acetylcholine
Transmitter substance (postganglionic nerve endings)	Acetylcholine	Norepinephrine (most cases); epinephrine and norepinephrine (adrenal medulla)
		Acetylcholine for sweat glands and blood vessels of skeletal muscles
Blocking drugs (postganglionic nerve endings)	Cholinergic blocking agents (atropine)	Adrenergic blocking agents Alpha-phentolamine Beta-propranolol

(2) the **neuroeffector junction** from a neuron to an effector organ. In this mechanism the arrival of an action potential at a nerve terminal starts the release of the neurotransmitter. The hormone or mediator then acts as a messenger by which nerve cells communicate information to the structures they innervate. The neurotransmitter exerts its influence primarily at the junctional spaces, (synaptic junction or neuroeffector junction) to facilitate the transmission of impulses to their final destination, which is usually the transmitter. Many drugs also act selectively at these junctions (Figure 18-3).

TYPES OF NEUROHUMORAL TRANSMISSION

The neurohormones acetylcholine and norepinephrine are responsible for neurohumoral transmission. Nerves that contain acetylcholine are called *cholinergic neurons,* and they are involved in cholinergic transmission. Nerves that contain norepinephrine or epinephrine (from adrenal medulla) are known as *adrenergic neurons,* and they are associated with adrenergic transmission.

In neurohumoral transmission the sequence of events includes (1) biosynthesis, (2) storage, (3) release, (4) action, and (5) inactivation of the mediator. Many autonomic drugs affect one of these individual events so it is essential to understand the basic mechanisms involved in this complicated process. These drugs have been useful in treating many patients afflicted with autonomic disorders.

Cholinergic Transmission

Synthesis and storage. Acetylcholine is synthesized in a reaction catalyzed by the enzyme choline acetylase (choline acetyltransferase) in the cytoplasm of the nerve terminal:

$$\text{Acetyl coenzyme A + Choline} \underset{\text{Acetylcholinesterase}}{\overset{\text{Choline acetylase}}{\rightleftharpoons}}$$
$$\textbf{Acetylcholine + Coenzyme A}$$

Once synthesized, the acetylcholine is stored in packets called synaptic vesicles or granules, which are located in the nerve terminal (see Figure 18-4, *B*).

Release and action. The arrival of an action potential at the nerve ending causes the vesicle to approach the membrane and release the acetylcholine molecules into the synaptic cleft or space. Calcium ions must be present for an efficient release. Once free, the acetylcholine diffuses across the synaptic or junctional cleft and attaches itself to specialized receptors (postjunctional sites) on the membrane of the next neuron or neuroeffector. The binding of acetylcholine to the receptor increases the permeability of the membrane to sodium and potassium ions; thus a depolarizing action finally results in excitation or inhibition of neural, muscular, or glandular activity (see Figure 18-4, *A* and *B*).

Cholinergic receptors. The cholinergic receptor sites that are stimulated by acetylcholine are either nicotinic or muscarinic. **Nicotinic (N) receptors** appear in the ganglia of both the parasympathetic and sympathetic fibers, the adrenal medulla, and the skeletal (striated) muscle that is supplied by the somatic motor system. **Muscarinic (M) receptors** are located in the smooth muscle, cardiac muscle, and glands of the parasympathetic fibers and the effector organs of the cholinergic sympathetic fibers. The N and M receptors are shown in Figure 18-5.

Inactivation. Once acetylcholine has exerted its effect on the postjunctional sites, the excess amount is inactivated rapidly by the enzyme acetylcholinesterase (AChE). The metabolites formed in this reaction are chemically inactive and are the same compounds from which acetylcholine is formed. Inactivation of this neurohormone is shown as a reverse action in the preceding formula (see Figure 18-4, *B*).

Adrenergic Transmission

The term "catecholamine" refers to a group of chemically related compounds: norepinephrine (noradrenalin), epinephrine (adrenaline), and dopamine. They are all involved in some aspect of adrenergic transmission.

Synthesis and storage. The catecholamines produced by the sympathetic nervous system include norepinephrine and epinephrine. The complex pathway for synthesis of these neurotransmitters is mediated by different enzymes located in the postganglionic nerve terminals and in the chromaffin cells of the adrenal medullary glands. The production of norepinephrine and epinephrine proceeds through the following steps:

$$\text{Tyrosine} \xrightarrow{\overset{\text{Tyrosine}}{\text{hydroxylase}}} \text{Dopa} \xrightarrow{\overset{\text{Dopa}}{\text{decarboxylase}}}$$

$$\text{Dopamine} \xrightarrow{\overset{\text{Dopamine}}{\beta\text{-hydroxylase}}} \text{Norepinephrine} \xrightarrow{\overset{\text{Methyl}}{\text{transferase}}}$$

epinephrine

The formation of norepinephrine is initiated by tyrosine, which an amino acid derived from proteins in the diet. When tyrosine enters the cytoplasm of the nerve terminal, it is converted into dopa, which in turn is decarboxylated to dopamine. Dopamine is then taken up into the storage vesicles, or granules, where it is transformed into the neurotransmitter norepinephrine by the enzyme dopamine β-hydroxylase. Figure 18-6 shows the steps of the synthetic process. In the adrenal medullary gland, the enzyme methyl transferases convert norepinephrine to epinephrine. On stimulation, both epinephrine and norepinephrine are released from the adrenal medulla and carried by the circulation to all parts of the body. The autonomic drugs may inhibit the rate of formation of norepinephrine.

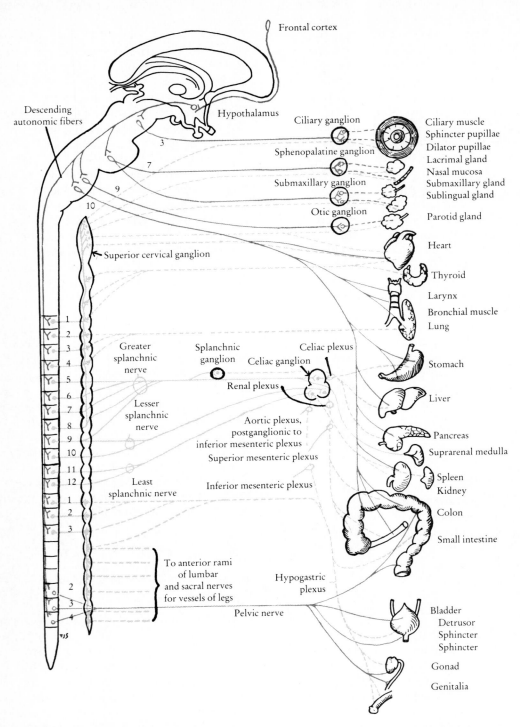

FIGURE 18-3 Sympathetic division of the autonomic nervous system. *CiG,* Ciliary ganglion; *SpG,* sphenopalatine ganglion; *SCG,* superior cervical ganglion; *OG,* otic ganglion; *SG,* submandibular ganglion; *CG,* celiac ganglion; *SMG,* superior mesenteric ganglion; *IMG,* inferior mesenteric ganglion; *PP,* pelvic plexus.

(From Conway-Rutkowski, BL: Carini and Owens' neurological and neurosurgical nursing, ed 8, St Louis, 1982, The CV Mosby Co.)

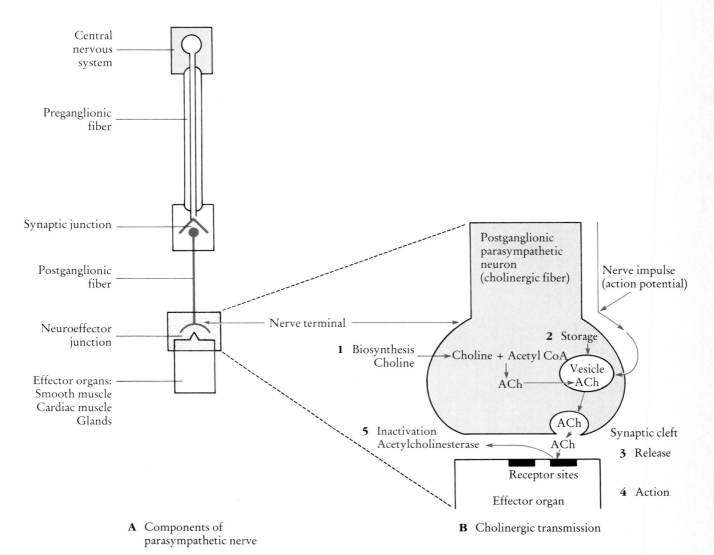

A Components of parasympathetic nerve

B Cholinergic transmission

FIGURE 18-4 **A,** Schematic representation to show the relationship between a neuron in the central nervous system, a neuron in a peripheral ganglion, and an effector organ supplied by the parasympathetic nerve. Note that the *synaptic junction* occurs as a space (cleft) or connection between the preganglionic fiber and the postganglionic fiber, and the *neuroeffector junction* occurs as a connection between the postganglionic fiber and the effector organs. These junctions act as important sites of neurohumoral transmission. **B,** *Cholinergic transmission.* Schematic diagram of parasympathetic postganglionic neuron showing steps in cholinergic transmission at the neuroeffector junction. *1, Biosynthesis* of acetylcholine (ACh): Choline is taken up by the nerve terminal, and it interacts with acetyl coenzyme A to synthesize ACh. *2, Storage:* Following synthesis, ACh is stored in the vesicle until the arrival of a nerve impulse. *3, Release:* An action potential at the nerve terminal causes the vesicle to attach itself to the membrane and release ACh. The neurohormone then diffuses across the synaptic cleft and combines with the receptors on the effector cell. *4, Action:* The interaction of ACh with the receptor sites results in a motor response. *5, Inactivation* of ACh: At the synaptic cleft, ACh is hydrolyzed by the enzyme acetylcholinesterase.

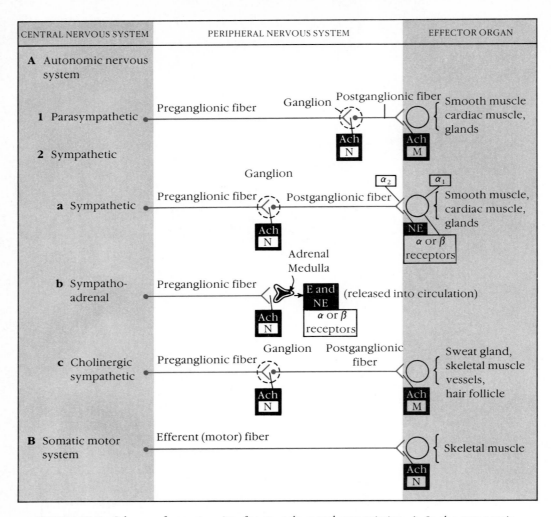

FIGURE 18-5 Schema of receptor sites for neurohumoral transmission. **A,** In the autonomic nervous system, the preganglionic fibers of both the parasympathetic and sympathetic divisions synapse in the ganglia of the postganglionic fibers and the adrenal medulla. The release of acetylcholine *(ACh)* by terminals of preganglionic fibers interacts with or stimulates nicotinic *(N)* receptors in the membrane of the postganglionic neurons or adrenal medullary cells. *1,* In the parasympathetic system, the terminals of the postganglionic fibers release acetylcholine and interact with muscarinic *(M)* sites in the membrane of smooth muscle, cardiac muscle, and glands. *2,* In the sympathetic system, there are three types of postganglionic fibers: *a.* The *sympathetic* neuron—releases norepinephrine *(NE)* and activates alpha (α) or beta (β) receptors in the membrane of smooth muscle, cardiac muscle, and glands. *b.* The *sympathoadrenal* neuron of the adrenal medulla—secretes norepinephrine and epinephrine *(E),* which are circulated in the blood to all parts of the body to activate alpha or beta receptors. *c.* The *cholinergic sympathetic* neuron—releases acetylcholine and interacts with muscarinic *(M)* sites on sweat glands and skeletal muscle vessels. **B,** The somatic motor nervous system has a single fiber whose terminals release acetylcholine and activates nicotinic *(N)* receptor sites on the skeletal muscle.

Release. The arrival of an action potential at the nerve terminal of the postganglionic fibers causes the vesicles to fuse with the cell membrane and release the stored supply of norepinephrine into the junctional cleft. Calcium ions must be present to enhance the release of norepinephrine from the vesicles. The free form of norepinephrine then diffuses across the cleft to the receptor sites on the postjunctional membrane of neuroeffector cells (smooth muscle, cardiac muscle, or glands). (See Figure 18-6.)

Action. Once the norepinephrine combines with either the alpha or beta receptor sites on the membrane of

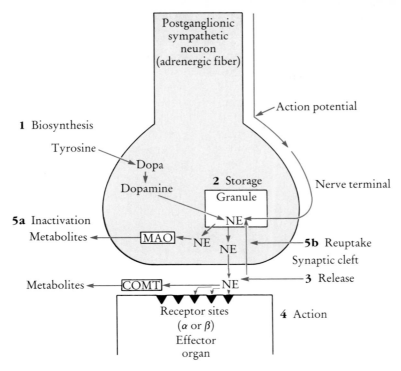

FIGURE 18-6 *Adrenergic transmission.* Schematic diagram of sympathetic postganglionic neuron showing steps in adrenergic transmission at the neuroeffector junction. *1, Biosynthesis* of norepinephrine (NE): Tyrosine is taken up by the nerve terminal and converted to dopamine, which after transport into the storage granule is finally synthesized into NE. *2, Storage:* Following synthesis, NE is stored in the granule until the arrival of a nerve impulse. *3, Release:* Action potential along the neuron stimulates release of NE from the granule; NE then diffuses into the synaptic cleft to the receptor site of the effector cell. *4, Action:* The interaction of NE with the receptor sites (α or β) results in a motor response. *5a, Inactivation of NE:* Enzymatic metabolism of NE occurs within the neuron by action of the enzyme monamine oxidase (MAO) or outside the neuron by the enzyme catechol-O-methyltransferase (COMT). *5b, Reuptake* of NE: reuptake into the nerve terminal and reentry into the storage granule constitute another method of removal of NE.

the neuroeffector cells, a series of chemical and electrical events produces either an excitatory or an inhibitory effect. The alpha receptor activation is primarily responsible for excitatory response, although it results in intestinal relaxation. By contrast, beta receptor activation is usually inhibitory except in the myocardial cells, where norepinephrine produces an excitatory effect.

Adrenergic receptors. The adrenergic receptor sites that are stimulated by the endogenous catecholamines—norepinephrine, epinephrine, and dopamine—are classified as alpha and beta receptors. Both classes have two subtypes. The alpha receptors are identified by neuronal location: (1) alpha$_1$ sites are located on the postsynaptic effector cells and (2) alpha$_2$ sites appear on the presynaptic nerve terminals, controlling the amount of norepinephrine release that operates through a negative feedback mechanism. By contrast, the beta receptors are designated by organ location: (1) beta$_1$ receptors are located primarily in the heart and (2) beta$_2$ receptors appear in

the smooth muscle of the bronchioles, arterioles, and various other visceral organs in the body. Dopaminergic receptors have been identified in the brain and on certain blood vessels (coronary, renal, and mesenteric vessels). (See Figure 18-5 and Table 18-2 for alpha and beta receptors.)

Inactivation. Once norepinephrine has performed its adrenergic function, its action must be rapidly stopped to prevent prolongation of its effects, which could lead to a loss of regulatory control of visceral function. The inactivation of norepinephrine occurs by (1) enzymatic transformation, (2) reuptake into nerve terminals, and (3) diffusion.

Catecholamines are metabolized by two enzymes, monoamine oxidase (MAO) and catechol-O-methyltransferase (COMT). Free norepinephrine *within* the cytoplasm of the nerve terminal is metabolized by MAO, which is stored in the mitochondria of sympathetic neurons. COMT, which is located *outside* the neuron or at the synaptic cleft, participates in the inactivation or metabolism of norepinephrine outside the neuron.

The *reuptake* mechanism plays a more significant role than enzymatic tranformation in catecholamine inactivation. In the reuptake process norepinephrine is removed by the active transport ("amine pump") from the junctional sites (synaptic and neuroeffector junctions) and is returned to the sympathetic nerve terminal and storage vesicles. Thus this mechanism provides a means other than the synthetic process for maintaining an adequate supply of norepinephrine.

Finally, a small portion of norepinephrine released at the synaptic cleft may be picked up by the circulation and metabolized elsewhere in the body. This is known as the diffusion process. Figure 18-6 portrays the steps in adrenergic transmission.

GENERAL ACTIONS OF AUTONOMIC TRANSMITTERS

In 1933 Dale and co-workers determined the chemical differences between fibers that release acetylcholine (**cholinergic** fibers) and those that release norepinephrine and epinephrine (**adrenergic** fibers). In the autonomic nervous system, all the preganglionic fibers originate in the central nervous system and synapse with the ganglia of the postganglionic fibers. The terminals of all the preganglionic fibers release acetylcholine and interact with nicotinic receptors in the membrane of the postganglionic fibers or the adrenal medulla.

In the parasympathetic system the terminals of the postganglionic fibers also release acetylcholine and interact with muscarinic receptors in the membrane of the smooth muscle, cardiac muscle, and glands.

In the sympathetic nervous system there are three different kinds of postganglionic neurons: (1) The sympathetic neuron, the major type, releases norepinephrine and activates either alpha or beta receptors in the membrane of the smooth muscle, cardiac muscle, and glands. (2) The sympathoadrenal neuron, in which the preganglionic fiber synapses with a nodified sympathetic ganglion, the adrenal medulla, releases mostly epinephrine and a small amount of norepinephrine, which are secreted into the circulation and carried to all parts of the body. (3) The cholinergic sympathetic neuron releases acetylcholine and stimulates muscarinic receptor sites on the sweat glands to produce swelling and on the blood vessels in skeletal muscle to increase vasodilation and enhance blood flow.

In the somatic (sensory) nervous system a single neuron, the efferent (motor) fiber, releases acetylcholine and interacts with the nicotinic sites on the skeletal muscle membrane. The autonomic drugs play an important role by enhancing or inhibiting physiologic activity at these sites of neurohumoral transmission (see Figure 18-5 and Table 18-2).

SUMMARY

The primary function of the autonomic nervous system is to control and integrate many physiologic tasks necessary to preserve internal homeostasis, emergency mechanisms, and repair. Its activities are integrated by a number of centers within the central nervous system: the hypothalamus, medulla oblongata, midbrain, limbic system, cerebellum, and cerebral cortex. The autonomic nervous system innervates the smooth muscles, cardiac muscles, and glands. It is composed of two divisions, the parasympathetic and the sympathetic; their actions oppose and balance each other.

1. Although both systems are present in the body, only one will predominate at any given time.
2. If a nervous system function is blocked, the opposite effect will take precedence.
3. Drugs are available to stimulate or block either system.

Functions stimulated by the parasympathetic system are chiefly those concerned with digestion, excretion, near vision, cardiac deceleration, and anabolism. Functions stimulated by the sympathetic system are primarily those concerned with the expenditure of energy and are called into play by physical or emotional stress.

Nerve impulse transmission is caused by the activity of chemical substances called *neurotransmitters:* acetylcholine and the catecholamines. Nerve fibers that synthesize and liberate acetylcholine are known as *cholinergic* fibers; those that synthesize and secrete norepinephrine and epinephrine are called *adrenergic* fibers.

For the nurse to achieve an understanding of the pharmacology of autonomic drugs a basic knowledge of the anatomy and physiology of the autonomic nervous system is essential. This information helps to predict the effects of drugs that stimulate or block autonomic function.

KEY TERMS

adrenergic, page 368
autonomic nervous system, page 357
cholinergic, page 368
conduction, page 362
feedback control mechanism, page 358
muscarinic receptors, page 363
neuroeffector junction, page 363
neurohormone, page 362
neurohumoral transmission, page 362
nicotinic receptors, page 363
reflex arc, page 357
reflex act, page 357
somatic nervous system, page 358
synaptic junction, page 362

BIBLIOGRAPHY

Avery GS, editor: Drug treatment principles and practice of clinical pharmacology and therapeutics, ed 3, Sydney, Australia, 1987, Adis Press.

Bhagat BD: Mode of action of autonomic drugs, Flushing, NY, 1979, Graceway Publishing Co.

Conway-Rutkowski BL: Carini and Owen's neurological and neurosurgical nursing, ed 8, St. Louis, 1982, The CV Mosby Co.

Gilman AG and others, editors: Goodman and Gilman's the pharmacological basis of therapeutics, ed 7, New York, 1985, Macmillan Publishing Co.

Guyton AC: Textbook of medical physiology, ed 7, Philadelphia, 1986, WB Saunders Company

Noback C and Deramarest R: The nervous system: introduction and review, ed 3, New York, 1986, McGraw-Hill Book Co.

CHAPTER
19

Drugs Affecting the Parasympathetic Nervous System

OBJECTIVES

After studying this chapter, the student will be able to:

1. Explain the difference between the muscarinic and nicotinic actions of acetylcholine.

2. Describe the side effects/adverse reactions of cholinergic, cholinergic blocking, and synthetic antispasmotic agents.

3. Describe the physiologic effects of the belladonna alkaloids.

4. List the physiologic effects of nicotine.

5. Describe the use of ganglionic blocking drugs.

6. Discuss nursing considerations for agents affecting the parasympathetic nervous system.

Autonomic Drugs

The autonomic drugs mimic, intensify, or block the effects of the parasympathetic and sympathetic divisions of the autonomic nervous system. They are divided into the following groups:

1. **Cholinergic (parasympathomimetic)** drugs, such as bethanechol, that act like mediators of the parasympathetic nervous system
2. **Cholinergic blocking (parasympatholytic** or anticholinergic) drugs, such as atropine, that block the action of the parasympathetic nervous system
3. **Adrenergic (sympathomimetic)** drugs, such as norepinephrine and epinephrine, that act like mediators of the sympathetic nervous system or the adrenal medulla, respectively
4. **Adrenergic blocking (sympatholytic)** drugs, such as propranolol, that block the action of the sympathetic nervous system

CHOLINERGIC (PARASYMPATHOMIMETIC) DRUGS

As previously mentioned, acetylcholine plays an important role in transmission of nerve impulses in both the parasympathetic and sympathetic divisions of the autonomic nervous system.

Acetylcholine has two major actions on the nervous system: (1) it has stimulant effects on the ganglia, adrenal medulla, and skeletal muscle, and (2) it has stimulant effects at postganglionic nerve endings in cardiac muscle, smooth muscle, and glands. The first action resembles the effects of nicotine and is referred to as the "nicotinic effect" of acetylcholine. The second action of acetylcholine at the postganglionic nerve endings is like that of muscarine (an alkaloid obtained from the toadstool *Amanita muscaria*) and is referred to as the **muscarinic effect** of acetylcholine. (See Table 19-1; Figure 18-5 shows nicotinic [N] and muscarinic [M] sites.)

Drugs that bring about effects in the body similar to those produced by acetylcholine are called *cholinergic drugs*. These agents are also called *parasympathomimetics* because they mimic the action produced by stimulation of the parasympathetic nervous system.

Cholinergic fibers are widespread: they are present in heart, spleen, uterus, vas deferens, colon, and the vessels of the skin and muscles. Cholinergic fibers probably are present in many more tissues of the body. In the gastrointestinal tract parasympathetic innervation predominates: it stimulates both motor and secretory action.

Although acetylcholine is important physiologically, it has no therapeutic value because (1) its actions are very brief owing to rapid hydrolysis by acetylcholinesterase and (2) no selective purpose can be achieved through its use, since it has several sites of action.

Cholinergic drugs may be obtained from plant sources or synthesized. The synthetic drugs are more stable and have a more selective action on particular organs. The two groups of cholinergic drugs available are (1) *direct acting* and (2) *indirect acting. Direct-acting drugs combine directly with the cholinergic receptors in postsynaptic*

membranes innervated by parasympathetic neurons and evoke effects similar to those produced by acetylcholine. By contrast, instead of a direct effect on receptors, *indirect-acting drugs act primarily on the enzyme by inhibiting the action of cholinesterase (acetylcholinesterase)* that normally degrades acetylcholine. This results in an accumulation of acetylcholine at all the sites where it is liberated (see Figure 18-4, B). By rendering the enzymatic action ineffective, the anticholinesterase drugs cause a prolonged and intensified cholinergic response at the various effector sites.

Cholinergic drugs are used for the following purposes:

1. To stimulate the intestine and bladder postoperatively
2. To lower intraocular pressure in clients with glaucoma
3. To promote salivation and sweating
4. To dilate peripheral blood vessels during vasospasm
5. To terminate **curarization**
6. To treat myasthenia gravis symptomatically*

The therapeutic effectiveness of cholinergic drugs depends primarily on their muscarinic action, but some of them also possess nicotinic action. This nicotinic action usually requires doses much larger than those used therapeutically. However, some drugs may exhibit more nicotinic than muscarinic effects.

The ideal cholinergic or anticholinesterase drug would:

1. Mimic or inhibit the effect of acetylcholine on a particular structure or organ

*Cholinergic but not parasympathomimetic action involves the somatic nervous system, innervating skeletal muscle.

TABLE 19-1   Muscarinic and Nicotinic Actions of Acetylcholine

	Muscarinic action	Nicotinic actions
Cardiovascular		
Blood vessels	Dilation	Constriction ⎫
Heart rate	Slowed	Increased ⎬ With large doses after atropine
Blood pressure	Decreased	Increased ⎭
Gastrointestinal		
Tone	Increased	Increased
Motility	Increased	Increased
Sphincters	Relaxed	—
Glandular secretions	Increased salivary, lacrimal, intestinal, and sweat secretion	Initial stimulation, then inhibition of salivary and bronchial secretions
Skeletal muscle	—	Stimulated
Autonomic ganglia	—	Stimulated
Eye	Pupil constriction Decreased accommodation	—
Blocking agent	Atropine	Tubocurarine
Remarks	Effects increase as dosage increases	Increased dosage inhibits effects and causes receptor blockade

2. Be effective when administered orally
3. Be more stable and less easily inactivated than the drugs now available
4. Produce a therapeutic effect with minimal side effects

Although these ideal drugs are not yet available, progress is being made in this direction.

Cholinergic drugs used primarily to lower intraocular pressure are discussed in Chapter 43. These include pilocarpine and carbachol. Table 19-2 lists the prominent cholinergic and anticholinesterase drugs.

DIRECT-ACTING CHOLINERGIC DRUGS (CHOLINE ESTERS)

Drugs that are chemically similar to the neurotransmitter acetylcholine include bethanechol, carbachol, and methacholine. All compounds in this group are quaternary amines and so they are poorly absorbed orally. Their actions are comparable to those of the physiologic mediator acetylcholine, but they are longer acting. The side effects of these drugs are a consequence of parasympathetic stimulation. They include bradycardia, hypotension, sweating, salivation, vomiting, diarrhea, and intestinal cramps.

bethanechol chloride (Duvoid, Myotonachol, Urecholine)

Mechanism of action. Bethanechol is a synthetic choline ester with actions similar to those of acetylcholine. It produces the effects of stimulation of the parasympathetic

nervous system. It has predominant muscarinic action with particular selectivity on the detrusor muscle of the urinary bladder and smooth muscle of the gastrointestinal tract. Hence contraction of the smooth muscle of the bladder is sufficiently strong to initiate micturition and empty the urinary bladder. Also, in the gastrointestinal tract, the drug stimulates gastric motility, increases gastric tone, and often restores impaired peristaltic activity of the esophagus, stomach, and intestine. It also promotes defecation. Unlike acetylcholine, bethanechol is not destroyed by cholinesterase, and therefore its effects are more prolonged than that of the natural neurotransmitter. Therapeutic test doses in normal human subjects have little effect on heart rate, blood pressure, or peripheral circulation.

Indications. Bethanechol chloride has been approved in the United States for the treatment of postoperative and postpartum nonobstructive urinary retention and for neurogenic atony of the urinary bladder associated with retention. Although not indicated on its U.S. product labeling, it is often used to relieve postoperative abdominal distention and gastric atony or stasis and reflux esophagitis associated with decreased pressure of lower esophageal sphincter.

Pharmacokinetics

Absorption. Although it is poorly absorbed from the gastrointestinal tract, bethanechol chloride is effective orally.

Distribution. It is widely distributed to organs innervated by the parasympathetic nervous system. Onset of action is within 30 to 90 minutes after oral administration,

TABLE 19-2   Prominent Cholinergic Agents Including the Anticholinesterase Drugs

Generic name	Trade name	Single adult dose	Usual route of administration
ambenonium*	Mytelase	5-25 mg	Oral
bethanechol	Urecholine	10-30 mg	Oral
			Sublingual
		2.5-5 mg	Subcutaneous
isoflurophate*	Floropryl	Thin strip (0.5 cm) of 0.025%	Topical (eye) ointment
neostigmine*	Prostigmin		
bromide	Bromide	15 mg	Oral
methylsulfate	Methylsulfate	0.5 mg (1-2 mg)	Intramuscular or subcutaneous
physostigmine*	Eserine	1 drop, 0.25-0.5% solution	Topical (eye)
physostigmine*	Antilirium	0.5 mg-2 mg	IM or IV
pilocarpine		1 drop, 0.5%-4% solution	Topical (eye)
pyridostigmine*	Mestinon	Highly variable	Oral

*Effects to be expected are similar to those that can be expected from stimulation of the parasympathetic nervous system (see Table 19-3). Drugs are listed in alphabetical order. The majority of drugs mentioned are administered in the form of their salts.

peak effect within 1 hour, and duration of action up to 6 hours, depending on the dose administered. If administered subcutaneously, the onset of action is within 5 to 15 minutes, peak effect within 15 to 30 minutes, and duration of action approximately 2 hours.

Excretion. Currently unknown

Side effects/adverse reactions. See Table 19-3.

Significant drug interactions. No significant drug interactions have been reported in the United States Pharmacopeia. However, the nurse should be aware of the following possibilities when bethanechol is given with the drugs listed below:

Drug	Possible Effect and Management
other cholinergics or anticholinesterase medications	Enhances cholinergic effects and perhaps toxicity. Monitor closely for adverse effects or, if possible, avoid this combination of medications.
ganglionic blocking agents	May result in severe abdominal distress followed by a precipitous fall in blood pressure. Avoid this combination if possible.
procainamide or quinidine	Cholinergic effects may be antagonized. Monitor closely.

Dosage and administration
Oral

Adults. 10-50 mg orally, 2 to 4 times daily. For treatment of gastroesophageal reflux, 10-25 mg orally, 4 times daily, after meals and at bedtime.

Children. 0.2 mg/kg body weight or 6.7 mg/m² of body surface, 3 times a day.

Parenteral

Adults. 5 mg *subcutaneously,* 3 or 4 times a day when needed.

Children. 0.15-0.2 mg/kg body weight or 5-6.7 mg/m² of body surface, 3 times a day. *(Subcutaneous use only.)*

Pregnancy safety. FDA category C.

NURSING CONSIDERATIONS

Assessment. Bethanechol should not be used after gastrointestinal anastomosis until healing has occurred. It is contraindicated when peptic ulcer, peritonitis, or an inflammatory disease is present.

Its use is also contraindicated during pregnancy or in clients with coronary disease, hyperthyroidism, asthma, and gastrointestinal or urinary obstruction.

Intervention. Administer bethanechol on an empty stomach to minimize the possibility of nausea and vomiting.

Bethanechol is to be parenterally administered only subcutaneously. Do not administer intramuscularly or intravenously because severe symptoms of cholinergic overstimulation (flushing of the skin, headache, severe hypotension, hypothermia, bradycardia, nausea and vomiting, abdominal cramps, bloody diarrhea, shock, or cardiac arrest) may occur.

TABLE 19-3 Side Effects/Adverse Reactions of Drugs Affecting the Parasympathetic Nervous System

Drug(s)	Side effects*	Adverse reactions†
CHOLINERGIC bethanechol chloride	More frequent: with high dosages, unsteadiness; faintness; nausea or vomiting; headache; flushed skin; abdominal pains or upset; increased salivation and sweating Less frequent: diarrhea; increased urination; blurred or disturbed vision; gas complaints	Rare and usually reported with subcutaneous injection: difficulty in breathing, shortness of breath, feeling of pressure in the chest In overdosage or in patients hypersensitive to drug: hypotension; profuse and bloody diarrhea; shock; possibly sudden cardiac arrest.
CHOLINERGIC BLOCKING (PARASYMPATHOLYTIC) atropine	More frequent: inhibition of sweating; constipation; complaints of dry mouth, throat, and skin Less frequent: abdominal distention; blurred vision; inhibition of lactation; urinary retention or dysuria; sedation; headache; photophobia; drowsiness; weakness; nausea or vomiting	Less frequent or rare: urticaria; dermatitis; eye pain from increased intraocular pressure Overdosage/toxicity: blurred vision; ataxia; confusion; disorientation; severe dryness of mouth, throat, and nose area; hyperpyrexia; hallucinations; restlessness; delirium; tachycardia; difficulty in breathing

*If side effects continue, increase, or disturb the patient, the physician should be informed.
†If adverse reactions occur, the physician should be contacted because medical intervention may be necessary.

Continued.

TABLE 19-3   Side Effects/Adverse Reactions of Drugs Affecting the Parasympathetic Nervous System—cont'd

Drug(s)	Side effects*	Adverse reactions†
scopolamine	Same as atropine, plus euphoria; amnesia, insomnia or increased drowsiness reported more often with scopolamine	Dilated and fixed pupil on side where disk was applied have been reported with use of transdermal disk behind the ear. To avoid extensive neurologic exams, unconscious individuals appearing with above symptoms should be checked first for the use of a disk behind the ear. If the disk is removed, this syndrome usually abates within 2 weeks. To avoid misdiagnosis, drops of 1% pilocarpine solution may be instilled in the eye; this will reverse the nonneurogenic dilated pupil.
SYNTHETIC ANTISPASMODICS		
dicyclomine (Bentyl, Antispas)	More frequent: abdominal distention, headache, dizziness Less frequent: nausea, vomiting, sedation, nervousness, decreased sexual ability, blurred or disturbed vision, confusion (especially in older clients) Rare: inhibition of sweating, tachycardia, dry mouth	More frequent: usually constipation (especially in older clients) Less frequent: dysuria Rare: dermatitis
glycopyrrolate (Robinul)	More frequent: dry mouth, nose, throat, and skin Less frequent/rare: the following may occur more often if high doses are given: abdominal distention, blurred vision, constipation, decreased lactation, inhibition of sweating, dysuria, sedation, headache, amnesia (especially in older clients) photophobia, nausea, vomiting, insomnia, weakness, decrease in sexual ability	Rarely reported: faintness, hypotension, dizziness, eye pain, dermatitis Overdosage: respiratory difficulties; severe muscle weakness; extreme tiredness; drowsiness or a paradoxical effect of increased excitability, nervousness, restlessness; tachycardia; warm, dry, and red flushing of skin
clidinium (Quarzan)	More frequent: dry mouth, nose, throat and skin Less frequent: abdominal distention, blurred vision, constipation, decreased lactation, insomnia, nausea, vomiting, increased weakness, headache, drowsiness, dysuria (especially in elderly men), inhibition of sweating, decrease in sexual ability	Rare: faintness, hypotension (especially in older clients); dermatitis Overdosage: same as glycopyrrolate
GANGLIONIC BLOCKING DRUGS		
trimethaphan camsylate (Arfonad)	Side effects are dose related: loss of appetite, nausea, vomiting, constipation, dilated pupil, dry mouth, impotency, pruritis, hives, hypotension, increased heart rate, urinary retention, and use may precipitate angina attack	Overdosage: severe hypotension, respiratory arrest

*If side effects continue, increase, or disturb the patient, the physician should be informed.
†If adverse reactions occur, the physician should be contacted because medical intervention may be necessary.

Education. Instruct the client to move slowly from a lying to a sitting or standing position because orthostatic hypotension is a common effect of bethanechol.

Evaluation. Observe the client closely for side effects or adverse reactions, particularly with subcutaneous administration. Monitor vital signs and carefully check respiration for 30 to 60 minutes after injection. Keep available 0.6 mg atropine in a syringe to counteract severe side effects.

Evaluate the effectiveness of the drug by monitoring

USE OF BETHANECHOL WITH CLIENTS HAVING NEUROGENIC BLADDER

Bethanechol is frequently used as an adjunct therapy in clients with chronic neurogenic bladder. After several baseline measurements of residual urine volume, the adult client is administered 7.5 to 10 mg of bethanechol chloride subcutaneously every 4 hours. Twelve hours after the first dose of bethanechol, the client is asked to void, and a residual urine volume is measured. If the amount of residual urine is less than the baseline volume, the drug is continued for another 24 hours. At that time the drug's effectiveness is again evaluated by another residual urine volume measurement. If this, too, is below the baseline volume, the drug is continued for another 24 to 48 hours on the "every 4 hour" schedule. After that period, the dosage should be decreased to 5 to 7.5 mg every 4 hours. If measured residual urine volume continues to be below baseline amounts, the dosage is changed to an oral form, 50 to 100 mg every 4 hours. According to the client's response, the dosage interval may be gradually increased and the dosage decreased.

intake and output, or residual urine volumes if applicable, when administering bethanechol for postoperative urinary retention.

If the bladder sphincter fails to relax as the urinary bladder contracts in response to bethanechol administration, urine may be forced up the ureter into the kidney. If the client has bacteriuria, this reflux of urine into the kidney may cause a kidney infection. Intake and output must be carefully monitored in these clients.

INDIRECT-ACTING CHOLINERGIC DRUGS (ANTICHOLINESTERASES OR CHOLINESTERASE INHIBITORS)

The indirect-acting cholinergic drugs are called anticholinesterases because they inhibit the action of the enzyme cholinesterase, thereby prolonging the effect of acetylcholine. Anticholinesterase agents (e.g., neostigmine, physostigmine) exert their influence on both muscarinic and nicotinic sites. They are used in the treatment of myasthenia gravis and glaucoma. (See Chapters 17 and 43 respectively.) Certain compounds in this group are considered to be potent agents for chemical warfare. Physostigmine salicylate is used for overdosage and anticholinergic substance toxicity. See discussion about tricyclic antidepressant overdosage treatment in Chapter 16.

Drugs Used for Treatment of Myasthenia Gravis

Myasthenia gravis is a condition characterized by weakness of the skeletal muscles innervated by the somatic efferent fibers. Since the disease affects cholinergic transmission, the anticholinesterase drugs are used because they elevate the concentration of acetylcholine at the myoneural junctions. The prolonged activity of the neurohormone at these sites results in a dramatic increase in muscle strength and function. There is a more extensive discussion of myasthenia gravis and its treatment in Chapter 17. (See also Figure 18-5, B, for site of action.)

CHOLINERGIC BLOCKING (PARASYMPATHOLYTIC) DRUGS
MUSCARINIC CHOLINERGIC BLOCKING (ANTIMUSCARINIC) DRUGS

The cholinergic blocking or parasympatholytic drugs, have many important uses in medicine. More specifically, these agents are called **muscarinic blocking** drugs or **antimuscarinic** drugs because they block the muscarinic effects of acetylcholine. When the nerve fiber is stimulated, the acetylcholine liberated from the terminal is unable to bind to the receptor site and fails to produce a cholinergic effect. Thus these agents also are referred to as anticholinergic drugs. (See Figure 18-5, *A1,* for muscarinic [M] sites.)

Belladonna Alkaloids

The best known muscarinic cholinergic blocking drugs are the belladonna alkaloids. The major drugs in this class are atropine and scopolamine.

A number of plants belonging to the potato family *(Solanaceae)* contain similar alkaloids. *Atropa belladonna* (deadly nightshade), *Hyoscyamus niger* (henbane), *Datura stramonium* (jimson weed or thorn apple), and several species of *Scopolia* also contain belladonna alkaloids. The principle alkaloids of these plants are atropine, scopolamine (hyoscine), and hyoscyamine.

Atropine is the prototype of the antimuscarinic drugs. It has been in use for over half a century and continues to be a popular drug because of its therapeutic effectiveness.

atropine sulfate (Atropine Sulfate, Buf-Opto Atropine, Isopto Atropine, Murocoll)

Mechanism of action. As a competitive antagonist, atropine acts by occupying the muscarinic (M) receptor sites, thereby preventing or reducing the muscarinic response of acetylcholine (see Figure 18-5, *A1* and *2c*). The drug-receptor complex is formed at the neuroeffector junctions of smooth muscle, cardiac muscle, and exocrine glands.

Atropine has very little effect on the actions of acetylcholine at nicotinic receptor sites. So at autonomic ganglia, where transmission normally involves the action of acetylcholine, relatively high doses of atropine are required to produce even a partial block. At the neuromuscular junctions of the somatic nervous system, where the receptors are exclusively nicotinic, extremely high doses of atropine are required to produce any degree of block. See Figure 18-5, *A* for nicotinic (N) sites on the ganglia or parasympathetic and sympathetic nerve divisions, and Figure 18-5, *B* for N site on effector organ (skeletal muscle) of somatic motor system. Atropine can produce a wide range of pharmacologic effects because a vast distribution of parasympathetic cholinergic nerves normally exists in the body. Furthermore, drug activity is dose-dependent. Small doses depress salivary and bronchial secretions and sweating. Large doses dilate the pupils, inhibit accommodation of the eyes, and increase heart rate by blocking vagal effects of the heart. Larger doses inhibit micturition and decrease the tone and motility of the gut by inhibiting parasympathetic control of both the urinary bladder and the gastrointestinal tract. In addition, still larger doses are required to inhibit gastric secretion and motility.

Pharmacologic properties

Eye. The pupil is dilated (mydriasis), and the ciliary muscle (muscle of accommodation) is relaxed (cycloplegia). The sphincter muscle of the iris and the ciliary muscle are both innervated by cholinergic nerve fibers and therefore are affected by atropine. Since the sphincter muscle is unable to contract normally, the radial muscle of the iris causes the pupil to dilate. *Pupil dilation may reduce outflow of aqueous humor, causing a rise in intraocular pressure. This is a hazardous situation for patients with glaucoma.* These effects in the eye are brought about by both local and systemic administration of atropine, although the usual single therapeutic dose of atropine given orally or parenterally has little effect on the eye. After the pupil is dilated, photophobia occurs, and when the drug has reached its full effect, the usual reflexes to light and accommodation disappear.

Systemic absorption of ophthalmic medications resulting in undesirable side effects or adverse reactions has been reported with atropine and a number of other eye preparations. When the patient exhibits such effects, ophthalmic preparations should be included in the review of the patient's current medications; an ophthalmic preparation may be the offending agent (Medical Letter, 1982; Wong, 1980).

Skin and mucous membranes. Since the *sweat glands of the skin* are supplied by sympathetic cholinergic nerves, atropine decreases or abolishes their activity. This causes the skin to become hot and dry. Further, since the flow of secretions from *glands lining the respiratory tract* is reduced, drying of the mucous membranes of the mouth, nose, pharynx, and bronchi occurs. Patients who have been given atropine, particularly for preoperative preparation, often complain of a dry mouth and thirst. Some of this discomfort may be relieved by frequent rinsing of the mouth.

Respiratory system. Secretions of the nose, pharynx, and bronchial tubes are decreased. The muscles of the bronchial tubes relax, and the airway widens to ease breathing. Atropine and scopolamine are less effective than epinephrine as bronchodilators and are seldom used for asthma.

Cardiovascular system

Heart. When low doses are given or an intravenous dose is administered slowly, the cardiac rate is temporarily and slightly slowed because of the central action of the drug on the cardiac center in the medulla **(paradoxical bradycardia).** Larger doses given rapidly intravenously will block the vagal effect on the SA and AV nodes and cause an increased heart rate.

Blood vessels. In therapeutic doses atropine has little or no effect on blood pressure. This is expected because most vascular beds lack significant cholinergic innervation. However, large (and sometimes ordinary) doses cause vasodilation of vessels in the skin of the face and neck. This may result from a direct dilator action or from histamine release. Reddening of the face and neck is seen, especially after large or toxic doses.

Gastrointestinal tract

Gastric glands. It appears that the amount and character of the gastric secretion are little affected by atropine given in ordinary therapeutic doses. The secretion of acid in the stomach is presumably less under vagal control than under hormonal or chemical control. The effect of atropine on the secretion of the pancreas and intestinal glands is not therapeutically significant.

Smooth muscle. Atropine and other belladonna alkaloids decrease tone and peristalsis in the stomach and small and large intestine. Atropine does not affect the secretion of bile, but it exerts a mildly antispasmodic effect in the gallbladder and bile ducts.

Urinary tract. The drug relaxes the ureter, especially when it has been in a state of spasm. Therapeutic doses decrease the tone of the fundus of the urinary bladder. When the detrusor muscle is hypertonic, it is relaxed by atropine. Also, the constriction of the internal sphincter can produce urinary retention.

Central nervous system. Atropine has prominent effects on the central nervous system and in large doses causes excitement and maniacal behavior. These behavioral effects suggest the existence of important cholinergic pathways and receptors within the central nervous system.

Cerebrum. Small or moderate doses of atropine have little or no cerebral effect. Large or toxic doses cause the patient to become restless, wakeful, and talkative. This condition may develop into delirium and finally stupor and coma. The exalted, excited stage has sometimes been called a "belladonna jag." A rise in temperature is sometimes seen, especially in infants and young children. This is probably the result of suppression of sweating rather than action on the heat-regulating center.

Atropine has been used to diminish tremor in Parkinson's disease. It probably reduces cholinergic synaptic transmission.

Medulla. Therapeutic doses of atropine stimulate the

respiratory center and make breathing faster and sometimes deeper. When respiration is seriously depressed, atropine is not always reliable as a stimulant; in fact, it may deepen the depression. Large doses stimulate respiration, but they can also cause respiratory failure and death.

Small doses stimulate the vagus center in the medulla, causing primary slowing of the heart. The vasoconstrictor center is stimulated briefly and then depressed. Because depression follows soon after stimulation, atropine has been called a borderline stimulant of the central nervous system.

Topical effects. There is a slight amount of absorption when atropine or belladonna is applied to the skin, especially if it is an oily or alcoholic preparation or in the form of a plaster.

Indications. Treatment of irritable bowel syndrome, spastic biliary tract disorders, genitourinary disorders; antidote for cholinergic toxicity from excessive amounts of cholinesterase inhibitors, muscarinics, or gamophosphate pesticide poisoning. Also used to treat sinus bradycardia and Parkinson's disease, to prevent excessive salivation and respiratory tract secretions (preanesthetic), and as an adjunctive medication for peptic ulcers and for gastrointestinal radiography.

Pharmacokinetics

Absorption. Readily absorbed from oral and parenteral administration; also absorbed from mucous membranes.

Distribution. After oral administration, the maximum effect is reached within 1 hour, duration of action is 4 to 6 hours. It is widely distributed in fluids of the body and easily passes the placental barrier to the blood of the fetus and the blood-brain barrier.

Metabolism. Primarily in the liver, approximately 13% to 50% of atropine is excreted unchanged in the urine.

Excretion. Kidneys

Side effects/adverse reactions. See Table 19-3.

Significant drug interactions. The following effects may occur when atropine (and other belladonna alkaloids) are given with the drugs listed below:

Drug	Possible Effect and Management
antacids or antidiarrheal agents	May reduce absorption and therapeutic effectiveness of atropine. Space medications at least 1 hour apart.
other antimuscarinics and monoamine oxidase (MAO) inhibitors	Increase in antimuscarinic effects reported. Monitor, because dosage adjustment may be necessary.
digitalis glycosides	The decrease in gastrointestinal tract motility may lead to an increased absorption of digoxin tablets, leading to increased serum level and toxicity. Monitor the client.
ketoconazole	Increase in gastrointestinal pH by atropine may result in reduced absorption of ketoconazole. Atropine should be administered preferably 2 hours after ketoconazole.

Drug	Possible Effect and Management
potassium chloride, especially wax matrix formulations	Increased contact with gastrointestinal tract may result in mucosal irritation and lesions. Liquid formulations of potassium should be considered a replacement for the wax matrix formulation in this situation.

Dosage and administration

Oral

Adults. Antimuscarinic effect, 0.3-1.2 mg orally every 4 to 6 hr; to prevent excessive salivation and production of respiratory tract secretions in anesthesia, dosage is 2 mg orally; in Parkinson's disease, 0.1-0.25 mg orally 4 times daily.

Children. Antimuscarinic, 0.01mg/kg body weight (do not exceed 0.4 mg) or 0.3 mg/m^2 of body surface, every 4-6 hr.

Parenteral

Adults

Antimuscarinic, 0.4-0.6 mg given IM, IV, or SC, every 4-6 hr.

Bradycardia, 0.4-1 mg every 1-2 hr intravenously as needed, up to a maximum of 2 mg.

To prevent excessive salivation and production of respiratory tract secretions in anesthesia, 0.2-0.6 mg IM given 30-60 min before surgery.

Antidote to:

Cholinesterase inhibitor toxicity, 2-4mg IV initially. May repeat 2 mg every 5-10 min until muscarinic symptoms disappear or toxicity to atropine occurs.

Muscarinic toxicity such as in mushroom poisoning, 1-2 mg IM every hour, until respiratory effects improve.

Organophosphate pesticide toxicity, 1-2 mg IM or IV, may repeat in 20-30 min after the cyanosis is diminished. Dosage is usually continued for several days until definite improvement is substantiated.

Children

Antimuscarinic, 0.01 mg/kg body weight SC (do not exceed 0.4 mg) or 0.3 mg/m^2 of body surface, every 4-6 hr.

Dysrhythmias (such as bradycardia), 0.01-0.03 mg/kg body weight.

To prevent excessive salivation and production of respiratory tract secretions in anesthesia or to prevent dysrhythmias induced by succinylocholine or surgical procedure, give atropine subcutaneously as follows:

Child up to 3 kg in weight:	0.1 mg
7 to 9 kg in weight:	0.2 mg
12 to 16 kg in weight:	0.3 mg
20 to 27 kg in weight:	0.4 mg
32 kg in weight:	0.5 mg
41 kg in weight:	0.6 mg

Antidote for cholinesterase inhibitor toxicity: 1 mg initially IV or IM, then 0.5-1 mg every 5-10 min until muscarinic symptoms disappear or toxicity to atropine occurs.

Pregnancy safety. FDA category B

Special considerations. The use of atropine (or belladonna alkaloids) should be avoided in patients with a medical history of severe cardiac disease, reflux esophagitis, gastrointestinal tract obstructive disease states or intestinal atony, urinary retention, prostatic hypertrophy, or myasthenia gravis.

NURSING CONSIDERATIONS

Assessment. Use with caution in elderly clients and children under 6 years of age because they are more susceptible to adverse reactions. Toxicity may occur in the elderly even when the drug is prescribed within the normal adult dosage range.

Do not use in patients with open-angle glaucoma, urinary and gastrointestinal obstruction, ulcerative colitis, asthma, renal or hepatic disease, or myasthenia gravis.

Administer carefully in systemic forms to clients with chronic pulmonary disease because bronchial secretions may be sufficiently decreased to result in bronchial plugs.

Use with caution in infants, clients with Down's syndrome, and pediatric clients with spastic paralysis and brain damage because they tend to be more sensitive to the drug's effects.

Intervention. Administer oral preparations 30 to 60 minutes before meals.

Administer antacids or antidiarrheal medications at least 1 hour after the administration of atropine.

Education. Inform client of possible side effects, and warn against operating a car or other machinery; blurred vision or dizziness may occur.

Advise the client about the use of sugarless gum and candy, ice, or saliva substitutes to relieve dry mouth.

Instruct the client to avoid alcohol and other CNS depressants while taking atropine.

Inform client using ophthalmic preparation that his or her vision will be impaired for a few days. Client should protect eyes by wearing dark glasses. Also, client's ability to judge distance will be impaired; therefore client should avoid driving a car or operating machinery. Drug should be discontinued if signs of local irritation or follicular conjunctivitis occur. This may happen after prolonged periods of ophthalmic therapy.

Counsel the client involved in long-term use to follow a consistent dental hygiene program, including semiannual visits to the dentist because the decreased salivary flow promotes caries, buccal candidiasis, and peridontal disease.

Instruct the client to avoid exposure to high environmental temperatures, exercising in warm, humid weather, or prolonged hot baths. These activities may lead to heat prostration. The client should report any fever to the physician because the medication may have to be discontinued.

Evaluation. Monitor pulse, which is a sensitive indicator of client's reponse to atropine. Also be alert to any change in blood pressure, temperature, and respiration, particularly after intravenous administration. Report any significant changes to physician.

Monitor client for urinary output and bowel regularity. Notify physician of any significant changes.

Observe elderly clients for excitement, agitation, and delirium. Assess for constipation, dryness of mouth, and, in the elderly male client, urinary retention.

For additional atropine preparations see Chapters 40, 41, and 43.

scopolamine (Transderm-Scop, Transderm-V)
scopolamine hydrobromide (Triptone, Isopto Hyoscine)

Mechanism of action. See the preceding discussion of atropine for mechanism of action. Its peripheral effects are similar to atropine, but it differs in its effects on the central nervous system. At therapeutic doses, it depresses the CNS and causes drowsiness, euphoria, memory loss, relaxation, sleep, and relief of fear. It does not increase blood pressure or respiration.

Indications. Used in the treatment of irritable bowel syndrome; renal and ureteral colic; dysrhythmias induced during surgery owing to increased vagal stimulation; and postencephalitic parkinsonism and paralysis agitans. Because of its depressant action on vestibular function, it is used for motion sickness to prevent nausea and vomiting. It is used as a general anesthesia adjunct, as a preanesthetic medication, to check secretions, and to prevent laryngospasm, and for its sedative (twilight sleep) and amnesic effects. It has also been used, along with opioid analgesics, in cardiopulmonary bypass patients to avoid the risk of inducing severe hypotension or collapse with the use of deep and prolonged anesthesia.

Pharmacokinetics. Same as atropine. The transdermal dosage form produces its antiemetic effects for up to 72 hours.

Side effects/adverse reactions. See Table 19-3.

Significant drug interactions. Same as atropine, plus, concurrent use of scopalamine with other CNS depressants may result in increased CNS depression effects. Clients should be monitored closely.

Dosage and administration

Oral

Adults. Antiemetic: 0.25-0.8 mg orally given 1 hour before desired effect is required.

Children. Not determined. Individualized by physician.

Parenteral

Adults

Antimuscarinic: 0.3-0.6 mg IM, IV, or SC given as a single dose.

To prevent or reduce salivation and respiratory tract secretions in anesthesia, 0.2-0.6 mg IM is given 30-60 min before induction with anesthesia.

Amnesic effect: 0.32-0.65 mg IM, IV, or SC.

Children

Antimuscarinic or antiemetic: administer 0.006 mg/kg of body weight or 0.2 mg/m^2 of body surface, IM, IV, or SC.

To prevent or reduce salivation and respiratory tract secretions in anesthesia, give the following dosage 45-60 minutes IM, before induction of anesthesia:

Child less than 4 months old, not recommended

From 4-7 months old, 0.1 mg

From 7 months to 3 years old, 0.15 mg

From 3-8 years old, 0.2 mg

From 8-12 years old, 0.3 mg

Transdermal

Adults. One transdermal patch (0.5 mg) applied behind the ear 4 hours before desired effect is required.

Pregnancy safety. FDA category C

NURSING CONSIDERATIONS

For the transdermal application of scopolamine, instruct the client to wash and dry hands before and after application of the patch. It is to be applied to the hairless skin area behind the ear. It is not to be applied over abrasions or rashes. Alert the client that drowsiness and dilated pupils (photophobia and blurred vision) may occur, and if they occur, tasks such as driving or mowing the lawn may be hazardous.

If scopolamine has been administered as part of a preoperative medication for an outpatient or ambulatory procedure, caution the client before discharge about the effects on memory and motor tasks. These effects may persist for a few hours.

See the discussion of atropine sulfate.

Synthetic Substitutes for Atropine (Antispasmodics)

The usefulness of atropine is limited by the fact that it is a complex drug and produces effects in a number of organs or tissues simultaneously. When it is administered for its antispasmodic effects, it also produces prolonged effects in the eye, causing dilated pupils and blurred vision. It also causes dry mouth and possibly rapid heart rate. When the antispasmodic effect is desired, other effects become side effects, which may be distinctly undesirable.

A large number of drugs have been synthesized in an effort to capture the antispasmodic effect of atropine without its other effects. Drugs of this type are frequently used to relieve hypertonicity and hypersecretion in the stomach and to treat patients with gastric and duodenal ulcers.

Many products are marketed as antispasmodic and anticholinergic agents, but their formulations are either modifications of a belladonna alkaloid or include one or more of the natural alkaloids as their active ingredients. The pharmacologic properties are therefore similar to the previously reviewed substances and will not be repeated here (see Table 19-4). The more commonly used or newer systemic agents—dicyclomine (Bentyl), a glycopyrrolate (Robinul), and clidinium bromide (Quarzan)—will be discussed.

dicyclomine (Bentyl, Antispas, Bentylol✦, and others)

Mechanism of action. Not known. It has been postulated that it produces both a local and direct effect on

TABLE 19-4 Selected Anticholinergic Agents Containing Specific Alkaloids*

Alkaloid formation†	Trade name
hyoscyamine	Cystospaz Cystospaz-M Levsinex Timecaps Levsin Anaspaz
hyoscyamine and scopolamine	Bellafoline
scopolamine	Triptone Transderm-Scop Transderm-V
atropine, hyoscyamine, scopolamine and phenobarbital	Bellastal Donnatal Barbidonna Barophen Kinesed Donnatal Extentabs
atropine and phenobarbital	Antrocol
belladonna and butabarbital	Butibel
belladonna and phenobarbital	Belap Chardonna-2
hyoscyamine and phenobarbital	Levsin-PB Anaspaz PB
hyoscyamine, scopolamine and phenobarbital	Belledenal Belledenal-S Belladenal Spacetabs

*Specific alkaloids include the active alkaloids of belladonna, such as hyoscyamine, atropine, and scopolamine.

†The alkaloid formulation lists the active ingredients as marketed under the various trade names. Individual salts, strengths, and dosing intervals may vary according to the manufacturer's instructions.

smooth muscle, resulting in a decreased tone and motility of gastrointestinal tract. It only appears to produce the typical antimuscarinic effect when administered in large doses.

Indications. Treatment of the irritable bowel syndrome.

Pharmacokinetics. Little has been determined about this product. It is rapidly absorbed after oral or parenteral administration, and about 50% of the dose is excreted by the kidneys and the other 50% in the feces.

Side effects/adverse reactions. See Table 19-3.

Significant drug interactions. The following effects may occur when dicyclomine is given with the drugs listed below:

Drug	Possible Effect and Management
other antimuscarinics or monoamine oxidase (MAO) inhibitors	Increased antimuscarinic effects reported. Reduced dosage or discontinuance of one product may be necessary.
antacids or antidiarrheal preparations	Reduced absorption of dicyclomine. These drugs should be administered at least 1 to 2 hours apart.
potassium chloride, especially wax matrix formulations	Increased gastrointestinal tract irritation and lesions may result. Liquid potassium preparations should be considered as an alternative.

Dosage and administration
Oral
Adults. 10-20 mg orally 3 or 4 times daily. Dosage may be adjusted according to response, up to a maximum of 160 mg/day.
Children
Less than 6 months old, not recommended.
6 months to 2 years old, 5-10 mg orally (syrup available, 5mg/tsp) 3 or 4 times daily; adjust as necessary.
2 years old and older, 10 mg orally 3 or 4 times daily; adjust as necessary.
Parenteral
Adults. 20 mg IM, every 4 to 6 hours. *Do not administer intravenously.*
Children. Not established.
Pregnancy safety. Not established.

NURSING CONSIDERATIONS

Administer with food or milk to minimize gastric distress.

Do not administer within 1 to 2 hours of antacids or antidiarrheal medications.

The syrup form may be diluted with equal parts of water to make administration easier.

When administering the parenteral form, ensure that the client is lying or sitting down because they could experience some temporary lightheadness.

For further discussion of nursing considerations, see discussion of atropine sulfate.

glycopyrrolate (Robinul, Robinul Forte)

Mechanism of action. This is a synthetic antimuscarinic product with effects similar to atropine. Unlike atropine, it is unable to easily cross lipid membranes (such as blood-brain barrier) and therefore has minimal central nervous system side effects. It also appears to be less likely to produce pupillary or ocular eye effects.

Indications. Antimuscarinic to prevent or reduce hypersecretions and arrhythmias induced during anesthesia; to prevent or reduce toxicities induced by cholinesterase inhibitors (neostigmine or pyridostigmine).

Pharmacokinetics

Absorption. Orally about 10% to 25% of a dose is absorbed

Onset of action. Intravenous dose within 1 minute

Time to peak effect. Intramuscular within 30 to 45 minutes

Duration of action. Vagal blocking action lasts from 2 to 3 hours, while the **antisialagogue** effect, the inhibition of the flow of saliva, may last up to 7 hours

Excretion. Kidneys

Side effects/adverse reactions. See Table 19-3.

Significant drug interactions. Same as atropine; see previous section. In addition, administering cyclopropane with glycopyrrolate IV may result in ventricular arrhythmias. To reduce this possibility, give smaller dosages of glycopyrrolate IV (0.1 mg or less) and monitor client closely.

Dosage and administration
Oral
Adults. For treatment of peptic ulcer, 1-2 mg orally 2 or 3 times daily and when necessary, 2 mg at bedtime; then reduce to 1 mg twice daily or adjust dosage according to client's response and tolerance. The elderly individual may be more sensitive to this dosage, so a lower dosage schedule should be considered.
Children. Not established.
Parenteral
Adults. Antimuscarinic:
For treatment of peptic ulcer, 0.1-0.2 mg IM or IV every 4 hours if necessary, up to a maximum of 4 doses per 24 hr.
To prevent or reduce excessive salivation and respiratory tract secretions or gastric hypersecretory situations during anesthesia, 4.4 μg/kg of body weight is given 30-60 min before anesthesia.
For dysrhythmias during anesthesia or in surgery, 0.1 mg IV is given at 2-3 min intervals, as necessary.

As a cholinergic adjunctive medication, 0.2 mg IV is given for each 1 mg of neostigmine or 5 mg of pyridostigmine. This may be given together in the same syringe.

Children

Peptic ulcer, Not determined

To prevent or reduce excessive salivation and respiratory tract secretions or gastric hypersecretory situations during anesthesia, 4.4-8.8 μg/kg body weight IM is given 30-60 min before anesthesia.

For dysrhythmias during anesthesia or in surgery, 4.4 μg/kg of body weight IV given every 2 or 3 min, as necessary.

As a cholinergic adjunctive medication, 0.2 mg IV is given for each 1 mg of neostigmine or 5 mg of pyridostigmine. This may be given together in the same syringe.

Pregnancy safety. FDA category B

NURSING CONSIDERATIONS

Alert the client to have ophthalmic examinations for intraocular pressure periodically. Intraocular pressure may become elevated because of the mydriasis produced by the drug.

See atropine sulfate discussion for additional nursing considerations.

clidinium (Quarzan)

Mechanism of action. Clidinium is a synthetic product related to the belladonna alkaloids, especially atropine. It competitively antagonizes acetylcholine at the postganglionic parasympathetic receptor sites in both smooth muscles and the secretory glands, thus reducing gastrointestinal motility and gastric acid secretion. Ganglionic blockade may be produced if high doses of clidinium are given. Unlike atropine, it produces few, if any, CNS side effects or alterations on the eye.

Indications. Adjunctive treatment for peptic ulcers.

Pharmacokinetics

Absorption. Orally about 10% to 25% of a dose is absorbed

Onset of action. Within 1 hour

Duration of action. Up to 3 hours

Metabolism. Liver

Excretion. Kidneys primarily, some in feces

Side effects/adverse reactions. See Table 19-3.

Significant drug interactions. Same as atropine.

Dosage and administration. Oral: Adults: 2.5-5 mg 3 or 4 times daily, before meals and at bedtime. Adjust dosage according to individual's response. Elderly: 2.5 mg orally 3 times a day, before meals. Children: not determined.

Pregnancy safety. Not established

NURSING CONSIDERATIONS

Administer ½ to 1 hour before meals to enhance absorption.

The client should have intraocular pressure determinations done periodically. Intraocular pressure increases because of the mydriatic effect of the drug.

For further nursing considerations, see atropine sulfate discussion.

Ganglionic Drugs

The major neurotransmitter of all autonomic ganglia is acetylcholine. This includes ganglionic synapses of both the parasympathetic and sympathetic nervous system. Acetylcholine activates the nicotinic receptor at the ganglionic sites, which is unlike that of the nicotinic receptors on the effector organ, the skeletal muscle. Thus stimulation of the preganglionic neuron results in the release of acetylcholine from its terminal. Acetylcholine then activates the nicotinic receptors on the ganglia of the postganglionic parasympathetic or sympathetic neurons, or adrenal medulla. This interaction ultimately generates a nerve impulse down the postganglionic fibers to produce specific effects on smooth muscle, cardiac muscle, and glands (see Figure 18-2). Ganglionic stimulation influences nerve impulse transmission to the entire autonomic nervous system, and because of such pervasive activity ganglionic drugs have limited therapeutic value.

The drugs that affect nicotinic or cholinergic receptor sites on autonomic ganglia are (1) ganglionic stimulating drugs and (2) ganglionic blocking drugs.

GANGLIONIC STIMULATING DRUGS
NICOTINE

Nicotine is a liquid alkaloid, freely soluble in water. It turns brown on exposure to air and is the chief alkaloid in tobacco.

Nicotine has no therapeutic use but is of great pharmacologic interest and toxicologic importance. Its use in experiments performed on animals has helped to increase understanding of the autonomic nervous system.

Nicotine is readily absorbed from the gastrointestinal tract, respiratory mucous membrane, and skin.

Pharmacologic Effects

Nicotine may produce a variety of complex and often unpredictable effects in the body. Many actions are dose related, with generally small doses inducing activation or stimulation and larger doses producing a decreased or depressed response. Because nicotine acts on multiple systems within the body, the ultimate response may be the sum of the different stimulation and depressant actions of this chemical.

At the autonomic ganglia, nicotine temporarily stimulates all sympathetic and parasympathetic ganglia. This is followed by depression, which tends to last longer than the period of stimulation. Its effects on skeletal muscle is similar to its effects on the ganglia; that is, a depressant phase follows stimulation. During the depressant phase nicotine exerts a curare-like action on skeletal muscle.

Nicotine stimulates the central nervous system, especially the medullary centers (respiratory, emetic, and vasomotor). Large doses may cause tremor and convulsions. Stimulation is followed by depression. Death may result from respiratory failure, although it may be caused more by the curare-like action of nicotine on nerve endings in the diaphragm, rather than by action on the respiratory center.

The actions and effects of nicotine on the cardiovascular system are complex. The rate of the heart is frequently slowed at first, but later may be accelerated above normal. Various disturbances in rhythm have been observed. The small blood vessels in peripheral parts of the body constrict but may later dilate, and the blood pressure will fall; this occurs in nicotine poisoning. Nicotine also has an antidiuretic action.

Repeated administration of nicotine causes tolerance to develop to some of its effects.

Toxicity

Nicotine has both short- and long-term toxic effects that are extremely important to the health care professional. Nicotine toxicity has resulted from misuse of insecticides containing nicotine, which at times has led to the death of the individual. And, because nicotine is a major ingredient in tobacco products, both acute toxicity (with ingestion of such products by small children) and chronic toxicity are well documented. See the box below for acute symptoms of toxicity.

Tobacco Smoking and Nicotine

Burning of tobacco can generate approximately 4,000 compounds in a gaseous and a particulate or particle phase. Gas phase substances include carbon monoxide, carbon dioxide, hydrogen cyanide, ammonia, volatile nitrosamines, and many other substances. The particulate phase contains mainly nicotine, water, and tar. Known carcinogens have been identified as etiologic factors in a variety of neoplastic diseases, such as cancer of the bladder, lung, buccal cavity, esophagus, and pancreas. Other smoking-related illnesses include pulmonary emphysema, chronic bronchitis, coronary heart disease, and myocardial infarction. Chronic dyspepsia may develop in

heavy smokers, and clients with gastric ulcer are usually advised to avoid overindulgence. Of considerable importance is the fact that smokers absorb sufficient nicotine to exert a variety of effects on the autonomic nervous system.

In individuals with peripheral vascular disease such as thromboangiitis obliterans (Buerger's disease), nicotine is generally believed to be a contributing factor in the disease and may cause spasms of the peripheral blood vessels and thus reduce the blood flow through the affected vessels. Vasospasm in the retinal blood vessels of the eye, associated with smoking of tobacco, is thought to cause serious disturbance of vision.

Passive smoking, the inhalation of cigarette smoke by nonsmokers, also has harmful effects. The fetus of a smoking mother may have a low birth weight and increased congenital abnormalities. Children of parents who smoke have an increased incidence of sudden infant death syndrome, an increased incidence of respiratory infections and allergic reactions, and an increased likelihood of becoming smokers. Nonsmoking adults exposed to smokers have increased symptoms as in those with chronic heart or lung disease, and higher rates of cancer are found in nonsmoking spouses.

The addictive component of tobacco is nicotine (Houghton, 1986). Many drugs are reported to interact with nicotine and at least two, theophylline and propranolol, have very significant interactions requiring an increased dosage in smokers to produce their therapeutic effect. Referral may be made to the literature on smoking for additional information on both direct and indirect drug interactions with smoking and other related smoking issues.

nicotine gum (Nicorette)

Nicotine is available in a resin for use in smoking cessation programs. The nicotine resin is in the form of

---

ACUTE SYMPTOMS OF NICOTINE TOXICITY

Increased flow of saliva
Nausea and vomiting
Abdominal cramps
Diarrhea
Confusion
Cold sweat
Fainting
Hypotension
Tachycardia
Prostration and collapse
Convulsions may occur.
Death results from respiratory failure.

chewing gum and provides a source of nicotine for the nicotine-dependent client who is undergoing acute cigarette withdrawal. When the client has a strong urge to smoke, he or she chews a stick of gum, which relieves the physical symptoms of nicotine withdrawal. The number of pieces of gum chewed is gradually reduced over a 2- to 3-month period.

Mechanism of action. See discussion of pharmacologic effects of nicotine.

Indications. Adjunct treatment for nicotine dependence.

Pharmacokinetics

Absorption. Through buccal mucosa, slower than if inhaled while smoking

Metabolism. Primarily hepatic, small amounts in kidney and lung

Half-life. 30 to 60 minutes

Elimination. Renal, 10% to 20% unchanged, the remainder as metabolites; excreted in breast milk.

Side effects/adverse reactions. See Table 19-5.

Significant drug interactions. The following effects may occur when nicotine is given with the drugs listed below:

Drug	Possible Effect and Management
insulin	May increase effect of insulin by increasing absorption; dosage reduction may be necessary.
propoxyphene, proprandol, possibly other beta-adrenergic blocking agents or xanthine bronchodilators	Smoking cessation may increase therapeutic effects by decreasing metabolism; dosage reduction may be necessary.

Dosage and administration. Oral: 2 mg as a chewing gum, repeated as needed to curb the client's urge to smoke, up to 30 pieces of gum/day maximum. The gum should be chewed intermittently and very slowly when the client has the urge to smoke. Most clients require about 10 pieces of gum per day when treatment is begun.

Pregnancy safety. FDA category X

NURSING CONSIDERATIONS

The amount of nicotine released depends on the rate of chewing and amount of time the saliva is in contact with the gum.

Overdose of nicotine may be fatal.

Gum may damage dental work. Instruct the client to discontinue use and consult with physician or dentist if gum sticks to dental work.

The client should *not* smoke while being treated with nicotine gum.

Using hard sugarless candy may help reduce mucosal discomfort.

The use of nicotine gum must be combined with a supervised program for smoking cessation and used under medical supervision.

Nicotine gum should not be used for longer than 6 months.

GANGLIONIC BLOCKING DRUGS

Ganglionic blocking drugs block transmission of both sympathetic and parasympathetic nerve impulses at the nicotinic receptors on the ganglia. The parent compound of this group of drugs is a quaternary ammonium compound called tetraethylammonium chloride. It is not good for treatment of hypertension because of its short duration of action, its ineffectiveness when given orally, and its distressing side effects.

In 1950 the methonium derivatives were introduced, and hexamethonium chloride became the drug of choice in managing severe and malignant hypertension. Despite the difficulties in managing individuals receiving hexamethonium because of its erratic absorption and action and severe side effects, its use demonstrated that severe hypertension could be controlled. Since 1961, the ganglionic blocking agents have been seldom used. Newer antihypertensive drugs that have more selective action and fewer severe side effects are preferred. However, the student should be aware of these products because some

TABLE 19-5 Side Effects/Adverse Reactions of Nicotine Gum (Nicorette)

Side effects*	Adverse effects†
More frequent: Belching, fast heart beat, mild headache, increased appetite, increased watering of mouth, sore mouth or throat. Less frequent: Constipation, coughing, dizziness or light headedness, dry mouth, hiccups, hoarseness, laxative effect, loss of appetite, irritability, indigestion, trouble sleeping	More frequent: Injury to mouth, teeth, or dental work Rare: Irregular heartbeat Early signs of overdose: Nausea and vomiting, severe increased watering of the mouth, severe abdominal pain, diarrhea, cold sweat, severe headache, severe dizziness, disturbed hearing and vision, confusion, and severe weakness Late signs of overdose: Fainting, hypotension, difficulty breathing, fast, weak, or irregular pulse; convulsions

*If side effects continue, increase, or disturb the patient, the physician should be informed.
†If adverse reactions occur, the physician should be contacted because medical intervention may be necessary.

NURSES AND SMOKING

Nurses, besides having the most prolonged contact with clients and their families, have the knowledge and skills to teach them about the hazards of smoking. Unfortunately, nurses continue to smoke at a frequency higher than other health professionals. In the United States, although 64% of physicians and 61% of dentists who have smoked in the past have stopped smoking, only 36% of nurses have stopped. This is particularly important because Dalton (1986) found that currently smoking nurses were less likely to agree that smoking was a major cause of cancer and other health problems and to counsel clients about those hazards. Nurses need to be role models and thus should decrease their smoking habits if they are to contribute to a change in the public's smoking behaviors.

An effective program of smoking cessation should incorporate acceptance, support, specific information, and regular opportunities for monitoring progress. Strecher (1985) found that even a minimal-contact smoking cessation program, including a brief practitioner consultation with self-help manuals conducted in health care settings, produced significant reductions in cigarette smoking.

Besides educating and counseling clients and their families about the benefits of smoking cessation, nurses can participate in community antismoking activities. Such activities include supporting clean indoor air acts, supporting no-smoking areas on public transportation and teaching health education courses in schools.

---

physicians may select trimethaphan as an alternative for clients resistent to the effects of sodium nitroprusside. Other physicians may use a ganglionic blocking agent such as trimethaphan for the treatment of a hypertensive crises in individuals with an acute dissecting aortic aneurysm. The two ganglionic blocking agents available are mecamylamine hydrochloride (Inversine tablets) and trimethaphan camsylate (Arfonad injection). Since mecamylamine has many side effects and is not considered a first line drug in the treatment of hypertension, read the package insert or current USP-DI for additional information on this product.

trimethaphan camsylate (Arfonad)

Mechanism of action. Ganglionic blocking agents lower arterial pressure by blocking the action of acetylcholine on the ganglion cells. This results in reduced transmission of impulses from preganglionic to postganglionic fibers in both sympathetic and parasympathetic nerves. Blocking transmission of impulses through the sympathetic ganglia abolishes vasoconstrictor tone; the blood vessels dilate and arterial pressure falls.

Indication. Treatment of hypertension
Pharmacokinetics
Administration. Intravenous infusion
Onset of action. Immediate
Duration of effect. 10 to 15 minutes
Metabolism. Probably by pseudocholinesterase
Excretion. Kidneys (unchanged)
Side effects/adverse reactions. See Table 19-3.
Significant drug interactions. The following effects may occur when trimethaphan is given with the drugs listed below:

Drug	Possible Effect and Management
ambenonium or neostigmine or pyridostigmine	The antimyasthenic effects of these drugs will be blocked, leading to increased weakness and inability to swallow. Avoid concurrent administration of trimethaphan with these medications.
antibiotics and sulfonamides	Do not use ganglionic blockers in individuals with chronic pyelonephritis being treated with these medications. Trimethaphan may reduce renal blood flow and urine output or cause urinary retention.

Dosage and administration. Parenteral
Adults
Hypertensive emergency, initially, 0.5 mg to 1 mg/minute by intravenous infusion. Adjust dosage according to client response. Maintenance dosage, 1 to 15 mg/minute by intravenous infusion.
To control blood pressure during surgery: Initially, 3 to 4 mg/minute, adjust as necessary. Maintenance dose is 0.2 to 6 mg/minute by intravenous infusion.
Elderly. May be more sensitive to this drug so a lower dosage with close monitoring is indicated.
Children. Initially 0.1 mg/minute, adjusted according to individual response, by intravenous infusion.
Pregnancy safety. FDA category not classified but this drug is not recommended during pregnancy

---

NURSING CONSIDERATIONS

Assessment. Use with caution for children and elderly clients, who tend to be more sensitive to its hypotensive effects.

Use with caution for clients with anemia, Addison's disease, diabetes, hepatic or renal disease, cardiovascular or cerebrovascular insufficiency, and for clients taking other antihypotensive or steroid medications.

Intervention. Clients receiving trimethaphan camsylate should be in an intensive care setting for appropriate monitoring. Emergency equipment should be available in the event of respiratory arrest.

The solution should be diluted with dextrose 5% injection only and administered by infusion pump to ensure a precise regulation of the flow rate. The prepared intravenous solution is stable at room temperature for 24 hours.

The client should be in a supine position to avoid cerebral anoxia.

Oral antihypertensive therapy should be started as soon as possible because a pseudotolerance to the drug may occur in some individuals.

If used for controlled hypotension during surgery, the drug should be discontinued before the wound is closed to allow the client's blood pressure to return to normal.

Evaluation. Monitor the client's blood pressure and respiratory function frequently.

KEY TERMS

adrenergic, page 370
adrenergic blocking, page 370
antimuscarinic, page 375
antisialagogue, page 380
cholinergic, page 370
cholinergic blocking, page 370
curarization, page 371
muscarinic, page 371
muscarinic blocking, page 375
paradoxical bradycardia, page 376
parasympatholytic, page 370
parasympathomimetic, page 370
sympatholytic, page 370
sympathomimetic, page 370

BIBLIOGRAPHY

American Hospital Formulary Service: AHFS drug information 86, Betheseda, Md, 1986, American Society of Hospital Pharmacists.

Baucke SL: Seeing eye to eye on physostigmine, J Post Anesth Nurs 2(1):51, 1987.

Black T: Smoking in pregnancy revisited, Midwifery 1(3):135, 1985.

Booth K and Faulker A: Links between nurses and cigarette smoking? Nurse Educ Today 6(4):176, 1986.

Chapman KR and others: Anticholinergic therapy in asthma and chronic bronchitis, Hosp. Formul. 17(5):686, 1982.

Dalgas P: Understanding drugs that affect the autonomic nervous system, Nursing '85 15(10):58, 1985.

Dalton JA and Swenson I: Nurses and smoking: role modeling and counseling behaviors, Oncology Nurs Forum 13(2):45, 1986.

Dalton J and Swenson I: Nurses—the professionals who can't quit, Am J Nurs 83(8):1149, 1983.

Fernandez E: Update on the pharmacologic approach to asthma: anticholinergics, corticosteroids, and cromolyn sodium. Part 2, Respir Ther 14(5):29, 1984.

Fraulini KE and Gorski DW: Don't let perioperative medications put you in a spin, Nursing '83 13(12):26, 1983.

Garvey JP: Breaking the habit, Occupa Health Saf 37(3):124, 1985.

Gelizia VJ: Pharmacotherapy of memory loss in the geriatric patient, Drug Intell Clin Pharm 18(10):784, 1984.

Gever LN: Anticholinergics. . . and what to teach your patient about them, Nursing '84 14(9):64, 1984.

Gever LN: Cholinergics: a concise review, Nursing '84 14(5)41, 1984.

Goodman L and Gilman A, editors: Goodman and Gilman's The pharmacological Basis of Therapeutics, ed 7, New York, 1985, Macmillan Publishing Co.

Johnson BE and others: Effect of inhaled glycopyrrolate and atropine in asthma precipitated by exercise and cold air inhalation, Chest 85(3):325, 1984.

Marks R and others: Sexual side effects, RN 46(2):34, 1983.

Mennies JH: Smoking: the physiological effects, Am J Nurs 83(8):1142, 1983.

Miller K: Atropine, Emergency 18(4):12, 1986.

Reeder TM: Direct cerebrospinal fluid infusion of bethanechol chloride in Alzheimer's disease: use of an implantable continuous infusion devise (Urecholine), J Neurosurg Nurs 17(3):184, 1985.

Reeder TM: Alzheimer's disease: using direct drug infusion to the central nervous system (bethanechol chloride), AORN J 44(2):222, 1986.

Rose DD: Review of anticholinergic drugs: their use and safe omittance in preoperative medications, AANA J 52(4):401, 1984.

Seifert R and others: Use of anticholinergics in the nursing home: an empirical study and review, Drug Intell Clin Pharm 17(6):470, 1983.

Spencer JK: Nurses and cigarette smoking: a literature review, J Adv Nurs 8(3):237, 1983.

Strecher VJ and others: Evaluation of a minimal-contact smoking cessation program in a health care setting, Patient Educ Couns 7(4):395, 1985.

Todd B: Central anticholinergic syndrome. Geriatric Nurs 5(2):117, 1984.

United States Pharmacopeial Convention: USP DI: drug information for the health care provider, Rockville, Md, 1987, The Convention.

Drugs Affecting the Sympathetic Nervous System

ADRENERGIC (SYMPATHOMIMETIC) DRUGS

The agents that enhance the effects of sympathetic nervous system are called **sympathomimetic drugs** because they mimic the effects of sympathetic nerve stimulation. The drugs are designed to produce activities that are similar to those of the neurotransmitters. The sympathomimetic drugs are also called adrenergic drugs. There are three types of adrenergic drugs: (1) direct-acting, (2) indirect-acting, and (3) dual-acting (direct and indirect) agents.

DIRECT-ACTING ADRENERGIC DRUGS
Catecholamines

The three naturally occurring catecholamines in the body—dopamine, norepinephrine, and epinephrine—are synthesized by the sympathetic nervous system. (For information on adrenergic transmission see Figure 18-6, *2,* and the discussion in Chapter 18.)

In the past there were confusing and conflicting reports that the effects of sympathetic nerve stimulation and the effects of epinephrine injection did not always correspond. In the mid-1940s it was shown that epinephrine had a twin, norepinephrine. The recognition that these were separate substances occurring naturally in the body helped clear up the confusion. With further research one more catecholamine has been positively identified—

dopamine. Dopamine is a precursor of norepinephrine and epinephrine. However, dopamine has a transmitter role of its own in certain portions of the central nervous system. Epinephrine acts mainly as an emergency hormone; norepinephrine, on the other hand, is an important transmitter of nerve impulses. It is also an intermediary in epinephrine biosynthesis.

The catecholamines depend on their ability to interact *directly* with adrenergic receptors (alpha and beta) and are called *direct-acting* drugs. Thus the response of these agents is mediated by directly stimulating the adrenergic receptors. In the sympathetic nervous system the adrenergic effector cells contained two distinct receptors, the alpha (α) and beta (β) receptors.

There is evidence that the alpha receptors appear on two locations. The alpha$_2$ receptors are found on the presynaptic nerve endings or terminals and are called presynaptic (prejunctional) receptors. It has been suggested that the function of the presynaptic receptor is associated with the control of the amount of transmitter released per nerve impulse. The rate of transmitter synthesized can be regulated by a feedback mechanism. Thus when the concentration of transmitter released from the nerve terminal into the synaptic cleft reaches a high level, it can stimulate the presynaptic receptors and prevent the further release of the transmitter. This kind of feedback prevents excessive and prolonged stimulation of the postsynaptic cell. The postsynaptic receptors, which are located on the effector organs, are known as alpha$_1$ or alpha (see Figure 18-6).

The beta receptors are subdivided on the basis of their responses to drugs. Beta$_1$ receptors are located mainly in the heart, and beta$_2$ receptors mediate the actions of catecholamines on bronchioles and arterial smooth muscles.

Norepinephrine acts mainly on alpha receptors and may cause pure vasoconstriction. Epinephrine acts on both alpha and beta receptors and produces a mixture of vasodilation and vasoconstriction. Isoproterenol, a synthetic catecholamine, acts only on beta receptors. For a discussion of receptor sensitivity see the box above.

The most important alpha adrenergic activities in humans are (1) vasoconstriction of arterioles in the skin and splanchnic area, resulting in a rise in blood pressure, (2) pupil dilation, and (3) relaxation of the gut. Beta adrenergic activity includes (1) cardiac acceleration and increased contractility, (2) vasodilation of arterioles supplying skeletal muscles, (3) bronchial relaxation, and (4) uterine relaxation. The effects of both alpha and beta stimulation result from a summation of action where they are interrelated. That is, a change in blood pressure will depend on the degree of vasoconstriction in the skin and splanchnic area *and* the extent of vasodilation in skeletal muscles, along with changes in heart rate. Large arteries and veins contain both alpha and beta receptors; the heart

---

ADRENERGIC RECEPTOR SENSITIVITIES

RECEPTOR	SENSITIVITIES
Alpha$_1$ (α_1)	Epinephrine is equal to or more potent than norepinephrine, which is more potent than isoproterenol.
Alpha$_2$ (α_2)	Epinephrine may be more or less potent than norepinephrine (depending on tissues involved). Isoproterenol is ineffective.
Beta$_1$ (β_1)	Isoproterenol is more potent than epinephrine. Epinephrine and norepinephrine are approximately equivalent in action.
Beta$_2$ (β_2)	Isoproterenol is equivalent to or more potent than epinephrine. Epinephrine is much more potent than norepinephrine.

---

contains only beta receptors (Table 20-1).

Although there are specific drugs that stimulate the alpha or beta receptors, there are also drugs that selectively block alpha or beta receptors. These agents work at peripheral autonomic sites, which distinguishes them from ganglionic blocking agents that act at the ganglia. The adrenergic blocking agents include both alpha and beta blockers. In the United States in 1968 a beta receptor blocking agent, propranolol, became available for clinical use.

As catecholamines, norepinephrine and epinephrine are important neurohormones in neural and endocrine integration. They are always present in arterial blood, although the amount varies widely during any one day. Certain physiologic stimuli such as stress and exercise significantly increase blood levels of catecholamine.

Studies indicate that the major sources of circulating norepinephrine are stimulated sympathetic nerve endings. Organs that receive a large fraction of blood and possess large numbers of sympathetic nerve endings contain the greatest amount of catecholamines. (Examples of such organs are the heart and blood vessels.) Thus the number of sympathetic nerve endings or adrenergic nerves to various organs determines the magnitude of response of these organs to increased levels or injections of catecholamines.

Pharmacologic Effects

Catecholamines produce a variety of physiologic responses.

Cardiac effects. Epinephrine and norepinephrine produce almost the same cardiac responses when injected. These responses follow.

TABLE 20-1   Adrenergic Receptor Stimulation

Effector organs	Receptor type	Adrenergic response
HEART		
Cardiac muscle (atria, ventricles)	β_1	Increased force of contraction
Sinoatrial node	β_1	Increased heart rate
Atrioventricular node	β_1	Increased conduction velocity; shortened refractory period
Conduction tissue	β_1	
BLOOD VESSELS		
Arterioles (smooth muscle)		
Coronary	α, β_2, dopaminergic	Constriction, dilation
Cerebral	α	Constriction
Pulmonary	α, β_2	Constriction, dilation
Mesenteric visceral	α, β_2, dopaminergic	Constriction, dilation
Renal	α, β_2, dopaminergic	Constriction, dilation
Skin, mucosa	α	Constriction
Skeletal muscle	α, β_2	Constriction, dilation
Veins	α_1, β_2	Constriction, dilation
LUNG		
Bronchial smooth muscle	β_2	Bronchodilation (relaxation)
Bronchial glands	α_1, β_2	Inhibition
GASTROINTESTINAL TRACT		
Smooth muscle (motility, tone)	α_2, β_2	Decrease
Sphincter	α	Contraction
Secretion	?	Inhibition
Gallbladder and ducts	—	Relaxation
LIVER	β_2	Glycogenolysis, gluconeogenesis
SPLEEN CAPSULE	α, β_2	Contraction, relaxation
PANCREAS: INSULIN SECRETION	α	Decrease
ADIPOSE TISSUE	β_1	Lipolysis
URINARY BLADDER		
Detrusor muscle	β_1	Relaxation
Sphincter	α	Contraction
KIDNEY URETER	α	Contraction
KIDNEY SECRETION (RENIN)	β_2	Increase
UTERUS		
Pregnant	α	Contraction
Nonpregnant	β_2	Relaxation
SEX ORGANS, male	α	Ejaculation
SKIN		
Pilomotor muscles	α	Contraction
Sweat glands	Cholinergic	Increased secretion
EYE		
Radial muscle, iris (pupil size)	α_1	Contraction–pupil dilation (mydriasis)
Ciliary muscle	β	Relaxation for far vision

Marked increase in myocardial contraction (positive inotropic effect). This increase is the result of increased influx of calcium into cardiac fibers. The strong myocardial contractions result in more complete emptying of the ventricles and an increase in cardiac work and oxygen consumption. The strong contractions brought about by isoproterenol and epinephrine also increase cardiac output, or volume. Norepinephrine, on the other hand, may not alter cardiac output and may even decrease it slightly. This effect of norepinephrine is believed to result from its potent vasoconstricting action, which increases resistance to ejection of blood from the heart. The increased work of the heart to move the blood against increased pressure is "pressure work" rather than "volume work."

It has been shown experimentally and clinically that 0.5 mg of epinephrine injected into arterial or venous blood and circulated by cardiac compression or massage may stimulate spontaneous and vigorous cardiac contractions. Even though the heart is in ventricular fibrillation, epinephrine increases fibrillation vigor and frequently promotes successful electric defibrillation of the individual. In these situations the drug may be injected repeatedly. However, epinephrine cannot be used repeatedly to improve the function of a failing heart (congestive heart failure), since it increases oxygen consumption by cardiac muscle. It can also cause anginal pain in clients with angina pectoris because it increases cardiac oxygen demand. Therefore, although it increases coronary blood flow, its use is contraindicated for patients with angina.

The production of strong contractions provides the rationale for the use of epinephrine in cardiac arrest.

Marked increase in cardiac rate (positive chronotropic effect). Acceleration of heart rate by the catecholamines is the result of the increased rate of membrane depolarization in the pacemaker cells in the sinus node during diastole. Action potential threshold is reached sooner, pacemaker cells fire more often, and heart rate increases.

Norepinephrine, with its predominantly alpha adrenergic activity, may not produce as severe a tachycardia as epinephrine. The increased vasoconstriction and increased blood pressure may cause a reflex bradycardia. Dosage and patient variables affect these responses. Isoproterenol usually produces a tachycardia, since its direct and reflex effects act in the same direction.

Increase in atrioventricular conduction (positive dromotropic effect). Because epinephrine increases atrioventricular conduction, some cardiologists use it in the treatment of heart block.

Purkinje fiber effects. Catecholamines may produce spontaneous firing of Purkinje fibers, which may cause them to exhibit pacemaker activity. This effect may cause ventricular extrasystoles and increase the susceptibility of ventricular muscle to fibrillation. These effects are more likely to occur with epinephrine than norepinephrine.

Blood pressure and blood flow effects. Vascular effects of the catecholamines depend on the dose and the vascular bed affected. Low doses of epinephrine may decrease total peripheral vascular resistance and so decrease blood pressure. In large doses epinephrine activates alpha receptors in the greater peripheral vascular system, which increases resistance and increases blood pressure. Norepinephrine elevates blood pressure by increasing peripheral resistance and decreasing blood flow through skeletal muscles.

Norepinephrine is a vasoconstrictor and increases total peripheral resistance. Isoproterenol is not a vasoconstrictor but a pure vasodilator; epinephrine is both a vasoconstrictor and vasodilator, with vasodilation being greater in its overall net effects. For example, during great stress the release of epinephrine from the adrenal medulla constricts blood vessels in the skin and splanchnic areas but dilates those of skeletal muscles, thus shunting blood to the areas needed for "fight or flight" responses.

There is greater renal artery constriction and resistance with epinephrine than with norepinephrine. In large doses epinephrine may actually stop blood flow through some nephrons (up to 40%) and stimulate release of antidiuretic hormone (ADH), thereby reducing urinary excretion.

Central nervous system effects. Epinephrine and isoproterenol in sufficient amounts can lead to alertness, tremulousness, respiratory stimulation, and anxiety. Norepinephrine is less likely to cause anxiety and tremulousness. Beneficial cerebral effects from epinephrine and norepinephrine in cases of hypotension are thought to be the result of increased systemic pressure with a resultant improvement in cerebral blood flow.

Smooth muscle effects. Generally, the catecholamines relax nonvascular smooth muscles. Smooth muscle of the gastrointestinal tract is relaxed, and amplitude and tone of intestinal peristalsis are reduced. This may retard propulsion of food and gastrointestinal emptying. However, with therapeutic doses this effect rarely occurs in humans.

The musculature of the splenic capsule is stimulated, causing increasing contractions of that organ. The increased contractions increase the number of circulating red cells and blood viscosity. This effect is not of great significance in humans.

In some situations smooth muscle of some organs reacts like vascular smooth muscle and contracts. For example, radial and sphincter muscles of the iris contract, and the smooth muscle that inserts into the lids may contract, giving rise to the widened, staring eyes seen in sympathetically stimulated individuals.

In the urinary bladder epinephrine causes trigone and sphincter contraction and detrusor relaxation with a delay in the desire to void.

Bronchodilator effects. Catecholamines dilate bronchial smooth muscle. Isoproterenol is a more active bronchodilator than epinephrine, and epinephrine is a stronger bronchodilator than norepinephrine. Epinephrine also constricts bronchial vessels and inhibits bronchial secretions, which accounts for its time-honored use in the treatment of acute bronchial asthma.

Effect on glands. Epinephrine may increase the amount of viscid saliva excreted, but as a rule sympathomimetics decrease secretion and produce a dry mouth. Catecholamines may produce local sweating on the palms of the hands and in the axillary and genital areas. The exact mechanism for these effects is not clear.

Metabolic effects. Epinephrine inhibits insulin secretion. Catecholamines have antagonistic effects on gluconeogenesis, and they decrease liver and skeletal muscle glycogen and increase lipolysis in adipose tissue. The result of these effects is a rise in blood sugar and an increase in free fatty acids. Thus in response to stress ("fight or flight" response) there can be an abundant supply of fuel and energy.

Catecholamines also have a **calorigenic effect** (capable of generating heat, which increases oxygen consumption) resulting from the sum of the preceding effects. Norepinephrine's action in relation to these effects is weaker than that of epinephrine or isoproterenol.

Other effects. Catecholamines cause a decrease in circulating eosinophils. The mechanism of this action is unknown.

epinephrine (Adrenalin)

Epinephrine is available in solutions for inhalation or nebulization, parenteral and ophthalmic administration. Many bronchodilator aerosols are available over the counter in solutions containing up to 1% of the epinephrine base. For example:

epinephrine inhalation aerosol (Bronkaid Mist, Bronkaid Mistometer✚, Primatene Mist Solution, Dysne-Inhal✚)

epinephrine bitartrate inhalation aerosol (Asthma Haler, Medihaler-Epi, Primatene Mist Suspension)

racepinephrine inhalation solution (AsthmaNefrin, Vaponefrin)

Parenteral dosage forms and ophthalmic solutions are ordered by prescription only:

epinephrine injection (Adrenalin, EpiPen Auto-Injector)

sterile epinephrine suspension (Sus-Phrine)

Ophthalmic epinephrine is discussed in Chapter 43.

Mechanism of action. Epinephrine is a direct-acting catecholamine that is naturally released from the adrenal medulla in response to sympathoadrenal stimulation. It also is prepared synthetically. Epinephrine stimulates alpha, beta$_1$, and beta$_2$ receptors. Its primary action is on the beta receptors of the heart, the smooth muscle of the bronchi, and the blood vessels. The beta$_1$ action stimulates the heart by increasing heart rate, force of myocardial contraction, and cardiac output. The beta$_2$ action on the smooth muscle of the bronchioles produces bronchodilation, thereby increasing tidal volume and vital capacity of the lung. Stimulation of alpha receptors constricts arterioles of the bronchioles and inhibits histamine release, thus reducing nasal congestion and edema. In contrast, beta$_2$ adrenergic activity of the smooth muscle of arterioles causes vasodilation.

Another effect of epinephrine is alpha activity, which results in contraction of the radial muscle in the iris, causing dilation of the pupil **(mydriasis).** Constriction of the blood vessels in the skin also is activated by alpha activity. The detrusor muscle in the urinary bladder contains beta receptors and is relaxed by epinephrine. Last, the uterine muscle contains both alpha and beta receptors, and epinephrine promotes muscle relaxation. (See "epinephrine"—Table 20-2.)

Indications

1. Used for symptomatic treatment of bronchial asthma and other obstructive pulmonary diseases, such as chronic bronchitis and emphysema that cause bronchospasm.

2. Used for symptomatic relief of acute hypersensitivity reactions. Indicated in the emergency treatment of acute anaphylactic shock and severe acute reactions to drugs, animal serums, insect stings, and other allergens to relieve bronchospasm, urticaria, hives, angioneurotic edema, and swelling of nasal mucosa. Pulmonary congestion is also alleviated by constriction of mucosal blood vessels.

3. Used as an adjunct with local anesthetics. Concurrent administration of epinephrine with local anesthetics reduces circulation to the site, which results in a slowing of vascular absorption. This promotes a local effect of the anesthetic and also prolongs its duration of action, thus reducing the risk of anesthetic toxicity.

4. Administered as a hemostatic agent to control superficial bleeding from arterioles and capillaries in the skin, mucous membranes, or other tissues.

5. Used in management of simple, open-angle glaucoma by reducing intraocular pressure; also indicated for relieving ocular congestion.

6. Used to treat cardiac arrest such as AV block with syncopal seizures. On occasion it may be given by intracardiac injection in acute attacks of ventricular standstill, after physical measures and electrical defibrillation have failed. Since epinephrine increases the amplitude of the fibrillatory waves, it may make the heart more responsive to the direct current (DC) shock. Therefore, after injection of epinephrine, the patient may again be given DC shock. The drug is not to be used in cardiac failure or in hemorrhagic, traumatic, or cardiogenic shock.

Pharmacokinetics

Absorption. Should not be given orally because it is rapidly metabolized in the mucosa of the gastrointestinal

TABLE 20-2   Direct Adrenergic Drug Effects—Catecholamine Type

	epinephrine (α, β_1, β_2)	isoproterenol (β_1, β_2)	norepinephrine (α, β_1)
Trade names	Adrenalin	Isuprel	Noradrenalin Levophed
Mode of action			
Alpha receptors	Stimulates	N.S.*	Stimulates
Beta receptors	Stimulates	Stimulates	Stimulates the heart
Effects			
Cardiovascular			
Myocardium	Increases strength of contractions Increases cardiac output	Like epinephrine	Slows rate reflexly
Pacemaker cells	Increases heart rate Increases irritability May cause dysrhythmias	Like epinephrine	Stimulates—like epinephrine
Coronary vessels	Dilates—increases blood flow	Like epinephrine	Dilates
Blood pressure	Increases (depending on dose)	Decreases diastolic Slightly increases systolic	Increases
Bronchi	Relaxes; dilates bronchi Improves airway	Potent bronchodilator—more effective than epinephrine	Relaxes less than epinephrine
Blood vessels			
Skeletal muscle	Dilates—increases blood flow	Dilates—increases blood flow	—
Kidney	Constricts—decreases blood flow	N.S.	Constricts—decreases blood flow
Gastrointestinal tract	Relaxes smooth muscle Inhibits peristalsis	N.S.	Like epinephrine
Metabolic	Increases oxygen consumption Mobilizes glycogen Causes hyperglycemia	N.S.	Increases metabolic rate but less than epinephrine
Remarks	Tolerance does not develop	Infiltration into tissues may cause necrosis and sloughing	Infiltration into tissues may cause necrosis and sloughing
Uses	Widely used for allergic states and with local anesthetics Given by injection or inhalation	Heart failure Asthma	To elevate blood pressure, given by slow intravenous infusion

*N.S., Not significant.

tract and liver, so serum levels achieved would be inadequate. Absorption from subcutaneous injection is also slow because of intense local vasoconstriction. (Heat and massage have been used to increase the rate of absorption from subcutaneous administration.) It is absorbed well from intramuscular administration.

Distribution. Rapid onset of action, from 3 to 5 minutes by inhalation or between 6 and 15 minutes when given subcutaneously. The duration of action of epinephrine is short, so, depending on the dose given and the indication, repeated doses may be scheduled for 5 to 10 minutes later (as in severe anaphylaxis, asthma, or cardiac arrest) or may be repeated in 20 minutes to 4 hours in more stabilized situations.

Metabolism. Liver

Excretion. Kidneys

Side effects/adverse reactions. See Table 20-3.

Significant drug interactions. The following interactions may occur when epinephrine is given with the drugs listed below.

Drug	**Possible Effect and Management**
anesthetics, such as cyclopropane, halothane and trichloroethylene	May sensitize the heart, increasing risk of severe dysrhythmias. Monitor closely because a reduction in epinephrine (sympathomimetics) is usually necessary.
local parenteral anesthetics	When used in end artery areas, such as fingers, toes, or penis, the reduced blood supply to the area may result in ischemia and gangrene. Use very cautiously in such areas and monitor closely.

TABLE 20-3   Side Effects/Adverse Reactions of Adrenergic (Sympathomimetic) Drugs

Drug	Side effects*	Adverse reactions†
epinephrine (Adrenalin)	More frequent: Systemic reactions—increased nervousness, restlessness; insomnia Less frequent: Elevation of blood pressure, tachycardia, tremors, sweating, nausea, vomiting, pallor, weakness. Inhalation reactions: Bronchial irritation and coughing (usually with high doses), dry mouth and throat, headaches, red or flushing face or skin	Chills, fever, dizziness, chest pain or pressure, severe headaches, severe hypertension, seizures, increased anxiety and nervousness, dilated pupils or blurred vision, respiratory difficulties (shortness of breath), severe tremors and pounding heart rate, either unusually fast or slow heartbeat, may result in cerebrovascular accident, tachyarrhythmias, or myocardial infarction (above are signs of overdosage)
isoproterenol (Isuprel)	Similar to epinephrine with the following exceptions: Inhalation and sublingual dosage forms may induce a pink to red discoloration of the saliva; this is an expected color alteration and it is not necessary to report it to physician.	Dizziness, chest pain or pressure, severe headache, increased anxiety and nervousness, trembling, palor, severe hypertension, rapid heart beat, dysrythmias
norepinephrine (Levophed)	Less frequent: Increased nervousness or anxiety, dizziness, palor, tremors, insomnia, headaches, pounding heart rate, swelling of thyroid gland in neck.	Rare: Extravasation leading to severe vasoconstriction, ischemia and necrosis—this requires immediate therapeutic intervention to prevent sloughing of tissue and gangrene; cardiac dysrhythmias, bradycardia, and allergic reactions (usually to sodium bisulfite in preparation) Overdosage: Severe hypertension and headaches, convulsions, vomiting, unusually slow heart rate

*If side effects continue, increase, or disturb the client, inform the physician.
†If adverse reactions occur, contact physician, since medical intervention may be necessary.

Drug	Possible Effect and Management
beta-adrenergic receptor blocking agents, including ophthalmics	Therapeutic effects of both agents may be inhibited. With bronchodilators having both alpha and beta stimulating effects (epinephrine), with beta receptor blockade, stimulation of alpha receptors may result in hypertension, severe bradycardia with possibly heart block. If possible, avoid concurrent administration or if absolutely necessary, monitor closely.
digitalis glycosides	Digitalis sensitizes the myocardium to the effects of epinephrine; the additive effect of the catecholamine may precipitate ectopic pacemaker activity.
ergotamine or ergoloid mesylates	Concurrent use may produce severe hypertension, peripheral vascular ischemia, and gangrene. Avoid this combination.
maprotiline or tricyclic antidepressants	May cause dysrhythmias, tachycardia, and hypertension or hyperpyrexia.

Dosage and administration
Parenteral
Bronchodilator
Adults: SC: 0.2-0.5 mg every 20 min to 4 hr as needed, with dosage increase up to a maximum of 1 mg/dose.

Children: SC: 0.01 mg/kg or 0.3 mg/m² repeated every 15 min for 2 doses every 4 hr as needed, up to a maximum of 0.5 mg/dose.

Anaphylaxis

Adults: IM: 0.2-0.5 mg repeated every 10-15 min, as needed, with dosage increase up to a maximum of 1 mg/dose.

Children: SC: 0.01 mg/kg or 0.3 mg/m², repeated every 15 min for 2 doses, then every 4 hr as needed; in severe cases, dosage may be increased up to 0.5 mg/dose.

Cardiac stimulant

Adults: IV or intracardiac injection, 0.5 ml (0.5 mg) or 0.1-1 mg (base) diluted to 10 ml with sodium chloride injection given to restore myocardial contractility. After intracardiac administration, external cardiac massage should be applied to enhance drug entry into coronary circulation.

Endotracheal tube instillation dosage is 1 mg (base) for cardiac resuscitation.

Children: IV or intracardiac, 0.005-0.01mg/kg or 0.15-

0.3 mg/m², repeat every 5 min or follow with an IV infusion at initial rate of 0.0001 mg/kg/min. Rate may be increased in increments of 0.0001 mg/kg/min if necessary to a maximum of 0.0015 mg/kg/min.

Anesthetic (local) adjunct

Adults and children: Intraspinal 0.2-0.4 ml (0.2-0.4 mg) added to anesthetic spinal mixture.

With local anesthetic: 0.1-0.2 mg in a 1:200,000 to 1:20,000 solution.

Auto-injection. Usually prescribed for individuals with history of insect stings and anaphylaxis. For emergency self-treatment of anaphylaxis. IM auto-injectors containing 0.5 mg/ml will deliver a dose of 0.15 mg on injection. The injector containing 1 mg/ml delivers a single dose of 0.3 mg.

Parenteral suspension (Sus-Phrine)

Bronchodilator

Adults: SC 0.5 mg initially, followed by 0.5 mg-1.5 mg every 6 hr as necessary.

Children: SC 0.025 mg/kg or 0.625 mg/m². Dose may be repeated in 6 hr. If child weighs 30 kg or less, the maximum single dose is 0.75 mg.

Inhalation

Bronchodilator. 1:100 (1%) solution administration by aerosol or nebulizer. Proper dose is automatically dispensed by the metered nebulizer when various preparations are used. Allow 1-5 min between inhalations to avoid excessive amounts of the drug. Least possible number of inhalations should be used.

Topical

Nasal decongestant. 1-2 drops (0.1%) solution every 4-6 hours.

Antihemorrhagic. 0.002%-0.1% (1:50,000 to 1:1000) solution of epinephrine applied locally.

Pregnancy safety. FDA category C

NURSING CONSIDERATIONS

Assessment. This drug should not be used by individuals with narrow-angle glaucoma, coronary insufficiency, shock, organic brain damage, or by those who are receiving general anesthesia with cyclopropane or halothane.

Use with caution in elderly clients and those with cardiovascular disease, hypertension, hyperthyroidism, or psychosis. Pulmonary edema, which can be fatal, may occur because of peripheral constriction.

Use with caution in clients with bronchial asthma or emphysema who also have degenerative heart disease. Clients with coronary insufficiency may develop anginal pain.

Intervention. Avoid overdosage, particularly inadvertent intravenous administration of the usual SC dosages, which may cause extreme hypertension. Cerebrovascular hemorrhage may result, particularly in the elderly client.

Read labels very carefully; epinephrine ophthalmic, nasal, and topical solutions must not be injected.

Store medication in tight, light-resistant container at a temperature between 15° and 30° C (59° and 86° F). Do not use if solution is pink or brown in color or contains a precipitate. This color change is caused by oxidation of the drug; multiple use vials in which air is injected to withdraw the solution are more prone to this change.

Parenteral administration. Carefully recheck solution strength, dosage, and route of administration of drug. Avoid medication errors by not confusing the 1:100 solution with the 1:1000 solution. Overdosage has resulted in fatalities.

Use a small syringe (tuberculin syringe) to assure accuracy in measurement of parenteral injection. Aspirate syringe before parenteral injection (subcutaneous and intramuscular) to prevent intravenous injection that can result in sudden hypertension.

Rotate site of injection to prevent tissue necrosis caused by vasoconstriction. Also, massage injection site to promote absorption of drug.

When administering a sterile epinephrine suspension, do so immediately after withdrawing the solution from the vial to avoid the suspension settling.

1:1000 solution must be diluted with 10-ml sodium chloride injection before intravenous or intracardiac administration.

Inhalation. Epinephrine and other beta adrenergic agents may be used interchangeably; however allow 4 hours between doses when changing from one to another. Do not administer concurrently.

Nasal administration. To prevent drug from entering the throat, instill nose drops with head low in lateral position. Rinse nose dropper with hot water to prevent contamination of medication.

Ophthalmic administration. Administer drug at bedtime or following a miotic to minimize discomfort, blurred vision, and sensitivity to light caused by mydriasis.

Education. Caution the client against the repeated or prolonged use of epinephrine, which can cause *tolerance* or "epinephrine fastness." If the drug is withheld 12 hours to several days, its effectiveness usually returns.

Emergency auto-injection. Remind the client that the medication requires a physician's prescription.

Instruct client to consult physician or pharmacist before taking any over-the-counter drug concurrently with epinephrine.

Review with client in detail the operation of the Epi-Pen auto-injector. The package insert *must* be read carefully.

Remind the client that the auto-injector contains the drug that the client injects intramuscularly in the anteriolateral region of the thigh or the deltoid part of the arm. Instruct client *not* to inject drug into buttock because of the increased risk of infection owing to fecal contaminants on the skin.

Emphasize importance of keeping the drug on hand in case of emergency and that the drug should be stored in a dark, cool place to prevent deterioration.

Caution client to check the auto-injector to make sure the solution is neither brown in color nor contains a precipitate. If so, the drug must be discarded.

Inhalation. Teach the client how to use the metered dose nebulizer. (See box on p. 395.)

Instruct client to take pulse rate before inhalation therapy. Allow 2 minutes between doses, and do not administer more frequently than required to relieve symptoms. Excessive repeated use may cause paradoxical bronchospasm.

To prevent drug tolerance, caution client not to overuse drug. Instruct client to notify physician if symptoms are not relieved. Symptoms should be relieved in 20 minutes.

Instruct client to rinse mouth with water to prevent mucosal absorption of drug.

Teach client with history of allergic reaction or bronchial asthma how to self-inject epinephrine subcutaneously in case of emergency.

Nasal administration. Inform client that this route of application may produce a stinging sensation.

Forewarn client that rebound congestion may occur with prolonged use, which may cause rhinitis. Nose drops should not be used for more than 3 to 5 days.

Ophthalmic administration. Alert client that lightheadedness, increased perspiration and heart rate, trembling, and pallor are signs of systemic absorption. These symptoms may be avoided by limiting the amount of medication that enters the systemic circulation by proper instillation of eyedrops. Instruct the client to create a pocket for the solution by gently pinching the skin below the lower eyelid and pulling it away from the eye. Place a drop of the solution in the pocket and hold it open for 1 or 2 seconds to allow the solution to settle. Have the client look down and then gently release the lower eyelid. Press just under the inner corner of the eye for 1 minute. This obstructs the nasolacrimal duct and minimizes the absorption of the drug into the bloodstream.

Instruct client who wears soft contact lenses to consult with physician regarding concurrent use of ophthalmic epinephrine instillations.

Instruct client to discontinue drug and notify physician if signs of hypersensitivity develop (itching, edema of lids, discharge from lids).

Advise client that after initial administration, stinging of the eyes and headache may occur but, with continued drug use, these symptoms disappear. Notify physician if these symptoms, which may be controlled by lower dosage, persist.

Recommend to the client that intraocular pressure determinations should be scheduled periodically.

The client should be alerted that after long-term use of epinephrine, brownish pigment deposits caused by oxidation of the drug may occur in the eyelids and conjunctiva or as large dark casts in the lacrimal sac or nasolacrimal duct. These may be mistaken as foreign objects in the eye. The casts may be removed by irrigation.

Evaluation. Since epinephrine increases blood glucose levels, observe individuals with diabetes for loss of diabetic control.

During intravenous administration, monitor blood pressure, observe electrocardiogram (ECG) results, and monitor pulse continuously until stabilized.

Observe client for urinary hesitancy, changes in mental activity, and pallor. Report symptoms to physician.

isoproterenol hydrochloride (Isuprel, Norisodrine, Vapa-Iso)
isoproterenol sulfate (Medihaler-Iso, Norisodrine Sulfate)

Mechanism of action. Isoproterenol, a synthetic catecholamine, is a nonselective beta adrenegic drug. This means that it stimulates $beta_1$ and $beta_2$ adrenergic receptors. The $beta_1$ receptor activity produces an increase in force of myocardial contraction and heart rate. The $beta_2$ receptor response of the smooth muscle of the bronchi, skeletal muscle, gastrointestinal tract, and blood vessels of the splanchnic bed causes a relaxation of these organs. More important, isoproterenol can greatly relax the smaller bronchi and may even dilate the trachea and main bronchi. This drug also stimulates insulin secretion and releases free fatty acid.

Hemodynamically, the $beta_1$ activity of the heart increases cardiac output and venous return to the heart. Moreover, peripheral vascular resistance is reduced and, in normal individuals, causes a significant drop in blood pressure with excessive dosage (see Table 20-2).

Indications

1. Used as cardiac stimulant in cardiac arrest, Adams-Stokes syndrome, atrioventricular (AV) block, and carotid sinus hypersensitivity.
2. May be used as adjunct therapy in treatment of cardiogenic shock.
3. Relieves bronchospasm associated with bronchial asthma, pulmonary emphysema, and bronchitis.

Pharmacokinetics

Absorption. Readily absorbed when given parenterally or as an aerosol. Absorption of sublingual isoproterenol is erratic and unreliable.

Onset of action. Rapidly absorbed following inhalation or parenteral administration

Duration of action. Usually up to 1 hour after oral inhalation for bronchodilator effect. For a few minutes

---

METERED DOSE BRONCHODILATOR INHALATION TECHNIQUE

It is important that the client be instructed in the correct use of a metered dose nebulizer before it is needed to relieve an asthma attack. If used incorrectly, the dose may be dispersed into the air or even swallowed. Since only 10% of an inhaled dose reaches the lungs under the best of conditions, the ability to use the metered dose nebulizer appropriately is essential for the client.

A placebo nebulizer should be used for demonstration. This will enable the client to repeat the demonstration a number of times until the nebulizer can be easily and correctly used.

1. Shake the container for 2 to 5 seconds.
2. Hold the nebulizer with the drug container upside down.
3. Place the mouthpiece in the mouth, closing lips tightly around it.
4. Exhale steadily and completely through nose.
5. Inhale slowly and deeply, and at the same time press the container down on the mouthpiece.
6. Hold breath for as long as possible before exhaling.
7. Wait several seconds.
8. Repeat steps 1 through 6 above.
9. If no relief is achieved after 5 minutes and condition worsens, contact physician.

Advise client that rinsing the mouth after using the nebulizer prevents systemic absorption and minimizes dryness of the mouth. The mouthpiece should be rinsed at least once daily to avoid clogging. Stress the importance of keeping the equipment clean to prevent infection. If using a refillable nebulizer, do not place more than a day's supply of drug in nebulizer. Change solution daily.

Clients with asthma benefit greatly from the use of sympathomimetic inhalers; however, they should be discouraged from using over-the-counter inhalers because of the nonselective beta-agonist drug effect of the epinephrine base. The nurse needs to recognize the possibility of misuse and the consequences of abuse in order to successfully help the client with inhalant drug therapy.

---

avoid concurrent administration of epinephrine and isoproterenol due to the possibility of increased additive effects and cardiotoxicity. When the action of one medication is considered complete (usually 4 hours), the second one may be implemented.

Dosage and administration

Cardiac standstill and dysrhythmias

Adults

IV: initial—0.02-0.06 mg (1-3 ml of diluted solution 1:50,000), then 0.01-0.2 mg (0.5-10 ml of diluted solution).

IV infusion: 5 μg/min (1.25 ml) of a diluted solution containing 2 mg in 500 ml of dextrose 5% in water.

IM: initial—0.2 mg (1 ml of 1:5000 solution undiluted), then 0.02-1 mg (0.1-5 ml).

SC: initial—0.2 mg (1 ml of 1:5000 solution undiluted), then 0.15-0.2 mg (0.75-1 ml) as needed.

Children. Not determined; individualized by physician.

Intracardiac

Adults. 0.02 mg (0.1 ml) of an undiluted 1:5000 solution, adjusted and repeated as needed.

Bronchodilator

Sublingual

Adults: 10-15 mg 3 to 4 times/day; maximum dosage is 60 mg/day.

Children: 5-10 mg 3 times a day

Inhaler. Isoproterenol hydrochloride inhalation aerosal/isoproterenol inhalation solution:

Adults: Follow individual manufacturer's instructions carefully. Generally, a metered-dose nebulizer (120 or 131 μg/inhalation)—1 inhalation is administered which may be repeated in 1-to-5 min if necessary, 4 to 6 times daily. In bronchospasm of chronic obstructive lung disease (COPD), the second dose should be given 3-4 hr after the initial dose.

Children: Oral inhalation of a 0.5% nebulized solution (5 to 15 deep inhalations). If necessary, may repeat in 5-10 min. Dosage may be repeated up to 5 times daily.

Pregnancy safety. FDA category C

NURSING CONSIDERATIONS

Assessment. Use with great caution in patients with cardiovascular disorders such as coronary insufficiency and hypertension, hyperthyroidism, glaucoma, diabetes, or sensitivity to sympathomimetic amines. Excessive use may decrease effectiveness.

Intervention. Read labels carefully; solution for oral inhalation must not be administered intravenously.

Intravenous administration. Before therapy, hypovolemia should be corrected if possible.

Plan nursing care so that the client is constantly attend-

---

after IV administration; up to 2 hours after subcutaneous or sublingual adminstration.

Metabolism. Gastrointestinal tract, liver, and lungs.

Excretion. Urine within 15 to 24 hours.

Side effects/adverse reactions. See Table 20-3.

Significant drug interactions. With the exception of monoamine oxidase (MAO) inhibitors and local-parenteral anesthetic interactions, the drug interactions with isoproterenol are similar to those listed under epinephrine. Use with MAO inhibitors may lead to a hypertensive crisis. Beta blockers may block therapeutic effect. In addition,

ed while receiving the drug. Never leave the client unattended during the infusion.

Use a two-bottle setup so that an intravenous infusion can be kept running if this drug is discontinued. Use an infusion pump to precisely regulate infusion rate.

Record baseline blood pressure and pulse before starting therapy. During infusion, check blood pressure every 2 minutes until stabilized, then every 5 minutes during drug administration. Adjust the flow rate to maintain blood pressure, usually at systolic 80 to 100 mm Hg or in hypertensive clients, 30 to 40 mm Hg below preexisting blood pressure. Monitor ECG pattern and central venous pressure, as well as urine volume and blood gases for clients in shock. Follow physicians guidelines for titrating flow in relation to heart rate, central venous pressure, blood pressure, ECG changes, and volume of urine flow. If precordial pain occurs, stop drug.

If heart rate exceeds 110 beats/minute, physician usually will prescribe a slower infusion rate or temporarily discontinue drug. With doses that cause a heart rate of 130 beats/minute, anticipate the development of ventricular dysrhythmias. Intravenous isoproterenol frequently causes dysrhythmias in clients with heart disease. Have oxygen and other resuscitative equipment available.

Monitor respiratory pattern and lung sounds during administration.

Education

Oral/sublingual administration. Instruct patient to allow sublingual tablet to dissolve under tongue without swallowing saliva until tablet is completely dissolved. Swallowing drug with saliva causes epigastric pain. Instruct patient to rinse mouth thoroughly with water between sublingual doses. Prolonged use can cause tooth decay.

Instruct patient to swallow sustained-release tablets whole and not chew.

Oral inhalation. Instruct the client to use oral inhalation correctly. (See box on p. 395.) The instructions for the metered powder nebulizer are the same as for metered dose nebulizer except that deep inhalation is not necessary.

The client should allow 1 to 5 minutes between first and second inhalations. Advise the client that there should be no more than six inhalations in an hour in any 24-hour period. If the client needs more than three aerosol treatments within a 24-hour period, the physician should be contacted.

Advise patient that drug may turn sputum and saliva pink.

Warn patient of overuse since tolerance can develop and sudden deaths have been reported. Instruct patient to notify physician if prescribed doses are not producing desired relief or if there are adverse effects.

Store drug in tight light-resistant container. Do not use if precipitate or discoloration is present (solutions be-

come pink or brownish pink on exposure to light, air, heat, or on contact with metal or alkali).

Evaluation. Discontinue medication if severe paradoxical airway resistance develops: institute alternative therapy.

Isoproterenol may increase blood glucose levels. Observe individuals with diabetes for loss of diabetic control. Dosage of insulin or hypoglycemic agents may need to be increased.

norepinephrine bitartrate (Levophed Bitartrate)

Mechanism of action. Norepinephrine is a direct-acting sympathomimetic amine that is identical to the body catecholamine synthesized in the postganglionic nerve ending of the sympathetic nervous system. This agent has a high affinity for the alpha receptors. Since the blood vessels of the skin and mucous membrane contain only alpha receptors, norepinephrine produces a powerful constriction in these tissues. In addition, the blood vessels (both arteriolar and venous beds) in the visceral organs, including the kidneys, contain predominantly alpha receptors. Consequently, norepinephrine causes vasoconstriction and a reduced blood flow through the kidneys and other visceral organs. This agent also activates beta$_1$ receptors in the heart and exerts a powerful increase in the force of myocardial contraction. The end result, however, is either no change or a decrease in the cardiac output because of a reflex slowing of the heart. Thus the main therapeutic effect results from peripheral anteriolar vasoconstriction in all vascular beds. Both systolic and diastolic pressures are elevated, causing an increase in mean arterial pressure. Of importance during shock is constriction of the venous capacitance vessels, which reduces splanchnic and renal blood flow. This is brought about by severe restriction of tissue perfusion in these regions. In presistent hypotension after blood volume deficit has been corrected, norepinephrine helps to raise the blood pressure to an optimal level and establishes a more adequate circulation (see Table 20-2).

Indications

1. Selectively employed for restoring blood pressure in certain acute hypotensive states such as sympathectomy, pheochromocytomectomy, spinal anesthesia, poliomyelitis, myocardial infarction, blood transfusion reaction, septicemia, and drug reactions. When this drug is used to treat hypotension associated with an acute myocardial infarction, an increase in cardiac output and oxygen demand plus the possiblity of inducing dysrhythmias may offset the benefits of using the drug to increase blood pressure. This would have to be carefully considered when selecting norepinephrine for use in such conditions.

2. Adjunct therapy in cardiac arrest and profound hy-

potension. *Since the advent of dopamine, the use of norepinephrine to treat shock has declined significantly.* It is usually prescribed for patients whose shock produces severe hypotension and vasodilation of the peripheral blood vessels.

Pharmacokinetics

Absorption. Oral norepinephrine is destroyed in the gastrointestinal tract, whereas subcutaneous norepinephrine is poorly absorbed. Therefore norepinephrine is only administered by intravenous infusion.

Onset of action. Immediate or rapid by intravenous infusion

Distribution. Mainly concentrates in sympathetic tissues

Metabolism. In liver, other tissues, and by reuptake into the sympathetic nerves

Duration of action. Approximately 1 to 2 minutes after an intravenous infusion is discontinued

Excretion. Kidneys

Side-effects/adverse reactions. See Table 20-3.

Significant drug interactions. See epinephrine. In addition, when given concurrently with doxapram, central nervous system stimulation and blood pressure may increase from the effects of both drugs. Monitor closely because dosage adjustments may be necessary. Also, when given concurrently with methyldopa, the hypotensive action of methyldopa is decreased while the hypertensive effect of norepinephrine may be enhanced. If norepinephrine is given to individuals receiving methyldopa, initiate with very small doses with close monitoring.

Dosage and administration

Hypotension

Adults. IV infusion, initially 8 to 12 μg/minute; adjusting dosage as necessary to raise and maintain the desired pressure; maintenance: 2 to 4 μg/minute, titrated according to patient's needs

Children

Acute hypotension: intravenous infusion given at 2 μg/minute or 2 mg/m^2/minute; adjust dosage as necessary to raise and maintain the desired pressure

Severe hypotension of cardiac arrest: intravenous infusion, initially 0.1 μg/kg/minute; adjust dosage as necessary to raise and maintain blood pressure

Pregnancy safety. Not established

NURSING CONSIDERATIONS

Assessment. Do not use in patients who are in hypovolemic states except as an emergency measure to maintain cerebral and coronary artery blood flow.

Do not give to patients with mesenteric or peripheral vascular thrombosis because of risk of extending ischemia.

Use with extreme caution in patients receiving mono-

amine oxidase inhibitors and tricyclic antidepressants because prolonged hypotension may result.

Do not give during general anesthesia when halogenated hydrocarbons (halothane) are administered. It is also contraindicated in profound hypoxia or hypercapnia and pregnancy.

Intervention. Be aware of the importance of maintaining adequate blood volume before administering norepinephrine. Blood should be administered separately. This is to prevent tissue ischemia that can result from the vasoconstrictive effect of the drug.

Administer norepinephrine only intravenously; its vasoconstrictor effect prohibits intramuscular or subcutaneous administration.

Anticipate that infusion will be administered through a plastic catheter deep into a large vein to minimize risk of extravasation. The veins of the leg are not recommended because of poor circulation, which can result in occlusive vascular disease. Do not use catheter tie-in setup because venous stasis around tubing can occur.

During infusion, adjust dosage according to physician's guidelines. This includes the client's response, with particular attention to urinary output, respiration, blood pressure, pulse, and observation of extremities for color and temperature (for peripheral ischemia). These parameters must be accurately recorded to attain precise titration of drug.

If extravasation occurs, the area should be quickly infiltrated with 5 to 10 mg of phentolamine in 10 to 15 ml of sodium chloride with a fine-gauge needle to dilate blood vessels. Have phentolamine ready.

Norepinephrine should be diluted with 5% dextrose in distilled water or 5% dextrose in sodium chloride solution because the dextrose prevents a significant loss of potency by oxidation. To prevent sloughing of the skin secondary to extravasation, 5 to 10 mg of phentolamine may be added to every liter of norepinephrine solution.

Anticipate the addition of heparin to infusion solution to prevent thrombosis of infused vein in clients with severe hypotension following myocardial infarction.

Store medication by protecting it from light. Since the solution deteriorates after 24 hours, discard it after that time. Do not use solution if it is discolored or if precipitate is present.

Evaluation. Never leave client unattended during infusion. Inspect the infusion site for extravasation every 10 to 15 minutes. If extravasation occurs, notify the physician immediately.

Observe client for blanching along route of infused vein and for cold, hard swelling around injection site. Have available phentolamine, which may be used at site of extravasation to dilate blood vessels.

Monitor by ECG; reduce or discontinue medication if cardiac dysrhythmia occurs.

Observe client for mentation (cerebral circulation), temperature of extremities, and color of earlobes, lips, and nail beds.

Monitor intake and output. After prolonged use of the drug a decrease in urinary output may indicate necrosis of the kidney.

Monitor for signs of sulfite sensitivity: (See boxed material.)

Discontinue therapy gradually by slowing infusion rate, and continue to monitor patient and vital signs to ensure circulatory adequacy.

IMPORTANT: See also nursing considerations under isoproterenol, intravenous administration.

Drugs Used for Circulatory Shock

In any instance of shock, treatment must be directed to the cause. A main concern is the need to improve circulation so that enough oxygen is available for tissue perfusion. Hypoxia that denotes impaired tissue perfusion may result from inadequate pumping action of the heart, decreased blood volume, decreased peripheral resistance of arterial vessels, or increased size of the venous bed.

During circulatory shock the autonomic nervous system plays an essential compensatory role in an attempt to restore normal circulation. Therefore many sympathomimetic drugs are used to manage this condition. Although there are other agents, the five drugs that are widely used for circulatory shock are dopamine, epinephrine, and norepinephrine, which are all vasopressors, and dobutamine and isoproterenol, which possess cardiogenic activity. Amrinone, which has positive inotropic and vasodilator effects, can also be used for clients with congestive heart failure that are not responsive to standard therapy. Milrinone, an analogue of amrinone, is under clinical investigation as possibly having fewer side effects than amrinone, as well as having both intravenous and oral administration activity. These are preliminary reports that will require extensive clinical trials and evaluation before the drug is marketed.

Vasopressors have strong alpha activity, and dopamine produces less vasoconstriction than epinephrine and norepinephrine. Dobutamine and isoproterenol are important for improving cardiac output because of their capability to stimulate beta$_1$ receptors in the heart. Most of the agents are nonselective beta acting drugs, but norepinephrine lacks beta$_2$ activity and amrinone does not appear to have beta agonist effects. Also, with the exception of isoproterenol and amrinone, all of them stimulate alpha receptors. (See drug monographs for epinephrine, norepinephrine, and isoproterenol.)

amrinone (Inocor)

Mechanism of action. This has not been fully identified. It increases force and velocity of myocardial tissues resulting in a positive inotropic effect. Experiments indicate that amrinone inhibits cyclic adenosine monophosphate (cAMP) phosphodiesterase activity, which in turn increases cellular cAMP concentration. The exact role of amrinone in producing the inotoropic activity is not fully known. Amrinone appears to produce a direct relaxant effect on the vascular smooth muscle, resulting in vasodilation.

Indications. Used to treat congestive heart failure in individuals who do not respond to standard therapies, such as digitalis glycosides, diuretics, and vasodilators.

Pharmacokinetics

Administration. Intravenous

Time to peak action. Within 10 minutes

Duration of effect. Dose-related. If 0.75 mg/kg is administered, duration of action is approximately 30 minutes. If 3 mg/kg is administered, duration is approximately 120 minutes.

Half-life. By intravenous infusion, nearly 5.8 hours. By intravenous injection, approximately 3.6 hours

Metabolism. Liver

Excretion. Kidneys primarily, some fecal.

Side effects/adverse reactions. See Table 20-4.

Significant drug interactions. Inotropic effects are additive to those of digitalis.

Dosage and administration

Adults. 0.74 mg/kg IV, given slowly over 2 to 3 minutes; if necessary, may repeat in 30 minutes. Maintenance: intravenous infusion, 5 to 10 μg/kg/minute, individualize dose according to clinical response. Maximum dosage is 10 mg/kg/day, but in several reports, dosages up to 18 mg/kg/day were given for short time periods.

Children. Dosage not established

Pregnancy safety: FDA category C

NURSING CONSIDERATIONS

Assessment. Do not use amrinone in clients with severe aortic or pulmonic valvular disease.

Use with caution in clients with impaired hepatic or renal function.

Amrinone may aggravate outflow tract obstruction in hypertrophic subaortic stenosis; use with caution.

Amrinone is not recommended for use during the acute phase of postmyocardial infarction.

Intervention. Examine the solution for color changes and/or precipitation. Amrinone is incompatible with dextrose because it loses its potency. Do not mix with furosemide or inject it into the same tubing because it precipitates.

For direct intravenous administration, it may be administered undiluted. Mix with sodium chloride solutions for continuous intravenous infusion. Use prepared solution within 24 hours.

Administer slowly intravenous, over 2 to 3 minutes, to minimize pain and burning at the injection site. Avoid extravasation.

Education. Tell the client to move slowly from a sitting or lying position to a more upright position because of the drug's hypotensive effects.

Evaluation. Blood pressure and pulse should be monitored to assess hypotensive and dysrhythmic effects of the drug. In addition, assess cardiac index and pulmonary wedge pressure if warranted. Assess central venous pressure, urine output, body weight, and the status of any orthopnea, dyspnea, and fatigue to evaluate the drug's effectiveness and the client's progress.

Assess platelet counts before and frequently during therapy. Observe for unusual bleeding and bruising, which are clinical signs of thrombocytopenia. The drug may be discontinued if the platelet count falls below 150,000/mm.

Because hepatotoxicity is a possibility, liver function studies are usually done and the client is monitored for clinical signs of jaundice. These signs include yellowish skin and/or sclera, dark urine, and pruritis.

Report nausea and vomiting to the physician. It may be severe enough to require that the drug be discontinued.

If the drug is monitored through plasma concentrations, the therapeutic range is 0.5 to 7 μg/ml, but optimal level is about 3 μg/ml.

Monitor for sulfite sensitivity (see box below).

SULFITE SENSITIVITY

Sulfite is contained in the commercially available formulations of:
 amrinone
 dopamine
 meteraminol
 methoxamine
 norepinephrine
 phenylephrine
They should not be administered to individuals with a known sensitivity to sulfite agents (sulfur dioxide, potassium or sodium bisulfite, potassium or sodium metasulfite, sodium sulfite).
 Symptoms of sulfite sensitivity include:
 Skin: clamminess, flushed, pruritis, urticaria, cyanosis
 Respiratory: bronchospasm, shortness of breath, wheezing, laryngeal edema, respiratory arrest
 Cardiovascular: hypotension, syncope
 CNS: severe dizziness, loss of consciousness
 Anaphylaxis, death

---

dobutamine hydrochloride (Dobutrex)

Mechanism of action. Dobutamine is a synthetic catecholamine that acts directly on the heart muscle to increase the force of myocardial contraction. This response is attributed to the direct stimulation of the beta$_1$ adrenergic receptors of the heart. At the same time dobutamine produces comparatively little increase in heart rate or peripheral vascular resistance. By enhancing stroke volume, this agent is an effective positive inotropic drug. Because of its minimal influence on heart rate and blood pressure (both major determinants of myocardial oxygen demand), it is valuable for use in individuals with low cardiac output syndrome. In contrast to dopamine, which also is capable of increasing myocardial contractility, dobutamine does not produce renal vasodilation. In a comparative study of dobutamine and dopamine, the improvement in peripheral blood flow, urine flow, and sodium excretion noted with the use of dobutamine was probably caused by the elevation in cardiac output.

Indications

1. Dobutamine is administered intravenously in the *short-term* management of clients requiring inotropic support. It is used to strengthen the decompensated heart in individuals with the low cardiac output syndrome.
2. It is currently used in the short-term treatment of acute and chronic (low cardiac output) congestive heart failure. Its beneficial effects are a progressive increase in cardiac output and a decrease in pulmonary capillary wedge pressure, thereby improving ventricular contraction.
3. Dobutamine also is used to promote myocardial performance after cardiac surgical procedures such as cardiopulmonary bypass.

    In a surgical procedure such as cardiopulmonary bypass, the concomitant use of sodium nitroprusside and dobutamine is often beneficial. It results in a higher cardiac output and a lower pulmonary capillary wedge pressure than when either drug is used alone. Because of the vasodilating effect of nitroprusside, the decrease in peripheral resistance lessens the workload on the heart.
4. In clients with acute myocardial infarction, the drug has been recommended only when congestive heart failure is also present. If cardiogenic shock also is present, hypovolemia should be corrected by administration of a suitable plasma volume expander before dobutamine treatment is given.

Pharmacokinetics

Absorption. Must be given parenterally for rapid absorption.

Duration of effect. Onset of action within 1 to 2 minutes; 10 minutes. The plasma half life is 2 minutes.

Metabolism. Rapid metabolism by liver.

Excretion. Urine.

Side effects/adverse reactions. See Table 20-4.
Significant drug interactions. None listed
Dosage and administration
Adults. Intravenous infusion, 2.5 to 15 µg/kg/minute.
Children. Dosage not determined.
Pregnancy safety. Not established.

NURSING CONSIDERATIONS

Assessment. Use cautiously in clients with tachycardia and increased blood pressure. Safety of use of this drug is not established when used after myocardial infarction. There is concern that a drug which increases the force of myocardial contraction and heart rate may intensify the ischemia by increasing the size of the infarction.

Note that dobutamine is contraindicated in idiopathic hypertrophic subaortic stenosis.

Intervention. Administer using an infusion pump or other device to control the rate of flow. Adjust dosage based on the clinical response of the client as for norepinephrine and isoproterenol. (See nursing considerations for intravenous administration of isoproterenol.) The concentration of dobutamine solution for administration should not exceed 5 mg of dobutamine per milliliter.

Intravenous solution remains stable for 24 hours. A color change during this period indicates some oxidation, but there is no loss of potency during the first 24 hours.

Dobutamine is incompatible with alkaline solutions and should not be mixed with products such as 5% sodium bicarbonate injection. Check for drug incompatibilities when considering administration through an intravenous line with other drugs.

Evaluation. During therapy, the electrocardiogram and blood pressure should be continuously monitored. If

TABLE 20-4   Side Effects/Adverse Reactions of Cardiotonic and Cardiac Stimulant Drugs

Drug	Side effects*	Adverse reactions†
amrinone (Inocor)	Less frequent: Fever, nausea, vomiting, abdominal pain, decrease in taste perception	Less frequent: Dizziness (hypotension), dysrhythmias Rare: Local pain at site of injection, angina or chest pain, unusual bruising or bleeding episodes (the thrombocytopenia that usually occurs after high dosages or chronic therapy is not usually symptomatic), jaundice
dobutamine (Dobutrex)	Less frequent: Nausea, headaches	Less frequent: Angina or chest pain, respiratory distress (shortness of breath), tachycardia, palpitation, increased heart rate and blood pressure, premature ventricular beats
dopamine HCl (Intropin)	More frequent: Headaches, nausea or vomiting Less frequent: Increased anxiety, nervousness, or restlessness	More frequent: Angina or chest pain, respiratory difficulties, decreased blood pressure, irregular or ecotopic heart beats (usually with high doses), tachycardia, palpitations Less frequent: Hypertension; decreased heart rate (unusually slow). Administration of chronic high dosages, or low doses in patients with peripheral vascular disease, may result in peripheral vasoconstriction, which may result in ischemia, necrosis, and gangrene; monitor for skin color changes in hands or feet, very cold hands or feet, complaints of numbness, tingling or pain in fingers or toes. In sulfite-containing preparations, allergic reactions have been reported: flushing of skin; rash; hives; pruritus; edema of face, lips, or eyelids; respiratory difficulties; dizziness; faintness.

*If side effects continue, increase, or disturb the client, inform the physician.
†If adverse reactions occur, the physician should be contacted because medical intervention may be necessary.

possible, the pulmonary capillary wedge pressure and cardiac output also should be monitored to ensure safe infusion of the drug. If the client responds by an increase in the heart rate (30 beats/minute or more) and an increase in systolic blood pressure (50 mm Hg or greater) during the course of treatment, a reduction of dosage usually reverses these adverse effects because the drug is rapidly metabolized.

Monitor intake and output. Increased urine output indicates improved cardiac output and urinary perfusion. NOTE: Clients with atrial fibrillation and rapid ventricular response should be treated with a digitalis preparation before dobutamine therapy.

Continue to observe client carefully after drug therapy is discontinued. The duration of action of the drug is brief, and the beneficial effects of the drug may be quickly terminated.

dopamine hydrochloride (Intropin)

Mechanism of action. Dopamine is a catecholamine that occurs as an immediate precursor of norepinephrine (see Figure 18-6). It acts both directly and indirectly by releasing norepinephrine. It then stimulates dopaminergic receptors, beta$_1$ receptors, and, in high doses, alpha receptors. Actually, receptor activity depends on the amount of drug administered.

Unlike norepinephrine, in low doses (usually 0.5 to 2 mcg/kg/minute) this drug is unique because it acts mainly on dopaminergic receptors to cause vasodilation of the renal and mesenteric arteries. Renal vasodilation increases renal blood flow with usually a greater amount of urine and sodium excretion. This prevents kidney failure secondary to shock. It is important that the dopaminergic receptors are not blocked by either alpha or beta blocking agents.

In low to moderate doses (usually 2 to 10 mcg/kg/minute), dopamine acts directly on the beta$_1$ receptors on the myocardium and indirectly by releasing norepinephrine from its neuronal storage sites in the sympathetic neuron. These actions increase myocardial contractility and stroke volume, thereby increasing cardiac output. Systolic blood pressure and pulse pressure may increase with either no effect or a slight elevation in diastolic blood pressure. Nevertheless, total peripheral resistance is usually unchanged. Coronary blood flow and myocardial oxygen consumption increase. However, heart rate increases only slightly at low doses.

In higher doses, alpha adrenergic receptors are stimulated, increasing peripheral resistance. Because of a rise in cardiac output, blood pressure increases. As a consequence, a high dose level may reduce urinary output, eliminating the benefit of vasodilation because the renal artery becomes constricted.

From the therapeutic standpoint, it is important to note that dopamine causes vasodilation in the renal, mesenteric, coronary, and cerebral blood vessels. These vasodilatory properties suggest that they may be attributed to the presence of specific dopamine receptors. Therefore, unlike norepinephrine, this agent helps alleviate inadequate tissue perfusion through the vital splanchnic organ systems. The combination of cardiac and circulatory effects has led to dopamine's successful use in the treatment of circulatory shock and refractory heart failure.

Indications. Used to correct hemodynamic imbalances associated with shock syndrome caused by myocardial infarction, trauma, endotoxic septicemia, open heart surgery, renal failure, and chronic cardiac decompensation (as in congestive heart failure).

Pharmacokinetics

Administration. Must be by intravenous infusion

Duration of effect. Rapid onset of action (2 to 5 minutes) and a short duration of action (5 to 10 minutes).

Distribution. It is widely distributed in the body but does not cross the blood-brain barrier.

Metabolism. Rapid metabolism by liver, kidney, plasma, by monoamine oxidase and catechol-O-methyltransferase (COMT) to inactive substances.

Excretion. Urine

Side effects/adverse reactions. See Table 20-4.

Significant drug interactions. With the exception of local-parenteral anesthetics, the interactions are similar to epinephrine. Also, if given concurrently with doxapram, blood pressure may increase. Monitor closely because dosage adjustments may be necessary.

Dosage and administration

Adults. Intravenous infusion started at 1 to 5 μg/kg/minute. Increase as necessary by 1 to 4 μg/kg/minute at 10 to 30 minute intervals.

For chronic refractory CHF: IV infusion administered at 0.5 to 2 mcg/kg/minute. If necessary, increase rate gradually until desired effects are achieved.

In occlusive vascular disease: IV infusion, at 1 mcg/kg/minute, increase as necessary until desired effects are achieved.

In seriously ill patients: IV infusion at 5 mcg/kg/minute, increase in 5 to 10 mcg/kg/minute increments (up to 20 to 50 mcg/kg/minute) until desired response is achieved.

Children. Not determined.

Pregnancy safety. FDA category C

NURSING CONSIDERATIONS

Assessment. Use cautiously in individuals with occlusive vascular disease such as Buerger's or Raynaud's disease, atherosclerosis, diabetic endarteritis, and arterial embolism.

Note that dopamine is contraindicated in pheochromocytoma, tachydysrhythmias, and ventricular fibrillation.

See also nursing considerations for dobutamine.

Intervention. Note that before dopamine therapy, hypovolemia should be corrected, if possible.

For precautions and care regarding extravasation, see norepinephrine nursing considerations. Have available a syringe with phentolamine mesylate (Regitine), 5 mg in 10 ml saline for use in extravasation (physician order).

Medication should be diluted immediately before administration. After dilution it is stable for 24 hours. However, dopamine is incompatible with sodium bicarbonate and other alkaline intravenous solutions; it will turn pink-violet.

Use an intravenous infusion device to regulate flow so that the dosage can be precisely titrated.

Evaluation. During infusion, adjust dosage according to physician's guidelines. This includes the client's response, with particular attention to urinary output, blood pressure, pulse, and observation of extremities for color and temperature (for peripheral ischemia). These parameters must be accurately recorded to attain precise titration of drug.

If a marked decrease in pulse pressure (disproportionate rise in diastolic pressure) is observed, decrease the infusion rate. Continue to observe patient for further evidence of vasoconstrictor activity. Decrease medication or stop temporarily and notify physician if the following occurs: reduced urine flow without hypotension, increasing tachycardia, dysrhythmia, and marked decrease in pulse pressure.

Monitor for sulfite sensitivity (see box on p. 399).

When appropriate, decrease the dosage gradually to prevent severe hypotension.

Administering the dopamine and dextrose injection to a client with subclinical or overt diabetes may exacerbate the diabetic condition.

INDIRECT- AND DUAL-ACTING ADRENERGIC DRUGS

The direct-acting adrenergic drugs—the catecholamines—act directly on alpha and beta receptors to stimulate adrenergic response. The indirect-acting adrenergic drugs act indirectly on receptors by first triggering the release of the catecholamines norepinephrine and epinephrine from their storage sites; these neurotransmitters then activate the alpha and beta receptors. Finally, the *dual-acting* adrenergic drugs have both indirect and direct effects. These drugs have many and varied uses in medicine.

ephedrine (Ephedrine Sulfate, Vatronol)

Mechanism of action. Ephedrine has both a direct and an indirect sympathomimetic action. It acts indirectly by stimulating release of norepinephrine from presynaptic nerve terminals. It acts directly on both alpha and beta receptors. Like epinephrine and norepinephrine, ephedrine has positive inotropic (myocardial stimulation) and chronotropic (increased heart rate) activities, but it is a less effective vasoconstrictor. However, it does raise the blood pressure and is used for this purpose during spinal anesthesia and to treat orthostatic hypotension.

Parenteral ephedrine has been used in hypotensive clients who do not respond to fluid replacement, position changes, and specific antidotes in the case of drug overdosage. Be aware though, if severe peripheral vasoconstriction is present; ephedrine may be ineffective and may actually worsen the situation. (See Table 20-5 for drug effects.)

Indications

1. Used to produce bronchodilation in the treatment of milder forms of bronchial asthma, since ephedrine is useful in preventing acute attacks. Epinephrine is preferable when attacks are acute because of its more rapid effect.

2. Used to relieve nasal mucosal congestion. As an ingredient in nasal drops, jellies, and sprays, ephedrine relieves acute congestion of hay fever, sinusitis, head colds, and vasomotor rhinitis. Shrinkage of mucous membranes begins immediately and lasts for several hours. Vasodilation does not ordinarily follow vasoconstriction, as may occur after administration of epinephrine.

3. Used as a pressor agent in hypotensive states during spinal anesthesia or after sympathectomy.

4. Although also indicated for the treatment of enuresis, Adams-Stokes syndrome with complete heart block, and myasthenia gravis, the availability of more effective agents for these conditions has largely replaced ephedrine.

Pharmacokinetics

Absorption. Rapid after oral, IM or SC administration

Distribution. Onset of action for bronchodilation occurs within 15 to 60 minutes with oral dosage form; within 10 to 20 minutes with intramuscular dosage form. Duration of action is 3 to 5 hours following oral dosage form; 30 to 60 minutes following IM or SC injections of 25 to 50 mg doses. The pressor effects and cardiac responses following parenteral administration usually occur within 60 minutes.

Metabolism. Liver

Excretion. Kidneys

Side effects/adverse reactions. See Table 20-6.

Significant drug interactions. The following interactions may occur when ephedrine is given with the drugs listed on p. 404:

TABLE 20-5 Indirect- and Dual-Acting Adrenergic Drug Effects

Receptors, action sites	Ephedrine	Phenylephrine	Mephentermine	Metaraminol	Methoxamine
Trade names	Ephedrine Sulfate	Neo-Synephrine	Wyamine	Aramine Pressonex	Vasoxyl
Mode of action					
Alpha receptors	Stimulates	Stimulates	Stimulates	Stimulates	Stimulates
Beta receptors	Stimulates More prolonged but less intense action than epinephrine	N.S.*			
Effects					
Cardiovascular					
Myocardium	Variable	N.S. Bradycardia may occur reflexly	Increases contractility and rate May cause bradycardia	Some increase in contractility Bradycardia may occur	— Reflex bradycardia may occur
Pacemaker cells	N.S.	N.S.	N.S.	—	—
Coronary vessels	Dilates— increases blood flow	Dilates— increases blood flow	Dilates— increases blood flow	—	—
Blood pressure	Increases	Increases	Increases	Increases	Increases
Bronchi	Dilates	Dilates but less than epi- nephrine	Dilates but less than epi- nephrine	N.S.	
Cerebral effects	Stimulating action	N.S.	N.S.	—	—
Blood vessels Skeletal muscle	N.S.	—†	N.S.	N.S.	Decreases blood flow
Kidney	Constricts	Constricts	Constricts but less than ephedrine	Constricts— decreases blood flow	
Gastrointestinal tract	Decreases peristalsis	Decreases motility	Relaxes smooth muscle— inhibits	Some inhibition	Inhibits
Metabolic	Increases metabolic rate	Some increase in metabolic rate	N.S.	N.S.	N.S.
Remarks	Serious dysrhythmias may occur if used with digitalis			Prolonged duration of action; cumulative effects may occur—give drug slowly	
	Can be given orally			May cause tissue sloughing—do not give subcutaneously	
Uses	Vasopressor Allergic states Nasal decongestant Enuresis Myasthenia gravis	Nasal decongestant Vasopressor Paroxysmal atrial tachycardia Mydriatic	Vasopressor	Vasopressor	Vasopressor Paroxysmal atrial tachycardia

*N.S., Not significant.

†Effect is slight, nonexistent, or unknown in humans.

Drug	**Possible Effect and Management**
adrenocorticoids, glucocorticoid, chronic therapy with corticotropin	Ephedrine may increase metabolism of glucocorticoids. Monitor closely because dosage adjustments may be necessary.
urinary alkalizers (antacids containing calcium and/or magnesium, citrates, sodium bicarbonate, and carbonic anhydrase inhibitors)	Alkalinization of the urine decreases excretion of ephedrine. An increase in duration of action and perhaps, ephedrine toxicity may occur. Monitor closely for increased nervousness, inability to sleep at night, and increased irritability or excitability because dosage adjustments may be necessary.
beta adrenergic blocking agents, including ophthalmic preparations	Therapeutic effects of both agents may decrease. An increase in alpha adrenergic activity may result in hypertension, increased bradycardia with the possibility of heart block. If possible, avoid concurrent administration of these drugs. If necessary, monitor closely because therapeutic interventions may be necessary.
digitalis glycosides and anesthetics, inhalation of hydrocarbons such as chloroform, enflurane, halothane and others	Increases risk of inducing serious cardiac dysrhythmias (such as severe ventricular dysrhythmias). If necessary to use concurrently, monitor closely with electrocardiographic readings because therapeutic interventions may be necessary.
ergotamine and ergoloid mesylates	Increased vasoconstriction, severe hypertension, and peripheral vascular ischemia and gangrene may occur. Avoid use of this combination.
maprotiline or tricyclic antidepressants	May decrease blood pressure response to ephedrine. Monitor closely or, if possible, another agent should be considered for administration.
monoamine oxidase (MAO) inhibitors	May result in a serious reaction because of the release of accumulated neurotransmitters into the synapse area, resulting in headaches, dysrhythmias, vomiting, severe hypertension and/or high fevers. Avoid concurrent administration of these drugs because ephedrine should not be given during or within 2 weeks after the administration of an MAO inhibitor.

Dosage and administration
Bronchodilator, decongestant (nasal) or CNS stimulant
Adults. Oral, SC, IM, or slow IV: 25 to 50 mg every 3 or 4 hours as needed
Children. Oral, SC, IM, or slow IV: 3 mg/kg or 100 mg/m^2 a day divided into 4 to 6 doses
Vasopressor effects
Adults. IM or SC, 25 to 50 mg. Repeat if necessary. Slow IV, 5 to 25 mg. This dose may be repeated if necessary in 5 to 10 minutes. Maximum dosage: 150 mg/24 hours
Children. Same as for bronchodilator

Intranasal. For decongestion, several drops of a 0.5% to 1% solution may be applied topically and repeated every 4 hours if necessary.
Pregnancy safety. FDA category C

NURSING CONSIDERATIONS

Assessment. Use with caution in clients with hypertension, hyperthyroidism, prostatic hypertrophy, and diabetes mellitus.

Do not use in clients with severe hypertension, narrow-angle glaucoma, or history of hypersensitivity to sympathomimetic drugs or with those receiving digitalis or MAO inhibitor therapy.

Intervention. Administer only if the solution is clear; discard any unused portion.

If possible, administer a few hours before bedtime and avoid administering at night to help prevent insomnia.

Education. Advise client not to take over-the-counter drugs unless physician is consulted first.

Caution client not to overuse drug because tolerance may develop. It may be necessary to withhold medication for several days to restore effectiveness. Instruct client to follow correct dosage and report any side effects or adverse reactions immediately to the physician. Also, advise client not to swallow nosedrops so as to avoid systemic effects.

Evaluation. During intravenous administration, closely monitor blood pressure repeatedly during first 5 minutes, then check every 3 to 5 minutes until it is stable. *Never leave client unattended during intravenous administration.*

Monitor intake and output, and advise client to report any difficulty in urinating (particularly older male patients).

phenylephrine systemic (Neo-Synephrine injection)
phenylephrine nasal (Neo-Synephrine nasal jelly, Alconefrin, Allerest, Coricidin, Neo-Synephrine, Sinarest nasal solutions)

Phenylephrine is also contained in many combination cough-cold, antihistamine and decongestant, and ophthalmic preparations.

Mechanism of action. While phenylephrine is a dual-acting agent, its primary effects are stimulation of the alpha receptors, resulting in vasoconstriction, and an increase in both diastolic and systolic blood pressures. The drug has little effect on the beta$_1$ receptors of the heart. Its vasoconstricting action is more prolonged than that of epinephrine. For this reason it is often used to treat hypotension caused by myocardial infarction, orthostatic hypotension, and hypotension resulting from loss of vasomotor tone from spinal anesthesia. It is not effective in

TABLE 20-6 Side Effects/Adverse Reactions of Indirect and Dual-Acting Adrenergic Drugs

Drug	Side effects*	Adverse reactions†
ephedrine	Similar to epinephrine—ephedrine not available in aerosol dosage forms so coughing, respiratory difficulties from local irritation are not reported with ephedrine	Similar to epinephrine with addition of mood changes and hallucinations; pallor, pounding heart rate, and bradycardia have not been reported with ephedrine
phenylephrine (Neo-Synephrine Injection)	Less frequent: Anxiety, restlessness, dizziness, tremors, difficult breathing, pallor, increased weakness	Less frequent: Angina or chest pain, allergic reactions reported with preparations containing sulfites (see description under dopamine adverse reactions). Overdosage: Persistent headache, decreased heart rate, hypertension, feeling of congestion in head, tachycardia, vomiting, tingling sensations in hands or feet
mephentermine sulfate (Wyamine sulfate)	Less frequent: Increased anxiety or nervousness, restlessness, tachycardia	Rare: Irregular heart rate, usually in patients with heart problems, convulsions. Overdosage: CNS adverse effects of visual hallucinations, paranoia, psychosis, severe headaches and hypertension also reported; vomiting. On discontinuance of drug, CNS adverse effects disappear.
metaraminol (Aramine)	None noted in USP DI, but monitor for anxiety, restlessness, increased weakness, headaches, nausea and vomiting	Rapid administration may produce cardiac dysrhythmias, pulmonary edema, and cardiac arrest; follow dosage administration recommendations carefully. Rare: Pallor and ischemia at injection site if extravasation occurs; abscess; pain, redness, and swelling at injection site. Overdosage: Severe elevation of blood pressure; convulsions; dysrhythmias. For preparations containing sulfites, allergic reactions may occur (see description under dopamine adverse effects).
methoxamine HCl (Vasoxyl)	Less frequent: Sweating and urinary urgency with high doses	Less frequent: Severe headaches, hypertension, persistent vomiting. High dosages: Bradycardia; for preparations containing sulfites, allergic reactions may occur (see description under dopamine adverse effects

*If side effects continue, increase, or disturb the client, the physician should be informed.
†If adverse reactions occur, the physician should be contacted because medical intervention may be necessary.

shock caused by loss of blood volume.

It is a synthetic adrenergic drug chemically related to epinephrine, norepinephrine, and ephedrine. Phenylephrine hydrochloride is relatively nontoxic, exhibits fewer side effects than epinephrine, and has longer-lasting therapeutic effects. It has little or no effect on the central nervous system.

Phenylephrine has little inotropic or chronotropic effect. It does cause a reflex bradycardia as a result of its ability to elevate the blood pressure, which stimulates the baroreceptors and vagal activity. For this reason it had been used to treat paroxysmal supraventricular tachycardia, but today it has been replaced by more effective and safer drugs.

When applied topically to mucous membranes, it reduces swelling and congestion by constricting the small blood vessels. It is useful in the treatment of sinusitis, vasomotor rhinitis, and hay fever. It is sometimes combined with local anesthetics to retard their systemic absorption and to prolong their action.

Phenylephrine hydrochloride is used as a mydriatic for certain conditions in which dilation of the pupil is desired without cycloplegia (paralysis of the ciliary muscle).

Indications
Used to prevent and/or treat acute hypotension induced during anesthesia, shock, or drug-induced hypotension
Used as vasoconstrictor in regional anesthesia
Applied intranasally for congestion caused by colds, hay fever, sinusitis, or allergies

Ophthalmically, used as a mydriatic, ophthalmic decongestant, and for ophthalmoscopic examinations; also used to treat uveitis

Pharmacokinetics

Absorption. Orally, irregularly absorbed. Nasal decongestion may result in 15 minutes, lasting 2 to 4 hours.

Distribution. To produce vasopressor effects:

IV, an immediate effect with a duration of action of 15 to 20 minutes

IM, effect occurs within 10 to 15 minutes, duration of effect is from ½ to 2 hours

SC, effect occurs within 10 to 15 minutes, duration of effect is from 50 to 60 minutes

Metabolism. Partially in gastrointestinal tract tissues and in the liver by the enzyme monoamine oxidase

Excretion. Not identified

Side effects/adverse reactions. See Table 20-6.

Significant drug interactions. The following interactions may occur when phenylephrine is given with the drugs listed below:

Drug	Possible Effect and Management
alpha receptor–blocking agents	May reduce or block the vasopressor effect of phenylephrine.
anesthetics, inhalation of hydrocarbons such as chloroform, enflurane, halothane and others, plus digitalis glycosides	Increases risk of inducing serious cardiac dysrhythmias. If necessary to use concurrently, monitor closely with electrocardiographic readings because therapeutic interventions may be necessary.
ergotamine and ergoloid mesylates	Increases vasoconstriction; severe hypertension and peripheral vascular ischemia and gangrene may occur. This combined use is not recommended.
doxapram	The vasopressor effects of either or both drugs may increase. Monitor closely since dosage adjustments may be necessary.
maprotiline or tricyclic antidepressants	May potentiate cardiovascular effects of phenylephrine, such as dysrhythmias, increase heart rate, and cause severe hypertension and elevated body temperature. Monitor closely.
methyldopa	May decrease hypotensive effects or increase vasopressor response to phenylephrine. If used concurrently smaller initial dosages of phenylephrine should be given with close monitoring.
monoamine oxidase (MAO) inhibitors	Release of accumulated neurotransmitters into the synapse area, may cause headaches, dysrhythmias, vomiting, severe hypertension, and/or high fevers. Avoid concurrent administration of these drugs because phenylephrine should not be given during or within 2 weeks after the administration of an MAO inhibitor.

Dosage and administration

Hypotension

Adults

IM or SC: initially, 2-5 mg of 1% solution. Maximum is 5 mg. If necessary, may be repeated every 10-15 minutes.

IV: 0.2 mg from a diluted solution (0.1%). Repeat in 15 minutes if necessary.

IV infusion: Initial, 100-180 μg/min until blood pressure is stabilized. (Solution contains 10 mg of phenylephrine to 500 ml 5% dextrose injection or 0.9% sodium chloride injection.) When the client is stabilized, give 40-60 μg/min.

Children. IM or SC, 0.1 mg/kg of body weight or 3 mg/m² of body surface. Repeat in 1-2 hr if necessary. For hypotension during spinal anesthesia, give 44-88 μg/kg/body weight, IM or SC.

To prolong spinal anesthesia. Add 2-5 mg to anesthetic solution (adult dosage).

Intranasal

Nasal jelly (0.5%). Adults: Small amount placed into each nostril every 3 or 4 hr as necessary.

Nasal solution or spray (0.25% to 0.5%)

Adults: 2 or 3 drops or 1 or 2 sprays in each nostril every 3 or 4 hr as necessary.

Children: 6 to 12 years (0.25%): 2 or 3 drops every 3-4 hr as necessary.

Spray (0.25%): 1 or 2 sprays every 3-4 hr as necessary. Less than 6 years (0.125%): 2 or 3 drops every 3-4 hr as necessary.

Nasal decongestant. Oral, 10 mg every 3-4 hr as necessary.

Ophthalmic preparations

Ophthalmoscopy

Adults (2.5% solution): 1 drop to conjunctiva. Repeat once in 15-30 min if necessary.

Children (2.5% solution): 1 drop to conjunctiva. Repeat once in 15-30 min if necessary.

Mydriasis and vasoconstriction

Adults. 1 drop topically to conjunctiva of a 2.5% to 10% solution. If necessary, may repeat in 1 hour.

Children. 1 drop of a 2.5% solution topically to conjunctiva. If necessary, may repeat in 1 hour.

Pregnancy safety. FDA category C

NURSING CONSIDERATIONS

Assessment. Use with caution in individuals with hyperthyroidism, hypertension, diabetes mellitus, ischemic cardiac disease, cerebral arteriosclerosis, or with those undergoing MAO inhibitor therapy.

Do not use in clients with narrow-angle glaucoma (ophthalmic preparations), severe coronary disease, severe hypertension, or ventricular tachycardia.

Intervention. After use, wash nasal tips and droppers with hot water to prevent contamination of solution; eye droppers should not touch the eye or any other surface.

Solutions and jelly lose potency with exposure to air, strong light, or heat. Keep container tightly sealed and away from light. Discard if solution is dark brown or contains a precipitate.

If nasal or ophthalmic preparations are administered to clients with hypertension, timing of the doses should not be at end of dosing periods of the antihypertensive drugs when therapeutic levels of antihypertensive medications are low.

Nasal preparations. Before administration of drug, instruct client to blow nose to clear nasal passages.

Drops: Instill by having client tilt head back and remain in position a few minutes to permit medication to spread through nose.

Spray: Have head upright, and squeeze bottle firmly and quickly to produce spray into each nostril; after 3 to 5 minutes blow nose and repeat.

Jelly: Place in each nostril and sniff well into nose.

IV administration. See nursing considerations under norepinephrine for intravenous administration.

Have phentolamine available to treat hypertensive emergencies.

Education. Instruct client not to swallow solutions or jelly, in order to avoid systemic effects.

Emphasize to client importance of adhering to drug regimen. Consult physician about any modification—dose, time interval, and others.

Alert client that dizziness and drowsiness are common side effects of the drug and activities should be modified to consider those effects. Advise client to avoid the ingestion of alcohol and other CNS depressants that would increase the severity of these effects.

Instruct the client to swallow the extended-release capsules whole.

Tell the client that phenylephrine inhibits salivation, and long-term use promotes caries, gum disease, and oral candidiasis. Regular dental checkups are advised.

Ophthalmic preparations. Instruct client to apply pressure to lacrimal sac during administration of eye drops and for 1 or 2 minutes after instillation.

Caution client about burning and stinging sensation after instillation of drops. Inform client that after instillation of drops, pupils will be dilated and may be sensitive to light.

Notify physician if sensitivity persists beyond 12 hours after discontinuation of drug.

The client with contact lenses should consult the physician for specific instructions.

Evaluation. Monitor for sulfite sensitivity (see box on p. 399).

Pediatric clients are more likely to be sensitive to the vasopressor effects. Elderly clients may demonstrate confusion, sedation, hypotension, dryness of mouth, and urinary retention.

The blood pressure of clients with hypertension should be monitored carefully while they are receiving nasal or ophthalmic preparations of phenylephrine. Any signs of angina should be reported to the physician immediately.

Observe client for rebound miosis (congestion) after topical administration.

mephentermine sulfate (Wyamine sulfate)

Mechanism of action. Mephentermine's effects are similar to those of ephedrine, but it produces more cerebral stimulation.

Mephentermine is a dual-acting (primarily) sympathomimetic. It releases catecholamines from storage sites in the heart and other tissues (indirect action). Therefore it tends to bring about both alpha and beta stimulating effects, including inotropic and chronotropic effects on the heart. Since mephentermine improves cardiac contraction and mobilizes blood from venous pools, thereby increasing cardiac output, it acts as a peripheral vasoconstrictor. (See Table 20-5)

Indications

1. Used as a pressor agent in the treatment of hypotension secondary to ganglionic blockade or spinal anesthesia.
2. Used as an emergency measure in therapy of shock secondary to hemorrhage until blood and blood substitutes become available. In this use, mephentermine has been largely replaced by more effective and safer drugs.

Pharmacokinetics. Administered parenterally. IM: onset of action within 5 to 15 minutes; duration of action is 1 to 4 hours. IV: nearly immediate in action; duration of action is 15 to 30 minutes.

Metabolism. Liver

Excretion. Kidneys

Side effects/adverse reactions. See Table 20-6.

Significant drug interactions. The following interactions may occur when mephentermine is given with the drugs listed below.

Drug	**Possible Effect and Management**
anesthetics, inhalation of hydrocarbons such as chloroform, enflurane, halothane and others, plus Digitalis glycosides	Increase risk of inducing serious cardiac dysrhythmias. If used concurrently, monitor closely with electrocardiographic readings because therapeutic interventions may be necessary.
maprotiline or tricyclic antidepressants	May decrease blood pressure response to mephentermine. Monitor closely.
beta adrenergic blocking agents	May result in decreased therapeutic effects of both drugs. An increase in alpha adrenergic activity may result in hyper-

Drug	Possible Effect and Management
	tension, increased bradycardia, and the possibility of heart block. If possible, avoid concurrent drug administration. If necessary, monitor closely because therapeutic interventions may be necessary.
doxapram	The vasopressor effects of either or both drugs may increase. Also possible to increase CNS stimulation. Monitor closely because dosage adjustments may be necessary.
ergotamine and ergoloid mesylates	Increased vasoconstriction, severe hypertension and peripheral vascular ischemia and gangrene may occur. Combined use is not recommended.
monoamine oxidase (MAO) inhibitors	The release of accumulated neurotransmitters into synapse area may cause headaches, dysrhythmias, vomiting, severe hypertension and/or high fevers. Avoid concurrent administration of these drugs because phenylephrine should not be given during or within 2 weeks after the administration of an MAO inhibitor.
sympathomimetics	When administered with other sympathomimetics, enhances CNS stimulation and possibly causes an increase in cardiovascular side effects. Monitor closely.

Dosage and administration. For hypotension:

Adults: 30 to 45 mg IV in a single injection. Repeat doses of 30 mg as needed to maintain blood pressure. IV infusion, add 600 mg of mephentermine to 500 ml of 5% dextrose in water. Rate of administration is determined by physician according to individual's response to the infusion.

Children: IM or IV, 0.4 mg/kg body weight or 12 mg/m² of body surface as a single dose. If necessary, it may be repeated. IV infusion, same as adult.

Pregnancy safety. Not established

NURSING CONSIDERATIONS

Assessment. Use cautiously in individuals with arteriosclerosis, hypertension, cardiovascular disease, hyperthyroidism, and chronically ill patients.

Drug may cause uterine contraction; therefore it should not be administered to pregnant women. The drug is contraindicated in individuals receiving MAO inhibitors, anesthetics (cyclopropane, halothane), or chlorpromazine.

Intervention. Administer using an infusion device to precisely regulate dosage according to the response of the client.

Evaluation. Monitor closely blood pressure, pulse, ECG, central venous pressure, and urinary output. The

blood pressure and pulse should be checked every 2 minutes until stabilized, then every 5 to 15 minutes thereafter during therapy. The blood pressure should be maintained at slightly less than the client's normal blood pressure. In clients with hypertension, maintain at 30 to 40 mm Hg below usual blood pressure.

Observe client for possible development of tolerance if repeated injections are administered. Note that blood volume replacement must be instituted as soon as possible in treatment of secondary shock.

metaraminol (Aramine)

Mechanism of action. Metaraminol is a vasopressor agent with both direct (primarily) and indirect effects on the sympathetic system. It acts indirectly by releasing norepinephrine from tissues and storage sites and directly as a neurohormone. Metaraminol has positive inotropic effects. Since it constricts blood vessels, increases peripheral resistance, elevates both systolic and diastolic blood pressure, and improves cardiac contractility and cerebral, coronary, and renal blood flow, the drug is used for the treatment of shock.

Since metaraminol exhibits beta as well as alpha adrenergic activity, it is often effective in raising blood pressure when alpha adrenergic agents are ineffective. This may be because of its ability to bring about more effective venous flow. It does not appear to cause dysrhythmias. It generally lacks CNS stimulatory effects. (See Table 20-5.) Although similar to norepinephrine in action, it is generally considered a less potent drug.

Indications. Used for hypotensive states occurring with spinal anesthesia. Also administered for the prevention and treatment of acute hypotension associated with surgery, drug-induced reactions, and shock.

Pharmacokinetics. Parenteral only. IV: onset is within 1 to 2 minutes; duration of action is approximately 20 minutes. SC or IM: onset of action is 10 minutes (IM) or 5 to 20 minutes (SC). Duration of action is approximately 60 minutes (IM and SC).

Metabolism. Liver

Excretion. Bile and kidneys

Side effects/adverse reactions. See Table 20-6.

Significant drug interactions. The following interactions may occur when metaraminol is given with the drugs listed below:

Drug	Possible Effect and Management
anesthetics, inhalation of hydrocarbons such as chloroform, enflurane, halothane and others, plus digitalis glycosides	Increases risk of inducing serious cardiac dysrhythmias. If necessary to use concurrently, monitor client closely with electrocardiographic readings because therapeutic interventions may be necessary.
alpha adrenergic blocking agents	May decrease the vasopressor effects of metaraminol.

Drug	Possible Effect and Management
beta adrenergic blocking agents	Therapeutic effects of both drugs may decrease. An increase in alpha adrenergic activity may result in hypertension and increase bradycardia with the possibility of heart block. If possible, avoid concurrent administration of these drugs. If necessary, monitor closely because therapeutic interventions may be necessary.
doxapram	The vasopressor effects of either or both drugs may increase. Monitor closely because dosage adjustments may be necessary.
ergotamine and ergoloid mesylates	Increased vasoconstriction, severe hypertension, and peripheral vascular ischemia and gangrene may occur. Combined use is not recommended.
maprotiline or tricyclic antidepressants	Cardiovascular side effects may occur, such as dysrhythmias, increased heart rate, and possibly severe hypertension or hyperpyrexia.
guanadrel or guanethidine	If given during or within 5 days of discontinuing guanethidine, hypertension may occur. The pressor effect of metaraminol is enhanced, but the antihypertensive effect of guanadrel or guanethidine is decreased. Hypertension and cardiac dysrhythmias may be induced. Monitor closely.
monoamine oxidase (MAO) inhibitors	The release of accumulated neurotransmitters into synapse area may result in headaches, dysrhythmias, vomiting, severe hypertension and/or high fevers. Avoid concurrent administration of these drugs because metaraminol should not be given during or within 2 weeks after the administration of an MAO inhibitor.

Dosage and administration. Parenteral only.

Adults

SC, IM to prevent hypotension. Administer 2 to 10 mg. To avoid cumulative effects, wait 10 minutes before giving additional doses.

IV infusion, 15 to 100 mg in 500 ml of sodium chloride injection (0.9%) or 5% dextrose in water. Administer at rate determined by physician to maintain the desired blood pressure response.

Direct IV injection for severe shock, 0.5 to 5 mg followed by the infusion described above.

Children

SC, IM, 0.1 mg/kg body weight or 3 mg/m^2 of body surface.

IV infusion, 0.4 mg/kg body weight or 12 mg/m^2 body surface. Dilution contains 1 mg in 25 ml of 0.9% sodium chloride solution or 5% dextrose in water. Administer at rate determined by physician to maintain the desired blood pressure response.

Direct IV injection for severe shock, 0.01 mg/kg body weight or 300 μg/m^2 body surface.

Pregnancy safety. Not established.

NURSING CONSIDERATIONS

Assessment. Use drug with caution in individuals with hypertension, peripheral vascular disease, thyroid disease, diabetes mellitus, cirrhosis of liver, and in individuals taking digitalis or MAO inhibitors.

Do not use in individuals with cyclopropane or halothane anesthesia or with those hypersensitive to metaraminol.

Intervention. Subcutaneous injection is rarely given since it causes tissue necrosis. Moreover, avoid extravasation during intravenous infusion. Monitor closely to prevent injury to local tissue and necrosis. The use of larger veins may be helpful during infusion. Have on hand phentolamine (decreases pressor effect) and atropine (for bradycardia).

Metaraminol must be diluted before administration. Once diluted, it should be used within 24 hours. Because metaraminol is incompatible with many drugs, it should not be administered in a solution containing other medications.

Evaluation. Closely monitor blood pressure every 2 to 5 min during infusion (client must be constantly attended). Since the drug has a prolonged effect, adjust flow rate carefully to avoid a cumulative response. Before terminating infusion, reduce flow rate gradually to avoid abrupt withdrawal of drug, which otherwise may result in severe hypotension. If possible, correct plasma volume before starting therapy. Continue to monitor blood pressure closely after the drug has been discontinued. If severe hypotension occurs, the drug should be resumed quickly.

Monitor for cardiac arrhythmias.

Monitor intake and output; also monitor sodium and potassium loss because clients with cirrhosis of liver may suffer from diuresis.

Monitor for sulfite sensitivity (see box on p. 399).

---

methoxamine hydrochloride (Vasoxyl)

Mechanism of action. Methoxamine is an alpha adrenergic stimulator that appears to be devoid of beta receptor activity. Therefore it is almost exclusively a vasoconstrictor. The direct-acting sympathomimetic agent is pharmacologically related to phenylephrine. Since it has no stimulating effect on the heart, the rise in blood pressure causes a reflex bradycardia. This effect makes it useful in treating paroxysmal supraventricular tachycardia. (See Table 20-5.)

Indications

1. Used to restore or maintain blood pressure during anesthesia
2. Used to terminate paroxysmal supraventricular tachycardia

Pharmacokinetics. Parenteral drug. IV administration: effects are immediate; duration of action as a vasopressor is 5 to 15 minutes. IM: effects seen within 15 to 20 minutes; duration of effects are 60 to 90 minutes. Metabolism and excretion routes: unknown.

Side effects/adverse reactions. See Table 20-6.

Significant drug interactions. The following interactions may occur when methoxamine is given with the drugs listed below.

Drug	Possible Effect and Management
alpha adrenergic blocking agents	May decrease the vasopressor effects of methoxamine.
maprotiline or tricyclic antidepressants	May increase cardiovascular adverse effects of methoxamine, resulting in dysrhythmias, increased heart rate, possibly severe hypertension or hyperpyrexia. Methoxamine should not be given concurrently or within 1 week of a tricyclic antidepressant.
digitalis glycoside	Increases risk of cardiac toxicity. Avoid if possible. If must be given, monitor closely with electrocardiographic monitoring.
ergoloid mesylate or ergotamine	Increased vasoconstriction, severe hypertension, and peripheral vascular ischemia and gangrene may occur. Combined use is not recommended.
doxapram	The vasopressor effects of either or both drugs may increase. Monitor closely because dosage adjustments may be necessary.

Dosage and administration. As vasopressor:

Adults. 10 to 15 mg IM or 3 to 5 mg given slowly by direct IV. Maximum: IM, 20 mg as a single injection up to a maximum of 60 mg in 24 hours; IV, up to 10 mg as a single injection.

Children. IM, 0.25 mg/kg body weight or 7.5 mg/m^2 of body surface; IV, 0.08 mg/kg body weight or 2.5 mg/m^2 body surface.

Pregnancy safety. FDA category C.

NURSING CONSIDERATIONS

Assessment. Use cautiously in clients with hyperthyroidism, pheochromocytoma, or hypertension and also following parenteral injection of ergot alkaloids.

Do not use in combination with local anesthetics to prolong their action and in clients with cardiovascular disease.

Intervention. Intramuscular doses may need to be repeated. If so, allow sufficient time for previous injection to have taken effect before considering administering another.

Administer IV slowly if the systolic pressure falls below 60 or in another emergency.

Evaluation. Monitor the blood pressure (BP) and pulse continuously during therapy and titrate the dose accordingly. The BP should be maintained at slightly less than the client's normal blood pressure. In clients with hypertension, maintain at 30 to 40 mm Hg below usual BP. Observe client for severe bradycardia with rhythm strips. Have atropine available if bradycardia occurs. Monitor intake and output because output increases when normal blood pressure levels occur (if the client is not hypovolemic). Observe client for sudden changes of blood pressure after the drug is terminated.

Monitor for sulfite sensitivity (see box on p. 399).

ADRENERGIC BLOCKING (SYMPATHOLYTIC) DRUGS
ALPHA ADRENERGIC BLOCKING DRUGS

Most **alpha adrenergic blocking agents** are competitive blockers; that is, they compete with the catecholamines at receptor sites and inhibit adrenergic sympathetic stimulation. They are more effective against the action of circulating catecholamines than against catecholamines released from storage sites in the neurons. These drugs may be obtained from natural sources, such as ergot and its derivatives, or they may be synthesized.

The alpha adrenergic blocking agents fall into three categories:

1. Noncompetitive, long-acting antagonists (e.g., phenoxybenzamine): action persists for several days or weeks because a stable bond is formed between a specific component of the drug and the alpha receptor site.
2. Competitive, short-acting antagonists (e.g., phentolamine, tolazoline): the blocking action is reversible and competitive at the alpha receptor site and the effects last only several hours.
3. Ergot alkaloids: usually act as partial alpha adrenergic antagonists. However, the drugs produce primarily a spasmogenic effect on smooth muscle of blood vessels, thereby causing vasoconstriction.

Noncompetitive, Long-Acting Antagonists
phenoxybenzamine (Dibenzyline)

Mechanism of action. Phenoxybenzamine is a long-acting alpha adrenergic blocking agent. The agent abolishes or decreases the receptiveness of alpha receptors to adrenergic stimuli. Its effects are mainly those of vasodilation and inhibition of vasospasm.

Since phenoxybenzamine competes with the catecholamines, it is also useful in decreasing the blood pressure of patients with pheochromocytoma. It does not block sympathetic impulses on the heart and therefore does not directly impair cardiac output. It has mild antihistaminic activity and may dry out nasal passages.

Indications. Used in the management of pheochromocytoma: preoperative preparation of client for surgery, chronic treatment of individuals with malignant pheochromocytoma, and individuals for whom surgery of pheochromocytoma is contraindicated.

Pharmacokinetics

Absorption. Oral absorption of the drug is variable

Distribution. Onset of action occurs in 2 hours. The drug can persist for 3 or 4 days since it forms a stable bond with the receptor. The half-life is about 24 hours.

Excretion. Kidney and bile

Side effects/adverse reactions. See Table 20-7.

Significant drug interactions. When phenoxybenzamine is given with other sympathomimetics, such as epinephrine, metaraminol, methoxamine and phenylephrine, the results may be as follows:

1. Blocking of the alpha adrenergic receptor effects of epinephrine, which may result in severe hypotension and increased tachycardia
2. Decrease in the vasopressor effects of metaraminol
3. Blocking of the vasopressor effect of methoxamine, resulting in severe hypotension
4. Decrease in the vasopressor effect to phenylephrine

Avoid concurrent drug administration if at all possible.

Dosage and administration

Adults. Initially, 10 mg twice daily orally; may increase by 10 mg every other day until the desired effect is noted. Maintenance: 20 to 40 mg two or three times daily.

Children. Initially, 0.2 mg/kg body weight orally or 6 mg/m^2 body surface, up to a maximum of 10 mg, given once daily; dosage may be increased every 4 days until the desired effect is noted. Maintenance: 0.4 mg to 1.2 mg/kg body weight or 12 to 36 mg/m^2 body surface daily, given in 3 or 4 divided doses.

Pregnancy safety. Not established

NURSING CONSIDERATIONS

Assessment. Use with caution in clients with renal insufficiency, marked cerebral or coronary arteriosclerosis, and respiratory infections.

Do not use in clients with compensated congestive failure because it will cause angina and congestive heart failure, or in conditions when a decrease in blood pressure might be dangerous, such as cerebrovascular insufficiency.

Intervention. Administer the oral drug with milk to reduce gastric irritation.

Adjust dosage according to the clinical response and level of urinary catecholamines.

Increase dosage gradually from the lowest therapeutic dose, but the increments should be no more frequent than every 4 days.

Treat overdosage by intravenous infusion of norepi-

TABLE 20-7　Side Effects/Adverse Reactions of Adrenergic Blocking Drugs

Drug	Side effects*	Adverse reactions†
phenoxybenzamine (Dibenzyline)	More frequent: Dizziness (postural hypotension), miosis, tachycardia, nasal congestion. Less frequent: Lethargy, confusion, dry mouth, headache, weakness, inhibition of ejaculation	None noted in USP DI but monitor closely, especially if patient is receiving large doses
phentolamine HCl (Regitine, Rogitine♣)	More frequent: Diarrhea, dizziness (postural hypotension), nausea, vomiting, abdominal pain Less frequent: Nasal congestion, flushing	More frequent: Tachycardia Less frequent: Increased weakness, fainting. Rare (following parenteral): Angina or chest pain, respiratory distress, myocardial infarction, cerebrovascular accident (confusion, severe headache, loss of coordination, slurred speech)
tolazoline (Priscoline)	None noted in USP-DI; monitor closely since most adverse effects are serious.	More frequent: Gastrointestinal bleeding, systemic alkalosis (hypochloremic), hypotension, thrombocytopenia, oliguria or acute renal failure Less frequent: Nausea, vomiting or diarrhea, skin flushing, piloerection, tachycardia

*If side effects continue, increase, or disturb the client, the physician should be informed.

†If adverse reactions occur, the physician should be contacted because medical intervention may be necessary.

nephrine. Do not use epinephrine since it will cause a further drop in blood pressure.

Education. Advise client to make position changes slowly (from recumbent to upright posture) to prevent orthostatic hypotension. Instruct client to dangle legs and exercise feet for a few minutes at the bedside before standing. If faintness or weakness occurs, a head-low position should be assumed or the person must lie down immediately. Physician may prescribe support stockings to help prevent orthostatic hypotension.

Advise the client to modify activities if dizziness and/or drowsiness occur.

Advise the client that because the drug inhibits salivary flow and thus promotes the development of caries, peridontal disease, and buccal candidiasis, regular dental checkups are required. Dryness of the mouth can be relieved by ice chips and sugarless gum.

Warn client against using any other drug, particularly over-the-counter sympathomimetics without consulting the physician.

An effect of this drug can be inhibition of ejaculation, which should be reported to the physician.

Evaluation. Monitor blood pressure and pulse rate both in recumbent and standing positions during period of dosage adjustment, particularly when dosage is increased. Observe client for signs of hypotension and tachycardia. Inform client that these signs usually disappear with continued therapy. However, with the vasodilation associated with exercise, drinking alcohol, or eating a large meal, these signs may recur.

Clients with pheochromocytoma will note decreases in blood pressure, pulse, and sweating that are signs of therapeutic effectiveness.

Competitive, Short-Acting Antagonists
phentolamine hydrochloride (Regitine, Rogitine✶)

Mechanism of action. Phentolamine is an alpha adrenergic blocking agent. It competitively blocks alpha$_2$ (presynaptic) and alpha$_1$ (postsynaptic) receptors. The action occurs at both arterial and venous vessels. This direct relaxation of vascular smooth muscle lowers total peripheral resistance. Accordingly, hypertension is inhibited when there are excessive levels of epinephrine and norepinephrine. It also decreases pulmonary vascular resistance. Phentolamine exerts a histamine-like action that enhances the secretion of hydrochloric acid and pepsin. It also stimulates beta receptors, which increases heart rate and cardiac output.

Indications
1. Used to prevent or control hypertensive episodes in the patient with pheochromocytoma
2. Used to reverse the vasoconstrictive action of an overdose or excessive response to injected norepi-

nephrine (Levophed) or dopamine. The subcutaneous injection of phentolamine following extravasation of intravenous norepinephrine or dopamine will prevent tissue necrosis if prompt action is taken. Use after dopamine extravasation is investigational at this time.
3. Phentolamine is used in the diagnosis of pheochromocytoma. Since this tumor secretes large amounts of catecholamines, which elevate blood pressure, a marked fall in blood pressure after administration of phentolamine suggests the presence of pheochromocytoma. However, this test lacks precision. A false-positive test may occur if the patient recently received a sedative, narcotic, or antihypertensive drug. (Measurement of urinary catecholamines provides a more accurate diagnosis.)

Pharmacokinetics
Absorption. Poorly absorbed; only approximately 20% of the drug is active following oral administration. Preferred method of administration is parenteral. Phentolamine test if positive: peak effects are seen within 20 minutes (IM) or 2 minutes (IV); duration of action is 30 to 45 minutes (IM) and 15 to 30 minutes (IV).

Metabolism and excretion. Unknown; only about 10% of drug found in urine after parenteral administration

Side effects/adverse reactions. See Table 20-7.

Significant drug interactions. Same as phenoxybenzamine.

Dosage and administration
Adults
Phentolamine test: 5 mg IV

Antiadrenergic preoperative: 5 mg IV 1 to 2 hours before surgery, may be repeated if needed; during surgery, 5 mg IV or 0.5 mg to 1 mg/min by intravenous infusion.

Children
Phentolamine test: 3 mg (IM) or 1 mg or 0.1 mg/kg body weight or 3 mg/m^2 body surface (IV)

Antiadrenergic preoperative: 1 mg or 0.1 mg/kg body weight or 3 mg/m^2 body surface area (IM or IV) given 1 to 2 hours before surgery, may be repeated if needed; during surgery, 1 mg or 0.1 mg/kg body weight or 3 mg/m^2 body surface area, adjust as necessary according to patient response.

Pregnancy safety. Not established.

NURSING CONSIDERATIONS

Assessment. Use with caution in clients with coronary artery disease, gastritis, and peptic ulcer.

Do not use in clients with hypersensitivity to phentolamine or in those with a history of myocardial infarction.

Intervention. During intravenous administration, individual must be in supine position.

Test for pheochromocytoma: Before test, withhold all medications for 24 to 72 hours. The client is placed in a supine position in a quiet, nonstimulating environment. The blood pressure is taken every 10 minutes for at least 30 minutes until the blood pressure is stabilized at basal level. After the physician administers the drug, the blood pressure is taken at 30-second intervals for first 3 minutes, then at 1-minute intervals for next 7 minutes. Positive test results indicated by a drop in systolic pressure of at least 35 mm Hg and diastolic pressure of 25 mm Hg, suggests the presence of pheochromocytoma. The blood pressure returns to pretest levels in 15 to 30 minutes.

When phentolamine is used to prevent sloughing of tissue following IV administration of norepinephrine, 10 mg may be added to every liter of intravenous fluids containing norepinephrine without affecting its vasopressor effect. If extravasation has already occurred, 5 to 10 mg of phentolamine in 10 ml of 0.9% sodium chloride injection should be immediately infiltrated into the affected area. However, this treatment is ineffective if 12 or more hours have passed since the extravasation.

Education. After therapy, advise client to rise slowly from bed and remain in sitting position for a few minutes before standing upright, to prevent orthostatic hypotension.

Evaluation. Monitor blood pressure and pulse every 2 minutes until stabilized.

tolazoline (Priscoline)

Mechanism of action. Like phentolamine, tolazoline produces a moderately effective competitive alpha adrenergic blocking action. However, tolazoline is considerably less potent. It acts as a vasodilator by a direct relaxant effect on vascular smooth muscle. It reduces pulmonary arterial pressure and peripheral vascular resistance.

Indications. Used to treat persistent pulmonary hypertension in the newborn when systemic arterial levels of oxygen cannot be maintained by oxygen supplementation and/or mechanical ventilation machines

Pharmacokinetics. Parenteral administration: onset of action is within ½ hour of inital dose. Half-life in neonates is 3 to 10 hours. Excretion: Kidneys, mainly unchanged.

Side effects/adverse reactions. See Table 20-7.

Significant drug interactions. None noted.

Dosage and administration. Given parenterally

Children. 1 to 2 mg/kg body weight (IV) initially via a scalp vein over a 5 to 10 minute period. Maintenance: 1 to 2 mg/kg body weight by IV infusion per hour; when arterial blood gases appear to be remaining stable, the drug may be gradually withdrawn.

NURSING CONSIDERATIONS

Assessment. Tolazoline should not be used when systemic hypotension (systolic blood pressure less than 40 mm Hg) exists.

Caution must be used when administering in the presence of acidosis or mitral stenosis.

Intervention. Administered only in pediatric or neonatal intensive care units where respiratory support is immediately available.

Use an infusion pump or micro drip regulator for administration to allow for precise flow regulation.

Pretreatment with antacids may be necessary to prevent stress ulcers secondary to the increase in gastric secretion caused by the drug.

Evaluation. Monitor the client's response to the drug through ECG, blood gases, blood pressure, and pulse rates. Also observe serum electrolyte levels, particularly sodium and potassium levels.

To monitor for gastrointestinal bleeding, perform a hematest of gastric aspirates.

ergot alkaloids:
dihydroergotamine mesylate (D.H.E. 45)
ergoloid mesylates (Hydergine, Hydergine LC, Deapril-ST)
ergotamine tartrate (Ergomar, Ergostat, Gynergen✶)
ergotamine tartrate and caffeine (Cafergot, Cafertabs, Cafetrate)
methysergide maleate (Sansert)

Mechanism of action. For many years the ergot alkaloids were the only alpha adrenergic blocking agents available. Ergot is a fungus that grows on rye, and when it is hydrolyzed, many of its derivatives dissociate to yield lysergic acid diethylamide (LSD). These alkaloids have diverse and somewhat contradictory effects. The ergot alkaloids listed here are alpha adrenergic blockers; however not all ergot derivatives are alpha adrenergic blockers. With the exception of ergoloid mesylates, all of the ergot alkaloids may be used to treat migraine and other vascular headaches. The exact mechanism of action of ergoloid mesylates is unknown but they increase cerebral blood flow and metabolism in the brain, and so are used to treat cerebrovascular insufficiency. The other ergot alkaloids stimulate smooth muscle, especially of the blood vessels and the uterus, so they decrease the cerebral blood supply.

The early phase of a migraine attack is associated with constriction of the cranial blood vessels. It is characterized by visual symptoms and malaise and appears as a warning or "aura" of an oncoming attack. This is followed by the painful phase of a migraine headache that results in cranial vasodilation. The increase in blood flow in the vessels produces pulsations that appear to be the source of the pain. The ergot alkaloids act as alpha adrenergic blocking agents and depress the central vasomotor center. They cause vasoconstriction of cranial blood vessels during the vasodilation phase, thereby reducing the pulsation thought to be responsible for the headache. The drugs also possess antiserotonin activity. Abnormalities in the metabolism of serotonin may play a role in the migraine syndrome. Serum levels of serotonin have been found to drop spontaneously just before a migraine attack. In addition, during the attack an increased quantity of serotonin metabolites are excreted in the urine. Evidence exists that the drugs that act favorably in alleviating migraine influence serotonin metabolism. Methysergide acts as a serotonin inhibitor, which may function as a "headache" substance that lowers the pain threshold. It also acts as a potent vasoconstrictor. (See Chapter 38 for serotonin activity.)

Indications
1. Used for treatment of vascular headaches, such as migraine and cluster headaches. The drug must be given early in an attack; it does not prevent migraine attacks (dihydroergotamine mesylate and ergotamine tartrate).
2. Used for treatment of cerebrovascular insufficiency (ergoloid mesylates).
3. Used for prevention of vascular headaches, such as migraine and cluster headaches (methysergide maleate).

Pharmacokinetics
Absorption
dihydroergotamine—administered parenterally
ergoloid mesylates—slowly and erratically absorbed from gastrointestinal tract
ergotamine tartrate and ergotamine tartrate and caffeine—oral, without caffeine, slow and erratic. Caffeine is said to aid oral absorption. Aerosol dosage form, well absorbed.
methysergide—good absorption
Onset of action
dihydroergotamine mesylate—IM, 15 to 30 minutes; IV, within 5 minutes
ergoloid mesylates—response usually seen within 3 to 4 weeks or longer
ergotamine tartrate and ergotamine tartrate and caffeine—within 1 to 2 hours
methysergide maleate—24 to 48 hours
Duration of action
dihydroergotamine mesylate—IM, 3 to 4 hours
methysergide maleate—within 24 to 48 hours
Half-life
dihydroergotamine mesylate—within 1.3 to 3.9 hours
ergoloid mesylates—3.5 hours

ergotamine tartrate and ergotamine tartrate and caffeine—about 2 hours
Metabolism. Liver
Excretion
dihydroergotamine mesylate—kidney
ergotamine tartrate and ergotamine tartrate and caffeine—bile
methysergide maleate—kidney
Side effects/adverse reactions. See Table 20-8.
Significant drug interactions. When ergot alkaloids are given with other ergot alkaloids, vasopressors or vasoconstrictors, the combination may result in increased vasoconstriction, ischemia, and possibly gangrene. Avoid this drug combination.

Dosage and administration
dihydroergotamine mesylate
Adults
IM: 1 mg at start of attack; repeat dosage of 1 mg every hour as needed up to 3 mg per migraine attack or 6 mg a week.
IV: 1 mg at start of attack; if needed, give 1 mg in an hour up to 2 mg per migraine attack or 6 mg a week.
ergoloid mesylates
Adults. 1 to 2 mg orally or sublingually, three times daily.
ergotamine tartrate
Adults. 2 mg orally initially, may repeat in ½ hour if needed, maximum is 6 mg per day or 10 mg in 1 week. Sublingual dosage: 1 mg initially, may repeat in ½ to 1 hour if necessary; if repeat dose is needed, at beginning of next attack, start with the larger dose; maximum for initial dose is 5 mg; maximum per week is 10 mg.
Children. For adolescents and older children, sublingually, 1 mg dose; repeat in ½ hour if necessary.
ergotamine tartrate and caffeine
Adults. Oral dosage (tablets or capsules): see sublingual dosage for ergotamine tartrate. Suppositories: one rectally initially; if necessary, a second suppository may be inserted in 1 hour; maximum is 2 suppositories per migraine attack or 5 suppositories in 1 week.
methysergide maleate
Adults. 4 to 6 mg orally in divided doses, taken with milk or meals.
Pregnancy safety. FDA category X for ergotamine tartrate and ergotamine tartrate and caffeine during pregnancy; other drugs unclassified but may also represent a risk if used during pregnancy.

NURSING CONSIDERATIONS

Assessment. Do not use in clients with pulmonary or collagen diseases, valvular heart disorders, and debilitated states.

TABLE 20-8   Side Effects/Adverse Reactions of Ergot Alkaloids

Drug(s)	Side effects*	Adverse reactions†
dihydroergotamine (D.H.E. 45)	Less frequent: Nausea, vomiting, headache, dizziness	Less frequent: Pruritus, edema of lower extremities, leg weakness Rare: Red colored blisters on hands or feet might be the first indication of gangrene; bradycardia or tachycardia Overdosage: Vasoconstriction leading to numbness, tingling and perhaps pain in the fingers, toes, arms, legs, face or back; cold hands and feet If headaches persist after medication is stopped, medical intervention is necessary.
ergoloid mesylates (hydergine, hydergine LC, Deapril-ST)	Less frequent: Dizziness (postural hypotension), sedation, bradycardia, rash, sublingual usage-soreness under tongue reported	Overdosage: Headaches, flushing, anorexia, nausea, vomiting, abdominal cramps, nasal congestion, impaired vision, dizziness, fainting
ergotamine tartrate (Ergomar, Ergostat, Gynergen♣) ergotamine tartrate and caffeine (Cafergot, Cafertabs, Cafetrate)	More frequent: Diarrhea, nausea, vomiting, dizziness	More frequent: Edema of lower extremities (feet, lower legs), numbness or tingling feelings in toes, fingers, or face Dose-related: Peripheral vasoconstriction or vasospasms (pruritus, cold hands or feet, leg weakness, pain in arms, legs or lower back) Less frequent: Confusion, visual disturbances, angina or chest pain, red colored blisters on hands or feet might be early sign of gangrene; abdominal pain and gas Acute overdosage: Bradycardia or tachycardia, increased weakness, confusion, abdominal pain, gas or bloating, shortness of breath Chronic overdosage: Depression; headaches; nausea or vomiting that persists or is severe; pain in arms, legs, or lower back (severe); increased weakness; cold hands or feet If headaches persist after medication is stopped, medical intervention is necessary.
methysergide maleate (Sansert)	More frequent: Diarrhea, dizziness, (postural hypotension), sedation, nausea, vomiting or abdominal pain Less frequent: Ataxia, depression or insomnia	More frequent: Pruritus, leg weakness, feelings of numbness or tingling sensations in fingers, toes, or face Less frequent: Visual disturbances, increased excitability, distortions of body image, hallucinations, nightmares, difficulty in thinking, anxiety.

*If side effects continue, increase, or disturb client, the physician should be informed.
†If adverse reactions occur, the physician should be contacted because medical intervention may be necessary.

Continued.

TABLE 20-8   Side Effects/Adverse Reactions of Ergot Alkaloids—cont'd

Drug(s)	Side effects*	Adverse reactions†
methysergide maleate (Sansert)—cont'd		Overdosage: Severe dizziness, unusual excitability, pale and cold extremities (hands or feet) Monitor for signs of fibrosis, a rare but serious complication. Large blood vessel fibrosis: edema of hands or ankles, cold hands and feet, complaints of leg cramps or pain in lower back Pleuropulmonary fibrosis: dyspnea, chest pain, fever Retroperitoneal fibrosis: ureteral obstruction; fever, flank or groin pain, anorexia, weight loss, dysuria or painful urination

*If side effects continue, increase, or disturb client, the physician should be informed.
†If adverse reactions occur, the physician should be contacted because medical intervention may be necessary.

Intervention. Administer oral dosage of methysergide with food to minimize gastrointestinal irritation.

Because there is a potential for serious side effects with methysergide, client should be advised to keep clinical appointments so that blood count, sedimentation rate, renal function, pulmonary function, and cardiac status may be assessed.

Methysergide is not administered continuously for more than 6 months; a drug-free period of 3 to 4 weeks must occur before the drug is restarted. Advise client to withdraw drug gradually over 2 to 3-week period to prevent "headache rebound" resulting from abrupt drug withdrawal. If the drug does not provide a therapeutic response after a 3-week trial period, it is unlikely that longer administration will be of benefit.

Education. Tell client to take initial dose of drug during early part of migraine attack, during "aura" (visual field defects, scintillating scotomas, paresthesia, and nausea). The client then should lie down in a quiet, dark room for several hours. Assure the client that the quality of relief is related to the promptness with which the medication is started after the onset of symptoms.

Warn client to take drug exactly as prescribed. Prolonged use or overdose can cause circulatory impairment (ergot poisoning): numbness, tingling sensation, weakness, intermittent claudication, cyanosis of extremities, muscle pain and coldness of extremities. Report symptoms immediately to physician. If not corrected, gangrene may develop. Severe peripheral vasoconstriction may be treated by administering intravenous sodium nitroprusside. Discontinuing the drug for 2 to 3 days may relieve these symptoms.

Instruct the client to avoid alcohol ingestion because it aggravates the headache.

Counseling should be provided for smoking cessation since nicotine increases the peripheral vasoconstriction effects of the drug. For the same reason, clients should be instructed to avoid exposure to cold.

Tell the client of the signs and symptoms of infection with the caution to report these to the physician as infection increases the sensitivity to the drug.

Warn female clients of childbearing age not to use ergot alkaloids because of potential oxytocic effects during pregnancy.

Clients with migraine may require assistance to identify physical and emotional stresses that cause migraine attack. Relaxation techniques, adequate rest, and avoidance of stressful situations may alleviate the severity or frequency of attacks.

Instruct the client in the proper method of taking sublingual tablets, including the avoidance of eating, drinking, and smoking until the tablet is completely dissolved.

Evaluation. Palpate peripheral pulses at monthly intervals to detect ergotism as early as possible.

Do not use drug in clients with occlusive peripheral vascular disease, renal or hepatic diseases, hypertension, severe pruritis, arteriosclerosis, coronary artery disease, infectious states, or malnutrition, or in children or pregnant women.

• • •

Methysergide. Nursing considerations with methysergide include the following, as well as those already listed.

An allergic reaction to the dye tartrazine (FD&C yellow No. 5) contained in methysergide tablets frequently occurs in clients also allergic to aspirin.

Regular examination must be performed by physician for possible development of fibrotic (formation of tissue) and vascular complications. Retroperitoneal fibrosis, as well as cardiac fibrosis, has been noted in a small number of patients. Often these conditions regress when the drug is discontinued.

Instruct client how to limit weight gain by checking for edema (daily weight) and by maintaining low salt intake and low caloric diet. Inform client of possible occurrence of postural hypotension. Position changes from recumbent to upright position should be made slowly to avoid dizziness or fainting. Alert the client to the possible need to modify activities if dizziness and drowsiness occur as side effects.

BETA ADRENERGIC BLOCKING AGENTS

    acebutolol (Sectral)
    atenolol (Tenormin)
    esmolol HC1 (Brevibloc)
    labetalol (Normodyne, Trandate)
    metoprolol (Lopressor, Apo-Metoprolol✦,
    Betaloc✦)
    nadolol (Corgard)
    oxyprenolol✦ (Trasicor✦)
    pindolol (Visken)
    propranolol (Inderal, Inderal LA, Apo-Propranolol✦,
    Detensol✦)
    timolol (Blocadren)

Beta blockers inhibit the beta receptors by competing with the catecholamines at the effector site.

Beta adrenergic blocking agents are differentiated into two subclasses: beta$_1$ and beta$_2$ blockers. They are also identified as follows:

1. Drugs that selectively inhibit only one type of receptor—beta$_1$ or beta$_2$—are called either *selective beta$_1$* or *selective beta$_2$ blocking agents*. Beta$_1$ selective antagonists are also frequently referred to as *cardioselective blockers* because these agents block the beta$_1$ receptors in the heart.
2. Drugs that inhibit both types of receptors, beta$_1$ in the heart and beta$_2$ in the smooth muscle of the bronchioles and blood vessels, are referred to as *nonselective beta adrenergic blocking agents*.

The more important beta adrenergic blocking drugs that occur in each classification are:

a. Selective beta$_1$ adrenergic blocking agents (cardioselective), which include atenolol and metoprolol
b. Selective beta$_2$ adrenergic blocking agents. See Chapter 37, "Mucolytics and Bronchodilators."
c. Nonselective beta adrenergic blocking agents (beta$_1$ and beta$_2$ blockers), which are nadolol, pindolol, propranolol, and timolol

Mechanism of action. Beta adrenergic blocking agents compete with beta adrenergic agonists (e.g., catecholamines) for available beta receptor sites that are located on the membrane of (1) cardiac muscle, (2) smooth muscle

of bronchi, and (3) smooth muscle of blood vessels. As previously described, beta receptors appear to exist as two subclasses: beta$_1$ and beta$_2$. The cardiac muscle contains beta$_1$ receptors, and the smooth muscle of the bronchi and blood vessels contain primarily beta$_2$ receptors. Acebutolol, atenolol, and metroprolol selectively inhibit beta$_1$ activity. Labetalol, nadolol, oxyprenolol, pindolol, propranolol, and timolol are nonselective inhibitors, that is, they block both beta$_1$ and beta$_2$ receptors. Pharmacologically, the beta$_1$ adrenergic blocking action in the heart decreases heart rate, conduction velocity, mycardial contractility, and cardiac output.

The antiangina effects produced by the beta-blockers are primarily caused by their ability to lower the myocardial oxygen requirements. Their antihypertensive actions are not specifically identified, but these effects may result from a decrease in cardiac output, a diminished sympathetic outflow from the vasomotor center in the brain to the peripheral blood vessels, and an inhibition of renin release by the kidney (the latter with labetalol). The result is a decrease in peripheral vascular resistance that lowers blood pressure.

To prevent a recurrence of a mycardial infarction, beta blockers are used for their antidysrhythmic effect plus their ability to decrease the myocardial oxygen demands on the heart. The latter effect may reduce the progression of ischemia and its severity on the heart.

In regard to the prevention of vascular headaches, exact effects are unknown but it has been theorized that beta blocking agents, such as propranolol, act on the membrane of the smooth muscle of cerebral vessels, inhibiting vasodilation and arteriolar spasms.

Intrinsic sympathomimetic activity (ISA) is exhibited mainly by pindolol and slightly by acetutolol and timolol. ISA or partial beta agonist (stimulation) activity along with beta blocking effects were initially believed to be advantageous when compared with agents that only possess beta blocking effects. It was projected that fewer serious side effects would occur with such agents, but clinically, the significance of this property has not been proved.

Propranolol is also capable of exerting a quinidine-like or anesthetic-like membrane function, which may affect cardiac action potential and depresses cardiac function. This effect was once connected to the antidysrhythmic effect of these drugs but now is no longer considered important because very high dosages (in excess of therapeutic) are necessary to produce this activity.

Beta adrenergic blocking agents are effective antidysrhythmic agents, blocking stimulation activity at the cardiac pacemaker sites.

Indications. Used to treat chronic angina pectoris; to prevent and/or treat cardiac dysrhythmias; to treat hypertension; to prevent a second myocardial infarction; to prevent vascular headaches; as an adjunct to thyrotoxicosis therapy; as an antianxiety and antitremor agent.

Pharmacokinetics. See Table 20-9.

Side effects/adverse reactions. See Table 20-10.

Significant drug interactions. The following interactions are possible when beta adrenergic blocking agents are given with the drugs listed below:

Drug	Possible Effect and Management
oral hypoglycemic agents or insulin	May cause hyperglycemia or hypoglycemia. Symptoms of hypoglycemia, such as increased heart rate and blood pressure, may be blocked, thus making it difficult to monitor. Monitoring of blood glucose levels and dosage adjustments of the hypoglycemic agent may be necessary.
calcium channel blocking agents or clonidine	May result in potentiated antihypertensive effects; monitor closely. If therapy with a beta adrenergic blocking agent and clonidine is to be discontinued, taper the dose of the beta blocker gradually over several days. When it is discontinued, the clonidine may then be tapered and discontinued also over several days. Closely monitor blood pressure throughout this procedure.
monoamine oxidase (MAO) inhibitors	Do not use this combination; severe hypertension may result, even up to 14 days after the MAO inhibitor is discontinued.
sympathomimetics	The effects of both drugs may be reduced or blocked (sympathomimetics with beta activity). In sympathomimetics with both alpha and beta activity, beta blockade may result in increased alpha effects; i.e., hypertension, severe bradycardia, and possibly heart block. Labetalol may be used if combination therapy is necessary because it has alpha blocking effects. In sympathomimetic drugs with beta adrenergic activity, the beta blocking agent may cancel the beta$_1$ cardiac activity of dopamine or dobutamine; or the beta$_2$ bronchodilating effects of isoproterenol, metaproterenol.
xanthines (aminophylline or theophylline)	Therapeutic response of both drugs may be reduced or blocked. May also result in theophylline accumulation in the body. Monitor closely when this drug combination is prescribed.

TABLE 20-9   Pharmacokinetic Differences of Beta-Adrenergic Blocking Agents

Drug	Primary effect	Time to peak effect (hr)	Half-life (hr)	Beta blocking plasma concentration	Metabolism	Excretion (% unchanged)
acebutolol	Beta-$_1$†	N/A‡	3-4 metabolite 8-13	0.2-2 µg/ml	Liver	Bile/feces (50%-60%) Kidneys (85%-100%)
atenolol	Beta-$_1$†	2-4	6-7 (renal impairment- 16-27 or more)	0.2-5 µg/ml	Liver (some)	
esmolol	Beta-$_1$†	Steady state 5 minutes with loading dose, 30 minutes with infusion)	9 minutes	N/A	Esterases in red blood cells	Kidneys
labetalol	Beta-$_1$ Beta-$_2$	oral, 2-4 IV, 5 minutes	Oral 6-8 IV approx 5	0.7-3 µg/ml	Liver	Kidneys (55%-60%)
metoprolol	Beta-$_1$†	oral, 1-2 IV, 20 minutes	3-7	50-100 ng/ml	Liver	Kidneys
nadolol	Beta-$_1$ Beta-$_2$	4	10-24	50-100 ng/ml	None	Kidneys (70%)
oxprenolol♣	Beta-$_1$ Beta-$_2$	N/A	1.3-1.5	N/A	Liver	Kidneys (less than 5%)
pindolol	Beta-$_1$ Beta-$_2$	1-2	3-4 (Liver impairment 2½-30 hr) (Renal impairment 3-11½ hr) (7-15 hr in elderly)	5-15 ng/ml	Liver	Kidneys (40%)
propranolol	Beta-$_1$ Beta-$_2$	1½	3-5	50-100 ng/ml	Liver	Kidneys (1%)
timolol	Beta-$_1$ Beta-$_2$	1-2	4	5-10 ng/ml	Liver	Kidneys (20%)

*Data from Frishman, WH, Kafka, KR, and Meltzer, AH: Antianginal agents. II β-Blockers, Hosp Formul 21(1):62, 1986.

†Selectivity for cardiac beta-$_1$ receptors decreases with increases in dosages.

‡N/A, Not available.

TABLE 20-10 Beta-Adrenergic Blocking Agents: Side Effects/Adverse Reactions

Drug	Side effects*	Adverse reactions†
acebutolol (Sectral)	More frequent: Fatigue, decrease in sexual potency Less frequent: Diarrhea or constipation, anxiety, headache, nightmares, abdominal discomfort, insomnia, frequent urination, dizziness	Less frequent: Respiratory difficulties, cold hands or feet, chest pain, depression, rash, edema of extremities, bradycardia (usually less than 50 beats/min) Overdosage: Bradycardia, severe dizziness, fainting, respiratory difficulties, blue coloration of nails or palms, convulsions, cardiac failure may occur
atenolol (Tenormin)	More frequent: Decrease in sexual potency Less frequent: Diarrhea, dizziness, nausea, vomiting, headaches, fatigue	Less frequent: Respiratory difficulties, cold hands or feet, depression, bradycardia (usually less than 50 beats/min) Overdosage: See acebutolol
esmolol HCl (Brevibloc)	More frequent: Sweating, hypotension, nausea, inflammation at site of injection, dizziness, sedation Less frequent: Headache, fatigue, agitation, vomiting, dry mouth, constipation, abdominal distress	Less frequent: Respiratory difficulties, peripheral ischemia (pallor, cold hands or feet), bradycardia (usually less than 50 beats/min), symptomatic hypotension may require dosage changes or discontinuance, urinary retention, visual disturbances, fever Overdosage: Bradycardia, bronchospasms, congestive heart failure
labetalol (Normodyne, Trandate)	More frequent: Decrease in sexual potency Less frequent: Taste alterations, dizziness, drowsiness, headache, pruritus, tingling or numbness on scalp or skin, abdominal distress, nasal congestion, fatigue	Less frequent: Respiratory difficulties, elevated temperature or sore throat (leukopenia), irregular heart rate, depression, edema of lower extremities Overdosage: Same as acebutolol with exception of blue fingernails or palms
metoprolol (Lopressor, Apo-Metoprolol♣, Betaloc♣)	More frequent: Decrease in sexual potency, dizziness, fatigue Less frequent: diarrhea	More frequent: Depression Less frequent: Respiratory difficulties, elevated temperature or sore throat (leukopenia), irregular heart rate, edema of lower extremities, increased bleeding or bruising (thrombocytopenia), bradycardia (usually less than 50 beats/min) Overdosage: Same as acebutolol
nadolol (Corgard)	More frequent: Decrease in sexual potency Less frequent: Constipation, dizziness, fatigue	More frequent: Bradycardia (usually less than 50 beats/min) Less frequent: Respiratory difficulties, depression, rash, cold hands and feet Overdosage: Same as acebutolol
oxyprenolol♣ (Trasicor♣)	More frequent: Decrease in sexual potency, dizziness, slight sedation, insomnia, fatigue Less frquent: Increased anxiety or nervousness, constipation or diarrhea, headache, nightmares, tingling of fingers and toes, abdominal discomfort	More frequent: Edema of lower extremities Less frequent: Respiratory difficulties, chest pain, hallucinations, cold hands and feet, dysrhythmia, rash Overdosage: Same as acebutolol; tachycardia and elevated blood pressure may occur
pindolol (Visken)	More frequent: Increased anxiety and nervousness, decrease in sexual potency, fatigue, insomnia, dizziness Less frequent: diarrhea, pruritus, nightmares, nausea and vomiting, abdominal discomfort, paresthesia	More frequent: Pain in back or joints, edema of lower extremities Less frequent: Respiratory difficulties, rash, hallucinations, dysrhythmias, cold hands or feet, chest pain

*If side effects continue, increase, or disturb client, the physician should be informed.
†If adverse reactions occur, the physician should be contacted because medical intervention may be necessary.

Continued.

TABLE 20-10   Beta-Adrenergic Blocking Agents: Side Effects/Adverse Reactions—cont'd

Drug	Side effects*	Adverse reactions†
pindolol (Visken)—cont'd		Overdosage: Same as acebutolol with exception of the blue fingernails or palms, tachycardia and elevated blood pressure may occur
propranolol (Inderal, Inderal LA, Apo-Propranolol✢, Detensol✢)	More frequent: Decrease in sexual potency, fatigue, nausea and vomiting, paresthesia, insomnia, dizziness, slight sedation (high doses) Less frequent: Increased anxiety or nervousness, constipation, headaches, nightmares, abdominal discomfort	More frequent: Depression, bradycardia (usually less than 50 beats/min) Less frequent: Respiratory difficulties, hallucinations, cold hands or feet, chest pain, rash, edema of lower extremities Overdosage: Same as acebutolol
timolol (Blocadren)	More frequent: Decrease in sexual potency Less frequent: Dizziness, fatigue, headaches, pruritus	Less frequent: Respiratory difficulties, cold hands or feet, dysrhythmia, bradycardia (usually less than 50 beats/min) Overdosage: Same as acebutolol

*If side effects continue, increase, or disturb client, the physician should be informed.

†If adverse reactions occur, the physician should be contacted because medical intervention may be necessary.

Dosage and administration

acebutolol (Sectral)

Adults

Antidysrhythmic: 200 mg orally twice daily or adjust dosage according to patient response.

Antihypertensive: 400 mg orally daily as single dose or divided into two daily doses. Adjust dosage as necessary.

Elderly. Elderly persons may be more or less responsive to this medication. Monitor closely. Maximum daily dose should not be greater than 800 mg per day.

Children. Not determined.

atenolol (Tenormin)

Adults

Antianginic: 50 mg orally daily to start. If necessary, dosage may be increased to 100 mg after 1 week of therapy. Some patients have required up to 200 mg/day to produce the desired effect.

Antihypertensive: 25 to 50 mg orally daily. If necessary, dosage may be increased to 50 mg to 100 mg/day after 2 weeks of initial therapy.

Elderly. Same as above.

Children. Not determined.

esmolol HCl (Brevibloc). Intravenous injection for infusion only.

Adults. Begin with 500 μg/kg loading dose IV infused over 1 minute; then 50 μg/kg/minute for 4 minutes. If response is inadequate, repeat loading dose and increase maintenance dose by 50 μg to 100 μg/kg/minute over 4 minutes. These steps are repeated until desired effects are observed. Close supervision and titration of the drug should follow the manufacturer's recommendations.

labetalol (Normodyne, Trandate)

Adults. Antihypertensive. 100 mg orally twice daily. Dosage may be increased in 100 mg increments every 2

or 3 days until a therapeutic response is noted. Maintenance: 200 mg to 400 mg orally twice daily. (If side effects of nausea or dizziness occur, the daily dosage of this drug may be divided into three doses.)

Elderly. Same as acebutolol

Children. Not determined.

metroprolol (Lopressor, Apo-Metoprolol✢, Betaloc✢)

Adults

Antianginic or antihypertensive: 100 mg orally in single or divided dosage. May increase at weekly intervals up to a maximum of 450 mg/day, if necessary.

To prevent second or recurrent myocardial infarction: 50 mg orally about 15 minutes after the last intravenous dose or when the clinical situation justifies a change in the dosage form. Continue dosage for 2 days (48 hours) then adjust the dosage to 100 mg orally twice daily for 3 months or up to 1 to 3 years.

Elderly. Same as acebutolol

Children. Not determined

metoprolol tartrate extended-release tablets (Betaloc Durules✢ Lopresor SR✢). These are not available yet in the United States.

Adults. 100 to 400 mg orally daily.

metoprolol tartrate injection (Lopressor)

Adults. To prevent a recurrence of myocardial infarction. Treat early with 5 mg given rapid IV, every 2 minutes for three doses.

Elderly. Same as acebutolol

Children. Not determined

nadolol (Corgard)

Adults

Antianginic: 40 mg orally daily to start. Increase dosage by 40 mg to 80 mg at 3- to 7-day periods as necessary.

Maximum daily dosage is 240 mg/day.

Antihypertensive: 40 mg orally daily to start. Increase dosage by 40 to 80 mg at 7-day periods as necessary. Maximum daily dosage is 320 mg.

Elderly. Same as acebutolol

Children. Not determined.

oxyprenolol✢ (Trasicor✢). Not available in United States

Adults. Antihypertensive. 20 mg orally three times daily. Dosage may be increased by 60 mg/day, every 1 to 2 weeks as necessary. Maximum is 480 mg/day.

Elderly. Same as acebutolol

Children. Not determined

oxyprenolol HCl extended-release tablets✢ (Slow-Trasicor✢)

Adults. 80 mg or 160 mg orally, taken daily in the morning.

pindolol (Visken)

Adults. Antihypertensive. 5 mg orally twice a day to start. Dosage may be increased by 10 mg/day at 2- to 3-week intervals, if necessary. Maintenance: usually 5 mg three times a day; Once proper dosage is reached, once-a-day dosing may be instituted. Maximum is 60 mg/day.

Elderly. Same as acebutolol

Children. Not determined.

propranolol (Inderal, Inderal LA, Apo-Propranolol✢, Detensol✢)

Adults

Antiangina: 10 to 20 mg orally, 3 or 4 times a day. Dosage may be increased slowly every 3 to 7 days to a maximum of 320 mg per day, if necessary.

Antidysrhythmic: 10 mg to 30 mg orally 3 or 4 times daily. Adjust dosage as necessary.

Antihypertensive: 40 mg orally twice daily. Increase dosage slowly as necessary up to a maximum of 640 mg/day.

Hypertrophic subaortic stenosis: adjunctive therapy, 20 to 40 mg orally 3 or 4 times a day. Adjust dosage as necessary.

Prevention of reoccurrence of myocardial infarction: 180 mg to 240 mg daily in divided dosages.

Pheochromocytoma therapy: adjunctive, 20 mg orally three times daily to 40 mg 3 or 4 times a day for 3 days before surgery. Administer alpha-blocking agents before starting the beta adrenergic blockade. In cases of inoperable tumors, administer 30 mg to 160 mg in divided dosages, daily.

Prevention of vascular headaches: 20 mg orally four times a day to start. Dosage may be increased gradually up to a maximum of 240 mg/day, if necessary.

Elderly. Same as acebutolol

Children. 0.5 mg to 1 mg/kg/body weight orally in two to four divided doses to start. Adjust dosage according to individual response to treat hypertension or to prevent supraventricular tachycardia. Maintenance: 2 to 4 mg/kg/day orally in two divided dosages.

propranolol HCl injection (Inderal)

Adults. Antidysrhythmic. 1 to 3 mg intravenously given at rate of 1 mg per minute. May be repeated after 2 minutes and if necessary, again after 4 hours. In surgery, an IV dose of one-tenth the oral dose may be administered to temporarily replace PO dose.

Elderly. Same as acebutolol

Children. Not determined

timolol (Blocadren)

Adults

Antihypertensive: 10 mg orally twice a day to start. Increase dosage at 7-day intervals as necessary. Maintenance: 20 mg to 40 mg orally in 2 to 4 divided doses.

To prevent recurrence of myocardial infarction: 10 mg orally, twice daily. Start therapy 1 to 4 weeks after the infarction.

Elderly. Same as acebutolol

Children. Not determined.

Pregnancy safety. FDA category C—atenolol, labetalol, nadolol, propranolol and timolol; FDA category B—acebutolol, metoprolol, and pindolol

Precautions to consider

Bronchospasm. Blockade of the beta$_2$ receptors of the bronchial smooth muscle leads to bronchoconstriction. This effect is particularly hazardous for individuals with chronic obstructive pulmonary disease (asthma, bronchitis, and emphysema). Thus there is less risk of inducing bronchospasm in these clients when a cardioselective beta blocker (beta$_1$ blocker) is used.

Diabetes and hypoglycemia. Beta$_2$ adrenergic blockade prevents the appearance of the warning signs and symptoms (sweating, increased heart rate, and anxiety) of acute hypoglycemia. Since these agents mask the appearance of the warning signs of hypoglycemia, they should be used with caution in diabetic individuals who take insulin or hypoglycemic drugs. Atenolol, a selective beta$_1$ adrenergic blocker, does not potentiate insulin-induced hypoglycemia.

Thyrotoxicosis. Since these drugs may mask clinical signs of hyperthyroidism (e.g., tachycardia), they give a false impression of improvement of hyperthyroidism. Abrupt withdrawal of the drug will exacerbate symptoms of hyperthyroidism, and therefore therapy should be discontinued gradually.

Congestive heart failure. The risk of decreasing myocardial contraction, thus increasing the risk of heart failure must be considered when selecting a beta blocking agent. Long-term use of beta adrenergic blockers may aggravate congestive heart failure because of decreased cardiac output. If a beta blocking agent is necessary for a client with stabilized congestive heart failure, labetolol or drugs with ISA activity such as pindolol at low dosages may be the agents of choice. Monitor these clients closely.

Mental depression. Exacerbation of depression has been reported in clients with depression or with a history of depression and so they should be closely monitored if placed on a beta blocking agent.

NURSING CONSIDERATIONS

Assessment. Always check the apical pulse rate before administering drug. If it is slower than 60 beats/min or rate is irregular, hold drug and call physician immediately. Also check and report significant variations in blood pressure. Low parameters indicate overdosage.

Use with caution in clients with diabetes mellitus. By blocking adrenergic responses and thus preventing catecholamine-induced glycogenolysis, insulin can produce insulin-induced hypoglycemia without the appearance of its signs and symptoms (diaphoresis, increased pulse rate, and blood pressure changes). Blood glucose levels will help determine adjustment of insulin dosage.

Use with caution in clients with nonallergic bronchospasm (emphysema, bronchitis), since the drug can block beta$_2$ receptors in bronchial smooth muscle and has the potential to precipitate bronchoconstriction.

Intervention. To minimize variations in absorption, be consistent in administering oral beta blocking agents with regard to taking it with food or on an empty stomach. Although the manufacturer recommends giving the drug before meals and at bedtime, there is disagreement about whether food enhances or delays bioavailability.

Notify anesthesiologist if client is scheduled for surgery and is receiving a beta blocker.

Note that the drug must be withdrawn slowly. Otherwise client will suffer from abrupt withdrawal syndrome: tremors, sweating, severe headache, malaise, palpitation, rebound hypertension, life-threatening dysrhythmias, myocardial infarction (in patients with cardiac problems

---

WITHDRAWAL OF A BETA BLOCKING AGENT

Withdraw beta adrenergic blocking agents slowly by tapering or lowering the dose over 3 to 14 days. Withdrawal from nadolol usually requires 2 weeks because of its long half-life.

Advise client to avoid vigorous physical exercises or activity during this time to decrease the risk of a reinfarction or cardiac dysrhythmia.

If withdrawal signs occur (angina or chest pain, sweating, tachycardia, respiratory distress), temporarily reinstitute the beta blocking agent to stabilize the client, then slowly lower the dose with close supervision.

---

and angina pectoris), and hyperthyroidism in patients with thyrotoxicosis.

If drug is to be discontinued, reduce dosage over a 1- to 2-week period. It may be recommended that the drug be withdrawn well before surgery. In individuals with pheochromocytoma, drug is usually not discontinued before surgery. When administering labetalol the client should be in a supine position during injection and for 3 hours afterward. Increase client's activity and move client to an upright position gradually.

Education. Instruct client to take own pulse rate before each dose; also, withhold medication and inform physician if pulse rate drops below 60 beats/minute.

Counsel client not to alter established drug regimen prescribed by physician. The drug controls but does not cure, so lifetime compliance is necessary. Medication should be taken even if the client feels well, and the client should always have an adequate supply of drug available so that strict compliance is observed. Advise the client of the hazards of untreated hypertension.

Emphasize the importance of keeping appointments for periodic laboratory tests.

Advise the client to carry medical identification to alert health professionals in an emergency situation that a beta blocker is being taken.

Caution the client not to take over-the-counter medications, especially decongestants and cough and cold medications, but to consult with the health care provider.

While the drug is being withdrawn, advise the client to avoid physical exertion to reduce the risk of myocardial infarction and/or dysrhythmias.

Instruct client to restrict sodium intake to prevent unnecessary fluid retention.

Caution patient to avoid cold temperatures because they have an increased sensitivity to cold. Painful, cold, and tender hands and feet are a sign of impaired circulation. Take peripheral pulse to monitor decrease in peripheral circulation.

Advise hypertensive clients to make position changes slowly to prevent lightheadedness and dizziness. Alcohol ingestion, standing still for long periods, exercise, and hot weather enhance the orthostatic hypotensive effects of the drug. If the problem continues to exist, notify physician. Drowsiness and dizziness are common side effects, so caution client about operating a car or hazardous equipment.

In angina pectoris, exercise tolerance should increase and pain should be reduced with drug. Caution client to avoid overexertion because there has been pain reduction. Instruct client to inform physician if adequate relief is not obtained from the drug.

Instruct client to monitor weight and to report to physician the possible signs of congestive heart failure: weight gain of 3 to 4 pounds a day, dyspnea, cough, fatigue, rapid pulse, and anxiety. (Weight gains of 1 pound represents approximately 500 ml of retained fluid; 4 pounds of weight gain represents about a half gallon of retained fluids.)

Evaluation. With intravenous administration, monitor ECG, blood pressure, and pulmonary wedge pressure. Have available atropine (for bradycardia), vasopressors (for hypotension), and bronchodilators (for bronchoconstriction). Institute oral therapy as soon as tolerated.

Note if there is a considerable slowing of the pulse rate. Notify physician to avoid bradycardia. Beta blocking action can result in cardiac standstill.

Measure intake and output, and weigh client daily to determine presence of fluid retention. Fluid retention can cause dyspnea, orthopnea, nocturnal cough, pulmonary rales, distended neck veins, and edema, which are all signs of impending congestive heart failure. Report weight gain to physician.

Monitor effectiveness of drug therapy by evaluating frequency of anginal attacks and exercise tolerance: a reduction in blood pressure will indicate effectiveness when drug is used as an antihypertensive.

Monitor the client for signs of mental depression, a common adverse effect of beta blocking agents.

Monitor closely hypertensive individuals who have congestive heart failure that is controlled by digitalis and diuretics. The effects of digitalis and beta blockers are additive in depressing AV conduction. Discontinue therapy if cardiac failure continues with digitalis administration. Cardiac failure may be precipitated because of drug-depressed myocardial contractility.

Observe client for possible signs of thryotoxicosis, since the drug may mask clinical signs of hyperthyroidism.

In individuals with renal and hepatic impairment, monitor for signs of excessive drug accumulation.

KEY TERMS

BIBLIOGRAPHY

Abdulla AM: On vasoactive drugs in cardiogenic shock, Emerg Med 15(2):28, 1983.

Abundis J: Hazards of metered-dose bronchodilator inhalers, JEN 11(5):262, 1985.

American Society of Hospital Pharmacists: American hospital formulary service drug information '87, Betheseda, Md, 1987, American Society of Hospital Pharmacists, Inc.

Armstrong C: Effects of maternal beta sympathomimetic therapy on the neonate, Neonatal Network 4(3):6, 1985.

Arnold CL and others: Critical evaluation of beta blockers, Hosp Formul 18(3):299, 1983.

Au BG and others: Drug therapy and dosage adjustment in asthma, Respir Care 31(5):415, 1986.

Bassan MM and others: The additive antianginal action of oral isosorbide dinitrate in patients receiving propranolol: magnitude and duration of effect, Chest 83(2):233, 1983.

Bayliff CD: Dopamine and dobutamine: using them safely and effectively, Can Crit Care Nurs J 2(3):13, 1985.

Biddle C: Eyedrops: more side effects than meet the eye, RN 49(6):46, 1986.

Border WA: Recent advances in beta-blocker therapy for hypertension, Hosp Formul 19(12):1120, 1984.

Borders CR: What's new in cardiac inotropes, Patient Care 15(6):69, 1981.

Brevibloc (esmolol HC1), Du Pont Critical Care, Inc, Package insert 43004, January 1987.

Burns-Stewart SM: Nodolol (Congard), Home Healthcare Nurse 1(1):8, 1983.

Carter BL: Labetalol (Trandate, Glaxo, Inc.; Normodyne, Schering Corp.), Drug Intell Clin Pharm 17(10):704, 1983.

Conner CS: Labetalol: an alpha- and beta blocker, Drug Intell Clin Pharm 17(7-8):543, 1983.

Crowe DW: The beta and calcium channel blockers, Top Emerg Med 8(1):26, 1986.

Crumpler CP and others: Beta-adrenergic blocking agents, Hosp Formul 17(5):723, 1983.

Daley KA and others: Glucagon: a first line drug for cardiotoxicity caused by beta blockade, JEN 12(6):387, 1986.

Dalgas P: Understanding drugs that affect the autonomic nervous system, Nursing '85 15(10):58, 1985.

Downie RL: Obstructive airway disease, Top Emerg Med 8(4):13, 1987.

Eberts MA: Advances in the pharmacologic management of angina pectoris, J Cardiovasc Nurs 1(1):15, 1986.

Fernandez E: Update on the pharmacologic approach to asthma: xanthine and adrenergic bronchodilators. Part I, Respir Ther 14(4):42, 1984.

Frishman WH: Beta blockade, facts and fallacies, Emergency Med 14(10):217, 1982.

Frishman WH, Kafka KR and Meltzer AH: Antianginal agents. II B-blockers, Hosp Formul 21(1):62, 1986.

Gever LN: Treat shock with dopamine, Nursing '86 16(3):93, 1986.

Gever LN: Dopamine: guidelines for safe administration, Nursing '83 13(6):30, 1983.

Gever LN: Administering epinephrine in an emergency, Nursing '85 15(6):65, 1985.

Goodman LS and Gilman A, eds: Goodman and Gilman's the pharmacological basis of therapeutics, ed 7, New York, 1985, Macmillan, Inc.

Herlihy, JT and others: Adrenergic receptors, Crit Care Nurse 6(2):16, 1986.

Johnson GP and Johnson BC: B-blockers, Amer J Nurs 83(7):1034, 1983.

Johnson WE and others: Recent advances in critical care pharmacology: treatment of myocardial ischemia. Part I, Hosp Formul 19(7):350, 1984.

Kelly HW: When and how to use bronchdilaors, Respir Ther 14(2):47, 1984.

Kirilloff, LH and Tibbals SG: Drugs for asthma: a complete guide, Amer J Nurs 83(1):55, 1983.

Kochansky SW: Epinephrine: use, adverse effects, and dosage calculation, AORN J 43(4):852, 1986.

Labson LH: What role for beta blockers in MI? Patient Care 17(12):17, 1983.

Labson LH: Angina: which drug when? Patient Care 18(1):23, 1984.

LeBoeuf MB: Using vasoactive infusions in pediatric critical care, Crit Care Nurs 4(5):60, 1984.

Lirette M and others: Management of the woman in pre-term labor, Perinat Neonat 10(1):30, 1986.

Ludwikowski KLK: PPA: an innocent over-the-counter drug? Phenylpropanolamine hydrochloride, Pediatr Nurs 10(6):387, 1984.

Malek-Ahmadi P: B-blocker interactions: pitfalls of coadministration with antidepressants, Consultant 26(8):167, 1986.

Manoguerra AS: Beta blockers, Emergency 15(4):32, 1983.

Maree SM: Beta adrenergic blockers: pharmacological and anesthetic considerations, AANA J 52(2):145, 1984.

McCoy CA: Acute adrenergic reaction after accidental nasal instillation of metaproterenol, JEN 12(1):7, 1986.

McGraw JP: A graphic solution to the calculation of dopamine and other vasoactive drug dosages, J Emerg Nurs 13(3):172, 1987.

McKenney JM: Alternative pharmacologic approaches to the initial management of hypertension, Drug Intell Clin Pharm 19(9):629, 1985.

Melmon KL: Getting the most out of antihypertensives, Emerg Med 18(2):80, 1986.

Miller K: Epinenephrine, Emergency 18(6):10, 1986.

Mills GA and others: B-blockers and glucose control, Drug Intell Clin Pharm 19(4):246, 1985.

Moore AJ and Ingram J: Calculating the rate of dopamine, Nurs Times 79(19):34, 1983.

Moore LC and others: An on-the-spot guide to antihypertensive drugs, Nursing '86 16(1):54, 1986.

Munroe WP and others: Systemic side effects associated with the ophthalmic administration of timolol, Drug Intell Clin Pharm 19(2):85, 1985.

Norsen L: Using emergency drugs correctly. Part I, Nurs Life 5(5):12, 1985.

Owens GR: Newer pharmaceuticals in respiratory therapy, Respir Ther 15(5):12, 1985.

Pas DA and others: Beta-blocker agents: an update, JEN 12(1):18, 1986.

Pepper GA: Labeltalol: an alpha- and beta-adrenergic receptor blocker, Nurse Pract 10(7):39, 1985.

Rackow EC: Of shock and vasoactive drugs, Emerg Med 16(1):115, 1984.

Rice V: Shock management: pharmacologic intervention. Part II, Crit Care Nurse 5(1):42, 1985.

Rimar JM: Albuterol: a selective beta 2 bronchodilator, MCN 11(3):169, 1986.

Rosenberg JM and Kirschenbaum HL: What to watch out for with alpha-adrenergic blockers, RN 46(12):46, 1983.

Rotmensch HH and others: Prophylactic use of beta-adrenergic blockade in survivors of myocardial infarction, Heart Lung 13(4):366, 1984.

Russell RO Jr: Protection of ischemic myocardium during and after convalescence from acute myocardium infarction, Chest 85(2):248, 1984.

Salem RB and others: Depression from beta-adrenergic-blocking drugs, Drug Intell Clin Pharm 18(9):741, 1984.

Salmenpera M and others: Hemodynamic responses to beta-adrenergic blockade with metoprolol and pindolol after coronary artery bypass surgery, Chest 83(5):739, 1983.

Scheidt S: Beta-blockers: varying mechanisms of action mean broad antiarrhythmic uses, Consultant 23(2):295, 1983.

Scholz H: Inotropic drugs in the treatment of heart failure, Hosp Pract 19(5):57, 1984.

Seligman M and others: Use of adrenergic agents in the critically ill patient, Hosp Formul 22(4):348, 1987.

Shapiro DB: Migraine prophylaxis: the effective role of B-blockers, Consultant 27(1):117, 1987.

Simkin P: Stress, pain, and catecholamines in labor: a review. Part I, Birth 13(4):227, 1986.

Sjogren ER: Metoprol tartate (Lopressor IV), Crit Care Nurse 5(1):90, 1985.

Stiell G and others: Adrenergic agents in acute asthma: valuable new alternatives, Ann Emerg Med 12(8):493, 1983.

Stowers RG: Akathisia: diagnosis and treatment with low-dose propanolol, Physician Assist 9(7):96, 1985.

Taplin NE: Medical management of coronary heart disease: cardiovascular drug therapy, Occup Health Nurs 32(11):570, 1984.

Taylor RA and others: Reversible airway obstruction: inhaled B2-bronchodilators as first-line therapy, Consultant 27(4):134, 1987.

United States Pharmacopeia Convention: Drug information for the health care provider, ed 7, Rockville, Md, 1987, The Convention, Inc.

Vidt RG B-blockers: Choosing the best one for cardiac conditions and hypertension, Consultant 27(3):128, 1987.

Vlasses PH and others: The role of B-blocking agents following myocardial infarction, Drug Intell Clin Pharm 19(7-8):581, 1985.

Weintraub, M and others: Oxyprenlol: a nonselective beta blocking agent with intrinsic sympathomimetic activity, Hosp Formul 19(5):359, 1984.

Weintraub M and Standish R: Milrinone shows potential for the long term treatment of congestive heart failure, Hosp Formul 19(1):25, l984.

Wiltse O: For your logbook—dopamine, Emergency 19(3):19, 1987.

Wood AJJ: How the B-blockers differ: a pharmacologic comparison, Drug Therapy 8(2):59, 1983.

Wright C: Managing stable angina pectoris: nitroglycerin, beta blockers and risk reduction, Nurse Pract 9(2):54, 1984.

Wulf BG and others: Cardio-pulmonary arrest—asystole: a review of the medications used to restart the heart, Plast Surg Nurs 6(2):73, 1986.

Zaritsky A and Chernow B: Catecholamines in critical care medicine, CCQ 6(3):39, 1983.

Zatuchi J: Bradycardia and hypotension after propranolol Hcl and verapamil, Heart Lung 14(1):94, 1985.

CHAPTER

21

Skeletal Muscle Relaxants

OBJECTIVES

After studying this chapter, the student will be able to:

1. Describe the physiology of muscle movement and motor nerve response.
2. Differentiate between muscle spasm and spasticity.
3. Compare the manifestations of the two primary types of muscle spasticity.
4. Compare the action of central-acting and direct-acting skeletal muscle relaxants.
5. Summarize the drug interactions associated with skeletal muscle relaxants.
6. Use nursing considerations specific to skeletal muscle relaxants in planning care for clients receiving these agents.

Skeletal muscles are affected by many different pharmacologic substances. Their effects may be at the neuromuscular junction or at different levels in the central nervous system, i.e., at the brain or spinal cord.

NEUROMUSCULAR JUNCTION

Skeletal muscles are striated (striped) muscles attached to the skeleton. They are usually under voluntary control. These muscles produce body movements, maintain body position against the force of gravity, and counteract environmental stressors such as wind. A muscle is made of numerous muscle cells or muscle fibers. Each muscle cell is connected to only one motor nerve fiber, but each of the nerve fibers is connected to several muscle cells. Therefore stimulation of one nerve fiber will cause stimulation and activation of a group of muscle cells. The region where a motor nerve fiber makes functional contact with a skeletal muscle fiber (synaptic contact) is known as the neuromuscular junction.

SKELETAL MUSCLE SPASM AND SPASTICITY

Skeletal muscle **spasms** result when there is an involuntary contraction of a muscle or group of muscles that is accompanied by pain or limited function. Most skeletal muscle spasms are caused by local injuries, but some may result from low calcium levels or epileptic myoclonic seizures. Each type of spasm is treated according to its etiology.

Skeletal muscle injuries are usually self-limiting and can be treated with rest; physical therapy; immobility by use of casts, neck collars, crutches, or arm slings; or whirlpool baths. With tissue damage and edema, however, antiinflammatory drugs may be used.

Central skeletal muscle relaxants are used mainly for conditions in which muscle spasms do not quickly respond to other forms of therapy. Such conditions include musculoskeletal strains and sprains, trauma, and cervical or lumbar radiculopathy as a result of degenerative osteoarthritis, herniated disk, spondylolysis, or laminectomy. Unlike diazepam, the centrally acting drug, baclofen, which is used for skeletal muscle spasticity, has not been found useful in the treatment of muscle spasms.

Skeletal muscle spasticity is characterized by skeletal muscle hyperactivity. Skeletal muscle spasticity happens when gamma motor neurons, which tonically control muscle spindle contractile activity, become hyperactive.

There are two primary types of muscle spasticity: spinal and cerebral. **Spinal spasticity** can be identified by a marked loss of inhibitory influences with hyperactive tendon stretch reflexes, clonus (alternate contraction and relaxation of muscles), primitive flexion withdrawal reflexes, and a flexed posture. Varying degrees of spasticity of the bladder and bowel can also be seen. **Cerebral spasticity** has less reflex excitability, increased muscle tone, and no primitive flexion withdrawal reflexes or flexed posture. **Dystonia** may also be present in such individuals with cerebral spasticity.

Muscle spasticity is most commonly seen in clients with central nervous system injuries and strokes. Moderate to severe spasticity can be seen in two thirds of clients with multiple sclerosis. Individuals with cerebral palsy and rare neurologic disorders can also have muscle spasticity, but it is seen less frequently in these instances.

Central-acting and direct-acting skeletal muscle relaxants are the drugs of choice in the treatment of muscle spasticity. These drugs include baclofen, diazepam, and dantrolene. They are more effective in the treatment of spinal spasticity than cerebral spasticity. However, optimal therapy cannot be achieved in the treatment of either unless physical therapy is given concurrently.

CENTRAL-ACTING SKELETAL MUSCLE RELAXANTS
Mechanism of Action

The exact mechanism of action of the central skeletal muscle relaxants is not known. Action results from CNS depression in the brain (brainstem, thalamus, and basal ganglia) and spinal cord. This CNS depression results in relaxation of striated muscle spasm.

Removal of the central nervous depressive action from the skeletal muscle relaxation action of the central-acting skeletal muscle relaxants is not possible at this time. As a result these drugs create the side effects of drowsiness, blurred vision, lightheadedness, headache, and feelings of weakness, lassitude, and lethargy that make their long-term use undesirable.

The Nurse's Role in Central-Acting Skeletal Muscle Relaxant Therapy

Assessment. The drugs should be used cautiously in the presence of hepatic or renal dysfunction and in pregnant women. The FDA disapproves of prolonged administration of these drugs and discourages their use for periods longer than 3 weeks.

Use with extreme caution with clients with peptic ulcer disease.

Intervention. The drugs should be administered with meals or milk to prevent the side effects of nausea, vomiting, heartburn, and abdominal distress associated with large doses.

Education. Tell individuals taking these agents to avoid activities that require mental alertness, judgment, and physical coordination, such as operating dangerous machinery or driving an automobile.

Tell the client that alcohol and other CNS depressants will increase the CNS effects of these drugs.

Because many clients have postural hypotension with these medications, clients should be cautioned about standing suddenly and instructed to rise slowly, in keeping with individual physical limitations.

The drugs used primarily as antispastic agents are baclofen, diazepam, and dantrolene. Dantrolene is a direct-acting skeletal muscle relaxant (peripheral action); it is discussed later in this chapter.

baclofen (Lioresal)

Mechanism of action. Baclofen is an analogue of the inhibitory neurotransmitter gamma-aminobutyric acid (GABA). Baclofen acts at a spinal level, where it inhibits monosynaptic and polysynaptic transmission, although its exact mechanism of action is unknown.

Indications. Treatment of spasticity resulting from multiple sclerosis or from injuries to the spinal cord. It has been used investigationally to treat trigeminal neuralgia.

Pharmacokinetics

Absorption. Good but may vary with different individuals. Reportedly absorption decreases with an increase in dosage.

Time to peak concentration. 2 to 3 hours

Onset of action. Variable effects may occur in hours or up to weeks

Half-life. 2.5 to 4 hours

Therapeutic serum level. 80 to 400 ng/ml

Metabolism. Liver (15% only)

Excretion. Kidneys (between 70% to 85% of a dose is excreted unchanged)

Side effects/adverse reactions. See Table 21-1.

Significant drug interactions. The combination of baclofen and alcohol or other CNS depressants may result in enhanced CNS depressant effects and hypotension. Monitor closely because reduction in dosage of one or both drugs may be necessary.

Dosage and administration. 5 mg orally two or three times daily, increased by 5 mg per dose every three days, until desired response is achieved, not to exceed 80 mg/day.

Pregnancy safety. Not established

NURSING CONSIDERATIONS

Intervention. The dosage should be increased gradually to therapeutic dosages to decrease the incidence of adverse effects.

A gradual reduction in dosage over a period of 2 weeks is recommended, since abrupt withdrawal may cause hallucinations, paranoia, nightmares, confusion, and rebound spasticity.

Education. Tell the client that maximum benefit of the medication may not be reached for 1 to 2 months.

If abrupt withdrawal is required, instruct the client that hallucinations and rebound spasticity may occur.

See also general discussion of the nurse's role.

Evaluation. Administration of baclofen may increase the client's blood glucose levels, thus requiring an adjustment of the insulin dosage during therapy and when baclofen therapy is stopped.

Observe for increased seizure activity in patients with epilepsy because the seizure threshold may be lowered. Monitor the client's clinical state and EEG results during therapy.

diazepam (Valium, Apo-Diazepam✿, E-Pam✿)

Mechanism of action. The mechanism of action is unknown. Diazepam appears to act primarily by inhibiting afferent monosynaptic and polysynaptic pathways. It may also directly suppress muscle function at the neuromuscular synapse.

Indications. See Chapter 13 for a more complete description.

1. Treatment of skeletal muscle spasm caused by reflex spasm to local pathologic conditions, such as inflammation of muscle and joints or secondary to trauma.
2. Treatment of spasticity caused by upper motor neuron disorders (cerebral palsy and paraplegia), paraplegia, athetosis, tetanus, and the stiff-man syndrome (to overcome the widespread chronic muscular rigidity, pain, and skeletal muscle spasms).

Pharmacokinetics. See Chapter 13.

Side effects/adverse reactions. See Chapter 13.

Significant drug interactions. See Chapter 13.

Dosage and administration. See Table 21-4.

Pregnancy safety. FDA Category D.

NURSING CONSIDERATIONS

Assessment. Baseline vital signs should be assessed before diazepam is given and then frequently after the injection.

Intervention. Diazepam is insoluble in water, and so the parenteral form is prepared in a specific solvent. Do not mix or dilute parenteral dosages with other fluids or add to intravenous fluids.

Administer intramuscular injections slowly and deeply into a large muscle to diminish local irritation.

Administer intravenous diazepam slowly, at least 1 minute for each 5 mg of the drug to prevent apnea, hypotension, bradycardia, or cardiac arrest. After receiving a parenteral dosage, the client should be observed and

TABLE 21-1 Side Effects/Adverse Reactions of Baclofen

	Side effects*	Adverse reactions†
baclofen (Lioresal)	More frequent: Transient drowsiness, vertigo, confusion, sleepiness, increased weakness, muscle weakness, nausea Less frequent: Diarrhea, stomach pain or upset, ataxia, headache, euphoria, insomnia, slurred speech, paresthesia, muscle stiffness, increased excitability, fatigue, constipation, dysuria, increased urgency to urinate, urinary incontinence, sexual difficulties in males, congested nasal passages, anorexia, edema of ankles, hypotension, tachycardia, weight gain	Rare: Fainting spells; chest pain; blood or dark coloration of urine; CNS alterations, such as hallucination (auditory and visual); depression; mood changes; tinnitus Overdosage: Visual disturbances (e.g., blurred or double vision), convulsions, respiratory difficulties, severe muscle weakness, vomiting

*If side effects continue, increase, or disturb the client, the physician should be informed.
†If adverse reactions occur, the physician should be contacted because medical intervention may be necessary.

should stay in bed for at least 3 hours. Resuscitative equipment should be available.

To avoid phlebitis and venous thrombosis, small veins on the back of the hand and wrist should not be used for intravenous administration.

To minimize the occurrence of thrombophlebitis following intravenous administration of diazepam, flush the vein with a 1 ml of saline per 1 mg of diazepam.

Continuous intravenous infusion is not recommended because diazepam may precipitate in the infusion bag and the medication may be adsorbed to the plastic of infusion bags and tubing. If the drug cannot be administered by direct intravenous infusion, it may be injected through the intravenous tubing, but the injection should be as close as possible to the insertion point.

Education. Diazepam crosses the placental barrier and has been associated with causing cleft lip in infants. The risks versus the benefits should be considered in the pregnant client. It is also excreted in breast milk.

See also general discussion of the nurse's role in central-acting skeletal muscle relaxant therapy.

Evaluation. Clients undergoing long-term therapy can become physically dependent on the drug and show signs and symptoms of withdrawal when the drug is discontinued.

carisoprodol (Rela, Soma, Sopradol✳)
chlorphenesin carbamate (Maolate)

chlorzoxazone (Paraflex)
cyclobenzaprine (Flexeril)
metaxalone (Skelaxin)
methocarbamol (Robaxin, Marbaxin)
orphenadrine HCl (Disipal)
orphenadrine citrate extended-release (Norflex, Orflagen)

Muscle spasms are treated with central-acting skeletal muscle relaxants that are analogs to various antianxiety medications. They include the drugs listed here.

Mechanism of action. The exact mechanism of action of these drugs has not been determined. All of the drugs have an action in the central nervous system. It is believed the muscle relaxant effects of many of these drugs may be related to this CNS-depressant activity.

Indications. Adjunct treatment for skeletal muscle spasms along with rest and physical therapy. Methocarbamol had been indicated for the control of tetanus spasms, but it has been replaced by diazepam.

Pharmacokinetics. See Table 21-2.

Side effects/adverse reactions. See Table 21-3.

Significant drug interactions. When a skeletal muscle relaxant is given with alcohol, CNS depressants, or opioid analgesics, enhanced CNS depressant effects may occur. Monitor closely because the dosage of one or both drugs should be reduced.

Dosage and administration. See Table 21-4.

Pregnancy safety. Not established

TABLE 21-2   Pharmacokinetics of Central-Acting Skeletal Muscle Relaxants

Drug	Onset of action	Time to peak concentration (hr)*	Peak serum concentration*	Duration of action (hrs)	Half-life (hrs)	Metabolism/ Excretion
carisoprodol	½ hr	4 (350 mg)	4-7 µg/ml	4-6	8	liver/kidneys
chlorphenesin	N/A	1 to 3	3.8-17 µg/ml (800 mg)	N/A	2.5-5	liver/kidneys
chlorzoxazone	within 60 min	1 to 2	10-30 µg/ml (750 mg)	3-4	1-2	liver/kidneys
cyclobenzaprine	within 60 min	3 to 8	15-25 ng/ml (10 mg)	12-24	24-72	GI and liver/kidneys
metaxalone	60 min	2 (800 mg)	295 µg/ml (800 mg)	N/A	2-3	liver/kidneys
methocarbamol	PO, within 30 minutes	2 (2 g)	16µg/ml (2 g)	N/A	0.9-2.2	may be liver/kidneys and feces
	IV, immediate	nearly immediate	19µg/ml (1 g)	N/A		
orphenadrine citrate extended release	within 60 min	6 to 8 (100 mg)	60-120 ng/ml (100 mg)	12	14†	liver/kidneys and feces
IM	5 min	½ (60 mg)				
IV	immediate	immediate				
orphenadrine HCl	within 60 min	3 (50mg)	110-210 ng/ml (100 mg)	8	14†	liver/kidneys and feces

*Single dose
†Parent drug half-life. Metabolites may range between 2 and 25 hours.

TABLE 21-3 Side Effects/Adverse Reactions of Other Centrally-Acting Skeletal Muscle Relaxants

Drug	Side effects*	Adverse reactions†
carisoprodol	More frequent: Drowsiness Less frequent: Hiccups, vomiting, stomach distress, ataxia, headache, tremors, insomnia, dizziness (postural hypotension), increased excitability, nervousness, or irritability.	Less frequent: Fainting spells, fever, allergic reaction (skin rash, pruritis, edema of face, lips or tongue, respiratory difficulties, or burning eyes), depression, tachycardia
chlorphenesin carbamate	Less frequent: Sleepiness, dizziness	Rare: Fever, skin rash, pruritus, sore throat, increased bleeding tendencies or bruising, fatigue
chlorzoxazone	More frequent: Sleepiness, dizziness Less frequent: Abdominal distress, diarrhea, stomach gas, nausea, vomiting, constipation, headache, increased excitability, nervousness, restlessness	Rare: Dark or bloody stools; rash; pruritus; edema of face, lips, or tongue; sore throat; elevated temperature; increased bleeding tendencies; bruising; fatigue
cyclobenzaprine	More frequent: Dizziness, sleepiness, dry mouth Less frequent: Blurred vision, headaches, nausea, paresthesias, difficulty speaking, insomnia, taste alterations, tremors, abdominal distress, constipation, uncommon fatigue, unusual pounding pulse, and muscle weakness	Rare: Ataxia, confusion, depression, tinnitus, dysuria, allergic reaction (rash, pruritus, edema of face, lips, or tongue), jaundice Overdosage: Severe drowsiness, respiratory difficulties, dysrhythmias, hallucinations, altered body temperature, convulsions, muscle stiffness, vomiting, severe restlessness
metaxalone	More frequent: Abdominal distress, nausea or vomiting, dizziness, sleepiness, headaches, increased excitability, restlessness	Rare: Skin rash, pruritus, sore throat, fever, increased bleeding tendencies or bruising, unusual fatigue, jaundice
methocarbamol	More frequent: Visual disturbances (double, blurred vision), sleepiness, dizziness Less frequent: Nausea, vomiting, ataxia, headaches, increased muscle weakness	Less frequent: Fever, rash, pruritus, nasal congestion, bloodshot eyes If IV dosage form is administered too fast, bradycardia and unusual eye movements are seen.
orphenadrine	Less frequent: Abdominal distress, visual disturbances (blurred, double vision), disorientation, sleepiness, headaches, tremors, constipation, dizziness, increased excitability, nervousness	Less frequent: Fainting spells, tachycardia

*If side effects continue, increase, or disturb the client, the physician should be informed.
†If adverse reactions occur, the physician should be contacted because medical intervention may be necessary.

NURSING CONSIDERATIONS

carisoprodol (Rela, Soma, Sopradol). Rela tablets contain a yellow dye, tartrazine, which may cause an allergic reaction, particularly in clients who are allergic to aspirin.

Allergic or idiosyncratic reactions usually appear by the fourth dose.

Carisoprodol crosses the placental barrier and is found in the milk of lactating mothers at levels two to four times the maternal plasma concentration, causing sedation and gastrointestinal distress in the infant. Risk and benefit should be considered before using this drug for a pregnant or lactating client.

See general discussion of the nurse's role in central-acting skeletal muscle relaxant therapy.

chlorphenesin carbomate (Maolate). Maolate tablets contain a yellow dye, tartrazine, which may cause an allergic reaction, particularly in clients with an allergy to aspirin.

Watch for sensitivity reactions. Hold dose, and notify the physician if unusual reactions occur.

Observe for unusual bleeding and indications of blood dyscrasias.

Safety when used for longer than 8 weeks has not been determined.

See also general discussion of the nurse's role in central-acting skeletal muscle relaxant therapy.

chlorzoxazone (Paraflex). Chlorzoxazone is contraindicated in individuals with hepatic disease. Liver function studies should be monitored closely during therapy because hepatotoxicity is a possible side effect.

Tell the client that the drug may discolor the urine orange or purple-red.

See the discussion of the nurse's role in central-acting skeletal muscle relaxant therapy.

diazepam (Valium). See previous section and Chapter 13.

metaxalone (Skelaxin). Metaxalone is contraindicated in individuals with renal and hepatic disease. Monitor liver function studies.

TABLE 21-4   Dosage and Administration of Central-Acting Muscle Relaxants

Drug	Adults	Children
baclofen (Lioresal)	5 mg orally 2 to 3 times daily, increase by 5 mg/dose every 3 days until desired response is achieved	Not determined
carisoprodol (Rela, Soma)	350 mg orally 4 times daily	Less than age 5, not determined; 5 to 12 years old, 6.25 mg/kg body weight orally, 4 times daily
chlorphenesine carbamate (Maolate)	Initially, 800 mg orally 3 times daily; may be later decreased to 400 mg 4 times daily (or less) to maintain desired effect	Not determined
chlorzoxazone (Paraflex, Parafon, Forte DSC)	250 to 750 mg orally 3 or 4 times daily (usual initial dose is 500 mg 3 or 4 times daily); adjust according to individual response	20 mg/kg body weight or 600 mg/m² body surface area, given in 3 or 4 divided doses daily, or 125 to 500 mg 3 or 4 times daily based on child's weight and age
cyclobenzaprine (Flexeril)	20 to 40 mg daily, in divided doses, orally (usual dose 10 mg 3 times daily)	Not determined
diazepam (Valium)	*Oral:* 2-10 mg 3 or 4 times daily *Parenteral:* 5-10 mg IM or IV initially, repeated every 3-4 hr as necessary. For tetanus, larger doses may be required.	1-2.5 mg 3 or 4 times daily (not for use in children less than 6 months of age) Up to 0.25 mg/kg slowly
metaxalone (Skelaxin)	800 mg orally, 3 or 4 times daily	Not determined
methocarbamol (Robaxin, Marbaxin)	*Oral* initially: 1.5 g orally 4 times daily for 2-3 days; if condition is severe, may increase divided dosage to 8 g daily. Maintenance therapy: 750 mg orally every 4 hr or 1 g 4 times daily or 1.5 g 3 times daily. Adjunct therapy for tetanus, dosage depends on clinical response; up to 24 g daily via nasogastric tube has been administered. *Parenteral:* 1-3 g IM or IV daily for 3 days. After 2 drug-free days, the drug may be repeated, if necessary. Adjunct therapy for tetanus, 1 or 2 g IV, an additional dose may be given by IV infusion. Total initial dose is up to 3 g. Dosage may be repeated every 6 hr as necessary. Maximum dosage, do not exceed 3 g/day for more than 3 days except in the treatment of tetanus	Not determined Not determined Adjunct therapy for tetanus, 15 mg/kg body weight IV every 6 hr
orphenadrine (Disipal, Norflex)	*Oral:* 50 mg 3 times daily for plain tablets, 100 mg twice daily for extended-release dosage form, 250 mg/day maximum daily dose *Parenteral:* 60 mg IM or IV every 12 hr, when necessary	Not determined Not determined

Monitor blood studies because leucopenia and hemolytic anemia may occur.

Be aware that metaxalone is not recommended for individuals with epilepsy.

Clinitest and Benedict's solution may give a false positive reading in urine tests of clients taking metaxalone. Use Clinistix, Diastix, or Testape instead.

Caution client to notify prescriber if skin rash or yellowish discoloration of skin or eyes occurs (signs of liver-related jaundice).

See also discussion of the nurse's role in central-acting skeletal muscle relaxant therapy.

methocarbamol (Robaxin, Marbaxin). Be aware that methocarbamol is not recommended for individuals receiving anticholinesterase agents or for those who have epilepsy or who are in renal failure (because this may increase preexisting acidosis and urea retention).

Have epinephrine, injectable steroids, and/or injectable antihistamines available for intravenous injection to treat syncope should it occur. Anaphylactic reaction has occurred after (IM) and intravenous administration.

Have client recumbent during intravenous infusion and remain recumbent 10 to 15 minutes after infusion to decrease the incidence of adverse effects such as syncope, hypotension, and bradycardia.

Do not give subcutaneously. Administer deep (IM) injection to decrease local irritation. Avoid intravenous extravasation; thrombophlebitis, pain, and tissue sloughing may result.

The intravenous infusion should not be refrigerated. In addition, its compatibility with other solutions is limited; see a specialized reference before mixing. It may be diluted in normal saline or 5% dextrose in water, but do not dilute to more than 10 ml (1 g) in 250 ml.

If administering intravenous undiluted, inject at a rate not greater than 3 ml/minute.

Note that tablets may be crushed and suspended in water or saline for administration via a nasogastric tube.

Advise client to notify the prescriber if skin rash, itching, fever, or nasal congestion occurs.

Tell client that urine, if it is standing, may darken to green, black, or brown.

See also discussion of the nurse's role in central-acting skeletal muscle relaxant therapy.

orphenadrine (Disipal). Use with caution in individuals with cardiac decompensation, coronary insufficiency, cardiac dysrhythmias, or tachycardia.

Note that orphenadrine is contraindicated in clients with glaucoma, prostatic hypertrophy, obstruction of the neck of the bladder, and myasthenia gravis.

Periodic blood, urine, and liver function studies should be done with prolonged therapy.

Discuss side effects with the client.

See also discussion of the nurse's role in central-acting skeletal muscle relaxant therapy.

DIRECT-ACTING SKELETAL MUSCLE RELAXANT

dantrolene (Dantrium)

Mechanism of action

Treatment of malignant hyperthermia (see Chapter 13)—dantrolene acts directly on skeletal muscles to produce skeletal muscle relaxation by inhibiting the release of calcium from the sarcoplasmic reticulum to the myoplasm, resulting in decreased muscle response to the action potential and decreased muscle contraction.

Antispastic agent—dantrolene's direct effect on skeletal muscle dissociates the excitation-contraction coupling. This effect is probably induced by the interference with calcium ion release from the sarcoplasmic reticulum. Dantrolene reduces both monosynaptic- and polysnaptic-induced muscle contractions.

Indications

1. Used for the prevention and treatment of malignant hyperthermia.
2. Used for the treatment of spasticity, especially upper motor neuron disorders, such as multiple sclerosis,

cerebral palsy, spinal cord insults, and cerebrovascular accident (CVA).

Pharmacokinetics. Available orally and parenterally.

Oral absorption. Fair, about 35% of dose is absorbed

Onset of action. Spasticity of upper motor neurons, 1 week or more

Half-life. Oral, 8.7 hours (100-mg dose); IV, 5 hours

Time to peak concentration. 5 hours (oral dose)

Therapeutic serum level. 300 to 1100 ng/ml, variable with the individual

Metabolism. Liver

Excretion. Kidneys

Side effects/adverse reactions. See Table 21-5.

Significant drug interactions. The following effects may occur when dantrolene is given with the drugs listed below:

1. When given for short-term use (1-3 days) or chronic use with alcohol or CNS depressants: enhanced CNS depression may occur. Dosage of one or both drugs may need to be decreased. Monitor closely.
2. When given for chronic use only with hepatotoxic drugs: the risk of inducing liver toxicity increases. Women over 35 years of age taking estrogen products are at particular risk for this toxicity.
3. IV dantrolene for malignant hyperthermia only, with calcium channel-blocking agents: avoid this combination while attempting management of a malignant hyperthermic emergency. In animals this combination has caused ventricular fibrillation, severe hypokalemia, and cardiovascular collapse. Although this interaction is not documented in humans, concurrent administration of this combination of drugs is not recommended.

Dosage and administration. See Table 21-6.

Pregnancy safety. Not established

NURSING CONSIDERATIONS

Assessment. Dantrolene should not be administered to clients with active hepatic disease.

Use caution in clients with impaired cardiac, renal, hepatic, or pulmonary function.

The precautions do not apply to the short-term intravenous use of dantrolene to treat malignant hyperthermia.

Careful assessment of the client is particularly important when dantrolene has been prescribed for spasticity. Because there is no way of knowing if a client will benefit without a clinical trial, the observations of the relief of spasticity are critical. The decision for long-term use of dantrolene depends on the balance between the drug-induced weakness and other adverse effects and the beneficial effects of the drug. Paraplegic clients may not consider the adverse effect of weakness as detrimental as

TABLE 21-5   Side Effects/Adverse Reactions of Direct-Acting Skeletal Muscle Relaxants

Drug	Side effects*	Adverse reactions†
dantrolene (Dantrium)	More frequent: With short-term (1-3 days use) or chronic oral intake of dantrolene: mild diarrhea, dizziness, sleepiness, feelings of uncomfortableness or unusual fatigue, muscle weakness (not of respiratory muscles), nausea, or vomiting. Less frequent: Abdominal pain or discomfort With chronic administration of drug only: visual disturbances, headache, slurred speech, insomnia, increased nervousness, chills, fever, mild constipation, dysphagia, increased urgency to urinate, urinary incontinence, anorexia, decrease in urinary output.	Less frequent: With short-term (1-3 days use) or chronic oral usage: severe diarrhea, respiratory difficulty, or depression, With chronic administration of drug only: Chest pain, severe constipation (may result in distention or appearance of bowel obstruction), dark or bloody urine, depression, disorientation, convulsions, dysuria, phlebitis of leg or foot, allergic skin reaction, and jaundice

*If side effects continue, increase, or disturb the client, the physician should be informed.
†If adverse reactions occur, the physician should be contacted because medical intervention may be necessary.

TABLE 21-6   Dosage and Administration of Dantrolene

Adults	Children
FOR MUSCLE SPASTICITY:	
Orally, 25 mg initially; increase by 25 mg/day every 4-7 days until therapeutic response is achieved or until the dosage of 100 mg 4 times a day is reached	0.5 mg/kg body weight orally twice daily initially; increase by 0.5 mg/kg daily every 4-7 days until therapeutic response is achieved or until dosage of 3 mg/kg body weight 4 times/day is reached. Do not use dosages over 400 mg daily.
ACUTE MALIGNANT HYPERTHERMIC REACTION (ADJUNCT):	
IV push of a minimum of 1 mg/kg body weight; continue this dose until symptoms abate or until maximum cumulative dose of 10 mg/kg body weight is reached. If symptoms recur, dosage may be repeated. After IV therapy, usually 4-8 mg/kg body weight is administered orally in 4 divided doses daily for 24-72 hr.	See usual adult dose
AS PROPHYLAXIS FOR MALIGNANT HYPERTHERMIC CRISIS:	
4-8 mg/kg body weight given orally in 3 or 4 divided doses daily for 24-48 hr before surgery. Give last dose 3-4 hr before surgery with small amount of water. Intravenous infusion, 2.5 mg/kg over 1 hour before anesthesia.	See usual adult dose

spasticity. Ambulatory clients who use spasticity to remain upright or balance are not candidates for datrolene therapy.

Intervention. The contents of the capsule may be mixed with fruit juice for oral administration to a client unable to swallow capsules. Administer immediately after mixing.

When intravenous dantrolene is used to treat malignant hyperthermia, use of all anesthetic agents is discontinued, oxygen is administered, metabolic acidosis and fluid and electrolyte imbalances are corrected, and the client is cooled.

Reconstitute intravenous dantrolene with 60 ml of sterile water for injection without a bacteriostatic agent and shake the mixture until it is clear. Use within 6 hours of preparation.

Oral dantrolene may be given after the intravenous dose to prevent recurrence of symptoms.

Avoid extravasation of intravenous dantrolene. It is painful and irritating to the tissue because of the high pH of the solution.

Education. Caution clients that photosensitivity is possible with dantrolene, so they should avoid exposure to the sun.

Instruct client that the therapeutic effects may not become evident until a week after the usual initial oral dose. However, improvement should be seen within 45 days or the drug should be discontinued.

Regular visits to the physician should be encouraged for assessment of progress and to monitor for side effects with blood studies.

For other nursing considerations, see the nurse's role in central-acting skeletal muscle relaxant therapy.

Evaluation. When dantrolene has been administered to prevent malignant hyperthermia, carefully monitor the client postoperatively for possible delayed effects of the drug (Table 21-5).

The client receiving long-term therapy should be monitored for blood cell counts and hepatic and renal functioning.

The risk of hepatoxicity is greater in clients with previous liver disease, those taking 800 mg daily in the short-term therapy or 200 mg daily for longer than 2 months, and women over 35 concurrently receiving estrogen therapy.

Hepatitis most frequently occurs between 3 and 12 months into therapy and is generally preceded by gastrointestinal symptoms such as anorexia, nausea, and vomiting. Side effects may be minimized by starting with low dosages and increasing them gradually.

With short-term use, diarrhea may be a concern and may be severe enough to discontinue therapy. In chronic use, constipation may occur and health teaching should focus on its prevention.

KEY TERMS

cerebral spasticity, page 426
dystonia, page 426
spasms, page 425
spinal spasticity, page 426

BIBLIOGRAPHY

American Hospital Formulary Service: AHFS drug information '87, Bethesda, Md, 1987, American Society of Hospital Pharmacists, Inc.

Elenbaas JK: Centrally acting oral skeletal muscle relaxants, Am J Hosp Pharm 30(10):1313, 1980.

Gilman AG and others: Goodman and Gillman's the pharmacological basis of therapeutics, ed 7, New York, 1985, Macmillan Publishing Co.

Glenn MB and others: Antispasticity medications in the patient with traumatic brain injury, J Head Trauma Rehabil 1(2):71, 1986.

Rice GPA: Pharmacotherapy of spasticity: some theoretical and practical considerations, Can J Neurol Sci 14(3) (suppl):510, 1987.

United States Pharmacopeial Convention: Drug information for the health care provider, ed 7, Rockville, Md, 1987, The Convention.

Wahlquist G: Evaluation and primary management of spasticity, Nurse Pract 12(3):27, 1987.

Young RR and Delwaide PJ: Drug therapy—spasticity. Part 1, New Engl J Med 304(1):28, 1981.

Young RR and Delwaide PJ: Drug therapy—spasticity. Part 2, New Engl J Med 304(2):96, 1981.

UNIT VI

Drugs Affecting the Cardiovascular System

Overview of the Cardiovascular System

The development of **microelectrode** techniques and sophisticated recordings has resulted in new knowledge and greater understanding of cardiac activity. The resulting anatomic, electophysiologic, and pharmacologic information has permitted greater precision in diagnosing and treating cardiac disease, particularly the dysrhythmias. Along with these advances has been the increased use of electrocardiographic monitoring of acutely ill patients and those with known or suspected cardiovascular disorders. In addition, the nurse's clinical role has expanded and now includes care of patients on monitoring equipment. This requires the nurse to recognize and understand abnormal electrocardiographic patterns and in some cases to begin therapy, including pharmacologic therapy, to prevent serious complications and unnecessary deaths. Therefore nurses must understand the electrical and physiologic properties of the heart and the effects drugs have on cardiac activity to keep their knowledge current and their nursing care therapeutically effective.

Microelectrode techniques have grown increasingly sophisticated and helped provide greater understanding of the electrical properties of cardiac fibers and of what causes various cardiac disorders. Fortunately, these advances have led to the discovery of new drugs that are useful in treating cardiac conditions.

Cardiac drugs largely affect three major tissues of the

heart: cardiac muscle (myocardium), conduction system, and coronary vessels. In this chapter the normal function of these structures is discussed. The physiologic properties of these structures and the drug groups used therapeutically are summarized in Table 22-1.

THE HEART

The heart is a hollow muscular organ that consists of two main pumping chambers: the right ventricle, which is linked with the pulmonary circulation, and the left ventricle, which is connected to the systemic circulation. The cardiac muscle or myocardium is the largest and most important structure of the heart. As a **contractile** muscle, under normal conditions it can adapt its performance by adjusting the cardiac output according to the body's needs. However, when the heart cannot produce a variable output, the therapeutic use of digitalis or cardiac glycosides (i.e., the digitalis drugs) produces changes at the cellular level. A description of myocardial ultrastructure and the contractile process facilitates an understanding of the basic mechanisms in cardiac glycoside action.

CARDIAC MUSCLE

The pumping action of the heart depends on the ability of the cardiac muscle to contract. The myocardium is composed of many interconnected branching fibers or cells that form the walls of the two **atria** and two **ventricles** of the heart. Each individual myocardial fiber contains a nucleus in the middle and a plasma membrane (cell membrane), the sarcolemma (Figure 22-1, *1* and *2*). By joining end to end, the cells form a long fiber, with each cell separated from the other by a plasma membrane called the **intercalated disk.** This disk is believed to provide sites of low electrical resistance to permit the spread of exciting impulses throughout the cardiac muscle.

Each individual muscle fiber (cell) comprises a group of multiple parallel **myofibrils,** and each myofibril is arranged end to end in a series of repeating units called the *sarcomere.* By light microscope examination, the muscle fiber reveals its most characteristic feature, alternating light and dark bands. These bands result from crossing of the multiple parallel myofibrils, which are aligned in register with one another (Figure 22-1, *3*).

At the level known as the Z line, the sarcolemma of the muscle fiber interlocks (**invaginates**) at its end with the sacromere to form the transverse sarcotubule or T system, which penetrates deeply into the cell. Furthermore, internal membranes form an extensive network called the **sarcoplasmic reticulum.** This structure encircles groups of myofibrils and makes contact with the sarcotubules. The tremendous energy requirements for cardiac muscle contraction may be seen by the great numbers of mitochondria lined up in long chains between the myofibrils (Figure 22-1, *3*). Figure 22-1, *4*, shows the sacromere, which is the basic unit of contraction in the heart. It lies between two successive Z lines and in part of the myofibril. The sarcomere consists of dark bands called A bands and lighter I bands.

The end unit of the myofibril is the myofilament. The darkness of the A band results from the thicker myosin filaments, and the lightness of the I bands reflects the thinner actin filaments. Cross-bridges, which are small projections that extend from the sides of the myosin filament, appear along the entire length of the thick filament. The interaction between these crossbridges of myosin and the active sites of actin produces contraction. In the sarcomere the H zone represents the middle, less dense portion of the A band, and the myosin filament runs the entire length of this band. The I band, on the other hand, is divided by the Z line. The actin filament runs through the whole I band and terminates at the H zone. This arrangement is shown in Figure 22-1, *5*.

Myocardial Contraction

During the past decade our understanding of the fundamental mechanisms governing contraction of cardiac muscle in both normal and pathologic states has increased tremendously. Yet some aspects of this complicat-

TABLE 22-1   Effect of Cardiac Drug Groups on Cardiac Tissues

Cardiac tissue	Physiologic property	Drug group	Pharmacologic action
Cardiac muscle (myocardium)	Force of myocardial contraction (Frank-Starling's law)	Cardiac glycosides	Positive inotropic effect—increases cardiac output
Sarcomere (functional unit)	Contractility and conductivity		
Cardiac conduction system	Automaticity (rhythm and rate) Conductivity	Antidysrhythmic drugs Calcium channel blockers	Converts to normal sinus rhythm or abolishes dysrhythmia
Coronary arteries	Nutritional blood flow to myocardium and other cardiac structures	Antianginal drugs Calcium channel blockers	Coronary vasodilation or lessens work of the heart

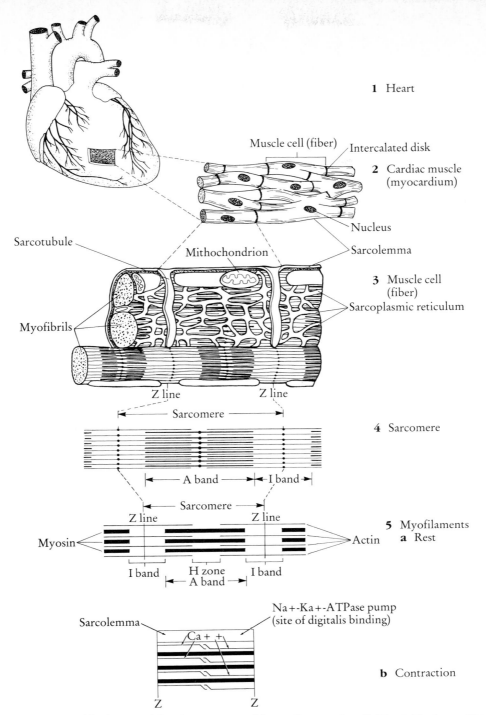

1 Heart

Muscle cell (fiber)
Intercalated disk

2 Cardiac muscle
(myocardium)

Nucleus

Sarcolemma

Sarcotubule

Mithochondrion

3 Muscle cell
(fiber)

Sarcoplasmic reticulum

Myofibrils

Z line   Z line

Sarcomere

4 Sarcomere

A band   I band

Sarcomere

Z line   Z line

5 Myofilaments
a Rest

Myosin   Actin

I band   H zone   I band
A band

Na+-Ka+-ATPase pump
(site of digitalis binding)

Sarcolemma

Ca+ +

b Contraction

Z   Z

FIGURE 22-1   The heart and the ultrastructure of the cardiac muscle cell (fiber). The heart *(1)* is mainly a muscular organ. The enlargement of the square illustrates a portion of the cardiac muscle (myocardium) *(2)* that is composed of myocardial cells. Each cell contains a centrally located nucleus and a limiting plasma membrane (sarcolemma), which forms the intercalated disk at the termination of each cell. An individual muscle cell (fiber) *(3)* consists of multiple parallel myofibrils. Each myofibril is arranged longitudinally in a series of light and dark repeating units, and the content of a unit is called a sarcomere. At the Z line, the sarcolemma invaginates to form the **transverse sarcotubules** or T system. An extensive network, called the sarcoplasmic reticulum, encircles groups of myofibrils and makes contact with the sarcotubules. The sarcoplasmic reticulum contains a high concentration of calcium ions. The mitochondria appear in long chains between the myofibrils. The sarcomere *(4)* is the unit of muscle contraction. It is composed of two types of bands, the A band and the I band. The latter is divided by the Z line. Myofilaments *(5)* of the sarcomere include the thin filament, actin, and the thick filament, myosin. The dark appearance of the A band is caused by the myosin and the lighter appearance of the I band by the actin. Here, the sarcomere is at rest *(a)*. On contraction *(b)* the sarcomere shortens so that the thick filaments approach the Z line and the width of the H zone narrows between the thin filaments. Calcium ions are needed for systolic contractions.

CARDIOVASCULAR TERMINOLOGY

Automaticity the ability to initiate an impulse

Cardiac output the amount of blood pumped by the heart per minute (cardiac output = heart rate × stroke volume)

Conductivity the ability to conduct or transmit the impulse

Depolarization an electrical impulse that results in contraction of muscle (for example, QRS interval represents the contraction of ventricular muscle).

Diastole a period of heart relaxation

Electrocardiogram (ECG or EKG) a graphic record of the electric currents produced by the heart

Excitability the ability to respond to an impulse

Myocarditis inflammation of heart muscle

Pericarditis inflammation of thin membrane sac that surrounds the heart

Repolarization the recovery phase following muscle contraction (for example, T wave represents recovery of ventricle muscle)

Stenosis the narrowing or stricture of an opening (for example, valve stenosis)

Stroke volume the amount of blood ejected with each contraction of the left ventricle

Systole the period of contraction in the heart (for example, atrial systole is contraction of the atria; ventricular systole is contraction of the ventricles)

Valvular insufficiency valve does not close properly; permits flow of blood in the wrong direction

ed process are still unknown. Cardiac muscle contraction begins with a rapid change in the cell membrane's electrical charge. This electrical current spreads to the interior of the cell where it causes release of calcium ions from the sarcoplasmic reticulum. The calcium ions then initiate the chemical events of contraction. The overall process for controlling cardiac muscle contraction, called **excitation-contraction coupling,** involves electrical excitation, mechanical activation, and contractile mechanisms.

Electrical excitation. Cardiac muscle contraction begins with electrical excitation or stimulus of the myocardial fiber. The source of electricity in the heart is found in the charges of *ion concentration*—mainly sodium, potassium, and calcium ions—across the cardiac cell membrane of the sarcolemma.

The **action potential** or rapid change in membrane potential, that produces the ion changes, occurs in the membrane of the myocardial cell. The *resting state* of an inactive muscle cell in the ventricle is created by the *difference* in electrical charge across the sarcolemma. In this case the inside of the cell is negative with respect to the cell's outside, which is positively charged. Because the

sarcolemma separates these opposite charges, the membrane in effect is *polarized.* At rest, the extracellular environment is rich in sodium ions (Na^+) and the intracellular environment in potassium ions (K^+), with calcium ion (Ca^{++}) concentration in the region of the sarcolemma and where it invaginates on the sarcotuble (see single myocardial fiber, Figure 22-2, *B*).

The cardiac action potential is divided into two stages: depolarization and repolarization. These stages are subdivided into five phases of ionic changes. The *resting potential* of an inactive myocardial cell is called *phase 4;* in this phase the membrane is polarized with a charge of approximately −90 millivolts (mv). At this voltage the interior of the cell is negative with respect to the cell's exterior. During this time the membrane cannot be penetrated by ions. However, any stimulus that changes the resting membrane potential to a critical value, called the *threshold,* can generate an action potential. (Follow Figure 22-2, *A,* for steps of the action potential.) Threshold is reached when the voltage becomes a fall in membrane potential. Thus the potential difference of the membrane is quickly lost and in fact results from the *fast inward current of sodium ions (fast channel)* and becomes pos-

COMMON CARDIAC DYSRHYTHMIAS

Heart block—impaired impulse conduction through the heart; usually the impaired conduction occurs between atria and ventricles

First-degree heart block—conduction time is prolonged but all impulses are conducted from atria to ventricles

Second-degree heart block—some but not all atrial impulses are conducted to ventricles

Third-degree heart block—no atrial impulses are conducted to ventricles

Ectopic beats—a contraction of the heart that originates some place other than the sinoatrial node

Extrasystole "premature beat"—a premature contraction of the heart that arises independent of the normal rhythm

Tachycardia—unusually rapid heart rate (usually over 100 beats/minute in adult)

Bradycardia—unusually slow heart rate (usually less than 60 beats/minute in adult)

Atrial flutter—extremely rapid rate of atrial contraction; may be 200 to 350 beats/minute

Atrial fibrillation—rapid and incoordinated contraction of the atria

Ventricular fibrillation—rapid and incoordinated contraction of the ventricles. Because of the incoordination of contractions, there is little or no effective pumping of blood; death will result if not immediately treated.

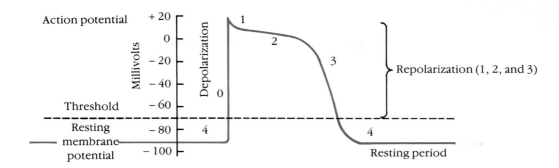

A

Depolarization

Phase 0—membrane becomes permiable to Na⁺, which rapidly flows into the cell

Repolarization

Phase 1—membrane potential becomes slightly positive because of the rapid influx of Na⁺

Phase 2—slow inward flow of Ca⁺⁺ and outward flow of K⁺

Phase 3—rapid outward flow of K⁺

Resting period

Phase 4—cell membrane actively transports Na⁺ outside and K⁺ inside, returning cell membrane to state of polarization

B

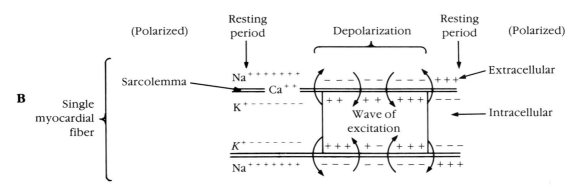

FIGURE 22-2 A, Action potential of a single myocardial fiber (cell). **B,** Ionic exchanges that occur across the cell membrane of a single myocardial fiber during an action potential.

itively charged to +20 mv. This sudden initial upstroke is *depolarization* and is designated as *phase 0* of the action potential. Phase 0 in the ventricular muscle is the contraction phase and is represented by QRS on the surface electrocardiogram. Soon after, the *repolarization* period occurs, and this process has three phases. The beginning of *phase 1* is the overshoot, and it makes a brief change toward repolarization. *Phase 2* is a slow period that forms

a plateau with a *slow inward current of calcium ions (slow channel)* and outward flow of potassium ion. *Calcium ion entry into the cell is essential for the excitation-contraction coupling mechanism*, which will be explained later. *Phase 3* is accomplished by rapid potassium ion efflux from the cell. Following repolarization, *phase 4* recovery or resting period ensues, whereby the cell membrane *actively* transports sodium ion outside and potassium ions inside, returning the cell membrane to a state of rest or polarization. These cation exchanges during recovery require the energy-utilizing transport mechanism of the Na^+-K^+-ATPase pump. The adenosine triphosphatase (ATPase) pump, which is powered by oxygen, is an enzyme that is located in the cell membrane or sarcolemma; it furnishes the energy needed for active transport to return sodium ions and potassium ions to their original resting positions at the membrane. Digitalis plays a key role at this site. By binding to the sarcolemma Na^+-K^+-ATPase pump, digitalis inhibits the return of sodium ions and potassium ions to their resting positions. Consequently, digitalis allows more sodium ions and calcium ions to enter the cell to strengthen myocardial contraction. However, it is also thought that if an excessive amount of these ions appears intracellularly, digitalis toxicity may occur (see Figure 22-2).

Mechanical activation. As previously stated, the unit that contracts is the sarcomere. It consists of two contractile proteins, actin and myosin. Myosin, the thicker filament, contains the **ATPase enzyme system** that is needed to **hydrolyze** ATP. Hydrolysis is required to provide the energy for contraction. ATP is synthesized in the mitochondria, which are normally abundant in cardiac muscle. Actin, the thin filament, is involved with calcium ion activity. These two filaments combine to help effect cardiac contraction.

Contraction is initiated when the nerve impulse reaches the myocardial cell and travels along the sarcolemma of the muscle fiber. As the depolarization wave spreads along the sarcotubules, it arrives at the sarcoplasmic reticulum, causing the release of its large quantities of calcium ions. These ions then bind to special receptors on the actin filaments. Hence the plateau, which is phase 2 of the action potential, is reached through the slow inward calcium current flow (slow channel). *Calcium ion movement is the chief component that links or couples electrical excitation of the sarcolemma with muscle activation of the myofilaments in the sarcomere.* Thus *mechanical activation* finally is accomplished when calcium ions bind to troponin, a regulator protein located on the actin filaments. This, in turn, then mediates the interaction of actin and myosin.

Contractile mechanism. As soon as the actin filaments are activated by the calcium ions, the myosin filaments immediately become attracted to the active sites of the actin filament. This interaction pulls the actin along the immobile myosin filaments toward the center of the A band, thus shortening the sarcomere and producing muscle contraction. In this process the lengths of individual filaments remain unchanged. The I band narrows as the thick filaments approach the Z line, and the H zone narrows between the ends of the thin filaments when they meet at the center of the sarcomere (Figure 22-1, *5a* and *b*). The greater the quantity of calcium ions delivered to

troponin, the faster the rate and numbers of interactions between actin and myosin. As a result of this response, the development of tension and contractility is increased.

When magnesium is present, ATP is cleaved by myosin ATPase. This reaction releases the energy needed to perform work. *The conversion of chemical energy to mechanical energy by ATP plays an essential role in energizing muscle shortening.* In other words, it provides the energy so the actin-myosin filaments move and produce muscle contraction. Although this is a somewhat simplified explanation of the contractile mechanism, it illustrates the important events pertinent to understanding cardiotonic drug action.

Finally, muscle relaxation depends on removing calcium ions from the sarcomere. The **calcium pump ATPase** (located in the walls of the sarcoplasmic reticulum) actively returns calcium ions to the sarcoplasmic reticulum and the sarcolemma, thereby allowing the actin-myosin filaments of the sarcomere to return to their resting positions.

In the normal heart *Frank-Starling's law of the heart* holds. This states that the longer the muscle fibers are at the end of diastole, the more forceful the contraction will be during systole. This law applies only when the muscle fiber is lengthened within physiologic limits. If a diseased heart is dilated and the fibers are stretched to a critical point beyond their limits of extensibility, the force of contraction and cardiac output are both diminished and ineffective. Thus the functional significance of Frank-Starling's law is that effective cardiac output can be brought about only by adequate relaxation and refilling of cardiac chambers after each myocardial contraction.

CARDIAC CONDUCTION SYSTEM

The effective pumping action of the heart depends on the regularity of events occurring in the cardiac cycle. Each cycle consists of a period of relaxation called *diastole* followed by a period of contraction known as *systole.* The *rhythm* and *rate* of the cardiac cycle are regulated by the conduction system, which has the ability to initiate and transmit the electrical impulses needed to stimulate contraction of the cardiac muscle.

The conduction system is made up of the following structures: (1) sinoatrial (SA) node, (2) internodal pathways, (3) atrioventricular (AV) node, (4) bundle of His, (5) right and left bundle branches, and (6) Purkinje fibers. The Purkinje fibers penetrate the endocardium and end in the myocardial cells. The AV node and the His area form the *AV junction,* which extends from the atrial fibers, through the AV node, to the **bifurcation** of the bundle of His. When referring to this region, the term "AV junction" is considered to be more accurate than "AV node" (Figure 22-3).

In the normal heart the SA node initiates the heartbeat.

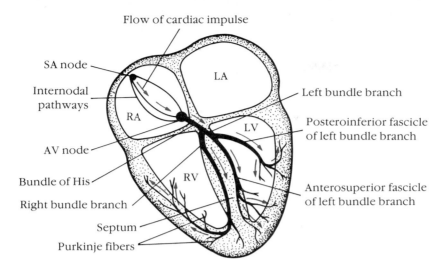

Flow of cardiac impulse

SA node

Internodal pathways

RA

LA

AV node

Bundle of His

Right bundle branch

Septum

Purkinje fibers

RV

LV

Left bundle branch

Posteroinferior fascicle of left bundle branch

Anterosuperior fascicle of left bundle branch

FIGURE 22-3 Conduction system of the heart. The cardiac impulse is initiated at the SA node and is transmitted through the internodal pathways to the two atria, resulting in atrial contraction. At the AV node, the electrical impulse is delayed. Conduction then speeds up at the bundle of His, with the impulse traveling through the right bundle branch and the left bundle branch continuing through the posteroinferior fascicle and anterosuperior fascicle of the latter bundle branch. Finally, the arrival of impulses at the Purkinje fiber results in their distribution to all parts of both ventricles, whereupon excitation, ventricular contraction is produced. *RA,* Right atrium; *RV,* right ventricle; *LA,* left atrium; *LV,* left ventricle.

(Modified from Andreoli, K, and others: Comprehensive cardiac care, ed 5, St Louis, 1983, The CV Mosby Co.)

The impulses generated here are then conducted through the **internodal pathways** to the "working" fibers of the atrial myocardium, producing atrial contraction. When the impulses move through the AV node, electrical conduction is delayed. However, at the bundle of His, conduction speeds up and the impulses travel through the right bundle branch and the left bundle branch, then through the posteroinferior and anterosuperior fascicles of the left bundle branch. The transmission of impulses at the Purkinje fibers, which consist of tiny fibrils that spread around the ventricles and connect directly with the myocardial cells, is very rapid. Finally, the simultaneous depolarization of both ventricles produces ventricular contraction, whereupon the cardiac output propels a volume of blood through the pulmonary artery and aorta.

Electrophysiologic Properties

The coordinated pumping action of the heart is initiated and regulated by the specialized fibers of the conduction system. The individual fibers of this system possess three basic **eletrophysiologic** properties: (1) automaticity, (2) conductivity, and (3) refractoriness.

Automaticity. The specialized fibers of the conduction system have the inherent ability to *spontaneously initiate* an electrical impulse without any external stimuli. This is the most fundamental mechanism of impulse formation, and the cells that possess this property of automaticity or self-excitation are called pacemaker cells. They are found in specialized conducting tissues such as the SA node, the AV node, and the His-Purkinje system. Normally, the impulse of the heart is spontaneously and regularly initiated at the pacemaker cells of the SA node. During resting potential (phase 4), the membrane of the cell depolarizes itself—spontaneously and gradually—until it reaches threshold and an action potential occurs. The slow depolarization of the membrane in the resting state is called spontaneous diastolic depolarization, or phase 4 depolarization, and defines automaticity. Thus the membrane of pacemaker cells is never at rest, and this property is attributed to the continuous influx of sodium ions into the interior of the cells, which readily drives the membrane to threshold. The resting potential of automatic pacemaker cells differs from that of the nonautomatic myocardial cells. After full repolarization, the membrane of myocardial cells maintains a steady resting potential until an external stimulus causes it to achieve threshold. To summarize, automaticity is a property of fibers of the conduction system that normally controls heart rhythm; it is not a feature of "working" muscle—atria and ventricles. However, under pathologic conditions, myocardial cells do have the potential to exhibit spontaneous depolarization.

The spontaneous excitation of pacemaker cells establishes the normal rhythm of the heart. The regularity of such pacemaking activity is termed *rhythmicity.* Under normal circumstances, only one functional pacemaker, the SA node, predominates because it has the highest frequency of depolarization. The normal rate of impulse formation is about 72 beats/minute. If the SA node decreases its rate of impulse formation to a level below the AV junction (40 to 60 beats/minute), then the AV junction becomes the primary pacemaker of the heart and will drive the heart at about 40 beats/minute.

Conductivity. Conductivity refers to the ability to transmit an action potential or nerve impulse from cell to cell. The property of conductivity therefore exists not only in the cells of the conduction system but also in the cardiac musculature. The speed of impulse conduction varies as it passes from one tissue to another in the heart. It is slowest in the AV node and fastest in the Purkinje fibers. The marked delay of conduction at the AV node allows more time for ventricular filling. On the other hand, the rapid depolarization of Purkinje fibers creates an instantaneous spread of impulses from the terminals to the ventricular muscles. Simultaneous activation of the musculature is essential for producing powerful ventricular contraction.

Velocity of conduction. The speed with which electrical activity is spread within the sinus node is quite slow, about 0.05 m/second. The impulse then spreads out rapidly over the atrial musculature at a rate of about 1.0 m/second. When the impulse reaches the AV node, a delay of about 0.05 m/second occurs and atrial systole takes place. The impulse then spreads rapidly, 2 to 4 m/second, along the right and left bundle branches and Purkinje fibers. Studies indicate that no more than 22 msec may elapse during this time. This rapid activation of contractile elements evokes a synchronous contraction of the ventricles.

The velocity of conduction is determined by the size of the resting potential of the cell membrane and the rate of rise of phase 0 of the action potential. This defines membrane responsiveness. Antidysrhythmic drugs may affect conduction by slowing phase 0 depolarization rate, thereby decreasing membrane responsiveness.

Refractoriness. Cardiac tissue is refractory to stimulation during the initial phase of systole (contraction). Throughout most of repolarization, the cell cannot respond to a stimulus. The *effective refractory period* represents that period in the cardiac cycle during which a stimulus, no matter how strong, fails to produce an action potential. Antidysrhythmic drugs can lengthen or shorten the refractory period of cardiac tissues by influencing the level of responsiveness of the cell membrane. Following the effective refractory period and as repolarization nears completion, a *relative refractory period* occurs. This is defined as that period during which a propagated action potential can be elicited, provided the stimulus is stronger than normally required in diastole. When this happens, the fiber is stimulated to contract prematurely.

Autonomic Nervous System Control

Although the conduction system possesses the inherent ability for spontaneous, rhythmic initiation of the cardiac impulse, the autonomic nervous system has an important role in the regulation of the rate, rhythm, and force of myocardial contraction of the heart. The heart is innervated by both the parasympathetic and sympathetic nerves. Vagal nerve fibers of the parasympathetic branch are found primarily in the SA node, atrial muscles, and AV node, whereas the sympathetic fibers innervate the SA node, AV node, and the atrial and ventricular muscles.

Vagal stimulation to the heart is mediated by the release of the acetylcholine, a neurohormone that acts on the muscarinic receptors to decrease heart rate and is also believed to decrease ventricular contraction. The main effect of acetylcholine on the AV node is to slow the rate of conduction and lengthen the refractory period. By contrast, sympathetic fiber stimulation is mediated by the release of norepinephrine, which acts specifically on the beta$_1$ receptors in the cardiac tissue. Circulating epinephrine from the adrenal medulla may also elicit cardiac responses. By acting on the beta adrenergic receptors, norepinephrine and epinephrine increase both heart rate and force of myocardial contraction. They also increase conduction velocity and shorten the refractory period of the AV node. Epinephrine has a very potent effect on the heart. In large doses its direct effect on the electrophysiologic properties of cardiac tissue can create cardiac dysrhythmias. Normally, the heartbeat is under the continuous influence of both parasympathetic and sympathetic control, so that the resting heart rate is the result of their opposing influences.

Electrocardiogram

Electrocardiograms are graphic representations of the sequence of cardiac excitation. Nurses caring for patients on monitor equipment should be able to detect and interpret changes in the cardiac rate or rhythm or in the conduction of the wave of electric activity or excitation. The electrocardiogram (ECG) is a useful tool in determining the therapeutic effectiveness of certain drugs. Drugs used to treat cardiovascular disease may alter the electric activity of the heart. The ECG may provide the earliest objective evidence of a drug's effectiveness or its toxic manifestations. A knowledgeable and observant nurse can use the information obtained from the ECG to assess the effectiveness of drug therapy for cardiac dysrhythmias.

Electric activity always precedes mechanical contraction. Immediately after a wave of electric activity moves through atrial muscle, the muscle contracts and blood flows from the atria into the ventricles. (See Figure 22-4 for the graphic illustration of the normal ECG.) The P wave is produced by a wave of excitation through the atria (atrial depolarization). The onset of the P wave follows

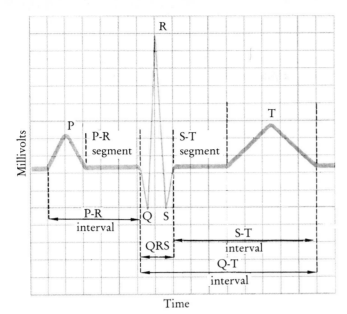

FIGURE 22-4 Graphic representation of the normal electrocardiogram. Vertical lines represent time, each square represents 0.04 second, and every five squares (set off by heavy black lines) represents 0.20 second. The normal P-R interval is less than 0.20 second; the average is 0.16 second. The average P wave lasts 0.08 second; the QRS complex is 0.08 second; the S-T segment is 0.12 second; the T wave is 0.16 second; and the Q-T interval is 0.32 to 0.40 seconds if heart rate is 65 to 95 beats/minute. Each horizontal line represents voltage; every five squares equals 0.5 millivolt.

the firing of the SA node. After the P wave, a short pause or interval (PR interval) occurs while the electric activity is transmitted to the AV node, conduction tissue, and ventricles. The ECG now records the QRS complex, or ventricular depolarization. This leads to contraction of the ventricles. Repolarization, or recovery, of the ventricles is indicated by the T wave. Atrial recovery or repolarization does not show on the ECG because it is hidden in the QRS complex.

PHYSIOLOGY OF FAST AND SLOW CHANNELS OF CARDIOVASCULAR FIBERS

To understand the clinical application of the new class of drugs known as calcium channel blockers, one must review the normal physiology of the fast and slow channels that exist in the membrane of the cardiovascular fibers. The cell membrane is composed of two types of channels that are controlled by "gates." When opened, they allow the movement of an inward current of (1) *sodium ions* through the *fast channels* and (2) *calcium ions* through the *slow channels* into the cell, depending on the type of fibers involved. These channels appear in the cell membrane of three types of cardiovascular fibers. The heart contains two types: (1) fast-channel fibers, which appear in the myocardial cells of the atria and ventricles and the Purkinje fibers and (2) slow-channel fibers, which occur in the SA node and the AV node. Last, the third type, slow fibers, are present in the smooth muscle of the coronary and peripheral arterial vessels.

In this mechanism, the role of calcium ions is essential in affecting three physiologic processes:

1. Increasing the strength of myocardial contraction (fast fibers)
2. Enhancing automaticity and conduction speed (slow fibers)
3. Vasoconstriction of coronary arteries and peripheral arterioles (slow fibers)

As previously described, the action potential that generates excitation-contraction coupling in the *fast fibers* consists of five phases. Depolarization (phase 0) results from an electrical stimulus that produces a fast inward current of sodium ion (fast channel). This is then followed by repolarization, which begins with a short phase 1, but more importantly, phase 2, the plateau phase, produces a slow inward current of calcium ions into the cell (slow channel). The influx of calcium ions is responsible for linking electrical excitation to myocardial contraction (excitation-contraction coupling) required to promote the sliding of actin and myosin filaments for myocardial contraction (positive intropic effect). Rapid repolarization occurs during phase 3, and finally, phase 4 reestablishes the resting state. (See configuration of action potential in Figure 22-2, *A*).

In the slow fibers of the SA and AV nodes, the action potential consists of only three phases. The principal distinguishing feature of the pacemaker fiber resides in phase 4. A slow spontaneous depolarization occurs that requires no external stimulus and is termed "diastolic depolarization." This is responsible for automaticity. Also, unlike the fast fibers of the myocardium, depolarization (or phase 0) is achieved by the slower current carried by both calcium ions and sodium ions through the slow channels of nodal cells. Thus phase 0 results in a slower conduction velocity in nodal cells than in myocardial cells. Calcium channel blockers inhibit these slow channels. Repolarization is more gradual and involves only phase 3. The membrane then finally returns to phase 4. (See Figure 22-5.)

The smooth muscle of blood vessels depends primarily on the presence of calcium ions to initiate and sustain contraction. The main source of calcium ions in cardiac muscle cells is the sarcoplasmic reticulum. In the action potential for smooth muscle, it is believed that the onset of depolarization (phase 0) is caused mainly by calcium ions rather than by sodium ions. Calcium ions enter the smooth muscle cell through slow channels, and it is the

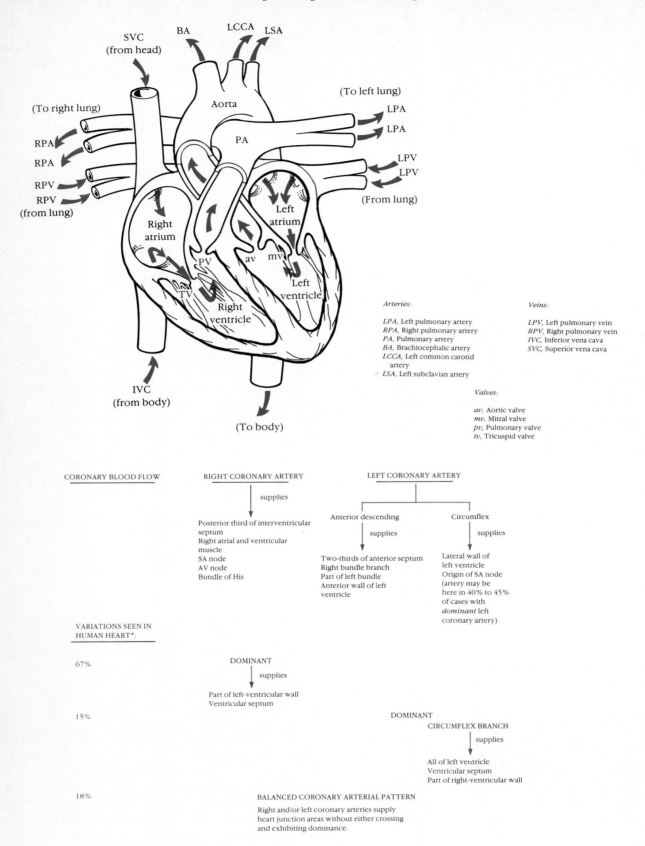

Arteries:

LPA, Left pulmonary artery
RPA, Right pulmonary artery
PA, Pulmonary artery
BA, Brachiocephalic artery
LCCA, Left common carotid artery
LSA, Left subclavian artery

Veins:

LPV, Left pulmonary vein
RPV, Right pulmonary vein
IVC, Inferior vena cava
SVC, Superior vena cava

Valves:

av, Aortic valve
mv, Mitral valve
pv, Pulmonary valve
tv, Tricuspid valve

CORONARY BLOOD FLOW

RIGHT CORONARY ARTERY

↓ supplies

Posterior third of interventricular septum
Right atrial and ventricular muscle
SA node
AV node
Bundle of His

LEFT CORONARY ARTERY

Anterior descending

↓ supplies

Two-thirds of anterior septum
Right bundle branch
Part of left bundle
Anterior wall of left ventricle

Circumflex

↓ supplies

Lateral wall of left ventricle
Origin of SA node (artery may be here in 40% to 45% of cases with *dominant* left coronary artery)

VARIATIONS SEEN IN HUMAN HEART*:

67%

DOMINANT

↓ supplies

Part of left-ventricular wall
Ventricular septum

15%

DOMINANT

CIRCUMFLEX BRANCH

↓ supplies

All of left ventricle
Ventricular septum
Part of right-ventricular wall

18%

BALANCED CORONARY ARTERIAL PATTERN

Right and/or left coronary arteries supply heart junction areas without either crossing and exhibiting dominance.

*Percentages from Netter, F.: Heart: the Ciba collection of medical illustrations, volume 5, p 17, 1974.

ANATOMY:

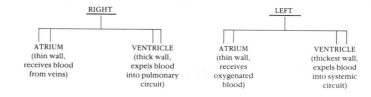

	RIGHT		LEFT	
	ATRIUM (thin wall, receives blood from veins)	VENTRICLE (thick wall, expels blood into pulmonary circuit)	ATRIUM (thin wall, receives oxygenated blood)	VENTRICLE (thickest wall, expels blood into systemic circuit)

MAJOR VESSELS:
1. Superior vena cava—blood returned from head and arms
2. Inferior vena cava—blood returned from internal organs and legs

1. Pulmonary artery—carries blood from right heart to lungs

1. Pulmonary veins, two right and two left—return blood to heart from lungs

1. Aorta—carries oxygenated blood to systemic circulation

MAJOR VALVES: Tricuspid—the entry port of right ventricle
Functions—to prevent backflow of blood from ventricle to atrium
Pulmonary valve—the exit port of right ventricle
Functions—to prevent backflow of blood from artery to ventricle

Biscuspid (mitral)—the entry port of left ventricle
Functions—to prevent backflow of blood from ventricles to atrium
Aortic valve—exit port of left ventricle
Functions—to prevent backflow of blood from artery to ventricle

CONDUCTION SYSTEM:

SA node (pacemaker) - - - - - - - - - - - - - - - → Atrial muscle contraction
↓
Atrial muscle
↓
AV node ———┐
          AV bundle ——————————————→ Left bundle branch
          ↓   ↓
     Right bundle branch   Purkinje fibers
          ↓   ↓
     Purkinje fibers   Ventricular muscle
          ↓
     Ventricular muscle
                    ↓
                Contraction

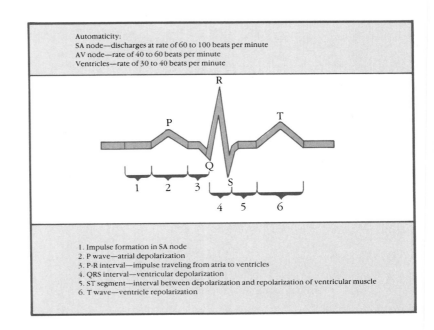

Automaticity:
SA node—discharges at rate of 60 to 100 beats per minute
AV node—rate of 40 to 60 beats per minute
Ventricles—rate of 30 to 40 beats per minute

1. Impulse formation in SA node
2. P wave—atrial depolarization
3. P-R interval—impulse traveling from atria to ventricles
4. QRS interval—ventricular depolarization
5. ST segment—interval between depolarization and repolarization of ventricular muscle
6. T wave—ventricle repolarization

rise in free calcium ion concentration that is considered to be the primary event in excitation-contraction coupling that is responsible for increasing muscle tone and vaso-constriction. In addition, activation of smooth muscle can reduce the caliber of small vessels markedly as is apparent from the "spasm" that may occur in coronary vessels. The calcium channel blockers (specifically verapamil, ne-fidipine, and diltiazem) are capable of blocking the slow calcium ion influx in smooth muscle of blood vessels, thereby producing relaxation.

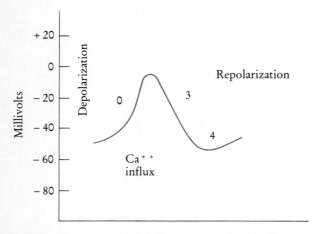

FIGURE 22-5 Action potential of a slow channel fiber, the SA node. It consists of 3 phases. Unlike the fast fibers of myocardial cells, depolarization phase 0 is attributed primarily to Ca^{++} inflow through slow channels of the cell membrane. Repolarization involves only phase 3, which is followed by phase 4

CORONARY VASCULAR SUPPLY OF THE HEART

The entire blood supply to the myocardium is provided by the right and left coronary arteries, which arise from the base of the aorta (Figure 22-6). The right atrium and ventricle are supplied with blood from the right coronary artery. The left coronary artery divides into the anterior (descending) branch and the circumflex branch and supplies blood to the left atrium and ventricle. These main coronary vessels continue to divide, forming numerous branches. The result is a profuse network of coronary vessels. The major arterial vessels are located on the external surface of the ventricles. Arterial branches penetrate the myocardium toward the endocardial surface.

Increased oxygen delivery to the myocardium is supported almost exclusively by increased coronary blood flow. When there is increased demand for oxygen and nutrients by body tissues, the heart must increase its output. At the same time, the heart muscle itself must be supplied with enough oxygen and nutrients to replace the energy expended. In other words, a balance must be maintained between energy expenditure and energy restoration.

During systole the myocardial contraction compresses the coronary vascular bed. This restricts coronary inflow but increases coronary outflow. Coronary inflow in the left ventricle occurs primarily during diastole when the ventricles have relaxed and the coronary vessels are no longer compressed. Blood is driven through the coronary arteries by aortic pressure perfusing the myocardium.

A change in heart rate is accomplished by shortening or

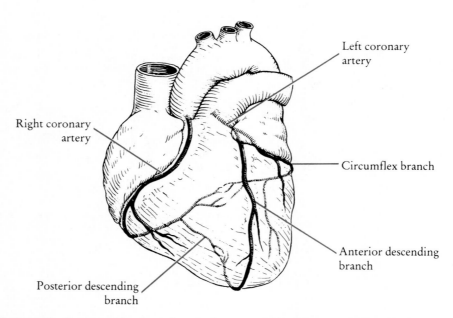

FIGURE 22-6 Coronary blood supply to the heart. Dark shaded vessels are those located on the external surface of the ventricles; light shaded vessels show penetration of arterial branches toward the endocardial surface.

lengthening diastole. With tachycardia the increased number of systolic contractions per minute reduces the time available for diastole and coronary inflow. An increase also occurs in the metabolic needs of the rapidly beating heart. Normally, coronary dilation occurs in an attempt to meet increased metabolic demand and to overcome restricted blood inflow. With bradycardia, the decreased number of systolic contractions per minute prolongs the diastolic period. Resistance to coronary flow and metabolic requirements of the myocardium are reduced.

Whenever the delivery of oxygen to the myocardium is inadequate to meet the heart's oxygen consumption needs, myocardial ischemia occurs. One of the major causes of ischemia is coronary artery disease.

KEY TERMS

action potential, page 440
ATPase enzyme system, page 442
atria, page 438
bifurcation, page 442
calcium pump ATPase, page 442
contractile, page 438
electrophysiologic, page 443
excitation-contraction coupling, page 440
hydrolyze, page 442
intercalated disk, page 438
internodal pathways, page 443
invaginates, page 438
microelectrode, page 437
myofibrils, page 438
sarcoplasmic reticulum, page 438
transverse sarcotubules, page 439
ventricles, page 438

BIBLIOGRAPHY

Andreoli K and others: Comprehensive cardiac care: a text for nurses, physicians, and other health practitioners, ed 5, St Louis, 1983, The CV Mosby Co.

Anthony CP and Thibodeau GA: Textbook of anatomy and physiology, ed 11, St Louis, 1983, The CV Mosby Co.

Berne R and Levy M: Cardiovascular physiology, ed 4, St Louis, 1981, The CV Mosby Co.

Bowman W and Rand M: Textbook of pharmacology, ed 2, London, 1980, Blackwell Scientific Publications, Inc.

Braunwalk E and others (editors): Harrison's principles of internal medicine, ed 11, New York, 1987, McGraw-Hill Book Co.

Goldberger E: Textbook of clinical cardiology, St Louis, 1982, The CV Mosby Co.

Gilman AG and others (editors): Goodman and Gilman's the pharmacological basis of therapeutics, ed 7, New York, 1985, Macmillan Publishing Co.

Guyton AC: Human physiology and mechanisms of disease, ed 4, Philadelphia, 1987, WB Saunders Co.

Netter FF: Heart: the Ciba Collection of medical illustrations, vol 5, Rochester, 1974, Case-Hoyt Corp.

Schwab MC and Bramah NS: Nifedipine: pharmacologic properties and clinical use, Hosp Formul 20(1):85, 1985.

Stone PH and others: Calcium channel blocking agents in the treatment of cardiovascular disorders. Part II. Hemodynamic effects and clinical applications, Ann Intern Med 93:886, 1980.

CHAPTER
23

Cardiac Glycosides

Drugs may change the force of myocardial contraction and the rate and rhythm of the heart. Pharmacologic terms that have specific meaning for the actions of drugs on the cardiovascular system include the following: "inotropic," "chronotropic," and "dromotropic" effects.

Drugs with an *inotropic* (Gr. *inos,* fiber; *tropikos,* a turning or influence) effect influence myocardial contractility. If the drug has a *positive inotropic effect,* it strengthens or increases the force of myocardial contraction (e.g., digitalis, dobutamine, dopamine, epinephrine, and isoproterenol). A drug with a *negative inotropic effect* weakens or decreases the force of myocardial contraction (e.g., lidocaine, quinidine, and propranolol).

Drugs with *chronotropic* (Gr. *chronos,* time) action affect the rate of the heart. If the drug accelerates the heart rate by increasing the rate of impulse formation in the sinoatrial (SA) node, it has a *positive chronotropic effect* (e.g., norepinephrine). A *negative chronotropic drug* has the opposite effect and slows the heart rate by decreasing impulse formation (e.g., acetylcholine).

When drugs have a *dromotropic* (Gr. *dromos,* a course) effect, they affect conduction velocity through the specialized conducting tissues. A drug having a *positive dromotropic action* speeds conduction (e.g., phenytoin). A drug with *negative dromotropic action* delays conduction (e.g., verapamil).

Drugs in the digitalis group are among the oldest drugs known as therapeutic agents for treatment of heart failure.

The effects of digitalis glycosides are twofold. They

increase the strength of contraction (positive inotrope) and alter the electrophysiologic properties of the heart by slowing the heart rate and slowing conduction velocity. Other agents may produce varying effects with the same objective of treating heart failure. To better understand the beneficial and toxic effects of the digitalis glycosides and other agents, we will first outline the mechanisms of heart failure.

HEART FAILURE

Heart failure or pump failure is a pathologic state in which the weakened myocardium is unable to pump sufficient blood from the ventricles (e.g., cardiac output) to sustain normal circulation required to meet the metabolic demands of the body organs. The etiologic factors of heart failure are listed in Table 23-1. Despite the etiology, depressed myocardial contractility is primarily the underlying cause of heart failure. Therefore, in heart failure, it is

important to identify and remove the cause, correct problems, and then treat the heart failure state, as follows:

1. Remove excess water and salt in the body. Sodium restrictions, reduction of physical activity, and initiation of diuretic and/or digitalis glycoside therapy are the usual measures taken.
2. Enhance myocardial contraction. The positive inotropic effect of digitalis has been related to excitation-contraction coupling. (See Chapter 22 for explanation of this phenomenon.)

The nurse should be aware that drugs may exacerbate or precipitate congestive heart failure (see box, p. 452). Also, many drugs contain sodium; their use must be considered with a salt-restricted diet. (See Table 23-2.)

Heart failure appears to be associated with a defect in excitation-contraction coupling, and in some individuals dysfunction of *contractile proteins* may occur as an additional abnormality. Ineffective calcium pumping by the sarcoplasmic reticulum may alter the normal relaxation process. Furthermore, the mitochondria—*not* the sarcoplasmic reticulum—may act as the dominant calcium uptake storage site. If so, less calcium is available for release from the sarcoplasmic reticulum to activate contraction. Thus the amount of coupling is reduced, and depressed myocardial contractility ensues.

With regard to dysfunction of contractile proteins in heart failure, attention has been focused on abnormal energy utilization. Some workers have shown that the activity of myosin adenosine triphosphatase (ATPase) is decreased. When the activity of this enzyme is reduced in heart failure, the interaction between actin-myosin filaments is reduced in intensity, and thus the force of contractility is lowered.

TABLE 23-1 Etiology of Heart Failure

Organic heart disorders	Extracardiac causes
Systemic hypertension	Anemia
Rheumatic fever	Liver disease
Infective endocarditis	Renal disease
Myocardial infarction	Hormonal disorders
Cardiac dysrhythmia	
Valvular disorders	
Pulmonary embolism	

TABLE 23-2 Sodium Content of Selected Prescription and Over-the-counter Medications

Medications	Sodium/unit	Sodium/maximum daily dose (adult)
ANTIBIOTICS		
carbenicillin disodium (Geopen, Pyopen)	108-150 mg/g	4.5 to 6.3 g/42 g
ticarcillin injection (Ticar)	120-150 mg/g	2.9 to 3.6 g/24 g
ampicillin sodium (Polycillin-N, Omnipen-N, and others)	62-78 mg/g	1 to 1.2 g/16 g
cephalosporins		
cefamandole naftate (Mandol)	77 mg/g	0.9 g/12 g
ceftriaxone sodium (Rocephin)	83 mg/g	0.33 g/4 g
cephradine injection (Velosef)	136 mg/g	1 g/8 g
moxalactam disodium (Moxam, Oxalactam)	88 mg/g	0.53 g/6 g
OVER-THE-COUNTER MEDICATIONS		
Alka-Seltzer Effervescent Pain Reliever and Antacid Tablets	0.5 g/tablet	
Bromo-Seltzer powder	0.76 g/capful	
Eno Powder	0.8 g/tsp	
Rolaids	53 mg/tablet	
Soda Mint Tablets	90 mg/tablet	

DRUGS THAT MAY PRECIPITATE OR EXACERBATE HEART FAILURE

DRUGS THAT CAUSE SODIUM AND WATER RETENTION

corticosteroids (cortisone, hydrocortisone, fludrocortisone or Florinef, desoxycorticosterone)
androgens
estrogens
diazoxide (Proglycem, Hyperstat)
guanethidine (Ismelin)
methyldopa (Aldomet)
phenylbutazone (Butazolidin, Butazolidin-Alka)

DRUGS THAT CAUSE OSMOTIC ACTIVITY THAT MAY RESULT IN INTRAVASCULAR VOLUME OVERLOAD

albumin
mannitol
urea
hypertonic glucose or saline

An important consequence of inadequate performance of the myocardium is hemodynamic alterations. Then compensatory mechanisms are activated, and incomplete emptying of the heart during ventricular systole eventually allows blood to accumulate inside the heart chambers, causing dilation or enlargement of the heart.

During this process, blood backs up into the atria. In the left atrium, this can lead to pulmonary congestion; in the right atrium, systemic congestion, including ascites, may occur. During the interim, the heart attempts to pump the blood forward in the circulation, but instead the increased fluid in the left ventricle produces stretching of the myocardial fibers and dilation of the ventricles.

Athletes commonly have cardiac hypertrophy, which is an enlargement of cardiac muscle and of the ventricular chambers. Thus the overall effectiveness of the heart as a pump is increased. Frank-Starling's law states that an increase in the length of the heart's muscle fibers results in increased contraction and cardiac output. This stretching of cardiac muscle results from increased preload, that is, an increased amount of blood returned to the heart and entering the heart chambers. Therefore the more the cardiac muscles are stretched during diastole, the greater the contraction in systole.

Congestive heart failure is a myocardial dysfunction resulting in a decreased cardiac output. Regardless of the primary cause, the result is that preload can increase until a massive overload results. The ventricles are unable to meet the needs for contraction or pumping. Mechanisms to compensate, involving sympathoadrenergic stimulation, may occur as the body attempts to maintain an adequate cardiac output. But the increased heart rate and peripheral vascular resistance also elevate the heart's demand for oxygen, thus further contributing to myocardial dysfunction. The inability to obtain adequate cardiac output is referred to as myocardial insufficiency or cardiac decompensation. Furthermore, chronic progressive ventricular failure generally leads to congestive heart failure, which means that the heart's ability to contract decreases to the extent that the heart pumps out less blood than it receives. Subsequently, myocardial infarction produces circulatory failure.

A decrease in cardiac output means less blood is in the blood vessels, and the body's various organs are receiving less blood. The kidneys respond by retaining more water and electrolytes, producing fluid retention and electrolyte disturbances. This is called right-sided heart failure (or cor pulmonale), and the clinical signs include jugular vein distention, hepatomegaly, ascites, and peripheral edema. On the other hand, left-sided heart failure leads to fluid accumulation in the lungs—pulmonary edema—producing dyspnea as well as interference with oxygen and carbon dioxide exchange. Failure of one side of the heart is usually followed by failure of the other side, which produces total heart failure (See Figure 23-1).

In summary, the failing heart may show increases in both preload (increased blood volume return to the heart chambers) and afterload (the increased pressure in the aorta that the ventricle muscles must overcome to open the aortic valve and push blood through). The decrease in renal perfusion just described may activate the renin-angiotensin-aldosterone (RAA) feedback mechanism. Then sodium and water are retained and intravascular volume and blood flow back to the heart increase. In less serious situations, this is usually enough to maintain arterial blood pressure, thus turning off the RAA system. But in individuals who have conditions bordering on heart failure, this can produce a frank decompensation or acute heart failure. The increase in circulatory blood volume increases the demands on the heart, which may result in acute pulmonary edema. Thus cardiotonic drugs such as digitalis glycosides (to increase contractility), diuretics (to reduce increased blood volume and edema), vasodilators (nitrates that pool blood in the extremities thus reducing blood return or preload, and arterial vasodilators that decrease arterial resistance, reducing afterload), and angiotensin II inhibitors (to decrease arterial resistance, afterload, and secretion of aldosterone) are all important drugs in the treatment of heart failure. In this chapter, the discussion will focus on digitalis glycosides and amrinone (Inocor).

DIGITALIS GLYCOSIDES

The story of the origin of digitalis is interesting in that it demonstrates an herbal remedy that, although used for

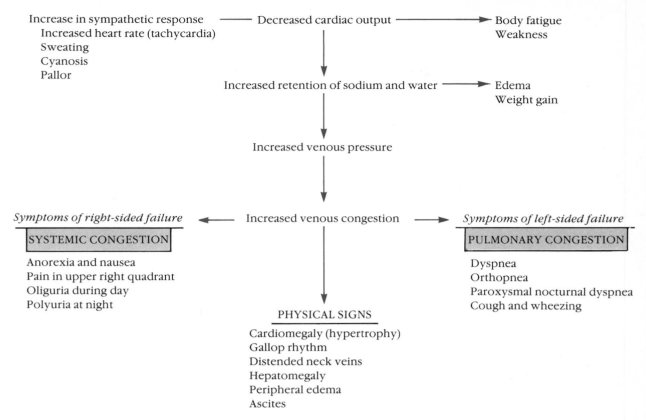

FIGURE 23-1. Signs and symptoms of heart failure.

hundreds of years by common people, was shunned for many years by the medical profession as too toxic. Digitalis (the "housewife's recipe") was prepared by farmers and housewives for dropsy. Over 400 years ago, Dr. Leonhard Fuchs recommended that physicians use it "to scatter the dropsy, to relieve swelling of the liver, and even to bring on menstrual flow" (Silverman, 1942). Dr. Fuchs was a botanist-physician, and at that time, the medical profession paid little attention to a "mere flower picker."

Digitalis was finally admitted to the London Pharmacopeia in 1722. Foxglove (digitalis) was promoted by William Salmon as a miraculous cure for consumption (tuberculosis). Because it was difficult to differentiate between tuberculosis and dropsy (edema of the chest, heart failure), it is now believed that Salmon was actually treating dropsy instead of consumption.

The popularity of digitalis among the medical profession was shaken by Dr. Salerne. Salerne, a French scientist, decided to test the drug's toxicity by force-feeding two healthy turkeys with as much digitalis as they were able to swallow. Within 4 hours, the turkeys were incapacitated; in several days they lost a tremendous amount of weight and died. Salerne examined the turkeys and found that internal organs (heart, lungs, liver) had shriveled and were thoroughly dry. When the medical community heard this, use of digitalis ceased because "no doctor

worthy of the name cared to use a drug that killed so horribly" (Silverman, 1942).

In the mid-1700s, a female patient shared an old family recipe for curing dropsy with Dr. William Withering. This spurred Dr. Withering to use digitalis with his dropsy patients and after spending 10 years studying digitalis, he published his conclusions, *An Account of the Foxglove*. This remarkable publication stressed instructions that are still valid today, that is, the necessity of individualizing dosage according to the patient's response.

The digitalis glycosides belong to many different botanical families. The action of each is fundamentally the same, so that the description for digitalis, with minor differences, will apply to all. The principal forms will be discussed here.

deslanoside (Cedilanid-D)
digitoxin (Crystodigin)
digoxin (Lanoxin, Novodigoxin✷, SK-Digoxin, Lanoxicaps)

Mechanism of action. Digitalis affects cardiac function through two important mechanisms:

1. Positive inotropic action. Influences the mechanical performance of the heart by increasing the strength of myocardial contraction.
2. Negative chronotropic and negative dromotropic ac-

tions. Involve alteration of electrophysiologic properties such as automaticity, conduction velocity, and refractory period.

Positive inotropic action. The main function of digitalis is inotropic. The increased myocardial contractility is associated with more efficient use of available energy. If the failing heart is enlarged, the positive inotropic action of digitalis can cause the myocardium to beat more forcefully, thereby increasing cardiac output and decreasing oxygen use. Thus the improved pumping action of the heart in patients with congestive heart failure may reach levels that approach normal because the net effect is not only reduced heart size but also decreased venous pressure to relieve edema. The positive inotropic mechanism is not precisely known. However, one theory asserts that digitalis is directly bound to sites on the myocardial cell membrane (sarcolemma), where it *inhibits the action of membrane-bound $Na^+ - K^+ - ATPase$ enzyme.* Normally, this enzyme hydrolyzes ATP to provide the energy for the $Na^+ - K^+$ pump needed to release Na^+ and transport K^+ into the cardiac cell during repolarization. By binding specifically to $Na^+ - K^+ - ATPase$, digitalis inhibits the active transport of $Na+$ and $K+$ (see Figure 22-1, 5*a* and *b*). Then intracellular $Na+$ accumulates, which stimulates the release of large quantities of free calcium ion from the sarcoplasmic reticulum. The *free calcium ion* is essential for *linking the electrical excitation of the cell membrane to the mechanical contraction of the myocardial cell,* a mechanism known as *excitation-contraction coupling.* Thus, more free calcium ion produces a greater degree of coupling of actin and myosin to form actinomyosin, which results in more forceful myocardial contraction with a concomitant increase in cardiac output. Inhibition of $Na^+ - K^+ - ATPase$ pump activity is projected to be the mechanism by which the cardiac glycosides increase myocardial contraction without causing increased oxygen consumption. (See "Myocardial Contraction" under "Cardiac Muscle" in Chapter 22)

Negative chronotropic and negative dromotropic actions. Digitalis has negative chronotropic (decreased heart rate) and negative dromotropic (slowed conduction velocity) effects because it can alter three electrophysiologic properties of cardiac tissues:

1. *Automaticity.* Cardiac tissue has the inherent ability to initiate and propagate an impulse without external stimulation. This property affects the rate and rhythm of the heart. Low to moderate doses of digitalis slow the heart rate because the SA node depolarizes less frequently. On the other hand, toxic concentrations of digitalis can directly increase automaticity. This increases the rate of both action potentials and spontaneous depolarization. This is one of the mechanisms responsible for digitalis-induced ectopic pacemakers. Toxic doses of digitalis may sig-

nificantly increase impulse formation in latent or potential pacemaker tissue, causing dysrhythmia.

2. *Conduction velocity.* All concentrations of digitalis decrease conduction velocity. The AV conduction velocity is slowed both by the direct action of digitalis and by increased vagal action. The ECG shows a prolonged P-R interval, and in toxic doses the drug can lead to increased heart block. (See Figure 23-2.)

3. *The refractory period* effects of digitalis vary in different parts of the heart. If the refractory period in the ventricles is reduced, nearly toxic amounts of digitalis are required. A prolonged refractory period occurs in the AV conduction system, which is very sensitive to digitalis action. This action is partly direct and partly caused by increased vagal tone. Toxic doses of digitalis may prolong the refractory period and depress conduction in the AV conduction system until complete heart block may occur.

Congestive heart failure. A heart in failure is no longer capable of supplying body tissue with adequate oxygen and nutrients or of removing metabolic waste products.

The positive inotropic effect of digitalis that results in increased myocardial contractility benefits the patient with a failing heart. The increased force of systolic contraction causes the ventricles to empty more completely. Also, a slower heart rate permits more complete filling, which results in the following:

1. Venous pressure falls, and the pulmonary and systemic congestion and their accompanying signs and symptoms are either diminished or completely abolished.

2. Coronary circulation is enhanced, myocardial oxygen demand is reduced, and the supply of oxygen and nutrients to the myocardium is improved.

3. Heart size is often decreased toward normal.

Some cardiac glycosides have a true but mild diuretic effect. However, marked diuresis in the edematous patient primarily results from improved heart action, improved circulation to all body tissue, and improved tissue and organ function including renal function. When digitalis is effective, the patient is noticeably improved and has an increased sense of well-being.

Atrial fibrillation. During atrial fibrillation several hundred impulses originate from the atria, but only a fraction of them are transmitted through the AV node. (See Figure 23-3 for electrocardiographic pattern of atrial fibrillation.) Digitalis is ideal for slowing the ventricular rate because it increases the refractory period of the AV node and also slows conduction at this site. It is important to know that the *purpose of using digitalis in atrial fibrillation is to slow the ventricular rate,* to reduce the possibility of inducing ventricular tachycardia. It also may prevent or eliminate cardiac failure. Digitalis does not con-

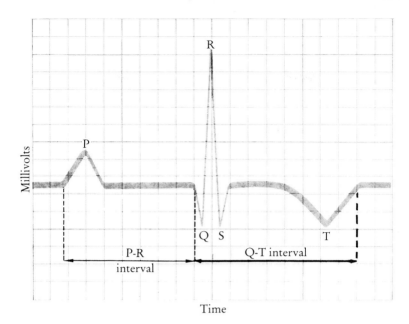

FIGURE 23-2. Representation of typical effects of digitalization on the electric activity of the heart as shown on the electrocardiogram. Note the prolonged P-R interval, the shortened Q-T interval, and the T wave inversion.

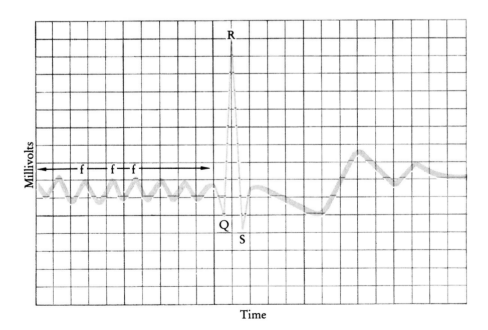

FIGURE 23-3. Graphic representation of atrial fibrillation as seen on the electrocardiographic monitor or tracing paper. No true P waves are noted; but f (fibrillation) waves consisting of rapid, small, and irregular waves are noted. The QRS complex is normal in configuration and duration but occurs irregularly.

vert the fibrillating atria into normally contracting ones.

Indications

1. Treatment of congestive heart failure
2. Treatment or prevention of cardiac arrhythmias, especially atrial fibrillation, atrial flutter, and paroxysmal atrial tachycardia

Pharmacokinetics. Absorption: digoxin's bioavailability is approximately 60% to 80% with tablets, 70% to 85% with the elixir, and 90% to 100% with the capsule dosage form.

Digitoxin is very lipophilic, so it is almost completely absorbed orally.

Deslanoside is only available in parenteral form.

The cardiac glycosides can be categorized into two main groups: rapid-acting agents and long-acting agents. See Table 23-3 for specific pharmacokinetic information.

Side effects/adverse reactions. See Table 23-4.

Significant drug interactions. The following interactions may occur when digitalis glycosides are given with the drugs listed below:

Drug	Possible Effect and Management
adrenocorticoids (corticosteroids), mineralocorticosteroids, amphotericin B (parenteral), ACTH, or potassium-depleting diuretics	The potential for inducing hypokalemia with these medications may, if used concurrently with digitalis preparations, increase the possibility of digitalis toxicity. Monitor potassium levels closely.
antacids (especially aluminum and magnesium types)	May decrease digitalis glycoside absorption 25% to 35%. Space medications apart, preferably giving digitalis glycoside 1 to 2 hours before antacids.

Drug	Possible Effect and Management
antidysrhythmic agents, injectable calcium salts, succinylcholine, or sympathomimetics	Concurrent administration may enhance risk of cardiac dysrhythmias. Avoid concurrent use whenever possible; if concurrent use is necessary, monitor closely with electrocardiographic monitoring.
calcium channel-blocking agents (verapamil, diltiazem)	Concurrent use may cause severe bradycardia. Monitor closely since digitalis glycoside dosage may need to be reduced.
indomethacin	In premature neonate, the renal excretion of digitalis glycosides may be reduced, leading to increased serum levels and possibly toxicity. Reduce digitalis glycoside dosage by 50% when indomethacin is started. Monitor closely for both therapeutic and toxic effects and make dosage adjustments accordingly.
magnesium sulfate injection	Use with extreme caution in individuals receiving digitalis. Alterations in cardiac conduction and heart block may result. Monitor closely.
potassium salts	Although potassium salts are commonly prescribed to treat hypokalemia, especially when clients are also taking a digitalis glycoside, potassium salts are not indicated in patients with severe heart block who are receiving digitalis. Hyperkalemia may be very dangerous in such individuals.

A number of other drugs have been reported to have moderate to significant potential for drug interaction with

TABLE 23-3   Pharmacokinetic Parameters of Cardiac Glycosides

Drug	Administration route	Onset of action	Peak effect (hr).	Plasma half-life	Duration of action (days)	Therapectic plasam level (nanogram/ml)	Metabolism	Excretion
RAPID ACTING								
deslanoside (Cedilanid D)	IV	10-30 min	1-3	33-36 hr	2-5	—		Kidney
digoxin (Lanoxin, Manoxin, SK-Digoxin)	IV	5-30 min	1-4	32-48 hr	6	0.5-2	Liver	Biliary (slight) Kidney (50%-70% unchanged)
	Oral	½-2 hr	2-6	32-48 hr	6	0.5-2	Liver	Same as above
LONG ACTING								
digitoxin (Crystodigin, Purodigin)	Oral	1-4 hr	8-14	5-9 days	14	13-25	Liver	Kidney (metabolites)

TABLE 23-4   Side Effects/Adverse Reactions of Cardiotonic Drugs

Drug(s)	Side effects*	Adverse reactions†

digitalis glycosides:
   deslanoside (Cedilanid-D)
   digitoxin (Crystodigin, Purodigin)
   digoxin (Lanoxin, Novodigoxin♣, Lanoxicaps)
	Nausea, vomiting, dysrhythmias	Infants and children: first symptoms are cardiac dysrhythmias
		Older children and adults: first symptoms are usually upset stomach, anorexia, bradycardia, and stomach pain
		Nausea, vomiting, and perhaps dysrhythmias may occur. If necessary, discontinue the digitalis glycoside until the cause is determined. Other symptoms of toxicity include diarrhea, increased weakness, blurred vision or complaints of visual disturbances (such as seeing a yellow, green, or white halo around objects or lights), confusion, headaches, skin rash or hives.

digoxin immune Fab (ovine) (Digibind)		Close monitoring is necessary, since withdrawal of digitalis may result in a decreased cardiac output, congestive heart failure, and hypokalemia. Allergic reactions, while not yet reported, are possible, especially in persons allergic to sheep proteins. An increase in ventricular rate may be seen in patients with atrial fibrillation.
amrinone (Inocor)	Infrequent or rare: nausea, vomiting, abdominal pain, increased temperature, taste blindness	Infrequent or rare: Hypotension, arrhythmias, unusual bruising (thrombocytopenia), chest pain, burning at injection site, jaundice

*If side effects continue, increase, or disturb the patient, inform the physician.
†If adverse reactions occur, contact the physician because medical intervention may be necessary.

digoxin. The following drugs should be given 1 to 2 hours before or after digoxin: cholestyramine, erythromycin, kaolin-pectin, metoclopramide, spironolactone, tetracycline, thyroid, and verapamil. Digoxin should be given first and the client monitored carefully for signs of therapeutic response or toxicity. Regular measurement of serum digoxin levels is also recommended. (Shinn, 1985).

A quinidine and digitalis drug interaction has also been reported. With combined use quinidine elevates the serum digitalis level; therefore the digitalis dose should be reduced to prevent toxicity and the client observed for clinical and ECG signs of toxicity and serum digitalis level. Syncope is a side effect of quinidine.

Although glycoside serum levels are of limited value in establishing therapeutic serum levels, they are sometimes helpful as an indicator of toxicity.

Dosage and administration. See Table 23-5. Also, the student should be aware of the following issues:

Bioavailability. Bioavailability (discussed in more detail in Chapter 4) refers to the amount of the administered drug that is usable in the target tissue. Bioavailability must be considered when a client is transferred from a parenteral form to the oral form of a cardiac glycoside. Usually dosage adjustment is required to compensate for the pharmacokinetic differences of the drug. However, there is an exception: both digoxin injection and the liquid-filled, soft capsules of digoxin have the same bioavailability.

Digitalization. **Digitalization** is the saturation of body tissues with enough digitalis glycoside to cause the signs and symptoms of heart failure to disappear. Although nomograms and formula calculations are available to estimate digoxin dosage based on lean body weight and renal function, most physicians still prescribe digoxin according to body weight of the client. (See dosage chart, Table 23-5.) However, digitalis glycosides have a very narrow therapeutic index, i.e., the therapeutic dose is very close to the toxic dose. Many clients have digitalis toxicity, so it is vital for the nurse to monitor, and to teach the client to watch for, signs and symptoms of improvement and of drug toxicity. Drug serum levels should also be monitored. There are essentially two methods of digitalization: the rapid (fast) method, which requires hospitalization of the client, and the slow method, which is usually prescribed in an ambulatory setting.

The rapid digitalization method is reserved for the client in acute distress from heart failure. If the client has not

TABLE 23-5   Dosage and Administration of Cardiac Glycosides

Drug	Route	Dosage range Digitalizing (loading)	Maintenance
deslanoside (Cedilanid-D)	IV	*Adults:* 1.6 mg as single injection or 0.8 mg initially and repeated after 4 hours *Children* (over 3 yr): 0.0225 mg/kg given in 2 or 3 divided doses at 3- or 4-hr intervals	
	IM	*Adults:* 0.8 mg given 2 times at 2 sites	
digitoxin (Crystodigin, Purodigin)	IV	*Adults:* 1.2-1.6 mg in divided doses (0.6 mg initially then 0.2-0.4 mg every 4-6 hr as needed) *Children* (2 to 12 yr): 0.03 mg/kg in 3 or 4 divided doses every 6 hr *Newborn to older infant:* 0.022 mg/kg or greater (check package insert) in divided doses	0.1-0.2 mg daily ¹⁄₁₀ of digitalizing dose
	Oral	*Adults:* RAPID: 0.6 mg initially, followed in 4-6 hrs by 0.4 mg and then 0.2 mg every 4-6 hr SLOW: 0.2 mg 2 times a day for 4 days *Children:* Not recommended	0.05-0.3 mg/day (common dose 0.15 mg)
digoxin (Lanoxicaps, Lanoxin, Masoxin, SK-Digoxin)	IV	*Adults:* 0.4-0.6 mg initially then 0.1-0.3 mg every 4-8 hr as needed; not to exceed 1 mg daily	0.125-0.5 mg daily as a single dose or in divided doses daily
	IV	*Children:* premature infant: RAPID: 15 -25 μg/kg—give about ½ dose at once and remainder in fractional doses at 4-8 hr intervals Full-term infant: RAPID: 20-30 μg/kg—give about ½ dose at once and remainder in fractional doses at 4-8 hr intervals Infant (1-24 months): RAPID: 30-50 μg/kg—give about ½ dose at once and remainder in fractional doses at 4-8 hr intervals	20%-30% of loading dose daily in divided doses 20%-35% of loading dose daily in divided doses 25%-35% of loading dose daily
	IV	*Children:* 2 to 5 yr—25-35 μg/kg 5 to 10 yr—15-30 μg/kg Over 10 yr—8-12 μg/kg Give about ½ dose at once and remainder in fractional doses at 4-8 hr intervals	25%-35% of loading dose in divided doses 2 or 3 times a day 25%-35% of loading dose once a day
	Oral	*Adults:* RAPID: 0.75-1.25 mg divided into 2 or more doses, each administered at 6-8 hr intervals SLOW: 0.125-0.5 mg once a day for 7 days *Children:* 2 to 10 yr: 0.03-0.04 mg/kg in divided doses every 6-8 hr	0.125-0.5 mg once a day 20%-30% of digitalizing dose daily

previously received any digitalis glycoside, then intravenous digoxin or deslanoside is given in divided doses in a 24-hour period. The goal of treatment is to obtain the maximum therapeutic effect of the glycoside as rapidly as possible. With this method, the drug toxicities will quickly become evident, while the client is in the controlled environment of the hospital unit. An advantage is that the toxicities can be easily correlated to a specific drug concentration. For example, the physician decides to digitalize an individual with a total dose of 1.0 mg digoxin intravenously. He or she prescribes digoxin 0.5 mg IV now and 0.25 mg IV every 6 hours for two doses for a total of 1.0 mg. The nurse is expected to observe the client for signs and symptoms of digitalis toxicity and also for clinical signs of improvement. If the client demonstrates digitalis toxicity after the 1.0 mg dose, the physician would know that this person was not able to tolerate a 1.0 mg total dose and in the future would avoid any dosage regimen that might reach this level.

The slow method of digitalization is generally used in less acute situations in the ambulatory setting. The length of time before an individual is fully digitalized is much longer than with the rapid method. The physician may prescribe an oral maintenance dose of digitalis daily, and the client would not be fully digitalized until approximately the fifth half-life of the drug. Digoxin, which has a

36-hour half-life, would take 7 1/2 days for digitalization, while digitoxin (with a half-life of 7 1/2 days) would require over a month.

The advantages of the slow method include (1) the individual may be treated on an outpatient basis, (2) it is a safer method, (3) close monitoring is not required, and (4) the doses may be taken orally. The disadvantages are (1) the extended length of time before the individual is digitalized and (2) the difficulty of determining when digitalis toxicity occurs since the onset of symptoms may be very gradual.

Digitalis toxicity. Almost every type of dysrhythmia can be produced by digitalis toxicity. The type of dysrhythmia produced varies with the age of the client and other factors. Premature ventricular contractions and bigeminal rhythm (two beats and a pause) are common signs of digitalis toxicity in adults, whereas children tend to develop **ectopic** nodal or atrial **beats.** Digitalis-induced dysrhythmias are caused by depression of the SA and AV nodes of the heart. This results in various conduction disturbances (first- or second-degree heart block or complete heart block). Digitalis may also cause increased myocardial automaticity, producing **extrasystoles** or **tachycardias.**

Nurses must be aware of the presdisposing factors to digitalis toxicity. The presence of any of these factors in clients indicates the need for close observation for signs and symptoms of digitalis intoxication.

1. Potassium loss. Hypokalemia (low potassium levels) can increase digitalis cardiotoxicity. Since potassium inhibits the excitability of the heart, *a depletion of body or myocardial potassium increases cardiac excitability.* Low extracellular potassium is synergistic with digitalis and enhances ectopic pacemaker activity (dysrhythmias). The following are causes of potassium loss:
   a. Hypokalemia occurs if large amounts of body fluids are lost as a result of vomiting, diarrhea, gastric suctioning, or diuresis from administration of diuretics. The use of various diuretic agents (carbonic-anhydrase inhibitors, ammonium chloride, and thiazide preparations) induces potassium diuresis along with sodium and water diuresis.
   b. Poor dietary intake or severe dietary restrictions decreasing electrolyte intake can cause loss of potassium.
   c. Adrenal steroids cause potassium loss and sodium retention.
   d. Surgical procedures associated with severe electrolyte disturbances such as abdominoperineal resection, colostomy, ileostomy, colectomy, and ureterosigmoidostomy can cause loss of potassium.
   e. Use of potassium-free intravenous fluids can cause hypokalemia.

2. Hypercalcemia. Excess calcium in the presence of digitalis may cause sinus bradycardia, atrioventricular conduction block, and ectopic dysrhythmia.
3. Pathologic conditions. Kidney, liver, and severe heart disease are major factors in digitalis toxicity. Approximately 80% of digoxin is excreted by the kidneys, whereas approximately 90% of digitoxin is first metabolized by the liver. Therefore, in a clinical setting, the physician may choose digitoxin as the drug of choice for a client in renal failure, because of its mode of excretion, that is, liver metabolism. For a client with liver impairment, the physician may select digoxin as the drug of choice, mainly because it does not rely on the liver for metabolism before excretion. The long half-life of digitoxin is a disadvantage in treatment. If the client should develop digitalis toxicity, the half-life of digoxin may increase from 36 hours to 120 hours, whereas the half-life of digitoxin increases from 120 to 210 hours (Bennett, 1977).

Pregnancy safety. digoxin, FDA category A; digitoxin, deslanoside, FDA category C

Antidote for Digitalis Glycosides

digoxin immune Fab(ovine) for injection (Digibind)

This drug is an antidote for severe digitalis glycoside toxicity.

Mechanism of action. Digoxin immune Fab(ovine) binds and makes complex molecules with digoxin or digitoxin in the serum. These molecules are then excreted by the kidneys. As more tissue digoxin is released into the serum to maintain an equilibrium, it will be bound and removed by this product, which results in lower levels of digoxin in serum and body tissues.

Indications. Treatment of life-threatening digoxin or digitoxin overdose

Pharmacokinetics

Onset of action. Less than 1 minute

Half-life. 15 to 20 hours

Initial signs of improvement in digitalis toxicity. In 15 to 30 minutes after administration, up to several hours

Excretion. Kidneys

Side effects/adverse reactions. See Table 23-4.

Significant drug interactions. None reported

Dosage and administration

Adults. Dosage may be calculated on the amount of digoxin or digitoxin consumed or it may be based on steady-state serum levels. Usually a 40-mg dose of digoxin immune Fab(ovine) will bind approximately 0.6 mg of digoxin or digitoxin. The formulas in Table 23-5 may be applied to determine the dose of the antidote.

Pregnancy safety. FDA category C

MISCELLANEOUS AGENT

amrinone (Inocor)

Mechanism of action. While its full mechanism is unknown, amrinone has positive inotropic effects and vasodilation activity. It does not inhibit Na^+-K^+-ATPase activity, but it does appear to increase cellular concentrations of cyclic AMP. It reduces preload and afterload by its direct effect on vascular smooth muscle.

Indication. Treatment of congestive heart failure, especially for individuals not responsive to digitalis glycosides, diuretics, or vasodilators.

Pharmacokinetics (parenteral dosage form)

Time to peak effect. Approximately 10 minutes after intravenous injection

Duration of action. Dose related: 0.75 mg/kg, approximately 1/2 hour; 3 mg/kg, approximately 2 hours

Half-life. Rapid intravenous injection, approximately 3.6 hours; intravenous infusion, approximately 5.8 hours

Metabolism. Liver

Excretion. Kidneys (approximately 63%), feces (18%)

Side effects/adverse reactions. See Table 23-4.

Significant drug interactions. None reported

Dosage and administration

Adults. Initially, 0.75 mg/kg intravenously over 2 to 3 minutes. If necessary, dose may be repeated after 30 minutes. Maintenance dose, 0.005 to 0.01 mg/kg by intravenous infusion per minute. Dosage is adjusted according to therapeutic response.

Children. Not established

Pregnancy safety. FDA category C

NURSING CONSIDERATIONS

Assessment. Use drug cautiously when the following conditions are noted:

- Dysrhythmias. They may be caused by underlying heart disease or reflect digitalis intoxication; drug should be withheld if the latter occurs.
- Progression of AV block. Incomplete AV block may progress to advanced or complete heart block in digitalizing patients; this means that heart failure may need to be managed by other measures.
- Hypothyroidism, myocardial damage, renal disease, and severe respiratory disease. These clinical conditions may require lower doses of digitoxin because of its delayed excretion.
- Elderly clients. Because of their small body mass (i.e., lean body weight) and frequent renal impairments, elderly clients must be given the drug cautiously.
- Electrolyte imbalances. Electrolyte imbalances require lower doses of digitalis glycoside.
    1. Potassium ion depletion increases risk of serious dysrhythmias and tends to diminish the positive ionotropic effect of the drug. Potassium supplements are recommended.
    2. Exercise great caution in giving drug to clients with hypercalcemia, to avoid dysrhythmia.

The use of digitalis glycosides is contraindicated in individuals with ventricular tachycardia, heart block, and hypersensitivity to any digitalis preparation. In addition, digitoxin is contraindicated in patients with beriberi heart disease.

Intervention. Rapid-acting digoxin is the most commonly prescribed form of a digitalis glycoside used in the coronary care unit (CCU). It may be given intravenously, intramuscularly, or orally.

- Administer intravenously as an undiluted digoxin (0.25 mg/ml) slowly at 0.25 mg/minute. Avoid rapid administration to prevent pulmonary edema. The drug may be administered in diluted form. Administer intravenously with caution to clients with hypertension since it temporarily causes an increase in blood pressure.
- Make intramuscular injections deep into large muscle mass and follow with massage. This route is infrequently used because of erratic absorption and intense pain lasting for several days. Also, there is a potential for tissue necrosis to occur at the injection site.
- The maintenance dose may be given orally if the client can tolerate food; otherwise intravenous injections are required. *Do not administer* oral preparation with meals having a high fiber content. Studies with digoxin show that the drug binds with the fiber, thereby reducing the amount of medication available for absorption from the gut. Advise the client to take drug after meals.

Be aware that digitoxin, though infrequently used, can be given undiluted intravenously (slowly) or orally to avoid pulmonary edema.

Oral administration is more consistently absorbed and is safer for individuals with renal disease because the metabolites excreted in the urine are inactive and do not affect the half-life of a digitalis glycoside.

Education. Advise clients who are not hospitalized to report weight gain of 1 to 2 pounds a day. Caution clients to avoid licorice because it can induce sodium and water retention.

Instruct client to take digitalis at the same time each day, precisely as prescribed. Do not skip or double a dose if missed. Also, do not change brand of drug when prescription is refilled. If using an elixir form of the drug, the dose should be determined using the special dropper that comes with the preparation. Caution client not to take other medications without prior approval of physician.

Advise the client to carry a medical identification and to alert health professionals unfamiliar with his or her drug regimen that the drug is being taken.

CHAPTER 24

Antidysrhythmics

CARDIAC DYSRHYTHMIAS

Cardiac **dysrhythmia** may be defined as any deviation from the normal rhythm of the heartbeat. Dysrhythmia is caused by some disorder that modifies the electrophysiologic properties of the cells of the conduction system or cardiac muscle cells.

Antidysrhythmic drugs are used for the treatment and prevention of disorders of cardiac rhythm. Disturbances in cardiac rhythm result from some abnormality in the electrophysiologic properties of the cells of the specialized conduction system or the heart muscle. Dysrhythmias often develop in individuals about 4 to 72 hours after myocardial infarction ("heart attack"). In addition, abnormal rhythm may occur in those recovering from cardiac surgery or in clients with coronary heart disease. Also, individuals with extracardiac disorders, such as pheochromocytoma, electrolyte imbalance, or thyroid disease, generally have some abnormal cardiac rhythms.

DISORDERS IN CARDIAC ELECTROPHYSIOLOGY

Disorders of cardiac rhythm arise as a result of (1) abnormality in spontaneous initiation of an impulse or **automaticity** or (2) abnormality in impulse conduction or **conductivity.** In some conditions, a combination of both processes may occur.

Abnormality in automaticity. A disturbance in automaticity may alter the heart's rate, rhythm, or site of origin of impulse formation. When the rate of pacemaker activity is affected, a decrease in automaticity of the SA node produces sinus bradycardia, whereas an increase in automaticity of the SA node results in sinus tachycardia. On the other hand, a shift in the site of origin of impulse formation can generate an abnormal pacemaker or an ectopic focus. In an ectopic beat, the impulse originates from an abnormal focus or site, resulting in activation of some part of the heart other than the SA node. This is called an **ectopic pacemaker.** It may discharge at either a regular or an irregular rhythm. It occurs because the cardiac fibers depolarize more frequently than the SA node. Consequently, abnormal automaticity may develop in cells that usually do not initiate impulses, for example, atrial or ventricular cells. Clinical disorders such as hypoxia or ischemia can activate sympathetic receptors that in turn become centers to initiate impulses. In addition, ischemic sites can cause impulse disturbances in automaticity and also in conductivity, and both manifestations are responsible for ectopic beats. The ectopic beats are classified as **escape beats,** premature beats or extrasystoles, and **ectopic tachydysrhythmia.**

Abnormality in conductivity. Altered conduction of the cardiac impulse probably accounts for more dysrhythmias than a change in automaticity. A disturbance in conductivity may be caused by (1) delay or block of impulse conduction or (2) the reentry phenomenon.

Delay or block of impulse conduction. Normally, the SA and AV nodes are poor conductors of impulse transmission. Under abnormal circumstances, conduction of an atrial impulse to the ventricles may be delayed or blocked in the AV node or structures beyond this region in the conduction pathway. However, impaired impulse transmission generally appears in the AV node or junction and occurs in varying degrees of block. In the first-degree AV block the impulses from the SA node pass through to the ventricles very slowly, and this is noted by a prolonged P-R interval on the ECG. In the second-degree block some atrial beats fail to pass into the ventricles. Finally, in the third-degree block or complete heart block, no impulses reach the ventricle, in which case the Purkinje fibers initiate their own spontaneous depolarization at a very slow rate. This results in independent ventricular and atrial rhythms referred to as **ventricular "escape."**

Reentry phenomenon. **Reentry phenomenon** is the mechanism responsible for initiating ectopic beats. A necessary condition for reentry is **unidirectional block.** Normally, when an impulse travels down the Purkinje fiber, it spreads along two branches. When it enters the connecting branch the impulses are extinguished at the point of collision in the center (Figure 24-1 *A*). At the same time, other impulses that begin laterally from the Purkinje fibers activate ventricular muscle tissue. In an abnormal situation the impulse descending from the central Purkinje fiber travels down the left branch normally

but in the right branch encounters a block as a result of ischemia or injury (Figure 24-1 *B*). This is a unidirectional block, because the impulse is capable of passing in one direction but not in the other. As a result, in the right branch, where the impulse is blocked in the forward direction at the site of injury, a retrograde or reverse impulse from the ventricular tissue penetrates or *reenters* the depressed region from the other direction, provided that the pathway proximal to the block is no longer refractory. When the effective refractory period of the blocked area is over, *reentry* of the impulse from the ventricular muscle into this site causes the impulse to circulate or recycle repetitively through the loop, resulting in a circus-type movement that produces dysrhythmia.

As shown in Figure 24-1, *C,* reentry is abolished by certain drug groups such as I-A, IV, and possibly II, which are explained later in this chapter. *The drugs that decrease or slow conduction velocity can convert unidirectional block to a two-way or bidirectional block.* As the impulses traveling in the antegrade or forward direction and those appearing in a retrograde or reverse direction are blocked at the injured site, the reentry pathway is interrupted, thereby abolishing the ectopic beats. In Figure 24-1 *D,* the conditions required for preventing reentry by another mechanism are also illustrated. *The Group I-B drugs, which either increase or have no effect on conduction velocity, eliminate reentry by stopping unidirectional block entirely.* Consequently the normal impulse conduction along the right and left branches of the Purkinje fibers is again restored.

• • •

In recent years an increasing number of antidysrhythmic drugs have required classification into categories based on their fundamental mode of action on cardiac muscle. Such a grouping of antidysrhythmic mechanisms should prove of value in predicting the drug's therapeutic efficacy, as well as its potential toxic effects in a given clinical cardiac condition. Drugs belonging to a particular class do not necessarily possess actions that are identical in every respect. In some cases a given agent may have subsidiary properties (extracardiac effects) that alter the basic electrophysiologic actions on the cardiac muscle. The currently available antidysrhythmic drugs are classified into four categories according to their mechanisms of action (Table 24-1). However, these drugs have one major electrophysiologic property in common: they all have the ability to suppress automaticity. Group I compounds are subdivided into groups I-A, I-B, or I-C to reflect the similar electrophysiologic effects of each subgroup. Group I-A drugs include disopyramide, procainamide, and quinidine, all of which decrease conduction velocity and prolong the action potential. Group I-B drugs such as lidocaine, phenytoin, tocainide, and mexiletine either in-

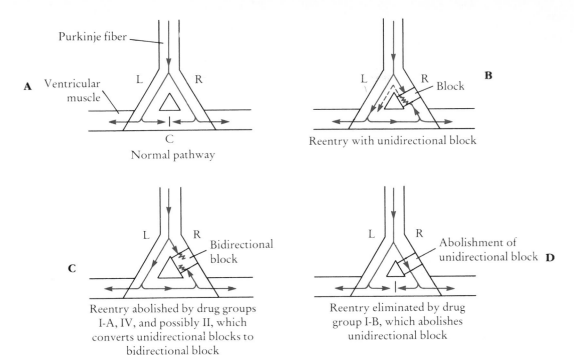

FIGURE 24-1 Reentry phenomenon. Diagrammatic illustration of unidirectional block in reentry showing a branched Purkinje fiber terminating on the ventricular muscle. **A,** In the normal pathway, the impulse travels down the Purkinje fiber and is conducted along the left *(L)* and right *(R)* branches. In the connecting branch, the impulses are extinguished at the point of collision in the center *(C)*. The propagation of impulses that travel laterally along the Purkinje fiber results in activation of the ventricular muscle. **B,** In the abnormal situation, the impulse in the left branch descends normally from the central Purkinje fiber, but in the right branch the impulse encounters a block caused by ischemia or injury. This is a *unidirectional block* because the impulse is capable of passing in the left branch but not in the right. Therefore this block creates a condition for *reentry.* As a result, the antegrade impulse is still blocked in the forward direction, but a retrograde impulse from the ventricular tissue pentrates or *reenters* the injured site from the other direction. As long as the pathway proximal to the block is no longer refractory. *reentry* of the impulse can occur, and by recycling repetitively through the loop, a circus type of movement is established, resulting in dysrhythmia. In **C,** reentry is abolished by drug groups I-A, IV, and possibly II because of a decrease in conduction velocity. Thus these agents convert unidirectional block into bidirectional block by inhibiting the flow of impulses from two directions—the antegrade or forward direction and the retrograde or reverse direction, thereby abolishing the ectopic beats. In **D,** reentry is eliminated by drug group I-B, which, by either increasing or not affecting conduction velocity, abolishes the unidirectional block. This process leads to restoration of normal impulse conduction, a condition that enhances the removal of ectopic beats.

crease or have no effect on conduction velocity. Group I-C drug flecainide also has little effect on conduction velocity. Propranolol is considered a group II drug because of its beta-adrenergic blocking action. The principal action of bretylium, a group III compound, is antiadrenergic. Unlike the other drug in this category, it has a decidedly positive inotropic action, and it prolongs repolarization. Amiodarone increases the refractory period and increases the P-R interval, QRS complex, and Q-T interval, contrary to the typical effects of bretylium. The last category, which is identified as group IV agents, is characterized by a selective calcium antagonistic action.

For this reason, verapamil is classified independently of other conventional compounds and is discussed in Chapter 26. (See Table 24-1 for comparative electrophysiologic properties of antidysrhythmic drugs.)

GROUP I-A DRUGS

The pharmacologic effects of procainamide, quinidine, and disopyramide are similar. **Quinidine** has been more widely used, but procainamide offers an advantage when parenteral therapy is required. Disopyramide appears to have fewer adverse effects.

TABLE 24-1   Classification and Comparative Electrophysiologic Properties of Antidysrhythmic Drugs

Group	I-A		I-B		I-C	II	III	IV
	disopyramide	procainamide quinidine	lidocaine phenytoin	tocainide mexiletine	flecainide encainide	propranolol	bretylium amiodarone	verapamil
Electrophysiologic effects*								
Automaticity	↓	↓	↓	→ or ↓	↓	↓	↓ or ↑	↓
Conduction velocity	→ or ↓	↓	→ or ↑	→	↓	↓	→ or ↑	→ or ↓
Effective refractory period	→ or ↑	↑	↓	↑ or ↓	→↑	↓	↑	→ or ↑
Inotropic effect	↓	↓	→	→ or ↓	→ or ↓	↓	↓ or ↑	↓
Autonomic effect	Vagolytic action	Vagolytic action	No vagolytic action	No vagolytic action	No vagolytic effect	Beta adrenergic blocking action	Adrenergic blocking action	
ECG effects†								
P-R interval	→ or ↑	→ or ↑	→	→	↑	→ or ↑	↑ or →	↑
QRS complex	→ or ↑	↑	→	→	↑	→	↑ or →	→
Q-T interval	↑	↑	→ or ↓	→ or ↓	→	↓	↑ or →	→
Hemodynamic effects								
Cardiac output	↓	↓	→ or ↓	→	→ or ↓	↓		
Blood pressure	↓	↓	→ or ↓	↓ or ↑	→ or ↑	→ or ↓	↓	

* ↑, Increased; ↓, decreased; →, no change.
† P-R interval refers to conduction through the AV node. QRS complex indicates intraventricular conduction. Q-T interval refers to repolarization phase of the action potential.

ANTIDYSRHYTHMIC CLASSIFICATION

Group I drugs—generally inhibit the fast sodium channel in cardiac muscle, resulting in an increased refractory period

(Subclasses I-A, I-B, and I-C further define the differences between the drugs. See Table 24-1.)

Group II drugs—beta-adrenergic blocking agents that reduce adrenergic stimulation on the heart

Group III drugs—generally do not affect depolarization but work by prolonging cardiac repolarization

Group IV drugs—block the slow calcium channel, resulting in depression of myocardial and smooth muscle contraction, decreased automaticity, and, perhaps, decreased conduction velocity.

---

disopryamide phosphate (Norpace)
disopyramide phosphate extended-release capsules (Norpace CR), Rythmodan✿ and Rythmodan-LA✿

Mechanism of action
Direct effects
Excitability: decreases; it inhibits cation exchange at the membrane (sodium ion influx and potassium ion efflux), thus depressing cell membrane responsiveness.

Automaticity: decreases the rate of diastolic depolarization (phase 4) and elevates the threshold potential (voltage takes longer to shift toward 0 millivolts) so that more current is needed to fire the cell (see Figure 24-2). Thus the velocity of depolarization (phase 0) is delayed, particularly at ectopic sites, which the drug is able to suppress or abolish. This property permits the SA node to reestablish control as a pacemaker of the heart.

Conduction velocity: slowed; depolarization (phase 0) is delayed, and action potential duration is prolonged in the myocardial tissue but not in the AV node, whose rate is essentially unchanged.

Effective refractory period: prolonged in atrial and ventricular fibers; this abolishes reentrant dysrhythmias by converting unidirectional block into bidirectional block (see Figure 24-1: quinidine).

Indirect effect. This involves anticholinergic (antimuscarinic) action that is evident in the gastrointestinal and urogenital systems. The reduced cardiac output caused by depressed myocardial contractility may contribute to the development of hypotension, which could reach serious proportions during therapy.

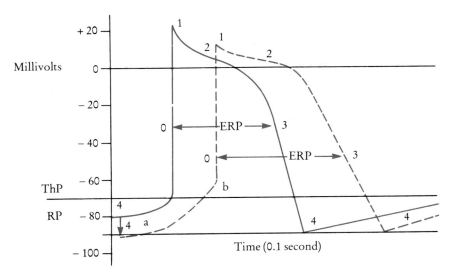

FIGURE 24-2 The effect of quinidine on resting membrane potential of a single Purkinje fiber. The solid line depicts the normal Purkinje fiber during the phases *(0 to 4)* of the action potential: the broken lines show how quinidine alters the action potential of the Purkinje fiber. The use of quinidine suppresses automaticity by effecting a decrease in the rate of depolarization from the resting potential *(RP)* during diastole (phase 4) shown at *a* and an increase in the threshold potential *(ThP)* toward O millivolts (mV) indicated at *b*. The effective refractory period *(ERP)* is also prolonged with the use of quinidine.

(Modified from Mason DT and others: Clin Pharmacol Therap 11:460, 1970.)

Indications
1. Treatment of premature (ectopic) ventricular contractions of both unifocal and multifocal origin.
2. Suppression and prevention of paired premature ventricular contractions and ventricular tachycardia.

Pharmacokinetics. See Table 24-2.

Side effects/adverse reactions. See Table 24-3.

Significant drug interactions. The following interactions may occur when disopyramide is given with the drugs listed below:

Drug	Possible Effect and Management
Other antiarrhythmic agents, such as diltiazem, flecainide, lidocaine, procainamide, beta-adrenergic blocking agents, quinidine, tocainide, or verapamil	Monitor closely for prolonged electrophysiologic conduction and decreased cardiac output. Beta-adrenergic blocking agents may exacerbate heart failure, especially in individuals with compromised ventricular function. Do not administer disopyramide concurrently or within 48 hours before or 24 hours after verapamil, since fatalities have been reported.
pimozide	Concurrent therapy may reduce serum levels of disopyramide below therapeutic effectiveness range. Monitor therapeutic effects and serum levels closely.

Dosage and administration. Dosage is individualized according to response and tolerance.

Adults. ORAL: Loading dose is 300 mg; then maintenance dose is 150 mg every 6 hours; usual dose is 400 to 800 mg/day in 4 divided doses. Individuals weighing less than 50 kg (110 pounds), dose is 100 mg every 6 hours preceded by a loading dose, of 200 mg if necessary.

Elderly. Usually require a reduction in dosage, since they are more sensitive to the effects produced by the usual adult dosage.

Children. Divide the following total daily doses by 4 and give orally, every 6 hours.

Less than 1 year old: 10 to 30 mg/kg body weight
1 to 4 years old: 10 to 20 mg/kg body weight
4 to 12 years old: 10 to 15 mg/kg body weight
12 to 18 years old: 6 to 15 mg/kg body weight

Disopyramide phosphate extended-release capsules

Adults. ORAL: 300 mg every 12 hours given as maintenance dose. Do not use as initial dose.

Pregnancy safety. Not established

NURSING CONSIDERATIONS

Assessment. Despite the fact that little effect has been shown on the AV nodal conduction time, do not use this drug in clients with greater than first-degree block. Drug should be discontinued if second- or third-degree block occurs during therapy. The P-R interval will be prolonged.

Do not use in clients with cardiogenic shock or known hypersensitivity to the drug.

TABLE 24-2 Pharmacokinetics of Antidysrhythmic Drugs

Drug	Onset of action (oral dosage)	Duration of action	Half-life (hr)	Therapeutic serum level (μg/ml)	Toxic serum levels (μg/ml)	Metabolism	Excretion
GROUP I-A DRUGS							
disopyramide	0.5-3.5 hr	1.5-8.5 hr	7	2-4	9	Liver	Kidneys
procainamide	0.5 hr	3 hr	2.5-4.5	4-8	12	Liver	Kidneys
quinidine	0.5 hr	6-8 hr	6	3-6	8	Liver	Kidneys
GROUP I-B DRUGS							
lidocaine	IV: 45-90 sec	10-20 min	1-2	1.5-5	5	Liver	Kidneys
	IM 5-15 min	60-90 min					
tocainide	—	8 hr	15	3-10	10	Liver	Kidneys
mexiletine	0.5-2 hr	—	10-12	0.5-2	May occur at therapeutic serum level	Liver	Liver, kidneys
GROUP I-C DRUGS							
flecainide	1-6 hr	—	12-27	0.2-1	1	Liver	Kidneys, feces
encainide	1-3 hr	—	1-2 (has active metabolites)	—	—	Liver	Kidneys, feces
GROUP II DRUGS							
propranolol	30 min	3-5 hr	2-3	0.05-0.1	—	Liver	Kidneys (<1%)
GROUP III DRUGS							
bretylium	IV; 5-120 min IM: 20-120 min	6-24 hr	4-17	—	—	—	Kidneys
amiodarone	2-180 days	Variable	Initial: 2.5-10 days Terminal: 26-107 days	1-2.5	May occur at therapeutic serum level	Liver	Liver

A baseline assessment of the client should involve blood glucose determination, blood pressure status, ECG, serum potassium levels, intraocular pressure, and hepatic and renal function.

Clients with preexisting closed-angle glaucoma should receive disopyramide only if cholinergic eye drops are also administered to control the ocular anticholinergic effects of the drug. The drops should be administered with caution to clients with a family history of angle closure glaucoma.

Intervention. Administer on an empty stomach, either 1 hour before or 2 hours after meals.

Education. Instruct client to make position changes slowly from recumbent posture if hypotension should occur.

Advise client about possibility of dry mouth, which can be relieved by hard candy, gum, or frequent clear water rinses. Recommend regular dental checkups for the prevention of caries and periodontal disease. Also, avoid alcoholic beverages.

Emphasize the importance of not skipping or stopping medication without consulting physician since adverse cardiac effects may occur upon sudden withdrawal.

Instruct patient to weigh daily to monitor fluid retention. Report to physician a weight gain of 2 or more pounds. Observe for edema.

TABLE 24-3 Side Effects/Adverse Reactions of Antidysrhythmic Drugs

Drug	Side effects*	Adverse reactions†
GROUP I-A DRUGS		
disopyramide (Norpace, Norpace CR, Rythmodan♣, Rhythmodan-LA♣)	Most frequent: Dry mouth, dry throat Less frequent: Dry eyes and nose, abdominal pain, gas, blurred vision, constipation, anorexia, urinary frequency, decrease in sexual potency	Most frequent: Difficulty in urination Less frequent: Edema of lower extremities, bradycardia, tachycardia, rapid weight gain, confusion, chest pain, dyspnea, dizziness, hypotension Rare: Depression, hypoglycemia (increased anxiety, chills, cold sweats, confusion, pale skin, headaches, nausea, increased heartbeat, shakiness, ataxia), sore throat, elevated temperature, jaundice; may precipitate acute glaucoma in susceptible individuals
procainamide (Pronestyl, Procan SR, Procamide, Procan, Pronestyl-SR)	Most frequent: Diarrhea, anorexia (especially with daily dosages greater than 4 g) Less frequent: Dizziness	Less frequent: Elevated temperature, chills, swollen or painful joints, pleuritic pain, skin rash, pruritus (caused by an allergic reaction or drug-induced systemic lupus erythematosus–like syndrome) Rare: Confusion, depression, psychosis, hallucinations; increased weakness; elevated fever; sore mouth, gums, or throat; unusual bleeding or bruising
quinidine (Quinaglute, Apo-Quinidine♣, Duraquin, Cardioquin, Cin-Quin, Quinora, Sk-Quinidine Sulfate, Quinidex)	Most frequent: bitter taste, diarrhea, anorexia, nausea, vomiting, abdominal pain or cramps, cutaneous flushing, pruritus Less frequent: confusion	Less frequent: Visual changes or blurred vision, severe headaches, tinnitus, hearing loss, fainting, hypotension, elevated temperature, rash, hives, difficult breathing, dizziness Rare: Unusual bleeding tendencies, tachycardia, increased weakness
GROUP I-B DRUGS		
lidocaine (Xylocaine, Xylocard♣, LidoPen)	Less frequent or rare: Pain at injection site At serum levels between 1.5 and 6 μg/ml: increased anxiety or nervousness, dizziness, sedation, sensations of cold, heat, or numbness.	Rare: Shortness of breath, pruritus, rash, edema Overdosage, serum levels between 6 and 8 μg/ml: Visual disturbances (blurred or double vision), nausea, vomiting, tinnitus, tremors Serum levels above 8 μg/ml: Severe dizziness, breathing difficulties, convulsions, bradycardia
tocainide (Tonocard)	Most frequent: dizziness, anorexia, nausea Less frequent: confusion, headaches, anxiety, paresthesias of fingers and toes, rash, increased sweating, vomiting	Less frequent: Tremors Rare: Cough, breathing difficulties (pneumonitis, pulmonary fibrosis, pulmonary edema, and pneumonia may occur 3 to 18 weeks after starting therapy), increased temperature, chills, sore throat, premature ventricular contractions, unusual bleeding tendencies
mexiletine (Mexitil)	Most frequent: Dizziness, anxiety, hand tremors, trembling, ataxia, nausea, vomiting, gas Less frequent: Confusion, diarrhea or constipation, headache, paresthesia of fingers and toes, tinnitus, rash, slurred speech, insomnia, increased weakness, blurred vision	Less frequent: Chest pain, breathing difficulties, fast or irregular heartbeats (PVCs) Rare: Elevated temperature, chills, sore throat, increased bleeding tendencies, convulsions

*If side effects continue, increase, or disturb the client, inform the physician.
†If adverse effects occur, contact physician because medical intervention may be necessary.

Continued.

TABLE 24-3   Side Effects/Adverse Reactions of Antidysrhythmic Drugs—cont'd

Drug	Side effects*	Adverse reactions†
GROUP I-C DRUGS		
flecainide (Tambocor)	Most frequent: Blurred vision, dizziness Less frequent: Nervousness, depression, constipation, headache, nausea, vomiting, rash, abdominal pain, anorexia, increased weakness	Less frequent: Chest pain, irregular heartbeats, breathing difficulties, edema of lower extremities, tremors, shaking.
encainide (Enkaid)	Less frequent: Visual disturbances, dizziness, headache, increased weakness, nausea, arm or leg pain, rash	Less frequent: Chest pain, fast or irregular heartbeats (induction of new ventricular arrhythmias) Rare: Breathing difficulties, edema of lower extremities, tremors
GROUP II DRUGS: SEE CHAPTER 23		
GROUP III DRUGS		
bretylium tosylate (Bretylol, Bretylatem♣)	Less frequent: Nausea, vomiting Rare: Chest pain, dizziness, hypotension, sensation of pressure in the chest	Rare: Breathing difficulties, bradycardia, elevated temperature, and impairment of renal function
amiodarone hydrochloride (Cordarone)	Most frequent: Constipation, headache, anorexia that might lead to severe weight loss, nausea, vomiting Less frequent: Bitter or metallic taste in mouth, decreased sexual potency in males, dizziness, facial flushing	Most frequent: Cough, breathing difficulties, elevated temperature (pulmonary fibrosis, interstitial pneumonitis), difficulty in ambulating, paresthesia of fingers or toes; hand tremors, shaking, arm or leg weakness, ataxia (neurotoxicity), photosensitivity Less frequent: In continuous usage of over 1 year, blue-gray skin coloring on face, neck, and arms, especially in fair-skinned clients; blurred vision or blue-green halos around objects; dry eyes; corneal deposits; cold skin sensation; dry, puffy skin; weight gain; increased tiredness; anxiety; insomnia; altered sensitivity to heat; increased sweating; unusual weight loss (hyperthyroidism may occur); scrotum pain and swelling; edema of lower extremities, irregular heart beats or new arrhythmias; sinus bradycardia; pulmonary fibrosis; hepatic toxicity

*If side effects continue, increase, or disturb the client, inform the physician.
†If adverse effects occur, contact physician because medical intervention may be necessary.

Caution the client about driving or other hazardous activities, since blurred vision and dizziness may occur.

Alert clients about the hypoglycemic effects of the drug, particularly clients with diabetes. Teach signs and symptoms of hypoglycemia; if they occur, instruct the client to take a form of sugar and notify the physician.

Caution the client that heat intolerance and reduced perspiration will occur and to avoid exertion and hot weather.

Constipation, may result from the anticholinergic effects of the drug. Instruct clients about high-fiber diet, increased fluid intake, moderate exercise, and regular bowel patterning.

Evaluation. Monitor blood pressure carefully; drug should be discontinued if severe hypotension, bradycardia, or congestive heart failure becomes worse. The symp-

toms of congestive heart failure are difficulty in breathing, shortness of breath, weight gain, distended neck veins, and pulmonary rales.

Monitor ECG intervals carefully to avoid cardiac toxicity. The following signs are indications for drug withdrawal:
- If QRS complex widens more than 25%
- If Q-T interval is prolonged more than 25% (use another antidysrhythmic agent)
- If P-R interval severely increases (dosage should be reduced)

ECG monitoring is essential for clients with severe cardiac disease, hypertension, or renal or hepatic impairment.

Monitor serum potassium level; it should be normal to achieve optimal effect. Toxic reactions are enhanced by excessive potassium levels.

Measure intake and output, particularly in patients with impaired renal function or prostatic hypertrophy. Urinary retention may require stopping use of the drug.

Observe clients with myasthenia gravis closely, since the drug's antimuscarinic properties may precipitate a myasthenic crisis.

procainamide hydrochloride (Promine, Procan, Procan SR, Pronestyl, Pronestyl-SR)

Mechanism of action. With the exception of slowing conduction in the bundle of His and prolonging of the refractory period in the atria, the direct electrophysiologic properties are the same as for disopyramide. In addition, contractility of the heart is usually not decreased unless myocardial damage exists. Also, alpha adrenergic blockade does not occur. (See Table 24-1.)

Indications
1. Treatment of premature ventricular contractions (PVCs), ventricular tachycardia, atrial fibrillation, and paroxysmal atrial tachycardia
2. Treatment of cardiac dysrhythmias associated with anesthesia and surgery

Pharmacokinetics. See Table 24-2.

Side effects/adverse reactions. See Table 24-3.

Significant drug interactions. The following interactions may occur when procainamide is given with the drugs listed below.

Drug	Possible Effect and Management
other antiarrhythmic agents	Monitor for enhanced or additive cardiac effects.
antihypertensives	Increased hypotension has been reported, especially when parenteral (intravenous) procainamide is given with antihypertensive agents. Monitor closely, since dosage adjustments may be necessary.
antimyasthenia agents	The effect of antimyasthenic agents on skeletal muscle may be blocked by the antimuscarinic effects of procainamide. Monitor closely, since dosage adjustments of the antimyasthenic agent may be required.
neuromuscular blocking agents	Concurrent use may result in enhanced neuromuscular blockade. Monitor closely since reversal of blockade may be prolonged.
pimozide	Prolonged Q-T intervals and cardiac dysrhythmias may be reported with concurrent use. Monitor closely, preferably with an ECG, since intervention may be necessary.

Dosage and administration
Adults. ORAL:
Ventricular tachycardia. 1 g as initial dose, followed by 6.25 mg/kg every 3 hours.

Atrial fibrillation and paroxysmal atrial tachycardia. 1.25 g as initial dose, followed by 0.75 g in 1 hour if no ECG changes are seen. Additional doses of 0.5 to 1 g every 2 hours until normal rhythm occurs.

Maintenance dose. 0.5 to 1 g every 4 to 6 hours.

Adults. PARENTERAL:
IM. 500 mg to 1 g repeated every 4 to 8 hours.

IV. Direct intravenous injection: 100 mg every 5 minute given slowly at a rate of 25 to 50 mg/min until dysrhythmia is controlled or until a maximum dosage of 1 g has been administered.

IV infusion. 20 to 25 mg/min of a diluted solution over a 30 minute period to a maximum of 600 mg; then maintain on 2 to 6 mg/min schedule if needed.

Procainamide hydrochloride extended-release tablets

Adults

Atrial dysrhythmia: maintenance, 1 g every 6 hours.

Ventricular dysrhythmia: maintenance, 12.5 mg/kg every 6 hours.

Pregnancy safety. FDA category C

NURSING CONSIDERATIONS

Assessment. Drug is contraindicated for use in second- and third-degree block, complete heart block, myasthenia gravis, and hypersensitivity to the drug.

Intervention. To initiate intravenous therapy, the drug should be diluted in 5% dextrose to facilitate control of the dosage range; the dose should be administered at a rate not greater than 25 to 50 mg/minute by direct intravenous administration or infusion. Also, intravenous therapy is limited to use in hospitals where monitoring facilities are available.

Once prepared, the solution is stable for 24 hours at room temperature or 7 days if refrigerated. Procainamide is physically incompatible with many substances; check specific references when considering mixing with other drugs.

Administer oral dosage on an empty stomach with a full glass of water to promote absorption. To lessen gastrointestinal irritation, drug may be taken with or immediately after meals.

Use with caution:
- In atrial fibrillation or flutter, the ventricular rate may increase suddenly since atrial rate is slowed.
- Embolization may result from dislodgement of mural thrombi caused by forceful contraction of the atrium with conversion to sinus rhythm.
- Hepatic and renal impairment may cause drug accumulation, leading to toxicity.

Education. Urge client on long-term therapy to keep appointments for periodic laboratory work: lupus erythematosus (LE) test, antinuclear antibody (ANA) titers, blood counts, hepatic and renal functions; and plasma procainamide and N-acetyprocainamide (NAPA) determinations. This is particularly important in clients with congestive heart failure, those with hepatic or renal function impairment, or those changing from regular oral to extended-release preparation of the drug. Symptoms of systemic lupus erythematosus (polyarthralgia, cough, fever, and pleuritic pain) should be reported to the prescriber so that the drug can be discontinued.

Counsel clients to report symptoms such as unusual bleeding and/or bruising; sore mouth, gums, or throat; fever; rash; or symptoms of an upper respiratory tract infection to the prescriber.

The antimuscarinic effects may decrease salivary flow and lead to the development of caries and gum disease. Instruct clients in proper oral hygiene, including the use of toothbrushes and dental floss. Regular dental checkups are also advised.

Some clients, particularly elderly clients, may be prone to dizziness. Alert them that driving and operating other mechanical equipment might be hazardous.

Advise the client to continue to take the medication even though feeling well. Instruct the client that if a regular oral preparation dose is missed but remembered within 2 hours, to take it (within 4 hours for extended-release form), if a missed dose is remembered after this time it should *not be taken*. Instruct the client not to double up on doses. Alert the client not to discontinue the medication without consulting the physician, since a gradual withdrawal may be necessary to prevent worsening the condition.

Recommend that the client carry medical identification. The client should be instructed to alert health professionals, including dentists, that he or she is taking procainamide.

The oral forms of procainamide are hygroscopic (they will absorb moisture). Advise the client to keep them tightly closed in their original container and not to transfer them to other less tightly sealed containers or to leave them exposed to air.

Caution the client receiving the extended-release form of the medication that the dose is contained in a wax matrix that may be detected in the stools. This has no effect on the drug's absorption.

Evaluation. Monitor (qualified personnel only) intravenous administration constantly, and observe the following:

- Infusion pump: maintain desired flow rate. Keep patient in supine position. Avoid rapid administration to prevent "speed shock" (irregular pulse, tight feeling in chest, flushed face, headache, loss of consciousness, shock, cardiac arrest).
- ECG: discontinue therapy if QRS complex is widened greater than 50% and P-R interval is prolonged.

- Arterial blood pressure: during loading dose take every 5 minutes; if blood pressure drops more than 15 mm Hg, discontinue infusion. Have pressor solutions available: dopamine or norepinephrine to treat hypotension. Elderly clients are more apt to exhibit hypotension.

Procainamide preparations contain sulfite and should not be used by clients with known sensitivity to sulfite agents. Symptoms of sulfite sensitivity include skin rash, itching, clamminess, shortness of breath, wheezing, cyanosis, hypotension, anaphylaxis, and respiratory arrest.

quinidine gluconate (Duraquin, Quinaglute)
quinidine polygalacturonate (Cardioquin)
quinidine sulfate (Cin-Quin, Quinora, SK- Quinidine Sulfate, Quinidex, Apo-Quinidine✱)

Mechanism of action. The main effect of quinidine results from its direct action on the cardiac cell membrane. Quinidine alters such electrophysiologic properties as automaticity, excitability, conduction velocity, and effective refractory period. The drug stabilizes the cell membrane by preventing ready movement of sodium and potassium across this cellular barrier. Thus the inhibition of cation exchange results in a decrease in the rate of diastolic depolarization from resting potential during phase 4 and an increase in the threshold potential (the voltage shifts toward 0 mv) (Figure 24-1). By decreasing impulse generation at ectopic sites in the atria, AV junction, and Purkinje fibers, quinidine suppresses or abolishes dysrhythmias. Fortunately, abnormal or ectopic pacemaker tissue appears to be more sensitive to quinidine than normal pacemaker tissue (SA node). This permits the SA node to reestablish control over impulse formation in the heart. Again, by preventing exchange of ions across the cell membrane, quinidine depresses the excitability of both atrial and ventricular myocardium, an important attribute in counteracting dysrhythmia. In addition, the drug slows conduction velocity in all cardiac tissues, namely atria and ventricles, including the specialized conduction system. Widening of the QRS complex indicates a decrease in intraventricular conduction, and lengthening of the P-R interval represents slower conduction through the AV node, which are changes observed on the ECG when quinidine is used. Thus caution must be used when the drug is given to individuals with intraventricular conduction disorders. Perhaps the most significant action of quinidine is its ability to prolong the effective refractory period of atrial and ventricular fibers. A delay in completion of repolarization probably exerts an important antifibrillatory action. The tissue remains refractory for a period of time after full restoration of the resting membrane potential. This property is believed to influence the conversion of unidirectional block to bidirectional block, thereby abolishing the reentry type of dysrhythmia (see Figure 24-1, *C,* and Table 24-1).

The indirect anticholinergic effect of quinidine inhibits vagal action on the SA and AV nodes. This atropine-like effect permits the sinus node to accelerate and often may provoke a dangerous sinus tachycardia. Therefore digitalis, which slows conduction at the AV node, usually is administered before quinidine to prevent ventricular acceleration when one is attempting to convert atrial fibrillation to normal sinus rhythm. Finally, the chief noncardiac action of quinidine is peripheral vasodilation which results from quinidine's alpha-adrenergic blocking effect on vascular smooth muscle. The combined effect of a decrease in peripheral vascular resistance and a reduced cardiac output caused by depressed myocardial contractility contributes to the development of hypotension, a condition that may reach serious proportions during quinidine therapy.

Indications. Management of premature atrial and ventricular contraction, paroxysmal AV junctional rhythm, atrial flutter and fibrillation, paroxysmal ventricular tachycardia not associated with complete heart block, and maintenance therapy after electrical conversion of atrial fibrillation and/or flutter.

Pharmacokinetics. See Table 24-2.

Side effects/adverse reactions. See Table 24-3.

Significant drug interactions. The following interactions may occur when quinidine is given with the drugs listed below.

Drug	Possible Effect and Management
antidysrhythmic agents, phenothiazines, alkaloids	May result in enhanced cardiac response. Monitor closely.
anticoagulants, such as coumarin or indandione formulations	Monitor for increased hypoprothrombinemia. It may be necessary to adjust anticoagulant dosage both during therapy and after quinidine therapy is discontinued.
neuromuscular blocking agents	Monitor for increased or enhanced blocking effects, especially in the postsurgical client.
pimozide	Prolonged Q-T intervals and cardiac dysrhythmias may be reported with concurrent use. Monitor closely, preferably with an ECG, since intervention may be necessary.
urinary alkalizers, such as carbonic anhydrase inhibitors, citrus fruit juices in large amounts, antacids	May result in increased reabsorption of quinidine and elevated serum levels; dosage adjustments may be necessary.

Dosage and administration. The quinidine salts have different percentages of active drug: quinidine gluconate, 62% active drug; quinidine polygalacturonate, 60% active

drug; quinidine sulfate, 83% active drug. Because of this they are not interchangeable without appropriate dosage adjustment. See Table 24-4.

Pregnancy safety. FDA category C

NURSING CONSIDERATIONS

Assessment. Do not use in clients with atrioventricular block, AV conduction defects, congestive heart failure, hypotension, and myasthenia gravis (because of the drug's weak curare-like action).

Clients sensitive to quinine may also be sensitive to quinidine.

Intervention. To determine if the client may have an idiosyncratic response or hypersensitivity to quinidine, give a test dose of 200 mg orally a few hours before the initiation of therapy. A parenteral dose of 200 mg is also administered before intramuscular or intravenous therapy if time permits. Observe the client for fever, acute asthma, angioedema, and anaphylactic shock. **Cinchonism** may also be manifested by headache, dizziness, fever, tinnitus, nausea, tremor, and visual disturbances.

Administer oral preparation on an empty stomach 1 to 2 hours after meals with a full glass of water to promote absorption. However, quinidine may be given with food to decrease gastric distress. Avoid administering with antacids because they may increase urinary pH and so increase the potential for quinidine toxicity.

Education. Instruct the client to report any symptoms of rash, ringing in the ears, or visual disturbances.

Caution client to immediately report feeling of faintness (see "quinidine syncope" in a subsequent nursing consideration). Also, examine buccal mucosa for petechial hemorrhage. If bleeding occurs, report immediately. The drug will be contraindicated because of possible thrombocytopenic purpura.

Advise the client to have regular dental checkups and to practice good dental hygiene since the antimuscarinic effects of the drug inhibit salivary flow and so contribute to caries and gum disease, particularly in the elderly.

Recommend that the client carry medical identification. Caution the client to alert health professionals that he or she is taking quinidine.

Evaluation. Use caution during intravenous administration because of possible vasodilation, depressed cardiac contraction, and cardiovascular collapse, which may lead to profound shock. NOTE: The intravenous route is seldom used. Continuously monitor both the ECG and the systemic arterial blood pressure during and immediately after pareneteral administration. Toxic effects include widening of QRS complex in excess of 25%, abolition of P waves, and ventricular extrasystoles. Notify physician immediately.

TABLE 24-4   Dosage and Administration for Quinidine Salts

Drug	Adults	Children
QUINIDINE SULFATE		
Oral dosage		
Premature atrial and ventricular contractions	200-300 mg 3 to 4 times a day	6 mg/kg or 180 mg/m²/24 hr in 5 divided doses
Paroxsysmal supraventricular tachycardia	400-600 mg every 2 or 3 hours until paroxysm is terminated	Same as above
Artial fibrillation conversion (controlled by digitalis before quinidine therapy)	200 mg every 2-3 hours for 5 to 8 doses; then increase daily up to 3-4 g/day until normal sinus rhythm is restored or toxicity occurs	Same as above
Maintenance therapy following electrical conversion of atrial fibrillation or flutter	200-300 mg 3 or 4 times a day	Same as above
QUINIDINE SULFATE EXTENDED-RELEASE TABLETS		
Oral dosage	300-600 mg every 8-12 hr as needed or tolerated	Not recommended for children
QUINIDINE GLUCONATE		
Dosage individualized according to patients response Oral dosage (maintenance and prophylaxis)	324-660 mg every 6-12 hr	Not recommended for children
QUINIDINE GLUCONATE INJECTION		
Intramuscular dosage	600 mg for loading dose, then 400 mg repeated up to 12 times a day if necessary	IV infusion 800 mg is added to 40 ml of 5% Dextrose in water and administered at a slow rate of infusion (1 ml/min). Monitor ECG and blood pressure.
QUINIDINE POLYGALACTURONATE		
Oral dosage	Initial: 275-825 mg every 3-4 hr for 3 or 4 doses, and then increase dose by 137.5 to 275 mg every third or fourth dose until rhythm is restored or toxic effects occur Maintenance: 275 mg 2 or 3 times a day as needed	8.25 mg/kg or 247.5 mg/m² 5 times daily, orally

Check plasma quinidine levels carefully. Be aware that concomitant administration with digitalis (digoxin) readily induces toxicity because the two drugs lead to an excessively high plasma concentration of digoxin (less digoxin is excreted by the kidney).

Monitor intake and output, blood counts, serum electrolyte determinations, and kidney and liver function tests during prolonged therapy. The effect of quinidine is reduced if hypokalemia is present.

Use quinidine with caution in clients with atrial fibrillation or flutter. The vagal blocking effect of the drug may increase the number of atrial beats conducted across the AV junction, resulting in sudden acceleration in ventricular rate. *Prior administration of digitalis slows AV conduction and reduces the hazard of ventricular tachycardia.* Monitor ECG and blood serum levels of the two drugs to avoid toxicity. Reduction in digoxin dosage is suggested when quinidine is given simultaneously.

Be alert to premature ventricular contractions not noted before drug administration (appears as an ectopic foci by reentry phenomenon) because they may lead to ventricular tachycardia or fibrillation and subsequently to cardiac standstill (asystole).

Note that another form of ventricular disorder can cause "quinidine syncope." It produces ventricular tachycardia or fibrillation, causing a decrease in cardiac output and thereby diminishing blood flow to the brain. The symptoms are feeling of faintness, loss of consciousness, and ultimately sudden death.

GROUP I-B DRUGS

The group I-B drugs are lidocaine and phenytoin. These drugs differ from group I-A drugs in that they either increase or have no effect on conduction velocity. Lidocaine is particularly useful for acute ventricular dysrhythmias. It must be administered parenterally. Despite the fact that phenytoin is not approved by the FDA for this use, it is commonly used in the therapy of digitalis-induced dysrhythmias.

lidocaine hydrochloride (LidoPen, Xylocaine, Xylocard♣)

Mechanism of action. Lidocaine is better known and extensively used as a local and topical anesthetic agent. Systemically, it is now commonly used as an antidysrhythmic agent, especially for ventricular dysrhythmias seen after cardiac surgery or an acute myocardial infarction.

Lidocaine exerts its most important cardiac effect by depressing excessive automaticity of ectopic pacemakers in the His-Purkinje fibers. Thus it is useful in suppressing premature ventricular contractions, a dysrhythmia that may be provoked by hypoxic or ischemic cells in myocardial infarction. Ischemia is a condition that favors the development of an ectopic pacemaker, discharging faster than the normal pacemaker in the SA node. In some cardiac disorders, premature ventricular contractions may eventually precipitate ventricular tachycardia or fibrillation. Therefore it is essential to provide effective treatment immediately.

In contrast to the findings with quinidine and procainamide, lidocaine has little, if any, effect on conduction velocity (phase 0) or on the effective refractory period in the AV node and the Purkinje fibers. The absence of these properties possibly prevents reentry types of dysrhythmia. For this reason the drug may play a part in improving AV conduction in the digitalis-intoxicated heart. Also, the potential for development of heart block, cardiac asystole, or ventricular ectopic rhythm is minimized with the use of lidocaine. On the ECG the P-R or Q-T intervals may not shorten, and the QRS is not prolonged. Unlike quinidine and procainamide, lidocaine has no **vagolytic** properties nor does it influence cardiac output and arterial pressure. Also, it does not depress myocardial contractility and thereby provides no potential for the development of congestive heart failure. Since it exerts limited if any effect on the SA node and atrial myocardium, the drug has no use in the treatment of supraventricular tachycardias. Because electric activities are primarily limited to the ventricular cells, the major use of lidocaine is in abolishing ventricular dysrhythmias. (See Table 24-1 and Figure 24-1, *D.*)

Indications. Treatment of ventricular arrhythmias

Pharmacokinetics. See Table 24-2.

Side effects/adverse reactions. See Table 24-3.

Significant drug interactions. Administration of lidocaine with hydantoin anticonvulsants may result in enhanced cardiac depressant response; also, hydantoin anticonvulsants may reduce lidocaine serum concentration by increasing liver metabolism.

Dosage and administration. See Table 24-5.

Pregnancy safety. FDA category B

TABLE 24-5 Dosage and Administration of Lidocaine

Route	Adults	Elderly	Children
IV bolus	1.0 mg/kg or 50-100 mg administered at a rate of 25-50 mg/min; repeat in 5 min if necessary; no more than 200-300 mg should be given over 1 hr.	Patients over 65 should initially receive half the dose and recommended rate of infusion noted for adult. Dosage should be adjusted as necessary and tolerated by patient.	1 mg/kg body weight initially as loading dose, administered at rate of 25-50 mg/min. If necessary, repeat dosage in 5 min but do not exceed total dose of 3 mg/kg.
IV infusion	Following a loading dose; 20-50 μg/kg/min infused at a rate of 1-4 mg/min		Following loading dose, a continous infusion is usually given at rate of 20-50 μg/kg body weight/min (usually 30 μg). Administer at rate of 1-4 mg/min.
IM	4.3 mg/kg or 300 mg initially; may repeat if necessary in 60-90 min.		Not established.

NURSING CONSIDERATIONS

Assessment. Do not administer lidocaine to clients with severe degrees of sinoatrial, atrioventricular, or intraventricular block, **Adams-Stokes syndrome** (sudden recurring episodes of loss of consciousness, caused by transient interruption of cardiac output by incomplete or complete heart block), **Wolff-Parkinson-White syndrome** (a supraventricular tachycardia), and known history of hypersensitivity to amide type of local anesthetics.

Use with caution in individuals with hypovolemia, shock, and all forms of heart block.

Use with caution and in lower doses in individuals with congestive heart failure or reduced cardiac output and in the elderly.

To prevent toxicity in clients with impaired renal and hepatic function, employ caution with prolonged use since the drug is metabolized mainly in the liver and excreted by the kidney.

Its use in pregnancy is not established. Administer only when potential benefits outweigh potential hazards to the fetus. Not recommended for pediatric usage.

Intervention. Recheck drug label; only lidocaine hydrochloride *without preservatives or epinephrine*, which specifically reads "IV use for cardiac dysrhythmias," should be administered. Preparations intended for use as an anesthetic contain epinephrine and *should not* be used for treating dysrhythmias. Intravenous infusions of lidocaine are usually prepared by adding 1 g of lidocaine to 1 L of 5% dextrose solution for a 1 mg/ml solution. Solution is stable for 24 hours. Do not add to blood transfusions.

For intravenous route, use a precision intravenous volume control set for continuous infusion. Monitor rate of flow prescribed by the physician, usually at no more than 4 mg/minute. Terminate intravenous infusion as soon as cardiac rhythm is stable or signs of toxicity develop.

Have resuscitative equipment and drugs available to treat adverse reactions involving cardiovascular system, respiratory system, and CNS.

Note that intravenous infusions are rarely continued beyond 24 hours. The client is then given an oral antidysrhythmic agent for maintenance therapy.

When using bolus administration, if the loading dose does not provide the desired therapeutic effect within 5 minutes, administer a second dose one half to one third of the initial dose. However, give no more than 200 to 300 mg within a 1 hour period.

Use deltoid muscle for intramuscular site because therapeutic blood levels are reached faster than in gluteus or lateral thigh muscles. Aspirate to ensure that intravascular injection will be avoided. Self-administration, however, is accomplished in the thigh and without aspiration. Intramuscular use may increase creatinine phosphokinase levels and interfere with diagnostic enzyme tests for myocardial infarction. Intramuscular administration is only for instances in which ECG is not available and the risk/benefit ratio has been considered by the physician.

Following initial use, discard partially used solutions of lidocaine that contain no preservatives.

To avoid more serious ventricular dysrhythmias or complete heart block in patients with sinus bradycardia or incomplete heart block, anticipate administration of isoproterenol or electric pacing to accelerate heart rate before lidocaine administration.

In clients over 65 or in those with congestive heart failure or renal or hepatic function impairment, consider reducing the dose and rate of infusion by one half and then adjusting it in response to the client's condition.

Measure serum lidocaine levels to minimize the chance of toxicity if high-dose infusions are used or if the client is receiving other drugs that might affect lidocaine clearance.

Education. Instruct the client on the procedure for self-injection and have client state and demonstrate the procedure. The client should ensure that the medication is always readily available and that it is not out of date. If symptoms of heart attack occur, instruct the client to contact physician immediately. Client should not administer the medication unless instructed to do so by the physician. To administer, client removes safety cap, places black end of the cylinder on thickest part of thigh, and presses hard; client should feel a needle stick. The needle is held in place for a slow count of 10 and then area is massaged for a slow count of 10. Instruct the client not to drive after administering the drug unless there is no other alternative.

Evaluation. Constant ECG monitoring is essential for intravenous administration and recommended during intramuscular administration to observe for signs of toxicity. Monitor ECG and blood pressure to avoid potential overdosage and toxicity. If excessive cardiac depression occurs, such as prolongation of P-R interval, QRS complex, or aggravation of dysrhythmias, stop infusion immediately.

Observe client for adverse signs of lidocaine (see box).

If the intravenous administration should run for more than 24 hours, observe for local thrombophlebitis and assess the client for the risk of accumulation.

phenytoin (Dilantin)

Phenytoin is not approved by the FDA as an antidysrhythmic agent group I-B, but it is commonly used to treat digitalis-induced atrial and ventricular dysrhythmias. It has been found to be ineffective in dysrhythmias not produced by digitalis toxicity. This drug has been approved for use as an anticonvulsant (see Chapter 14).

Mechanism of action. Phenytoin may stabilize the sodium influx in Purkinje fibers of the heart, decrease abnormal ventricular automaticity, decrease the refractory period, and cause no change or an increase in the conduction rate through the atrioventricular tissues and Purkinje fibers. (See Table 24-1.)

Pharmacokinetics, side effects/adverse reactions, and significant drug interactions are noted in Chapter 14.

Dosage and administration. Digitalis-induced dysrhythmias: usually 50 to 100 mg intravenously every 10 to 15 minutes as needed to stop the dysrhythmia or until toxicity appears. Do not exceed a dose of 15 mg/kg. Intravenous administration must be slow, usually at 25 to 50 mg/minute. For elderly patients, the dosage is reduced and the rate of intravenous injection should be 25 to 50 mg over 2 to 3 minutes (USP-DI, 1987).

Pregnancy safety. Not established

NURSING CONSIDERATIONS

Intervention. Follow manufacturer's instructions for preparing drug for parenteral use (see dosage and administration, Chapter 14).

Administer slowly intravenously to prevent toxicity. Do not exceed 50 mg/minute infusion rate. Consult laboratory reports for therapeutic serum levels and for blood sugar levels in clients with diabetes mellitus, since drug tends to cause hyperglycemia.

Since phenytoin is so highly alkaline, administer oral preparation with at least half a glass of milk or water or with meals to minimize gastric irritation.

Do not use in clients with hypersensitivity to phenytoin: skin rash may occur; seizures may be caused by hypoglycemia. Also, sinus bradycardia, incomplete heart block, hepatic dysfunction, and hematologic disorders may result. (See Chapter 14 for additional information.)

Evaluation. Closely monitor blood pressure, respiration, and ECG during intravenous administration to avoid bradycardia and hypotension. Have appropriate antidotal medications and resuscitative equipment available.

Observe client closely for drug toxicity, which may occur early in the elderly or in those with impaired liver function. Use caution in individuals with hepatic or renal dysfunction, hypotension, alcoholism, respiratory disorders, diabetes mellitus, and pancreatic adenoma.

See also The Nurse's Role in Hydantoin Therapy, Chapter 14.

tocainide (Tonocard)

Tocainide has been called an oral lidocaine, and chemically it is related to lidocaine. Dysrhythmias responsive to parenteral lidocaine are usually responsive to tocainide.

Mechanism of action. Tocainide decreases automaticity in the Purkinje fibers; blocks the fast sodium channel in cardiac muscle, thus decreasing fiber excitability by raising the threshold of the action potential. It has no autonomic or vagolytic effects.

Indications. Treatment and prevention of ventricular arrhythmias

Pharmacokinetics. See Table 24-2.

Side effects/adverse reactions. See Table 24-3.

Significant drug interactions. None reported

Dosage and administration

Adults. 400 mg orally every 8 hours. Adjust dosage as necessary. Maintenance: 1200 to 1800 mg orally daily, in three divided doses.

Elderly. Should receive smaller doses, since they may be more sensitive to this product. Dosage may be adjusted according to patient's response and the development of side effects or toxicity.

Children. Dosage not established

Pregnancy safety. FDA category C

NURSING CONSIDERATIONS

Assessment. Determine that client is not sensitive to amide-type anesthetics and has no AV block or preexisting second- or third-degree block without a ventricular pacemaker.

Note whether client has congestive heart failure or renal or hepatic function impairment, since tocainide must be used cautiously, with intensive monitoring, in such clients.

Intervention. Administer with food or milk to reduce gastric distress.

If the client has adverse reactions shortly after taking a dose of tocainide, lower each individual dose but administer with greater frequency. If the dysrhythmia returns before the next scheduled dose, a higher dosage or more frequent dosing should be considered.

ADVERSE EFFECTS RELATED TO SERUM CONCENTRATIONS OF LIDOCAINE

1.5 to 6 μg/ml: anxiety, nervousness, drowsiness, dizziness, sensations of cold, heat or numbness

6-8 μg/ml: tremors, twitching, blurred or double vision, nausea, vomiting, tinnitus

>8 μg/ml: dyspnea, severe dizziness, loss of consciousness, bradycardia, convulsions

Education. Instruct the client to take medication even though he or she feels well. Doses should not be missed and should be evenly spaced. If a forgotten dose is remembered within 4 hours, it should be taken. If a longer interval has passed, dose is not to be taken until the next scheduled time.

Advise the client to maintain regular visits to the physician to monitor progress. Recommend that a medical identification card be carried or a bracelet worn.

Alert the client that dizziness may occur and that caution should be taken when driving or operating other mechanical equipment. The elderly client might be at increased risk for falling.

Instruct client to report signs and symptoms of leukopenia and thrombocytopenia (evidence of infection, delayed healing, fever, chills, sore throat, unusual bleeding, and/or bruising). If these symptoms occur, the client should postpone dental work and should be instructed to use toothbrushes, dental floss, and toothpicks cautiously.

Evaluation. Take blood counts and ECG before therapy and at periodic intervals, to detect bone marrow suppression and medication effectiveness. Chest x-ray examinations are required at the first sign of pulmonary complications, such as pneumonia, pulmonary edema, or pulmonary fibrosis.

If the client evidences tremor, it may be an indication that the highest tolerable dose has been reached.

mexiletine (Mexitil)

Mechanism of action. Mexiletine is similar to tocainide.
Indications. Treatment and prevention of ventricular dysrhythmias
Pharmacokinetics. See Table 24-2.
Side effects/adverse reactions. See Table 24-3.
Significant drug interactions. None reported
Dosage and administration
Adults

Initial dose: 200 mg orally every 8 hours. If necessary, increase dosage by 50 to 100 mg every 2 or 3 days.
Loading dose: 400 mg orally followed by 200 mg every 8 hours to rapidly control ventricular arrhythmias.
Some individuals' symptoms may be controlled on twice daily dosage, while other clients may require four times a day dosing. This is determined on an individual basis.
Maximum recommended: 1200 mg/day if administered every 8 hours or 900 mg/day when administered every 12 hours.
Children. Not established
Pregnancy safety. FDA category C

NURSING CONSIDERATIONS

See tocainide (p. 477–478).

GROUP I-C DRUGS
flecainide (Tambocor)

Mechanism of action. Flecainide depresses the rate of depolarization of the action potential (phase 0); has little effect on repolarization; decreases excitability, conduction velocity, and automaticity because of its effects on the atria, AV node, His-Purkinje fibers, and intraventricular conduction.

Indications. Treatment of ventricular dysrhythmias, especially for symptomatic, life-threatening dysrhythmias such as ventricular tachycardia, and frequent premature ventricular contractions (PVCs), of both unifocal and multifocal origin.

Pharmacokinetics. See Table 24-2.
Side effects/adverse reactions. See Table 24-3.
Significant drug interactions. Administration of flecainide with other antidysrhythmic agents may result in enhanced cardiac effects. In individuals with hypotensive ventricular tachycardia, irreversible ventricular tachycardia or ventricular fibrillation has been reported. Avoid concurrent use.

Dosage and adminstration
Adults

Initial: 100 mg orally every 12 hours. Increase by increments of 50 mg twice a day, every 4 days if necessary.
Maintenance: for sustained ventricular tachycardia, administer up to 150 mg orally, every 12 hours. For symptomatic ventricular tachycardia (nonsustained) or premature ventricular complexes or couplets, administer up to 200 mg orally, every 12 hours.
Usual maximum per day: Sustained ventricular tachycardia—400 mg daily; symptomatic ventricular tachycardia (nonsustained), premature ventricular complexes or couplets—600 mg daily; Clients with existing congestive heart failure—400 mg daily.
Children. Dosage not established
Pregnancy safety. FDA category C

NURSING CONSIDERATIONS

Nursing considerations are essentially the same as for tocainide, except pulmonary symptoms such as pneumonia and pulmonary fibrosis are not a concern with flecainide.

encainide (Enkaid)

Mechanism of action. Encainide is similar to flecainide except the electrophysiologic effects appear to be greater in ischemic tissue than in normal cardiac tissue.

Indications. Treatment of ventricular dysrhythmias, especially for symptomatic, life-threatening dysrhythmias such as sustained ventricular tachycardia. Also treatment of symptomatic ventricular tachycardia (nonsustained)

and persistent premature ventricular contractions.
Pharmacokinetics. See Table 24-2.
Side effects/adverse reactions. See Table 24-3.
Significant drug interactions. None
Dosage and administration

Adults

Initial: 25 mg orally every 8 hours. If necessary, after 3 to 5 days of therapy, increase to 35 mg every 8 hours. Further increases should be scheduled at 3 to 5 day intervals, to a maximum of 50 mg every 8 hours.

Twice daily dosage has been used in some clients. Do not exceed 75 mg/dose and schedule every 12 hours. Other individuals may require dosing every 6 hours, so dosing schedules should be individualized.

Dosage should be decreased in those with severe renal impairment. See package insert or USP-DI for appropriate dosing schedules for renal impairment.

Children. Dosage not established.
Pregnancy safety. FDA category B

NURSING CONSIDERATIONS

Assess for new or increasing arrhythmias. These usually occur within the first week of therapy, especially when the dosage exceeds 200 mg/day.

Other nursing considerations are similar to those for flecainide.

GROUP II DRUGS

propranolol hydrochloride (Inderal)

Propranolol, a beta-adrenergic blocking agent; is used to control cardiac dysrhythmias caused by excessive sympathetic nerve activity. The principal action of propranolol is associated with its ability to inhibit adrenergic stimulation of the heart. Therefore dysrhythmias caused by increased sympathetic discharge (hyperthyroidism) are effectively blocked by the beta-adrenergic action of propranolol. (See drug monograph in Chapter 20 and Table 24-1.)

GROUP III DRUGS

The electrophysiologic properties of drugs in this group differ markedly from the drugs previously discussed.

bretylium tosylate (Bretylol, Bretylate✲)

Mechanism of action. Unlike other antiarrhythmic agents, bretylium does not suppress automaticity. In addition, it has no effect on conduction velocity. The only direct electrophysiologic action on the heart appears to be prolongation of the action potential and a lengthening of the effective refractory period. It is believed that this mechanism helps to terminate dysrhythmias caused by the reentry phenomenon. As an antidysrhythmic agent, the significant effect of bretylium is related primarily to its adrenergic blocking action. The drug is taken up and concentrated in the adrenergic nerve terminals, where, after an initial release of norepinephrine, it prevents any further release. This sympatholytic action significantly increases the threshold, producing an antifibrillatory response in the ventricles. The drug exerts no influence on vagal reflexes. Furthermore, unlike other drugs in this category, bretylium produces a positive inotropic effect, increasing myocardial contractility. With long-term treatment, the drug shows increased responsiveness to circulating epinephrine and norepinephrine, which may account for the increased myocardial contractility. (See Table 24-1.)

Pharmacokinetics. See Table 24-2.
Side effects/adverse reactions. See Table 24-3.
Siginificant drug interactions. Do not give digitalis glycosides to clients receiving bretylium. The initial release of norepinephrine produced by bretylium may increase digitalis toxicity.

Dosage and administration. Only the intravenous and intramuscular forms are available in the United States.

Intravenous infusion. Adults:

For life-threatening ventricular fibrillation: initially 5 mg/kg of undiluted solution, then 10 mg/kg every 15 to 30 minutes if needed to a total of 30 mg/kg in 24 hours.

For unstable ventricular tachycardia: administer intravenous infusion (diluted solution) of 5 to 10 mg/kg over 10 to 30 minutes. May be repeated every 6 hours. A constant infusion may be administered at a rate of 1 to 2 mg/minute.

For other ventricular arrhythmias: Initially administer a diluted intravenous solution at a rate of 5 to 10 mg/kg over 10 to 30 minutes. If necessary, this dose may be repeated in 1 to 2 hours. Maintenance: Administer diluted intravenous solution at a rate of 5 to 10 mg/kg over 10 to 30 minutes. If necessary, repeat every 6 to 8 hours. Alternatively a constant infusion may be administered at a rate of 1 to 2 mg/minute.

Intramuscular injection. Adults: Give 5 to 10 mg/kg of undiluted bretylium. Repeat dose after 1 or 2 hours if needed. Maintenance dose given every 6 to 8 hours.

Pregnancy safety. Not established

NURSING CONSIDERATIONS

Administer bretylium to clients in an area that is adequately staffed by qualified personnel and equipped with appropriate facilities for constant ECG monitoring and use of emergency equipment.

Closely monitor ECG and blood pressure. Keep client in supine position during therapy until tolerance to the hypotensive effect of the drug occurs. This may take a few days.

Anticipate the possible development of transient hypertension and dysrhythmias during the early stage of therapy. This is caused by the initial release of norepinephrine from adrenergic nerve terminals.

Rotate intramuscular injection site. Do not administer more than 5 ml at one site. Necrosis, muscle atrophy, or fibrosis may occur if injection is given at the same site. Note that intramuscular injection is rarely used.

Bretylium is generally discontinued in 3 to 5 days and an alternate antidysrhythmic agent may be substituted if indicated.

Do not administer digitalis glycosides simultaneously with bretylium because increased incidence of dysrhythmias may occur as a result of digitalis toxicity.

Administer slowly intravenously to prevent nausea and vomiting.

amiodarone hydrochloride (Cordarone)

Mechanism of action. Amiodarone hydrochloride increases the refractory period in all cardiac tissues by a direct effect on the tissues. It decreases automaticity, prolongs AV conduction, and decreases the automaticity of fibers in the Purkinje system. It also causes adrenergic and calcium channel inhibition.

Indications. Prevention and treatment of ventricular dysrhythmias, especially unstable ventricular tachycardia or ventricular fibrillation.

Pharmacokinetics. See Table 24-2.

Side effects/adverse reactions. See Table 24-3.

Significant drug interactions. The following drug interactions may occur when amiodarone is given with the drugs listed below.

Drug	Possible Effect and Management
other antidysrhythmic agents	May increase cardiac effects and the risk of inducing tachyarrhythmias. It also increases serum levels of quinidine, procainamide, flecainide, and phenytoin. If amiodarone must be given with Group I antidysrhythmic agents, reduce the dose of the Group I antidysrhythmic drug by 30% to 50% several days after starting amiodarone and gradually withdraw the Group I drug. If additional treatment with amiodarone is necessary, start therapy at half the usual recommended dosage.
anticoagulants, coumarin	May increase anticoagulant effect. Dose of anticoagulant should be reduced by one third to one half of the dose when adding amiodarone

Drug	Possible Effect and Management
	to the client's drug regimen. Also, prothrombin times should be closely monitored.
digitalis glycosides	May increase the serum level of digoxin and other digitalis glycosides, resulting in toxicity. Digitalis glycosides should be stopped or the dose reduced to 50% whenever amiodarone is given. Monitor serum levels closely. May also see additive effects of both drugs on the SA and AV nodes.
phenytoin	May result in increased serum levels of phenytoin, possibly resulting in toxicity. Monitor serum levels of phenytoin.

Dosage and administration. Amiodarone has a delayed onset of action, a complex dosing schedule and some very serious adverse effects, so this drug is usually used only when other, safer agents are ineffective or they cannot be tolerated by the client.

Adults. For ventricular dysrhythmias. Initially, a loading dose of 800 to 1.6 g orally daily for 1 to 3 weeks (sometimes longer), until a therapeutic response is noted or side effects appear. If stomach upset occurs or the dosage is greater than 1 g daily, the dose should be divided and given after meals. When therapeutic control of the dysrhythmia occurs or excessive side effects are noted, the dose should be reduced to 600 to 800 mg daily for 1 month. Afterward, decrease dosage to lowest effective dose. Maintenance: 232.5 mg orally daily; adjust dosage as necessary.

Children. Initially, a loading dose of 10 mg/kg/day, or 465 mg/m^2/day for 10 days, or until a therapeutic response is noted or side effects appear. Then decrease the dose to 5 mg/kg/day or 232.5 mg/m^2/day for several weeks and gradually taper the dose down to the lowest effective dose. Maintenance: 2.5 mg/kg/day or 116 mg/m^2/day orally.

Pregnancy safety. FDA category C

NURSING CONSIDERATIONS

Assessment. Determine that client does not have AV block, preexisting second- or third-degree block without a pacemaker, or syncope as a result of severe bradycardia unless controlled by a pacemaker. Use caution if the client has congestive heart failure or impaired hepatic or thyroid function.

Intervention. Begin the loading dose phase at the beginning of amiodarone therapy in the hospital, because of the difficulty in adjusting dosage and the potential for adverse effects, such as neurotoxicity and ocular, pulmonary, and thyroid toxicity.

Since gastrointestinal disturbances occur in 25% of clients during loading, take care to minimize these as much as possible. Instruct clients to eat a high-fiber diet and increase fluid intake, unless contraindicated, to prevent constipation. Administer with food or milk to decrease nausea. Make efforts to stimulate appetite to counteract anorexia.

Education. Instruct client to continue the medication even if he or she is feeling well. If a dose is missed, the client should be advised not to take it at all, to avoid doubling up on doses. If two or three doses are missed, instruct the client to contact the physician.

Instruct client to maintain regular contact with the physician to monitor drug use. Advise the client to carry medical identification at all times. Instruct client to alert health professionals unfamiliar with the medication regimen to the amiodarone administration.

Photosensitivity is a potential adverse effect with this drug. Caution client to avoid exposure to the sun and to wear sun protective clothing and sun-screening lotions. In addition, a blue-gray coloration of the skin occurs with long-term use (over 1 year) and affects sun-exposed parts of the body, such as face, neck, and arms, and those with fair skin.

Alert clients to report any of the following signs and symptoms to the physician: cough, dyspnea, fever (pulmonary toxicity); ataxia, numbness, tingling, weakness, or spasm of extremities (neurotoxicity); blurred vision or increased sensitivity of the eyes to light (ocular toxicity); unusual weight gain or loss, increased sensitivity to heat or cold (thyroid toxicity); pain and swelling of the scrotum; jaundice (hepatic toxicity); or swelling of the feet and lower legs (congestive heart failure).

Evaluation. Perform ECG, thyroid function studies, liver function studies (SGPT, SGOT, and serum alkaline phosphatase), chest x-rays, examinations and pulmonary studies before the initiation of therapy and periodically thereafter. Ophthalmologic examinations should be done initially, and if eye symptoms occur. Pulmonary fibrosis may occur in 10% to 30% of the clients receiving long-term amiodarone therapy. Because this is usually reversible if detected early enough, chest x-ray examinations every 3 months are recommended.

KEY TERMS

Adams-Stokes syndrome, page 476
automaticity, page 463
cinchonism, page 473
conductivity, page 463
dysrhythmia, page 463
ectopic pacemaker, page 464
ectopic tachydysrhythmia, page 464
escape beats, page 464
quinidine, page 465
reentry phenomenon, page 464

unidirectional block, page 464
vagolytic, page 475
ventricular escape, page 464
Wolff-Parkinson-White syndrome, page 476

BIBLIOGRAPHY

American Hospital Formulary Service: AHFS drug information '87, Bethesda, Md, 1987, American Society of Hospital Pharmacists, Inc.

Benchimol A: New drugs for treating cardiac arrhythmias, Postgrad Med 69(1):77, 1981.

Canada AT and others: Amiodarone for tachyarrhythmias: pharmacology, kinetics, and efficacy, Drug Intell Clin Pharm 17(2):100, 1983.

Carlstedt BC and Stanaszek, WF: Cardiac arrhythmias, US Pharmacist 11(1):43, 1986.

Catalano JT: Antiarrhythmic medications classified by their autonomic properties, Crit Care Nurse 6(3):44, 1986.

Dance D and others: Nursing assessment and care of children with complications of congenital heart disease, Heart Lung 14(3):209, 1985.

Falk RH: Lorcainide: a comparative trial with quinidine gluconate in patients with previously untreated ventricular arrhythmias, Chest 86(4):537, 1984.

Garson A Jr: The six most common acute cardiac dysrhythmias in children: ventricular dysrhythmia and drug treatment of acute dysrhythmia in children. Part 3, Appl Cardiol 12(5):16, 1984.

Gever LN: Giving procainamide safely, Nursing '84 14(5):116, 1984.

Gilman AG and others: Goodman and Gilman's the pharmacological basis of therapeutics, ed 7, New York, 1985, Macmillan Publishing Co.

Hasegawa GR: Tocainide: a new oral antiarrhythmic, Drug Intell Clin Pharm 19 (7/8):514, 1985.

Huang SK and Marcus FI: Flecainide and encainide, Hosp Ther 12(8):33, 1987.

Kastrup EK and Olin BR: Facts and comparisons, drug information, St Louis, 1987, JB Lippincott Co.

Kent JM: Maximizing safety in antiarrhythmic use, Patient Care 18(20):14, 1984.

Kent, JM: Treating ventricular arrhythmias, Patient Care 19(7):29, 1985.

Luceri RM and others: The drug treatment of atrial arrythmias, Hosp Formul 20(3):322, 1985.

Miller K: Lidocaine, Emergency 18(3):14, 1986.

Moser SA and others: Get ready: the new antiarrhythmias are coming, Nursing '85 15(9):56, 1985.

Nikolic G: Lidocaine bradycardia, Heart Lung 13(3):79, 1984.

Pepper, GA: Tocainide (Tonocard) for ventricular arrhythmias, Nurse Pract 10(4):36, 1985.

Pepper GA: New antiarrhythmic agents, Nurse Pract 11(7):62, 1986.

Podrid PJ: Antiarrhythmic drug therapy: benefits and hazards. Part I, Chest 88(3):453, 1985.

Podrid PJ: Antiarrhythmic drug therapy: benefits and hazards. Part 2, Chest 88(4):618, 1985.

Pohl JEF: Flecainide: a possible advance in antiarrhythmic therapy, Intensive Care Nurs 1(2):111, 1985.

Rosenberg JM and others: What to watch out for with lidocaine, RN 47(10):61, 1984.

Rossi L: Nursing care for survivors of sudden cardiac death, Nurs Clin No Amer 19(3):411, 1984.

Royster RL and others: Recent advances in cardiac care pharmacology. II. Newer drugs in antiarrhythmic therapy, part 2, Hosp Formul 19(9):801, 1984.

Schrader BJ and others: Mexiletine: a new type 1 antiarrhythmic agent, Drug Intell Clin Pharm 20(4):255, 1986.

Scherer P: New drugs of 1985: in theory and practice, Am J Nurs 86(4):406, 1986.

Scordo K: Cardiac dysrhythmias: recognizing the ones that matter, Nursinglife 4(5):33, 1986.

Sloskey GE: Drug Reviews-Amiodarone: a unique antiarrhythmic agent, Clin Pharm 2(7-8):330, 1983.

Smith GH: Flecainide: a new class 1c antidysrhythmic, Drug Intell Clin Pharm 19(10):703, 1985.

Strang JM and others: Treatment of prehospital refractory ventricular fibrillation with bretylium tosylate, Ann Emerg Med 13(4):234, 1984.

Thielbar S: Antiarrhythmic drug therapy: an overview, Crit Care Quart 7(2):21, 1984.

United States Pharmacopeial Convention: Drug information for the health care provider, ed 7, Rockville, Md, 1987, The Convention, Inc.

Venkatesh N and others: Antiarrhythmic agents: interactions when new and old drugs are combined, Consultant 25(16):108, 1985.

Wehmeyer AE and others: Encainide: a new antiarrhythmic agent, Drug Intell Clin Pharm 20(1):9, 1986.

Weintraub M and Standish R: Flecainide: a new orally active antiarrhythmic agent, Hosp Formul 19(7):541, 1984.

Woosley RL and Funck-Brentano C: Overview of the clinical pharmacology of antiarrythmic drugs, Am Cardiol 61:61A, 1988.

CHAPTER 25

Antihypertensives

HYPERTENSION

Hypertension is a circulatory disease characterized by a sustained elevation of the systemic arterial pressure. It is the most common cardiovascular community health problem, affecting approximately 30 million Americans. Untreated hypertension or subtherapeutic treatment of hypertension increases the risk of stroke, cerebral hemorrhage, congestive heart failure, coronary heart disease, and renal failure, yet hypertension is rarely listed as the cause of death. Clients with elevated blood pressure are frequently asymptomatic. Because there is a potential for a steady progression of secondary organ damage that may become fatal, untreated hypertension is known as the "silent killer."

The diagnosis and treatment of hypertension have varied considerably over the years, which has resulted in a great deal of misunderstanding. The National High Blood Pressure Coordinating Committee, which is associated with the National Institutes of Health, is a leading group that reviews hypertension data and makes recommendations concerning diagnosis and treatment. **High blood pressure** is now defined as a systolic blood pressure over 140 mm Hg and/or a diastolic blood pressure greater than 90 mm Hg. An average of two or more diastolic or systolic blood pressures taken on at least two or more occasions is necessary to diagnose a patient as hypertensive. Persons with a blood pressure equivalent to or greater than 140/90 should be treated to reduce the risk for premature death and disability (Joint National Committee on the Detection, Evaluation, and Treatment of High Blood Pressure, 1988).

Obtaining a careful and detailed drug history before diagnosis is very important, since many over-the-counter (OTC) and prescription medications may increase blood pressure or interfere with the effectiveness of the antihypertensive agent. Oral contraceptives (estrogen-containing agents), corticosteroids, nonsteroidal antiinflammatory agents, antidepressants, nasal decongestants, and appetite-suppressing agents are typical examples of interfering substances.

Controversy exists as to when the physician should start antihypertensive medications, especially in clients with a diastolic blood pressure between 90 and 94 mm Hg. In such cases, the long-term adverse effects of the medica-

tions are a particular concern. Clients 50 years or older with mild hypertension should receive the antihypertensive agents, since studies indicate a decrease in cardiovascular mortality and morbidity in this age group.

CLASSIFICATION

In **essential, idiopathic,** or **primary hypertension** the specific cause of the hypertension is unknown. This group accounts for approximately 90% of cases. **Secondary hypertension,** affecting approximately 10% of cases, may be a symptom of pheochromocytoma, toxemia of pregnancy, or renal artery disease or may result from use of specific medications. If the cause of secondary

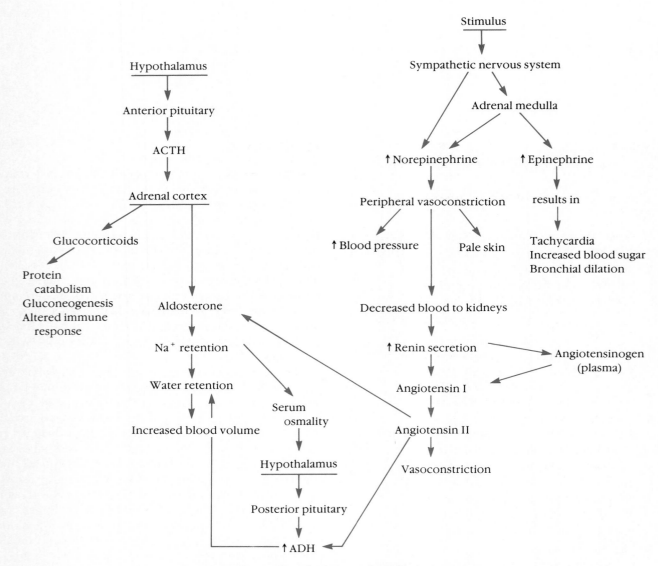

FIGURE 25-1. Physiologic control of blood pressure.

hypertension is corrected, the blood pressure will usually return to normal.

PHYSIOLOGIC CONTROL OF BLOOD PRESSURE

Control of blood pressure involves a complex interaction between the nervous, hormonal, and renal systems, since all play a part in regulating arterial blood pressure (see Figure 25-1).

The body has two primary mechanisms to control blood pressure:

1. **Baroreceptor reflex**—a rapid-acting system
2. **Renin-angiotensin-aldosterone mechanism**— a long-acting system

Baroreceptor Reflex

The baroreceptors or pressoreceptors are spray-type nerve endings located in the walls of the internal carotid arteries and the aortic arch. Sensory receptors rapidly respond to changes in blood pressure. Any elevation in pressure stretches the receptors, which causes an impulse to be transmitted along the afferent neuron (vagus nerve) to the vasomotor center in the medulla of the brain. The vasomotor center responds to the impulse by causing (1) a decrease in heart rate and force of myocardial contraction, which lowers cardiac output, and (2) vasodilation of peripheral vessels, which decreases total peripheral resistance. The subsequent reduction in blood pressure is attributed to the reflex activity of the baroreceptor mechanism.

This reflex functions as a rapidly acting system for short-term control of blood pressure. It has been demonstrated that over a prolonged period the rate of firing of the baroreceptors diminishes even if the blood pressure remains elevated. Therefore in hypertension it has been speculated that these receptors are "reset" to maintain a higher level of blood pressure.

Sympathetic nervous system. The sympathetic nervous system is mediated by two hormones: norepinephrine and epinephrine. Stimulation of the postganglionic adrenergic nerve terminals causes the release of norepinephrine, while activation of the adrenal medulla results in secretion of mostly epinephrine and only a small amount of norepinephrine. Both of these adrenal medullary hormones influence the activity of the heart and blood vessels.

Norepinephrine acts mainly on alpha adrenergic receptors, and epinephrine acts on both alpha and beta adrenergic receptors. The alpha adrenergic receptors are located in most of the arterioles. The affinity of norepinephrine for these receptors produces vasoconstriction, with a resultant increase in blood pressure. The beta$_1$ adrenergic receptors prevalent in the heart are also activated by norepinephrine. This response increases both the heart rate and the force of myocardial contraction, thereby indirectly causing an elevation in blood pressure.

On the other hand, because it produces dilation of blood vessels, epinephrine does not cause any increase in peripheral resistance. However, epinephrine does produce a considerable increase in heart rate and force of myocardial contraction, so the elevation in cardiac output indirectly raises the blood pressure. (See box for basic blood pressure equations.)

Renin-Angiotensin-Aldosterone System

The renin-angiotensin-aldosterone system (see Figure 25-2) regulates blood pressure by increasing or decreasing the blood volume through kidney function. The initiating factor is renin, an enzyme secreted by the juxtaglomerular cells located in the afferent arteriolar walls of the nephron. When blood flow through the kidneys is reduced, renal arterial pressure is reduced, which causes release of renin into the circulation. Here, renin catalyzes the cleavage of a plasma protein to form angiotensin I. Subsequently, in the small vessels of the lung, angiotensin I is converted by angiotensin-converting enzyme (ACE) to angiotensin II.

Angiotensin II is one of the most potent **vasoconstrictors** known. It is particularly effective in constricting arterioles, which increases peripheral resistance and raises blood pressure. In addition, angiotensin II acts on the adrenal cortex to stimulate the secretion of aldosterone, a hormone that promotes reabsorption of sodium by the kidneys. The increased sodium elevates the osmotic pressure in the plasma, causing a release of antidiuretic hormone from the hypothalamus. Angiotensin II acts on the kidney tubules to promote reabsorption of water.

Excessive fluid retention is controlled by the negative-feedback mechanism operating within this system so that fluid balance is restored to a normal level. Thus the renin-angiotensin-aldosterone system involves slow adjustments to changes in fluid volume.

The kidneys are by far the most important organs in the body for long-term regulation of blood pressure. When the operation of the urinary system fails, increased pe-

---

BASIC BLOOD PRESSURE EQUATIONS

Blood pressure = Cardiac output × Peripheral resistance
Cardiac output = Stroke volume × Heart rate
Mean arterial pressure = Cardiac output × Peripheral resistance

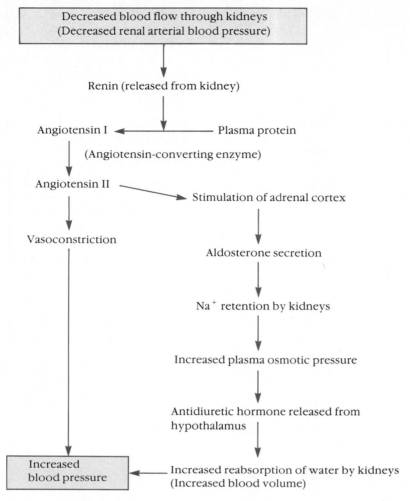

FIGURE 25-2   Renin-angiotensin-aldosterone system.

ripheral resistance and retention of fluid volume produce a combination of hypertensive effects, which keep blood pressure constantly elevated.

THE NURSE'S ROLE IN ANTIHYPERTENSIVE THERAPY

Client participation in antihypertensive therapy (see Table 25-1) is essential for control of blood pressure. The client needs to understand that hypertension is usually asymptomatic and that therapy does not cure but only controls hypertension. Long-term therapy is necessary to prevent the morbidity and mortality secondary to hypertension. Compliance with an individualized antihypertensive regimen is associated with a good prognosis and normal life-style.

Nonpharmacologic approaches are legitimate interventions. They may be used independently in mild hypertension and always as an adjunct to drug therapy for clients with moderate to severe hypertension. Adherence by the client to a prescribed nonpharmacologic regimen may allow reduction of medication dosage and of subsequent side effects. These measures include weight control, sodium restriction, elimination or limited consumption of alcohol and tobacco, reduction of dietary saturated fats, a regular exercise program, and behavior modification to promote relaxation.

Antihypertensive medications, like all medications, should be stored away from children, in a tightly closed container at room temperature (preferably between 15° and 30° C [59° and 86° F]) unless otherwise indicated by the manufacturer.

DRUG THERAPY

Careful use of antihypertensive drugs can effectively control the blood pressure in a majority of hypertensive individuals with less risk of serious complications and intolerable side effects. However, antihypertensive drug therapy remains empirical, since essential hypertension is

TABLE 25-1 Pharmacokinetic Overview of Selected Antihypertensive Drugs

Generic name	Trade name	Absorption, metabolism, and excretion	Serum half-life	Onset of action	Peak effect	Duration of effect
CENTRAL-ACTING ADRENERGIC INHIBITORS						
clonidine	Catapres Dixarit♣	Absorption: good Metabolism: liver Excretion: urine primarily, some in bile	12.7 (range: 6-23 hr In clients with renal dysfunction: 25-37 hr	½-1 hr	2-4 hr	up to 8 hr
methyldopa	Aldomet Apo-Methyldopa♣ Dopamet♣ Medimet-250♣	Absorption: approximately 50% orally Metabolism: converted centrally to alpha methylnorepinephrine in liver Excretion: urine (20% - 55% unchanged) and feces (unabsorbed drug)	Normally biphasic: alpha: 1.7 hr beta: 7-16 hr. Anuric alpha 3.6 hr	2 hrs	Single dose (po or IV): 4-6 hours Multiple doses: 2-3 days	Variable Oral: 12-24 hr (single dose); 24-48 hr (multiple dose) IV: 10-16 hr.
guanabenz	Wytensin	Absorption: 75% orally; has low bioavailability because of first-pass metabolism Metabolism: liver Excretion: urine and feces	6 hr	Within 1 hr for single dose	2-4 hr	12 hr (single dose)
PERIPHERAL ADRENERGIC INHIBITOR DRUGS						
guanethidine	Ismelin Apo-Guanethidine♣ Visutensil♣	Absorption: variable, with continued dosing between 3%-30% of oral dose absorbed Metabolism: liver Excretion: urine (25%-50% unchanged)	Alpha: 1-2 days Beta: 5-10 days	—	Single dose: within 8 hr Multiple doses: 1-3 wk	Multiple doses: when drug stopped, blood pressure returns to pretreatment level in 1-3 wk

Continued.

TABLE 25-1 Pharmacokinetic Overview of Selected Antihypertensive Drugs—cont'd

Generic name	Trade name	Absorption, metabolism, and excretion	Serum half-life	Onset of action	Peak effect	Duration of effect
guanadrel	Hylorel	Absorption: good Metabolism: liver Excretion: urine (85%)	Variable: approximately 10 hr	2 hr (single dose)	4-6 hr (single dose)	9 hr (range: 4-14 hr, after single dose)
RAUWOLFIA DERIVATIVES						
reserpine	Serpasil Sandril Novoreserpine♣ Reserfia♣	Absorption: good Metabolism: liver Excretion: feces (60% mostly unchanged in 4 days) and urine (8%)	Initial: 4.5 hr Chronic dosing: 45-168 hr Anuria chronic dosing: 87-323 hr.	Several days to 3 wk with multiple dosing Catecholamine depletion: 1 hr after single dose	Oral, multiple dosing: 3-6 wk Catecholamine depletion: 24 hr	Oral: 1-6 wk
ALPHA ADRENERGIC BLOCKING DRUGS						
prazosin	Minipress Hypovase♣	Absorption: good, bioavailability 50%-85% Metabolism: liver Excretion: mainly bile and feces; also urine (6%-10%)	2-3 hr; not altered in renal dysfunction; congestive heart failure: 6-8 hr	Within 2 hours	Single dose: 2-4 hrs multiple doses: 3-4 wks Congestive heart failure: 1 hr	Single dose: Up to 10 hr Congestive heart failure: 6 hrs
VASODILATOR DRUGS						
diazoxide	Hyperstat Parenteral	Absorption: IV Metabolism: liver Excretion: kidneys (50% unchanged)	28 hr (range: 21-36 hr) Anuric: 20-53 hr	1 min following IV push	2-5 min	2-12 hr
hydralazine	Apresoline	Absorption: orally, good bioavailability (30%-50%) Metabolism: liver Excretion: urine	0.44-0.47 hr (2-4 hr half-life of metabolite) Antihypertensive half-life much longer	Oral: 45 min IV: 10-20 min	Oral: 1 hr IV: 15-30 min	Oral and IV: 3-8 hr
minoxidil	Loniten	Absorption: orally, good Metabolism: liver Excretion: urine (97%)	2.8-4.2 hr for drug and metabolites	½ hr	Single dose: 2-3 hr	1-2 days, up to 75 hr

TABLE 25-1   Pharmacokinetic Overview of Selected Antihypertensive Drugs—cont'd

Generic name	Trade name	Absorption, metabolism, and excretion	Serum half-life	Onset of action	Peak effect	Duration of effect
sodium nitro-prusside	Nipride Parenteral Nitropress Parenteral	Absorption: IV from infusion solution only Metabolism: erythrocytes convert to cyanide; liver converts cyanide to thiocyanate Excretion: urine	Minutes; thiocyanate: 7 days	Nearly immediate	Nearly immediate	1-10 min after infusion discontinued

ANGIOTENSIN II INHIBITOR DRUGS

Generic name	Trade name	Absorption, metabolism, and excretion	Serum half-life	Onset of action	Peak effect	Duration of effect
captopril	Capoten	Absorption: good (75% from gastrointestinal tract, but this will be reduced by 30%-40% if food is present) Metabolism: liver Excretion: urine (40%- 50% unchanged)	Less than 3 hr; more in renal impairment	Single dose: 15-60 min	1- 1½ hr, full effect may take several weeks to achieve	6-12 hr (dose related)
enalapril	Vasotec	Absorption: 60% orally; not affected by food Metabolism: liver, to enalaprilat, an active metabolite Excretion: urine (60%: 20% enalapril, 40% enalaprilat) fecal (33%: 6% enalapril, 27% enalaprilat)	metabolite: 11 hr	Single dose: 1 hr	4-6 hr although full effect may take several weeks of therapy	Minimum of 24 hr

GANGLIONIC BLOCKING AGENTS

Generic name	Trade name	Absorption, metabolism, and excretion	Serum half-life	Onset of action	Peak effect	Duration of effect
mecamylamine	Inversine	Absorption: orally, almost complete Excretion: urine, mostly unchanged	—	½-2 hr	—	6-12 hr or greater

Continued.

TABLE 25-1   Pharmacokinetic Overview of Selected Antihypertensive Drugs—cont'd

Generic name	Trade name	Absorption, metabolism, and excretion	Serum half-life	Onset of action	Peak effect	Duration of effect
trimethaphan camsylate	Arfonad Parenteral	Metabolism possibly by pseudocholinesterase Excretion: urine, mostly unchanged	—	Immediate	—	10-15 min
MONOAMINE OXIDASE INHIBITING DRUG						
pargyline	Eutonyl Eudatin✼	Absorption: good Metabolism: liver Excretion: urine	—	—	4 days to 3 wk after starting drug	Up to 3 wk after drug discontinued
TYROSINE HYDROXYLASE INHIBITOR DRUG						
metryosine	Demser	Absorption: good Metabolism: minimum Excretion: urine	3.4-3.7 hr	—	2-3 days	2-3 days for blood pressure to return to pretreatment level after drug is discontinued; 3-4 days for development of urinary catecholamines

a disease of unknown origin and the mechanism of action of many antihypertensive drugs also remains unknown. The ideal antihypertensive drug should:

1. Maintain blood pressure within normal limits for various body positions.
2. Maintain or improve blood flow, without compromising tissue perfusion or blood supply to the brain.
3. Reduce the work load on the heart.
4. Have no undesirable side effects.
5. Permit long-term administration without development of tolerance.

Stepped-Care Regimen

Medications used for the control of hypertension are generally prescribed on the basis of the stepped-care approach. The **stepped-care regimen** follows a rational method of treatment. This plan is a progressive approach, which begins therapy with administration of a single drug, increases the dosage of that drug, and then, in sequential order, gradually adds more potent agents when the need for more intensive therapy is indicated (see Figure 25-3).

Of importance is that the treatment be designed individually, according to the therapeutic response of the client. The stepped-care regimen is also applied to adolescents and children.

The advantage of the stepped-care regimen is that it provides direction for treatment of clients with mild to severe hypertension. Nonpharmacologic approaches are beneficial for persons with mild to severe hypertension and are usually included in the client's teaching plan. Step 1 offers diuretics, beta-blocking agents, calcium antago-

---

REBOUND HYPERTENSION

Rebound hypertension is the problem associated with abrupt withdrawal or discontinuation of antihypertensive medications. The blood pressure usually returns to at least the pretreatment level or above, along with symptoms of sympathetic system hyperactivity (sweating, anxiety, tachycardia, insomnia, muscle pain, etc.).

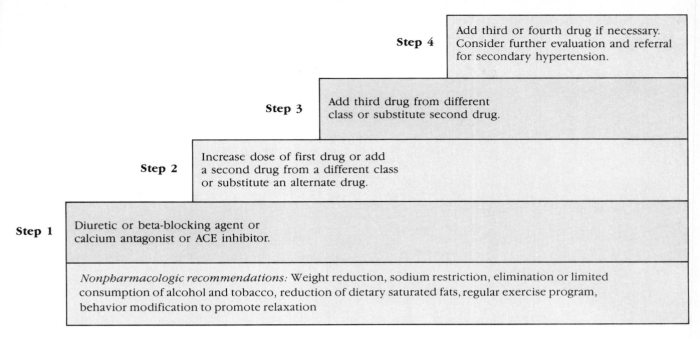

FIGURE 25-3 Stepped-care regimen for hypertension.

nists, or ACE inhibitors as useful, first-line drugs. This allows for flexibility in drug selection for an individual client. If after 1 to 3 months of therapy, the client's response to the medication is considered inadequate, then the prescriber may increase the dose of the first drug to the maximum recommended for it, substitute a second drug, or add a second drug from a different classification (step 2).

Whichever drug is selected, it is started in small doses and is increased gradually until the therapeutic goal is achieved. In addition, the diuretic dosage may have to be adjusted to prevent fluid retention. Steps 3 and 4 provide for the addition of drugs from other classes or the substitution of a third or fourth drug if necessary. If blood pressure control is still not achieved, then further clinical evaluation and/or referral to a specialist is recommended.

The major antihypertensive agents used are listed by drug category in Figure 25-3. Diuretics are the preferred initial therapy in clients over 50 years of age and also in black clients. Blacks do not respond as well as whites do to beta blockers or the ACE inhibitors as monotherapy, but in combination therapies they usually respond equivalently to whites. Calcium antagonists are usually very effective agents in the elderly. Beta blockers may be the first step for younger clients with tachycardia and marked lability of blood pressure, although ACE inhibitors and diuretics are also usually effective as single agents (McKenney, 1985).

Pregnancy

Hypertension during pregnancy is a serious condition that requires early detection and treatment. It has been estimated that 20% of maternal deaths and approximately 25,000 of stillborn/neonatal deaths are caused by hypertension during pregnancy (Chobanian, 1982).

Hypertension during pregnancy may result from preeclampsia (a hypertension induced by pregnancy) or essential hypertension. Preeclampsia is usually treated empirically or with antihypertensive therapy (Joint National Committee on the Detection, Evaluation, and Treatment of High Blood Pressure, 1988) to reduce the possibility of eclampsia, a true hypertensive emergency characterized by convulsions and coma.

Although antihypertensive therapy has resulted in an increase in fetal survival, the therapies of choice are debatable and depend mainly on the prescribing physician. If antihypertensive therapy is necessary, methyldopa, hydralazine, and beta-blocking agents have been reported to be effective. Avoid ACE inhibitors because an increase

---

CALCIUM ANTAGONISTS

diltiazem (Cardizem SR): orally, 60-120 mg 2 times a day
nicardipine (Cardene): orally, 20 mg 3 times a day, increased as necessary
verapamil (Calan, Isoptin): orally, 80 mg 3-4 times daily, increased as necessary
For additional information, see Chapter 26.

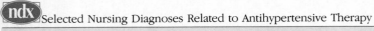

Nursing diagnosis	Outcome criteria	Nursing interventions
Knowledge deficit related to newly prescribed or altered antihypertensive drug therapy	Client will describe hypertension, how drug therapy relates to condition, how and when to take medications, common drug interactions, particularly with OTC drugs, safety precautions, common side effects and which are reportable, storage requirements of drugs, and will monitor effectiveness of drug therapy with sequential blood pressure readings.	Assess learning needs and learning readiness Plan with client and family for achievement of realistic goals Provide information to meet outcome criteria
Noncompliance with medication regimen	Client will self-administer medicaions safely and accurately.	Check refill frequency to determine compliance. Explore with client reasons for noncompliance and take appropriate teaching/counseling interventions. Provide needed drug information concerning rationales for specific client's hypertensive status. Emphasize that drug therapy does not cure but controls hypertension and possible need for lifelong therapy. Discuss possibility of rebound hypertension with noncompliance.
Sexual dysfunction related to antihypertensive drug therapy	Client will describe nature of dysfunction, consult with prescriber for dosage reduction or drug substitution, and resume sexual activity.	Assess for causative factors. Encourage client to share concerns. Provide health teaching and referral when needed. Encourage return to sexual activity.

in fetal mortality in pregnant animals has been reported. The calcium channel blockers are effective in controlling severe hypertension in late pregnancy, but they may cause a decrease in uterine contractions during labor. Avoid nitroprusside, since it may affect fetal thyroid function. Advise mothers receiving continuous antihypertensive therapy not to breast feed, since most of the agents are transferred to breast milk.

Sexual Dysfunction

Sexual dysfunction is a common complication of hypertensive medications and may be manifested in males as decreased libido, impotence, impaired or retrograde ejaculation, and gynecomastia and in females as decreased libido, decreased vaginal lubrication, and inability to achieve orgasm. Such symptoms may lead to the client's poor compliance with the drug regimen. The nature of the disorder and a knowledge of the effects associated with different antihypertensive agents (see Table 25-2) will assist in determining the cause of the symptoms. Frequently, a dosage reduction or the substitution of another drug will alleviate the problem.

Surgical Clients

Clients scheduled for elective surgery should receive their antihypertensive medications up to the time of surgery and as soon afterward as possible. Parenteral diuretics, adrenergic inhibitors, and vasodilators are available for clients unable to take oral medications. Such preparations should be used to prevent rebound hypertension, especially if the client was taking an adrenergic inhibitor before surgery.

The client's electrolyte status should be carefully checked before surgery. If hypokalemia is detected, it should be corrected before the scheduled operation. The anesthesiologist should always be completely informed about the client's medication regimen; this is vital information that may alter the medications or the monitoring methods used.

Children

The goal of therapy for hypertensive children and adolescents is to reduce the blood pressure without adverse effects that limit compliance or interfere with normal growth and development. The type of intervention will be determined by the causative factors, the presence of complications, and the degree of hypertension. Nonpharmacologic measures (weight control, reduction of dietary sodium, exercise, avoidance of smoking and alcohol, and reduction of saturated fat) are strongly recommended. If children do not respond to nonpharmacologic measures or if their blood pressures place them at risk for organ damage, then pharmacologic therapy should be considered.

Pharmacologic interventions for children also follow the stepped approach, which includes diuretics, adrenergic inhibiting agents, and vasodilators. Continued assessment of the child and family is necessary to ensure satisfactory blood pressure control and compliance with the therapeutic program, whether pharmacologic or nonpharmacologic.

Elderly Clients

A significant proportion of those over 65 years of age have elevated systolic or diastolic blood pressure or both, which increases their risk of cardiovascular morbidity and mortality. Nonpharmacologic means of blood pressure reduction (weight reduction if necessary and dietary sodium restriction) are indicated.

Antihypertensive drugs should be started with smaller than usual doses, increased with smaller dosages, and scheduled at less frequent intervals with the elderly, since they are more sensitive to volume depletion and sympathetic inhibition than younger clients. They commonly have impaired cardiovascular reflexes, which makes them more susceptible to hypotension.

In clients with isolated systolic hypertension who are treated with antihypertensive drugs, the systolic pressure should be cautiously decreased to 140 to 160 mm Hg. Only if this level is tolerated without side effects should consideration be given to further lowering the value.

The elderly client's response to both nonpharmacologic and pharmacologic therapies should be monitored closely.

• • •

The antihypertensive drugs currently used to reduce blood pressure are classified into four major categories: **diuretics, sympathetic depressant** (sympatholytic) **agents, vasodilators,** and **angiotensin II inhibitors.** The sites of action of the various antihypertensive drugs are shown in Figure 25-4.

DIURETIC DRUGS

Diuretic drugs play a vital role in lowering blood pressure. They are currently used as an initial drug in managing mild hypertension, or they may be administered in combination with other antihypertensive agents.

The use of diuretics results in a loss of excess salt and water from the body by renal excretion. The decrease in plasma and extracellular fluid volume subsequently depresses vascular reactivity to sympathetic stimulation. Thus volume depletion, plus a direct effect on the arterioles that produces vasodilation, results in lowering of the blood pressure.

This response then causes an initial decline of cardiac output followed by a decrease in peripheral resistance and a lowering of blood pressure. (See Figure 25-4.)

The **thiazides** and related sulfonamide diuretics, such as chlorthalidone and metolazone, when used in maximum therapeutic doses, are moderately effective in decreasing blood pressure. Therefore they can be used alone for individuals with mild hypertension. By contrast, many of the other types of antihypertensive agents, when used alone, produce a gradual retention of sodium and water with resultant expansion of plasma fluid volume. This process then tends to diminish the effectiveness of the antihypertensive agent. For this reason thiazides are given concomitantly to prevent fluid retention.

Loop diuretics, such as furosemide and ethacrynic acid, are powerful drugs that cause excessive loss of potassium and water. Since these drugs produce fewer antihypertensive effects, they should be given to clients with complicated renal insufficiency or to individuals who cannot take other diuretics.

The **potassium-sparing agents,** such as spironolactone and triamterene, are useful in counteracting potassium loss induced by other diuretics. They promote sodium and water loss without accompanying loss of potassium. These drugs are indicated for management of hyperaldosteronism and renal vascular hypertension when clients are resistant to other diuretics. (See Chapter 33 for drug monographs of diuretic drugs. See box for examples of diuretic drugs.)

BETA BLOCKING AGENTS

Beta adrenergic blocking agents (see box on p. 495) have been successfully used to treat cardiovascular disorders, including hypertension. These drugs decrease cardiac output and inhibit renin secretion, which results in a lowering of blood pressure. Beta blocking drugs compete with epinephrine for available beta receptor sites, thus inhibiting typical organ or tissue response to beta stimulation.

For additional information about this category of drugs, see Chapter 20.

ADRENERGIC INHIBITING (SYMPATHOLYTIC) AGENTS

Adrenergic inhibiting agents, the most effective antihypertensive drugs, modify the function of the sympathetic nervous system.

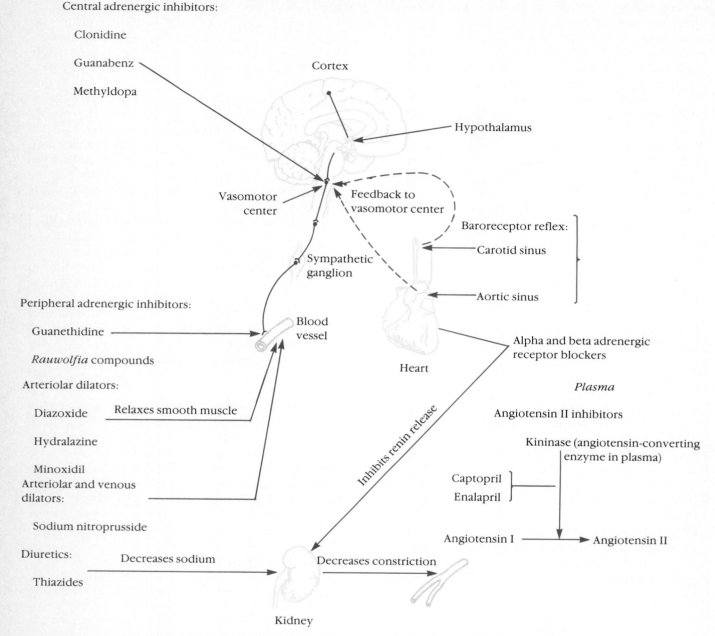

FIGURE 25-4   Site and method of action of various antihypertensive drugs based on reported clinical and experimental evidence.

The heart, blood vessels, and kidneys influence arterial pressure through various reflex mechanisms. Sympathetic stimulation increases heart rate and force of myocardial contraction, constricts arterioles (resistance vessels) and venules (capacitance vessels), and releases renin from the kidney. These agents generally are effective in reducing blood pressure and preventing serious cardiovascular complications. The sites at which these drugs modify sympathetic nervous system activity vary widely and usually involve complex mechanisms.

Many of these drugs are believed to have multiple sites of action or have unknown mechanisms of action. For clarification, the drugs are characterized by their primary proposed site of action.

CENTRALLY ACTING ADRENERGIC INHIBITORS

The centrally acting agents clonidine, methyldopa, and guanabenz are effective step 2 antihypertensives, especially when combined with a diuretic. When given as a single

SELECTED DIURETIC DRUGS FOR HYPERTENSION

GENERIC NAME	TRADE NAME
Single agents:	
chlorothiazide	Diuril
hydrochlorothiazide	HydroDiuril
	Esidrex
	Diuchlor H✤
	Natrimax✤
chlorthalidone	Hygroton
	Apo-Clorthalidone✤
	Novothalidone✤
metolazone	Zaroxolyn
triamterene	Dyrenium
	Dytac✤
spironolactone	Aldactone
	Novospiroton✤
furosemide	Lasix
	Furoside✤
	Neo-Renal✤
ethacrynic acid	Edecrin
	Hydromedin✤
Hydrochlorothiazide (HCT) combination agents:	
HCT, 25 mg, plus spironolactone, 25 mg	Aldactazide
HCT, 25 mg, plus triamterene, 50 mg	Dyazide
HCT, 50 mg, plus triamterene, 75 mg	Maxzide

SELECTED BETA ADRENERGIC BLOCKING AGENTS

GENERIC NAME	TRADE NAME
Beta$_1$ adrenergic (cardioselective) blocking agents:	
acebutolol	Sectral
atenolol	Tenormin
	Atenol✤
	Premormine✤
metoprolol	Lopressor
	Apo-Metoprolol✤
	Betaloc✤
Beta$_1$ and beta$_2$ adrenergic (nonselective) blocking agents:	
labetalol	Normodyne
	Trandate
nadolol	Corgard
pindolol	Visken
propranolol	Inderal
	Inderal LA
	Novopranol✤
	PMS Propranolol✤
timolol	Blocadren
	Betim✤
	Temserin✤

agent, clonidine and methyldopa (guanabenz to a lesser extent) usually produce sodium and water retention. If they are combined with a diuretic, their antihypertensive effect is enhanced.

clonidine hydrochloride (Catapres)

Mechanism of action. Clonidine reduces systolic and diastolic blood pressure by suppressing sympathetic outflow from the brain. Stimulation of the alpha$_2$ receptors in the central nervous system (especially the medulla oblongata) decreases sympathetic outflow of norepinephrine from the brain to the heart, kidneys, and peripheral vascular system. This lowers blood pressure primarily by decreasing cardiac output rather than peripheral vascular resistance. The depressed cardiac output is the result of a reduction in both heart rate and stroke volume. Consequently, this action can cause bradycardia.

The decreased sympathetic outflow to the kidneys reduces renal vascular resistance and thus preserves renal blood flow. Hence, renin activity is suppressed. The decreased cardiac output, however, produces sodium retention and edema does occur. This, unfortunately, can reduce the antihypertensive effect of clonidine, and therefore a diuretic is needed to correct the extracellular fluid volume retention.

Indication. Antihypertensive
Pharmacokinetics. See Table 25-1.
Side effects/adverse reactions. See Table 25-2.
Significant drug interactions. The following interactions may occur when clonidine is given with the drugs listed below:

Drug	Possible Effect and Management
Beta adrenergic blocking agents	Concurrent administration with clonidine may lead to loss of blood pressure control. Additive bradycardia effects may also occur. Monitor closely. If the physician wants to discontinue both drugs in a client, the beta blocking agent should be stopped first. Discontinuing clonidine first may increase the risk of inducing a withdrawal hypertensive crisis.

TABLE 25-2   Side Effects/Adverse Reactions of Antihypertensive Agents

Drug(s)	Side effects*	Adverse reactions†
centrally acting adrenergic inhibitors (clonidine, methyldopa, guanabenz)	More frequent: dizziness, drowsiness, dry mouth, headache (methyldopa primarily) Less common: nausea, vomiting, headache, impotence, decreased sexual drive, impaired ejaculation Clonidine: anorexia, constipation, insomnia, postural hypotension Methyldopa: diarrhea, paresthesia, rash, bradycardia, nasal congestion	clonidine/methyldopa: edema, depression, vivid nightmares or dreams, irregular or slow heartbeat
peripheral adrenergic inhibiting drugs (guanethidine, guanadrel)	More frequent: orthostatic hypotension, weakness, impaired ejaculation; guanethidine: diarrhea, bradycardia, stuffy nose Less common: increased urination at night, muscle pain or tremors, dry mouth, headaches, impotence, decreased libido; guanethidine: alopecia, blurred vision, ptosis of eyelids, nausea, vomiting, rash	Fluid retention, edema, angina guanadrel: severe dizziness, bradycardia, pinpoint pupils
reserpine	More frequent: nausea, vomiting, anorexia, diarrhea, dizziness, dry mouth, stuffy nose Less common: fluid retention, especially of lower extremities; sexual dysfunctions: impotence, decreased sexual drive, impaired ejaculation	Abdominal cramps, black stools or hematemesis (peptic ulcer reactivation); chest pain, bradycardia; headaches; bronchospasms (shortness of breath); weakness, drowsiness, lack of ability to concentrate, increased nervousness; nightmares, mental depression that may persist for months after drug is discontinued and has been reportedly severe enough to lead to suicide
alpha adrenergic blocking drug (prazosin)	More frequent: weakness, nausea, vomiting, headache, drowsiness	Orthostatic hypotension, chest pain (angina), edema of lower extremities, irregular heartbeat, syncope, shortness of breath, incontinence, paresthesia, impotence, priapism
vasodilators (diazoxide, hydralazine, minoxidil)	diazoxide: abdominal cramps, changes in taste perception; with continued use, increased hair growth on arms, legs, back, and forehead; complaints of stiffness, trembling of hands and fingers hydralazine: constipation, nausea, anorexia, vomiting, diarrhea, headache, rapid or irregular heartbeat, dizziness, facial flushing, stuffy nose, irritated eyes minoxidil: excessive hair growth, usually on face, arms, and back, headache, breast tenderness in males and females	All: salt and water retention, increased weight gain, chest pain (angina) diazoxide: tachycardia, chest pain from ischemia to myocardial infarction, rash, fever (allergic reaction), confusion, hyperglycemia hydralazine: hepatoxicity; blisters, sore throat, joint pain, chest pain (SLE-like syndrome); weakness, hypersensitivity, numbness, tingling in hands/feet (peripheral neuritis) minoxidil: skin rash, itching (allergy), flushing, tachycardia or irregular heartbeat, pericardial effusion that may progress to cardiac tamponade
angiotensin II inhibitor drugs (captopril, enalapril)	More frequent: loss of taste (which usually returns in several months, even if therapy is continued; enalapril: weakness, nausea, diarrhea, cough, headache	Reversible renal failure, proteinuria; skin rash, hypotension; chest pain, difficult breathing; swelling of face, mouth, hands, or feet (angioedema); fever, chills, sore throat
ganglionic blocking drugs (mecamylamine, trimethaphan)	Dose-related effects, dilated pupil, constipation that may lead to paralytic ileus, drowsiness, weakness, dry mouth, nausea and vomiting, anorexia, decreased sexual ability	All: orthostatic hypotension, urinary retention mecamylamine: confusion, depression, mania, tremors, shortness of breath (interstitial pulmonary edema and fibrosis) trimethaphan: hypersensitivity and hematologic reactions

TABLE 25-2   Side Effects/Adverse Reactions of Antihypertensive Agents—cont'd

Drug(s)	Side effects*	Adverse reactions†
monoamine oxidase inhibiting drug (pargyline hydrochloride)	More frequent: urinary retention, orthostatic hypotension, drowsiness, dry mouth, constipation Less common: increased appetite, weight gain, photosensitivity, trembling, chills, nightmares, restlessness, insomnia or muscle twitching while asleep (from CNS stimulation)	Diarrhea, tachycardia, orthostatic hypotension, edema, chest pain, fever, severe headache, nausea and vomiting or stiff neck (possibility of hypertensive crisis); hallucinations; hepatitis
tyrosine hydroxylase inhibitor drug (metyrosine)	More frequent: drowsiness, which generally decreases after first week of therapy	Severe diarrhea, drooling, trembling and shaking of hands/fingers (extrapyramidal effects), bloody urine or painful urination (crystalluria), skin rash, pruritus, shortness of breath (allergic effect), edema, muscle spasms of neck and back, shuffling walk or jerky movements of head, face, mouth, and neck (parkinsonism, trismus)

*If side effects continue, increase, or disturb the patient, inform the physician.
†If adverse reactions occur, contact physician since medical intervention may be necessary.

Drug	Possible Effect and Management
Tricyclic antidepressants	The antihypertensive effectiveness of clonidine may be reduced. This usually occurs in the first or second week of therapy. Monitor closely since dosage adjustments and/or alternate hypotensive agents may need to be considered as alternative options by the physician.

Dosage and administration
Adults
Initial. Give 100μg (0.1 mg) twice daily, increased every 2 to 4 days by 100 to 200 μg (0.1 or 0.2 mg) as necessary to control blood pressure.

Maintenance. Give 100 or 200 μg (0.1 or 0.2 mg) two to four times daily.

Nonemergency, severe hypertensive episode. Loading dose method may be ordered. Give 200 μg (0.2 mg) initially orally followed by 100 μg (0.1 mg) hourly until the diastolic pressure is under control or a maximum of 800 μg (0.8 mg) has been given. Then a maintenance dosage schedule is begun.

Vascular headaches (migraine), prophylactic use. Give 25 μg (0.025 mg) orally two to four times a day or up to 50 μg (0.05 mg) three times daily.

Dysmenorrhea. Give 25 μg (0.025 mg) orally twice daily for 2 weeks before and during menses.

Menopause. Give 25 to 75 μg (0.025 to 0.075 mg) orally twice daily.

The box gives information on additional uses of clonidine.

ADDITIONAL USES OF CLONIDINE

Clonidine has several additional uses that are not currently approved in the United States. It is being used as a prophylactic treatment to prevent migraines, to treat dysmenorrhea, and also to treat flushing that occurs during menopause. Another interesting use is during opiate withdrawal, especially in clients who had been receiving methadone. Clonidine reportedly reduces the symptoms of opiate withdrawal during the detoxification process (Washington and others, 1979; Schwinghammer, 1982). (See Chapter 12.)

Children. Dosage has not been established.

Catapres-TTS (a clonidine transdermal therapeutic system). Clonidine is available in various strengths (0.1, 0.2, or 0.3 mg) programmed to deliver the specified strength daily for 1 week. The system is composed of four layers of film that contain a drug reservoir of clonidine, a membrane that controls the rate of drug delivery, an adhesive layer that also contains clonidine to initially saturate the skin site, and a top backing or cover layer.

The system was formulated for the drug to flow from a higher concentration to the lower concentration in the body, which is limited by the rate-controlling membrane layer. It takes approximately 2 to 3 days to reach a therapeutic clonidine serum level on initial application, whereas replacing the system weekly at a new body site will maintain the therapeutic serum level.

Pregnancy safety. FDA Category C

NURSING CONSIDERATIONS

Assessment. Do not administer to the client with abnormal vaginal bleeding of undetermined origin, ovarian cyst, mental depression, or active thrombophlebitis.

Intervention. When applying clonidine using the transdermal system, select a hairless intact area of the patient's upper arm or torso. Reapply once every 7 days on a different skin site. If the system loosens, cover it with an adhesive overlay from the drug package to ensure good adhesion.

Reduce dosages gradually over 2 to 4 days or preferably longer (1- to 2-week period) to prevent rebound hypertension.

With noncompliant clients, consultation with the prescribing physician may result in a change from oral to the transdermal therapeutic system or another antihypertensive drug because of the risk of rebound hypertension.

Education. Emphasize the importance of periodic follow-up visits so that the clonidine level and blood pressure are closely monitored. Be explicit in instructions concerning the serious consequences of missing a dose or abrupt cessation of the drug. Clients with serious side effects should immediately report the problem to the physician so that the dosage may be adjusted or the drug may be withdrawn gradually over a period of 2 to 4 days. Abrupt withdrawal, including omission of sequential doses, can result in hypertensive crisis within 8 to 24 hours. The symptoms of hypertensive crisis are anxiety, sweating, tachycardia, insomnia, salivation, muscle pain, and stomach pain.

Instruct client to keep an adequate supply of the drug at all times, particularly during travel.

Instruct client to take last dose before bedtime to ensure continuous blood pressure control during the night.

Instruct client to make position changes slowly even though clonidine does not usually cause postural hypotention. Client should move slowly from recumbent to upright position and dangle feet from edge of bed to prevent dizziness and fainting. The elderly client may be more sensitive to postural hypotension.

Use with caution in patients with coronary insufficiency, recent myocardial infarction, cerebrovascular disease, chronic renal failure, Raynaud's disease, history of mental depression, or hepatic function impairment.

Inform client of the possible side effects, particularly dry mouth (use saliva substitutes—VAOraLube, Orex, sugarless gum, or sour hard candy) and sedative effects, which require caution in operating a car or other machinery.

Advise client on long-term therapy to have a periodic eye examination (every 6 to 12 months) to avoid possible retinal degeneration. This has occurred in rats to which clonidine has been administered.

Instruct client to carry medical identification card or Medic Alert.

Warn client not to take OTC medication without consulting the physician.

Caution client about the increased sedative effects of alcohol, barbiturates, and other CNS depressants during clonidine therapy particularly if the individual is operating machinery.

Evaluation. Closely monitor blood pressure and pulse during initiation of therapy and continue to observe these parameters until dosage is properly titrated. Blood pressure should decrease within 30 to 60 minutes after administration and may persist for 8 hours.

Weigh patient daily for 3 to 4 days after initiation of therapy, since weight gain may occur because of sodium retention and edema. If fluid retention does not disappear, it may be necessary to add a diuretic to the regimen.

Observe patient for drug tolerance. Physician may increase dosage or add a diuretic to obtain the required antihypertensive response.

Blood pressure control may be impaired when taken concurrently with tricyclic antidepressants and beta adrenergic blocking agents. If taken concurrently, beta blockers should be discontinued before clonidine to decrease the risk of hypertensive crisis caused by clonidine withdrawal.

Closely monitor patient with a history of mental depression because the drug may intensify this condition.

methyldopa (Aldomet)
methyldopate hydrochloride injection (Parenteral Aldomet)

Mechanism of action. Although the exact hypotensive mechanism is unknown, the current theory is that methyldopa is converted to alpha methylnorepinephrine in centrally located adrenergic neurons. Alpha methylnorepinephrine lowers arterial blood pressure by stimulating the central alpha adrenergic inhibiting receptors. The result is a reduction in norepinephrine (sympathetic) outflow to the heart, kidneys, and peripheral vasculature. A reduction in total peripheral resistance and plasma renin levels may also contribute to the hypotensive effect.

Methyldopate hydrochloride is hydrolyzed to methyldopa in the body, which then must undergo the previous theoretical process to produce the hypotensive effect. The antihypertensive effect produced by the parenteral dosage form begins in approximately 4 to 6 hours, so it should not be used as the primary single agent in a hypertensive emergency. Faster acting agents such as nitroprusside or diazoxide are parenteral antihypertensive agents indicated for an emergency situation.

Indication. Antihypertensive
Pharmacokinetics. See Table 25-1.
Side effects/adverse reactions. See Table 25-2.

Significant drug interactions. The following interactions may occur when methyldopa is given with the drugs listed below:

Drug	**Possible Effect and Management**
methotrimeprazine	An additive hypotensive effect may occur. This combination should be avoided.
monoamine oxidase (MAO) inhibitors	Hyperexcitability, hallucinations, headache, and hypertension reported with this combination. If alternate therapies are unacceptable and this combination is prescribed, monitor very closely.
sympathomimetics (norepinephrine, phenylephrine, and others)	A decrease in methyldopa's antihypertensive effect is reported. If necessary to use sympathomimetics, the physician should prescribe very small doses of the sympathomimetic agent. Monitor closely.

Dosage and administration

Adults Initial. Give 250 mg orally two to three times daily for 2 days. Dosage increases should be instituted after 2 days of therapy, according to the individual client's response.

Maintenance. Give 500 to 2000 mg/day, divided into two to four individual dosages. Maximum daily dosage is 3 g/day.

Children. Initially give 10 mg/kg body weight or 300 mg/m^2 of body surface in two to four divided doses. Increase at 2-day intervals according to client's response, up to 65 mg/kg or 3 g/day, whichever is less.

Parenteral methyldopa

Adults. Intravenous infusion of 250 to 500 mg in dextrose 5% injection (100 ml) is given over a 30- to 60-minute period, every 6 hours as needed. Maximum dose is 1 g every 6 to 12 hours.

Children. Intravenous infusion of 5 to 10 mg/kg body weight in dextrose 5% injection is given over a 30- to 60-minute period every 6 hours, as needed, up to 65 mg/kg or 3 g/day, whichever is less.

Pregnancy safety. Not established

NURSING CONSIDERATIONS

Assessment. Use with caution in clients with previous liver disease or in those suffering from severe renal impairment.

Do not use in clients with acute hepatic disease, acute hepatitis, cirrhosis of liver, and hypersensitivity to methyldopa.

Risks and benefits must be considered in childbearing and lactating women.

Intervention. Dosage increases should be initiated with the evening dose to minimize the effects of sedation.

Intramuscular or subcutaneous administration is not recommended because of unreliable absorption.

When changing a client from parenteral to oral form, the same dosage is used.

Administer intravenous infusion over 30 to 60 minutes.

Education. Emphasize to the client the importance of keeping clinical laboratory visits. Methyldopa hepatotoxicity (reversible) may occasionally develop 2 to 4 weeks after initiation of therapy. The flulike symptoms are chills, fever, headache, anorexia, fatigue, arthralgia, enlarged liver, and pruritus. Physician will prescribe liver function tests; if they are positive, therapy will be discontinued.

Caution client to avoid prolonged standing in one position or strenuous exercise to prevent orthostatic hypotension. Instruct client to avoid sudden position changes.

Inform client that urine may darken. It may first turn red, then brown and black when it comes in contact with a hypoclorite toilet bleaching agent. Assure client that this reaction is harmless.

Inform client of possible drowsiness, which requires caution in operating a car or other machinery.

Instruct client to carry medical identification card or Medic Alert.

Warn client not to take OTC medications without consulting the physician.

Caution patient about increased sedative effects of alcohol, barbiturates, and other CNS depressants.

Evaluation. Take blood pressure and pulse as prescribed during initiation of therapy and continue until drug dosage is properly titrated. Take blood pressure at regular intervals with client in lying, sitting, and standing positions.

Observe client for drug tolerance, which may occur during second or third month of therapy.

Note that physician may prescribe an increase in dosage in the evening to minimize daytime sedation. Observe client for drug-induced depression and report symptom to physician.

Observe client for side effects, especially unexplained fever and immediately report any to the physician.

If unexplained fever or rash occurs, obtain liver function studies (e.g., SGOT, bilirubin) especially during the first 2 or 3 months of therapy. If present, discontinue drug permanently to avoid drug-induced hepatitis.

Hemolytic anemia may occur in 4% of clients with possible fatal complications. Before drug therapy, physician will prescribe a complete blood count and direct Coombs' test. These tests should be done periodically during treatment. Positive Coombs' test may or may not indicate hemolytic anemia. With prolonged use of methyldopa, 10% to 20% of patients develop a positive direct Coombs' test; this is not a contraindication to further use of the drug. With a positive Coombs' test with resultant hemolytic anemia, physician should discontinue therapy. If a blood transfusion is needed, both direct and indirect Coomb's test should be performed. Positive tests may interfere with the cross matching of blood.

If reversible leukopenia occurs, drug therapy should be discontinued.

Monitor intake and output and weigh daily. Report fluid retention to the physician.

guanabenz acetate (Wytensin)

Mechanism of action. The mechanism of action of guanabenz acetate is the same as clonidine; however, with guanabenz there is no fluid retention. In clinical trials of 6 to 30 months, hypertensive clients whose blood pressure was controlled with guanabenz actually lost 1 to 4 pounds. The mechanism of this weight loss is not known. In addition, plasma renin activity may be unchanged or decreased during long-term therapy. Cardiac output remains unchanged. The antihypertensive effect occurs without major changes in peripheral resistance. Nevertheless, peripheral resistance does eventually decrease with continued therapy. There is no evidence that tolerance develops to the hypotensive effect of this drug.

Indication. Antihypertensive

Pharmacokinetics. See Table 25-2.

Side effects/adverse reactions. See Table 25-3.

Significant drug interactions. Although the potential for drug interactions with guanabenz exists, no major drug interactions have been identified so far.

Dosage and administration

Adults. Initial dose is 4 mg orally twice daily, increased if necessary every 1 to 2 weeks by increments of 4 to 8 mg/day, up to a maximum of 32 mg/day.

Children. Dosage is not established.

Pregnancy safety. FDA Category C

NURSING CONSIDERATIONS

Assessment. Guanabenz should be used during pregnancy only if the benefits outweigh the potential risk to the fetus. This agent may have adverse effects on the fetus when administered to pregnant women. In animal studies an increase in skeletal abnormalities has been observed, along with increased fetal loss and diminished body weight of the neonate. Always inquire if the female client is pregnant or has plans to be.

Do not use in patients who have hypersensitivity to guanabenz.

Intervention. The last dose of each day should be taken at bedtime to ensure overnight control of blood pressure.

Guanabenz is usually not discontinued before surgery; however, the anesthesiologist must be aware that the client is receiving the drug.

Education. Emphasize the importance of periodic follow-up visits so that the guanabenz dosage and blood pressure are monitored.

Caution client against abrupt withdrawal of drug. The possibility of withdrawal syndrome should be considered, although rebound hypertension does not generally occur.

Inform client of the possible side effects, particularly dry mouth, and sedative effects, which require caution in operating a car or other machinery.

Instruct client to take last dose before bedtime to ensure continuous blood pressure control during the night.

Instruct client to carry medical identification card or Medic Alert.

Warn client not to take OTC medication without consulting the physician.

Caution client about the increased sedative effects of alcohol, barbiturates, and other central nervous system depressants.

Evaluation. Closely monitor blood pressure and pulse during the initiation of therapy and until the dosage is properly titrated.

Closely observe clients with severe hepatic or renal failure, severe coronary insufficiency, recent myocardial infarction, or cerebrovascular disease.

PERIPHERAL ADRENERGIC INHIBITOR DRUGS
guanethidine sulfate (Ismelin)

Mechanism of action. Guanethidine sulfate is a powerful antihypertensive drug that acts as a postganglionic adrenergic neuron blocking agent. Guanethidine enters the storage vesicles of the adrenergic nerve terminal, where it gradually displaces the stored norepinephrine. The subsequent depletion of norepinephrine inhibits transmission of nerve impulses at the neuroeffector junction. Although there is no significant change in peripheral resistance, the drug reduces blood pressure by decreasing vascular tone, primarily at the venous side and secondarily at the arterial side of the circulatory system. This lowers venous return, which reduces cardiac output. Consequently, a proportional decrease in cerebral, splanchnic, and renal blood flow results.

The venous pooling of blood is responsible for orthostatic hypotension. The reduction in blood pressure is noticeably greater with the client in the standing position than in the recumbent position. The salt and water retention that increases plasma volume is probably caused by hemodynamic effects, such as reduced renal plasma flow and glomerular filtration rate. This is why tolerance to the drug may occur. The heart rate, however, is generally slowed. The adrenergic blocking action of guanethidine increases gastrointestinal motility, frequently causing diarrhea. It is speculated that this response may possibly be attributed to parasympathetic predominance. The drug does not affect the catecholamines in the adrenal medulla. In contrast, it may cause the release of catecholamines from a pheochromocytoma, thus producing a hypertensive crisis.

Indication. Antihypertensive
Pharmacokinetics. See Table 25-2.
Side effects/adverse reactions. See Table 25-2.
Significant drug interactions. The following interactions may occur when methyldopa is given with the drugs listed below:

Drug	Possible Effect and Management
oral antidiabetic medications or insulin	May result in an increased hypoglycemic effect. Monitor closely and communicate with physician since dosage adjustments may be necessary.
minoxidil	Concurrent use with guanethidine is not recommended since antihypertensive effects may be potentiated.
monoamine oxidase (MAO) inhibitors	Severe hypertension may result. It is recommended that MAO inhibitors be discontinued for a minimum of 1 week before starting guanethidine.
metaraminol, norepinephrine, and possibly other sympathomimetics	The antihypertensive effectiveness of guanethidine may be reduced. Metaraminol and guanethidine concurrently may result in cardiac arrhythmias, severe prolonged hypertension, or a hypertensive crisis. If it is absolutely necessary to use this combination, the smallest dose possible should be prescribed with very close patient monitoring.
tricyclic antidepressants, loxapine, thioxanthenes, and possibly other psychotropic medications	May reduce the antihypertensive effect of guanethidine by blocking its access to the adrenergic nerve site. Monitor closely since dosage adjustments or alternate antidepressant medications on a trial basis may be ordered by the physician.

Dosage and administration
Adults
Ambulatory clients. Initial dose is 10 or 12.5 mg orally daily, increased by 10- or 12.5-mg increments at 5- to 7-day intervals, as necessary. Maintenance dose is 25 to 50 mg orally daily.

Hospitalized clients. Initial dose is 25 to 50 mg orally daily, increased by 25- to 50-mg increments at daily or every other day intervals, as necessary.

Children. Dosage is 200 μg (0.2 mg)/kg or 6 mg/m² body surface area orally daily. Increase by same amount daily at 7- to 10-day intervals, as necessary for blood pressure control.

Pregnancy safety. Not established

NURSING CONSIDERATIONS

Assessment. Anticipate that hospitalized clients will receive a higher initial dosage than ambulatory clients because they can be watched more carefully.

Use with caution in a client with a history of bronchial asthma, which may be precipitated because of hypersensitivity to catecholamine depletion.

Use with caution in a client with peptic ulcer or colitis because depletion of norepinephrine may increase parasympathetic tone.

Do not use in clients who are hypersensitive to guanethidine or have pheochromocytoma or frank congestive heart failure not caused by hypertension. (See use of MAOI under drug interactions.)

Cautious use is indicated in a client with severe renal disease (nitrogen retention, increased BUN levels), coronary insufficiency, recent myocardial infarction, cerebrovascular disease, congestive heart failure, sinus bradycardia, impaired hepatic function, diabetes mellitus, or fever.

Intervention. The most frequent problem with guanethidine is orthostatic hypotension. As a baseline for comparison, take blood pressure readings before initiation of drug therapy; continue to keep a record of client's blood pressures while in the supine and standing positions during therapy. The hypotensive effect of the drug is greater with the client in the upright position than in the supine position. Therefore dosage adjustment of guanethidine is determined by blood pressure taken first while the client is in the supine position, then again after client has been standing for 10 minutes or performing mild exercise. If there is *no decrease* from the previous levels, an increase in dosage is indicated. Dosage should be reduced when the client has (1) normal supine blood pressure, (2) excessive fall in orthostatic pressure, or (3) severe diarrhea.

Note that guanethidine has a long duration of action as well as a prolonged half-life. Also, the full therapeutic benefits may not be noticed for 1 to 3 weeks. This means that dosage increase, when needed, is made at intervals of 5 to 7 days.

Education. Forewarn client that orthostatic hypotension (dizziness, lightheadedness, or syncope) occurs frequently and is prominent when rising from sleep or making rapid position changes. Instruct client to change position gradually. Venous return to the heart can be increased by flexing arms and legs slowly before sitting or standing. Some physicians prescribe that the client don elastic stockings before getting out of bed. During dosage adjustment, the hospitalized client should receive help when getting out of bed.

Inform client that orthostatic hypotension is aggravated by hot showers or baths, hot weather, prolonged standing, physical exercise, and alcohol ingestion. During an episode of orthostatic hypotension, caution client to sit or lie down at the first sign of dizziness or weakness.

Instruct client to report any signs of diarrhea. If it persists, physician may order an anticholinergic agent (atropine), paregoric, or a kaolin-pectin preparation. Guanethidine may be discontinued, or the dosage may be reduced. Note the state of hydration of the client, and check the level of electrolyte balance during this episode.

Evaluation. Closely monitor client receiving long-term therapy because the effects of guanethidine are cumulative. Periodic liver and kidney function tests and blood counts should be performed.

Monitor intake and output, observing for reduced urine volume, particularly in clients with limited cardiac or renal function. Weigh patient daily, and watch for signs of edema or fluid retention. Report increased weight (2 pounds or more) to physician.

Carefully monitor the client's pulse rate. If bradycardia occurs, report readings to physician.

Observe clients with diabetes receiving antidiabetic therapy since guanethidine may produce additive hypoglycemic effects.

Alert client to inform surgeons, anesthesiologists, and dentists that he or she is taking guanethidine before any intrusive procedures are considered.

Emphasize the importance of drug compliance. Report side effects so that the physician can modify drug regimen without discontinuing medication. Also, advise client to avoid emotional encounters or any other form of stress.

Instruct client not to take any other medication or over-the-counter drugs, which may contain sympathomimetic agents, without consulting the physician.

Stress the importance of keeping follow-up appointments to the physician's office.

Instruct client to carry medical identification card or Medic Alert.

guanadrel sulfate (Hylorel)

Mechanism of action. Same as guanethidine.
Indication. Antihypertensive.
Pharmacokinetics. See Table 25-1.
Side effects/adverse reactions. See Table 25-2.
Significant drug interactions. Metaraminol and other sympathomimetics; monoamine oxidase inhibitors (MAOI); and tricyclic antidepressants, loxapine, thioxanthenes, and psychotropic agents may cause drug interactions; see under guanethidine.

In addition, trimeprazine may reduce the antihypertensive effect of guanadrel by displacement and blocking guanadrel's access to the adrenergic neuron. Monitor closely.

Dosage and administration
Adults
Initial. Dosage is 5 mg orally twice daily. Dosage may be increased at daily, weekly, or monthly intervals, as necessary for blood pressure control.

Maintenance. Dosage is 20 to 75 mg orally per day, in two to four divided doses.
Children. Dosage is not established.
Pregnancy safety. FDA Category B

NURSING CONSIDERATIONS

See discussion of guanethidine.

Rauwolfia Derivatives
reserpine (Sandril, Serpasil, Rau-Sed, Reserpoid)

Rauwolfia derivatives are alkaloids obtained primarily from *Rauwolfia serpentina,* a shrub endemic to India and various tropical areas of the world. The major alkaloid reserpine was isolated in 1952, and it is still used for its antihypertensive effect. Other *Rauwolfia* alkaloids have different chemical structures, but in general they have similar actions, uses, and cautions. Since reserpine is the most commonly prescribed alkaloid, it will serve as the prototype for this category of drugs. Other available *Rauwolfia* derivatives include alseroxylon (Rauwiloid), deserpidine (Harmonyl), *Rauwolfia serpentina* (Raudixin, Rauverid, Wolfina), and rescinnamine (Moderil).

Mechanism of action. Blood pressure is lowered by reserpine (*Rauwolfia* alkaloids) by depleting the storage sites of norepinephrine in the peripheral postganglionic adrenergic neuron. Studies indicate that *Rauwolfia* compounds alter the ability of storage granules in nerve cells to take up and bind norepinephrine. Without adequate norepinephrine available for release, discharges of nerve impulses from the peripheral sympathetic neurons, which supply the smooth muscle of arterioles, produce little or no effect on these blood vessels. The resultant vascular relaxation decreases peripheral resistance, thereby reducing blood pressure. These compounds also decrease heart rate and thus lower cardiac output. In addition, they decrease plasma renin activity.

Depletion of brain norepinephrine and serotonin may account for the sedative action of reserpine. The antihypertensive effect, however, appears to be mainly caused by the peripheral adrenergic blockade, which results in peripheral pooling of blood and a reduction in cardiac output.

Although some CNS effects may be involved in the antihypertensive action, the central nervous system is not currently believed to be the major site of action for the *Rauwolfia* alkaloids.

Indication. Antihypertensive
Pharmacokinetics. See Table 25-1.

Side effects/adverse reactions. See Table 25-2.

Significant drug interactions. The following interactions may occur when reserpine is given with the drugs listed below:

Drug	Possible Effect and Management
CNS depressants and/or alcohol	Enhanced CNS depressant effects. Monitor closely.
MAO inhibitors	May result in hyperpyrexia and hypertension (moderate to severe or even crisis level). Concurrent administration is not recommended. Patients receiving MAO inhibitors should be taken off this medication for at least 1 week before a *Rauwolfia* alkaloid is started.

Dosage and administration

Adults. Give 100 to 250 μg (0.1 to 0.25 mg) orally daily.

Children. Give 5 to 20 μg (0.005 to 0.02 mg)/kg or 150 to 600 μg (0.15 to 0.6 mg)/m² body surface in one or two divided daily doses.

For administration of the less commonly used *Rauwolfia* alkaloid preparations, see package inserts.

Pregnancy safety. FDA Category D

NURSING CONSIDERATIONS

Assessment. Use with extreme caution in clients with history of mental depression. Discontinue therapy at the first sign of despondency; otherwise continued therapy could result in suicide or cardiovascular effects.

Use cautiously in clients with a history of gallstones, to prevent biliary colic, or with a history of renal insufficiency (diuretic is usually required), to avoid difficulty in adjusting to lower blood pressure levels.

Use cautiously in clients with cerebral hemorrhage (severe hypotension may be precipitated with parenteral doses greater than 0.5 mg), epilepsy, cardiac damage, asthma, chronic sinusitis, parkinsonism, and pheochromocytoma.

Do not use in clients with mental depression (particularly with suicidal tendencies), ulcerative colitis, and acute peptic ulcers or those who are hypersensitive to *Rauwolfia* derivatives.

Intervention. Administer oral medications with meals or with milk or other food to minimize gastric irritation, since drug increases gastric secretions.

Note that the *Rauwolfia* derivatives have a slow onset of action and a long duration of action, so therapeutic benefits may take about 2 weeks to develop. Action may persist for approximately 1 month after discontinuation of therapy. If client requires general anesthesia, discontinue drug 1 month before surgery, including dental surgery.

Education. Although orthostatic hypotension does not usually occur, advise client to make position changes slowly to avoid potential dizziness and fainting. Because of the sedative effect of the drug, caution client about operating dangerous or hazardous machinery.

Advise client not to take alcohol or other CNS depressants.

Teach the client or a responsible member of the family the possible side effects that may occur and that should be reported to the physician. Mental depression (anorexia, self-depreciation, detached attitude, and impotence) may lead to suicide. This usually occurs in clients who receive a high dosage.

If nasal stuffiness occurs, nasal decongestants or other OTC preparations containing sympathomimetics should not be used without first consulting the physician. Dry mouth may be relieved by rinsing with warm water, OTC saliva substitutes (VAOraLube, Xero-Lube), sugarless gum, or sour hard candy. Consult physician before using any of these compounds.

Emphasize the importance of drug compliance even if the client is feeling well. Instruct client not to discontinue the drug suddenly but to report unpleasant side effects to the physician. Also stress the need for medical follow-up visits.

Instruct client to carry medical identification card or Medic Alert.

Evaluation. Monitor the client's blood pressure and pulse rate frequently and compare with baseline readings, particularly before parenteral administration. A decrease in blood pressure may be a result of bradycardia.

Weigh client daily. Excessive weight gain indicates fluid retention, which should be reported to the physician.

ALPHA ADRENERGIC BLOCKING DRUGS

The alpha adrenergic blocking agents used in the management of hypertension include phenoxybenzamine, phentolamine, and prazosin. Phenoxybenzamine and phentolamine are alpha blockers that are relatively nonselective because they antagonize responses mediated by both alpha$_1$ and alpha$_2$ receptors. Hence, they lower blood pressure by preventing norepinephrine from activating alpha$_1$ receptors on vascular smooth muscle to produce vasoconstriction. See Chapter 20 for monographs of phenoxybenzamine and phentolamine. Prazosin is more selective in its activity and is classed as an alpha$_1$ adrenergic blocking agent.

prazosin hydrochloride (Minipress)

Mechanism of action. Prazosin reduces blood pressure by decreasing peripheral vascular resistance.

Although several mechanisms of action have been proposed, some aspects of how prazosin produces a hypotensive effect are still not completely understood. According to the current hypothesis, prazosin is an alpha$_1$ adrenergic blocking agent. By selectively blocking the postsynaptic alpha receptors on the vascular smooth muscle of both the arterioles and the veins, prazosin inhibits the action of norepinephrine when the sympathetic nerves are stimulated. This blocking action causes a decrease in peripheral vascular resistance, lowering blood pressure, especially diastolic blood pressure. Prazosin usually has little effect on cardiac output. In clients with congestive heart failure, prazosin may increase cardiac output by decreasing systemic and pulmonary venous pressure.

Indication. Antihypertensive

Pharmacokinetics. See Table 25-1.

Side effects/adverse reactions. See Table 25-2.

Significant drug interactions. There are no known major drug interactions to date.

Dosage and administration

Adults

Initial. Give 1 mg orally two or three times daily.

Maintenance. Give 6 to 15 mg daily, in divided doses.

Children. Children under 7 years old are given 250 µg (0.25 mg) orally, two or three times daily. Children 7 to 12 years old are given 500 µg (0.5 mg) orally two or three times daily.

Pregnancy safety. Not established

NURSING CONSIDERATIONS

Assessment. Use caution in clients with angina pectoris or severe cardiac disease.

Clients with impaired renal function may require lower doses.

Intervention. Syncope along with dizziness, light-headedness, or sudden loss of consciousness may occur, generally within ½ to 1½ hours following an initial dose of prazosin "first-dose hypotensive reaction" or a rapid dose increase of the drug. These symptoms may also appear when other antihypertensive agents are added to the regimen. Occasionally, the syncopal episode is preceded by severe tachycardia (heart rate of 120 to 160 beats/min). To minimize this reaction, limit initial dose to 1 mg, then increase dosage slowly. When adding a diuretic or other antihypertensive agent, reduce prazosin to 1 or 2 mg and then increase dosage as needed.

It is recommended that the initial dose be administered at bedtime to minimize the "first-dose hypotensive reaction."

Education. Inform client of "first-dose hypotensive reaction."

Instruct client to avoid rapid postural changes, particularly from recumbent to upright positions. Also, if dizziness occurs, client should lie down. This effect tends to disappear with continued use of the drug or dosage reduction. Inform client not to drive or operate hazardous machinery during the early period of adjustment to drug therapy. Note that the full effect of the drug may not be achieved for 4 to 6 weeks.

Teach client to take daily weight and report any increase to the physician. Prazosin tends to increase fluid retention. Also, instruct client to minimize sodium intake.

Emphasize the importance of drug compliance and keeping physician's appointments. If tolerance to prazosin develops, ineffectiveness usually occurs within several months and the physician will need to alter the drug regimen. Inform client not to take any other drugs without first consulting the physician. This includes OTC medications that contain sympathomimetic agents used for a cold, cough, or allergic condition.

Evaluation. Monitor blood pressure and pulse rate frequently and observe for sudden drop in blood pressure and tachycardia.

VASODILATOR DRUGS

The vasodilator drugs exhibit a direct action on the smooth muscle walls of the arterioles and/or veins, thereby lowering peripheral resistance and blood pressure. Although various theories have been proposed, the mechanism of action, at least in part, involves the direct relaxation of vascular smooth muscle by stimulation of the calcium-binding process. The drop in blood pressure stimulates the sympathetic nervous system and activates the baroreceptor reflexes, increasing heart rate and cardiac output. This also increases renin release. Therefore combined therapy is recommended. To inhibit sympathetic reflex response use of a beta adrenergic blocker such as propranolol has been advocated, along with a diuretic to alleviate sodium and water retention that occurs during vasodilator therapy.

There are two types of vasodilators: (1) arteriolar dilators, such as diazoxide, hydralazine, and minoxidil, which exert a selective effect on arterioles, and (2) arteriolar and venous dilators, such as sodium nitroprusside, which lower blood pressure by acting on both arteriolar resistance vessels and venous capacitance vessels.

ARTERIOLAR DILATOR DRUGS
diazoxide (Hyperstat IV)

Mechanism of action. The antihypertensive action results from direct relaxation of smooth muscles in the peripheral arterioles, which causes a decrease in peripheral resistance. The drug does not affect the venous capacitance vessels. As blood pressure is reduced, a reflex increase in heart rate and cardiac output occurs, with resultant maintenance of coronary and cerebral blood flow. This cardiovascular reflex mechanism also inhibits the development of orthostatic hypotension. Diazoxide also causes retention of sodium and water the produces increased plasma renin activity. Since tolerance usually develops, the drug is frequently given with a diuretic.

When administered intravenously, diazoxide is a potent antihypertensive agent. However, the oral form (Proglycem) produces only a slight decrease in blood pressure. Its main action is to stimulate hyperglycemia and decrease plasma insulin levels by suppressing insulin release. (See Chapter 48.)

Indications
1. Diazoxide is administered intravenously to reduce blood pressure promptly in *hypertensive emergencies* such as malignant hypertension, hypertensive encephalopathy, impaired renal function (acute or chronic glomerulonephritis), and eclampsia, when an urgent decrease in diastolic pressure is required. Drug is administered to hospitalized clients.
2. Intravenous diazoxide is ineffective in reducing elevated blood pressure in clients with pheochromocytoma. Also, because of its adverse effects, the drug is not used for chronic treatment of hypertension.

Pharmacokinetics. See Table 25-1.

Side effects/adverse reactions. See Table 25-2.

Significant drug interactions. Diazoxide given concurrently with other antihypertensive medications or peripheral vasodilators may result in a severe hypotensive reaction. If concurrent use is necessary, smaller doses may be indicated. The patient should be monitored closely for several hours for hypotension.

Dosage and administration

Adults. Administer up to 150 mg (or 1 to 3 mg/kg of body weight) intravenously within 10 to 30 seconds. Repeat dose in 5 to 15 minutes if necessary, up to a maximum of 1.2 g/day. Following the emergency period, give diazoxide for several days, until the ordered oral hypertensive agent is effective.

Children. Give dose of 1 to 3 mg/kg of body weight or 30 to 90 mg/m^2 body surface intravenously. Repeat dose if necessary in 5 to 15 minutes.

Pregnancy safety. FDA category C

NURSING CONSIDERATIONS

Assessment. Clients who are unable to tolerate thiazide diuretics or sulfonamide-type medications may also show intolerance to diazoxide.

Use with caution in clients with impaired cerebral or cardiac circulation since an abrupt drop in blood pressure may seriously reduce blood flow to these organs.

Intervention. Intravenous diazoxide should be administered only in a peripheral vein through an established IV line to avoid cardiac disrhythmias.

Avoid extravasation because the solution is alkaline and will cause cellulitis and pain of the tissue. If extravasation occurs, treat with cold packs.

Place client in recumbent position during therapy and keep in same position for at least 30 minutes after injection. If a diuretic such as furosemide (Lasix) is administered, the diuretic generally is given ½ to 1 hour before diazoxide. Have client remain supine for 8 to 10 hours because of additive hypotensive effect.

The entire dose should be given by rapid intravenous injection (in less than 30 seconds). Slower administration may result in reduced effect or decreased duration of effect.

Notify physician of signs of abdominal distention, absence of bowel sounds, or constipation.

Simultaneous use of anticoagulants with diazoxide may require reduction in dosage of the former because of increased anticoagulant effects.

Administer injection cautiously to clients who are treated concurrently with methyldopa, reserpine, or peripheral vasodilator agents, especially hydralazine, nitrites, and papaverine-like compounds.

Do not use intravenous injection of diazoxide in the treatment of compensatory hypertension, such as aortic coarctation or anteriovenous shunt. Diazoxide should not be administered to clients who are hypersensitive to this agent, other thiazides, or sulfonamides unless the potential benefits outweigh the risk.

Evaluation. Monitor blood pressure every 5 minutes until stable, then every hour during the duration of drug action. Before ending surveillance, take blood pressure with client standing. Take pulse before and during therapy. If tachycardia occurs with intravenous administration, report immediately to the physician.

Because of sodium and water retention, weigh client daily. Measure intake and output, and report weight gain to the physician. Diuretic may be indicated. After repeated injections, observe client closely for signs of congestive heart failure (edema, dyspnea, cough, pulmonary rales, distended neck veins, and fatigue).

Before intravenous diazoxide administration and during treatment, monitor blood and urinary glucose levels, serum electrolytes, and complete blood counts. (Hypokalemia potentiates hyperglycemia.) The long half-life of diazoxide requires that client with hyperglycemia be observed up to 7 days, until blood sugar level is stabilized.

Hyperglycemia usually occurs in most clients, especially when injections are repeated; closely monitor blood glucose levels, particularly in individuals with diabetes mellitus. In some instances insulin may be indicated.

hydralazine hydrochloride (Apresoline)

Mechanism of action. Hydralazine hydrochloride is thought to produce its hypotensive effects by direct relaxation of vascular smooth muscle, particularly the arteries and arterioles, with little effect on veins. Thus arteriolar vasodilation reduces peripheral resistance. Consequently, renal blood flow is increased, providing an advantage to clients with renal failure. Hydralazine also maintains cerebral blood flow and produces sodium and water retention. However, the resultant hypotension is thought to stimulate the baroreceptor reflex, causing an increase in heart rate and cardiac output. Unfortunately, this response offsets the antihypertensive effects of the drug.

This development of tolerance to the antihypertensive action may be offset by the addition of a diuretic to the drug regimen. The diuretic enhances the antihypertensive effect and reduces the potential for increased cardiac output and fluid retention.

Hydralazine decreases diastolic pressure more than systolic. It also increases plasma renin activity.

Indications. Antihypertensive

Pharmacokinetics. See Table 25-1.

Side effects/adverse reactions. See Table 25-2.

Significant drug interactions. Hydralazine and diazoxide used concurrently may result in a severe hypotensive effect. If given together, monitor client for at least several hours for this effect.

Dosage and administration

Oral. Hypertension or congestive heart failure:

Adults. Give 40 mg daily for 2 to 4 days, then 100 mg for the remainder of the first week. Give 200 mg orally daily thereafter in two to four divided doses. Once control is achieved, determine and use lowest effective dosage.

Children. Give 750 μg (0.75 mg)/kg body weight or 25 mg/m^2 body surface daily, divided into two to four doses. Increase the dosage slowly over 1 to 4 weeks as necessary, up to a maximum of 7.5 mg/kg or 300 mg/day.

Parenteral. Hypertension:

Adults. Give 10 to 40 mg intramuscularly or intravenously. Repeat if necessary.

Children. Give 1.7 to 3.5 mg/kg or 50 to 100 mg/m^2 body surface daily, divided in four to six doses.

Pregnancy safety. FDA Category C

NURSING CONSIDERATIONS

Assessment. Use with caution in clients with coronary artery disease, mitral valvular disease, cerebrovascular accidents, or advanced renal disease. Also, cautious use is advised in clients taking monoamine oxidase inhibitors.

Tartrazine sensitivity may cause allergic-type reactions (bronchial asthma) in susceptible individuals who take apresoline 10 and 100 mg tablets that contain tartrazine (FD and C Yellow No. 5).

Hydralazine hydrochloride is contraindicated in coronary artery disease in which anginal attacks may be intensified, rheumatic mitral valvular disease that may precipitate congestive heart failure, and hypersensitivity to hydralazine.

Before initiation of hydralazine therapy, complete blood count, antinuclear antibody titer test, and lupus erythematosus (LE) cell preparation tests may be performed. Repeat these tests periodically if client is receiving prolonged therapy.

Clients with impaired renal function may require lower doses.

Intervention. Use the parenteral form as quickly as possible after drawing through a needle. The drug changes color after contact with a metal filter.

Administer drug with meals or food; this minimizes first-pass metabolism of drug in the intestinal wall, thereby enhancing bioavailability.

Education. Teach client the importance of taking medication at the same time each day and to take it exactly as prescribed by the physician, even when feeling well. Inform client that drug should not be discontinued even if side effects occur; instead, the physician should be contacted. This agent should be discontinued gradually; otherwise abrupt withdrawal will precipitate a sudden rise in blood pressure and heart failure.

Emphasize to the client the importance of keeping clinical appointments, including those involving laboratory studies. Following long-term administration of hydralazine, drug tolerance may develop, necessitating adjustment of drug regimen.

Inform client that palpitations and headache may occur during the early stages of oral administration, but these symptoms usually subside with continued therapy. Usually, a beta blocker such as propranolol may be prescribed to prevent reflex tachycardia.

Instruct client to report any signs of peripheral neuritis (numbness, tingling, and paresthesias) so that pyridoxine (vitamin B$_6$) may be prescribed to combat the antipyridoxine response of hydralazine.

Since orthostatic hypotension may occur, advise client to make position changes slowly. Also, inform client to avoid standing still for long periods of time, taking hot baths or showers, and doing strenuous exercise.

Warn client against operating potentially hazardous machinery, since dizziness or faintness may occur.

Instruct client to carry medical identification card or Medic Alert.

Evaluation. Closely monitor blood pressure and pulse rate of clients receiving parenteral hydralazine. Measure every 5 minutes until stabilized; continue to check frequently (about every 10 to 15 minutes) during therapy.

Monitor intake and output during parenteral therapy; output may be increased with improved renal blood flow.

Weigh client daily to check for edema. Report to physician any gain in weight. Also, advise client to reduce salt intake.

Observe mental status of client. Report to physician any signs of anxiety or mental depression; this condition may indicate cerebral ischemia.

Lupus erythematosus cell preparation tests are indicated if client develops fever, sore throat, arthralgia, chest pain, and chronic malaise. Systemic lupus erythematosis (SLE)–like syndrome may occur in clients receiving higher doses (more than 200 mg/day), in slow acetylators, and in patients with renal impairment. Discontinue drug if tests are positive.

To evaluate for blood dyscrasias obtain periodic blood counts during prolonged therapy; discontinue hydralazine if abnormalities develop.

With simultaneous use of parenteral diazoxide, observe client for several hours to assess for profound hypotension.

minoxidil (Loniten)

Mechanism of action. Minoxidil is a potent and orally effective direct-acting peripheral vasodilator. It reduces elevated systolic and diastolic blood pressure by decreasing peripheral vascular resistance in the arteriolar vessels, with little effect on veins. This agent does not have any influence on vasomotor reflexes; therefore it does not cause orthostatic hypotension.

The vasodilator effect of minoxidil is considerably greater than that of hydralazine. Like other vasodilators, minoxidil causes a reflex increase in cardiac output, induces sodium retention, promotes development of edema, and increases plasma renin activity.

Indications
1. Minoxidil is used in *severe* hypertension that is refractory to the conventional antihypertensive agents. Thus it is not considered to be a primary drug for management of severe hypertension. Because of the serious adverse effects, minoxidil is indicated for use in severe hypertension associated with target organ damage such as chronic renal failure.
2. Concomitant administration of a beta adrenergic blocking agent such as propranolol is necessary to prevent severe reflex tachycardia. Also, administration of a diuretic agent is essential to counteract sodium and water retention.

Pharmacokinetics. See Table 25-1.

Side effects/adverse reactions. See Table 25-2.

Significant drug interactions. The following interactions may occur when minoxidil is given with the drugs listed at the top of the page:

Drug	Possible Effect and Management
guanethidine	This combination is not recommended since antihypertensive effects may be potentiated.
diazoxide, nitrates, or nitroprusside	This combination may result in severe hypotensive reaction. Monitor patient closely for several hours if given concurrently.

Dosage and administration
Adults
Initial. Give 5 mg orally daily, increasing in 100% increments as necessary (10 mg, 20 mg, 40 mg, etc.). It is usually recommended that dosage increases be on a minimum 3-day schedule, but in selected cases increases can be made on every 6 hours with close monitoring of the patient.

Maintenance. Give 10 to 40 mg orally daily, in a single or in a divided dosage schedule

Children up to 12 years old
Initial. Give 200 µg (0.2 mg)/kg body weight daily in a single dose. Increases may be made of 100, 150, and 200 µg/kg, to a maximum of 50 mg/day.

Maintenance. Give 250 µg (0.25 mg) to 1 mg/kg daily in a single dose or divided dosage schedule. Maximum is 50 mg/day.

Pregnancy safety. FDA Category C

NURSING CONSIDERATIONS

Assessment. Inquire if client is pregnant or has plans for pregnancy, since no adequate studies have been conducted to determine the risk to fetus.

Do not use in clients with pheochromocytoma (minoxidil may stimulate catecholamine secretion from tumor).

Use minoxidil cautiously in clients with recent myocardial infarction (of 1 month or less), since drug may further limit blood flow to myocardium. Report signs of chest, arm, or shoulder pain.

Education. Teach client to count radial pulse rate for 1 minute before taking minoxidil. Report to physician an increase of 20 or more beats/min above normal.

Instruct client receiving combination therapy to take each medication at the proper time and not to mix them. A diuretic is given to reduce salt and fluid retention, and a beta blocker is given to control reflex tachycardia. Combined therapy is indicated to increase drug's effectiveness and to minimize side effects by lowering the dose of minoxidil.

Inform client that if a dose is missed, it may be taken a few hours later. However, a missed dose should not be made up the next day; instead the regular dosing schedule should be resumed. Consult the physician if there is a question.

Emphasize the importance of drug compliance despite uncomfortable side effects. Inform client that minoxidil is a powerful drug for reducing blood pressure and by relaxing small blood vessels, more blood flow protects vital organs (heart, kidney, and brain). Alert client not to discontinue drug without notifying the physician, since abrupt withdrawal will cause rebound hypertension.

Inform client that hypertrichosis will likely occur (incidence is 80%) 3 to 6 weeks after starting therapy. This involves elongation, thickening, and increased pigmentation of fine body hair over the temples, eyebrows, sideburns, malar area, shoulders, back, legs, and forearms. This side effect is particularly troublesome to women. Condition is reversible within 2 to 6 months following discontinuation of therapy. No endocrine abnormalities have been found to account for this distressing effect. Hair remover (depilatory creams) or shaving may be effective in removing unwanted hair.

Tell client that minoxidil may be taken with or without food. Advise client against salt intake, and request that dietitian provide information regarding diet.

Inform client that if difficulty in breathing occurs, especially when lying down, to notify the physician since this may mean impending congestive heart failure.

Advise client not to take other drugs including OTC agents without first consulting the physician.

Instruct client to carry medical identification card or Medic Alert.

Evaluation. When minoxidil is first administered, clients, particularly those who have been receiving guanethidine, should be monitored in a hospital setting to prevent too rapid a decrease in blood pressure.

Take blood pressure and pulse rate before administering minoxidil and use these parameters as a guideline to determine progress. During therapy, monitor blood pressure and pulse rate regularly. Report to physician any sharp drop in blood pressure, which can precipitate cerebrovascular accident and myocardial infarction.

Monitor weight gain, intake and output, and edema. Inform physician of an increase in weight (3 or 4 pounds/day) so that fluid retention can be corrected. Client also should monitor weight at home.

Monitor electrolyte balance, especially potassium level if client is receiving a diuretic, which may produce an increase in serum potassium loss. Replacement therapy should be instituted.

Watch for pericardial effusion with or without tamponade, since this may occur in about 3% of clients not receiving dialysis. This requires more vigorous diuretic therapy, or if pericardiocentesis does not alleviate condition, discontinuation of minoxidil.

Observe for anginal symptoms or tachycardia which

can then be relieved by concomitant administration of a beta adrenergic blocker.

Closely supervise clients with renal failure or those receiving dialysis to prevent exacerbation of renal failure or precipitation of cardiac failure. Lower dose of minoxidil is indicated.

ARTERIOLAR AND VENOUS DILATOR DRUGS
sodium nitroprusside (Nipride, Nitropress)

Mechanism of action. Sodium nitroprusside is a potent direct-acting vasodilator agent that greatly reduces arterial blood pressure. This drug relaxes both arteriolar and venous smooth muscles. Because of the latter effect, more venous pooling of blood occurs when the client is upright. Consequently, there is no increase in venous return of blood to the heart. In addition, sodium nitroprusside produces a slight increase in heart rate and a mild decrease in cardiac output. It also enhances the secretion of renin.

Nitroprusside reduces cardiac load; that is, the decrease in systemic resistance results in a reduction in preload and afterload, thus improving cardiac output in the client with congestive heart failure.

Indications
1. Rapid reduction of blood pressure
2. Cardiac load–reducing agent: treatment of congestive heart failure and adjunct treatment of myocardial infarction and valvular regurgitation

Pharmacokinetics. See Table 25-1.

Side effects/adverse reactions. See Table 25-2.

Significant drug interactions. No major interactions are noted at this time.

Dosage and administration

Adults. Mix contents of vial in dextrose 5% injection only. Administer by intravenous infusion, 0.5 μg (0.0005 mg)/kg/min. Slowly increase in increments of 0.5 μg according to patient response. Usual dose is 3 μg/kg/min, although dosage may range up to 10 μg/kg/min or a total dose of 3.5 mg/kg.

Children. Give 1.4 μg (0.0014 mg)/kg/min. Adjust dosage as needed.

Pregnancy safety. FDA Category C

NURSING CONSIDERATIONS

Assessment. Do not use drug in clients with inadequate cerebral circulation or compensatory hypertension (e.g., arteriovenous shunt or aortic coarctation).

Intervention. After preparing intravenous solution, promptly wrap container in aluminum foil or other opaque material (brown paper bag) to protect drug from light. Use fresh solution and do not keep longer than 24 hours. Freshly prepared solution has a faint brown tinge;

discard if it is highly colored (e.g., blue, green, or dark red).

Administer infusion using a microdrip regulator or an automatic infusion pump. These devices must be available to allow precise measurement of the flow rate as prescribed by physician. Do not add other drugs to the nitroprusside infusion.

Raising the head of the client's bed will increase the hypotensive effect of the drug.

Because sodium nitroprusside is converted to thiocyanate, monitor blood thiocyanate level when infusion is continued for more than 72 hours, especially in clients with renal dysfunction. If blood thiocyanate level exceeds 10 mg/dl, the infusion should be discontinued or decreased to prevent toxicity.

Be aware that client's therapy will be changed to oral antihypertensive agents as soon as response occurs.

As oral therapy is instituted, the client will require lower doses of nitroprusside.

Evaluation. Monitor blood pressure every half minute when infusion is first started to avoid rapid hypotension. Later, check it every 5 minutes. Facilities and personnel must be adequate for this purpose; intensive care facilities are recommended.

Observe client for precipitous drop in blood pressure, which may occur in large doses. Do not allow infusion rate to exceed 10 μg/kg/min. If adequate reduction in blood pressure does not occur in 10 minutes, the drug should be discontinued.

Monitor intake and output.

Monitor client for thiocyanate toxicity (tinnitus, blurred vision, and delirium). With prolonged treatment and overdosage, a potential for cyanide intoxication exists. (Note that nitroprusside is metabolized first to cyanide, then to thiocyanate.) In the event of cyanide toxicity (coma, dilated pupils, pink color, shallow respirations, imperceptible pulse rate, distant heart sounds, hypotension, and absent reflexes), discontinue nitroprusside. The treatment for overdosage is as follows: administer amyl nitrite inhalations for 15 to 30 seconds each minute; inject sodium nitrite 3% solution intravenously at a rate not to exceed 2.5 to 5.0 ml/min up to a total dose of 10 to 15 ml; then administer sodium thiosulfate intravenously, 12.5 g/50 ml of 5% dextrose in water over a 10-minute period. If symptoms of overdosage reappear, repeat sodium nitrite and sodium thiosulfate injections at half the preceding doses. Continue to observe client for several hours to prevent the recurrence of signs of overdosage.

Observe infusion site for swelling or pain. If extravasation occurs, readjust infusion as required.

ANGIOTENSIN II INHIBITOR DRUGS

Angiotensin II antagonists inhibit the action of the renin-angiotensin-aldosterone system. The importance of this system in maintaining blood pressure and sodium and fluid balance is now well accepted. (see Figure 25-2 for normal activation of the renin-angiotensin-aldosterone system.)

It is apparent that a disturbance of the basic function of the renin-angiotensin-aldosterone system can cause hypertension. Further, a damaged kidney that cannot regulate its renin release through normal feedback mechanisms may easily cause an elevation in blood pressure in certain individuals. Fortunately, this evidence has given rise to a new concept in the pharmacologic treatment of hypertension. More importantly, it has led to the development of a new class of drugs, the angiotensin II inhibitors. Captopril and enalapril maleate are the two currently marketed angiotensin-converting enzyme inhibitors in the United States.

captopril (Capoten)

Mechanism of action. Captopril reduces blood pressure primarily through suppression of the renin-angiotensin-aldosterone system. By inhibiting the action of the angiotensin-converting enzyme (ACE), captopril prevents the conversion of angiotensin I to angiotensin II (see Figure 25-4). Angiotensin II is a powerful vasoconstrictor that raises blood pressure and also causes aldosterone release, which contributes to sodium and water retention. Thus, by inhibiting the action of ACE, captopril decreases the angiotensin II level, which in turn produces the following: (1) a decrease in vascular tone, thereby directly lowering blood pressure, (2) inhibition of aldosterone release, reducing sodium and water reabsorption; the resultant excretion of fluid is thought to cause only a secondary reduction in blood pressure (decrease in aldosterone secretion does lead to a slight elevation in serum potassium), and (3) an increase in plasma renin activity, caused by a loss of negative feedback on renin release.

Blood pressure is lowered to about the same extent in patients in supine and upright positions. Although orthostatic hypotension and tachycardia are uncommon, they may occur in volume-depleted individuals.

Long-term studies have shown that in clients with severe, treatment-resistant congestive heart failure, captopril enhances cardiac output by reducing ventricular afterload and possibly preload.

Indications
1. Antihypertensive
2. Congestive heart failure (cardiac load–reducing agent)

Pharmacokinetics. See Table 25-1.

Side effects/adverse reactions. See Table 25-2.

Significant drug interactions. The following interactions may occur when captopril is given with the drugs listed on the next page:

Drug	Possible Effect and Management
diuretics	If client receiving captopril is given a diuretic, a very severe hypotensive episode may occur within 3 hours of the first diuretic dose. To reduce this reaction either discontinue the diuretic 1 week before or increase the salt intake of the patient for 1 week before initiating the captopril. Generally, this reaction does not recur with continued dosing, and the diuretic may be given later, if necessary.
potassium-sparing diuretics, low-salt milk, potassium supplements, or potassium-containing medications and salt substitutes	Monitor for hyperkalemia. Frequently measure and closely monitor serum electrolytes, especially potassium.

Dosage and administration
Adults

Antihypertensive. Initially give 12.5 mg orally two or three times daily. Dose may be increased in 1 to 2 weeks to 25 mg three times daily.

Congestive heart failure. Initially give 12.5 mg orally three times daily; increase daily if necessary up to 50 mg three times daily. Increments higher than this should not be started for at least 2 weeks. (If patients have sodium and fluid depletion, reduce initial dose to 6.25 to 12.5 mg two or three times daily.)

For maintenance give 25 to 100 mg orally, two or three times daily.

Children

Antihypertensive or to reduce cardiac load. Give initial dose of 300 μg (0.3 mg)/kg orally three times daily. If necessary to increase, add increments of 300 μg (0.3 mg)/kg after 8 to 24 hours until the minimum effective dose is reached.

Pregnancy safety. FDA Category C.

NURSING CONSIDERATIONS

Assessment. Be aware that captopril is not used as a primary (first-line) drug because of its serious side effects. It is reserved for individuals who have not responded to "triple-drug antihypertensive therapy" (diuretic, beta blocker, and vasodilator) or who have developed serious side effects from this treatment.

Clients with reduced renal function may require lower or less frequent doses.

Intervention. Before initiating therapy, the current antihypertensive regimen should have been discontinued for at least 1 week. All other medications need physician approval.

Administer drug 1 hour before meals to enhance absorption.

Clients with renal disease, particularly those with renal artery stenosis, may have an increase in BUN and serum creatinine levels. Reduce dosage of captopril or discontinue diuretic therapy if necessary.

Neutropenia and agranulocytosis have also been observed. Some neutropenic clients develop systemic or oral cavity infections. Most appear to have complex medical histories such as advanced renal failure, systemic lupus erythematosus, or other autoimmune/collagen disorders. Therefore a few of these individuals may be receiving multiple concomitant drug therapy, including immunosuppressive therapy. An elevation in potassium level may occur because of depressed aldosterone levels. Monitor serum potassium level. Serum sodium levels should also be monitored.

During the first 4 weeks of therapy, skin rash occurs in approximately 10% of clients. Dosage reduction or cessation or administration of an antihistamine usually causes the rash to disappear.

Education. Inform client that the full therapeutic benefits of the drug will not be noticed until several weeks of therapy. Therefore, emphasize the importance of drug compliance. Report side effects so that physician can modify drug regimen without discontinuing medication. Also, advise client to avoid emotional encounters or any forms of stress.

Advise client that signs of infection (e.g., sore throat or fever) should be reported to the physician. Also, easy bruising or bleeding (possible agranulocytosis) should be reported. If taste impairment (dysgeusia) occurs, it generally disappears in 2 or 3 months, but it may cause weight loss. Provide the client with nutritional guidance.

Instruct client not to use potassium supplements or substances containing large amounts of potassium (i.e., salt substitutes or low-sodium milk, which may contain up to 60 mEq potassium/L) without physician approval.

Caution clients with heart failure to increase their physical activity slowly in response to decreased chest pain.

Evaluation. Before beginning therapy, obtain white blood cell and differential counts and continue every 2 weeks for first 3 months of therapy and periodically thereafter. Instruct client to report any sign of infection (e.g., sore throat, fever), which indicates possible neutropenia or edema associated with proteinuria and nephrotic syndrome.

Proteinuria associated with nephrotic syndrome may occur, particularly in clients with previous renal disease. Before beginning therapy, perform urinary protein determinations and continue at monthly intervals for the first 9 months, then monitor periodically thereafter. If proteinuria is greater than 1 g/day, drug should be discontinued unless benefits outweigh risks.

Monitor blood pressure closely because a precipitous fall can occur in 1 to 3 hours, particularly in clients who have been receiving salt-restricted diets, diuretics, or dialysis. Vomiting, diarrhea, and dehydration can intensify hypotension. The client is to discontinue salt-restricted diet. Monitor pulse rate. If bradycardia occurs, report readings to physician.

enalapril (Vasotec)

Mechanism of action. The action of enalapril is due to an active metabolite, enalaprilat. Like captopril, enalapril inhibits angiotensin-converting enzyme activity. It is antihypertensive even in low-renin hypertension and is believed to reduce the breakdown of bradykinin (a potent vasodilator).

Indication. Antihypertensive

Pharmacokinetics. See Table 25-1.

Side effects/adverse reactions. See Table 25-2.

Significant drug interactions. The drug interactions are the same as for captopril.

Dosage and administration

Adults.

Antihypertensive. Initially give 5 mg daily orally. Increase if necessary. In patients who are salt and fluid depleted (because of diuretics or renal failure), reduce the initial dose to 2.5 mg.

For maintenance give 10 to 40 mg orally daily, in a single or twice daily dosage.

Congestive heart failure. Initially give 2.5 mg orally daily. Increase according to patient response. For maintenance give 10 to 40 mg orally in a single or twice daily dosage.

Children. Dosage is not established.

Pregnancy safety. FDA Category C

NURSING CONSIDERATIONS

See discussion of captopril.

ADDITIONAL ANTIHYPERTENSIVE AGENTS
GANGLIONIC BLOCKING DRUGS

The ganglionic blocking drugs, trimethaphan camsylate (Arfonad) and mecamylamine (Inversine), are available in the United States. Their use as antihypertensive agents is limited because of their action in blocking both parasympathetic and sympathetic ganglia, which may result in many serious adverse effects (see Table 25-3). Whenever possible today, the newer, more selective, and safer agents have supplanted these drugs.

Their antihypertensive action depends on the sympathetic ganglia blockade, which results in a decrease in peripheral resistance, cardiac output, and stroke volume. Mecamylamine is an oral preparation, and trimethaphan camsylate is a parenteral drug. Today some physicians use the ganglionic blocking agents as an alternative to sodium nitroprusside in clients who are resistant or nonresponsive to nitroprusside. They may also select the ganglionic blocking agents for use in hypertensive crisis in clients with an acute dissecting aortic aneurysm. (See Chapter 19 for description of these drugs.)

MONOAMINE OXIDASE INHIBITING DRUG
pargyline hydrochloride (Eutonyl)

Mechanism of action. The monoamine oxidase (MAO) inhibitors lower blood pressure by blocking the release of norepinephrine at the sympathetic neuroeffector junctions, thereby interfering with vasoconstriction. MAO is an enzyme active in the metabolic breakdown of catecholamines (norepinephrine, dopamine, and serotonin) within the adrenergic nerve terminals (see figure 18-5). By blocking the enzyme action, MAO inhibitors actually increase the amount of norepinephrine in the adrenergic nerve endings. Because these drugs interfere with the transmission of the sympathetic nerve impulse, they reduce peripheral resistance and decrease blood pressure.

Since safer and more effective drugs are now available for the treatment of hypertension, there is no reason to use MAO inhibitors for this purpose. Nevertheless, this group of drugs does have a place in the management of mental depression.

Indication. Treatment of moderate to severe depression.

Pharmacokinetics. See Table 25-1.

Side effects/adverse reactions. See Table 25-2.

Significant drug interactions. The following interactions may occur when pargyline is given with the drugs listed below:

Drug	Possible Effect and Management
alcohol or CNS depressants local anesthetics containing phenylephrine or cocaine	methotrimeprazine May enhance CNS depressant effects. Also, possible tyramine content in alcohol may result in a hypertensive effect. Advise patient to avoid alcohol or CNS depressants unless prescribed or approved by their physician.
spinal anesthetics	Avoid concurrent use since severe hypertensive episode may occur.
oral antidiabetic agents or insulin	Hypotension may be enhanced. For elective surgery with spinal anesthesia, discontinue pargyline at least 10 days before surgery.

Drug	Possible Effect and Management
antihistamines or antimuscarinics (especially atropine)	Enhanced hypoglycemia effects may result. Dosage adjustment of the antidiabetic drug may be required.
	Enhanced antimuscarinic side effect may occur and should be closely watched for. Paralytic ileus may occur with this combination. Also, the CNS depressant action of the antihistamines may be enhanced and prolonged. Monitor closely.

Dosage and administration

Adults

Initial. Give 25 mg orally daily. This may be increased in 10-mg increments every 7 days until appropriate response is noted.

Maintenance. Give 25 to 50 mg daily. Maximum limit is 200 mg/day.

Children. Dosage is not established for children under 12 years old.

Pregnancy safety. Not established

NURSING CONSIDERATIONS

Assessment. Use with caution in clients with renal impairment, hepatic disease, and also in elderly persons, who may be more sensitive to the hypotensive effects.

Use of pargyline is contraindicated in clients with advanced renal failure, pheochromocytoma, parkinsonism, or hyperexcitability.

Intervention. Drug should be discontinued 2 weeks before elective surgery to prevent augmentation of hypotensive effects of anesthetic agent. If drug is discontinued for a period of time, reinstitute medication at a lower dosage level.

In emergency surgery the preoperative medications or narcotics should be reduced by one fourth or one fifth the usual amount.

It is recommended that the drug be taken in the morning to reduce interference with nighttime sleep. The hypotensive effect is especially pronounced when the client is standing.

Education. Instruct client to report symptoms of orthostatic hypotension (dizziness, palpitation, fainting, weakness) that may require dosage adjustment. Tell client to lie down immediately. To prevent orthostatic hypotension, advise client to rise slowly from supine position and to dangle feet at the bedside before standing. Also, hot showers or baths should be avoided, as well as standing in one position.

Instruct client to keep clinical appointments and laboratory checkups at prescribed intervals. Liver function determinations and renal function tests should be performed periodically. Monitor intake, output, and BUN in clients with impaired renal function. Physician will check for pargyline tolerance, which can develop rapidly.

Advise client to take drug in morning to avoid interference with nighttime sleep. Inform client not to take any other drug without consulting the physician while taking pargyline. This includes alcohol, which is not recommended.

Emphasize the importance of abstaining from tyramine-rich foods. Obtain a printed list of foods to be omitted from the diet. Foods high in tyramine are involved with aging, protein breakdown, and putrefaction. These include aged cheese: cheddar, Gruyère, Brie, Camembert, blue, Gouda, mozzarella, Parmesan, provolone, Romano, and Roquefort; wines: Chianti, sherry, sauterne, and Riesling; beer; ale; meat: aged game, canned liver meats with yeast extracts, and chicken liver; fish (salted, dried): herring, cod, capelin, and pickled herring; other foods: sour cream, yogurt, soy sauce, vanilla, chocolate, cola drinks, canned figs, raisins, salad dressings, homemade bread containing yeast, and fava beans. Excessive intake of these foods can lead to hypertensive crises (marked increase in blood pressure, occipital headache, stiffness and soreness of neck, dilated pupils, photophobia, constricting chest pain, nausea, vomiting, sweating, palpitations, tachycardia or bradycardia).

Inform client that mouth dryness may be relieved with ice chips, sour hard candy, sugarless chewing gum, or a saliva substitute (VA-Ora Lube, Moistir, Xero-Lube).

Teach client to keep a daily record of weight and to check ankles for peripheral edema. Report weight gain of 3 pounds or more.

Advise client with angina not to increase physical activity since pargyline may suppress anginal pain and create euphoria.

Advise client that drowsiness is possible and caution against operating machinery or driving until response to drug is ascertained.

Evaluation. Monitor pulse rate and blood pressure frequently while client is in a standing position to help establish drug dosage.

Monitor client with diabetes by checking urine sugar levels; dosage adjustment of antidiabetic medication usually is required.

TYROSINE HYDROXYLASE INHIBITOR DRUG
metyrosine (Demser)

Mechanism of action. Metyrosine blocks the activity of tyrosine hydroxylase, the enzyme necessary to convert tyrosine to dopa. This is the first biosynthetic step in the formation of catecholamines. (See Chapter 20 for biosynthesis of epinephrine and norephinephrine.) As a result the synthesis of endogenous levels of catecholamines is reduced, lowering blood pressure. The successful inhibition of tyrosine hydroxylase by metyrosine usually is measured as a decrease in urinary excretion of catecholamines and their metabolites.

Indications

1. Used in treatment of patients with pheochromocytoma to reduce blood pressure. In this condition there is an excessive amount of circulating catecholamines, resulting from hypersecretion of tumors, usually located in the medulla of one or both adrenal glands or even outside the glands. If possible, the treatment of choice is surgical removal of the tumors.
2. Used for preoperative preparation of clients for pheochromocytoma surgery.
3. Used to manage clients when surgery is contraindicated or to treat individuals with chronic malignant pheochromocytoma. This drug is not recommended for the control of essential hypertension.

Pharmacokinetics. See Table 25-1.

Side effects/adverse reactions. See Table 25-2.

Significant drug interactions. No major interactions have been noted.

Dosage and administration

Adults

Initial. Give 250 mg four times daily orally. Dose may be increased as necessary by 250 to 500 mg/day increments.

Maintenance. Give 2 to 3 g orally daily in four divided daily doses, up to a maximum of 4 g/day.

Children. Dosage is not established.

Pregnancy safety. Not established

NURSING CONSIDERATIONS

Assessment. Use drug with caution in individuals with renal or hepatic impairment.

Do not use drug in clients known to be hypersensitive to metyrosine. Also, the safety of the drug in pregnant women and nursing mothers has not been established.

Intervention. After surgery, maintain adequate intravascular fluid volume to avoid problems associated with vasodilation and hypotension.

Notify physician if drooling, speech difficulty, stiffness of jaw, tremors, disorientation, diarrhea, or painful urination occurs. If metyrosine is stopped, insomnia may appear as a troublesome symptom.

Education. Instruct client to increase daily fluid intake to achieve a urine volume of 2000 ml or more a day, to minimize the risk of developing crystalluria. Because

metyrosine will crystallize as needles or rods, routine examination of the urine should be performed. If crystalluria occurs or persists, the drug should be discontinued or dosage decreased.

Advise clients that sedation usually occurs but subsides after several days of drug therapy. Warn individual against engaging in activities requiring mental alertness and operating machinery.

Caution client against taking alcohol or other CNS depressants.

Evaluation. Take blood pressure frequently and during surgery monitor ECG continuously to detect dysrhythmias or hypertensive crises. Have available lidocaine and alpha adrenergic blocking agent phentolamine.

Monitor urinary catecholamine measurements since physician will prescribe test before therapy and at periodic intervals for clients on long-term therapy. Initial dosage will be adjusted on the basis of these results.

KEY TERMS

angiotensin II inhibitors, page 493
baroreceptor reflex, page 485
diuretics, page 493
essential hypertension, page 484
high blood pressure, page 483
hypertension, page 483
idiopathic hypertension, page 484
loop diuretics, page 493
potassium-sparing agents, page 493
primary hypertension, page 484
renin-angiotensin-aldosterone mechanism, page 485
secondary hypertension, page 484
stepped-care regimen, page 490
sympathetic depressant agents, page 493
thiazides, page 493
vasoconstrictors, page 485
vasodilators, page 493

BIBLIOGRAPHY

AHFS Drug Information 86, American Hospital Formulary Service, Bethesda, Md, 1986, American Society of Hospital Pharmacists, Inc.

Andreoli, KG: Self-concept and health beliefs in compliant and noncompliant hypertensive patients, Nurs Res 30:323, Nov/Dec 1981.

Border, WA: Recent advances in beta-blocker therapy for hypertension, Hosp Form 19:1120, 1984.

Borreson, RE: The case for reserpine in hypertension, Hosp Form 20:719, June 1985.

Carter, BL: Labetalol (Trandate, Glaxo, Inc.; Normodyne, Schering Corp.), Drug Intell Clin Pharm 17:704, 1983.

Chesley, LC: Hypertensive disorders in pregnancy, Drug Ther (Hosp), p 10, April 1977.

Chobanian, AV: Hypertension, Clin Symp 34(5):3, 1982.

Drayer, JIM, and Weber, MA: Should antihypertensive therapy be modified prior to surgery? Drug Ther (Hosp), p 63, May 1981.

Ferguson, RK, and Vlasses, PH: The ACE inhibitors: clinical pharmacology of captopril and enalapril, Hosp Form 21:46, Jan 1986.

Goodman and Gilman's the pharmacological basis of therapeutics, ed 7, New York, 1985, Macmillan Publishing Co.

Haines, CM, and Ward, GW: Recent trends in public knowledge, attitudes, and reported behavior with respect to high blood pressure, Pub Health Rep 96:514, 1981.

Hill, MN, and Cunningham, SG: New recommendations for high blood pressure control: guidelines for all NPs, Nurse Practitioner 10:35, July 1985.

Hinds, C: A hypertension survey: respondents' knowledge of high blood pressure, Int Nurs Rev 30(1):12, 1983.

Hou, S, and Madias, N: Antihypertensive medications: minoxidil and captopril, Hosp Form 18:1059, 1983.

Hubbell, FA, and Weber, MA: Adverse effects of sudden withdrawal of antihypertensive medication, Postgrad Med 68(2):129, 1980.

Joint National Committee on the Detection, Evaluation, and Treatment of High Blood Pressure: The 1988 report of the Joint National Committee on Detection, Evaluation, and Treatment of High Blood Pressure, Arch Intern Med 148(5):1023, 1988.

Kaplan, NM: Disarming a killer: how to lower pregnancy-induced hypertension, Current Prescribing, p 41, March 1977.

Kelly, KL: Beta blockers in hypertension, Drug Therapy Reviews, Am J Hosp Pharm 33:1284, Dec 1976.

Kirshenbaum, HL, and Rosenberg, JM: Guanethidine and reserpine, RN 47:31, Dec 1984.

Lam, YWF, and others: Calcium channel blockers and treatment of hypertension, Drug Intell Clin Pharm 20:187, March 1986.

Linas, SL, and Nies, AS: Minoxidil, Ann Intern Med 94:61, 1981.

Malatestinic, WN, ed: Enalapril maleate—an angiotensin-converting enzyme inhibitor, Saint Margaret Hospital Drug Information Bulletin 12(2 and 3):5, 1986.

McKenney, JM: Alternative pharmacologic approaches to the initial management of hypertension, Drug Intell Clin Pharm 19:629, Sept 1985.

McMahon, M, and Palmer, RM: Exercise and hypertension, Med Clin North Am 69(1):57, 1985.

Melmon, KL: Getting the most out of antihypertensives, Emerg Med, p 51, Jan 30, 1986.

Mroczek, WJ: Selected recent and future antihypertensive agents, Hosp Form, p 840, Nov 1980.

Murphy, DH: Treatment of mild hypertension: new results on MRFIT sodium, Am Pharm, NS25(3):39, 1985.

Onesti, G, and Brest, A, eds: Hypertension: mechanisms, diagnosis and treatment, Philadelphia, 1978, F.A. Davis Co.

Pepper, GA: Labetalol: an alpha- and beta-adrenergic receptor blocker, Nurse Practitioner 10(7):39, 1985.

Perez-Stable, E, and others: Mild hypertension: treat all patients? Patient Care 17(14):171, 1983.

Reichgott, MJ, and others: The nurse practitioner's role in complex patient management: hypertension, J Natl Med Assoc 75:1197, 1983.

Sasso, MS: Nitroprusside for hypertensive emergencies, MCN 8:265, 1983.

Schwinghammer, T: Drug withdrawal syndromes, U.S. Pharmacist, p 35, March 1982.

Sloan, RS: Achieving compliance to a reduced sodium diet, Nurse Practitioner 10(2):24, 1985.

Smith, S: Drugs and hypertension, Nursing Times 80:37, Feb 20, 1985.

Sparacino, J: Blood pressure, stress and mental health, Nurs Res 31:89, March/April 1982.

Sparacino, J, and others: Psychological correlates of blood pressure: a closer examination of hostility, anxiety and engagement, Nurs Res 31:143, May/June 1982.

Sternberg, EB, and others: Drugs that induce hypertension: a discussion of mechanism, Dateline Hypertension (National Hypertension Information Network) 2(4):1, 1984.

Stevenson, JG, and Umstead, GS: Sexual dysfunction due to antihypertensive agents, Drug Intell Clin Pharm 18:113, Feb 1984.

Swartz, SL: Stabilizing malignant hypertension, Patient Care 17:159, May 30, 1983.

Taylor, DL: Renal hypertension, Nursing '83 13:44, Oct 1983.

United States Pharmacopeial Convention: Drug information for the health care provider, ed 6, Rockville, Md, 1986, United States Pharmacopeial Convention, Inc.

Wallin, JD, and O'Neill, Jr, WM: Labetalol, current research and therapeutic status, Arch Intern Med 143:485, March 1983.

Weintraub, M, and Evans, P: Labetalol: an alpha-beta blocker for treatment of hypertension, Hosp Form 19:295, 1984.

Wroblewski, JJ: New and old agents offer range of options, Drug Topics p 56, Feb 6, 1984.

CHAPTER
26

Calcium Channel Blockers

One of the newer subclassifications of cardiac drugs is the **calcium channel blockers,** discovered in 1969 by Flackenstein of West Germany.

Although these compounds have diverse chemical structures, they all share a basic electrophysiologic property—they block the inward movement of calcium through the slow channels of the cell membranes of cardiac and smooth muscle cells. (See Chapter 22 for a discussion of the physiology of fast and slow channels of cardiovascular fibers.) This activity, however, varies according to the specific type of cardiovascular cells involved. The three types of tissues or cells are:

1. Cardiac muscle or **myocardium** (heart)
2. Cardiac conduction system—SA node and AV nodes
3. Vascular smooth muscle
   a. Coronary arteries and arterioles
   b. Peripheral arterioles

Cardiac muscle or myocardium. Calcium channel blockers *decrease the force of myocardial contraction* by blocking the inward flow of calcium ions through the slow channels of the cell membrane during phase 2 (or plateau phase) of the action potential. The diminished entry of calcium ions into the cells thereby fails to trigger the release of large amounts of calcium from the sarcoplasmic reticulum within the cell. This free calcium is needed for excitation-contraction coupling, an event that activates contraction by allowing cross-bridges to form between the actin and myosin filaments. The force of the heart's contraction is determined by the number of actin and myosin crossbridges formed within the sarcomere. Decreasing the amount of calcium ion released from the sarcoplasmic reticulum causes fewer actin and myosin crossbridges to be formed, and the force of contraction then decreases, producing a negative inotropic effect.

Cardiac conduction system (SA and AV nodes). In these tissues calcium channel blockers *decrease automaticity in the SA node* and *decrease conduction in the AV node.* Automaticity means that a cell depolarizes spontaneously and initiates an action potential without an external stimulus. Automaticity is a normal characteristic of the SA nodal cells. Depolarization (or phase 0) of the action potential is normally generated by the inward calcium ion current through the slow channels. Thus the agents that can block the inward calcium ion current across the cell membrane of SA nodal tissue decrease the rate of depolarization and depress automaticity. The result is a decrease in heart rate (negative chronotropic effect). Similarly, an agent that decreases calcium ion influx across the cell membrane of the AV node slows AV nodal conduction (negative dromotropic effect) and prolongs AV refractoriness. When AV conduction is prolonged, fewer atrial impulses reach the ventricles. Diltiazem depresses SA nodal automaticity while verapamil slows AV conduction, so verapamil is used to treat supraventricular tachycardia.

Vascular smooth muscle. The smooth muscle of the coronary and peripheral vessels has a significant influence on the hemodynamics of circulation. Calcium channel blockers effectively inhibit calcium ion influx through the slow channels of the membrane of smooth muscle cells. They thereby depress interaction between actin and myosin, resulting in a *decrease in force of smooth muscle contraction.* As a consequence, coronary artery dilation occurs, which lowers coronary resistance and improves blood flow through collateral vessels, as well as oxygen delivery to ischemic areas of the heart. Hence drugs with these actions are useful in the treatment of angina pectoris. Calcium channel blockers also *inhibit the contraction of smooth muscle of the peripheral arterioles.* This results in widespread reduction in **peripheral vascular resistance** (resistance to blood flow through the body) and blood pressure. The hemodynamic change reduces afterload, which also decreases oxygen demands of the heart. This indirectly provides a beneficial effect in the management of angina.

• • •

The calcium blockers that have met with FDA approval include diltiazem, nifedipine, and verapamil. All three of these agents are effective in dilating coronary vessels. However, each drug has additional actions that make it different from the others. Verapamil has been shown to be effective as a dysrhythmic and an antianginal agent. It prolongs AV conduction time and depresses myocardial

contraction. It can also lower blood pressure by dilating the systemic blood vessels and decreasing the oxygen demands of the heart. Because of its pronounced effect on the peripheral vascular bed, nifedipine causes the greatest fall in blood pressure. However, it exerts minimal cardiac depressant action. The action of diltiazem is largely restricted to dilating the coronary blood vessels.

Presently, the calcium channel blockers are being investigated as antihypertensive agents. A calcium channel blocker called nimodipine is also being studied for the possibility of preventing a stroke resulting from cerebral spasm that follows a stroke initially caused by a ruptured aneurysm. (For the role of calcium see the discussion in Chapter 22 of myocardial contraction: excitation-contraction coupling.)

diltiazem hydrochloride (Cardizem)

Mechanism of action. The therapeutic benefits of diltiazem are believed to be related to its ability to prevent the influx of calcium ions through the slow channels of the membrane of myocardial muscle and vascular smooth muscle during membrane depolarization. The slowed calcium ion influx reduces vascular tone and mildly decreases the force of myocardial contraction. Dilation of coronary arteries and arterioles is achieved, thereby improving oxygen supply to myocardial tissue and ultimately inhibiting **coronary artery spasm.** Further, dilation of peripheral arterioles reduces **cardiac afterload** (peripheral resistance), a hemodynamic function that also lessens oxygen requirements of the myocardial tissue. This property probably alleviates chronic stable angina. Diltiazem also decreases SA nodal function and AV nodal conduction because of inhibited influx of calcium ions to the SA and AV nodes. The inhibitory effects decrease heart rate and reduce myocardial contraction.

Indications
1. Treatment of coronary artery spasm (Prinzmetal's or variant angina).
2. Treatment of chronic stable angina (increases exercise tolerance).
3. Treatment of hypertension (experimental).

TABLE 26-1   Comparison of Effects of Calcium Channel Blocking Agents

	Diltiazem	Nifedipine	Verapamil
Heart rate	0/--*	+	−/+
AV node conduction	--	0/−	---
Myocardial contractility	0/−	0/−	--
Myocardial oxygen demand	--	--	--
Cardiac output	0/+	+	−/+
Coronary vasodilator	+	+	+
Peripheral vasodilator	+	++	+

*−, decrease; +, increase; −/+, variable effect; 0, no effect.

Pharmacokinetics. See Table 26-2.

Side effects/adverse reactions. See Table 26-3.

Significant drug interactions. The following interactions may occur when diltiazem is given with the drugs listed below.

Drug	Possible Effect and Management
beta adrenergic blocking agents, including ophthalmic preparations	Monitor closely for bradycardia, hypotension, and heart failure, which may be symptoms of prolonged AV conduction. In clients with impaired cardiac function, avoid concurrent use if possible; if a calcium antagonist is necessary, nifedipine would be the agent of choice.
carbamazepine, quinidine, prazosin, or theophylline	Metabolism of these drugs may be impaired by calcium channel blockers, leading to increased serum levels and possibly toxicity. Monitor serum levels closely.
digitalis glycosides	Increased serum levels of digitalis glycosides have been reported, so monitor digoxin serum levels closely whenever a calcium blocking agent is started or discontinued or when dosage is changed. Also, watch for prolonged AV conduction, increased bradycardia, or AV blocks, especially during the initial week of therapy. A dosage decrease for digoxin may be necessary.
disopyramide	Use extreme caution when administering disopyramide with diltiazem or verapamil. It is recommended that disopyramide not be given 2 days before or 1 day after the administration of verapamil or diltiazem because of additive negative inotropic effects, which in some instances have caused fatalities.

Dosage and administration

Adults. Give 30 mg orally three or four times daily for angina. Increase dosage at 1- to 2-day intervals until optimum response is obtained. Maximum daily dosage is 360 mg.

Elderly clients may be more sensitive to this drug, so monitor closely.

Children. Dosage is not established.

Pregnancy safety. FDA Category C

TABLE 26-2 Pharmacokinetics of Calcium Channel Blocking Agents

Drug	Onset of action (min)	Time to peak concentration (hr)	Therapeutic serum level (μg/ml)	Half-life (hr)	Duration of action (hr)	Metabolism	Excretion
diltiazem (Cardizem)	30	2-3	0.04-0.3	Biphasic: Short phase: ½ Long phase: 3-5	4-8	Liver—has active metabolite desacetyldiltiazem	Kidneys and bile
nifedipine (Procardia)	Orally 20 (more rapid when given sublingually)	½-1	0.025-0.1	Biphaspic: Short phase: 2½-3 Long phase: 5	4-8	Liver	Kidneys (80%) feces (20%)
verapamil (Calan, Isoptin)	Oral: 60-120 IV: 1-5	1-2	0.08-0.3	Oral, single dose: 2.8-7.4 Regular dose scheduling: 4½-12 IV: biphasic Short phase: 4 min Long phase: 2-5	IV: 2 Oral regular: 8-10 Oral extended release: 24	Liver—has active metabolite norverapamil	Kidneys and feces

TABLE 26-3   Side Effects/Adverse Reactions of Calcium Channel Blocking Agents

Drug	Side effects*	Adverse reactions†
diltiazem (Cardizem)	Less frequent: dizziness, headaches, nausea, skin flushing or rash	Less frequent: edema of extremities, allergic skin reaction, shortness of breath or wheezing, severe hypotension, bradycardia
nifedipine (Procardia)	More frequent: dizziness, headaches, nausea, feelings of warmth or flushing Less frequent: constipation, abdominal cramping, anxiety or mood changes	Most frequent: edema of extremities Less frequent: shortness of breath; tachycardia; tender, bleeding, or swollen gums; chest pain; hypotension; allergic skin rash
verapamil (Calan, Isoptin)	Less frequent: constipation, dizziness, feelings of warmth or flushing, headache, nausea, increased weakness	Less frequent: shortness of breath, tachycardia, edema of extremities, bradycardia

*If side effects continue, increase, or disturb the patient, inform the physician.
†If adverse reactions occur, contact physician, because medical intervention may be necessary.

NURSING CONSIDERATIONS

Assessment. Do not use drug for individuals with sick sinus syndrome in the presence of a functioning ventricular pacemaker; hypotension (less than 90 mm Hg systolic); and second- or third-degree heart block unless cardiac pacemaker is in place.

Ask the client if she is pregnant or plans to be. Test in laboratory animals have resulted in teratogenic effects.

Intervention. Administer oral dosage on an empty stomach to promote rapid absorption. Take pulse before each dose; withhold dose and report to the physician if rate is 50 or below.

Instruct client to perform meticulous daily dental hygiene with regular dental examinations and cleaning, since this may reduce the incidence or severity of gingivitis and gingival hyperplasia.

Education. Since drug may be coadministered with sublingual nitroglycerin and other nitrates, instruct client to keep a record of nitroglycerin and report promptly if changes occur in previous pattern (increased frequency, duration, and severity of anginal attacks). The symptoms may develop when starting diltiazem or increasing its dose. (Nitroglycerin is used to abort acute angina attacks.)

Instruct the client to change from a sitting or lying position to a standing position cautiously to avoid orthostatic hypotension. Advise client to avoid alcohol to prevent dizziness and hypotension.

Emphasize the importance of regular visits to physician to check progress during therapy.

Teach client to take a pulse appropriately and report a heart rate less than 50. Instruct client to report headaches, rashes, nausea, and vomiting, as well as edema and weight gain (may indicate congestive heart failure).

If a dose is missed, advise the client to take it as soon as remembered, unless it is almost time for the next dose, in which case, it should be omitted.

Instruct client in a program of vigorous plaque control and regular dental care to minimize gingival hyperplasia (a rare side effect).

If diltiazem is taken as an antihypertensive, instruct the client to take the medication even if feeling well, since lifelong therapy may be required. Compliance may be ascertained by monitoring refill frequency. Advise on the hazards of untreated hypertension and the need for decreased sodium intake and weight control. Caution the client to check with the physician before taking other medications, particularly OTC sympathomimetics, such as Neo-Synephrine nose drops.

Evaluation. Monitor blood pressure and pulse rate, particularly if the drug is coadministered with a beta adrenergic blocking agent. Observe ECG for prolonged P-R interval, which is caused by slowing of AV conduction.

nifedipine (Procardia)

Mechanism of action. The action of nifedipine is generally the same as that of diltiazem. One major difference is that nifedipine has a more powerful vasodilating effect on the coronary arteries and arterioles as well as on the peripheral arterioles. Thus, when arterial pressure is reduced, a reflex response is stimulated, causing a small increase in heart rate and a mild elevation in the force of myocardial contraction. Despite this response, the reduced total peripheral resistance (cardiac afterload) lessens the myocardial oxygen demand. This probably accounts for the drug's effectiveness in treating chronic stable angina and hypertension. In addition, unlike the other members of its class, nifedipine has no tendency to slow the SA nodal activity or prolong AV nodal conduction.

Indications
1. Management of classic angina (chronic stable angina or effort angina).
2. Treatment of vasospastic angina (Prinzmetal's, variant or at-rest angina).

3. Control of hypertension (investigational).
Pharmacokinetics. See Table 26-2.
Side effects/adverse reactions. See Table 26-3.
Significant drug interactions. See discussion of diltiazem. Also, closely monitor clients receiving phenytoin or cimetidine together with nifedipine; elevated levels of both phenytoin and nifedipine have been reported.

Dosage and administration

Adults. Initially give 10 mg orally, three times per day for angina. Dosage is gradually increased over 7 to 14 days as needed and tolerated.

Elderly clients may be more sensitive to this drug, so monitor closely.

Maximum daily dosage is 180 mg daily, although daily dosages greater than 120 mg are rarely necessary.

Children. Dosage is not established.

Special instructions. In clients unable to swallow, the contents of a nifedipine capsule may be administered buccally or sublingually. This method of administration also produces a more rapid effect than the oral administration. Dosage is equivalent to the oral dosage.

Pregnancy safety. FDA Category C.

NURSING CONSIDERATIONS

Assessment. Determine that the client does not have severe hypotension, Wolff-Parkinson-White syndrome (anomalous atrioventricular excitation), or sick sinus syndrome unless the client has an artificial ventricular pacemaker, since nefedipine is contraindicated in these cases.

Intervention. Record the baseline radial pulse, blood pressure, and ECG before starting nifedipine therapy or adjusting the dosage.

Alert client that there may be an increase in the frequency, duration, and severity of anginal attacks when nifedipine is introduced or dosage increased. Withdrawal of beta blocker therapy increases the risk of anginal attack when nifedipine therapy is started.

Congestive heart failure may occasionally occur after initiation of nifedipine therapy, particularly in those also receiving beta blocking agents. If beta blockers are withdrawn before nifedipine therapy, taper dosage gradually. Abrupt withdrawal may provoke angina, especially when nifedipine is started.

Education. Instruct client to take medication as prescribed. This means that dosage should not be omitted, increased, or decreased or dosage interval changed without consulting physician. Be aware that discontinuation of nifedipine should be gradual, with close medical supervision, to prevent severe hypotensive effects or other side effects.

Since drug may be coadministered with sublingual nitroglycerin and other nitrates, instruct client to keep a record of nitroglycerin use and to report promptly if changes occur in previous anginal pattern.

Inform client that the drug may cause an increase in heart rate. Flushing, headache, nausea, and dizziness, particularly in elderly persons, are frequent side effects, and these symptoms should be reported to the physician if they interfere with activities of daily living.

Evaluation. Drug may cause excessive hypotension in an occasional client when therapy is introduced or dosage is subsequently increased. Monitor blood pressure carefully in both lying and upright positions (to rule out orthostatic hypotension) during titration period, particularly if individual is also taking other drugs known to lower blood pressure.

Peripheral edema, primarily in lower extremities, may develop because of peripheral vasodilation. Diuretics may be indicated.

verapamil hydrochloride (Calan, Isoptin)

Mechanism of action. See discussion of types of cardiac tissue.

Indications

1. Treatment of chronic stable angina and to relieve angina at rest.
2. Parenteral verapamil indicated for treatment of supraventricular tachyarrhythmias; may also be used for temporary control of rapid ventricular rate in atrial flutter or atrial fibrillation.
3. Control of hypertension.

Pharmacokinetics. See Table 26-2.
Side effects/adverse reactions. See Table 26-3.
Significant drug interactions. See discussion of diltiazem.

Dosage and administration. Angina pectoris, supraventricular tachyarrhythmias, hypertension:

IV

Adults

Initial dose: 5 to 10 mg (0.075 to 0.15 mg/kg body weight) given as an IV bolus over 2 minute period.

Repeat dose: 10 mg (0.15 mg/kg body weight) 30 minutes following first dose, if the initial response is not adequate. In older patients, administer slowly (at least 3 minutes).

Children

Up to 1 year: 0.1 to 0.2 mg/kg body weight over 2 minutes.

1 to 15 years: 0.1 to 0.3 mg/kg over period of 2 minutes. Repeat dose if necessary 30 minutes afterward. Maximum total dose is 5 mg.

Oral

Adults. Give initial dose of 80 mg orally three or four times per day. Increase dosage daily or weekly as needed and tolerated. The total daily required dosage usually ranges from 240 to 480 mg.

Elderly clients may be more sensitive to this drug, so monitor closely.

Children. Dosage is not established.

Pregnancy safety. FDA Category C

NURSING CONSIDERATIONS

Assessment. Use drug with caution in clients with SA node dysfunction since verapamil depresses automaticity of the SA node.

Use with caution when digitalis preparation is administered concurrently. Verapamil can produce digitalis toxicity because it decreases urinary excretion of the cardiac glycoside.

Do not use in individuals with severe hypotension, cardiogenic shock, or second- or third-degree AV block; do not use in sick sinus syndrome, severe congestive heart failure, and IV administration of beta blocking agents unless a cardiac pacemaker is in place.

Intervention. Inspect the parenteral drug preparation; discard if cloudy. Administer initial intravenous dosage in a treatment center with appropriate facilities for monitoring and resuscitation. Give slowly as a direct injection over at least 2 minutes (in the elderly, not less than 3 minutes). Monitor with ECG.

Avoid repeated doses in clients with hepatic or renal failure since intravenous dose may prolong duration of effects. If repeated injections are required, closely monitor blood pressure and P-R interval, and use smaller doses.

Education. Instruct client to remain in recumbent position following IV bolus for at least 1 hour to diminish hypotensive effects.

Instruct client receiving verapamil at home to take radial pulse before each dose and report an irregular pulse or one lower than 50. Warn client about signs of dizziness or light-headedness during early treatment period. Warn client to avoid driving or operating dangerous equipment. Instruct client to report edema and weight gain, since they may indicate congestive heart failure. If drug must be discontinued, withdraw gradually by decreasing dosage 25% each day.

Emphasize the importance of recording the need for nitroglycerin. Both frequency and type of activity should be noted so the physician can determine dosage regimen for verapamil. If anginal pain is not reduced by this drug, notify the physician.

Stress the importance of keeping appointments for periodic evaluation of cardiac status and verapamil effectiveness.

Instruct the client to change from a sitting or lying position to a standing position cautiously because of the hypotensive effects of the drug. Advise client to avoid alcohol to prevent dizziness and hypotension.

INVESTIGATIONAL DRUGS

nitrendipine (Baypress)—Type II calcium channel blocking agent; a potent vasodilator without electrophysiologic effects

nicardipine—similar to nifedipine in action

Instruct the client to increase dietary fiber, fluid intake, and moderate exercise unless contraindicated, since constipation is a side effect of this drug.

Evaluation. Monitor intake and output during intravenous and early oral-maintenance therapy. Impairment of renal function prolongs duration of action, thereby increasing potential for toxicity.

Monitor the P-R interval since the drug prolongs AV conduction. Note that the P-R interval is proportional to serum concentration of drug. Reduce dosage or discontinue drug to prevent second- or third-degree AV block or bundle branch block.

Monitor client for depressed myocardial contractility or AV conduction when beta adrenergic blockers are administered concomitantly with verapamil.

Perform liver function studies periodically during long-term verapamil therapy.

KEY TERMS

BIBLIOGRAPHY

American Hospital Formulary Service: AHFS Drug Information '87, Bethesda, Md, 1987, American Society of Hospital Pharmacists, Inc.

Baky, SH, and others: Verapamil hydrochloride: pharmacologic properties and therapeutic utility, Hosp Formul 19(8):671, 1984.

Barner, HB: Calcium-entry bockers in cardioplegia, Appl Cardiol 14(1):31, 1986.

Bussey, HI, and Talbert, RL: Evaluations of new indications, promising uses of calcium-channel blocking agents, Pharmacotherapy 4(3):137, 1984.

Clark, RE, and others: Use of nifedipine during cardiac surgery for improved myocardial protection, Am J Med 78(suppl 2B):6, 1985.

Field, G, and others: Diltiazem: pharmacologic properties and therapeutic uses, Hosp Formul 20(7):814, 1985.

Fischer, RG, and others: Calcium channel blockers, Pediatr Nurs 12(5):379, 1986.

Iliopoulou, A, and others: Acute haemodynamic effects of a new calcium antagonist, nicardipine, in man: a comparison with nifedipine, Br J Clin Pharmacol 15:59, 1983.

Kastrup, EK, and Olin, BR: Facts and comparisons, drug information, Philadelphia, 1987, JB Lippincott Co.

Kupersmith, J, and others: Calcium channel blockers: pharmacologic basis for therapeutic properties, Hosp Formul 20(2):184, 1985.

Labson, LH: Understanding calcium entry blockers, Patient Care 18(5):52, 1984.

Labson, LH: Using calcium entry blockers, Patient Care 18(15):87, 1984.

Lake, CL: Calcium blockers and vasodilators, Curr Rev Recov Room Nurses 8(7):50, 1986.

Lam, YWF, and others: Calcium channel blockers and treatment of hypertension, Drug Intell Clin Pharmacol 20(3):187, 1986.

McCarron, DA: Calcium in the pathogenesis and therapy of human hypertension, Am J Med 78(suppl 2B):27, 1985.

Meltzer, AH, and others: Antianginal agents: calcium-entry blockers, Hosp Formul 21(3):299, 1986.

Piepho, RW: The calcium antagonists, mechanisms of action and pharmacologic effects, Drug Therapy 8(1):69, 1983.

Pierce, CH: Heart drugs: how calcium antagonists interact with cardiac glycosides, Consultant 26(9):82, 1986.

Rimar, JM: Verapamil for fetal supraventricular tachycardia, MCN 10(5):345, 1985.

Rossen, JD: Calcium antagonists: an overview, Appl Cardiol 13(3):13, 1985.

Schab, MC, and others: Nifedipine: pharmacologic properties and clinical use, Hosp Formul 20(1):85, 1985.

Shapiro, W: Calcium channel blockers: actions on the heart and uses in ischemic heart disease, Consultant 24(12):150, 1984.

Shinn, AF, ed: Evaluations of drug interations, St Louis, 1985, The CV Mosby Co.

Simpson, R: Verapamil and nifedipine in the treatment of coronary artery spasm and angina pectoris, Hosp Formul 19(6):461, 1984.

Stone, KS, and others: Understanding the calcium channel blockers, Heart-Lung 13(5):563, 1984.

Stowe, HO: Reviews of calcium-blockers, Nurse Pract 11(4):57, 1986.

Taplin, NE: Medical management of coronary heart disease: cardiovascular drug therapy, Occup Health Nurs 32(11):570, 1984.

Touloukin, JE: Calcium channel blocking agents: physiologic basis of nursing interventions, Heart-Lung 14(4):342, 1985.

United States Pharmacopeial Convention: Drug information for the health care provider, ed 7, Rockville, Md, 1987, US Pharmacopeial Convention, Inc.

Weiner, DA: Calcium channel blockers, Med Clin North Am 72(1):83, 1988.

Willerson, JT: New directions in the use of calcium channel blockers, Am J Med 78(suppl 2B):1, 1985.

Young, GP: Calcium channel blockers in emergency medicine, Ann Emerg Med 13(9):712, 1984.

Zatuchni, J: Bradycardia and hypotension after proprandol HCl and verapamil. Heart-Lung 14(1):94, 1988.

CHAPTER

27

Vasodilators

OBJECTIVES

After studying this chapter, the student will be able to:

1. Discuss the etiology of angina pectoris and differentiate between the three types of angina pectoris.

2. Identify the three therapeutic objectives for the use of antianginal agents.

3. Compare the effects of nitrates, beta blockers, and calcium blocking agents on the heart.

4. Discuss the mechanism of action, side effects/adverse reactions, significant drug interactions, and dosages for nitrates.

5. Explain the transdermal system for the administration of nitroglycerin.

6. Discuss cyclandelate, isoxsuprine, nylidrin, and papaverine as agents used in the treatment of peripheral vascular disease.

7. Implement nursing considerations in the administration of vasodilators.

The drugs reviewed in this chapter produce peripheral vasodilation by relaxing smooth muscle in the blood vessel walls. For example, nitrates are effective for treatment of angina pectoris because of their effect on the veins **(capacitance blood vessels)** and arteries **(resistance blood vessels)**. The pooling of blood in the veins decreases the amount of blood returned to the heart (preload), which reduces left ventricular end-diastolic volume. This decrease in blood return may help reduce the myocardial oxygen demand. Chest pain induced by angina pectoris largely results from an inadequate supply of oxygen to the heart (see box).

The miscellaneous vasodilators used for **peripheral occlusive arterial disease** have generally been very discouraging. Many of the drugs discussed in this section have been awarded the possibly effective rating by the U.S. Food and Drug Administration. Substantial evidence of effectiveness would need to be submitted in order to upgrade this rating to effective.

ANTIANGINAL DRUGS

Antianginal drugs are used to treat the pathologic condition known as angina pectoris.

The term **angina pectoris** refers to **intermittent myocardial ischemia** (temporary interference with the flow of blood, oxygen, and nutrients to heart muscle). Angina is characterized by pain below the sternum. The pain usually occurs with exercise or stress and is relieved

TYPES OF ANGINA PECTORIS

CLASSIC (STABLE OR EFFORT) ANGINA

Pain usually associated with coronary arteriosclerosis. The attack can be precipitated by exertion or stress (e.g., cold, fear, emotion) and by eating. The pain lasts about 15 minutes and disappears with rest or nitrates.

UNSTABLE (CRESCENDO OR PREINFARCTION) ANGINA

A progressive form of angina whereby pain occurs more frequently and becomes more severe in time. The attack may appear during rest and may last longer, with less relief with antianginal drugs. These individuals eventually show signs and symptoms of impending myocardial infarction or coronary failure.

VARIANT (PRINZMETAL'S OR VASOSPASTIC) ANGINA

Pain that may be associated with spasms of the coronary arteries and that usually occurs in the presence of coronary stenosis. The pain often happens during rest without any cause. Its occurrence follows a regular pattern (e.g., it appears at the same time during the night). Dysrhythmias often accompany the attack, and the ECG shows an elevation in the S-T segment during the anginal episode.

by rest. Angina pectoris occurs when the work load on the heart is too great and oxygen delivery is inadequate. Coronary flow is very responsive to oxygen requirements of the heart. Inadequate oxygenation of the heart implies that coronary blood flow is less than the amount actually needed. Therefore angina pectoris is usually associated with myocardial ischemia. When coronary blood flow is inadequate, hypoxia causes an accumulation of pain-producing substances such as lactic acid (anaerobic metabolite) and other chemical irritants such as potassium ions, kinins, and prostaglandins. These products then stimulate the cardiac sensory nerve endings, which transmit impulses to the central nervous system to produce the typical anginal pain response.

Inadequate oxygenation may be caused by coronary atherosclerosis or vasomotor spasm of the coronary vessels. Other causes of anginal pain may be pulmonary hypertension and valvular heart disease. Individuals with severe anemia, even with minimal coronary artery disease, may suffer from anginal attacks because of inadequate oxygen supply. The presence of carbon monoxide hemoglobin (**carboxyhemoglobin**) in smokers, who have reduced amounts of available blood oxygen, is another factor in causing angina pectoris.

Drug therapy of angina pectoris is based on the belief that relaxation of coronary smooth muscle will bring about coronary vasodilation, which in turn will improve

blood flow to the heart. However, coronary arteries narrowed by disorders such as sclerosis and calcification cannot respond to any coronary vasodilator.

There are three therapeutic objectives for the use of antianginal agents:

1. To decrease the duration and intensity of pain during an attack
2. To prophylactically decrease frequency of attacks and improve work capacity even though angina may occur
3. To prevent or delay the onset of myocardial infarction

Although evidence exists that the first objective may be achieved, less evidence exists that the second objective can be attained, and no real proof exists that the third objective is attainable. The ideal antianginal drug would:

1. Establish a balance between coronary blood flow and the metabolic demands of the heart
2. Have a local rather than a systemic effect (It would act directly on coronary vessels to promote coronary vasodilation with no effects on other organ systems.)
3. Promote oxygen extraction by the heart from arterial flow
4. Be effective when taken orally, and have sustained action
5. Have absence of tolerance

Currently, no drug meets these criteria. Drugs presently available provide only temporary relief. Evidence is increasing that the nitrates exert their effect not so much by coronary vasodilation but by lowering blood pressure and decreasing venous return and cardiac work.

See the box on p. 524 for a comparison of the effects of nitrates, beta blockers, and calcium blocking agents.

NITRATES

amyl nitrite inhalant
erythrityl tetranitrate (Cardilate)
isosorbide dinitrate (Isordil, Sorbitrate, Coronex✽, Sorbitrate SA)
nitroglycerin sublingual tablet (Nitrostat, Nitrostabilin✽)
nitroglycerin extended-release buccal tablet (Nitrogard)
nitroglycerin lingual aerosol (Nitrolingual)
nitroglycerin oral, extended-release capsules (Nitro-Bid, Nitrobon)
nitroglycerin oral, extended-release tablets (Nitronet, Klavikordal)
nitroglycerin parenteral injection (Nitro-Bid, Nitrol, Tridil)
nitroglycerin ointment (Nitro-Bid, Nitrostat, Nitrol, Nitrong)

COMPARISON OF EFFECTS OF NITRATES, BETA BLOCKERS, AND CALCIUM BLOCKING AGENTS

	NITRATES	BETA BLOCKERS	CALCIUM BLOCKING AGENTS
Systolic blood pressure	(−)	(−)	(−)
Ventricular volume	(−)	(+)	(−) or (0)
Heart rate	(+)	(−)	(−), (+), or (0)
Myocardial contractility	(0)	(−)	(−)
Coronary blood flow	(+)	(+) or (0)	(+)
Coronary vessel resistance	(−)	(+) or (0)	(−)
Coronary spasms	(−)	(+) or (0)	(−)
Collateral flow of blood	(+)	(0)	(−)

(−), decreased; (+), increased; (0), no change.

nitroglycerin transdermal topical systems (Nitrodisc, Nitro-Dur, Transderm-Nitro, Deponit)

pentaerythritol tetranitrate tablet (Pentol, Peritrate, Pentylan)

pentaerythritol tetranitrate extended-release capsules (Duotrate, Pentraspan SR)

pentaerythritol tetranitrate extended-release tablet (Pentol SA, Peritrate SA)

Mechanism of action. Nitrates reduce myocardial oxygen demand by causing peripheral vasodilation. They especially dilate venous capacitance and arterial resistance vessels. The arterial dilation results in a more efficient distribution of blood in the myocardium. The antihypertensive effect of nitrates also is a result of peripheral vasodilation.

Amyl nitrite had been used to treat acute angina attacks, but it has been replaced by the other, safer nitrate dosage forms. Although not approved by FDA labeling in the United States, amyl nitrite has been used as an antidote for cyanide poisoning and in cardiac function tests to assess reserve cardiac function. It has also been abused and used as a sexual stimulant or euphoric agent, but it is very toxic and should not be used for these purposes.

Indications
1. To reduce pain of angina—erythrityl tetranitrate, isosorbide dinitrate, nitroglycerin, pentaerythritol tetranitrate
2. As an antihypertensive—nitroglycerin injection
3. As a cardiac load-reducing agent—nitroglycerin
4. Congestive heart failure associated with myocardial infarction

Pharmacokinetics. See Table 27-1.

Side effects/adverse reactions. See Table 27-2.

Significant drug interactions. Administration of nitrates with alcohol (medium to extreme amounts), antihypertensives, or other vasodilators may result in enhanced hypotensive effects. Avoid concurrent use if possible; if not, monitor closely since dosage reductions may be necessary.

Dosage and administration. See Table 27-3 and box below and on p. 527.

Pregnancy safety. FDA category C

NURSING CONSIDERATIONS

Assessment. Although it is rare, patients intolerant of one nitrate may show intolerance to other nitrates.

Intervention. Dosage must be adjusted to needs and tolerance of the individual client.

Following long-term or high-dose administration, dosage should be reduced gradually to prevent possible withdrawal rebound angina.

NITROGLYCERIN CONTENT AND AVERAGE AMOUNT DELIVERED IN 24 HOURS

DOSAGE FORM	NITROGLYCERIN CONTENT (mg)	AVERAGE AMOUNT OF NITROGLYCERIN DELIVERED (mg)
Nitro-Dur 2.5	26	2.5
Nitro-Dur 5	51	5
Nitro-Dur 7.5	77	7.5
Nitro-Dur 10	104	10
Nitrodisc 5	16	5
Nitrodisc 10	32	10
Transderm-Nitro 5	25	5
Transderm-Nitro 10	50	10

TABLE 27-1 Pharmacokinetics of Nitrates

Drug	Onset of action (min)	Duration of action (hr)	Metabolism	Excretion
erythrityl tetranitrate				
Oral tablet	15-30	Up to 6	Liver	Kidneys
Chewable tablet	5	2-3		
Sublingual tablet	5	2-3		
isosorbide dinitrate				
Oral tablet/capsule	15-40	4-6	Liver	Kidneys
Chewable tablet	2-5	1-2		
Extended release	30	12		
Sublingual	2-5	1-2		
nitroglycerin				
Sublingual	1-3	½-1	Liver	Kidneys
Extended release (buccal)	3	5		
Lingual aerosol	2-4	—		
IV infusion	Immediate	Several minutes		
Ointment	30	4-8		
Transdermal	30	18-24		
Extended release tablet/capsule	40	8-12		
pentaerythritol tetranitrate				
Tablet	30	4-5	Liver	Kidneys
Extended release tablet and capsule	Slow	12		

TABLE 27-2 Side Effects/Adverse Reactions of Nitrates

Side effects*	Adverse reactions†
Most frequent: dizziness (orthostatic hypotension), headaches, nausea or vomiting, agitation, facial flushing, increased pulse rate	Rare or infrequent: dry mouth, rash, prolonged headaches, blurred vision
Less frequent (topical forms): red, tender sites	Overdose effects: usually in the following sequence: bluish tinge to lips, fingernails, and palms of hands; severe dizziness or fainting spells; feeling of increased pressure in head; respiratory shortness; increased weakness; weak, fast heart rate; elevated temperature; convulsions

*If side effects continue, increase, or disturb the patient, inform the physician.
†If adverse reactions occur, contact physician, because medical intervention may be necessary.

Store stock supply of drug in original container that is tightly closed with tight metal screw cap. Federal regulation requires that the sublingual form of nitroglycerin be dispensed in the original unopened manufacturer's container.

Education. Instruct client to avoid alcoholic beverages while taking nitrates because of a shocklike syndrome (flushing, weakness, pallor, hypotension, and syncope) that may occur.

Inform client about the importance of learning to iden-

tify stressful situations that precipitate anginal attacks. These include emotional stress, overeating, smoking, temperature extremes, and sudden increase in physical activity. The client should receive support to modify behaviors that precipitate anginal attacks.

When nitrates are used to prevent angina in the buccal, lingual, sublingual, and chewable oral forms, instruct the client to take the drug 5 to 10 minutes before the occurrence of the anticipated stressor.

Instruct client to report to physician if blurring of

TABLE 27-3   Dosage and Administration of Nitrates

Drug	Adults	Children
erythrityl tetranitrate (Cardilate)	*Capsules and tablets:* 5-20 mg orally, sublingually, or buccally, three or four times daily. Adjust dosage as necessary, to a maximum of 100 mg/day. *Chewable form:* 10 mg orally three or four times daily. Adjust dosage as necessary to a maximum of 100 mg/day.	Not established
isosorbide dinitrate (Isordil, Sorbitrate, Coronex✦, Sorbitrate SA)	*Capsules and tablets:* 5-20 mg orally every 6 hr. Adjust dosage as necessary. (Range is usually 5-40 mg four times daily; 10-20 mg four times daily is most common.) *Chewable tablets:* 5 mg, chewed well and swallowed, every 2 or 3 hr. Adjust dosage as necessary. Hold chewed tablet in mouth 1-2 min before swallowing. *Sublingual tablets:* 2.5-5 mg sublingually or buccally, every 2 or 3 hr as needed. *Extended-release tablets or capsules:* 40-80 mg orally every 8-12 hr.	Not established
nitroglycerin	*Sublingual tablet:* 150-600 µg (0.15-0.6 mg) sublingually or buccally, repeated at 5-min intervals if necessary. If relief is not obtained following three tablets (or 15 min), immediately contact physician or transport individual to a hospital. Maximum dose is 10 mg/day. *Extended-release buccal tablet:* 1 mg dissolved bucally every 5 hr during waking hours. Adjust dosage as necessary. *Lingual aerosol:* Apply one or two metered doses on or under tongue. Dose may be repeated at 5-min intervals up to a total of three doses. If relief is not obtained, contact a physician or transport individual to a hospital. Maximum daily dose is 1.2 mg. Each metered dose is equivalent to 400 µg (0.4 mg). *Oral, extended-release capsules:* 2.5, 6.5, or 9 mg orally every 12 hr. Dosage may be increased to every 8 hr, if necessary. *Oral, extended-release tablets:* 1.3, 2.6, or 6.5 mg every 12 hr. Dosage may be increased to every 8 hr if necessary. *Parenteral injection:* Intravenous infusion—initial 5 µg/min increased in increments of 5 µg/min at 3- to 5-min intervals until desired effect is obtained. If no response is seen at 20 µg/min, increase by 10 µg/min and then 20 µg/min. When partial blood pressure response is observed, reduce size of dosage increments and lengthen interval between increases. (This preparation is not for direct injection. Follow manufacturer's instructions carefully.) *Ointment:* Apply 1-2 inches (15-30 mg) to skin every 8 hours and at bedtime. If angina occurs before 8 hr elapse, drug may be applied every 6 hr. Maximum is 5 inches (75 mg) per application. *Transdermal topical system:* Apply a transdermal unit to intact skin every 24 hr. Dosage adjustments are instituted by changing the dose to the next larger dose or by using a combination of the units. Many dosages are available. See the package insert for additional information.	Not established
pentaerythritol tetranitrate	*Tablet:* 10-20 mg orally, four times daily. Increase dosage as necessary to a maximum of 160 mg/day. *Extended-release capsules/tablets:* 30-80 mg orally twice daily. Increase dosage as necessary to a maximum of 160 mg/day.	Not established

vision, dry mouth, or severe headaches occur. These are signs of overdosage that require immediate attention.

Inform client about the inactivation of nitroglycerin by exposure to air, heat, and moisture. It is generally recommended that unused tablets be discarded 6 months after the bottle is opened. The length of time of potency appears to vary with the manufacturer. Read drug insert.

After the bottle is opened, do not leave cotton or package insert in container; these articles may absorb some of the drug, which results in less potent tablets.

Open stock bottle and transfer a week's supply of tablets in an amber-colored *glass* bottle with metal cap. Be sure hands are dry since moisture hastens deterioration of the drug. Also, allow bottle to warm to room temperature before tablets are removed to prevent condensation of water on tablets if they are cold.

To avoid body heat, the drug should not be carried close to the body; carry it in jacket pocket or handbag.

Usually potency of drug is indicated by a burning or stinging sensation under the tongue. However, the newer, more stable preparations may not produce this effect.

Evaluation. Tolerance has been reported and is manifested by a lack of pain relief following the usual dose. Nitrates may be discontinued for several days until tolerance is lost and then the drug is reinstated.

Special considerations for dosage forms

Intravenous infusion. Use special nitroglycerin disposable infusion sets provided by manufacturer. They are made of non–polyvinyl chloride plastic to minimize the loss of nitroglycerin. Polyvinyl chloride (PVC) plastic may adsorb up to 40% to 80% of the nitroglycerin from a diluted solution of infusion. Therefore use glass intravenous bottles or manufacturer's administration set provided. Observe aseptic technique during procedure.

The drug is not to be used as a direct intravenous infusion. Dilute with 5% dextrose injection USP or 0.9% injection USP before infusion. Since the concentration and/or volume of the drug varies, carefully follow the dosage instructions of the manufacturer. Be aware that switching from a standard (PVC) set to a special (non-PVC) set is likely to affect the dosage—the PVC set requires a higher dosage, which would be excessive if changed to a non-PVC set. In addition, *do not mix nitroglycerin with other medications.*

To titrate dosage for desired hemodynamic function, monitor blood pressure, heart rate, and pulmonary capillary wedge pressure continuously until the correct dose is obtained. Clients with normal or low capillary wedge pressure are likely to be sensitive to hypotensive effects of intravenous nitroglycerin.

Sublingual tablets. Instruct the client to sit or lie down and take the medication on the first indication of an oncoming anginal attack. This prevents postural hypotension that results from the drug. The signs and symptoms include dizziness, syncope, and weakness.

Explain to the client that the tablet should be placed under the tongue or in the buccal pouch and allowed to dissolve; tablet is not to be swallowed. Avoid eating, drinking, smoking while the drug dissolves.

Dosage may be repeated at 5-minute intervals for three doses if necessary. If pain in not relieved in 15 minutes, the physician should be notified. For hospitalized individual, dispense a specific number of tablets (about 25) at the bedside, placed in an appropriate container and properly labeled.

Instruct client to keep a record of frequency of anginal attacks, precipitating factors, number of tablets used, and occurrence of side effects.

Warn client of transient headaches, which usually last 5 to 20 minutes following sublingual administration. Report to physician if the headache persists. Headache may disappear within several days to weeks if the drug is continued. The headache may be relieved by aspirin or acetaminophen or a temporary reduction of the nitrate dosage.

Buccal extended-release tablets. Instruct the client to place the tablet between the upper lip and gum to dis-

solve, above the incisors if food or drink is to be taken with 3 to 5 hours. Caution against using at bedtime since aspiration is a risk. The tablet may be replaced if it is accidentally swallowed.

Chewable tablets. Instruct the client to chew the tablet well and to hold it in the mouth for 2 minutes before swallowing.

Oral sustained-release tablets or capsules. Administer on an empty stomach (1 hour before or 2 hours after meals) with a full glass of water and swallow medication whole.

TRANSDERMAL NITROGLYCERIN SYSTEMS

Since the transdermal nitroglycerin delivery systems are quite popular, the nurse should be familiar with several issues and concerns associated with these products. Three systems are currently available, and the actual amount of nitroglycerin delivered by each system can vary, depending on the system and the individual client's skin absorption of the nitroglycerin.

Each system has a different mechanism of drug delivery. For example, Nitrodisc contains nitroglycerin mixed in a solid polymer similar to silicone. The drug is absorbed through the skin from this polymer, which also contains a cosolvent to enhance skin penetration.

Nitro-Dur contains a gel-like matrix surrounded by fluid. Nitroglyerin moves from the matrix to the fluid to the skin.

Transderm-Nitro contains a semipermeable membrane between the drug supply and the skin. The membrane is actually the controlling factor for the drug delivery. (See Figure 27-1.)

Drug absorption in all systems is by passive diffusion and is based on processes relating to heat transfer (or Fick's law of diffusion) (see Black [1985] for further details).

The three systems are not interchangeable, since the patch size, nitroglycerin content, and average amount of nitroglycerin delivered in 24 hours can differ (see box on p. 524). Although many individuals are reportedly controlled or have responded to this dosage form, other clients do not achieve adequate therapeutic blood levels or a clinically significant therapeutic response. Some researchers (e.g., Parker, 1985) believe maintaining stable nitroglycerin serum levels over 24 hours is not always desirable, since tolerance to the drug and the need to increase dosages would occur. Parker has suggested that intermittent use of transdermal products, such as application for 12 to 16 hours and then removal for the night, would result in prolonged clinical results without the development of significant drug tolerance.

Research and studies are ongoing in this area, and manufacturers are continuing their search for better methods of delivering their drug products.

Nitrodisc type   Nitro-Dur type   Transderm-Nitro type

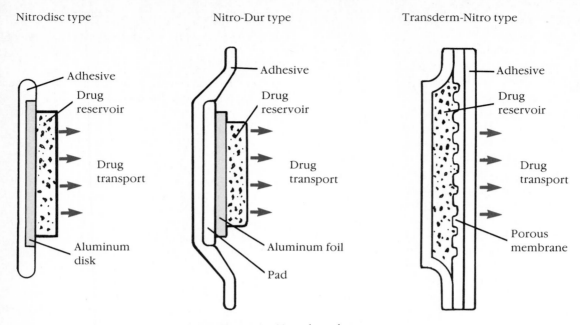

FIGURE 27-1 Transdermal systems.

Alert the client to notify the physician if undigested tablets are found in stools.

Lingual aerosol. When administering, do not shake the can. Hold the can vertically and spray it onto or under the client's tongue.

Instruct the client not to inhale the spray and not to swallow immediately.

Ointment. Take baseline blood pressure and heart rate with the client in a sitting position, after having been at rest for 10 minutes. Repeat the vital signs 1 hour after drug administration and report them to physician. An appropriate dosage produces a 10 mm Hg fall in blood pressure or 10-beat rise in heart rate with the patient in a resting position.

Squeeze prescribed dose onto a specially designed dose-measuring applicator supplied with the package. *Avoid use of fingers* to spread ointment. Apply in a thin, uniform layer to premarked 6-square-inch surface on clean, dry, nonhairy skin area of chest, abdomen, anterior aspect of thigh, or forearm. Rotate sites to prevent inflammation. Also, wash off last application. Do not massage or rub in ointment because rapid absorption will interfere with the drug's sustained action. Last, cover area with a transparent wrap and secure with tape.

If medication is to be terminated, dosage and frequency of application are reduced gradually over a 4- to 6-week period to avoid withdrawal responses (pain or severe myocardial ischemia).

Store nitroglycerin ointment in a cool place and in the original container with the tube tightly capped.

Instruct the client not to change dosage or medication without consulting the physician and to report to the phy-

sician regularly for cardiac function monitoring.

Transdermal systems. Remove the old system and apply the new one at the same time each day. The system should be applied to clean, dry, and hairless skin areas of the chest, shoulder, or inside of the upper arm. Avoid skin folds, areas distal to the knee or elbow, and irritated or excessively scarred areas. Rotate application sites to prevent irritation.

Apply a new system if the current one becomes loosened.

Do not trim the units, since this will alter the dosage.

DRUGS FOR PERIPHERAL OCCLUSIVE ARTERIAL DISEASE

The use of vasodilators in chronic occlusive arterial disease or peripheral vascular disease has been discouraging. Adrenergic blocking agents are frequently used to treat peripheral vascular diseases. Because several drugs that are not adrenergic blocking agents have had some success in treating these disorders, they are also included.

The FDA rating for these drugs is possibly effective for the treatment of peripheral vascular diseases.

cyclandelate (Cyclospasmol)

Mechanism of action. Cyclandelate produces a direct relaxation effect on the smooth muscles of peripheral arterial walls. It increases peripheral circulation of the extremities and digits and elevates skin temperature of the extremities.

Indications
1. Possibly effective for treatment of peripheral vascular disease or cerebrovascular insufficiency.
2. Adjunctive therapy in Raynaud's disease, thrombophlebitis, intermittent claudication, and arteriosclerosis obliterans.

Pharmacokinetics. Cyclandelate is well absorbed orally. Peak effect after single dose occurs within 1½ hours. Therapeutic improvement occurs slowly, over a period of several weeks.

Side effects/adverse reactions. Side effects include gas; heartburn; nausea or abdominal pain; dizziness; facial flushing; headaches; increased rapid heart rate; paresthesia of fingers, toes, or face; increased weakness; and unusual sweating. If these effects continue, increase, or disturb the client, inform the physician.

Significant drug interactions. No significant drug interactions have been reported.

Dosage and administration

Adults. Cyclandelate, 1.2 to 1.6 g orally in divided doses, is given before meals and at bedtime. When clinical effects are noted, reduce dosage by 200 mg amounts until a maintenance dose of 400 to 800 mg orally, in two to four divided doses is achieved.

Children. Dosage is not established.

Pregnancy safety. Not established

NURSING CONSIDERATIONS

Assessment. Before administration of cyclandelate, ascertain that client does not have severe cerebrovascular disease and has not recently had a myocardial infarction or severe coronary artery disease. Because it has a greater vasodilating effect on peripheral vessels than those of coronary or cerebral areas, cyclandelate may reduce blood flow and so increase ischemia in those areas.

Intervention. Administer with milk, food, or antacids to prevent gastrointestinal distress.

Education. Alert the client that symptoms such as flushing of the face, dizziness, weakness, headache, and rapid heart rate usually disappear after a few weeks of taking the medication.

Instruct the client to move slowly upright from a sitting or lying position because of the drug's hypotensive effects.

Advise clients to avoid smoking, since nicotine's vasoconstrictive properties are counterproductive to the use of cyclandelate.

Evaluation. Monitor blood pressure in lying, sitting, and standing positions to detect hypotension.

isoxsuprine hydrochloride (Vasodilan, Vasoprine)

Mechanism of action. Isoxsuprine produces a direct relaxation effect on the smooth muscles of peripheral

arterial walls located within skeletal muscle. It has little effect on cutaneous flow of blood. It was believed to be a beta adrenergic stimulant, but its effects are not reversed by beta adrenergic blocking agents. It also stimulates the heart and relaxes the uterus. Heart rate and peripheral vascular resistance decrease while cardiac output increases.

Indications
1. Possibly effective for the treatment of peripheral vascular disease or cerebrovascular insufficiency
2. May relieve symptoms of Raynaud's disease, arteriosclerosis obliterans, and thromboangitis obliterans (Buerger's disease).

Pharmacokinetics

Absorption. Absorption of isoxsuprine is good from the gastrointestinal tract.

Duration of action. Isoxsuprine's duration of action is 1¼ hours. In neonates duration or action ranges from 1½ to 3 hours for near-term babies to 6 to 8 hours for less mature babies.

Onset of action. Onset of action for oral administration of isoxsuprine is 1 hour. For intravenous administration it is 10 minutes.

Metabolism. Isoxsuprine is partially metabolized in the blood.

Excretion. Isoxsuprine is excreted in the kidneys.

Side effects/adverse reactions. If nausea or vomiting (usually dose related, occurring most often with parenteral form) continues, increases, or disturbs the client, inform the physician.

If the following adverse reactions occur, contact the physician, since medical intervention may be necessary:
    Rare: chest pain, respiratory difficulties, rash
    Dose-related, occurring most often with parenteral forms: dizziness, hypotension, increased or irregular heart rate, pulmonary edema

Significant drug interactions. There are no significant drug interactions with isoxsuprine.

Dosage and administration

Adults. In the tablet form 10 to 20 mg is given orally three or four times daily. The parenteral form is not available in the United States. Intramuscularly, 5 to 10 mg is given two or three times daily.

Pregnancy safety. Not established

NURSING CONSIDERATIONS

See discussion under cyclandelate.

nylidrin hydrochloride (Arlidin, PMS Nylidrin✣)

Mechanism of action. Nylidrin may have both a direct effect and a beta adrenergic stimulation effect on skeletal arteries and arterioles, resulting in vasodilation.

Indications
1. Possibly effective for the treatment of peripheral vascular disease or cerebrovascular insufficiency.
2. Treatment of frostbite, thrombophlebitis, diabetic vascular disease, night leg cramps, Raynaud's disease, arteriosclerosis obliterans, thromboangiitis obliterans, and circulatory problems of the inner ear.

Pharmacokinetics
Absorption. Absorption of nylidrin is good.
Onset of action. Onset of action for nylidrin is within 10 minutes.
Time to peak effect. Nylidrin reaches its peak effect in 30 minutes.
Duration of action. Nylidrin's action lasts 2 hours.
Side effects/adverse reactions. Side effects include facial flushing, complaints of feeling chilly, headache, nausea and vomiting, anxiety, and tremors. If side effects continue, increase, or disturb the client, inform the physician.

If the following adverse reactions occur, contact the physician, since medical intervention may be necessary:
Less frequent: dizziness; rapid, irregular heart rate; increased weakness
Overdose signs: blurred vision, chest pain, increased fever, metallic taste in mouth, decreased urination
Significant drug interactions. There are no significant drug interactions with nylidrin.

Dosage and administration
Adults. Adult dose of nylidrin is 3 to 12 mg orally three or four times daily.
Pregnancy safety. Not established

NURSING CONSIDERATIONS

Time doses so that the last dose is not at bedtime. On occasion, palpitations may cause insomnia. See discussion of cyclandelate for further nursing considerations.

papaverine hydrochloride (Cerebid, Cerespan, Pavabid)

Papaverine is an old drug that was exempted from the FDA's review on drug effectiveness. However, the advisory committee of the FDA, the Peripheral and Central Nervous System Drug Review Committee, reported that papaverine has vasodilator effects but was not proved to be effective for its claimed indications, namely, smooth muscle relaxation.
Mechanism of action. Papaverine relaxes smooth muscle.

Indications
1. Cerebral and peripheral ischemia.

2. Visceral spasms. It has limited use in therapeutic practice today.

Pharmacokinetics
Absorption. Tablet absorption of papaverine is variable and undependable, with approximately 54% absorbed. Extended-release dosage forms have poor absorption.
Half-life. Papaverine has a half-life of ½ to 2 hours but can vary as long as up to 24 hours.
Metabolism. Papaverine is metabolized by the liver.
Excretion. Papaverine is excreted by the kidneys.
Side effects/adverse reactions. Side effects of injectable dosage forms include dizziness (hypotension), facial flushing, increased heart rate, and deep, labored breathing. If side effects continue, increase, or disturb the client, inform the physician.

If the following adverse reactions occur, contact the physician, since medical intervention may be necessary:
Rare: jaundice
Injectable form: redness, tenderness, or pain at the injection site
Overdose signs: blurred vision, diplopia, sleepiness, increased tiredness
Significant drug interactions. There are no significant drug interactions with papaverines.

Dosage and administration
Adults.
Tablets. Papaverine tablets, 100 to 300 mg, are given orally three to five times per day.
Capsules. Papaverine capsules, 75 to 300 mg, are given orally three to five times daily.
Extended-release capsules or tablets. Extended-release papaverine, 150 mg, is given orally every 12 hours. Dosage may be increased to 150 mg every 8 hours or 300 mg every 12 hours if necessary.
Injection. Intraarterial papaverine, 40 mg, is given over 1 to 2 minutes. Intramuscular or intravenous papaverine, 30 to 120 mg, is given every 3 hours over 1 to 2 minutes.
Children. Intramuscular or intravenous papaverine, 1.5 mg/kg body weight, is given four times daily.
Pregnancy safety. FDA Category C

NURSING CONSIDERATIONS

Observe the client for gastrointestinal distress or yellowing of the sclera of the eyes and of the skin as symptoms of hepatotoxicity. Hepatic function studies may be indicated.

Take periodic intraocular pressure measurements in clients with glaucoma who are also receiving papaverine.

See discussion of cyclandelate for further nursing considerations.

OTHER VASODILATING AGENTS

Sodium nitroprusside, hydralazine, and minoxidil are other potent vasodilators. They exhibit their effects primarily by direct relaxation of vascular smooth muscle, particularly the arteries and arterioles. Hydralazine and minoxidil have little effect on veins. These three agents are used primarily for their hypotensive effects and are discussed in detail in Chapter 25.

KEY TERMS

angina pectoris, page 522
capacitance blood vessels, page 522
carboxyhemoglobin, page 523
classic angina, page 523
crescendo angina, page 523
effort angina, page 523
intermittent myocardial ischemia, page 522
peripheral occlusive arterial disease, page 522
preinfarction angina, page 523
Prinzmetal's angina, page 523
resistance blood vessels, page 522
stable angina, page 523
unstable angina, page 523
variant angina, page 523
vasospastic angina, page 523

BIBLIOGRAPHY

Abramowicz, M, Nitroglycerin patches, Med Lett Drugs Therapeut 26(664):59, 1984.

Abrams, J: Nitrates, Med Clin North Am 72(1):1, 1988.

American Hospital Formulary Service: AHFS drug information '87, Bethesda, Md, 1987, American Society of Hospital Pharmacists, Inc.

Bera, MD: Experience brief, transdermal nitroglycerin patches, Hosp Formul 20(4):514, 1985.

Black, CD: Concepts and principles involved in transdermal drug delivery. In Rayment, CM, chairperson: Recent controversies involving transdermal nitroglycerin delivery systems. Symposium presented at the ASHP Midyear Clinical Meeting, New Orleans, 1985.

Brown, BG, and others: Nitroglycerin: mechanism of action, Physician Assist 8(1):47, 1984.

Bruni, PJ: Criticism of nitroglycerin patches continues to mount, Patient Care 19(1):151, 1985.

Chatterjee, K: Options for the failing heart: vasodilators for added effect . . . reduction of systemic vascular resistance, Emerg Med 16(15):51, 1984.

Coffman, JD: New drug therapy for peripheral vascular disease, Med Clin North Am 72(1):259, 1988.

Cohn, JN: Treatment by modification of circulatory dynamics . . . vasodilator drugs. Hosp Pract 19(8):37, 1984.

Conner, CS, and others: Transdermal nitroglycerin: a reevaluation, Drug Intell Clin Pharm 18(11):889, 1984.

Deans, KW, and others: Nitrates in the treatment of coronary artery disease, J Cardiovasc Nurs 1(1):81, 1986.

Doyle, JE: Treatment modalities in peripheral vascular disease, Nurs Clin North Am 21(2):241, 1986.

Eberts, MA: Advances of pharmacologic management of angina pectoris, J Cardiovasc Nurs 1(1):15, 1986.

Johnston, WE, and others: Recent advances in critical care pharmacology: treatment of myocardial ischemia, Hosp 1984.

Kafka, KR, and others: Antianginal agents: ischemic heart disease and the role of nitrates, I, Hosp Formul 20(11):1144, 1985.

Kastrup, EK, and Olin BR: Facts and comparisons, drug information, Philadelphia, 1987, JB Lippincott Co.

Kleinhenz, TJ: The inside story on preload and afterload, Nursing '85 15(5):50, 1985.

Labson, LH: Angina: which drug when? Patient Care 18(1):23, 1984.

Logue, RB: Use of intravenous nitroglycerin in ischemic heart disease, Pract Cardiol 11(6):37, 1985.

Miller, ED, Jr: Cardiac drugs—old and new, Curr Rev Recov Room Nurses 7(10):75, 1985.

Miller, K: Nitroglycerin, Emergency 18(7):14, 1986.

Parker, J: Nitrate tolerance. In Frishman, WH, ed: A symposium: transdermal nitroglycerin-maximizing therapeutic efficacy, Am J Cardiol 56(17):281, 1985.

Scheidt, SS: Do the transdermal nitroglycerin systems work? In Rayment, CM, chairperson: Recent controversies involving transdermal nitroglycerin delivery systems. Symposium presented at the ASHP Midyear Clinical Meeting, New Orleans, 1985.

Sjogren, ER: Transdermal nitroglycerin systems: ending the confusion (or . . . "can I show you something in a Nitro-Dur 5?"), Crit Care Nurse 4(2):38, 1984.

Thomas, MG, and others: Antianginal efficacy of nitroglycerin patches: the jury is still out, Hosp Formul 21(9):918, 1986.

Todd, B: Transdermal nitroglycerin ointment and patches, Geriatr Nurs 7(3):152, 1986.

United States Pharmacopeial Convention: Drug information for the health care provider, ed 7, Rockville, Md, 1987, US Pharmacopeial Convention, Inc.

Weinhardt, JA: Making the most of topical nitroglycerin, RN 48(12):38, 1985.

UNIT VII

Drugs Affecting the Blood

CHAPTER

28

Overview of the Blood

OBJECTIVES

After studying this chapter, the student will be able to:

1. Describe the functions of blood in the body.
2. List the three types of blood cells and their function.
3. Compare and contrast the five types of white blood cells.
4. Describe the role of platelets in blood clotting in the body.
5. Name the three major blood proteins and their function.

Blood is the major transport system in the body. It is also vitally important for the proper functioning and regulation of a human body. Pumped by the heart, blood carries nutrients and oxygen from the digestive and respiratory systems to cells throughout the entire body. In addition, it picks up waste products from body cells and delivers them to the proper system for excretion, usually the liver, kidneys, and lungs. Hormones, enzymes, buffers, and many other biochemical substances are also transported by the blood from one site in the body to the receptors or target cells.

Blood also helps regulate body heat by absorbing and transporting heat from the body core where it can be more easily dispersed.

BLOOD VOLUME

Blood is composed of billions of cells and a fluid portion called **plasma.** While blood volume can vary from person to person, the average blood volume in a normal adult is approximately 5000 ml (5 L). Of this volume, 3000 ml is usually plasma, and the remainder is red blood cells.

Hematocrit is the percent of cells in the blood, or the blood viscosity. For example, if a person has a hematocrit of 40, then 40% of the blood volume is cells, with the remainder being plasma. Hematocrit is measured by a laboratory test performed on a blood sample. The higher the hematocrit, the greater the blood viscosity. For example, persons with **polycythemia** may have a hematocrit of 60 or 70, because of an excessive number of red blood corpuscles. Increased blood viscosity can retard blood flow through blood vessels, resulting in headaches, fatigue, weakness, dyspnea, and perhaps an enlarged spleen and increased basal metabolism.

BLOOD COMPOSITION

Blood is composed of three types of blood cells: (1) red blood cells, or **erythrocytes,** which transport oxygen and carbon dioxide; (2) **leukocytes,** or white blood cells, which defend the body against bacteria and infections; and (3) **platelets,** or **thrombocytes,** which are necessary for blood coagulation. Proteins such as serum albumin, globulins, and fibrinogen are also present in the blood.

Plasma may contain thousands of other substances, such as glucose, electrolytes, vitamins, hormones, and waste products. This discussion on blood, however, is limited to blood cells, blood proteins, and blood groups, or types.

BLOOD CELLS

Red blood cells. Red blood cells (RBCs, erythrocytes) are small and disk shaped. They are the cells present in the largest quantities in the bloodstream. Their life span is approximately 120 days. The major function of red blood cells is to carry **hemoglobin** within the cell. Each hemoglobin molecule contains four iron atoms, which combine with four oxygen molecules to transport oxygen from the lungs to the tissues. Hemoglobin can also combine with carbon dioxide and carry it from the cells to the lungs for excretion. It also serves as an acid-base buffering system in whole blood.

After birth, red blood cells are produced by the bone marrow. They are manufactured by most bones in early life, but after 20 years of age most red blood cells are produced in the bone marrow of the vertebrae, sternum, ribs, and ilia.

Males have more hemoglobin in their blood than females do. Generally, most normal men have between 14 to 16 g/dl, while women have a range of 12 to 24 g/dl. A person with a hemoglobin below 10 is usually diagnosed as having **anemia.** Anemias are classified according to both the size and the number of functional red blood cells in the blood.

Red blood cells are rapidly formed and destroyed in the body. It has been estimated that over 100 million red blood cells are produced every minute during adulthood. The normal healthy adult has between 4.5 and 5.5 million cells/mm^3 of blood. The body balances production versus destruction of these cells to maintain a relatively constant body level of red blood cells. The exact body mechanism for this is unknown.

It is known that the rate of red cell production can be increased if a considerable decrease in red blood cells occurs or tissue hypoxia develops. Then the kidneys will be stimulated to increase secretion of **erythropoietin,** a hormone. Erythropoietin increases red cell production by stimulating the bone marrow. With maximum bone marrow stimulation, red blood cell production can be increased nearly seven times over normal.

The bone marrow needs adequate supplies of vitamin B_{12}, iron, and other substances to make new red blood cells. A deficiency in absorption of vitamin B_{12} from the gastric tract, caused by a lack of intrinsic factor (see Chapter 40), can lead to pernicious anemia.

Anemias can also be induced by increased red cell destruction, such as occurs in infections and cancer (malignancies) or from bone marrow suppression caused by radiation therapy and many cancer chemotherapeutic agents. (See box on p. 537 for a selected list of drugs that cause bone marrow depression.)

Leukocytes. There are five types of leukocytes (white blood cells) found in the blood. They are classified according to the presence or absence of granules in the cell cytoplasm. The granular leukocytes are **neutrophils, eosinophils,** and **basophils,** while the nongranular leukocytes are **lymphocytes** and **monocytes.** The granular leukocytes have two or more nuclear lobes, so they are referred to as polymorphonuclear leukocytes or "polys."

Blood in a normal person usually contains between 5000 and 9000 leukocytes. (See box below for approximate percentages for each type.) A differential count may be ordered by the physician to aid in diagnosis. For example, in acute appendicitis, the percentage of neutrophils increases, as does the total leukocyte count.

Leukocytes are produced primarily in the bone marrow. Lymphocytes are produced mainly in lymph tissues and organs, such as the spleen, thymus, tonsils, and various other lymphoid tissue in the bone marrow, gastrointestinal tract, and elsewhere.

Several terms are important to understand. **Leukopenia** refers to a decrease in the number of leukocytes present, while **leukocytosis** is an increased number of leukocytes.

DIFFERENTIAL NORMAL LEUKOCYTE COUNT

Neutrophils, polymorphonuclear	62%
Eosinophils, polymorphonuclear	2.3%
Basophils, polymorphonuclear	0.4%
Monocytes	5.3%
Lymphocytes	30%

From Guyton, AC: Textbook of medical physiology, ed 7, Philadelphia, 1986, WB Saunders Co.

DRUGS THAT CAUSE BONE MARROW DEPRESSION

amphotericin B, systemic (Fungizone)
antithyroid medications
azathioprine (Imuran)
busulfan (Myleran)
carmustine (BCNU; BiCNU)
chlorambucil (Leukeran)
chloramphenicol (Chloromycetin)
cisplatin (Platinol, Platinol-AQ✿)
colchicine
cyclophosphamide (Cytoxan, Procytox✿)
cytarabine (Ara-C, Cytosar✿)
dacarbazine (DTIC✿, DTIC-Dome)
dactinomycin (Actinomycin-D, Cosmegen)
daunorubicin (Cerubidine)
doxorubicin (Adriamycin RDF)
etoposide (VePesid, VP-16)
floxuridine (FUDR)
flucytosine (Ancobon, 5-FC, Ancotil✿)
fluorouracil, systemic (5-FU, Adrucil)
hydroxyurea (Hydrea)
interferon (Roferon-A, Intron A)
lomustine (CCNU, CeeNU)
mechlorethamine, systemic (Mustargen, nitrogen mustard)
melphalan (Alkeran, L-PAM)
mercaptopurine (Purinethol)
methotrexate (Abitrexate, Mexate)
mitomycin (Mutamycin)
pentamidine (Pentam, Lomidine✿)
plicamycin (Mithracin, mithramycin)
procarbazine (Matulane, natulan✿)
sodium iodide I 131 (Iodotope)
sodium phosphate P 32
streptozocin (Zanosar)
thioguanine (Lanvis✿)
thiotepa
uracil mustard
vinblastine (Velban, Velbe✿)
vincristine (Oncovin)
zidovudine (Retrovir)

Neutrophils, monocytes, lymphocytes, and basophils are very mobile. They can leave the capillaries and migrate to organisms or foreign particles that have entered the body. The neutrophils and monocytes will ingest and destroy the invaders through a process known as **phagocytosis.** Lymphocytes defend the body against bacteria, fungus, and viruses by forming B-lymphocytes or T-lymphocytes. (See Chapter 64 for an overview of the immune system.)

Eosinophils are considered weak phagocytes and have limited mobility. An increased level is usually seen with allergic reactions or a cell injury caused by parasites (e.g., hookworm).

The life span of granulocytes is estimated to be 4 to 8 hours in the bloodstream and 3 to 5 days in body tissues. If involved in ingestion of invading organisms, this life span can be reduced to only a few hours, because during this process they are also destroyed. Monocytes also have a short life span in blood, but in the body tissues, they can live for months or even years if not destroyed by phagocytosis. Monocytes in the tissues often increase in size to become tissue macrophages, so they often provide a first line of defense against tissue infections.

Platelets. Platelets (thrombocytes) are small, round or oval, colorless cells produced by the bone marrow. They have a life span of 5 to 8 days. A normal platelet level in the blood is between 150,000 and 350,000/mm³.

Platelets are key substances for blood clotting in the body. If a blood vessel is injured and blood is escaping, platelets will quickly congregate at the site and clump together to form a plug to stop the bleeding. If the wound is large, platelets will set off a series of chemical reactions within the body to form a clot and seal the injury. (See Chapter 29 for detailed information on the clotting mechanisms.)

Persons with a low quantity of platelets have **thrombocytopenia.** Such persons tend to bleed, and their skin usually displays small purple spots, hence the name thrombocytopenic purpura. Bleeding problems usually do not occur until the platelets are below 50,000/mm³. Thrombocytopenia is often induced by irradiation injury to the bone marrow or from aplasia of the bone marrow induced by specific drugs.

BLOOD PROTEINS

The blood contains three major proteins: **albumin, globulins,** and **fibrinogen.** Albumin is responsible for the osmotic pressure gradient produced at the capillary membrane. This prevents plasma fluid from leaving the capillaries to enter the interstitial spaces.

Globulins are divided into alpha, beta, and gamma globulins. Gamma globulin and perhaps beta globulin (to a lesser extent) help to protect the body against infections. Gamma globulin is involved with humoral immunity.

Alpha and beta globulins are also believed to perform other functions, such as transportation of certain substances in the blood by reversibly combining with them. They may also be a substrate to form other substances.

Fibrinogen is necessary for blood clotting. A discussion is found in Chapter 29.

BLOOD GROUPS OR TYPES

Blood type refers to the type of antigen located on red blood cell membranes. Although many antigens have been identified, antigens A, B, and Rh are the most important blood antigens involved with blood transfusions and newborn survival. Every person belongs to one of the four blood groups and, in addition, is also Rh positive or Rh negative. The ABO blood groups are:

Type A: A antigen on red blood cells (while the plasma has antibody B)

Type B: B antigen on red blood cells (while the plasma has antibody A)

Type AB: A antigen and B antigen on red blood cells (no antibodies)

Type O: neither A nor B antigens on red blood cells (plasma contains A and B antibodies)

Persons with type A blood can safely receive blood from A and O donors. Persons with type B blood can safely receive blood from type B and O donors. People with AB blood are known as the universal recipients, because their blood is compatible with types AB, A, B, and O. Before transfusion, however, cross matching of the blood is necessary since other agglutinins may be present. Type O persons can only receive type O blood, but they are called the universal donors since they can donate blood to anyone. (See Chapter 29 for additional information on blood transfusion.)

A person who is Rh positive carries Rh antigen on the red blood cells. One who is Rh negative does not have any Rh antigens on the red blood cells. Approximately 85% of the population is Rh positive. Rh factor is particularly important when an Rh-negative woman is impregnated by an Rh-positive man. The mother may have antibodies against the Rh antigen that can cross the placenta and attack the fetus should its blood be Rh positive. If this occurs, the infant may develop jaundice or be dead on delivery.

An Rh-negative woman could acquire Rh antibodies via blood transfusions. It is also possible for her to develop them if fetal blood enters her bloodstream during childbirth or miscarriage. Regardless, the first pregnancy usually has less risk associated with it than subsequent pregnancies. Physicians can reduce this danger by administering an anti-Rh antibody (Gamulin Rh, RhoGAM, HypRho-D) to Rh-negative woman after each pregnancy. This will prevent their systems from making antibodies to Rh-positive blood. Rh-negative women who have a spontaneous or induced abortion or a termination of an ectopic pregnancy of up to and including 12 weeks gestation are given a micro dose of immune globulin (MICRhoGAM, Mini-Gamulin Rh) if the father is Rh positive.

KEY TERMS

albumin, page 537

anemia, page 536

basophils, page 536

eosinophils, page 536

erythrocytes, page 536

erythropoietin, page 536

fibrinogen, page 537

globulins, page 537

hemoglobin, page 536

hematocrit, page 535

leukocytes, page 536

leukocytosis, page 536

leukopenia, page 536

lymphocytes, page 536

monocytes, page 536

neutrophils, page 536

phagocytosis, page 537

plasma, page 535

platelets, page 536

polycythemia, page 536

thrombocytes, page 536

thrombocytopenia, page 537

BIBLIOGRAPHY

Guyton, AC: Textbook of medical physiology, ed 7, Philadelphia, 1986, WB Saunders Co.

Guyton, AC: Human physiology and mechanisms of disease, ed 4, Philadelphia, 1987, WB Saunders Co.

Kastrup, EK, ed: Facts and comparisons, Philadelphia, 1988, JB Lippincott Co.

Thibodeau, G: Anatomy and physiology, St Louis, 1988, The CV Mosby Co.

United States Pharmacopeial Convention: Drug information for the health care provider, ed 8, Rockville, Md, 1988, US Pharmacopeial Convention, Incorporated.

CHAPTER

29

Anticoagulant, Thrombolytic, Antihemophilic, and Hemostatic Drugs; Blood and Blood Components

OBJECTIVES

After studying this chapter, the student will be able to:

1. Describe the physiologic response that occurs with an injury to a blood vessel.

2. Identify the disease processes that require the administration of drugs to inhibit clotting.

3. Differentiate between the mechanisms of action of parenteral and oral anticoagulant agents.

4. Discuss the nursing assessments, interventions, client education, and evaluative methods concerned with the administration of anticoagulants.

5. Discuss the use of protamine sulfate and vitamin K as anticoagulant antagonists.

6. Differentiate between the actions or thrombolytic and anticoagulant drugs on blood clots.

7. Discuss drugs that may be successfully used in treating hemophilia.

8. Discuss the appropriate nursing assessments and interventions needed before, during, and following the administration of blood components.

This chapter concerns drugs and substances that affect blood clotting, preformed thrombi, and blood administration.

Normally, blood clotting functions as a defense mechanism that is constantly available for protection against excessive hemorrhage. However, the development of a **thrombus** (clot) in a blood vessel can obstruct blood flow and cause an infarction with resultant tissue necrosis. An **embolus,** a mass of undissolved matter that breaks off from the thrombus, can travel in the blood vessel and lodge in areas of the body; this can cause death. By contrast, a defect in the blood clotting mechanism may lead to excessive bleeding or hemorrhage, even after a minor injury.

Both thrombotic and hemorrhagic disorders can be treated with drugs. The following discussion describes the blood clotting mechanism and provides a rationale for use of various groups of therapeutic agents.

MECHANISMS AFFECTING BLOOD COAGULATION
HEMOSTATIC MECHANISM

Hemostasis is a process that spontaneously stops blood loss from damaged blood vessels. Blood is normally fluid while circulating in the vessels, but with vessel injury, it rapidly clots at the site of injury.

After any injury to a blood vessel, hemostasis is achieved by three sequential steps: (1) blood vessels constrict to retard blood flow from the injured area, (2) platelet plugs form to temporarily seal the leaking small arteries and veins, and (3) blood coagulates to plug openings within the damaged vessels and wounds to prevent further bleeding.

Blood vessel constriction. Immediately after a blood vessel is injured, vascular constriction occurs as a reflex reponse. This response instantly slows the flow of blood from the ruptured vessel.

Platelet plug formation. Following injury to a blood vessel, interruption of the continuity of its endothelial lining exposes the collagen (a fibrous protein) in the underlying connective tissue. Immediately, platelets adhere to the exposed collagen to form a dense aggregate, a process known as **platelet adhesion.** This attachment triggers the release of adenosine diphosphate (ADP), which causes the outer surface of the platelets to become extremely sticky so that other adjacent platelets adhere to one another at the damaged site (platelet aggregation). This process eventually forms the **platelet plug.** Because this plug is relatively unstable, it can stop bleeding quickly as long as the damage to the vessel is minute. However, for long-term effectiveness, the platelet plug must be reinforced with fibrin. This involves a chemical mechanism called blood coagulation.

Blood coagulation. Blood coagulation is the final stage of a complex series of events in hemostasis. The process ultimately results in the formation of a stable fibrin clot, which is composed of a meshwork of fibrin threads that entraps platelets, blood cells, and plasma. Thus the physical formation of a *blood clot* or *thrombus* plays a key role in hemostasis by permanently closing the hole in the injured vessel to prevent further bleeding.

The chemical events in the blood coagulation mechanism involve two distinct pathways: the intrinsic pathway and the extrinsic pathway.

Intrinsic pathway. Because all the chemical substances involved in coagulation are normally found in the circulating blood, this pathway is referred to as the intrinsic system of coagulation. In this pathway, activation of specific blood coagulation factors is initiated by injury to the endothelial lining of the blood vessel wall. When blood contacts the exposed underlying collagen, this activates the Hageman factor (factor XII) by enzymatically converting it to the active form (factor XIIa). The simultaneous damage of platelets also causes the release of platelet phospholipid (platelet factor 3), which is required later in the coagulation process. Factor XIIa then activates factor XI to XIa. The reaction of factor XIa with factor IX requires calcium ions to form activated factor IX. In the presence of calcium ions and platelet phospholipid, factor IXa interacts with factor VIII and thrombin to form a complex. This combination then speeds up the activation of factor X. Factor Xa combines with factor V, calcium ions, and platelet phospholipid to form a complex known as the prothrombin activator (factor IIa). Factor IIa initiates the cleavage of prothrombin to form thrombin, which then enzymatically converts fibrinogen into fibrin, forming an unstable clot. The final step involves the action of factor XIII (a fibrin-stabilizing factor), thrombin, and calcium ions, which catalyze the formation of a stronger, stable fibrin clot. Figure 29-1 summarizes the main events of the intrinsic pathway.

Extrinsic pathway. The extrinsic pathway is activated by trauma to the vascular wall or to the tissues outside the blood vessels. In this pathway, clotting occurs when products of tissue damage gain access to the blood. The tissue factor thromboplastin is released and becomes part of a complex with factor VII and calcium ions. This combination of components activates factor X, which is the step at which the extrinsic pathway converges with the intrinsic pathway; coagulation then continues through a common route with the resultant formation of a final stable clot. (See Figure 29-1 for the extrinsic pathway and Table 29-1 for a listing of blood coagulation factors.)

The final pathway common to both the intrinsic and the extrinsic coagulation systems begins with the activation of factor X and ends in the formation of fibrin. Both systems function simultaneously in the body. The lack of a normal factor in either system will usually result in a blood disorder.

BLOOD COAGULATION ABNORMALITIES

Diseases associated with abnormal clotting vessels cause many deaths. It is estimated that over a million persons suffer from thrombosis or embolism in the United States each year. Diseases caused by intravascular clotting include some of the major causes of death from cardiovascular sources—coronary occlusion and cerebrovascular accidents. Drugs that inhibit clotting are therefore important.

Local trauma, vascular stasis, and systemic alterations in coagulability of blood are considered the main factors in the initiation of thrombosis. Basically, coagulation mechanisms are responsible for forming two kinds of thrombi: arterial thrombi and venous thrombi. Arterial thrombi are most frequently associated with atherosclerotic plaques, high blood pressure, and turbulent blood flow that damages the endothelial lining of the blood vessel and causes platelets to stick and aggregate in the arterial system. Arterial thrombi are mostly platelets, and their formation is associated with the intrinsic pathway of the coagulation mechanism.

Venous thrombi occur most often in areas where blood flow is reduced or static. This appears to initiate clotting and produces a thrombus in the venous system. Its formation involves the extrinsic pathway of the coagulation mechanism. Current anticoagulants are more effective in preventing venous rather than arterial thrombi.

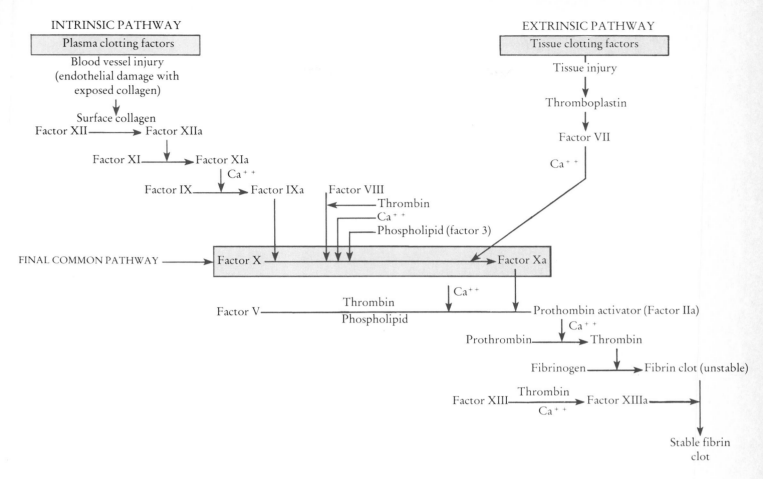

FIGURE 29-1 Coagulation mechanism showing the steps in the intrinsic pathway and the extrinsic pathway for initiating blood clotting. The protein factors are present in plasma as inactive precursors. The letter *a* following a Roman numeral indicates an activated factor. See Table 29-1 for synonyms of coagulation factors. The final common pathway is common to both the intrinsic and extrinsic coagulation systems. This begins with the activation of factor X and ends in the formation of a stable fibrin clot.

ANTICOAGULANT DRUGS

Anticoagulant therapy is primarily prophylatic. These agents act by preventing (1) fibrin deposits, (2) extension of a thrombus, and (3) thromboembolic complications. Long-term anticoagulant therapy remains controversial. Nevertheless, there is evidence that anticoagulant therapy reduces the incidence of thrombosis and therefore prolongs life.

Anticoagulation therapy is directed toward preventing intravascular thrombosis by decreasing blood coagulability. This therapy has no direct effect on a blood clot that has already formed or on ischemic tissue injured by an inadequate blood supply because of the clot.

There are two main groups of anticoagulant drugs: (1) parenteral anticoagulant drugs and (2) oral anticoagulant drugs. For effective anticoagulant therapy with both types, the manner of use is important. They can be used to complement each other. In some instances the administration

TABLE 29-1   Blood Coagulation Factors and Synonyms

Factor	Name or synonym
I	Fibrinogen
II	Prothrombin
III	Tissue thromboplastin
IV	Calcium
V	Proaccelerin (labile factor, accelerator globulin)
VII	Proconvertin (stable factor, serum prothrombin conversion accelerator [SPCA]
VIII	Antihemophilic factor (AHF)
IX	Plasma thromboplastin component, Christmas factor
X	Stuart-Power factor
XI	Plasma thromboplastin antecedent (PTA)
XII	Hageman factor
XIII	Fibrin stabilizing factor

of both parenteral (heparin) and one of the synthetic oral anticoagulants is started simultaneously. The heparin is discontinued as soon as the prothrombin time has been sufficiently reduced and the oral compound is producing a full therapeutic effect. Heparin is needed when a rapid anticoagulant effect is required or when adequate facilities for determining the prothrombin time are unavailable (this prevents the use of one of the synthetic anticoagulants).

Heparin is usually given in a hospital setting. Oral anticoagulants are given inside and outside hospital settings.

PARENTERAL ANTICOAGULANT DRUGS

heparin sodium (Liquaemin, Hepalean✱, Unihep✱)
heparin calcium (Calciparine, Calcilean✱)

Heparin was found first in the liver and subsequently in the lungs and intestinal mucosa. It is formed in especially large amounts in the mast cells of these tissues. It has also been found in the tunica intima of blood vessels. Heparin for injection is obtained from beef lung and the mucosal lining of pig intestine.

Mechanism of action. Heparin produces its anticoagulant effect by combining with antithrombin III (heparin cofactor), a naturally occurring anticlotting factor in the plasma. This compound is unrelated to factor III (tissue thromboplastin), which is involved in blood coagulation. The binding of heparin with antithrombin III forms a complex that acts at multiple sites in the normal coagulation system. It inactivates factors IX, X, XI, and XII. Inactivation of factor Xa of the intrinsic and extrinsic pathways prevents the conversion of prothrombin to thrombin, thereby inhibiting the formation of fibrin from fibrinogen. Furthermore, by preventing the activation of factor XIII (fibrin stabilizing factor), heparin also prevents the formation of a stable fibrin clot. The drug does not have fibrinolytic activity. This means that it will not dissolve existing clots but can prevent the extension of existing clots.

The normal function of antithrombin III is to maintain intravascular fluidity of the blood. Thromboembolism frequently occurs in individuals with acquired or congenital deficiency of this plasma protein. Therefore, in the absence of antithrombin III, heparin is unable to perform its anticoagulating effect.

Indications

1. Used in the prevention and treatment of all types of thromboses and emboli.
2. Administered to patients with disseminated intravascular coagulation (DIC).
3. Used prophylactically to prevent clotting in surgery of the heart or blood vessels.
4. Used during blood transfusions and in hemodialysis to prevent blood clotting.
5. Drug of choice for sudden arterial occlusion, since its action is immediate and readily reversible if surgery becomes necessary.
6. Used in thrombophlebitis; heparin is superior to the coumarin drugs in preventing pulmonary complications.
7. Used to treat thrombophlebitis during pregnancy, since it does not cross the placental barrier and is not excreted in breast milk.
8. Used before oral anticoagulants when rapid anticoagulant action is desired (Table 29-2).

Pharmacokinetics. The large molecular size and polarity of heparin prevents gastrointestinal absorption. Therefore it is given only by the parenteral route for rapid absorption.

Onset of action. Intravenous injection—immediate; subcutaneous—usually within 20 to 60 minutes.

Half-life. Dosage dependent, averages 1.5 hours (range 1 to 6 hours).

Protein binding. Very high.

Metabolism. Liver.

Excretion. Kidneys.

Side effects/adverse reactions. See Table 29-3.

Significant drug interactions

Drug	Possible Effect and Management
aspirin or sulfin-pyrazone	Increased risk of bleeding because of platelet inhibition by these drugs. Also, large doses of aspirin may produce hypoprothrombinemia. Either drug increases the risk of toxicity due to its potential of producing gastrointestinal ulceration and bleeding. If possible, avoid this combination therapy. If necessary to give concurrently, monitor closely.

TABLE 29-2   Comparison of Characteristics of Anticoagulant Drugs

	Heparin	Coumarin and indanedione derivative
Onset of action	Immediate	Slow (24 to 48 hours)
Route of administration	Parenteral	Oral
Duration of action	Short (less than 4 hours)	Long (approximately 2 to 5 days)
Laboratory test for dosage control	APTT,* clotting time	Prothrombin time
Antidote	Protamine sulfate	Vitamin K, whole blood, or plasma
Cost	Expensive	Inexpensive

*APTT, activated partial thromboplastin time.

TABLE 29-3. Anticoagulant Agents: Side Effects/Adverse Reactions

Drug	Side effects*	Adverse reactions†
heparin		Less frequent or rare: chest pain, chills, elevated temperature, respiratory difficulties, wheezing, rash, pruritus, hives, increase in nasal secretions (allergic reaction), anaphylaxis, paresthesis of hands or feet, blue tinge on arms or legs, increased or persistent erections Early signs of overdosage: increased bruising, nosebleeds, excessive bleeding from minor cuts, wounds, brushing of teeth, or menstrual period Internal bleeding signs: stomach pain or swelling, backaches, bloody urine, bloody or black stools, dizziness, severe persistent headaches, swollen, stiff, or painful vomiting or coughing up of blood Following 6 months or more of therapy: rib or back pain, height decrease (osteoporosis), alopecia At site of injection: hematoma or blood accumulation under the skin, pain, local skin reaction such as irritation, peeling, or sloughing
anisindione		The following effects, though not yet reported with this drug, were reported with phenindione, another indanedione derivative, and may also be seen with this product: edema of face or lower extremities, unexpected weight gain, leukopenia, agranulocytosis, liver toxicity, diarrhea, nausea, vomiting, severe abdominal distress, alopecia, visual disturbances, and mouth sores.
dicumarol	More frequent: stomach gas Less frequent: anorexia, alopecia	More frequent: diarrhea Less frequent or rare: leukopenia, liver toxicity, nausea, vomiting, mouth sores, agranulocytosis
phenprocoumon	Less frequent: alopecia	Less frequent or rare: unexpected weight gain, blue-purple discoloration on toes, painful toes, leukopenia, agranulocytosis, liver toxicity, diarrhea, nausea or vomiting, abdominal cramps or distress, rash, hives, pruritus, mouth sores
warfarin	Less frequent: alopecia	Less frequent or rare: same as phenprocoumon

*If side effects continue, increase, or disturb the patient, inform the physician.
†If adverse reactions occur, contact the physician, as medical intervention may be necessary.

Drug	Possible Effect and Management
azlocillin, parenteral carbenicillin, dextran, dipyridamole, divalproex, mezlocillin piperacillin, ticarcillin or valproic acid	Increased risk of bleeding tendencies due to platelet inhibition induced by any of these drugs. Avoid concurrent therapy if possible. If necessary to give concurrently, monitor closely.
cefamandole, cefoperazone, moxalactam, or plicamycin	Increased risk of bleeding and hemorrhage possible with these drugs. These agents can cause hypoprothrombinemia and platelet inhibition, and moxalactam reportedly causes irreversible platelet damage. Avoid concurrent therapy if possible. If necessary to give concurrently, monitor closely.
methimazole or propylthiouracil	May produce a hypoprothrombinemic effect that can increase the anticoagulant effect of heparin. If necessary to give concurrently, monitor closely.
probenecid	May prolong and enhance heparin's anticoagulant effects. If necessary to give concurrently, monitor closely.
streptokinase or urokinase	Increased risk of bleeding and hemorrhage possible with this combination. Avoid concurrent usage. Some studies indicate that heparin should be given before or after thrombolytic therapy with these agents.

Dosage and administration. Dosage is expressed in USP heparin units in the United States. In Canada, dosage may be expressed in USP units or in International Units (IU).* The following recommended dosages will be given in USP units. Also, 1 mg of sodium heparin is no longer equivalent to 100 USP units. The strength of sodium heparin is labeled in USP units/ml.

Dosage is based on 150-pound (68-kg) body weight (adult).

*USP heparin units are not equivalent to International Units. Since the potency may vary between USP and IU, the student should review the current package insert for dosage instructions whenever packages are labeled in International Units.

Adults

Deep SC

Initial: 10,000 to 20,000 USP units (usually preceded by intravenous loading dose of 5000 USP units).

Maintenance: 8000 to 10,000 USP units every 8 hours or 15,000 to 20,000 USP units every 12 hours.

Intermittent IV injection. Initial: 10,000 USP units followed by 5000 to 10,000 units every 4 to 6 hours.

Continuous IV infusion. Initial bolus dose: 5000 USP units direct IV; then maintain on 20,000 to 40,000 USP units/day in 1000 ml of isotonic sodium chloride solution.

Prophylaxis of postoperative thromboembolism. SC: 5000 USP units 2 hours before surgery, then 5000 USP units every 8 to 12 hours for 7 days or until patient is ambulatory.

Open heart surgery. IV: 150 to 400 units/kg.

Disseminated intravascular coagulation. Give 50 to 100 USP units/kg every 4 hours by intravenous bolus or infusion. If no improvement is noted within 4 to 8 hours, the medication should be discontinued.

Children. IV

Initial: 50 USP units/kg.

Maintenance: 50 to 100 USP units/kg every 4 hours.

Disseminated intravascular coagulation. Give 25 to 50 USP units/kg every 4 hours. If no improvement is noted within 4 to 8 hours, the medication should be discontinued.

•   •   •

Heparin dosage is closely monitored with coagulation tests: activated partial thromboplastin time (APTT) or the Lee-White whole blood clotting time (WBCT). The heparin dosage should be adjusted to maintain the APTT between one and one-half to two times the normal control level, whereas the WBCT should be at approximately two and one-half to three times the control value.

Pregnancy safety. FDA category C.

NURSING CONSIDERATIONS

Assessment. The client should be assessed to determine that heparin is not contraindicated by preexisting conditions such as:

- Blood dyscrasias, liver disease (with hypoprothrombinemia), kidney disease, peptic ulcer, chronic ulcerative colitis, and active bleeding.
- Individuals undergoing eye, spinal cord, or brain surgery, since even minor bleeding may cause serious consequences.
- Individuals with continuous drainage of the stomach or small intestine, threatened abortion, subacute endocarditis, severe hypertension, or hypersensitivity to the drug.

Caution must be used in administering heparin to clients with any condition in which hemorrhage is possible. Use cautiously in individuals with mild hepatic or renal disease or in cases of alcoholism.

A baseline assessment should consist of an activated partial thromboplastin time (APTT) or a Lee-White whole blood clotting time (WBCT), a platelet count, and a hematocrit evaluation.

Anticipate that each dose of heparin will be individualized after the physician has evaluated the APTT or WBCT. Check to be sure that these tests are performed as ordered (before each IV or SC injection) and the results are reported promptly.

Clients over the age of 60, especially women, are more susceptible to the hemorrhagic effects of heparin.

Intervention. Heparin comes in many concentrations: carefully check the vial and the physician's order. Be alert that the heparin-lock flush solution maintains patency of the indwelling venipuncture unit and that it is not used for systemic anticoagulation.

For subcutaneous administration, use a small-gauge (25 to 27) ⅜ to ⅝ inch needle. Use a "bunching" technique (pulling the fatty layer away from the underlying tissue) or Z-track method. Inject the heparin deep into the fatty tissue above the iliac crest or into the abdominal fat layer. Avoid the umbilical veins by avoiding a 2-inch radius around the umbilicus. This distance should be maintained from scars and lesions. Do not aspirate and *do not massage the injection site.* Hold the needle in place for 10 seconds after administration and withdraw gently to minimize bruising. Apply direct pressure for 1 to 2 minutes if needed. Rotate sites to prevent the formation of hematomas. Document the location of injection sites graphically. Intramuscular injection is not recommended because it causes hematomas, irritation, and pain at the injection site and because it causes erratic absorption.

A loading dose usually precedes a continuous infusion. This IV dose may be given undiluted over at least a minute.

For continuous IV infusion of heparin, use an infusion pump or a volume control unit so that the flow rate and fluid volume of the drug can be precisely controlled. Check the system frequently to prevent overdosage or underdosage. Never piggyback other drugs into an intravenous line containing heparin, as many other drugs inactivate heparin.

For clients on intermittent heparin dosage, subcutaneously or via heparin lock, the blood samples for the APTT should be drawn ½ hour before the next dose to avoid a falsely high APTT. This false reading can also be avoided for the client with a continuous heparin infusion by drawing the sample from the arm opposite the infusion.

Although controversy exists on whether normal saline or diluted heparin solutions (10 to 100 units of heparin sodium per milliliter should be used to irrigate and maintain patency of the indwelling venipuncture device, the nurse should be aware that the purpose of the device is to maintain an open intravenous line so that ordered intermittent drugs, intravenous solutions, or both may be administered through this line. Therefore, within each clinical practice setting, obtain information about the accepted (usually medically approved) practices or policies concerning the solution to be used and how often the device should be flushed if not in frequent use; then closely monitor the unit for patency.

If heparin solution is being used to maintain the patency of an indwelling venipuncture device, usually 1 ml of heparin lock flush solution will be effective for 4 to 8 hours. If the device is being used to administer a drug that is incompatible with heparin, the device should be flushed with sterile water or 0.9% sodium chloride for injection before and after the drug is given. Inject the heparin lock flush solution after the second flush. If the device is being used to obtain blood samples for laboratory analysis and heparin might alter the results of the test, the heparin solution should be cleared from the device by aspirating and discarding 1 ml of solution from the device before the blood sample is taken. After the blood sample is drawn, the device is again filled with 1 ml of heparin lock flush solution.

Heparin is to be stopped immediately if the client complains of a chill, low back pain (sign of abdominal bleeding), or spontaneous bleeding. Notify the physician and have on hand protamine sulfate. In some cases it may be necessary to give whole blood or plasma.

Alert other staff that the client is receiving heparin (i.e., sign over the client's bed). Pressure should be applied to venipuncture and injection sites to minimize bruising. These invasive procedures should be avoided if at all possible. Consult with the physician regarding a change from intramuscular administration to other routes of administration while the client is receiving heparin.

Education. Instruct client to use a soft toothbrush for oral hygiene and an electric razor to avoid activities with a potential for injury.

Alert client not to use over-the-counter preparations containing ibuprofen, aspirin, and other salicylates. Teach the client how to read over-the-counter drug labels.

Alert client to signs of bleeding: nosebleeds, bleeding gums, petechiae, purpura, ecchymotic areas, tarry stools, hematuria, and hematemesis. Advise client to report these signs to the physician immediately.

Advise client to alert any other health care providers, such as dentists, that the drug is being taken. A medical alert bracelet or card should be carried.

Caution female clients with heavy menstrual flow; however, heparin therapy is not contraindicated if bleeding is not excessive.

Inform client of diuresis beginning 36 to 48 hours after

initial dose of heparin and lasting 36 to 48 hours following termination of therapy.

Advise client that alopecia may occur several months following heparin therapy and that the condition is reversible on discontinuation of drug.

Evaluation. Adjust heparin dosage to maintain the APTT between one and one-half and two and one-half times normal control level and WBCT between two and one-half and three times the control value, with client remaining free of signs of hemorrhage. Any value under or over this range should be reported to the physician immediately.

Test stools for occult blood daily to determine hidden bleeding.

Monitor platelet count and examine patient for possible thrombocytopenia, which may be associated with arterial thrombosis or "white clot" syndrome. Perform hematocrit tests frequently.

Be aware of the possibility of "heparin resistance" in conditions associated with infection, thrombophlebitis, fever, pleurisy, cancer, myocardial infarction, and extensive surgery.

Be aware that abrupt withdrawal of heparin may precipitate an increase in coagulability; usually a full dose of heparin is followed by oral anticoagulants for prophylaxis. Thus there generally is an overlap of both drugs for 3 to 5 days while heparin is being tapered off.

PARENTERAL ANTICOAGULANT ANTAGONIST
protamine sulfate (heparin antidote)

Protamine sulfate is a proteinlike substance derived from the sperm and mature testes of the salmon and other fish. Protamine alone is a very weak anticoagulant but will prolong clotting time; it is an antithromboplastin but is not as active as heparin. When protamine is given in conjunction with heparin, they form a combination, and each neutralizes the anticoagulant activity of the other. Because protamine is a basic protein (many free amino groups), it is able to combine with the sulfuric acids of heparin and inactivate them.

Mechanism of action. See preceding discussion. A study indicates that combining protamine and heparin dissociates the heparin–antithrombin III complex, thus reducing the anticoagulant action of heparin.

Indications. Treatment of heparin overdose and toxicity; used to neutralize the effects of heparin administered during the extracorporeal circulation involved in cardiac or arterial surgery or dialysis.

Pharmacokinetics. Administered intravenously only.

Onset of action. Within ½ to 1 minute.

Duration of action. Usually 2 hours.

Side effects/adverse reactions. See Table 29-3.

Significant drug interactions. None.

Dosage and administration. Protamine sulfate is administered intravenously. In the treatment of heparin overdosage, the extent of the overdosage can be determined from the amount of heparin given over the previous 3 or 4 hours.

The dosage ratio is 1 mg protamine to neutralize approximately 90 USP units of heparin activity derived from lung tissue or about 115 USP units of heparin activity derived from intestinal mucosa. Do not exceed 50 mg of protamine in any 10-minute period; if given 30 minutes after heparin, decrease dosage by 50%.

Children. See usual adult dosing.

Pregnancy safety. Not established.

NURSING CONSIDERATIONS

Intervention. Protamine sulfate is to be administered by a physician. The drug should be administered slowly intravenously — over 1 to 3 minutes — not more than 50 mg in any 10-minute period. Too rapid administration may cause dyspnea and shock. Emergency equipment should be available.

Evaluation. Observe client for spontaneous bleeding or heparin "rebound" (the effects of heparin last longer than the effects of protamine) following procedures involving extracorporeal circulation such as cardiac or arterial surgery or dialysis. This may occur as long as 18 hours after the initial neutralization of the heparin.

Monitor WBCT or APTT to determine protamine efficacy and dosage.

ORAL ANTICOAGULANT DRUGS

There are two major types of oral anticoagulant drugs: coumarins and indanediones.

Coumarins

     dicumoral (Dicumoral)
     phenprocoumon (Liquamar)
     warfarin sodium (Coumadin, Panwarfin, Marevan✿, Warfilone✿)

Indanediones

     anisindione (Miradon)

Mechanism of action. Both the coumarin and the indanedione derivatives interfere with liver synthesis of the vitamin K–dependent clotting factors. Thus they depress the synthesis of factors X, IX, VII, and II (prothrombin). Factor VII is depleted quickly; the sequential depletion of factors IX, X, and II follows. These agents do not affect established clots but do prevent further extension of formed clots, thereby diminishing the potential for secondary thromboembolic complications.

Indications

1. Prophylactic therapy and treatment of venous thrombosis and pulmonary embolism.
2. Prophylaxis against thromboembolism for individuals with chronic atrial fibrillation and myocardial infarction.

The major advantages associated with these drugs are that they are effective with oral administration and they need to be given only once a day when the maintenance dose has been established. (See Table 29-2.)

Pharmacokinetics

Absorption. Anisindione, phenprocoumon and warfarin are well absorbed from the gastrointestinal tract. Dicumarol absorption is slow, incomplete, and erratic from the gastrointestinal tract.

Distribution

Protein binding. Highly protein-bound (approximately 99%). (See Table 29-4 for additional pharmacokinetic information.)

         Liver.

         Kidneys.

Side effects/adverse reactions. See Table 29-3.

Significant drug interactions. See Table 29-5.

Dosage and administration. See Table 29-4.

Pregnancy safety. Not established. Both coumarin and indandione derivatives cross the placenta and should not be used during pregnancy. Fetal abnormalities and facial anomalies have been reported. Many physicians believe oral anticoagulants should not be used during pregnancy. If an anticoagulant is necessary, heparin is the drug of choice since it does not cross the placenta.

NURSING CONSIDERATIONS

Assessment. Use cautiously in individuals with allergic disorders, hazardous occupations, conditions that may increase prothrombin time (collagen diseases, disorders of the pancreas, alcoholism, hepatic and renal insufficiency), and conditions that may decrease prothrombin time (hypothyroidism, diabetes mellitus, hyperlipidemia, and hypercholesterolemia).

Contraindications include hemorrhagic tendencies, aneurysm, hemophilia, open ulcerative or visceral carcinoma, colitis, diarrhea, severe hypertension, recent surgery of spinal cord, brain, or eye, suspicion of cerebrovascular hemorrhage, subacute bacterial endocarditis, regional block anethesia, and vitamin C deficiency.

Before therapy, inquire if client is pregnant and inform her of the potential risk of congenital malformations.

Intervention. Be aware that the onset of action of oral anticoagulants is slow; therefore, heparin sodium is usually given during the first few days of treatment. Blood for prothrombin time should be drawn within 5 hours of intravenous heparin administration.

TABLE 29-4   Pharmacokinetic Activity and Dosage and Administration of Oral Anticoagulants

Generic/trade name	Onset of action (days)	Duration of action (days)	Half-life (days)	Dosage and administration
COUMARIN				
dicumarol (Dicumarol)*	1-5	2-10	1-4 (dose dependent)	Adult: 25-200 mg daily orally, as indicated by prothrombin time Children: not established
phenprocoumon (Liquamar)	2-3	7-14	6-7	Adult: 0.75-6 mg daily orally, as indicated by prothrombin time Children: not established
warfarin sodium (Coumadin)	½-3	2-5	1.5-2.5	Adult: 10-15 mg orally for 2-4 days; then 2-10 mg daily, as indicated by prothrombin time Children: not established Injectable dosage form: same dosage as oral
INDANEDIONES				
anisindione (Miradon)	2-3	1-3	3-5	Adult: 25-250 mg orally daily, as indicated by prothrombin time Children: not established

*Dicumarol activity is variable.

TABLE 29-5   Significant Drug Interactions of Oral Anticoagulants

Since the oral anticoagulants have a great potential for causing drug interactions, clients must be cautioned against taking any drug, including nonprescription or over-the-counter medications, and making significant dietary changes, without prior consultation with their physicians.

The following drugs prolong prothrombin time, thus increasing the anticoagulant effect. They often require a dosage reduction.

allopurinol	dextrothyroxine	phenytoin‡
amiodarone	diflunisal	piperacillin
anabolic steroids	dipyridamole†	plicamycin
androgens	disulfiram	propylthiouracil
aspirin	erythromycins	quinidine
azlocillin	fenoprofen	salicylates
cefamandole	gemfibrozil	sulfinpyrazone
cefoperazone	indomethacin	sulfonamides
chloral hydrate*	mefenamic acid	sulindac
chloramphenicol	methimazole	thyroid hormone
cimetidine	metronidazole	urokinase
clofibrate	moxalactam	
danazol	nalidixic acid	
dextran	phenylbutazone	

The following drugs decrease prothrombin time, thus decreasing the anticoagulant effect. An increase in anticoagulant dosage is often necessary.

antidiabetic agents§
barbiturates
carbamazepine
cholestyramine
colestipol
contraceptives, oral
estramustine
estrogens
ethchlorvynol
glutethimide
griseofulvin
primidone
rifampin
vitamin K

*Usually occurs during first 2 weeks of therapy. With chronic concurrent therapy, the increase in anticoagulant effect may return to normal or even demonstrate a decreased activity.

†Occurs usually with doses of dipyridamole over 400 mg/day.

‡Increased anticoagulant effect occurs initially. With chronic concurrent therapy the increased anticoagulant effect may demonstrate a decreased activity. May also see a decrease in metabolism of phenytoin, possibly leading to increased serum levels and toxicity.

§Oral antidiabetic agents may initially increase anticoagulant effects, but with long-term concurrent therapy, such effects may decrease. Also, the decrease in metabolism of the antidiabetic agent may increase serum levels, prolonged half-life, hypoglycemia, and toxicity.

Terminate therapy gradually over a 3- or 4-week period to prevent rebound thromboembolic complications.

Education. Once maintenance therapy is established and client is discharged, stress the importance of adherence to schedule of laboratory procedures and physician's appointments. Prothrombin time should be performed from intervals of 1 to 4 weeks, depending on dosage. Also, periodic urinalysis, blood counts, stool guaiac, and liver function tests should be performed.

Instruct client to carry an identification card that lists the client's and physician's names and phone numbers and the name and dosage of the oral anticoagulant drug.

Emphasize the importance of not taking any other medication, especially ibuprofen, aspirin, and other salicylates, without checking with the physician, since so many drugs interact with anticoagulant agents. Also, alcoholic individuals should be closely monitored because of potential for noncompliance to drug regimen.

Instruct client to stop medication and notify physician if bleeding occurs: nosebleeds, bleeding gums (use soft toothbrush), bloody sputum, hematuria (red, brown, or cloudy urine), red or black stools, petechiae, purpura, ecchymotic areas, abdominal or lumbar swelling (retroperitoneal bleeding), or severe headaches (intracranial bleeding).

Advise self-protection from injury.

Instruct client to note usual (normal) menstrual flow and, when prolonged or excessive, to notify physician.

Vitamin K_1 (phytonadione) should be readily accessible if bleeding occurs. Outpatients should carry vitamin K_1 with them and, after first consulting with the physician, take 1 to 10 mg at once if bleeding occurs. Statistics show that bleeding occurs in approximately 10% of all patients on long-term anticoagulant therapy; however, fatalities are rare.

Tell client taking phenindione that urine, when alkaline, may turn orange-red.

Advise client to use an electric razor rather than a razor blade when shaving.

Advise client of proper diet because prothrombin time is shortened by a high-fat diet or vitamin K–rich foods such as broccoli, asparagus, cabbage, cauliflower, lettuce, turnip greens, spinach, fish, liver, green tea, or coffee.

Advise client to inform dentist of medication if dental procedures are to be performed.

Instruct client not to cross legs or wear garments (girdles, knee-high stockings, or garters) that would promote venous stasis in persons with potential venous thrombosis or thrombophlebitis.

Evaluation. Anticipate that dosage is based on prothrombin time. Check to be sure that this test is performed as ordered, and report results to the physician immediately. The therapeutic aim for clients undergoing anticoagulant therapy is to produce a prolongation of the prothrombin time within one and one-half to two times the control.

ORAL ANTICOAGULANT ANTAGONIST
Vitamin K

menadiol sodium diphosphate (Synkayvite)
phytonadione (Mephyton, AquaMephyton, Konakion)

Mechanism of action. Vitamin K is essential to the hepatic synthesis of prothrombin (Factor II) and factors VII, IX, and X. It contributes to the activation of an enzyme necessary to the formation of prothrombin. Deficiency of vitamin K leads to hypoprothrobinemia and hemorrhage.

Indications. Vitamin K is used to prevent and treat hypoprothrombinemia. Prothrombin deficiency may occur because of inadequate absorption of vitamin K from the intestine (usually caused by biliary disease in which bile fails to enter the intestine) or because of destruction of intestinal organisms, which may occur with antibiotic therapy. It is also seen in the newborn, in which case it is probably caused by the fact that the intestinal organisms have not yet become established. It may result from therapy with certain anticoagulants.

Vitamin K is useful only in conditions in which the prolonged bleeding time is caused by a low concentration of prothrombin in the blood and not by damaged liver cells. Vitamin K is routinely administered to newborns to help prevent hemorrhage. Although prothrombin levels may be normal at birth, they decline until about the sixth day, when the liver is able to form prothrombin. Vitamin K may be given to the mother before delivery.

Vitamin K is also indicated in the preoperative preparation of individuals with deficient prothrombin, particularly those with obstructive jaundice. In addition, it is given as an antidote for overdosage of oral anticoagulants. It is important to measure prothrombin activity of the blood frequently when the client is receiving a preparation of vitamin K. Parenteral preparations should be administered if for some reason the intestinal absorption is impaired.

Pharmacokinetics. Natural vitamin K is normally synthesized by the intestinal flora. When synthetic forms of vitamin K are administered, the pharmacokinetics are as follows.

Absorption. Good. The absorption of phytonadione requires bile salts.

Onset of action

menadiol sodium diphosphate injectable. 8 to 24 hours.

phytonadione. Oral: 6 to 12 hours. Injectable: 1 to 2 hours. Hemorrhage is usually under control within 3 to 6 hours, whereas normal prothrombin levels are achieved within 12 to 14 hours.

Metabolism. Liver.

Excretion. Kidneys and bile.

Side effects/adverse reactions. Less frequently reported are facial flushing, taste alterations, and redness or pain at injection site.

Significant drug interactions

Drug	Possible Effect and Management
oral anticoagulants	Decreases effectiveness of the oral anticoagulant (generally used to treat overdose or toxicity with oral anticoagulants).
primaquine	May increase potential for toxicity. If drugs must be given concurrently, monitor closely.

Dosage and administration. As antidote to drug-induced hypothrombinemia.

menadiol sodium diphosphate tablets (Synkayvite)

Adults. 5 to 10 mg orally daily.

Children. Same as adult.

menadiol sodium diphosphate injectable

Adults. 5 to 15 mg intramuscular or subcutaneous, once or twice daily.

Children. 5 to 10 mg intramuscular or subcutaneous, once or twice daily.

phytonadione (Mephyton tablets or AquaMephyton injection)

Adults. 2.5 to 10 mg orally or parenterally (intramuscular or subcutaneous), up to 25 mg. The oral dose may be repeated between 12 and 48 hours if necessary. The injectable may be repeated between 6 and 8 hours if necessary.

Children. 5 to 10 mg orally. Injectable: 1 to 2 mg intramuscular or subcutaneous (infants); 5 to 10 mg intramuscular or subcutaneous (children).

NURSING CONSIDERATIONS

Assessment. Monitor prothombin time as a baseline measurement and throughout vitamin K therapy to evaluate response.

Intervention. Because vitamin K has a delayed onset, the administration of plasma or fresh whole blood may be necessary with severe bleeding.

Administer by slow intravenous infusion, over 2 to 3 hours. Protect the infusion container from light by wrapping it in aluminum foil.

Evaluation. During intravenous infusion, observe for signs of side effects such as flushing, weakness, and hypotension, and report them to the physician.

THROMBOLYTIC (FIBRINOLYTIC) AGENTS

Thrombolytic (fibrinolytic) drugs are used to treat acute thromboembolic disorders. They dissolve clots and are used in a hospital setting only by physicians who are experienced in the management of diseases caused by thrombosis. The thrombolytic drugs dissolve thrombi after their formation, unlike the coagulants, which prevent their extension. Thrombolytic enzyme therapy alters the hemostatic capability of the client more profoundly than does anticoagulant therapy. Consequently, when bleeding occurs, it is more severe and very difficult to control.

streptokinase (Streptase, Kabikinase)
urokinase (Abbokinase, Ukidan✤)

Mechanism of action. These agents dissolve clots via the endogenous fibrinolytic system. Both streptokinase

---

ATLEPLASE, RECOMBINANT (ACTIVASE, A TISSUE PLASMINOGEN ACTIVATOR [tPA]

Atleplase, recombinant, was marketed in 1988 for the emergency treatment of acute myocardial infarctions (MI). This clot-dissolving agent is administered intravenously, as soon as possible after an acute MI. This enzyme binds to fibrin-plasminogen at the site of the arterial clot, thus converting plasminogen to plasmin. Plasmin will digest the fibrin strands of the clot, thus breaking up the thrombus that is blocking the coronary artery.

The increase in oxygen flow to the area will help prevent any permanent heart muscle damage. Ventricular contractions improve, thus reducing the potential for congestive heart failure, a common and serious complication of a massive myocardial infarction.

Alteplase is most effective when given within 4 to 6 hours of the onset of MI symptoms. The benefits to patients receiving this drug after 6 hours are still under investigation. The most common complication is bleeding, both internal (gastrointestinal tract, genitourinary tract, retroperitoneal or intracranial sites) or surface sites (venous cutdowns, arterial punctures, or recent puncture sites). The major drug interactions are therefore concerned with drugs that affect bleeding or platelet function, such as aspirin, heparin, dipyridamole, coumarin, and others. Concurrent usage increases the risk of bleeding episodes.

The usual dose is 100 mg intravenously, given in divided doses (i.e., 60 mg in the first hour, 20 mg the second and third hours).

---

and urokinase can activate plasminogen. When injected, streptokinase combines with plasminogen, a circulating protein in the blood, to form a complex that is then converted to plasmin (fibrinolysin). The plasmin in turn functions as an enzyme that degrades fibrin threads (the mesh of the clot) as well as the fibrinogen, thereby causing lysis of the blood clot. Urokinase activates plasminogen by cleaving peptide bonds at two different sites. It then follows the same pathway as streptokinase in degrading the blood clot. (See Figure 29-1 for site of action: fibrin and fibrinogen.)

Indications

1. Used for lysis of acute massive pulmonary emboli.
2. Used for treatment of deep venous thrombosis involving extensive thrombi of deep veins—popliteal and proximal vessels.
3. Used for arterial thrombosis or embolism. Not used for arterial emboli emanating from left side of heart (e.g., in mitral stenosis with atrial fibrillation) because new emboli may develop.

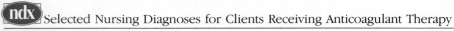

Nursing diagnosis	Outcome criteria	Nursing interventions
Tissue perfusion, alteration in: reduced blood flow (prevention and treatment of thromboembolic disorders)	Clotting studies are maintained within therapeutic range; PTT is prolonged to 1.5-2 times the control (heparin). PT is prolonged to 1.5-2 times the control (warfarin). Extension of the thrombus or embolization of thrombi does not occur.	Monitor clotting studies as ordered. Administer anticoagulent therapy and assess effectiveness. Monitor vital signs and blood pressure every 4 hours. Report immediately any change in vital signs or decrease in blood pressure. Auscultate breath sounds every 4 hours. Report the development of rales. Assess for other developments of pulmonary emboli, in addition to above, such as dyspnea, cough, or hemoptysis. Apply antiembolism stockings as ordered. Measure calf dimension, bilaterally; compare and record every 8 hours.
Injury, potential for hemorrhage	No signs of hemorrhage occur.	Administer heparin SC rather than IM to prevent hematoma formation. Inject into lower abdomen using a small-gauge needle (25-27); do not massage injection sites. Rotate sites. All personnel should be alerted that the client is on anticoagulant therapy. Venipunctures and injections should be kept to a minimum and pressure applied to prevent bleeding when they are done. Observe client for excessive bruising, bleeding gums, nosebleed, blood in urine and/or secretions, and report.
Knowledge deficit related to medication regime	Client will describe underlying condition and how the drug relates to the condition, how and when to take the medication, common drug interactions, safety precautions, common side effects, and which of these warrant reporting. Self-administer warfarin safely and accurately.	Assess learning needs and learning readiness. Plan with client for the achievement of realistic goals. Provide information to meet outcome criteria. Caution the client to use a soft toothbrush and an electric razor. Recommend to client that all health care personnel be informed of anticoagulant therapy before treatment. Advise on the importance of having blood studies done as ordered. Instruct client on the need to report any signs of bleeding.

4. Administered to clear occluded arteriovenous cannulas.

5. Employed for lysis of thrombi that obstruct coronary arteries. Presently, studies are being conducted in an attempt to evaluate use in the treatment of myocardial infarction. It is still not known if thrombolytic therapy results in the salvage of myocardial tissue or if it reduces the mortality rate.

Pharmacokinetics. Drugs are given intravenously or intraarterially.

Half-life

streptokinase. 11 to 13 minutes initially. Half-life may later increase up to 83 minutes. (A short half-life usually results from antibodies in the system from previous streptococci infections.)

urokinase. Up to 20 minutes.

Duration of effect. When agents are discontinued, the fibrinolytic effect usually disappears within a couple of hours. The thrombin time will return to less than double the normal value within 4 hours. Although rare, prolonged prothrombin times of 12-24 hours have been reported.

Excretion. Kidneys, bile.

Side effects/adverse reactions. See Table 29-6.

Significant drug interactions. See Table 29-7.

TABLE 29-6 Thrombolytic Agents: Adverse Reactions

Drug	Adverse reactions*
streptokinase and urokinase	Most frequent: stomach pain or swelling, backache, bloody urine, bloody or black stools, constipation, coughing up of blood, severe headaches, dizziness, swollen, stiff, or painful joints, painful or stiff muscles, nosebleeds, excessive bleeding from vagina, vomiting of blood or substances that look like coffee grounds, tachycardia, bradycardia, oozing of blood from cuts or scratches. Elevated temperature is more frequent with streptokinase than urokinase. Less frequent with streptokinase but rare with urokinase are flushed red skin, mild headaches or muscle pain, nausea, rash, pruritus, hives, respiratory difficulties. Rare: for streptokinase only: severe and/or sudden hypotension, shortness of breath, chest tightness, severe wheezing, or edema of eyes, face, lips, or tongue (anaphylaxis or a severe allergic reaction)

*If adverse reactions occur, contact physician because medical intervention may be necessary.

TABLE 29-7 Thrombolytic Agents: Drug Interactions

Drug	Possible effect and management
aminocaproic acid or other antifibrinolytic drugs	May inhibit effectiveness of thrombolytic agents. Reserve such drugs to treat severe bleeding induced by the thrombolytic agents.
anticoagulants (oral) or heparin	Increased risk of bleeding and hemorrhage. If possible, avoid concurrent drug administration. Anticoagulants may be given before or after thrombolytic therapy.
antiinflammatory agents, nonsteroidal, aspirin, or sulfinpyrazone	Inhibition of platelet aggregation may increase potential for gastrointestinal ulceration and bleeding. Avoid concurrent drug administration.
azlocillin, parenteral, carbenicillin, dextran, dipyridamole, divalproex, mezlocillin, pipercillin, ticarcillin, valproic acid	These drugs inhibit platelet aggregation; if used concurrently with the thrombolytic agents, they may increase the risk of severe bleeding and hemorrhage. Avoid concurrent drug administration.
cefamandole, cefoperazone, moxalactam, or plicamycin	May cause hypoprothrombinemia and platelet aggregation. Moxalactam can also cause irreversible platelet damage. Use of these drugs is not recommended because of increased risk of hemorrhage.

Dosage and administration

streptokinase for injection (Streptase, Kabikinase)
Adults
For arterial or deep vein thrombosis or pulmonary embolism: 250,000 IU initially as loading dose given over 30 minutes. Then administer 100,000 IU hourly as a continuous infusion.
For coronary artery thrombosis: 20,000 IU initially via an intraarterial catheter, followed by 2000 IU/min.
To clear an arteriovenous cannula: 100,000 to 250,000 IU instilled slowly into occluded arteriovenous cannula limb.
Children. Not established.

urokinase for injection (Abbokinase, Ukidan✸)
Adults
For acute pulmonary embolism: 4400 IU IV/kg initially over 10 minutes, followed by 4400 IU/kg/hr.

For coronary artery thrombosis: 6000 IU/min via an intraarterial line. Lysis of a coronary artery thrombus usually requires an average total dose of 500,000 IU. Usually the medication is given for up to 2 hours.
To clear an IV catheter: instill 1 ml of a 5000 IU/ml dose of urokinase into the catheter.
Children. Not established.
Pregnancy safety. Streptokinase, FDA category A; urokinase, FDA category B.

NURSING CONSIDERATIONS

Assessment. Note that thrombolytic therapy is contraindicated in individuals with recent (past 2 months) cerebrovascular accident or intracranial or intraspinal surgery, active internal bleeding, and intracranial neoplasm.

Use with caution in high-risk clients with recent (within past 10 days) surgery, obstetric delivery, serious gastrointestinal bleeding, organ biopsy, previous puncture of noncompressible vessels, recent trauma including cardiopulmonary resuscitation, severe, uncontrolled hypertension, suspected left heart thrombus involving mitral stenosis with atrial fibrillation, subacute bacterial endocarditis, hemostatic defects including secondary to severe hepatic and renal disease, pregnancy, diabetic hemorrhagic retinopathy, evidence of cerebrovascular disease, other conditions in which bleeding causes a significant hazard or would be difficult to control because of its location, septic thrombosis, or serious infection at the site of occluded atrioventricular cannula.

Before thrombolytic therapy, thrombin time (TT), activated partial thromboplastin time (APTT), prothrombin time (PT), and hematocrit and platelet count must be performed.

Intervention. Thrombolytic therapy is administered only by a physician who is experienced in management of thrombotic diseases and where skilled personnel and laboratory resources are available. Also, typed and crossmatched whole blood and packed red cells should be available in case of hemorrhage.

Follow manufacturer's instructions when reconstituting and diluting drug to minimize flocculation (i.e., fibrin formation):

- *Streptokinase.* Slowly add 5 ml of sodium chloride injection or 5% dextrose injection, directing the stream toward the side of the vial rather than into the powder. Do not shake the vial but gently roll and tilt it for reconstitution (i.e., returning a substance altered for storage nearly to its original state). Note that shaking may cause foaming and increase flocculation. Then slowly dilute the entire contents of the vial to a total of 45 ml or, if necessary, up to 500 ml in 45 ml increments. If solution is not used soon after reconstitution, store at 2° to 4° C, and use within 24 hours. Note that a patient with a recent streptococcal infection may require a higher loading dose because of higher resistance levels.
- *Urokinase.* Add 5.2 ml of sterile water (not bacteriostatic water) for injection immediately before use. Then for intravenous infusion, dilute reconstituted powder with 0.9% sodium chloride injection to a total volume of 195 ml. Discard the unused portion of the reconstituted material.

Do not administer by intramuscular injection because of the danger of hematoma. In addition, use venipuncture sites as seldom as possible, and perform this procedure with care. Maintain pressure dressings at the site for at least 30 minutes, and check frequently for bleeding.

Start streptokinase therapy as soon as possible after the thrombotic event, preferably within 7 days. If after 4 hours of therapy, thrombin time is less than one and one-half times the normal control value, discontinue therapy.

For arteriovenous cannula occlusion, administer heparinized saline solution to clear the cannula. If adequate flow is not reestablished, use streptokinase.

To prevent bruising during therapy, avoid unnecessary handling of patient. The side rails of the client's bed should be padded.

Following completion of thrombolytic therapy, begin continuous intravenous infusion of heparin (without a loading dose) when thrombin time has decreased to less than twice the normal control value (usually within 4 hours after completion of the infusion). Use an infusion pump for heparin. Later give the client oral anticoagulant therapy, a procedure that prevents the recurrence of thrombosis.

Evaluation. Observe client carefully during early phase of therapy for allergic reactions. With urokinase, relatively mild reactions (e.g., bronchospasm, skin rash) are reported. Streptokinase may produce more serious reactions and possibly anaphylaxis. (See allergic effects under side effects/adverse reactions.) If allergic manifestations occur, discontinue infusion and treat with epinephrine, antihistamines, and corticosteroids. If fever occurs, treat symptomatically with acetaminophen.

Monitor vital signs frequently (i.e., pulse rate, temperature, respiratory rate, and blood pressure), at least every 4 hours. To avoid possible dislodgment of deep vein thrombi, do not take blood pressure in the lower extremities.

Monitor client carefully for bleeding: every 15 minutes for the first hour, every 30 minutes for the next 8 hours, and every 4 hours until therapy is discontinued. The physician should be notified immediately if bleeding occurs.

Observe extremities and palpate pulses of affected extremities every hour. The physician should be notified immediately if there are signs of circulatory impairment.

In addition to observing for overt bleeding, observe client for internal bleeding—bloody sputum, hematuria, hematemesis, dark stools (i.e., guaiac positive), flank and abdominal pain, and neurologic changes. For uncontrollable bleeding, stop treatment and administer whole blood (fresh blood if available), packed red cells, cryoprecipitate or fresh-frozen plasma, and aminocaproic acid.

Observe client carefully for dysrhythmias during and after intracoronary infusion of streptokinase. Rapid lysis of coronary thrombi has caused atrial and ventricular dysrhythmias.

Continue to observe client for bleeding during and

after treatment. Because the thrombolytic effects of the drug last for several hours, the sites of invasive devices are common areas for hematoma formation.

Following therapy, monitor fibrinogen levels—which are decreased by thrombolytic agents—until they return to normal.

ANTIHEMOPHILIC AGENTS

Hemophilia is a hereditary disorder caused by a deficiency of one or more plasma protein clotting factors. This condition usually leads to persistent and uncontrollable hemorrhage after even minor injury. The symptoms include excessive bleeding from wounds and hemorrhage into joints, urinary tract, and on occasion the central nervous system. There are two types of hemophilia: hemophilia A, the classic type, in which factor VIII activity is deficient, and hemophilia B, or Christmas disease, in which factor IX complex activity is deficient. In recent years a correct diagnosis of the coagulation disorder has led to specific factor replacement therapy, and this medical advance has resulted in effective management of the client at home.

factor VIII (Factorate, Hemofil-T, Humafac, Koāte, Profilate)

Mechanism of action. In the intrinsic pathway of the coagulation mechanism, antihemophilic factor (AHF), or factor VIII, is required for the transformation of prothrombin to thrombin. In the treatment of hemophilia A administration of factor VIII is based on replacement of this missing plasma clotting factor. Thus AHF specifically corrects or prevents bleeding episodes in individuals with only hemophilia A.

Indications. See preceding.

Pharmacokinetics. When administered intravenously, factor VIII is rapidly cleared from the plasma following administration.

Half-life. Average 4 hours (range 4 to 24 hours).

Side effects/adverse reactions

Side effects. Mild allergic reactions, bronchospasm, elevated temperature, chills, or rash may occur.

Adverse reactions. Many of the following reactions may be directly related to the rate of infusion: headache, increased heart rate, tingling of fingers, fainting, lethargy, sedation, hypotension, back pain, nausea or vomiting, visual disturbances, chest constriction.

Significant drug interactions. None.

Dosage and administration. Dosage of factor VIII must be individualized according to the individual's weight, severity of the deficiency, and the amount of hemorrhage. The prophylactic dose is 250 units/day for clients weighing less than 50 kg and 500 units/day for heavier individuals. During hemorrhage, the dosage is adjusted so that a level of at least 40% of normal can produce hemostasis. Clients who develop inhibitors to factor VIII may not respond to factor VIII therapy. After careful evaluation of the client, the administration of anti-inhibitor coagulant complex, which reduces factor VIII inhibitors, may be indicated to correct this condition.

Pregnancy safety. Not established.

NURSING CONSIDERATIONS

Assessment. Weigh the benefits of antihemophilic factor against the risk of hepatitis associated with its administration.

Obtain baseline values of coagulation studies and vital signs before administering antihemophilic factor. If the pulse increases significantly, reduce the rate of the administration or stop the drug.

Intervention. Vaccinate the client against hepatitis B, as ordered, using hepatitis B vaccine inactivated. Since factor VIII is prepared from human plasma, the risk of transmitting hepatitis exists.

Refrigerate the concentrate, but do not freeze it until ready for use. Do not refrigerate after reconstitution, as the active ingredient may precipitate. Warm the concentrate and diluent to room temperature before reconstitution. Gently rotate (do not shake) vial containing the concentrate and diluent until it is completely dissolved. This may take as long as 5 to 10 minutes. Since the antihemophilic factor is filtered before administration, the active components would be filtered out if it is not fully dissolved. Although antihemophilic factor remains stable for 24 hours at room temperature after reconstitution, it should be used within 3 hours. Do not mix with other medications.

Antihemophilic factor is for intravenous infusion only. Use only plastic syringes to prepare for administration, since the solution adheres to the ground surfaces of glass syringes.

Evaluation. Monitor vital signs over the course of the drug's administration. Adverse effects are related to the rate of administration. Periodic coagulation studies will determine the efficacy of the drug with each client.

antiinhibitor coagulant complex (Autoplex, Feiba VH Immuna)

Antiinhibitor coagulant complex is made from pooled human plasma. It contains variable quantities of clotting factors and kinin system factors and has been standardized to help correct clotting time in factor VIII–deficient individuals or to treat factor VIII–deficient individuals who have plasma-containing inhibitors to factor VIII.

Mechanism of action. See preceding discussion.

Indications. For individuals with factor VIII inhibitors who are bleeding or are being prepared for surgery. Approximately 10% of factor VIII–deficient individuals have inhibitors to factor VIII present. Generally clients with factor VIII inhibitor levels greater than 10 Bethesda units are treated with this product.

Pharmacokinetics. Not available.

Side effects/adverse reactions. Allergic reactions and hypersensitivity (increased temperature, chills, rash, blood pressure alterations, and anaphylaxis reported). If administered too rapidly, recipient may experience flushing, headache, and changes in blood pressure and rate. These are warnings to slow down or stop the infusion until symptoms disappear.

Significant drug interactions. Concurrent administration with epsilon-aminocaproic acid or tranexamic acid is not recommended.

Dosage and administration. By intravenous infusion only. The recommended dose varies from 25 to 100 units/kg, depending on site and severity of the hemorrhage. Check current package insert for specific recommendations.

Pregnancy safety. FDA category C.

factor IX complex (Konȳne H.Ti, Profilnine, Proplex SX-T)

Factor IX Complex is a purified plasma fraction prepared from pooled units of plasma. It contains factors II, VII, IX, and X, which are known as the vitamin K coagulation factors. This agent is used for therapy in individuals with a deficiency of these factors during hemorrhage or before surgery. It is also indicated for hemophilia B in which factor IX is deficient.

Mechanism of action. See preceding discussion.

Indications. Factor IX complex is used to prevent or control bleeding in individuals with factor IX deficiency. It is also used to treat clients with bleeding problems who have inhibitors to Factor VIII and will reverse hemorrhage induced by coumarin anticoagulants.

Pharmacokinetics

Half-life. Approximately 24 hours.

Side effects/adverse reactions. Thrombosis or disseminated intravascular coagulation (DIC) has occurred. Factor IX should not be used in individuals undergoing elective surgery, since they are at a greater risk for thrombosis.

Chills and fever have been reported, especially when large doses are given. Also, if the intravenous infusion is given too rapidly, headache, flushing, rash, nausea, vomiting, sedation, lethargy, elevated temperature, and tingling have been reported. The infusion should be stopped, and in most clients it can be resumed at a much slower rate.

Significant drug interactions. None.

Dosage and administration. By intravenous injection (slowly) or intravenous infusion. The dosage is individualized according to the client's coagulation assay, which is performed before treatment. Check current package insert for specific recommendations. To reverse bleeding induced by coumarin anticoagulants, a dose of 15 units/kg is usually administered.

Pregnancy safety. Not established.

NURSING CONSIDERATIONS

The considerations are as for factor VIII, except for instructions for preparation.

Factor IX is administered intravenously or by intravenous infusion only at a rate not to exceed 3 ml/min. Warm diluent to room temperature before reconstitution. Gently rotate mixture in vial until it is completely dissolved, or the active components will be filtered out when it is administered through the filter needle. Although stable for 12 hours at room temperature, it should be used within 3 hours of reconstitution. Do not refrigerate reconstituted preparation, since the active ingredients may precipitate.

HEMOSTATIC AGENTS

Hemostatic agents are compounds used to hasten clot formation to reduce bleeding. The purpose of these agents is to control rapid loss of blood.

SYSTEMIC HEMOSTATICS

aminocaproic acid (Amicar, Epsikapron♣)

Mechanism of action. Aminocaproic acid is a synthetic compound that inhibits fibrinolysis when excessive bleeding occurs. This drug acts as a competitive antagonist of plasminogen, preventing the generation of plasmin and thereby inhibiting the dissolution of clots. To a lesser degree, it may inhibit plasmin (fibrinolysin) by noncompetitive mechanisms.

Indications. Used in the treatment of fibrinolysis-induced hemorrhage such as fibrinolytic bleeding following heart surgery, prostatectomy, nephrectomy, and hematologic disorders such as aplastic anemia, hepatic cirrhosis, and neoplastic disease states. It has also been used as a specific antidote for an overdose of thrombolytic drugs such as streptokinase and urokinase, even though this use is not approved.

Pharmacokinetics

Absorption. Good following oral administration.

Time to peak concentration. Within 2 hours after one oral dose.

Therapeutic serum concentration. 130 μ/ml to inhibit systemic hyperfibrinolysis.

Side effects/adverse reactions. See Table 29-8.

Significant drug interactions. None.

Dosage and administration

aminocaproic acid syrup/tablets

Adults. 5 g orally initially, followed by 1 g (tablet or syrup) or 1.25 g (syrup) hourly for up to 8 hours or until the desired response is achieved. Maximum dose is 30 g/24 hours.

Children. 100 mg/kg or 3 g/m² initially, followed by 33.3 mg/kg or 1 g/m²; do not exceed 18 g/m²/24 hours.

aminocaproic acid injection

Adults. 4 or 5 g by intravenous infusion given over 1 hour, then 1 g/hr may be given for up to 8 hours or until the desired response is obtained. Maximum is up to 30 g/24 hr.

Children. 100 mg/kg or 3 g/m² initially by intravenous infusion over 1 hour, followed by a continuous infusion of 33.3 mg/kg or 1 g/m²/hr. Do not exceed 18 g/m²/24 hours.

Pregnancy safety. Not established.

NURSING CONSIDERATIONS

Assessment. Aminocaproic acid is contraindicated for use in clients with active intravascular clotting. It is used cautiously in individuals with cardiac, hepatic, or renal disease or those with a predisposition to thrombosis.

Assess baseline vital signs and coagulation studies initially and periodically during administration.

Intervention. Dilute before administering intravenously. Administer slowly, since too rapid infusion may result in hypotension or bradycardia. Take care with insertion and positioning of the infusion needle to minimize thrombophlebitis.

Evaluation. Monitor client for signs of thromboembolic complications such as thrombophlebitis, pulmonary embolus, myocardial infarction, and cerebrovascular accident.

tranexamic acid (Cyclocapron)

Mechanism of action. At regular dosages tranexamic acid is a competitive inhibitor of plasminogen activation; at high doses, it is a noncompetitive inhibitor of plasmin. Its effects are similar to aminocaproic acid, but it is approximately 10 times more potent in vitro.

Indications. Used for short periods (such as 2 to 8 days) in clients with hemophilia to prevent or reduce bleeding episodes. Also used during and after tooth extraction in clients with hemophilia.

Pharmacokinetics

Absorption. Fair after oral administration (approximately 30% to 50% absorbed).

Peak plasma level. 3 hours after a 1 g oral dose, reaching 8 mg/l level; following a 2 g dose, a 15 mg/l level is achieved.

Duration of action. In tissues approximately 1.7 hours; in serum, 7 or 8 hours.

Excretion. Kidneys.

Side effects/adverse reactions. Nausea, vomiting, or diarrhea may occur but will usually disappear if dosage is reduced. Giddiness or dizziness is reported infrequently. With intravenous injection, hypotension may be observed if injection is given too rapidly.

Significant drug interactions. None.

Dosage and administration. For dental extractions in clients with hemophilia, give 10 mg/kg intravenously before surgery; after surgery, give 25 mg/kg orally three or four times a day for 2 to 8 days. An alternative method is to give 25 mg/kg orally three or four times a day, starting 1 day before surgery; then follow the recommendations listed previously for after surgery.

For clients with renal impairment, follow dosage recommendations as described in manufacturer's literature.

Pregnancy safety. Not established.

TOPICAL HEMOSTATICS

absorbable gelatin sponge (Gelfoam)

Absorbable gelatin sponge is a specially prepared form of

TABLE 29-8   Aminocaproic Acid: Side Effects/Adverse Reactions

Drug	Side effects*	Adverse reactions†
aminocaproic acid (Amicar, Epsika-pron✿)	Headache, dizziness, nausea, abdominal pain, diarrhea, bloodshot eyes, tinnitus, rash, and stuffy nose	Complaints of weakness or severe muscle pain; decreased urination; edema of face, feet, or lower legs; or unusual weight increase (renal failure); slow or irregular heart rate or increased weakness usually results from too fast drug administration

*If side effects continue, increase, or disturb the patient, inform the physician.
†If adverse reactions occur, contact physician because medical intervention may be necessary.

nonantigenic gelatin that is capable of holding many times its weight in whole blood. It is used in thin strips to control capillary bleeding and may be left in place in a surgical wound. It is completely absorbed in 4 to 6 weeks. It should be well moistened with isotonic saline solution or thrombin solution before it is applied to a bleeding surface. Its presence does not induce excessive scar formation. Sterile technique must be used to avoid infection.

Mechanism of action. When inserted into cavities or tissue spaces, the gelatin sponge reduces bleeding by acting as a tampon. The contact with the sponge damages platelets, liberating thromboplastin that is needed for clot formation.

This product completely dissolves within 2 to 5 days when applied to bleeding areas on skin or in nose, rectum, or vagina.

Indications. Surgical procedures as adjunct to hemostasis when bleeding is not controlled by ligature or when such methods are impractical. Also used by dentists to aid in hemostasis and in open prostatic surgery. Insertion of the gelatin sponge in the prostatic cavity promotes hemostasis.

Pharmacokinetics. See preceding discussion.

Side effects/adverse reactions. May provide site for infection. Monitor closely.

Significant drug interactions. None.

Dosage and administration. Available in different sizes and diameters. Application instructions and size depend on area to be treated.

NURSING CONSIDERATIONS

Monitor client for signs of infection or recurrent bleeding.

absorbable gelatin film (Gelfilm)

A sterile absorbable gelatin film (Gelfilm) is also available for specific indications, as in neurosurgery, thoracic, or ocular surgery. When implanted in tissues, the rate of absorption could range from 1 to 6 months, depending on the site of implantation and the size of the film implanted. This product is useful as a dural substitute (neurosurgery) or to repair pleural defects during thoracic surgery.

absorbable gelatin powder (Gelfoam)

A sterile absorbable gelatin powder (Gelfoam) is also available to promote hemostasis. This powder can be made into a paste to control bleeding from bone areas when standard procedures such as ligatures are ineffective or not practical. It is also used to treat chronic leg ulcers and decubitus ulcers.

oxidized cellulose (Novocell, Oxycel, Surgicel)

Oxidized cellulose is a specially treated form of surgical gauze or cotton that exerts a hemostatic effect but is absorbable when buried in the tissues.

Mechanism of action. The hemostatic action is caused by the formation of an artificial clot by cellulosic acid. Absorption of oxidized cellulose occurs between the second and the seventh days following implantation, although absorption of large amounts of blood-soaked material may take 6 weeks or longer. Oxidized cellulose is valuable in controlling bleeding in surgery of organs such as the liver, pancreas, spleen, kidney, thyroid, and prostate. Its hemostatic action is not increased by the addition of other hemostatic agents. It should not be used as a surface dressing except for the control of bleeding, because cellulosic acid inhibits the growth of epithelial tissue. Since it interferes with bone regeneration, it should not be implanted in fractures.

Indications. See preceding discussion.

Pharmacokinetics. See preceding discussion.

Side effects/adverse reactions. Serious adverse reactions are related to site of application, amount used, and pressure applied to blood vessel or specific area. Careful application and monitoring are necessary to reduce complications such as obstruction, necrosis, and stenosis. When used following nasal polyp removal or hemorroidectomy, a burning sensation has been reported. Headache, stinging, and sneezing may also occur.

Significant drug interactions. None.

Dosage and administration. Use sterile techniques in applying or inserting the cellulose. Do not moisten.

Pregnancy safety. Not established.

microfibrillar collagen hemostat (Avitene)

Mechanism of action. This is an absorbable topical hemostatic substance that, when placed on a bleeding surface, will attract platelets and platelet aggregation in the area, forming a thrombi.

Indications. Adjunct to hemostasis during surgery when ligature or standard procedures are not effective or impractical.

Pharmacokinetics. See preceding discussion.

Side effects/adverse reactions. Adhesions, allergic or foreign body reactions, hematomas, or infections such as abscesses may occur. Monitor closely, as these conditions may cause serious problems.

Significant drug interactions. None.

Dosage and administration. Generally it is applied directly on the source of bleeding in a dry form. Do not moisten or wet this substance, and do not resterilize it. Apply pressure over the area with a dry sponge for a minute or more. Use dry forceps to handle, as it will adhere to wet gloves or instruments. Do not use gloved fingers to apply the necessary pressure.

Pregnancy safety. Not established.

negatol (Negatan)

Negatol (Negatan) is a colloid preparation used as a styptic (astringent and hemostatic) to control minor bleeding from the vagina, cervix, and vulva. It does not control bleeding from large blood vessels. A 1:10 dilution is applied in the vagina. To avoid soiling of clothing, a perineal pad is usually worn by the patient.

thrombin (Thrombinar, Thrombostat)

Thrombin is a hemostatic agent prepared as a sterile powder obtained from bovine prothrombin that has been treated with thromboplastin in the presence of calcium.

Mechanism of action. Thrombin catalyzes the conversion of fibrinogen to fibrin. It has several additional mechanisms, which may include stimulating the release reaction and aggregation of platelets.

Indications. Topically to treat capillary bleeding. It has been used during various surgeries with absorbable gelatin sponge for hemostasis.

Pharmacokinetics. Usually 2 US units are needed to clot 1 ml of oxalated human plasma.*

Side effects/adverse reactions. Some febrile reactions and an allergic type reaction when used for epistaxis have been reported.

Significant drug interactions. None.

Dosage and administration. May be applied topically as a powder or solution. Concentration of the preparation varies with its use. See package insert.

Pregnancy safety. Not established.

NURSING CONSIDERATIONS

Assessment. Ascertain whether the client is sensitive to bovine products.

Intervention. Do not inject thrombin into large blood vessels, since extensive intravascular clotting and even death may result.

Sponge — do not wipe — all blood from recipient surface before applying the thrombin as a powder or a solution. If applied as a powder, it may need to be pulverized with a sterile instrument before use. Do not sponge once the thrombin is applied to avoid disturbing the clotting.

Thrombin may be used in association with absorbable gelatin foam. In this case, the saturated sponge is applied to the bleeding area for 10 to 15 seconds to promote hemostasis.

Following reconstitution, use solution within a few hours or freeze and use within 48 hours.

Evaluation. Monitor client for recurrent bleeding.

---

*One US unit is equivalent to 1 National Institute of Health (NIH) unit.

BLOOD AND BLOOD COMPONENTS

The bloodstream is the main mode of transport and distribution in the body. As such, it functions to deliver vital nutrients, water, and oxygen from the digestive and respiratory systems to all body parts. Wastes are retrieved for excretion by the bloodstream. In the kidneys, the bloodstream provides the hydrostatic pressure necessary to create urine as an excretory vehicle for those waste products. It conveys hormones from endocrine glands and enzymes, vitamins, buffers, and other biochemical substances to target areas. The bloodstream buffers and regulates the body's heat-exchange processes by absorbing and transferring core body heat to the surface for dissipation, and it buffers the body's acid-base balance. The bloodstream also carries components such as platelets, blood cells, and antibodies to sites where a sudden need for these exists, as in hemorrhage, inflammation, or infection. It creates oncotic or colloid osmotic pressure to regulate the volume of interstitial fluids. It also transports therapeutic additives such as medications, fluids, electrolytes, and nutrients to their respective sites of action.

ABNORMAL STATES OF BLOOD COMPONENTS

Normally, a thrifty bodily balance is maintained between the production and loss, attrition, or excretion of all components that comprise the bloodstream. Pathology results from a disturbance in production or an excessive loss or excretion of one or more components. Hemorrhage results in a generally impoverished bloodstream and may significantly alter many body functions. Impaired production or increased destruction of any one component may impinge on one or more functions. All this is a matter of degree. If the impairment is minor or is detected early, correction of the cause and replenishment by natural or therapeutic means may restore functioning. Naturally harmful or foreign substances also may build up in the bloodstream when excretory systems fail (e.g., renal failure) or when metabolizing capabilities fail (e.g., liver failure). Some examples follow.

Depending on the individual's size and preexisting blood integrity, acute whole blood loss of more than 500 ml is manifested by signs of anemia. Chronic, gradual, unnoticed blood loss from gastrointestinal tract malignancy, ulcers, or hemorrhoids may be compensated for naturally, or iron deficiency anemia may develop. Signs of anemia usually reflect the true importance of red blood cell loss. Deficiencies in intake or functioning of certain essential nutritional elements may result in iron deficiency anemia or one of the megaloblastic anemias, which usually are caused by deficiencies in vitamin B_{12} or folic acid. A pathologic overabundance of erythrocytes can be compensation for long-standing hypoxia from pulmonary or cardiac disease, certain tumors, or polycythemia vera.

Delayed or disordered production of erythrocytes (aplastic anemia) may result from disorders of the reticuloendothelial system, primarily the bone marrow, which is responsible for their systematic production. The bone marrow is particularly vulnerable to certain drugs, poisons, and antineoplastic agents. On the other hand, too-rapid destruction of erythrocytes can lead to hemolytic anemia.

Leukocytes also are lost in hemorrhage, but reductions in their numbers most often are associated with certain specific conditions. Each of the five types of white blood cells—neutrophils, eosinophils, basophils, lymphocytes, and monocytes—is associated with different disorders. For example, abnormally low neutrophil counts are associated with certain aplastic diseases, as well as with acute reactions to such drugs as sulfonamides, propylthioracil, and chloramphenicol. Excessively high neutrophil counts primarily are found with bacterial infections, as well as with some inflammatory disorders, leukemia, and hyperplastic disorders.

Thrombocytes also may be present in inadequate numbers because of their rapid destruction, typically caused by idiopathic thrombocytopenia purpura. Conversely, excessive platelet counts are associated most often with hyperplastic disorders, iron deficiency anemia, splenectomy, and chronic inflammatory conditions such as tuberculosis. Other factors crucial to the clotting process may be absent in hemophilia and similar disorders.

Losses of the liquid portion of the blood can create dehydration problems, impede metabolic processes that function only through use of hydrogen or oxygen molecules, or subvert hydrodynamic and hydraulic processes.

In addition to hemorrhage, plasma proteins may be lost through burn wounds or wound drainage or may be insufficient because adequate available substrates such as amino acids are lacking. The results vary, depending on the type of plasma protein, and may include deficiencies in immune status, blood viscosity, or colloid osmotic pressure (oncotic pressure).

BLOOD AND BLOOD COMPONENT REPLACEMENT THERAPIES

Therapy to replace all or certain components of the bloodstream is a common practice in most health facilities. Since blood is considered a tissue, transfusions are technically tissue transplants. The usual treatment of choice is replacement of the sole blood component that is deficient rather than whole blood, since the body is better able to replace intravascular fluids than formed elements of the blood. Transfusing only the depleted blood fraction serves two other purposes: (1) it prevents the fluid overload in high-risk individuals such as the elderly and those with cardiovascular or renal disease, and (2) it more effi-

ciently uses the remaining blood fractions for other clients needs. Table 29-9 outlines indications for this therapy. When a client is to receive blood, the nurse is largely responsible for its safe administration.

NURSING CONSIDERATIONS

Assessment. Take client history regarding previous transfusions and the client's response to them. Report any history of an adverse reaction to the physician and the blood bank.

Gather baseline data about the client's blood studies and vital signs before administration and observe the general appearance and demeanor of the client.

Intervention. Administer blood components promptly to ensure that the transfused product is fresh, uncoagulated, and without toxic breakdown products. Before administration, the product should remain out of the blood bank's refrigerator and untransfused for no longer than 30 minutes. Refrigeration in the standard hospital units or home refrigerator will not prevent deterioration. Blood and blood components must not lie unused at the nursing station but must be returned to the blood bank refrigerator if not administered within half an hour. A unit of whole blood or packed RBCs cannot be returned to a blood bank if it has been out of a monitored environment (1° to 6° C) for more than 30 minutes. Whole blood or packed red blood cells should be transfused within 2 hours, 4 hours at the most.

Since incompatibility is a possibility, especially after multiple doses of these products, take such precautions as scrupulously comparing the product ordered and the label on the product before administration. Often the worst adverse reactions to blood transfusions result from misidentification of the blood or client. Although procedures of various institutions vary, at least two persons, often two registered nurses, must verify the identification of blood product and client. Client identification must match, as well as the prescriber's name, blood type, Rh factor, and unit number. Note Venereal Disease Research Laboratories' (VDRL) information and expiration date. Compare the client's identifying armband or tag to the label on the container.

Nurses should be aware of transfusion hazards in certain blood-type combinations. Careful typing and cross-matching help to prevent serious complications (see "Nursing Considerations"). ABO antigen-antibody reactions result from the following and must be avoided:

Recipient's Blood Type	Should Not Receive
A	Type B or AB
B	Type A or AB
O	Any except type O

TABLE 29-9   Indications for Common Blood Component Therapies

Component	Indications
Whole blood	Hemorrhage, hypovolemic shock
Fresh whole blood	Multiple transfusions, exchange transfusions; priming agent for hemodialysis machines (normal saline also may be used)
Packed red blood cells	Transfused when whole blood could result in circulatory overload
Deglycerolized or washed red cells	Transfused when hypersensitivity reactions are likely; as in immunosuppressed patients and those with history of reactions or extreme hypersensitivity
Fresh-frozen plasma (FFP)	Clotting deficiencies, especially factors V and VII; blood volume expansion in burns, shock, or protein deficiencies (believed to be overused for these deficiencies)
Plasma exchange (plasmapheresis): blood drawn off, cleansed, and components returned	Immune-related disorders: multiple myeloma, glomerulonephritis, systemic lupus erythematosus, rheumatoid arthritis, myasthenia gravis
Plasma expanders (Dextran—large polysaccharide polymer)	Temporary volume expansion in hemorrhagic shock states (sole use for Dextran 70 or 75); not a substitute for blood or plasma NOTE: Unexplained adverse reactions (1983) within minutes of administration of Dextran 40 or 70 included dyspnea, flushing, rash, fever, oliguria, dysrhythmias and most frequently, hypotension. Three deaths occurred. Injection of 20 ml of Dextran 1 over 2 minutes before other Dextran infusions decreased incidence of severe side effects
Granulocytes	Granulocyte counts below 500
Platelets	Platelet counts at or below $20,000/mm^3$
Cryoprecipitate (fresh-frozen plasma precipitate; contains factors I and VIII)	Hemophilia, fibrinogen deficiency, von Willebrand's disease
Antihemophilic factor (AHF) concentrate Factor VII	Treatment of hemophilia; preferred over FFP
Factor IX complex	Hemophilia B; deficiencies of clotting factors II, VII, X; coumarin overdose
Plasma protein fraction (PPF)	Hypovolemic shock; protein replacement; burns; adult respiratory distress syndrome, dehydration, and hypoalbuminemia; as additive to complement packed cells when necessary
Fibrinogen	When fibrinogen levels insufficient for adequate control of bleeding
Albumin	Blood volume expansion by oncotic pressure; serum levels less than 3.5 g/dl reduction, prevention of cerebral edema
Gamma globulins	Exposure to hepatitis; to prevent complications of mumps

Recipient's Blood Type	Reactions with Multiple Transfusions
A	Type O
B	Type O
AB	Type A, B, or O

Immediately report to the blood bank any discrepancies between the information on the compatibility tag, the unit of blood, and the physician's order on the clinical record; blood that is past its expiration date; or any signs of contamination.

Hypersensitivity is also common, since most of these products are essentially foreign proteins. Exceptions include autologous transfusions collected previously from the patient's own blood or transfusions of inert, synthetic products. Twenty-five milligrams of diphenhydramine in-

jected into blood transfusion tubing before the transfusion or taken orally is recommended to prevent allergic reactions.

Return the product to the blood bank or laboratory if the contents appear unusual because of discoloration, gas bubbles, or an overfull (gaseous) appearance. Mix the contents by gently upending the container once or twice, taking care not to bruise or damage blood cells or other fragile components by squeezing or agitating the bag carelessly.

Note that many of these agents require the concomitant use of a 170 μg filter incorporated into the transfusion tubing to remove the debris and tiny clots found in the blood. Check the filter often to ensure that it is not clogged and slowing the transfusion. If the rate of transfusion is too slow, it may be necessary to use a filter with a larger surface area. This may also be necessary when administering packed RBCs because of the viscosity of the product. Access to the vein should be provided by a needle no smaller than 19 gauge and fresh tubing. For adults with small veins and for children, a 22- or 23-gauge needle is recommended. A normal saline solution should be hung in tandem with the blood product using a Y-set multiple lead tubing. Use the saline solution to flush the tubing before connecting it to the insertion site. Using straight tubing limits the possibility of stopping the transfusion while keeping the vein open if the client has an untoward response to the blood. Piggybacking on an established intravenous line increases the risk of contamination, especially with the administration of multiple units of blood.

Infuse approximately 60 ml of saline through the tubing before and after the transfusion. Do not use dextrose and other solutions with red blood cell products, since they may react with the product in the tubing to clump cells and cause hemolysis.

When inserting the spike of the administration set into the port of the blood bag, guide it straight into the container to avoid puncturing the side of the bag.

Note that infusion pumps specifically for maintaining transfusion rates are safe and reliable when used with appropriate tubing and filters. Raising the height of the container or applying a pressure sleeve to the bag (at pressures up to 300 mm Hg) is also useful to maintain transfusion flows at prescribed rates. Higher pressures may burst the bag.

To maintain the prescribed infusion rate, agitate the blood by inverting the bag frequently during administration.

If a rapid transfusion is to be made through a CVP line, a blood-warming device (up to 37° C or 98.6° F) will be necessary.

Do not administer any medications through the same tubing while any blood products are infusing.

Documentation should include the client's baseline vital signs before the transfusion was started; the signatures of the two persons who identified the client and the blood product; the blood product administered; the time the transfusion was started and completed; the total volume of fluid transfused, listing the starter solution separately; the client's response to the transfusion; and any nursing intervention taken in response to an adverse response to the blood.

Be aware that the risks of nursing personnel contracting diseases such as acquired immune deficiency syndrome (AIDS) or hepatitis when accidentally injected with pooled blood, especially repeatedly, are not entirely known. Therefore, take care when manipulating these products and their equipment.

Education. Explain the transfusion procedure to the client, especially the reason it has been ordered. Many elderly clients associate blood transfusion with being critically ill and may be upset about the need for a blood transfusion. Ensure that a consent form for the procedure has been signed.

Instruct the client to report any symptoms of an adverse reaction, such as nausea, chills, burning sensations, or headache.

Evaluation. As administration begins, observe the client closely for reactions for 15 minutes or more while the flow rate is kept at 20 to 30 drops/min. Assess vital signs several times during the first 15 minutes. If reactions occur, stop the transfusion and administer prescribed corrective measures. Symptoms of reactions may include:

- Apprehension; restlessness; flushed skin; increased pulse and respiratory rates; burning sensations; fever; chills; dyspnea; chest, head or back pain; shock—hemolysis (possible blood type incompatibility)
- Rash; swellings of the skin, face, or throat; pruritus; shock—hypersensitivity reaction
- Fever and chills starting 1 hour after administration and lasting up to 10 hours—febrile reaction
- Nausea, weakness, jaundice considerably later—possible viral hepatitis
- Fever and chills, hypotension, vomiting, abdominal pain, bloody diarrhea—bacterial contamination
- Dyspnea, tight chest, cough with basilar rales, pulmonary edema—circulatory overload
- Cyanosis, dyspnea, abrupt onset of localized pain, shock—air embolism
- Frequent assessment of the needle insertion site is essential, since absorption of infiltrated blood is very slow.

If no symptoms of reactions appear after the first 15 minutes, the flow rate may be calculated and set so that therapy is concluded in 1½ to 2 hours (volumes usually are between 250 and 500 ml). Continue monitoring vital signs and observing for symptoms throughout administration.

One unit of whole blood typically raises the average adult's hemoglobin level by 1 to 1.5 g/dl and the hematocrit by 2% to 3%.

KEY TERMS

embolus, page 539
hemostasis, page 539
platelet adhesion, page 540
platelet plug, page 540
thrombus, page 539

BIBLIOGRAPHY

American Hospital Formulary Service: AFHS Drug Information '87, Bethesda, 1987, American Society of Hospital Pharmacists, Inc.

Berkman, S.A.: The spectrum of transfusion reactions, Hosp. Pract. 19(6):205, 1984.

Camesas, A.M.: Anticoagulation and cardiovascular disease: determining therapeutic options, Hosp. Formul. 20(12):1238, 1985.

Cooper, J.W., Jr.: Anticoagulant drug interactions. 1. Nurs. Homes 34(5):17, 1985.

Cooper, J.W., Jr.: Anticoagulant drug interactions. 2. Nurs. Homes 34(6):15, 1985.

Cunliffe, M.T., and others: How to clear catheter clots with urokinase, Nursing 16(12):40, 1986.

Cygenski, J.M., and others: The case for heparin flush, Am. J. Nurs. 87(6):796, 1987.

Davis, K.G.: The blood story. IV. Adverse reactions to blood transfusion, Aust. Nurses J. 15(6):40, 1986.

Davis, K.G.: The blood story. III. The storage and administration of blood and blood products, Aust. Nurses J. 15(5):40, 1985.

Davis, R.B.: Anticoagulation therapy: rationale and guidelines in thromboembolic disorders, Consultant 25(8):47, 1985.

Elguidi, A.S., and others: Pulmonary embolism: evaluation and management, Hosp. Formul. 21(6):688, 1986.

Gever, L.N.: Embolex: to prevent a double post-op danger . . . DVT and pulmonary embolism, Nursing '86 16(5):73, 1986.

Gever, L.N.: Anticoagulants: and what to teach your patient about them, Nursing '84 14(11):64, 1984.

Gever, L.N.: Stopping bleeding with aminocaproic acid, Nursing '84 14(9):8, 1984.

Gilman, A.G., and others: Goodman & Gillman's The pharmacological basis of therapeutics, ed. 7, New York, 1985, Macmillan Publishing Co.

Goodwin, S.A.: Drug-induced coagulation alterations, CCQ 7(4):1, 1985.

Hall, J.R., and others: Urokinase therapy for massive pulmonary embolism, CCQ 7(4):69, 1985.

Herfindal, E.T., and Hirshman, J.L.: Clinical pharmacy and therapeutics, ed. 3, Baltimore, 1984, Williams & Wilkins.

Hirsh, J., and others: Treatment of venous thromboembolism. Chest 89(5):426S, 1986.

Hull, R.D., and others: Prophylaxis of venous thromboembolism: an overview, Chest 89(5):374S, 1986.

Jaques, L.B.: The new understanding of the drug heparin, Chest 88(5):751, 1985.

Jowett, N.I., and others: Do indwelling cannulae on coronary units need a heparin flush?, Intensive Care Nurs. 2(1):16, 1986.

Kafer, E.R., and others: Using blood components, part 2, Emerg Med. 17(14):46, 1985.

King, N.H.: Controlling bleeding when the platelet count drops, RN 47(8):25, 1984.

Kloch, S.M., and others: Oral medications affecting blood coagulation, Plast. Surg. Nurs. 4(2):52, 1984.

Lancier, W.C., and others: How to administer blood components to children, MCN 12(3):178, 1987.

Masoorli, S.T., and Piercy, S.: A lifesaving guide to blood products, RN 47(9):32, 1984.

McConnell, E.A.: APIT and PT: the tests of time, Nursing 16(5):47, 1986.

McMahan, B.E.: Why deep vein thrombosis is so dangerous, RN 50(1):20, 1987.

McVan, B.W.: How we give blood transfusions at home, RN 50(8):79, 1987.

Moake, J.L., and others: Thrombotic disorders, Clin. Symp. 37(4):3, 1985.

Murphy, M.: Blood component theory, Emergency 16(3):58, 1984.

PDR: Physicians' desk reference, ed. 41: Oradell, N.J., 1987, Medical Economics Co., Inc.

Peck, N.L.: Action STAT! Blood transfusion reaction, Nursing 17(1):33, 1987.

Phillips, A.: Are blood transfusions really safe?, Nursing 17(6):63, 1987.

Querin, J.J., and Stahl, L.D.: 12 simple steps for successful blood transfusions, Nursing 13(11):34, 1983.

Rimar, J.M.: Heparin, MCN 10(3):197, 1985.

Royal Melbourne Pharmacy Department, Amalgamated Melbourne and Essendon Hospitals: Oral anticoagulants—advice to patients, Aust. Nurses J. 16(8):52, 1987.

Sacher, R.A.: Hemostasis and hypercoagulability: laboratory tests for cost-effective evaluation, Consultant 26(11):60, 1987.

Sipperly, M.E.: Thrombolytic therapy update, Crit. Care Nurse 5(6):30, 1985.

Todd, B.: Use heparin safely, Geriatr. Nurse 8(4):48, 1987.

Turpie, A.G.G., and others: Venous thromboembolism: current concepts, part 2, Hosp. Med. 20(11):13, 1984.

United States Pharmacopeial Convention: Drug information for the health care provider, ed. 7, Rockville, Md., 1987, U.S. Pharmacopeial Convention, Inc.

Vanbree, N.S., and others: Clinical evaluation of three techniques for administering low-dose heparin, Nurs. Res. 33(1):15, 1984.

Vitello-Ciccini, J.: Thrombolytic therapy-urokinase, J. Cardiovascul. Nurs. 1(2):59, 1987.

Weinstein, S.M.: Thrombolytic therapy, NITA 9(1):31, 1986.

Antihyperlipidemic Drugs

OBJECTIVES

After studying this chapter, the student will be able to:

1. Define hyperlipidemia and describe the pathophysiology of this condition.

2. Identify the four types of lipoproteins and differentiate according to their lipid content.

3. Discuss the importance of combining dietary modifications with drug therapy to treat hyperlipidemia.

4. Utilize the appropriate nursing considerations with clients receiving antihyperlipidemic agents.

Antihyperlipidemic or antilipemic drugs are used along with dietary modifications to modify a condition known as **hyperlipidemia.** This is a metabolic disorder characterized by increased concentrations of cholesterol and triglycerides, two of the major serum lipids in the body.

Both clinical and experimental studies offer evidence that an important relationship exists between **atherosclerosis** and high levels of circulating triglycerides and cholesterol. Atherosclerosis is a disorder involving the large- and medium-sized arteries. Lipids are deposited in the lining of these blood vessels, eventually producing degenerative changes and obstructing blood flow. Atherosclerosis is a causative factor in coronary artery disease and myocardial infarction, in cerebral arterial disease that results in senility or cerebrovascular accidents, in peripheral arterial occlusive disease (which may cause gangrene and loss of limb), and in renal arterial insufficiency. It is also a factor in hypertension. Therefore there is intensive research to develop more effective and safer antihyperlipidemic drugs. If serum lipid or blood lipid levels could be controlled within normal limits, the development and progression of atherosclerosis might be inhibited or prevented.

That a positive relationship exists between high serum lipid levels and atherosclerosis is controversial. Some individuals with high serum lipid levels have no objective evidence of atherosclerosis, whereas others with marked atherosclerotic signs and symptoms have normal serum lipid levels. However, more persons with high blood lipid levels have atherosclerosis than those with so-called normal blood lipid levels. Consequently, some researchers and clinicians believe that if lipid levels can be controlled, so can the atherosclerotic process. At the present time the available antihyperlipidemic drugs are also controversial, and their place in drug therapy requires more long-term critical studies. None of the antihyperlipidemic or antilipemic drugs is thought to have any effect on reversing the atherosclerotic process once it has begun. Means of preventing atherosclerosis remain obscure. Multicausative factors are undoubtedly involved and include dietary saturated fats, faulty fat metabolism, genetic influence, and other factors as yet unknown.

HYPERLIPIDEMIC DISORDERS

Lipid compounds do not circulate freely in the bloodstream but rather are bound to plasma proteins (albumin, globulin), which act as carriers. These complexes are called **lipoproteins.** Hyperlipoproteinemia is always associated with an increased concentration of one or more lipoproteins, particularly cholesterol.

Classification of lipoproteins. Lipoprotein complexes are classified according to their densities and electrophoretic mobilities. Paper electrophoresis is a process by which the blood lipid fraction is separated and identified; it includes alpha (most mobile of the moving particles), beta, and prebeta (least mobile of the moving particles) lipoproteins. The density of lipoproteins varies with the proportion of lipid to protein. The larger the size of the particle, the lower the density.

The major groups of lipoproteins are classified into four types and are listed according to their lipid composition:

1. **Chylomicrons.** The chylomicrons are the largest particles and the least dense of the lipoproteins. They consist of 85% to 95% triglycerides and 3% to 5% cholesterol. In a normal person they are produced in the small intestine during absorption of a fatty meal and are cleared from the bloodstream by the enzyme lipoprotein lipase after 12 to 14 hours. A deficiency of the enzyme is rare, but when present, it results in increased levels of chylomicrons, causing a disease called exogenous hyperlipoproteinemia. This condition is usually found in children, but it may also be induced by alcoholism. Therapy is aimed at keeping the diet low in fat. Chylomicrons lack eletrophoretic mobility.

2. **Very low-density lipoproteins (VLDLs).** VLDLs or prebeta lipoproteins, contain a large amount of triglycerides (64% to 80%) and 7% to 14% cholesterol, which is formed in the liver from endogenous fat sources.

3. **Low-density lipoproteins (LDLs).** LDLs, or beta lipoproteins, contain the major portion of cholesterol in blood and may be considered the most harmful. They consist of 40% to 50% cholesterol and 7% to 10% triglycerides. An elevation of LDL levels suggests that an individual has a high potential risk for developing atherosclerosis.

4. **High-density lipoproteins (HDLs).** HDLs, or alpha lipoproteins, which are the smallest and most dense of lipoproteins, contain about 17% to 20% cholesterol and 1% to 7% triglycerides. HDL appears to be beneficial. The higher the HDL levels, the lower the potential risk for developing cardiovascular disease. HDL is protective because it picks up cholesterol and triglycerides from the body cells of membranes and carries them back to the liver, where they are metabolized and then excreted. This transport mechanism prevents the accumulation of lipids in the arterial walls, thereby providing protection against the development of coronary artery disease. It has now been found that physical exercise is beneficial because it elevates the HDL levels.

At present the lipid disorders are classified into six types, each of which may be identified by a generic name (Table 30-1). Table 30-1 also lists the elevation of the lipoprotein pattern and the treatment of each type. Although the incidence is rare, it is important to describe briefly the existence of intermediate-density lipoproteins (IDLs) or broad-beta lipoproteins. As VLDL loses its triglycerides, it is converted into IDL and then into LDL, with a resultant chemical composition between the two lipoproteins. IDL consists of an elevation of endogenous triglycerides and carries about 30% cholesterol. Like VLDL, it tends to be atherogenic. Normally, IDL is not found in plasma in significant amounts.

Many drugs may affect serum levels of LDL cholesterol, HDL cholesterol, and triglycerides; Table 30-2 contains a listing.

Government review and guidelines. In the early 1980s, a random sample survey of physicians was conducted by the National Heart, Lung and Blood Institute. The survey revealed that 50% to 75% of physicians surveyed failed to provide diet instructions or prescribe drugs for clients with high serum cholesterol levels, persons at high risk for coronary artery disease (CAD) or stroke. This indicated clearly the need for more definitive educational programs for both health care professionals and the general public.

Then in 1985, the National Institute of Health organized the National Cholesterol Education Program. A primary goal of this program was to have all Americans 20 years old or older tested for total cholesterol levels. Those found to be at high risk for CAD would be advised to obtain medical help. Guidelines were developed and criteria for identification, treatment, and monitoring of individuals were issued in 1987 (See box on p. 565 for NIH adult recommendations of risk classification and cholesterol levels).

TABLE 30-1   Classification and Treatment of Hyperlipidemic Disorders

Type	Generic name	Elevated lipoprotein pattern	Elevated Cholesterol	Elevated Triglycides	Incidence	Treatment Diet	Treatment Drugs
I	Exogenous hyperli-pemia	Chylomi-crons		↑	Rare	Very low fat: 25-35 g/day; high carbohy-drate	None
IIa	Familial hypercholes-terolemia	LDL (beta lipo-pro-teins)	↑		Com-mon	Low cholesterol (300 mg/day); low saturated fat; high un-saturated fat	cholestyramine, colestipol, dex-trothyroxine, neomycin, nico-tinic acid, pro-bucol, sitosterols
IIb	Combined hyperlipo-proteinemia	LDL + VLDL	↑	↑	Com-mon	Low cholesterol; high unsatu-rated fat; re-duce obesity	nicotinic acid, pro-bucol
III	Broad-beta hyperlip-idemia (familial dysbeta-lipoprotei-nemia)	IDL (broad-beta lipo-proteins	↑	↑	Rare	See IIb	clofibrate, nicotinic acid
IV	Endogenous hyperli-pemia	VLDL (pre-beta lipo-proteins)		↑	Com-mon	Low carbohy-drate; high unsaturated fat; low cho-lesterol and alcohol; re-duce obesity	clofibrate, gemfi-brozil, nicotinic acid
V	Mixed hyperlipemia	VLDL + chylomi-crons	↑	↑	Rare	Low fat and car-bohydrate; high protein; low alcohol	clofibrate, nicotinic acid

TABLE 30-2   Drugs and Serum Lipids

Drug(s)	LDL cholesterol	HDL cholesterol	Triglycerides
barbiturates	+*	+	
beta blocking agents (with exception of labetalol)		−	+
corticosteroids	+		+
oral contraceptives	+		−
phenytoin		+	
phenothiazines	+		
thiazide diuretics	+		+

*+, Increase; −, decrease.

Treatment recommendations are based on the client's cholesterol level and the presence of CAD or two other risk factors, such as smoking, hypertension, family history of CAD, male sex, obesity, and lack of exercise. Borderline individuals with CAD or at least two other risk factors present were advised to have an LDL cholesterol level performed. The primary goals are as follows:

1. Individuals with borderline total cholesterol (200 to 239 mg/dl) with no CAD or less than two risk factors should receive dietary instructions and be reevalu-

ated in 1 year. The minimum goal is to lower their LDL cholesterol to below 160 mg/dl.
2. Individuals with borderline cholesterol results and CAD or two or more risk factors, with an LDL cho-lesterol up to 160 mg/dl, should be given dietary instructions and additional advice if necessary for risk factors that are present. Their goal is to lower the LDL cholesterol to less than 130 mg/dl by diet.
3. Individuals at high risk should have an LDL choles-terol level performed. If CAD or at least two other

---

NIH ADULT RECOMMENDATIONS OF RISK CLASSIFICATION AND CHOLESTEROL LEVELS

RISK	TOTAL CHOLESTEROL (mg/dl)	LDL CHOLESTEROL (mg/dl)
Desirable	Below 200	Below 130
Borderline/high risk	200-239	130-159
High risk	240 or greater	160 or greater

---

risk factors are present and their LDL cholesterol level is up to 190 mg/dl, then medication is indicated to lower the LDL cholesterol level to less than 130 mg/dl. If the individual did not have CAD or less than two risk factors, then the goal is to lower the LDL cholesterol level to less than 160 mg/dl.

The student is referred to the reference by Naito (1987) for a detailed review of drug application, current drug application, and management.

Antihyperlipidemic agents offer the client a pharmacologic method for reducing serum lipid levels and ideally reducing the risk of atherosclerosis with its many complications. Use of antihyperlipidemic agents is reserved for clients who have specifically been identified at significant increased risk (see box above) and are unable to satisfactorily lower their serum lipid levels through exercise, diet, and other nondrug methods. Drug therapy for these clients augments their therapy aimed at lowering serum lipids and cardiovascular risk.

BILE ACID SEQUESTERING AGENTS

cholestyramine (Questran)
colestipol hydrochloride (Colestid)

Mechanism of action. Cholestyramine and colestipol are nonabsorbable anion-exchange resins. They are also called bile acid sequestrants. These drugs are used for their cholesterol-lowering effects. Cholesterol is the major precursor of bile acids that normally are secreted from the gallbladder and liver into the small intestine. Here, the bile acids perform two functions: (1) they emulsify fat present in food to facilitate chemical digestion and (2) they are required for absorption of lipids (including fat-soluble vitamins A, D, E, and K). After their physiologic performance, the major portion of the bile acids is returned to the liver.

As anion-exchange resins, these drugs combine with bile acids in the intestine, thus preventing their absorption and producing an insoluble complex that is excreted in the feces. To compensate for the loss of bile acids removed by the drugs, the liver increases the rate of oxidation of cholesterol by converting more sterol to bile acids. Subsequently, the long-term fecal loss of bile acids causes a reduction of serum cholesterol levels and low-density (beta) lipoprotein.

In individuals with partial biliary obstruction, excess bile acids may be deposited in the dermal tissues, resulting in pruritus. Since cholestyramine increases fecal bile acid excretion, it can alleviate this condition.

Indications. Both cholestyramine and colestipol are used in the treatment of hyperlipidemia of the primary hypercholesterolemia type (type IIa). Cholestyramine is also indicated as an antidiarrheal agent for diahrrea caused by bile acids (not for common diahrrea), an antipruritic (for pruritus caused by cholestasis), and an antidote for negatively charged and other medications (e.g., digoxin, oral penicillins, tetracyclines, and thyroid medication).

Pharmacokinetics

Absorption. These drugs are not absorbed from the gastrointestinal tract.

Onset of action. Usually within 24 to 48 hours after initiation of therapy a decrease in plasma cholesterol concentration is noted.

Time to peak effect. With cholestyramine, plasma cholesterol levels may continue to fall for up to a year. After the initial decrease, plasma cholesterol levels in some individuals may increase to previous levels or even exceed these levels with continued therapy. Close monitoring for effectiveness is necessary.

Diarrhea induced by increased bile acids will respond to cholestyramine within 24 hours, whereas pruritus caused by cholestasis usually takes 1 to 3 weeks of therapy before a response is noted.

Colestipol's peak effect is noted within 1 month. After the initial decrease in cholesterol, some clients may exhibit an increased cholesterol level that equals or surpasses the previous level.

Duration of action. After withdrawal of cholestyramine, plasma cholesterol levels will increase in about 2 to 4 weeks. Pruritus will return in about 1 to 2 weeks after discontinuance of the medication.

Side effects/adverse reactions. See Table 30-3.

Significant drug interactions

Drug	Possible Effect and Management
oral anticoagulants, coumarins or indanediones	Concurrent usage significantly decreases absorption of oral anticoagulants and vitamin K. Coumarins may reduce effectiveness of the anticoagulant while indanediones may enhance anticoagulant effects. It is suggested that oral anticoagulants be administered at least 6 hours before cholestyramine or colestipol. Monitor prothrombin time frequently and closely, since dosage adjustments may be necessary.

TABLE 30-3   Antihyperlipidemic Agents: Side Effects/Adverse Reactions

Drug	Side effects*	Adverse reactions†
BILE ACID SEQUESTERING AGENT:		
cholestyramine	Most frequent: gas or indigestion, nausea or vomiting, abdominal pain Less frequent: diarrhea, bloated or distended stomach	Most frequent: constipation Rare: severe abdominal pain with nausea and vomiting (gallstones, pancreatitis), increased weight loss, black stools (gastrointestinal bleeding or peptic ulcers)
clofibrate	Most frequent: diarrhea, nausea Less frequent and rare: tenderness or muscle pain, muscle cramping, increased fatigue, impotence, headache, increased appetite or weight gain, abdominal pain or gas, vomiting, mouth and lip sores	Rare: edema of lower extremities; decreased, painful, or bloody urination; chest pain; respiratory difficulties; increased temperature; chills; sore throat; irregular heart rate; severe abdominal pain with nausea and vomiting
colestipol	Less frequent: distended stomach, gas, diarrhea, nausea or vomiting, abdominal pain	Most frequent: constipation Rare: same as cholestyramine
dextrothyroxine		Rare: chest pain; increased, very fast, or irregular heart rate; abdominal pain with nausea and vomiting Drug overdose: appetite changes, altered menstrual cycle, diarrhea, increased temperature, hand tremors, headache, increased heat sensitivity, increased anxiety, leg cramps, shortness of breath, rash, pruritus, insomnia, tachycardia, increased sweating, flushing, vomiting, weight loss, increased urination
gemfibrozil	Less frequent: muscle ache and cramping, nausea or vomiting, rash, diarrhea, abdominal gas, pain or distress	Rare: increased temperature, chills, sore throat, severe abdominal pain with nausea and vomiting (gallstones)
niacin (nicotinic acid)	Less frequent: increased feelings of warmth, flushing or red skin on face and neck, headache With high doses: diarrhea, dizziness, dry skin, nausea or vomiting, abdominal pain	Rare: skin rash, pruritus, wheezing (seen mostly after intravenous administration—anaphylactic reaction) High doses may be associated with: elevated serum glucose levels, hyperuricemia, dysrhythmias, liver toxicity
probucol	Most frequent: increased gas production, diarrhea, nausea and vomiting, abdominal pain or distress Less frequent: dizziness; headache; paresthesia of fingers, toes, or face	Rare: edema of face, hands, feet, or mouth (angioneurotic edema)
ENZYME INHIBITOR		
lovastatin	Most frequent: increased gas, stomach pain or cramps, rash, constipation or diarrhea, nausea, headaches	Need to monitor its usage to determine additional side effects or adverse reactions

*If side effects continue, increase, or disturb the client, inform the physician.
†If adverse reactions occur, contact physician, since medical intervention may be necessary.

Drug	Possible Effect and Management	Drug	Possible Effect and Management
digitalis glycosides, especially digitoxin	Half-life of digitalis glycosides as well as gastrointestinal absorption may be reduced. It is recommended that cholestyramine or colestipol be administered at least 8 hours after digoxin to reduce the potential for interactions. Also, if cholestyramine or colestipol is discontinued with a client also taking a digitalis product, monitor the individual closely for digitalis toxicity.	oral penicillin G, oral tetracyclines, or oral vancomycin	Decreased absorption of antibiotics has been reported. Give such medications several hours before or after cholestyramine or colestipol. Whenever possible, give antibiotics first.
		Thyroid hormones	Decreased absorption of thyroid products is reported. Give thyroid first on the medication administration schedule, then give cholestyramine or colestipol several hours later.

Dosage and administration
cholestyramine

Adults. For hyperlipidemia or pruritus give 4 g initially orally, three times daily, before meals. Dosage may be adjusted according to individual's response. For maintenance give 4 g orally three or four times daily, before meals and at bedtime. Maximum daily dosage for antihyperlipidemia is 24 to 32 g, for antipruritus it is up to 16 g.

Children. Dosage is not established for children up to 6 years old. For those 6 to 12 years old give 80 mg/kg orally or 2.35 g/m^2 orally, three times daily. For children over 12 years old use adult schedule.

colestipol hydrocholoride (oral suspension)

Adults. For hyperlipidemia give 15 to 30 g orally before meals in two to four divided dosages.

Children. Dosage is not established.

Pregnancy safety. Not established.

NURSING CONSIDERATIONS

Assessment. Ascertain whether client has a preexisting condition for which the drug would be used with great caution or contraindicated.

Use with caution in clients with gastrointestinal disorders, especially in individuals with clinically symptomatic coronary artery disease, osteoporosis, bleeding disorders, steatorrhea, hemorrhoids, and impaired renal function and with the elderly.

These drugs are contraindicated for use in clients who have hypersensitivity to bile acid sequestrants and complete biliary obstruction. Safe use by pregnant women, lactating mothers, and children is not established.

Determine baseline serum cholesterol and triglyceride levels before drug therapy, and continue to monitor them periodically at regular intervals.

Intervention. Administer the drug before meals.

Mix powder by sprinkling it on the surface of 2 to 6 ounces of a preferred liquid or semiliquid (e.g., beverages, hot cereals, thin soups, pulpy fruit) to increase palatability of the drug. Allow drug to sit on the surface of the liquid for 1 to 2 minutes before stirring to prevent lumpiness. Be sure the drug is thoroughly mixed, since it does not dissolve. Incomplete mixing of the dry form may result in mucosal irritation and esophageal impaction, or it may be accidentally inhaled.

Rinse the glass or cup with a small amount of liquid and have the client drink it to ensure the complete dose is taken.

Because resins interfere with absorption of other drugs when taken concurrently, administer the other drugs 1 hour before or 4 to 6 hours following cholestyramine or colestipol.

Education. Warn client that sudden withdrawal of res-

ins could lead to uninhibited absorption of other drugs taken concomitantly, resulting in overdosage or toxicity.

Usually, supplemental parenteral or water-miscible vitamins A, D, E, and K and also folic acid are prescribed to avoid vitamin deficiencies in clients receiving long-term therapy. Instruct individual to report immediately early symptoms of bleeding: petechiae, ecchymoses, bleeding from mucous membranes of gums or nose, or tarry stools (which indicate hypoprothrombinemia). Administration of vitamin K$_1$ (parenteral) and vitamin K$_2$ (oral) may be necessary.

Encourage client to observe bowel habits and to adhere to a high-bulk diet (e.g., grains, fruits, raw vegetables) and an increased fluid intake as adjunctive therapy to the drug. If constipation occurs, dosage may be lowered to prevent fecal impaction, or a stool softener or laxative may be prescribed. Instruct individual to report gastrointestinal symptoms to the physician: gastric distress, nausea and vomiting (pancreatitis), unusual weight loss (steatorrhea), and sudden back pain (osteoporosis in postmenopausal women).

Evaluation. Monitor serum cholesterol and triglycerides at regular intervals. Drug is withdrawn if response is unsatisfactory after 3 months of therapy.

Monitor cardiac glycoside levels in clients receiving both drugs simultaneously. To avoid toxicity, adjust dosage of cardiotonic glycoside before discontinuing anion-exchange resin.

clofibrate (Atromid-S, Claripex✦, Novofibrate✦)

Mechanism of action. Clofibrate is more effective in reducing very low–density lipoproteins (VLDLs) rich in triglycerides than in lowering low-density lipoproteins (LDLs) high in cholesterol. The exact mode of action of the drug is unknown, but it appears to block synthesis of triglycerides in the liver by increasing catabolism of VLDLs to LDLs. In addition, the drug inhibits early cholesterol formation in the liver and promotes fecal excretion of the neutral sterols. Clofibrate also possesses platelet-inhibiting effect (e.g., decreases platelet adhesiveness), but this action is not significant enough to warrant its use as an antiplatelet drug.

Indications. Treatment of hyperlipidemia (type III)

Pharmacokinetics

Absorption. Slowly but well absorbed orally

Distribution

Protein binding. Very high

Time to peak plasma concentration. 2 to 6 hours following a dose

Time to peak effect. With long-term therapy, within 3 weeks

Onset of action. Reduction of plasma VLDL concentrations is seen within 2 to 5 days.

Half-life. Half-life for a single dose in a healthy individual is 6 to 25 hours; for a single dose in an anuric individual it is 113 hours; and at steady state in a healthy individual half-life is 54 hours.

Metabolism. Liver and gastrointestinal tract

Excretion. Kidneys

Side effects/adverse reactions. See Table 30-3.

Significant drug interactions. When clofibrate is given with oral anticoagulants, coumarin- or indanedione-type, an increased anticoagulant effect is reported. Monitor prothrombin times closely, since the anticoagulant dosage may need to be decreased significantly.

Dosage and administration

Adults. Clofibrate dosage for hyperlipidemia is 1.5 to 2 g orally daily in two to four divided doses. Maximum dosage is usually 2 g/day.

For the adult with impaired renal or liver function clofibrate dosage should be reduced significantly. In individuals with cirrhosis, recommended dosage is 50% of usual adult dosage.

Children. Dosage is not established.

Pregnancy safety. Not established.

NURSING CONSIDERATIONS

Assessment. Perform appropriate laboratory studies, and obtain personal family and complete health history. Because of genetic tendency of the disease, children and other family members should be screened for abnormal lipid levels.

Inquire if client is pregnant. Strict birth control measures must be observed to prevent damage to the fetus. Drug must be withdrawn at least 2 months before conception.

Use with caution in clients with peptic ulcer because the drug may reactivate a previous ulcer.

Do not use in clients who are pregnant and in lactating women, in individuals with clinically significant hepatic or renal dysfunction, and in individuals with primary biliary cirrhosis because drug may raise the already elevated cholesterol level.

Intervention. Administer drug with meals to prevent gastric distress.

Control diabetes mellitus and hypothyroidism if present.

Education. Before initiating clofibrate therapy, advise client to adhere to diet prescribed by physician. The diet is usually low in fats, cholesterol, and/or sugars. Encourage weight reduction and physical exercise.

During the first and second months of therapy, a decrease in serum lipid levels indicates a therapeutic response. Warn client that a paradoxic rise may occur in 2 or 3 months, but afterward a further decrease is customary.

Instruct client to keep clinical appointments. If serum cholesterol and triglyceride levels are not lowered within

3 months, discontinue drug therapy. Initially, these levels are performed every 2 weeks for the first few months and then at monthly intervals.

Advise client to report flu-like symptoms (muscular aching, soreness, cramping). This condition may be remedied by dosage reduction. Instruct individual to check with physician about alcohol intake since its use may be restricted to prevent hypertriglyceridemia.

There is no substantial evidence that the drug reduces the incidence of coronary artery disease or fatal myocardial infarction. Further, an increased incidence of cardiac dysrhythmias, thromboembolism, intermittent claudication, and angina has been reported in clients treated with clofibrate.

Evaluation. Since clofibrate may increase the risk of biliary diseases such as cholelithiasis and cholecystitis, perform appropriate diagnostic tests if signs and symptoms of biliary disease occur.

Evaluate both liver and renal function tests, complete blood counts to detect anemia or leukopenia (fever, chills, sore throat), and blood sugar tests. In diabetic individuals, drug may produce hyperglycemia and glycosuria. Withdraw drug if any of the test results are abnormal.

Use with caution in clients with a history of jaundice or hepatic disease since the drug may cause hepatic impairment. An elevation of serum transaminase levels and abnormal results of other liver function tests require withdrawal of the drug.

dextrothyroxine (Choloxin)

Mechanism of action. Dextrothyroxine's mechanism of action as an antihyperlipidemic agent is not fully understood. Dextrothyroxine appears to act in the liver to increase formation of LDL and, to a greater extent, to increase the breakdown of LDL. The result is an increased excretion of cholesterol and bile acids via bile into the feces, which results in a decrease in serum cholesterol and LDL.

A definite relationship exists between thyroid function and serum cholesterol levels. Hypothyroidism is associated with high serum cholesterol levels, and administration of thyroid hormones lowers serum cholesterol. Dextrothyroxine apparently stimulates the liver to increase the rate of oxidation of cholesterol, and it promotes biliary excretion of cholesterol and its byproducts.

Indications. Dextrothyroxine is used for hyperlipidemia (type IIa) in conjunction with other medications.

In the past it was used to treat hypothyroidism in individuals with known cardiac disease who could not tolerate other thyroid preparations. Today this usage is not prevalent because safer and more effective agents are available.

Pharmacokinetics

Absorption. 25% of drug absorbed from the gastrointestinal tract

Distribution
Protein binding. High

Peak effect. As an antihyperlipidemic agent, 1 to 2 months

Duration of action. 6 weeks to 3 months after the drug is withdrawn

Metabolism. Liver

Excretion. Kidneys and feces

Side effects/adverse reactions. See Table 30-3.

Significant drug interactions

Drug	Possible Effect and Management
oral anticoagulants, coumarins, or indanediones	Action of oral anticoagulant may be potentiated. Monitor prothrombin times closely and adjust oral anticoagulant dosage as necessary.
cholestyramine or colestipol	Concurrent administration may reduce absorption of dextrothyroxine. Administer dextrothyroxine approximately 4 to 5 hours before or after cholestyramine or colestipol.

Dosage and administration
Adults. For hyperlipidemia initially give dextrothyroxine, 1 to 2 mg/day orally. Increase by 1-mg to 2-mg increments per month to minimum effective dose. Maximum dosage recommended is 8 mg/day.

Children. Give 0.05 mg/kg orally or 1.5 mg/m^2 orally daily. Increase by 0.05 mg/kg increments at monthly intervals up to the minimum effective dosage. Maximum dosage recommended is 4 mg/day. Maintenance dosage for children is 0.1 mg/kg or 3 mg/m^2 orally daily.

Elderly. Use caution in dosages for elderly persons, since they are much more sensitive to thyroid hormones. Monitor therapy closely.

Pregnancy safety. Not established

NURSING CONSIDERATIONS

Assessment. Perform appropriate laboratory studies, and obtain personal family and complete health history. Because of genetic tendency of the disease, children and other family members should be screened for abnormal lipid levels.

Inquire if client is pregnant. Strict birth control measures must be observed to prevent damage to the fetus. Drug must be withdrawn at least 2 months before conception.

Do not administer drug to clients with organic disease (e.g., angina pectoris, history of myocardial infarction, cardiac dysrhythmias, congestive heart failure, rheumatic heart disease), hypertensive states (other than mild, labile systolic hypertension), liver or kidney disease, or history of iodism. Also, do not give to pregnant women, lactating mothers, or as treatment for obesity (i.e., the large doses that are required may produce life-threatening toxicity).

Use with caution with elderly clients who may be more sensitive to thyroid hormones.

Intervention. Discontinue dextrothyroxine at least 2 weeks before surgery to reduce the potential for precipitating cardiac dysrhythmias during operative procedure.

In clients receiving digitalis, do not give more than 4 mg/day of dextrothyroxine to prevent danger of increasing myocardial oxygen requirement. Also, closely monitor effects of both drugs.

Control diabetes mellitus and hypothyroidism if present.

Education. Before initiating dextrothyroxine therapy, advise client to adhere to diet prescribed by physician. The diet is usually low in fats, cholesterol, and/or sugars. Encourage weight reduction and physical exercise.

Instruct the client to keep clinical appointments so that physician can check progress. Also, laboratory values will show that a decrease in cholesterol levels may not occur until 2 to 4 weeks after initiation of drug therapy; maximum decrease occurs about 2 or 3 months later. During therapy, determine serum lipid values at monthly intervals. If response is inadequate after 3 months of therapy, discontinue drug.

Advise client to immediately report the following side effects: chest pain, palpitation, headache, sweating, diarrhea, nocturnal coughing, and dyspnea. Also, report promptly signs of iodism: stomatitis, bronchitis, laryngitis, coryza, brassy taste, conjunctivitis, acneiform rash, and pruritus. Side effects may not occur for 6 weeks.

Evaluation. The drug may increase blood sugar levels and therefore in diabetic individuals, an increase in antidiabetic drugs or a decrease in dextrothyroxine may be required. Loss of diabetic control is noted by the following symptoms: glycosuria, polydipsia, and polyuria.

gemfibrozil (Lopid)

Mechanism of action. Gemfibrozil is a lipid-lowering agent that primarily decreases serum triglycerides found in very low–density lipoprotein (VLDL). It also variably lowers total serum cholesterol that occurs in low-density lipoprotein (LDL) fractions. In the process, the drug provides a beneficial effect by increasing high-density lipoprotein (HDL) concentrations that may inhibit the progression of atherosclerosis. The mechanism of this complicated action has not been established. It may involve an inhibition of peripheral lipolysis and a decrease in hepatic extraction of free fatty acids, which result in reduction of triglyceride production. In addition, the drug may accelerate turnover and removal of cholesterol from the liver, which is ultimately excreted in the feces.

Indication. Treatment of hyperlipidemia (type IV)

Pharmacokinetics
Absorption. Well absorbed from the gastrointestinal tract

Distribution

Time to peak concentration. 1 to 2 hours

Onset of action. Reduces serum VLDL levels within 2 to 5 days

Time to peak effect. Gemfibrozil produces a major decrease in serum VLDL levels in 4 weeks. More decreases may occur over several more months.

Half-life. Half-life for a single dose is 1.5 hours. Half-life for long-term treatment is 1.3 hours.

Metabolism. Liver

Excretion. Kidneys and feces

Side effects/adverse reactions. See Table 30-3

Significant drug interactions. See discussion of clofibrate.

Dosage and administration

Adults. Give 1.2 g (range 900 to 1500 mg) orally daily in two divided doses (preferably before breakfast and supper).

Children. Dosage is not established.

Pregnancy safety. FDA Category B

NURSING CONSIDERATIONS

Gemfibrozil has chemical, pharmacologic, and clinical effects that are similar to those of clofibrate. See discussion of clofibrate for nursing considerations.

niacin (nicotinic acid, Diacin, Niac, Nicobid, Nico-400)

Niacin is a water-soluble vitamin that can lower serum cholesterol and triglyceride levels. It is used as an adjunct to other therapies only, because its vasodilating and other side effects limit its usefulness.

Mechanism of action. Niacin interferes with triglyceride synthesis, which ultimately lowers hepatic secretion of VLDL. The decrease in VLDL concentration subsequently leads to a reduction in circulating levels of LDL, with a resultant lowering of cholesterol concentration. In fact, plasma triglyceride levels decrease within a few hours following the administration of nicotinic acid, and a reduction of cholesterol levels occurs several days after drug therapy. Since nicotinic acid inhibits lipolysis in adipose tissue, it lowers the plasma concentration of free fatty acids, which actually is the main source of synthesis of triglycerides in the liver.

Indications. Niacin is used as adjunctive therapy in the treatment of both hypertriglyceridemias and hypercholesterolemia (types IIa, IIb, III, IV, or V). It is also used to prevent and treat niacin (vitamin B$_3$) deficiency.

Pharmacokinetics
Absorption. Good

Half-life. Approximately 45 minutes

Onset of action. Reduction in cholesterol levels occurs several days after oral doses are begun. Reduction in triglyceride levels occurs several hours after oral doses are begun.

Metabolism. Liver

Excretion. Kidneys

Side effects/adverse reactions. See Table 30-3.

Significant drug interactions. None

Dosage and administration

Adults. As an antihyperlipidemic agent 100 mg is given initially orally three times daily. Dosage may be increased by 300-mg increments every 4 to 7 days as needed.

Maintenance. For maintenance 1 to 2 g is given orally three times daily. Maximum dosage is 6 g/day.

Pregnancy safety. FDA Category C

NURSING CONSIDERATIONS

Assessment. The drug should be used cautiously in individuals with allergies and peptic ulcers, since nicotinic acid causes a release of histamine and stimulates hydrochloric acid secretion.

The drug is contraindicated for use in individuals with hepatic dysfunction, active peptic ulcer, hemorrhagic diathesis, glaucoma, chronic diarrhea, and gout.

Intervention. Giving the drug with meals or with antacids may reduce the incidence and severity of side effects. Prolonged treatment with niacin has resulted in hepatic disease.

Instruct client to swallow the extended-release form whole, without chewing or crushing. The powder within the capsule may be mixed with jam or applesauce for ease of administration.

Education. Advise the client to adhere to dietary regimen—low cholesterol and low saturated fats.

Instruct client to maintain clinical appointments so that serum cholesterol and triglycerides may be monitored on a periodic basis.

Alert the client that numerous and often disagreeable side effects may occur from nicotinic acid. Common side effects include severe gastrointestinal upset, flushing, pruritus, nervousness, and urticaria.

probucol (Lorelco)

Mechanism of action. Probucol appears to be effective in reducing cholesterol levels in individuals with elevated concentrations of low-density lipoproteins (LDLs). The drug is believed to act by inhibiting the earlier stages of cholesterol synthesis, but it does not affect the latter stages of its production. In addition, probucol enhances excretion of bile acids in feces and slightly inhibits absorption of dietary cholesterol.

Indication. Treatment of hyperlipidemia (type IIa)

Pharmacokinetics

Absorption. Oral absorption is variable and limited.

Distribution. Probucol tends to accumulate in fatty tissue with prolonged therapy.

Time to peak serum concentration. Peak serum concentration occurs after 3 or 4 months of treatment.

Time to peak effect. Peak effect usually occurs 20 to 50 days after starting treatment. Clinical response is usually noted within 1 to 3 months.

Half-life. 12 hours to more than 500 hours.

Excretion. Probucol is excreted as bile (in feces). Little of the drug is excreted by the kidneys.

Side effects/adverse reactions. See Table 30-3.

Significant drug interactions. None

Dosage and administration

Adults. Give 500 mg orally twice daily with breakfast and supper.

Children. Dosage is not established.

Pregnancy safety. Not established

NURSING CONSIDERATIONS

Assessment. Administer drug to individuals who do not respond adequately to dietary management and weight reduction. Do not give probucol to clients with evidence of myocardial damage or any indication of ventricular dysrhythmias or to those with primary biliary cirrhosis since probucol increases cholesterol concentrations.

Education. If medication is given, adherence to a low-cholesterol and low-fat diet and physical exercise should continue.

Instruct individual to take drug with food to minimize gastric irritation.

Evaluation. Determine cholesterol levels before therapy; reduction in level should occur 2 to 3 months following drug administration. Also, perform serum triglyceride levels during therapy. Change medication if serum cholesterol and triglyceride levels are not reduced within the first 3 to 4 months.

Animal studies have shown that a marked prolongation of the Q-T interval and syncope can occur. Perform ECG before drug therapy, then periodically thereafter (e.g., 6 months, then after 1 year). If prolongation of Q-T interval is not corrected, change to another drug.

ENZYME INHIBITOR

lovastatin (Mevacor)

Lovastatin is a recently released agent that is highly effective in lowering serum cholesterol levels.

Mechanism of action. Lovastatin inhibits liver synthesis of cholesterol and has been effective in lowering both normal and increased LDL cholesterol serum concentrations.

Indications. Lovastatin is used as an adjunct to dietary measures for clients with primary hypercholesterolemia (types IIa and IIb), especially when dietary measures and other nonpharmacologic methods are unsuccessful.

Pharmacokinetics

Absorption. Variable and low, orally.

Distribution. Protein-bound distribution of lovastatin is high. Peak serum levels for drug and active metabolites are reached within 2 to 4 hours.

Excretion. Feces, kidneys (lesser amount)

Side effects/adverse reactions. See Table 30-3.

Significant drug interactions. None

Dosage and administration. The client should be on a standard cholesterol-lowering diet before and during administration of this drug.

Adults. Give 20 mg orally daily with the evening meal. Increase dosage as necessary according to client's response to therapy, up to a maximum of 80 mg/day. Dosage adjustments should be instituted at monthly or even longer intervals.

Pregnancy safety. FDA Category X

NURSING CONSIDERATIONS

As with other antihyperlipidemic medications, an appropriate diet, exercise, and weight reduction in obese clients should be instituted along with drug therapy.

Lovastatin may elevate creatine phosphokinase and transaminase levels. Do not administer to clients with active liver disease or unexplained persistent elevations of serum transaminases.

• • •

Antihyperlipidemic effects of the drugs discussed in this chapter are summarized in Table 30-4.

KEY TERMS

atherosclerosis, page 562
chylomicrons, page 563
high-density lipoproteins (HDLs), page 563
hyperlipidemia, page 562
lipoproteins, page 563
low-density lipoproteins (LDLs), page 563
very low–density lipoproteins (VLDLs), page 563

BIBLIOGRAPHY

Allison, SK, and Allison, KL: Drug treatment of lipid disorders, U.S. Pharmacist 10(12):44-52, 1985.

Drugs Affecting the Blood

TABLE 30-4 Summary of Comparison of Antihyperlipidemic Effects

Drug	Effect on lipids		Effect on lipoproteins			Typical response	Indications with diet control
	Cholesterol	Triglycerides	VLDL	LDL	HDL		
cholestyramine	−*	0 or slight +	0 or +	−	0 or +	Decreases cholesterol 20%-40%	Type IIa
colestipol	−	0 or slight +	+	−	0 or +	Decreases cholesterol 20%-40%	Type IIa
clofibrate	−	− (greatest effect)	−	0 or −	0 or +	Lowers triglycerides; only slight decrease in cholesterol	Type III
dextrothyroxine	−	0	0 or −	−	0		Type IIa
gemfibrozil	−	−	−	0 or −	+	Decreases triglycerides; only slight decrease in cholesterol; increases HDL	Type IV
niacin	−	−	−	−	+	Decreases triglycerides and cholesterol 10%-20%	Types II, III, IV, and V
probucol	−	0 or +	+ or −	−	−	Decreases cholesterol 12%-25%; also decreases HDL	Type IIa
lovastatin	−	−	−	−	+	LDL cholesterol levels reduced 19%-39%, total cholesterol levels reduced 18%-34%	Types IIa and IIb

*+, Increased; −, decreased; 0, no change. Typical response was approximated with individual taking drug while concurrently on specified diet.

American Hospital Formulary Service: AHFS drug information '87, Bethesda, Md, 1987, American Society of Hospital Pharmacists, Inc.

Burke, MD: Cholesterol, triglyceride, and lipoprotein studies: strategies for clinical use, Postgrad Med 67(3):263-273, 1980.

Cholesterol guidelines issued by expert panel, Pharmacy Weekly 26(40):161-162, 1987.

Cholesterol-lowering agent approved for U.S. market, Clin Pharm 6(11):824, 1987.

Gilman, AG, and others: Goodman & Gilman's the pharmacological basis of therapeutics, ed 7, New York, 1985, Macmillan Publishing Co.

Ginsberg, HN, and others: Treatment of common lipoprotein disorders, Physician Assist 10(4):122, 1986.

Hartshorn, JC, and others: Treatment of hyperlipidemia with gemfibrozil, J Cardiovasc Nurs 1(4):76, 1987.

Hoeg, JM, and others: An approach to the management of hyperlipoproteinemia, JAMA 255(4):512-521, 1986.

Labson, LH: Lipids: lowering elevated serum levels, Pt Care 19(5):49, 1985.

Mevacor (Lovastatin/MSD) prescribing information sheet. DC7489500, West Point, Pa, issued Aug 1987, Merck Sharp & Dohme.

Naito, HK: Reducing cardiac deaths with hypolipidemic drugs, Postgrad Med 82(6):102-112, 1987.

United States Pharmacopeial Convention: Drug information for the health care provider, ed 7, Rockville, Md, 1987, U.S. Pharmacopeial Convention, Inc.

CHAPTER 31

Antihemorrheologic Agent

OBJECTIVES

After studying this chapter, the student will be able to:

1. Define the science of hemorrheology.
2. Discuss the mechanism of action of pentoxifylline.
3. Identify side effects/adverse reactions of pentoxifylline.
4. Apply nursing considerations to the client receiving pentoxifylline.

Hemorrheology is a science that deals with the deformation and flow properties of blood under physiologic and pathophysiologic conditions. Because arteriosclerosis reduces blood flow to tissues distal to the obstruction, blood viscosity is elevated, thereby diminishing the flow of blood still further. In addition, the impaired blood flow at the microcirculatory level affects the normal capacity of the red blood cells to flex as they enter the narrowed capillary lumen, which has a mean diameter smaller than the erythrocytes.

A major function of red blood cells is to transport hemoglobin that carries oxygen, which during the metabolic process is converted to energy for muscle movement such as walking. Accordingly, the decreased flexibility of the red blood cells and the elevated blood viscosity are responsible for diminishing tissue oxygenation. Hence, during exercise the demand for an increase in blood flow and tissue oxygenation may result in claudication, thereby limiting the distance a person can walk.

Intermittent claudication is a syndrome that results from an insufficient blood supply to skeletal muscles in the legs. Reduced microcirculatory blood flow causes ischemia and pain. This syndrome is a common complication of atherosclerosis and is characteristic of **Buerger's disease.** While walking, these individuals have first pain, and then cramps and weakness in muscles.

pentoxifylline (Trental)

Pentoxifylline represents an important concept in the therapy of peripheral vascular disorders because the ability of vasodilators to improve blood flow by dilation of rigid, arteriosclerotic blood vessels is somewhat limited. Further, because capillary walls lack smooth muscle, dilation by this group of drugs is often unlikely to occur.

Mechanism of action. Pentoxifylline improves hemorrheologic disorders in the microcirculation, which involves the flow of blood through the fine vessels (arterioles, capillaries, and venules). Although the mechanism of action of pentoxifylline is not completely clear, current evidence shows that the drug possesses several properties to improve microcirculatory blood flow to ischemic tissues:

1. It restores red blood cell flexibility, probably by its inhibition of phosphodiesterase, which results in an increase in cyclic AMP in red blood cells.
2. It lowers blood viscosity by decreasing fibrinogen concentrations and inhibiting aggregation of red blood cells and platelets.

The result is increased microcirculatory blood flow and oxygenation of tissues.

Indications
1. An adjunct treatment (to surgery) for peripheral vascular disease
2. Intermittent claudication that results from chronic occlusive arterial disease of the limbs

Pharmacokinetics
Absorption. Good
Onset of action with long-term dosing. 2 to 4 weeks
Half-life. Drug: 0.4 to 0.8 hour; metabolites: 1 to 1.6 hours
Peak concentration in blood. 2 to 4 hours
Metabolism. Red blood cells and liver
Excretion. Kidneys and feces
Side effects/adverse reactions. Less frequent side effects are dizziness, headaches, abdominal distress, nausea, and vomiting. Rare adverse reactions are chest pain and an irregular heart rate. With an overdose the client experiences increased sedation, flushing of skin, feeling of faintness, increased excitability, or convulsions.
Significant drug interactions. None
Dosage and administration. For adults give 400 mg orally three times daily with meals. If undesirable side effects occur, such as gastrointestinal upset or CNS disturbances, the dosage should be decreased to 400 mg twice daily.
Pregnancy safety. FDA Category C

NURSING CONSIDERATIONS

Assessment. Since pentoxifylline is a xanthine derivative, do not administer to clients with an intolerance to other xanthine derivatives such as caffeine, theophylline, or theobromine.

Intervention. Administer with food, milk, or antacids to decrease gastrointestinal distress. If gastrointestinal side effects persist, notify the physician to consider a reduction in the dosage.

Education. Instruct client to swallow extended-release tablets whole without crushing or chewing.

Instruct the client that improvement in the clinical status may not occur before 8 weeks of therapy and that it is essential for the medication to be taken as prescribed until discontinued by the physician.

Advise smoking cessation since nicotine constricts the blood vessels and defeats the purpose of the medication. The client should receive support in smoking avoidance through group or individual counseling.

Evaluation. Monitor blood pressure periodically in clients receiving concurrent antihypertensive therapy. Small decreases in blood pressure have been noted in clients receiving pentoxifylline alone, so a reduction of the hypotensive agent might be indicated.

Monitor the client with peripheral vascular disease for an improvement in walking distance and duration. Assess the client with cerebrovascular disease for memory loss, disorientation, motor impairment, dizziness, and frequency of transient ischemic attacks.

KEY TERMS

Buerger's disease, page 573
hemorrheology, page 573
intermittent claudication, page 573

BIBLIOGRAPHY

American Hospital Formulary Service: AHFS drug information '87, Bethesda, Md, 1987, American Society of Hospital Pharmacists, Inc.

Baker, DE, and others: Pentoxifylline: a new agent for intermittent claudication. Drug Intell Clin Pharm 19(5):345, 1985.

Campbell, RK, and others: Trental: a new medication for peripheral vascular disorders, Diabetes Educ 10(2):66, 1984.

Kastrup, EK, and Olin, BR: Facts and comparisons, drug information, Philadelphia, 1987, JB Lippincott Co.

Pepper, GA: New drug for intermittent claudication...pentoxifylline (Trental), Nurse Pract 10(5):54, 1985.

United States Pharmacopeial Convention: Drug information for the health care provider, ed 7, Rockville, Md, 1987, US Pharmacopeial Convention, Inc.

Weintraub, M, and others: Pentoxifylline: a new medication for intermittent claudication, Hosp Formul 19(2):117, 1984.

UNIT VIII

Drugs Affecting the Urinary System

CHAPTER

32

Overview of the Urinary System

OBJECTIVES

After studying this chapter, the student will be able to:

1. Describe the anatomy and physiology of the urinary system.
2. Identify the functions of the various segments of the nephron.
3. Describe the major functions of the kidneys.
4. Describe the site and primary effects of antidiuretic hormone and aldosterone on the nephrons.

The urinary system is composed of organs that manufacture and excrete urine from the body: two kidneys, two ureters, the bladder, and the urethra (see Figure 32-1). Urine formed in the kidneys flows through the ureters to the bladder, where it is stored. When approximately 250 ml of urine is collected, the bladder expansion will result in a feeling of distention and a desire to void. The urine flows from the bladder into the urethra to be expelled from the body.

In the male the urethra is surrounded by the prostate gland; it then passes through fibrous tissue connected to the pubic bones and terminates at the urinary meatus, or tip of the penis (see Figure 32-2). The male urethra serves a dual purpose, that is, the elimination of urine from the body and semen transport. In the female the urethra is the final vehicle for urination (see Figure 32-3).

The kidneys regulate homeostasis in the body; that is, they are responsible for the maintenance of body fluids, electrolytes, and acid-base balance in addition to elimination of body waste, urea, and urine. The primary focus of this chapter will be the kidneys.

ANATOMY AND PHYSIOLOGY OF THE KIDNEY

The kidney is composed of millions of individual units called nephrons. Each nephron consists of a glomerulus and a tubular system. The volume and composition of urine as a result of concentration and dilution depend on

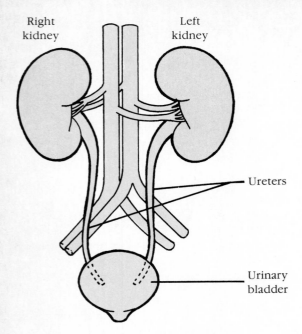

FIGURE 32-1   Urinary system.

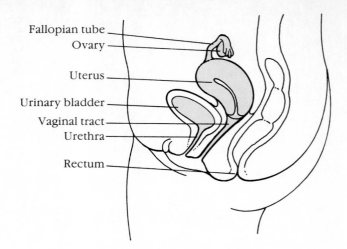

FIGURE 32-3   Female urethra.

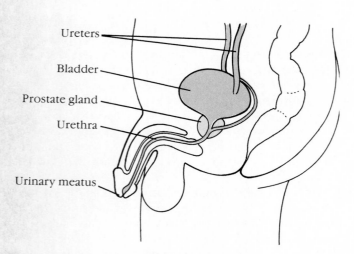

FIGURE 32-2   Male urethra.

three major processes in the kidney: glomerular filtration, tubular reabsorption, and tubular secretion.

Glomerular filtration. **Glomerular filtration** occurs as a result of plasma flowing across a capillary bed called the **glomerulus.** The heart works to create pressure in the blood vessels, which in turn provides the force necessary to accomplish glomerular filtration. Blood flow to the kidney is 1200 ml/min, which is 20% to 25% of cardiac output. The blood pressure within the glomerular capillaries is about 60% of arterial pressure. Systemic blood pressure has to be significantly reduced before glomerular filtration is greatly altered. Usually some degree of

filtration will exist if the mean blood pressure remains above 50 mm Hg. Maintenance of glomerular hydrostatic pressure is aided by the ability of the afferent and efferent arterioles to effectively alter vessel resistance. In the absence of disease the glomerular membrane does not filter plasma proteins greater than 100 angstroms (Å), such as hemoglobin and albumin and the small amount of protein-bound substances. The glomerular filtrate is otherwise almost identical to plasma. The rate of filtration in an average adult is approximately 125 ml/min; 99% of this tubular filtrate is ultimately reabsorbed throughout the tubule.

Tubular reabsorption. Tubular reabsorption involves both active and passive transport of substances into the tubular epithelial cell and into the extracellular fluid compartment. Passive transport or diffusion through the tubular membrane occurs because of a difference in concentration of particles **(osmotic gradient)** or electrical charge **(electromagnetic gradient).**

In the proximal tubule, sodium is *actively* transported across the tubular cell membrane from tubule filtrate. Chloride follows passively because of an electromagnetic gradient. Water, in turn, follows passively in response to an osmotic gradient established by sodium chloride solute. Then diffusion of 60% of urea content occurs to maintain a chemical gradient. Depending on the amount of a drug in ionized or nonionized form and the pH of the tubular fluid, weak acids and weak bases may be reabsorbed by diffusion.

For almost every substance that is actively transported across the membrane, there is a maximum rate at which the transport mechanism can function. This is called the **tubular transport maximum.** For example, the tubular transport maximum for glucose averages 320 mg/min for most adults. If the tubular load becomes greater than 320 mg/min, then the excess will not be reabsorbed but will appear in the urine. Every substance that has a tubular transport maximum also has a **threshold concentration** that is the plasma concentration below which none of the substance appears in the urine and above which progressively larger quantities appear.

Tubular secretion. Tubular secretion affects the composition of urine by allowing compounds such as penicillin, probenecid, methotrexate, and thiazides to enter into tubular fluid from peritubular or interstitial capillaries. This is accomplished via specific transport mechanisms for secretion of organic acids, organic bases, and ethylenediaminetetraacetic acid (EDTA) in the proximal tubule. Other very important examples of tubular secretion include that of the hydrogen ion, ammonia, and potassium.

Proximal tubule. Most of the glomerular filtrate is reabsorbed in the proximal tubule and returned to the bloodstream. Approximately 60% to 70% of salt and water is reabsorbed rapidly, maintaining nearly the same osmolality between tubular fluid and interstitial fluid at the end of the proximal tubule **(isotonic).** The general mechanism for sodium, chloride, water, and urea reabsorption is under tubular reabsorption with respect to gradient transport. There are *no* dilutional or concentration changes of these ions in the proximal tubule.

Other substances reabsorbed in the proximal tubule include glucose, amino acids, phosphate, uric acid, and a major portion of potassium. Nearly 90% of bicarbonate in tubular filtrate is reabsorbed as carbon dioxide if hydrogen ion is secreted in the tubular lumen. Plasma carbon dioxide is hydrolyzed in the tubular cell to form carbonic acid, which dissociates to give bicarbonate and hydrogen ion. This reversible reaction is catalyzed by carbonic anhydrase. The hydrogen ion secreted into the lumen combines with bicarbonate of the glomerular filtrate to form carbonic acid in the lumen. This again dissociates to give water and carbon dioxide, which are reabsorbed. This reaction is again catalyzed at both steps by carbonic anhydrase. Proximal tubule reabsorption is usually constant in spite of moderate changes in glomerular filtration rate.

Descending loop of Henle. This portion of the nephron is permeable to water; water is passively taken up to equilibrate medullary interstitial osmolality. This produces a **hypertonic** (more concentrated) filtrate at the tip of the loop of Henle, the papilla. There is very low sodium and urea permeability in this segment.

Ascending loop of Henle. Water permeability is almost nil in the ascending limb of the loop of Henle, whereas sodium and chloride permeability is high. Approximately 20% to 25% of sodium load in glomerular filtrate is reabsorbed and sodium *passively* follows. Consequently, two very important situations occur. The concentration of tubular filtrates becomes very dilute, or **hypotonic;** this is often termed "free water production." Meanwhile, the medullary interstitium becomes hypertonic, which is nec-

essary to the concentration capacity of the countercurrent multiplier. The concentration gradient established across the tubular epithelium becomes multiplied in a longitudinal direction, resulting in a large osmotic gradient between the isosmotic renal cortex and the hyperosmotic medulla and papilla. The ascending limb of the loop of Henle is not responsive to any hormones as are other segments.

Distal convoluted tubule. Between 5% and 10% of sodium reabsorption *actively* takes place in the distal tubule. This uptake is largely determined by the presence of a hormone called aldosterone. When the extracellular fluid volume is decreased, the renin-angiotensin system is involved, stimulating the release of aldosterone. Increased levels of aldosterone act to increase the active reabsorption of sodium. Although an increase in potassium secretion is seen, a simple sodium-potassium exchange pump is no longer recognized.

Collecting duct. The hypotonic fluid entering the collecting duct may be altered in the medullary portion by the presence of antidiuretic hormone (ADH). Fluid is lost because of the osmotic gradient set up by hypertonic medullary interstitium. Thus the collecting duct is responsible for urine concentration.

NEPHRON FUNCTIONS

SITE	MAJOR FUNCTIONS
Glomerulus	Filtration
Proximal tubule	Reabsorption of glucose, potassium, sodium, amino acids, water, and nutrients; remaining fluid isotonic
Loop of Henle	Sodium and chloride reabsorbed in ascending loop. Countercurrent mechanism produces decrease in osmolality of filtrate in ascending loop of Henle; that is, sodium chloride is transported into the body but not water. Filtrate leaves loop of Henle as hypotonic urine.
Distal tubule	Sodium and bicarbonate reabsorbed. Potassium, hydrogen, and ammonia may be secreted. ADH necessary to reabsorb water at this site. Filtrate leaves distal tubule as hypotonic urine.
Collecting duct	ADH, if present, will reabsorb water at this site. Urine may be hypertonic. If ADH is unavailable or not functioning, dilute urine (hypotonic) may be excreted.

SUMMARY OF MAJOR KIDNEY FUNCTIONS

1. The kidneys excrete metabolic by-products of the body, especially nitrogenous-type substances such as urea.

2. The kidneys maintain electrolyte homeostasis (sodium, potassium, chloride, etc.) and body fluids. Sodium is actively reabsorbed in the proximal tubules (approximately 65%) and ascending loop of Henle (27%). Approximately 8% sodium reaches the distal tubules, and the rate of reabsorption here depends on the presence of aldosterone. If large quantities of aldosterone are present, sodium is reabsorbed. A lack of aldosterone will result in elimination of sodium in the urine. Generally, healthy kidneys excrete the daily sodium intake. See Figure 32-4 and box for nephron functions. Potassium is also reabsorbed from the proximal tubules and loop of Henle in percentages equivalent to sodium. Thus approximately 8% of the filtered potassium reaches the distal tubules. Aldosterone controls potassium secretion; that is, in its presence, sodium is reabsorbed and potassium is secreted in the distal tubules. The daily potassium intake is generally excreted daily in the kidneys.

3. ADH (vasopressin), synthesized in the hypothalamus and stored in the posterior pituitary gland, is a water-conserving hormone. When plasma osmolarity increases as a result of dehydration or water deprivation, osmoreceptors in the supraoptic area of the hypothalamus will stimulate the release of ADH. The released ADH will act at the distal tubule and collecting duct to reabsorb water to increase plasma volume, thus lowering plasma osmolality. Urine output is more concentrated and also decreased.

4. Acid-base control is in the kidneys. The kidneys are one of three pH control mechanisms in the body; the others are blood buffering and the respiratory adjustment mechanism. As the blood pH becomes more acidic, the kidneys will respond by increasing the renal tubule excretion of hydrogen and ammonia, which results in an increase in blood bicarbonate and an increase in pH (toward normal). This is an effective method of adjusting hydrogen ions within the system.

5. The hormone erythropoietin is synthesized in the kidneys. A decrease in red blood cells below normal, or tissue hypoxia, will stimulate an increased release of

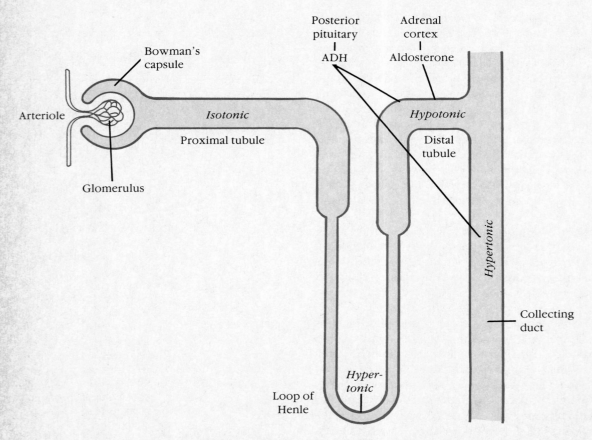

FIGURE 32-4 Functioning of nephron.

erythropoietin from the kidneys. The increased serum concentration of erythropoietin will stimulate the bone marrow to increase its production of red blood cells, so that the red blood cell average is restored to normal.

KEY TERMS

electromagnetic gradient, page 578
glomerular filtration, page 578
glomerulus, page 578
hypertonic, page 579
hypotonic, page 579

isotonic, page 579
osmotic gradient, page 578
threshold concentration, page 579
tubular transport maximum, page 578

BIBLIOGRAPHY

Anthony, CP, and Thibodeau, GA: Textbook of anatomy and physiology, ed 11, St Louis, 1982, The CV Mosby Co.

Braunwalk, E, and others, eds: Harrison's principles of internal medicine, ed 11, New York, 1987, McGraw-Hill Co.

Guyton, AC: Human physiology and mechanisms of disease, ed 4, Philadelphia, 1987, WB Saunders Co.

Diuretics

Diuretics are among the most commonly used medications. They represent the mainstay in the treatment of hypertension (see also Chapter 25) and are an integral part of drug therapies in edematous conditions such as cirrhosis, nephrotic syndrome, and congestive heart failure. Diuretics influence water and electrolyte balance, particularly sodium, in the body. This action is exerted on tubular function of the kidney rather than on glomerular filtration. It generally involves the inhibition of solute reabsorption and thus water reabsorption, since water passively diffuses across the tubular membrane when sodium transport occurs. This inhibition results in a diuresis, or loss of body water by urination.

Diuretics have their primary effect on tubular function in the nephron. Understanding their action requires knowledge of the events that take place along each of the tubular segments. (See Chapter 32.)

Therapeutically, drug selection is best understood if each diuretic is presented according to the major site of action. This approach does not preclude drug effect at other sites in the nephron. Figure 33-1 shows the various sites of action of diuretic groups by means of water and electrolyte transport system in a kidney nephron.

PROXIMAL TUBULE DIURETICS
CARBONIC ANHYDRASE INHIBITORS

acetazolamide (Diamox, Dazamide, Acetazolam✤, Apo-Acetazolamide✤)

Acetazolamide is the prototype of the proximal tubule agents that are sulfonamides. These drugs act primarily to

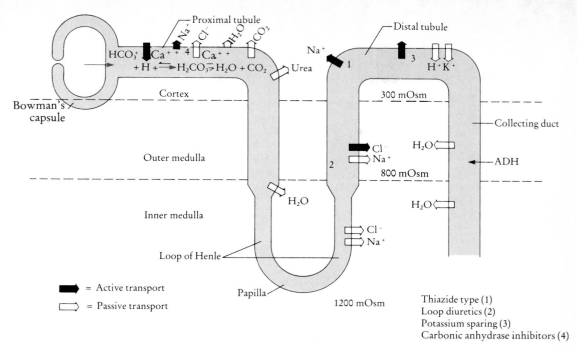

FIGURE 33-1   Diuretics. Site of action by means of water and electrolyte transport.

reduce the volume of sequestered fluids, especially of the aqueous humor.

Mechanism of action. Acetazolamide inhibits the action of the enzyme **carbonic anhydrase,** which in turn prevents the reabsorption of bicarbonate ions from the proximal tubules. These bicarbonate ions then act to increase tubular osmotic pressure, causing osmotic diuresis. With long-term use, however, the diuretic effect of these drugs is lost. Therefore acetazolamide is used primarily to produce an alkaline urine, which helps increase excretion of weakly acidic drugs in cases of drug overdose.

Acetazolamide is widely used as an antiglaucoma agent because it lowers intraocular pressure by decreasing production of aqueous humor by over 50%. This will be discussed in Chapter 43.

Indications

1. Treatment of open-angle glaucoma.
2. Adjunct treatment with anticonvulsants to manage absence seizures (petit mal), generalized tonic-clonic seizures (grand mal), mixed seizure patterns, and myoclonic seizures. It has been found to be especially useful for women who experience an increase in seizures during their menstrual periods (intermittent therapy used).
3. Also used to treat altitude sickness. Orally, acetazolamide decreases the incidence and severity of symptoms of altitude sickness in mountain climbers.

Pharmacokinetics

Absorption. Acetazolamide is absorbed well.

Half-life. Half-life for acetazolamide (tablets) is 10 to 15 hours.

Time to peak concentration. Peak concentration is reached 2 to 4 hours following a 500-mg dose and 8 to 12 hours after a 500-mg extended-release capsule.

Peak serum concentration. Acetazolamide reaches a serum concentration of 12 to 27 μg/ml following a 500-mg tablet dose; 6 μg/ml after a 500-mg extended-release capsule.

Excretion. Acetazolamide is excreted by the kidneys.

Side effects/adverse reactions. See Table 33-1.

Significant drug interactions. The following interactions may occur when acetazolamide is given with the drugs listed below.

Drug	**Possible Effect and Management**
amphetamines, mecamylamine, or quinidine	Because of alkalinization of urine, the excretion of these drugs is decreased. Therefore increased serum levels and toxicity may be seen. Avoid concurrent drug administration with mecamylamine. Dosage adjustments may be necessary with the other two drugs whenever a carbonic anhydrase inhibitor is started, dosage is changed, or medication is discontinued.
methenamine	Alkaline urine will reduce the effectiveness of methenamine. Avoid concurrent usage.

Dosage and administration. See Table 33-2.

Pregnancy safety. Not established

TABLE 33-1   Side Effects/Adverse Reactions of Diuretics

Drug	Side effects*	Adverse reactions†
Proximal tubule diuretics: acetazolamide (Diamox, etc.)	Most frequent: moderate headaches Less frequent/rare: alopecia, rash on arms and face	Most frequent: increased nervousness, anorexia, nausea or vomiting, depression, tremors Less frequent/rare: severe or sudden headaches; sudden ataxia; pain in chest, groin, calves, or legs; slurred speech; visual disturbances; respiratory difficulties
Diluting segment diuretics: thiazide and thiazide-type drugs (see Table 33-3)	Less frequent: impotence, diarrhea, postural hypotension, skin photosensitivity, anorexia, abdominal distress	Most frequent: dry mouth; increased thirst; mood or mental alterations; pain or cramping in muscles; increased weakness, nausea, or vomiting; dysrhythmias or weak pulse (electrolyte imbalance) Rare: abdominal or joint pain, sore throat, and elevated temperature, jaundice, increased bleeding tendencies
Loop diuretics: bumetanide ethacrynic acid furosemide	Most frequent: postural hypotension ethacrynic acid only: diarrhea, anorexia (dose-related effects) Less frequent: blurred vision, headaches, abdominal cramping or pain bumetanide: chest pain, diarrhea, anorexia, premature ejaculation ethacrynic acid: confusion, anxiety furosemide: diarrhea, skin photosensitivity, anorexia	Less frequent: weak pulse Rare: abdominal or joint pain, hives or allergic reaction, sore throat, elevated temperature, nausea, vomiting, increased bleeding episodes, jaundice, tinnitus or loss of hearing ethacrynic acid: bloody urine or black stools associated with injection
Distal tubule diuretics/potassium-sparing diuretics: amiloride spironolactone triamterene	Most frequent (spironolactone): nausea, vomiting, abdominal cramps, diarrhea Less frequent: dizziness, dry mouth, sedation, increased thirst, loss of energy, (caused by hyponatremia), headache amiloride: constipation, muscle cramps, abdominal distress, decreased sexual activity triamterene: skin photosensitivity, abdominal distress spironolactone: gynecomastia (dose related), clumsiness, decreased sexual activity	Most frequent: signs of hyperkalemia—increased weakness; heavy feeling in legs; increased anxiety; respiratory difficulties; paresthesias of hands, feet, or lips; dysrhythmias Rare: rash, pruritus, shortness of breath triamterene: red tongue, (patient may complain of burning sensation), cracks at corners of mouth, increased weakness, flank pain, sore throat, elevated temperature, increased bleeding episodes
Osmotic diuretics: Parenteral: mannitol urea	Most frequent mannitol: headache, increased urination, nausea, vomiting, dry mouth urea: nausea or vomiting Less frequent mannitol: visual disturbances, dizziness, rash urea: headaches	Less frequent (urea): inadvertent intravascular or intraperitoneal administration may result in abdominal pain, weakness, myometrial necrosis, and dehydration Rare: confusion, muscle cramping or pain, paresthesias in hands or feet, increased weakness, legs feel heavy and weak, dysrhythmias mannitol: chest pain; chills; elevated temperature; confusion; tachycardia; dysrhythmias; pain or cramping of muscles; paresthesias, pain, or weakness in hands and feet; convulsions; tremors; increased weakness; legs feel heavy and weak; respiratory difficulties; dysuria; redness; pain or swelling at injection site; edema of lower extremities
Oral: glycerin	Most frequent: headache, nausea or vomiting Less frequent: dry mouth, increased thirst, diarrhea, dizziness	Less frequent: confusion Rare: dysrhythmias
isosorbide	Nausea, vomiting, abdominal distress, hiccoughs, rash, dizziness, lethargy, increased irritability	Disorientation, syncope

*If side effects continue, increase, or disturb the client, inform the physician.
†If adverse reactions occur, contact the physician, since medical intervention may be necessary.

TABLE 33-2　Acetazolamide Dosage and Administration

Form	Adults	Children
acetazolamide tablets	Glaucoma (open-angle): 250 mg orally 1-4 times daily initially, then titrate to client response for maintenance dose	Glaucoma: 10-15 mg/kg (range 8-30 mg) orally, or 300-900 mg/m² daily in divided doses
	Anticonvulsant: 8-30 mg/kg daily (average initial dose: 10 mg); administer in 3 or 4 oral divided doses daily; usual dose is 375 mg/day	Anticonvulsant: see adult dose
	Altitude sickness: 250 mg orally 2-4 times daily	
acetazolamide extended-release capsules	Glaucoma: 500 mg orally morning and evening	
	Altitude sickness: 500 mg orally once or twice daily	
acetazolamide sodium injection	Glaucoma: for rapid lowering of intraocular pressure, 500 mg IV or, alternatively, 250 mg IV and 250 mg IM; may be repeated in 2-4 hr in acute circumstances or oral acetazolamide may be started, depending on individual's response	Glaucoma: 5-10 mg/kg IV (preferred) or IM every 6 hr

NURSING CONSIDERATIONS

Assessment. Ascertain whether the client has diabetes or a familial history of diabetes because acetazolamide has caused elevations of blood glucose and glycosuria in these clients.

Do not give acetazolamide to clients allergic to sulfonamides.

Note that elderly clients are especially susceptible to excessive diuresis and may be unable to tolerate the usual adult doses.

Intervention. Reconstituting acetazolamide with at least 5 ml sterile water is necessary before parenteral use. Discard it after 24 hours of reconstitution since it contains no preservatives.

Administer the oral forms of acetazolamide with meals or with antacids such as Maalox to decrease gastrointestinal distress.

For clients unable to tolerate tablets for oral administration, crush acetazolamide tablets and mix with a flavored syrup such as chocolate or cherry. Although up to 500 mg may be prepared in 5 ml syrup, it is more palatable if only 250 mg/5 ml is used. Refrigeration also increases palatability but not stability of the preparation; use within a week of preparation. Mixing the drug with fruit juices and elixirs is not as satisfactory.

Planning a high fluid intake for the client with gout or **hypercalciuria** (excessive calcium in the urine) is necessary because of the risk of renal calculi.

Establish dosing schedules that minimize the inconvenience of diuresis for the client.

When this drug is used in diuretic therapy, consult the physician and dietitian to provide a high-potassium diet.

Acetazolamide is used to prevent or minimize high altitude sickness, but it is not a substitute for rapid descent if the climber manifests signs of pulmonary or cerebral edema.

Education. Oral and intravenous routes of administration are preferred, but if the drug is to be given intramuscularly, alert the client that the injection will be painful because of the drug's alkalinity.

Alert the client that constipation is common with diuretic therapy and may be prevented or minimized by adequate fluid intake, high-fiber diet, and moderate exercise if these are not contraindicated by the client's health status.

Instruct the client to move gradually from a sitting or lying position to a more upright one to prevent lightheadedness caused by orthostatic hypotension.

Caution the client that the ability to accomplish tasks requiring mental alertness and physical coordination may be impaired.

Advise the client that dryness of the mouth may occur, but its discomfort may be minimized by the use of sugarless hard candies and frequent mouth rinses. Advise the client to get regular dental checkups to monitor caries and gum disease development that may occur as the result of xerostomia.

Although the sensation of "not feeling well" is common with the drug, malaise should be reported to the physician so that monitoring for acidosis, blood dyscrasias, or hypokalemia may be done.

Advise the client to notify the physician if paresthesias (numbness, tingling, or burning) of the mouth occur.

Instruct the client and the family member who shops for and prepares the food about a high-potassium diet in keeping with the client's usual dietary patterns.

Advise the client to consult the physician before switching brands or using a generic formulation of acetazolamide because bioequivalence problems have been noted.

Evaluation. Observe the client for signs of allergic reaction and photosensitivity.

Weigh the client daily. A rapid loss of body water (which may cause hypotension) will be reflected in a rapid weight loss.

Monitor intake and output and electrolytes, especially serum potassium levels.

Do complete blood cell counts periodically to monitor for blood dyscrasias. Monitor blood and urine sugar levels for clients with diabetes or those at risk for diabetes.

DILUTING SEGMENT DIURETICS
THIAZIDE AND THIAZIDE-TYPE DRUGS

chlorothiazide (Diuril), hydrochlorothiazide (Hydro-Diuril, Esidrix, Oretic), metolazone (Zaroxolyn)*

The thiazides, the major diuretics active within the diluting segments of the kidney, are synthetic drugs chemically related to the sulfonamides.

Hydrochlorothiazide is one of the most commonly used thiazides. Since quinethazone, metolazone, and chlorthalidone—other common diluting segment diuretics—are pharmacologically and structurally similar to the thiazides, all of the diluting segment diuretics will be described collectively as the **thiazide-type diuretics.** Important differences will be mentioned later. Table 33-3 presents these diuretics and their dosages.

Mechanism of action. The primary action and site of action appear to be inhibition of sodium reabsorption at

*See also Table 33-3.

TABLE 33-3   Diuretic Dosages and Administration

Generic/trade name	Age	Usual daily dosage
THIAZIDE AND THIAZIDE-TYPE DIURETICS		
bendroflumethiazide (Naturetin)	Adults	Diuretic, 2.5-10 mg orally once or twice daily or once per day for 3-5 days/wk. Maintenance, 2.5-5 mg daily or once every other day or once a day for 3-5 days/wk. Antihypertensive, 2.5-20 mg orally daily in 1 or 2 divided doses; adjust dosage as necessary. Elderly may be more sensitive to adult dosages, so monitor closely.
	Children	Diuretic, up to 0.4 mg/kg or 12 mg/m^2 daily orally, in 1 or 2 divided doses. Maintenance, 0.05-0.1 mg/kg or 1.5-3 mg/m^2 daily. Antihypertensive, 0.05-0.4 mg/kg or 1.5-12 mg/m^2 daily, in single or 2 divided doses; adjust dosage as necessary.
benzthiazide (Aquatag, Exna, Hydrex)	Adults	Diuretic, 25-100 mg orally twice daily, once every other day, or once daily for 3-5 day/wk. Antihypertensive, 50-200 mg orally daily in 1 or 2 divided doses. Adjust dosage as necessary. Elderly may be more sensitive to adult dosages, so monitor closely.
	Children	0.9-3.9 mg/kg or 30-120 mg/m^2 daily in single or divided doses.
chlorothiazide (Diuril, SK-Chlorothiazide)	Adults	Diuretic, 250 mg orally, every 6-12 hr; injectable form is same. Antihypertensive, 250 mg to 1 g daily, as single or divided doses; adjust dosage according to response. Injectable form; 500 mg to 1 g IV daily as a single dose or in 2 divided doses. Elderly may be more sensitive to adult dosages, so monitor closely.
	Children	Up to 6 mo old, 10-30 mg/kg orally as single dose or in 2 divided doses daily; adjust dose as necessary. 6 mo and older, 10-20 mg/kg orally daily as a single dose or in two divided doses daily; adjust dose as necessary. Injectable form not recommended.
chlorthalidone (Apo-Chlorthalidone♣, Hygroton, Thalitone, Uridon♣)	Adults	Diuretic, 25-100 mg orally daily; or 100-200 mg once every other day, or once daily for 3 days/wk. Antihypertensive, 25-100 mg orally daily; adjust dosage as necessary. Elderly may be more sensitive to adult dosages, so monitor closely.
	Children	2 mg/kg or 60 mg/m^2 orally once daily for 3 days/wk. Adjust dosage as necessary.
cyclothiazide (Anhydron, Fluidil)	Adults	Diuretic, 1-2 mg orally daily, every other day, or once daily for 2-3 day/wk. Antihypertensive, 2 mg orally daily; adjust dosage as necessary (up to 6 mg daily in divided doses). Elderly may be more sensitive to adult dosage, so monitor closely.
	Children	0.02-0.04 mg/kg or 0.6-1.2 mg/m^2 orally daily. Adjust dosage as necessary.
hydrochlorothiazide (Esidrix, Hydro-Diuril, Apo-Hydro♣, Nefrol♣, Oretic)	Adults	Diuretic, 25-100 mg orally once or twice daily, every other day or once daily for 3-5 days/wk. Antihypertensive, 25-100 mg daily in 1 or 2 divided doses; adjust dosage as necessary. Elderly may be more sensitive to adult dosages, so monitor closely.

TABLE 33-3 Diuretic Dosages and Administration—cont'd

Generic/trade name	Age	Usual daily dosage
	Children	1-2 mg/kg or 30-60 mg/m² orally in 1 or 2 divided doses; adjust dosage as necessary. (Infants less than 6 mo old may receive up to 3 mg/kg daily.)
hydroflumethiazide (Diucardin, Saluron)	Adults	Diuretic, 25-100 mg orally 1 or 2 times daily, once every other day, or once daily for 3-5 days/wk. Antihypertensive, 50-100 mg daily in 1 or 2 divided doses; adjust dosage as necessary. Elderly may be more sensitive to adult dosages, so monitor closely. Maximum daily dosage is 200 mg in divided dosages.
	Children	1 mg/kg or 30 mg/m² orally daily; adjust dosage as necessary.
methyclothiazide (Aquatensen, Enduron, Duretic✿)	Adults	Diuretic, 2.5-10 mg orally daily, once every other day, or once daily for 3-5 days/wk. Antihypertensive, 2.5-10 mg orally daily; adjust dosage as necessary. Elderly may be more sensitive to adult dosages, so monitor closely.
	Children	0.05-0.2 mg/kg or 1.5-6 mg/m² orally daily; adjust dosage as necessary.
metolazone (Diulo, Zaroxolyn)	Adults	Diuretic, 5-20 mg orally daily. Antihypertensive, 2.5-5 mg orally daily; adjust dosage as necessary. Elderly may be more sensitive to adult dosages, so monitor closely.
	Children	Not established.
polythiazide (Renese)	Adults	Diuretic, 1-4 mg orally daily, once every other day, or once daily for 3 to 5 days/wk. Antihypertensive, 2-4 mg daily orally; adjust dosage as necessary. Elderly may be more sensitive to adult dosages, so monitor closely.
	Children	0.02-0.08 mg/kg or 0.5-2.5 mg/m² daily; adjust dosage as necessary.
quinethazone (Aquamox✿, Hydromox)	Adults	Diuretic, 50-200 mg orally as single dose or in 2 divided doses daily; adjust dose as necessary. Elderly may be more sensitive to adult dosages, so monitor closely.
	Children	Not established.
trichlormethiazide (Naqua, Metahydrin)	Adults	Diuretic, 1-4 mg orally daily, once every other day, or once daily for 3-5 days/wk. Antihypertensive, 2-4 mg orally daily; adjust dosage as necessary. Elderly may be more sensitive to adult dosages, so monitor closely.
	Children	0.07 mg/kg or 2 mg/m² orally daily as a single dose or in 2 divided doses; adjust dosage as necessary.
LOOP DIURETICS		
bumetanide (Bumex)	Adults	0.5-2 mg orally daily; adjust dosage as necessary by adding a second or third dose, every 4-5 hr. An alternative schedule of dosing on alternate days may also be used. Maximum is 10 mg daily. Injectable form; 0.5-1 mg IV or IM, may repeat at 2-3 hr intervals, if necessary, up to 10 mg daily. Elderly may be more sensitive to adult dosages, so monitor closely.
	Children	Not established
ethacrynic acid (Edecrin)	Adult	Diuretic, 50-100 mg orally daily in single or divided doses; may increase by 25-50 mg daily, as needed up to 400 mg maximum/day; maintenance, usually 50-200 mg daily. Injectable form; diuretic, 50 mg or 0.5-1 mg/kg IV; may repeat in 2-4 hr if needed; if client is responsive, dosage may be repeated every 4-6 hr thereafter; in emergencies, dosage may be repeated every hour; maximum dosage is 100 mg daily. Elderly may be more sensitive to adult dosages, so monitor closely.
	Children	Diuretic, 25 mg orally daily; adjust dosage by 25 mg/day as necessary; do not use in infants. Injectable form; 1 mg/kg IV.
furosemide (Lasix, Furoside✿)	Adults	Diuretic, 20-80 mg orally initially. Increase dosage by 20-40 mg at 6-8 hr intervals if necessary. Maintenance dose as determined by adjustments, may be given as a single daily dose, divided into 2 or 3 doses, given once daily every other day, or given once daily for 2-4 consecutive days out of each week. Antihypertensive, 40 mg orally initially twice daily. Increase dosage as necessary to achieve desired results. Maximum daily dosage is 600 mg. Elderly may be more sensitive to adult dosages, so monitor closely. (Note that in chronic renal failure doses have been increased up to 4 g daily to achieve desired results.)
	Children	Diuretic, 2 mg/kg orally as a single dose. Increase dose by 1-2 mg /kg every 6-8 hr until desired results are achieved. Although dosages as large as 5 mg/kg have been used in children with nephrotic syndrome, dosages above 6 mg/kg daily are not recommended.

Continued.

TABLE 33-3 Diuretic Dosages and Administration—cont'd

Generic/trade name	Age	Usual daily dosage
DISTAL TUBULE DIURETICS/POTASSIUM-SPARING DIURETICS		
amiloride (Midamor)	Adults	Diuretic or antihypertensive, 5-10 mg orally daily; adjust dosage as necessary up to a maximum of 20 mg daily. Elderly may be more sensitive to adult dosages so monitor closely.
	Children	Not established.
spironolactone (Aldactone, Novospiroton✦, Sincomen✦)	Adults	Diuretic for edema as a result of congestive heart failure, cirrhosis, or nephrotic syndrome, 25-200 mg orally in 2-4 divided doses for at least 5 days. Maintenance, 75-400 mg daily orally in 2-4 divided doses.
		Antihypertensive, 50-100 mg orally initially as a single dose or in 2-4 divided doses for approximately 14 days. Then gradually adjust dosage as necessary up to 200 mg daily.
		For primary hyperaldosteronism, 100-400 mg orally daily in 2-4 divided doses before surgery. For individuals unable to undergo surgery, lower dosages are used for longer-term maintenance.
		Diagnostic tool for primary hyperaldosteronism Long test: 400 mg orally daily in 2-4 divided doses for 3-4 wk. Short test: 400 mg orally in 2-4 divided dosages for 4 days.
		For hypokalemia caused by diuretics, 25-100 mg daily as single dose or divided into 2-4 doses.
		Elderly may be more sensitive to adult dosages, so monitor closely. Maximum daily dosage is 400 mg.
	Children	Diuretic or antihypertensive, 1-3 mg/kg or 30-90 mg/m² orally as single dose or in 2-4 divided doses; adjust dosage as necessary after 5 days. Dosage increments may be increased up to 3 times the starting initial dose.
triamterene (Dyrenium)	Adults	Diuretic, 25-100 mg orally daily; adult dosage as necessary to achieve desired results. Maximum is 300 mg daily. Elderly may be more sensitive to adult dosages, so monitor closely.
	Children	Diuretic, 2-4 mg/kg or 120 mg/m² orally daily or on alternatie days in divided doses. Maintenance, increase to 6 mg/kg orally daily or adjust according to the individual's response to a maximum of 300 mg/day in divided dosages.
OSMOTIC DIURETICS		
Parenteral preparations mannitol (Osmitrol✦)	Adults	Diuretic, IV infusion 50-100 g (as 5%-25% solution), given at a rate to establish a urine flow of approximately 30-50 ml/hr.
		Cerebral edema or increased intracranial pressure or glaucoma, 1.5-2 g/kg in a 15%-25% solution given as an IV infusion over ½-1 hr. (If client is small or debilitated, a dose of 500 mg/kg may be adequate.)
		Adjunct to remove toxic substances, IV infusion of 50-200 g (as 5%-25% solution) given to establish and maintain a urine flow of 100-500 ml/hr.
		Antihemolytic, 2.5% bladder-irrigating solution during transurethral prostatic resection.
		Maximum dosage daily is 6 g/kg.
	Children	Diuretic, IV infusion, 2 g/kg or 60 g/m² as a 15%-20% solution, given over 2-6 hr.
		Cerebral edema, increased intracranial pressure, or glaucoma, IV, 1-2 g/kg or 30-60 g/m² as a 15%-20% solution, given over ½-1 hr. In small or debilitated clients, a dose of 500 mg/kg may be adequate.
		Adjunct to remove toxic substances, up to 2 g/kg or 60 g/m² as a 5%-10% solution given as IV infusion.
urea	Adults	Diuretic or antiglaucoma agent, 500 mg-1.5 g/kg as 30% solution in 5% or 10% dextrose injection administered as an IV infusion at a rate of 60 drops (4-6 ml)/min over ½-2 hr. Maximum dose is up to 2 g/kg in 24 hr.
	Children	If 2 yr or older, see adult dosage. For 2 yr and younger, 100 mg to 1.5 g/kg as a 30% solution in 5% or 10% dextrose injectable, administered as IV infusion at a rate of 60 drops (4-6 ml)/min over ½-2 hr.
ORAL PREPARATIONS		
glycerin	Adults	1-1.5 g/kg orally as single dose. Additional doses of 500 mg/kg may be given every 6 hr if necessary.
	Children	1-1.5 g/kg orally or 40 g/m² orally as a single dose. May be repeated in 4-8 hr if necessary.
isosorbide	Adults	1.5 g/kg orally initially. Range is 1-3 g/kg 2-4 times per day as necessary.
	Children	Not established.

the cortical diluting segment of the nephron, including portions of the thick ascending loop of Henle and the distal convoluted tubule. The role of these drugs in carbonic anhydrase inhibition is minor. They are less potent than the loop diuretics, since the maximum portion of the sodium load they can affect at the distal tubule is less than 10% of the glomerular filtrate. The thiazide-type diuretics therefore primarily promote the excretion of sodium, chloride, and water. Especially important is their ability to impair free water clearance with no effect on concentration ability. The initial natriuretic effect lasts for about 1 week and then resets at a lower level. This diuretic tolerance occurs because of increased aldosterone levels and a decreased sodium load at the distal tubule. The mechanisms of antihypertensive action are unknown, but they are believed to be of both extrarenal and renal origins and perhaps an altered sodium balance in the body.

When an increased sodium load is presented to the distal tubule, there is a corresponding increase in potassium secretion. In addition, as the extracellular fluid volume decreases, plasma renin activity and aldosterone levels increase, with resulting potassium loss. See Figure 33-2 for the body's adaptation to extracellular volume depletion. Potassium is one of the most common electrolytes lost, with loss occurring in up to 40% of clients. This loss is dose related; that is, it occurs more frequently with the larger diuretic doses, with the long-acting type of

diuretics (e.g., chlorthalidone), and in individuals with a high sodium intake (Herfindal and Hirschman, 1984). However, in many cases, the loss is intermittent and neither harmful nor clinically observable. Potassium loss may be a serious threat in those who are taking digitalis preparations, since it can precipitate serious dysrhythmias as a result of digitalis toxicity. Hypokalemia may predispose the client with cirrhosis to hepatic encephalopathy and coma.

Usually health care providers caution clients with prescribed thiazide therapy to increase their dietary intake of potassium (see box for foods high in potassium). If hypokalemia occurs, the physician may prescribe oral potassium preparations or, if urgent replacement is necessary, intravenous potassium chloride administration. Potassium loss may also be reversed by the addition of a potassium-sparing diuretic that acts to inhibit potassium loss at the distal tubule.

However, potassium replacement is usually not necessary in 80% to 90% of individuals taking the thiazide diuretics, particularly in the treatment of nonedematous states. It should be remembered that potassium replacement may be dangerous in the elderly, in renal dysfunction, and when used in combination with potassium-sparing diuretics, since dangerously high serum potassium levels may occur.

The thiazide-type diuretics are noted to increase serum

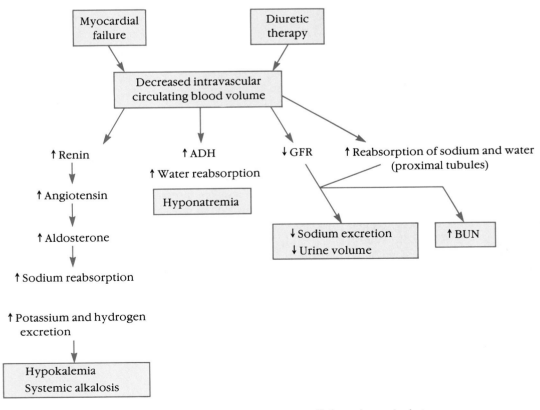

FIGURE 33-2 Body adaptation to extracellular volume depletion.

FOODS RICH IN POTASSIUM

FOOD	AMOUNT	POTASSIUM (mg)	FOOD	AMOUNT	POTASSIUM (mg)
Apricots			Prunes		
Fresh	1	105	Dried	1 cup	1200
Canned in water	1 cup	465	Juice, canned or	1 cup	706
Dried, uncooked	1 cup	1791	bottled		
Avocado	1	1369	Raisins	1 cup	1089
Banana	1	471	Lima beans, frozen,	1 cup	694
Figs			cooked		
Fresh	1	116	Beets, sliced,	1 cup	532
Canned in heavy	1 cup	258	cooked		
syrup			Brussels sprouts,	1 cup	494
Dried, uncooked	1 cup	1418	cooked		
Grapefruit			Peanuts roasted in	1 ounce	200
Canned in water	1 cup	322	oil		
Fresh	½	312	Potato		
Juice, canned,	1 cup	378	Baked	1	610
unsweetened			Boiled	1	515
Melon, fresh	1 cup	494	Spinach		
cantalope			Cooked, fresh	1 cup	838
Orange			Canned	1 cup	709
Fresh	1	237	From frozen	1 cup	566
Juice, frozen, diluted	1 cup	474	Squash		
Peaches			Acorn, baked	1 cup	896
Fresh	1	171	Hubbard, mashed	1 cup	504
Canned in water	1 cup	241	Winter, mashed	1 cup	895
Dried	1 cup	1594	Zucchini, canned	1 cup	622
Pears			Sweet potato, baked	1	397
Fresh	1	208	Tomato	1	297
Canned in juice	1 cup	238	Tomato juice,	1 cup	535
Dried	1 cup	959	canned		

From Burtis, G, Davis, J, and Martin, S: Applied nutrition and diet therapy, Philadelphia, 1988, WB Saunders Co.

uric acid in 40% of men (less often in women). The 1 to 2 mg/dl increase in serum uric acid is persistent and probably results from inhibition of tubular secretion of uric acid. However, this effect is reversible when the drugs are discontinued. In the absence of gout or genetic predisposition the hyperuricemia is usually no problem and requires no treatment. However, in a client with a history of gout the use of allopurinol or probenecid is suggested, to counteract any elevation of serum uric acid.

Hyperglycemia or impaired glucose tolerance has been reported with the thiazide-type and loop diuretics. This effect is reported most often in the elderly, and the thiazides can precipitate diabetes in individuals with overt and subclinical disease patterns. The thiazide diuretics are not contraindicated in diabetic clients because if hyperglycemia is noted it can usually be controlled by diet alterations or increasing the insulin dose. When hyperglycemia does occur in the nondiabetic client, many physicians prefer to try another type of diuretic such as furosemide to see if the problem can be reduced or alleviated.

The thiazide diuretics and perhaps furosemide have been associated with increasing serum levels of cholesterol and triglycerides, approximately 6% to 8% and 15% to 17%, respectively. Since elevated serum lipids are associated with an increase in coronary heart disease, it is important that serum lipids be monitored and perhaps a specific dietary approach or weight loss program be implemented if necessary.

Indications
1. Edema that may be associated with congestive heart failure

2. Cirrhosis with ascites
3. Some types of renal impairment, such as nephrotic syndrome, acute glomerulonephritis, and chronic renal failure

Pharmacokinetics

Absorption. Absorption of thiazide and thiazide-type diuretics is good.

Excretion. Thiazide and thiazide-type diuretics are excreted by the kidneys.

For half-life, onset of action, peak effect, and duration of action, see Table 33-4.

Side effects/adverse reactions. See Table 33-1.

Significant drug interactions. The following interactions may occur when thiazide and thiazide-type diuretics are given with the drugs listed below.

Drug	Possible Effect and Management
adrenocorticoids, glucocorticoid, mineralocorticoid, corticotropin (ACTH)	Electrolyte disturbances such as hypokalemia and sodium retention may occur. Diuretic effects may also be decreased. Monitor closely if concurrent therapy is necessary. Frequent electrolyte serum levels should be done, since potassium supplements may be necessary.
digitalis glycosides	Increased risk of digitalis toxicity in presence of hypokalemia. Monitor closely.
lithium	Not recommended. Increased risk of lithium toxicity possible because of decreased lithium excretion. Also, lithium has potential for nephrotoxic side effects. Avoid this combination.
methenamine	Thiazides may cause an alkaline urine that would decrease the effectiveness of methenamine. Avoid this combination.

Dosage and administration. See Table 33-3.

Pregnancy safety. Not established

NURSING CONSIDERATIONS

Assessment. Do not give thiazide and thiazide-type diuretics to people who are allergic to sulfonamides, since there may be a cross-sensitivity.

They are contraindicated or given carefully to pregnant women, since they cross the placental barrier.

Check creatinine clearance for elderly clients before administering thiazide-type diuretics.

Intervention. To reverse hypokalemia add foods rich in potassium to the diet (see p. 590). Liquid potassium for oral use, although unpleasant tasting, may be disguised in cold juices and taken with food. Tomato juice is not recommended for this purpose because it is high in sodium content. Enteric-coated potassium tablets should be avoided because they have been implicated in ulcerations of the gastrointestinal tract lining.

Discontinue thiazides before parathyroid function tests are performed, since they may alter serum calcium concentrations.

As with other diuretics, plan dosing schedules to minimize the inconvenience of diuresis for the client.

Education. Teach clients that thiazides may make them feel unusually tired. While taking these drugs, they also need to know how to take their pulse rate before taking digitalis medications. If the pulse rate is less than 60 beats/min or is irregular, digitalis medications should be discontinued and the physician notified. Nausea, vomiting, and anorexia are even earlier signs of digitalis toxicity that nurses and clients should recognize.

Clients should understand that diuretic drugs, if prescribed for a chronic condition, need to be taken as an integral part of their life-style. Compliance may be enhanced when nurses observe closely client's self-medicating habits and verbally reinforce them.

As with acetazolamide, the client should receive instruction related to the prevention and minimization of the effects of xerostomia, constipation, and orthostatic hypotension. Signs and symptoms of electrolyte imbalances and blood dyscrasias should be taught with proper referral to the physician.

Instruct clients to eat foods rich in potassium if a supplement is not prescribed (see p. 590).

Evaluation. Since hypokalemia is possible, monitor laboratory reports of serum potassium levels. Monitoring is particularly important when digitalis compounds are part of the regimen, since hypokalemia primes clients taking digitalis preparations for toxic cardiac effects of the digitalis, such as bradycardia or ventricular irritability.

Latent diabetes or gout may occasionally occur; laboratory reports should be monitored for hyperglycemia or hyperuricemia.

Observe the client for signs and symptoms of fluid and electrolyte imbalances: hypovolemia, hyponatremia, hypokalemia, hypocalcemia, hypochloremia, and hypomagnesemia (see box, p. 594).

LOOP DIURETICS
bumetanide (Bumex), ethacrynic acid (Edecrin), furosemide (Lasix, Furoside❀, Apo-Furosemide❀)

Bumetanide, furosemide, and ethacrynic acid are the classic examples of the loop diuretics, so called because they exert their action in the loop of Henle. These drugs for the most part are very similar to the thiazide-type diuretics in pharmacology and in the side effects they produce. Furosemide and ethacrynic acid exhibit their major effect by inhibiting active *chloride* transport in the thick portion of the ascending limb of the loop of Henle. The resulting passive sodium transport is also inhibited. The maximal effect of the loop diuretics is their indirect influence on urine concentration rather than on urine

TABLE 33-4   Diuretic Pharmacokinetics

Drug	Onset of action (hr)	Peak effect (hr)	Duration of action (hr)	Equivalent dose (mg)
DILUTING SEGMENT DIURETICS (THIAZIDE AND THIAZIDE-TYPE DIURETICS)				
bendroflumethiazide (Naturetin)	1-2	6-12	>18	5
benzthiazide (Exna, Hydrex)	2	4-6	12-18	50
chlorothiazide (Diuril, SK-Chlorothiazide)	2	4	6-12	500
chlorthalidone (Apo-Chlorthalidone♣, Hygroton, Thalitone)	2	2	24-72	64
cyclothiazide (Anhydron, Fluidil)	Within 6	7-12	18-24	2
hydrochlorothiazide (Esidrix, HydroDiuril, Oreton)	2	4	6-12	50
hydroflumethiazide (Diucardin, Saluron)	1-2	3-4	18-24	50
methyclothiazide (Aquatensen, Duretic♣)	2	6	>24	5
metolazone (Diulo, Zaroxolyn)	1	2	12-24	5
polythiazide (Renese)	2	6	24-48	2
quinethazone (Aquamox♣, Hydromox)	2	6	18-24	50
trichlormethiazide (Metahydrin, Naqua)	2	6	24	2
LOOP DIURETICS				
bumetanide (Bumex)	½-1 within minutes (IV)	1-2 ¼-½ (IV)	4 (usual dosages) 4-6 (higher dosages) 3½-4 (IV dose)	0.5-2 (PO) 0.5-1 (IV)
ethacrynic acid (Edecrin)	½ (PO); approx. 5 min (IV)	2 (PO); ¼-½ (IV)	6-8 (PO) 2 (IV)	50-100 (PO) 50 (IV)
furosemide (Lasix, Furoside♣)	½-1 (PO); 5 min (IV)	1-2 (PO);' ⅓-1 (IV)	6-8 (PO) 2 (IV)	20-80 20-40
DISTAL TUBULE DIURETICS OR POTASSIUM-SPARING DIURETICS				
amiloride (Midamor)	Within 2	6-10	24	5-20*
spironolactone (Aldactone, Novospiroton♣, Sincomen♣)	24-48	48-72	48-72	25-200*
triamterene (Dyrenium)	2-4	24-48	7-9	25-100*

*Daily dose range.

dilution. Furosemide and ethacrynic acid are more potent diuretics than the thiazides because they have the potential for altering 20% to 25% of the filtered sodium load, which is presented to the ascending limb of the loop of Henle. The loop diuretics do not inhibit carbonic anhydrase, except when furosemide is administered in very high doses. Carbohydrate intolerance may occur but is less frequent. Rather than the hypocalciuric effect of the thiazides, the loop diuretics (particularly furosemide) promote calcium excretion. Furosemide in combination with normal saline infusion is the treatment of choice in hypercalcemia. Ethacrynic acid has little or no direct effect on glomerular filtration rate, whereas furosemide exhibits a renal vasodilator effect, resulting in less vascular resistance and increased renal blood flow. Furosemide is therefore useful in renal failure, although it is contraindicated in anuria. Bumetanide inhibits sodium reabsorption in the ascending limb of the loop of Henle, as shown by marked reduction of free-water clearance during hydration and tubular free-water reabsorption during dehydration. Reabsorption of chloride in the ascending loop is also blocked by bumetanide, which may have an additional action in the proximal tubule. Since phosphate reabsorption takes place largely in the proximal tubule, phosphaturia during bumetanide-induced diuresis indicates this additional action. This proximal tubular activity does not seem to be related to an inhibition of carbonic anhydrase. Bumetanide does not appear to have a noticeable action on the distal tubule. It decreases uric acid excretion and increases serum uric acid.

The loop diuretics also differ from the thiazides in that they have an infinite dose-response curve. Increasing the dose continues to produce greater responses; hence they are referred to as "high-ceiling" diuretics.

Mechanism of action. See previous section.

Indications

1. Treatment of edema associated with congestive heart failure, adjunct therapy in acute pulmonary edema, and adjunct therapy in renal disease
2. Treatment of hypertension, especially as adjuncts or in combination with other therapies
3. Ethacrynic acid used for short-term treatment of ascites

Pharmacokinetics

For half-life, onset of action, peak effect, and duration of action, see Table 33-4.

Absorption. Oral absorption of the loop diuretics is fair to good.

Protein binding. Protein binding by the loop diuretics is high to very high.

Metabolism. The loop diuretics are metabolized by the liver.

Excretion. The loop diuretics are excreted by the kidneys and bile.

Side effects/adverse reactions. See Table 33-1.

Significant drug interactions. The following interactions may occur when loop diuretics are given with the drugs listed below.

Drug	Possible Effect and Management
adrenocorticoids, amphotericin B injectable	See thiazide drug interactions. Avoid concurrent therapy. Increases risk for ototoxicity, nephrotoxicity, and electrolyte imbalance (especially hypokalemia). If given concurrently, monitor closely with frequent electrolyte serum testing.
lithium	See discussion of thiazide drug interactions.
nephrotoxic medications or other ototoxic medications	Increases risks for ototoxicity and nephrotoxicity (especially in clients with renal impairment). Avoid concurrent and even sequential drug administration.

Dosage and administration. See Table 33-3.

Pregnancy safety. FDA Category C for bumetanide and furosemide; not established for ethacrynic acid.

NURSING CONSIDERATIONS

Assessment. Recommend against using loop diuretics in the presence of anuria and liver dysfunction. With bumetanide and furosemide, there may be cross hypersensitivity to sulfonamides.

Note precautions if the client is also receiving the following medications:

- Aminoglycoside antibiotics: watch for tinnitus, vertigo, or hearing difficulties.
- Digitalis compounds, corticosteroids, or corticotropin: review serum electrolyte reports closely.
- Cephalothin, cephaloridine, or lithium: watch for diminished urinary output and other signs of nephrotoxicity.

Intervention. Use of the intramuscular route can produce temporary pain at the site, so oral or intravenous routes are preferable.

Administer these drugs so that onset and peak of action will coincide with access to toilet facilities.

Administer with food if gastrointestinal upset occurs with oral forms.

When administering oral solutions, use the calibrated dropper provided by the manufacturer for accurate dosages.

For bumetanide and furosemide, administer intravenous injection slowly over 2 minutes. Administer ethacrynic acid intravenously at a controlled rate over 30 minutes.

Because many glass ampules are required to be broken to prepare large dosages of furosemide intravenous infusions, there is the possibility of glass fragments occurring in the solution. Use filter to remove these particles during intravenous administration.

Education. Caution the client to move carefully from sitting or lying positions to upright ones because of positional hypotension. Alcohol ingestion, hot weather, and standing for long periods also increase the risk of orthostatic hypotension.

Instruct the client in the symptoms of electrolyte imbalances (see box, p. 594), particularly hypokalemia. Provide dietary counseling so the client will know which foods are rich in potassium.

Checking refills of the medication prescription provides a basis for client counseling for compliance with the regimen and also provides the opportunity for appropriate feedback. Caution clients about switching brands of furosemide because differences in bioavailability occur between them.

Photosensitivity is a problem for some clients taking furosemide; caution them to avoid prolonged exposure to the sun or sunlamps. Encourage clients to use sun-blocking lotion and cover themselves with clothing.

Evaluation. Closely monitor clients, especially the elderly, for blood pressure changes; postural hypotension; dehydration (e.g., body weight loss of more than 2 pounds/day); allergic reactions (rashes); nausea, vomiting, and diarrhea; and serum potassium deficiency.

Monitor carefully clients who may be experiencing potassium loss through other causes, such as vomiting, diarrhea, diaphoresis, gastrointestinal drainage, or paracentesis for signs and symptoms of hypokalemia.

Check reports of serum electrolytes, uric acid, blood and urine glucose tests, and BUN levels for abnormalities.

Excessive doses or too frequent administration can lead to prolonged water loss, electrolyte depletion, dehydration, reduction in blood volume, and circulatory collapse, with the possibility of vascular thrombosis and embolism, especially in elderly clients.

Be aware that hypokalemia can occur. Prevention of hypokalemia requires particular attention to the following conditions: individuals receiving digitalis and diuretics for congestive heart failure, hepatic cirrhosis and ascites; states of aldosterone excess with normal renal function; potassium-losing nephropathy; and certain diarrheal states.

Measure serum potassium levels periodically and add potassium supplements or potassium-sparing diuretics if necessary. Periodic determination of other electrolytes is advised in clients with high doses for prolonged periods, particularly in those on low-salt diets.

Be aware that hyperuricemia may occur; reversible elevation of BUN and creatinine levels may occur, especially in association with dehydration and particularly in clients with renal insufficiency.

Periodically determine blood sugar, particularly in clients with diabetes or suspected latent diabetes.

DISTAL TUBULE DIURETICS/POTASSIUM-SPARING DIURETICS

amiloride (Midamor), spironolactone (Sincomen✦, Aldactone), triamterene (Dyrenium)

Mechanism of action. These three **potassium-sparing diuretics** will be considered together because many of their actions are similar. Important differences among them will be noted. They are generally considered weak diuretics that act at the distal renal tubules, but they are primarily considered useful when combined with other potassium-losing diuretics. Amiloride is a salt of a moderately strong base; spironolactone is an aldosterone antagonist; and triamterene directly inhibits reabsorption of sodium and water and yet retains potassium at the distal tubule. Any of the three agents may be used when it is necessary to restore or preserve the normal serum potassium level if other concurrent diuretic therapy challenges it and when potassium supplementation by medication or

---

SIGNS AND SYMPTOMS OF FLUID AND ELECTROLYTE IMBALANCES ASSOCIATED WITH DIURETIC THERAPY

Hypovolemia: hypotension, weak pulse, tachycardia, clammy skin, rapid respirations, and reduced urinary output

Hyponatremia: low serum sodium levels (normal range 135 to 145 mEq/L), lethargy, disorientation, muscle tenseness, seizures, and coma

Hypokalemia: low serum potassium levels (normal range 3.5 to 5.0 mEq/L), weakness, abnormal ECG, postural hypotension, and flaccid paralysis

Hypocalcemia: low serum calcium levels (normal range 8.4 to 10.2 mg/dl), irritability, vomiting, diarrhea, twitching, hyperactive reflexes, cardiac dysrhythmias, tetany, and seizures

Hypochloremia: low blood chloride levels (normal range 100 to 110 mEq/L)

Hypomagnesemia: low serum magnesium levels (normal range 1.3 to 2.1 mEq/L), nausea and vomiting, lethargy, muscle weakness, tremors, and tetany

WITH POTASSIUM-SPARING DIURETICS, BE ALERT FOR:

Hyperkalemia: above-normal values for potassium serum levels, nausea, diarrhea, muscle weakness, postural hypotension, and ECG changes

---

diet is inappropriate. They are highly effective for this purpose. Thus these drugs are usually administered as an adjunct to diuretic therapy. If prescribed singly, however, their efficacy may actually result in an undesirable and rapidly developing hyperkalemia.

Amiloride is not an aldosterone antagonist, and it is chemically unrelated to any other diuretic in use. It acts to block sodium-potassium exchange in the distal renal tubule with resultant increases in sodium and chloride excretion and with decreased potassium and hydrogen excretion. Its action leaves glomerular filtration rate and renal blood flow unchanged.

Spironolactone is a synthetic steroidal compound used to antagonize the effect of aldosterone by competitively binding to the protein that permits potassium secretion at the distal tubule. This response is directly related to the amount of circulating aldosterone in the serum. Spironolactone produces a very mild diuresis of sodium and water at the distal tubule by means of this mechanism. It does not interfere with renal tubule transport of sodium and chloride and does not inhibit carbonic anhydrase.

Triamterene directly depresses the renal tubular transport of sodium in the distal tubule independent of the presence of aldosterone. Excretion of sodium, chloride, bicarbonate, magnesium, and calcium is increased. The increased loss of bicarbonate, which may slightly alkalinize the urine, is not a result of carbonic anhydrase inhibition. The decreased serum bicarbonate levels can produce metabolic acidosis. More important is the ability of triamterene to decrease the secretion of potassium at the distal tubule. Unlike the thiazide-type diuretics, triamterene does not inhibit uric acid excretion, although elevated serum levels have been reported, particularly in clients with a history of gout. Cardiac output is decreased, as is the glomerular filtration rate, which may result in an increased BUN level and a decreased creatinine clearance rate.

Indications

1. Adjunct in the treatment of edema and hypertension
2. Diagnosis and treatment of primary hyperaldosteronism
3. Prevention and treatment of hypokalemia

Pharmacokinetics. For half-life, onset of action, peak concentration, and duration of action, see Table 33-4.

Absorption. Amiloride absorption is low (15% to 20%). Spironolactone absorption is good. Triamterene absorption is variable (30% to 70%).

Metabolism. Amiloride is not metabolized. Spironolactone and triamterene are metabolized by the liver.

Excretion. Amiloride and spironolactone are excreted primarily by the kidneys and then feces and bile; triamterene is excreted primarily by bile and then the kidneys.

Side effects/adverse reactions. See Table 33-1.

Significant drug interactions. The following interactions may occur when potassium-sparing diuretics are given with the drugs listed below.

Drug	Possible Effect and Management
lithium	See discussion of thiazide drug interactions
blood from blood bank; captopril, cyclosporine, or other potassium-sparing diuretics; enalapril; low-salt milk; potassium-containing medications; or potassium supplements	May increase potassium levels and result in hyperkalemia. Monitor closely.
for spironolactone only: carbenoxolone	Spironolactone may inhibit both the therapeutic effects (ulcer healing) and side effects of carbenoxolone. Avoid concurrent drug administration.

Dosage and administration. See Table 33-3.

Pregnancy safety. FDA Category B for amiloride; FDA category not established for spironolactone and triamterene.

NURSING CONSIDERATIONS

Assessment. Before giving these compounds, ascertain that the client has no related drug history of hypersensitivity or hyperkalemia.

Intervention. Administering these drugs with food or milk may allay some gastrointestinal symptoms and possibly enhance bioavailability.

Deal with discomforting side effects such as dry mouth, thirst, or drowsiness if they arise.

Plan nursing measures common to diuretic agents, for example, measurements of fluid intake and output, daily weight changes, vital signs and heart rhythm, assessment of postural hypotension, weakness, or confusion.

Monitor closely for hyperkalemia when transfusing blood. Whole blood may contain up to 30 mEq of potassium per liter; this may be doubled if blood has been stored more than 10 days.

Education. The client should be counseled to avoid excessively stringent low-salt diets and relatively concentrated potassium intake in the form of citrus juices, cola beverages, low-sodium milk, some salt substitutes, and other potassium supplements.

Evaluation. Evaluate compliance with the client frequently. Especially at first, be alert to an irregular heartbeat (often the first clinical sign of hyperkalemia) or peaked T waves on ECG. Other warning signs of hyperkalemia are confusion, tingling in the extremities, difficulty in breathing, unexplained anxiety, fatigue, and physical weakness. Serum electrolyte determinations and an ECG are probably indicated if these occur.

Check laboratory reports closely, especially if the client is taking other similar drugs or potassium-rich foods. Rapidly increased serum potassium levels may occur. Act immediately to reverse hyperkalemia if serum potassium level exceeds 6 to 6.5 mEq/L and anticipate treatment with sodium bicarbonate, with glucose and regular insulin preparations, or with other therapy.

If the client is receiving spironolactone, remain sensitive to cues that he or she may be concerned about body image changes that may threaten sexual identity.

Note that when triamterene is being given, a complete blood count is probably indicated if the client has an unexplained sore throat, mouth ulcerations, or fever, indications of a possible blood dyscrasia.

OSMOTIC DIURETICS

mannitol (Osmitrol✣), urea (Ureaphil), glycerin (Glyrol, Osmoglyn), isosorbide (Ismotic)

Osmotic diuretics include mannitol and urea parenterally and glycerin and isosorbide orally. The two parenteral agents cause diuresis by adding to the solutes already present in the tubular fluid; they are particularly effective in increasing osmotic pressure there because they are not reabsorbed by the tubules. Thus more water is pulled into tubular fluid, and less sodium, chloride, and water are reabsorbed by the kidneys in an effort to equalize the higher solute content. These excesses are then excreted in the urine.

The oral agents are primarily used to reduce intraocular pressure, before and after intraocular surgery or to interrupt an acute attack of glaucoma.

Mechanism of action. See previous section.

Indications. For oral agents, see previous section. Parenteral agents are used to treat cerebral edema and secondary glaucoma when other methods have been unsuccessful. Mannitol has also been used to increase urinary excretion of toxic substances (salicylates, barbiturates, lithium, bromides), as an irrigating preparation to prevent hemolysis and hemoglobin accumulation during transurethral prostatic resection, and as an adjunct to other therapies in the treatment of edema in acute renal failure.

Pharmacokinetics

Parenteral agents

Metabolism. Very little if any mannitol is metabolized in the liver. Urea is partially metabolized in the gastrointestinal tract to ammonia and carbon dioxide, which may be resynthesized into urea.

Half-life. Mannitol has a half-life of approximately 100 minutes (up to 36 hours in acute renal failure). Urea has a half-life of approximately 1.17 hours.

Onset of action. Mannitol's diuresis effect takes place in 1 to 3 hours; lowering of cerebrospinal and intraocular fluid pressure occur within 15 min. Lowering of intracranial and intraocular pressure with urea occurs within 10 minutes.

Time to peak effect. The peak effect for mannitol in lowering intraocular pressure occurs ½ to 1 hour after administration. For urea it occurs in 1 to 2 hours.

Duration of action. Mannitol lowers cerebrospinal fluid for 3 to 8 hours after the injection is stopped; it lowers intraocular pressure for 4 to 8 hours. Urea promotes diuresis for 3 to 10 hours after the infusion is stopped; it lowers cerebrospinal fluid pressure for 3 to 10 hours after stopping the infusion; and it lowers intraocular pressure for 5 to 6 hours.

Excretion. Both mannitol and urea are excreted by the kidneys.

Oral agents

Absorption. Glycerin absorption is good.

Onset of action. Glycerin lowers intraocular pressure within 10 minutes.

Time to peak effect. Glycerin achieves its peak effect in lowering intraocular pressure within 1 to 1½ hours.

Duration of action. Glycerin's effect lasts approximately 5 hours.

Metabolism. Glycerin is metabolized by the liver.

Excretion. Glycerin is excreted by the kidneys.

•   •   •

Isosorbide pharmacokinetics are not available.

Side effects/adverse reactions. See Table 33-1.

Significant drug interactions. For glycerin, isosorbide, and urea there are no drug interactions. Mannitol when given with digitalis glycosides may increase the risk of digitalis toxicity as a result of hypokalemia. If given concurrently, monitor closely.

Dosage and administration. See Table 33-3.

Pregnancy safety. Mannitol and urea are FDA Category C. Glycerin is FDA Category C. FDA Category is not established for isosorbide.

NURSING CONSIDERATIONS

Assessment. Ascertain that the client does not have preexisting congestive heart failure, severe dehydration, or pulmonary or renal disease for which osmotic diuretics are contraindicated. Intracranial bleeding, except during craniotomy, would negate the use for mannitol and urea.

Recommend that baseline serum electrolyte and renal function determinations be performed if they have not been done, and monitor the results.

Mannitol is different from the drug mannitol hexanitrate. Do not confuse them.

Intervention. If the adequacy of renal function is suspect before the administration of mannitol, a test dose is recommended. It is given as an intravenous infusion over 3 to 5 minutes. Urine flow should increase to at least 30 to 50 ml/hr for 2 to 3 hours after this or a second test dose. If it does not, mannitol should be withheld and the client reevaluated.

Infuse mannitol and urea separately from other drugs and blood. Crystalization in solution is common; it may be countered by warming the solution until crystals are invisible and by inserting a filter in the line any time this drug is infused.

Avoid extravasation of urea and mannitol; observe the intravenous site periodically for tissue inflammation, irritation, and necrosis.

With urea, use large veins for infusion. With both urea and mannitol, avoid using lower extremity intravenous sites since phlebitis and thrombosis may occur, particularly in the elderly.

Do not infuse urea more rapidly than 4 ml/minute because hemolysis and cerebral vasomotor symptoms may occur.

To assist in the prevention and relief of headache caused by cerebral dehydration, have the client lie down during and after the administration of these drugs.

Use an indwelling catheter with comatose clients to ensure urinary drainage. The use of a urometer that allows for precise measurement of output is important because the therapy is based on evaluation of accurate intake and output.

When these drugs are administered preoperatively, the dosing schedule should be: glycerin, isosorbide, and mannitol, 1 to 1½ hours before surgery; and urea, 1 hour before surgery if for the reduction of intraocular pressure or at the time of scalp incision during intracranial surgery.

Glycerin and isosorbide may be mixed with iced unsweetened fruit juice and sipped through a straw to increase palatability.

With repeated doses of these drugs, maintain adequate fluid and electrolyte balance.

Education. Prepare the client for the diuresis that will occur with these drugs. Provide for the convenience, comfort, and privacy of the client.

Advise client taking glycerin and isosorbide for the reduction of intraocular pressure to visit the physician regularly for intraocular pressure monitoring.

Evaluation. Since these are potent osmotic drugs, alertness to rapidly changing client conditions is essential: frequent assessment of urinary output and vital signs for changing intravascular volume, pulmonary edema, or hemoconcentration.

Monitor fluid and electrolyte balance, particularly serum and urine potassium and sodium levels. When urea is administered, BUN determinations should be done before and frequently during intravenous administration. If the BUN exceeds 75 mg/dl or if there is no diuresis within 1 to 2 hours, slow or stop the infusion and have the client reevaluated.

If the osmotic diuretics are administered for reduction of intraocular pressure, monitor the pressure closely.

DIURETIC COMBINATIONS

As mentioned previously, a thiazide diuretic may be combined with a potassium-sparing diuretic. Fixed-dose combinations are commercially available (see box) that may provide additional diuretic activity and decrease the potassium depletion characteristic of the thiazide diuretics.

KEY TERMS

carbonic anhydrase, page 583
hypercalciuria, page 585
hyperkalemia, page 594
hypocalcemia, page 594
hypochloremia, page 594
hypokalemia, page 594

EXAMPLES OF FIXED-DOSE DIURETIC COMBINATIONS

TRADE NAME	CONTENTS
Moduretic	amiloride HCl, 5 mg; hydrochlorthiazide, 50 mg
Aldactazide 25/25	spironolactone, 25 mg; hydrochlorothiazide, 25 mg
Aldactazide 50/50	spironolactone, 50 mg; hydrochlorothiazide, 50 mg
Dyazide	triamterene, 50 mg; hydrochlorothiazide, 25 mg
Maxzide	triamterene, 75 mg; hydrochlorothiazide, 50 mg
Maxzide-25	triamterene, 37.5 mg; hydrochlorothiazide, 25 mg

---

hypomagnesemia, page 594
hyponatremia, page 594
hypovolemia, page 594
osmotic diuretics, page 595
potassium-sparing diuretics, page 594
thiazide-type diuretics, page 586

BIBLIOGRAPHY

American Hospital Formulary Service: AHFS drug information '87, Bethesda, Md, 1987, American Society of Hospital Pharmacists, Inc.

Brater, DC: Clinical use of loop diuretics, Hosp Formul 18(10):962, 1983.

Brater, DC: Clinical use of thiazide diuretics, Hosp Formul 18(8):788, 1983.

Brater, DC: Sites and mechanisms of action of diuretics, Hosp Formul 18(3):309, 1983.

Brater, DC: Clinical use of diuretics. V. Logical combinations of diuretics: prescribing guidelines, Hosp Formul 19(6):485, 1984.

Brater, DC: Clinical utility of the potassium-sparing diuretics, Hosp Formul 19(1):79, 1984.

Brater, DC: Clinical use of diuretics: Nondiuretic uses of nondiuretic agents, part 6, Hosp Formul 20(1):62, 1985.

Brest, AN: Diuretic drug therapy in cardiac failure, Hosp Formul 17(6):804, 1982.

Brest, AN: Clinical considerations in diuretic drug therapy, Physician Assist 9(10):121, 1985.

Burgess, KE: Recognizing and responding to increased I.C.P., Nursinglife 5(2):33, 1985.

Burtis, G, Davis, J, and Martin, S: Applied nutrition and diet therapy, Philadelphia, 1988, WB Saunders Co.

Chobanian, AV: Options for the failing heart: diuretics with caution . . . the kidney and its role in diuresis, Emerg Med 16(15):37, 1984.

Cutler, RE: Antihypertensive therapy: a hard look at the agents we use, Consultant 24(3):321, 1984.

Eddins, B: A review of the pathophysiologic basis of end stage renal disease, J Nephrol Nurs 1(2):85, 1984.

Eilers, MA: Pharmacologic therapeutic modalities: osmotic and diuretic agents . . . rapid intervention to reverse elevated intracranial pressure, CCQ 5(4):44, 1983.

Franciosa, JA, and others: Intervening effectively in early CHF, Patient Care 21(2):39, 1987.

Gever, LN: Bumetanide: the latest loop diuretic, Nursing '87 17(4):115, 1987.

Gever, LN: Acetazolamide: the diverse diuretic, Nursing '84 14(12):12, 1984.

Gever, LN: Thiazide diuretics: minimizing their adverse effects, Nursing '84 14(2):72, 1984.

Guyton, AC: Textbook of medical physiology, ed 7, Philadelphia, 1986, WB Saunders Co.

Halpern, JS, and others: Furosemide . . . drug update, J Emerg Nurs 8(6):311, 1982.

Halstenson, CE, and others: Bumetanide: a new loop diuretic, Drug Intell Clin Pharm 17(11):786, 1983.

Herfindal, ET, and Hirschman, JL: Clinical pharmacy and therapeutics, ed 3, Baltimore, 1984, The Williams & Wilkins Co.

Hill, MN: Diuretics for mild hypertension: still the best choice? Nursing '87 17(9):62, 1987.

Hutcheon, DE, and Martinez, JC: A decade of developments in diuretic drug therapy, J Clin Pharmacol 26(8):567, 1986.

Kastrup, EK, and Olin, BR: Facts and comparisons: drug information, Philadelphia, 1987, JB Lippincott Co.

Katcher, BS, and others: Applied therapeutics: the clinical use of drugs, ed 3, San Francisco, 1983, Applied Therapeutics, Inc.

Kirschenbaum, HL, and others: What to watch out for with thiazides, RN 46(7):28, 1983.

Klassen, DK, and others: Thiazide therapy: possible complications and how to avoid them, Consultant 25(17):106, 1985.

Klein, AE: When potassium therapy is needed, Patient Care 16(16):63, 1982.

Lamy, PP: Side effects of diuretics: a danger for aged, J Gerontol Nurs 11(6):44, 1985.

Lumb, PD: Use and abuse of diuretics in the immediate postoperative period, Curr Rev Recov Room Nurses 5(9):67, 1983.

McCauley, K, and others: Your detailed guide to drugs for C.H.F., Nursing 14(5):46, 1984.

McGillicuddy, JE: Cerebral protection: pathophysiology and treatment of increased intracranial pressure, Chest 87(1):85, 1985.

McKenny, JM: Alternative pharmacologic approaches to the initial management of hypertension, Drug Intell Clin Pharmacol 19(9):629, 1985.

Melmon, KL: Getting the most out of antihypertensives, Emerg Med 18(2):80, 1986.

Meyer, SK, and others: Digitalis and diuretics: prescribing for the elderly, part 4, Hosp Formul 20(6):708, 1985.

Miller, K: Mannitol conscious, Emergency 18(10):17, 1986.

Paige, DM: Manual of clinical nutrition, ed 2, St Louis, 1987, The CV Mosby Co.

Pennington, AT, and Church, HN, eds: Bowes and Church's food values of portions commonly used, ed 14, Philadelphia, 1985, JB Lippincott Co.

Rosenberg, JM, and others: What to watch out for with nonthiazides, RN 46(8):41, 1983.

Shreeve, C: Controlling edema . . . potassium-sparing diuretics, Nurs Mirror 157(18):49, 1983.

Smith, S: How drugs act: diuretic agents, Nurs Times 83(23):53, 1987.

United States Pharmacopeial Convention: Drug information for the health care provider, ed 7, Rockville, Md, 1987, US Pharmacopeial Convention, Inc.

Webster, M: Trends and controversies in head-trauma care, Nursinglife 4(6):46, 1984.

CHAPTER
34

Antimicrobials for Urinary Tract Infections

OBJECTIVES

After studying this chapter, the student will be able to:

1. Discuss the prevalence and risk factors associated with urinary tract infections.

2. Describe the principles of preventive therapy for urinary tract infections.

3. Describe nursing interventions in antimicrobial therapy related to urinary tract infections.

4. Discuss the role of antibiotics, sulfonamides, urinary antiseptics, and urinary tract analgesics in urinary tract infections.

5. Describe the mechanism of action, indications, pharmacokinetics, dosages, and side effects/adverse reactions of common agents used in the treatment of urinary tract infections.

6. Apply appropriate nursing considerations for clients receiving drug therapy for urinary tract infections.

Urinary tract infections (UTIs) include a variety of clinical conditions, such as cystitis, pyelonephritis, prostatitis, urethritis, and catheter-related bacteriuria. The incidence of UTIs increases with age and results in nearly 6 million physician office visits annually and approximately 20% of all prescribed antibiotics. Nearly 40% of UTIs are caused by **nosocomial infection,** that is, acquired in an institutional setting such as a hospital or nursing home, with such infections often resulting in or harboring resistant organisms. The incidence of **bacteriuria** (the presence of bacteria in the urine) in women between the ages of 20 and 50 years increases with advancing age more so than with men. Usually in men, UTI is associated with inflammation of the prostate gland **(prostatitis),** prostate hypertrophy leading to urinary retention, or urinary tract instrumentation.

Important predisposing risk factors for UTIs need to be assessed in clients (see box). UTIs occur in approximately 25% of individuals who have an indwelling urethral catheter. It has been stated that the risk of a catheterized client developing a UTI is nearly 5% per day (Stamm and Turck, 1987). In the past it was believed that chronic renal failure was the result of UTIs. It was also thought that if UTI occurred during pregnancy, it may have resulted in low birth weight and infants with congenital defects. These beliefs have been discounted by many researchers (Critchley and Robson, 1987), but one must be aware that

PREDISPOSING RISK FACTORS FOR UTIs

RISK FACTORS	FREQUENCY
Diabetes	20%
Indwelling catheter (closed system)	37%-50%
Condom catheter	50%
Urologic disease (congenital)	57%
Nephrolithiasis	85%
Indwelling catheter (open system)	98%

Data from Goldstein, EJC: Consultant Pharmacist 2(suppl A):3-7, 1987.

there is an increased risk of developing acute pyelone-phritis in untreated, asymptomatic UTIs (30%). Also, infants and young children with intrarenal reflux and adults with abnormal kidneys or urinary tracts are definitely at risk for developing renal failure from untreated UTIs. Because of the risks from UTIs it is recommended that all clients with symptomatic or asymptomatic UTI be treated with the appropriate antimicrobial medication.

Many oral and parenteral antimicrobial agents are commonly used to treat UTIs. Before selecting an agent, the physician should try to identify the microorganism and determine its antimicrobial sensitivity. The most common bacteria-causing UTIs include *Esherichia coli, Klebsiella,* species, *Proteus* species, *Pseudomonas* species, and other gram-negative organisms. The goal is to eliminate the causative agent with an appropriate drug regimen. To do this, short-term treatment (3 to 7 days) is usually prescribed for the client with an acute UTI, whereas clients with recurrent UTIs are often treated with low-dose, long-term drug therapy. The primary agents used are penicillins, cephalosporins, sulfonamides, urinary tract antiseptics (nitrofurantoin, methenamine mandelate, nalidixic acid, and cinoxacin), aztreonam, and norfloxacin. For simplification, this chapter will divide the agents into antibiotics, antiseptics, monobactams and fluoroquinolones, and analgesics.

THE NURSE'S ROLE IN ANTIMICROBIAL THERAPY FOR CLIENTS WITH URINARY TRACT INFECTIONS

Assessment. Initial assessment of the client provides baseline information and includes history of past UTIs and the signs and symptoms of the current UTI. Drug allergies, concurrent drug therapy, and altered function of any body system may affect the drug therapy. Specific considerations will be discussed for each class of antimicrobial drug later in the chapter and in Chapter 61.

Intervention. Nursing interventions relative to antimicrobial drug therapy are discussed in greater detail in Chapter 61. Generally, these interventions relate to (1) assistance in the identification of the infecting organism, (2) actual administration of the drug, (3) assessment of the client's response to the drug, (4) client education, and (5) prevention and treatment of adverse responses, including pharmacologic and chemical drug-drug interactions.

Obtaining urine specimens to determine the causative organism for UTI is frequently the nurse's responsibility. Through client education, most clients can obtain a clean-catch urine sample of appropriate quantity and quality for laboratory testing. The physician will specify whether a midstream clean-catch or catheterized specimen is required. In either case it is essential that the procedure be done appropriately to ensure the most accurate results. A basic nursing text should be consulted for these procedures. Specimens for culture should be taken directly to the laboratory to prevent death of the suspect organisms and to prevent the growth of contaminating ones.

If an antimicrobial agent is ordered before the infecting organism has been identified, it is important that the urine sample for initial culture be obtained before the administration of the first dose of the drug. With subsequent specimens for culture, it is important to describe the client's antimicrobial regimen for the laboratory, since the selection and interpretation of laboratory tests often depend on this information.

Because around-the-clock administration of antimicrobial drugs at prescribed dosage intervals is required for maintaining therapeutic blood levels of these drugs, it is the nurse's responsibility to see that this is accomplished. This is done by providing the necessary client education, which may entail awakening sleeping clients and ensuring that tests or therapies do not interrupt the dosage.

Education. Clients should be taught the principles of antimicrobial therapy so that these drugs can be self-administered safely. The necessity of adherence to an inconvenient around-the-clock schedule may require special counseling. Compliance for the full course of therapy is essential to prevent the possible development of resistant strains of microorganisms. "Leftover" antimicrobial medications should not be used for new bouts of infection; rather, medical attention should be sought. For specific instructions for each drug, refer to the text.

Instruct the client to avoid coffee, tea, juices with high citric acid content, cola, alcohol, chocolate, and spices, which often irritate a sensitive bladder.

The client should be taught health practices that may reduce the chance of developing another UTI (see box).

Evaluation. Evaluation of the client for therapeutic responses to antimicrobial agents is a primary nursing responsibility. A decrease in the severity or a disappearance of the clinical and laboratory manifestations of the UTI indicates a positive response to antimicrobial therapy. Documentation should include the client's health status relating to fever, chills, flank pain, and nausea and vomiting; frequency and urgency of urination; dysuria; costovertebral tenderness; gross hematuria and pyuria; and general well-being. Urinalysis should be monitored for WBCs, RBCs, casts, protein, crystals, and bacteria. Urine culture and sensitivity examinations should indicate the drug's efficacy. CBCs should also be monitored. Serum antibiotic concentrations can be monitored through the course of therapy to assess for therapeutic and toxic levels of specific antimicrobials.

In addition to monitoring the therapeutic effects of these antimicrobials, the nurse must assess the client for the development of common side effects/adverse reactions of individual drugs. (See discussions of specific drugs for these effects.)

ANTIBIOTICS

The primary antibiotics used to treat UTIs include ampicillin, amoxicillin, and the cephalosporins and sulfonamides. They are used to treat microorganisms such as *E. coli* that are sensitive to their antibacterial action. Ampi-

---

CLIENT EDUCATION TO REDUCE OCCURRENCE OF UTIs

UTIs frequently occur as a result of contamination of the lower urinary tract with perineal bacteria. Preventive measures attempt to reduce perineal bacteria and prevent bacteria from entering the lower urinary tract. Client education should focus on these two measures and include the following instructions:

1. Good perineal hygiene helps reduce bacterial growth.
2. Female clients should always wipe from the front to the back to prevent contamination of the urinary tract with fecal bacteria.
3. Emptying the bladder soon after intercourse helps wash out bacteria that may have entered the urethra.
4. Cotton undergarments (or synthetics with a cotton crotch) that "breathe" are preferred to synthetics that foster bacterial growth.
5. Drinking six to eight glasses of fluids per day and urinating often help to cleanse the urinary tract of bacteria.

---

ndx Selected Nursing Diagnoses for Clients Receiving Urinary Tract Antiinfectives

Nursing diagnosis	Outcome criteria	Nursing interventions
Infection, potential for	Prevention of infection or resolution of symptoms of infection: Temperature remains within the normal range.	Monitor and record temperature at least every 4 hours. Report elevations.
	WBC remains within the normal range.	Monitor WBCs. Report significant changes.
	Urine cultures demonstrate no pathogens.	Culture urine as ordered and monitor results.
	Urine is clear and odorless.	Use strict aseptic technique when inserting urinary catheters.
	Fluid intake of 3000 ml/24 hr.	Encourage a fluid intake of at least 3000 ml daily.
Knowledge deficit related to medication regimen	Client will describe underlying conditions and how the drug relates to the condition, how and when to take the medication, common drug interactions, safety precautions, common side effects/adverse reactions, and which of these warrant reporting.	Assess learning needs and learning readiness. Plan with client for the achievement of realistic goals. Provide information to meet outcome criteria. Administer medication with food or milk to decrease GI distress. Alert client that medication may cause a discoloration of the urine.
	Self-administer medication safely and accurately.	Instruct client to take medication as ordered and to consult with the physician if no improvement is seen within a few days.

cillin causes a maculopapular rash in approximately 10% to 15% of the clients; therefore amoxicillin combined with potassium clavulanate (a beta lactamase inhibitor) appears to have an advantage over ampicillin. That is, the incidence of rash is less, and the presence of potassium clavulanate has reduced the development of resistant organisms. Thus the effectiveness of this product is reportedly equivalent to or better than the sulfonamides. Many cephalosporins are also effective in treating UTIs (see Chapter 61).

sulfonamides

Sulfonamides are among the most widely used antibacterial agents in the world, particularly for UTI. All the sulfonamides used therapeutically are synthetically produced and contain the para-aminobenzene-sulfonamide group, which gives them their common characteristics. See Table 34-1 for a list of sulfonamides in current clinical practice.

Mechanism of action. The sulfonamides are primarily **bacteriostatic** (that is, they inhibit bacterial growth) in concentrations that are normally useful in controlling infections in the human being rather than **bacteriocidal** (that is, causing cell death). They are structurally similar to para-aminobenzoic acid (PABA), and they inhibit a bacterial enzyme (dihydropteroate synthetase) that is necessary to incorporate PABA into dihydrofolic acid. By blocking the synthesis of dihydrofolic acid, a decrease in tetrahydrofolic acid results, which interferes with the synthesis of purines, thymidine, and DNA in the microorganism. Therefore, the bacteria most sensitive to sulfonamides are those that synthesize their own folic acid. The presence of pus, necrotic tissue, and serum interferes with the activities of the sulfonamides, since PABA is present in such materials. Among the microorganisms highly susceptible to sulfonamides are group A beta hemolytic streptococci, pneumococci, *Neisseria meningitidis, N. gonorrhoeae, E. coli, Pasteurella pestis, Bacillus anthracis, Shigella* species, *Haemophilus influenzae,* and *Pneumocystis carinii.*

Indications
1. Treatment of sensitive, bacterial UTIs
2. Treatment of otitis media (caused by *H. influenzae*), bronchitis (caused by *H. influenzae* or *Streptococ-*

TABLE 34-1 Sulfonamides

Generic/trade name	Dosage	
	Adults	Children
sulfacytine (Renoquid)	500 mg initially, then 250 mg every 6 hr for 10 days; maximum daily dose is 2 g	Not recommended children older than 14 yrs—see adult dose
sulfamethoxazole (Gantanol, Methoxanol)	2-3 g daily	Infants less than 1 mo, do not use; 1 mo and older, 50-60 mg/kg (maximum is 2 g) initially, then 25-30 mg/kg every 12 hr (maximum is 75 mg/kg daily)
sulfamethoxazole and trimethoprim (Bactrim, Cotrim, Septra, Protrin♣)	800 mg sulfamethoxazole, 160 mg trimethoprim every 12 hr	Children: up to 40 mg/kg body weight; 20 mg sulfamethoxazole and 4 mg trimethoprim/kg every 12 hr Children 40 kg and over: adult dose
Injectible dosage form	IV infusion, 10-12.5 mg sulfamethoxazole and 2-2.5 mg trimethoprim/kg every 6 hr, or 13.3-16.7 mg sulfamethoxazole and 2.7-3.3 mg trimethoprim/kg every 8 hr, or 20-25 mg sulfamethoxazole and 4-5 mg trimethoprim/kg every 12 hr	Not for use in infants under 1 mo old; otherwise, adult dosage
sulfisoxazole (Gantrisin, Novosoxazole♣)	2-4 g orally initially, then 750 mg to 1.5 g every 4 hr or 1-2 g every 6 hr; maximum daily dose is 12 g day	Not for use in infants less then 1 mo old; infants 1 mo old and older; orally, 75 mg/kg or 2 g/m² initially, then 25 mg/kg or 667 mg/m² every 4 hr; maximum daily dose should not exceed 6 g
sulfisoxazole diolamine injection (Gantrisin)	IM, 50 mg/kg or 1.125 g/m² initially, then 33.3 mg/kg or 750 mg/m² every 8 hr	Do not use in infants less than 1 mo old; infants 1 mo old and older: see adult dose

cus pneumoniae), enteritis (caused by *Shigella flexneria* and *S. somnei*), meningitis (adjunct or preventive; caused by *H. influenzae* and *N. meningitidis*), pneumonia (caused by *P. carinii*) in immunocompromised clients, and other sensitive bacterial infections

Pharmacokinetics

Absorption. Good

Half-life

sulfacytine: 4 hours

sulfamethoxazole: 6 to 12 hours, longer in end-stage renal disease (20 to 50 hours)

sulfisoxazole: 3 to 7 hours, longer in end-stage renal disease (6 to 12 hours)

Time to peak urine concentration. ½ hour

Time to peak serum concentration. 2 to 4 hours for sulfamethoxazole and sulfisoxazole

Metabolism. Acetylation is the major process by which the sulfonamides are metabolically inactivated. This change is probably caused by the action of the liver. Acetylation is important to the physician when choosing a drug: the acetylated forms are believed to be nontherapeutic, and they may produce toxic symptoms.

Excretion. Excretion of the sulfonamides occurs chiefly by way of the kidney, where both the free and the acetylated forms of the drug are filtered through the glomerulus. Most sulfonamides are reabsorbed to some extent in the kidney. Some of the sulfonamides, and especially their acetyl derivatives, are relatively insoluble in neutral or acid media, so as the kidney concentrates the urine, which becomes more acid, there is some danger that sulfonamide will precipitate, causing crystalluria, hematuria, and even renal shutdown. The forcing of fluids to keep the urine dilute helps to keep a number of the sulfonamides from precipitating in the urine. However, sulfonamide precipitation is no longer a great clinical problem. Newer sulfonamides, such as sulfisoxazole and sulfacetamide, are quite soluble even in acid urine. The problem of solubility in the urine can also be dealt with by administration of combinations of small doses of two or three different sulfonamides. In this way the saturation point of each is not reached, and each drug remains in solution. The "insoluble" sulfonamides are poorly absorbed from the gastrointestinal tract and are excreted largely in the feces. Their action is mainly on intestinal flora; they are used to inhibit bacterial growth in the colon.

Side effects/adverse reactions. See Table 34-2.

Significant drug interactions

Drug	Possible Effect and Management
para-aminobenzoic acid (PABA)	Bacteria absorb PABA, antagonizing therapeutic effects of sulfonamides. Avoid concurrent administration.
anticoagulants, such as coumarin or indanedione derivatives; anticonvulsants (hydantoin); oral antidiabetic agents, or methotrexate	These agents are highly protein bound; concurrent drug administration may displace them from their protein-binding sites, resulting in increased serum levels and possible toxicity. Metabolism of these agents may also be inhibited by sulfonamides. Monitor closely for signs of toxicity, indicating need for dosage adjustments.
bone marrow suppressants	Increased potential for toxicity. If concurrent therapy is necessary, monitor closely.
hemolytics, other	Increased potential for toxicity. Monitor closely.
hepatotoxic medications	Increased risk of inducing liver toxicity. Closely monitor for signs of liver toxicity.
methenamine	Methenamine requires an acid urine to be active and effective. It may precipitate if given with a sulfonamide and result in crystalluria. Do not administer concurrently.

Dosage and administration. See Table 34-1.

Pregnancy safety. Not established

NURSING CONSIDERATIONS

In addition to instituting the nursing measures common to all types of antimicrobial therapy, the nurse should observe these considerations for individuals receiving sulfonamides.

Assessment. Although cross-sensitization is not as severe as among penicillins, it is safer to avoid all sulfonamides in clients who develop hypersensitivity to any one agent. Cross-sensitivity also exists with some diuretics, such as actazolamide and the thiazides, and with sulfonylurea antidiabetic agents, so the nurse should obtain an accurate history of the client's sensitivities.

Avoid sulfonamides in clients with hepatic and renal dysfunction, blood dyscrasias, allergies, and asthma.

Administration of sulfonamides is contraindicated during the last trimester of pregnancy, in nursing mothers, and in infants.

Intervention. Administer sulfonamides on an empty stomach with a full glass of water to enhance absorption. However, if the common adverse reaction of nausea and vomiting occurs, administer with food to decrease gastrointestinal distress.

Do not administer sulfonamides with antacids because the latter inhibit their action by decreasing absorption.

Education. Instruct the client that it is important that a full course of drug therapy be completed, even though the client may feel better after several days of therapy.

TABLE 34-2 Agents for UTIs: Side Effects/Adverse Reactions

Drug	Side effects*	Adverse reactions†
SULFONAMIDES		
sulfacytine (Renoquid) sulfamethoxazole (Gantanol), with trimethoprim (Bactrim, Cotrim, Septra, Protrin♣, Apo-Sulfatrim♣) sulfisoxazole (Gantrisin, Novosoxazole♣)	Most frequent: diarrhea, anorexia, headaches, dizziness, nausea, or vomiting	Most frequent: pruritus, rash Less frequent: muscle and joint pain; increased temperature; sore throat; increased bleeding tendencies; pallor; red, blistering, or peeling skin (**Stevens-Johnson syndrome**); weakness, jaundice Rare: bloody urine, pain on urination, low back pain, swelling or edema in neck (thyroid dysfunction)
URINARY TRACT ANTISEPTICS		
cinoxacin (Cinobac, Cinobactin♣)	Less frequent/rare: nausea, rash, pruritus, swelling, diarrhea, anorexia, abdominal distress, vomiting	Less frequent/rare: photosensitivity (eye), tinnitus, insomnia, headache, dizziness
methenamine mandelate (Mandelamine), methenamine hippurate (Hiprex, Urex, Hip-Rex♣)	Less frequent: nausea, rash, abdominal distress	Less frequent: bloody urine, low back pain, painful urination
nalidixic acid (NegGram)	Most frequent: diarrhea, nausea or vomiting, rash, pruritus, headache Less frequent: dizziness, sedation, skin photosensitivity	Most frequent: visual disturbances, (changes in color vision or double vision, halos encircling lights, etc.) Rare: jaundice, severe abdominal distress, light-colored stools, dark urine (cholestatic jaundice); mental alterations, hallucinations, convulsions, (CNS toxicity usually with very high doses); sore throat, elevated temperature, increased bleeding tendencies, increased weakness, pale skin (blood dyscrasias)
nitrofurantoin (Furadantin, Macrodantin, Novofuran♣, Apo-Nitrofurantoin♣)	Most frequent: abdominal distress, diarrhea, anorexia, nausea, or vomiting Less frequent: rash, itching	Most frequent: chest pain, chills, increased temperature, respiratory difficulties, cough (pneumonitis) Less frequent: dizziness, sedation, headache, pale skin, increased weakness, paresthesias Rare: jaundice
MONOBACTAMS AND FLUOROQUINOLONES		
aztreonam (Azactam)	Less frequent/rare: stomach distress, dizziness, nausea or vomiting, diarrhea, double vision, vaginal itching, tinnitus	Less frequent: rash, pruritus Rare: convulsions, confusion, jaundice of skin or eyes
norfloxacin (Noroxin)	Most frequent: drowsiness, anorexia, nausea, or vomiting Less frequent/rare: abdominal distress; bloody urine; low back pain; painful urination (crystalluria); diarrhea; constipation; dry mouth; skin rash; swollen, painful joints; insomnia	Most frequent: dizziness, headache (CNS toxicity) Less frequent: depression Rare: visual disturbances, eye photosensitivity
URINARY TRACT ANALGESIC		
phenazopyridine (Azo-Standard, Phenazo♣, Pyridium, Pyronium♣)	Client complains of dizziness, headache, abdominal pain, cramps, or gas	Skin discoloration (blue to purple tint on skin caused by methemoglobinemia), rash, increased weakness (hemolytic anemia), jaundice

*If side effects continue, increase, or disturb the client inform the physician.
†If adverse reactions occur, contact physician, since medical intervention may be necessary.

Instruct the client to observe for and report any dermatologic reactions after initiation of the sulfonamide. Fever may occur after 7 to 10 days of therapy, indicating a serum-sickness–like reaction. It may be accompanied by joint pain, urticaria, and leukopenia. All these responses are indications for discontinuation of the drug and physician referral.

Advise the client to avoid exposure to the sun and sunlamps because skin photosensitivity may be present.

Alert clients with diabetes that sulfonamides may cause false urine sugar and urine ketone test results.

Evaluation. Because renal toxicity may present a potentially serious problem, monitor the hospitalized client's urinary output and ensure that it amounts to at least 1500 ml in 24 hours. Maintenance of urinary output at this level decreases the tendency for crystals to form. Individuals who are not hospitalized should be instructed to drink at least 3 quarts of fluids per day. Liquids and vitamins that produce acid urine should be avoided. The urine should be visually examined for the presence of crystals, and in long-term sulfonamide therapy periodic urinalysis should be done to determine if crystals are present.

Carefully observe the client for toxic effects, such as rash, sore throat, or purpura. Instruct nonhospitalized individuals to report these symptoms to their physicians and to discontinue taking the drug. In prolonged sulfonamide therapy, periodic blood counts should be performed to assess the occurrence of hematologic side effects (anemia, granulocytopenia, and thrombocytopenia).

URINARY TRACT ANTISEPTICS (ANTIBACTERIAL)

Cinoxacin, nitrofurantoin, nalidixic acid, and methenamine mandelate are the primary urinary tract antiseptics. Urinary tract antiseptics, although given simultaneously, are drugs that exert antibacterial activity in the urine but have little or no systemic antibacterial effects. Their usefulness is limited to the treatment of UTIs. Table 34-2 lists the urinary tract antiseptics that are currently used in medical practice.

cinoxacin (Cinobac, Cinobactin✦)

Mechanism of action. Inhibits replication of bacterial DNA; bactericidal in urine

Indications. Treatment of UTIs caused by *E. coli, K. pneumoniae* and other *Klebsiella* species, *Enterobacter, Proteus mirabilis,* and *P. vulgaris*

Pharmacokinetics

Absorption. Very good orally

Distribution. Although serum levels are generally low, urinary levels of cinoxacin are high. This substance crosses the placenta.

Metabolism. Liver

Time to peak serum levels. 2 to 3 hours

Peak serum levels. Serum levels of cinoxacin can reach 15 μg/ml after a 250-mg dose and up to 28 μg/ml after a 500-mg dose. They may drop to 1 to 2 μg/ml in 6 hours. Peak serum levels decrease if cinoxacin is administered with food.

Peak urine levels. Urine levels of cinoxacin can reach 900 μg/ml. Average levels are approximately 300 μg/ml during the first 4 hours and usually decrease to approximately 100 μg/ml during the second 4 hours.

Excretion. Kidneys

Side effects/adverse reactions. See Table 34-2.

Significant drug interactions. None

Dosage and administration. See Table 34-3.

Pregnancy safety. FDA Category B

methenamine mandelate (Mandelamine)
methenamine hippurate (Hiprex, Urex, Hip-Rex✦)

Mechanism of action. Methenamine, which is used to treat UTIs, combines the action of methenamine and mandelic acid or hippurate acid salts. Its effectiveness depends on the release of formaldehyde, which requires an acid medium. Acids released from the mandelate or hippurate salts contribute to this acidity. Formaldehyde may be bactericidal or bacteriostatic, and its effects are believed to be the result of denaturation of bacteria protein. It is ineffective if the urine is alkaline. Because of its fairly wide bacterial spectrum, low toxicity, and a low incidence of resistance, methenamine has often been the drug of choice in long-term suppression of infections.

Indications. Prevention or treatment of bacterial UTIs.

Pharmacokinetics

Absorption. Good

Time to peak urinary formaldehyde levels. At a urinary pH of 5.6, methenamine reaches peak urinary formaldehyde level in ½ to 1½ hours; methenamine hippurate reaches its peak in 2 hours; and methenamine mandelate (enteric coated) reaches its peak in 3 to 8 hours.

Excretion. Kidneys

Side effects/adverse reactions. See Table 34-2.

Significant drug interactions

TABLE 34-3 Cinoxacin: Dosage and Administration

Adults	Children
250 mg orally every 6 hr or 500 mg orally every 12 hr for 1-2 wk. Individuals with impaired renal function require a dosage reduction (see package insert).	Less than 12 yr old: not recommended. 12 yr and older, see adult dosage.

TABLE 34-4   Methenamine: Dosage and Administration

	Adults	Children
methenamine	1 g orally every 6 hr up to maximum of 12 g daily	Less than 6 yr, 18.3 mg/kg every 6 hr; 6-12 yr, 500 mg orally every 6 hr; 12 yr and older, see adult dosage
methenamine hippurate tablets, methenamine mandelate solution/suspension/enteric-coated tablets	1 g every 12 hr up to maximum of 4 g/day	6-12 yr, 500 mg to 1 g every 12 hr; 12 yr and older, see adult dosage

Drug	Possible Effect and Management
urinary alkalizers, such as antacids (calcium and/or magnesium), carbonic anhydrase inhibitors, citrates, sodium bicarbonate, or thiazide diuretics	May result in an alkaline urine, thus inhibiting methenamine's conversion to formaldehyde and rendering it ineffective. Avoid concurrent drug administration.
sulfonamides	In acid urine, the formaldehyde produced may precipitate with certain sulfonamides, which increases the potential for crystalluria. Avoid concurrent drug administration.

Dosage and administration. See Table 34-4.
Pregnancy safety. FDA Category C

nalidixic acid (NegGram)

Mechanism of action. Nalidixic acid is believed to inhibit bacterial DNA synthesis by interfering with polymerization of DNA. Resistance usually develops rapidly during treatment with this drug.

Indications. Treatment of UTIs caused by *E. coli, Proteus* species, *Klebsiella* species, and *Enterobacter* species

Pharmacokinetics
Absorption. Good
Time to peak serum levels. 1 to 2 hours
Time to peak urine levels. 3 to 4 hours
Half-life
Serum. With normal renal function, approximately 1.2 to 2.5 hours; with renal impairment, up to 21 hours
Urine. 6 hours
Metabolism. Liver, with approximately 30% converted to an active metabolite, hydroxynalidixic acid
Excretion. Kidneys
Side effects/adverse reactions. See Table 34-2.
Significant drug interactions. When nalidixic acid is given with oral anticoagulants (coumarin or indandione type), warfarin (Coumadin) and dicumarol may be dislodged from their protein binding sites, resulting in enhanced anticoagulant effects. Dosage adjustments may

be necessary. Monitor closely if concurrent therapy is necessary.
Dosage and administration. See Table 34-5.
Pregnancy safety. Not established

nitrofurantoin (Furadantin, Macrodantin, Novofuran✽, Apo-Nitrofurantoin✽)

Mechanism of action. Nitrofurantoin's mechanism of action is unknown, but it is believed to interfere with bacterial enzymes. Depending on urine concentration, nitrofurantoin may be bacteriostatic or bactericidal.

Indications. Treatment of urinary tract infections with organisms such as *E. coli, S. aureus, Klebsiella* species, *Enterobacter* species, and *Proteus* species
Pharmacokinetics
Absorption. Completely absorbed in the small intestine following oral administration
Half-life. 20 minutes to 1 hour (prolonged in renal disease)
Metabolism. 50% to 70% metabolized in body tissues
Excretion. 30% to 50% excreted by kidney; may also be excreted in bile
Side effects/adverse reactions. See Table 34-2.
Significant drug interactions

TABLE 34-5   Nalidixic Acid: Dosage and Administration

Adults	Children
1 g orally every 6 hr for 7-14 days; maintenance dosage: 500 mg orally every 6 hr; maximum dosage: 4 g/day, although there have been reports of using up to 6 g/day (The health care provider should be aware that incidence of side effects usually increases with high dosages.)	Infants less than 3 mo old, not recommended; infants and children 3 mo and older, initially 13.75 mg/kg orally every 6 hr for 7-14 days; maintenance: 8.25 mg/kg orally every 6 hr

Drug	Possible Effect and Management
other hemolytic agents	Increased possibility of toxic side effects. Monitor closely if concurrent therapy is necessary.
neurotoxic medications	Increased risk of inducing neurotoxicity. Monitor closely if concurrent therapy is necessary.
probenecid or sulfinpyrazone	Tubular secretion of nitrofurantoin will be inhibited, leading to increased serum levels and possibly toxicity. A decrease in urinary concentrations and effectiveness may also result. Dosage adjustment of probenecid may be required. Monitor closely.

Dosage and administration. See Table 34-6.
Pregnancy safety. Not established

• • •

The following nursing considerations include both general ones for all urinary antiseptics and specific ones for particular antiseptics.

NURSING CONSIDERATIONS

Assessment. The nurse should ascertain whether the client has preexisting hepatic or renal function impairment because urinary antiseptics are used cautiously in such instances.

Photophobia may occur during cinoxacin use. The client should be advised to avoid bright sunlight and to wear sunglasses.

There is a possibility of photosensitivity with nalidixic acid during therapy and for up to 3 months after it is discontinued. The client should be cautioned to avoid exposure to sunlight and sunlamps.

Clients with diabetes should use Clinistix, Diastix, or Testape to test for glucosuria because nitrofurantoin and nalidixic acid may produce a false-positive result with Clinitest.

The client taking nitrofurantoin should be told that urine may have a brown color.

TABLE 34-6 Nitrofurantoin
Capsules/Suspension/Tablets: Dosage and
Administration

Adults	Children
50-100 mg orally every 6 hr or 1.25-1.75 mg/kg every 6 hr; maximum daily dosage up to 600 mg/day or 10 mg/kg daily	Infants less than 1 mo, do not use (risk of inducing hemolytic anemia is high); 1 mo and older, 1.25-1.75 mg/kg every 6 hr

Nitrofurantoin is discolored by alkalies and strong light. The client should also avoid metal pill boxes unless they are stainless steel or aluminum because the drug decomposes on contact with other metals.

The client should be assessed for an intolerance to either nalidixic acid or cinoxacin since cross-sensitivity may occur.

Intervention. Acidification of the urine inhibits the growth of many urinary tract microorganisms and thereby enhances the effects of several urinary antiseptics. Thus, when encouraging clients with UTIs to consume large volumes of fluids, the selection of fluids should be those that increase urine acidity, such as cranberry juice (see box, next page) or prune juice. Vitamin C will also acidify the urine and can enhance antiinfective therapy. Methenamine is most effective when the urine pH is 5.5 or less. Urine pH is easily monitored at the bedside by commercially available test strips.

Compliance can be increased by suggesting cranberry sauce if the client considers cranberry juice unpalatable. Most fruits, particularly citrus fruits and juices, milk and other dairy products, and other alkalinizing foods should be avoided. Alka-seltzer and sodium bicarbonate, which alkalinize the urine, should be avoided.

Urinary antiseptics may be administered on an empty stomach or, if gastric distress is a concern, with food or just after meals.

If oral solutions are used, the nurse should ensure that they are shaken well and administered with the calibrated device provided by the manufacturer.

Education. The client should be instructed to complete a full course of therapy even if marked improvement occurs within a few days. If no such improvement occurs, the physician should be notified.

The client should be told that dizziness and drowsiness may occur with these drugs and that these symptoms should be reported to the physician. Driving and other activities requiring alertness should be avoided until there is resolution of symptoms.

Evaluation. The client's progress should be monitored periodically by urinalysis and objective and subjective signs and symptoms.

MONOBACTAMS AND FLUOROQUINOLONES

New classes of antibiotics, the monobactams (aztreonam) and fluoroquinolones (norfloxacin), are potent drugs released in 1987 for the treatment of UTIs. Aztreonam is effective against many gram-negative bacteria and appears to be a safer agent than aminoglycoside therapy in the seriously ill. At present, it is only available in an injectable form. Norfloxacin is an oral antibiotic that has a broad spectrum of action against both gram-positive and gram-negative bacteria, including *Pseudomonas aeruginosa* and many drug-resistant bacteria species.

aztreonam (Azactam)

Mechanism of action. Aztreonam inhibits bacterial cell wall synthesis, which usually results in lysis of the bacterial cell and death. Stable in the presence of bacterial beta lactamases, it is effective in treating infections caused by drug-resistant or virulent pathogens. Its activity is mainly against aerobic-type gram-negative bacteria.

Indications. As a secondary agent in treatment of moderately severe systemic infections and UTIs.

Pharmacokinetics

Absorption. Intramuscular; completely absorbed

Time to peak serum levels. Intramuscular, approximately 0.6 to 1.3 hours

Time to peak bile concentration. Intravenous, approximately 2.4 hours

Peak serum levels. Intramuscular peak serum levels of 20 to 25 μg/ml and 40 to 45 μg/ml are reached after an intramuscular dose of 500 mg and 1 g, respectively. Intravenous peak serum levels of 40 to 60 μg/ml, 100 to 125 μg/ml, and 240 μg/ml are reached 5 minutes after intravenous injection of 500 mg, 1 g, and 2 g, respectively. Following a 30-minute intravenous infusion, peak serum levels of 55 to 65 μg/ml, 90 to 165 μg/ml, and 205 to 255 μg/ml after half administration of an intravenous infusion of 500 mg, 1 g, and 2 g, respectively.

Peak bile concentration. Approximately 43 μg/ml after a 1-g intravenous dose

Urine concentrations. Urine concentration is approximately 500 mg/ml and 1200 μg/ml about 2 hours after an intramuscular dose of 500 mg and 1 g, respectively. Urine concentration is approximately 1100 μg/ml, 3500 μg/ml, and 6600 μg/ml about 2 hours after a 30-minute intravenous infusion of 500 mg, 1 g, and 2 g, respectively.

Metabolism. Only 6% to 16% is metabolized; most is excreted unchanged in the urine.

THE ROLE OF CRANBERRY JUICE IN UTIs

Although cranberry juice has traditionally been recommended to help prevent and treat UTIs, its role in the treatment of UTIs remains controversial. It has been felt that cranberry juice served to acidify the urine, which created a less favorable environment for bacterial growth. However, very large quantities of juice must be consumed to adequately lower the urine pH (Kinney and Blount, 1979). Cranberry juice has also been shown to reduce bacterial adherence to mucosal surfaces (Sobota, 1984), an important prerequisite for UTI, which may explain its efficacy in treatment. Cranberry juice should not be taken during sulfonamide therapy since the sulfonamide drugs require an alkaline urine to achieve maximum effectiveness.

Excretion. Kidneys (60% to 75%) and bile/feces (up to 12%)

Side effects/adverse reactions. See Table 34-2.
Significant drug interactions. None
Dosage and administration. See Table 34-7.
Pregnancy safety. FDA Category B

NURSING CONSIDERATIONS

The following nursing considerations are in addition to the general nursing considerations for urinary antiseptics.

When administering aztreonam intravenously, the nurse should give the bolus over 3 to 5 minutes, or, as an intermittent infusion, in 50-100 ml of fluid over 20 to 60 minutes.

The nurse should observe the intravenous site for the development of phlebitis.

When giving aztreonam intramuscularly, use large muscle masses rather than the deltoid muscle. Observe the intramuscular sites for pain and swelling.

norfloxacin (Noroxin)

Mechanism of action. Norfloxacin's mechanism of action is unknown. It is believed to inhibit DNA coiling reaction; it inhibits relaxation of supercoiled DNA; and it promotes the breakage of DNA double strands in bacteria. At low concentrations it is bacteriostatic; at high concentrations it is bactericidal.

Indication. Treatment of UTIs

Pharmacokinetics

Absorption. Rapid, incomplete (30% to 40%)

Time to peak serum levels. 1 to 2 hours

Average peak serum concentration. Approximately 1.4 to 1.6 μg/ml 1 to 2 hours after a single 400-mg dose; approximately 2.5 μg/ml 1 to 2 hours after a single 800-mg dose.

TABLE 34-7   Aztreonam: Dosage and Administration

Adults	Children
For systemic, moderately severe infections, 1-2 g every 8-12 hr	Not established
For life-threatening, severe systemic infections, 2 g every 6-8 hr	
For UTIs, 500 mg to 1 g every 8-12 hr	
Maximum daily dosage: 8 g	
Individuals with impaired renal function require a dosage reduction (see package insert).	

Urine concentration. In individuals with normal renal function, urine concentration is 98 to 200 μg/ml or more, 2 to 3 hours after a single 400-mg dose. The urine levels will remain above 30 μg/ml for at least 12 hours. In individuals with impaired renal function, described as a glomerular filtration rate of less than 10 ml/min, norfloxacin urine concentration will be approximately 20 to 25 μg/ml after a 400-mg dose.

Half-life. Normal renal function: elderly, 4 hours; other clients, 3 to 4 hours. Impaired renal function (creatinine clearance equal to or less than 30 ml/min): 6.5 to 8.3 hours.

Metabolism. Liver

Excretion. Kidneys (approximately 40% to 50%); bile/feces (28% to 30%)

Side effects/adverse reactions. See Table 34-2.

Significant drug interactions. When norfloxacin is given with antacids, a reduction in absorption of norfloxacin may occur. Administer antacids at least 2 hours after or 1 hour before norfloxacin.

Dosage and administration. See Table 34-8.

Pregnancy safety. FDA category C

TABLE 34-8 Norfloxacin: Dosage and Administration

Adults	Children
Uncomplicated UTIs: 400 mg orally every 12 hr for 72 hr Complicated UTIs: 400 mg every 12 hr for 10-21 days Maximum daily dosage: 800 mg Impaired renal function: reduce dosage to usually 400 mg daily for 7-10 days (uncomplicated cases) or 21 days (complicated cases)	Not recommended

Nearly 90% of an oral dose is excreted renally in 24 hours.

Side effects/adverse reactions. See Table 34-2.

Significant drug interactions. None

Dosage and administration. Adults are given 200 mg orally three times daily after meals. Children are given 4 mg/kg orally, three times daily with food.

Pregnancy safety. FDA Category B

NURSING CONSIDERATIONS

The following nursing considerations are in addition to the general nursing considerations for urinary antiseptics.

Determine whether the client has a sensitivity to nalidixic acid or cinoxacin because there is the possibility of cross-sensitivity with this drug.

Dizziness may occur with norfloxacin. The client should be told to modify activities that require alertness and coordination, such as driving.

Instruct the client to avoid taking antacids at the same time as norfloxacin or within 2 hours of norfloxacin.

URINARY TRACT ANALGESIC

phenazopyridine (Azo-Standard, Pyridium, Pyronium✱)

Mechanism of action. Phenazopyridine's mechanism of action is unknown, but it appears to provide a topical analgesic or local anesthetic effect on the mucosa of the urinary tract.

Indications. Phenazopyridine is used for urinary tract irritation, such as pain on urination, urinary frequency, and burning on urination. It is only indicated for short-term use because the underlying reason for the irritation should be determined and treated appropriately.

Pharmacokinetics

Metabolism. Liver and other body tissues

Excretion. Phenazopyridine is excreted by the kidneys.

NURSING CONSIDERATIONS

Assessment. Phenazopyridine is contraindicated in clients with impaired renal and hepatic function.

Intervention. Phenazopyridine should be used in conjunction with an antimicrobial or urinary antiseptic to treat the underlying cause of the irritation.

Education. The client should be told that the urine will become reddish orange and may stain clothing.

The client should be instructed to observe for yellow color of the skin and sclera. This may indicate an accumulation of the drug owing to renal impairment. Discontinue drug and notify the physician.

Clients with diabetes should use Clinistix, Diastix, or TesTape to test for glucosuria because Clinitest may give a false-positive result with this drug.

Evaluation. Phenazopyridine may be discontinued after 3 days if the client no longer has discomfort.

KEY TERMS

bacteriocidal, page 602
bacteriostatic, page 602
bacteriuria, page 599
nosocomial infection, page 599
prostatitis, page 599
Stevens-Johnson syndrome, page 604

BIBLIOGRAPHY

American Hospital Formulary Service: AHFS drug information '87, Bethesda, Md, 1987, American Society of Hospital Pharmacists, Inc.

Bjork, DT, and others: Urinary tract infections with antibiotic resistant organisms in catheterized nursing home patients, Infect Control 5(4):173, 1984.

Brodoff, AS: Alleviating stubborn UTI in women, Patient Care 18(6):176, 1984.

Burgener, S: Justification of closed intermittent urinary catheter irrigation/instillation: a review of current research and practice, J Adv Nurs 12(2):229, 1987.

Conti, MT, and others: Preventing UTIs: what works? Am J Nurs 87(3):307, 1987.

Critchley, JA, and Robson, JS: Renal diseases. In TM, Speight, TM: Avery's drug treatment, ed 3, Baltimore, 1987, Adis Press.

Cunha, BA: Nosocomial urinary tract infections . . . causes . . . diagnosis . . . control measures . . . treatment, Heart Lung 11(6):545, 1982.

Cunha, BA: Single-dose treatment of urinary tract infections, Physician Assist 7(8):105, 1983.

D'Arcy, PF: Nitrofurantoin, Drug Intell Clin Pharm 19(7/8):540, 1985.

Erwin, WG, and others: Geriatric pharmacology: the treatment of urinary tract infections. III, Hosp Formul 20(3):339, 1985.

Goldstein, EJC: Urinary tract infections in the elderly patient: An overview, Consultant Pharmacist 2(suppl A):3-7, 1987.

Hatch, K: Cinoxacin for urinary tract infections, AUAA J 3(3):10, 1983.

Hooton, T, and others: Up-to-date advice on managing urethritis, Patient Care 21(3):93, 1987.

Jackson, EA, and others: New drug evaluations . . . cinoxacin, Drug Intell Clin Pharm 16(12):916, 1982.

Kinney, AB, and Blount, M: Effect of cranberry juice on urinary pH, Nurs Res 28(5):287, 1979.

Latham, RH: Acute lower urinary tract infection in women, Hosp Med 22(8):77, 1986.

McNellis, D: The role of antibiotics in the management of infections associated with pregnancy, Fam Commun Health 6(3):13, 1983.

Miller, S: Management of urinary tract infection in a college population, Physician Assist 8(1):94, 1984.

Owen, JA, Jr: Cinoxacin: an antibacterial agent for the treatment of urinary tract infection, Hosp Formul 18(3):248, 1983.

Peterson, H: Pearls for managing the problem, Patient Care 19(13):133, 1985.

Peterson, H: Microbes and antibiotics in UTI today, Patient Care 19(12):51, 1985.

Prentice, RD, and others: Treatment of lower urinary tract infections with single-dose trimethoprim-sulfamethoxazole, J Fam Pract, 20(6):551-557, 1985.

Quinlan, MW: UTI: helping your patients control it once and for all, RN 47(3):38, 1984.

Sheahan, SL, and others: Understanding urinary tract infection in women: the first step to controlling it, Nursing '82 12(11):68, 1982.

Simpson, RA: Systemic and local antimicrobial agents in the prevention of catheter-associated bacteriuria and its consequences, Infect Control (Suppl) 7(2):100, 1986.

Sobota, AE: Inhibition of bacterial adherence by cranberry juice: potential use for the treatment of urinary tract infections, J Urol 131(5):1013, 1984.

Stamm, WE, and Turck, M: Urinary tract infection, pyelonephritis and related conditions. In Braunwald, E, and others, (eds): Harrison's principles of internal medicine, ed 11, New York, 1987, McGraw-Hill Book Co.

Stein, G: New antimicrobial therapy for treatment of urinary tract infections in the elderly, Consultant Pharmacist, 2 (suppl A):12-16, 1987.

Tideksaar, R: Infections in the elderly: diagnosis and treatment, part 1, Physician Assist 11(2):17, 1987.

CHAPTER 35

Drug Therapy for Renal System Dysfunction

Many potentially toxic drugs are excreted by the kidneys unchanged or as active metabolites of the parent drug. If individuals with impaired renal function receive standard drug dosages on standard schedules, the drugs may accumulate in the system because of reduced excretion, resulting in elevated serum levels, extended drug half-life, and toxicity. Therefore it is important for the health care provider to evaluate and monitor clients with impaired renal function because drug dosages or time intervals frequently need to be adjusted.

ACUTE VERSUS CHRONIC RENAL FAILURE

Acute renal failure, or a rapid decline in renal function, occurs in approximately 5% of all hospitalized individuals. Primary causes include trauma, pregnancy, renal ischemia as a result of surgery, severe hemorrhage, severe volume depletion, and shock. In some instances, nephrotoxic agents such as heavy metals and aminoglycosides may also induce acute renal failure. If recognized early and treated promptly, acute renal failure may be reversed before acute tubular necrosis or permanent damage occurs.

On the other hand, **chronic renal failure** (CRF) is usually the result of an irreversible kidney injury that results in permanent nephron or renal mass loss. The most common causes of CRF are glomerulonephritis, diabetes mellitus, hypertension, polycystic kidney disease, and other diseases that may lead to destruction or impaired functioning of the kidneys. Individuals with CRF may be treated conservatively initially, but eventually **hemodialysis, peritoneal dialysis,** or organ transplantation may be necessary. Since the focus of this book is pharmacology, this chapter will concentrate on the therapeutic regimen and recommendations for drug dosage adjustments in these clients with impaired renal function.

SIGNS AND SYMPTOMS OF RENAL FAILURE OR INSUFFICIENCY

One of the more common signs of acute renal failure is a marked alteration in the expected urine output, usually a significant reduction (< 400 ml/day) of urine output. Signs of acute renal failure, in the presence of reduced urine production, are usually the result of fluid overload: edema, weight gain, weakness, hypertension, and tachycardia.

The most common complaints with CRF are increasing weakness, fatigue, and lethargy. Gastrointestinal signs include anorexia, gastrointestinal distress, nausea, vomiting, thirst, and weight loss. Paresthesias, peripheral neuropathy, convulsions, and neuromuscular irritability may also occur. On examination, the client may appear pale and dehydrated and have an increased respiratory rate and uremic breath. Hypertension with retinopathy, cardiac hypertrophy, pulmonary edema, or pericarditis may often be present.

A detailed client history, thorough physical examination, urinalysis, and blood chemistry levels are important for assessment, diagnosis, and determination of an appropriate treatment plan. The degree of renal impairment is usually estimated by reviewing the serum creatinine and blood, urea, nitrogen (BUN) levels. Elevated levels indicate a decrease in renal clearance, which, of course, predisposes the individual to drug toxicity.

MEASUREMENT OF RENAL FUNCTION

Many formulas and nomograms are available to determine the client's approximate creatinine clearance and the appropriate dosage adjustment necessary to minimize the possibility of toxicity. Although BUN levels (normal 8 to 25 mg/dl) and creatinine serum levels (normal 0.7 to 1.5 mg/dl) are usually ordered, the BUN is directly related to protein metabolism and thus it is a nonspecific test for renal function. The creatinine level, which is related to muscle mass, is independent of protein consumption and is a more accurate measure of renal function than is the BUN. A review of the formulas and nomograms is not within the purview of this chapter; therefore the interested reader is referred to the bibliography for further study.

SPECIAL NEEDS OF THE CLIENT

The individual in CRF has special dietary, electrolyte, and fluid requirements. In general, dietary protein is usually restricted to 0.5 to 1 g/kg of lean body weight daily. This limitation will reduce the incidence of **azotemia** (build up of urea in the blood), hyperkalemia, and acidosis. Fluid intake is based on daily losses and metabolic needs. Dietary sodium is restricted to approximately 4 g/day. Potassium, magnesium, and phosphorus are also restricted. Often, an aluminum hydroxide gel is prescribed to decrease phosphate absorption from the gastrointestinal tract. The reduced excretion of phosphates, magnesium, and potassium from the kidneys in chronic renal failure can lead to elevated serum levels or hypermagnesemia, hyperkalemia, and hyperphosphatemia, which in turn lead to hypocalcemia and osteosclerosis. Thus dietary restrictions are absolutely necessary. Calcium supplements and vitamin D are often prescribed for these clients to reduce or prevent hyperparathyroidism and bone disease. Magnesium levels are kept somewhat in check by client avoidance of magnesium-containing antacids and laxatives.

Production of red blood cells **(erythropoiesis),** which is usually decreased in CRF, leads to anemia, weakness, and fatigue. Iron therapy may be prescribed for those clients with iron deficiency anemia resulting from chronic blood loss; folic acid, vitamin C, and soluble B-complex vitamins are often given to replace substances usually lost during dialysis. Therefore it is not unusual to care for CRF clients with many dietary and fluid restrictions, as well as prescriptions for vitamins, calcium, specific antacids, and additional drugs as necessary.

SELECTED DRUG MODIFICATIONS IN RENAL FAILURE

As previously mentioned, BUN and serum creatinine are waste products excreted by the kidneys. Serum levels of these substances are used to measure renal function. Unfortunately, neither test is useful in discovering early renal impairment because abnormal levels do not appear until 50% or more of renal function is impaired. Fortunately, our kidneys are functional even if 90% of the glomerular filtration rate is lost. However, the continuing progressive loss may result in **end-stage renal disease,** which then leads to the need for hemodialysis, peritoneal dialysis, or even organ transplantation.

Normal values may vary from laboratory to laboratory, but in general a normal BUN ranges between 5 and 25 mg/dl, while the range of serum creatinine, which varies with age, is usually between 0.6 and 1.3 mg/dl. The most reliable test is the creatinine clearance test, but since it is difficult to collect accurately all urine excreted for a 24-hour period, many clinicians use a formula to estimate creatinine clearance whereas others may prefer to use a nomogram. The formulas most commonly used are noted in the box. The mean endogenous creatinine clearance in an adult is usually between 90 and 130 ml/min/1.73 m² body surface per 24 hours. Therefore reductions in this quantity signify impairment of renal function. (See box for usual ranges for grading renal impairment.)

Another important factor in evaluating drug blood levels in clients with renal failure or renal impairment is an assessment of serum albumin and total protein for the client. Serum protein is decreased in individuals with renal insufficiency, and this can alter the interpretation of serum levels of drugs that are protein bound (90% or more) in the normal person. Individuals with a lower albumin or protein value may have a drug concentration in the low range that appears to be therapeutic. This is possible if the laboratory does not differentiate between the bound and unbound drug in their testing. Lower protein levels may lead to a higher unbound concentration of the drug (the active form), thus producing an adequate therapeutic response.

DOSING METHODS

In individuals with renal insufficiency or impairment, the drug dosage may be decreased (dosage reduction method) while maintaining the usual interval, or the dosage may be the usually prescribed dose, but the interval between doses is lengthened (interval extension method). Usually the dosage reduction method is preferred for drugs that require a constant blood therapeutic level. For most clients receiving a loading dose, the dose is similar to the dose given to a client without renal impairment. This permits a therapeutically desirable blood level that is then maintained by one of the above dosing methods.

Table 35-1 gives typical dosing recommendations for selected medications along with a list of drugs that may or may not be removed by hemodialysis or peritoneal dialysis. The reader is referred to the current package inserts or renal failure dosing guides for specific data. Table 35-2 lists the medications that are most commonly associated with inducing renal dysfunction.

ESTIMATION OF CREATININE CLEARANCE*

$$\text{Men:} \left[\frac{145 - \text{age}}{\text{Serum creatinine}} \right] - 3$$

Values for women are 85% of the above predicted value, or the following formula may be used:

$$\text{Women: } 0.85 \left[\frac{145 - \text{age}}{\text{Serum creatinine}} \right] - 3$$

*Values obtained are in ml/min/70 kg.

THE NURSE'S ROLE IN PHARMACOLOGIC THERAPIES FOR CLIENTS WITH RENAL SYSTEM DYSFUNCTION

Assessment. The initial assessment should include a history of recent weight changes, edema, malaise, increasing irritability or mental changes, metallic taste in the mouth, polyuria and nocturia (caused by reduced ability to concentrate urine), headache, dizziness, gastrointestinal disturbances, and hypertension. Because other body systems may be affected by renal dysfunction, a thorough multisystem assessment should be conducted.

Intervention. Fluid intake may be restricted. If so, fluid allotments should be planned with the client as to the type of fluids and time of intake to enhance the regimen's acceptability by the client and to maintain the client's feeling of control. Dietary sodium is usually restricted, and intake will need to be planned with the client, based on degree of restriction.

Drug therapy is based on each client's particular form of dysfunction and its cause. Because of the many body systems that are affected by renal dysfunction, several medications may be used. The more common agents are diuretics for control of fluid balance, edema, and hypertension and antibiotics to treat infection. Because altered renal function also alters pharmacokinetics of many drugs, dosages and dose intervals are adjusted based on the drug and degree of renal system dysfunction.

Education. The client should be instructed in the purpose of the medications, such as antihypertensives, diuretics, calcium supplements, vitamin D, and phosphate binders. In addition, the client should be told of the side effects and adverse reactions of any medications being taken because with increasing renal insufficiency of the client the margin of safety with any medication is diminished. Multiple drug therapy increases the chance of a drug interaction.

The stressors placed on the client with increasing renal insufficiency are multiple. Changes in life-style, body image, and the impact of the disease on the client require

---

TYPICAL GRADING FOR RENAL IMPAIRMENT USING CREATININE CLEARANCE

DEGREE OF RENAL FAILURE	CREATININE CLEARANCE
Normal	Men: 90-139 ml/min
	Women: 80-125 ml/min
Mild impairment	50-80 ml/min
Moderate impairment	10-50 ml/min
Severe impairment	<10 ml/min

Data from Bennett, WM, and others: Am J Kidney Dis 3(3):155, 1983.

TABLE 35-1   Selected Medications and Dosing Recommendations in Renal Insufficiency

| Medication | Dosage recommendation based on creatinine clearance (glomerular filtration rate [ml/min])* | | | Drug removal by hemodialysis or peritoneal dialysis† |
	>50	10-50	<10	
AMINOGLYCOSIDE ANTIBIOTICS				
amikacin (Amikin)	60-90 (q12h)	30-70 (q12h)	20-30 (q24h)	Yes (H,P)
gentamicin (Garamycin)	60-90 (q8-12h)	30-70 (q12h)	20-30 (q24h)	Yes (H,P)
tobramycin (Nebcin)	60-90 (q8-12h)	30-70 (q12h)	20-30 (q24h)	Yes (H,P)
CEPHALOSPORIN ANTIBIOTICS				
cefaclor (Ceclor)	100	50-100	33	Yes (H)
ceftriaxine (Rocephin)	45-100	10-45	5-10	Unknown
cephradine (Anspor, Velosef)	100	50	25	Yes (H,P)
CARDIOVASCULAR DRUGS				
digoxin (Lanoxin)	100	25-75	10-25	No (H,P)
OTHER DRUGS				
cimetidine (Tagamet)	100	75	50	No (H,P)
metoclopramide (Reglan)	100	75	50	Unknown

*Recommendations may use the percent of dosage adjustment and/or the suggested extension of the time interval. The above is based on the percentage of the usually recommended dose; intervals are only included when an extended interval is recommended with the dosage adjustment. Those without time interval extensions are given at the normal dose interval. For additional drugs based on time extension intervals, the reader is referred to Bennett, WM, and others (1983).
†Yes or No refers to the need for dose supplement following the procedure. Yes implies it is usually necessary; No implies it is usually not required. In overdose situations, however, hemodialysis (H) or peritoneal dialysis (P) may be used to lower body concentrations of the drug.

TABLE 35-2   Medications Associated with Renal Toxicity or Dysfunction

Medications	Possible toxicity or dysfunction
kanamycin, colistin, amikacin (rare), tobramycin (rare), gentamicin (rare), cephalothin, cephaloridine, lithium, amphotericin B, cisplatin	Damage and/or necrosis to renal tubules
penicillins, methoxyflurane, cephalothin, sulfonamides, nonsteroidal antiinflammatory drugs, allopurinol	Acute interstitial nephritis, vasculitis, etc.
trimethadione, paramethadione, gold, probenecid, lithium, heroin	Glomerular damage
Injectable antihypertensive drugs given to elderly, excessive dosages of low molecular weight dextran, diuretics, opioid medications	May induce acute ischemic renal failure

From Speight, TM: Avery's drug treatment, principles and practice of clinical pharmacology and therapeutics, ed 3, Baltimore, 1987, The Williams & Wilkins Co.

the nurse to exercise skill in the roles of support and education for the client and family.

Evaluation. Daily weights should be taken at the same time of day, with the same amount of clothing, and with the same scale. The client at home may be better able to establish a routine by weighing first thing in the morning after the first voiding and before dressing or eating. The daily weight can be evaluated in light of the 24-hour intake and output balance.

The fluid intake and output of the client should be accurately recorded on a 24-hour basis. The 24-hour balance should be calculated by subtracting the output from the intake. The balance, whether positive or negative, should relate to weight loss or gain at approximately 500 ml to the pound.

Serum BUN and creatinine levels should be monitored to ascertain the client's end-stage renal disease and to anticipate clinical signs and symptoms that would require nursing intervention and client education.

Serum potassium levels should be monitored daily. When the level exceeds 6 mEq/L, cardiovascular monitoring should become more intense. In addition to blood pressure and apical heart rate determinations, assessment by cardiac monitor is required.

Serum levels of calcium and phosphate should be monitored every 3 to 4 days, and the client should be clinically assessed for hypocalcemia and hyperphosphatemia as evidenced by irritability, muscular twitching, and tetany.

The client's arterial blood gases should be monitored. Clinically, the client should be observed for increased respiratory rate and depth and changes in mental status that would indicate impending metabolic acidosis.

CBCs should be taken periodically, and the client should be assessed for signs and symptoms of anemia that might necessitate interventions such as iron supplements and anabolic steroids or, in the extreme, transfusion of packed or frozen RBCs.

SUMMARY

In summary, renal system dysfunction may be a source of tremendous stress for the client and family, and it also presents a challenge for the nurse. Therapy is complicated by multiple drug therapy and altered pharmacokinetics. Drug interactions or adverse reactions may appear at any time and make close monitoring of drug effects and renal function by the nurse essential. In addition, nondrug therapy, such as diet modification and fluid restriction, and involvement of other body systems present additional areas for nursing intervention.

KEY TERMS

acute renal failure, page 611
azotemia, page 612
chronic renal failure, page 611
end-stage renal disease, page 612
erythropoiesis, page 612
hemodialysis, page 612
peritoneal dialysis, page 612

BIBLIOGRAPHY

Allaire, M: Implications of administering drugs in renal insufficiency, Focus Crit Care 13(1):46, 1986.

Banerjee, AK, and others: The management of acute renal failure in intensive care units, Intensive Care Nurs 2(2):84, 1986.

Bennett, W: Update on drugs in renal failure, Adv Nephrol 15:379, 1986.

Bennett, WM, and others: Drug prescribing in renal failure: dosing guidelines for adults, Am J Kidney Dis 3(3):155, 1983.

Braunwald, E, and others, eds: Harrison's principles of internal medicine, ed 11, New York, 1987, McGraw-Hill Book Co.

Butler, B: Protein restriction in renal disease: how much is enough? J Nephrol Nurs 3(1):27, 1986.

Chronic renal failure, Aust Nurses J 15(11):58, 1986.

Compher, CW: Nutrition assessment in chronic renal failure, Nutr Support Serv 5(8):18, 1985.

Eddins, B: A review of the pathophysiologic basis of end stage renal disease, J Nephrol Nurs 1(2):85, 1984.

Everett, B, and others: Kidney failure: the nephrotoxic potential of drugs and procedures, Consultant 25(6):76, 1985.

Johnson, D: Pathophysiology of renal failure, Crit Care Nurse 5(4):18, 1985.

Kasch, CR: Communication, adaptation, and the restoration of psychosocial competence: helping patients cope with chronic renal failure, ANNA J 11(11):14, 1984.

Katcher, BS, and others, eds: Applied therapeutics, ed 3, San Francisco, 1983, Applied Therapeutics, Inc.

Knoben, JE, and Anderson, PO: Handbook of clinical drug data, ed 5, Hamilton, Ill, 1986, Drug Intelligence Publications.

Krupp, MA, and others, eds: Current medical diagnosis and treatment, Norwalk, Conn, 1987, Appleton & Lange.

Lieurance, C: Adolescents with end stage renal disease: indications for nursing interventions, J Nephrol Nurs 2(1):34, 1985.

Mann, HJ, and others: Acute renal failure, Drug Intell Clin Pharmacol 20(6):421, 1986.

Myers, AR: Medicine, Media, Pa, 1986, Harwal Publishing Co.

Nace, SG: Use of analgesic medications in patients with renal failure, J Nephrol Nurs 2(4):185, 1985.

Nace, SG: Preventing adverse drug reactions in patients with renal failure, J Nephrol Nurs 2(3):125, 1985.

Nova, G: Dialyzable drugs, Am J Nurs 87(7):933, 1987.

O'Brein, ME, and others: Therapeutic options in end-stage renal disease: a preliminary report, ANNA J 13(6):313, 1986.

Outcome criteria and nursing diagnosis in ESRD patient care planning: conservative management. I, ANNA J 14(1):11, 1987.

Phillips, K: Psychological effects of chronic renal failure, Nurs Times 82(22):56, 1986.

Possible renal effects of nonsteroidal anti-inflammatory drugs, J Gerontol Nurs 11(12):38, 1985.

Pullman, TN, and others: Pathophysiology of chronic renal failure, Clin Symp 36(3):3, 1984.

Rounds, KA, and others: Social works and social support: living with chronic renal disease, Patient Educ Counseling 7(3):227, 1985.

Speight, TM: Avery's drug treatment, principles and practice of clinical pharmacology and therapeutics, ed 3, Baltimore, 1987, The Williams & Wilkins Co.

Spiegel, DM, and others: Acute renal failure, Postgrad Med 82(4):96, 1987.

Stark, JL, and Hunt, V: Helping your patient with chronic renal failure, Nurs 83 13(9):56, 1983.

Wallach, J: Interpretation of diagnostic tests, Boston, 1986, Little, Brown & Co.

UNIT IX

Drugs Affecting the Respiratory System

CHAPTERS

CHAPTER 36

Overview of the Respiratory System

The respiratory system includes all structures involved in the exchange of oxygen and carbon dioxide—such as the airway passages, the lungs, nasal cavities, pharynx, larynx, trachea, bronchi, bronchioles, pulmonary lobules with their alveoli, the diaphragm, and all muscles concerned with respiration itself.

The most urgent and critical need for maintaining life is a continued, uninterrupted supply of oxygen. Oxygen is supplied to the body through the process of respiration. **Respiration** is a term loosely used to describe three distinct but interrelated processes.

1. **Pulmonary ventilation,** which involves the movement of air into and out of the lungs

2. **Gas transport,** which involves the exchange of gases between the air in the lungs, the blood, and the cell

3. **Cellular respiration,** which involves the utilization of oxygen in the catabolism of energy-yielding substances for the production of energy

Respiration, one of the body's regulating systems, helps maintain physiologic dynamic equilibrium. It also compensates for rapid adjustment to changes in metabolic states.

The air passages permit air to flow from the external environment to pulmonary blood and modify the air taken in by warming and moistening it and removing noxious substances. Airway efficiency is determined by the following factors:

1. Shape and size of each portion of the respiratory tract (nasal cavity, pharynx, larynx, trachea, bronchi, bronchioles, alveolar sacs)
2. Presence of a ciliated, mucus-secreting, epithelial lining throughout most of the respiratory tract
3. Character and thickness of respiratory tract secretions
4. Compliance of the cartilaginous and bony supports
5. Pressure gradients
6. Traction on airway walls
7. Absence of foreign substances in the lumen of the respiratory tract

Any alteration of any of these factors will affect the ease with which air flows through the air passages. Congenital anomalies, injuries, allergies, or disease will cause air flow resistance if these factors are abnormally affected. Resistance occurs, for example, if there is stenosis or nar-

rowing of any portion of the respiratory tract, loss of cilia that ordinarily sweep out foreign substances, any thick or tenacious secretions, loss of elasticity, or presence of foreign objects.

RESPIRATORY TRACT SECRETIONS

The tracheobronchial tree, made up of repeated branching tubes, is a tubular airway that serves as a conduit for passage of air from the external environment to the alveolar-capillary exchange unit. The inner surface of the tracheobronchial tree is lined with ciliated columnar epithelium interspersed with **goblet cells.** The gelatinous mucus (gel layer) produced by goblet cells is normally discharged into the tubular lumen. In some obstructive pulmonary diseases, mucus secretion is greatly increased, thus making it difficult for the cilia to transport secretions along the airway (see Figure 36-1).

The **bronchial glands,** which are located in the submucosa of the tracheobronchial tree, secrete a relatively

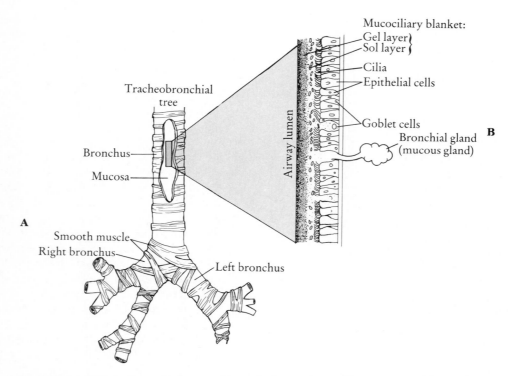

FIGURE 36-1 Tracheobronchial tree and bronchial smooth muscle. **A,** Diagram of the tracheobronchial tree illustrates the double helical or spiral arrangement of the bronchial smooth muscle along the bronchi. Cut-out section shows the inner lining or the mucosa of the bronchus. **B,** The elements of the mucosal lining are enlarged to show details of structures that contribute to the mucociliary blanket. Note that the cilia move in an upward direction toward the larynx. The goblet cells interspersed between the columnar epithelium produce a gelatinous mucus, called the gel layer, whereas the bronchial gland has a tubular duct to the lumen of the tracheobronchial tree through which it secretes a watery fluid, the sol layer. Thus the sol-gel layer forms the mucociliary blanket, a protective fluid film that bathes the ciliated epithelium of the tracheobronchial tree. The normal adult produces approximately 100 ml of respiratory secretions a day.

watery fluid (sol layer) through ducts leading to the surface of the ciliated epithelium. Under vagal (parasympathetic) control, the glands can be stimulated by irritant agents or aerosol drugs to release their contents into the lumen of the airway (see Figure 36-1, *B*).

The products of these two sources—goblet cells and bronchial glands—form the **sol-gel film** that makes up the **mucociliary blanket.** This protective blanket of fluid bathes the ciliated epithelium of the tracheobronchial tree. In addition, the cilia continuously propel the sol-gel film up toward the larynx along the respiratory tree. The normal adult produces approximately 100 ml of respiratory secretions per day, and swallows this material without being aware of it. The process of moving mucus along the tracheobronchial tree is called **mucokinesis.** The mucociliary blanket is a basic concern in most chronic obstructive pulmonary disease. The cilia must sustain appropriate function; a dry atmosphere causes the respiratory secretions to become thick and tenacious, which tends to interfere with ciliary movements. Thus adequate humidity should be maintained to prevent the change in the normal consistency of the respiratory secretions.

BRONCHIAL SMOOTH MUSCLE

Smooth muscle arrangement. An important structure of the tracheobronchial tree is the smooth muscle. The mass of muscle fibers along the bronchi progressively increases as it extends down toward the distal bronchioles. Isolated muscle fibers may be found as far down as the alveolar ducts. The smooth muscle fibers are arranged along the length of the tubular tree in a double helical or spiral pattern, and this formation profoundly influences the diameter or the lumen of the airways. Because of this structural feature, the effect of muscle contraction reduces both the caliber and the length of the bronchus (see Figure 36-1, *A*).

Nerve supply. The airway or tracheobronchial tree is innervated by the autonomic nervous system. The bronchial smooth muscle tone is influenced by the balance maintained between parasympathetic and sympathetic stimuli during rest. Activation of the parasympathetic fiber (vagus nerve) releases acetylcoline, which results in **bronchoconstriction** and narrowing of the airway. By contrast, the stimulation of the sympathetic fiber and the sympathoadrenal system releases epinephrine and norepinephrine from the adrenal medulla into circulation. Their action on the beta$_2$ receptor sites in the bronchial smooth muscle produces **bronchodilation** by means of smooth muscle relaxation.

Receptors. Several kinds of receptors are found along the bronchial airway. The release of acetylcholine activates muscarinic receptors during stimulation of the parasympathetic system, whereas the sympathetic system affects adrenergic receptors. Most of the adrenergic receptors present in the bronchial smooth muscle are beta$_2$ receptors that are stimulated mainly by epinephrine released from the adrenal medulla. Beta$_1$ receptors are also found, although the ratio of beta$_2$ to beta$_1$ receptors is approximately 3:1. Thus bronchial smooth muscle is supplied primarily by beta$_2$ receptors. The sympathomimetic drugs used principally as bronchodilators stimulate the beta$_2$ receptors. Because many of these agents are not purely selective in their pharmacologic effect, they also stimulate the beta$_1$ receptors in the heart, as well as alpha receptors in the lungs and peripheral arterioles. The side effects on the heart are increased cardiac output, tachycardia, and dysrhythmia. The presence of alpha receptors on the bronchial smooth muscle is relatively scarce, and their stimulation results in only mild bronchoconstriction.

Bronchodilation. The beta$_2$ adrenergic receptors mediate bronchodilation. This mechanism presumably is initiated by epinephrine released from the adrenal medulla and norepinephrine released from the peripheral sympathetic nerves. Also located in the cell membrane is an enzyme system known as adenyl cyclase. In the presence of magnesium ions, adenyl cyclase catalyzes the action of adenosine triphosphate (ATP) in the cytoplasm of the cell to produce cyclic 3'5' adenosine-monophosphate (cyclic 3'5' AMP or c3'5' AMP). Cyclic AMP then performs its important function, that is, inducing relaxation of bronchial smooth muscle or bronchodilation. The hormone epinephrine is designated as the "first messenger" and cyclic 3'5' AMP as the "second messenger." As a final action, cyclic 3'5' AMP is inactivated by an enzyme, phosphodiesterase, which catalyzes it to the inactive 5' AMP. This results in a fall in the cyclic 3'5' AMP level. The action of phosphodiesterase may be inhibited by a xanthine drug such as theophylline. As a consequence, the cyclic 3'5' AMP level remains elevated, thereby effecting smooth muscle dilation (see Figure 36-2).

Circulating catecholamines can exert their effects on beta$_1$, beta$_2$, and alpha receptors. Clients with asthma may have an abnormal reaction to both alpha and beta stimulation through a reduced cyclic AMP response, by an abnormally sensitive response to alpha stimulation, and by an exaggerated response to the muscarinic agonists via the vagal pathways. This exaggerated airway response may be due to the effects of a decrease in cyclic AMP, histamine effects on smooth muscle, the vagal reflex pathway, an increase in cyclic guanylic acid secondary to calcium influx, and histamine-induced release of the contents of mast cells. Bronchodilation is induced by circulating catecholamines or administration of a sympathomimetic agent.

Circulating catecholamines reach the lung via circulation and interact with the beta$_2$ adrenergic receptors in the cell membrane of the bronchial smooth muscle cell.

BRONCHIAL SMOOTH MUSCLE FIBER CELL

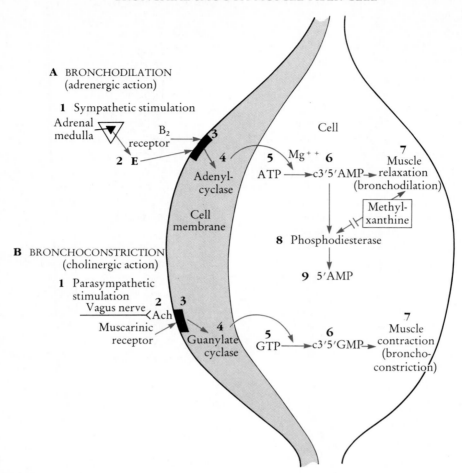

FIGURE 36-2   Mechanism of bronchial smooth muscle action. **A,** *Bronchodilation* involves the adrenergic action. The sequence is numbered from *1* through *9*. Sympathetic stimulation norepinephrine *(NE)*, releases epinephrine *(E)* and the "first messengers," from the adrenal medulla. The interaction of mainly epinephrine with the beta$_2$ receptor in the cell membrane activates adenyl cyclase, an enzyme also in the cell membrane. Adenyl cyclase catalyzes the conversion of adenosine triphosphate (ATP) to cyclic 3'5'AMP (c3'5'AMP) the "second messenger," which in some way induces muscle relaxation or bronchodilation. Magnesium (Mg^{++}) is required to promote the reaction. Normally, c3'5'AMP undergoes fairly rapid hydrolysis to inactive 5'AMP by the intracellular enzyme *phosphodiesterase*. Methylxanthine is capable of inhibiting the action of the enzyme *phosphodiesterase* so that the level of c3'5'AMP is increased and bronchodilation is prolonged. **B,** *Bronchoconstriction* involves cholinergic action. The sequence is numbered from *1* to *7*. The steps in this mechanism include the release of acetylcholine *(Ach)* following vagal nerve stimulation. Interaction of Ach with the muscarinic receptor in the cell membrane activates the enzyme guanylate cyclase, also found in the membrane. Guanylate cyclase catalyzes the reaction that converts guanosine triphosphate (GTP) to cyclic 3'5' guanosine monophosphate (c3'5'GMP). The production of c3'5'GMP causes muscle contraction or bronchoconstriction.

Bronchoconstriction. The bronchial smooth muscle is innervated by the parasympathetic fibers from the vagus nerve. Acetylcholine released from the terminal interacts with the muscarinic receptors on the membrane of the cell. Stimulation of the muscarinic receptor increases the activity of the enzyme guanylate cyclase in the membrane,

thereby promoting the rate of formation of cyclic 3'5' guanosine monophosphate (cyclic 3'5'GMP) from guanosine triphosphate (GTP). The cyclic GMP level affects the bronchial muscle by producing bronchoconstriction. In addition, alpha receptors found on the bronchial smooth muscle have a similar involvement with this mechanism. On

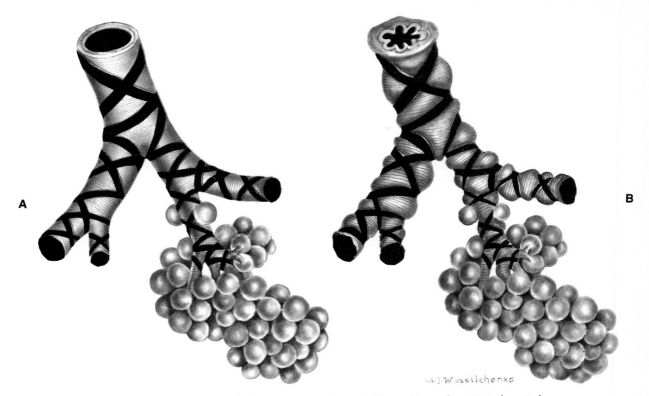

FIGURE 36-3 Mechanisms of obstruction in asthma. **A,** Normal bronchus. **B,** Asthmatic bronchus.

(From Whaley, LF and Wong, DL: Nursing care of infants and children, ed 3, St Louis, 1987, The CV Mosby Co.)

activation, the alpha receptors also increase the cyclic GMP level. Further, cyclic 3'5'GMP stimulates the release of chemical mediators from the mast cell during an asthmatic attack, and these mediators are responsible for causing bronchoconstriction (see Figure 36-2).

CONTROL OF RESPIRATION

Central control. The basic rhythm for respiration is initiated and maintained in the medullary rhythmicity area located beneath the lower part of the floor of the fourth ventricle in the medial half of the medulla. Neurons that control inspiration and expiration intermingle and discharge, or fire impulses alternately. However, signals from the spinal cord, the cerebral cortex and midbrain, the apneustic area of the pons, and the pneumotaxic area of the upper pons can enter the medullary rhythmicity area, modify the rhythm of respiration, and contribute to the normal pattern of respiration.

Normally, the human organism is unaware of the respiratory process. However, voluntary influence and control of breathing are possible. This is important when a client must learn to voluntarily control breathing patterns.

Peripheral control. The medullary rhythmicity area is also influenced by various sensory and peripheral stimuli, the vasomotor center, reflex mechanisms (e.g., the He-

ring-Breuer reflex), the chemo-receptors in the carotid and aortic bodies, and the baroreceptors in the carotid sinus and aortic arch. Fear, pain, stress, blood pressure, body temperature, and blood levels of oxygen and carbon dioxide can all modify the activity of the respiratory centers.

Humoral regulation of respiration is achieved primarily through changes in the concentrations of oxygen, carbon dioxide, or hydrogen ions in body fluids. In a healthy individual, carbon dioxide is the chief respiratory stimulant. An increase in the carbon dioxide tension of the blood directly stimulates the inspiratory and expiratory centers, which increases both the rate and depth of breathing. This results in a blowing off of carbon dioxide to keep the carbon dioxide tension of the blood constant. The pH of the blood is determined by the ratio of bicarbonate ion (HCO_3) to carbon dioxide. When the carbon dioxide content of the blood is increased, there is a subsequent increase in the formation of carbonic acid in the blood. This alters the bicarbonate/carbonic acid ratio from the normal value of 20:1 and results in acidosis. Conversely, a decrease in the carbon dioxide content of the blood results in alkalosis. Therefore respiration is important for regulating the pH of the blood by controlling the carbon dioxide tension of the blood.

Basically, changes in arterial oxygen concentration

have little, if any, direct effect on the respiratory center. However, if the arterial oxygen concentration falls below normal, the chemoreceptors in the carotid and aortic bodies are stimulated and in turn stimulate the respiratory center to increase alveolar ventilation. This mechanism operates primarily under abnormal conditions such as chronic obstructive pulmonary disease.

• • •

Some of the main groups of drugs used to maintain and restore the function of lung structure in the management of respiratory diseases may be classified according to their sites of tissue action. Thus the pharmacologic aspects associated with these drugs include the factors shown in Table 36-1.

AEROSOL THERAPY

Aerosol therapy is a form of topical pulmonary treatment. An **aerosol** is a suspension of fine liquid or solid particles dispersed in a gas or in solution. Dry powder inhalers are also available. Liquid or solid particles range in size from about 0.005 to 50 μm in diameter. Nebulizers are designed to deliver a maximum number of particles of a desired size. Thus aerosol therapy is delivered through nebulization. The terms "aerosol therapy" and "nebulization therapy" are often used interchangeably. Aerosol medication is inhaled as a fine mist deposited on the respiratory tract. This form of therapy promotes the following:

1. Bronchodilation and pulmonary decongestion
2. Loosening of secretions
3. Topical application of steroids
4. Moistening, cooling, or heating of inspired air

TABLE 36-1   Drug Groups in Management of Obstructive Pulmonary Disease and Cold Symptoms

Drug groups	Pharmacologic action
Bronchodilator agents	Act on beta-$_2$ receptors to produce bronchodilation
Nasal decongestants	Stimulate alpha receptors to produce vasoconstriction, which relieves nasal congestion
Cromolyn sodium	Mast cell stabilizing agent that inhibits release of histamine and other substances that cause hypersensitivity reactions
Corticosteroids (steroids)	Antiinflammatory, immuno-suppressant effects systemically; mechanism of action for local antiasthmatic effect unknown

The effectiveness of nebulization therapy depends on the number of droplets that can be suspended in an inhaled aerosol. The number that can be suspended is directly related to the size of the droplets. Small droplets can be suspended in greater numbers than large droplets. Smaller droplets (about 2 to 4 μm in diameter) are more likely to reach the periphery of the lungs—the alveolar ducts and sacs. Currently, in many institutions, ultrasonic nebulizers are used to treat bronchial constriction and pulmonary congestion. Larger droplets (8 to 15 μm in diameter) will be deposited primarily in the bronchioles and bronchi. Droplets of more than 40 μm will be deposited primarily in the upper airway (mouth, pharynx, trachea, and main bronchi).

Rate and depth of breathing are other factors that determine effectiveness of nebulization therapy. Rapid or shallow breathing decreases the number, as well as the retention, of droplets reaching the periphery of the lungs. Rapid breathing permits escape of significant amounts of fine droplets during expirations, although few droplets will escape if the breath is held long enough after deep inspiration to permit droplet deposit in the lung periphery. Small droplets are more effective for absorption of bronchodilators.

Almost all large droplets will be retained somewhere in the air passage. Large droplets are used for keeping large airways (nose, trachea) moist and for loosening secretions. Slow and deep breathing is required for proper lung aeration and penetration of the mist into peripheral lung areas. The breath should be held for a few seconds after a full inspiration.

Droplet size can be controlled by the amount of pressure used to force oxygen or room air through the solution to produce a mist. The tubing used, its length, and its number of bends affect turbulent flow and mist temperature. With most nebulizers maximum density of the inhaled mist is achieved by making the flow of mist as smooth and direct as possible. Nebulizers commonly used in hospitals produce similar mists. *A note of precaution:* drug reconcentration can occur with both jet and ultrasonic nebulizers if a humidity deficit occurs. Evaporation of water molecules causes a gradual increase in drug concentration in the droplets being returned to the fluid reservoir, thus increasing the risk of drug toxicity. Control of temperature and humidity can prevent this.

The main groups of drugs conventionally administered by aerosol include bronchodilators, cromolyn sodium, and steroid preparations. It is important to remember that the lung is an absorptive organ and thus is a route of access for drugs to enter the systemic circulation. For example, after inhalation anesthetic agents enter the blood, they exert their main effect on the central nervous system. Aerosol therapy, when used as a method of administering drugs, is supposed to minimize their side effects. Yet certain bronchodilator aerosols do produce cardiovascular effects simply because the drug may possess a property that adversely influences cardiac action after it is *absorbed* into the bloodstream.

KEY TERMS

aerosol, page 624
bronchial glands, page 620
bronchoconstriction, page 621
bronchodilation, page 621
cellular respiration, page 619
gas transport, page 619
goblet cells, page 620
mucociliary blanket, page 621
mucokinesis, page 621
pulmonary ventilation, page 619
respiration, page 619
sol-gel film, page 621

BIBLIOGRAPHY

Bogartz, LJ: Control of respiration: a review and update, Curr Rev Respir Ther 5(21):167, 1983.

Boushey, and others: The role of the parasympathetic system in the regulation of bronchial smooth muscle, EJ Respir Dis 65(S135):80, 1984.

Bullock, BL, and Rosendahl, PP: Patho-physiology, Boston, 1984, Little, Brown & Co.

Chatbum, RL, and others: A rational basis for humidity therapy, Respir Care 32(4):249, 1987.

Guyton, AC: Textbook of medical physiology, ed 7, Philadelphia, 1986, WB Saunders, Co.

Harper, RW: A guide to respiratory care: physiology and clinical application, Philadelphia, 1981, JB Lippincott Co.

Hedemark, LL, and others: Chemical regulation of respiration, Chest 82(4):488, 1982.

Knepil, J: The control of breathing . . . the neuronal and chemical control of breathing, Nurs Mirror 156(19):44, 1983.

Lehnert, BE, and Schachter, EN: The pharmacology of respiratory care, St Louis, 1980, The CV Mosby Co.

Mecca, R: The physiology and physics of ventilation. II, Curr Rev Recov Room Nurses 5(12):99, 1983.

Meurs, H, and others: Dynamics of the lymphocyte B-adrenergic system in patients with allergic bronchial asthma, EJ Respir Dis 65(S135):47, 1984.

Moser, KM, and Spragg, RG, eds: Respiratory emergencies, ed 2, St Louis, 1982, The CV Mosby Co.

Newhouse, M: Aerosol therapy in adult lung disease, Respir Technol 20(4):11, 1984.

Shapiro, BA, Harrison, RA, and Trout CA: Clinical application of respiratory care, ed 3, Chicago, 1985, Year Book Medical Publishers, Inc.

West, JB: Pulmonary pathophysiology, ed 3, Baltimore, 1987, The Williams & Wilkins Co.

CHAPTER 37

Mucokinetic and Bronchodilator Drugs

OBJECTIVES

After studying this chapter, the student will be able to:

1. Define mucokinetic agent.

2. Compare the advantages and disadvantages of water and saline as diluents.

3. State the purpose of administering mucolytic agents and appropriate nursing considerations.

4. Discuss the therapeutic goals of bronchodilator drugs.

5. Compare and contrast the sympathomimetic bronchodilator drugs.

6. Name drugs and beverages in the xanthine group.

7. Discuss the use of the xanthine derivatives in the treatment of asthma and appropriate client education.

8. Discuss the use of corticosteroid drugs in the treatment of asthma.

Mucokinetic drugs concerned with expectoration and bronchodilator drugs that maintain patency of the respiratory tract are the two main groups discussed in this chapter.

Mucokinetic Drugs

A **mucokinetic** agent is a compound that promotes the removal of abnormal or excessive respiratory tract secretions by thinning hyperviscous secretions, therefore allowing more effective ciliary action. These agents prevent sputum retention, which may result from abnormal ciliary activity, defects in airflow, or modification in cough effectiveness. Sputum (or phlegm) may be defined as an abnormal, viscous secretion that is an excretory product of the lower respiratory tree. It consists mainly of **mucus,** a proteinaceous material having a mucopolysaccharide as its major component. In addition, sputum contains deoxyribonucleic acid (DNA) molecules, which are derived from the breakdown of mucosal cells, leukocytes, and bacteria. These products are responsible for the characteristic heavy quality and yellow color of the sputum. The terms "sputum" and "mucus" should not be used interchangeably. **Sputum** is an abnormal secretion originating in the lower respiratory tract, whereas mucus is a normal secretion produced by the surface cells in the mucous membrane.

Individuals with respiratory disorders such as chronic bronchitis develop disturbances of the mucociliary blanket, which results in a significant impairment of the mucus clearance process. (See Chapter 36, Figure 36-1, *B*.) Consequently, mucus plugging and pathogenic colonization of microorganisms occur in the lower respiratory tract. These changes then lead to overproduction of thick, tenacious sputum. Thus the advantage provided by the mucokinetic drugs is that they alter the consistency of the sputum, thereby promoting the eventual expulsion of these secretions.

DILUENTS
Water

Water is the most commonly used diluent of respiratory secretions. Clients with chronic obstructive pulmonary disease frequently suffer from dehydration, thus respiratory secretions are retained. These secretions then become highly viscous in consistency and lead to widespread plug formation in the respiratory tree.

Water may be administered by ultrasonic nebulizer. Small amounts of water deposited on the gel layer of the respiratory tree appear to reduce the adhesive characteristics and general viscosity of the gelatinous substances found in this layer. Care is needed with clients receiving restricted fluid intake, since water can be absorbed through the inhalation route. (If fluid intake is being measured, water absorbed through the inhalation route must be added to the client's intake record.) If a client's fluid intake is not restricted, large amounts of water are usually encouraged to liquefy the respiratory secretions.

Saline Solutions

Normal saline (0.9% sodium chloride) is physiologic salt solution or isotonic solution that exerts the same osmotic pressure as plasma fluids. Therapy by nebulization is well tolerated, resulting in hydration of respiratory secretions. Hypotonic solution (0.45% sodium chloride) is thought to provide deeper penetration into the more distal airways or in the alveoli via the inhalation route, whereas inhalation or hypertonic solution (1.8% sodium chloride) stimulates a productive cough since the particles deposited on the respiratory mucosa are irritating. Hypertonic solution osmotically attracts fluid out of the mucosa and into the respiratory secretions, thereby promoting their excretion.

MUCOLYTIC DRUGS
acetylcysteine (Mucomyst, Airbron✢)

Mechanism of action. Acetylcysteine reduces the thickness and stickiness of purulent and nonpurulent pulmonary secretions by breaking up the linkages or bonds of mucoprotein molecules of the respiratory secretions

into smaller, more soluble, and less viscous strands. In addition to altering the molecular composition of the mucopolysaccharides, this drug also affects similar changes in the DNA molecule and cellular debris. The decrease in viscosity of bronchial secretions aids their removal by coughing, postural drainage, or suctioning.

Acetylcysteine reduces the extent of liver injury following acetaminophen overdose. This protective effect is thought to occur as a result of altered hepatic metabolism by acetylcysteine.

Indications
1. As an adjunct treatment for thick, viscid or abnormal mucus secretions in individuals with bronchopulmonary disease, cystic fibrosis or atelectasis caused by a mucus plug.
2. Diagnostic aid in various bronchial studies, such as bronchospirometry and bronchograms.
3. Treatment of acetaminophen overdose.

Pharmacokinetics

Absorption. From pulmonary epithelium; although most of the drug dose produces its effects locally, on the mucus in the lungs.

Metabolism. Liver.

Onset of action. Inhalation: within 60 seconds; direct instillation via intratracheal catheter: immediately.

Time to peak effect. Inhalation: within 5 to 10 minutes.

Side effects/adverse reactions. See Table 37-1.

Significant drug interactions. None.

Dosage and administration

Adults

Nebulization: Range is 1 to 10 ml of 20% solution or 2 to 20 ml of the 10% solution, every 2 to 6 hours. Nebulization is via a face mask, mouth piece, or tracheostomy.

Diagnostic aid: Instill by intratracheal or inhalation, 1 to 2 ml of a 20% solution or 2 to 4 ml of a 10% solution for two to three doses before procedure.

Treatment of acetaminophen overdose: Intravenous 300 mg/kg (not currently available in U.S.), given according to protocol, over approximately 20 hours. Orally (available in U.S.), 140 mg/kg initially, then 70 mg/kg every four hours for 17 doses.

Children. See adult dosage. For treatment of acetaminophen overdose, see adult dosages.

Pregnancy safety. FDA Category B.

NURSING CONSIDERATIONS

Assessment. Use acetylcysteine with caution in elderly and debilitated clients and with clients with asthma or severe respiratory insufficiency, because it may increase airway obstruction; bronchospasm may occur in susceptible clients.

TABLE 37-1   Side Effects/Adverse Reactions of Mucokinetic and Bronchodilator Drugs

Drug(s)	Side effects*	Adverse reactions†
acetylcysteine (Mucomyst, Airbron♣)	Less frequent: elevated temperature, sedation, nausea, or vomiting	Rare: respiratory difficulties, rash, or hives
epinephrine (Adrenalin, Bronkaid, and others)	Most frequent: increased nervousness, insomnia, tachycardia Less frequent: difficulty in urination, dizziness, headaches, hypotension, anorexia, nausea, pounding tachycardia, weakness, sweating, vomiting, dry mouth or throat (especially with inhalation products)	Rare: chest pain, breathing difficulties Overdose: blue discoloration of skin, chest pressure or pain, chills, elevated temperature, severe dizziness, hallucinations, severe hypertension, irregular heart rate, mood changes, severe headaches, convulsions, respiratory difficulties, tremors, increased anxiety, restlessness, visual changes, unusually fast or slow heart rate, increased weakness
isoproterenol (Isuprel, Aerolone, and others)	Most frequent: increased restlessness or anxiety, insomnia, saliva colored pink or red, and dry mouth or throat after use of inhalation products Less frequent: dizziness, flushing or red skin, headache, tremors, pounding heart rate, sweating, tachycardia, weakness, vomiting, hypertension, or hypotension	Rare: chest pressure or pain, irregular heart rate Overdose: similar to epinephrine with the exception of blue discoloration of skin, hallucinations, mood changes, respiratory difficulties, visual disturbances, bradycardia, and pale skin
isoetharine (Bronkosol and others)	Less frequent: dizziness, headaches, dry mouth and bad taste in mouth or throat after use of inhalation products, nausea, increased anxiety, pounding heart rate, tremors, insomnia, tachycardia, weakness, vomiting	Rare: increase in breathing difficulties Overdose: same as isoproterenol with exception of irregular heart rate
albuterol (Proventil, Ventolin)	Most frequent: nausea, increased anxiety, pounding heart rate, tremors, tachycardia Less frequent: sedation, difficulty in urination, dizziness, headaches, heartburn, cramping or twitching of muscles, pain at injection site, insomnia, increased sweating, vomiting, increased weakness, hypertension or hypotension, unusual taste in mouth.	Rare: chest pressure or pain, breathing difficulties Overdose: similar to isoproterenol with the exception of irregular heart rate and weakness
metaproterenol (Alupent, Metaprel)	Most frequent: increased anxiety or restlessness Less frequent: dizziness, headaches, hypertension, cramping or twitching of muscles, nausea, pounding heart rate, tremors, sweating, tachycardia, vomiting, and weakness	Rare: respiratory difficulties Overdose: same as isoproterenol
terbutaline (1rethaire, Brethine, Bricanyl)	Most frequent: tremors, increased anxiety or restlessness Less frequent: dizziness, sedation, headaches, hypertension, cramping or twitching of muscles, nausea, pounding heart rate, insomnia, sweating, tachycardia, vomiting, increased weakness, dry mouth or throat and unusual taste in mouth	Rare: chest pressure or pain, increase in respiratory difficulties. Overdose: same as isoetharine with addition of severe nausea and/or vomiting

*If side effects continue, increase, or disturb the patient, inform the physician.
†If adverse reactions occur, contact physician since medical intervention may be necessary.

TABLE 37-1 Side Effects/Adverse Reactions of Mucokinetic and Bronchodilator Drugs—cont'd

Drug(s)	Side effects*	Adverse reactions†
xanthine derivatives (aminophylline, dyphylline, oxtriphylline, and theophylline)	Most frequent: nausea, increased anxiety or restlessness Less frequent: rectal irritation with rectal dosage form only	Less frequent: gastric upset, vomiting Rare: rash or hives that usually occurs 12 to 24 hours after administration of aminophylline (thought to be due to ethylenediamine in aminophylline) Injectable aminophylline or theophylline, if given too fast IV: dizziness, tension, red skin or flushing, headaches, pounding heart rate, chest pain, and rapid breathing Overdosage or toxicity: levels above 20 μg/ml usually result in behavior changes, insomnia, headaches, flushing, dizziness, increased irritability, anorexia, severe nausea or vomiting, convulsions, abdominal cramping or pain, fast breathing, irregular heart rate, increased weakness, black stools or blood in stools or vomiting of dark material (dry blood) or blood, increased urgency for urination In the past, serum levels have been associated with specific side/adverse effects, such as levels >20 ug/ml (GI toxicity), levels >30 ug/ml (cardiac toxicity), and levels >40 ug/ml (convulsions). Studies such as Bertino & Walker (1987) indicate that clear differentiation of side effects with specific levels are not clearly defined; for example, they reported gastrointestinal symptoms at ranges of 21-46 ug/ml), convulsions at 21.6 ug/ml, and cardiac toxicity at ranges of 19.4 to 40 ug/ml. Therefore, monitoring by symptoms and serum levels is more important that relating toxicity to a specific serum level range only.
cromolyn sodium (Intal, Fivent✿)	Most frequent: hoarseness, cough Less frequent: dry mouth or throat, nasal congestion, sneezing, irritated throat, eye watering, bad taste in mouth from inhalation device	Less frequent: pain on urination, difficulty urinating, dizziness, severe headache, increased wheezing, pain or weak muscles or joints, nausea or vomiting, rash, hives, edema of lips and eyes, chest pressure, breathing difficulties, difficulty in swallowing
beclomethasone dipropionate (Vanceril, Beclovent) and other corticosteroids: dexamethasone, flunisolide, and triamcinolone	Most frequent: flunisolide: tachycardia, gastrointestinal distress, anorexia, cough without infection, dizziness, headaches, unpleasant taste in mouth; dexamethasone: gastrointestinal distress Less frequent/rare: cough without infection, dry nose or oral cavity, hoarseness; dexamethasone: insomnia, increased anxiety, increased appetite, and euphoria or false sense of wellbeing; flunisolide: feeling ill, shaky, or faint, increased appetite, and insomnia	Most frequent: oral fungal infection (candidiasis); dexamethasone and flunisolide: increased potential for developing infections Reported with flunisolide: development of respiratory tract infections, pruritis, rash, nausea, vomiting, respiratory difficulties, menstrual irregularities

Intervention. Ultrasonic nebulizers are recommended for administration of the drug. Hand nebulizers are discouraged because the output is too small and the fluid particles too large. The nebulized drug may be inhaled either directly or by the use of a plastic face mask, face tent, mouthpiece, or oxygen tent. The nebulizer may be used with an intermittent positive pressure breathing (IPPB) apparatus. When the drug is nebulized using a dry gas, it may become concentrated because of evaporation of the solution. The last remaining quarter of the drug can be diluted with an equal part of sterile water for injection to continue nebulization to ensure the client receives the appropriate dosage. After nebulization, the face should be washed with water to remove the sticky coating left by the drug.

The equipment should be cleaned immediately after use to prevent blockage of the fine parts and corrosion of the metal ones. Some clients may develop nausea and vomiting, but this may be due to the disagreeable odor of the nebulized drug and quantity of respiratory secretions eliminated. With the aid of these agents and postural drainage, most individuals can expectorate pulmonary secretions without further assistance; however, in the elderly or debilitated, suctioning may be indicated. Because of release of hydrogen sulfide, solutions of acetylcysteine will harden rubber and become discolored on contact with certain metals. Acetylcysteine solutions should be used with equipment made of glass, plastic, or stainless steel. If the vacuum seal has been broken on the bottle, the solution should be refrigerated to retard oxidation and then used within 48 hours.

When acetylcysteine is administered orally, it may be diluted in soft drinks or citrus juices. The diluted solution should be used within the hour.

Education. The client should clear the airway by coughing before the drug is administered by aerosol. Instruction should be given on the correct use of the nebulizer.

Evaluation. The frequency of the client's cough and its character should be monitored and documented. The character and quantity of expectorated material should be observed. Percussion and auscultation of the chest should be accomplished on a periodic basis.

Other Expectorants

Over the years, many other products have been used as expectorants in both prescription and over-the-counter medications. The FDA advisory review panel on nonprescription products did not find any to be effective (Feldman and Davidson, 1986). The products reviewed included ammonium chloride, guaifenesin (glyceryl guaiacolate), syrup of ipecac, beechwood creosote, potassium guaiacolsulfonate, terpin hydrate, peppermint oil, pine tar, turpentine oil, menthol, camphor, and sodium citrate. The review panel reported that the use of expectorants is

---

EXPECTORANTS IN CATEGORY III*
ammonium chloride beechwood creosote guaifenesin potassium guaiacolsulfonate syrup of ipecac terpin hydrate

*Safe but not proven to be effective. Recommended dosages and additional information available (Feldman and Davidson, 1986).

---

largely based on tradition, rather than scientific data to substantiate effectiveness. Therefore, a number of these products (see box) were classified as Category III or considered safe, but current information is not available to classify them as effective.

DRUGS THAT ANTAGONIZE BRONCHIAL SECRETIONS

Atropine, although not used as an expectorant, may be given cautiously to decrease secretions and excessive expectoration in certain forms of bronchitis.

Many remedies used to treat colds contain atropine. Morphine, codeine, and papaverine not only act as sedatives but also tend to dry the mucous membranes. In many cases the best treatment of a cold or inflammation of the respiratory mucous membranes is extra rest, forcing fluids, and eating simple but nutritious food.

Bronchodilator Drugs

Bronchodilator drugs are primarily used to treat chronic pulmonary diseases such as asthma, chronic bronchitis, and emphysema. Major causes of airway obstruction include:

1. Bronchial smooth muscle contraction (asthma)
2. Mucus hypersecretion (chronic bronchitis)
3. Mucosal edema or inflammation (chronic bronchitis)

There are three types of asthma: extrinsic, intrinsic, and a mixture of both. The mixture of both is the most common type of asthma seen in clinical practice. Table 37-2 compares extrinsic and intrinsic asthma.

The major drugs used in treatment of asthma include sympathomimetic drugs, theophylline, cromolyn sodium, and the corticosteroids. Figure 37-1 illustrates major sites of action for these drugs.

The principal agents used in the treatment of airway obstruction include sympathomimetic drugs and xanthine derivatives. Prophylactic antiasthmatic agents also prevent airway obstruction in individuals with certain

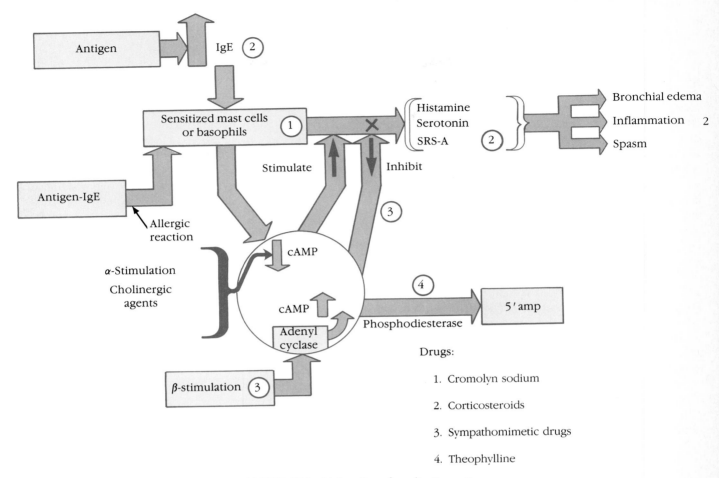

FIGURE 37-1 Major sites of medication action.

TABLE 37-2 Comparison of Intrinsic (Nonallergic) and Extrinsic (Allergic, Immunologic) Asthma

	Intrinsic	Extrinsic
Causative factors	Exercise, upper respiratory infection, irritants, cold air, fumes (cigarette smoking, chemicals), emotional factors	Pollens, molds, dust, animal hair, or dander
IgE levels	Normal	Increased
Skin test results	Negative	Positive
Family history of allergies	Negative	Positive
Age at onset	Middle age (over 35 years)	Childhood (5 years to teenage years)
Nasal symptoms	Presence of polyps	Hay fever
Aspirin* hypersensitivity	Often present	None

*If aspirin is a problem, other NSAI drugs may be also.

types of asthma. Most of these drugs enhance the production of cyclic 3'5' AMP in bronchial smooth muscle cells to affect bronchodilation. (See Figure 36-2.)

In the management of constricted airways the use of bronchodilator drugs includes the following therapeutic goals:

1. Maximal bronchial smooth muscle relaxation.
2. Prolonged activity of the drug.
3. Prevention of tachyphylaxis or development of tolerance to the beta-adrenergic agonists.
4. Production of minimal adverse adrenergic (sympathomimetic stimulation) effects or theophylline tox-

icity (Close monitoring and supervision of client dosing should reduce this potential for adverse effects.)

SYMPATHOMIMETIC DRUGS

Based on their receptor action, three groups of sympathomimetic drugs are recognized: (1) *nonselective adrenergic drugs* that have alpha, beta$_1$ (cardiac), and beta$_2$ (respiratory) activities (e.g., epinephrine); (2) *nonselective beta adrenergic drugs* with both beta$_1$ and beta$_2$ effects (e.g., isoproterenol); and (3) *selective beta$_2$ agents* (e.g., albuterol) that act primarily on beta$_2$ receptors in the lungs (bronchial smooth muscle).

NONSELECTIVE ADRENERGIC DRUGS

Nonselective adrenergic drugs such as epinephrine, ephedrine, and others possess both alpha- and beta-receptor stimulating properties. Alpha activity appears to mediate vasoconstriction to reduce mucosal edema, while beta$_2$ stimulation increases the level of cyclic 3'5' AMP, producing bronchodilation and vasodilation. In contrast, beta$_1$ receptor action causes unwanted cardiac side effects such as increases in heart rate and force of myocardial contraction. Undesirable effects on beta$_2$ receptors include muscle tremors, glycogenolysis, and gluconeogenesis. These products may also cause an increase in CNS stimulation.

epinephrine inhalation aerosol (Bronkaid Mist, Bronkoaid Mistometer✣, Primatene Mist Solution, Dysne-Inhal✣)
epinephrine inhalation solution (Adrenalin)
epinephrine bitartrate inhalation aerosol (AsthmaHaler, Bronkaid Mist Suspension, Medihaler-Epi, Primatene Mist Suspension)
racepinephrine inhalation solution (AsthmaNefrin, microNEFRIN, S-2 Inhalant, Vaponefrin)

Mechanism of action. Epinenephrine acts as a bronchodilator that stimulates beta$_2$ receptors in the lungs, resulting in relaxation of bronchial smooth muscle and alleviates bronchospasm, increases vital capacity and reduces airway resistance. It also inhibits the release of histamine and slow-reacting substances released during anaphylaxis. Also the bronchial vasoconstrictor effects of histamine are antagonized.

Indications. Treatment of bronchial asthma, bronchitis, and other pulmonary disease states and prevention of bronchospasm and bronchial asthma

Pharmacokinetics

Absorption

Inhalation: Only slight absorption with the usually prescribed dosages, can be increased if larger doses are given

IM or SC: rapid absorption

Onset of action. Within 3 to 5 minutes (inhalation); within 6 to 15 minutes (subcutaneous); variable (intramuscular)

Duration of action. Between 1 and 3 hours (inhalation); between 1 and 4 hours (intramuscular subcutaneous)

Metabolism. Liver and at sympathetic nerve endings

Excretion. Small amount via kidneys

Side effects/adverse reactions. See Table 37-1.

Significant drug interactions

1. Alpha-adrenergic blocking agents (such as prazosin, tolazoline, phenoxybenzamine, or phentolamine) or other medications with alpha-blocking properties (such as phenothiazines, thioxanthenes, haloperidol, loxapine, nicotine, dibenzamine) or fast-acting vasodilators (such as nitrites) may block the alpha-stimulating effects of epinephrine, which may result in severe hypotension and tachycardia. Monitor closely as medical interventions may be necessary.

2. Beta-adrenergic blocking agents (oral, parenteral, and ophthalmic) may reduce therapeutic effects of both agents. Also may result in hypertension, bradycardia, and possibly heart block. Avoid concurrent administration.

3. Digitalis glycosides (digoxin, digitoxin) may increase potential for cardiac arrhythmias. Monitor electrocardiogram if both drugs must be given concurrently.

4. Tricyclic antidepressants may increase potential for cardiac arrhythmias, tachycardia, hypertension, and hyperpyrexia. Avoid concurrent administration.

Dosage and administration

epinephrine inhalation aerosol

Adults. Bronchodilator: one inhalation (0.2-0.25 mg); may repeat in 1 to 2 minutes if needed, then every 4 hours

Children. Under 6 years old—individualized by physician; 6 years and older—see adult dosage

epinephrine inhalation solution

Adults. Bronchodilator: one inhalation of a 1% solution; may repeat in 1 to 2 minutes if necessary

Children. Under 6 years old—individualized by physician; 6 years and older—see adult dosage

epinephrine bitartrate inhalation aerosol

Adults. Bronchodilator: one inhalation (0.16 mg) initially; if necessary, may repeat in 1 minute, then every 4 hours thereafter

Children. Under 6 years old—individualized by physician; 6 years and older—see adult dosage

racepinephrine inhalation solution

Adults. Bronchodilator: two or three inhalations of a 2.25% solution; may repeat in 5 minutes if necessary, then may be administered 4 to 6 times per day. Nebulization via respirator: 5 ml of a 0.1% solution by oral inhalation over 15 minutes, every 3 to 4 hours

Children. Under 4 years old—individualized by physician; 4 years and older—see adult dosage

epinephrine injection

Adults. Bronchodilator: 0.2 to 0.5 mg subcutaneous, may repeat every 20 minutes up to 4 hours, if necessary; dosage may also be increased to 1 mg if needed

Children. Bronchodilator: 0.01 mg/kg or 0.3 mg/m^2 up to a maximum of 0.5 mg/dose; may repeat every 15 minutes for two doses, then ever 4 hours, as necessary

sterile epinephrine suspension (Sus-Phrine)

Adults. Bronchodilator: 0.5 mg subcutaneous initially, then 0.5 to 1.5 mg subcutaneous every 6 hours, as necessary

Children. 0.025 mg/kg or 0.625 mg/m^2, subcutaneous; if necessary, dosage may be repeated every 6 hours. If child weighs 30 kg or less, the maximum single dose is 0.75 mg

Pregnancy safety. FDA category C

NURSING CONSIDERATIONS

See drug monograph in Chapter 20.

NONSELECTIVE BETA ADRENERGIC DRUGS

The nonselective beta adrenergic drugs exhibit both beta$_2$ and beta$_1$ activities. Their main action is on the bronchial smooth muscle, as well as the heart.

isoproterenol inhalation solution (Aerolone, Vapo-Iso, Isuprel)
isoproterenol hydrochloride inhalation aerosol (Isuprel Mistometer, Norisodrine Aerotrol)

Mechanism of action. A potent bronchodilator with effects on both beta$_1$ and beta$_2$ receptors.

Indications. Treatment of bronchial asthma, bronchitis, and other pulmonary disease states

Pharmacokinetics

Onset of action

Inhalation: within 2 to 5 minutes

IV: immediate

Sublingual: within 15 to 30 minutes

Duration of action. Within ½ to 2 minutes (inhalation); less than 1 minute (IV); within 1 to 2 minutes (sublingual)

Metabolism. Liver, lungs, and other body tissues

Excretion. Kidneys, depending on route of administration: 40% to 50% if given IV, approximately 5% to 15% if given orally or by inhalation.

Side effects/adverse reactions. See Table 37-1.

Significant drug interactions. When isoproterenol is given concurrently in less than 5-minute intervals with corticosteroid aerosol, ipratropium aerosol, or other oth-er adrenergic bronchodilator aerosol, the risk of inducing a fluorocarbon toxicity is increased since the aerosols contain fluorocarbons. Advise clients to space such aerosol medications apart by, at least, 5 minutes.

Dosage and administration

isoproterenol inhalation solution

Adults

Bronchodilator: 6 to 12 inhalations of a 0.25% solution by oral inhalation. May be repeated at 15-minute intervals if needed, up to three doses. Do not exceed eight treatments in 24 hours

Treatment of acute bronchial asthmatic attack: 5 to 15 deep inhalations by oral inhalation of a 0.5% solution or 3 to 7 deep inhalations of a 1% solution. May be repeated once if needed, in 5 to 10 minutes. Do not exceed five treatments daily, if necessary

Treatment of bronchospasm in chronic obstructive lung disease: 5 to 15 deep inhalations of a 0.5% or 3 to 7 inhalations of a 1% solution by oral inhalation (hand nebulizer) every 3 to 4 hours

Intermittent positive-pressure breathing (IPPB): 2 ml of a 0.125% solution or 2.5 ml of a 0.1% solution by oral inhalation given over 10 to 20 minutes. This treatment may be repeated up to five times daily

Children

Bronchodilator: 6 to 12 inhalations of a 0.25% solution, may repeat in 15-minute intervals for three doses, if necessary. Do not exceed eight treatments in 24 hours.

Treatment of acute bronchial asthma: 5 to 15 deep inhalations of a 0.5% solution; may repeat once after 5 to 10 minutes. This treatment may be repeated up to five times daily.

Treatment of bronchospasm in chronic obstructive lung disease: Hand nebulizer: 5 to 15 deep inhalations orally of a 0.5% solution, every 3 to 4 hours. IPPB or nebulization by compressed air or oxygen: 2 ml of a 0.0625% solution or 2.5 ml of a 0.05% solution given over 10 to 15 minutes, up to five times daily

isoproterenol hydrochloride inhalation aerosol

Adults

Bronchodilator: Treatment of acute bronchial asthma: one inhalation (0.12 or 0.131 mg) initially; may repeat after 1 to 5 minutes if needed, up to four to six times a day

Treatment of bronchospasm in chronic obstructive lung disease: one inhalation orally, every 3 to 4 hours as needed

Children. See adult dosage.

isoproterenol sulfate inhalation aerosol

Adults. Bronchodilator: one inhalation (0.08 mg), may repeat in 2 to 5 minutes if needed, up to four to six times per day

Children. See adult dosage.

isoproterenol hydrochloride tablets (Isuprel)

Adults. Bronchodilator: 10 to 15 mg sublingually, three or four times a day, up to 60 mg maximum

Children. 5 to 10 mg sublingually, three times daily, up to 30 mg maximum

isoproterenol hydrochloride injection (Isuprel)

Adults. Bronchodilator for bronchospasm during administration of anesthesia: 10 to 20 μg (0.01 to 0.02 mg) intravenous. Repeat if necessary

Children. Individualize according to physician's order

Pregnancy safety. FDA category C

NURSING CONSIDERATIONS

See drug monograph in Chapter 20.

SELECTIVE BETA₂ RECEPTOR DRUGS

The high incidence of undesirable cardiotoxic effects caused by the beta₁ property of sympathomimetic agents has led to a search for a more specific beta₂ receptor agonist. There are two types: (1) the catecholamine beta₂ receptor agonist (e.g., isoetharine) and (2) the noncatecholamine beta₂ receptor agonist (e.g., albuterol, metaproterenol, and terbutaline).

Catecholamine Beta₂ Receptor Drugs

isoetharine inhalation solution (Bronkosol, Disorine, Dey-Lute Isoetharine)

isoetharine mesylate inhalation aerosol (Bronkometer)

Mechanism of action. Isoetharine is a direct-acting sympathomimetic catecholamine that selectively stimulates beta₂ receptors. Since it possesses a weak beta₁ response, there is less risk of cardiotonic side effects than is experienced with epinephrine and isoproterenol. Its beta₂ adrenergic-receptor activity relaxes bronchial smooth muscle, thereby relieving bronchospasm, increasing vital capacity, and decreasing resistance of bronchial airways. It may also inhibit antigen-induced release of histamine by stimulating the production of cyclic 3′5′ AMP, which stabilizes the mast cell.

Indications. See epinephrine.

Pharmacokinetics

Onset of action. Within 1 to 6 minutes

Time to peak effect. Within 15 to 60 minutes

Duration of action. Within 1 to 4 hours

Metabolism. Liver; also lungs, gastrointestinal tract, and other body tissues

Excretion. Kidneys

Side effects/adverse reactions. See Table 37-1.

Significant drug interactions. See isoproterenol.

Dosage and administration

isoetharine inhalation solution

Adults. Bronchodilator

Hand nebulizer: 3 to 7 inhalations of undiluted 1% solution; usual dose is four inhalations.

For recommended IPPB and oxygen aerosolization dosages: see current package insert or U.S.P.-D.I.

Children.. Not established

isoetharine mesylate inhalation aerosol (Bronkometer)

Adults. Bronchodilator: one inhalation orally, may repeat in 1 to 2 minutes if needed, then every 4 hours

Children. Not established

Pregnancy safety. FDA category C

NURSING CONSIDERATIONS

Assessment. Initially determine if the client has a preexisting condition in which the drug is used with caution: cardiovascular disease, such as hypertension, coronary artery disease, limited cardiac reserve; hyperthyroidism; and pheochromocytoma.

Intervention. Isoetharine may be administered by hand nebulizer, IPPB, and oxygen aerosolization. The use of IPPB is currently limited as a method of aerosol deposition. However, it is a convenient procedure for helping clients with airway obstruction to breathe deeply. The disadvantage is that the amount of drug lost in the room air and the apparatus is approximately 40% to 65%, and the amount of drug deposited in the lower airways is about 5% to 15%. IPPB is generally administered by the respiratory therapist.

Education. Instruct client in the use of the nebulizer.

Warn client to avoid contact of spray with eyes and to rinse mouth after therapy to prevent dryness and throat irritation.

Advise client to use inhalation therapy as prescribed since rapid relief encourages overuse. Thus tolerance to a bronchodilator agent may occur, with a potential for causing cumulative drug toxicity (e.g., palpitations, tachycardia, headache, dizziness, and nausea). Repeated use may cause paradoxical airway resistance, which produces sudden dyspnea. To relieve possible bronchospasm, the physician may discontinue therapy and have epinephrine available.

Instruct client to take no more than two inhalations at a time and to allow 1 to 2 minutes between inhalations. Also, encourage patient to increase fluid intake to aid in liquefaction of bronchial secretions.

Inform client that sputum may be rust-colored because of oxidation of medication.

Noncatecholamine Beta₂ Receptor Drugs

When compared with the catecholamine beta₂ receptor agonists, the noncatecholamine beta₂ receptor drugs have two advantages. They are a longer duration of activity and few cardiovascular side effects.

albuterol inhalation aerosol (Proventil, Ventolin)
albuterol inhalation solution (Ventolin✲)
albuterol sulfate for inhalation (Ventolin✲)
albuterol sulfate syrup (Proventil, Ventolin)
albuterol sulfate tablets (Proventil, Ventolin)
albuterol sulfate injection (Ventolin✲)

Mechanism of action. Albuterol is a sympathomimetic bronchodilator. It possesses a relatively selective specificity for beta₂ adrenergic receptors in the lungs and therefore is less likely to cause unwanted cardiovascular effects. Its interaction with the beta₂ receptor in the cell membrane of the bronchial smooth muscle stimulates the enzyme adenyl cyclase, which is also located in the membrane, to produce cyclic 3'5' AMP. The cyclic AMP thus formed mediates a response that is capable of relaxing the smooth muscle of the bronchi (see Figure 36-2), thus relieving bronchospasms and decreasing airway resistance. In addition, this mechanism causes relaxation of the smooth muscle of the uterus and blood vessels of the skeletal muscle. However, it has been reported that high doses of the drug administered intravenously would be required to inhibit uterine contractions to delay premature labor.

Indications. Same as epinephrine

Pharmacokinetics

Distribution

Inhalation
Onset of action: 15 minutes
Time to peak effect: 1 to 1½ hours after two inhalations
Duration of action: 3 to 4 hours
Oral
Onset of action: 30 minutes
Time to peak effect: within 2 to 3 hours
Duration of action: usually not > 6 hours
Metabolism. Liver
Excretion. Kidneys and feces
Side effects/adverse reactions. See Table 37-1.
Significant drug interactions. See isoproterenol. May also interact adversely with anesthetics, beta-adrenergic blocking agents, digitalis glycosides, tricyclic antidepressants, and MAO inhibitors. Monitor closely if concurrent administration is necessary.

Dosage and administration. Albuterol inhalation solution, albuterol sulfate for inhalation, and albuterol sulfate injection (Ventolin) are not available in the United States. Doses for these products are listed in the U.S.P.-D.I.

albuterol inhalation aerosol (Proventil, Ventolin)
Adults. Bronchodilator (oral inhalation): 180 μg (2 inhalations) every 4 to 6 hours. Note that for some patients a dose of 90 μg (1 inhalation) every 4 hours may be adequate
Children. 12 years or older: same as adults. Safety and dosage recommendations for children below the age of 12 years have not been established.

albuterol sulfate tablets and syrup
Adults. Bronchodilator: 2 to 6 mg orally three or four times a day initially. Increase dosage if necessary, up to an 8 mg maximum, four times a day
Elderly. 2 mg orally 3 or 4 times daily initially. Increase dosage as necessary and tolerated, up to 8 mg three or four times daily
Children
Under 2 years old—not established
2 to 6 years old—0.1 mg/kg 3 times daily, increasing as needed to 0.2 mg/kg 3 times daily; maximum: 4 mg 3 times daily
6 to 14 years old—2 mg 3 or 4 times daily initially; dosage may be increased as necessary and tolerated, up to a maximum of 24 mg daily, given in divided doses.
14 years and older—see adult dosage

albuterol solution for inhalation
Adults. 2.5 mg by nebulization 3-4 times daily
Children. Over 12: see adult dose; not recommended for children under 10

Pregnancy safety. FDA category C

NURSING CONSIDERATIONS

Assessment. Initially clients should be assessed for a previous intolerance to other sympathomimetic agents, since this may indicate an intolerance to albuterol.

Albuterol should be used with caution with clients with coronary insufficiency, hypertension, and pheochromocytoma. Clients with diabetes mellitus may need an increased dosage of insulin when receiving albuterol. It needs to be considered that clients with hyperthyroidism may have exaggerated response to albuterol.

Elderly clients are more susceptible to the drug's effects and usually require lower dosages.

Intervention. A mouthpiece or a face mask may be used to administer the inhalation solution through a nebulizer. The nebulizer may be used with compressed air or oxygen, 6 to 10 liters per minute. An average treatment lasts about 10 minutes.

Education. The client should be taught the correct use of the inhaler (Figure 37-2): shake the container thoroughly; exhale through nose; administer drug while inhaling deeply on the mouthpiece of the inhaler; hold

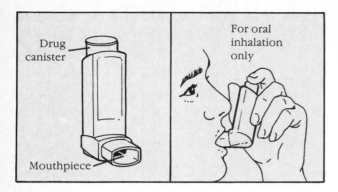

FIGURE 37-2. Inhaler.

breath for a few seconds; exhale slowly. Wait 2 minutes between inhalations. If a solution is being used that needs dilution, it should be diluted immediately before use.

Inform client that after long-term use, drug may have a shorter duration of action (1 to 2 hours). Report to physician failure to respond to usual dose, which may mean the development of drug tolerance. This may stimulate adverse effects such as cardiac arrest.

Advise client to rinse mouth after inhalation therapy to prevent dryness, throat irritation, and systemic absorption. If a bad taste occurs, it will gradually disappear with repeated usage.

Warn client that excessive use of aerosol may be harmful, causing paradoxical (rebound) bronchospasm, which means that the effects of the drug are no longer therapeutic. Stress the importance of not changing dosage or frequency without consulting physician.

Chest pain, extreme dizziness and lightheadedness, severe headache, palpitations, continuing tachycardia, dysrhythmias and hypertensive episodes should be reported to the physician.

Evaluation. Signs of the client's anxiety should decrease as breathing becomes more effective. Wheezing, if present, should also decrease. Signs of respiratory distress such as increased effort to breathe, increased use of accessory muscles, contraction of the abdominal muscles on expiration, and diaphoresis will decrease as the medication becomes effective. The client will respond subjectively if relief from the respiratory distress is felt.

metaproterenol sulfate inhalation aerosol (Alupent, Metaprel)
metaproterenol sulfate inhalation solution (Alupent, Metaprel)
metaproterenol sulfate syrup (Alupent, Metaprel)
metaproterenol sulfate tablets (Alupent, Metaprel)

Mechanism of action. Same as albuterol
Indications. Same as epinephrine

Pharmacokinetics
Distribution
Inhalation (aerosol)
Onset of action: 1 to 5 minutes
Time to peak effect: approximately 1 hour
Duration of action: 1 to 5 hours after single dose; approximately 1-2.5 hours after continuous dosing
Inhalation with nebulizer or IPPB:
Onset of action: within 5 to 30 minutes
Duration of action: 2 to 6 hours after single dose; 4 to 6 hours after continuous dosing
Oral dosage form
Onset of action: within 15 to 30 minutes
Time to peak effect: within 1 hour
Duration of action: up to 4 hours
Metabolism. Liver
Excretion. Kidneys
Side effects/adverse reactions. See Table 37-1.
Significant drug interactions. See albuterol, with the exception of tricyclic antidepressants and MAO inhibitors. Significant problems have not been reported with the latter two categories.
Dosage and administration. Bronchodilator:
Inhalation aerosol. Oral inhalation
Adults. 2 or 3 inhalations (1.3 or 1.95 mg) every 3 to 4 hours, not to exceed 12 inhalations (7.8 mg) day
Children. For those up to 12 years of age, use is not recommended
Inhalation solution for nebulizer or IPPB. See package insert or U.S.P.-D.I. for recommended dosages
Syrup. Oral
Adults. 20 mg three or four times a day.
Children. For those weighing up to 27 kg or 6 to 9 years: 10 mg three or four times a day; for children weighing over 27 kg or older than 9 years: see adult dose
Tablets
Adults. See metaproterenol sulfate syrup.
Children. See metaproterenol sulfate syrup.
Pregnancy safety. FDA category C

NURSING CONSIDERATIONS

See discussion under albuterol, p. 635.

terbutaline sulfate inhalation aerosol (Brethaire)
terbutaline sulfate tablets (Brethine, Bricanyl)
terbutaline sulfate injection (Brethine, Bricanyl)

Mechanism of action. Similar to albuterol and metaproterenol
Indications. Same as epinephrine
Pharmacokinetics
Distribution
Inhalation
Onset of action: in 5 to 30 minutes

Time to peak effect: in 1 to 2 hours
Duration of action: 3 to 6 hours
Oral
Onset of action: 30 minutes
Time to peak effect: in 2 to 3 hours
Duration of action: 4 to 8 hours
Parenteral
Onset of action: within 15 minutes
Time to peak effect: in ½ to 1 hour
Duration of action: 1.5 to 4 hours
Metabolism. Liver
Excretion. Kidneys
Side effects/adverse reactions. See Table 37-1.
Significant drug interactions. See albuterol.
Dosage and administration
terbutaline sulfate inhalation aerosol
Adults. Bronchdilator: 2 inhalations (0.4 mg) every 4 to 6 hours; separate each inhalation by one minute
Children. Under 12 years old—not established; over 12 years old—see adult dose
terbutaline sulfate tablets (Brethine, Bricanyl)
Adults. Bronchodilator: orally, 2.5 to 5 mg every 6 hours three times a day; maximum dosage is 15 mg/day.
Children. 12 to 15 years—2.5 mg three times a day, every 6 hours; under 12 years old—not established
terbutaline sulfate injection (Brethine, Bricanyl)
Adults. Bronchodilator: subcutaneous, 0.25 mg; repeat once 15 to 30 minutes later if needed. Do not exceed total dosage of 0.5 mg within a 4-hour period. Consider alternate therapy if client does not respond to second dose
Children. Under 12 years old—not established
Pregnancy safety. FDA category B

NURSING CONSIDERATIONS

See discussion under albuterol, p. 635.

XANTHINE DERIVATIVES

The xanthine group of drugs includes caffeine, theophylline, and theobromine. Beverages from the extracts of plants containing these alkaloids have been used by humans since ancient times. These drugs relax smooth muscle, particularly bronchial muscle, stimulate cardiac muscle and the central nervous system, and also produce diuresis probably through a combined action of increased renal perfusion and increased sodium and chloride ion excretion.

The drugs in this category are methylated forms of xanthines and referred to as methylxanthines. The effectiveness of these preparations as bronchodilators depends on their conversion to *theophylline,* which is the active constituent. Therefore with the exception of dyphylline, the

---

FACTORS AFFECTING THEOPHYLLINE'S THERAPEUTIC EFFECTS

May be increased by:
Age: elderly and newborn
Drugs: erythromycin, cimetidine, and oral contraceptives
Disease states: cirrhosis, pulmonary edema, congestive heart failure, and severe COPD
Diet: high carbohydrate
May be decreased by:
Substances: tobacco, marijuana
Drugs: corticosteroids (inconclusive data), phenobarbital
Diet: high protein
Age: adolescence

---

action of xanthine depends on the content of theophylline. Xanthines inhibit mast cell degranulation and the release of histamine and other mediators that are responsible for bronchoconstriction. Because they impede enzymatic action, the methylxanthines are also called phosphodiesterase inhibitors (see Figure 36-2).

Combinations of theophylline with iodides (Elixophyllin KI and others) and with ephedrine (Tedral and others) are not considered rational formulations (Hendeles and Weinberger, 1982), since the reported increase in toxicity is not balanced or offset by an increased therapeutic effect. Therefore, these products should be avoided because they do not offer an increase in beneficial effects.

Theophylline products, especially slow-release products, can vary in their rate of absorption and therapeutic effects. Some states, such as Florida, do not permit generic substitution for theophylline products.

Theophylline toxicity at levels above 20 μg/ml presents with different signs and symptoms. See Table 37-1 for reported side effects and adverse reactions. Also, dosage adjustment with theophylline is necessary under certain conditions. The box lists some of the most common ones to consider.

aminophylline (Amoline, Somophyllin, Phyllocontin, Aminophyllin, Palaron✤)
dyphylline (Dilor, Lufyllin, Protophylline✤, Droxine, Dyflex)
oxtriphylline (Choledyl, Apo-Oxtriphylline✤, Novotriphyl✤)
theophylline (Bronkodyl, Elixophyllin, Somophyllin-T, Aerolate, Slo-Phyllin Gyrocaps, Theo-Dur, and others)

Mechanism of action. Theophylline is the prototype of

the xanthine derivatives. It competitively inhibits the action of phosphodiesterase, the enzyme that degrades cyclic 3'5'AMP to the inactive form 5'AMP. Thus the resulting inhibition increases the level of intracellular cyclic 3'5'AMP, which mediates pharmacologic action such as relaxation of smooth muscle of bronchial airways and pulmonary blood vessels. This produces a reversal of bronchospasm and increases respiratory flow rates and vital capacity. (See Figure 36-2.)

Indications. For the treatment and prevention of bronchial asthma; treatment of bronchitis, pulmonary emphysema, and other chronic obstructive pulmonary diseases.

Pharmacokinetics

Absorption

Aminophylline, oxtriphylline, and theophylline

Oral: usually rapid for oral liquids and uncoated tablets. Enteric coated tablets give a delayed and at times, unreliable absorption. Extended-release dosage formulations—slow and for some products, complete. Other products have demonstrated unreliable absorption patterns

Retention enema: usually rapid absorption

Suppository: slow, unreliable absorption, especially if suppository is composed of hydrogenated vegetable oils

Dyphylline. Good oral absorption.

Time to peak levels

Aminophylline, oxtriphylline, and theophylline

Oral solution: 1 hour

Uncoated tablets: 2 hours

Chewable tablets: 1 to 1.5 hours

Enteric-coated tablets: 5 hours

Extended-release capsules and tablets: 4 to 7 hours

Retention enema: 1 to 2 hours

Dyphylline. Within 1 hour

Half-life

Aminophylline, oxtriphylline, and theophylline

Newborns up to six months old: >24 hours

Children over 6 months old: 2.6 to 4.8 hours

Adult nonsmoker, with uncomplicated asthma: 6.5 to 10.9 hours.

Smokers (from 1 to 2 packs a day): 4 to 5 hours; if client stops smoking, the normal pharmacokinetics for theophylline may not appear for 3 months up to 24 months

Elderly individuals with chronic obstructive pulmonary disease, cor pulmonale or other forms of heart failure, and liver dysfunction: in excess of 24 hours

Dyphylline. 2 to 2.5 hours

Metabolism. Aminophylline, oxtriphylline, and theophylline salts all release free theophylline in vivo. Theophylline is metabolized by the liver to caffeine. Caffeine concentrations may average about 30% of the theophylline concentration, but in neonates, it may be much great-

er than that. Caffeine does not accumulate in adults. Dyphylline: not metabolized.

Therapeutic serum levels

Bronchodilator effect: theophylline—between 10 and 20 µg/ml; dyphylline—not established

Respiratory stimulant: theophylline—between 5 and 10 µg/ml

Excretion. Theophylline—kidneys; dyphylline—kidneys

Side effects/adverse reactions. See Table 37-1.

Significant drug interactions

1. When xanthine products are given with phenytoin, primidone, or rifampin, increased metabolism of xanthines occurs. Decreased absorption of phenytoin, leading to low serum levels, may be seen with concurrent administration. Serum levels of both drugs should be closely monitored, since dosage adjustments may be necessary.

2. When xanthine products are given with beta-adrenergic blocking agents, therapeutic effects of both drugs may be inhibited. Concurrent use may also decrease theophylline excretion. Monitor closely as dosage adjustments may be necessary.

3. When xanthine products are given with cimetidine, erythromycin, or troleandomycin, they may decrease theophylline metabolism resulting in elevated serum levels of theophylline and possible toxicity. Monitor closely as dosage adjustments may be necessary.

4. When xanthine products are given to clients who smoke tobacco or marijuana, the metabolism of theophylline may increase, which may result in low serum theophylline levels. Dosage adjustments of 50% to 100% greater dosage has been required in smokers.

5. Alteration in effectiveness of estrogen-containing oral contraceptives may occur with concurrent use of theophylline.

Dosage and administration. The dosage for clients receiving theophylline preparations must be tailored to the medical circumstances in each case and in selected individuals must be monitored by measurement of serum theophylline concentration. *The efficacy of a theophylline preparation depends on the attainment of a serum concentration of 10 to 20 µg/ml.* The rapid intravenous administration of theophylline and its derivatives has caused severe and even fatal acute circulatory failure; therefore the drug should be administered slowly. (See Table 37-3 for the individual preparations and dosages of the various xanthine derivatives.) Since theophylline has a low therapeutic index, using caution when determining the dosage is essential. Also, specific dyphylline serum levels may be used to maintain therapy because serum theophylline levels will *not* measure dyphylline.

Hemoperfusion with resin or activated charcoal is now

TABLE 37-3   Dosage and Administration of Xanthine Derivatives

Drug	Dosage
aminophylline oral solution and tablets	See theophylline elixir
aminophylline enteric-coated tablets	Maintenance therapy: orally, the equivalent of anhydrous theophylline, 6 to 8 mg/kg up to a maximum of 400 mg daily, in divided dosages. If necessary, dosage may be increased 25% every 2 to 3 days until desired effect is achieved or maximum dose of 13 mg/kg or 900 mg/day is reached. If maximum dosage is utilized or exceeded, monitor with theophylline serum levels Children 12 years old and younger—not recommended
aminophylline extended-release tablets	See theophylline extended-release capsules
aminophylline injection	See theophylline and dextrose injection
dyphylline elixir, oral solution, and tablets	15 mg/kg orally every 6 hr, up to four times daily Children—must be individualized by physician
dyphylline extended-release tablets	400 mg orally every 8 hr Children—not established
dyphylline injection	500 mg IM initially, followed by 250 to 500 mg every 2 to 6 hr as indicated; maximum is 15 mg/kg every 6 hr Children—must be individualized by physician
oxtriphylline elixir, syrup, tablet	See theophylline elixir
oxtriphylline extended-release tablets	See theophylline extended-release capsules

theophylline elixir	*Adults*
	Acute attack, loading dose for individuals not receiving theophylline: 5 to 6 mg of anhydrous theophylline/kg. If client is receiving a theophylline product, obtain a theophylline serum level and dose appropriately. (Each 0.5 mg of theophylline/kg of lean body weight will produce a 1 μg/ml increase (range 0.5 to 1.6 μg) in serum theophylline. If unable to wait for the results of a serum theophylline level due to the client's urgent need for therapy, 2.5 mg/kg of anhydrous theophylline may be administered if no symptoms of theophylline toxicity are present. Additional dosages are given according to serum theophylline level reports
	Maintenance in an acute attack:
	    Smokers, young adults—4 mg/kg of anhydrous theophylline every 6 hours.
	    Elderly individuals and clients with cor pulmonale—2 mg/kg of anhydrous theophylline every 8 hours; not to exceed 400 mg anhydrous theophylline/24 hr.
	    Clients in congestive heart failure or liver impairment—2 mg/kg anhydrous theophylline every 12 hours; not to exceed 400 mg anhydrous theophylline/24 hr.
	    Healthy, nonsmoking adults—3 mg/kg anhydrous theophylline every 8 hours.
	Long-term therapy: 6 to 8 mg/kg of anhydrous theophylline up to a 400 mg/day maximum, given in three or four divided doses. Increase the dose 25% every two or three days up to a maximum dose of 13 mg/kg or 900 mg daily. If the maximum dosage is to be continued or exceeded, monitor closely with serum theophylline levels.
	Children
	Acute attack, loading dose for children (up to 16 years old) not receiving theophylline: give 5 to 6 mg/kg of anhydrous theophylline orally. If child is receiving theophylline, obtain a serum theophylline level, then dose on the same principle as described under adults. (0.5 mg = 1 μg/ml of serum theophylline). If unable to wait for the results of a serum theophylline level due to the child's urgent need for the drug, then give a single dose of 2.5 mg/kg of anhydrous theophylline.
	Maintenance in acute attack:
	    Infants up to 6 months old—give the following dose of anhydrous theophylline: (0.07) (age in weeks) + 1.7 = mg/kg every 8 hours.
	    Children 6 months to 12 months old—give the following dose of anhydrous theophylline: (0.05) (age in weeks) + 1.25 = mg/kg every 6 hours.
	    Children 1 to 9 years old—give the following dose of anhydrous theophylline; 5 mg/kg every 6 hours.
	    Children 12 to 16 years old—give the following dose of anhydrous theophylline: 3 mg/kg every 6 hours.

Continued.

TABLE 37-3   Dosage and Administration of Xanthine Derivatives—cont'd

Drug	Dosage
	Long-term therapy: The equivalent of anhydrous theophylline—16 mg/kg initially, up to a maximum of 400 mg daily in three or four divided doses (at 6 to 8 hour intervals); if necessary, dosage may be increased by 25% every two to three days up to the following maximum doses without measuring serum levels: Infants up to 12 months old—(0.3) (age in weeks) + 8 = dose in mg/kg/day. Children 1 to 9 years old—24 mg/kg/day. Children 9 to 12 years old—20 mg/kg/day. Adolescents 12 to 16 years old—18 mg/kg/day. Adolescents over 16 years old—13 mg/kg or 900 mg per day, whichever is smaller
theophylline oral solution, oral suspension, syrup; and tablets	See theophylline elixir
theophylline and dextrose injection	Check current package literature or U.S.P.–D.I. for detailed dosing information

used in the treatment of theophylline overdosage. It is indicated for individuals who develop a plasma theophylline level greater than 60 μg/ml within 4 hours following drug administration. In addition, it may be used for individuals with such risk factors as age (60 years or older), congestive heart failure, liver disease, theophylline half-life value of 24 hours, and a plasma theophylline concentration range of 30 to 50 μg/ml. Since these high-risk clients tend to clear the drug slowly from the body, they require immediate hemoperfusion before any seizures develop.

The bronchodilator effect of the xanthines depends on the theophylline concentration. The various xanthine preparations contain the following:

Drug	Percent of Anhydrous Theophylline Present
aminophylline anhydrous	86
aminophylline dihydrate	79
oxtriphylline	64
theophylline monohydrate	91
theophylline sodium glycinate	49
dyphylline	0

Pregnancy safety. Aminophylline, oxtriphylline, theophylline, and dyphylline—FDA category C

NURSING CONSIDERATIONS

Assessment. Use with caution in individuals with a history of peptic ulcers, since theophylline products may cause local gastrointestinal irritation. This condition can be aggravated when the serum theophylline level exceeds 20 μg/ml.

Exercise great caution in clients with severe cardiac disease, acute myocardial injury, cardiac dysrhythmias, congestive heart failure, or cor pulmonale, since circulatory impairment may cause very slow serum theophylline clearance. Also, individuals with severe hypoxemia, hypertension, hyperthyroidism, prostatic hypertrophy, diabetes mellitus, and renal and hepatic disease require cautious use of xanthines. In addition, use caution with young children and the elderly.

During pregnancy theophylline crosses the placenta; since teratogenic effects have been demonstrated in mice, the risk benefit to the fetus and mother must be considered. Also, dangerous levels of caffeine concentration in the neonate may occur, since the newborn is unable to metabolize this compound. The xanthines are excreted in breast milk, and toxicity may be exhibited by the neonate: tachycardia, jitteriness, irritability, gagging, and vomiting.

Smoking 1 to 2 packs a day decreases the serum half-life of theophylline and, consequently, smokers require larger doses of xanthines than nonsmokers. This effect may persist for months to years, even after the person has stopped smoking.

Xanthines are contraindicated in individuals with hypersensitivity to any of its components.

Intervention. Be aware of the following intravenous admixture incompatibilities:
- Do not mix theophylline in a syringe with other drugs; add it separately to the intravenous solution.
- When administering "piggyback," turn off the other intravenous solution already in place while giving drug.
- Do not mix with alkali-labile drugs such as epinephrine, norepinephrine, isoproterenol, or penicillin G.

Administer oral dosage on an empty stomach to promote faster absorption; to lessen local gastrointestinal irritation, give the drug with food. For chewable tablet form, client should chew tablets before swallowing; for enteric-coated tablet form, client should swallow tablet whole without crushing, breaking, or chewing; for extended-release form, patient should swallow tablet or capsule whole without breaking, crushing, or chewing. Also, contents of capsule may be mixed with 1 teaspoon of jelly, jam, or applesauce if too large to swallow.

To enhance absorption, schedule administration of rectal preparations when rectum is free of feces. Have client remain in recumbent position for 15 to 20 minutes. Administer before meal to enhance retention. Rectal suppositories are irritating to tissues, and absorption is unreliable. Although rectal retention enema provides rapid and more reliable absorption, it should be used only if client is unable to take oral preparations. Rectal preparations are also contraindicated if irritation or infection of the rectum or lower colon is present. If enemas are used, they should not be administered for more than 24 to 36 hours because of the irritating effect of the alkaline solution on the bowel wall.

Store medication in a tightly closed container at room temperature. Also follow manufacturer's directions regarding storage of suppositories, since some are stored at room temperature and others refrigerated.

Education. Caution client not to take over-the-counter remedies that contain ephedrine or other sympathomimetics for treatment of asthma or cough. Instruct individual to limit intake of xanthine-containing beverages, namely, coffee, tea, cocoa, and cola beverages. Also inform client to limit charcoal-broiled foods because charcoal increases theophylline elimination.

Warn elderly clients of possible dizziness during therapy and to take necessary precautions for safety.

If the client is taking the extended-release form of the drug, advise against changing brands unless prescribed by the physician, since the various brands may not be bioequivalent.

The client should notify the physician of any fever, flu-like symptoms, or diarrhea as the prescribed dosage may need to be changed.

Advise client to keep physician and laboratory appointments to check progress of therapy.

Evaluation. Anticipate adverse effects if serum theophylline level exceeds the normal serum therapeutic range of 10 to 20 μg/ml. Because of the variation in the metabolism of xanthines, constant monitoring of serum theophylline concentration and client response will prevent toxicity.

Be sure that intravenous administration is given slowly with volumeter infusion pump. Monitor vital signs and observe client for signs of toxicity such as hypotension, tachycardia, ventricular dysrhythmias, or convulsions. There may not be early, less severe signs of toxicity. Have available oxygen, respirator, and IV diazepam (for convulsions). Maintain airway, hydration, and normal temperature by tepid water sponges or hypothermic blanket for hyperpyrexia. Unconscious patient may require gastric lavage. Serum levels taken immediately before the next dose (trough concentrations) tend to be more consistent than peak serum levels. Accomplish pulmonary studies to assess the client's progress on the drug. Intake and output should also be monitored.

Observe children closely because they are more susceptible than adults to CNS effects (nervousness, restlessness, insomnia, hyperactive reflexes, twitching, and convulsions).

Monitor client during a change from one route of administration to another until dosage is regulated. Wait 4 to 6 hours after changing from intravenous to oral therapy and 12 hours when changing from rectal administration, since its absorption tends to be less consistent.

If client with status asthmaticus does not respond quickly to bronchodilating agents, additional medication such as corticosteroids will be required. Note positive responses to the medication, such as increased ease of respiration, decreased wheezing, and a decrease in the client's anxiety regarding the dyspnea.

PROPHYLACTIC ASTHMATIC DRUGS
cromolyn sodium (Intal, Fivent✤, and Sodium Cromoglycate)

Mechanism of action. A mast cell stabilizing agent that inhibits the release of histamine, leukotrienes, especially SRS-A, and other agents from the mast cell that causes hypersensitivity reactions. This may be mediated through an interference with calcium transport across the membrane of the mast cell. Cromolyn also provides a local protectant action on the gastrointestinal mucosa, thus aiding in preventing gastrointestinal allergies and perhaps, stopping the absorption of the allergic antigen.

Indications. Mast cell stablizer, asthma preventive, antiallergic

Pharmacokinetics

Absorption. Approximately 8% to 10% via the lungs through inhalation

Half-life. About 80 minutes

Excretion. Kidneys and bile

Side effects/adverse reactions. See Table 37-1

Dosage and administration

cromolyn sodium inhalation aerosol (Fivent✤, Intal)

Adults

To prevent bronchial asthma: two inhalations (1.6 mg) orally, four times daily. Adjust dosage as necessary

To prevent exercise-induced or allergen-induced bronchospasm: two inhalations (1.6 mg) orally approximately 10 to 15 minutes before exposure

Children. Under 5 years old—not established; 5 years and older—see adult dosage

ndx Selected Nursing Diagnoses for Clients Taking Bronchodilators (Xanthine Derivatives)

Nursing diagnosis	Outcome criteria	Nursing interventions
Airway clearance, ineffective, related to reversible airway obstruction	Coughs effectively and expectorates sputum Absence of abnormal breath sounds Normal sputum production Fluid intake of at least 3000 ml/24 hours	Assess respiratory status every 4 hours Assist client to turn, cough, and deep breathe as necessary Provide adequate humidification as ordered Monitor characteristics of sputum every 8 hours and record Encourage fluids to at least 3000 ml daily
Activity intolerance related to reversible airway obstruction	Increasing level of activity Pulse, respiration, and blood pressure remain with-in acceptable limits during activity	Plan with client for increasing levels of activity including activities which have priority for client Identify and limit the factors that decrease the client's tolerance for activity Monitor pulse rate, respiration, and blood pressure while increasing the level of activity
Knowledge deficit related to medication regimen	Client will describe underlying condition and how the drug relates to the condition, how and when to take the medication, common drug interactions, safety precautions, common side/adverse effects and which of those warrant reporting Self-administer medication safely and accurately	Administer oral forms with food to minimize gastrointestinal distress Emphasize the need for drug to be taken as prescribed around the clock Caution the client not to self-administer any over-the-counter drugs without consultation with the physician Advise the client to notify the physician if the usual dose fails to be therapeutic or if condition worsens after treatment Instruct the client to minimize ingestion of foods and beverages containing xanthine (coffee, chocolate, colas) Emphasize the need for ongoing contact with the physician for serum levels and evaluation

cromolyn sodium for inhalation, capsules, and solution (Intal)

Adults. To prevent bronchial asthma, 20 mg four times daily. Adjust dosage as necessary and tolerated, up to a maximum of 160 mg per day. To prevent exercise-induced or allergen-induced bronchospasm, 20 mg inhaled before exposure.

Children. Capsules: under 2 years old—not recommended; 2 years and older—see adult dosage

Pregnancy safety. FDA category B

NURSING CONSIDERATIONS

Assessment. Determine that the client does not have an intolerance to lactose, milk, or milk products, since this would prohibit the use of the inhalation capsule form of cromolyn; which contains a lactose base.

The inhalation aerosol may be contraindicated in clients with history of cardiac dysrhythmias or coronary artery disease because of the propellants in the aerosol.

Clients with pre-existing hepatic or renal impairment may require a reduction in dosage.

Intervention. Cromolyn helps prevent, but does not relieve asthma or bronchospasm attacks. If used during an acute attack, it may actually worsen the client's symptoms.

If the client is also using a bronchodilator inhaler, it should be used 15 minutes before the cromolyn inhalation.

Education. The client should be taught to rinse the mouth and gargle after an inhalation treatment to relieve the dryness of the mouth and throat, and the bad aftertaste.

If the client is using the aerosol, capsule, or solution dosage form for inhalation, the individual should be aware that instructions come with each preparation. The nurse should make sure the client can administer the drug correctly. Demonstration kits are available for the inhalation capsule dosage form. Caution clients using the aerosol form to avoid medication contact with the eyes. Inhalation capsules are to be used with a special inhaler; they are not effective if swallowed. The inhalation solution is to be used with a power-operated nebulizer, since the hand-held nebulizers do not provide sufficient force to administer the medication.

The client should be advised that it may be as long as 4 weeks before the drug is fully beneficial. Compliance with the regimen is necessary to achieve these results. It is also important to maintain any concurrent therapies, such as adrenocorticoids, until discontinued by the physician. If the client's condition does not improve or becomes worse, the physician should be notified.

Evaluation. A satisfactory response to cromolyn therapy is indicated by a reduction in the number of attacks, reduced cough, decreased sputum production, and/or a decreased need for other antiasthma drugs. Some clients show improvement in pulmonary function. These re sponses occur in 4 weeks of treatment. Only those clients showing improvement should continue to receive cromolyn.

CORTICOSTEROID DRUGS

Corticosteroid drugs are used in chronic asthma to decrease airway obstruction. As antiinflammatory agents, they stabilize the membranes of lysosomes, thus preventing the release of hydrolytic enzymes that produce the inflammatory process in the tissues. The exact mechanism in asthma is still poorly understood, but it does involve suppression of antibody formation that is responsible for provoking the asthmatic attack. In addition, corticosteroids potentiate an increase in cyclic AMP, a compound needed to promote bronchodilation. At the same time it is thought that they prevent the formation of cyclic GMP, which induces bronchial constriction.

Corticosteroids are used in conjunction with other drugs, in clients with asthma to treat **status asthmaticus,** which is life-threatening exacerbation of asthma associated with bronchospasm. Individuals with this condition are usually unresponsive to nonsteroid bronchodilators. Corticosteroids are also indicated for clients with severe chronic asthma when relief is difficult to obtain from other bronchodilating agents.

Steroids should not be used when other measures are available. Although maintenance programs of steroid therapy decrease the frequency of severe asthmatic attacks, they do not prevent all asthmatic episodes. Furthermore, it is not known whether all episodes of asthma could be prevented by continuous administration of large doses of these drugs. Actually, prolonged administration of large doses is associated with severe adverse effects that are permanent—osteoporosis, subcapsular cataracts, and stunting of growth in children. Other adverse effects caused by this group of drugs are usually reversible.

Daily administration of systemic corticosteroid therapy provides great therapeutic benefits, but the high incidence of adverse effects has led to the use of the alternate-day schedule of treatment. This regimen provides the best benefit/risk ratio for prolonged therapy because it mini-mizes the likelihood of unwanted side effects. The corticosteroids generally used have an intermediate-acting duration of action. These corticosteroids include prednisone, prednisolone, and methylprednisone (see Chapter 49 for details of these drugs).

Recently, the use of steroid aerosols has become increasingly popular. Topical corticosteroid therapy offers the possibility of limiting action at the site of application and thereby avoiding systemic effects. By chemically modifying the structural arrangement of the steroid molecule, several compounds were developed to diminish systemic absorption from the respiratory tract. One such topical agent is beclomethasone dipropionate (Vanceril), which offers the advantage of producing few systemic adverse effects, including that of limited or no adrenal suppression.

beclomethasone dipropionate (Vanceril Inhaler, Beclovent)

Mechanism of action. Beclomethasone, a synthetic corticosteroid chemically related to prednisolone, has high antiinflammatory activity.

Indications. Beclomethasone is indicated only for clients who require chronic treatment with corticosteroids for control of bronchial asthma in conjunction with other therapy. It may be used after bronchodilator or cromolyn failure when long-term steroid control is considered or when oral steroids are producing undesirable side effects.

Beclomethasone is used in clients not receiving systemic steroids (withheld because of concern of potential adverse reactions). It is also administered when nonsteroid measures inadequately control the disease; improvement in pulmonary function appears in 1 to 4 weeks.

When stable asthmatic clients who are dependent on systemic steroids take beclomethasone, management is difficult because of the slow recovery from impaired adrenal function. Suppression of adrenal function may last up to 1 year. Beclomethasone may be effective in managing these clients and may permit significant reduction in the oral corticosteroid dosage. The slow rate of withdrawal is emphasized. During withdrawal from systemic steriods some individuals exhibit symptoms of systemically active steroid withdrawal (e.g., joint and muscle pain, lassitude, and depression).

Pharmacokinetics. Because it is an inhalational agent, only a limited amount of systemic absorption occurs from respiratory and gastrointestinal tissues, with excretion in the feces and urine (less than 10%).

Side effects/adverse reactions. See Table 37-1.
Significant drug interactions. None
Dosage and administration
Beclomethasone dipropionate inhalation aerosol
Adults. Two inhalations orally, three or four times daily. For severe asthma, 12 to 16 sprays initially a day, then

decrease dosage according to client response. Maximum is 840 μg (or 20 metered sprays daily.)

Children. Under 6 years old—not established; 6 to 12 years old—one or two metered sprays (42 to 84 μg) three or four times daily (maximum is 10 sprays daily)

Pregnancy safety. Not established

NURSING CONSIDERATIONS

Assessment. Beclomethasone is contraindicated in clients with status asthmaticus or nonasthmatic bronchial conditions. Its use is not appropriate for asthma controlled by other medications, such as bronchodilators or other noncorticosteroids. Do not use for acute attack.

Intervention. If the client also uses a bronchodilator, it should be used 15 minutes before the beclomethasone inhalation.

Education. The client should hold the inhaled drug for a few seconds and allow a minute to elapse between each inhalation to increase its effectiveness. The nurse should ensure that the client is able to self-administer the inhaler.

The client should be told that fungal infections of the mouth may occur with inhalation of this drug. The mouth should be thoroughly examined daily for the presence of infection. In addition, tell the client that rinsing the mouth after each treatment and washing and drying the inhaler thoroughly after each use will help prevent infection.

Evaluation. If the client's response to the drug begins to diminish, the physician should be notified so that the dosage can be adjusted.

dexamethasone sodium phosphate (Decadron Phosphate)

Dexamethasone is used for allergic or inflammatory nasal conditions and nasal polyps (excluding polyps originating within the sinuses).

Adults should receive two sprays in each nostril two or three times a day; children should receive one or two sprays in each nostril two times a day, depending on age. Maximum daily dosage is 12 sprays per day for adults and 8 sprays per day for children.

The nurse should review with the client the instructions for use of the Decadron Turbinaire for nasal use. Immediately before using the spray, the client should be reminded to blow accumulated mucus and secretions from the nose and, while holding the breath, to press the cartridge to release one measured dose of medication. The client should not inhale but should hold the breath (to avoid systemic absorption by the lungs) for several seconds after applying the medication for its full nasal topical effectiveness. The client should be told not to blow the nose immediately after applying the medication.

Each cartridge delivers 170 metered nasal sprays; 12 sprays deliver about 1 mg of dexamethasone.

The most common side effects are nasal irritation and dryness. Headache, light-headedness, urticaria, nausea, epistaxis, rebound congestion, bronchial asthma, perforation of the nasal septum, and loss of the sense of smell have occurred. Signs of adrenal hypercorticism may occur, especially with overdose. (See drug monograph in Chapter 49.)

KEY TERMS

mucokinetic, page 626
mucus, page 626
sputum, page 626
status asthmaticus, page 643

BIBLIOGRAPHY

Aberman, A: (1986) Managing asthmatics, Emerg Med 18(8):26 (1986).

American Hospital Formulary Service—*AHFS Drug Information '87.* Bethesda: American Society of Hospital Pharmacists, Inc., 1987.

Bertino, JS and Walker, JW: Reassessment of theophylline toxicity, Arch Intern Med. 147(4):757–760, 1987.

Borders, CR: COPD: controlling bronchitis flareups, Patient Care 21(9):99, 1987.

Bowton, DL: Bronchodilator therapy, Curr Rev Respir Crit Care 9(8):62, 1987.

Boyd, G: Drugs and the respiratory system, Nursing '84 2(27):805, 1984.

Braunwald, E, and others (Editors): Harrison's Principles of Internal Medicine, ed 11, New York: McGraw-Hill Co, 1987.

Desmond, M: Plotting a course for asthma therapy, Patient Care 21(9):62, 1987.

Falliers, CJ: Inhalational steroids for asthma, Practical Cardiology 11(7):77-86, 1985.

Feldman, EG and Davidson, DE: Handbook of Nonprescription Drugs, ed 8, Washington: American Pharmaceutical Association and The National Professional Society of Pharmacists, 1986

Fernandez, E: Update on the pharmacologic approach to asthma: xanthine and adrenergic bronchodilators, part 1, Respir Ther 14(4):42, 1984.

Gilman, AG, and others: Goodman & Gillman's The Pharmacological Basis of Therapeutics, ed 7, New York: Macmillan Pub Co. 1985.

Haesoon, L, and others: Evaluation of inhalation aids of metered dose inhalers in asthmatic children, Chest 91(3):366, 1987.

Hendeles, L, and Weinberger, M: The Clinical Pharmacy of theophylline, Fla J Hosp Pharm 2(3):10-26, 1982.

Herfindal, ET, and Hirschman, JL: Clinical Pharmacy and Therapeutics, ed 3, Baltimore: Williams & Wilkins, 1984.

Kastrup, EK, and Olin, BR: Facts and Comparisons, Drug Information. St. Louis. JB Lippincott Co, 1987.

Keys, PA, and Keys, PW: Monitoring theophylline therapy, US Pharmacist 7(6):H-1-13, 1982.

Kirillof, LH, and others: Drugs for asthma: a complete guide . . . what you need to know to teach patients. Am J Nurs 83(1):55, 1983.

Konig, P: Cromolyn sodium: clinical applications and known mechanisms of action, Hosp Formul 19(8):711, 1984.

Newhouse, M: Aerosol therapy in adult lung disease, Respir Technol 20(4):11, 1984.

Newman, SP: Aerosol deposition considerations in inhalation therapy, Chest 88(2):152S, 1985.

Newman, SP, and others: The proper use of metered dose inhalers, Chest 86(3):342, 1984.

Owens, GR: Exercise-induced asthma: optimal testing methods and preventive measures, Consultant 27(3):23, 1987.

PDR: Physicians' desk reference, ed 41, Oradell, NJ: Medical Economics Co., Inc., 1987.

Petty, T: Drug strategies for airflow obstruction, Am J Nurs 87(2):180, 1987.

Rimar, JM: Albuterol: a selective beta$_2$ bronchodilator, MCN 11(3):169, 1986.

Self, TH, and Fuentes, RJ: Metered dose inhalers and extender devices, US Pharmacist 10(5)36-48, 1985.

Slaughter, RL, and others: Theophylline clearance in obese patients in relation to smoking and congestive heart failure. Drug Intell Clin Pharm 17(4):274, 1983.

Summer, WR: Status asthmaticus. Chest 87(1):87S, 1985.

Taylor, RA, and others: Reversible airways obstruction: inhaled B$_2$-bronchodilators as first-line therapy, Consultant 27(4):134, 1987.

Todd, B: Precautions in using bronchodilators, Geriatr Nurs 5(7):328, 1984.

United States Pharmacopeial Convention: *Drug Information for the Health Care Provider,* ed. 7, Rockville: US Pharmacopeial Convention, Inc., 1987.

Wabschall, JM: Nursing management of children during a mild to moderate asthma attack. JEN 12(3):134, 1986.

CHAPTER
38

Antihistamines, Antitussives, and Decongestants

OBJECTIVES

After studying this chapter, the student will be able to:

1. Describe how the body uses oxygen and the result of oxygen deprivation.

2. Identify nursing interventions applicable to each of the various methods of oxygen administration.

3. List the effects of carbon dioxide.

4. Discuss nursing considerations for the administration of respiratory stimulants and depressants.

5. Discuss antitussive agents and the proper method of administration.

6. Explain the three actions of histamine in the body.

7. Discuss common antihistamines and related nursing considerations.

DRUGS THAT AFFECT THE RESPIRATORY CENTER

THERAPEUTIC GASES

oxygen

Oxygen—a gas that is essential for life—is colorless, odorless, and tasteless. It is not flammable, but it supports combustion much more vigorously than does air.

Inspired air normally contains 20.9% oxygen, which, at an atmospheric pressure of 760 mm Hg, exerts a partial pressure (PO_2) or tension of 159 mm Hg. However, as oxygen passes through the bronchial airway, the inspired air becomes saturated with water vapor, which then reduces the PO_2 in the alveoli to approximately 100 mm Hg. Finally, the oxygen appears as arterial PO_2, a dissolved form of oxygen in the arterial blood. The PO_2 of arterial blood is normally above 80 mm Hg.

Oxygen must be continuously supplied to tissue cells, since no fiber or cell can remain without oxygen, or hypoxic, for very long and survive. The adult human brain consumes from 40 to 50 ml oxygen/minute. The cortex consumes more than the centers in the medulla or spinal cord. Cerebral oxygen consumption proceeds without pausing, and the replenishment of oxygen by the blood must be maintained continuously. Whenever any circulatory stress exists, cerebral blood flow tends to be preserved at the expense of other less vital organs. Of all the tissues affected by hypoxia, the brain is most susceptible to disruption of normal function and irreversible damage. An acute reduction of the PO_2 to 50 mm Hg decreases mental functioning, emotional stability, and finer muscular coordination. Further reduction of the PO_2 to 40 mm Hg produces impaired judgment, decreased pain perception, and impairment of muscular coordination. When the PO_2 is reduced to 32 mm Hg or less, unconsciousness and a progressive descending depression of the central nervous system ensue.

The kidneys are vital organs in which there must be considerable constancy of blood flow and oxygen supply. Oxygen consumption is greater in the renal cortex; renal medullary tissue has an oxygen consumption that is 15% less than that of the renal cortex. This difference is related to the variation in pressure gradient and to the fact that cortical flow is rapid while the medullary flow is slower. The renal cortex is highly dependent on oxygen, whereas the renal medulla can function relatively independently of the oxygen supply.

The rate of oxygen consumption by the kidneys is approximately 0.06 ml/g/minute, more than most other tissues. For each 100 ml of blood entering the kidney, 1.4 ml of oxygen is consumed. The oxygen consumed by the kidneys is primarily used for sodium reabsorption. When the renal arterial content falls to less than 55% of normal, renal vasoconstriction occurs. This response is believed to be mediated by chemoreceptors, which stimulate the vasomotor center to produce renal vasoconstriction. Renal vasoconstriction also occurs as a result of the action of ether, barbiturates, and other anesthetics. Renal blood flow is also decreased during periods of exercise. It is important to note that autoregulation of renal perfusion does occur.

In skeletal muscles oxygen consumption is related to blood flow. Oxygen consumption and blood flow are decreased when muscle is at rest and significantly increased during exercise.

Reduction of oxygen supply to the intestinal tract is regarded by some investigators as a key factor for inadequate splanchnic vascular compensation (splanchnic vasoconstriction) during hypotension. Inadequate oxygen supply impairs myocardial metabolism and function.

Arterial blood pressure determinations, when used alone, are unreliable indicators of the adequacy of tissue perfusion. Therefore arterial blood gas determinations should be obtained, since these results provide a more accurate and reliable indication of shifts in the partial pressures of oxygen and carbon dioxide. Severe hypoxia may produce changes in the ST segment and T wave of the ECG, dysrhythmias, ectopic beats, and myocardial infarction.

Indications. Oxygen is used in medicine chiefly to treat **hypoxia** (oxygen lack) and **hypoxemia** (diminished oxygen tension in the blood). Basically, the four types of hypoxia are the following:

1. **Hypoxic hypoxia**—produced by any condition causing a decrease in PO_2
2. **Ischemic hypoxia**—inadequate blood flow to an organ or tissue in the presence of a normal PO_2 and hemoglobin content
3. **Anemic hypoxia**—inadequate hemoglobin to carry O_2 in the presence of a normal PO_2
4. **Histotoxic hypoxia**—adequate PO_2 and hemoglobin, but inability of tissues to utilize oxygen delivered because of a toxic agent

Clinically, hypoxic hypoxia is the most common form of hypoxia. A variety of pathologic conditions result in hypoxic hypoxia, which makes the use of oxygen treatment necessary. Some of these conditions are hypoventilation, increased airway resistance, pneumothorax, respiratory center depression, abnormal ventilation/perfusion ratio, congenital cyanotic heart disease, decreased pulmonary compliance, and breathing oxygen-poor air. The use of oxygen is also indicated in (1) cardiac failure or decompensation and coronary occlusion and (2) anesthesia administration (to increase the safety of general anesthesia).

Administration. Oxygen is administered by inhalation. Various methods are used, each having advantages and disadvantages (Figure 38-1).

A *nasal catheter* is made of soft plastic. When used, it should be lubricated with water-soluble K-Y Jelly and passed through the nose until the tip is just above the epiglottis. This distance is usually the same as the distance from an individual's external nares to the tragus of the ear, minus 1 cm. The catheter should not be inserted so far that the client swallows oxygen, since this will cause stomach distention and abdominal discomfort. The catheter is fastened with tape to the forehead and/or nose. Flow rate varies according to individual need, but 4 to 8 L oxygen/minute of a 25% to 40% concentration of oxygen is commonly used. Since this form of therapy is very drying to the mucous membrane, the oxygen should be humidified. In addition, nasal and oral hygiene is important to maintain cleanliness and intact mucous membrane and to prevent infection and discomfort. Most clients receiving oxygen therapy are mouth breathers, and frequent mouth care is required to prevent sores. Nasal catheters become obstructed with encrusted secretions and must be removed and cleaned or replaced several times a day.

A *nasal cannula* is much more comfortable for the client than is a catheter. Cannulas have either single or double short prongs that are inserted into the lower part of the nostrils. They are less likely to become obstructed with secretions. Nasal and oral mucosa still require frequent attention. A flow of 1 to 6 L/minute of a 23% to 40% concentration of oxygen is adequate for many patients.

An *oxygen mask* is the most effective means of delivering needed oxygen. Oxygen concentrations up to 90%

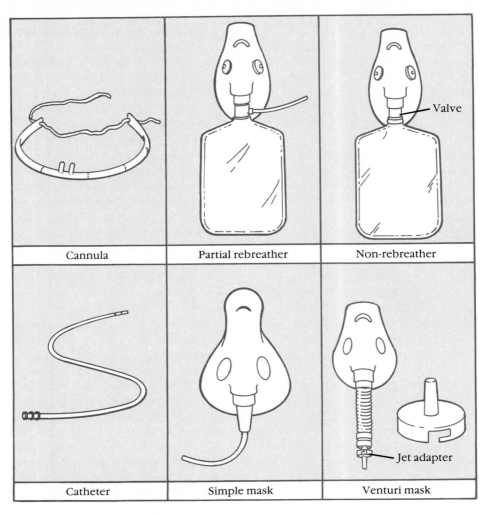

| Cannula | Partial rebreather | Non-rebreather |
| Catheter | Simple mask | Venturi mask |

FIGURE 38-1   Basic oxygen delivery systems.

can be administered by mask. To be effective, the mask must fit well over the nose and mouth; high flow rates can compensate to some extent for a poor fit. Masks are better tolerated when used intermittently or when disposable plastic masks are used. Only absolutely clean and uncontaminated rubber masks should be used, since they can be a source of nosocomial infection. There are two main types of oxygen masks: (1) those that deliver low concentrations of oxygen and (2) those that deliver high concentrations of oxygen.

A *simple face mask,* which is lightweight and disposable, is useful for short-term therapy of oxygen administration, such as in the early postoperative period or when intermittent oxygen therapy is required. The flow rate is only 6 to 10 L/minute at a low oxygen concentration of 35% to 60%. Since the mask is loose-fitting and can leak, simple face masks are suitable for individuals with carbon dioxide retention.

A *partial rebreathing mask* is a disposable, light-weight plastic face mask consisting of a reservoir bag and a partial rebreathing valve. It is commonly used by individuals who require oxygen. On expiration, only a portion of the exhaled air enters the reservoir. Accordingly, to prevent the rebreathing of carbon dioxide, the reservoir bag should deflate only slightly on inhalation. By this method a concentration of 60% to 90% of oxygen can be delivered at a flow rate of 10 L/minute.

A *nonrebreathing mask* is designed to fit tightly over the face and is usually made of rubber with a reservoir bag and a nonbreathing valve. On inhalation, oxygen flows into the bag and mask, and the one-way valve prevents exhaled air from flowing back into the bag. The expired air instead escapes through the one-way flap valve in the mask. The concentration of oxygen is 95%, which is high, and the flow is adjusted to keep the reservoir bag fully inflated. This type of mask is used for short-term therapy such as counteracting smoke inhalation. The rubber can become hot and sticky so that prolonged use can cause discomfort.

An *oxygen tent* is of limited value, particularly when it is necessary to open the canopy for monitoring vital signs and administering care to the client. The rate of flow is 20 L/minute at an oxygen concentration of 60%. Obviously, the oxygen concentration falls, making the flow difficult to control each time the tent is opened. Consequently, oxygen tents are now used less frequently.

The *Ventimask (Mix-O-Mask)* is a recent development originating from the Venturi mask. It is used for clients with chronic alveolar hypoventilation and carbon dioxide retention. Exact low-flow concentrations of oxygen are delivered to the individual. The Ventimask provides an air-oxygen mixture with the desired oxygen concentration. The size of the orifice to the mask determines the concentration of oxygen—24%, 28%, 35%, and 40% with flow rates of 4, 6, 8, and 10 L/minute, respectively. A thin elastic band holds the Ventimask in position and tends to cut into the skin behind the ears. A gauze padding under each side of the elastic band will alleviate this discomfort. The device must be removed when the client eats and may give the client a feeling of being smothered.

Most of the oxygen administered in hospitals for therapy is provided from a central source where it is stored as a gas or liquid oxygen. The gas is piped into a patient room at a standard pressure of 50 pounds per square inch (psi) at the gauge. Compressed oxygen is marketed in steel cylinders that are fitted with reducing valves for the delivery of the gas. The cylinders are usually color coded; green is used in the United States. Since the gas is under considerable pressure, the tanks must be handled carefully to prevent falling or jarring.

The effectiveness of oxygen administration depends on the carbon dioxide content of the blood. Individuals with chronic obstructive pulmonary disease (COPD) have difficulty with carbon dioxide and oxygen exchange and are subject to **hypercapnia** (high carbon dioxide content in the blood). Because of chronic hypercapnia, the medullary center of these individuals is relatively insensitive to stimulation of carbon dioxide; rather, a low PaO_2 serves as a stimulant to respiration. Caution must be used when attempting to prevent a greater accumulation of carbon dioxide. Toxic carbon dioxide levels may result in further depression of respiration and respiratory acidosis. The nurse should be alert to neurologic symptoms that indicate an accumulation of carbon dioxide. Symptoms may include drowsiness, mental confusion, paresthesias, and visual disturbances. The occurrence of carbon dioxide narcosis may be prevented by gradually increasing the concentration of oxygen administered.

Oxygen administration in the premature infant. Nurses caring for premature infants in incubators must be constantly aware of the danger of retrolental fibroplasia. This is a vascular proliferative disease of the retina that occurs in some premature infants who have had high concentrations of oxygen at birth.* The oxygen concentrations should be kept between 30% and 40%. Higher concentrations can be administered to cyanotic infants without increasing the danger of retrolental fibroplasia because it is PaO_2, not inspired PO_2, that is implicated in this disease. Therefore careful monitoring of arterial blood gases is essential. Some incubators are equipped with a safety valve that automatically releases any excess oxygen outside the chamber.

When orders for an infant include oxygen prn, the nurse must make certain that it is administered only as needed and at low concentrations rather than continuously. Frequently, the removal of a very small plug of mucus can clear the airway, thus enabling the infant to breathe oxygen without assistance.

Hyperbaric oxygen. In recent years hyperbaric oxygen has been used in the treatment of various conditions. In the treatment of infections caused by *Clostridium welchii,* the anaerobic bacillus producing gas gangrene, the intermittent use of hyperbaric oxygen has been valuable. It is believed that an increased oxygen pressure in the tissue may exert an inhibitory effect on enzyme systems of these bacteria. This same inhibitory effect may be implicated in the use of hyperbaric oxygen on other anaerobic microorganisms.

Hyperbaric oxygen has been used in the treatment of tetanus, but the results are less satisfactory than those obtained in the treatment of gas gangrene. Hyperbaric oxygen has also been used in certain circulatory disturbances. In shock, in which there is a generalized circulatory deficit, hyperbaric oxygen may be of some value. It has also been used in certain local circulatory disturbances such as various peripheral vascular diseases.

Helium-oxygen mixtures. Helium-oxygen mixtures have been used to treat obstructive types of dyspnea. Helium is an inert gas and so light that a mixture of 80% helium and 20% oxygen is only one third as heavy as air. Helium is only slightly soluble in body fluids and has a high rate of diffusion. Because of its low specific gravity, mixtures of this gas with oxygen can be breathed with less effort than either oxygen or air alone when air passages are obstructed. These mixtures are recommended for individuals with status asthmaticus, bronchiectasis, and emphysema, as well as during anesthesia for a client with respiratory tract obstruction.

Oxygen toxicity. Exposure to 100% oxygen for a period of 6 hours causes an inflammatory response with sub-

---

*Excessive oxygen constricts the developing retinal vessels of the eye. Consequently, normal vascularization is suppressed; since the endothelial cells become disorganized, they cause destruction of the immature retina. The result is blindness.

sequent destruction of the alveolocapillary membrane of the respiratory tract. Toxicity is often difficult to recognize, but the most common symptoms are substernal distress (ache or burning sensation behind the sternum), increase in respiratory distress, nausea, vomiting, restlessness, tremors, twitching, paresthesias, convulsions, and a dry, hacking cough.

NURSING CONSIDERATIONS

Assessment. Dyspnea or increased respiratory rate, may indicate the need for oxygen therapy. The best means of gauging the need for oxygen or the effectiveness of oxygen therapy is via arterial blood gas evaluations or pulse oximetry before and during therapy. The nurse should know normal blood gas values (see box) and recognize deviations. The goal of oxygen therapy is to achieve a PO_2 range between 60 to 80 mm Hg or oxygen saturation greater than 90%. In chronic carbon dioxide retention, the PO_2 may range between 55 to 60 mm Hg. Arterial blood gas analysis is required 30 minutes after the oxygen dosage is changed unless the oxygen saturation is being monitored.

Oxygen should be given with extreme caution to some clients. The client with COPD maintains respiratory drive by low oxygen tension. A high oxygen concentration in the blood causes the client to have reduced ventilation and result in acute acidosis and carbon dioxide narcosis. Arterial blood gas evaluations should be checked frequently with clients with COPD.

Intervention. To prevent dryness of nose and throat and respiratory complications, add sterile, distilled water to the humidifying device, and administer oxygen concentration and liter flow as prescribed. Because oxygen is a dry gas, adequate humidification is essential to the patient and must be monitored frequently.

Since oxygen supports combustion and combustible materials (linens, wooden furniture, plastic articles) burns with greater ease and intensity, smoking and using matches, woolen blankets, clothing, or electric equipment (radios, electric razors, hair dryers) that may cause sparks are strictly forbidden in rooms where oxygen is being administered. Also, post NO SMOKING signs on the individual's door and above the bed.

Because oxygen therapy is frequently administered to debilitated clients, take special care to prevent contamination of the equipment used in the administration of oxygen to prevent nosocomial infection. Nasal cannulas, Ventimasks, other masks, tubing, nebulizers, and other equipment exposed to moisture need to be changed daily. Nasal catheters should be changed every 8 to 12 hours.

Remove an oxygen mask periodically, if the client's condition permits, to dry, powder, and massage the skin around the mask.

Education. The equipment for oxygen administration should be shown to the client and family. Explain the procedure and the benefits of oxygen therapy.

Point out the importance of not smoking in the client's room to the client and visitors. (Since oxygen supports combustion, the possibility of fire always exists.)

Evaluation. Monitor the client's vital signs—pulse rate, blood pressure, and respiratory rate and pattern.

NORMAL VALUES FOR ARTERIAL BLOOD GASES

pH	7.36-7.44
$PaCO_2$	36-44 mm Hg
PaO_2	80-100 mm Hg
O_2 saturation	95% or above
HCO_3	22-26 mEq/L

PULSE OXIMETRY

A recent advance in monitoring for tissue hypoxia is the development of *pulse oximetry.* It has been called one of the most significant technologic advances ever made in monitoring the respiratory function of clients. Simply explained, pulse oximetry works by passing light of differing wavelengths through living tissue and analyzing the differences in absorption. Oxygenated hemoglobin absorbs light differently, and these variations in absorption serve as the basis of calculations that determine the presence and amount of oxygenated hemoglobin compared to nonoxygenated hemoglobin. This provides a continuous reading of arterial blood oxygen saturation. A saturation of 90 percent or greater is desired for clients. (This correlates with a PaO_2 of 60).

Current pulse oximeters work with a small probe (light source and detector), which may be placed on a client's ear, finger, toe, bridge of the nose, nasal septum, or temple. Pulse oximetry monitors are relatively inexpensive, noninvasive, safe, extremely accurate, require no calibration and provide almost instantaneous results. While initially used with clients during anesthesia, recovery, and critical care, the use of pulse oximetry is rapidly expanding as an immediate and safe method of determining tissue oxygenation in any client experiencing respiratory difficulties.

Also, observe level of consciousness, skin temperature, and color. Report any abnormal findings to the physician.

Examine the client and the equipment frequently to see if skin and mucous membrane in contact with the equipment are intact and without irritation; the equipment is patent, without leaks, and properly positioned; the flow rate is at the prescribed level; the humidifier contains solution; and, if an oxygen cylinder is being used, that it contains enough oxygen.

carbon dioxide

Carbon dioxide is a colorless, odorless gas that is heavier than air. Carbon dioxide used as a pharmacologic agent affects respiration, circulation, and the central nervous system. Inhalation of carbon dioxide for a short period of time increases both rate and depth of respiration unless the respiratory center is depressed by narcotics or disease.

Carbon dioxide stimulates cells of the sympathetic nervous system, the respiratory center, and the peripheral chemoreceptors. Carbon dioxide also depresses the cerebral cortex, myocardium, and smooth muscle of the peripheral blood vessels. Carbon dioxide may also interfere with nerve conduction and transmission. When carbon dioxide increases the rate and force of respiration, venous return to the heart is usually enhanced as a result of decreased peripheral resistance; there is improved rate and force of myocardial contraction and less likelihood of myocardial irritability and dysrythmias.

Too much carbon dioxide has a depressant effect and results in acidosis and unresponsiveness of the respiratory center to the gas. Therefore it is important that carbon dioxide be administered with caution.

Indications. The following are indications for use of carbon dioxide.

Carbon monoxide poisoning. A 5% to 7% concentration of carbon dioxide in oxygen is sometimes used in the treatment of carbon monoxide poisoning. Physiologically, carbon dioxide increases the rate of separation of carbon monoxide from carboxyhemoglobin.

General anesthesia. Most general anesthetics cause a reduction in response to carbon dioxide, which is reflected in central nervous system depression. The degree of depression is directly related to the depth of anesthesia. The more deeply the individual is anesthetized, the greater the depression of the central nervous system. Carbon dioxide initially speeds up anesthesia by increasing pulmonary ventilation. By lessening the sense of asphyxiation, it reduces struggling. In the postanesthesia period, it hastens the elimination of many anesthetics. Inhalation of 5% to 7% carbon dioxide increases cerebral blood flow by approximately 75%, primarily by dilation of cerebral vessels.

Respiratory depression. The use of carbon dioxide as a respiratory stimulant in the presence of depressed respiration is limited. When used, close monitoring of PaO_2 is important; if desired results are not obtained, it should be discontinued. Mechanical assistance to respiration and oxygen administration is the usual treatment in cases of respiratory depression.

Postoperative use. Occasionally, carbon dioxide is used postoperatively to increase ventilation and prevent atelectasis. Most investigators think the use of deep breathing exercises, coughing, frequent turning, tracheal suction, and intermittent positive pressure breathing produces better results. Carbon dioxide administration has also been used in the treatment of postoperative singultus (hiccups). Relief of singultus is apparently accomplished by stimulating the respiratory center, causing large excursions of the diaphragm that submerge spasmodic contractions of that muscle, thereby promoting regular contractions.

Administration. Carbon dioxide is kept in metal cylinders and vaporizes as it is delivered from the cylinder. When carbon dioxide is used for medical purposes, it is administered in combination with oxygen. A 5% to 10% concentration of carbon dioxide delivered through a tight-fitting face mask is inhaled by the client until the depth of respiration is definitely increased, which usually occurs within 3 minutes. For the postoperative individual, the procedure would be repeated every hour or two for the first 48 hours, and then several times a day for several days.

Another way of administering carbon dioxide is to allow the client to hyperventilate with a paper bag held over the face. Reinhaling expired air causes the carbon dioxide content to be continually increased.

Signs of carbon dioxide overdosage are dyspnea, breath-holding, markedly increased chest and abdominal movements, nausea, and increased systolic blood pressure. Administration of the gas should be discontinued when these symptoms appear. The administration of 5% carbon dioxide may produce severe mental depression, if given over an hour and a 10% concentration can lead to loss of consciousness within 10 minutes. The administration should be stopped as soon as the desired effects on the patient's respiration have been obtained.

DIRECT RESPIRATORY STIMULANTS

Direct respiratory stimulants come under a broader classification of central nervous system stimulants and are often referred to as **analeptics.** These drugs act directly on the medullary center to increase respiratory rate and tidal exchange. Although these drugs are available for stimulating depth of respiration and rate of respiration, airway management and support of ventilation are more effective in the treatment of respiratory depression. The mechanical support of ventilation is often superior to the use of drugs, since respiratory stimulants in large doses can cause convulsions.

Respiratory stimulants (analeptics) have in the past been advocated in the treatment of drug-induced respiratory depression, but since these drugs are not specific antagonists to sedatives or narcotics, their use in drug-induced respiratory depression is now considered obsolete. Indeed, repeated doses of an analeptic may potentiate the depressant effects of central nervous system depressants.

Analeptics have also been used to counteract respiratory depression caused by anesthetics or to shorten post-anesthetic recovery time. However, these methods of therapy are not recommended, since decreasing the concentration of the anesthetic agent in the blood is accomplished more effectively with mechanical ventilatory measures.

doxapram hydrochloride (Dopram)

Mechanism of action. Doxapram is a short-acting drug that stimulates all levels of the central nervous system. It stimulates the respiratory center in the medulla and the peripheral carotid chemoreceptors and the ventilatory response increases both tidal volume and oxygen uptake.

Indications. Treatment of respiratory depression induced by anesthesia or muscle relaxant medications; drug overdoses and in individuals with acute respiratory insufficiency, such as COPD. The latter use is temporary and used generally with mechanical ventilation.

Pharmacokinetics

Onset of action: within 20 to 40 seconds

Time to peak effect: 1 to 2 minutes

Duration of action: between 5 and 12 minutes

Excretion: feces

Side effects/adverse reactions. See Table 38-1

Significant drug interactions. When doxapram is given with monoamine oxidase inhibitors, such as procarbazine, furazolidone and pargyline or vasopressor agents, an increase in pressor effects is reported. Avoid concurrent usage or, if necessary, monitor closely as dosage adjustments may be necessary.

Dosage and administration

Adults

For post-anesthesia respiratory depression: 0.5 mg to 1 mg/kg IV (Do not exceed 1.5 mg/kg). If necessary, dosage may be repeated in 5 minute intervals up to a maximum total dosage of 2 mg/kg body weight

By intravenous infusion—give at a rate of 5 mg/minute initially until the desired response is noted, then decrease to 1 to 3 mg/minute. The maximum total dose is 4 mg/kg but do not exceed 300 mg

For drug-induced CNS depression:

TABLE 38-1   Side Effects and Adverse Reactions of Respiratory Drugs

Drug(s)	Side effects*	Adverse reactions†
doxapram HCl (Dopram)	Less frequent: cough, diarrhea, dizziness, confusion, headache, nausea, vomiting, sensation of warmth, sweating, urinary difficulties	Less frequent/rare: heaviness and/or pain in chest; very fast or irregular heart rate; redness or swelling at site of injection; fast, irregular breathing; wheezing; hemolysis of blood cells Overdosage: convulsions, hypertension, increase in deep tendon reflexes, tremors or ataxia, tachycardia
antihistamines: diphenhydramine HCl (Benylin, Benadryl) and others	Most frequent: constipation, decreased sweating, urinary difficulty or pain (in elderly males especially); sedation; visual disturbances; dry mouth, nose, or throat; photosensitivity; nausea; or vomiting Less frequent/rare: orthostatic hypotension, euphoria (especially with high doses in elderly), headaches, anxiety, weak hands or feet, sore mouth and tongue, abdominal pain or upset, increased excitability, muscle cramps	Rare: confusion especially in elderly receiving high doses, glaucoma (eye pain) in susceptible individuals, rash Overdose: ataxia; severe dry mouth, nose, or throat; respiratory difficulty; tachycardia; red, dry, flushing of skin; severe CNS depression; mood swings; toxic psychosis; hallucinations; convulsions; insomnia Withdrawal symptoms: increased nervousness, loss of balance, dysphagia, muscle spasms (especially face, neck, and back), increased excitability, stiff feeling in arms or legs, tremors and shaking of hands and fingers, extrapyramidal-type side effects, postural hypotension, insomnia, tachycardia

*If side effects continue, increase, or disturb the patient, inform the physician.
†If adverse reactions occur, contact physician since medical intervention may be necessary.

Initially—1 to 2 mg/kg IV as single dose. May repeat in 5 minutes. Maintenance—1 to 2 mg/kg IV every 60 to 120 minutes until desired response is achieved, up to a maximum total dose of 3 g per day. Before a second regimen is given, 24 hours from the initial dose should have elapsed

Intermittent IV infusion—give 1 to 3 mg/minute until the desired effect is achieved; if necessary, the infusion may be repeated after 30 to 120 minutes. Maximum infusion time is two hours—also, additional infusions are not suggested.

For acute respiratory insufficiency: 1 to 2 mg/minute up to 3 mg/minute as needed, given by intravenous infusion. Maximum infusion time is 2 hours. Additional infusions are not suggested.

Children. Under 12 years old—not recommended

Pregnancy safety. Not established

NURSING CONSIDERATIONS

Assessment. Do not use in individuals with known hypersensitivity to doxapram or in those with convulsive disorders, head injury, cerebrovascular accident, pulmonary embolism, severe hypertension, or pneumothorax. In children under 12 years and in pregnant women, safe use has not been established.

Administer cautiously in clients with cerebral edema, dysrhythmias, bronchial asthma, hyperthyroidism, peptic ulcer.

Check client for patent airway before drug administration.

Intervention. Mix drug with normal saline solution or dextrose in water; do not mix with alkaline solution such as 2.5% sodium thiopental or bicarbonate, since precipitate will result.

Have available intravenous short-acting barbiturates, oxygen, and resuscitative equipment in case of overdosage.

Too rapid a rate of infusion may result in hemolysis.

Avoid extravasation or use of a single injection site for prolonged periods, since thrombophlebitis may result.

Evaluation. Carefully monitor blood pressure, pulse rate, and deep tendon reflexes to avoid overdose. Observe client continuously during therapy. Maintain vigilance for at least 1 hour until client is alert and pharyngeal and laryngeal reflexes are completely restored.

Although doxapram may be considered safer than other agents in this category, it is not without side effects. Be alert for early signs of toxicity such as tachycardia, muscle tremor, or spasticity. Notify physician immediately if any of these occur. Drug should be discontinued if sudden hypotension or dyspnea develops.

Determination of arterial blood gases is essential before doxapram infusion in clients with COPD. During infusion, monitor at least every half hour.

REFLEX RESPIRATORY STIMULANTS

Ammonia is the only drug given by inhalation for its action as a reflex respiratory stimulant. In cases of fainting, aromatic spirits of ammonia is administered by inhaling the vapor. When given orally, 2 ml of aromatic ammonia spirits is diluted with at least 1 fluid ounce of water. Reflex stimulation of the medullary center occurs through peripheral irritation of sensory nerve receptors in the pharynx, esophagus, and stomach. The rate and depth of respiration are then increased through afferent messages to the respiratory control centers. Reflex stimulation of the vasomotor center results in a rise in blood pressure.

RESPIRATORY DEPRESSANTS

The most important respiratory depressants are the central depressants of the opium group and those of the barbiturate group of drugs. These agents depress the respiratory center, thereby making breathing slower and more shallow and lessening the irritability of the respiratory center. Respiratory depression, however, is seldom desirable or necessary, although it is sometimes unavoidable. It is frequently a side effect of otherwise very useful drugs. Occasionally, an opiate, such as codeine, is administered to inhibit the rate and depth of respiration for a painful or harmful cough. Too-high concentrations of carbon dioxide in inhalation mixtures may paradoxically act to depress respiration.

COUGH SUPPRESSANTS

Coughing is a protective reflex for clearing the respiratory tract of environmental irritants, foreign bodies, or accumulated secretions and thus should not be depressed indiscriminately. The afferent impulses that arise from irritated pharyngeal and laryngeal tissues initiate the cough reflex. Drugs act either by suppressing the cough center in the medulla oblongata or peripherally by lessening irritation of the respiratory tract. A cough is *productive* when irritants or secretions are removed from the respiratory tract; it is *nonproductive* when it is dry and irritating. Frequent and prolonged coughing should be diminished since it can be exhausting, painful, and taxing to the circulatory system and the elastic tissue of the respiratory system, particularly in the elderly and in young children. Some coughs occur primarily at night or when the individual is recumbent because of the accumulation of secretions, and some coughs occur in the morning on arising as a result of the gravitational movement of secretions. Coughing is under some voluntary control; a person can cough at will and at times can suppress coughing. However, coughing is usually initiated by a respiratory tract reflex, which, on irritation, sends an impulse to the cough center in the brain. Intake of fluids and inhalation of fully water-saturated vapors (steam) should be stressed as one of the most important means of producing increased amounts of mucus and thinning such secretions.

Treatment of the cough is secondary to treatment of the underlying disorder. Antitussives should not be given in situations in which retention of respiratory secretions or exudates may be harmful. The therapeutic objective is to decrease the intensity and frequency of the cough yet permit adequate elimination of tracheobronchial secretions and exudates. Medications that may be used to relieve the cough include narcotic and nonnarcotic antitussive agents.

NARCOTIC ANTITUSSIVE DRUGS

Narcotics such as morphine and hydromorphone, are potent suppressants of the cough reflex, but their clinical usefulness is limited by side effects. They inhibit the ciliary activity of the respiratory mucous membrane, depress respiration, and may cause bronchial constriction in allergic or asthmatic patients. In addition, they can cause drug dependence.

Codeine and hydrocodone exhibit less pronounced antitussive effects, but they also have fewer side effects. They are widely used. (See Chapter 11 for narcotic agents.)

NONNARCOTIC ANTITUSSIVE DRUGS

The instillation of a local anesthetic agent before various diagnostic techniques such as bronchoscopy has proved effective in suppressing the cough reflex. This has led to the investigation of other agents that exert a similar action. The clinical effectiveness of these drugs against pathologic cough still remains to be established. Newer nonnarcotic drugs in this group have fewer gastrointestinal side effects than do codeine and related compounds.

The medicating effect of these drugs is local, therefore they should not be followed by liquids of any sort for 30 to 35 minutes or the effect will be washed away.

benzonatate (Tessalon)

Mechanism of action. Benzonatate is chemically related to the local anesthetic tetracaine. It relieves coughing through a peripheral action involving selective anesthesia of stretch receptors in the lungs.

Indications. Symptomatic treatment of cough, without suppressing respiration

Pharmacokinetics

Distribution. Following oral administration; onset of action within 15 to 20 minutes with duration of action 3 to 8 hours

Side effects/adverse reactions

CNS. Drowsiness, headaches, dizziness

CV. Tightness or numbness in chest

GI. Nausea, constipation, abdominal upset

Other. Skin eruptions, chilling sensation, nasal congestion

Significant drug interactions. None

Dosage and administration. Adults and children over 10 years: 100 mg three times a day; maximum dose is 600 mg/per day. Children under 10 years: 8 mg/kg PO in 3-6 divided doses. Warning: do not chew capsules; doing so may produce a temporary mouth anesthesia.

Pregnancy safety. Not established

NURSING CONSIDERATIONS

Assessment. Assess from the client's history that there is no known hypersensitivity to the drug to be administered. Also determine cause of cough, since cough could indicate congestive heart failure or other disease.

Intervention. Nursing actions supportive of antitussives are deep breathing exercises, postural drainage, frequent change of position, limitation or cessation of smoking, maintenance of adequate humidity in the environment, and adequate hydration. The nurse should attempt to pinpoint the cause of the cough and then direct nursing measures toward the cause. Infections should be treated with pulmonary hygiene (cough, deep breathing, etc. as discussed above). If a specific stimulus for the cough can be identified, such as dust, smoking, or pollen, then attempts should be made to minimize exposure to these substances.

Education. The capsule should be swallowed whole. If it is chewed or dissolved in the mouth, temporary local anesthesia of the oral mucosa would result. Caution client about operating a car or other machinery, since drug may cause drowsiness or dizziness.

Evaluation. Clients should be observed for drowsiness and dizziness, nausea, gastrointestinal distress, constipation and rash.

Assess the client's cough as to whether it is productive or nonproductive. Chest pain associated with the cough should be noted. The intensity and frequency of the client's cough should diminish with the administration of the antitussive.

diphenhydramine HCl (Benylin, Benadryl, and others)

Mechanism of action. Depresses cough center in the medulla of the brain (antitussive effect). Also has antihistamine effects (blocks H_1 receptors), central antimuscarinic effect (antiparkinson action).

Indications. Antitussive, antihistamine, sedative-hypnotic effect, treatment of extrapyramidal side effects, prevents or treats nausea and vomiting of motion sickness.

Pharmacokinetics

Absorption. Good

Onset of action

Oral: within 15 to 60 minutes

IM: within 20 to 30 minutes

Time to peak concentration. Oral, within 1 to 4 hours

Half-life. 1 to 4 hours

Metabolism. Liver

Excretion. Kidneys

Side effects/adverse reactions. See Table 38-1.

Significant drug interactions. See antihistamine section in this chapter.

Dosage and administration

Adults

Antitussive (syrup): 25 mg orally, every 4 to 6 hours

Antihistamine (H_1 receptor): 25 to 50 mg orally, every 4 to 6 hours when necessary

Sedative-hypnotic: 50 mg ⅓ to ½ hour before bedtime

Antidyskinetic (or antiparkinson effects): 50 to 150 mg orally daily, in divided doses

Antiemetic or antivertigo effects: 25 to 50 mg orally one-half hour before traveling and before each meal, as necessary

Elderly may be more sensitive to the effects of this drug, therefore lower adult doses should be prescribed with close monitoring. If necessary and tolerated, the dosage may be increased.

Maximum daily dosage recommended for all indications except antitussive syrup effect is 300 mg daily, in divided dosages. For syrup, the maximum antitussive daily dosage is 100 mg per day, in divided dosages.

Children

Antihistamine (H_1 receptor): 1.25 mg/kg or 37.5 mg/m^2 orally every 4 to 6 hours. Maximum daily dose is 300 mg, or:

For children weighing up to 9.1 kg—6.25 to 12.5 mg orally, every 4 to 6 hours

For children 9.1 kg and over—12.5 to 25 mg orally every 4 to 6 hours

Antiemetic or antivertigo effects: 1 to 1.5 mg/kg orally every 6 hours as necessary. Maximum 300 mg per day.

Do not use in premature and full-term neonates.

Antitussive effect (syrup):

Under 2 years old—individualized by physician's order

2 to 6 years old—6.25 orally every 4 to 6 hours, maximum 25 mg in 24 hours

6 to 12 years old—12.5 mg orally every 4 to 6 hours, maximum 50 mg in 24 hours

diphenhydramine HCl injection

Adults

Antihistamine or antidyskinetic: IM or IV 10 to 50 mg every 2 to 3 hours

Antiemetic or antivertigo: IM or IV 10 mg initially, may increase to 20 to 50 mg every two or three hours

Children

Antihistamine (H_1 receptor) or antidyskinetic: 1.25 mg/kg IM or 37.5 mg/m^2 four times daily, up to a 300 mg per day maximum

Antiemetic or antivertigo agent: 1 to 1.5 mg/kg IM every 6 hours, up to 300 mg per day maximum

Do not use in premature and full-term neonates.

Pregnancy safety. Not established

NURSING CONSIDERATIONS

See discussion under benzonatate (p. 654).

dextromethorphan HBr (Mediquell, Sucrets Cough Control)

dextromethorphan in combination with cough syrups, antihistamines, expectorants, and benzocaine (Pertussin, Benylin DM, Vicks Cough Silencers, and others)

Mechanism of action. Depression of cough center in the medulla, as an antitussive, 15 to 30 mg of dextromethorphan is considered equivalent in effect to 8 to 15 mg of codeine

Indications. Antitussive for control of nonproductive coughs

Pharmacokinetics

Absorption. Rapidly absorbed from gastrointestinal tract

Onset of action. Within 15 to 30 minutes

Duration of effect. 3 to 6 hours

Side effects/adverse reactions. In usually recommended doses, side effects are minimal. Nausea and some dizziness have been reported. In overdosage in children, nausea, vomiting, blurred vision, ataxia, psychosis including hallucinations, insomnia, hysteria, edema and coma have been recorded. Thus far though, no fatalities have been reported.

Significant drug interactions. Use caution with MAO inhibitors.

Dosage and administration

Adults and children 12 years and older: 10 to 20 mg orally every 4 hours or, 30 mg every 6 to 8 hours, up to a maximum of 120 mg per day

Children 6 to 11 years old: 5 to 10 mg every 4 hours or 15 mg every 6 to 8 hours, not exceeding 60 mg per day

Children 2 to 5 years old: 2.5 to 5 mg every 4 hours or 7.5 mg every 6 to 8 hours, up to a maximum of 30 mg per day

Children under 2 years old: dosage should be individualized by the physician

Pregnancy safety. Not established

NURSING CONSIDERATIONS

As with other nonnarcotic antitussives, advise the client not to drink fluids for 30 to 35 minutes after taking the lozenge or chewable tablet or the effect will be washed away.

Advise the client also to consult with the physician if the cough persists for 7 days, or if other symptoms occur with the cough such as fever, rash, or continuing headache.

Many other products have been used as antitussive agents in various preparations but the FDA advisory review panel on nonprescription cold, cough, allergy, bronchodilator and antiasthmatic products has placed most of them in Category III, that is, more evidence is needed to prove their effectiveness. Some of the products in this category include noscapine, beechwood creosote, elm bark, cod liver oil, horehound and others.

NASAL DECONGESTANTS

Vasoconstricting drugs are most commonly used for their capacity to shrink the engorged nasal mucus membranes in mild upper respiratory infections. Many drugs are used exclusively as nasal vasoconstrictors. Because of their wide popular use and lack of serious hazard (when used topically), a large number of preparations have been provided by the pharmaceutical industry for direct sale to the public.

The FDA advisory review panel recommended the following products as safe and effective topical nasal decongestant products: ephedrine (0.5%), naphazoline hydrochloride (0.05%, 0.025%) (Privine), oxymetazoline hydrochloride (0.05%, 0.025%) (Afrin, Dristan Nasal Spray), phenylephrine hydrochloride (0.125%, 0.25%, 1%) (Neo-Synephrine), and xylometazoline hydrochloride (0.1%, 0.05%) (Otrivin). The oral decongestant products found safe and effective include phenylephrine (in Dristan), phenylpropanolamine (component in many products, such as Sinarest, Sine-Off, Sinutab, Comtrex), and pseu-

doephedrine (component in Ambenyl-D Cosanyl, Fedahist, and others). See Table 38-2 for recommended dosages for topical nasal decongestant products and oral decongestant products.

These drugs are adrenergic agents that act on alpha receptors of blood vessels in the nasal mucosa to produce mucosal constriction. Some nasal decongestant products also possess beta-stimulating effects, which may cause nervousness, restlessness, insomnia, irregular heart rate, and perhaps the adverse effect of vasodilation following vasoconstriction.

Nasal decongestant drugs are used to shrink engorged mucus membranes of the nose and to relieve nasal stuffiness. However, there is a tendency on the part of the public to misuse them by taking too large an amount and too frequently. This may result in "rebound" engorgement or swelling of the mucous membranes. Preservatives, antihistaminics, detergents, and antibiotics are sometimes added to the preparation of the decongestant. In some cases, reactions are believed to be caused by the additive rather than by the decongestant. Frequent interference with the vasomotor mechanism in the nose may do more harm than good, and there is always the possibility of spreading the infection deeper into the sinuses or to the middle ear. Sprays and nose drops are beneficial when used judiciously under the advice of a physician.

HISTAMINE
DISTRIBUTION

Histamine is a chemical mediator that occurs naturally in almost all body tissues. It is present in highest concentration in the skin, lung, and gastrointestinal tract. These structures are frequently exposed to environmental assaults and require protection against damage. When liberated from its cells, the free form of histamine plays an early transient role in the inflammatory process that defends the exposed tissues against injury.

In many tissues the chief site of production and storage of histamine occurs in the cytoplasmic granules of the mast cell or, in the case of blood, the basophil, which closely resembles the mast cell in function. The mast cells are small, ovoid-shaped structures widely distributed in the loose connective tissue. They are especially abundant along small blood vessels and along the bronchial smooth muscle cell, which appears to have the highest concentration of mast cells of any organ in the body. Both the mast cells and basophils make up the **mast-cell histamine pool.** A second major site of histamine production is known as the **nonmast pool** where the amine is stored in the cells of the epidermis, gastrointestinal mucosa, and the central nervous system. Although histamine is present in various foods and is synthesized by intestinal flora, the amount absorbed does not contribute to the body's stores of this amine.

TABLE 38-2 Recommended Dosage of Topical and Oral Nasal Decongestants

Drug/strength	Adults	Children (6 to 12 years old)
ephedrine, 0.5% (in Va-Tro-Nol nose drops and others)	2-3 drops every 4 hours	1-2 drops every 4 hours
naphazoline (Privine and other combinations)		
0.05%	1-2 drops or spray, every 6 hours	Not recommended
0.025%	—	1-2 drops every 6 hours
oxymetazoline (Afrin, Allerest, Dristan Long-Lasting Nasal Spray and others)		
0.05%	2-3 drops/spray twice daily	Not recommended
phenylephrine (Neo-Synephrine and others)	—	2-3 drops twice daily
1%	2-3 drops/spray every 4 hours	Not recommended
0.25%	Same as 1%	2-3 drops/spray every 4 hours
xylometazoline (Neo-Synephrine II and others)		
0.1%	2-3 drops/spray every 8-10 hours.	Not recommended
0.05%	Same as 0.1%	2-3 drops/spray every 8-10 hours

ORAL NASAL DECONGESTANTS
(USUALLY COMBINED WITH OTHER DRUG PRODUCTS)

phenylephrine	10 mg every 4 hours	5 mg every 4 hours
phenylpropanolamine	25 mg every 4 hours	12.5 mg every 4 hours
pseudoephedrine	60 mg every 6 hours	30 mg every 6 hours

PHARMACOLOGIC ACTIONS

The reactions mediated by histamine are attributed to receptor activity, which involves two distinct populations of receptors called H_1 and H_2 receptors. The principal actions of histamine include vascular effects mediated by H_1 and H_2 receptors of both arterioles and capillaries, smooth muscle effects of the bronchioles and the gastrointestinal tract as a result of activation of the H_2 receptors, and secretory glandular effects caused by H_2-receptor stimulation of the gastric mucosa (see Table 38-3)

Vascular effects. In the microcirculatory component of the cardiovascular system (arterioles, capillaries, venules) the liberation of histamine has been shown to involve both the H_1 and H_2 receptors. Stimulation of these receptors dilates the capillaries and venules, producing an increased localized blood flow, and promotes capillary permeability, allowing the escape of plasma protein and fluids through the capillary wall into the interstitial space. These are localized responses that result in erythema and swelling of the tissues. By activating the H_1 and H_2 receptors on the smooth muscles of the arterioles, histamine is also capable of eliciting a systemic response. In certain conditions it causes massive vasodilation of the arterioles, which can result in profound fall in blood pressure.

TABLE 38-3 Receptor-Mediating Effects of Histamine

Structure	Histamine receptors	Pharmacologic effects
Vascular system		
Capillary (Microcirculation)	H_1 and H_2	Dilation
		Increased permeability
Arteriole (Smooth muscle)	H_1 and H_2	Dilation
Smooth muscle		
Bronchial, bronchiolar	H_1	Contraction
Gastrointestinal	H_1	Contraction
Exocrine glands		
Gastric	H_2	Gastric acid secretion (HCl)
Epidermis	H_1	Triple response (flush, flare, wheal)
Adrenal medulla	—	Epinephrine and norepinephrine release
Central nervous system	H_1	Motion sickness

Smooth muscle effects. Although histamine exerts a powerful relaxing effect on the smooth muscle of the arterioles, it produces a contractile action on smooth muscles of many nonvascular organs, such as the bronchi and gastrointestinal tract. In sensitized individuals activation of the H_1 receptors of the lungs can cause marked bronchial muscle contraction that often progresses to dyspnea and leads to airway obstruction.

Exocrine glandular effects. Histamine stimulates the gastric, salivary, pancreatic, and lacrimal glands. The chief effect on human beings, however, is seen in the gastric glands. Stimulation of H_2 receptors in the exocrine glands of the stomach increases production of gastric acid secretions. Its high hydrochloric acid concentration is attributed to the activity of the parietal cells of the stomach and is implicated in the development of peptic ulcers.

Central nervous system effect. Histamine is also known to be present throughout the tissues of the brain. Its effects seem to involve both H_1- and H_2-receptor mediation. The activation of H_1 receptors of the semicircular canals is associated with motion sickness.

Triple response. An intradermal injection of histamine causes a series of reactions called the "triple response." This is characterized as a local action resulting from stimulation of H_1 receptors in the skin. Blood vessels (capillaries) immediately affected by the histamine dilate and produce a *flush,* or redness. Surrounding blood vessels then dilate to produce a *flare,* or diffuse redness. This reaction is probably the result of a neural mechanism— axon reflexes stimulate sensory nerves and their branches to produce dilation of blood vessels. Widely dilated blood vessels have increased permeability. There is an increase in tissue fluid or local edema, termed a *wheal.* Any chemical or mechanical injury to the skin can cause this triple response of flush, flare, and wheal. Therefore it is believed that histamine is released from injured skin. The triple response is believed to be one of the body's protective mechanisms, since increased permeability of blood vessels permits the passage of plasma proteins and white cells into the tissues.

PATHOLOGIC EFFECTS

Histamine as a chemical mediator is implicated in many pathologic disorders. Conditions for which drugs are used to counteract this compound are concerned with the hypersensitivity response known as the *allergic reaction.* Although four different types of hypersensitivity responses to immunologic injury exist, the type I-anaphylactic reaction is the one associated with the disorders caused by histamine release.

Individuals with type I-mediated hypersensitivity develop allergies as a result of sensitization to a foreign agent that may be ingested, inhaled, or injected. An incalculable number of these agents acting as antigens exist. They vary widely in that seasonal exposure to pollens, grasses, and weeds or nonseasonal agents such as house dust, feathers, molds, and other similar substances can develop different forms of allergic reactivity. Hypersensitivity to a variety of foods such as shellfish or strawberries requires ingestion of the antigen. Insects such as bees or wasps and even drugs, particularly penicillin, also possess allergic properties that may induce a severe response in hypersensitive individuals. Thus type I-anaphylactic hypersensitivity accounts for a substantial number of allergic disorders, and it involves a complex series of anomalies that range from mild urticaria to anaphylactic shock.

The mechanism of type I-anaphylactic reaction involves the attachment of an antigen (Ag) to an antibody (Ab), specifically immunoglobulin E (IgE), and this complex in turn becomes fixed to the mast cell. The pathologic manifestations of Ag-IgE interaction are caused by mast cell degranulation, resulting in the release of histamine and other mediators responsible for producing the allergic symptoms. The type I-anaphylactic reaction is responsible for various disorders, such as urticaria, atopy (allergic rhinitis, hay fever), food allergies, bronchial asthma, and systemic anaphylaxis.

Urticaria. **Urticaria** is a vascular reaction of the skin characterized by immediate formation of a wheal and flare accompanied by severe itching. Contact with an external irritant such as drugs or foods produces the Ag-IgE mediated response with resultant release of histamine from the mast cell into the skin. The local vasodilation produces the red flare, and the increased permeability of the capillaries leads to tissue swelling. These swellings are called "hives," and when giant hives occur they are known as *angioneurotic edema.* Antihistaminic drugs administered before exposure to the antigen will prevent this response.

Atopy. **Atopy** occurs in genetically susceptible individuals and is usually caused by seasonal pollen. This condition is manifested as an upper respiratory tract disorder known as *allergic rhinitis* (hay fever). Following the interaction of Ag-IgE antibody on the surface of the bronchial mast cells, histamine is released, producing local vascular dilation and increased capillary permeability. This change produces a rapid fluid leakage into the tissues of the nose, resulting in swelling of the nasal linings. In certain individuals antihistaminic therapy can prevent the edematous reaction if the drug is administered before antigenic exposure.

Food allergies. Food allergies involve intestinal immunoglobulin E (IgE)—mast cell responses to ingested antigens. If the upper gastrointestinal tract is affected, vomiting results; if the lower gastrointestinal tract is invaded, cramps and diarrhea occur. This condition also has been known to produce systemic anaphylaxis following ingestion of a large amount of antigen.

Bronchial asthma. When the inhaled antigen combines with the IgE antibody, stimulation of the mast cells triggers the release of mediators in the lower respiratory tract, usually in the bronchi and bronchioles. Histamine plays a minor role in this response because the slow-reacting substance of anaphylaxis (SRS-A) is a more potent mediator, causing long-term contraction of the bronchiolar smooth muscle. The difficulty in breathing may be relieved by a bronchodilator such as epinephrine. The administration of antihistaminic drugs actually has no value in relieving this condition, since more potent chemical mediators than histamine are responsible for causing the reaction.

Systemic anaphylaxis. **Systemic anaphylaxis** is a generalized reaction manifested as a life-threatening systemic condition. The Ag-IgE mediator response involves the basophils of the blood and the mast cells in the connective tissue. The most common precipitating causes of this response are drugs, particularly penicillin; insect stings (wasps and bees); and occasionally certain foods. The release of massive amounts of histamine into the circulation causes widespread vasodilation, resulting in a profound fall in blood pressure. The excessive dilation also allows plasma to leave the capillaries, and a loss of circulatory volume ensues. When the reaction is fatal, death is usually caused not only by shock but also by laryngeal edema. The symptoms of the latter condition include smooth muscle contraction of the bronchi and pharyngeal edema, which usually leads to asphyxiation. Since the mediators, SRS-A, also is released from the cells, spasm of the smooth muscle of the bronchioles elicits the asthmalike attack.

Antihistaminic drugs are less effective against systemic anaphylaxis because these agents do not antagonize the SRS-A mediator that causes the severe bronchoconstriction. Accordingly, a drug such as epinephrine, a broncho-dilator, is indicated for this life-threatening situation. The relief produced by this drug results from the beta$_2$-receptor action that relaxes bronchial smooth muscles.

Drug allergies frequently develop in susceptible individuals who show no adverse effects following the first dose of drug administration. However, a second or subsequent reexposure to even a minute amount of this same antigen may elicit an exaggerated IgE response either locally or systemically. Individuals who exhibit such reactions are said to be allergic to the drug. The IgE-mediated response, particularly with penicillin, may occur either in the skin, producing severe urticaria, or in the respiratory tract, causing bronchial asthma. On the other hand, even limited contact in certain sensitized individuals can produce a fatal systemic anaphylaxis. Some of the drugs that elicit an allergic response include penicillin, chloramphenicol, streptomycin, sulfonamides, aspirin, and phenacetin. Allergic reaction to penicillin account for nearly 100 deaths per year in the United States. Therefore, if an individual exhibits even the mildest sign of an allergic response, such as a slight skin rash, this symptom, should be reported immediately to the physician. In all probability the drug will be discontinued to avoid the possibility of an exaggerated type I hypersensitivity reaction. See Table 38-4 for symptoms of drug allergies involving various organ systems.

DOSAGE AND ADMINISTRATION

Gastric function testing. Client should fast for a minimum of 12 hours and be at rest under basal conditions. Use a nasogastric tube to obtain gastric contents. Client may swallow 300 ml of water; then the histamine dose of 0.01 mg/kg (equal to histamine phosphate 0.0275 mg/kg) is given subcutaneously. Monitor pulse rate and blood

TABLE 38-4 Common Manifestations of Drug-Induced Allergic Reactions

Tissue or organ	Symptom	Hapten commonly involved
Skin	Hives (urticuria) and generalized itching Rashes Exofoliative dermatitis (loss of superficial skin layers)	Penicillin, aspirin Barbiturates, sulfonamides, streptomycin Tetracycline, streptomycin, phenobarbital
Mucous membranes (particularly of nose and eye)	Inflammation, swelling, and excessive secretions	Sulfonamides, barbiturates
Respiratory tract	Difficulty in breathing	Penicillin, local anesthetics, aspirin, heroin
Vascular system	Fall in blood pressure	Penicillin, aspirin
Blood and blood-forming tissues*	Reduction in the number of one or more types of circulating blood cells	Aminopyrine (Pyramidon) Quinidine

From Levine, R: Pharmacology: drug actions and reactions, ed. 2, Copyright © 1978 by Little, Brown & Co. Used with the permission of Little, Brown & Co.
*The presence of an antibody that reacts specifically with the sensitizing drug has been demonstrated in the case of each of the drugs cited as well as for a number of other drugs. Such demonstrations provide proof that drug allergy can account for some disorders of blood and the blood-forming tissues.

pressure closely. Obtain four samples gastric contents, 15 minutes apart for analysis. The maximum effect from the histamine is usually seen in about ½ hour.

Pheochromocytoma. Before giving histamine, withdraw all antihypertensive drugs, sympathomimetics, sedatives and opioids for at least 24 hours—preferably for 3 days. Food is given routinely. The individual should be at rest in a supine position so that the blood pressure stabilizes. Then a cold pressure test* is performed; 30 minutes afterward, a slow intravenous infusion of 5% dextrose injection or normal saline is started. When blood pressure is stablized, a 2-hour collection of urine is obtained to test for catecholamines. Then histamine is given through the intravenous infusion and another 2-hour collection of urine is obtained for testing. Initial dose of histamine is 0.01 mg. Monitor blood pressure and pulse rate every 30 seconds for 15 minutes. If no response is noted, give a second dose of 0.05 mg.

Nearly all individuals will experience flushing, headache, and a decrease in blood pressure after the administration of the histamine. Within a couple of minutes, the blood pressure will increase. The package insert has further information on this test.

• • •

Both of these tests should be performed by and under the direction of a physician.

NURSING CONSIDERATIONS

Histamine should be used cautiously in individuals with any cardiac abnormality. The gastric histamine test is contraindicated in clients with a history of hypersensitivity to the drug, bronchial asthma, urticaria, or severe cardiac, pulmonary, or renal disease.

For the gastric histamine test, the drug is administered subcutaneously. Before the medication is injected, the plunger of the syringe should be drawn back to ensure that the needle is not in a blood vessel. Epinephrine should be available in case of inadvertent injection into a vessel.

The procedure and any anticipated effects of the histamine test should be explained to the client.

ANTIHISTAMINES

Antihistamines are drugs that compete with histamine for its receptor sites. With the discovery of two histamine receptors, H_1 and H_2, the antihistamines should be divid-

ed into the H_1-receptor antagonists and the H_2-receptor antagonists.

The H_2-receptor blocking agents, which include cimetidine (Tagamet), ranitidine (Zantac), and famotidine (Pepcid), are discussed in Chapter 40. These are valuable agents with a variety of indications, especially in the treatment or prevention of peptic ulcers (see Chapter 40).

H_1 RECEPTOR ANTAGONISTS

Antihistamines prevent the physiologic action of histamine. It is postulated that the antihistamines act by preventing histamine from reaching its site of action, that is, by competing for the receptors. The antihistamines of the H_1 type have the greatest therapeutic effect on nasal allergies, particularly on seasonal hay fever. They relieve symptoms better at the beginning of the hay fever season than during its height but fail to relieve the asthma that frequently accompanies hay fever. These preparations are palliative and do not immunize the individual or protect him over time against allergic reactions. Their benefits are therefore comparatively short-lived and provide only symptomatic relief. They must be regarded only as adjuncts to more specific methods of treatment. They do not begin to replace such remedies as epinephrine, ephedrine, and aminophylline. In acute asthmatic reactions the antihistamine drugs serve only as supplements to these remedies. Also, relief of various symptoms of allergy is obtained only while the drug is being taken. Antihistamines do not appear to have a cumulative action and can therefore be taken over a period of time.

Dozens of antihistamine drugs are available and generally differ from each other by potency, duration of action, and incidence of side effects, particularly sedation. It is often necessary to try different types of antihistamines to determine the appropriate one for a client. Many OTC preparations also contain antihistamines; some contain two or more different ones. Antihistamines are used in antitussive preparations, cough-cold products, nighttime sedation or OTC sleeping products, oral analgesic products, menstrual tablets, and many other products. The nurse and consumer should check ingredients of all medications they buy, recommend, consume, or administer. Often individuals experience unwanted side effects or are accidently overdosed since the same product may be available in several different medications they are consuming. Unfortunately, this is frequently overlooked in a clinical setting.

Mechanism of action. Antihistamines compete with histamine for H_1 receptors on various effector structures, such as smooth muscle of vascular system and bronchioles, lacrimal, salivary and respiratory mucosal glands. They do not inhibit histamine already attached to receptors. Thus these drugs are more effective if given before histamine is released.

---

*Cold pressure test is immersing one hand in cold water for 60 seconds and then measuring the rise in blood pressure. The increase in blood pressure after histamine is compared to the cold pressure test; it must exceed the water test to be indicative of pheochromocytoma.

Many H_1-receptor blocking agents also have anticholinergic effects, antiemetic, anti-motion sickness, and antivertigo properties. Many cross the blood-brain barrier to affect H_1 receptors in the brain, thus inducing sedation and perhaps, antitussive effects (diphenhydramine).

Indications. Treatment of allergies, vertigo, motion sickness, antitussive (diphenhydramine), sedative and local anesthetic effects in dentistry.

Pharmacokinetics. For diphenhydramine, see previous section.

Absorption. Good

Onset of action. Orally, within 15 to 60 minutes; rectally, dimenhydrinate within 30 to 45 minutes

Time to peak concentration
azatadine: 4 hours
brompheniramine: within 2 to 5 hours
chlorpheniramine: within 2 to 6 hours
clemastine: within 2 to 4 hours
triprolidine: 2 hours

Time to peak effect
bromphiramine: within 3 to 9 hours
chlorpheniramine: 6 hours
clemastine: within 5 to 7 hours
terfenadine: within 3 to 4 hours
triprolidine: within 2 to 3 hours

Elimination half-life
azatadine: 12 hours
brompheniramine: 25 hours
carbinoxamine: within 10-20 hours
chlorpheniramine: within 12 to 15 hours
terfenadine: 20.3 hours
triprolidine: within 3 to 3.3 hours

Duration of action. See box for chemical classification of H_1-receptor antagonists.
ethanolamine derivatives: within 6 to 8 hours
ethylenediamine derivatives: within 4 to 6 hours
pyrilamine: 8 hours
piperidine derivatives:
   azatadine: 12 hours
   cyproheptadine: 8 hours
phenindamine: within 4 to 6 hours
propylamine derivatives: within 4 to 25 hours
terfenadine: over 12 hours

Metabolism. Liver

Excretion. Kidneys (with terfenadine, mostly in feces)

Side effects/adverse reactions. See Table 38-1.

Significant drug interactions. When antihistamines are given with alcohol and CNS depressants, enhanced CNS depressant effects may be noted. If CNS depressant also has anticholinergic side effects, enhanced anticholinergic side effects may be seen. Monitor closely as interventions may be necessary.

When antihistamines are given with anticholinergic medications, psychotropics, and others, an enhanced CNS

CHEMICAL CLASSIFICATION OF H_1 RECEPTOR ANTAGONISTS

butyrophenone derivative: terfenadine (Seldane)
ethanolamine derivatives: brompheniramine (Dimetane); carbinoxamine (Clistin); dimenhydrinate (Dramamine, Travamine♣); diphenhydramine (Benadryl): doxylamine (Unisom Nighttime Sleep-Aid).
ethylenediamine derivatives: pyrilamine (Sominex); tripelennamine (PBZ)
piperidine derivatives: azatadine (Optimine); cyproheptadine (Periactin, Vimicon♣); diphenylpyraline (Hispril)
propylamine derivatives (alkylamines): brompheniramine (Dimetane); chlorpheniramine (Teldrin, Chlortrimeton); dexchlorpheniramine (Polaramine); triprolidine (Actidil)
Miscellaneous: phenindamine (Nolahist)

---

depressant effect may be noted (see above).

When antihistamines are given with monoamine oxidase (MAO) inhibitors, prolonged anticholinergic and CNS depression effects may result. Avoid concurrent drug administration.

Dosage and administration
azatadine (Optimine)
Adults. 1 to 2 mg orally every 8 to 12 hours.

Elderly may be more sensitive to the majority of antihistamines; therefore dosage reduction initially should be considered.

Children. Under 12 years old: not recommended; 12 years old and older: 0.5 mg to 1 mg twice daily as necessary

brompheniramine maleate elixir or tablets
Adults. 4 mg orally every 4 to 6 hours when necessary, up to a a maximum of 24 mg per day

Children. 0.5 mg/kg orally or 15 mg/m² daily, given in three or four divided dosages, as necessary. Children 2 to 6 years old: 1 mg orally every 4 to 6 hours when needed; 6 to 12 years old: 2 mg every 4 to 6 hours when needed; 12 years and older: see adult dosing

brompheniramine maleate extended-release tablets
Adults. 8 or 12 mg every 8 to 12 hours when necessary

Children. Under 6 years old: not recommended; 6 years old and older: 8 or 12 mg every 12 hours as necessary

brompheniramine maleate injection
Adults. 10 mg IM, IV, or SC every 8 to 12 hours when necessary; maximum is 40 mg daily

Children. Under 12 years old: IM, IV, SC, 0.125 mg/kg or 3.75 mg/m², three or four times daily as necessary; not recommended for neonates *carbinoxamine (Clistin)*

Adults. 4 to 8 mg orally every 6 to 8 hours as necessary

Children. 1 to 3 years old: 2 mg orally every 6 to 8 hours as necessary; 3 to 6 years old: 2 to 4 mg orally every 6 to 8 hours as necessary; 6 years and older: 4 to 6 mg every 6 to 8 hours as necessary; not recommended for neonates

chlorpheniramine syrup, tablets, chewable tablets

Adults. 4 mg orally every 4 to 6 hours when necessary; maximum daily dosage is 24 mg

Children. 0.0875 mg/kg orally or 2.5 mg/m^2 every 6 hours as necessary. Or: Children up to 6 years old: not recommended; 6 to 12 years old: 2 mg orally three or four times daily as necessary, not exceeding 12 mg in 24 hours

chlorpheniramine maleate extended-release capsules/tablets

Adults. 8 or 12 mg orally every 8 to 12 hours as necessary

Children. 12 years and older: 8 mg orally every 12 hours as necessary; under 12 years old: not recommended

chlorpheniramine maleate injection

Adults. 5 to 40 mg IM, IV or SC as single dose; maximum 40 mg in 24 hours

Children. 0.0875 mg/kg SC or 2.5 mg/m^2 SC every 6 hours as necessary

clemastine (Tavist)

Adults. 1.34 mg twice daily or 2.68 mg one to three times daily, up to a maximum of 8.04 mg daily

Children. Up to 12 years old: 0.67 mg orally to 1.34 mg orally every 8 to 12 hours when necessary; not recommended for neonates

cyproheptadine (Periactin, Vimicon)

Adults. 4 mg orally every 6 to 8 hours when necessary, up to 0.5 mg/kg of adult body weight daily

Children. 0.125 mg/kg or 4 mg/m^2 orally every 8 to 12 hours when necessary. Or: 2 to 6 years old: 2 mg orally every 8 to 12 hours when necessary, up to a maximum of 12 mg daily; 6 to 14 years old: 4 mg orally every 8 to 12 hours when necessary, up to a maximum of 16 mg daily

dexchlorpheniramine maleate tablet/syrup (Polaramine)

Adults. 2 mg orally every 4 to 6 hours when necessary

Children. Under 12 years old: 0.15 mg/kg or 4.5 mg/m^2 orally in four divided doses daily; or 0.5 mg to 1 mg every 4 to 6 hours when necessary

Not recommended for neonates

dexchlorpheniramine maleate extended-release tablets

Adults. 4 or 6 mg orally every 8 to 12 hours when necessary

Children. Not recommended

dimenhydrinate elixir/syrup/tablets (Dramamine, Gravol)

Adults. Antiemetic or antivertigo effect: 50 to 100 mg every four hours when necessary, up to a maximum of 400 mg daily

Children. Antiemetic or antivertigo effect: 5 mg/kg or 150 mg/m^2 orally in four divided doses when necessary. Do not exceed 300 mg daily. Or: 2 to 6 years old: 12.5 to 25 mg orally every 6 to 8 hours when necessary, up to a maximum of 75 mg daily; 6 to 12 years old: 25 to 50 mg orally every 6 to 8 hours when necessary, up to a maximum of 150 mg daily; not recommended for neonates.

dimenhydrinate injection

Adults. Antiemetic or antivertigo effect: 50 mg intramuscularly every 4 hours as necessary. Intravenous, 50 mg in 10 ml or normal saline injection (0.9% sodium chloride injection) given slowly over 2 minutes. If necessary, dose may be repeated every 4 hours.

Children. Antiemetic or antivertigo effect: 1.25 mg/kg or 37.5 mg/m^2 intramuscularly, every 6 hours when necessary, up to 300 mg daily; intravenously 1.25 mg/kg or 37.5 mg/m^2 in 10 ml of normal saline injection, given slowly over at least 2 minutes, every 6 hours when necessary. Do not exceed 300 mg daily.

dimenhydrinate suppositories (Nauseatol). Not available in U.S.

diphenydramine. See previous section.

diphenylpyraline HCl extended-release capsules (Hispril)

Adults. 5 mg orally every 12 hours when necessary

Children. Under 6 years old: not recommended; 6 years and older: 5 mg once daily as needed

doxylamine succinate tablets (Unisom Nighttime Sleep-Aid)

Adults

Antihistaminic: 12.5 to 25 mg orally every 4 to 6 hours when necessary.

Sedative-hypnotic: 25 mg orally 30 minutes before retiring; maximum adult daily dose is 150 mg

Children

Antihistaminic: under 6 years old—not recommended; 6 to 12 years old—6.25 mg to 12.5 mg orally every 4 to 6 hours when necessary

Sedative-hypnotic: not recommended

phenindamine tartrate tablets (Nolahist)

Adults. 25 mg orally every 4 to 6 hours as necessary; maximum daily dosage is 150 mg

Children. Under 6 years old: individualized by physician; 6 to 12 years old: 12.5 mg orally every 4 to 6 hours when necessary, up to 75 mg daily; 12 years and older: see adult dosing

pyrilamine maleate capsules/tablets (Sominex, Somnicaps)

Adults

Antihistaminic: 25 to 50 mg orally every 8 hours when necessary.

Sedative-hypnotic: 25 to 50 mg orally 20 to 30 minutes before retiring. Maximum daily dosage is 200 mg

Children

Antihistamic only: 2 to 6 years old—not recommended; 6 years and older—12.5 to 25 mg orally every 8 hours when necessary

Sedative-hypnotic: not recommended.

terfenadine tablets (Seldane)

Adults. Antihistamine: 60 mg orally every 8 to 12 hours when necessary. Terfenadine does not readily cross the blood-brain barrier; therefore the enhanced CNS depression and anticholinergic side effects seen generally with the antihistamines may not be as prominent with this product.

Children. Not established

tripelennamine citrate elixir/HCl tablets (PBZ)

Adults. Antihistamine: 25 to 50 mg orally every 4 to 6 hours when necessary; maximum daily dose is 600 mg

Children. 1.25 mg/kg or 37.5 mg/m² orally every 6 hours up to a maximum of 300 mg daily; not recommended for neonates

tripelennamine HCl extended-release tablets (PBS-SR)

Adults. 100 mg orally every 8 to 12 hours when necessary, up to a maximum of 600 mg daily

Children. Not recommended

triprolidine HCl syrup/tablets (Actidil)

Adults. Antihistamine: 2.5 mg orally every 6 to 8 hours when necessary, up to a maximum of 10 mg daily

Children. Antihistamine: 4 months to 2 years old—0.312 mg orally every 6 to 8 hours when necessary; 2 to 4 years old—0.625 mg orally every 6 to 8 hours when necessary; 4 to 6 years old—0.937 mg every 6 to 8 hours when necessary; 6 to 12 years old—1.25 mg orally every 6 to 8 hours when necessary, not recommended for neonates.

Pregnancy safety. Azatadine, brompheniramine, cyproheptadine, dexchlorpheniramine, dimenhydrinate, and triprolidine—FDA category B; carbinoxamine—FDA category C; doxylamine—not established; terfenadine—FDA category C

NURSING CONSIDERATIONS

Assessment. Take client medication history to determine if there is a previous intolerance to antihistamines.

Use antihistamines with caution in clients with asthma, since the drying effect may thicken secretions and diminish expectoration; prostatic hypertrophy or predisposition to urinary retention, because the urinary retention may be aggravated; or a predisposition to narrow-angle glaucoma, since the drug may precipitate an acute episode.

Intervention. In the administration of the parenteral form of brompheniramine, the concentrated solution (100 mg per mL) is not recommended for intravenous use. Do not break, crush, or chew sustain-release capsules or long-acting tablets.

Education. Advise the client who will be using antihistamines on a long-term basis to maintain dental hygiene by brushing and flossing because the diminished salivary flow resulting from antihistamines will contribute to caries and gum disease. Regular dental checkups should also be advised. The discomfort of the dryness of the mouth may be minimized by using ice, sugarless gum, or hard candy.

Drowsiness is a common effect of antihistamines. Caution the client about driving or using other hazardous equipment until the response to the drug has been ascertained. When the effect is known, then the client may modify life-style accordingly. Also, if the drowsiness is severe, another antihistamine may be prescribed.

Alert the client to the symptoms of blood dyscrasias, such as sore throat, fever, unusual bruising and bleeding, and tiredness, as these should be reported to the physician.

Caution the client about ingesting alcohol or CNS depressants because the effects of the drugs will be potentiated.

Inform the client that antihistamines may be taken with food or milk to minimize gastric distress.

If the client is taking antihistamines as prophylaxis of motion sickness, the dose should be taken 30 minutes to 1 to 2 hours before its effect is needed. The client taking antihistamines should alert the allergist if scheduled for allergy skin tests because these drugs interfere with the results.

Evaluation. Clients on long-term antihistamine therapy should have periodic blood counts to monitor for the development of blood dyscrasias.

Tolerance to some antihistamines may occur. If a tolerance develops, another antihistamine may be prescribed.

In the older child, a paradoxical response to the drug may occur and the child may exhibit hyperexcitability rather than the drowsiness that is usually seen.

With the elderly client, sedation and hypotension are more likely to occur, as well as the antimuscarinic effects of the drug, resulting in dryness of the mouth, or urinary retention, particularly in the male.

Closely monitor individuals with hypertension or cardiac or renal disease who are taking antihistamines.

INHIBITOR OF HISTAMINE RELEASE

See cromolyn sodium in previous chapter. Cromolyn sodium provides a local protective effect in the mucosal airways by inhibiting the granulation of pulmonary mast cells and thereby preventing the release of histamine and SRS-A.

SEROTONIN

Over a century ago scientists found that serum from coagulated blood contained a vasoconstrictor substance. During experiments involving the perfusion of isolated organs in blood, this substance appeared as an unwanted compound that had to be eliminated in order to obtain accurate laboratory results. In 1948 researchers at the Cleveland Clinic finally isolated the vasoconstrictor material and named it serotonin. One year later the active moiety of this complex was identified as 5-hydroxytryptamine (5-HT).

As with histamine, serotonin has no therapeutic application; however, its importance is related to the action of other drugs and several disease states.

Serotonin is widely distributed in nature, occurring in both plants and animals. It appears in fruits such as pineapples, bananas, strawberries, and tomatoes, as well as in various nuts. Its presence has been established in the salivary glands of the octopus and in the venom of the scorpion and wasp. It also appears in the stinging fluid of the common nettle. In human beings, serotonin occurs in various body tissues. The sites of endogenous serotonin are discussed in the next section.

CHEMISTRY

Synthesis. In human beings, the synthesis of serotonin begins with the essential dietary amino acid, tryptophan. Only two enzymatic steps are required to form serotonin in the tissues (Figure 38-2).

Metabolism. The inactivation of serotonin is not complex. The principal enzyme concerned with this process is monamine oxidase, which forms 5-hydroxyindoleacetic acid (5-HIAA). The compound is then excreted in the urine along with a much smaller amount of another metabolite, 5-hydroxytryptophol (5-HTOL). Normal excretion of 5-HIAA is 2 to 9 mg a day. However, the excretion levels in carcinoid syndrome may range from 50 to 500 mg a day. The 24-hour urine testing for 5-HIAA excretion level is of great diagnostic value in determining the presence of this clinical disorder.

Distribution. Serotonin appears primarily in three types of tissues in the body: (1) the largest fraction (90%) is synthesized and stored in the enterochromaffin cells of the gastrointestinal tract mucosa, particularly in the pylorus of the stomach and in the upper region of the small intestine; (2) a much smaller fraction is stored but not synthesized in platelets; on disintegration this fraction is released in serum and in the spleen; and (3) in the CNS the greatest concentration occurs in the hypothalmus,

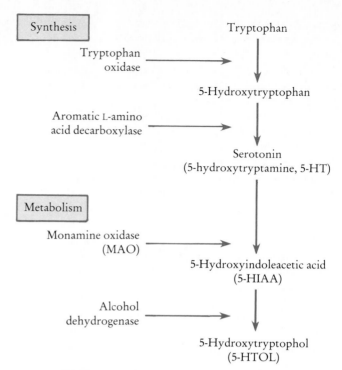

FIGURE 38-2   Synthesis and metabolism of serotonin.

midbrain, reticular formation, raphe (midline) regions of medulla and pons, and pineal gland. A neuron that releases serotonin is termed a **serotoninergic** or **tryptaminergic** fiber. Finally, only a very low concentration of serotonin appears in cells.

PHARMACOLOGIC ACTIONS

Serotonin appears to possess multiple pharmacologic actions, but because of discrepant experimental findings, this variability has caused much controversy. Despite the need for additional experimental analysis, it is now known that the primary function of serotonin is exerted on various smooth muscles and nerves. As previously stated, serotonin is not a therapeutic agent, but its more prominent effects are associated with its influence on other drugs and some disease states.

Gastrointestinal tract. Among the columnar epithelial cells of the stomach and intestine are located specialized cells that are stained by silver; therefore these structures are called **argentaffin** or enterochromaffin cells. The serotonin secreted by these cells is responsible for contraction of the gastrointestinal smooth muscle, thereby producing the peristaltic response.

Carcinoid syndrome is a condition that elicits a complex array of signs and symptoms mediated by humoral compounds released from malignant carcinoid tumors. Carcinoid tumors are best described as slowly growing neoplasms of enterochromaffin cells of the stomach, intestine, or bronchial trees. The overproduction of serotonin is an important biochemical reaction caused by these tumors; bradykinin and histamine also may be elaborated. Serotonin is responsible for causing this syndrome, which is characterized by paroxysmal flushing, hyperperistalsis, diarrhea, bronchoconstriction, and cardiac valvular lesions. The diagnosis of carcinoid syndrome is confirmed by the presence of excess 5-HT, which eventually is excreted in the urine as 5-HIAA. The normal daily urinary excretion is 2 to 9 mg in adults. Obviously this amount is greatly increased in the presence of carcinoid tumor.

Blood platelets. Serotonin is released from platelets during their breakdown within the circulation. This compound then activates receptors on the surface of other blood platelets, thereby promoting platelet aggregation. It has been suggested that through this mechanism the discharge of serotonin from platelets may contribute to the formation of pulmonary embolism.

Central nervous system. Serotonin is manufactured and stored in the neurons in the brain. The central action of the neuronal system appears to elicit primarily in *inhibitory* response from the specific nuclei of the brain. Researchers now postulate that altered function of serotoninergic pathways is a factor in various CNS dysfunctions. Serotonin synthesized in the pineal gland serves as a precursor for the synthesis of melatonin, a hormone that functions as a potent lightening agent in animals. Melatonin does not affect human skin and pigment.

Sleep. Serotonin-synthesizing cells are required for the induction of non-rapid-eye-movement (NREM) sleep (quiet brain, potentially excitable muscles) and the onset of REM sleep (active brain, rapid-eye movements, dreams, atonic muscles). Normal sleep depends on serotonin along with the combined functions of norepinephrine and cholinergic systems. The basic sleep pattern consists of four to six cycles that alternate between NREM and REM sleep. Destruction of the raphe nuclei results in insomnia. Other disorders of sleep are quite common; for example, **narcolepsy** is characterized by a sudden change from wakefulness directly to REM sleep.

Sleep hypnotics such as barbiturates tend to decrease REM sleep, which is an essential component of restful sleep. Also, the drug *p*-chlorophenylalanine inhibits formation of serotonin, and this depletion can cause prolonged wakefulness when administered to animals.

Pain perception. The serotoninergic neurons located in the raphe nuclei of the brainstem have axons that project to the spinal cord and forebrain. One important system related to the brain involves a substance called *beta-endorphin,* which is associated with neurons that interconnect various nuclei in the hypothalamus, limbic system, and thalamus. The *beta*-endorphin neurons mediate euphoric and emotional behavior. The thalamic nuclei mediates poorly localized deep pain, which is best influenced by opiates. The density of opiate receptors in the brain appears to be much greater in the medial and lateral thalamus. Many receptors are required to determine how addiction and withdrawal can be influenced.

Serotonin also is implicated in the action of morphine. Studies suggest that as tolerance develops toward this narcotic, the synthesis but not the accumulation of serotonin doubles. In addition, a decrease in brain serotonin level increases a person's sensitivity to painful stimuli, thus decreasing the analgesic effect of morphine.

Mental illness. CNS depression correlates with low levels of total brain serotonin. The enzyme monoamine oxidase metabolizes serotonin, resulting in a lower level of the transmitter (see Figure 38-2). Accordingly, a monoamine oxidase inhibitor (MAOI) blocks the degradation of serotonin and thereby increases the concentration level of the neurotransmitter in the brain. The antidepressant effects of MAOI drugs are discussed in Chapter 16. The tricyclic compounds also act as antidepressants, blocking the reuptake of serotonin and norepinephrine at the membrane of the neuron and thereby potentiating the action of the synapse. Reserpine, formerly an antipsychotic drug, is now used as an antihypertensive agent. Because it causes a prolonged depletion of serotonin and norepinephrine in the brain, reserpine is responsible for producing a tranquilizing effect (see Chapter 23).

ANTISEROTONINS

Antiserotonins, or serotonin antagonists, are considered complex compounds because they possess varying degrees of specificity, and thus the exact mechanism of action is unknown. In addition to performing serotonin-blocking activity, many other pharmacologic actions are involved in inhibiting responses to serotonin.

cyproheptadine (Periactin)

Cyproheptadine blocks serotonin activity in smooth muscle of blood vessels and the intestine and also has antihistaminic and possibly anticholinergic properties. It may produce weight gain in children because of stimulation of appetite through action in the hypothalamus. It is administered primarily for various allergic disorders. (See "antihistamines" and Figure 38-2.)

lysergic acid diethylamide (LSD)

The psychotomimetic properties of LSD were discovered in 1943 by Hoffman at a Swiss drug firm. Later, a team of researchers at Harvard University conducted a series of experiments on LSD; Timothy Leary, a collaborator, became interested in the effects of this drug and withdrew from the team to pursue independent studies. The validity of his findings were later questioned because of doubts about his use of the scientific approach. In the

1960s a psychedelic drug cult developed, and Leary became a staunch advocate of LSD use.

The basic mechanism underlying LSD's hallucinogenic properties is not known. Experts agree, however, that its profound effects on behavior are mediated through the central neurotransmitter, serotonin. Studies in the 1970s have suggested that the more powerful hallucinogenic drugs exert a dual function in the brain: they inhibit the action of serotonin and stimulate the norepinephrine system (see Chapter 9).

methysergide maleate (Sansert)

Although its mechanism of action is unknown, methysergide is both a potent antiserotonin and a vasoconstrictor agent. These properties apparently help to relieve migraine and other vascular headaches (see Chapter 20).

KEY TERMS

analeptics, page 651
anemic hypoxia, page 647
argentaffin, page 664
atopy, page 658
carcinoid syndrome, page 664
histotoxic hypoxia, page 647
hypercapnia, page 649
hypoxemia, page 647
hypoxia, page 647
hypoxic hypoxia, page 647
ischemic hypoxia, page 647
mast-cell histamine pool, page 656
narcolepsy, page 665
nonmast pool, page 656
serotoninergic, page 664
systemic anaphylaxis, page 659
tryptaminergic, page 664
urticaria, page 658

BIBLIOGRAPHY

Ambielli, M.P. (1983) A review of histamine 2-receptor antagonists, J Neurosurg Nurs 15(6):370.

American Hospital Formulary Service (1987) AHFS Drug Information '87. Bethesda: American Society of Hospital Pharmacists, Inc.

Braunwald, E. and others (editors) (1987) Harrison's Principles of Internal Medicine, ed. 11. New York: McGraw-Hill Company.

Carpenter, V.P. et al. (1985) Rantidine and cimetidine: a critical comparison, Hosp Formul 20(5):599.

Connell, J.T. et al. (1984) Efficacy of a timed-release antihistamine/decongestant tablet for symptoms of nasal allergy, Drug Intell Clin Pharm 18(3):244.

Feldman, E.G. & Davidson, D.E. (1986) Handbook of Nonprescription Drugs, ed. 8. Washington: American Pharmaceutical Association and The National Professional Society of Pharmacists.

Fuller, E. (1985) Helping patients pick cold remedies, Patient Care 19(15):24.

Gilman, A.G. and others (1985) Goodman & Gillman's The Pharmacological Basis of Therapeutics, ed. 7. New York: Macmillan Publishing Company.

Griffin, J.W. Jr. (1984) H2-blocker update . . . success of H2-receptor antagonists in ulcer disease, Hosp Formul 19(11):1032.

Kastrup, E.K. & Olin, B.R. (1987) Facts and Comparisons, Drug Information. St. Louis: J.B. Lippincott Company.

Krupp, M.A. and others (Editors) (1987) Current Medical Diagnosis & Treatment 1987. Norwalk, Connecticut: Appleton & Lange.

Kuhn, J.J. et al. (1982) Antitussive effects of guaifenesin in young adults with natural colds, Chest 82(6):713.

Labson, L.H. (1984) Perennial problems: "Doctor, I can't stand this itching!", Patient Care 18(17):89.

Pepper, G.A. (1987) OTCs vs. Rx for allergic rhinitis, Nurse Pract 12(6):58.

Pepper, G.A. (1986) OTC vs. Rx for coughs and colds, Nurse Pract 11(10):66.

Rumore, M.M. (1984) Clinical pharmacokinetics of chlorpheniramine, Drug Intell Clin Pharm 18(9):701.

Ryerson, G.G. et al. (1983) Safe use of oxygen therapy: a physiologic approach, part 2, Respir Ther 13(2):25.

United States Pharmacopeial Convention. (1987) Drug Information for the Health Care Provider, ed. 7. Rockville: U.S. Pharmacopeial Convention, Inc.

Vincent, J.L. et al. (1984) Ketanserin, a serotonin antagonist: administration in patients with acute respiratory failure, Chest 85(4):510.

UNIT X

Drugs Affecting the Gastrointestinal System

CHAPTER 39

Overview of the Gastrointestinal Tract

OBJECTIVES

After studying this chapter, the student will be able to:

1. Identify the major parts of the gastrointestinal tract.
2. Describe the functions of individual components of the gastrointestinal tract.
3. List the effects of parasympathetic and sympathetic enervation on the gastrointestinal tract.
4. Describe common disorders affecting the gastrointestinal tract.

Gastrointestinal disorders are the most common of human problems. Since the cause of many gastrointestinal diseases remains unclear, pharmacologic management is often directed at relieving symptoms rather than at control or cure.

The gastrointestinal system itself (see Figure 39-1) is made up of the alimentary canal or digestive tract, the biliary system, and the pancreas.

The **alimentary canal** extends from the mouth to the anus. Food substances entering the canal undergo mechanical and chemical changes called **digestion.** These changes permit nutrients to be absorbed and undigestible materials to be excreted by the body. Absorbed nutrients may be used as an energy source or stored (glycogen for glucose or fat for carbohydrate). Movements by the smooth muscle fibers surrounding the canal (1) mix the contents by segmental contractions and (2) move the mass through the tract by peristalsis.

The secretory and muscular activities of the gastrointestinal system are regulated by neural mechanisms. An interconnecting network of neurons is located in smooth muscle and secretory cells. This system is self-regulating; it is capable of controlling exocrine gland secretions and muscular contractions without any external influence.

By contrast, the external innervation of the gastrointestinal system is supplied by the divisions of the autonomic nervous system. Their major function is to correlate activ-

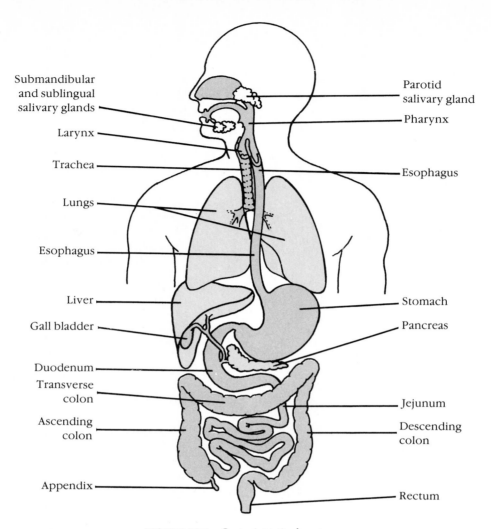

FIGURE 39-1 Gastrointestinal system.

ities between different regions of the gastrointestinal system and also between this system and other parts of the body.

The influence of the parasympathetic division is mediated by two branches of the vagus nerve. This division exerts an excitatory action, which increases digestive secretions and muscular activity. By contrast, the splanchnic nerves of the sympathetic division are primarily inhibitory, depressing digestive secretions and muscular activity. Under normal conditions, the two divisions of the autonomic nervous system maintain a delicate balance of control of functions.

Drugs affecting the gastrointestinal tract exert their action mainly on muscular and glandular tissues. The action may be directly on the smooth muscle and gland cells or indirectly on the autonomic nervous system. Drugs also may cause increased or decreased function, tone, emptying time, or peristaltic action of the stomach or bowel. In addition, they may be used to relieve enzyme deficiency, to counteract excess acidity or gas formation, to produce or prevent vomiting, or as diagnostic aids.

MOUTH (ORAL CAVITY)

The mouth, or oral cavity, is composed of the lips, cheeks, tongue, and hard and soft palates. The mouth functions as the starting point of the digestive process. Food is taken in, cut and ground between the teeth, and mixed with saliva. Saliva contains the enzyme amylase (ptyalin), which begins the process of chemical digestion.

Three pairs of salivary glands secrete saliva into ducts emptying into the mouth. The sublingual and submandibular salivary glands are located beneath the tongue; the largest pair, the parotid glands, are found in front of and slightly below the ears.

When the food bolus has been chewed and so mechanically reduced in the mouth, it is swallowed. Swallowing

(deglutition) is a complex process that begins as a voluntary movement but is continued as an involuntary muscular reflex as the food is propelled through the gastrointestinal tract.

Disorders affecting the mouth. Systemic diseases, nutritional deficiencies, and mechanical trauma can cause irritation or inflammation of buccal structures. Dental disorders (e.g., caries, gingivitis, and pyorrhea) and bacterial, viral, or fungal infections (e.g., candidiasis or herpes simplex) can affect the structures of the oral cavity, causing such symptoms as mouth blistering or other lesions, swelling, pain, and inflammation.

Agents acting on the oral cavity are discussed in Chapter 40.

PHARYNX

The pharynx (throat) is a tubelike passageway connecting the mouth and the esophagus. It is important in swallowing. Food and fluid pass through the pharynx into the esophagus. During this passage, the trachea is closed to prevent aspiration into the lungs.

Disorders affecting the pharynx. Like the mouth, the pharynx can be affected by various systemic diseases. It can become irritated and inflamed (e.g., from sinusitis or the "common cold") and treated symptomatically with an antiinflammatory agent. It can also become a locus of infection (e.g., with strep throat), requiring systemic antibiotic therapy.

ESOPHAGUS

The esophagus is a pliable muscular structure approximately 25 cm long that extends from the pharynx to the cardiac end of the stomach. It extends through the diaphragm as it drops from the thoracic cavity into the abdominal cavity.

The esophagus is considered the beginning of the digestive system proper, since the rest of the gastrointestinal tract organs function only in digestion and/or excretion.

The esophagus continues the process of swallowing and begins the **peristaltic process,** or the squeezing of the food bolus down the gastrointestinal tract by band contraction. The peristaltic band wave stimulates the lower esophageal sphincter, which closes to prevent gastroesophageal reflux and then returns the esophagus to its normal resting state.

Disorders affecting the esophagus. Esophageal disorders are characterized by retrosternal pain (heartburn) and difficulty in swallowing **(dysphagia).** The sources of the pain are numerous; some potential causes include diffuse esophageal spasm, achalasia, pyloric or duodenal ulcers, scleroderma, postural changes (bending forward), excessive alcohol ingestion, and nonspecific dysmotility.

However, heartburn commonly results from **reflux esophagitis,** in which the incompetent lower esophageal sphincter permits gastric contents to flow back into the esophagus, or from hiatal hernia, in which a part of the stomach protrudes into the diaphragm. One type of **hiatal hernia,** paraesophageal hernia, may be associated with esophageal obstruction and strangulation.

Difficulty in swallowing can be a symptom of esophageal obstruction, mechanical interference with or paralysis of the muscles of deglutition, neuromuscular incoordination, achalasia, carcinoma of the esophagus, anxiety states, hysteria, or schizophrenic hallucinations.

Inflammation of the esophagus can have many causes: reflux esophagitis associated with hiatal hernia, irritant ingestion, infection, peptic ulceration, prolonged gastric intubation, and uremia.

STOMACH

The stomach is a pouchlike structure lying below the diaphragm. It has three divisions: the fundus, the body, and the pylorus. Two sphincter muscles—the cardiac sphincter and the pyloric sphincter—regulate the stomach opening. Gastric glands secrete mucus and gastric juice, which is composed of enzymes and hydrochloric acid. They also produce intrinsic factor, a protein essential for absorption of vitamin B_{12}. Vitamin B_{12} in turn is needed for **erythropoiesis** (red blood cell formation).

The stomach functions as a temporary storage site for food as it is being digested. It also manufactures gastrin, a hormone that regulates enzyme production to facilitate digestion.

The stomachs of men and women differ, both in food storage capacity and size. Females have smaller and more slender stomachs. The stomach is capable of holding 1500 to 2000 ml. It distends after eating and gradually collapses as the food bolus moves out into the small intestine. Its churning action further breaks down the food bolus and mixes it with gastric juice to continue chemical digestion. A limited amount of nutrient and drug absorption takes place in the stomach.

The time required for digestion in the stomach depends on the amount of food eaten. Normal emptying time is 2 to 6 hours. However, the gastric emptying time may be affected by drug administration, physical activity of the individual, and body position during digestion. Gastric emptying time is a factor to consider in the timing of drug administration, since the presence of food may block the absorption of some drugs.

Disorders affecting the stomach. **Acute gastritis** is an inflammatory response of the stomach lining to ingestion of irritants, such as ethanol or nonsteroidal antiinflammatory agents, including aspirin. Symptoms include epigastric discomfort, nausea, abdominal tenderness, and gastrointestinal hemorrhage. Treatment consists of life-style modifications and drugs such as antacids, antiemetic agents, anticholinergics, and antihistamines (see Chapter 40).

Chronic gastritis is a degeneration of the gastric mucosa, but its causes are not well established. It is more common in women, and the incidence increases with age and excessive smoking and ethanol use. Symptoms are nonspecific but may include flatulence, epigastric fullness after meals, diarrhea, and bleeding. Treatment is the same as for acute gastritis.

Iron deficiency anemia and pernicious anemia may result from chronic gastritis. Treatment of symptoms with antacids, anticholinergics, and sedatives, as well as vitamin B_{12} if pernicious anemia is present, and elimination of possible causative or aggravating factors (e.g., aspirin use) comprise the usual therapeutic regimen.

Peptic ulcer disease is a broad term encompassing both gastric and duodenal ulcers. Although both types of ulcers produce a "break" in the gastric mucosa, the causes differ. With gastric ulcers, the ability of the gastric mucosa to protect and repair itself seems to be defective; in duodenal ulcers hypersecretion of gastric acid is responsible for the erosion of the gastric mucosa.

Duodenal ulcers are more common than gastric ulcers, accounting for nearly 80% of all peptic ulcers. Duodenal ulcers usually occur more frequently in younger persons. Overall, the reported incidence of peptic ulcers is much lower in females.

Pharmacologic treatment of peptic ulcer disease involves use of antacids, histamine-2 receptor antagonists, and sucralfate. However, nondrug treatment (diet and life-style modifications) are equally important. (See "Nursing considerations" in Chapter 40.) Hereditary factors, use of some drugs (e.g., aspirin and corticosteroids), psychic factors, stress, and diet have been implicated in the development of peptic ulcer disease.

LIVER

Immediately under the diaphragm and above the stomach is the largest gland in the body, the liver. It weighs approximately 1.5 kg. It is an extremely active and important organ that performs over 100 different functions.

The liver consists of two lobes composed of multitudes of lobules that function to remove toxins from the bloodstream, store nutrients such as iron and some vitamins, and secrete bile. Bile is transported, via the hepatic ducts, to the gallbladder for storage. In the intestine, bile aids in digestion, emulsification, and absorption of fat. Because it is normally alkaline, bile also functions to neutralize gastric acid in the duodenum.

Venous blood goes directly to the liver from the intestinal tract, so nutrients and absorbed drugs pass through the liver before reaching the systemic circulation. Thus the liver plays an active role in absorbing and metabolizing fats, carbohydrates, and proteins. It also stores vitamins A, B_{12}, and D and iron.

Some drugs are taken up by the liver, released into the bile, and then excreted in the feces. Other drugs move from the bile into the small intestine, where they are reabsorbed and recirculated. Still other drugs are transformed by the liver and excreted in the urine. In all of these cases the liver metabolizes the drug to make it more water soluble. This biotransformation changes the parent compound to a metabolite that may have greater, lesser, or equal activity. Cytochrome P-450 in the liver is responsible for biotransformation. There are also drugs that pass through the body and are secreted unchanged in the urine.

Disorders affecting the liver. Viral hepatitis, Laënnec's and postnecrotic cirrhosis, carcinoma, or chronic alcoholism causes damage to the liver and liver cell dysfunction.

GALLBLADDER

Lying on the undersurface of the liver is the gallbladder, a pear-shaped organ 7 to 10 cm long and 2.5 to 3.5 cm wide. The gallbladder can hold 30 to 50 ml of bile. It concentrates the bile and stores it until it is needed for digestion in the stomach and small intestine.

Disorders affecting the gallbladder. **Cholecystitis,** inflammation of the gallbladder, is often associated with the presence of gallstones **(cholelithiasis).** The stones lodge in the gallbladder neck or ducts, causing congestion and edema as bile builds up. This may be an acute or a chronic condition. Treatment of cholecystitis and cholelithiasis includes administration of analgesics, antispasmodics, and chenodeoxycholic acid.

Malignant tumors of the gallbladder are infrequent.

PANCREAS

The pancreas is a gland about 15 to 20 cm long and 5 cm wide. It weighs approximately 75 g. The gland has three major segments: the head (found in the curve of the duodenum), the body, and the tail (which touches or nearly touches the spleen). The role of the pancreas is twofold: the exocrine cells secrete the digestive enzymes found in pancreatic juice, and the endocrine cells help control carbohydrate metabolism with their production of glucagon and insulin.

Disorders affecting the pancreas. With the exception of diabetes mellitus, many pancreatic diseases have symptoms that are not readily diagnosed. Inflammation of the pancreas may be acute or chronic. Among the many causes are blockage of the pancreatic ducts, trauma to the pancreas, alcohol consumption, drug use, and tumors, cysts, or abscesses. Symptoms are nonspecific but ultimately include severe pain. Carcinoma of the pancreas is as difficult to diagnose as other pancreatic disorders.

SMALL INTESTINE

The small intestine is a coiled tube approximately 21 feet long. It consists of the duodenum, jejunum, and ileum. Within the small intestine the food bolus is thoroughly mixed with the digestive juices to complete the "breakdown" process. The intestinal mucosa then absorbs nutrients and drugs, which are filtered through the liver before entering the circulatory and lymphatic systems.

Disorders affecting the small intestine. Two disorders affecting the entire lower gastrointestinal tract are diarrhea and constipation. These are discussed in Chapter 41 along with the drugs used in their treatment.

Other disorders affecting the small intestine include obstruction, malabsorption syndrome, and blind loop syndrome. Symptomatic treatment is customary while the underlying causative factors are investigated.

LARGE INTESTINE

The cecum, colon, and rectum make-up the large intestine. The distal 2.5 cm of the rectum is known as the anal canal. The large intestine is approximately 5 feet long. It completes the digestive and absorptive processes. The large intestine is involved mainly with water absorption (from 1800 to 3000 ml/day) and synthesis of vitamin K. The lining of the large intestine secretes mucus to coat the undigested residue and protect the bowel lining. The undigestible residue is expelled through the reflex action known as **defecation.**

Disorders affecting the large intestine. Diarrhea and constipation, mentioned earlier and in Chapter 41, also affect the large intestine. Other disorders include diverticular disease, which has no specific therapy; ulcerative colitis, treated with life-style modifications, antidiarrheals, and steroids; carcinoma; and irritable bowel syndrome.

Hemorrhoids (varicosities of the external or internal hemorrhoidal veins) are common, with many kinds of drugs used in treatment (see Chapter 41).

KEY TERMS

alimentary canal, page 669
acute gastritis, page 671
cholecystitis, page 672
cholelithiasis, page 672
chronic gastritis, page 672
defecation, page 673
deglutition, page 671
digestion, page 669
dysphagia, page 671
erythropoiesis, page 671
hemorrhoids, page 673
hiatal hernia, page 671
peptic ulcer disease, page 672
peristaltic process, page 671
reflux esophagitis, page 671

BIBLIOGRAPHY

Berkow, R, editor-in-chief: The Merck manual, vol 1, ed 14, Rahway, NJ, 1982, Merck Sharp & Dohme Research Laboratories.

Bullock, BL, and Rosendahl, PP: Pathophysiology, Boston, 1984, Little, Brown & Co.

Diseases, The Nurse's Reference Library, Nursing 81 Books, Horsham, Penn, 1981, Intermed Communications, Inc.

Gitnick, MD, ed: Current gastroenterology, New York, 1984, John Wiley & Sons, Inc.

Given, BA, and Simmons, SJ: Gastroenterology in clinical nursing, ed 4, St Louis, 1984, The CV Mosby Co.

Price, SA, and Wilson, LM: Pathophysiology, ed 2, New York, 1982, McGraw-Hill Book Co.

Sleisenger, MH, and Fordtran, JS: Gastrointestinal disease: pathophysiology, diagnosis, management, Philadelphia, 1983, WB Saunders Co.

chapter 40

Drugs Affecting the Upper Gastrointestinal Tract

Drugs and Agents that Affect the Mouth

In general, drugs have little effect on the mouth. Good oral hygiene, which includes brushing properly after meals and at bedtime, flossing, and gum stimulation, has more influence on the tissues of the mouth than most medicines. Some clients may require more than two visits per year to their dentists for professional plaque removal. Many other mouth and throat preparations are available containing steroids, anesthetics, and antiseptics for various disorders of the oral cavity, including chapped lips, sun and fever blisters, inflammatory lesions, ulcerative lesions secondary to trauma, gingival lesions, teething pain, toothache, irritation caused by orthodontic appliances or dentures, and oral cavity abrasions.

MOUTHWASHES AND GARGLES

In 1984 Americans spent approximately $500 million for mouthwashes and gargles, a 10% increase over 1983. This increase is primarily a result of the introduction of products promoted to control plaque and reduce periodontal or gum disease.

Mouthwashes and gargles are dilute aromatic solutions that contain a sweetener and an artificial coloring agent. They may also contain an antiseptic (alcohol, cetylpyridinium chloride, phenol, povidone-iodine, carbamate peroxide), anesthetic (eugenol, clove oil), astringent (zinc chloride), and anticaries agent (sodium fluoride). Although several products claim to contain ingredients that reduce plaque formation, clinical trials have demonstrated success only with volatile oils and cetylpyridinium chloride alone or in combination with domiphene bromide. Commercial products that contain at least one of these active ingredients include Cepacol (cetylpyridinium chloride), Listerine (volatile oils), and Scope (cetylphyridinium chloride and domiphene bromide).

Mouthwashes are often used for **halitosis,** or "bad breath," or as gargles to treat colds or sore throats. They are generally not effective for such problems. Mouthwashes may improve mouth odor briefly, but if such a problem persists, the underlying cause needs to be identified and treated. For example, poor dental hygiene, various gum diseases, consumption of odorous products such as onions and garlic, postnasal drip, infections, tumors, diabetes, and many other disease states may produce bad breath.

Sore throats are usually caused by infection, most often viral rather than bacterial. Gargling cannot reach the site of infection, which is usually deep in the throat tissues. The FDA has prohibited manufacturers from claiming that their OTC products will prevent colds and sore throats or that the products will stop bad breath, because these are considered false claims (Cornacchia and Barrett, 1985).

Sodium chloride (½ tsp of salt to an 8-oz glass of warm water) has been recommended for use as a gargle and mouthwash. It is probably as effective, if not more effective, than some of the remedies sold today.

OXYGEN-RELEASING AGENTS

Hydrogen peroxide is a weak antibacterial agent used to clean wounds topically and orally. The antibacterial effect depends on the liberation of oxygen, which occurs when the peroxide comes in contact with the tissue enzyme **catalase.** The resulting **effervescence** (bubbling action) loosens pus and tissue debris, which helps reduce bacterial content. Hydrogen peroxide is usually used in a 1.5% to 3% solution for cleaning wounds or as a mouthwash. As a gargle, the 3% solution should be diluted with an equal amount of water before use.

A number of other oxygen-releasing products are commercially available. *Gly-oxide peroxide (Carbamide Peroxide)* in a 10% solution is used for treatment of canker sores, denture irritation, and irritation following orthodontic intervention. This preparation is applied directly to the affected area for a few minutes, and then the solution is expectorated.

Hydrogen peroxide gel (Peroxyl) is also available for minor mouth irritation and is applied and expectorated after use.

ALCOHOLIC MOUTHWASH WARNINGS

PEDIATRIC ALERT

The leading mouthwashes usually contain from 14% to 25% alcohol. Safety closures are not generally used with mouthwashes, so parents of young children should be cautioned to store such products (and drinking alcohol) in a safe area, preferably a locked cabinet. Young children appear to be extremely sensitive to alcohol-induced hypoglycemic effects; hypoglycemia requiring hospitalization has been reported after the consumption of only ½ to 1 oz of an alcoholic mouthwash in a 2-year-old (D'Arcy, 1985). The use of mouthwash in young children is not recommended since children often swallow the mouthwash rather than expectorate it after use.

ADULT USE

It is reported that 10% to 15% of alcoholics in detoxification units use nonbeverage alcohol (mouthwashes, hair tonics, and aftershave lotions with high alcohol contents) as a substitute for alcohol. Such products are easily accessible. Be alert for ingestion abuse of alcohol-containing external products (Egbert and others, 1985).

ANTIGINGIVITIS PRODUCT

An oral rinse containing 0.12% chlorhexidine gluconate (Peridex) was the first product approved for prevention of gingivitis. It has received the American Dental Association Council of Therapeutics' seal of acceptance for control of plaque and gingivitis (FDC Report, 1986).

FLUORIDATED MOUTHWASH

A number of fluoride-containing preparations, including mouthwash (Fluorigard), toothpaste, tablets, and solutions, are available for use as anticaries agents. The exact mechanism of action of fluoride in preventing caries is not fully understood; however, fluoride ions appear to exchange for hydroxyl or citrate (anion) ions and then settle in the anionic space in the surface of the enamel (Goodman and Gilman, 1985). This results in a harder outer layer of tooth enamel that is more resistant to demineralization.

Mouthwashes are generally used once a day (rinsed for a minute and expectorated), usually after brushing and flossing. Fluoridated mouthwashes have been used in communities with both limited fluoridated and unflouridated water supplies, and their use has been associated with a significant decrease in tooth decay. Such products are generally approved by the Council on Dental Therapeutics of the American Dental Association, and the packages bear its seal of approval.

ANTISEPTIC MOUTHWASH

Chloraseptic mouthwash contains phenol and sodium phenolate, which act as antimicrobial and anesthetic agents. In spray form, it is reported effective for treatment of sore throat (Gossel, 1986). It provides surface anesthesia when this is indicated for oropharyngeal discomfort, and it maintains oral hygiene. It is diluted with equal parts of water or sprayed full strength.

DENTIFRICES

A **dentifrice** is a substance used to aid in cleaning teeth. Ordinary dentifrice contains one or more mild abrasives, a foaming agent, and flavoring materials made into a powder or paste (toothpaste) to be used as an aid in the mechanical cleansing of accessible parts of the teeth.

The following ingredients, alone or mixed, are found in a number of dentifrices:

Glycerin	Pumice (flour)
Alcohol	Stannous fluoride
Sweetening agents	Soap
Propylene glycol	Sodium borate
Precipitated calcium carbonate	Milk of magnesia

The essential requirement of a toothpaste or cleaner is that it not injure the teeth or surrounding tissues. If toothpaste is not available, the patient can use a toothbrush and proper flossing techniques, since thorough mechanical cleansing of bacterial plaques and food debris is the primary objective.

Fluoride (stannous fluoride and sodium monofluorophosphate) dentifrices are effective anticaries agents. These products carry the American Dental Association Council on Dental Therapeutics seal to indicate its endorsement.

Dentifrices are also available for the treatment of hypersensitive teeth. Such products contain strontium chloride (Sensodyne, Thermodent) or potassium nitrate (Promise, Denquel). These products are not generally accepted as effective by the American Dental Association.

Others are said to remove or reduce the formation of tartar (calculus or plaque). Studies have not yet proven their effectiveness.

DRUGS USED TO TREAT ORAL INFECTION, INFLAMMATION, OR IRRITATION

nystatin (Mycostatin, Nilstat, Nadostine✸)
clotrimazole (Mycelex-G, Canesten, Myclo)

Mechanism of action. Nystatin is believed to attach to sterols in the fungal wall, increasing permeability of the cell membrane and resulting in loss of important cellular contents. Clotrimazole has the same action as nystatin. It inhibits oxidative enzyme activity, which may increase intracellular hydrogen peroxide to toxic levels and thus contribute to the destruction of the fungal cells and their contents. In addition, it inhibits fungal synthesis of triglycerides and phospholipids.

Indications. Nystatin and clotrimazole are used to treat oropharyngeal candidiasis.

Pharmacokinetics. Nystatin is not absorbed in the gastrointestinal tract and is excreted in the feces.

Orally, clotrimazole is poorly absorbed. When absorbed, it is metabolized in the liver to an inactive substance. Duration of action is approximately 3 hours. Excretion is fecal.

Side effects/adverse reactions. The most commonly reported side effects of clotrimazole and nystatin are nausea, vomiting, abdominal pain, and diarrhea.

Significant drug interactions. No interactions of clotrimazole or nystatin with other drugs have been reported.

Dosage and administration

Nystatin. Adults and children are given 400,000 to 600,000 units four times daily. Oral suspension should be swished in the mouth and retained as long as possible before swallowing. Lozenges should be allowed to dissolve slowly in the mouth (not for children under 5 years old).

FLUORIDE TOXICITY

Fluoride is capable of producing an acute toxic reaction that may be fatal if not treated promptly. A chronic toxic state resulting in mottling or discoloration of the tooth enamel and possible osteosclerosis has been reported. This effect may occur when excessive fluoride is consumed during childhood. In severe cases, the teeth appear as brown- to black-stained corroded areas. Fluoridated water supplies usually contain 1 ppm (part per million) of fluoride, which is accepted as a safe level that is effective in reducing the incidence of caries in permanent teeth. Health care professionals need to be aware of the amount of fluoride in their water supplies and to closely supervise the use of additional fluoride products by their clients.

Clotrimazole. Adults: one lozenge (10 mg) dissolved completely in mouth five times daily. Children over 4 years: see adult dosage. Children under 4 years: dosage not established.

Pregnancy safety. FDA category C

NURSING CONSIDERATIONS

Assessment. Improperly fitting dentures can be a source of inflammation.

Patients who have cancer or are taking immunosuppressive drugs, such as steroids, are particularly at risk for oral candidiasis.

Intervention. Brush teeth or have client brush teeth carefully before each dose is administered.

For infants and dependent patients, gently swab the medication on the oral mucosa.

When administering the oral suspension, shake well to ensure consistency in dosing. Protect the suspension from freezing. When preparing the oral suspension from powder, shake well and use immediately, since it contains no preservatives.

To improve retention within the mouth, nystatin can be administered in the form of flavored frozen water on a stick.

The nystatin vaginal tablet may also be used as a lozenge since its slow rate of dissolution prolongs contact with the oral mucosa.

Education. Instruct the client in good oral hygiene techniques. Inform the client that a yearly dental examination is recommended.

When using the suspension forms of nystatin, instruct the client to swish the medication around in the mouth and maintain contact with the mucosa for several minutes before swallowing. The client may also gargle the solution.

Provide a careful explanation to the client using the troche form (clotrimazole) that it is to be dissolved slowly (15 to 30 minutes) in the mouth. It is not to be chewed or swallowed whole. The client is to swallow the saliva. The troche may be cut in half to facilitate administration.

Instruct the client to continue the medicine for the full time of prescription and report to the prescriber if symptoms persist.

Before an initial course of antineoplastic chemotherapy, instruct the client to consult a dentist to complete any care needed, to avoid oral complications.

Evaluation. Instruct the client to continue therapy for 48 hours after symptoms have disappeared to prevent relapse.

Assess and document daily the size and condition of the affected areas of the mouth, using a tongue blade and flashlight.

ketoconazole (Nizoral)

Ketoconazole is a systemic antifungal agent that is also used in the treatment of oral fungal infections. See Chapter 60 for a complete discussion and nursing considerations.

SALIVA SUBSTITUTES

Saliva substitutes (Orex, Xero-Lube, Moi-stir, Salivart) are used to overcome dry mouth and throat. They are available as solutions in squirt bottles and as pump or aerosol sprays. They contain electrolytes (potassium phosphate, magnesium chloride, potassium chloride, calcium, and sodium), sodium fluoride, sorbitol, and carboxymethylcellulose as the base.

DRUGS USED TO TREAT MOUTH BLISTERING

Acute and chronic diseases contribute to mouth blistering and erosions. Acute viral diseases such as herpes simplex, herpes zoster, herpangina, and varicella have previously been treated only symptomatically. With the advent of acyclovir (Zovirax), a new era began with an antiviral agent that is effective against herpes simplex virus and varicella zoster virus, the viruses associated with skin manifestations. Acyclovir is available in topical, oral, and parenteral dosage forms and is covered in Chapter 60.

Skin blistering may also be caused by drug therapy (fixed or acute erythema multiforme types); in these cases treatment is directed at the underlying cause.

Mouth lesions or blistering (acute or chronic) may be caused by local irritation, medications, radiation, dental manipulations, or systemic disease. To properly treat, one must first identify the causative factor and then institute appropriate treatment.

Drugs that Affect the Stomach

Conditions of the stomach requiring drug therapy include hyperacidity, hypoacidity, ulcer disease, nausea, vomiting, and hypermotility. Some of the drugs used for these conditions are not unique in their treatment of gastric dysfunction but are members of other major groups of drugs, such an anticholinergic preparations, antihistamines, and antidepressants.

DRUGS USED TO TREAT GASTRIC HYPERACIDITY
ANTACIDS

Mechanism of action. Antacids are chemical compounds that buffer or neutralize hydrochloric acid in the stomach and thereby increase the gastric pH. The major ingredients in antacids include aluminum salts, calcium carbonate, magnesium salts, and sodium bicarbonate, alone or in combination.

Traditionally, the antacids have been termed nonsystemic or systemic. Nonsystemic indicates the almost negligible amount of drug absorbed into the circulation; activity occurs only locally within the gastrointestinal tract. The nonsystemic metal ion, however, is absorbed to some degree. The aluminum ion is absorbed the most and magnesium the least; calcium is absorbed slightly more than magnesium. Increased adverse effects from metal ion absorption occur in the presence of impaired renal function and long-term excessive use of calcium carbonate and magnesium hydroxide.

Indications. Antacids are indicated for the relief of symptoms associated with hyperacidity related to the diagnosis of peptic ulcer, gastritis, peptic esophagitis, gastric hyperacidity, heartburn, or hiatal hernia. The selection of an antacid is usually based on the following:

1. It must be an effective neutralizer of hydrochloric acid.
2. It should be relatively harmless to the client.
3. It should not produce diarrhea or constipation.
4. It should be economical and palatable, to improve patient compliance.

Pharmacokinetics. Antacids generally have a rapid onset of action. Their effects usually last 30 to 60 minutes, although magnesium compounds may have a prolonged effect. Only a small amount of the metal compound is absorbed (15% to 30%). The remainder is broken down via the digestive process and excreted via the feces.

Side effects/adverse reactions. See Table 40-1.

Significant drug interactions. The following interactions may occur when antacids are given with the drugs listed below.

Drug	Possible Effect and Management
ketoconazole	Increased gastric pH may decrease absorption of ketoconazole. Advise patients to take antacids at least several hours after ketoconazole.
mecamylamine	Effects of mecamylamine may be prolonged because an alkaline urine decreases its excretion. Concurrent administration should be avoided.
methenamine	An alkaline urine may decrease methenamine's effectiveness by prohibiting its conversion to formaldehyde. Concurrent administration is not recommended.
tetracyclines, oral	Antacids may complex with tetracyclines, decreasing their absorption in the gastrointestinal tract. Advise patients to take antacids at least 1 to 2 hours before or after tetracycline.
digitalis preparations	Antacids may decrease absorption of digitalis preparations, resulting in a decrease in serum concentration of digitalis. Space medications by at least 1 to 2 hours.

Drug	Possible Effect and Management
ion-exchange resin (e.g., sodium polystyrene sulfonate)	If aluminum-containing antacids are administered with an ion-exchange resin, the resin may also bind calcium and magnesium, producing anion absorption (as bicarbonate) and creating systemic alkalosis. This may be avoided by rectal administration of the resin.
phenothiazine	Magnesium trisilicate, aluminum hydroxide, and magnesium hydroxide gel antacids decrease plasma phenothiazine levels by decreasing absorption.
indomethacin	Indomethacin is adsorbed by antacids and kaolin, delaying the concentration peak and reducing bioavailability when administered simultaneously with antacids.
levodopa	Absorption of levodopa is increased threefold when antacid is given simultaneously, because raising the pH increases gastric emptying, placing more levodopa in the duodenum where it is absorbed readily. Therefore relapse or toxicity may occur if the client begins to use antacids while being treated with levodopa.
isoniazid	Aluminum antacids interfere with the absorption of isoniazid. Separate the administration of these drugs over 1 hour or administer a nonaluminum-containing antacid to prevent this interaction.
propranolol	Propranolol is significantly decreased in absorption when given with antacid gels. These drugs should be administered several hours apart.

Altered drug solubility, stability, and absorption with antacids. Many drugs are either weak acids or weak bases, and the pH of the stomach is an important factor in their absorption. Drugs that are weak acids are nonionized in the acidic environment of the stomach. These are lipid soluble and are absorbed by simple diffusion across the gastric mucosal cells. The administration of an antacid either with a weak acidic drug or shortly before or after its administration will raise the pH of the stomach contents, causing the formation of a more ionized drug that will not be absorbed to the degree the nonionized, lipid-soluble form was absorbed. A weakly basic drug is absorbed in a more alkaline medium. Changes in pH will modify drug solubility and stability, which also affect absorption.

As the pH of the gastric contents increases, alterations of absorption of weak acids and bases occur as a result of altering the degree of ionization in the following manner: for basic drugs absorption increases because as the pH increases as a result of antacid administration there is an increase in the nonionized concentration of basic drugs; for acidic drugs absorption decreases because as the pH increases there is a decrease in the nonionized concentration of acidic drugs.

Drugs that are weak bases include morphine sulfate, quinine, pseudoephedrine, antihistamines, amphet-

TABLE 40-1.   Antacid Side Effects/Adverse Reactions

Name	Side effects/adverse reactions
Aluminum aluminum carbonate (Basaljel) aluminum hydroxide (Alterna-GEL, Alu-Cap, Alu-Tab, Amphojel, Dialume) aluminum phosphate (Phosphaljel) aluminum/magnesium compounds (Aludrox, Gaviscon, Gelusil-M, Maalox, Mylanta)	Constipation (combination products with magnesium reduce this) Phosphate depletion via feces (including weakness, apnea, hemolytic anemia, tetany) Delay in gastric emptying Concretions (intestinal and renal) Encephalopathy from aluminum intoxication Impaired absorption of drugs such as digitalis, isoniazid, tetracycline Dialysis "dementia" (from CNS accumulation) Bone demineralization (osteomalacia, osteoporosis)
Bicarbonate sodium bicarbonate (Alka-Seltzer, Instant Metamucil)	Systemic alkalosis or sodium overload (elevated plasma pH and carbon dioxide, anorexia, mental confusion) Gastric acid hypersecretion ("acid rebound") Enhanced effects of amphetamines, quinidine, quinine
Calcium calcium carbonate (Tums)	Milk-alkali syndrome (including metabolic alkalosis, anorexia, nausea, vomiting, confusion, hypercalcemia, possibly renal impairment) Increased potential for calcium stone formation Nephrocalcinosis Gastric acid hypersecretion ("acid rebound") Antagonism of digitalis preparations Elevated serum and urine calcium levels Kidney failure Constipation Decreased phosphate levels (if dietary phosphate intake low)
Magnesium magnesium hydroxide (Milk of Magnesia) magnesium trisilicate	Diarrhea (combination products with aluminum reduce this) Decreased potassium levels (hypokalemia) Increased magnesium levels (hypermagnesemia) in clients with renal failure or severe kidney impairment (causing low blood pressure, nausea, vomiting, respiratory depression, CNS depression, coma)
Sodium sodium bicarbonate	Sodium overload or systemic alkalosis Salt and water retention (causing edema, ascites, effusion, hypertension) Metabolic alkalosis Milk-alkali syndrome (see under calcium) Gastric acid hypersecretion ("acid rebound")

amines, theophylline, tricyclic antidepressants, and quinidine. Examples of weak acids are isoniazid, barbiturates, nalidixic acid, nonsteroidal antiinflammatory agents, sulfonamides, salicylates, nitrofurantoin, and coumarins.

Additional drug interactions. Because antacids change the pH of the stomach, they cause the medication in enteric-coated tablets to be released into the stomach instead of the alkaline duodenum.

Dosage and administration. The amount of antacid necessary to neutralize hydrochloric acid depends on the individual, the condition being treated, and the buffering capability of the preparation used. The acid-neutralizing property of antacids varies, so the physician must select the proper dosage for the individual client.

The liquid and powder dosage forms have been found to be much more effective antacids than the tablet dosage formulations. Most tablets require chewing before swallowing to be effective.

Most major antacids contain 10 mg or less of sodium per recommended adult dose. Examples of antacids containing more than 10 mg per recommended adult dose include:

Alka-Seltzer Effervescent Pain Reliever & Antacid	551 mg sodium/tablet
Alka-Seltzer Effervescent Antacid	296 mg sodium/tablet
Bisodol Antacid Powder	157 mg sodium/tsp
Gaviscon Oral Suspension	12.9 mg sodium/5 ml
Gaviscon Chewable Tablets	19 mg sodium/tablet
Gaviscon-2 Chewable Tablets	36.8 mg sodium/tablet
Rolaids	53 mg sodium/tablet

Antacids given before meals have a duration of action of approximately 30 minutes (range 20 to 60 minutes). If the antacid is given after meals the duration may be prolonged up to 3 hours.

Specific recommendations. Duodenal ulcers require 75 to 150 mg of acid-neutralizing effect; gastric ulcers usually require 40 to 80 mEq (see Table 40-2; Zaenger, 1981).

TABLE 40-2   Acid-Neutralizing Capacity of Antacids

Antacids	Ingredients	Acid-neutralizing capacity	Dose to neutralize 80 mEq HCl
LIQUID PREPARATIONS			
		mEq/ml	*ml needed*
Aludrox	AlOH, MgOH	2.8	28
Amphojel	AlOH	1.9	42
Gelusil		2.4	33
Gelusil-II	AlOH, MgOH, simethicone	4.8	16.6
Gelusil-M		3	26.6
Maalox		2.7	29.6
Maalox Plus	AlOH, MgOH (plus: simethicone)	2.7	29.6
Maalox TC		5.7	14
Mylanta	AlOH, MgOH, simethicone	2.5	32
Mylanta-II		5.1	15.6
Phosphalgel	AlPO$_4$	0.4	200
TABLET PREPARATIONS			
		mEq per tablet	*Tablets needed*
Gelusil Chewable	AlOH, MgOH, simethicone	11	7.3
Gelusil-II Chewable		21	3.8
Maalox No. 1 Chewable		8.5	9.4
Maalox No. 2 Chewable	AlOH, MgOH	18	4.4
Maalox Plus Chewable		11.4	7
Mylanta Chewable	AlOH, MgOH, simethicone	11.5	7
Mylanta II Chewable		23	3.5
Riopan Tablet		13.5	5.9
Riopan Chewable Tablet	magaldrate (plus: simethicone)	13.5	5.9
Riopan Plus Chewable Tablet		13.5	5.9
Rolaids	Dihydroxyaluminum sodium carbonate	8	10
Titralac Tablet	Calcium carbonate, glycine	7.5	10.7

Adapted from Zaenger, P: Fl J Hosp Pharm 1(1):1, 1981; and Kutsop, JJ: Am Pharmacy N524(12):778, 1984.

The FDA has set a limit of 8 g/day as a recommended maximum dose for calcium carbonate, for a maximum period of 2 weeks. This is equivalent to 16 Tums tablets per day or approximately 10 Tums Extra Strength per day. Since Tums are frequently used for calcium supplementation as well as for an antacid, it is believed that many people exceed the FDA's recommendations, thus increasing the potential for producing many of the side effects or adverse reactions discussed.

Pregnancy safety. Antacids are generally considered safe if prolonged or high doses are avoided. FDA category is not established.

NURSING CONSIDERATIONS

Assessment. Do not give magnesium salts to clients in renal failure without careful assessment; if given, use low doses (50 mEq magnesium/day) under close monitoring and physician's supervision.

Intervention. The scheduling of dosing of antacid therapy is important. Antacids given immediately after meals will delay gastric emptying and the buffering effect. When given at 1 and 3 hours after meals and at bedtime, the gastric pH remains at about 3 throughout the day. Because of their ability to interact with numerous medications, scheduling in relation to other medications should be considered. Administer antacids 1 hour before or 2 hours after digoxin, tetracyclines, phenothiazines, and all enteric-coated medications. However, antacids combined with ibuprofen, indomethacin, phenylbutazone, potassium chloride supplements, reserpine, sulindac, and tolmetin can help to reduce the gastric distress that these drugs can cause.

Shake liquid preparations vigorously before administration to achieve a uniform suspension. When administering antacids via a nasogastric tube, assess the placement and patency of the tube before giving the medication and follow the dose with sufficient water to clear the tube.

Refrigerate antacids to make them more palatable. (Do not freeze.)

Do not administer calcium carbonate antacids with milk, milk products, or other foods or vitamin supplements high in vitamin D, since milk-alkali syndrome may occur.

Education. Discuss the sodium content and side effects of various antacids with the client (see p. 679). Inform clients that antacids differ in their sodium content, which can be significant for clients who are on low-sodium diets or who take antihypertensive drugs or diuretics. Instruct clients with hypertensive, cardiac, or renal disease to avoid antacids containing sodium, particularly if antacids are used frequently.

Inform clients that liquid antacids have superior neutralizing properties compared with tablets. However, clients who must frequently take liquid antacids may lose their desire for food or drink. For this reason chewable tablets followed by adequate water may be of value.

Instruct clients taking chewable antacid tablets to chew or pulverize the tablets thoroughly. The tablets will not mix well with water. A sip of water or milk will facilitate swallowing of tablets.

Stress compliance to antacid therapy schedules. Allow clients to take their own antacids while they are hospitalized to encourage compliance.

Caution clients about side effects, and instruct them to consult their physician if these occur.

Teach clients to check the expiration dates of the antacids, since the effectiveness of antacids decreases with age.

Teach clients to carefully check the name when purchasing OTC antacids. Names may be similar (Mylanta versus Mylanta II, Gelusil versus Gelusil II), but dosage requirements will differ.

Advise clients who self-medicate with antacids for recurring gastrointestinal symptoms to seek medical care, since they are treating the symptoms rather than the cause of the problem. Since antacids are all OTC drugs and there is no medically supervised restriction, clients may abuse or misuse antacids through self-medication.

Help clients to identify the source of gastric discomfort, such as overeating, tension, anxiety, or other emotional stress, since this may teach them to avoid the causes of discomfort and eliminate the need for antacid therapy.

Evaluation. Note the frequency and consistency of stools. If diarrhea occurs, it may be advantageous to change to another antacid, such as magnesium hydroxide with magnesium trisilicate or aluminum hydroxide. If constipation occurs, a magnesium hydroxide antacid or an increase in the intake of bran and roughage in the diet may be instituted.

Assess epigastric discomfort at the time of each dose and record the client's progress. Evaluation of antacid therapy is important. The client's subjective response to antacid therapy and the nurse's objective observations (e.g., frequency with which the client takes the antacid) can help determine the effectiveness of therapy. Monitor clients undergoing long-term aluminum antacid therapy regularly for serum phosphate levels.

Antacid Combinations

There are many antacid combinations; however, the antacid combination Gaviscon deserves particular attention because of its uniqueness and widespread use.

gaviscon

Gaviscon forms a viscous cohesive foam that floats on the surface of the stomach contents, neutralizing stomach acid. This helps protect the sensitive mucosa from irritation, because the foam precedes the stomach contents into the lower esophagus when reflux occurs.

The foam is caused by the alginic acid contained in the product. The other ingredients are aluminum hydroxide, magnesium trisilicate, and sodium bicarbonate. Gaviscon is available in two tablet strengths and a liquid suspension.

ANTIFLATULENTS

simethicone (Mylicon, Silain, Orol❀)

Simethicone acts in the stomach and intestines. This defoaming agent relieves flatulence by dispersing and preventing the formation of mucus-surrounded gas pockets in the gastrointestinal tract.

The approved clinical use is for relief of painful symptoms of gas in the gastrointestinal tract. Gas retention is a problem in conditions such as air swallowing, diverticulitis, functional dyspepsia, peptic ulcer, postoperative gaseous distention, and spastic or irritable colon.

The tablets are chewed thoroughly four times daily, after meals and at bedtime, and as needed for flatulence. Several antacid combination products contain simethicone.

DIGESTANTS

Digestants are drugs that promote the process of digestion in the gastrointestinal tract. Problems with digestion may be caused by a deficiency of hydrochloric acid, digestive substances, enzymes, or bile salts; organic disease states (stomach cancer, pernicious anemia, cholecystectomy); or possibly a reaction to emotional situations or stress.

Dilute hydrochloric acid (10% solution) was formerly used as a digestant but is rarely prescribed today. Instead betaine hydrochloride or glutamic acid hydrochloride (Acidulin) may be ordered. These preparations, available as tablets or capsules, usually release only a small amount of free hydrochloric acid in the stomach, but this is usually sufficient to treat many cases of gastric **achlorhydria** (the absence of hydrochloric acid). They must be given with a full glass of water.

Digestive enzymes are secreted by the mouth, stomach, small intestine, pancreas, and liver. They are necessary to process the digestion of food.

Pepsin is the stomach enzyme that reduces protein to smaller particles. It can be given alone or in combination with a hydrochloric acid source in hypochlorhydric or achlorhydric clients. Hydrochloric acid keeps the gastric pH below 4 and protects the proteolytic activity of pepsin. A pH of 1.5 to 2.5 is usually the optimal range. Pepsin is not considered a critial enzyme, because proteolytic enzymes released from the pancreas and intestine cause the same effects.

pancreatin

Pancreatin is a powdered substance obtained from the pancreas of the hog or ox. It contains principally pancreatic amylase, trypsin, and pancreatic lipase. Acid chyme entering the duodenum and vagal stimulation regulate pancreatic secretion, so that replacement therapy may be necessary for patients who have had vagal fibers surgically severed or surgical procedures that cause food to bypass the duodenum. Pancreatin and pancrelipase aid in the digestion and absorption of fats, carbohydrates, and triglycerides. In addition, replacement therapy is usually necessary in exocrine pancreatic enzyme deficiency states, chronic pancreatitis, cystic fibrosis, pancreatic tumors, pancreatic obstruction, and pancreatectomy. The drug is available in enteric-coated capsules to avoid destruction in the stomach.

The dosage for adults is 325 mg to 1 g daily in divided doses before meals, during meals, or within 1 hour after meals, with an extra dose taken with any food eaten between meals. In high doses this drug may cause nausea, diarrhea, hyperuricosuria, and hyperuricemia. To avoid temporary indigestion the client must maintain a dietary balance of fat, protein, and starch.

pancrelipase (Cotazym, Pancrease, Viokase, Ilozyme)

Pancrelipase is similar to other pancreatic enzyme preparations, but its lipase activity is greater and it can be given in lower doses to control **steatorrhea** (fatty stools). It is a concentrate of pancreatic enzymes from hogs. The dosage for adults is one to three capsules or tablets or one or two packets before or with meals or snacks. In extreme deficiency the dosage interval may be changed to hourly if no nausea or diarrhea develops. Because of its enteric-coated microsphere formulation, Pancrease resists gastric inactivation, so enzymes reach the duodenum to hydrolyze fats into glycerol and fatty acids, proteins into proteases, and starch into dextrins and sugars.

Indications
1. For use in clients with deficient secretion of exocrine pancreatic enzymes
2. For use as an enzyme replacement in cystic fibrosis, chronic pancreatitis, postpancreatectomy, pancreatic duct obstructions secondary to pancreatic carcinoma, and pancreatic insufficiency; and for the steatorrhea of malabsorption syndrome and following gastrectomy.

Side effects/adverse reactions. Nausea, abdominal cramps, and loose stool are possible side effects of pancrelipase.

Significant drug interactions. Calcium and magnesium antacids negate pancrelipase enzyme action. Serum iron response to oral iron therapy is decreased by pancreatic extracts.

Dosage and administration. One to three capsules or tablets are given before or with meals and snacks. Dose may be increased to 8 in cases of severe deficiency if no nausea, cramps, or diarrhea results. With the powder form 0.7 g is given with meals.

Pregnancy safety.

NURSING CONSIDERATIONS

Instruct the client to swallow enteric-coated tablets whole; do not crush or chew them.

Because pancretin is inactivated by gastric pepsin and acid pH, cimetidine or antacids (except for those containing calcium and magnesium) may be prescribed to be taken with it.

For children or adults who cannot swallow the capsules or tablets, sprinkle the powder from the opened capsule or the powdered form on food.

Instruct the client on the rationale for taking the pancreatic enzyme preparations. Also instruct client not to stop taking the medication without physician approval. Urge the client to adhere to the prescribed diet, since the dosage for pancrelipase is individualized and determined by the client's maldigestion and malabsorption and the fat content of the diet.

If capsules need to be opened to be administered, advise client to be careful not to spill the contents on hands or to inhale them, since this substance is very irritating to nasal membranes, respiratory tract, and skin. If side effects occur, have the client contact the physician.

ANTIEMETICS

Antiemetics are drugs given to relieve nausea and vomiting. Control of vomiting is important and often difficult. Numerous preparations have been used, but effective treatment usually depends on treating the cause. Vomiting may result from very different causes, including strong emotion, severe pain, increased intracranial pressure, and labyrinthine disturbances. Other causes include motion sickness, endocrine disturbances, toxic reaction to drugs, gastrointestinal disease, roentgenographic treatments, and chemotherapy.

Antiemetics may exert their effects on the vomiting center, the cerebral cortex, the chemoreceptor trigger zone, or the aural vestibular apparatus.

The following drugs are used as antiemetics:
1. Anticholinergics, such as scopolamine, reduce the excitability of labyrinth receptors, depress conduction in the vestibular cerebellar pathways, or prevent impulses from stimulating the chemoreceptor trigger zone.

2. Antihistamines H_1 affect neural labyrinth pathways. Examples include cyclizine (Marezine), dimenhydrinate (Dramamine), and diphenhydramine (Benadryl).

3. Phenothiazines, such as chlorpromazine and promethazine, and metoclopramide are dopamine antagonists. They act on the chemoreceptor trigger zone and on the vomiting center. These are the most effective antiemetics and often the drugs of choice.

4. Antacids relieve gastric irritation.

5. Miscellaneous drugs include diphenidol (Vontrol), which acts on the aural vestibular apparatus, and benzquinamide (Emete-Con), which acts on the chemoreceptor trigger zone. Steroids (dexamethasone, methylprednisolone) and cannabinoids (nabilone, THC) are also used.

Most of the drugs are discussed elsewhere in the text (see Index).

EMETIC (VOMITING) REFLEX

The **emetic center** is located in the medulla oblongata. Smells, various sights, and psychologically based responses from the cerebral cortex may all stimulate the emetic center. Disturbances of the stomach and of the vestibular apparatus can also activate the emetic center (see Figure 40-1). These stimuli involve vagal and/or sympathetic afferent nerve transmission. Dopamine is a primary neurotransmitter.

A chemoreceptor trigger zone is a relay station that can send messages to the emetic center. The chemoreceptor trigger zone detects irritating chemicals in the blood or cerebrospinal fluid. In itself, the chemoreceptor trigger zone is not able to induce vomiting.

Since the chemoreceptor trigger zone is located close to the respiratory center in the brain, it is difficult to completely control vomiting initiated from this site without affecting respiration. Various neurotransmitters are involved in this area. The cerebral cortex area is involved in anticipatory nausea and vomiting, that is, a conditioned response caused by a stimulus connected with a previous unpleasant experience. For example, a client receiving cancer chemotherapy that has resulted in vomiting might vomit at the sight of the hospital, even before treatment is given (Bergmann, 1986).

If the emetic center is activated by any of the stimuli mentioned, it sends impulses (via efferent nerves) to the diaphragm, stomach muscles, esophagus, and salivary glands, resulting in vomiting.

The proposed sites of action for antiemetics are reported in the box (Bergmann, 1986; Grunberg, 1982).

CANCER CHEMOTHERAPY–INDUCED VOMITING

Vomiting from cancer chemotherapy can be serious enough to limit the dosages of chemotherapeutic agents given to a client. Since antiemetics are usually more effective in preventing vomiting than they are in treating it, they should be administered prophylactically, before the

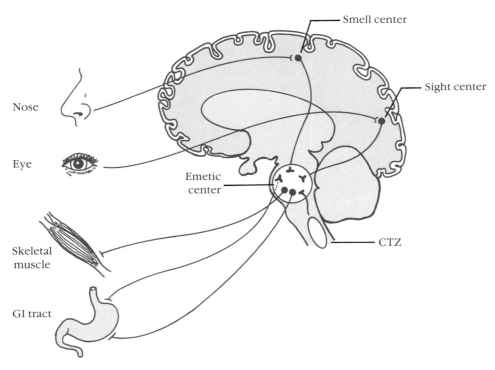

FIGURE 40-1 Sites activating the emetic center. *CTZ*, Chemoreceptor trigger zone.

PROPOSED SITES OF ACTION FOR ANTIEMETIC DRUGS

PROPOSED SITES	DRUGS
Emetic center	anticholinergic
	antihistamines
	thiethylperazine maleate*
Chemorecep- tor trigger zone	benzquinamide hydrochloride
	butyrophenones
	diphenidol hydrochloride*
	metoclopramide*
	phenothiazine
	thiethylperazine maleate*
	trimethobenzamide HCl
Cerebral cor- tex	cannabinoids (THC), nabilone (Cesa- met♣), dronabinol (Marinol)
	diazepam, lorazepam
	scopolamine*
	antihistamines
Peripheral	diphenidol hydrochloride*
	metoclopramide*
	scopolamine*
Unknown	corticosteroids

*Dual action.

chemotherapy administration. Also, chemotherapy-induced vomiting often requires several antiemetic agents with different sites of action for effectiveness—for example, metoclopramide and lorazepam; metoclopramide and dexamethasone; or prochlorperazine and dexamethasone (Bergmann, 1986). Combinations of rectal antiemetic suppositories are also under investigation.

NURSING CONSIDERATIONS

Assessment. Do not give antiemetics until the underlying cause of nausea has been established. For example, overdosage of drugs or increased intracranial pressure may cause nausea.

If antiemetic therapy is unavailable or cannot be given, provide a quiet environment, make the client comfortable, and give ice chips, a carbonated beverage, or hot tea to drink.

Intervention. Give antiemetics, such as prochlorperazine maleate, thiethylperazine maleate, trimethobenzamide, and metoclopramide, before the administration of chemotherapeutic agents. The time of administration of the antiemetic agent will depend on the chemotherapeutic regimen prescribed.

Education. Instruct the client that any hypersensitivity to these drugs necessitates discontinuance of the drug and reporting the effects to the physician.

Most antiemetics cause drowsiness as a side effect. Caution clients against performing hazardous tasks until the effects of the drug have subsided.

Caution clients against combining antiemetics with alcohol or any CNS depressants. The CNS depressant effects on the drug can be potentiated when these drugs are combined.

Vomiting during pregnancy can cause serious electrolyte imbalance and a nutritional deficit. Instruct the pregnant client to take small frequent meals or small snacks between meals.

metoclopramide (Reglan, Maxeran♣)

Mechanism of action. Metoclopramide is structurally similar to procaine and procainamide but without significant anesthetic or cardiac effects. The central action of metoclopramide in preventing or relieving nausea and emesis is by blockade of dopamine receptors in the chemoreceptor trigger zone. The peripheral mechanism is by improvement of orthograde motility of the upper gastrointestinal tract, increase of stomach peristaltic action, and overcoming the immobility, dilation, and reverse motility occurring with the vomiting reflex.

Indications

1. Adjunct for gastrointestinal radiologic examination. Parenteral metoclopramide facilitates small bowel intubation. It also hastens barium's transit through the upper gastrointestinal tract by its stimulation of gastric emptying and acceleration of intestinal transit.

2. Used for diabetic gastroparesis, gastroesophageal reflux, and parenterally, for prevention of nausea and vomiting secondary to emetogenic cancer chemotherapeutic agents.

Pharmacokinetics. The onset of action is ½ to 1 hour after administration of an oral dose, 10 to 15 minutes after an intramuscular dose, and within 3 minutes after an intravenous dose. Effects last up to 2 hours after an intravenous dose and 2 to 3 hours following oral administration. The half-life is 4 to 6 hours. The drug is moderately bound to protein.

Side effects/adverse reactions. See Table 40-3.

Significant drug interactions

Motility effects are antagonized by anticholinergic agents and narcotic analgesics.

Digoxin tablets, other than Lanoxin, may have decreased absorption.

The absorption of acetaminophen, aspirin, diazepam, alcohol, L-dopa, lithium, and tetracycline may be increased.

TABLE 40-3 Selected Antiemetics: Side Effects and Adverse Reactions

Drug	Side effects*	Adverse reactions†
metoclopramide (Reglan, Maxeran✿)	More frequent: loose stools, dizziness (orthostatic hypotension), sleepiness, nausea, vomiting, abdominal pain Less common: depression, insomnia, poor physical coordination	Anorexia, weight loss, difficulty in urination, hyperthermia, difficult breathing, chest pain, pruritus, leg weakness, paresthesia, hallucinations, visual disturbances, disassociation, change in cardiac rate, nightmares
diphenidol hydrochloride (Vontrol)	More frequent: sleepiness Less common: dry mouth, headache, insomnia, weakness, rash, dizziness, indigestion	Disorientation, delusion, hallucinations
thiethylperazine maleate (Torecan, Toresten✿)	More frequent: sleepiness, dry mouth Less common: hyperthermia, ringing of the ears, blurred vision, headache, edema of extremities and face	Extrapyramidal side effects, convulsions, orthostatic hypotension (usually after first intramuscular injection)
trimethobenzamide hydrochloride (Tigan, Xametina✿)	More frequent: sleepiness Less common: headache, loose stools, dizziness, muscle cramps, blurred vision	Seizures or severe vomiting, depression, tremors, weakness, sore throat, jaundice, back muscle pain
benzquinamide hydrochloride (Emete-Con)	More frequent: sleepiness, agitation, inability to sleep, headache Less common: dry mouth, increased sweating, increased salivation, hiccups, blurred vision	Extrapyramidal side effects (usually from large doses of the drug), hypotension or hypertension, dysrhythmias (especially with intravenous administration)
scopolamine transdermal (Transderm-Scop)	More frequent: constipation, dry skin, dry mucous membranes Less common: flatulence, blurred vision, dysphagia, photophobia, difficulty in urination, sleepiness, insomnia (paradoxic reaction with large doses)	Allergic reaction (rash, hives), glaucoma or eye pain caused by increased intraocular pressure

*If side effects continue, increase, or disturb the client, inform the physician.
†If adverse reactions occur, contact physician, since medical intervention may be necessary.

Extrapyramidal reactions have been reported more often in children and young adults, but high doses or combination therapy with other medications that cause extrapyramidal effects may increase the frequency and seriousness of this reaction. Metoclopramide is contraindicated for use in clients receiving other medications that produce extrapyramidal side effects.

Insulin dosing or time of administration may have to be adjusted to reflect metoclopramide's influence on food delivery to the intestine and the increased rate of its absorption. Monitor closely.

Dosage and administration

Adults. For diabetic gastroparesis or gastroesophageal reflux, oral dose is 10 mg 30 minutes before each meal and at bedtime. Check package insert for further instructions.

Intravenously, 10 mg is given to facilitate small bowel intubation if the biopsy tube has not passed the pylorus in 10 minutes.

Antiemetic (chemotherapy-induced emesis): 1 to 2 mg/kg IV 30 minutes before chemotherapy; may be repeated every 2 to 3 hours as necessary.

Children. Intravenous dose is 0.1 mg/kg in children under 6 years and 2.5 to 5 mg/kg in children 6 to 14 years old.

Pregnancy safety. FDA category B

NURSING CONSIDERATIONS

Assessment. Do not give metoclopramide to clients with epilepsy or pheochromocytoma, or those in whom stimulation of gastrointestinal motility is hazardous (e.g., those with gastrointestinal hemorrhage, perforation, or mechanical obstruction).

Clients with an intolerance to procaine and procainamide may experience cross-sensitivity.

Metoclopramide has not been approved for use during pregnancy; it crosses the blood-brain and placental barriers.

Intervention. Administer oral preparations 30 minutes before meals and at bedtime.

Administer intravenous injections slowly over 1 to 2 minutes. If metoclopramide is administered more rapidly, a brief episode of anxiety and restlessness will occur followed by drowsiness. Infusions should not be for a period of less than 15 minutes.

Keep solutions of the parenteral dosage for 48 hours after dilution; protect from light; discard unused portions after 48 hours.

Do not give in combination with drugs having extrapyramidal side effects (phenothiazines, butyrophenones, amoxapine, loxapine, metyrosine, and thioxanthenes).

Be aware that extrapyramidal side effects may be seen at therapeutic doses and are more likely in children and young adults.

Education. Because this drug can cause drowsiness, caution client against operating any potentially hazardous equipment.

Caution client against using alcohol or other CNS depressants with this drug.

Evaluation. Approximately 20% to 30% of clients experience side effects that are usually mild and reversible after the drug is withdrawn.

diphenidol hydrochloride (Vontrol)

Mechanism of action. Diphenidol controls nausea and vomiting by inhibiting the medullary chemoreceptor trigger zone. It controls vertigo by a specific antivertigo effect on the vestibular apparatus.

Indications
1. Recommended for the prevention and control of nausea and vomiting, the vertigo of Meniere's disease, labyrinthitis following middle or inner ear surgery, and motion sickness
2. Used to control postoperative vomiting, drug-induced vomiting, and vomiting resulting from radiation therapy

Pharmacokinetics

Absorption. Diphenidol is well absorbed after oral administration.

Half-life. Diphenidol has a half-life of 4 hours.

Elimination. Ninety percent of diphenidol is excreted by the kidneys

Side effects/adverse reations. See Table 40-3.

Significant drug interactions. When diphenidol is given with alcohol or other CNS depressants, the effects of either drug may be potentiated. One must monitor closely for enhanced CNS depressant effects.

Dosage and administration. Adult dosage for antiemesis and antivertigo is 25 to 50 mg orally, every 4 hours as needed.

Pregnancy safety. Not classified

NURSING CONSIDERATIONS

Assessment. Use diphenidol cautiously in clients with glaucoma or gastrointestinal or urinary obstruction.

Do not use diphenidol in the presence of renal failure.

Diphenidol contains tartrazine, which may cause allergic reactions in sensitive clients. There is an increased frequency of tartrazine sensitivity among asprin-sensitive individuals.

Because diphenidol may cause hallucinations, disorientation, and confusion, its administration should be limited to clients within the hospital setting. Assess the client's mental status before and during therapy.

Intervention. Administer diphenidol with food, water, or milk to decrease gastric irritation.

Education. Caution client against using alcohol or other CNS depressants with this drug.

Evaluation. The antiemetic effect may mask symptoms of an underlying disorder such as intestinal obstruction, brain tumor, or drug overdose.

thiethylperazine maleate (Torecan)

Mechanism of action. Thiethylperazine is a phenothiazine derivative. It acts as an antiemetic and antinauseant on the chemoreceptor trigger zone and vomiting center. Studies indicate that this drug is a more effective antiemetic than other phenothiazines.

Indication. Prevention of nausea and vomiting caused by anesthetics, radiation therapy, and chemotherapy

Pharmacokinetics. See discussion of phenothiazines in Chapter 16.

Side effects/adverse reactions. See Table 40-3.

Significant drug interactions. The following interactions may occur when thiethylperazine is given with the drugs listed below.

Drug	Possible Effect and Management
epinephrine	Avoid use of epinephrine to treat hypotension induced by thiethylperazine. Norepinephrine and phenylephrine are drugs of choice for this purpose.
phenothiazines	Monitor for increased potential for extrapyramidal reactions.

Dosage and administration

Adults. Thiethylperazine is given in a 10-mg dose one to three times daily orally, intramuscularly, or rectally.

Children. Thiethylperazine is not recommended for children under 12 years of age.

Pregnancy safety. Not classified

NURSING CONSIDERATIONS

Do not administer thiethylperazine intravenously since this may cause severe hypotension. (See additional considerations for phenothiazine drugs in Chapter 16.)

trimethobenzamide hydrochloride (Tigan)

Mechanism of action. Trimethobenzamide is believed to depress the chemoreceptor trigger zone in the medulla rather than the vomiting center directly.

Pharmacokinetics
Indications
1. Prevention or relief of nausea and vomiting caused by radiation sickness, infection, and operative procedures
2. Relief of nausea and vomiting caused by a number of other conditions

Side effects/adverse reactions. See Table 40-3.

Significant drug interactions. The following interactions may occur when trimethobenzamide is given with the drugs listed below.

Drug	Possible Effect and Management
alcohol, CNS depressants	May potentiate effects of either medication. Monitor closely. Avoid use of alcohol.
phenothiazines, barbiturates, belladonna	Has resulted in extrapyramidal reactions, opisthotonos, seizures, and coma. Closely supervise clients and take appropriate actions if adverse reactions occur.

Metabolism. Trimethobenzamide is metabolized in the liver.

Excretion. Trimethobenzamide is excreted in the urine.

Dosage and administration
Adults. Oral administration of trimethobenzamide is 250 mg three or four times per day. Rectally or intramuscularly, 200 mg is given three or four times per day.

Children. For children over 45 kg, 15 mg/kg is given orally per day, divided into three or four doses. For children weighing 15 to 45 kg, administer 100 to 200 mg oral or rectally three to four times per day. IM route is not recommended.

Pregnancy safety. Not classified.

NURSING CONSIDERATIONS

Be aware that trimethobenzamide is not recommended for use in children with viral illness, since it may contribute to development of Reye's syndrome, an acute encephalopathy.

Inject the drug deeply into the upper outer quadrant of the gluteal area to minimize injection site irritation.

Hypotension can occur in the surgical client when trimethobenzamide is administered parenterally. Assess blood pressure before administering the medication and frequently after it has been given.

Caution the client against using alcohol or other CNS depressants with this drug.

Suppositories contain 2% benzocaine (caution for allergic patients).

benzquinamide hydrochloride (Emete-Con)

Mechanism of action. Benzquinamide is believed to depress the chemoreceptor trigger zone to produce its antiemetic effects.

Indication. For prevention and treatment of nausea and vomiting associated with anesthetics and surgery in those clients in whom emesis would endanger the results of surgery or be harmful.

Pharmacokinetics
Metabolism. Benzquinamide is metabolized in the liver.

Excretion. Benzquinamide is excreted in the urine. Half-life is about 40 minutes in plasma.

Side effects/adverse reactions. See Table 40-3.

Significant drug interactions. No major interactions have been noted.

Dosage and administration
Deep intramuscular administration. Initially, 50 mg is given and repeated in 1 hour with subsequent doses every 3 to 4 hours as necessary.

Intravenous administration. A single dose of 25 mg is given slowly (1 ml over 30 seconds to 1 minute).

Pregnancy safety. Not classified

NURSING CONSIDERATIONS

Do not give benzquinamide intravenously to clients with cardiovascular disease or to those who demonstrate hypersensitivity (fever, urticaria) to the drug.

Use with caution in the elderly.

Medication may cause a dry mouth.

For best effect give drug about 15 minutes before expected emergence from anesthesia (this would be done by the anesthesiologist or anesthetist).

Reconstituted solutions remain potent for 14 days and need not be refrigerated.

scopolamine transdermal (Transderm-Scop)

Mechanism of action. Scopolamine acts either on the cortex or peripherally on maculae of the utriculus and saccule to decrease labyrinthine receptor excitability and depress the vestibular cerebellar pathway conduction.

Indication. Prevention of motion sickness
Pharmacokinetics
Metabolism. Scopolamine is metabolized in the liver.

Excretion. Scopolamine is excreted by the kidneys.
Side effects/adverse reactions. See Table 40-3.
Significant drug interactions

The decreased gastrointestinal tract motility and delay of gastric emptying time may decrease the absorption of other medications.

Anticholinergic/antimuscarinic drugs or CNS depressants may be potentiated.

Monoamine oxidase (MAO) inhibitors may increase antimuscarinic effects. They may also potentiate the effects of scopolamine by preventing its detoxification in the body (United States Pharmacopeial Convention, 1986).

Dosage and administration. Scopolamine is used in adults only. A four-layered film, 2.5 cm², contains 1.5 mg scopolamine that is released gradually from the adhesive matrix after application on the skin behind the ear. A priming dose is released to saturate the dermal binding site for scopolamine, thus bringing the plasma concentration to a steady-state level. The rate-controlling membrane of the matrix provides controlled release that maintains a constant plasma drug level. This film will deliver 0.5 mg of scopolamine over a 3-day period. It must be applied approximately 4 hours before the antiemetic effect is desired.

Pregnancy safety. FDA category C

NURSING CONSIDERATIONS

Assessment. Take precautions when clients have asthma, narrow-angle glaucoma, pyloric or intestinal obstruction, urinary tract obstruction, or diminished renal or hepatic function.

Do not use in children because of adverse effects.

Use cautiously, if at all, during pregnancy or for women who are breast-feeding.

Intervention. Apply the system at least 4 hours before therapeutic effect is desired.

Wash and dry the hands thoroughly before and after application of the system.

Apply to intact skin in the hairless area behind the ear.

Amnesic effects can occur with this drug. Protect the elderly client by raising the bedrails after the drug has been given.

Education. Warn client that operating machinery or driving a motorized vehicle is hazardous because of drowsiness, disorientation, and confusion.

Evaluation. Scopolamine may cause delirium, excitement, and disorientation before sedative effects occur. Consider client safety when this drug is given.

Be aware that clients can develop tolerance to the drug after prolonged use.

Cannabinoids

Delta-9-tetrahydrocannabinol (THC), an active ingredient of marijuana, has been used as an investigational drug in many studies involving cancer chemotherapy–induced vomiting. Clinical studies on the effectiveness of THC have been conflicting. It was found to be more effective than placebos and at least as effective as prochlorperazine

in some studies. Other studies reported that certain chemotherapeutic agents (cisplatin, mechlorethamine, and nitrosoureas) often produced a refractory nausea and vomiting that did not respond to THC or many other agents.

Significant CNS side effects including hallucinations, grand mal convulsions, and psychosis have also been reported. Teenagers and young adults seem to tolerate this drug much better than older adults (Frytak and Moertel, 1981). Absorption problems and lack of flexibility in the dosage schedule may be contributing factors to the large variable response in patients (Anderson and McGuire, 1981).

dronabinol (Marinol)

Dronabinol is the synthetic derivative of delta-9-tetrahydrocannabinol approved by the FDA in 1985 for the treatment of nausea and vomiting related to cancer chemotherapy. Since this drug is listed in the Controlled Substances Act, each individual state legislature must approve its use before it can be prescribed in that state.

Dosage and administration

Adults. 5 mg/m² by mouth 1 to 3 hours before the administration of chemotherapy, for 4 to 6 doses daily. Maximum dosage of 15 mg/m² per dose. Elderly are more sensitive.

Pregnancy safety. FDA category B

nabilone (Cesamet)

Nabilone is a synthetic derivative of cannabinoid (not THC) that was tested as an antiemetic in clients receiving cancer chemotherapy. It is reportedly more effective than placebos and prochlorperazine. It has an onset of action within ½ to 1 hour after an oral dose (2 mg). It peaks in 2 hours, and its effects last about 8 hours. Adverse effects include somnolence, dry mouth, dizziness, and a mild euphoric effect (Weintraub and Standish, 1983). Nabilone received FDA approval in the United States in December 1985. It has been available for use in the United Kingdom and Canada since the early 1980s.

Pregnancy safety. FDA category B

NURSING CONSIDERATIONS

Assess the client's mental status before and during therapy. Some clients report feelings of well-being and euphoria, others have transient psychoses characterized by hallucinations and depersonalization.

Before giving dronabinol, assess the client's intolerance to sesame oil since the gelatin capsule dosage form of dronabinol contains this substance.

Caution the client about performing tasks that require alertness, since sleepiness and dizziness are common adverse reactions.

Instruct the client to make position changes slowly, particularly from the recumbent to upright position, and to dangle feet from the edge of the bed to prevent dizziness and fainting, symptoms of orthostatic hypotension.

Instruct the client to avoid alcoholic beverages and other CNS depressants while taking cannabinoids.

Administer 1 to 3 hours before chemotherapy.

Corticosteroids

Corticosteroids have been reported to be effective for chemotherapy-induced nausea and vomiting when used in combination with other antiemetics. The mechanism of action is unknown, but it has been proposed that these drugs may inhibit prostaglandin synthesis, which may be involved in cancer chemotherapy–induced vomiting. Research has indicated that certain prostaglandins (especially the PGE series) can induce nausea and vomiting.

Many studies with corticosteroids have involved the use of dexamethasone or methylprednisolone. Antiemetic use is not yet an FDA-approved indication for the drugs. Their possible effectiveness as antiemetics was a serendipitous discovery—patients receiving various chemotherapeutic regimens had less nausea and vomiting when prednisone was one of the agents administered. Corticosteroids are not approved or generally recommended for common use.

Further trials in clients not responding to all other available antiemetic agents might be warranted with this class of medications (Ryan, 1983).

EMETIC AGENTS

Emetic drugs exert their effects on the same centers as antiemetic drugs but with the opposite effect. They are used to induce vomiting as part of the treatment for certain drug overdoses and poisonings.

apomorphine

Apomorphine, a product formulated by mixing morphine with dilute hydrochloric acid, is an agent with enhanced emetic effects and greatly reduced analgesic properties. Apomorphine is given parenterally as a single dose only. It directly stimulates the chemoreceptor trigger zone and may affect the vestibular centers, since client movement increases the individual's response to this product. It also stimulates dopamine receptors. Apomorphine may cause respiratory depression, increased salivation, hypotension, and sedation.

Subcutaneous administration produces vomiting on 90% of clients within 15 minutes (usually within 5 minutes). Sedative effects also occur within a few minutes and may last for several hours. When used early in treatment of an acute oral drug overdose, apomorphine produces emesis in 80% to 100% of clients with a recovery of gastrointestinal contents in the range of 3% to 92% (mean 31%). For client safety other measures—including gastric lavage, activated charcoal, and supportive measures—should also be instituted, since some toxic substances may remain in the gastrointestinal tract.

A glassful of water (approximately 240 ml) should be given with apomorphine to facilitate its action (young children should have less water).

Dosage and administration. Adults. Give 5 to 6 mg (range 2 to 10 mg) subcutaneously. Children. Give 0.07 to 1.0 mg/kg subcutaneously as a single dose.

Pregnancy safety. FDA category C

ipecac syrup

Ipecac syrup is an over-the-counter drug for home emergency treatment. Its major alkaloids are emetine and cephaeline, which stimulate the chemoreceptor trigger zone and irritate the gastric mucosa.

Approximately 90% of patients vomit within a half hour following oral drug administration; the average time for vomiting is 20 minutes. Although this product is generally given in the home, a poison control center or medical personnel should be called for advice before administration (see appendix for additional poisons and antidotes). However, if medical help is not available, one should still use this product.

Vomiting induced by ipecac syrup occurs in 80% to 99% of clients, and gastrointestinal contents recovered may range from up to 78% (mean 28%). Therefore clients need further monitoring and/or treatment, since not all the toxic substances are recovered from the gastrointestinal tract.

Although apomorphine is faster acting, ipecac syrup has the advantage of oral administration. Ipecac does not produce the CNS effects or respiratory depression reported with apomorphine.

Active alkaloids of ipecac include emetine, a cardiotoxic substance. Although administration of a single dose does not usually lead to major problems, serious complications including fatalities have resulted from chronic use of this product by persons with an eating disorder, such

---

WARNING!

Ipecac syrup is the only product to be used as an antiemetic. *Do not use ipecac fluidextract;* it is 14 times more concentrated than the syrup, and its use has resulted in serious injury and sometimes death. Although the fluidextract is no longer commercially produced in the United States, this product may still be on the shelves of some older pharmacies.

an anorexia or bulimia. Emetine is excreted very slowly so with repeated doses, ipecac accumulates in the body. It may produce systemic effects for months, even after the drug is discontinued.

Myopathy or muscle aching and weakness, especially in muscles of the neck and extremities, hyporeflexia, slurred speech, and dysphagia have been reported. Cardiotoxicity has caused some fatalities. The cardiac alterations include premature ventricular contractions, supraventricular tachycardia, inverted T waves, prolonged QT and PR intervals, QRS complex alterations, ventricular tachycardia and fibrillation, and cardiac arrest. Signs and symptoms may include precordial chest pain, hypotension, congestive heart failure, pericardial effusion, pulmonary edema, and dyspnea.

Dosage and administration. Adults and children over 12 years are given 30 ml (1 oz) orally. Children 1 to 12 years are given 15 ml orally. Children 6 months to 1 year are given 5 ml orally. For children under 6 months obtain professional advice before using.

If vomiting does not occur in 30 minutes, a second dose may be given. If vomiting does not occur 30 minutes after the second dose, then other measures should be used.

Pregnancy safety. Not classified

NURSING CONSIDERATIONS

Following administration of ipecac syrup, give a glassful (approximately 240 ml) of water. Less water or clear liquid should be given to younger children. Sometimes giving the water before the medication is more helpful in young or frightened children. If children will not drink water, carbonated sodas (clear) may be substituted. Do not give milk, since it will delay the emetic effect of this drug.

If the patient is conscious, drug-induced vomiting is usually preferable to gastric lavage, particularly in children, since aspiration of vomitus is less likely to occur. Nurses should employ the necessary measures to reduce the likelihood of aspiration of vomitus (e.g., proper positioning of patient). Occasionally, induction of vomiting may be facilitated by stimulating the pharynx, but time should not be wasted in repeated futile attempts.

CAUTION: Vomiting should never be induced in the client who is unconscious or who has depressed gag or cough reflexes. Vomiting may result in aspiration of gastric contents into the lungs, which may be fatal.

DRUGS USED TO TREAT PEPTIC ULCERS

Treatment of peptic ulcer disease includes the following drugs: antacids, anticholinergics, antidepressants, H_2 receptor antagonists, and **cytoprotective** agents (substances that protect cells from damage) such as sucralfate. In addition, use of anxiolytics and avoidance of smoking, ethyl alcohol, and other ulcerogenic substances are suggested.

CYTOPROTECTIVE AGENTS
sucralfate (Carafate, Sulcrate✲)

Mechanism of action. The aluminum complex of sucrose sulfate is believed to act as a locally active topical agent that hastens healing of the peptic ulcer by protecting the mucosa. The mechanism of action is thought to involve the formation of an ulcer-adherent complex with the fibrinogen in the ulcer crater that produces a protective, acid-resistant barrier.

Indications. Short-term (up to 8 weeks) duodenal ulcer treatment

Pharmacokinetics. Only 3% to 5% of sucrose sulfate is absorbed from the gastrointestinal tract. Excretion is primarily by the fecal route, with minute amounts secreted in the urine. The duration of action is about 5 hours.

Side effects/adverse reactions. The most common side effect is constipation. Other reported effects include diarrhea, nausea, gastric discomfort, indigestion, dry mouth, dizziness, drowsiness, back pain, rash, and itching.

Significant drug interactions

1. Because antacids may interfere with the sucralfate binding, they should be given either 30 minutes before or 1 hour after sucralfate administration.
2. Interference with absorption of fat-soluble vitamins makes vitamin depletion possible with long-term use.

Dosage and administration. For adults, give 1 g four times daily on empty stomach 1 hour before each meal and at bedtime. Therapy should continue for 4 to 8 weeks until healing is documented.

Pregnancy safety. FDA category B

NURSING CONSIDERATIONS

Administer to client with water on an empty stomach, 1 hour before meals and at bedtime.

If the client's regimen also includes antacids, they may be administered ½ hour before or 1 hour after the sucralfate.

Sucralfate therapy is not recommended for longer than 8 weeks.

Instruct client not to chew the tablet.

Encourage compliance with the regimen for at least 4 to 8 weeks, until healing has been documented by x-ray or endoscopic examination.

H₂ RECEPTOR ANTAGONISTS

Histamine is found in the mucosal cells of the gastrointestinal tract, extending from the stomach to the colon. The action of histamine is mediated through H_2 receptors and has been associated with gastric acid secretion. The major components of the gastric secretion of the stomach include hydrochloric acid (HCl) and **intrinsic factor** (IF), produced by the parietal (acid-forming) cells; pepsinogen, synthesized by the chief cells; and mucus. The principal function of mucus is to protect the epithelial cells of the gastrointestinal tract from attack by pepsin and irritation by the HCl secreted by the stomach. Pepsinogen, an enzyme, is the precursor of pepsin; HCl catalyzes the cleavage of pepsinogen to active pepsin by providing a low pH environment in which pepsin can initiate the digestion of proteins.

Gastric secretion is regulated by a neural mechanism, parasympathetic (vagus) fibers, and a hormonal mechanism, gastrin. Activation of the vagus nerve causes secretion of vast quantities of pepsinogen and HCl. In contrast, the hormonal mechanism involves the actual presence of food, which distends the stomach and stimulates the antral mucosa to release gastrin. This hormone is then absorbed into the blood and carried to the parietal cells and chief cells secreting HCl and pepsinogen, respectively. Histamine is believed to activate the gastric mucosa much the same as gastrin does. In addition, caffeine and alcohol are potent stimuli for gastrin release. When the acidity of the gastric juice is increased to a pH of 2, a negative feedback mechanism helps to block production of gastric secretion from the parietal and chief cells. Thus inhibition of gastric gland secretion plays an essential role in protecting the stomach against excessively acidic secretions, which are responsible for causing peptic ulcerations.

Normally the mucosal surface of the stomach and upper duodenum is protected from the irritation of gastric acid by a layer of mucus. If a circumscribed area of the mucosal surface is damaged and fails to repair rapidly, it may become eroded, forming an ulcer at one of these sites. When gastric acid comes in contact with this inflammatory region, pain may result. Moreover, clinical studies have suggested that esophageal, gastric, and duodenal ulcers (peptic ulcers) are associated with the excessive production of gastric acid.

Clinical evidence has shown that histamine released by severe injuries, particularly burns, may lead to the formation of peptic ulcers.

The H_2 receptor blocking agents include cimetidine (Tagamet), ranitidine (Zantac), famotidine (Pepcid), and nizatidine (Axid). They act to prevent histamine from stimulating the H_2 receptors located on the gastric parietal cells, thus resulting in a reduction in the volume of gastric acid secretion (from stimuli such as food, pentagastrin, histamine, caffeine, and insulin) and the concentration (acid content) of the secretions. All four drugs are presently considered to be equally potent and effective, although pharmacokinetics, side effects/adverse reactions, and drug interactions may differ.

> cimetidine (Tagamet)
> ranitidine (Zantac)
> famotidine (Pepcid)
> nizatidine (Axid)

Mechanism of action. See previous section.

Indications. Treatment and prevention of gastric ulcer, duodenal ulcer, gastroesophageal reflux (ranitidine), and hypersecretory gastric states.

Pharmacokinetics. See Table 40-4.

Side effects/adverse reactions. See Table 40-5.

Significant drug interactions. Since cimetidine, unlike the other H_2 receptor antagonists, inhibits the liver drug metabolism systems, the major drug interactions noted are with cimetidine. All of the H_2 receptor antagonists may exhibit a similar effect with ketoconazole and antacids.

TABLE 40-4 Pharmacokinetics of H_2 Receptor Antagonists

Drug	Absorption	Time to peak plasma level	Plasma half-life (hr)	Duration of action (hr)	Metabolism/excretion
cimetidine (Tagamet)	Very good orally, 60%-70%	45-90 min after oral dose	2-3	4-5	Liver/kidneys
famotidine (Pepcid)	Fair orally, 40%-45%	1-3 hr after oral dose	2.5-3.5	10-12	Liver/kidneys
nizatidine (Axid)	Very good orally, 90%	0.5-3 hr after oral dose	1-2	—	Liver (has active metabolite)/kidneys
ranitidine (Zantac)	Good orally, 50%	2-3 hr after oral dose	2.5-3	Up to 4 hr (basal and stimulated); up to 12 hr (nocturnal)	Liver/kidneys

TABLE 40-5   H$_2$ Receptor Antagonists: Major Side Effects/Adverse Reactions

Drug(s)	Side effects	Adverse reactions
cimetidine (Tagamet) famotidine (Pepcid) nizatidine (Axid) ranitidine (Zantac)	Less frequent: rash, diarrhea, constipation, dizziness, headaches, muscle pain (cimetidine, famotidine), stomach cramps or pain Cimetidine only: breast swelling or pain in males and females (with chronic therapy) Famotidine only: dry mouth or skin, anorexia, depression, nausea or vomiting, temporary loss of hair, taste alterations, decrease in libido	Rare: confusion, sore throat, elevated temperature, bruising (blood disorder), increased weakness, altered heart rate (slow, fast, irregular), chest pain (famotidine), eyelid edema (allergic reaction—famotidine)

Drug	Possible Effect and Management
anticoagulants, metoprolol, phenytoin, propranolol, or xanthines (exception: dyphylline)	May result in decreased metabolism and excretion of these medications. Since dosage adjustments may be necessary, blood concentration (for phenytoin and xanthines), prothrombin time (for anticoagulants), and blood pressure monitoring (for metoprolol and propranolol) are indicated.
antidepressants, tricyclic	May decrease metabolism of tricyclic antidepressant, causing an increased serum level and toxicity. Assess the client for signs of toxicity, and monitor for serum levels.
antacids	Concurrent use is often prescribed by physicians, but if the H$_2$ receptor antagonist is given concurrently with an antacid, absorption of the antagonist may be decreased. Give antacids at least 1 hour apart from these medications.
ketoconazole	An increase in gastrointestinal pH induced by the H$_2$ receptor antagonists may result in a reduced absorption of ketoconazole. Advise clients to take the H$_2$ receptor antagonist at least 2 hours after ketoconazole.

Dosage and administration. See Table 40-6.

Pregnancy safety. Cimetidine, not established; famotidine, FDA category B; nizatidine, FDA category C; ranitidine, FDA category B

NURSING CONSIDERATIONS

Assessment. Note that clients with impaired renal function require a reduction in dosage of cimetidine, famotidine, or ranitidine because of delayed excretion. The recommended dosage of cimetidine is 300 mg every 12 hours orally or parenterally. In clients with impaired liver function, a further reduction in dosage may be necessary. For clients undergoing hemodialysis, adjust the time of dosage so that the medication is administered at the end of the procedure, thus preventing a decrease in blood level of the drug. These agents are dialyzable.

Do not use the drugs for minor digestive complaints.

Before administering, rule out the potential existence of malignant gastrointestinal neoplasm.

Do not administer to nursing mothers, pregnant women, women of childbearing potential, and children under 16 years of age.

Intervention. Administer drug with meals, since food slows gastric emptying and prolongs the drug's effect. If prescribed, a bedtime dose protects the stomach from nocturnal hypersecretion of gastric acid. Give concomitant antacids to relieve acute ulcer pain 1 hour *before* or *after* administration of H$_2$ antagonist, to prevent drug interaction.

Note that the parenteral form of the drug is stable for 48 hours at room temperature. The intravenous solutions in which cimetidine and famotidine are compatible for dilution are 0.9% sodium chloride, dextrose (5%, 10%), lactated Ringer's, and 5% sodium bicarbonate.

Warn client that intramuscular administration may be painful.

Rapid intravenous bolus administration (less than 2 minutes) may result in cardiac dysrhythmias and hypotension.

Education. Instruct client to keep clinical and laboratory appointments as scheduled. Periodic evaluation of blood counts and renal and hepatic function tests are required during therapy.

Encourage the client with peptic ulcer disease to discontinue smoking or at least to discontinue smoking after the last dose of the day, since the effectiveness of H$_2$ antagonists to inhibit nocturnal gastric acid secretions is diminished by smoking.

Evaluation. Be aware that following long-term treatment (1 month or more), mild bilateral gynecomastia in males and galactorrhea in females have been observed in some clients taking cimetidine. This drug also may cause a reversible decline in sperm count or impotence. No such problems have been reported with ranitidine.

The use of ranitidine, which is metabolized in the liver, may cause elevated hepatic enzyme levels, especially serum glutamic-pyruvic transaminase (SGPT) level. Since ranitidine is potentially hepatotoxic, perform periodic hepatic studies. It is not advisable to prolong therapy;

TABLE 40-6   Dosage and Administration for H$_2$ Receptor Antagonists

Drug	Dosage recommendations
cimetidine (Tagamet)	*Oral* Adults: Duodenal ulcers: initially, 300 mg four times daily, with meals and at bedtime; or 400 mg twice daily, in the morning and at bedtime; or 800 mg at bedtime (1600 mg at bedtime has been used to heal ulcers larger than 1 cm in clients who are heavy smokers) Preventive therapy: 400 mg at bedtime. Gastric ulcer (benign): 300 mg four times daily, with meals and at bedtime Gastric hypersecretions: 300 mg four times daily, with meals and at bedtime; dosage adjustments are instituted as needed Clients with renal impairment: initially, 300 mg every 12 hr; increase dose as necessary, if tolerated by the client Maximum daily dose: usually up to 2.4 g, but in some hypersecretory conditions, dosages up to 10 g per day were used Children*: 20 to 40 mg/kg (base) four times daily, with meals and at bedtime *Parenteral* Adults: IM: 300 mg (base) every 6 to 8 hr IV: 300 mg (base), diluted with normal saline or a compatible solution, every 6 to 8 hr; administer over 2 min or more IV infusion solution: 300 mg (base) every 6 to 8 hours, mixed in a compatible solution, given over 15 to 20 min Clients with renal impairment: initial dose, 300 mg IV every 12 hr, adjusting to a more frequent schedule if tolerated Maximum daily dose: up to 2.4 g Children: IM: 5 to 10 mg/kg (base) every 6 to 8 hr IV: 5 to 10 mg/kg (base), diluted in a suitable intravenous solution, every 6 to 8 hr; administer over 2 min or more IV infusion: 5 to 10 mg/kg every 6 to 8 hours, after dilution in a suitable intravenous solution; administer over 15 to 20 min
famotidine (Pepcid)	*Oral* Adults: Peptic ulcer: initially, 40 mg at bedtime or 20 mg twice a day Preventive therapy: 20 mg at bedtime Gastric hypersecretion: 20 mg every 6 hours; adjust dose according to client's response to therapy and tolerance of the drug In very severe renal impairment (creatinine clearance less than 10 ml/min): limit dose to 20 mg at bedtime; adjust dose interval as necessary, since it may need to be increased to 36 to 48 hours Children: not established *Parenteral* Adults: IV: 20 mg every 12 hr after dilution with a compatible IV solution; administer 2 min or more IV infusion: 20 mg every 12 hr after dilution with a compatible IV solution; administer over 15 to 30 min Children: not established
nizatidine (Axid)	Adults: Duodenal ulcer: 300 mg orally at bedtime or 150 mg twice a day Preventive therapy: 150 mg orally at bedtime For clients with renal impairment: refer to a current reference or package insert for instructions Children: not established
ranitidine (Zantac)	*Oral* Adults: Peptic ulcer: initially, 150 mg (base) twice daily or 300 mg (base) at bedtime Preventive therapy: 150 mg (base) at bedtime Treatment of gastric hypersecretion: 150 mg (base) twice daily; adjust dose as necessary, up to 6 g/day

*Use of cimetidine in children under 16 years old is considered limited in practice; therefore the physician should weigh the benefit-to-risk factor when considering this product.

Continued.

TABLE 40-6   Dosage and Administration for H$_2$ Receptor Antagonists — cont'd

Drug	Dosage recommendations
	Treatment of gastroesophageal reflux: 150 mg (base) twice daily
	Clients with renal impairment (creatinine clearance less than 50 mg/min): 150 mg (base) daily; adjust dose as necessary according to client's tolerance of the medication
	Children: not established
	Parenteral
	Adults:
	IM: 50 mg (base) every 6 to 8 hr
	IV: 50 mg (base) every 6 to 8 hr, after dilution with an appropriate IV solution; administer over 5 min or more
	IV infusion: 50 mg (base) every 6 to 8 hr, after dilution in 100 ml of a compatible IV solution; administer over 15 to 20 min
	For clients with renal impairment, (creatinine clearance less than 50 ml/min): IV, 50 mg (base) every 18 to 24 hr, adjusting dose as necessary according to client's response and tolerance of the medication
	Maximum daily dose: up to 400 mg (base)
	Children: not established

most clients with active duodenal ulcers heal within 4 weeks, and the usefulness of further treatment is unknown.

Drugs that Affect the Gallbladder

chenodiol (Chenix, Chendol✴)

Chenodiol (chenodeoxycholic acid) is a normal bile acid synthesized in the liver. Cholesterol is broken down by bile acids and lecithin, so when the amount of cholesterol exceeds the capacity of bile acids and lecithin to perform this effect, crystallization and gallstones may result.

Mechanism of action. Chenodiol blocks liver synthesis of cholesterol, thus reducing biliary cholesterol levels and leading to gradual dissolving of floating, radiolucent cholesterol gallstones.

Indications. Chenodiol is indicated for the patient with radiolucent stones who has a well-opacified, functioning gallbladder, but who is at increased surgical risk for elective surgery because of systemic disease, age, or cardiovascular, renal, or respiratory disease.

Pharmacokinetics

Absorption. Chenodiol is absorbed in the small intestine.

Metabolism. Chenodiol is metabolized by the liver.

Excretion. Chenodiol is excreted in feces.

Side effects/adverse reactions. Dose-related diarrhea has been reported in 30% to 40% of patients taking chenodiol. It may occur with initial therapy or any time during the treatment period. Most cases of diarrhea are mild and tolerated, so they do not interfere with therapy. In 10% to 15% of clients, a dosage decrease and/or antidiarrheal agent may be required.

INVESTIGATIONAL DRUGS FOR PEPTIC ULCERS

Several drugs are under investigation for peptic ulcer disease, including misoprostol (Cytotec) and omeprazole. Misoprostol is a synthetic analogue of prostaglandin E$_1$ that has both a cytoprotective or coating effect on the mucosa and an acid, antisecretory effect. It is currently available in 36 countries, including Canada and Mexico.

Omeprazole is an extremely potent inhibitor of gastric acid secretion, because of its specific inhibition of the hydrogen-potassium ATPase enzyme that mediates the final transport of hydrogen ions in exchange for potassium ions by the parietal cells in the gastric lumen. Both drugs are under clinical investigation in the United States.

Other side effects of chenodiol include fecal urgency, cramps, heartburn, constipation, nausea, vomiting, anorexia, flatulence, and nonspecific abdominal pain.

Significant drug interactions

Cholestyramine and colestipol sequester bile acids, reducing the absorption of chenodiol. Products that adsorb bile acids (e.g., aluminum-based antacids) will also reduce absorption.

Estrogen therapy, oral contraceptives, and clofibrate may increase biliary cholesterol secretion, counteracting the effectiveness of this drug.

Dosage and administration

Adults. Give 13 to 16 mg/kg/day in two divided doses orally morning and night, beginning with 250 mg twice daily for 2 weeks and increasing by 250 mg/day each week thereafter until either maximum tolerated dose or recommended dose is attained.

Pregnancy safety. FDA category X

NURSING CONSIDERATIONS

Ultrasonography is a screening procedure for gallstone detection, but initiation and continuation of therapy are based on the results of oral cholecystograms.

Determine serum aminotransferase levels each month for 3 months and every 3 months thereafter (discontinue monitoring if over three times normal upper limits). Oral cholecystograms or ultrasonograms are needed at 6- and 9-month intervals to monitor response. The response to therapy may be noted on a cholecystogram or ultrasonogram taken 1 month after therapy is begun. Success usually occurs within 12 to 18 months. If no therapeutic response is achieved by 18 months the drug is discontinued; use beyond 24 months is not recommended. Stones recur within 5 years in about 50% of patients. Radiolucency and gallbladder function must be established before initiating another course of treatment.

Administer with food or milk, since the presence of bile and pancreatic juice in the intestine enhances dissolution.

Instruct the client about a high-fiber, low-fat diet and a weight reduction program if necessary.

Because therapy is long term, compliance may be a problem. Encourage the client through a relationship of trust and confidence.

KEY TERMS

achlorhydria, page 681
antiemetics, page 682
catalase, page 675
chemoreceptor trigger zone, page 683
cytoprotective, page 690
dentifrice, page 676
effervescence, page 675
emetic center, page 683
halitosis, page 675
intrinsic factor, page 691
pepsin, page 681
steatorrhea, page 682

BIBLIOGRAPHY

AHFS Drug Information 86, American Hospital Formulary Service, Bethesda, Md, 1986, American Society of Hospital Pharmacists, Inc.

Allbright, MS: Oral care for the cancer chemotherapy patient, Nursing Times 80(21):40, 1984.

American Pharmaceutical Association: Handbook of nonprescription drugs, ed 8, Washington, DC, 1986, American Pharmaceutical Association.

Anderson, PO, and McGuire, GG: Delta-9-tetrahydrocannabinol as an antiemetic, Am J Hosp Pharm 38:639, May 1981

Bergmann, KA: Managing chemotherapy-induced nausea and vomiting, Consultant Pharmacist, p 134, July/Aug 1986.

Berry-Opersteny, D, and Heusinkveld, KB: Prophylactic antiemetics for chemotherapy-associated nausea and vomiting, Cancer Nur 6(3):117, 1983.

Bersani, G: Oral care for cancer patients, Am J Nurs 83(4):533, 1983.

Bruckstein, AH: Peptic ulcer disease—new concepts, new and current therapeutics, Consultant 26(4):157, 1986.

Compendium of Pharmaceuticals & Specialities, 1986, Ottawa, 1986, Canadian Pharmaceutical Association.

Cornacchia, HJ, and Barrett, S: Consumer health: a guide to intelligent decisions, St Louis, 1985, The CV Mosby Co.

D'Arcy, PF: Hypoglycemia from alcoholic mouthwash: a warning, Pharmacy International 6(10):244, 1985.

Egbert, AM, and others: Alcoholics who drink mouthwash: the spectrum of nonbeverage alcohol use, J Stud Alcohol 46(6):473, 1985.

F.D.C. reports, trade and government memos, 8/18/86.

Fortner, CL, and others: Combination antiemetic therapy in the control of chemotherapy-induced emesis, Drug Intell Clin Pharmacol 19:21, 1985.

Frytak, S, and Moertel, CG: Management of nausea and vomiting in the cancer patient, JAMA 245(4):393, 1981.

Geyer, LN: I.V. metoclopramide: relief for cancer chemotherapy patients, Nurs 84 14(4):87, 1984.

Goodman and Gilman's the pharmacological basis of therapeutics, ed 7, New York, 1985, Macmillan Publishing Co.

Gossel, TA: The role of fluorides in preventing cavities, US Pharmacist 11:28, March 1986.

Griffin, JW: H$_2$-blocker update, Hosp Formul 19:1032, 1984.

Grunberg, SM: Grunberg discusses choice of appropriate antiemetic therapy. Highlights from a series of symposia held in comprehensive cancer centers, 1982, Biomedical Information Corporation Publishers.

Hoffman, RS, and others: Cancer: giving the elderly long-term care, Patient Care 17(20):105, 1983.

Howrie, DL, and others: Metochlopramide as an antiemetic agent in pediatric patients, Drug Intell Clin Pharmacol 20(2):122, 1985.

Kunkel, DB: The toxic emergency: the toxic toll of keeping thin, Emerg Med 17(1):176, 1985.

Kutsop, KK: Effectiveness of liquid antacids, Am Pharmacy NS24(12):778, 1984.

Marihuana for nausea and vomiting due to cancer chemotherapy, Med Let Drugs Therapeutics 22(10):41, 1980.

Patton, S: Easing the complications of chemotherapy: a matter of little victories, Nurs 84 14(2):58, 1984.

Physicians' desk reference for nonprescription drugs, Oradell, NJ, 1982, Medical Economics Co, Inc.

Physicians' desk reference, ed 40, Oradell, NJ, 1986, Medical Economics Co, Inc.

Rawls, DE, and Dyck, WP: Previewing new drugs, reviewing current therapy, Consultant 24(2):85, 1984.

Reich, SD: Metoclopramide: a brief review, Cancer Nurs 6(2):71, 1983.

Rimar, JM: Metoclopramide for enhancing lactation, MCN 11(2):93, 1986.

Rodman, MJ: An update on the new drugs you're dispensing now. RN 47(4):67, 1984.

Rovinski, CA: Therapeutic use of noninvestigational marijuana in cancer care, Cancer Nurs 6(2):141, 1983.

Rudy, CA: Oral THC approved and rescheduled, Drug Information Bulletin of St. Margaret Hospital of Hammond 12(7):23, 1986.

Ryan, GM: Steroids as antiemetics, Cancer Nurs 6(2):147, 1983.

Sasso, SC: Metoclopramide and cholasia, MCN 8(5):361, 1983.

Shaughnessy, AF: Potential uses for metoclopramide, Drug Intell Clin Pharmacol 19:723, 1985.

Smith, FP: Antiemetics combat both pre and post chemotherapy nausea and vomiting. Highlights from a series of symposia held in comprehensive cancer centers, 1982, Biomedical Information Corporation Publishers.

Schwinghammer, T: Antiemetic: choosing from the alternatives, Hosp Form 37:38, Jan 1980.

United States Pharmacopeial Convention: Drug information for the health care provider, ed 6, Rockville, Md, 1986, United States Pharmacopeial Convention, Inc., Mack Printing Co.

Weintraub, M, and Standish, R: Nabilone: an antiemetic for patients undergoing cancer chemotherapy, Hosp Form 40:1033, 1983.

Wilson, D: Make mouth care a must for your patients, RN 49(2):39, 1986.

Zaenger, P: The rational use of antacids in peptic ulcer disease, Fla J Hosp Pharm 1:1, Oct 1981.

Drugs Affecting the Lower Gastrointestinal Tract

Drugs that Affect the Intestine

LAXATIVES

Constipation is abnormally infrequent and difficult fecal evacuation. Each person has regular bowel movements, ranging from three per day to three per week. A subjective aspect of constipation is the individual's feeling or attitude of dissatisfaction regarding bowel function or pattern of elimination.

Chronic constipation is sometimes caused by organic disease, such as benign or malignant tumors or childhood Hirschsprung's disease, which obstructs the bowel; megacolon; metabolic abnormalities such as diabetes mellitus, hypercalcemia, hypothyroidism, uremia, porphyria; rectal disorders; diseases of the liver, gallbladder, muscles, and connective tissues; neurologic abnormalities, such as multiple sclerosis and Parkinson's disease; and pregnancy. Clients who suffer from disorders of the gastrointestinal tract frequently complain of constipation. On the other hand, many persons complain of constipation when no organic disease or lesion can be found. A number of factors may operate to cause constipation in such persons.

1. Faulty diet and faulty eating habits (A diet that provides inadequate bulk and residue will contribute to the development of constipation. The gastrointestinal tract should function normally if fluids and residue are supplied in sufficient quantities to keep the stool formed but soft.)

2. Failure to respond to the normal defecation impulses and insufficient time to permit the bowel to produce an evacuation
3. Sedentary habits and insufficient exercise (Bedridden clients may be constipated because of inactivity or unnatural position for defecation.) (Constipation, when not a result of organic causes, is generally attributable to the above three factors.)
4. The effect of drugs (The use of antacids, diuretics, morphine, tricyclic antidepressants, codeine, aluminum hydroxide, ganglionic blocking agents, and anticholinergics often leads to constipation as a side effect.)
5. Febrile states, psychosomatic disorders, anemias, and tension headaches (Constipation can be a symptom of both functional and organic disorders.)
6. Atonic and hypotonic conditions of the musculature of the colon (These may result from habitual use of cathartics.)

Classification. Laxatives are drugs given to induce defecation. They may be classified according to their source, site of action, degree of action, or mechanism of action. The latter two classifications will be described.

Degree of action
1. **Laxatives**—stimulate bowel movements, which are formed and usually unaccompanied by cramping
2. **Purgatives**—produce more frequent bowel movements, which are soft or liquid in nature and frequently accompanied by cramping

Mechanism of action
1. **Saline laxatives**—retain and increase water content of feces by virtue of osmotic qualities
2. **Stimulant laxatives**—increase peristalsis in the colon by irritating intramural sensory nerve plexi endings in the mucosa
3. **Bulk laxatives**—absorb water and increase the volume, bulk, and moisture of nonabsorbable intestinal contents, thereby distending the bowel and initiating reflex bowel activity
4. **Intestinal lubricants**—mechanically lubricate feces to facilitate defecation
5. **Emollients,** or **fecal softening agents**—act as dispersing wetting agents, facilitating mixture of water and fatty substances within the fecal mass; when a homogeneous mixture is produced, the feces become soft
6. **Hyperosmotic agents**—act by increasing the intraluminal osmotic pressure in the bowel; because they are not absorbed, they draw water into the intestine, resulting in an increased volume that stimulates peristalsis

Table 41-1 summarizes the traditional laxatives that can be bought without a prescription and two laxatives, Lactulose and GoLytely, that require a prescription.

Indications. Laxatives may be administered for the following purposes:

1. In preparation of abdominal viscera before roentgenographic examination or surgery

2. In cases of food and drug poisoning to promote the elimination of the offending substance from the gastrointestinal tract; saline cathartics considered useful for this purpose
3. To keep the stool soft when it is essential to avoid the irritation or straining that accompanies the passage of a hardened stool (after a myocardial infarction, a rectal disorder, irritated polyps in the bowel, or cases in which straining should be avoided, as after the repair of a hernia or after a cerebrovascular accident, episiotomy wound, thrombosed hemorrhoids, hemorrhoidectomy, perianal abscess)
4. To expel parasites and toxic anthelmintics; saline laxatives routinely prescribed
5. To secure a stool specimen to be examined for parasites; saline cathartic often preferred
6. To relieve constipation during pregnancy or the postnatal period
7. To overcome decreased intestinal motility caused by drugs

There are a number of conditions for which laxatives should be given with caution, if at all.

1. Inflammatory disorders of the alimentary tract, such as appendicitis, typhoid fever, and chronic ulcerative colitis
2. Cases of undiagnosed abdominal pain; should the pain be caused by an inflamed appendix, a laxative may bring about a rupture of the appendix by increasing intestinal peristalsis
3. After some operations such as repair of the perineum or rectum (for a time, at least)
4. Pregnancy, breast-feeding, and severe anemia; debilitated clients
5. Chronic constipation and spastic constipation
6. Bowel obstruction, hemorrhage, or intussusception

Pediatric laxative use. Since constipation is common in children, parents need to be informed about problems associated with indiscriminant use of laxatives (see box on laxative abuse). In children, emotions, environmental changes (new home, new school, new friends), dietary changes, and febrile illnesses may all contribute to or cause constipation. Adding or increasing fluids, vegetables, fruits, and bran products may be very helpful. Malt soup extract is often suggested for infants up to 2 months old. For older children, glycerin suppositories or docusate sodium may be appropriate.

Elderly laxative use. Elderly clients usually have multiple chronic (and perhaps some acute) illnesses that require several medications. In addition, the aging process, with its associated decline in physiologic functions, may contribute to the increased incidence of constipation in the elderly. An increase in fluid intake, a moderate exercise program, if permitted by the physician, and an increase in intake of bran products, vegetables, and fruit may all help to correct this problem. Because there may be many factors contributing to constipation, a complete

TABLE 41-1 Traditional Laxatives

	No prescription required					Prescription required
	Irritant contact stimulant type	Osmotic saline type	Stool softener surfactant or wetting agent type	High-fiber and bulk-forming type	Lubricant	Lactulose syrup/PEG 3350*
Disadvantages with repeated frequent (longterm) administration	Watery stools, griping	Watery stools, cramps	Unreliable results, may contribute to liver toxicity	Obstruction of narrowed lumen, some difficulty in chewing and swallowing	Anal leakage, lipid pneumonia	Early, transient flatulence and cramps; nausea reported
Increases rate of transit in small bowel	Yes	Yes	Yes	Yes	Unknown	Possibly
Causes net secretion of water and electrolytes in small bowel	Yes	Yes	Yes	Yes	No	No
Inhibits absorption in small bowel	Yes	Yes	Yes	Yes	Yes	Not reported
Increases mucosal permeability in small bowel	Yes	Not studied	Yes	Not reported	Not reported	No
Causes mucosal damage in small bowel	Yes	Not studied	Yes	Not reported	Not reported	No
Acts only in colon (not small bowel)	No	No	No	No	Yes	Yes
Indicated for long-term treatment	No	No	No	Probably	No	Yes—lactulose No—PEG 3350
Examples of type	anthraquinone, bisacodyl, phenolphthalein, caster oil, danthron	magnesium salts, MOM, sodium salts, glycerin	DSS, DCS Poloxamer 188	methylcellulose, karaya gum, sodium CMC, malt soup extract, psyllium seed, agar, plantago bran (unprocessed), polycarbophil	mineral oil	Chronulac (lactulose) CoLyte Go-LYTELY (PEG 3350)
Physical or chemical property responsible for action	Mucosal surface irritation to stimulate or increase intestinal motor function or activity	Hyperosmolar ingredients trap water in intestinal lumen; hypertonicity of colon increases liquid in colon; hyperosmotic or saline	Changes surface tension of fecal mass, provides increased penetration of colonic water; penetrates and softens fecal mass by wetting agents	Absorbs water on surface, increases soft fecal mass, adds bulk and moisture to feces causing distention and elimination	Coats over fecal mass, passes with ease, lubricates gastrointestinal tract and softens feces	Colon-specific increase in stool water content and stool softening by increase in osmotic pressure (hyperosmotic) and colon acidification

*PEG 3350, Polyethylene glycol electrolyte solution.

LAXATIVE ABUSE

Regular or excessive use of laxatives usually leads to laxative abuse. This syndrome takes several years to develop and is often undiagnosed. Laxative abuse may occur in conjunction with eating disorders, such as bulimia or anorexia. Symptoms are similar to other disease states, such as nephritis, diabetes insipidus, ulcerative colitis, or Addison's disease. The major complaints on hospital admission are diarrhea and abdominal cramps. More often than not, clients deny excessive laxative usage.

If chronic laxative abuse is not detected and the client is weaned off the laxative, permanent bowel damage, osteomalacia, and electrolyte imbalance may occur.

---

and thorough history by the health care professional is necessary. Laxative abuse (see box) is often reported with this age group.

Pregnancy and constipation. Constipation is commonly reported during pregnancy. It is usually caused by colon compression as a result of the increase in size of the uterus or a decrease in muscle tone and peristalsis. Also, vitamins containing iron and calcium are often prescribed for pregnant women, and such products tend to be constipating.

Laxatives used in pregnancy should be limited to emollients or bulk-forming laxatives. Most of the other laxatives have the potential for undesirable effects; for example, castor oil may induce premature labor, mineral oil may decrease absorption of fat-soluble vitamins, and osmotic agents may induce dangerous electrolyte alterations. One must advise the childbearing client about proper diet, adequate fluid intake, appropriate exercise programs, and the importance of discussing the problem with her physician. The FDA has labeled docusate sodium, danthron, and polyethylene glycol–electrolyte solution as pregnancy safety category C. Other laxatives are unclassified.

Side effects/adverse reactions. Side effects usually include abdominal cramping, nausea, diarrhea, and flatulence.

Adverse reactions that should be reported to the physician if they occur include allergic reactions, esophageal or intestinal obstruction, change in heart rate, disorientation, cramping of muscles, increased weakness, and skin rash.

Significant drug interactions

1. The high-fiber and bulk-forming laxatives may decrease the effects of antibiotics, anticoagulants, digitalis glycosides, or salicylates by binding with the drug or delaying its absorption. Separate administration by at least 2 hours.

2. Saline or osmotic laxatives that contain calcium may interact with the same drugs as the magnesium-containing antacids. Calcium or magnesium salts may interact with tetracycline, forming a nonabsorbable complex when administered within 1 to 2 hours of tetracycline. The diarrhea produced by these drugs may interfere with absorption.

3. Irritant/stimulant/contact laxatives such as bisacodyl oral tablets, which contain an enteric coating, will be prematurely released in the stomach when administered with antacids or dairy products, producing severe cramping in the stomach and duodenum.

4. Lubricant/emollient laxatives such as mineral oil may interfere with absorption of antibiotics, anticoagulants, oral contraceptives, digitalis glycosides, and fat-soluble vitamins when concurrently administered, thereby reducing their therapeutic effectiveness.

5. Mineral oil may decrease prothrombin levels.

6. Stool softener/surfactant or wetting agent laxatives may increase the absorption of mineral oil if administered together. Granuloma formation or tumorlike deposits in tissues are also reported.

7. Other laxatives such as danthron or phenolphthalein may have their absorption increased with the concurrent use of docusate, a stool softener.

NURSING CONSIDERATIONS

Assessment. Determine the client's bowel status by careful assessment. Defecation habits, dietary patterns, fluid intake, level of daily activity, and use of laxatives are important components of the nurse's assessment.

Do not use laxatives when an emergency surgical condition in the abdomen might be suspected, such as appendicitis, bowel obstruction, hemorrhage, or intussusception.

Intervention. Encourage nonpharmacologic interventions to relieve constipation. Depending on the client's health assessment, measures to relieve constipation include adding fresh fruits, vegetables, and whole grains to increase bulk to the diet; allowing for a calm, adequate, and routine time for defecation; ensuring a daily fluid intake of eight to ten glasses of water for adequate hydration; and increasing the amount of daily exercise.

When laxatives are indicated, use the mildest effective laxative.

Education. Instruct clients to forbid children free access to laxative preparations that are in a candylike form, chewing gum, or mint, since they are likely to regard them as ordinary candy or gum and take an overdose of the drug. Deaths have been reported from such accidents.

Encourage clients to avoid the laxative habit. Inform them that misuse or overuse may result in dependence on laxatives for routine bowel function. Instruct the client not to take laxatives unnecessarily. For example, some individuals believe that laxatives are to be taken to "clean out" the system, as a tonic, in the case of colds, or at the change of seasons.

Evaluation. Determine that the client has returned to his or her normal, adequate bowel pattern.

SALINE LAXATIVES

The saline laxatives are soluble salts that are only slightly absorbed from the alimentary canal. Because of their osmotic effect in the small intestine, these salts retain water and increase the water content of feces.

Mechanism of action. An isotonic saline solution inhibits absorption of water from the bowel and therefore increases the total fluid bulk. Peristalsis is increased, and several liquid or semiliquid stools result. A hypertonic saline solution causes diffusion of fluid from the blood in the wall (semipermeable membrane) of the bowel (small intestine) and into the lumen of the organ until the solution becomes isotonic.

The water in the intestinal lumen produces fluid accumulation and distention, leading to peristalsis and eventual evacuation of bowel contents. The laxative effect may be enhanced by the intestinal release of cholecystokinin (CCK). Diarrhea is created in the small intestine to overcome constipation in the colon. Laxation results in 30 minutes to 3 hours.

Indications. The saline laxatives are the laxative of choice for securing a stool specimen for examination, for fecal impactions, for use with certain anthelmintics, and in some cases of food and drug poisoning. Phosphate enemas are useful as preparations for a barium enema.

When the object is merely to empty the intestine, magnesium citrate, magnesium sulfate, sodium phosphate, or milk of magnesia is effective. Milk of magnesia (magnesium hydroxide) is the mildest of the salines and is often the cathartic of choice for children.

The sodium salts are contraindicated in cardiac clients or those on a low-sodium diet. The magnesium and potassium salts are contraindicated in clients with renal disease.

Side effects/adverse reactions. The intestinal membrane is not entirely impermeable to the passage of saline laxatives. Electrolyte disturbances have been reported with their long-term daily use. Some saline laxatives find their way into the general circulation only to be excreted by the kidney, in which case they act as saline diuretics. Hypertonic saline solutions in the bowel may result in so much fluid loss that little or no diuretic effect will be possible. Some saline laxatives contain up to 1 g or more of sodium per dose. Some ions may have a toxic effect in impaired renal function if they accumulate in the blood in sufficient quantity. This may occur with magnesium ions if a solution is retained in the intestine for a long time or if the client suffers from renal impairment. It may also occur when large doses of the salt are given intravenously. Magnesium acts as a depressant of the central nervous system and neuromuscular activity.

Dosage and administration. The following salts, when given for their laxative effect, are usually given orally. Certain of them may be given rectally as an enema. The salts tend to have a rapid action, especially if orally administered before breakfast. They may be taken at bedtime with food for early morning evacuation (food delays the effect). Clients sometimes complain of gaseous distention after taking saline laxatives. All preparations should be dissolved and accompanied by a liberal (8-oz) intake of water, since the salts do not readily leave the stomach and may cause vomiting unless well diluted.

When a salt such as magnesium sulfate is given, it should not only be dissolved in an adequate amount of water on an empty stomach but it should also be disguised in fruit juice, plain water (chilled), citrus-flavored carbonate beverage, or chipped ice.

magnesium sulfate (Epsom salt). Magnesium sulfate occurs as glassy, needlelike crystals or as a white powder. It is readily soluble in water. It has a bitter saline taste. The usual dose for laxative effect is 10 to 15 g in 8 ounces of water. Children over 6 are given 5 to 10 g in 8 ounces of water.

milk of magnesia; magnesium hydroxide mixture. Milk of magnesia (MOM) is also used as an antacid. In the stomach the magnesium hydroxide reacts with the hydrochloric acid to form magnesium chloride, which is responsible for the laxative effect. The usual dose for adults is 15 ml (½ fluid ounce) with additional liquids, although the range of dosage is 5 to 60 ml. Children are given one-fourth to one-half the adult dose, depending on the child's age.

magnesium citrate solution. Magnesium citrate solution is not very soluble, hence the need for a relatively large dose. It is not unpleasant to take because it is carbonated and flavored. The usual adult dose is 240 ml, and the usual dose for children 6 to 12 years old is 50 to 100 ml. Results occur in 30 minutes to 3 hours.

effervescent sodium phosphate. Effervescent sodium phosphate is made effervescent by the addition of sodium bicarbonate and citric and tartaric acids. The usual dose is 10 g.

A concentrated aqueous solution of sodium biphosphate and sodium phosphate is available under the name of Fleet Phospho-Soda. The usual adult dose as a laxative is 10 to 40 ml mixed with ½ glass of cold water. Children

6 to 10 years old are given 2.5 to 5 ml. It is also marketed in a disposable enema unit. It should be used cautiously in clients on low-sodium diets.

NURSING CONSIDERATIONS

Dosing may be made more palatable by following the dose with fruit juice or citrus-flavored soda.

If mixed from a solid, thoroughly dissolve the preparation before it is administered.

These laxatives have a quicker effect when taken on an empty stomach with a full glass of water. Since results occur within ½ to 3 hours, do not administer late in the day.

Use preparations that contain added sugar or sodium with caution in clients on sodium-restricted diets or with diabetes.

STIMULANT LAXATIVES

The principal members of the stimulant group of laxatives are botanical glycoside drugs obtained from the bark, seed pods, leaves, and roots of a number of plants. Cascara, senna, rhubarb, and aloe yield anthraquinones in the alkaline portion of the small intestine. These are absorbed and later secreted to produce irritation in the large intestine. These compounds are partially absorbed from the intestine.

Mechanism of action. The anthracene laxatives act in 6 to 24 hours. They exert their main action on the small and large intestines, which explains their tendency to produce cramping. Aloe and rhubarb are almost obsolete because of their irritating properties.

Indications. Stimulant laxatives are used in preparation for barium enemas, in some cases of acute constipation, and before a proctologic examination.

Side effects/adverse reactions. The side effects and adverse reactions of stimulant laxative abuse include hypokalemia, enteric loss of protein, and malabsorption. Senna, cascara sagrada, danthron, and aloe are passed through the breast milk, initiating laxation in the nursing infant. Their occasional use should be restricted to 1 week, since long-term abuse may lead to a poorly functioning large intestine. The stimulant laxatives may lead to mucous secretion and fluid evacuation. Table 41-2 compares the stimulant laxatives in use today. They may cause discoloration of the urine (yellow-brown in acid urine, pink to red in alkaline urine). Laxatives are habit forming; they should be used judiciously.

cascara sagrada

Cascara sagrada is obtained from the bark of the *Rhamnus purshiana,* a shrub or small tree, and was one of the most extensively used laxatives. Its action is mainly on the small and large bowel. Although its effects are comparatively mild, it does act by irritation. It is less likely to cause gripping than some of the other laxatives belonging to this group of compounds. The active ingredients reach the large bowel by way of the bloodstream, after absorption in the small bowel, as well as by passage along the alimentary tract. Bowel evacuation occurs in about 8 hours. Prolonged use leads to melanotic pigmentation in rectal mucosa, which is reversible 4 to 12 months after discontinuation of the drug.

TABLE 41-2   Oral Stimulant Laxatives

Generic name	Trade name	Therapeutic effect (hrs)	Stool consistency	Remarks
bisacodyl	Dulcolax	6-10	Soft	Not to be taken within 1 hr after ingestion of milk or antacids to prevent premature dissolving of enteric coating and gastrointestinal irritation
castor oil	Neoloid emulsion, Caster Oil	2-6	Watery	Chilling, mixing with fruit juice or carbonated drinks increases palatability
cascara sagrada	Cascara sagrada	6-10	Soft, formed	Gives a yellowish brown color to acid urine; reddish color to alkaline urine
phenolphthalein	Ex-Lax, Feen-A-Mint, Phenolax, Doxidan	6-10	Semifluid	Gives pink color to alkaline urine or feces; action may persist for 3-4 days; may cause skin eruptions as dermatitis
senna	X-prep, Senokot	6-12	Soft	Crude senna may cause urine discoloration like cascara

Dosage and administration

aromatic cascara fluidextract. Aromatic cascara fluidextract is prepared using magnesium oxide as a debitterizing agent to make it more palatable. Flavoring agents, sweeteners, and alcohol (18%) are also added. Each milliliter represents 1 g cascara sagrada. The presence of magnesium oxide decreases some bitter irritating substances and the laxative action, requiring a higher dose than the other preparations. The usual dose is 5 ml; range of dose is 5 to 15 ml. For infants up to 2 years the dose is 1 to 2 ml.

cascara tablets. Cascara is available in 325-mg tablets. The average adult dose is 325 (gr 5) to 650 mg.

senna

Senna is obtained from the dried leaves of the *Cassia acutifolia* plant. It produces a thorough bowel evacuation in 6 to 12 hours and is likely to be accompanied by abdominal pain or gripping. It may cause hemorrhagic gastritis and nephritis. Senna resembles cascara but is more powerful. It is found in the proprietary remedies Fletcher's Castoria and Black Draught.

Senna tea is an infusion of senna leaves made from a teaspoonful of leaves to a cup of hot water.

A powdered concentrate of senna (X-prep), obtained from the pod of the plant, is said to contain the desirable laxative components but to be free of the impurities that have been the cause of gripping. This compound is sold under the name of Senokot (tablets, syrup, suppositories, and granules). The usual adult bedtime dose of Senokot is two tablets, 1 suppository, or 1 teaspoon of the granules.

Dosage and administration

senna syrup. The usual adult dose is 10 to 15 ml orally at bedtime. For children the dose is as follows: 5 to 15 years is 5 to 10 ml; one-half this dose for 1 to 5 years; one-fourth the dose for 1 to 12 months.

senna fluidextract. The usual dose is 2 ml orally for adults.

castor oil (Unisoil✸)

Castor oil (oleum ricini) is obtained from the seeds of the castor bean, *Ricinus communis,* a plant that grows in India but that is also cultivated in a number of places with warm climates. Castor oil is a bland, colorless, emollient glyceride that passes through the stomach unchanged, but, like other fatty substances, it retards the emptying of the stomach. For this reason it is usually given when the stomach is empty. In the small intestine the oil is hydrolyzed by pancreatic lipase to glycerol and a hydroxy fatty acid, ricinoleic acid. This hydroxy fatty acid is responsible for irritation of the bowel, especially the small intestine. It rarely reaches the large intestine before causing irritation. Its irritating effect causes a rapid propulsion of contents from the small intestine, including any of the oil that may

have escaped hydrolysis. A therapeutic dose will produce several copious semiliquid stools in 2 to 6 hours, so it should not be given at bedtime. Some persons have little or no gripping or coliclike distress; others may experience considerable abdominal cramping and exhaustion. Clients who have an irritable bowel or lesions in the bowel may be made very ill.

The fluid nature of the stool is caused by the rapid passage of the fecal content rather than by a diffusion of fluid into the bowel. Castor oil tends to empty the bowel completely; hence, no evacuation is likely to occur for a day or so after its administration. The drug is excreted into the milk of nursing mothers.

Indications. Castor oil is used much less often today than formerly. It continues to be used in the preparation of certain clients who are to have a roentgenographic examination of abdominal viscera.

Dosage and administration. The usual adult dose of castor oil is 15 to 60 ml orally. Dose for children 2 years and older is 5 to 15 ml.

NURSING CONSIDERATIONS

Castor oil may be unpleasant and nauseating. This may be overcome by mixing with orange or other fruit juices or pharmaceutical mixtures (Neoloid) to emulsify and disguise the taste of the oil.

Castor oil is contraindicated in pregnancy. Its administration often results in engorgement of the pelvic area, which may reflexively stimulate the gravid uterus.

phenolphthalein tablets (Fructines-Vichy✸)

Phenolphthalein, a phenol derivative, is a synthetic substance. Its laxative action is similar to that of the anthracene group. It is a white powder insoluble in water but soluble in the juice of the intestine, where it exerts its relatively mild irritant action. Evacuation is produced in 6 to 8 hours, unaccompanied by gripping. It acts on both the small and the large bowels, particularly the latter. When given orally, part (15%) of the drug is absorbed and resecreted into the bile (enterohepatic), and thus a prolonged laxative action may be obtained for 3 to 4 days. If the urine and feces are alkaline, they will be pink-red in color from this drug.

Repeated large doses may cause cardiac and respiratory distress, nausea, and in some susceptible individuals an allergic skin rash (pink-purple color). In other cases a prolonged and excessive purgative effect may indicate individual idiosyncrasy.

Dosage and administration. The usual dose is 30 to 195 mg orally at bedtime.

Phenolphthalein is found in some proprietary preparations with other laxatives such as agar and liquid petrolatum, as well as with other irritant laxatives.

NURSING CONSIDERATIONS

Patients taking phenolphthalein laxatives may experience belching, cramping, loose stools, nausea, mucous secretion, fluid and electrolyte loss, and rectal skin irritation. The urine and feces may become pink.

bisacodyl (Dulcolax, Bisco-Lax)

Bisacodyl is a relatively nontoxic laxative agent that reflexly stimulates peristalsis on contact with the mucosa of the colon. Bisacodyl has been successful in the treatment of various types of constipation. In larger doses, it is also widely used for cleansing the bowel before some surgeries and before proctoscopic and roentgenographic examinations. Bisacodyl is insoluble in neutral or alkaline solution and should not be taken within 1 hour after antacids have been administered. It may cause abdominal cramps.

Dosage and administration. Oral adult dosage is 10 to 15 mg. The suppositories and enema act within 15 to 60 minutes, while the tablets produce evacuation of the bowel in 6 to 10 hours. The suppositories may cause a burning sensation and proctitis.

NURSING CONSIDERATIONS

Because biscodyl tablets are enteric coated instruct clients not to chew them, or administer them chipped.

Instruct clients to swallow bisacodyl tablets whole no sooner than 1 hour before or after ingestion of dairy products or antacids. Milk or antacids can break down the enteric coating, which can lead to gastric irritation, cramping, and vomiting.

BULK-FORMING LAXATIVES

Mechanism of action. The laxatives comprising this group are polycarbophil (Mitrolan) and other natural or semisynthetic cellulose derivatives made from agar, plantago seed, kelp, and plant gums. Often these products are combined with fecal softeners (Dialose) or stimulant laxatives (Dialose Plus). They may also be emulsified with liquid petrolatum (Petrogalar, Agoral), cascara, phenolphthalein, or milk of magnesia.

The mineral oil and agar emulsions are widely advertised but are of little value because the agar content is so small (2% to 6%). The laxative effect of these emulsions is usually caused by the addition of some other ingredient.

Hydrophilic colloids stimulate peristalsis by increasing bulk and so modifying the consistency of the stool. This mechanism of laxative action is normal stimulus and is one of the least harmful. These drugs do not interfere with absorption of food, but they can cause fecal impaction and obstruction, so it is important to administer them with adequate daily fluids (8 ounces per dose). The effect of these laxatives may not be apparent for 12 to 24 hours, and their full effect may not be achieved until the second or third day after administration. Some physicians maintain that bran and dried fruits (e.g., prunes and figs) exert the same effect, and they prefer to advise these foods rather than the bulk-forming laxatives. When moistened, they swell, forming a mass of material that passes through the intestine without being affected by the digestive juices. By their blandness and bulk they make the stool large and soft so that it is easily moved along the colon and into the rectum.

Indications. The bulk-forming or bulk-producing laxatives are often the first choice for constipation. They are also used in irritable bowel syndrome, diverticular disease, and postpartum constipation and in the elderly.

Side effects/adverse reactions. Flatulence and bulky stools may occur.

Significant drug interactions. The bulk-forming laxatives interact with salicylates, digitalis drugs, and other drugs by inhibiting their absorption from the gastrointestinal tract.

NURSING CONSIDERATIONS

Because there is a possibility of impaction or obstruction if fluid intake is not substantial, avoid use of bulk-forming laxatives in clients with stenosis, adhesions, or dysphagia.

Administer with a full glass of liquid (240 ml) plus additional liquid every day to avoid intestinal impaction.

Results may not occur for 12 hours to 3 days.

Some preparations contain sugar and sodium and so may not be used with clients for whom these substances are restricted.

polycarbophil calcium (Mitrolan)

Polycarbophil is used to normalize stools both in diarrhea and in constipation by restoring the normal moisture level and providing bulk in the intestinal tract. In diarrheal conditions the intestinal mucosa is unable to absorb the excess fecal water. This agent absorbs the water (up to 60 times its weight) by forming a gel in the intestinal lumen, thus creating formed stools. In constipation the agent retains water in the lumen.

Polycarbophil has a low sodium content, and each tablet contains 150 mg calcium. The maximum dosage of calcium recommended by the FDA is much higher than the 1800 mg a patient would receive by taking the maximum dosage of 12 tablets per day. Nevertheless, patients with hypercalcemia or those susceptible to hypercalcemia should not take this product without prior consultation with their physician.

Significant drug interactions. Decreased absorption of tetracyclines may occur if they are given concurrently with polycarbophil. The client should be counseled about this possibility.

NURSING CONSIDERATIONS

Instruct the client to follow each dose of polycarbophil calcium for constipation with at least 8 ounces of water or other liquid.

Instruct the client to thoroughly chew polycarbophil tablets before swallowing.

plantago seed (psyllium seed)

Plantago seed is the dried ripe seed of the *Plantago psyllium, Plantago indica,* or *Plantago ovata.* The small brown or blond seeds contain a mucilaginous material that swells in the presence of moisture to form a jellylike indigestible mass. Although the seeds swell, their ends remain sharp and may be the cause of irritation in the alimentary tract. At present, only the preparations of the extracted gums are available, and these have the advantage of causing less mechanical irritation.

Dosage and administration

psyllium hydrophilic mucilloid (Metamucil, Karacil✲). Psyllium hydrophilic mucilloid is a white- to cream-colored powder containing about 50% powdered mucilaginous portion (outer epidermis) of blond psyllium seeds and about 50% dextrose or sucrose. This mixture is used to treat constipation because it promotes the formation of a soft, water-retaining gelatinous residue in the lower bowel within 12 to 72 hours. In addition, it has a demulcent effect on inflamed mucosa. The dosage is 4 to 7 g, administered one to three times daily.

Sugar-free Metamucil contains aspartame (Nutra-Sweet). Products containing aspartame should not be given to clients on a phenylalanine-restricted diet.

methylcellulose (Cologel)

Methylcellulose is a synthetic hydrophilic colloid. It is a grayish white, fibrous powder that, in the presence of water, swells and produces a viscous, colloidal solution in the upper part of the alimentary tract.

Dosage and administration. Methylcellulose is available in liquid, tablets, capsules, and powder dosage forms. Whichever form is used, it is recommended that a full glass of water be given. Defecation usually occurs within 12 to 72 hours.

LUBRICANT LAXATIVES
mineral oil

Mechanism of action. Mineral oil (liquid petrolatum, MO) is a mixture of liquid hydrocarbons obtained from petroleum. The oil is not digested, and absorption is minimal. Mineral oil softens the fecal mass and prevents excessive absorption of water.

Indications
1. Especially useful when it is desirable to keep feces soft and when straining at stool must be reduced, as after abdominal surgery, rectal operations, prevention of hemorrhoidal tearing, repair of hernias, cerebrovascular or spinal cord accidents, aneurysm, or myocardial infarction
2. Useful for clients who have chronic constipation because of prolonged inactivity, as in the case of clients with orthopedic conditions

Side effects/adverse reactions. Some physicians object to the use of mineral oil on the basis that it dissolves (acts as a lipid solvent) certain of the fat-soluble vitamins (A, D, E, and K), food, and bile salts and inhibits their absorption. Others maintain that only the precursor to vitamin A (carotene) is so affected and that natural vitamin A is absorbed from the intestine in the presence of mineral oil. Another objection to its use is that in large doses it tends to leak or seep from the rectum, which may cause pruritus ani and interfere with healing of postoperative wounds in the region of the anus and perineum. Although absorption of mineral oil is limited, it is said to cause a chronic inflammatory reaction in tissues where it is found after absorption. Indiscriminate use by elderly or weak individuals should be discouraged. Mineral oil may also produce a lipid pneumonia if drops coating the pharynx enter the trachea.

Significant drug interactions. Concurrent use with fecal moistening agents should be avoided, since they increase absorption of mineral oil.

Dosage and administration

Adults. Doses range from 15 to 45 ml.

Children over 6 years. Doses range from 10 to 15 ml.

Mineral oil should not be given immediately after meals, since it may delay the passage of food from the stomach.

NURSING CONSIDERATIONS

Mineral oil is not recommended for children or the elderly, because they are more at risk for aspiration of droplets, which may result in lipid pneumonia.

Administer at bedtime for results in 6 to 8 hours.

Protect client's clothing, since there may be leakage of oil from the rectum.

Do not give mineral oil routinely to pregnant women,

since it decreases vitamin K availability to the fetus, resulting in hypoprothrombinemia and hemorrhagic disease.

Do not give mineral oil within 2 hours of meals or for prolonged periods, because it interferes with the absorption of dietary nutrients, particularly with the fat-soluble vitamins A, D, E, and K.

EMOLLIENT OR FECAL MOISTENING AGENTS (STOOL SOFTENERS, SURFACTANTS, OR WETTING SOLUTIONS)

Fecal moistening agents are constantly being improved and are commonly used for treatment of hard or dry stools.

Mechanism of action. The stool softener/surfactant or wetting agent type of laxatives has its site of action within the colonic epithelium. In this area, alterations in colonic transport produce increased mucosal secretion. There are several mechanisms that decrease colonic absorption, increase secretion, or both. These mechanisms are stimulation of adenyl cyclase, inhibition of sodium absorption, mucosal alterations or permeability, and stimulation of prostaglandin E.

docusate or dioctyl sodium sulfosuccinate (Colace, D-S-S, Doxinate)

Docusate acts like detergents. It permits water and fatty substances to penetrate and to be well mixed with the fecal material. Thus this agent promotes the formation of soft-formed stool (occasionally diarrhea) and is useful in the treatment of constipation. Formed stools are usually excreted in 1 to 3 days. Docusate is available in three different salt formulations: calcium (Surfak, D-C-S), potassium (Dialose, Diocto-K), and sodium (Colace, Regulex♣, DSS, Modane Soft).

Indications
1. Indicated for clients with rectal impaction, hemorrhoids, chronic constipation, postpartum constipation, and painful conditions of the rectum and anus
2. Used in treatment of clients who should avoid straining (e.g., with rectal surgery or myocardial infarction) at the time of defecation
3. Useful for bedridden clients, especially children

Side effects/adverse reactions. Docusate is said to have a wide margin of safety and some potential negligible adverse reactions.

Significant drug interactions. Concurrent use with mineral oil may promote absorption of the oil.

Dosage and administration. All of the following dosages should be given with a full glass of water.

sodium docusate
Adults and children over 12 years. Give 50 to 500 mg daily orally.

Children 6 to 12 years. Give 40 to 120 mg daily.
calcium docusate (Surfak)
Adults. Give one capsule daily (50 to 240 mg daily orally).
Children over 6 years. Give 50 to 150 mg daily.
Dialose or Kasof
Adults. Give 100 to 300 mg daily with a glass of water.
Children over 6 years. Give 100 mg at bedtime.

poloxamer 188 (Alaxin)

Poloxamer is another oral surface–acting agent with therapeutic properties similar to docusate.

Dosage and administration
Adults. Give 480 mg orally at bedtime.
Children. Give 240 to 480 mg orally at bedtime.

hyperosmotic suppository

Glycerin suppositories are available in adult, child, and infant sizes. They promote peristalsis through local irritation of the mucous membrane of the rectum. The adult dose is 3 g; for children under 6 years of age the dose is 1 to 1.5 g held high in the rectum for 15 minutes. The effects are achieved in 15 minutes to 1 hour.

BOWEL EVACUANT
PEG electrolyte gastrointestinal lavage solution (GoLYTELY)

Mechanism of action. This powder consists of polyethylene glycol and sodium salts (sulfate, bicarbonate, and chloride) with potassium chloride, which are dissolved in 4 L of water. Bowel movement occurs within 1 hour after oral administration, with bowel cleansing taking approximately 4 hours. The drug acts as an osmotic agent. Less stool is retained after its use, but the water or electrolyte balance does not change.

Indications. GoLYTELY is used for bowel cleansing before colonoscopy and before barium enema for radiologic examination.

Side effects/adverse reactions. There is a low incidence of nausea, vomiting, bloating, cramps, and abdominal fullness with GoLYTELY.

Dosage and administration. GoLYTELY is given orally, 4 L at a rate of 240 ml every 10 min (rapidly swallowed). Fasting 3 to 4 hours before use is necessary. Generally a midmorning examination permits 3 hours for consumption, followed by a 1-hour period for bowel movement. Only clear liquids are permitted following administration and before examination. Refrigeration of dissolved powder before use (up to 48 hours) is necessary.

Pregnancy safety. FDA category C

lactulose syrup (Chronulac, Cephulac, Duphalac♣)

Mechanism of action. The normal colonic bacteria

(Lactobacillus and *Bacteroides; Escherichia coli; Streptococcus faecalis)* metabolize lactulose syrup to organic acids, primarily lactic acid, plus small amounts of carbon dioxide, acetic acid, and formic acid. This produces a drop in pH (7 to 5) of the contents of the ascending colon and softening of the feces. There is also an increase in the number of osmotically active molecules because of the formation of low–molecular weight acids.

The drop in pH and the increased osmotic action combine to stimulate the colon's own propulsive activity. A stool of increased weight, volume, and moisture content results. This unique colon-specific laxative does not cause net secretion of water and electrolytes in the small intestine and does not inhibit absorption in the small bowel.

Pharmacokinetics. After oral administration only small amounts reach the blood. Urinary excretion is less than 3% and is complete in 24 hours. The drug works on the colon where transit time is slow. The laxative effect occurs 24 to 48 hours after administration.

Indications. Lactulose syrup is used in clients with a history of chronic constipation. It increases the number of bowel movements daily and the number of days on which bowel movements occur.

Side effects/adverse reactions. Dose-related flatulence and intestinal cramps, gas, belching, and extension (transient) are seen. Excessive doses may produce some diarrhea (hypokalemic) and nausea (caused by the sweet taste).

Significant drug interactions. The effectiveness of lactulose may be reduced if it is used concomitantly with an antibiotic that destroys the normal colonic bacteria. A nonabsorbed antibiotic such as neomycin destroys enough luminal colonic bacteria to interfere with lactulose. Most systemic, highly absorbable antibiotics do not affect the colonic bacteria in the lumen.

Dosage and administration. For adults give 1 to 2 tablespoons (15 to 30 ml) daily, increased in 5- and 10-ml increments to 60 ml daily following breakfast. Severe constipation and treatment with other laxatives plus enemas and suppositories may require an initial dose of 30 ml.

To reduce blood ammonia levels in portal systemic encephalopathy the initial dose is 30 to 45 ml, three to four times daily, adjusted to produce a fecal pH of 5 to 5.5 and two to three soft, formed stools daily.

NURSING CONSIDERATIONS

To make lactulose more palatable, mix it in water, juice, or milk.

Results may take 24 to 36 hours after administration of lactulose.

Use of lactulose during pregnancy has not been evaluated; therefore another type of laxative may be given under the physician's direction.

Lactulose use in diabetic clients may cause elevations in blood glucose levels; another type of laxative without galactose or lactose may be better.

Elderly and debilitated clients receiving lactulose for 6 months or more should have serum electrolytes (potassium, chloride, and carbon dioxide) periodically evaluated.

Since lactulose contains galactose (less than 2.2 g/15 ml), it is contraindicated in low-galactose diets.

The solution may darken on exposure to high temperature, but this will not change its therapeutic effect. Freezing does not alter the therapeutic effect.

ANTIDIARRHEALS

The term **diarrhea** describes the abnormal passage of stools with increased frequency, increased fluidity, or increased weight and increase in stool water excretion. Diarrhea is acute when it is of sudden onset in a previously healthy individual, lasts about 3 days to 3 weeks, is self-limiting, and resolves without sequelae. Morbid and mortal consequences are seen in malnourished populations, the elderly, infants, and debilitated persons. Chronic diarrhea lasts for over 3 to 4 weeks, with the recurring passage of diarrheal stools, fever, anorexia, nausea, vomiting, weight reduction, and chronic weakness. It is the result of multiple causative factors (see box). Chronic diarrhea necessitates definitive treatment directed to the organic cause or causes. The causes vary from psychogenic to neoplastic origins.

The objectives of treatment are to (1) replenish fluid and electrolyte loss, (2) ascertain, if possible, the cause or causes of diarrhea, (3) reduce the frequency of evacuation, (4) absorb toxins, (5) restore the intestinal flora, and (6) treat the underlying cause or causes.

Nonspecific treatment is directed at the increased stool frequency, which burdens daily life-style; the alleviation of abdominal cramps; the prevention of dehydration and metabolic acidosis from fluid and electrolyte loss; and the minimization of weight loss and nutritional deficits resulting from malabsorption. Specific treatment is directed at the cause or condition creating the diarrhea. (See the sample nursing diagnoses related to antidiarrheal medications, p. 709.)

Ideally, the nursing process lends itself to ascertaining the type or cause of diarrhea to be treated through careful individual client evaluation. Such evaluative questions for discovering the cause or causes may be used in assessing the following criteria:

Age of the client
Occupation
Duration of diarrhea (precipitating factors tantamount to onset)
Stool description (frequency of evacuation, rectal bleeding or black stool appearance, foul-smelling odor, light color, or greasy consistency)

CAUSES OF ACUTE AND CHRONIC DIARRHEA

CAUSES OF ACUTE DIARRHEA

A. Bacterial
  1. Invasive organisms
     a. *Campylobacter fetus (jejuni)*
     b. *Clostridium difficile*
     c. *Escherichia coli* (enteropathogenic)
     d. *Salmonella*
     e. *Shigella dysenteriae*
     f. Staphylococci
  2. Noninvasive toxigenic organisms
     a. Cholera *(Vibrio cholerae)* enterotoxin
     b. *Escherichia coli* (enterotoxigenic) toxin
  3. Food poisoning as toxin mediated
     a. *Bacillius cereus*
     b. *Clostridium perfringens*
     c. *Salmonella*
     d. *Staphylococcus aureus*
B. Viral
  1. Adenoviruses
  2. Coxsackievirus
  3. Coronaviruses
  4. Echoviruses
  5. Norwalk agent
  6. Rotavirus
C. Protozoal
  1. Amebic dysentery *(Entamoeba histolytica),* amebiasis
  2. Giardiasis *(Giardia lamblia)*
D. Drug induced
  1. Antacids (magnesium containing)
  2. Antiadrenergic antihypertensive
     a. Guanethidine
     b. Methyldopa
     c. Reserpine
  3. Antibiotics
     a. Ampicillin
     b. Cephalosporins
     c. Clindamycin (clindamycin colitis associated with toxin-producing *Clostridium difficile)*
     d. Chloramphenicol
     e. Erythromycin
     f. Lincomycin
     g. Metronidazole
     h. Neomycin
     i. Penicillin G
     j. Sulfonamides
     k. Tetracyclines
     l. Trimethoprim-sulfamethoxazole
  4. Antineoplastics
  5. Antitubercular agents
  6. Chenodeoxycholic acid—chenodiol
  7. Cholinergic agents
  8. Colchicine
  9. Digitalis
  10. Ethanol
  11. Ferrous sulfate
  12. Laxatives
  13. Nitrofurantoin
  14. Other osmotic agents
  15. Parasympathomimetic (alpha agonist) drugs
  16. Prostaglandin E
  17. Quinidine
  18. Sorbitol
E. Nutritional
  1. Allergy
  2. Ingestion without discretion (spices, fats, roughage, seeds, performed toxin)
F. Other
  1. Bile acids
  2. Carcinoma
  3. Diverticulitis
  4. Fatty acids
  5. Neurogenic
  6. Psychogenic
  7. Radiation therapy
  8. Regional and ulcerative colitis
  9. Stress

CAUSES OF CHRONIC DIARRHEA

A. Addison's disease
B. Diabetic enteropathy/neuropathy
C. Iatrogenic
  1. Bacterial overgrowth
  2. Postsurgical
D. Inflammatory bowel disease
  1. Chronic ulcerative and granulomatous colitis
  2. Crohn's enteritis
E. Irritable bowel syndrome
F. Malabsorption syndrome
G. Pancreatic adenoma—non–gastrin secreting, such as syndrome of watery diarrhea-hypokalemia-achlorhydria (WDHA)
H. Pancreatic insufficiency
I. Thyroid—hyperthyroidism
J. Tumors
  1. Carcinoma of colon and rectum
  2. Intestinal
  3. Lymphoma
  4. Polyposis
  5. Villous adenoma
K. Other
  1. Blind loops, ileostomy, colostomy
  2. Carcinoid syndrome
  3. Enteritis
  4. Gardner's syndrome
  5. Gastrointestinal hormones
  6. Gluten enteropathy

CAUSES OF ACUTE AND CHRONIC DIARRHEA—cont'd

7. Ileorectal anastomosis
8. Lactase deficiency (lactose intolerance)
9. Medullary carcinoma of thyroid
10. Radiotherapy
11. Scleroderma

12. Strictures
13. Tuberculosis
14. Uremia
15. Whipple's disease
16. Zollinger-Ellison syndrome

 Selected Nursing Diagnoses Related to Administration of Antidiarrheal Medications

Nursing diagnosis	Outcome criteria	Nursing interventions
Altered bowel elimination related to diarrhea	Decrease in number of stools to less than three per day Formed stools	Record frequency, number, consistency of stools. Encourage bland diet and liquids. Administer antidiarrheal agents as prescribed.
Potential for fluid volume depletion related to diarrhea	The client will: Maintain electrolytes within normal limits Maintain normal fluid balance Experience less diarrhea Maintain normal body weight	Monitor client's intake and output. Monitor bowel movements, recording diarrhea as output. Weigh client daily. Administer antidiarrheal agents as prescribed. Assess client for signs of dehydration. Encourage high fluid intake.
Potential alteration in comfort related to abdominal cramping and diarrhea	The client will: Verbalize comfort or pain relief Maintain ADL without disruption because of discomfort	Assess comfort status of client. Instruct client in appropriate diet to minimize intestinal cramping. Provide suggestions for nondrug pain management (positioning, activities, distraction). Administer antidiarrheal medications as prescribed. Consult physician if additional pain relief is needed.

Medication profile (prescribed and self-administered as OTC drugs)

Presence or absence of anorexia, weight reduction (involuntary), fever, abdominal tenderness, dehydration

Ingestion of foods, toxic substances, milk intake, alcohol use

Travel outside the United States

Symptom description (location)

Relief obtained, if any, and treatment modality

Chronic diseases, presence of acute or concurrent illness, emotional or behavioral problems

Fluid and electrolyte loss may cause tachycardia, postural hypotension, elevated hematocrit or blood urea nitrogen, and poor skin turgor. The stool specimen may reveal occult blood (gastrointestinal bleeding), fecal leukocytes, parasites, or fat. Endocrine diseases such as diabetes mellitus and hyperthyroidism should be considered. Hospitalization is needed for dehydration that would compromise a client with congestive heart failure or chronic renal disease, since this complicates fluid replacement efforts. If any child or infant is unable to consume oral replacement fluid, hospitalization is needed to replace fluids and maintain urine flow. Bed rest alone may reduce stool frequency. In addition to the child or infant, the elderly client with a poor medical history, a client with chronic illness (heart disease, asthma), and pregnant women are at risk from acute or chronic diarrhea.

Maintenance of fluid and electrolyte balance is the most important goal of supportive therapy in acute diarrhea. If left untreated, a loss of anions (bicarbonate, organic anions as short-chain fatty acids) will create a gain of hydrogen ions, resulting in metabolic acidosis. This gain will be exacerbated by the (often) concomitant ketoacidosis of starvation and acidosis of prerenal azotemia. As volume increases in diarrhea, a rise in sodium and chloride develops with a decrease in potassium concentration. The decreased contact time of the luminal contents with the mucosal surface decreases the passive secretion of potassium. The electrolyte composition of stool water will then be close to that of plasma. The electrolyte loss of sodium, potassium, chloride, and bicarbonate is the basis of therapy.

It is recommended that clear liquids (noncarbonated soft drinks, fruit juice, diluted and flavored gelatin, and apple juice) and a bland diet be continued for 1 to 2 days. According to the cause of the diarrhea, several different medications can be given along with bed rest. These include:

Activated attapulgite
Activated charcoal
Adsorbents
Aluminum hydroxide
Antibiotics (some)
Anticholinergic activity drugs
Antiemetics
Aspirin
Astringents
Belladonna alkaloids
Bismuth salts
Bulk-forming products (including polycarbophil)
Cholestyramine
Colestipol
Digestive enzymes
Electrolyte replacement
Kaolin and pectin
Lactobacillus cultures (intestinal flora modification)
Metronidazole
Narcotic derivations
Quinacrine
Sedatives
Smooth muscle relaxants
Steroids
Sulfasalazine
Tranquilizers (anxiolytics and cyclic antidepressants)

This section focuses on the drugs with a direct pharmacologic effect on the gastrointestinal tract. The drugs providing symptomatic therapy do not alter the pathophysiology of diarrhea and do not prevent electrolyte and fluid loss. The antidiarrheal agents diminish stool water by inhibiting intestinal fluid secretion or by increasing intestinal fluid absorption. Although these drugs decrease the number, consistency, and fluidity of the stool, there is no absolute clinical evidence that an effective antidiarrheal therapeutic benefit accrues to the client. However, there is a relief of the bothersome symptoms that interrupt daily routines.

Over-the-counter antidiarrheals may contain the following ingredients: limited amounts of opiates; adsorbents, such as bismuth salts, aluminum salts, kaolin, pectin, activated charcoal, activated and colloidal attapulgite, carageenan enzymes, belladonna alkaloids (hyoscyamine, hyoscine [scopolamine], atropine); homatropine; intestinal flora modifiers; carboxymethylcellulose, phenyl salic-

ylates, zinc sulfocarbonate, calcium salts (carbonate and hydroxide), salicylates. Inactive ingredients vary, but the nurse should be aware of the alcohol content variation (1.5% to 18%).

These antidiarrheal products have a warning not to use beyond 2 days, not to use if a fever is present, and not to use in infants or children under 3 years of age. The physician may modify these instructions.

The intractable diarrhea of infancy is traditionally treated with clear liquids and gradual reintroduction of milk or formula with the addition of oral elemental diets or total parenteral nutrition. The infant syndrome is described as loose stools, resulting in dehydration and a failure to thrive. Since newborn's total body weight is usually 75% water, a 10% or greater weight loss may occur if the infant has severe diarrhea. If an infant has eight to ten bowel movements in a 24-hour period, the fluid loss may cause circulatory collapse and renal impairment. Diarrhea in infants should be considered serious enough to refer the client to a physician for evaluation.

Persistent diarrhea in the elderly can result in fluid and electrolyte loss, dehydration, and perhaps more serious medical complications. Such clients should be referred to a physician.

ADSORBENTS

Adsorbents act by coating the walls of the gastrointestinal tract, adsorbing the bacteria or toxins causing the diarrhea and passing them out with the stools. Examples of drugs in this class not requiring a prescription are activated charcoal, aluminum hydroxide, bismuth salts, kaolin, pectin, and activated attapulgite. Colestipol and cholestyramine are anion exchange resins requiring a prescription.

Kaolin is a natural hydrated aluminum silicate that is relatively inert but carries the danger of obstruction; stools appear to be more formed with this agent. The adsorbents kaolin, pectin, activated charcoal, and attapulgite are recognized as safe in therapeutic doses. Pectin causes a decrease in the intestinal pH, which destroys bacterial growth because of the unfavorable acid medium. The anion exchange resins (colestipol and cholestyramine) have adsorbent affinity directed at acidic materials (e.g., bile acids). The bismuth salts are used as adsorbents, astringents, and protectives.

Generally the adsorbent preparations are taken after each loose bowel movement until the diarrhea has been controlled. Constipation may develop because of the large amounts of the adsorbent products that must be used.

Significant drug interactions. A caution with all the adsorbents is the interference with absorption of medications given concurrently (e.g., digoxin, clindamycin, lincomycin, and quinidine). The interactions are a function of their adsorbent properties. The drugs and nutrients adsorbed include a wide range of ingested substances. These may be decreased by administering the adsorbent 2 hours or more before or after a drug (except when used to inactivate a drug or desired poison for overdose therapy).

bismuth subsalicylate (Pepto-Bismol)

Bismuth subsalicylate is available in suspension and chewable tablets. The adult dosage is 30 ml or two tablets chewed or dissolved every 30 to 60 minutes up to eight doses. A dose of 2 ounces can be given every 6 hours to prevent pathogens from attaching themselves to the intestinal wall. This impedes their replication in the gut and inhibits intestinal secretion of fluids and electrolytes (see Chapter 40).

Significant drug interactions. Since bismuth subsalicylate is a salicylate and may be taken in large amounts to control the diarrhea, it will enhance the effects of oral anticoagulants (i.e., increased bleeding time, bruising). Methotrexate may be displaced from its protein binding sites, thus causing toxicity. Probenecid, an antigout agent, promotes the renal excretion of uric acid. When combined with bismuth subsalicylate the uricosuric effects of probenecid can be inhibited by the salicylate.

The salicylate may antagonize the effects of hypoglycemic agents. It could require a change in the dosage of the hypoglycemic agent.

NURSING CONSIDERATIONS

Exercise caution when giving bismuth subsalicylate to a client taking any of the following medications: oral anticoagulants, methotrexate, probenecid, nonsteroidal antiinflammatory agents, and hypoglycemic agents.

Pregnancy safety. Not established.

Do not give bismuth subsalicylate to those allergic to salicylates.

Warn clients that bismuth subsalicylate may cause their stools to become black.

activated charcoal (Charcocaps, Charcodote✤, charcoal)

Activated charcoal is indicated for the prevention and relief of intestinal gas and diarrhea and gastrointestinal distress associated with indigestion. It acts as an adsorbent and detoxicant of irritants. It may also adsorb medication, nutrients, and enzymes.

The activated vegetable charcoal is administered as two capsules repeated every 30 to 60 minutes as needed up to eight doses (16 Charcocaps) for treatment of diarrhea symptoms. Tablets may be chewed or dissolved in the mouth and followed by water.

kaolin with pectin (Kaopectate)

Kaolin with pectin is a suspension with 6 g kaolin and 130 mg pectin/30 ml; the dosage is 60 to 120 ml after each loose bowel movement.

Dosage and administration. Kaopectate concentrate is a peppermint-flavored liquid with 8.7 g kaolin and 190 mg pectin/30 ml; the dosage is 45 to 90 ml after each loose bowel movement. Kaopectate tablets contain 600 mg attapulgite per tablet; the dose is two tablets after each bowel movement.

cholestyramine (Questran)

Cholestyramine has a direct adsorbent affinity for acidic materials (e.g., bile acids). It is indicated as adjunctive therapy to diet in the treatment of hypercholesterolemia. It has also been used for diarrhea, but this is not an FDA-approved indication for this drug.

NURSING CONSIDERATIONS

Dissolve cholestyramine well in water or fruit juice before administration.

Cholestyramine may be difficult for the client to drink because of its unpleasant taste. It is best poured on the surface of the liquid and allowed to sit a few minutes to prevent lumps. It should be drunk immediately after mixing. Water should be added to residue to ensure that the full dose is taken. It may be given with soups or applesauce.

The client's CBC, serum cholesterol, triglycerides, electrolytes, and glucose level should be monitored while the client is taking this medication.

Elderly clients are more likely to experience gastrointestinal side effects, such as heartburn, nausea, and vomiting.

Clients often complain of constipation while taking cholestyramine. This can be averted by increasing the fluid intake, adding more roughage to the diet, or taking a stool softener. Often a stool softener is ordered when this drug is started.

This drug may decrease the levels of vitamins A, D, and K. Supplemental vitamins should be added to the diet.

ANTICHOLINERGICS

The belladonna alkaloids—atropine, hyoscyamine and hyoscine, and homatropine methylbromide—are found in antidiarrheal products often with the absorbents and other antidiarrheal agents as opium extracts. These are effective agents in treating diarrhea, but the recommended doses found in nonprescription products are somewhat ineffective. The higher effective doses have a narrow margin of safety in both children and adults.

The belladonna alkaloids, however, offer effectiveness in the treatment of diarrhea by causing a decrease in intestinal tone and peristalsis at doses of 0.6 to 1 mg of atropine sulfate, thus decreasing intestinal cramps and pain. The "cotton mouth" or "dry mouth" effect usually indicates therapeuticly effective drug levels when these doses are administered. This dose of atropine, however, requires a prescription.

The following warnings on these products should be heeded by the nurse: not to be used by persons having glaucoma or excessive pressure within the eye; not to be used by children under 6 years of age; discontinue use if blurring of vision, rapid pulse, or dizziness occurs; a dry mouth may occur, necessitating a lower dosage. These anticholinergics are also contraindicated in clients with urinary retention. They may precipitate ileus and the toxic megacolon of ulcerative colitis.

The following toxic effects of belladonna alkaloids are dose related: an increase in viscosity of bronchial mucus; bradycardia and tachycardia; obstructive uropathy. They are contraindicated in clients with heart disease, hypertension, hyperthyroidism, and prostatic hypertrophy.

Donnagel

Donnagel is a suspension of kaolin and pectin, with 0.105 mg hyoscyamine sulfate, 0.018 mg atropine sulfate, and 0.0060 mg hyoscine hydrobromide in each 30 ml. The dosage is 30 ml immediately and then 15 to 30 ml after each loose bowel movement.

Pregnancy safety. Not established.

OPIATES

The opiates (codeine and paregoric—Rx C-III) act by virtue of their constipative and sedative action. They lower the propulsive motility of the bowel, reduce pain, and relieve tenesmus (rectal spasms). The delay in transit time of food permits contact time of intestinal contents with the absorptive surface of the bowel, which increases the reabsorption of water and electrolytes and reduces stool frequency and net volume.

The anticholinergics and opium derivatives decrease the motility of the bowel. They should not be used when the cause of diarrhea is an invading organism (as toxigenic bacteria or pseudomembranous enterocolitis), because these drugs permit epithelial penetration and multiplication of the organism by decreasing the intestinal motility with the subsequent lowered excretion of the organisms and their toxins.

Codeine and paregoric cause depression and sedation. This factor must be considered if the client is taking other CNS depressant drugs because of the additive effects. The opiates are short acting; frequent administration (4- to 6-hour intervals) is needed to control the gastrointestinal smooth muscle function.

combination products

Parepectolin suspension contains 15 mg opium, equivalent to 3.7 ml paregoric/30 ml, with kaolin and pectin and 0.69% alcohol. The dosage is 15 to 30 ml after each loose bowel movement. This class V drug may not require a prescription.

Parelixir is a liquid containing 0.2 ml tincture of opium/30 ml with pectin in an 18% alcoholic elixir with fruit flavor. The dosage is 15 to 30 ml, administered three to four times daily. This class V drug may not require a prescription.

Dia-Quel liquid has 18 mg opium (4.5 ml paregoric)/30 ml homatropine and pectin in a 10% alcoholic base. The dosage is 15 to 30 ml, administered three to four times daily. This class V drug may not require a prescription.

Donnagel-PG suspension contains 24 mg powdered opium/30 ml with kaolin, pectin, hyoscyamine, atropine, hyoscine (scopolamine) and a 5% alcohol base. The dosage is 30 ml immediately and then 15 ml every 3 hours as needed for loose stools.

opium tincture, deodorized

Tincture of opium, a hydroalcoholic (19% alcohol) solution, contains 10% opium with an average dose of 0.6 ml four times daily. This is a class II prescription under the Controlled Substances Act.

paregoric

Paregoric (camphorated opium tincture) requires a prescription. It is a class III drug that is equivalent to 2 mg of morphine per 5 ml. It is important that the nurse not confuse opium tincture, deodorized (10 mg morphine equivalent/1 ml), and camphorated opium tincture (0.4 mg morphine equivalent/1 ml), because opium tincture, deodorized, has 25 times more of the morphine equivalent than camphorated opium tincture. Addiction liability has been reported with these preparations. When paregoric is combined with another product, it becomes a class V product when the combination contains no more than 100 mg of opium or 25 ml of paregoric/100 ml of the mixture. The adult dosage is 5 to 10 ml, one to four times daily. For children the dose is 0.25 to 0.5 ml/kg one to four times daily.

codeine

Codeine, a class II product, when administered at a dosage of 15 mg four times daily, has shown effective antidiarrheal properties, although a range of up to 120 mg daily is suggested.

INTESTINAL FLORA MODIFIERS

Intestinal flora modifiers are bacterial cultures that consist of viable *Lactobacillus* organisms. They suppress the growth of diarrhea-causing pathogens and reestablish the normal intestinal flora.

Lactobacillus acidophilus produces lactic acid in the gastrointestinal tract. This alteration creates an unfavorable environment for the overgrowth of pathogens, especially bacteria and fungi. The acidic media also aid in the development of favorable bacteria in the gastrointestinal tract.

The modifiers may be useful in the treatment of uncomplicated diarrhea (including that caused by antibiotic therapy) and acute fever blisters and canker sores. The nurse may consider the use of a diet rich in milk or buttermilk and yogurt and high lactose or dextrose, since this is equally effective in colonizing the intestine. Patients with milk allergies should not take any of these dairy products or intestinal flora modifiers.

Lactinex

Lactinex (*Lactobacillus acidophilus* and *Lactobacillus bulgaricus*) is available in tablets and granules. Both need to be refrigerated. The dosage for gastrointestinal disturbances is one packet of granules (or four tablets) added to or taken with cereal, food, milk, fruit juice, or water three or four times daily.

Bacid

Bacid capsules are *Lactobacillus acidophilus* in sodium carboxymethylcellulose. They should be administered with milk. The dosage is two capsules two to four times daily. A fruity odor may be apparent in the stools because of these drugs.

OTHER ANTIDIARRHEAL AGENTS

diphenoxylate hydrochloride (with added atropine sulfate) (Lomotil, Diarsed✦)

Diphenoxylate, a class V product, is a narcotic chemical analog of meperidine. It does not have analgesic effects. It inhibits intestinal propulsive motility by acting directly on intestinal smooth muscles and thus decreases transit time.

Pharmacokinetics. The half-life is about 2.5 hours (range 1.9 to 3.1 hours). Because of its short duration of action (3 to 4 hours), it is administered four times or more daily. Peak plasma concentrations are reached in 2 hours.

Indication. Diphenoxylate is used for effective adjunctive treatment of diarrhea.

Side effects/adverse reactions. Side effects include drowsiness, dizziness, tachycardia, dry mouth, hyperthermia, abdominal distress, rash, and agitation.

Significant drug interactions
1. The CNS depressant effects are potentiated by alcohol and other CNS depressant drugs.
2. Concurrent use with monoamine oxidase inhibitors (MAOIs) may precipitate hypertensive crisis because of the chemical similarity to meperidine.

3. Additive effects are seen with drugs that have anticholinergic/antimuscarinic effects because of the atropine present.

Dosage and administration

Adults. Give one to two tablets (5 to 10 ml) three or four times daily until control is achieved; then reduce dosage.

Children. Use liquid dosage form only with the calibrated dropper.

Use in children under 2 years is not recommended.

Children aged 2 years and older: 0.3 to 0.4 mg/kg body weight daily, in divided doses.

Pregnancy safety. FDA Category C

NURSING CONSIDERATIONS

Pediatric and geriatric clients are more susceptible to the respiratory depressant effects of diphenoxylate.

Children with Down syndrome are reported to be more susceptible to the toxic effects of atropine.

Monitor hepatic function in the client receiving long-term therapy.

Dehydration in clients may cause a variability in the response to diphenoxylate. Clients can have a delayed toxic response. In hospitalized clients electrolytes must be monitored and dehydration corrected. If the client is not hospitalized, fluid intake should be increased to prevent dehydration.

Diphenoxylate should not be given to clients with ulcerative colitis, because toxic megacolon can occur. If abdominal distention occurs, discontinue the drug.

Diphenoxylate use should be carefully monitored to observe if constipation, a potential side effect, occurs.

Caution clients about taking alcohol and CNS depressants with the drug. Instruct about its habit-forming potential.

Dizziness and drowsiness are common side effects. Caution the client regarding tasks that involve alertness.

Refer the client to a physician if diarrhea increases or fever develops.

loperamide hydrochloride (Imodium)

Mechanism of action. Loperamide is a synthetic oral antidiarrheal similar to diphenoxylate. It inhibits peristalsis in the intestinal wall, improving both stool frequency and consistency. The slowing of intestinal motility acts directly on the neuronal pathways of the intestinal wall. Loperamide also may inhibit intestinal secretion, producing a decrease in stool water excretion.

Pharmacokinetics. Peak plasma level of this highly protein-bound drug are highest within 5 hours after administration. Plasma half-life ranges from 7 to 15 hours, with elimination half-life up to 15 hours (11-hour average). One hour following an oral dose, 85% of lopera- mide is found in the gastrointestinal tract; 25% of a 4-mg dose is excreted in the feces within 3 days, while 1.3% is found in the urine as free drug and a glucuronide metab- olite.

Indications. Indications include symptomatic control of acute and chronic diarrhea (as in inflammatory bowel disease) and in ileostomy clients to decrease the volume of intestinal discharge resulting from the intestinal resec- tion. The results are prolonged intestinal transit time, increase in density and viscosity of discharge, and normal- ization of diarrheal-induced loss of fluid and electrolytes. It may be used in diarrhea secondary to radiation therapy of diarrhea following gastrointestinal surgery.

Side effects/adverse reactions. CNS fatigue and dizzi- ness are seen only when therapeutic doses are greatly exceeded. Drug-induced gastrointestinal side effects are difficult to separate from those of diarrhea itself (epigas- tric pain, abdominal cramps, nausea, dry mouth, vomit- ing, anorexia). Skin rash hypersensitivity has been report- ed. Overdose symptoms include CNS depression, consti- pation, gastrointestinal irritation, nausea, and vomiting. Naloxone may reverse the CNS depression, but the long duration of action of loperamide requires that the nurse monitor vital signs for a least 24 hours and repeat nalox- one (because of naloxone's short duration of action) when necessary for recurring symptoms. Fluid and elec- trolyte levels must also be carefully watched.

Dosage and administration

Adults. For acute diarrhea, 4 mg is given orally, then 2 mg after each loose stool, usually not exceeding eight capsules (16 mg) daily. The long duration of action lends itself to twice daily dosage. For chronic diarrhea, the dose begins as in acute diarrhea and is then titrated to individ- ual client needs. The dosage may be administered in a single dose (because of the long duration of action) or divided doses. Average daily maintenance dose is 4 to 8 mg, not exceeding 16 mg daily.

Children. The following are recommended dosages for children for the first day of treatment:

   2 to 5 years (13 to 20 kg): 1 mg three times daily
   5 to 8 years (20 to 30 kg): 2 mg twice daily
   8 to 12 years (greater than 30 kg): 2 mg three times daily

After the first day, children should receive 0.1 mg/kg fol- lowing each unformed stool. Dosage should not exceed the dosage recommended for the first day of therapy.

Pregnancy safety. FDA category B.

NURSING CONSIDERATIONS

Do not give antidiarrheal agents (e.g., diphenoxylate, loperamide, or narcotics) for acute diarrhea or traveler's diarrhea caused by bacteria (enterotoxin-producing strains of *Escherichia coli, Campylobacter jejuni, Salmo- nella,* or *Shigella*), parasites (*Giardia lamblia*), and vi- ruses (parvovirus or rotavirus), because these penetrate the intestinal wall if retained in the intestine and must be eliminated in the feces.

Do not use these agents in clients with antibiotic- induced pseudomembranous colitis (*Clostridium difficile* toxin).

If after 48 to 72 hours of therapy the symptoms of acute diarrhea have not clinically improved, if fever persists, or if blood or mucus appears in the stool, discontinue these agents and notify the physician.

Loperamide hydrochloride may be used to reduce the volume of ileostomy discharge and so decrease fluid and electrolyte loss.

CNS side effects are not as pronounced as with diphen- oxylate hydrochloride.

Dryness of the mouth can be relieved by increasing the fluid intake or rinsing the mouth frequently.

This drug is classified as a class V controlled drug. It can cause physical dependence if taken in high doses.

Since it can cause drowsiness, caution the client against operating any hazardous equipment or driving a car.

KEY TERMS

bulk laxatives, page 698
constipation, page 697
diarrhea, page 707
emollients, page 698
fecal softening agents, page 698
hyperosmotic agents, page 698
intestinal lubricants, page 698
laxatives, page 698
purgatives, page 698
saline laxatives, page 698
stimulant laxatives, page 698

BIBLIOGRAPHY

AHFS drug information 88, American hospital formulary service, Bethesda, Md, 1988, American Society of Hospital Pharmacists, Inc.

American Pharmaceutical Association: Handbook of nonpre- scription drugs, ed 8, Washington, DC, 1986, American Phar- maceutical Association.

Anderson, BJ: Tube feeding: is diarrhea inevitable? Am J Nurs 86:704, 1986.

Berkow, R, editor-in-chief: The Merck manual. General medi- cine, vol. 1, Rahway, NJ, 1982, Merck Sharp & Dohme Research Laboratories.

Brunton, LL: Laxatives. In Gilman, AG, and others,: The pharma- cological basis of therapeutics, ed 7, New York, 1985, Macmil- lan Publishing Co.

Coombs, BM: Laxatives as colonic preparation for barium ene- ma: the patient's viewpoint, Radiography 49(585):221, 1983.

Coralli, CH: Promoting health in international travel, Nurse Pract 10(10):28, 1985.

Davis, L: The use of castor oil to stimulate labor in patients with premature rupture of membranes, J Nurse-Midwifery 29(6):367, 1984.

DuPont, HL, and others: Prevention of traveler's diarrhea (emporiatric enteritis): prophylactic administration of subsalicylate bismuth, JAMA 243:237, 1980.

Egbert, AM, and others: J Stud Alcohol 46(6):473, 1985.

Ericsson, CD: Travelers diarrhea, precautions, prophylaxis and treatment, Consultant 24(4):195, 1984.

Feldman, M: Travelers' diarrhea, Am J Med Sci 288(3):136, 1984.

Gaginella, TS: Diarrhea: some new aspects of pharmacotherapy, Drug Intell Clin Pharmacol 17(12):914, 1983.

Gever, LN: Antidiarrheals: ensuring their safe use, Nurs '83 13(10):17, 1983.

Kunkel, DB: The toxic toll of keeping thin, Emerg Med 17(1):176, 1985.

Mager-O'Connor, E: How to identify and remedy fecal impactions, Geriatr Nurs 5(3):158, 1984.

Noble, JA and Grannis, FW, Jr: Acute esophageal obstruction by a psyllium-based bulk laxative (letter), Chest 86(5):800, 1984.

Physician's desk reference for nonprescription drugs, Oradell, NJ, 1982, Medical Economics Co, Inc.

Physicians Desk Reference, ed 40, Oradell, NJ, 1986, Medical Economics Co, Inc.

Ractoo, S, and Baumber, CD: Testing times, Nurs Mirror 156(24):26, 1983.

Royal Melbourne Hospital Pharmacy Dept: Laxatives, I, Aust Nurse 14(10):58, 1985.

Royal Melbourne Hospital Pharmacy Dept: Laxatives, II, Aust Nurse 14(11):42, 1985.

Schiller, LR, and others: Mechanism of antidiarrheal effects of loperamide, Gastroenterology 86(6):1475, 1984.

Schoen, AM: Tincture of opium (letter), N Engl J Med 310(17): 1124, 1984.

Thompson, WG: Laxatives: clinical pharmacology and rational use, Drugs 19(1):49, 1980.

Tuttobene, SA: A bowel prep that's easy to swallow, RN 47(3):52, 1984.

United States Pharmacopeial Convention: Drug information for the health care provider, ed 8, Rockville, Md, 1988, USP Convention Inc.

Woodward, WE, and Woodward, TE: Management of dehydrating diarrhea, Hosp Pract 21(3):60, 1986.

UNIT XI

Drugs Affecting the Visual and Auditory Systems

Overview of the Eye

The eye is the receptor organ for one of the most delicate and valuable senses—vision. Figure 42-1 shows the parts of the eye.

The **eyeball** has three layers or coats: the protective external layer (cornea and sclera), the middle layer (which contains choroid, iris, and ciliary body), and the light-sensitive retina.

The eyeball is protected in a deep depression of the skull called the orbit. It is moved in the orbit by six small extraocular muscles.

The anterior covering of the eye is the cornea. The cornea is normally transparent, so it allows light to enter the eye. The cornea has no blood vessels and receives its nutrition from the aqueous humor and its oxygen supply by diffusion from the air and surrounding structures. The corneal surface consists of a thin layer of epithelial cells, which are quite resistant to infection. However, an abraded cornea is very susceptible to infection. The cornea is also supplied with 60 to 80 sensory fibers that elicit pain whenever the corneal epithelium is damaged. Seriously injured corneal tissue is replaced by scar tissue, which is usually not transparent. Increased intraocular pressure results in loss of transparency.

The sclera, which is continuous with the cornea, is non-transparent; it is the white fibrous envelope of the eye.

The conjunctiva is the mucous membrane lining the anterior part of the sclera and the inner surfaces of each eyelid.

The iris gives the eye its brown, blue, gray, green, or hazel color. It surrounds the pupil; the sphincter and dila-

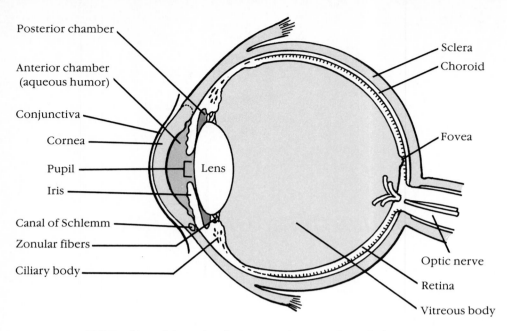

FIGURE 42-1   Schematic of a horizontal section through the eye.

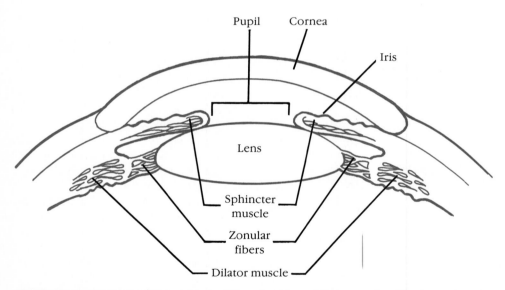

FIGURE 42-2   Accommodation and pupillary alterations. When zonular fibers contract, the pupil dilates, resulting in sharp distant vision and blurred near vision (unaccommodated eye). Parasympathetic stimulation accommodates the eye for near vision; the pupil constricts in response to contraction of the sphincter muscle. The zonular fibers are relaxed.
Pupillary diameter. Constriction (miosis): contraction of sphincter muscle (parasympathetic stimulation) alone or with relaxation of dilator muscle. Dilation (mydriasis): contraction of dilator muscle (sympathetic stimulation) alone or with relaxation of dilator muscle.

tor muscles in the iris alter pupil size. The sphincter muscle, which encircles the pupil, is parasympathetically innervated; the dilator muscle, which runs radially from the pupil to the iris periphery, is sympathetically innervated. Contraction of the sphincter muscle, either alone or with

relaxation of the dilator muscle, causes constriction of the pupil, or **miosis.** Contraction of the dilator muscle and relaxation of the sphincter muscle causes dilation of the pupil, or **mydriasis.** (See Figure 42-2.)

Drugs producing miosis (miotics) act by (1) interfering

with cholinesterase activity or (2) acting like acetylcholine at receptor sites in the sphincter muscle. Drugs producing mydriasis (mydriatics) act by (1) interfering with the action of acetylcholine or (2) stimulating sympathetic or adrenergic receptors. Pupil constriction normally occurs in bright light or when the eye is focusing on nearby objects. Pupil dilation normally occurs in dim light or when the eye is focusing on distant objects.

The lens is situated behind the iris. It is a transparent mass of uniformly arranged fibers encased in a thin elastic capsule. Its protein concentration is higher than that of any other tissue of the body.

The function of the lens is to ensure that the image on the retina is in sharp focus. The lens does this by changing shape **(accommodation).** This occurs readily in young persons, but with age the lens becomes more rigid. The ability to focus close objects is then lost, and the *near point* (the closest point that can be seen clearly) recedes. With age the lens may also lose its transparency and become opaque. This is known as a **cataract.** Unless it can be treated or removed surgically, blindness can occur. However, if the opaque (cataract) portion is located peripherally in the lens, vision is not compromised.

The lens has suspensory ligaments called zonular fibers around its edge, which connect with the ciliary body. Their tension helps to change the shape of the lens. In the unaccommodated eye, the ciliary muscle is relaxed and the zonular fibers are taut. For near vision the ciliary muscle fibers contract, and this relaxes the pull of the ligaments. Accommodation depends on two factors: (1) ciliary muscle contraction and (2) the ability of the lens to assume a more biconvex shape when tension on the ligaments is relaxed. The ciliary muscle is innervated by parasympathetic fibers. Paralysis of the ciliary muscle is termed **cycloplegia.**

Aqueous humor is formed by the ciliary body. It bathes and feeds the lens, iris, and posterior surface of the cornea. After it is formed, it flows forward between the lens and the iris into the anterior chamber. It drains out of the eye through drainage channels located near the junction of the cornea and sclera. A trabecular meshwork called the canals of Schlemm drains the aqueous humor into the venous system of the eye. (See Figure 42-3.)

The retina contains nerve endings plus the rods and cones that function as visual sensory receptors. It is connected to the brain by the optic nerve, which leaves the orbit through a bony canal in the posterior wall.

Eyelashes, eyelids, blinking, and tears all serve to protect the eye. Each eye has about 200 eyelashes. A blink reflex occurs whenever a foreign body touches the eyelashes. The lids close quickly to prevent the foreign substance from entering the eye. Blinking, which is bilateral, occurs every few seconds during waking hours. It keeps the corneal surface free of mucus and spreads the lacrimal fluid evenly over the cornea. Tears are secreted by lacrimal glands and contain lysozyme, a mucolytic enzyme with bactericidal action. Tears provide lubrication for lid movements. They wash away noxious agents. By forming a thin film over the cornea tears provide it with a good optical surface. Tear fluid is lost by evaporation and by draining into two small ducts (the lacrimal canaliculi) at the inner corners of the upper and lower eyelids.

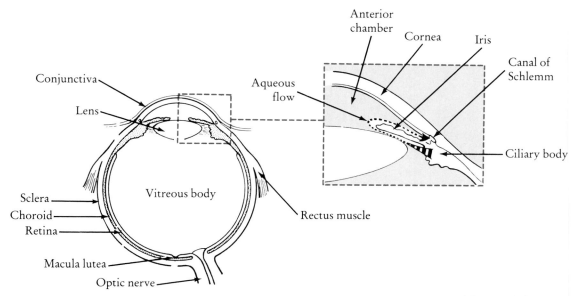

FIGURE 42-3 Diagram of a section of the eyeball showing the main structures of the eye and enlargement of the canal of Schlemm showing aqueous flow.

KEY TERMS

accommodation, p. 721
cataract, p. 721
cycloplegia, p. 721
eyeball, p. 719
miosis, p. 720
mydriasis, p. 720

BIBLIOGRAPHY

Anthony CP and Thibodeau GA: Textbook of anatomy and physiology, ed 12, St Louis, 1988, CV Mosby Co.

Gittinger JW: Ophthalmology, a clinical introduction, Boston, 1984, Little, Brown & Co.

Guyton AC: Human physiology and mechanisms of disease, ed 4, Philadelphia, 1987, WB Saunders Co.

CHAPTER
43

Ophthalmic Drugs

OBJECTIVES

After studying this chapter, the student will be able to:

1. Compare and contrast the antiglaucoma agents.
2. Discuss systemic effects of ocular drugs.
3. List antiinfective and antiinflammatory agents.
4. Discuss the various other ocular preparations and nursing considerations involved in their use.

Drugs used to treat eye disorders can be divided into three major groups: the antiglaucoma agents, the mydriatics and cycloplegics, and the antiinfective/antiinflammatory agents. Those groups of agents most likely to be encountered by the nurse in clinical practice are outlined in the box on p. 724. There are many other eye preparations, including ophthalmic diagnostic products, enzymes, irrigating solutions, eye washes, and hyperosmolar preparations. This chapter discusses the major groups and these other eye preparations, along with their major dosage and administration and other nursing considerations.

THE NURSE'S ROLE WITH DRUGS AFFECTING THE EYE

Assessment. Monitor the affected eye(s) on a daily basis for improvement in the condition for which the medication was prescribed.

Assess the redness, itching, swelling, and burning sensation that was not present before therapy started, which might be indicative of a hypersensitivity.

Systemic absorption may occur with eye drops and cause adverse systemic effects (see Table 43-7). Assess the client for ocular side effects/adverse reactions related to administration of systemic medications. (See Table 43-6.)

Intervention. In addition to developing a working knowledge of the ophthalmic agents available, the nurse must be especially aware of the special considerations in administering these drugs.

MAJOR CATEGORIES OF OPHTHALMIC AGENTS

Antiglaucoma agents
   Direct-acting miotics
   Indirect-acting miotics
   (Anticholinesterase inhibitors)
   Sympathomimetics
   Beta adrenergic blocking agents
   Carbonic anhydrase inhibitor agents
   Osmotic agents
Mydriatic and cycloplegic agents
Antiinfective/antiinflammatory agents
   Antibacterial
      Antibiotics
      Sulfonamides
   Antifungal
   Antiviral
   Antiseptics
   Corticosteroids
Anesthetics
Artificial tear solutions/lubricants
Antiallergic agents
Diagnostic aids
Enzyme preparations
Hyperosmolar preparation
Nonsteroidal antiinflammatory agents
Ophthalmic surgery aids
Irrigating solutions
Contact lens products

Ocular drugs are administered by topical application of a solution or ointment (see box, p. 725). Ocular solutions are sterile, are easily administered, and usually do not interfere with vision. Their main disadvantage is the short time the drug is in contact with the eye. Ocular ointments have the advantages of being quite comfortable on instillation and keeping the drug in longer contact with the eye for more prolonged effects. However, ointments form a film or haze over the eye that interferes with vision and causes a higher incidence of contact dermatitis than solutions. In addition, most ointments are not sterile.

Packs may also be used to apply drugs to the eye. These are cotton pledgets saturated with an ophthalmic solution and inserted into the inferior or superior cul-de-sac. Ocular drugs may also be administered by **iontophoresis,** subconjunctival (sub-Tenon's) injection, retrobulbar injection, and injection directly into the vitreous or anterior chamber of the eye.

Ocular gel formulations and Ocuserts provide new delivery systems for pilocarpine and perhaps other medications as well. The newer systems were developed to overcome some of the problems with conventional eye drops or ointments. Their longer duration of action improves client compliance and convenience and avoids the peak and valley response found with the previous solutions and ointments. It has been theorized that maintaining a steady pilocarpine release or range should reduce drug-induced adverse reactions and improve treatment outcome (Weintraub, 1985).

Education. Instruct the client and/or home care giver in proper administration of eye medications (see box, p. 725).

Caution the client to always check the bottle label for correct medication and concentration, such as 0.1% or 1%. This is an increasing concern, since many substances such as beauty aids and home products (glues) are now packaged in similar containers. Discard solutions that have become cloudy or darkened.

Store medications as directed on the label; some may need refrigeration. Once opened, most medications have a limited life (3 months or the end of the current illness). If stored longer, the medication is more likely to become contaminated.

The sterility of the preparation and/or dropper must be maintained. Do not allow the tube tip or dropper to touch anything, including the skin. Hold the dropper with the tip down. Never allow medication into the bulb of the dropper. Keep the container closed when not in use.

If two or more family members are using eye medications, each should have a separate vial to prevent cross-contamination.

Inform the client of signs of side effects/adverse reactions, as well as signs of progress. Advise client when to contact or return to the prescriber for assessment.

ANTIGLAUCOMA AGENTS

Glaucoma is an eye disease characterized chiefly by abnormally elevated intraocular pressure (IOP). This may result from excessive production of aqueous humor or from diminished ocular fluid outflow. Increased pressure, if sufficiently high and persistent, may lead to irreversible blindness.

There are three major types of glaucoma—primary, secondary, and congenital. Primary glaucoma includes narrow-angle (acute congestive) glaucoma and wide-angle (chronic simple) glaucoma. Clients with narrow-angle glaucoma have a shallow anterior chamber that may be a physiologic/anatomic predisposition. Drugs are needed to control the acute attack associated with narrow-angle glaucoma, followed usually by surgery (such as iridectomy or laser surgery). Wide-angle glaucoma has a gradual insidious onset, and its control depends on permanent drug therapy. Secondary glaucoma may result from previous eye disease or may follow cataract extrac-

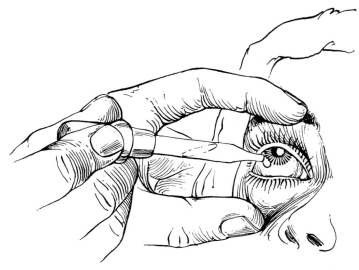

Instillation of drops into the lower lid of the eye before formation of the cul-de-sac.

tion. Therapy for secondary glaucoma is usually with drugs for an indefinite period. Congenital glaucoma requires surgical treatment.

Cholinergic and anticholinesterase drugs are used to treat glaucoma; selection of a drug is determined largely by the requirements of the individual.

MIOTIC AGENTS

Miotics, so called because they cause pupillary constriction, are topically applied agents useful in treating glaucoma and accommodative **esotropia** (crossed eyes). The parasympathomimetic miotic agents are cholinergic (minimizing the effects of acetylcholine at autonomic synapses or the neuroeffector junction of the parasympathetic nervous system) or anticholinergic (inactivating the enzyme cholinesterase by preventing hydrolysis of acetylcholine and thus prolonging the effect of acetylcholine). (See Table 43-1 for the pharmacokinetics of miotic agents.)

Side Effects/Adverse Reactions

The disadvantages to instillation of cholinergic and anticholinesterase drugs into the eye include the following.
1. Visual blurring, myopia, ciliary spasm, brow pain, and headache result from stimulation of accommodative ancillary muscles.
2. Miosis makes it difficult to adjust quickly to changes in illumination. This may be serious in elderly persons, since their light adaptation and visual acuity are often reduced. Nighttime is particularly hazardous for these individuals.
3. These drugs may cause irritation, conjunctivitis, blepharitis, dermatitis, and so on.

GUIDELINES FOR INSTALLATION OF EYEDROPS

Instillation of drops into the lower lid of the eye before formation of the cul-de-sac.

TO INSTILL EYEDROPS

Wash your hands.

Gently cleanse exudate from the eye, if necessary.

Ask the client to tilt the head toward the side of the affected eye.

Gently pull the lower eyelid down and ask the client to look up.

Instill the correct number of drops in the sac formed by the lower eyelid.

Gently apply pressure for 30 seconds to 1 minute over the inner canthus next to the nose to prevent absorption through the tear duct and premature drainage of the medication away from the eye.

Ask the client to gently close the eye, which distributes the solution. Warn against squeezing the eye tightly, which will force out the medication.

Wipe away any excess medication.

If both eyes are to be medicated, do the second instillation quickly before the patient begins to blink and tear as a reaction to the burning sensation occurring in the first eye medicated.

With children, follow the same procedure. The head may be stabilized by an assistant.

TO INSTILL EYE OINTMENT

The procedure is the same except instead of applying pressure to the inner canthus, gently massage the closed eye to distribute the medication.

TABLE 43-1   Pharmacokinetics of the Miotic Agents

Drug/strength	Indication	Onset of action*	Duration	Dose
DIRECT-ACTING				
carbachol (Isopto Carbachol, 1.5%, 2.25%, 3%)	Open-angle glaucoma	M, 2-5 min IOP, 4 hr	4-8 hr 8 hr	1 drop 1 to 3 times daily
pilocarpine HCL solution—Pilocar, Pilokair, Miocarpine♣, etc.; Nitrate solution—P.V. Carpine Liquifilm; Ocular System-Ocusert Pilo; HC1 Ophthalmic Gel—Pilopine HS	open- and closed-angle glaucoma; secondary glaucoma; during and after iridectomy; to neutralize mydriatics during eye examinations	M, solution 10-30 min IOP, peak action: Ocusert 1½-2 hr; solution usually within 75 min	4-8 hr 1 wk 4-14 hr	†
INDIRECT ACTING				
(anticholinesterases) demecarium (Humorsol, 0.125%, 0.25%)	Open- and closed-angle glaucoma; after iridectomy; to diagnose and treat accommodative esotropia	M, 15-60 min IOP, within 1 day (peak)	3-10 days 9 days or more	For glaucoma, 1 drop once or twice daily; for accommodative esotropia, see package insert for special instructions
echothiophate iodide (Phospholine Iodide, 0.03%, 0.06%, 0.125%, 0.25%)	Same as demecarium; in addition, used to treat secondary glaucoma	M, 10-30 min IOP, 1 day	7-28 days up to 28 days	‡
isoflurophate ophthalmic ointment (Floropryl, 0.025%)	Same as demecarium	M, 5-10 min IOP, 1 day	7-28 days 1 week or more	Apply thin strip from once every 3 days up to three times daily
physostigmine salicylate ophthalmic solution (Eserine, Isopto Eserine); physostigmine sulfate ointment (Eserine)	Open-angle glaucoma	M, 10-30 min	12-48 hr	Apply 1 cm ointment or 1 drop solution up to 3 times daily

*M, miotic effect; IOP, to reduce intraocular pressure.

†Dosage in acute glaucoma, 1 drop of 1% or 2% solution every 5 to 10 minutes for 6 doses, then 1 drop every 1 to 3 hours until pressure is reduced. Chronic (open-angle) glaucoma: 1 drop of 0.5% to 4% solution up to four times daily. Ocusert system: apply topically to conjunctiva once weekly. System delivers between 20 and 40 µg of pilocarpine per hour. Ophthalmic gel: apply approximately ½ inch strip of 4% gel topically to conjunctiva at bedtime.

‡To treat glaucoma, 1 drop of 0.03% to 0.25% to conjunctiva, once or twice daily. For accommodative esotropia, 1 drop of 0.03% to 0.125% solution once daily or every other day. As diagnostic agent for accommodative esotropia, 1 drop of 0.125% to conjunctiva once daily at bedtime for 14 to 21 days.

4. Cysts of the iris, synechiae, retinal detachments, obstruction of tear drainage, and even cataracts may develop with prolonged usage, especially with the long-acting anticholinesterases.

5. Tolerance and resistance may develop with any of the miotics.

6. Instillation must be frequent with the liquid and ointment forms.

7. Systemic side effects include salivation, nausea, vomiting, diarrhea, precipitation of asthmatic attack, fall in blood pressure, and other symptoms of parasympathetic stimulation (see Chapter 19).

8. Anticholinesterase drugs may cause spasm of the wink reflex, which is annoying to the individual.

9. Anticholinesterase agents (including those used to treat myasthenia gravis) lower plasma pseudocholinesterase activity. If an adjunctive skeletal muscle relaxant such as succinylcholine (a neuromuscular blocking agent) is used during surgery, respiratory and cardiovascular collapse will result. Because of their long duration of effects, the eye drops must be discontinued several weeks before surgery or electroshock therapy. Another depolarizing neuromuscular blocking agent is decamethonium bromide. Some nondepolarizing agents are metocurine iodide, tubocurarine, gallamine, and pancuronium bromide.

10. Cholinesterase inhibitors also interact with carbamate and organophosphate pesticides, causing additive sys-

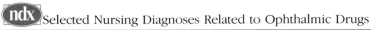

Nursing diagnosis	Outcome criteria	Interventions

Knowledge deficit related to new ophthalmic drug regimen	Client will:
	Express understanding of purpose, function, side effects/adverse reactions
	Demonstrate proper handling and administration
		Assess client's level of understanding.
		Determine educational needs of client.
		Instruct client in:
		  Purpose and function of medicine
		  Side effects/adverse reactions that may occur and appropriate response
		  Proper storage and handling
		  Correct method of administration
		  Systemic reactions that may occur with topically applied eye preparations
		Provide client with a list of possible drug interactions.

Anxiety related to possible decrease in or loss of vision	Client will: Verbalize fears and concerns	Assess client for perceptions and fears related to eye disorder. Encourage open communication about fears. Provide emotional support. Provide information related to effectiveness of drug therapy. Allay unwarranted fears.
Alteration in comfort related to ophthalmic disorder	Client will: Express a decrease in symptoms and discomfort	Closely assess the client's symptoms and level of comfort. Provide rest and limiting of eye activity (reading, etc.). Provide emotional support and encouragement.
Potential injury related to impaired vision	Client will: Maintain activity appropriate for level of vision without injury	Assess level of vision impairment. Provide safety measures as needed. Encourage client to adjust activities in accordance with client's level of vision.

temic effects from absorption through the respiratory tract or skin. Nursing intervention includes advising clients of the need for respiratory mask and frequent bathing and changes of clothing if these substances are encountered in the house, garden, or working/living environment or in treatment of head lice (malathion).

Two antidotes are available for overcoming effects caused by cholinergic stimulation—atropine and pralidoxime. Pralidoxime chloride (Protopam) is effective only against anticholinesterases that phosphorylate the enzyme. Given early enough, it reactivates the enzyme.

Cholinergic (Parasympathomimetic) Miotics (Direct Acting)

Cholinergic drugs are chemically related to acetylcholine, the neurotransmitter that mediates nerve impulse transmission at all cholinergic or parasympathetic nerve sites. Applied topically to the eye, cholinergic drugs (1) cause contraction of the sphincter muscle of the iris, resulting in pupil constriction (miosis), (2) cause spasms of the ciliary muscle and deepening of the anterior chamber, and (3) cause vasodilation of intraocular vessels (such as those in the iris) or where intraocular fluids leave the eye, leading to an increase in aqueous humor outflow. The ciliary muscle effect leaves the eye in accommodation of near vision.

The cholinergic agents have a duration of miotic action of approximately 4 to 8 hours (pilocarpine drops) or 2 to 8 hours (carbachol). These agents are very effective in many cases of chronic glaucoma. Their side effects are less severe and occur less frequently than those caused by anticholinesterase agents.

The cholinergic drugs are used to lower intraocular pressure in glaucoma and in accommodative esotropia. Unless the elevated pressure is lowered, the result is an impaired blood supply to the optic nerve, with eventual atrophy of the nerve and visual field loss. Contraction of the ciliary muscles and constriction of the pupil may widen the filtration angle and permit increased outflow of aqueous humor. Increased outflow may also result from dilation of collector channels and veins peripheral to the canal of Schlemm.

Clinical toxicity from overdosage or unusual sensitivity to these drugs is manifested by headache, salivation, sweating, abdominal discomfort, diarrhea, asthmatic attacks, and a fall in blood pressure.

Anticholinesterase Miotics (Indirect Acting)

Anticholinesterase drugs inhibit the enzymatic destruction of acetylcholine by inactivating cholinesterase. This permits acetylcholine to act on the iris sphincter and ciliary muscles, producing pupil constriction (miosis) and ciliary muscle contraction (accommodation).

Physostigmine and demecarium act on true cholinesterase. Echothiophate and isoflurophate depress both plasma (true cholinesterase) and erythrocyte cholinesterase.

The irreversible anticholinesterase drugs (echothiophate, isoflurophate) form stable complexes with cholinesterase and thus irreversibly impair the destructive function of the enzyme. Destruction of acetycholine then depends on synthesis of new enzymes.

Demecarium is more toxic than the other agents in this category, so it is not as commonly used. Although it is a reversible inhibitor, its prolonged action has results similar to the irreversible inhibitors. Isoflurophate is available only in an ointment formulation.

SYMPATHOMIMETIC AGENTS

The mechanism by which the topically applied adrenergic epinephrine acts is by contraction of the dilator muscle of the pupil. Mydriasis (pupillary dilation) is achieved within minutes following ophthalmic instillation and has a duration of action of several hours, during which time it lowers the intraocular pressure. These sympathomimetics decrease aqueous humor production (beta adrenergic effect) and increase its outflow (alpha adrenergic effect).

Sympathomimetic ophthalmic effects are pupil dilation, alpha adrenergic agonist effects (vasoconstriction and increased aqueous humor outflow), and beta adrenergic agonist effects (ciliary muscle relaxation and decreased aqueous humor formation). (See Table 43-2.)

The primary sympathomimetic agents are dipivefrin and epinephrine.

dipivefrin HCI ophthalmic solution (Propine 0.1%)

Mechanism of action. Dipivefrin is a prodrug of epinephrine. Enzymes in the eye will convert dipivefrin to epinephrine. The chemical modification creates a more lipophilic compound that facilitates absorption and penetration through the cornea into the anterior chamber of the eye. The penetration and absorption of dipivefrin are about 17 times greater than those of epinephrine. The epinephrine liberated from dipivefrin acts as an adrenergic agonist. It decreases the intraocular pressure by

TABLE 43-2 Drug Effects on Aqueous Humor

Drug	Decreases aqueous humor production	Increases aqueous humor drainage or outflow
SYMPATHOMIMETICS		
epinephrine	+++	++
dipivefrin	+++	++
BETA-BLOCKERS		
betaxolol	+++	U
levobunolol	+++	U
timolol	+++	+
DIRECT MIOTICS		
acetylcholine	+	+++
carbachol	+	+++
pilocarpine	+	+++
INDIRECT MIOTICS		
physostigmine	U	+++
demecarium	U	+++
echothiophate	U	+++
isoflurophate	U	+++
CARBONIC ANHYDRASE INHIBITORS		
acetazolamide	+++	U

+, low potential; +++, greatest potential; U, unknown

reducing aqueous humor production and enhancing aqueous outflow.

Indications. Treatment of open-angle glaucoma

Pharmacokinetics

Onset of effect. Within 1/2 hour

Peak effect. Within 60 minutes

Duration of action. Approximately 12 hours

Side effects/adverse reactions. Frequently reported is a burning or stinging sensation in the eye that is rarely troublesome. If the drug is absorbed, systemic effects of tachycardia, dysarrhythmias, and hypertension may occur.

Significant drug interactions. None significant

Dosage and administration. Administer 1 drop topically to the conjunctiva every 12 hours.

Pregnancy safety. FDA category B

NURSING CONSIDERATIONS

Dipivefrin is contraindicated in clients with narrow-angle glaucoma because pupil dilation may aggravate the condition. In aphakic clients (those devoid of a crystalline lens), dipivefrin or epinephrine may cause macular edema.

epinephrine ophthalmic solution (Epifrin, Glaucon in 0.1%, 0.25%, 0.5%, 1%, and 2%)

epinephrine bitartrate ophthalmic solution (Epitrate, 1% and 2%)

epinephryl borate ophthalmic solution (Epinal, Eppy/N in 0.25%, 0.5%, 1%, and 2%)

Mechanism of action. A direct-acting sympathomimetic agent, it decreases production of aqueous humor and increases its outflow. Epinephrine is also used as a surgical agent or antihemorrhagic mydriatic. It stimulates alpha adrenergic receptors in the conjunctiva, producing vasoconstriction and hemostasis of the small blood vessels. It contracts the dilator muscle of the pupil (alpha stimulating effect), which produces pupillary dilation.

Indications. Treatment of open-angle glaucoma and of topical hemorrhage in ocular surgery or to induce a mydriatic effect

Pharmacokinetics

Onset of effect. Vasoconstriction within 5 minutes, reduction of intraocular pressure within 1 hour

Time to peak effect. For reduction of intraocular pressure, between 4 and 8 hours

Duration of action. Intraocular pressure reduction—up to 24 hours. Vasoconstriction effect—usually less than 60 minutes.

Side effects/adverse reactions. Most frequently reported side effects (rarely troublesome) are headaches, pain in brow, stinging or burning sensation in the eye, or watering of the eye. Less often reported is eye pain. The

following adverse effects require a physician's attention: signs and symptoms of systemic absorption, such as tachycardia, palpitations, increased sweating, tremors, and lightheadedness. Visual disturbance such as blurred vision may indicate maculopathy (edema) in eyes without the crystalline lens (**aphakia**).

Significant drug interactions. Tricyclic antidepressants, H_1 antihistamines, and guanethidine potentiate the pressor response of epinephrine.

Exaggerated sympathomimetic effects occur with monoamine oxidase inhibitors.

Myocardial sensitization may occur with ophthalmic use of epinephrine before halothane general anesthesia.

Dosage and administration

Glaucoma. Instill 1 drop of Epitrate 1% or 2% solution, Epinal 0.5% to 1% solution, Epifrin 0.5% to 2% solution to conjunctiva twice daily.

As a surgical agent or for antihemorrhagic and/or mydriatic effect. 1 drop of 0.1% epinephrine ophthalmic solution only to conjunctiva for up to three doses or as needed to produce the specific effects.

Pregnancy safety. FDA category C

NURSING CONSIDERATIONS

Assessment. Watch for systemic effects such as tachycardia and elevated blood pressure, which may occasionally occur with its use. Other possible side effects include eye pain, ocular irritation, and tearing. There have also been reports of epinephrine causing macular edema.

Intervention. Discoloration or precepitation of epinephrine indicates oxidation to inactive products and the solution should be discarded.

Education. Warn client not to use the over the counter sympathomimetic drugs such as phenylephrine (an alpha agonist vasoconstrictor) with timolol ophthalmic drops (a beta blocker). The beta blocker eye drop may prevent the vasodilation, which opposes the alpha adrenergic vasoconstriction. Further, epinephrine or phenylephrine may be absorbed systemically to interact with beta blockers and MAO inhibitors.

Evaluation. Monitor the affected eye(s) on a daily basis for improvement.

BETA ADRENERGIC BLOCKING AGENTS

The beta blocking agents include betaxolol, levobunolol, and timolol. Betaxolol is a cardioselective (beta$_1$) blocking agent, whereas levobunolol and timolol are noncardioselective, that is, they can block both beta$_1$ and beta$_2$ adrenergic receptors. These agents reduce intraocular pressure in clients with or without glaucoma. The precise mechanism of action is not understood, but the effect may be related to the reduction of aqueous humor formation and to a minimal increase in outflow (reported with timolol).

betaxolol hydrochloride ophthalmic solution (Betoptic 0.5%)

Indications. Treatment of open-angle glaucoma and ocular hypertension; may be a drug of choice for clients with pulmonary disease because of its selective $beta_1$ blocking effects, although the nurse should still monitor for respiratory difficulties.

Pharmacokinetics
Onset of effect. Within ½ hour
Time to peak action. 2 hours
Duration of action. Following a single dose of medication, 12 hours

Side effects/adverse reactions. May frequently produce stinging sensation in eye. Less often reported is photosensitivity or eye irritation. Physician intervention is necessary if severe irritation or inflammation occurs in the eye. If drug is systemically absorbed, depression, confusion, bradycardia, insomnia, increased weakness, wheezing, or respiratory difficulties may be seen.

Significant drug interactions. None noted
Dosage and administration. Instill 1 drop of 0.5% solution to conjunctiva, twice daily.
Pregnancy safety. FDA category C

levobunolol hydrochloride ophthalmic solution (Betagan 0.5%)

Indications. Treatment of open-angle glaucoma and ocular hypertension
Pharmacokinetics
Onset of effect. Within 60 minutes
Time to peak action. Between 2 and 6 hours
Duration of effect. The lowering of intraocular pressure may be maintained for up to 1 day after a single dose administration

Side effects/adverse reactions. Burning or stinging sensation in the eye is infrequently reported and rarely troublesome. The following adverse effects require medical intervention if they occur. Rare adverse effects include severe eye inflammation or irritation, visual disturbances, rash, pruritus, or allergic reaction. Signs and symptoms of systemic absorption may include chest pain, ataxia, depression, confusion, lightheadedness, headaches, bradycardia or tachycardia, nausea, vomiting, edema of feet, ankles, or lower extremities, increased weakness, and wheezing or respiratory difficulties.

Significant drug interactions. None reported.
Dosage and administration. Instill 1 drop to conjunctiva once or twice daily.
Pregnancy safety. FDA category C

Timolol maleate ophthalmic solution (Timoptic 0.25 and 0.5%)

Indications. Treatment of open-angle glaucoma, ocular hypertension, secondary glaucoma, and glaucoma in aphakic eyes
Pharmacokinetics
Onset of effect. Within 1/2 hour
Time to peak action. Between 1 and 2 hours
Duration of effect. Up to 24 hours after a single dose.

Side effects/adverse reactions. Same as levobunolol. In addition, the following systemic effects have also been reported: increased anxiety, decreased libido, diarrhea, hallucinations, abdominal distress, and pain.

Dosage and administration. Instill 1 drop to conjunctiva once or twice daily.
Pregnancy safety. FDA category C

NURSING CONSIDERATIONS

Usually these agents are well tolerated with occasional signs of mild ocular irritation. Local hypersensitivity (rash) occurs rarely. A slight reduction of resting heart rate may occur, and acute bronchospasm in clients with bronchospastic disease has been reported.

There is sufficient absorption from the conjunctiva and nasopharynx to produce systemic nonselective beta adrenergic ($beta_1$ and $beta_2$) effects such as cardiopulmonary complications and exacerbation of asthma. Use caution in administering beta adrenergic blocking agents to clients who have bronchial asthma, heart disease, sinus bradycardia or greater than first-degree heart block, cardiogenic shock, right ventricular failure caused by pulmonary hypertension, or congestive heart failure. Also see nursing considerations for beta adrenergic blocking agents in Chapter 20.

CARBONIC ANHYDRASE INHIBITOR AGENTS

The three carbonic anhydrase inhibitors include acetazolamide, dichlorphenamide, and methazolamide. Acetazolamide, the most widely used drug of this class, is the focus of this discussion.

Mechanism of action. The carbonic anhydrase inhibitors are sulfonamides (nonbacteriostatic). The mechanism of action is incompletely understood, but they lower intraocular pressure by decreasing the aqueous production to half of its baseline measurement. This mechanism may be attributed to the decrease of bicarbonate ion concentration in aqueous humor ocular fluids and the resulting systemic metabolic acidosis.

Indications. Treatment of open-angle, secondary, and angle-closure glaucoma.

Pharmacokinetics. See Table 43-3.

Side effects/adverse reactions. The most frequent side effects are rarely troublesome. They include diarrhea, feeling of discomfort, diuresis, anorexia, metallic taste in mouth, nausea, vomiting, tingling or numbness (paresthesia) of fingers, hands, toes, feet, mouth, or anus, and weight loss. Physician intervention is necessary if client has the signs and symptoms of acidosis, blood dyscrasias, or hypokalemia.

Significant drug interactions. The following interactions may occur when carbonic anhydrase inhibitors are given with the drugs listed below.

Drug	Possible Effect and Management
amphetamines, quinidine, mecamylamine	carbonic anhydrase inhibitors decrease excretion of these drugs because of alkalinization of the urine, and they may increase their therapeutic and side effects and prolong their duration of effect. Avoid concurrent use of mecamylamine. Monitor closely, since dosage adjustments are usually necessary with other medications.
methenamine	carbonic anhydrase inhibitors reduce the effectiveness of methenamine because of alkalinization of urine, which prevents conversion of methenamine to formaldehyde. Concurrent drug administration is not recommended.

Dosage and administration. Acetazolamide tablets (Ak-Zol, Diamox, Dazamide):

Adults

Open-angle glaucoma. Initially—250 mg orally up to four times daily. Maintenance—titrate according to client's response.

TABLE 43-3 Pharmacokinetics of Carbonic Anhydrase Inhibitors

	acetazolamide	dichlorphenamide	methazolamide
Half-life Peak effects	Tablet: 10-15 hr 1 tablet: 2-4 hr Sustained action tablet: 8-12 hr 15 min IV	2-4 hr	14 hr 6-8 hr
Onset of action	Tablet: 1-1½ hr Capsule: 2 hr 2 min IV	30-60 min	2-4 hr
Duration of action	Tablet: 8-12 hr Capsule: 18-24 hr 4-5 hr IV	6-12 hr	10-18 hr

Secondary glaucoma. 250 mg orally every 4 hours; adjust dose according to client's response.

Malignant (ciliary block) glaucoma. 250 mg orally four times daily.

Children

Glaucoma. 8 to 30 mg/kg orally (usually 10 to 15 mg/kg), or 300 to 900 mg/m^2 daily, given in divided doses.

Pregnancy safety. Not established

NURSING CONSIDERATIONS

Assessment. Recall that these drugs cause some decrease in renal blood flow and glomerular filtration rate, which produces an increased excretion of sodium, potassium, bicarbonate, and water alkaline diuresis. Monitor appropriate serum concentrations.

Reactions to sulfonamide agents (thiazide diuretic, oral sulfonylureas), will raise an index of suspicion for cross allergenicity and hypersensitivity. Contraindications include clients with decreased sodium/potassium serum levels (because of increased drug plasma levels) and hepatic and renal dysfunction (potential for renal calculi formation).

Education. Consider use of potassium supplements by client or suggest dietary sources of potassium for client.

Evaluation. Monitor the affected eye(s) on a daily basis for improvement.

OSMOTIC AGENTS

Osmotic agents are given intravenously or orally to reduce the intraocular pressure. These agents generally do not cross the blood aqueous barrier into the anterior chamber of the eye and are rarely found in ocular humor.

The osmotherapeutic agents (glycerin and mannitol) create ocular hypotension by producing an osmotic gradient (making the blood hypertonic relative to the intraocular fluids). This gradient forces the water from the aqueous and vitreous humors into the bloodstream. The effect on the eye is reduction of volume of intraocular fluid, producing a decrease in intraocular pressure.

glycerin oral solution (Glyrol, Osmoglyn)
glycerin ophthalmic solution (Ophthalgan)

Glycerin is given orally before iridectomy to reduce intraocular pressure in individuals with acute narrow-angle glaucoma. It is used preoperatively and postoperatively in conditions such as congenital glaucoma, retinal detachment, cataract extraction, and keratoplasty (corneal transplant). It may also be used in some secondary glaucomas.

A local anesthetic (1 to 2 drops) is administered before use of glycerin ophthalmic solution because of pain and irritation from glycerin instillation.

Indications. Glucose (Glucose-40 Ophthalmic ointment) is indicated for topical osmotherapy to reduce corneal edema. This 40% ointment is used two to six times daily.

Pharmacokinetics

Oral glycerin

Onset of effect. Reduces intraocular pressure within 10 minutes

Time to peak action. 1 to 1½ hours

Duration of effect. 5 hours

Metabolism. Liver

Excretion. Kidneys

Side effects/adverse reactions. Reported side effects (rarely troublesome) include headaches, nausea, vomiting, diarrhea, dry mouth, increased thirst, and lightheadedness. Physician intervention is necessary for confusion or irregular heart rate.

Significant drug interactions. None

Dosage and administration

Oral. 1 to 1.5 g/kg before surgery for adults and children. Additional doses of 500 mg/kg (children) up to 1.5 g/kg (adults) may be administered in 4 to 8 hours, if necessary.

Ophthalmic glycerin. Instill 1 or 2 drops before examination to reduce edema, clear the cornea, and improve visualization for ophthalmoscopic gonioscopic examination.

NURSING CONSIDERATIONS

Assessment. Use glycerin cautiously in clients with cardiac, renal, or hepatic disease. The shift in body water may cause pulmonary edema or congestive heart failure. Elderly clients may be subject to dehydration because of a mild diuretic action. Diabetic individuals receiving glycerin should be carefully observed for symptoms of acidosis, since the metabolism of glycerin to carbohydrates may cause transient hyperglycemia and glycosuria.

Intervention. Flavor glycerin with lemon or lime juice, pour over cracked ice, and have the client sip it through a straw to decrease the incidence of nausea and vomiting.

Education. Headache is the result of cerebral dehydration. To relieve it have the client lie down during and after oral administration of glycerin.

Evaluation. Monitor the affected eye(s) on a daily basis for improvement.

isosorbide (Ismotic 45% Solution)

Indications. Isosorbide is an oral osmotic agent used for emergency treatment of acute angle-closure glaucoma

and for conditions requiring rapid reduction of intraocular pressure. Isosorbide is available as a 45% solution.

Pharmacokinetics

Onset of action. 10 to 30 minutes

Peak effect. Within 1 to 1½ hours

Duration of action. 5 to 6 hours

Side effects/adverse reactions. Nausea, vomiting, headaches, confusion, and disorientation have been reported.

Significant drug interactions. None

Dosage and administration

Initial dosage. 1.5 g/kg, with a dosage range of 1 to 3 g/kg, given two to four times daily if necessary.

Pregnancy safety. FDA category B

NURSING CONSIDERATIONS

Prepare as for oral glycerin to increase palatability. Isosorbide is contraindicated in clients with dehydration, pulmonary edema, hemorrhagic glaucoma, and anuria caused by kidney disease.

mannitol injection (Osmitrol✳)

Mannitol has osmotic and diuretic properties. It is available in 5%, 10%, 15%, 20%, and 25% solutions.

Mechanism of action. See discussion for osmotic agents p. 731.

Indications. Treatment of ocular hypertension, edema, and cerebral edema and promotion of urinary excretion of selected toxic substances, such as salicylates, barbiturates, and bromides

Pharmacokinetics

Onset of effect. Diuretic effect, 1 to 3 hours; reduction of intraocular fluid pressure or cerebrospinal pressure, within 15 minutes

Time to peak action (reduction in intraocular pressure). ½ to 1 hour after starting infusion

Duration of effect. Reduction of intraocular pressure, 4 to 8 hours

Reduction of cerebrospinal fluid pressure, 3 to 8 hours after infusion is stopped

Both pressures will increase in about 12 hours after a mannitol infusion is discontinued.

Metabolism. Liver (slightly)

Excretion. Kidneys

Side effects/adverse reactions. The following side effects are rarely troublesome: dry mouth, thirst, headache, nausea, vomiting, increased frequency of urination, lightheadedness, rash, and blurred vision. Physician intervention is necessary if client has chest pain, tachycardia, elevated temperature, chills, confusion, irregular heart rate, muscle cramping or pain, paresthesia in hands or feet, convulsions, tremors, increased weakness, pulmonary congestions, difficulty urinating, or edema of lower extremities.

Significant drug interactions. When mannitol is given concurrently with digitalis glycosides, an increase in digitalis toxicity may result. Monitor closely.

Dosage and administration

Adults. To treat cerebral edema, elevated intracranial pressure, or glaucoma: 1.5 to 2 g/kg by intravenous infusion given over 1/2 to 1 hour. (Usually a 15% to 25% solution is used.) Small clients or very debilitated persons may require only a 500 mg/kg dosage. Maximum daily dose, 6 g/kg.

Children. 1 to 2 g/kg by intravenous infusion or 30 to 60 g/m^2 (15% to 20% preparation) given over ½ to 1 hour.

Pregnancy safety. FDA category C

NURSING CONSIDERATIONS

If the solution has crystallized, warming will return the crystals to solution. Monitor clients receiving mannitol carefully for fluid and electrolyte balance (hypervolemia), urinary output, and vital signs, since mannitol produces more diuresis than urea.

urea, sterile (Ureaphil)

Mechanism of action. See osmotic agents, p. 731.

Indications. Treatment of cerebral edema, secondary glaucoma, and malignant glaucoma

Pharmacokinetics

Onset of action. Reduces intraocular and intracranial pressure within 10 minutes of starting an infusion

Time to peak action. 1 to 2 hours

Duration of effect

Diuretic effect, 3 to 10 hours after infusion is discontinued

Reduction in intraocular pressure, 5 to 6 hours

A rebound effect can occur approximately 12 hours after urea is stopped.

Half-life. 1.17 hours

Metabolism. Gastrointestinal tract (partially).

Excretion. Kidneys

Side effects/adverse reactions. Side effects (rarely troublesome) include dry mouth, increased thirst, headache, nausea, vomiting, lightheadedness, and skin blemishes. Physician intervention is necessary if client has visual disturbances, severe headaches, confusion, tachycardia, elevated temperature, increased anxiety, irregular heart rate, muscle cramping, paresthesia of hands or feet, convul-

sions, tremors, increased weakness, or redness or swelling at injection site.

Significant drug interactions. None

Dosage and administration

Adults. Diuretic or to treat glaucoma: 500 mg to 1.5 g/kg by intravenous infusion (a 30% solution in 5% or 10% dextrose injection), given at a rate of 60 drops (4 to 6 ml) per minute over 1/2 to 2 hours. Maximum daily dose is 2 g/kg/day.

Children. 2 years and older, see adult dose. Less than 2 years old, 100 mg to 1.5 g/kg. Preparation of solution and administration are the same as for adults.

Pregnancy safety. FDA category C

NURSING CONSIDERATIONS

Assessment. Urea is contraindicated in clients with severe dehydration, active intracranial bleeding (except during craniotomy), and hepatic and renal impairment.

Assess BUN before and frequently during intravenous administration. If it becomes elevated to 75 to 100 mg/100 ml, slow infusion rate or discontinue infusion.

Monitor vital signs and fluid intake and output.

Evaluate serum electrolyte concentrations, especially sodium and potassium, and renal function studies.

Intervention. Preparation for administration varies from product to product depending on the manufacturer. Consult package insert.

Do not infuse at a rate greater that 4 ml/minute, since it may result in hemolysis and cerebral vasomotor symptoms.

Use urea as soon as it is reconstituted. Discard any unused solution.

Do not infuse into veins of lower extremities, since phlebitis and thrombosis may occur, especially in the elderly.

To prevent tissue irritation and necrosis at the injection site, avoid extravasation.

If the client has difficulty urinating or is comatose, insert an indwelling urethral catheter.

If there is a need to concurrently administer urea and blood, do not administer through the same intravenous administration set.

Education. Prepare the client for the anticipated diuresis. Explain to the client that urea is usually administered 60 minutes before ocular surgery to reduce intraocular pressure.

MYDRIATIC AND CYCLOPLEGIC AGENTS

These topically applied autonomic drugs can cause dilation of pupils (**mydriasis**) and paralysis of accommodation **(cycloplegia).** Both sympathomimetic and para-sympatholytic agents can cause mydriasis, by different mechanisms of action. The effects of these agents depend on the patient's age, race, and color of iris. Mydriatic agents evoke less of a response in persons with heavily pigmented (dark) irides than in those with lighter pigmented (blue) irides. Thus blacks tend to respond less to the agents than whites.

ANTICHOLINERGIC (PARASYMPATHOLYTIC) AGENTS

Mechanism of action. Anticholinergic agents block acetylcholine stimulation of the sphincter muscle of the iris and the accommodative muscle of the ciliary body.

Indications

Treatment of inflammations such as uveitis and keratitis to relieve ocular pain by relaxing inflamed intraocular muscles by putting the eye at rest

Relaxation of ciliary muscle for accurate measurement of refractive errors, which permits proper lens determination for eyeglasses

Preoperative and postoperative use in intraocular surgery

Pharmacokinetics. See Table 43-4.

Side effects/adverse reactions. Locally, anticholinergics may cause stinging or an increase in intraocular pressure. With chronic use, allergic lid reactions, red eye, and various eye irritation injuries may be induced.

If absorbed systemically, mild to serious adverse reactions may result, such as dryness of the mouth, inhibition of sweating, flushing, tachycardia, ataxia, hallucinations, psychiatric and behavioral problems, fever, delirium, convulsions, respiratory depression, and coma. Deaths have been recorded in children after systemic absorption.

Pupillary dilation from either local or systemic administration can precipitate acute glaucoma in predisposed persons. If unrecognized or untreated, this can result in blindness.

Significant drug interactions. None

Dosage and administration. Atropine sulfate ophthalmic solution (Atropair, Isopto Atropine):

Adults

Mydriatic. Preoperatively instill 1 drop of 1% solution along with 1 drop of a 2.5% or 10% phenylephrine solution. Postoperatively, instill 1 drop (1% or 2% solution) to conjunctiva one to three times daily.

ANTICHOLINERGIC EFFECTS ON THE EYE

The circular smooth muscles of the iris, which constrict the pupil, are innervated by parasympathetic fibers from the oculomotor (third cranial) nerve. Anticholinergics (parasympatholytics) block the effects of the neurohormonal mediator, acetylcholine. This leaves the pupil (radial fibers of the iris) under the unopposed influence of its sympathetic, or adrenergic, nerve supply, and pupil dilation occurs. The oculomotor nerve also supplies the ciliary muscle. Contraction of this muscle slackens the suspensory ligament of the lens and allows the lens to become more convex. Accommodation for near vision depends on the ciliary muscle's ability to contract.

Uveitis. Instill 1 drop (1% solution) to conjunctiva up to three times daily.

Children

Cycloplegic refraction. Instill 1 drop of the following concentrations three times daily for 1 to 3 days before scheduled refraction.

Less than 12 months old, 0.125% solution

1 to 5 years old, 0.25% solution

5 years and older with blue irides, 0.25% solution

5 years and older with dark irides, 0.5% to 1% solution

Uveitis. Instill 1 drop (0.125% to 1% solution) to conjunctiva one to three times daily.

Postoperative mydriasis. Instill 1 drop (0.5% solution) to conjunctiva one to three times daily.

Pregnancy safety. FDA category C

NURSING CONSIDERATIONS

Assessment. Atropine is contraindicated in clients with glaucoma. Dilation of the pupil causes a narrowing of the iridocorneal angle where the canal of Schlemm is located. This restricts drainage of intraocular fluids, although secretion continues and intraocular pressure rises. This may precipitate an attack of acute glaucoma.

Education. Instruct clients that the next instillation should be omitted if side effects (dryness of mouth, tachycardia) are present. Alert client that during therapy he

---

TABLE 43-4 Anticholinergic (parasympatholytic) agents (Mydriatics): Approximate Maximum Range of Effects

	Maximal mydriasis	Usual recovery time	Maximal cycloplegia	Usual recovery time
atropine	30-40 min	7-12 days	Several hr	6-12 days
cyclopentolate	30-60 min	1 day	25-60 min	¼-1 day
homatropine	40-60 min	1-3 days	30-60 min	1-3 days
scopolamine	15-30 min	3-7 days	30-60 min	3-7 days
tropicamide	20-40 min	6 hr	20-35 min	6 hr

may be unable to focus (blurred vision) on nearby objects and will be unusually sensitive to light. Dark glasses should be worn to decrease this photophobia. The eye will be accommodated for distant vision.

Since atropine is highly toxic, store it in a safe place out of the reach of children.

cyclopentolate hydrochloride ophthalmic solution (Ak-Pentolate, Cyclogyl, Minims Cyclopentolate✹)

Dosage and administration
Adults
Cycloplegic refraction. Instill 1 drop (1% or 2% solution) to conjunctiva. Repeat in 5 minutes. Schedule refraction for approximately 40 to 50 minutes following the second dose.

Uveitis. Instill 1 drop (0.5% to 1% solution) to conjunctiva three or four times daily. For ophthalmoscopic examination: Instill 1 drop (1% or 2% solution) and repeat it once, in 5 minutes.

Children
Cycloplegic refraction. Premature and small infants, instill 1 drop (0.5% solution) to conjunctiva as single dose. Other children, instill 1 drop (1% or 2% solution) to conjunctiva. Repeat in 5 minutes and schedule examination for 40 to 50 minutes after the second dose.

Uveitis. Instill 1 drop (0.5% to 1% solution) to conjunctiva three or four times daily.

For ophthalmoscopic examination. Instill 1 drop (0.5% or 1% solution) to conjunctiva.

Neonates. Do not use concentrations above 0.5%.

Pregnancy safety. Not established

homatropine hydrobromide ophthalmic solution (Isopto Homatropine, Minims Homatropine✹)

Dosage and administration
Adults
Cycloplegic refraction. Instill 1 drop (2% or 5% solution) to conjunctiva every 5 to 10 minutes for two to five doses before refraction.

Uveitis. Instill 1 drop (2% or 5% solution) to conjunctiva two or three times daily.

Children
Cycloplegic refraction. Instill 1 drop (1% or 2% solution) every 10 minutes for three to five doses before refraction.

Uveitis. Instill 1 drop (1% or 2% solution) to conjunctiva two or three times daily.

Pregnancy safety. Not established

scopolamine hydrobromide ophthalmic solution (Isopto Hyoscine)

Dosage and administration
Adults
Mydriasis for diagnostic procedures. Instill 1 drop (0.25% solution) to conjunctiva as necessary.

Uveitis. Instill 1 drop (0.25% solution) to conjunctiva up to three times daily.

Posterior synechiae. Instill 1 drop (0.25% solution) to conjunctiva every minute for 5 doses. If necessary to enhance the mydriatic effect of this drug, instill 1 drop of 10% phenylephrine solution every minute for three doses.

Preoperative and postoperative iridocyclitis. Instill 1 drop (0.25% solution) to conjunctiva one to four times daily as necessary.

Children
Cycloplegic refraction. Instill 1 drop (0.25% solution) to conjunctiva twice daily for 2 days before refraction.

Uveitis. Instill 1 drop (0.25% solution) to conjunctiva one to three times daily.

Preoperative and postoperative iridocyclitis and mydriasis in diagnostic procedures. See adult doses.

Pregnancy safety. Not established

tropicamide ophthalmic solution (Mydriacyl, Minims Tropicamide✹)

Dosage and administration
Adults
Cycloplegic refraction. Instill 1 drop (1% solution) to conjunctiva; repeat in 5 minutes.

Fundus eye examination. Instill 1 drop (0.5% solution) to conjunctiva approximately 15 to 20 minutes before examination.

Children
Cycloplegic refraction. Instill 1 drop (0.5% or 1% solution) to conjunctiva; repeat in 5 minutes.

Fundus eye examination. See adult dose recommendations.

Pregnancy safety. Not established

ADRENERGIC (SYMPATHOMIMETIC) AGENTS

Adrenergic agents mimic (direct acting) or potentiate (indirect acting) the action of epinephrine on the dilator muscle of the iris. Mydriasis and decreased congestion of conjunctival blood vessels are produced when these drugs are applied topically to the eye. Six adrenergic drugs are used in ophthalmology—epinephrine (see p. 729), phenylephrine, oxymetazoline, hydroxyamphetamine, naphazoline, and tetrahydrozoline.

Adrenergic drugs applied topically to the eye elicit the following sympathetic responses:
1. Mydriasis brought about by contraction of the radial or dilator muscle of the eye
2. Constriction of conjunctival blood vessels
3. Slight relaxation of the ciliary muscle
4. Decreased formation of aqueous humor and increased outflow with a resultant drop in intraocular pressure

Mechanism of action. Exactly how these effects are

produced remains uncertain, but there is some evidence that alpha adrenergic receptors are present in the outflow mechanism of the eye. When stimulated, they increase outflow of aqueous humor. It has also been shown experimentally that vasoconstriction decreases the rate of aqueous humor formation.

Indications. Adrenergic drugs are used to treat wide-angle glaucoma and glaucoma secondary to uveitis, to produce mydriasis for ocular examination, and to relieve congestion and hyperemia. Adrenergic drugs are contraindicated in the treatment of narrow-angle glaucoma or abraded cornea since dilation of the pupil will further restrict ocular fluid outflow and this may cause an acute attack of glaucoma.

Pharmacokinetics. See discussion of pharmacokinetics of adrenergic agents, Chapter 20.

Side effects/adverse reactions. Serious systemic side effects from these drugs are unusual, but care must be taken in patients with cardiovascular disease, since tachycardia and elevated blood pressure can occur with these agents.

Significant drug interactions. As with other sympathomimetic amines, the potential exists for drug interactions between these adrenergic drugs and monoamine oxidase inhibitors, creating exaggerated adrenergic effects. The potentiation of adrenergic pressor effects is increased with the use of the tricyclic antidepressants.

See Table 43-5 for trade names, duration of action, and market availability

Dosage and administration. See Table 43-5.

Pregnancy safety. Epinephrine, phenylephrine, and naphazoline—FDA category C; others—not established

ANTIINFECTIVE/ANTIINFLAMMATORY AGENTS

In treatment of ocular infections, the drug of choice and the dose required should be determined by laboratory isolation of the offending organism. The initial culture from the infected area is obtained before any antiinfective/antiinflammatory agent is applied. However, treatment is not withheld if the time required to make these determinations may cause increased severity of infection and if the type of infection (for example, most cases of conjunctivitis, which tend to be self-limiting) does not warrant the expense of laboratory analysis. Prophylactic use of antiinfective/antiinflammatory agents in general is useless, wasteful, and potentially dangerous. A large proportion of the inflammatory diseases seen in ophthalmology is caused by viruses or other agents that are not susceptible to any currently available antiinfective agents. Obviously, the use of these agents in such situations is unwarranted.

Most antiinfective agents do not readily penetrate the eye when applied. However, some drugs will penetrate the inflamed eye when the blood-aqueous barrier is decreased by injury or inflammation. Topically applied antiinfective agents can cause sensitivity reactions (stinging, itching, angioneurotic edema, urticaria, dermatitis). Individuals sensitized to one drug may show cross reac-

TABLE 43-5   Trade Names, Duration, Availability, Strength, and Dosage and Administration for Ophthalmic Mydriatic-Vasoconstrictor Drugs

Name	Duration of action (hours)	Availability	Strength (% solution)	Dosage and administration
epinephrine	1-3	Prescription	0.1	1 or 2 drops into eye, repeat once if necessary
hydroxyamphetamine (Paredrine 1%)	1-2	Prescription	1.0	1 or 2 drops into conjunctival sac
naphazoline (Allerest, Clear Eyes, Vaso Clear, Albalon, others)	2-3	Over-the-counter	0.012 0.02 0.03 0.05	1 or 2 drops into conjunctival sac
		Prescription	0.1	
oxymetazoline (Ocu Clear)	< 6	Over-the-counter	0.025	1 or 2 drops into affected eye every 6 hours
phenylephrine (Isopto-Frin, Neo-Synephrine, others)	0.5-1.5 5-7	Over-the-counter Prescription	0.12 2.5 10.0	1 or 2 drops (only 1 drop for 10% solution) into eye
tetrahydrozoline (Visine, Collyrium with Tetrahydrozoline, Murine Plus, others)	2-3	Over-the-counter	0.05	1 or 2 drops 2 to 4 times a day

tions to chemically related drugs. Topical application of antiinfective agents also interferes with the normal flora of the eye, which may encourage growth of other organisms.

Eye infections require prompt treatment to help prevent spread of infection. Severe infections may damage the eye and impair vision. Solutions are preferred for treatment of eye infections, since ointment bases often tend to interfere with healing.

ANTIBACTERIALS

Antibiotics

All systemic antibiotics are used at indicated times to treat external ocular and intraocular infections. To avoid possible sensitization to common systemic antiinfective drugs and to discourage development of resistant strains of offending organisms, the antibiotic of choice is not given systemically. Rather, these agents are administered topically, subconjunctivally, intrauveally, or intravenously.

Selection of an antibiotic for ocular infection is based on (1) clinical experience, (2) nature and sensitivity of the organisms most commonly causing the condition, (3) the disease itself, (4) sensitivity and response of the client, and (5) laboratory results.

Some of the common ocular infections treated with antibiotics include the following.

conjunctivitis—Acute inflammation of the conjunctiva (the mucous membrane lining the back of the lids and the front of the eye, except for the cornea) resulting from bacterial invasion or viral infection. It is a common sign in severe colds. "Pink eye" is the acute contagious epidemic form of conjunctivitis usually caused by *Haemophilus* organisms. Symptoms include redness and burning of the eye, lacrimation, itching, and at times photophobia. Conjunctivitis is usually self-limiting. The eye should be protected from light.

hordeolum (sty)—An acute localized infection of the eyelash follicles and the glands of the anterior lid margin, resulting in the formation of a small abscess or cyst.

chalazion—Infection of the meibomian (sebaceous) glands of the eyelids. A hard cyst may form from blockage of the ducts.

blepharitis—Inflammation of the margins of the eyelid resulting from bacterial infection or allergy. Symptoms are crusting, irritation of the eye, and red and edematous lid margins.

keratitis—Corneal inflammation caused by bacterial infection; herpes simplex keratitis is caused by viral infection.

uveitis—Infection of the uveal tract, or the vascular layer of the eye, which includes the iris, ciliary body, and choroid.

endophthalmitis (bacteria)—Inner structure eye inflammation.

bacitracin ophthalmic ointment (Baciguent)
bacitracin zinc

Bacitracin is rarely used systemically because of its nephrotoxic effects. It is particularly useful in treating

TABLE 43-6 Ocular Side Effects Induced by Systemic Medications

Drug	Possible ocular side effect induced
allopurinol	Retinal hemorrhage, exudative lesions
aspirin	Allergic dermatitis including keratitis and conjunctivitis
barbiturates	Nystagmus
busulfan	Cataracts
cannabis, marijuana	Nystagmus, conjunctivitis, double vision
chloral hydrate	Eyelid edema, conjunctivitis, miosis
chloroquine	Lenticular and corneal opacity, retinopathy
clomiphene citrate	Blurred vision, light flashes
clonidine	Miosis
corticosteroids	Cataracts, increased intraocular pressure, papilledema
diazoxide	Oculogyric crisis
digitalis glycosides	Scotomas, optic neuritis
ethyl alcohol	Nystagmus
guanethidine	Miosis, ptosis, blurred vision
hydralazine	Lacrimation, blurred vision
ibuprofen	Altered color vision, blurred vision
indomethacin	Mydriasis, retinopathy
isoniazid	Optic neuritis
lithium carbonate	Exophthalmos
nitroglycerin	Transient elevations in intraocular pressure
opiates	Miosis, nystagmus
phenothiazines	Corneal and conjunctival deposits, cataracts, retinopathy, oculogyric crisis
phenytoin	Nystagmus
quinine	Blurring of vision, optic neuritis, blindness (reversible)
thiazide diuretics	Acute transient myopia, yellow coloring of vision
vincristine	Ptosis, paresis of extraocular muscles
vitamin A overdose or toxicity	Papilledema, increased intraocular pressure
vitamin D toxicity	Calcium deposits in cornea

surface superficial infections caused by gram-positive bacteria (it inhibits protein synthesis). Bacitracin does penetrate the conjunctiva or the cornea slightly, but in therapeutic amounts it is nonirritating to the eye, is excreted in the nasolacrimal system, and produces no systemic effects.

A broader spectrum of antimicrobial activity is produced when bacitracin is used in combination with gramicidin, neomycin, and polymyxin (Neosporin, Neo-polycin) than when it is used alone. Bacitracin is preferable to neomycin for topical use, since fewer organisms are resistant to it, allergic reactions occur less frequently, and sensitization is avoided. It may impede corneal wound healing, and the ointment form will cause a temporary clouding or haze. Prolonged use may lead to overgrowth of nonsusceptible microorganisms.

Thimerosal and silver nitrate (both of which are heavy metals) will inactivate bacitracin; therefore concurrent use is not advisable. Ophthalmic bacitracin is available as an ointment containing 500 units/g of suitable base and as a powder containing 10,000 and 50,000 units for making solutions for topical use. Ointment is instilled into the lower conjunctival sac of the affected eye one to three times daily or more often. Ointment preparations are stable for about 1 year at room temperature.

chloramphenicol ophthalmic ointment (Chloroptic, Isopto Fenicol✳, Chloroptic)
chloramphenicol ophthalmic solution (Chloroptic, Isopto Fenicol✳)
chloramphenicol for ophthalmic solution (Chloromycetin)

Mechanism of action. A bacteriostatic, chloramphenicol prevents peptide bond formation and protein synthesis in a wide variety of gram-positive and gram-negative organisms. Thus it is an extremely useful drug for superficial intraocular infections.

Side effects/adverse reactions. Side effects are usually rare. Burning and stinging on instillation have been reported. Irreversible aplastic anemia has not been reported with this dosage form of chloramphenicol, although it would be prudent to monitor for blood dyscrasias. One must observe for symptoms of sore throat, elevated temperature, increased bleeding episodes, increased weakness, and indicative changes in the complete blood count.

Dosage and administration

Ointment dosage form

Adults. Apply a thin strip of ointment (1% solution) to the conjunctiva every 3 hours, or more often if necessary.

Solution

Adults. Instill 1 drop into conjunctiva every 1 to 4 hours.

Children. See adult dosage.
Pregnancy safety. Not established

NURSING CONSIDERATIONS

Avoid prolonged (over 3 days) or frequent use. Chloramphenicol has been implicated in the development of aplastic anemia after prolonged use.

erythromycin ophthalmic ointment (Ilotycin)

Mechanism of action. Erythromycin ophthalmic ointment is a bacteriostatic agent, but in high concentrations against very susceptible organisms it may be bactericidal.

Indications. Treatment of neonatal conjunctivitis caused by *Chlamydia trachomatis;* prevention of ophthalmia neonatorum (against *Neisseria gonorrhoeae* or *C. trachomatis*) and other ocular infections caused by susceptible organisms

TABLE 43-7   Adverse Systemic Effects from Ophthalmic Drugs

Ophthalmic drug	Reported adverse effect
ANTIMICROBIAL AGENTS	
chloromycetin eye drops	Aplastic anemia
sulfacetamide eye drops	Stevens-Johnson syndrome, systemic lupus erythematosus
ANTICHOLINERGIC DRUGS	
atropine eye drops	Tachycardia, elevated temperature, fever, delirium
cyclopentolate	Convulsions, hallucinations
scopolamine eye drops	Acute psychosis
ANTIGLAUCOMA MEDICATIONS	
beta blocking agents (timolol)	Bradycardia, syncope, low blood pressure, asthmatic attack, congestive heart failure, hallucinations, loss of appetite, headaches, nausea, weakness, depression
anticholinesterase (echothiophate)	Asthmatic attack, systemic cholinergic effects
parasympathomimetic (pilocarpine)	Nausea, stomach pain, increased sweating, salivation, tremors, bradycardia, lightheadedness
SYMPATHOMIMETIC MEDICATIONS	
phenylephrine (10%)	Severe hypertension, cerebral hemorrhage, dysrhythmias, myocardial infarction
epinephrine eyedrops	Tremors, increased sweating, headaches, hypertension

Modified from Abramowicz M, ed: Adverse systemic effects from ophthalmic drugs, Med Lett Drugs Ther 24(610):53, 1982.

Side effects/adverse reactions. None
Dosage and administration

Adults

Ocular infections. Apply a thin ointment strip to conjunctiva daily or more often if necessary.

Children

Ophthalmia neonatorum. Apply a thin ointment strip to conjunctiva following delivery.

Pregnancy safety. Not established

neomycin, polymyxin B sulfate, and bacitracin ophthalmic ointment (Mycitracin, Neosporin)

While all three agents have been or are available as single ophthalmic drugs, reports of sensitization to the individual drug have somewhat limited their usefulness. The combination dosage form provides a bactericidal effect against many gram-positive and gram-negative organisms. It is indicated for the treatment of superficial ocular infections caused by susceptible organisms. A small ointment (1% solution) strip is usually applied to the conjunctiva every 3 to 4 hours.

tetracycline hydrochloride ophthalmic ointment and suspension (Achromycin)
chlortetracycline hydrochloride ophthalmic ointment (Aureomycin)

The tetracyclines are used topically to treat superficial infections of the cornea and conjunctiva. Generally they are bacteriostatic rather than bactericidal; they have a broad antimicrobial spectrum. Organisms resistant to one tetracycline are usually resistant to the others. Trachoma may be treated with both topical and oral tetracycline therapy for 60 days or more. The tetracyclines have been recommended for prophylaxis of gonorrheal ophthalmia neonatorum, since they produce a lower incidence of conjunctivitis and less irritation of the eye than does silver nitrate. Topical tetracyclines rarely cause adverse reactions.

Aminoglycosides

gentamicin sulfate (Garamycin, Genoptic)

Gentamicin is effective against a wide variety of gram-negative and gram-positive organisms. It is particularly useful against *Pseudomonas, Proteus,* and *Klebsiella* organisms and *Escherichia coli,* as well as staphylococci and streptococci that have developed resistance to other antibiotics. It is applied as an ointment two or three times daily, or 1 drop of solution is applied every 4 to 8 hours and excreted by the nasolacrimal apparatus. Penetration occurs with epithelial damage.

tobramycin (Tobrex)

This water-soluble aminoglycoside is used topically on a wide variety of culture-verified gram-positive and gram-negative external ophthalmic pathogens. It is particularly valuable for treating gentamicin-resistant infections.

Among the pathogens affected by the aminoglycoside are the staphylococci, streptococci, *Pseudomonas, Escherichia coli, Klebsiella, Enterobacter, Proteus, Haemophilus influenzae, Moraxella, Acinetobacter,* and some *Neisseria.* Adverse reactions include ocular toxicity and hypersensitivity including lid itching, swelling, and conjunctival erythema. When topical aminoglycosides are used concurrently with systemic aminoglycosides, the total serum concentration will be affected and should be monitored. Systemic toxicity from absorption may occur from excessive use.

The dose for mild to moderate infection is 2 drops in the affected eye every 4 hours. For severe infections 2 drops are instilled hourly in the eye until improvement is seen, and then the dose is reduced before the drops are discontinued. The solution is incompatible with tetracycline therapy because it contains tyloxacol, a formaldehyde polymer used as a surfactant.

Sulfonamides

sulfacetamide sodium ophthalmic ointment (Bleph-10, Cetamide, Sulamyd)
sulfacetamide sodium ophthalmic solution (Bleph-10, Isopto Cetamide, Sulfamyd, Sulfex✶)
sulfisoxazole diolamine ophthalmic ointment and solution (Gantrisin)

These bacteriostatic antiinfective agents block the synthesis of dihydrofolic acid and decrease the quantity of active tetrahydrofolic acid, a necessary cofactor to synthesize purines, thymidine, and DNA in specific bacterial organisms. Their effectiveness is antagonized by the presence of para-aminobenzoic acid (PABA) or its derivatives procaine and tetracaine.

The presence of purulent drainage or exudate interferes with the action of the sulfonamides, since the purulent matter contains para-aminobenzoic acid. Any lid exudate should be removed before instillation of the drugs.

Since the activity of sulfacetamide may be inhibited by ophthalmic anesthetics, the drugs are applied 30 to 60 minutes apart. They are physically incompatible with thimerosal and silver preparations.

Before administration the client should check to see that the solution has not darkened in color; if it has darkened, it should be discarded. Solutions are instilled 1 drop every 1 or 2 hours initially, with increased time intervals based on response. Instillation of the drops may cause some mild pain and discomfort. The ointments are applied one to three times a day and at bedtime.

Sulfisoxazole is available in 4% ophthalmic solution and a 4% ophthalmic ointment. It is applied topically to the conjunctiva three or more times daily.

Sulfacetamide is available only for topical use as a 10% ointment or a 10%, 15%, or 30% solution. It is preferred over other sulfa drugs used systemically. It may cause local irritation. Intraocular penetration is variable.

ANTIFUNGAL AGENTS

natamycin ophthalmic suspension (Natacyn)

Natamycin is used in treatment of fungal blepharitis, fungal conjunctivitis, and fungal keratitis. By binding to steroids in the cell membrane of the fungus, natamycin produces an altered membrane permeability and causes loss of the cellular constituents. It is mainly retained in the conjunctival area; significant drug levels in the ocular fluids are not usually achieved. It is not systemically absorbed. Natamycin may cause irritation of the eye. One drop of the 5% solution is instilled into the conjunctiva every 1 to 2 hours initially. The dose is gradually tapered to 1 drop every 3 or 4 hours after the first 3 to 4 days of therapy.

ANTIVIRAL AGENTS

Three antiviral ophthalmic preparations are on the market: idoxuridine, vidarabine, and trifluridine.

idoxuridine ophthalmic ointment/solution (Stoxil, Herplex)

Mechanism of action. Idoxuridine resembles thymidine, a substance necessary for viral DNA. Thus it replaces it and inhibits the replication of the viral DNA.

Indications. Treatment of herpes simplex virus keratitis

Side effects/adverse reactions. May increase flow of tears from the eye. Physician intervention is necessary if client reports photosensitivity, blurred vision or visual disturbances, or eye irritations that were not present before therapy.

Dosage and administration

Adults

Herpes simplex virus keratitis. Solution—instill 1 drop hourly during waking hours and every 2 hours during the night or 1 drop every minute for five doses. Repeat this dosage schedule every 4 hours day and night. When improvement is seen, dosage may be decreased to 1 drop every 2 hours during waking hours and every 4 hours during the night. Ointment—apply a thin strip every 4 hours (five times daily) during waking hours.

Children. See adult dosage.
Pregnancy safety. Not established.

trifluridine ophthalmic solution (Viroptic)

Mechanism of action. See idoxuridine.
Indications. See idoxuridine. In addition, it is used to treat herpes simplex virus keratoconjunctivitis.
Side effects/adverse reactions. Frequent but usually not troublesome side effects include burning or stinging of the eyes. Hypersensitivity reaction, evidenced by redness, swelling, or eye irritation not present before therapy, is rarely reported, but it requires physician intervention.

Dosage and administration
Adults. Instill 1 drop (1% solution) into conjunctiva every 2 hours during waking hours. Maximum daily dose is 9 drops. Continue therapy until cornea is reepithelialized. Then reduce dosage to 1 drop every 4 hours during waking hours (minimum of 5 drops per day) for 1 week.
Pregnancy safety. Not established.

NURSING CONSIDERATIONS

Use trifluridine only when clinical diagnosis is positive for herpetic keratitis. The possibility of viral resistance may follow multiple exposure. There is also the possibility that mutagenic agents may cause genetic damage. The oncogenic potential is unknown at this time. It is not prescribed for pregnant women or nursing mothers unless the potential benefits outweigh the potential risks.

vidarabine ophthalmic ointment (Vira-A)

Mechanism of action. The antiviral mechanism of action is not established for this agent, but it appears to interfere with early steps of viral DNA synthesis. Activity is directed against herpes simplex (types 1 and 2), varicella-zoster, and vaccinia viruses. The deaminated metabolite arabinosylhypoxanthine (Ara-Hx) has less antiviral activity than the parent compound vidarabine. An epithelial defect in the cornea permits trace amounts of the parent and metabolite to be found in the aqueous humor. Systemic absorption is not expected after ocular administration or by swallowing lacrimal secretions as a result of deamination in gastrointestinal tract secretions.

Indications. Treatment of herpes simplex virus keratitis and keratoconjunctivitis

Side effects/adverse reactions. Increased tear flow and a sensation of something being in the eye have been reported. Physician intervention is necessary if client has photosensitivity, redness, eye swelling or increased eye irritation not present before treatment.

Dosage and administration
Adults. Apply a thin ointment strip to conjunctiva every 3 hours five times daily. Continue therapy until cornea is completely reepithelialized. Then decrease dosage to twice daily for 7 to 10 days.
Pregnancy safety. Not established.

ANTISEPTICS

Many antiseptics used to treat surface infections of the eye before the advent of antibiotics are now obsolete. Not only were many of these drugs relatively ineffective, they also delayed healing and in some cases caused permanent damage to the eye. Antiseptic solutions are employed in ophthalmology for irrigation, dissolution of secretions, and precipitation of mucus and in certain instances in which specific antimicrobial agents cannot be used. A 2.2% boric acid solution is used as an irrigant; this concentration is thought to be isotonic with tear fluid.

Inorganic mercuric salts such as yellow mercuric oxide ophthalmic ointment (1% to 2%), thimerosal (Merthiolate), and ammoniated mercury formerly served as bacteriostatic agents. Today they are seldom used, since they do not completely sterilize, spores are resistant to them, and they are irritating to the eye.

silver nitrate

Two drops of a solution of 1% silver nitrate in each eye is routinely employed immediately after birth as a prophylaxis against gonorrheal ophthalmia neonatorum. In many states this is required by law. The gonococci are particularly susceptible to silver salts. Liberated silver ions precipitate bacterial proteins. Silver nitrate is preferred to effective antibiotic agents, since these may sensitize the client and silver nitrate has stood the test of time. Inactivation by bacitracin is seen. Silver nitrate ophthalmic solution is available in collapsible capsules containing about 5 drops of a 1% solution. The solution should be in contact with the conjunctival sac for not less than 30 seconds to produce a mild chemical conjunctivitis. Irrigation following use is not recommended.

CORTICOSTEROIDS

Many corticosteroids are available for ophthalmic use as topical solutions, suspensions, or ointments. They include betamethasone (Betnesol♣), dexamethasone (Maxidex, Decadron), fluorometholone (FML S.O.P., FML♣), hydrocortisone (Cortamed♣), medrysone (HMS Liquifilm), and prednisolone (Pred-Forte, Predair-A). These are available in varying strengths and in combination with various antibiotics or mydriatics.

Indications. Treatment of allergic and inflammatory ophthalmic disorders of the conjunctiva, cornea, and anterior segment of the eye.

Side effects/adverse reactions. Burning or eye watering rarely occur and are not generally bothersome. Physician intervention is usually necessary when blurred vision or visual disturbances, eye pain, headaches, ptosis, or enlarged pupils occur.

Dosage and administration. See USP DI or current package inserts for dosing information.

Pregnancy safety. Prednisolone, fluorometholone, and medrysone—FDA category C; others—not established.

NURSING CONSIDERATIONS

Assessment. Ophthalmic corticosteroid therapy is not used for pyogenic (pus-producing) inflammations of the eye, since corticosteroids decrease defense mechanisms and reduce resistance to pathogenic organisms.

Corticosteroid therapy is not recommended for minor corneal abrasions. Steroids may actually increase ocular susceptibility to fungous infection. When steroids are used for various eye conditions, they should be used for a limited time only and the eye should be checked for increased intraocular pressure.

Corticosteroids may diminish the resistance to infection and may also mask the allergic reactions or hypersensitivity reactions to other drugs.

Intervention. The glucocorticoids used in ophthalmology may be applied topically, injected into the conjunctiva, or given systemically to diminish leukocyte infiltration where inflammation exists.

Education. Instruct the client to shake the ophthalmic suspensions well before use for adequate dispersion of the active ingredients. Caution the client not to stop the medication without consulting the physician. Inflammation recrudescence secondary to abrupt cessation of ophthalmic steroid administration may be overcome by dose frequency reduction (from every 3 hours, to every 6 hours, to 3 times daily, to twice daily, to once daily, and to every other day) or by decreasing the percentage strengths and using the above schedule.

TOPICAL ANESTHETIC AGENTS

Mechanism of action. Local anesthetics stabilize neuronal membranes so that they become less permeable to ions; this prevents initiation and transmission of nerve impulses. It is theorized that sodium ion permeability is limited by the closing of pores through which the sodium ions move in the nerve cell membrane lipid layer.

Indications. Local anesthetics are used to prevent pain (deep anesthesia) during surgical procedures (removal of sutures and foreign bodies), tonometry, and examinations.

Pharmacokinetics. The local anesthetics have rapid onset (within 20 seconds) and last for 15 to 20 minutes.

proparacaine hydrochloride (Ophthaine, Ophthetic, Alcaine)

Proparacaine is similar to tetracaine. A 0.5% solution is administered by topical instillation. Anesthesia is produced within 20 seconds and lasts for 15 minutes. It is relatively free from the burning and discomfort of other anesthetics and is highly toxic if it enters the systemic circulation. Allergic contact dermatitis, softening and erosion of corneal epithelium, pupillary dilation, cycloplegia, conjunctival congestion and hemorrhage, and stromal edema have been reported.

tetracaine hydrochloride (Pontocaine)

Tetracaine is used topically in a 0.5% ointment and solution for rapid, brief, superficial anesthesia. It is a widely used local ocular anesthetic. One to two drops of a 0.5% solution of tetracaine will produce anesthesia within 30 seconds; the client may feel a burning or stinging sensation. The anesthetic effect lasts for 10 to 25 minutes. Tetracaine can cause epithelial damage and systemic toxicity; therefore it is not recommended for prolonged home use by clients. It is physically incompatible with the mercury or silver salts often found in ophthalmic products.

NURSING CONSIDERATIONS

The practice of repeatedly applying such an anesthetic to an eye after removal of a foreign body is to be condemned. Besides delaying wound healing, this can produce sensitivity, permanent corneal opacification, visual loss, or perforation of the cornea.

Question the client about past experiences with anesthetics to determine if a hypersensitivity reaction occurred. Those local anesthetics that produce systemic toxicity are manifested as central nervous system excitation followed by CNS and cardiovascular depression. Patching the anesthetized eye is prudent, since the blink reflex is lost and protection of the cornea from debris and irritants is then needed.

OTHER OPHTHALMIC PREPARATIONS

ARTIFICIAL TEAR SOLUTIONS AND OCULAR LUBRICANTS

Lubricants or artificial tears are used to provide moisture and lubrication in diseases in which tear production is deficient, to lubricate artificial eyes and moisten contact lenses, to remove debris, and to protect the cornea during procedures on the eye. These agents are also incorporated into ophthalmic preparations to prolong the contact time of topically applied drugs.

Such products have a balanced salt solution (equivalent to 0.9% sodium chloride), buffers to adjust pH, highly viscous agents (methylcellulose, propylene glycol, gelatin, dextran, and others) to extend eye contact time, and preservatives to maintain sterility. These products are usually administered three or four times a day.

An artificial tear insert (Lacrisert) was devised to extend the effect of the preparation. It is usually inserted daily or at most twice a day for selected clients.

Ointment preparations are also used as ocular lubricants. They will help protect the eye (such as during and following eye surgery) and lubricate the eye. They are particularly valuable for nighttime use. Examples include Lacri-Lube, Duratears, and Hypo Tears.

ANTIALLERGIC AGENTS
cromolyn sodium (Opticrom)

Mechanism of action. In animals cromolyn sodium inhibits degranulation of sensitized mast cells occurring after exposure to a specific antigen. This mast cell release inhibition prevents the mediators of inflammation (histamine and slow-releasing substance of anaphylaxis) from producing their characteristic effects.

Indications. Used for allergic eye disorders (vernal and allergic keratoconjunctivitis, papillary conjunctivitis, keratitis) that have symptoms of itching, tearing, redness, and discharge.

Pharmacokinetics. Absorption is 0.03% (from eye).

Side effects/adverse reactions. Stinging and burning of eyes may occur.

Dosage and administration. Concomitant corticosteroids may be necessary.

Adults and children (over 4 years old). Instill 1 drop in each affected eye four to six times a day at regular intervals for up to 6 weeks.

Pregnancy safety. FDA category B.

NURSING CONSIDERATIONS

Assessment. Be aware that some transient burning or stinging may occur because of the solution vehicle (phenylethyl alcohol).

Intervention. Refrigerate drug, keep out of direct sunlight, and discard unused portion after 4 weeks.

Education. Remind client to remove soft contact lenses before the first instillation of drops and resume wearing them only after drug discontinuation.

Evaluation. Note that signs and symptoms of relief will appear within days but that treatment at regular intervals for as long as 6 weeks may be required.

DIAGNOSTIC AIDS
fluorescein sodium (AK-Fluor, Fluorescite, Ful-Glo, Fluor-I-Strip, etc.)

Fluorescein is a nontoxic water-soluble dye that is used as a diagnostic aid. When applied to the cornea, it stains corneal lesions or ulcers a bright green; foreign bodies appear surrounded by a green ring. These effects permit detection of corneal epithelial defects caused by injury or infection and location of foreign bodies in the eye. The dye is also used in fitting hard contact lenses. Areas that lack fluorescein-stained tears will appear black under ultraviolet light, indicating the contact lens is touching the cornea at those areas. Fluorescein is used in retinal photography to determine retinal vascular status and to identify defects in the retinal pigment epithelium. In addition, it may be used to test lacrimal apparatus patency; if after the dye is instilled into the eye it appears in the nasal secretions, the nasolacrimal drainage system is open.

Injection is used in ophthalmic angiography to examine the fundus, vasculature of the iris, and aqueous flow, to make differential diagnosis of cancerous and noncancerous tumors, and to determine time for circulation in the eye.

Side effects/adverse reactions. Nausea, headache, abdominal distress, vomiting, hypotension, hypersensitivity reactions, and anaphylaxis have been reported following injection.

Dosage and administration

Topical solution. To detect foreign bodies and corneal abrasions; instill 1 or 2 drops of 2% solution.

Strip application and injection. Check a current drug reference for instructions.

ENZYME PREPARATION

chymotrypsin (Alpha Chymar, Zolyse, Catarase)

This proteolytic enzyme is used in selected cases to facilitate cataract extraction. It is injected behind the iris into the posterior chamber where it dissolves the filaments or zonules that hold the lens, thereby facilitating intracapsular lens extraction. This effect is usually obtained in 1 to 2 minutes with 0.2 to 0.5 ml of a freshly prepared 1:5000 solution. Chymotrypsin may cause a transient postoperative glaucoma lasting about 1 week, which can be relieved by the use of pilocarpine. Acids, alcohol, alkalies, antiseptics, blood, detergents, and serum inactivate this enzyme. It is inhibited by chloramphenicol and isoflurophate. Epinephrine inactivates it in 1 hour.

It is available in ampules containing 150, 300, or 750 units (proteolytic activity) in lyophilized enzyme dissolved in 2 to 10 ml of diluent.

HYPEROSMOLAR PREPARATION

sodium chloride ointment (Muro-128) and solution (Adsorbonac)

This 5% ointment and 2% or 5% solution are used to reduce the corneal edema that occurs in certain corneal dystrophies and after cataract extraction. It is also used as an aid in gonioscopy, funduscopy, and biomicroscopy. The dose is 1 to 2 drops in affected eye(s) every 3 to 4 hours as directed. The ointment is applied once a day.

NONSTEROIDAL ANTIINFLAMMATORY AGENT

flurbiprofen sodium (Ocufen)

Fluribiprofen is a topical nonsteroidal antiinflammatory agent used to inhibit intraoperative miosis. Minor symptoms of transient burning and stinging may occur on instillation into the eye. Systemic absorption is possible, so the nurse should monitor for increased bleeding tendencies. Concurrent administration of acetylcholine and carbachol is avoided, since both drugs may be ineffective if used in clients receiving flurbiprofen. One drop (0.03% solution) is instilled every 30 minutes starting 2 hours before surgery. Maximum dosage is 4 drops.

Pregnancy safety. FDA category C.

OPHTHALMIC SURGERY AIDS

sodium hyaluronate (Healon, Amuisc)

Sodium hyaluronate, a purified viscoelastic gel, is used during anterior segment and vitreous procedures in cataract surgery (intracapsular and extracapsular). During intraocular lens implantation it is used to coat the instruments and the lens before insertion. A dose of 0.5 ml in the anterior chamber before insertion of the new lens delivery protects the corneal endothelium from damage when a cataractous lens is being removed. Other indications include glaucoma filtration surgery and corneal transplant surgery. Sodium hyaluronate is also used as a vitreous replacement after retinal detachment surgery and vitrectomy.

IRRIGATING SOLUTIONS

The sterile isotonic external irrigating solutions are used in tonometry, fluorescein procedures, removal of foreign material, and gonoscopy and to cleanse and soothe eyes of patients wearing hard contact lenses. These external products do not require a prescription and are available in drops, irrigations, and eyewashes. Examples of irrigating solutions include BSS Plus, Surgisol, and Lavoptik Eye Wash.

KEY TERMS

aphakia, page 729
blepharitis, page 737
chalazion, page 737
conjunctivitis, page 737
cycloplegia, page 734
endophthamitis, page 737
esotropia, page 725
glaucoma, page 724
hordeolum, page 737
iontophoresis, page 724
keratitis, page 737
miotics, page 725
mydriasis, page 733
uveitis, page 737

BIBLIOGRAPHY

Abramowicz M, ed: Adverse systemic effects from ophthalmic drugs, Med Lett 24(610):53, 1982.

Cascella PJ: Topical administration of eye medications, US Pharmacist 12(3):54, 1987.

Kastrup EK, ed: Facts and Comparisons, St. Louis, 1988, JB Lippincott Co.

Koetting JF: Ocular and visual side effects of drugs—a reconsideration, J Am Pharmaceutical Assoc NS 15 10:558, 1975.

Lesar TS and others: Antimicrobial drug delivery to the eye, Drug Intell Clin Pharm 19(9):642, 1985.

Roberts AM and others: et al Corticosteroid therapy of opthalmologic diseases. Part 7, Hosp Pract 19(2):181, 1984.

Schwinghammer TL and Britton HL: Adverse effects of drugs on the eye, US Pharmacist 4(1):49, 1979.

Todd B: Using eye drops and ointments safely, Geriatr Nurs 4(1):53, 1983.

United States Pharmacopeial Convention: Drug Information for the Health Care Provider, ed 8, Rockville, Md, 1988, The Convention.

Weintraub M and Evans P: Pilocarpine: the method is the message, Hosp Formul 20(2):177, 1985.

Whitton S: Trends in ophthalmic surgery, Today's OR Nurse 6(12):26, 1984.

Wuest JR: Advising consumers on eye preparations. Part II. OTC drugs for use in the eye, Fla Pharm J 51(11):10, 1987.

Overview of the Ear

ANATOMY AND PHYSIOLOGY

The ear consists of three sections or parts: external ear, middle ear, and inner ear (see Figure 44-1).

The *external ear* has two divisions, the outer ear or pinna and the external auditory canal. The external auditory canal leads to the eardrum or **tympanic membrane,** a thin transparent partition of tissue between the canal and the middle ear. The function of the external ear is to receive and transmit auditory sounds to the eardrum. The eardrum protects the middle ear from foreign substances and transmits sound to the bones of the middle ear.

The *middle ear* is an air-filled cavity that contains three small bones called the **auditory ossicles.** The ossicles are the **malleus** (hammer), **incus** (anvil), and **stapes** (stirrup). The tip of the malleus is attached to the surface of the tympanic membrane. Its head is attached to the incus, which in turn is attached to the stapes. The ossicles amplify and transmit sound waves to the inner ear. The middle ear is also directly connected to the nasopharynx by the **eustachian** (auditory) **tube.** The eustachian tube is usually collapsed except when the individual swallows, chews, yawns, or moves the jaw. This tube equalizes air pressure on both sides of the eardrum, to prevent the eardrum from rupturing. On airline flights pressure changes are relieved by action of the eustachian tube when the individual chews gum, yawns, or swallows deliberately.

The *inner ear,* also referred to as the **labyrinth**

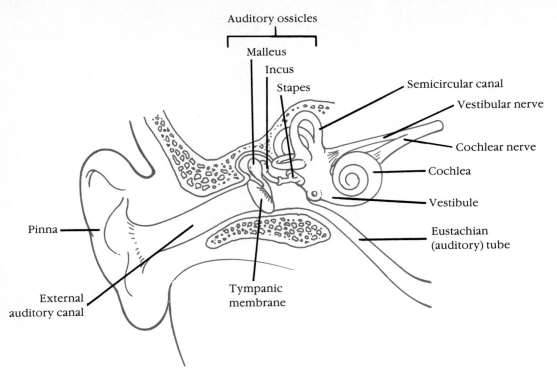

FIGURE 44-1 Ear anatomy.

because of its series of canals, has two main divisions. The bony labyrinth consists of the **vestibule, cochlea,** and **semicircular canals,** and the membranous labyrinth consists of a series of sacs and tubes within the bony labyrinth. The cochlea is the primary organ of hearing, and the vestibular apparatus is necessary to maintain equilibrium and balance. (See Figure 44-1.)

COMMON EAR DISORDERS

The most common ear disorders include infections of the ear (bacterial or fungal), earwax accumulation, and various other painful or distressing conditions. Many ear disorders are minor and easily treated or are self-limiting. Persistent pain or ear problems should be professionally evaluated since some untreated disorders can lead to hearing loss.

External ear disorders usually include trauma, such as lacerations or scrapes to the skin. These are often minor and heal with time. If the injury results in bleeding and perhaps a hematoma, a physician referral is necessary. Localized infections of the hair follicles resulting in boils may occur. Clients with recurring boils and small boils that do not respond to good hygiene and topical compresses should be referred to a physician for evaluation and possibly systemic antibiotics.

Dermatitis of the ear, itching, local redness, weeping,

or drainage are also reported. Such conditions must be individually evaluated, since the causes can vary from inflammation induced by seborrhea, psoriasis, or contact dermatitis to head trauma producing ear discharge. Self-medication should be discouraged when infection is suspected or in the presence of known injuries of the ear or whenever drainage, pain, and dizziness are present.

Middle ear disorders are never treated with over-the-counter medications. Most commonly reported problems are infections of the middle ear, such as otitis media. This most often occurs in children, although with adults chronic otitis media may be caused by a nasopharyngeal tumor. Pain, fever, malaise, pressure, a sensation of fullness in the ear and hearing loss are common symptoms. Clients with such conditions should be treated promptly by a physician. Acute tympanic membrane perforation from foreign objects or from water sports (such as diving or water skiing) will result in a multitude of symptoms, if untreated. Pain at the time of injury that subsides, a diminished hearing acuity, tinnitus, nausea, vertigo, and otitis media or mastoiditis may be noted. A physician's examination is vital when a perforated tympanic membrane is suspected.

Inner ear disorders: Loss of hearing, especially unilateral hearing loss, may result from viral infection of the inner ear. Hearing deficits may be caused by genetic diseases or slowly progressive diseases such as otosclerosis or Meniere's disease. Untreated external and middle ear infections may also affect hearing and the functioning of the inner ear.

KEY TERMS

auditory ossicles, page 745
cochlea, page 746
eustachian tube, page 745
incus, page 745
labyrinth, page 745

malleus, page 745
semicircular canals, page 746
stapes, page 745
tympanic membrane, page 745
vestibule, page 746

BIBLIOGRAPHY

Anthony CP and Thibodeau GA: Textbook of anatomy and physiology, ed 12, St Louis, 1987, Times Mirror/Mosby College Publishing.

Guyton AC: Human physiology and mechanisms of disease, ed 4, Philadelphia, 1987, WB Saunders Co.

Auditory Drugs

ANTIBIOTIC EAR PREPARATIONS

Chloramphenicol (Chloromycetin Otic, Pentamycetin✚) is a broad-spectrum antibiotic (bacteriostatic) solution used to treat infections of the external auditory canal surface. Organisms susceptible to chloramphenicol usually include *Staphylococcus aureus, Escherichia coli, Pseudomonas aeruginosa, Enterobacter aerogenes, Haemophilus influenzae,* and others. However, if the client has an inner ear infection, systemic antibiotics would be indicated.

The possible side effects produced by chloramphenicol are burning, redness, rash, swelling, or other signs of topical irritation that were not present before the start of therapy. These would indicate a hypersensitivity reaction. Usual dosage for adults and children is 2 or 3 drops inserted in the ear canal every 6 to 8 hours.

Gentamicin sulfate otic solution (Geramycin) is a bactericidal antibiotic, another antibiotic that is not presently available in the otic preparation in the United States. Although not FDA approved, physicians sometimes use the ophthalmic preparation marketed in the United States for otic infections.

STEROID AND ANTIBIOTIC COMBINATIONS

The steroid hydrocortisone is most commonly combined with antibiotics, such as neomycin sulfate and polymyxin B sulfate, for treatment of superficial bacterial infections in the external auditory canal. Hydrocortisone is included for its antiinflammatory, antipruritic, and antiallergy effects. The antibiotics are used primarily for their antibacterial action. These products also may be used to treat mastoidectomy cavity infections caused by susceptible organisms, including *S. aureus, P. aeruginosa, E. coli, Klebsiella* species, and others. See Table 45-1 for examples of steroid and antibiotic combinations.

MISCELLANEOUS PREPARATIONS

A wide variety of both single and combination products is used to treat ear wax, inflammation, bacterial or fungal infections, ear pain, and other minor or superficial problems associated primarily with the external ear canal. More serious problems such as an earache secondary to an upper respiratory tract infection, ear discharge or drainage, persistent or recurrent otitis, or ear pain caused by recent injury or head trauma require a physician's thorough evaluation and intervention to prevent complications. In such cases systemic medications with or without ear preparations are usually necessary.

Although most over-the-counter otic preparations are considered safe and effective, health care professionals should advise clients to see a physician if symptoms do not improve within several days of using these preparations or if an adverse reaction occurs. (See Tables 45-2 and 45-3.)

THE NURSE'S ROLE WITH DRUGS AFFECTING THE EAR

Assessment. Before initiation of therapy, assess hearing and extent of symptoms (ear ache, pain, erythrema, vertigo, discharge, and others) that may be present.

To identify areas for education, assess client for improper hygiene or health practices that may contribute to the development of infections.

Intervention. Ear drops are more comfortably tolerated if they are warmed (if not contraindicated) before instillation. This can be achieved by running warm water over the side of the bottle without the label or immersing the bottle in warm water in a medicine cup. Even carrying the bottle in a pocket for half an hour or so will take the chill off the drops.

To prepare for the instillation of ear drops cleanse any drainage present from the ear and position the client so that the ear to be medicated is facing upward.

TABLE 45-1 Steroid and Antibiotic Otic Preparations

Ingredients	Trade name
Solution of hydrocortisone 1%, 3.5 mg neomycin sulfate, and 10,000 units of polymyxin B sulfate/ml	Cortisporin Otic Drotic Oretega Otic M Otocort
Solution of hydrocortisone 0.5% and 10,000 units of polymyxin B sulfate/ml	Otobiotic Otic Pyocidin Otic
Suspension of hydrocortisone 1%, 3.5 mg neomycin sulfate, and 10,000 units of polymyxin B sulfate/ml	Cortisporin Otic Otocort
Suspension of hydrocortisone acetate 1%, 3.3 mg neomycin, and 3 mg colistin/ml	Coly-Mycin S Otic

TABLE 45-2 Over-the-Counter Ear Preparations

Ingredients	Trade name	Use
boric acid 2.75% in isopropyl alcohol	Aurocaine 2 Auro-Dri Dri/Ear Ear Dry Swim Ear	Antibacterial preparation, commonly used after bathing or swimming to prevent excessive water accumulation and infection
chloroxylenol and acetic acid with benzalkonium chloride and glycerin	Aurinol Ear Drops Benzodyne Drops Halogen Ear Drops	Antibacterial, antifungal, in an acid medium. Increasing acidity of external auditory canal results in an undesirable site for bacteria growth, especially *Pseudomonas*
carbamide peroxide 6.5% in glycerin, anhydrous glycerin, solution of 10% triethanolamine with 0.5% chlorobutanol in propylene glycol	Cerumenex Drops	Agent to emulsify and aid in removal of ear wax
solution of 2% acetic acid in aluminum acetate solution	Borofair Otic BurOtic Otic Domeboro	Antibacterial or antifungal in acid medium

TABLE 45-3   Miscellaneous Prescription Otic Preparations

Ingredients	Trade name	Use
Solution of 1% hydrocortisone, 1% pramoxine, and 0.1% chloroxylenol; also propylene glycol, acetic acid, and benzalkonium	Ear-Eze Otic-HC Ear Drops Tega-Otic	Antibacterial, anti-fungal, local anesthetic, antiinflammatory products
Solution of 1% hydrocortisone, 2% acetic acid, 3% propylene glycol diacetate, and 0.02% benzethonium chloride	VoSol HC Otic	Antiinflammatory, antibacterial, or anti-fungal in an acid medium
Solution of 1.4% benzocaine, 5.4% antipyrine, glycerin, and oxyquinoline sulfate	Allergen Ear Drops Auralgan Otic Auromid Auroto Otic Earocol Ear Drops	Local anesthetic, analgesic, emollient
6.5% carbamide peroxide in glycerin and/or propylene glycol	Debrox Drops Murine Ear Drops Auro Ear Drops	Treatment of ear wax

The instillation of ear drops requires a knowledge of anatomic structure across the life span, since the shape of the auditory canal of a young child is different from that of an adult. In children 3 years of age or younger, gently pull the pinna of the ear slightly down and back to instill eardrops. In older children and adults, hold the pinna up and back. Gentle massage of the area immediately anterior to the ear will facilitate the entry of the drops into the ear canal.

Education. Instruct the client to remain on his side for 5 minutes. A small cotton pledget may be gently inserted into the ear canal, if desired.

Instruct the client and/or family member in the appropriate ear drop instillation method based on the client's age.

Evaluation. Monitor the client's affected ear(s) for improvement of the condition for which the ear drops are being administered.

Monitor for possible hypersensitivity to the ear drops, evidenced by burning, redness, and swelling. If hypersensitivity occurs, discontinue drops and notify the prescriber.

DRUG-INDUCED OTOXICITY

Many medications have reportedly caused **ototoxicity** in humans. The ototoxicity may affect the person's hearing (auditory or cochlear function), balance (vestibular function), or both. The most common symptom reported is **tinnitus,** a ringing or buzzing sound in the ears.

Cochlear ototoxicity causes a progressive or continuing hearing loss. Loss of the highest tones occurs first, then progresses to affect the lowest tones. Because of this slow progression, most clients are not aware that it is occurring. Vestibular damage may be indicated by dizziness, ataxia, and difficulty with equilibrium. The person may

feel as though the room is in motion **(vertigo).** Ototoxicity is usually bilateral and may be reversible, but it can become irreversible if not recognized early enough to stop the offending medications. Most drug-induced ototoxicity is associated with the use of aminoglycosides. Table 45-4 notes the potential ototoxic effects of selected aminoglycosides. Table 45-5 lists other drugs reported to induce ototoxicity.

NURSING CONSIDERATIONS

Assessment. Assess hearing function before starting therapy with an ototoxic drug.

Concurrent administration of more than one ototoxic drug may increase the potential for hearing loss.

Use caution when administering ototoxic drugs in clients with any condition that may increase their risk of auditory drugs. An example is the client with renal failure,

TABLE 45-4   Potential Ototoxic Effects of Aminoglycoside

Drug	Cochlear	Vestibular
amikacin	++	+
gentamicin	+	++
kanamycin	+++	+
neomycin	++++	+
netilmicin	+	++
sisomicin	+	++
streptomycin	+	+++
tobramycin (Nebcin)	+	++

From Knoben JE and Anderson PO: Handbook of clinical drug data, ed 6, Hamilton, Ill., 1988, Drug Intelligence Publications, Inc.
+, low potential; ++++, greatest potential

TABLE 45-5 Selected Drugs Reported to Cause Ototoxicity

Drug	Comments
Antibiotics aminoglycosides	See Table 48-4
erythromycin lactobionate IV	When administered in high doses (4 g/day), hearing loss (usually reversible) has been reported.
minocycline (Minocin)	Vestibular toxicity including dizziness, lightheadedness, and ataxia reported. Studies indicate that women are more susceptible than men. Toxicity is reversible if drug is stopped.
vancomycin (Vancocin)	Tinnitus usually precedes hearing loss, which may be either transient or permanent. This drug appears to affect the auditory portion of the eighth cranial nerve. It should not be given concurrently with other known ototoxic medications.
Diuretics ethacrynic acid (Edecrin) and furosemide (Lasix)	Both transient and permanent hearing loss have been reported with high-dose, parenteral administration. Concurrent administration with other ototoxic drugs may increase the potential for hearing loss.
Cardiac drugs quinidine	Tinnitus, vertigo, and transient hearing loss have been reported with this drug. Irreversible hearing loss is rare.
Analgesics NSAIDs aspirin	Salicylates, especially in high doses, can cause tinnitus, vertigo, and hearing loss. Generally it is considered reversible if drug is reduced or discontinued, although some cases of irreversible hearing loss are documented.
indomethacin (Indocin), ibuprofen (Motrin), others	NSAIDs have reportedly caused tinnitus, vertigo, and transient hearing loss.
Antineoplastic agents bleomycin, cisplatin, dactinomycin, mechlorethamine	Ototoxicity is reported when these drugs are given in high dosages, especially in persons with renal impairment or those receiving other ototoxic drugs. Tinnitus, vertigo, and transient high tone deafness have been documented. These effects may be reversible or irreversible.

which alters the elimination of aminoglycosides and may result in ototoxic serum levels.

Intervention. Serum levels of some drugs may be monitored to help detect the development of dangerously high blood levels. When given intravenously, aminoglycosides should be administered over 30 to 60 minutes to avoid high peak levels.

Education. Instruct clients to report tinnitus or any other hearing impairment immediately. Auditory damage is usually reversible if the causative drug is discontinued.

Evaluation. Monitor the client's ability to hear by observing for cues indicative of increasing hearing loss (inappropriate responses to others' conversation, speaking loudly, moving closer to others when they speak) and noting client's comments of not being able to hear or understand what others are saying. Report indications of increased hearing loss to the prescriber.

KEY TERMS

ototoxicity, page 750
tinnitus, page 750
vertigo, page 750

BIBLIOGRAPHY

Castiglia PT and others: Focus: nonsuppurative otitis media, Pediatr Nurs 9(6):427, 1983.

Davidson DE: Handbook of nonprescription drugs, ed 8, Washington DC, 1986, American Pharmaceutical Association and The National Professional Society of Pharmacists.

Fischer RG: Drug management of otitis media, Pediatr Nurs 11(6):474, 1985.

Hughes MF: External otitis: managing its dermatologic and otic problems, Consultant 24(5):113, 1984.

Kastrup EK, ed: Facts and comparisons drug information, St Louis: 1988, JB Lippincott Co.

Knoben JE and Anderson PO: Handbook of clinical drug data, ed 5, Hamilton, Ill, 1986 Drug Intelligence Publications, Inc.

Lamb C: Otitis media: selecting the therapy, Patient Care 17(15):108, 1983.

Richman E: Swimmer's ear: timely management tips, Patient Care 21(10):28, 1987.

Sloan RW: Practical geriatric therapeutics, Oradell, NJ, 1986, Medical Economics Inc.

United States Pharmacopeial Convention: Drug information for the health care provider, ed 8, Rockville, Md, 1988, The Convention.

UNIT XII

Drugs Affecting the Endocrine System

CHAPTER
46

Overview of the Endocrine System

OBJECTIVES

After studying this chapter, the student will be able to:

1. Define hormones and explain their functions.

2. List the primary hormones released from the anterior and posterior pituitary.

3. Describe the effects of the thyroid hormones on the body.

4. Discuss the functioning of the parathyroid glands in relationship to calcium and vitamin D.

5. Describe the functions of the three hormones released from the adrenal glands.

6. Compare the effects of insulin and glucagon on blood sugar levels.

HORMONES

The **hormones** are natural chemical substances that act after being secreted into the bloodstream from the endocrine glands. They have specific, well-defined physiologic effects on metabolism. The list of major hormones includes the products of the secretions from the anterior and posterior pituitary glands, the thyroid hormones, parathyroid hormone, insulin and glucagon from the pancreas, epinephrine and norepinephrine from the adrenal medulla, several potent steroids from the adrenal cortex, and the gonadal hormones of both sexes.

The major types of hormones are the steroid hormones and the amino acid-derived hormones. Steroid hormones are those substances secreted by the adrenal gland and the sex glands. They are bound in the plasma to transport proteins. Their physiologic effect begins when the steroid enters the cell, with subsequent binding to the specific cytosol or nuclear protein receptor.

Hormones from the various endocrine glands work together to regulate vital processes, including the following:

1. Secretory and motor activities of the digestive track

2. Energy production

3. Composition and volume of extracellular fluid

4. Adaptation, such as acclimatization and immunity

5. Growth and development
6. Reproduction and lactation

Hormones may exert their effects by controlling the formation or destruction of an intracellular regulator such as cyclic 3'5' adenosine monophosphate (cyclic AMP), controlling protein synthesis, or controlling membrane permeability and the movement of ions and other substances. The effect of a hormone depends on its interaction with a receptor and is determined by the level of the circulating active hormone.

To maintain the internal environment, hormone secretion must be controlled. This is achieved by a self-regulating series of events known as "negative feedback"; that is, a hormone produces a physiologic effect that, when it is strong enough, inhibits further secretion of that hormone, thereby inhibiting the physiologic effect. Increased hormonal secretions may be evoked in response to stimuli from the external environment; cessation of external stimuli ends the internal secretion response (Figure 46-1).

Hormones are not "used up" in exerting their physiologic effects but must be inactivated or excreted if the internal environment is to remain stable. Inactivation occurs enzymatically in the blood or intercellular spaces, in the liver or kidney, or in the target tissues. Excretion of hormones is primarily via the urine and to a lesser extent the bile.

Most hormones are destroyed rapidly, having a half-life in blood of 10 to 30 minutes. However, some, such as the catecholamines, have a half-life of seconds, and thyroid hormones have a half-life measured in days. Some hormones exert their physiologic effects immediately; others require minutes or hours before their effects occur. In addition, some effects end immediately when the hormone disappears from the circulation. Other responses may persist for hours after hormone concentrations have returned to basal levels. The exposure of a tissue to an active hormone also is controlled by that hormone's pathway for metabolism, including molecular alterations, consumption at the site of action, and hepatorenal excretion. This wide range of onset and duration of hormonal activity contributes to the flexibility of the endocrine system.

One of the major developments of this century in the fields of biology and medicine has been the recognition and isolation, purification, and chemical and cellular understanding of most known hormones. In addition, once their chemical structure is known, duplicating hormones

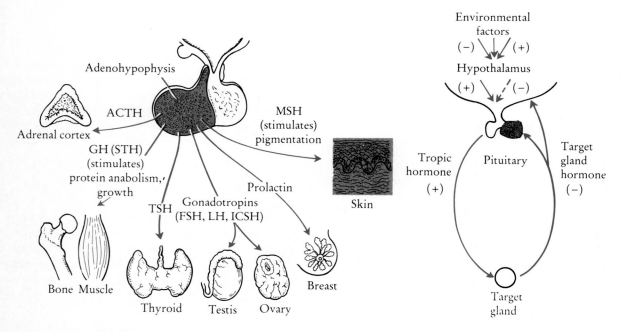

FIGURE 46-1 Various internal and external environmental factors may inhibit or stimulate the hypothalamus to secrete inhibitory (−) or releasing (+) factors to control output of hormones from anterior pituitary and ultimate hormone release from target glands. Hormone secretion from target glands (adrenal cortex, thyroid, etc.), on reaching a critical level, have inhibitory effect on secretion of tropic hormones by anterior pituitary and releasing factors (RF) by the hypothalamus. *ACTH,* Adrenocorticotropic hormone; *GH,* growth hormone; *STH,* somatotropin hormone; *TSH,* thyroid-stimulating hormone; *FSH,* follicle-stimulating hormone; *LH,* luteinizing hormone; *ICSH,* interstitial cell-stimulating hormone; *MSH,* melanocyte-stimulating hormone.

by chemical synthesis becomes theoretically possible. This had been accomplished for some but not all hormones.

In medicine, hormones generally are used in three ways: (1) for replacement therapy, exemplified by use of insulin for diabetes or adrenal steroids in Addison's disease; (2) for pharmacologic effects beyond replacement, as in the use of larger than endogenous doses of adrenal steroids for their antiinflammatory effects; and (3) for endocrine diagnostic testing.

Research in endocrinology has advanced the concept of specific receptors within or on the surface of cells. This has led to knowledge of hormone specificity and the essential cellular mechanisms involved in the hormone-receptor complex. The recognition and activation properties found in the hormone-receptor complex come from different receptor molecular sites. Only specific receptor material binds a hormone and begins its activity; the hormone has no effect on other tissues that do not carry specific receptors. Alterations in either hormone secretion or hormone receptor responses may culminate in endocrine disease states. Certain cell surface receptors may become antigenic and develop antibodies that accelerate receptor destruction, block receptor function, or mimic the action of the target tissue. Among the receptor-like disorders, referred to as antireceptor autoimmune diseases, are myasthenia gravis, Graves' disease, insulin-resistant diabetes mellitus, and bronchial asthma.

PITUITARY GLAND

The hormones of the pituitary gland exert an important effect in regulating the secretion of other hormones. The pituitary body is about the size of a pea and occupies a niche in the sella turcica of the sphenoid bone. It consists of an anterior lobe (adenohypophysis), a posterior lobe (neurohypophysis), and a smaller pars intermedia composed of secreting cells. The anterior lobe is particularly important in sustaining life. The function of the pars intermedia is not well known.

REGULATION OF ANTERIOR PITUITARY FUNCTION

The pituitary and target glands have a negative feedback relationship. A tropic hormone from the pituitary stimulates the target gland to secrete a hormone that inhibits further secretion of the tropic hormone by the pituitary. When the serum concentration of the target gland hormone falls below a certain level, the pituitary again secretes the tropic hormone until the target gland produces enough hormone to inhibit the pituitary secretion. However, the negative feedback concept alone is not enough to account for changes in serum levels of target gland hormones, especially those caused by changes in the external environment. Thus the central nervous system is

believed to play a decisive role in regulating pituitary function to meet environmental demands.

The discovery of various hypothalamic-releasing factors is of great research interest. These factors cause the release of inhibition of the various hormones from the anterior pituitary. Among these releasing factors are thyroid-stimulating hormone releasing factor, corticotropin-releasing factor, growth hormone releasing hormone, growth hormone inhibitory hormone (somatostatin), luteinizing hormone releasing hormone and prolactin inhibitory factor.

ANTERIOR PITUITARY HORMONES

The number of hormones secreted by the anterior pituitary gland is unknown, but at least seven extracts have been prepared in a relatively pure state, and they have definite specific action.

1. A growth factor influences the development of the body. It promotes skeletal, visceral, and general growth. Acromegaly, gigantism, and dwarfism are associated with pathologic conditions of the anterior lobe of the pituitary gland.

   Growth hormone (somatotropin, somatropin, somatotropic hormone, STH) has been obtained as a small crystalline protein, but thus far the growth hormone has found no established place in medicine except in documented clinical and laboratory evidence of growth hormone deficiency. Its use in various clinical conditions is largely experimental. It tends to increase the blood sugar and antagonize insulin, and it may be the "diabetogenic" hormone postulated in the past.

2. **Follicle-stimulating hormone (FSH)** stimulates the growth and maturation of the ovarian follicle, which in turn brings on the characteristic changes of estrus (menstruation in women). This hormone also stimulates spermatogenesis in the male. FSH appears to be a protein or is associated with a protein, but this human pituitary gonadotropin has not yet been obtained in a highly purified form.

3. **Luteinizing hormone (LH),** also known as the interstitial cell-stimulating hormone (ICSH), together with FSH (Pergonal), causes maturation of the graafian follicles, ovulation, and the secretion of estrogen in the female. It causes spermatogenesis, androgen formation, and growth of interstitial tissue in the male. Luteinizing hormone also promotes the formation of the corpus luteum in the female.

4. **Thyrotropic hormone (TSH)** is necessary for normal development and function of the thyroid gland. If too much is present, it is known to produce hyperthyroidism and increase the size of the gland in laboratory animals.

5. A **lactogenic factor** (prolactin or mammotropin) plays a part in proliferation and secretion of the mammary glands of mammals. This may be identical to the hormone responsible for the development of the corpus luteum. In its absence the corpus luteum fails to produce progesterone.

6. **Adrenocorticotropic hormone (corticotropin or ACTH)** stimulates the cortex of the adrenal gland.

7. **Melanocyte-stimulating hormone (intermedin or MSH)** is probably produced in the intermediate lobe. Its

physiologic role is unknown, but when injected in human beings, it will darken the skin.

The hormones produced by the anterior lobe of the pituitary gland are important physiologically, but only recently have purified preparations been available, at least for clinical study; and such preparations are both expensive and limited in supply. They may have become useful in combating certain disorders in the future, however, as chemically defined preparations become available.

POSTERIOR PITUITARY HORMONES

Two hormones obtained from the posterior lobe of the pituitary gland have been identified and chemically analyzed. These compounds, **oxytocin** and **vasopressin** (antidiuretic hormone), are both peptides, and each contains eight amino acids. It has proved possible to synthesize them chemically. Availability of these hormones in pure form has clarified their mechanism of action and has allowed better control of their therapeutic use. For example, a certain overlap of pharmacologic action exists even in the pure preparation; pure oxytocin has some vasopressor activity, and vice versa. The antidiuretic potency of vasopressin is much greater than its pressor potency. While vasopressin is available in a natural state, synthetic formulations, such as lypressin and desmopressin have been developed; and they act primarily as ADH. They have very little, if any, pressor or oxytoxic activity.

Oxytocin is discussed in Chapter 53.

THYROID GLAND

The thyroid gland, one of the most richly vascularized tissues of the body, secretes three hormones essential for proper regulation of metabolism: **thyroxine (T_4), triiodothyronine (T_3)**, and **calcitonin.** Because of its role in calcium metabolism, calcitonin is discussed later with the parathyroid gland hormones. (See Chapter 48.)

The thyroid gland is composed of at least two types of cells: follicular, which produce T_3 and T_4; and parafollicular, the source of calcitonin.

THYROID HORMONES

The large amount of iodine in thyroid hormones and the availability of radioactive iodine have led to detailed knowledge about thyroid physiology and its role in metabolism. Iodine is essential for thyroid hormone synthesis. About 1 mg of iodine per week is required, most of which is ingested in food, water, and iodized table salt. About two thirds of this iodine is reduced in the gastrointestinal tract, enters the circulation as iodide, and is excreted into the urine. The remaining third is taken up by the thyroid gland for hormone synthesis. This process is aided by the "iodide pump," which takes up the iodide from the extracellular fluid, traps it, and concentrates it to many times that found in plasma. The ratio of iodide in the thyroid gland to that in the serum is expressed as the T/S ratio; normally this ratio is 20:1. In hypoactivity the ratio may be 10:1; in hyperactivity it may be as great as 250:1.

Thyroglobulin is synthesized first. It contains thyrosine, an amino acid that reacts with iodine to form thyroid hormones. The thyroglobulin-thyroid hormone complex is stored in the follicles of the thyroid gland and is called "colloid." About 30% of the thyroid mass is stored thyroglobulin, which contains enough thyroid hormone to meet normal requirements for 2 to 3 months without any further synthesis.

Normally, thyroglobulin is not released into the circulation but undergoes proteolytic digestion (a coupling reaction), which releases the active thyroid hormones T_3 and T_4. Hormone synthesis—iodine trapping, iodination and proteolysis of thyroglobulin, and hormone release—is controlled by the thyroid-stimulating hormone (thyrotropin, TSH) from the beta cells of the anterior pituitary gland. Thyroid secretion is maintained by this TSH secretion. Decreased serum levels of T_4 and T_3 stimulate thyrotropin-releasing hormone (TRH) from the hypothalamus, which stimulates the pituitary gland to secrete TSH, which in turn stimulates release of thyroxin from thyroglobulin.

TSH secretion is negatively regulated by T_4 and T_3, which directly inhibit the pituitary gland's thyrotopic cells. An increase in free, unbound thyroid hormone causes a decrease in TSH secretion and inhibits TRH production, and a decrease in the free unbound hormone causes an increase in TSH secretion and stimulates TRH production—a negative feedback mechanism.

Physiologic Effects of Thyroid Hormones

The precise physiologic role of the thyroid hormones is not yet known, although several hormonal actions have been identified and studied. Three generalizations can be made about thyroid hormones:

1. They have a diffuse effect and do not seem to have any specific target organ effect; no special cells or tissues appear to be particularly affected by the thyroid hormones.

2. Their long delay in onset of action and their prolonged action rule them out as minute-to-minute regulators of physiologic function. Instead, their role is more likely to be that of establishing and maintaining long-term functions such as growth, maturation, and adaptation.

3. They are not necessary for survival, although reduced levels can affect quality of life.

Thyroxine and triiodothyronine appear to have the

same physiologic actions, although T_3 is far more potent than T_4.

Thyroid hormones have the following physiologic effects:

1. *Growth and maturation.* A normal, functioning thyroid is essential for normal growth. Thyroid hormones stimulate production of messenger ribonucleic acid (RNA) molecules, which are involved in the synthesis of various proteins, thus facilitating growth and development. The hormones must be present in the right amounts for growth to occur at the normal rate. In children who are hypothyroid, rate of growth is retarded, which may lead to shortness of stature. Conversely, children who are hyperthyroid may have excessive skeletal growth and become taller than they otherwise would. If there is premature closing of the epiphyses because of accelerated bone maturation, however, stunting of growth results. In the adult, excess thyroid hormone causes increased demineralization of bone and increased loss of calcium and phosphate.

   Cells in the interstitial tissue between follicles of the thyroid gland produce calcitonin; the effect of this hormone is to reduce the blood calcium ion concentration, the exact opposite effect of parathyroid hormone. Calcitonin is essential for bone formation in children, since it promotes deposition of calcium. In the adult, calcitonin has a very weak effect on plasma concentration, since absorption and deposition of calcium are slow in the adult and calcitonin effects are rapidly overridden by parathyroid hormone.

2. *Central nervous system function.* At time of birth through the first year of life, thyroid hormone must be present for normal development of the cerebrum; if the hormone is not present, irreversible mental retardation occurs. In the adult, hypothyroidism causes listlessness, a general dulling of mental capacity, decreased sensory capacity, slow speech, impaired memory, and somnolence. Hyperthyroidism in the adult results in hyperexcitability, irritability, restlessness, exaggerated responses to environmental stimuli, and emotional instability. Psychosis can occur in either hypo- or hyperthyroidism.

3. *Basal metabolic rate.* Thyroid hormones increase oxygen consumption in most cells of the body with the exception of the lungs, spleen, gastric smooth muscle, the gonads, and accessory sex organs. In hypothyroidism the basal metabolic rate is subnormal; in hyperthyroidism it may be 40% to 60% above normal.

4. *Carbohydrate and lipid metabolism.* Thyroid hormones accelerate glucose catabolism, increase cholesterol synthesis, and enhance the liver's ability to excrete cholesterol in the bile. Since the effect on cholesterol excretion is greater than that on cholesterol synthesis, the result is a decrease in plasma cholesterol level. The hormones also stimulate the mobilization of fatty acids from adipose tissue. The hypothyroid individual will have an elevated serum cholesterol level and increased blood levels of phospholipids and triglycerides.

5. *Protein metabolism.* Thyroid hormones are essential for the development of protein mass. In hypothyroidism both the synthesis and the breakdown of protein are diminished, but the effect on protein synthesis is more profound. In addition, deposition of mucoproteins occurs in subcutaneous spaces, which osmotically attracts water, causing "puffiness." In hyperthyroidism increased catabolism of protein, or breakdown of muscle mass, and increased nitrogen excretion occur.

6. *Gastrointestinal function.* Thyroid hormones increase gastrointestinal motility, absorption of food, and secretion of digestive juices. Hypothyroidism decreases both intestinal absorption and secretion of pancreatic enzymes. Constipation also may occur.

7. *Water and electrolyte balance.* In thyroid hormone deficiency, water and electrolytes accumulate in subcutaneous spaces; administering a thyroid hormone results in diuresis and a loss of fluid and electrolytes from the subcutaneous spaces.

8. *Cardiovascular function.* Since the thyroid hormones increase metabolism, the tissues have an increased need for oxygen and nutrients, which in turn demands increased blood flow. In hyperthyroidism these effects cause increased cardiac output, increased pulse pressure, and tachycardia. If these effects are prolonged, cardiac hypertrophy and even high-output myocardial failure may occur. Opposite effects occur in hypothyroidism.

9. *Muscle function.* Moderate increases in thyroid hormone makes muscle react with vigor; large increases result in muscle weakness because of excess protein catabolism. A characteristic sign of hyperthyroidism is a fine muscle tremor. Hypothyroidism causes the muscles to be sluggish.

10. *Temperature regulation.* Thyroid hormones must be present for an increase in heat production or a decrease in heat loss to occur. Although the hormones do not initiate the physiologic response to cold, they appear to magnify the body's response to catecholamine effects, which innervate the sympathetic system during cold exposure. Hypothyroidism causes decreased tolerance to cold.

11. *Lactation.* Thyroid hormone is necessary for normal milk production; without thyroid hormone, fat content of milk and total milk production are greatly reduced.

12. *Reproduction.* Thyroid hormone is required for normal rhythmicity in the reproductive cycle.

THYROID GLAND DISORDERS
Goiter

The synthesis of the thyroid hormones and their maintenance in the blood in adequate amounts depend largely on an adequate intake of iodine. Iodine ingested by way of food or water is changed into iodide and is stored in the thyroid gland before reaching the circulation. Prolonged iodine deficiency in the diet results in enlargement of the thyroid gland, known as a simple goiter. When thyroid hormones fail to be synthesized because of a lack of iodine, the anterior lobe of the pituitary is stimulated to increase the secretion of thyrotropic hormone, which in turn causes hypertrophy and hyperplasia of the gland. The enlarged thyroid then removes residual traces of iodine from the blood. This type of goiter (simple or nontoxic) can be prevented by providing an adequate supply of iodine for young persons. Iodine is not abundant in most foods except fish and seafoods, and iodized salt is frequently the primary source for iodine in areas where seafood is expensive or not readily available.

Hypothyroidism

Clients with primary hypothyroidism have decreased T_3 and T_4 levels and an elevated TSH level. Those with pituitary (secondary) hypothyroidism have decreased levels of T_3, T_4, and TSH but normal levels of TRH, whereas those with hypothalamic (tertiary) hypothyroidism have decreased levels of T_3, T_4, and TSH and normal levels of TRH.

The TSH test, the most sensitive index of hypothyroidism, is elevated in primary hypothyroidism and depressed in secondary hypothyroidism. The free thyroxine index (FTI = $TT_4 \times RT_3U$) is depressed in clients with both primary and secondary hypothyroidism but elevated in clients with hyperthyroidism. The T_3 resin uptake (RT_3U) is depressed in pregnancy and in clients with primary and secondary hypothyroidism but elevated in clients with hyperthyroidism. The serum T_3 level is depressed in both secondary and primary hypothyroidism but elevated in hyperthyroid states and T_3 thyrotoxicosis. The total T_4 (TT_4 Murphy-Pattee) is elevated in pregnancy and hyperthyroidism but depressed in both primary and secondary hypothyroidism. The free T_4 (unbound) is depressed in both primary and secondary hypothyroid states but is elevated in hyperthyroid states.

In children, normal skeletal growth is evidence of adequate therapy; an increase in serum alkaline phosphatase indicates that growth will occur. In cretinism (see below), thyroid hormone levels equal to or above those required for the adult must be established immediately after birth to prevent permanent mental and physical retardation. Treatment of the older cretin will not reverse the mental retardation that has already occurred. Clients with hypothyroidism need to be informed of their lifelong need for replacement therapy.

Cretinism. Hypothyroidism in the young child is known as **cretinism** and is characterized by cessation of physical and mental development, which leads to dwarfism and idiocy. Clients with cretinism usually have thick, coarse skin; a thick tongue; gaping mouth; protruding abdomen; thick, short legs, poorly developed hands and feet; and weak musculature. This condition may result from faulty development or atrophy of the thyroid gland during fetal life. Failure of development of the gland may be caused by lack of iodine in the mother.

Myxedema. Severe hypothyroidism in the adult is called **myxedema** (acid mucopolysaccharide accumulation). When it is the last stage of a long-standing, inadequately treated or untreated hypothyroidism, coma appears, accompanied by hypotension, hypoventilation, hypothermia, bradycardia, hyponatremia, and hypoglycemia. The development of myxedema is usually insidious and causes gradual retardation of physical and mental functions. There is gradual infiltration of the skin and loss of facial lines and facial expression (a puffy, expressionless face). The formation of subcutaneous connective tissue causes the hands and face to appear puffy and swollen. The basal metabolic rate becomes subnormal, the skin is cold and dry, the hair becomes scanty and coarse, movements become sluggish, cardiac output is reduced, and the patient becomes hypersensitive to cold.

Hyperthyroidism (Thyrotoxicosis)

Excessive formation of the thyroid hormones and their escape into the circulation result in a toxic state called **thyrotoxicosis.** This occurs in the condition known as diffuse toxic goiter, or exophthalmic goiter (Graves' disease), or in some forms of adenomatous goiters.

Primary hyperthyroidism is characterized by elevated levels of T_3 and T_4 and decreased level of TSH. In pituitary (secondary) hyperthyroidism levels of T_3, T_4, and TSH increase.

Hyperthyroidism leads to symptoms quite different from those seen in myxedema. The metabolic rate is increased, sometimes as much as +60 or more. The body temperature frequently is above normal, the pulse rate is fast, and the client complains of feeling too warm. Other symptoms include restlessness, anxiety, emotional instability, muscle tremor and weakness, sweating, and exophthalmos. The increased thyroxine levels may cause cardiomegaly, tachycardia, congestive heart failure, hepatic alterations (necrosis, dysfunction, fatty changes), lymphoid hyperplasia, osteoporosis, pretibial myxedema, and neurologic irritability. In *thyroid storm* sudden onset of hyperthyroid symptoms occurs, especially those affecting the nervous and cardiovascular systems, because of elevated thyroxine levels.

Before the advent of antithyroid drugs, treatment was limited to a subtotal resection of the hyperactive gland. Propylthiouracil is the most commonly used antithyroid medication. However, antithyroid drugs provide less rapid control of hyperthyroidism than do surgical measures. Radioactive therapy is used primarily in treatment of middle-age and elderly clients.

PARATHYROID GLANDS

Lying just above and behind the thyroid gland are bean-shaped glands known as the parathyroids. Humans have two pairs. The adult glands consist of encapsulated masses of cells, between which are abundant adipocytes and vascular channels. The primary function of the parathyroids is to maintain adequate levels of calcium in the extracellular fluid. Parathyroid hormone has multiple effects, ultimately culminating in mobilization of calcium from bone. It also reduces phosphate concentration, permitting more calcium to be mobilized.

PARATHYROID HORMONES

Parathyroid hormone (PTH) is a polypeptide. The active component has a half-life of 30 minutes; the inactive component, 7 to 10 days. PTH circulates in elevated concentrations in clients with hyperplastic parathyroid glands as a result of diminished calcium levels, as found in persons with impaired renal function or intestinal malabsorption. These elevated PTH levels may cause metabolic bone disease, including osteoporosis and osteomalacia.

The mechanism of PTH action in the bone or kidney is incompletely understood. Some researchers suggest that PTH receptor-binding and adenylate cyclase activity are coupled events subject to down regulation of the receptors. Patients with hyperparathyroidism may be resistant to PTH action on kidney and bone. The decreased number of these receptors, not their altered affinity, produces a reduction in PTH-stimulated adenylate cyclase activity.

Cholesterol-derived provitamin D is converted to vitamin D_3 by action of sunlight on the skin. The vitamin is also present as a milk additive. Along with PTH, vitamin D_3 is converted to its active form in the kidney. It is involved in calcium, phosphate, and magnesium metabolism in bone and the gastrointestinal tract.

Primary hyperparathyroidism is the most common parathyroid disorder. Generally it is caused by adenomas, chief cell hyperplasia, or hypertrophy. PTH elevations produce altered function of renal tubular cells, bone cells, and gastrointestinal tract mucosa. Elevated levels of calcium and increased bone resorption with the development of renal calculi occurs, generally, in hyperparathyroidism. In secondary hyperparathyroidism, an overactive parathyroid gland causes increased calcium excretion and possibly kidney stones, but generally, serum calcium levels remain stable due to an effective feedback mechanism.

Hypoparathyroidism leads to manifestations of hypocalcemia and tetany, the symptoms of which include muscle spasms, convulsions, gradual paralysis with dyspnea, and death from exhaustion. Before death, gastrointestinal hemorrhages and hematemesis frequently occur. At death the intestinal mucosa is congested, and the calcium content of the heart, kidney, and other tissues is increased.

The symptoms of tetany are relieved by administration of calcium salts. Large doses of vitamin D also help to relieve tetany and to restore the normal calcium level in the blood. The client is hospitalized, since frequent assessment of blood calcium and phosphate levels is essential.

ADRENAL GLANDS

The adrenal glands are located just above the kidneys. They consist of two parts, the inner medulla and the outer cortex.

The adrenal cortex synthesizes three important classes of hormones: the **glucocorticoids** (cortisol), **mineralocorticoids** (primarily aldosterone), and **androgens** (primarily dehydroepiandrosterone). The glucocorticoids are synthesized primarily in the zona fasciculata and are under the control of ACTH from the pituitary gland. Although the basal production rate averages 30 mg every 24 hours, under stressful conditions (trauma, major surgery, infection) there is a reserve capacity production of up to 300 mg daily. Increases in glucocorticoid production may be related to proportional increases in release of ACTH by the pituitary.

The mineralocorticoids are synthesized specifically in the zona glomerulosa. Production is primarily under the control of both the renin-angiotensin axis system (discussed later) and the blood potassium level. The production of aldosterone is stimulated by salt depletion and causes sodium retention in the kidney at the distal convoluted tubule to preserve the extracellular fluid volume.

The androgens are synthesized in the zona fasciculata and the zona reticularis and essentially control growth of the hair follicles in the skin.

Normally a reaction to serious stress causes a prompt and noticeable increase in cortisol and aldosterone production; these hormones operate together to maintain the cardiovascular tone essential for survival. A client under stress who has impaired ability to produce these hormones incurs the risk of developing acute adrenal crisis. The production of cortisol is under the control of a continous feedback mechanism involving the pituitary and ACTH production, which is in turn inhibited by the circulating cortisol levels. Stress is a stimulus to override this inhibition and initiates secretion of corticotropin-releasing factor, which culminates in ACTH release and activation of the adrenal cortex, leading to an increased production of cortisol.

MINERALOCORTICOIDS: ALDOSTERONE

Aldosterone is the primary mineralocorticoid in humans. It is synthesized in the adrenal zona glomerulosa, which is the outer edge of the adrenocortical tissue below the adrenal capsule. Aldosterone production is maintained primarily by the renin-angiotensin system and the concentration of circulating serum potassium. A drop in the circulating arterial volume stimulates volume receptors in the juxtaglomerular apparatus. As a result, renin (a proteolytic enzyme) is produced and acts on angiotensinogen, which is synthesized by the liver to form angiotensin I. When the angiotensin I passes through the pulmonary circulation, two amino acids are cleared from it to form angiotensin. Angiotensin II stimulates the adrenal zona glomerulosa to produce aldosterone. Aldosterone promotes sodium reabsorption in the kidney at the distal convoluted tubule to preserve extracellular fluid volume. In the normal client, aldosterone secretion is stimulated by a decrease in circulating volume (loss of blood, excessive diuresis, low salt intake, etc.) and increased potassium levels. Aldosterone secretion is suppressed by an elevation of sodium levels in the blood (e.g., by excessive dietary salt intake). It restricts the loss of sodium and its accompanying anions, chloride and bicarbonate, and thereby helps maintain extracellular fluid volume. It also maintains acid-base and potassium balance.

In adrenal insufficiency, aldosterone deficit occurs, sodium reabsorption is inhibited, and potassium excretion decreases. Hyperkalemia and mild acidosis occur. In adrenalectomy the loss of aldosterone leads to an overall reduction of sodium reabsorption and a powerful and uncontrolled loss of extracellular fluid. Plasma volume drops, and a state of hypovolemic shock may ensue. This may cause death unless a mineralocorticoid, salt, and water are administered. In excessive doses, aldosterone increases potassium excretion, and unless dietary intake compensates for the loss, hypokalemia results. Acidification of the urine then occurs, leading to metabolic alkalosis.

Aldosterone is much more potent in its electrolyte effects than desoxycorticosterone, though it has not yet established a therapeutic status comparable to that of desoxycorticosterone. Its use has been limited because of its cost and relative unavailability and because it must be administered intramuscularly.

The amount of aldosterone secreted by the adrenal cortex apparently is affected by the concentration of sodium in body fluids rather than by the stimulation of the adrenal cortex by ACTH.

PANCREAS

The pancreas is a gland that lies transversely across the posterior wall of the abdomen. It secretes a limpid, colorless fluid that digests proteins, fats, and carbohydrates.

It also produces internal secretions— **insulin** and **glucagon**—that affect blood sugar levels.

Insulin is a hormone secreted by the beta cells of the islets of Langerhans in the pancreas. On hydrolysis, this hormone yields several amino acids. In its crystalline state it appears to be chemically linked with certain metals (zinc, nickel, cadmium, or cobalt). Normal pancreatic tissue is rich in zinc, which may be significant to the natural storage of the hormone. Insulin consists of two polypeptide chains and contains 48 amino acids, the exact sequence of which is known. Insulin is stored in the beta cells as a larger protein known as *proinsulin*.

Since relatively small amounts of insulin are necessary in the body tissues, it is thought that insulin acts as a catalyst in cellular metabolism.

Carbohydrate metabolism is controlled by a finely balanced interaction of several endocrine factors (adrenal, anterior pituitary, thyroid, insulin), but the particular phase of carbohydrate metabolism that is affected by insulin is not entirely known. When insulin is injected subcutaneously, however, it produces a rapid lowering of the blood sugar. This effect is produced in both diabetic and nondiabetic persons. Moderate amounts of insulin in the diabetic animal promote the storage of carbohydrate in the liver and also in the muscle cells, particularly after the feeding of carbohydrate. In the normal animal the deposit of muscle glycogen also increases, but apparently the level of liver glycogen does not. In both diabetic and nondiabetic persons the oxygen consumption increases and the respiratory quotient rises.

Glucagon, like insulin, is a pancreatic extract and is thought to oppose the action of insulin. Glucagon is a product of the alpha cells of the islets of Langerhans. Glucagon acts primarily by mobilizing hepatic glycogen and converting it to glucose, which produces an elevation of the concentration of glucose in the blood.

DIABETES MELLITUS

Diabetes mellitus is a heterogenous metabolic disease characterized particularly by an inability to use carbohydrate. Insulin action is ineffective at the tissue site, or not enough insulin is available. Obesity, certain drugs, viruses, autoimmune phenomena, genetic predisposition, and age may have roles in its development. The blood sugar becomes elevated, and when it exceeds a certain amount, the excess is secreted by the kidney (glycosuria). Symptoms include increased appetite (polyphagia), thirst (polydipsia), weight loss, increased urine output (polyuria), weakness (fatigue), and itching such as pruritus vulvae.

In diabetes mellitus, glycogen fails to store in the liver, although the conversion of glycogen back to glucose or the formation of glucose from other substances (gluconeogenesis) is not necessarily impaired. As a result, the level of blood sugar rapidly rises. This derangement of carbohydrate metabolism results in an abnormally high metabolism of proteins and fats. The ketone bodies, which result from oxidation of fatty acids, accumulate faster than the muscle cells can oxidize them, resulting in ketosis and acidosis. The course of untreated diabetes mellitus is progressive. The symptoms of diabetic coma and acidosis are directly or indirectly the result of the accumulation of acetone, beta-hydroxybutyric acid, and diacetic acid. Respirations become rapid and deep, the breath has an odor of acetone, the blood sugar is elevated, the client becomes dehydrated, and stupor and coma develop unless treatment is started promptly.

The long-term complications of diabetes mellitus can lead to an increase in morbidity and mortality. Some of the most commonly associated problems are peripheral atherosclerosis, which may result in coronary artery disease, infections, gangrene, or strokes; diabetic retinopathy which can include vitreal hemorrhage, retinal detachment, and blindness; renal disease, peripheral sensory neuropathy, and cardiomyopathy leading to heart failure are also reported.

Diabetes mellitus usually is treated with exogenous insulin, diet, and exercise. Glucose and insulin promote the formation and retention of glycogen in the liver, and the oxidation of fat in the liver is arrested. Therefore the rate of formation of acetone bodies is slowed and the acidosis is checked. Other supportive measures, such as restoring the fluid and electrolyte balance of the body, are very important in its treatment.

Diabetic therapy includes (1) the synthesis of human insulin by bacteria genetically altered by recombinant DNA technology, (2) islet-cell and/or pancreas transplantation, and (3) external and implanted continuous insulin infusion pumps.

KEY TERMS

adrenocorticotropic hormone, corticotropin (ACTH), page 757
aldosterone, page 762
androgens, page 761
calcitonin, page 758
cretinism, page 760
follicle-stimulating hormone (FSH), page 757
glucagon, page 762
glucocorticoids, page 761
growth hormone, somatotropic hormone (GH or STH), page 757
hormones, page 755
insulin, page 762
intermedin, page 757
lactogenic factor, page 757
luteinizing hormone (LH), page 757
melanocyte-stimulating hormone (MSH), page 757

mineralocorticoids, page 761
myxedema, page 760
oxytocin, page 758
parathyroid hormone (PTH), page 761
somatotropin, page 757
somatropin, page 757
thyrotoxicosis, page 760
thyrotropic hormone (TSH), page 757
thyroxine (T$_4$), page 758
triiodothyronine (T$_3$), page 758
vasopressin, page 758

BIBLIOGRAPHY

Anthony, CP, and Thibodeau, GA: Textbook of anatomy and physiology, 12th ed, St. Louis: Times Mirror/Mosby College Publishing, 1987.

Biecher, M: Antireceptor autoimmune diseases, part 2, Diagn Med 6(7):39, 1983.

Brewer, J: The anatomy and physiology of the pancreas, SGA J 8(3):38, 1986.

Claman, HN: Glucocorticosteroids: anti-inflammatory mechanisms, part 1, Hosp Pract 18(7):123, 1983.

Claman, HN: Glucocorticosteroids: the clinical responses, part 2, Hosp Pract 18(7):143, 1983.

Groer, MW, and Shekleton, ME: Basic pathophysiology: a conceptual approach, 2nd ed, St. Louis: The CV Mosby Co, 1983.

Guyton, AC: Human physiology and mechanisms of disease, 4th ed, Philadelphia: WB Saunders Co, 1987.

Herlihy, B: Endocrine physiology (pituitary hormones), Crit Care Nurse 3(5):111, 1983.

Kupperman, HS: Hypothyroidism, Physician Assist 10(3):60, 1986.

Larson, CA: The critical path of adrenocortical insufficiency, Nursing 14(10):66, 1984.

Leebaw, WF, and others: Endocrine problems: effects of aging on normal and abnormal function, Consultant 24(7):165, 1984.

Mathewson, MK: Thyroid disorder, Crit Care Nurse 7(1):74, 1987.

Mathewson, MK: Antidiuretic hormone, Crit Care Nurse 6(5):88, 1986.

Maxwell, M: The endocrine system, Nurs Mirror 157(5):23, 1983.

McConnell, EA: Assessing the thyroid, Nursing 15(5):60, 1985.

Miller, SM: Action and assessment of parathyrin, a calcium regulating hormone, J Med Technol 3(6):335, 1986.

Palmieri, MJ: Pathophysiology of the pancreas . . . certification review, SGA J 9(3):134, 1987.

Schoeff, L: Antidiuretic hormone and water regulation, J Med Technol 3(6):342, 1986.

Simkins, ME: Diagnosis: hyperparathyroidism, Point View 20(4):16, 1983.

Taylor, DL: Hypoglycemia: physiology, signs, and symptoms, Nursinglife 7(1):36, 1987.

Tyson, JE: Reproductive endocrinology: new problems call for new solutions, Diagn Med 7(4):24, 1984.

Verbalis, JG, and others: Hypopituitarism, Top Emerg Med 5(4):74, 1984.

CHAPTER 47

Drugs Affecting the Pituitary

OBJECTIVES

After studying this chapter, the student will be able to:

1. Describe the primary functions of the anterior and posterior pituitary hormones.

2. Describe the effects of somatrem and somatropin.

3. List the effects of vasopressin.

4. Apply nursing considerations to the client receiving drugs affecting the pituitary.

There are a variety of preparations available that affect the hypothalamus and pituitary gland. They are generally used as replacement therapy for hormone deficiency; drug therapy for specific disorders, using such preparations to produce a therapeutic hormonal response; and diagnostic aids to determine hypofunctional or hyperfunctional hormone states.

A number of hormones have been identified, and many have been synthesized, including the following: growth hormone–releasing hormone (GRH), growth hormone-inhibiting hormone (Somatostatin), thyrotropin-releasing hormone (TRH), corticotropin-releasing hormone (CRH), gonadotropin-releasing hormone (GnRH), and prolactin-inhibiting hormone (PIH or dopamine). Also, six anterior pituitary hormones and two posterior pituitary hormones have been identified. The anterior pituitary hormones include growth hormone (GH), thyrotropin (TSH), adrenocorticotropin (ACTH), follicle-stimulating hormone (FSH), luteinizing hormone (LH) and prolactin. The posterior pituitary hormones are vasopressin and oxytocin.

This chapter covers specific agents affecting the hypothalamus and pituitary. It does not discuss formulations that directly affect or involve the pancreas, thyroid, parathyroid, and adrenal cortex. These latter formulations are discussed in the chapters devoted to these areas.

Of the above-mentioned hormones, gonadotropin-releasing hormone (gonadorelin) is discussed in Chapter 51, while thyrotropin-releasing hormone (TRH) and corticotropic-releasing hormone (CRH) are discussed in

Chapters 48 and 49. While a true hormone with prolactin-inhibiting effects has not been identified, the substance is believed to be dopamine. Bromocriptine, a drug with dopamine-agonist properties, is reviewed in Chapters 17 and 53.

Of the remaining two substances, the **growth hormone–releasing hormone (GHRH)** has been identified in vivo but is still under investigation. This substance has been found to stimulate the release of growth hormone after intranasal application. If it is marketed, it will be used to test clients with growth hormone deficiency, thus testing the responsiveness of the anterior pituitary gland.

The **growth hormone–inhibiting hormone (somatostatin)** was obtained from human cadaver pituitaries, but its distribution in the United States was stopped in 1985. **Creutzfeldt-Jakob disease** (a neurotropic virus) that is very rare in young people, was diagnosed in some clients and resulted in the death of several clients 5 to 7 years after receiving this product. Therefore human-derived preparations are now replaced by a biosynthetic hormone grown through recombinant DNA technology. This product (somatrem) is considered equivalent to the pituitary human growth hormone in effectiveness.

ANTERIOR PITUITARY HORMONES

somatrem (Protropin)

Somatrem contains the identical sequence of the pituitary-derived human growth hormone plus one additional amino acid, methionine. In tests it has been demonstrated to be therapeutically equivalent to somatotropin, or the human growth hormone from the pituitary.

Mechanism of action. Somatrem stimulates the release of **somatomedins** (hormones that are synthesized in the liver and elsewhere), in response to the growth hormone. It is believed most of the actions of somatrem are related to the effects of the somatomedins, which include stimulation of growth by their effect on organ size and growth of long bones and by an increase in the number and size of muscle tissue cells. Therefore a major pharmacologic consequence of somatrem use is an increase in longitudinal growth, whereas a deficiency in growth hormone usually results in **dwarfism.**

Somatrem also has metabolic effects—that is, it impairs glucose uptake, and antagonizes the effects of insulin; increases lipolysis; promotes cellular growth by retaining phosphorus and potassium and enhances protein synthesis by increased nitrogen retention.

Indications. For the treatment of growth failure in children caused by a pituitary growth hormone deficiency

Pharmacokinetics
Parenteral dosage (IM or SC)

Half-life. 20 to 30 minutes, but the effects of this product are longer acting

Metabolism. Liver

Excretion. Less than 1% (approximately 0.1% of a dose) by the kidneys.

Side effects/adverse reactions. Antibodies to somatrem have been reported in 30% to 40% of treated clients during the first 3 to 6 months of therapy, but only 5% of the clients develop neutralizing antibodies. It is rare that a client does not respond to therapy.

Pain and edema have been reported at the site of injection.

Excessive doses may produce **gigantism** in children, so before the drug is used, growth failure must be carefully documented and dosages and individual responses closely monitored.

Hypothyroidism has been rarely reported.

Significant drug interactions. When somatrem is given concurrently with adrenocorticoids, glucocorticoids, or corticotropin (ACTH), the growth response effects of somatrem may be impaired. ACTH should not be given concurrently and if it is necessary to treat with an adrenocorticoid agent, the daily dosages should be limited. For example, the total daily dose per square meter of body area should not be greater than cortisone (12.5–18.8 mg); hydrocortisone (10–15 mg); methylprednisolone (2 to 3 mg); prednisone or prednisolone (2.5 to 3.75 mg); betamethasone (300–450 mcg) and dexamethasone (375–563 μg)

Dosage and administration
somatrem for injection (Protropin)

Children. Administer 0.05 to 0.1 IU/kg intramuscularly every other day or three times weekly. (A minimum of 48 hours between doses is recommended.) Monitor growth rate response in 6 months to determine if dosage adjustment is necessary.

Pregnancy safety. Not established

NURSING CONSIDERATIONS

Assessment. Ascertain that the client does not have a malignancy, especially an intracranial tumor. Somatrem is also contraindicated in clients with closed epiphyses or those with a known sensitivity to benzyl alcohol such as neonates. Use with caution in clients with diabetes mellitus or untreated hypothyroidism.

Obtain baseline data by bone age determinations, thyroid function studies, and blood glucose determinations. Monitor these data periodically during therapy.

Intervention. Prepare the drug for parenteral use by diluting with 10 ml of the diluent provided by the manufacturer. Do not shake the vial; rotate it gently between the palms of the hands until the solution is clear. Use within 7 days following preparation. Store in the refrigerator.

Education. Advise the client of the importance of regular visits to the physician for the monitoring of blood and urine studies.

Evaluation. Increases in the growth pattern should occur.

Pain and swelling has occurred at the site of injection. After several months of therapy, antibodies to somatrem may be formed in some clients. These rarely reduce the response to therapy.

Monitor for signs of hypothyroidism, which has been reported in less than 5% of clients with hypopituitarism receiving somatrem therapy.

somatropin

A new growth hormone product—somatropin, recombinant DNA origin, for injection—was released in 1988. Because this product is identical to the amino acid sequence of human growth hormone, the development of antibodies and resistance is considerably less. The mechanism of action, indications and other properties of this product are similar to somatrem. The recommended dosage is up to 0.06 mg/kg (0.16 IU/kg) three times weekly.

POSTERIOR PITUITARY HORMONES

The two hormones from the posterior lobe of the pituitary gland are oxytocin and vasopressin (ADH, or antidiuretic hormone). Oxytocin will be discussed in Chapter 53; only vasopressin is discussed in this chapter.

vasopressin (Pitressin)

Mechanism of action. Antidiuretic hormone effect includes increasing water reabsorption in the collecting ducts of the nephron, resulting in a decreased urine volume with a higher osmolarity. Vasopressin stimulates peristalsis through a direct effect on gastrointestinal motility. Thus it has been used for abdominal distention due to bowel gas. It also increases secretion of corticotropin, growth hormone, and follicle-stimulating hormone. At larger doses, it causes vasoconstriction.

Indications. Vasopressin is used to treat insufficient antidiuretic hormone release centrally, in other words, to treat the symptoms of **diabetes insipidus** resulting from true deficiency of ADH. It is not effective for polyuria induced by renal impairment, nephrogenic diabetes insipidus, psychogenic diabetes insipidus, or drug-induced (lithium or demeclocycline) diabetes insipidus.

Vasopressin is also used to treat abdominal distention or gas, especially before abdominal x-rays or postoperatively.

Pharmacokinetics

Absorption. Intramuscular absorption may be erratic; intranasal absorption is poor. While usually given subcutaneously, it may be administered intravenously or intra-arterially. The vasopressin tannate oil suspension dosage form should only be administered intramuscularly.

Half-life. 10 to 20 minutes

Duration of action. Vasopressin aqueous—2 to 8 hours; vasopressin tannate in oil—between 1 and 3 days

Metabolism. Liver and kidneys

Excretion. Kidneys

Side effects/adverse reactions. See Table 47-1.

Significant drug interactions. None reported

Dosage and administration

vasopressin injection, aqueous (Pitressin)

Adults. 5 to 10 units intramuscularly or subcutaneously two or three times a day when needed to treat central diabetes insipidus. For abdominal gas and distention: 5 units intramuscularly initially. If necessary, the next dose may be increased to 10 units. The dose may be repeated every 3 to 4 hours as necessary. Prior to abdominal roentgenography (x-rays): 10 units intramuscularly or subcutaneously approximately 2 ½ hours before the planned x-rays.

Children. Treatment of central diabetes insipidus: 2.5 to 10 units intramuscularly or subcutaneously, three or four times daily. Use as a peristaltic stimulant must be individualized by the prescribing physician.

sterile vasopressin tannate oil suspension (Pitressin)

Adults. 1.5 to 5 units intramuscularly every 1 to 3 days for central diabetes insipidus

TABLE 47-1 Side Effects/Adverse Reactions of Vasopressin (Pitressin)

Drug	Side effects*	Adverse reactions†
vasopressin (Pitressin)	Most frequent: pain at injection site (usually with tannate dosage form) Less frequent: stomach gas and pain, diarrhea, dizziness, increased pressure for bowel evacuation, nausea, vomiting, tremors, sweating, pallor.	Rare: chest pain due to angina or myocardial infarction, increased or continuing headaches, confusion, coma, convulsions, weight gain, drowsiness, urinary difficulties (usually due to water retention or intoxication, occurs more with tannate dosage form). Allergic type reactions include elevated temperature; rash; pruritus; hives; edema of face, hands, feet or mouth; wheezing or respiratory difficulties

*If side effects continue, increase, or disturb the patient, inform the physician.
†If adverse reactions occur, contact physician as medical intervention may be necessary.

Children. 1.25 to 2.5 units, every 1 to 3 days for central diabetes insipidus

Pregnancy safety. Not established

NURSING CONSIDERATIONS

Assessment. Use with caution in clients with angina, myocardial infarction, inadequate coronary circulation, and hypertension.

Use with caution in elderly clients because of the risk of water intoxication and hyponatremia. Avoid use if at all possible in clients with chronic nephritis with nitrogen retention.

Obtain a baseline ECG.

Intervention. Note that the spontaneous disappearance of side effects such as skin blanching, abdominal cramps, and nausea may be hastened by concomitant administration of 1 or 2 glasses of water.

Be aware that vasopressin tannate cannot be given intravenously. Prolonged rotation and shaking of the ampule is necessary so that all of the particles are included in the suspension. Failure to shake the ampule thoroughly can result in inaccurate dosage and inadequate therapeutic response. Tannate injection is indicated only for treatment of diabetes insipidus.

To allow for a precise intravenous or intra-arterial flow rate, administer the vasopressin aqueous injection by an infusion pump. Avoid extravasation for tissue necrosis and gangrene may result.

If the drug is administered to relieve the client's abdominal distention due to flatus, use a rectal tube following the injection to enhance the action of the drug.

Education. Warn the client that the side effects of paleness, nausea, abdominal or stomach cramps, or vomiting may occur. Drinking one or two glasses of H_2O at the time of drug administration may help reduce the occurrence of the side effects. If they do occur, they are not serious and generally will disappear within minutes.

Evaluation. Obtain fluid and electrolyte determinations periodically during therapy. Monitor the specific gravity of the client's urine as well as the intake and output and daily weights to evaluate the drug's effectiveness. Monitor blood pressure; hypertension may occur, or in the case of nonresponse to the drug, hypotension.

Be alert for early signs of water toxicity, and withdraw drug and restrict fluid intake until specific gravity of urine is at least 1.015 and polyuria occurs.

Assess whether the client has obtained relief from abdominal distention, e.g. the passage of flatus and stool, as a result of the drug.

There should be a diminished urinary output.

KEY TERMS

BIBLIOGRAPHY

American Hospital Formulary Service Drug Information '88: Betheseda, Maryland: American Society of Hospital Pharmacists, Inc, 1988.

Black, PM: Diagnosis: pituitary tumor, Hosp Med 21(10):43, 1985.

Cohen, KL: Pituitary function tests: simple ways to evaluate possibly complex conditions, Consultant 24(12):41, 1984.

Fode, NC, and others: Pituitary tumors and hypertension: implications for neurosurgical nurses, J Neurosurg Nurs 15(1):33, 1983.

Fuller, E: Growing up . . . and up . . . with hGH . . . use of biosynthetic human growth hormone, Patient Care 18(16):18, 1984.

Hall, MB: New heights for growth hormone-deficient children, Nurse Pract 7(10):26, 1982.

Huff, BB (managing editor): Physicians' Desk Reference, ed 42, Oradell, Medical Economics Company, Inc, 1988.

Kastrup, EK (editor): Facts and Comparisons, St. Louis, JB Lippincott Co, 1988.

Katzung, BG: Basic and Clinical Pharmacology, ed 3, Norwalk, Connecticut, Appleton & Lange, 1987.

Nachtigall, LE: Sheehan's syndrome, Hosp Med 19(10):120, 1983.

Stachura, ME. Human growth hormone: use and potential abuse, Hosp Formul 22(1):48, 1987.

U.S. Pharmacopeia Convention Drug Information for the Health Care Provider, ed 8, Rockville, Maryland: US Pharmacopeia Convention, Inc, 1988.

Verbalis, JG, and others: Hypopituitarism, Top Emerg Med 5(4):74, 1984.

Volner, JS: Endocrine dysfunction associated with pituitary adenomas and pituitary surgery, J Neurosurg Nurs 15(6):325, 1983.

48

Drugs Affecting the Parathyroid and Thyroid

OBJECTIVES

After studying this chapter, the student will be able to:

1. Describe the clinical complications associated with hypothyroidism, hyperthyroidism, and hyperparathyroidism.

2. Describe the dose and action of calcium and vitamin D_2 products in the treatment of hypoparathyroidism.

3. Describe the primary therapy and the agents available to treat hypothyroidism.

4. Name two diagnostic agents used to assess thyroid function.

5. Describe the actions of iodine (iodide ion), radioactive iodine, and thioamide drugs in treating hyperthyroidism.

6. Apply nursing considerations to the client receiving drugs affecting the parathyroid or thyroid gland.

A number of medications are available to treat the various conditions of the thyroid and parathyroid glands.

PARATHYROID

With hypoparathyroidism (idiopathic), serum calcium levels are decreased while serum phosphate levels are increased. Usually vitamin D levels are low. The administration of vitamin D (25,000 units or more, three times weekly) and calcium supplements usually will restore the calcium and phosphorus levels to normal. Calcitriol (Rocaltrol) is an active metabolite form of vitamin D that is also used to elevate serum calcium levels. See Table 48-1 for drugs used to treat hypoparathyroidism.

Primary hyperparathyroidism causes excessive serum and urinary levels of calcium. While the urine phosphate is high, the serum level is low to normal. This can lead to renal stones, bone pain with skeletal lesions, and possibly pathologic fractures. Since **adenomas** or tumors may be causing this syndrome, usually surgery is the primary treatment. In clients with mild hypercalcemia or mild hyperparathyroidism, a thorough examination by a physician would determine whether or not surgery was indicated. High serum levels of calcium may require immediate treatment. See Table 48-2 for typical recommendations for treatment of hypercalcemia.

TABLE 48-1   Drugs Used to Treat Hypoparathyroidism

Drug(s)	Purpose/dose
PTH (oral)	Not available Severe hypocalcemia—calcium gluconate 10%, intravenously until symptoms of tetany are relieved or serum calcium levels are above 7.5 mg/dl. Start oral calcium supplements as soon as possible. Mild to moderate hypocalcemia—restrict phosphate absorption with aluminum hydroxide–binding preparations. A 1-to-2 oral intake of calcium (elemental) is usually sufficient. If calcium serum level is below 7.5 mg/dl, then administer vitamin D to maintain an adequate serum calcium level. See box for comparisons for calcium preparations.
vitamin D_2 (ergo-calciferol)	Inactive. It requires activation by liver 25-hydroxylation and by kidneys 1-alpha hydroxylase. Also need bile salts for improved absorption in the gut. Usual dose is 50 to 100,000 units daily. This is least expensive formulation, but its onset of action is slow (2 weeks or more) and duration of action is long (16-18 weeks after it is discontinued).
dihydrotachysterol (DHT) (Hytaker-ol) capsules	Needs only liver 25-hydroxylation to activate. While more expensive than vitamin D_2, it has a rapid onset of action (within 2 hours) duration is 7 to 15 days. Dose is 0.2-2.5 mg/day (average dose is 0.5 mg). May be preferred for postoperative hypocalcemic tetany.
calcitriol (Rocaltrol)	Active drug. Rapid onset, 1 to 3 days duration. More expensive. Dose 0.25 μg initially (range 0.5 to 1 μg), increased in 2- to 4-week periods.
calcediol (Calderol)	Active drug. Has a metabolite with a long half-life of 16 days. Onset of action is faster than vitamin D_2 but slower than DHT. Dose is 50 to 100 μg/day.

TABLE 48-2   Recommendations for Treatment of Hypercalcemia

Method	Special comments
INHIBITION OF BONE RESORPTION	
mithramycin	Lowers serum calcium within 1 to 2 days after single dose of 25 to 50 μg/kg injection. Maximum effect seen within 2 to 5 days. This is a toxic drug that is usually reserved for use when other therapies have been unsuccessful.
calcitonin	Usual dosages of 4 MRC units/kg may induce serum calcium decreases of 1 to 2 mg/dl. Produces maximum effect in 6 to 9 hours. Used to treat Paget's disease.
INCREASE IN CALCIUM EXCRETION	
hydration	Hydrate client with normal saline. This can reduce serum calcium by 2 to 3 mg/dl. Monitor for fluid overload and electrolyte disturbances. (Not therapy of choice for client with heart failure or compromised cardiac function.)
furosemide diuretic	Used with administration of large quantities of normal saline hydration, usual dose is 100 mg every 2 hours. Monitor electrolytes closely because replacement electrolytes may be necessary.
DECREASE CALCIUM ABSORPTION	
oral phosphates	250 mg every 6 hours orally if phosphorous level is low. Correcting hypophosphatemia usually lowers calcium serum levels. May cause diarrhea and compromise renal function. Monitor closely.
OTHER MECHANISMS	
glucocorticoids, such as prednisone or hydrocortisone.	They decrease calcium absorption, increase calcium excretion, and inhibit the effects of vitamin D.

THYROID
THYROID PREPARATIONS

thyroid tablets (various manufacturers)
levothyroxine sodium tablets (Synthroid, L-thyroxine, Levothroid, Eltroxin✲)
liothyronine sodium tablets (Cytomel)
liotrix tablets (Euthroid, Thyrolar)
thyroglobulin tablets (Proloid)

Practitioners have agreed that individuals with hypothyroidism need thyroid replacement therapy. However, there is disagreement about which preparation is best for substitution therapy. For many years, natural or **desiccated** thyroid has served admirably for replacement therapy, and it is still considered to be satisfactory for many clients. A major problem with desiccated thyroid is that its potency varies among different brands of the preparation. The rate at which it loses its potency also varies. No requirement for metabolic potency exists, and prepara-

CALCIUM SUPPLEMENTS

The activity of calcium depends on calcium ion (elemental) content. The following calcium salts are listed by milli-grams per gram, milliequivalents per gram, and percent of calcium in the preparation.

CALCIUM PREPARATION	CALCIUM mg/g	CALCIUM mEq/g	PERCENT OF CALCIUM
calcium carbonate	400	20.0	40
calcium chloride	272	13.6	27.2
calcium citrate	211	10.5	21.1
calcium gluceptate	82	4.1	8.2
calcium gluconate	90	4.5	9
calcium lactate	130	6.5	13
calcium phosphate			
dibasic	230	11.5	23
tribasic	380	19	38

When low-percentage preparations are used, larger quantities of the drug are necessary to provide adequate calcium supplementation. For example, if the physician desired 1 g of elemental calcium from either calcium carbonate or calcium lactate preparations, it would require 2.5 g of calcium carbonate or nearly 7 g of calcium lactate to provide the calcium ordered. Other considerations would include client acceptance—that is, taste, tolerance, side effects, etc.

---

tions may not contain enough metabolically active substance to produce the desired therapeutic effect, even though the drug meets USP requirements. This has led to the present lack of popularity of natural thyroid products.

Thyroid USP is mainly derived from hog thyroid glands, although cattle and sheep thyroid glands have also been used. Thyroglobulin (Proloid) is an extract of hog thyroid gland, whereas levothyroxine sodium, liothyronine, and liotrix are synthetic thyroid replacement products. The question as to which preparation is superior has not yet been fully answered, but the synthetic preparations have a higher standardization in potency. See Table 48-3 for dose equivalents of selected thyroid products.

In the plasma, about 95% of the hormone is thyroxine, and the remainder is liothyronine. Approximately 99% of the hormones are protein bound (thyroxine-binding globulin, TBG) and may be expressed as iodide; thus the term *protein-bound iodide* (PBI). The normal PBI concentration is 4 to 8 μg/dl plasma. T_4 is bound more firmly than T_3; this permits a more rapid entry of T_3 into the cells.

The goal of treatment of clients with hypothyroidism or **myxedema** is to eliminate their symptoms (see box for clinical features of hyperthyroidism versus hypothyroidism) and to restore them to a normal emotional and physical state. Clinical response is more important than blood hormone level. However, laboratory assessments of T_3, T_4, serum cholesterol, and TSH levels are used as criteria for adequacy of therapy.

Mechanism of action. While not completely understood, thyroid hormones have both anabolic and catabolic effects; therefore they are involved in metabolism, growth, and development (especially development of the central nervous system in infants).

Thyroid hormone concentrations are regulated by the hypothalamic–anterior pituitary and thyroid body feedback mechanism.

Indications. Treatment of hypothyroidism; treatment and prevention of goiter; treatment and prevention of thyroid carcinoma; for thyroid function diagnostic tests

Pharmacokinetics

Absorption. Thyroid, thyroglobulin, and levothyroxine sodium: incomplete and variable; liothyronine: completely absorbed; liotrix is combination of levothyroxine and liothyronine, so absorption is between above values

Protein binding. Very high

TABLE 48-3   Dose Equivalents of Some Thyroid Products

Product	Dosage
thyroid, USP	60 mg
thyroglobulin	60 mg
levothyroxine	100 μg (0.1 mg) or less
liothyronine	25 μg (0.025 mg)
liotrix—levothyrtoxine (T_4) and liothyronine (T_3), 4:1 ratio	
T_4	50 to 60 μg
T_3	12.5 to 15 μg

CLINICAL FEATURES OF HYPERTHYROIDISM VERSUS HYPOTHYROIDISM

	HYPERTHYROIDISM	HYPOTHYROIDISM
Eyes	Prominent	Eyelids edematous, **ptosis**
Hair	Thin, fine texture	Dry, brittle, thin
Temperature	Intolerance to heat	Intolerance to cold
Weight	Appetite increases, weight loss	Appetite decreases, weight gain
Emotional	Increased nervousness, irritability, insomnia	Lethargic, depressed, increase in sleeping needs
Gastrointestinal	Diarrhea	Constipation
Neuromuscular	Fast deep-tendon reflexes	Slow or delayed deep-tendon reflexes
Extremities	Hot, moist skin	Cold, dry skin

Time to peak effect. Thyroid, thyroglobulin, levothyroxine: 3 to 4 weeks; liothyronine: 1 to 3 days

Duration of effect after withdrawal of long-term therapy. Thyroid, thyroglobulin, levothyroxine: 1 to 3 weeks; liothyronine: up to 3 days

Metabolism. Same as endogenous thyroid hormone—some in peripheral tissues, smaller amounts metabolized in liver, excreted in bile

Side effects/adverse reactions. See Table 48-4.

Significant drug interactions. When thyroid hormone preparations are given concurrently with the following drugs, the interactions listed may occur.

Drug	Possible Effect and Management
anticoagulants, oral (coumarin or indandione)	May alter the therapeutic effects of the oral anticoagulant. An increase in thyroid hormone may require a decrease in anticoagulant oral dosage. Monitor coagulation time closely, utilizing the prothrombin time (PT) test.
sympathomimetics	The effects of one or both medications may be increased. May result in an increased risk of coronary insufficiency if individual has coronary artery disease, or, if a thyroid preparation is given with tricyclic antidepressants, an increase in cardiac arrhythmias may result. Monitor closely, since dosage adjustments may be necessary.
cholestyramine or colestipol	May bind thyroid hormones, delaying or decreasing their absorption from the gastrointestinal tract. A 4- to 5-hour interval is recommended between administration of these drugs.

Dosage and administration
levothyroxine sodium tablets

Adults

Mild hypothyroidism: orally, 50 μg (0.05 mg) daily; may increase at 3- to 4-week intervals with increments of 25 to 50 μg (0.025 to 0.05 mg) as necessary

Severe hypothyroidism: orally, 12.5 to 25 μg (0.0125 to 0.025 mg) daily; may increase at 3- to 4-week intervals with increments of 25 μg (0.025 mg) as necessary

Maintenance: 75 to 125 μg (0.075 to 0.125 mg) orally daily or 1.5 μg/kg daily, as a single dose

Elderly: The initial dose is usually 12.5 to 25 μg (0.125 to 0.025 mg) daily. Maintenance dosage is usually 75 μg (0.075 mg) daily.

Maximum adult daily dosage: usually 150 μg (0.15 mg) per day. If client fails to respond to this dosage, it probably indicates the physician should review the findings and consider ordering additional tests to confirm the diagnosis.

Children

Less than 6 months: 5 to 6 μg/kg orally or 25 to 50 μg daily

6 to 12 months: 5 to 6 μg/kg orally or 50 to 75 μg daily

1 to 5 years old: 3 to 5 μg/kg orally or 75 to 100 μg daily

6 to 12 years old: 4 to 5 μg/kg or 100 to 150 μg daily

Over 12 years old: 1 to 3 μg/kg orally until adult dosage is reached (usually 150 μg to 200 μg per day)

Premature infants (weighing less than 2000 g or at risk for heart failure): 25 μg (0.025 mg) initial dose that may be increased if necessary, to 50 μg (0.05 mg) daily in 4 to 6 weeks

TABLE 48-4   Thyroid Preparations: Side Effects/Adverse Reactions

Side effects*	Adverse reactions†
Side effects are dose related and individualized by patient response. They may occur more rapidly with liothyronine than with the other products because it has a faster onset of action.	
The following are generally signs of under-dosage (hypothyroidism): dysmenorrhea, ataxia, coldness, dry skin, constipation, lethargy, headaches, drowsiness, tiredness, weight gain, muscle aching.	Rare: severe headaches, allergic skin rash Hyperthyroidism or overdosage: alterations in appetite and menstrual periods, elevated temperature, diarrhea, hand tremors, increased irritability, leg cramps, increased nervousness, tachycardia, irregular heart rate, increased sensitivity to heat, chest pain, respiratory difficulties, increased sweating, vomiting, weight loss, drowsiness

*If side effects continue, increase, or disturb the patient, inform the physician.
†If adverse reactions occur, contact physician since medical intervention may be necessary.

levothyroxine sodium for injection

Adults

Hypothyroidism: 50 to 100 μg (0.05 to 0.1 mg) IM or IV daily.

Myxedema stupor or comatose: 200 to 500 μg (0.2 to 0.5 mg) initially intravenously, even in the geriatric patient. If improvement is not noted by second day, an additional 100 to 200 μg (0.1 to 0.3 mg) may be given. Continuous daily administration would depend on client's response and tolerance for the medication. Switch to oral dosage form as soon as possible. Clients with cardiovascular disease may require smaller dosages.

Children. Approximately 75% of the usual oral pediatric dose, IV or IM.

liothyronine sodium tablets

Adults

Mild hypothyroidism: orally, 25 μg (0.025 mg) daily; may increase in increments of 12.5 to 25 μg (0.0125 or 0.025 mg) daily every 1 to 2 weeks, if necessary

Myxedema: orally, 2.5 to 5 μg (0.0025 to 0.005 mg) daily; may increase in 5- to 10-μg increments every 1 to 2 weeks. After 25 μg daily is reached, increments may be increased by 12.5 to 25 μg (0.0125 to 0.025 mg) every 1 to 2 weeks as tolerated.

Simple goiter (nontoxic): initially, 5 μg (0.005 mg) orally daily; may increase every 1 to 2 weeks by 5- to 10-μg increments if necessary. When 25 μg per day is reached, increments may follow the previous schedule.

Elderly and clients with cardiovascular disease: initial dose is 5 μg (0.005 mg); increment increases are 5 μg every 2 weeks if necessary.

Children. Cretinism: not recommended

liotrix tablets

Adults

Hypothyroidism without myxedema: initially, 50 μg (0.05 mg) orally of levothyroxine and 12.5 μg (0.0125 mg) of liothyronine or 60 μg (0.06 mg) of leothyroxine and 15 μg (0.015 mg) of liothyronine daily. Increases may be instituted monthly in like amounts, until the desired response is achieved.

Myxedema or hypothyroidism with cardiovascular disease: 12.5 (0.0125 mg) of levothyroxine and 3.1 μg (0.0031 mg) of liothyronine daily orally. Increases may be instituted at 2- to 3-week intervals in like amounts, until the desired response is achieved.

Maintenance: 50 to 100 μg (0.05 to 0.1 mg) of levothyroxine and 12.5 to 25 μg (0.0125 to 0.025 mg) of liothyronine orally daily

Elderly: initial dosage is 25% to 50% of the usual adult dosage. It may be doubled at 6- to 8-week intervals until the desired response is achieved.

Children

Cretinism or severe hypothyroidism: see usual adult dose for myxedema

Hypothyroidism: use adult dosage for hypothyroidism with myxedema

Increment increases in children should be instituted at 2-week intervals. Base dosage on the results of thyroid function tests.

thyroglobulin tablets

Adults

Hypothyroidism without myxedema: 32 mg orally daily; may be increased at 1- to 2-week intervals if necessary

Maintenance: 65 to 160 mg orally daily

Myxedema or hypothyroidism with cardiovascular disease: 16 to 32 mg orally daily; may increase in like amounts every 2 weeks, if necessary

Maintenance: 65 to 160 mg orally daily

Children

Cretinism or severe hypothyroidism: see adult dosage for myxedema

Hypothyroidism: see adult dosage for hypothyroidism without myxedema

Always base dosages on results of the thyroid function testing.

thyroid tablets

Adults

Hypothyroidism without myxedema: initially, 60 mg orally daily; may increase at 60-mg increments monthly if necessary

Maintenance: 60 to 120 mg orally daily

Myxedema or hypothyroidism with cardiovascular disease: Initially, 15 mg orally daily; may be increased to 30 mg after 2 weeks and 60 mg daily, after 2 more weeks. Assess the drug's effects closely; if necessary, increase dosage to 120 mg orally daily.

Maintenance: 60 to 120 mg orally daily

Elderly: 7.5 to 15 mg initially orally daily. If necessary, this dose may be doubled in 6 to 8 weeks.

Children

Cretinism or severe hypothyroidism: see adult dose for myxedema

Hypothyroidism: see adult dose for hypothyroidism without myxedema.

Always base dosage on results of thyroid function tests.

In congenital hypothyroidism, levothyroxine is usually considered the drug of choice.

Pregnancy safety. FDA category A.

NURSING CONSIDERATIONS

Assessment. Use with care in elderly clients, because they are more sensitive to the effects of thyroid hormones. A 25% reduction in the dose of the thyroid hormone replacement may be required for clients over 60 years of age.

Carefully consider use of thyroid hormonal therapy if the client has preexisting adrenocortical or pituitary insufficiency (thyroid hormonal replacement increases physiologic need for adrenocortical hormone), cardiovascular disease (too rapid thyroid hormonal replacement increases metabolic demand), history of hyperthyroidism, or thyrotoxicosis.

In cases of chronic hypothyroidism or myxedema, an increased sensitivity may exist. Start the client on the lowest possible dosage, with increases in the dosage titrated in accordance with the client's clinical response and laboratory data.

Intervention. Since hypothyroid clients respond rapidly to replacement doses, therapy is begun with a small dose and gradually increased over several weeks until the optimal clinical response is obtained. Once the maintenance dose has been established, it is taken or given daily, preferably before breakfast.

It is recommended that levothyroxine be taken on an empty stomach. In its parenteral form, levothyroxine sodium is reconstituted with 5 ml of sodium chloride injection (without preservative) to a solution of 100 μg (0.1 mg)/ml. It should be reconstituted immediately before use.

Education. Lifelong therapy is a possibility with thyroid hormonal replacement. Counsel the client accordingly. This means regular consultations with the physician to monitor effectiveness of the therapy as well as compliance with the prescribed regimen. To simulate the natural process of the body, the client should take the dosage at the same time every day. Morning administration will help to prevent insomnia.

Inform the client that if a dose is missed, it is to be taken as soon as possible. If it is close to the next day's dose, caution the client not to take the dose, since this will have the effect of doubling doses. Contact the physician if two or more consecutive doses are missed.

Tell the client to alert other health care providers as to the thyroid hormonal replacement—particularly if any kind of surgery is required, including dental surgery. A medical identification should be worn.

Advise the client to consult with the physician before taking other medications concurrently with thyroid replacement.

Advise the client to inform the physician if the pulse rate increases or if palpitations or chest pain occur. Irritability, nervousness, heat intolerance, and excessive sweating may indicate a need for a reduction in dosage; however, insomnia is usually the earliest sign. If such symptoms occur, withdrawal of the drug may be indicated for a few days before it is resumed at a lower dose.

Alert parents of a pediatric client that partial hair loss sometimes occurs during the first few months of therapy with children, but it is temporary and the hair will usually return, even if hormonal replacement is continued.

Advise the client not to change brands of thyroid replacement therapy, since different brands of the drug are not bioequivalent.

Evaluation. Assess the client for a decrease in the symptoms of hypothyroidism: weight loss, loss of constipation, and increased activity levels, appetite, sense of well-being, and pulse rate should be seen. Laboratory reports should indicate normal T_3 and T_4 levels.

Monitor thyroid function studies before and throughout therapy. Such studies may include free T_4 index determinations, TSH determinations, T_3 or T_4 resin uptake determinations, and total serum T_3 and T_4 determinations. Assess pediatric clients periodically for growth, bone age, and psychomotor development.

Monitor baseline apical pulse and blood pressure before and periodically during therapy. If the resting pulse is over 100, hold the dose and notify the physician. For clients with preexisting cardiovascular disease, observe closely for ischemia and tachyarrhythmias.

DIAGNOSTIC TESTING FOR HYPOTHYROIDISM

Protirelin (Thypinone, Relefact TRH) and thyrotropin (thyroid-stimulating hormone, TSH) are diagnostic agents used to assess thyroid function. See Table 48-5 for a comparison of the tests. The thyroid-stimulating hormone (TSH) test is a very sensitive test used to diagnose hypothyroidism. The thyroid-releasing hormone (TRH) test measures the pituitary's response to TRH. For example, in hypothalamic hypothyroidism, the pituitary responds slowly to exogenous TRH and produces a slow but rising TSH. In clients with primary hypothyroidism, TSH basal levels are increased, and the pituitary is hyperreactive to TRH stimulation. If the client has hypothyroidism resulting from hypopituitarism, no response to TRH is expected. Therefore the TRH test can differentiate a primary from a secondary hypothyroidism and also differentiate hypopituitary from hypothalamic hypothryroidism. (See box for physiology of thyroid gland and its hormones.)

ANTITHYROID AGENTS

An antithyroid drug is a chemical agent that lowers the basal metabolic rate by interfering with the formation, release, or action of the hormones made by the thyroid gland. Those that interfere with the synthesis of the thyroid hormones are known as **goitrogens.** A variety of compounds are included in this category of antithyroid drugs, but only iodine (iodide ion), radioactive iodine, and thioamide derivatives are discussed here.

Iodine, Iodides

Iodine is the oldest of the antithyroid drugs. Although a small amount of iodine is necessary for normal thyroid function and to synthesize thyroid hormones, the response of the client with **thyrotoxicosis** is prompt inhibition of thyroid release from the hyperfunctioning thyroid gland.

Thyroid-iodide pump

Iodide enters the body from the diet and is rapidly absorbed into the bloodstream. Approximately one third of it is removed from the blood by the iodide pump in the thyroid. The initial iodide removed from the blood is usually sodium or potassium iodide. The enzyme **perioxidase** converts the iodides to iodine, which is then used to form **monoiodotyrosine (MIT)** and **diiodotyrosine**

(**DIT),** which are the components of T_3 and T_4. The synthesized hormones (T_3, T_4) are stored within **thyroglobulin** until they are released into the blood circulation. These activities involve a complex negative feedback mechanism between the thyroid gland and the hypothalmus-pituitary gland. Low levels of circulating thyroid hormone increase the release of thyroid-stimulating hormone (TSH) from the pituitary and appear to influence the secretion of thyrotropin-releasing factor (TRF) from the hypothalamus. Increased levels of TSH increase iodide trapping by the gland, which results in an increase in synthesis and circulating thyroid hormones. As thyroid hormone levels increase, the hypothalmic and pituitary centers stop the release of TRF and TSH. This process will be repeated if the thyroid hormone levels decrease again, in response to the declining levels of circulating thyroid hormones. (See box below.)

Although iodides are used to synthesize thyroid hormones, an excess of iodides, as previously used to treat hyperthyroidism since the 1940s, will block thyroid hormone synthesis and release and will also decrease the vascularity of the thyroid gland. Although the mechanism of effect is unknown, the inhibition of thyroid hormone release for several weeks will lead to an increase in TSH secretion that can overcome this blockade. Thus, large

---

TABLE 48-5 Diagnostic Testing for Hypothyroidism

Origin of deficiency	Level of TSH	TSH levels following TRH testing
Thyroid gland	Increased	Very increased
Pituitary gland	Decreased	No response
Hypothalamus	Increase	Slow response
Hyperthyroid	Decreased	No response

PHYSIOLOGY OF INFLUENCES ON THE THYROID GLAND: A FEEDBACK MECHANISM

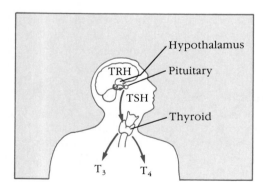

When serum levels of T_3 and T_4 are increased, the release of TRH from the hypothalamus and TSH from the anterior pituitary gland is reduced, thus inhibiting their effects on the thyroid gland.

When serum levels of T_3 and T_4 are decreased, TRH release triggers the release of TSH from the pituitary. TSH effects on the thyroid are an increase in the size and number of follicular cells in the thyroid, thus increasing their ability to absorb iodide, and an increase in thyroglobulin breakdown, which releases T_3 and T_4 hormones from the thyroid gland into the bloodstream, thus increasing blood levels of the thyroid hormones.

doses of iodides are generally used for 7 to 14 days before thyroid surgery in order to decrease the thyroid's size and vascularity, resulting in diminished blood loss and a less complicated surgical procedure.

Radioactive iodine (RAI) is preferred for clients who are poor surgical risks, such as debilitated clients, those with advanced cardiac disease, and elderly clients. It is also used for clients who have not responded adequately to drug therapy or who have had recurrent hyperthyroidism after surgery. The primary disadvantage of using surgery or RAI therapy, in addition to the risk involved with surgery and postsurgical complications, is the induction of hypothyroidism.

Iodine Products

strong iodine solution (Lugol's solution)
sodium iodide
potassium iodide

Mechanism of action. See above.
Indications

To protect the thyroid gland from radiation before and after the administration of radioactive isotopes of iodine or in radiation emergencies

May be used with an antithyroid drug in clients with hyperthyroidism in preparation for thyroidectomy

Pharmacokinetics. Effects noted within 24 to 48 hours; maximum effects achieved within 10 to 14 days of continuous therapy

Side effects/adverse reactions. See Table 48-6.
Significant drug interactions. When iodide products are given concurrently with the following drugs, the interactions listed may occur.

Drug	Possible Effect and Management
antithyroid drugs	May increase the hypothyroid and goitrogenic effects of the drugs. Monitor closely.
diuretics, potassium-conserving type	If these diuretics are used concurrently with potassium iodide, increased levels of potassium may result in hyperkalemia, cardiac arrhythmias, or cardiac arrest. Monitor serum potassium levels closely.
lithium	The hypothyroid and goitrogenic effects of both drugs may be potentiated. Obtain and monitor baseline thyroid status periodically to plan appropriate interventions.

TABLE 48-6   Antithyroid Agents: Significant Side Effects and Adverse Reactions

Drug(s)	Side effects*	Adverse reactions†
iodine or iodide products	Diarrhea, nausea, vomiting, abdominal pain	Most frequent: skin rash, swelling or tenderness of the salivary gland Rare: bloody or black colored stools (due to GI bleeding), irregular heart rate, paresthesias of hands or feet, increased tiredness, leg weakness, confusion (due to potassium toxicity), increased temperature (hypersensitivity), edema of neck or throat With prolonged usage: severe headaches, sore gums or teeth, increased salivation, burning in mouth or throat, metallic taste in mouth
sodium iodide I 131 (Iodotope)	Less frequent: sore throat, neck swelling or pain, loss of taste (temporary), nausea, vomiting, painful salivary glands	After treatment for hyperthyroidism: increased or unusual irritability or tiredness After treatment of thyroid carcinoma: fever, sore throat, and chills (due to leukopenia), increased bleeding episodes (due to thrombocytopenia) Signs of hypothyroidism may follow treatment, including changes in menstrual cycle, increased clumsiness, cold feelings, sedation, dry, puffy skin, headaches, muscle aching, temporary dryness or thinning of hair, increased weakness, and unusual weight gain.
thioamide derivatives: methimazole tablets, propylthiouracil tablets	Most frequent (3% to 5%): rash or pruritus Less frequent: dizziness, loss of taste, nausea, vomiting, paresthesias, abdominal pain	Less frequent: elevated temperature, chills or sore throat, overall feeling of discomfort or weakness (may be agranulocytosis, leukopenia, or lupus-like syndrome), jaundice of skin and eyes (due to cholestatic hepatitis) Rare: edema of feet or lower legs, backache, unusual increases or decreases in urination (nephritis), joint pain, swollen lymph nodes, increased bleeding tendencies or bruising Signs of overdosage or hypothyroidism: see above Signs of thyrotoxicosis or subtherapeutic therapy: fever, diarrhea, increased irritability, weakness, tachycardia, vomiting

*If side effects continue, increase, or disturb the patient, inform the physician.
†If adverse reactions occur, contact physician since medical intervention may be necessary.

Dosage and administration

strong iodine solution (not listed in USP-DI). Adult oral dosage recommended (Kastrup, 1988) for individuals with hyperthyroidism, pre-surgery: give 2 to 6 drops of strong iodine solution, three times daily for 10 days before surgery. Be certain to dilute this preparation with water or fruit juices to improve taste and client acceptance.

sodium iodide injection (not listed in USP-DI). 10% in 10-ml ampules (Kastrup, 1988); adjunct therapy in managing a thyroid crisis, give 2 g intravenously daily

potassium iodide syrup (Pima), tablets (Iosat, Thyro-Block), oral solution, and enteric-coated tablets. Also referred to as SSKI and KI. The USP-DI does not recommend the use of enteric-coated potassium iodide tablets because of their association with small-bowel lesions. Oral solution/syrup/tablet dosage:

Adults

To protect the thyroid gland from radiation: 100 to 150 mg orally for 24 hours before, and for 3 to 10 days after, exposure to radioactive iodine isotopes

Pre-thyroidectomy: 5 drops of 1 g/ml solution (approximately 250 mg) three times daily for 10 days prior to surgery. This is usually given with an antithyroid drug.

Maximum dosage: up to 12 g daily

Children

To protect the thyroid gland from radiation: infants up to 12 months old—65 mg orally daily for 10 days, after exposure to radioactive iodine isotopes; children 1 year and older—130 mg orally daily for 10 days, after exposure to radioactive iodine isotopes

Pre-thyroidectomy: see adult dosage

Pregnancy safety. FDA category C

NURSING CONSIDERATIONS

Assessment. Thyroid function studies should be monitored before and periodically during therapy.

Be aware that iodine products are contraindicated in hyperkalemic states and in clients receiving lithium therapy, since lithium has synergistic hyperthyroid activity, resulting in hypothyroidism. Checking serum potassium levels is advisable before administering iodine products.

Note that pulmonary edema and pulmonary tuberculosis are contraindications to the use of iodines.

Be aware that iodine therapy during pregnancy can cause abnormal thyroid function or goiter in the newborn.

Iodine products are contraindicated in clients sensitive to them. Initial assessment should determine if the client is allergic to seafood, since this may be indicative of a cross-sensitivity to iodine. The earliest symptoms of the hypersensitivity are irritation and swelling of the eyelids.

Intervention. Dilute Lugol's solution and saturated solutions of sodium or potassium in one-third to one-half glass of fruit juice, carbonated beverage, or another substance to improve taste. Administer after meals to minimize gastric irritation.

Dilute the liquid dose of SSKI with fruit juice, water, or milk. Since the medication evaporates rapidly, do not leave open to air for long periods before administration.

Administer iodides through a straw to prevent discoloration of the teeth.

Education. Instruct the client to discontinue use and notify the physician if any of the following occur: fever, skin rash, metallic brassy taste, swelling of the neck and throat, burning soreness of gums and teeth, head cold symptoms, or severe gastrointestinal distress. These symptoms are characteristic of chronic iodide poisoning.

Instruct the client to consult with the physician regarding the use of iodized salt and seafood in the diet. Iodine-rich foods, such as soybeans, cabbage, kale, and other green leafy vegetables may need to be restricted.

Caution the client to maintain the prescribed dosage. Missing doses may precipitate a thyroid storm. Instruct the client to consult with the prescriber before taking over-the-counter cold remedies, because some contain iodides.

Evaluation. A decrease in the symptoms of hyperthyroidism should occur. For clients receiving the drug as part of a preoperative course of therapy, there should be a decrease in the size and vascularity of the thyroid.

radioactive iodine, sodium iodide I 131 (Iodotope)

Sodium iodide I 131 is a radioactive isotope of iodine.

Mechanism of action. Iodine accumulates and is retained in thyroid tissue. Radioiodine, if localized in large enough doses in the thyroid, will selectively damage or destroy thyroid tissue.

Indications

Treatment of hyperthyroidism

Treatment of thyroid carcinoma

Testing of thyroid function, diagnosis of suspected hyperthyroidism, and, perhaps, thyroid imaging (although today sodium iodide I 123 and sodium pertechnetate Tc 99m are preferred for thyroid imaging because they expose the client to lower radiation dosages)

Pharmacokinetics

Absorption. Good from gastrointestinal tract

Onset of therapeutic effect. Within 2 to 4 weeks

Time to peak therapeutic effect. Between 2 and 4 months

Time to peak diagnostic effect. 4 to 24 hours

Biologic half-life. 138 days

Excretion. Kidneys (65% to 90%) within 24 hours; feces and salivary excretion are secondary; up to 20% may appear in breast milk in 24 hours

Half-life. 8.06 days. Principal types of radiation are beta (90%) and gamma rays.

For diagnostic use. In a euthyroid patient, 10% to 25% of administered I 131 concentrates in the thyroid gland, with a half-life of 7.6 days. The balance (75% to 90%) is in the extracellular fluid, with a half-life of approximately 0.34 day.

For therapeutic use. In hyperthyroidism, 60% of I 131 concentrates in the thyroid gland, with a half-life of approximately 6 (ranges from 1 to 8) days. The balance (40%) is in the extracellular fluid, with a half-life of approximately 0.34 day.

Side effects/adverse reactions. See Table 48-6.

Significant drug interactions. Although other medications may reduce the thyroid uptake of I 131, this interaction was not noted to be highly significant by the USP-DI. Nevertheless, the nurse should be aware of the potential interferences present if the client is also taking adrenocorticoids, iodine-containing foods or drugs, salicylates, thyroid preparations, or thyroid-blocking agents, such as strong iodine solution or potassium iodide.

Dosage and administration

sodium iodide I 131 capsules

Adults

Diagnostic purposes, for thyroid uptake and imaging: 5 to 100 microcuries orally

Localization of thyroid metastases: 1 to 10 millicuries orally

To treat hyperthyroidism: 4 to 10 millicuries orally (Note that toxic nodular goiter and perhaps some other conditions may require a larger dose.)

Antineoplastic therapy: 100 to 150 millicuries orally to ablate normal thyroid tissue; follow up therapy is usually between 100 and 200 millicuries, orally

Children. Individualized by the physician

sodium iodide I 131 solution. See sodium iodide I 131 capsules.

Pregnancy safety. FDA category C

NURSING CONSIDERATIONS

Assessment. Thyroid function studies should be performed before and after therapy.

Do not give radioactive iodine to pregnant women or nursing mothers. In a patient with childbearing potential, therapy begins the first few days after the onset of menses.

Intervention. The client should take nothing by mouth after midnight before a morning dose, because food slows the absorption of the drug.

To avoid exposure to the radioactive products of the iodine, wear rubber gloves when giving I 131 to clients and when disposing of their excreta.

If the dose is administered for hyperthyroidism, institute full radiation precautions for 24 hours. If the dose is for cancer of the thyroid, isolate the client for 3 days. Pregnant women, be they personnel or visitors, should not have contact with the client. Use disposable utensils with the client. Increase the fluid intake of the client to 2500 ml/daily to enhance excretion of the isotope. Consult with nuclear medicine personnel as to limitations for individual staff contact with the client.

Education. Instruct the client in appropriate methods for disposal of urine and feces until radiation precautions are no longer needed.

If the client is discharged but radiation precautions are still necessary, ensure that the client receives specific instructions for visitor contact and disposal of utensils and excreta from the personnel in the nuclear medicine department.

Evaluation. Assess post-therapy thyroid function with serum thyroxine examinations.

Thioamide Derivatives (Antithyroid Agents)

methimazole (thiamazole) tablets (Tapazole)
propylthiouracil tablets (Propyl-Thyracil✦)

Mechanism of action. Both drugs inhibit the synthesis of thyroid hormone by inhibition of iodide into tyrosine and the coupling of iodotyrosines. They do not affect exogenous thyroid hormones. Propylthiouracil (not methimazole) also inhibits the conversion of thyroxine (T_4) to triiodothyronine (T_3), which may make it more effective for treatment of a thyroid crisis or storm.

Indications. Treatment of hyperthyroidism, prior to surgery or radiotherapy, or as adjunct therapy for treatment of thyrotoxicosis or thyroid storm (propylthiouracil preferred for latter indication)

Pharmacokinetics

Absorption. Very good (70% to 80%)

Half-life. Methimazole is variable (4 to 14 hours); propylthiouracil is 1 to 2 hours in normal individual and approximately 8.5 hours in anuric patient

Onset of action. Clinically with propylthiouracil: within 10 to 20 days

Time to peak effect. Propylthiouracil: within 2 to 10 weeks

Metabolism. Liver

Excretion. Kidneys

Side effects/adverse reactions. See Table 48-6.

Significant drug interactions. Administration of methimazole or propylthiouracil concurrently with iodinate glycerol, lithium, or potassium iodide may result in potentiation of hypothyroid and goitrogenic effects. Monitor closely.

Dosage and administration

methimazole tablets (Tapazole)

Adults. Hyperthyroidism:

Initially for mild cases: 15 mg orally daily, divided into three doses given at 8-hour intervals for 6 to 8 weeks or until the client is euthyroid

For moderate to severe cases: 30 to 40 mg orally daily, divided into three doses given at 8-hour intervals for 6 to 8 weeks or until the client is euthyroid

For severe hyperthyroidism: 60 mg orally daily divided into three doses, given at 8-hour intervals for 6 to 8 weeks or until the client is euthyroid

Maintenance: 5 to 30 mg orally in two or three divided doses daily

Thyrotoxic crisis: 15 to 20 mg orally, every 4 hours for 24 hours; use as adjunct to other therapies

Children. Hyperthyroidism:

Initially: 0.4 mg/kg orally daily, divided into three doses, at 8-hour intervals

Maintenance: 0.2 mg/kg orally daily, divided into three doses, at 8-hour intervals

propylthiouracil tablets (Propyl-Thyracil)

Adults. Hyperthyroidism:

Initially: 300 to 1200 mg orally daily, divided into three doses at 8-hour intervals (or four doses at 6-hour intervals), until the client is euthyroid (Clients with severe cases may need up to 2 g per day.)

ndx Selected Nursing Diagnoses for Clients Receiving Thyroid Drugs

Nursing diagnosis	Outcome criteria	Nursing interventions
Knowledge deficit related to thyroid dysfunction	Client will: Express understanding of normal thyroid function and the effects of altered thyroid function	Assess client's level of understanding. Determine educational needs of client and family. Instruct client in function of the thyroid gland and thyroid hormones. Instruct client in specific effects related to client's alteration in thyroid function. Provide opportunity for client to ask questions and verbalize concerns.
Knowledge deficit related to drug regimen (thyroid drug)	Client will: Understand the purpose of drug therapy and recognize side/adverse effects of the medication	Teach the client: Purpose and action of the drug Proper administration The need for continued therapy throughout lifetime, even after euthyroid state is obtained Signs and symptoms of hypothyroidism and hyperthyroidism Side effects/adverse reactions Provide the client with a list of drugs or conditions that interact with or alter the drug requirements. Explain the benefit of wearing or carrying a medical identification tag, bracelet, or card.
Alteration in body image related to thyroid dysfunction	Client and family will: Express concerns regarding body image changes Understand basis for body changes related to thyroid function and recognize the benefit of drug therapy	Assess the client and family for perceptions and concerns related to body image. Encourage open communication and talking about perceived body image. Encourage adequate rest periods. Adjust calorie intake and diet to changing client needs. Encourage a high-bulk diet, fluids, and exercise to prevent or limit constipation. Encourage good grooming and attractive dress to promote self-confidence and positive self-image. Administer thyroid drugs as prescribed.
Altered nutrition related to altered metabolic needs	Client will: Maintain a stable body weight Show evidence of maintaining a well-balanced diet	Assess normal dietary patterns. Instruct client to monitor his or her weight weekly. Instruct client to adjust diet to match caloric needs. Assist client in planning meals and dietary modifications.
Potential for impaired skin integrity related to altered thyroid function	Client will: Maintain intact skin Demonstrate proper skin care	Assess skin for dryness, itching, or altered integrity. Monitor client for development of skin disruption. Keep skin clean and well lubricated, Apply moisturizer as needed. Use skin massage and position changes. Instruct client in proper skin care.

Maintenance: 50 to 800 mg orally daily in two to four divided dosages

Thyrotoxic crisis: 200 to 400 mg orally every 4 hours for the first 24 hours, then decrease dosage as crisis subsides; this is used as adjunct to other therapies

Children

Initially, children 6 to 10 years old: 50 to 300 mg orally in two or three divided dosages

Children 10 years and older: 150 to 600 mg orally daily, divided into three doses at 8-hour intervals

Neonatal thyrotoxicosis: 10 mg/kg orally daily, in divided doses

Pregnancy safety. FDA category D

NURSING CONSIDERATIONS

Assessment. Monitor thyroid function studies prior to and periodically during therapy.

Concomitant thyroid administration during thioamide therapy in the hyperthyroid pregnant woman may avert hypothyroidism in the mother and fetus.

Intervention. Administer with meals to minimize gastric irritation.

Use the smallest effective dose (less than 300 mg daily) for pregnant clients. Propylthiouracil crosses the placental barrier; therefore large doses can cause goiter in the newborn or cretinism in the fetus.

Education. Instruct clients that if they develop sore throat, a head cold, skin eruptions, or malaise, they should report these symptoms immediately to their physicians, since these symptoms signal the onset of agranulocytosis. It may occur too quickly to be determined by periodic blood testing.

Instruct the client to consult with the prescriber as to the restriction of iodized salt and seafood. Caution against taking over-the-counter medications because many contain iodine preparations.

Advise breast-feeding mothers not to take this drug, since it is excreted in the milk.

Evaluation. Take a complete blood count periodically during therapy to detect blood dyscrasias such as agranulocytosis, leukopenia, or thrombocytopenia. Propylthiouracil may reduce thrombin and result in bleeding; monitor prothrombin time during therapy.

KEY TERMS

adenomas, page 768
desiccated, page 769
diiodotyrosine (DIT), page 774
goitrogens, page 774
monoiodotyrosine (MIT), page 774
myxedema, page 770
perioxidase, page 774

primary hyperparathyroidism, page 768
ptosis, page 771
thyroglobulin, page 774
thyrotoxicosis, page 774

BIBLIOGRAPHY

Balkin, MS: A guide to thyroid function tests, Emerg Med 15(3):116, 1983.

Blonde, L, and others: Answers to questions on hypothyroidism, Hosp Med 20(7):13, 1984.

Braunwald, E, and others, eds: Harrison's principles of internal medicine, ed 11, New York, 1987, McGraw-Hill Book Co.

Brown, SL: Practical points in the postanesthesia assessment and care of the patient having a thyroidectomy, J Post Anesth Nurs 1(3):191, 1986.

Bullock, BL, and Rosendahl, PP: Pathophysiology, ed 2, Glenview, Ill, 1988, Scott, Foresman & Co.

Coody, D: Congenital hypothyroidism: etiology, diagnosis, treatment and follow-up of infants, Pediatr. Nurs. 10(5):342, 1984.

DeRubertis, FR: Hypocalcemia: etiology and management, Hosp Med 21(3):88, 1985.

Dunn, JT: Treating hypothyroidism: what are our therapeutic choices? Hosp Formul 21(4):456, 1986.

Durie, M: The thyroid gland, Nursing '83 2(13):365, 1983.

Evanier, D: Look for these clues to thyrotoxicosis, Patient Care 17(7):143, 1983.

Evanier, D: Is your patient in thyroid storm? Patient Care 18(5):191, 1984.

Frost, GJ: Congenital hypothyroidism, Midwife Health Visit Community Nurse 21(10):358, 1985.

Herfindal, ET, and Hirschman, JL: Clinical pharmacy and therapeutics, ed 3, Baltimore, 1984, The Williams & Wilkins Co.

Huff, BB, ed: Physicians' Desk Reference, ed 42, Oradell, NJ, 1988, Medical Economics Co., Inc.

Kastrup, EK, ed: Facts and comparisons, St Louis, 1988, JB Lippincott Co.

Katcher, BS, and others: Applied therapeutics: the clinical use of drugs, ed 3, San Francisco, 1983, Applied Therapeutics, Inc.

Katzung, BG: Basic and clinical pharmacology, ed 3, Norwalk, Conn, 1987, Appleton & Lange.

Krupp, MA, and others, eds: Current medical diagnosis and treatment, Norwalk, Conn, 1987, Appleton & Lange.

Kupperman, HS: Hypothyroidism, Physician Assist 10(3):60, 1986.

Leebaw, WF, and others: Endocrine problems: effects of aging on normal and abnormal function, Consultant 24(7):165, 1984.

Levin, RM: Sick euthyroid syndrome, Hosp Pract 21(6):110C, 1986.

Mathewson, MK: Thyroid disorder, Crit Care Nurse 7(1):74, 1987.

Ray, RA, and others: RIA in thyroid function testing, Diag Med 7(5):55, 1984.

Simkins, ME: Diagnosis: hyperparathyroidism, Point View 20(4):16, 1983.

U.S. Pharmacopeial Convention: Drug information for the health care provider, ed 8, Rockville, Md, 1988, U.S. Pharmacopeial Convention, Inc.

CHAPTER
49

Drugs Affecting the Adrenal Cortex

OBJECTIVES

After studying this chapter, the student will be able to:

1. Compare and contrast glucocorticoids and mineralocorticoids.

2. Describe the major pharmacological effects of the corticosteroids.

3. Describe five significant drug interactions (including management) of the glucocorticoids.

4. Describe the advantages for an alternate day regimen schedule.

5. Describe a recommended method for corticosteroid drug withdrawal.

6. Name six symptoms relating to rapid corticosteroid withdrawal.

7. Name four major adverse effects associated with the use of adrenocorticoids.

8. Apply nursing considerations for drug therapy to the care of clients receiving agents affecting the adrenal cortex.

All the adrenocortical hormones, and the synthetic analogs of even higher potency, are commercially available. The generic name for these hormones and analogs is **corticosteroids.**

Some corticosteroids, such as cortisol, have a profound effect on carbohydrate metabolism, whereas aldosterone primarily affects mineral (or electrolyte) and water metabolism. Therefore corticosteroids are divided into two classes, **glucocorticoids** and **mineralocorticoids** (halogenated glucocorticoids).

Biosynthesis of corticosteroids. Cholesterol, which is used for the biosynthesis of corticosteroids, is synthesized and stored in the adrenal cortex. The adrenal cortex also obtains cholesterol from the blood. This cholesterol may be from dietary sources or synthesized by the liver.

Synthesis of corticosteroids depends on the ACTH secreted by the pituitary. The predominant action of ACTH on the adrenal cortex is synthesis of corticosteroids and secretion of glucocorticoids. The exact mechanism for these events is not known.

The release of ACTH by the pituitary is believed to be stimulated by the corticotropin-releasing hormone (CRH) from the hypothalamus, although CRH has not yet been chemically identified. Some evidence suggests that the corticosteroids can inhibit the adrenal glucocorticoid system by inhibiting the release of CRH from the hypothalamus and by inhibiting the release of ACTH from the pituitary.

GLUCOCORTICOIDS

Glucocorticoid rhythms. Two rhythms appear to influence glucocorticoid function: circadian (daily) rhythm and ultradian rhythm. **Circadian rhythm** appears to be controlled by the dark/light and sleep/wakefulness cycles. Normal persons sleeping in the dark at night will have increased plasma cortisol levels in the early morning hours that reach a peak after they are awake. These levels then slowly fall to very low levels in the evening and during the early phase of sleep. The importance of this rhythm is emphasized by the finding that corticosteroid therapy is more potent when given at midnight than when given at noon.

Ultradian rhythms are periodic or intermittent functions with frequencies higher than once every 24 hours. In human beings, four to eight adrenal glucocorticoid bursts occur each 24 hours, which may follow bursts in CRH and ACTH releases. These bursts are clustered close together and are very pronounced during the circadian rise in plasma glucocorticoid levels in the early hours of the morning. At other times they may be so widely spaced that adrenal secretion is zero. Consequently the adrenal cortex secretes glucocorticoids only about 25% of the time in unstressed individuals.

Pharmacologic actions. Glucocorticoids have the following pharmacologic actions:

1. *Antiinflammatory action.* Glucocorticoids, especially cortisol in larger than normal dosages, can stabilize lysosomal membranes and prevent release of proteolytic enzymes during inflammation. They can also potentiate vasoconstrictor effects.

2. *Maintenance of normal blood pressure.* Glucocorticoids potentiate the vasoconstrictor action of norepinephrine. When glucocorticoids are absent, the vasoconstricting action of the catecholamines is diminished, and blood pressure falls.

3. *Carbohydrate and protein metabolism.* Glucocorticoids help to maintain the blood sugar level and liver and muscle glycogen content. They facilitate breakdown of protein in muscle and extrahepatic tissues, which leads to increased plasma amino acid levels. Glucocorticoids increase the trapping of amino acids by the liver and stimulate the deamination of amino acids. They also increase the activity of enzymes important to gluconeogenesis and inhibit glycolytic enzymes. This can produce hyperglycemia and glycosuria. They are diabetogenic. These effects can aggravate diabetes, bring on latent diabetes, and cause insulin resistance. Inhibition of protein synthesis can delay wound healing and cause muscle wasting and osteoporosis. In young persons these effects can inhibit growth.

4. *Fat metabolism.* Glucocorticoids promote mobilization of fatty acids from adipose tissue. This increases the concentration of fatty acids in the plasma and their use for energy. Despite this effect, clients taking glucocorticoids may accumulate fat stores (rounded face, buffalo hump). The effect of glucocorticoids on fat metabolism is complex and little known.

5. *Thymolytic, lympholytic, and eosinopenic actions.* Glucocorticoids can cause atrophy of the thymus and decrease the number of lymphocytes, plasma cells, and eosinophils in blood. They also decrease the rate of conversion of lymphocytes into antibodies. These effects ultimately can interfere with the immune and allergic responses. This, along with their antiinflammatory action, makes them useful **immunosuppressants** for delaying rejection in clients with organ or tissue transplants, as well as useful **antiallergenics** for the treatment of acute allergic reactions such as urticaria, bronchial asthma, and anaphylactic shock. However, steroids can be a source of danger in infections by limiting useful protective inflammation. These hormones also inhibit activity of the lymphatic system, causing lymphopenia and reduction in size of enlarged lymph nodes.

6. *Stress effects.* During stressful situations, corticosteroids are suddenly released, which is believed to be a protective mechanism. The corticosteroids support blood pressure and increase blood sugar to provide energy for emergency actions such as running. This is known as the "fight-or-flight" phenomenon. Clients with decreased adrenal function require increased amounts of steroids during stressful periods such as surgery. Without steroid administration, hypotension and shock tend to occur. (See Figure 49-1.)

During stress, epinephrine and norepinephrine also are released from the adrenal medulla, and these catecholamines have a synergistic action with the corticosteroids. However, there is disagreement about the physiologic usefulness of the steroids during stress.

Mechanism of action. ACTH, or corticotropin, stimulates the synthesis of adrenal steroids by combining with a receptor in the adrenal cell plasma membrane in clients with a normal adrenal cortex function or in clients with a adrenocortical insufficiency secondary to corticotropin deficiency.

The released adrenocorticoids can cross cell membranes and combine with specific receptors in the cytoplasm. The complexes may then enter the cell nucleus, bind to DNA, and ultimately affect protein synthesis.

Indications. Replacement therapy for adrenocortical insufficiency. Also used to treat severe allergic reactions; anaphylactic reactions not responsive to other therapies; collagen disorders such as systemic lupus erythematosus, carditis, and systemic dermatomyositis **(polymyositis);** treatment of dermatologic conditions, gastrointestinal disorders, hematologic disorders, treatment of hypercalcemia associated with neoplasms, adjunct treatment for neo-

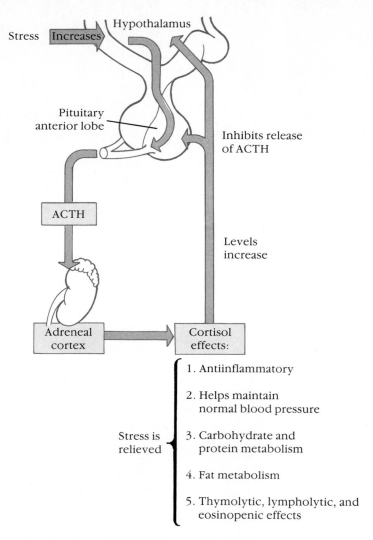

Stress [Increases] Hypothalamus

Pituitary
anterior lobe

Inhibits release
of ACTH

ACTH

Levels
increase

Adreneal
cortex

Cortisol
effects:

1. Antiinflammatory

2. Helps maintain
   normal blood pressure

Stress is   3. Carbohydrate and
relieved   protein metabolism

4. Fat metabolism

5. Thymolytic, lympholytic, and
   eosinopenic effects

FIGURE 49-1   Glucocorticoid secretion.

plastic disease, nephrotic syndrome, neurologic disease, ophthalmic disorders, respiratory disorders, rheumatic disorders, and treatment of shock.

Pharmacokinetics

Absorption. Very good orally

Parenteral (intramuscular)—soluble esters (sodium phosphate, sodium succinate), rapidly absorbed; less soluble derivatives (acetate, acetonide, diacetate, hexacetonide, tebutate), slow but will be completely absorbed.

Topical—soluble esters, less rapidly absorbed; less soluble derivatives, slow but completely absorbed.

Rectal—approximately 20% absorbed normally; if rectal tissue is inflamed, absorption may increase up to 50%.

Metabolism. Mainly liver, also some by tissues and kid-

neys. Cortisone and prednisone need to be metabolized to their active metabolites, which are hydrocortisone and prednisolone, respectively. The fluorinated adrenocorticoids are more slowly metabolized than the other drugs.

For onset of action, peak effect, and duration of action, see Table 49-1.

For relative potency of the major short-acting, intermediate-acting and long-acting adrenocroticoids, see Table 49-2.

Excretion. Metabolism in the body, excretion of inactive metabolites in the kidneys.

Side effects/adverse reactions. See Table 49-3.

Significant drug interactions

The following interactions may occur when corticosteroids are given concurrently with the drugs listed below.

TABLE 49-1   Pharmacology of Adrenocorticoids/Corticotropin

Drug (route)	Onset of action	Peak effect	Duration of action
betamethasone (PO)	—	1-2 hr	3.25 days
sodium phosphate (IM, IV)	Rapid	—	—
acetate/sodium phosphate (IM)	1-3 hr	—	7 days
(IA) (IS)	—	—	7-14 days
(IL) (ST)	—	—	7 days
corticotropin repository (IM)	—	—	12-24 hours
zinc hydroxide (IM)	—	—	2 days
cortisone acetate (PO)	Rapid	—	30-36 hours
(IM)	Slower	20-48 hr	—
dexamethasone (PO)	—	1-2 hr	66 hours
acetate (IM)	—	8 hr	6 days
(IA) (ST) (IL)	—	—	1-3 weeks
sodium phosphate (IV)	Rapid	—	—
(IM)	Rapid	—	—
(IA) (IS) (IL) (ST)	—	—	72 hr to 3 wk
hydrocortisone (PO)	—	1 hr	30-36 hr
(IM)	—	4-8 hr	—
Rectal enema (retention)	3-5 days	—	—
acetate (IA) (IS) (IB) (IL) (ST)	—	1-2 days	3-28 days
rectal foam	5-7 days	—	—
cypionate (PO)	Slow	1-2 hr	—
sodium phosphate (IV)	Rapid	—	—
(IM)	Rapid	1 hr	Varies
sodium succinate (IV)	Rapid	—	—
(IM)	Rapid	1 hr	Varies
methylprednisolone (PO)	—	1-2 hr	30-36 hr
acetate (IM)	6-48 hr	4-8 days	1-4 wk
(IA) (IL) (ST)	Very slow	7 days	1-5 wk
sodium succinate (IV)	Rapid	—	—
(IM)	Rapid	—	—
paramethasone acetate (PO)	—	1-2 hr	2 days
prednisolone (PO)	—	1-2 hr	30-36 hr
acetate (IM)	Slow	—	—
acetate/sodium phosphate (IM)	—	—	Up to 4 wk
(IB) (IS) (IA) (ST)	—	—	3-28 days
sodium phosphate (IV)	Rapid	1 hr	—
(IM)	Rapid	1 hr	
(IA) (IL) (ST)	—	—	3-21 days
tebutate (IA) (IL) (ST)	1-2 days	—	7-21 days
prednisone (PO)	—	1-2 hr	30-36 hr

Abbreviations: —, specific times not listed in USP-DI (1988); *PO*, orally; *IA*, intra-articularly; *IB*, intrabursal; *IL*, intralesion; *IM*, intramuscularly; *IS*, intrasynorial; *ST*, in soft tissue.

Continued.

TABLE 49-1   Pharmacology of Adrenocorticoids/Corticotropin—cont'd

Drug (route)	Onset of action	Peak effect	Duration of action
triamcinolone (po)	—	1-2 hr	52 hr
acetonide (IM)	Slow	—	1-6 wk
(IB) (IA) (IS) (IL) (ST)	—	—	Several weeks
diacetate (po)	—	1-2 hr	—
(IM)	Slow	—	4-28 days
(IL)	—	—	1-2 wk
(IA) (IS) (ST)	—	—	1-8 wk
hexacetonide	—	—	3-4 wk
(IA) (IL)			

TABLE 49-2   Relative Potency and Half-Lives of Major Adrenocorticoids

Adrenocorticoids	Equivalent glucocorticoid dose (mg)*	Relative glucocorticoid potency†	Relative mineralocorticoid potency‡	Half-life (hrs) Serum	Half-life (hrs) Tissue
SHORT-ACTING					
cortisone	25	0.8	2	0.5	8-12
hydrocortisone	20	1	2	1.5-2	8-12
INTERMEDIATE					
methylprednisolone	4	5	0§	>3.5	18-36
prednisolone	5	4	1	2.1-3.5	18-36
prednisone	5	4	1	3.4-3.8	18-36
triamcinolone	4	5	0§	2->5	18-36
LONG-ACTING					
betamethasone	0.6	20-30	0§	3-5	36-54
dexamethasone	0.5-0.75	20-30	0§	3-4.5	36-54
paramethasone	2	10	0§	3-4.5	36-54

*Approximate dosages, applies to oral and IV only.
†Refers to antiinflammatory, immunosuppressant, and metabolic-type effects.
‡Potassium excretion, sodium and water retention.
§Some hypokalemia and/or sodium and water retention may occur. This depends on individual and dosage administered.

Drug	Possible Effect and Management
aminoglutethimide	Aminoglutethimide suppresses adrenal function, therefore do not administer corticotropin concurrently. When aminoglutethimide is given, glucocorticoid supplements are often prescribed. Be aware that aminoglutethimide can increase the metabolism of dexamethasone, reducing its half-life significantly. Hydrocortisone is recommended though, because its metabolism does not appear to be affected by aminoglutethimide.
amphotericin B parenteral	May result in severe hypokalemia. If given concurrently, monitor serum potassium levels closely. May also decrease the adrenal gland response to corticotropin.
antidiabetic drugs (oral) or insulin	Glucocorticoids may elevate serum glucose levels (both during therapy and after, if the glucocorticoid is stopped); therefore a dosage adjustment of one or both drugs may be necessary.

Drug	Possible Effect and Management
digitalis products	May result in increased potential of toxicity (dysrhythmias) associated with hypokalemia.
diuretics	The sodium- and fluid-retaining effects of the adrenocorticoids may reduce the effectiveness of the diuretic agents. Monitor closely for edema and fluid retention. Potassium depleting diuretics given with adrenocorticoids may result in severe hypokalemia. Monitor potassium serum levels. The effects of potassium-sparing diuretics may be decreased. Monitor serum potassium levels and patient response closely.
liver enzyme-inducing agents	Agents such as glucocorticoids, barbiturates, carbamazepine, phenytoin, and others may decrease the adrenocorticoid effect because of increased metabolism. Dosage adjustment may be necessary. Monitor closely.

TABLE 49-3 Side Effects/Adverse Reactions of Adrenocorticoids/Corticotropin

Side effects*	Adverse reactions†
Most frequent: Euphoria, increase in appetite, insomnia, restlessness, increased anxiety, gas. With triamcinolone: anorexia. Less frequent/rare: Hyper or hypopigmentation, (hypo most likely at injection sites), hypotension, headache, increased hair growth on body or face. After intranasal administration—red flushing of face, nosebleeds. Following intraarticular injection—increase in joint pains that may persist for 48 hours.	Lowers resistance to infections (bacterial, viral, fungal, and parasitic). May also mask symptoms of infections making it difficult to diagnose (at pharmacologic dosages). At replacement dosages for adrenocorticoid insufficiency, major adverse effects rarely occur if patient is closely monitored and dosage is adjusted according to individual's need (at physiologic dosages). Less frequent: Visual disturbances (cataracts, diabetes), increased urination or thirst (diabetes), decreased growth in children Rectal dosage form—bleeding, blistering, pain or itching caused by local irritation or allergic reaction Rare: Mental changes including depression, mania, psychoses, paranoia, disorientation, and other psychic disturbances possible At injection site—redness, swelling, rash caused by allergic reaction, or pain, tingling, or numbness at site of injection If **"pulse" therapy**, i.e., rapid IV administration of high dosages, is used: Seizures, severe hypotension, rash or hives, respiratory difficulties, wheezing, shortness of breath. Hypertension, tachycardia, and redness of face also reported. Chronic or long term therapy: Abdominal pains (may be caused by peptic ulcer formation or pancreatitis), acne, black tarry stools (GI bleeding), round face (Cushing's syndrome), hip or shoulder pain. Hypertension, edema of feet or lower legs and weight gain reported because of sodium and water retention. Muscle cramping or pain, increased weakness, irregular heart rate caused by potassium loss. Nausea, vomiting, muscle weakness, menstrual alterations, bone pain, increased bruising, wounds difficult to heal.

*If side effects continue, increase, or disturb the patient, the physician should be informed.
†If adverse reactions occur, contact the physician, since medical intervention may be necessary.

Drug	Possible Effect and Management	Drug	Possible Effect and Management
mitotane	Mitotane will decrease the adrenal gland's response to corticotropin. Avoid concurrent use. Adrenocorticoids are usually necessary during mitotane administration because mitotane suppresses adrenocortical function. Usually higher than normal doses of glucocorticoids are needed.		above certain levels, such as daily doses of prednisone or prednisolone above 2.5 to 3.75 mg/m² of body surface. For dosages for other glucocorticoids, the reader is referred to a current USP-DI, volume 1.
potassium supplements	These reduce the effect of either or both medications on serum potassium levels. Monitor serum levels if given concurrently.	vaccines, live virus and other immunizations	Generally, immunizations are not recommended for patients receiving pharmacologic or immunosuppressant doses of glucocorticoids. Since corticosteroids inhibit antibody response, the immunization effect will be reduced or ineffective and the client may develop neurologic complications. Avoid concurrent use. If live virus vaccines are given to individuals receiving immunosuppressant glucocorticoid therapy, the client may develop the viral disease or at least, have a reduced response to the vaccine. Avoid if at all possible. Also, do not administer the oral polio vaccine to persons in close contact with a person receiving immunosuppressant glucocorticoid therapy.
ritodrine	When ritodrine is given to inhibit premature labor in the pregnant woman and the long-acting glucocorticoids are given to enhance fetal lung maturity, the result may be pulmonary edema in the mother and if not detected and treated, death. Monitor pregnant women closely for first signs of pulmonary edema (shallow, rapid, difficult breathing; anxiety; restlessness; increased heart rate and blood pressure; enlarged peripheral and neck veins; edema of extremities; lung rales; and diaphoresis).		
somatrem or somatropin	The growth response to somatrem or somatropin may be inhibited with concurrent chronic therapy with corticotropin or with daily doses of glucocorticoids		

betamethasone syrup (Celestone)
betamethasone tablets (Betnelan, Celestone)
betamethasone extended-release tablets
(Celestone)—not available in the U.S.
betamethasone sodium phosphate effervescent
tablets (Betnesol)—not available in the U.S.
betamethasone sodium phosphate injection (B-S-P,
Betnesol, Celestone Phosphate, Prelestone,
Selestoject)
sterile betamethasone sodium phosphate and
betamethasone acetate suspension (Celestone
Soluspan)
betamethasone sodium phosphate enema (Betnesol)
betamethasone syrup/tablets

Adults. 600 μg (0.6 mg) orally to a maximum of 7.2 mg daily as a single dose or in divided doses.

Children. For adrenocortical insufficiency—17.5 μg (0.0175 mg)/kg orally or 500 μg (0.5 mg)/m² daily, given in three divided doses.

For other indications. 62.5 to 250 μg (0.625 to 0.25 mg)/kg orally or 1.875 to 7.5 mg/m² daily, given in 3 or 4 divided doses. Dosage is determined by the severity of the condition and patient response.

betamethasone sodium phosphate injection

Adults. Intramuscularly or intravenously, administer up to 9 mg of betamethasone base (which is equivalent to 12 mg of betamethasone sodium phosphate) daily. **Intraarticular, intralesional,** or soft tissue injections—same dosage as above, may be repeated as necessary.

Children. Adrenocortical insufficiency—Intramuscularly, 17.5 μg (0.0175 mg) base/kg or 500 μg (0.5 mg) base/m² daily, given in 3 divided doses every third day; or 5.8 to 8.75 μg (0.0058 to 0.00875 mg) base/kg or 166 to 250 μg (0.166 to 0.25 mg) base/m² daily. Other indications—Intramuscularly, 20.8 to 125 μg (0.028 to 0.125 mg) base/kg or 625 μg (0.625 mg) to 3.75 mg base/m² every 12 to 24 hours.

sterile betamethasone sodium phosphate and
betamethasone acetate suspension

Adults. Intramuscularly, 500 μg (0.5 mg) to 9 mg daily. Intraarticular, 1.5 to 12 mg, depending on joint size. May be repeated if necessary. Intrabursal, 6 mg. Repeat if necessary. Intradermal or intralesional, 1.2 mg/cm² of affected skin area, up to total amount of 6 mg. May be repeated at weekly intervals if necessary.

Children. Not established
Pregnancy safety. Not established

corticotropin for injection (Acthar)
repository corticotropin injection (Acthar Gel, H P
Acthar Gel)
sterile corticotropin zinc hydroxide suspension
(Cortrophin Zinc)

Adults. To determine pituitary-adrenal function (diagnostic acid)—Administer intravenous infusion of 10 to 25 USP units in 500 mg of 5% dextrose injection, over 8 hours. Therapeutically, intramuscular is preferred parenteral route although it may be given subcutaneously, 40 to 80 USP units daily. Dosage and frequency may be adjusted according to the disease state treated and patient response. Multiple sclerosis (acute exacerbation)—Intramuscular, 80 to 120 USP units daily for 14 to 21 days.

Children. Intramuscular, 1.5 USP units/kg or 50 USP units/m² daily, as a single dose or in divided doses. Intravenous or subcutaneous, 1.6 USP units/kg or 50 USP units/m² daily, given in 3 or 4 divided doses.

repository corticoptropin injection

Adults. Therapeutically, intramuscular (preferred) or subcutaneous, 40 to 80 USP units every 24 to 72 hours. Multiple sclerosis (acute exacerbation)—80 to 120 USP units daily for 14 to 21 days.

Children. Therapeutically, intramuscular (preferred) or subcutaneous, 0.8 USP units/kg or 25 USP units/m² daily, given as a single dose or divided into two.

sterile corticotropin zinc hydroxide suspension

Adults. Therapeutically, intramuscular 40 USP units every 12 to 24 hours.
Children. Not established
Pregnancy safety. FDA category C

cortisone acetate tablets (Cortelan, Cortistab)

Adults. 25 to 300 mg orally as single dose or in divided doses.

Children. For adrenocortical insufficiency—700 μg (0.7 mg)/kg or 20 to 25 mg/m² orally daily, in divided doses. For other indications—2.5 to 10 mg/kg or 75 to 300 mg/m² orally daily as single dose or in divided doses. Adjust dose according to condition and individual's response to medication.

sterile cortisone acetate suspension

Adults. 20 to 300 mg intramuscular daily.
Children. For adrenocortical insufficiency—700 μg (0.7 mg)/kg or 37.5 mg/m² intramuscular a day every third day, or 233.33 to 350 μg (0.2333 to 0.350 mg)/kg or 12.5 mg/m² once daily. Adjust dose according to condition and individual's response to medication.
Pregnancy safety. Not established

dexamethasone elixir (Decadron, Hexadrol)
dexamethasone oral solution
dexamethasone tablet (Decadron, Deronil,
Dexasone✱)

Adults. 500 μg (0.5 mg) to 9 mg orally daily as single dose or in divided doses. The dexamethasone suppression test:
1. For Cushing's syndrome—give 1 mg orally as a single dose at 11 PM or give 500 μg (0.5 mg) every 6 hours for 2 days.

2. To distinguish Cushing's syndrome from pituitary ACTH excess from other causes—give 2 mg orally every 6 hours for 2 days.
3. Depression diagnosis—administer 1 mg orally at 11 PM. Plasma cortisol and/or urinary 17-hydroxycorticoids are measured to determine the effect of dexamethasone on ACTH secretion.
4. To treat cerebral edema in a recurrent or inoperable brain tumor—give 2 mg orally, two or three times daily following the use of the injectable dexamethasone.

Children. For adrenocortical insufficiency—23.3 μg (0.023 mg)/kg or 670 μg (0.67 mg)/m^2 orally daily, in three divided doses. For other indications—83.3 to 333.3 μg (0.083 to 0.333 mg)/kg or 2.5 to 10 mg/m^2 orally daily, in three or four divided doses.

sterile dexamethasone acetate suspension (Dalaone DP, Decadron LA, Dexon LA)

Adults. For intraarticular or soft tissue injection—administer 4 to 16 mg of dexamethasone (base). If necessary, may repeat at 1 to 3 week intervals. Intralesion, 800 μg (0.8 mg) to 1.6 mg per injection site. May repeat if necessary. Intramuscularly, 8 to 16 mg of dexamethasone (base). If necessary, may repeat in 1 to 3 weeks.

Children. Not established

dexamethasone sodium phosphate injection (Dalalone, Decadron Phosphate, Hexadrol Phosphate)

Adults. Intraarticular, intralesional, or for soft tissue injections—200 μg (0.2 mg) to 6 mg of dexamethasone; repeat at 3- to 21-day intervals if needed. Intramuscular or intravenous, 500 μg (0.5 mg) to 9 mg daily. For cerebral edema—initially, 10 mg intravenous, followed by 4 mg intramuscular every 6 hours until the symptoms decrease. Dosage may be decreased after 2 to 4 days and eventually discontinued over a 5- to 7-day period, unless a brain tumor is present. Maintenance for a recurrent or an inoperable brain tumor—intramuscular, 2 mg 2 or 3 times daily initially. Adjust according to patient's response to therapy. Septic shock—see box at right. Intravenous, 20 mg initially, followed by 3 mg/kg/24 hours via an intravenous infusion; or intravenous, 2 to 6 mg/kg as a single dose or intravenous, 40 mg as single dose given every 2 to 6 hours as necessary or intravenous, 1 mg/kg as a single dose.

Maximum prescribing limit is usually 80 mg daily.

Children. For adrenocortical insufficiency—23.3 μg (0.023 mg)/kg or 670 μg (0.67 mg)/m^2 intramuscular daily, given in three divided doses every third day. Or 7.76 to 11.65 μg (0.00776 to 0.01165 mg)/kg or 233 to 335 μg (0.233 to 0.335 mg)/m^2 once daily. For other indications—27.76 to 166.65 μg (0.02776 to 0.16665 mg)/kg or 0.833 to 5 mg/m^2 intramuscular every 12 to 24 hours. Adjust dosage according to client's condition and re-

sponse to the medication.

Pregnancy safety. Not established

hydrocortisone tablets (Cortef, Hydrocortone) hydrocortisone cypionate oral suspension (Cortef)

Adults. 20 to 240 mg orally as single dose or divided doses daily.

Children. For adrenocortical insufficiency—560 μg (0.56 mg)/kg or 15 to 20 mg/m^2 orally daily, as a single dose or in divided doses. For other indications—2 to 8 mg/kg or 60 to 240 mg/m^2 orally daily, as a single dose or in divided doses.

sterile hydrocortisone suspension

Adults. 15 to 240 mg intramuscular daily.

Children. For adrenocortical insufficiency—560 μg (0.56 mg)/kg or 30 to 37.5 mg/m^2 intramuscular daily, every third day or 186 to 280 μg (0.186 to 0.28 mg)/kg or

---

SEPTIC SHOCK

Septic shock usually results from a gram-negative bacteremia that leads to circulatory insufficiency. The inadequate tissue perfusion generally results in hypotension, oliguria, tachycardia, elevated temperature, and tachypnea.

MECHANISM

Septic shock may be caused by bacterial substances that interact with body cell membranes and systems, especially coagulation and the complement system, resulting in injury to cells and alterations in blood flow in the body.

TREATMENT

Treatment may consist of volume replacement, antibiotics, surgery (if client has an abscessed or necrotic bowel or organs/tissues), vasoconstricting agents (dopamine, norepinephrine, or levarterenol), diuretics and glucocorticosteroids (steroids). Use of steroids is somewhat controversial but several published studies have reported a benefit with their use if used early in the treatment of shock.

STEROID BENEFICAL EFFECTS

Beneficial effects of steroids include protecting cellular membranes from injury, decreasing platelet aggregation, reducing extracellular release of leukocyte enzymes, and preventing the formation of vasoactive substances in the body.

10 to 12.5 mg/m² daily. Other indications—666 μg (0.666 mg) to 4 mg/kg or 20 to 120 mg/m² intramuscular every 12 to 24 hours.

sterile hydrocortisone acetate suspension (Biosone, Hydrocortistab)

Adults. Intraarticular, intralesional, or soft tissue injections, 5 to 75 mg dosage. May be repeated at 2- to 3-week intervals if necessary.
Children. Not established

hydrocortisone sodium phosphate injection (Efcortesol, Hydrocortone phosphate)

Adults. 100 to 500 mg intramuscular, intravenous, or subcutaneous. If necessary, may be repeated every 2 to 6 hours.
Children. For adrenocortical insufficiency—186 to 280 μg (0.186 to 0.28 mg)/kg or 10 to 12 mg/m² intramuscular or intravenous a day, given in three divided doses. For other indications—666 μg (0.666 mg) to 4 mg/kg or 20 to 120 mg/m² intramuscular, every 12 to 24 hours.

hydrocortisone sodium succinate for injection (A-hydroCort, Solu-Cortef)

Adults. Initially, 100 to 500 mg intramuscular or intravenous. May be repeated every 2 to 6 hours if necessary.
Give initial intravenous dose over a minimum of 30 seconds (for 100 mg) to 10 minutes (for 500 mg or greater). Maintenance dose if necessary, should be at least 25 mg/day.
Children. For adrenocortical insufficiency—186 to 280 μg (0.186 to 0.28 mg)/kg or 10 to 12 mg/m² intramuscular or intravenous daily, given in three divided dosages.
For other indications. 666 μg (0.666 mg) to 4 mg/kg or 20 to 120 mg/m² intramuscular, every 12 to 24 hours.

hydrocortisone enema (Cortenema, Hycort)

Adults. 100 mg rectally nightly for 21 days, or until clinical improvement is noted.
Children. Not established.

hydrocortisone acetate rectal aerosol (Colifoam, Cortifoam)

Adults. 90 mg (one applicator) rectally, once or twice a day for 2 to 3 weeks. Decrease frequency to every other day thereafter.
Children. Not established
Pregnancy safety. Not established

methylprednisolone tablets (Medrol, Medrone✱)

Adults. 4 to 48 mg orally daily, as single dose or in divided doses. In multiple sclerosis—administer 200 mg orally daily for 7 days, then 80 mg every other day for 30 days.

Children. For adrenocortical insufficiency—117 μg (0.117 mg)/kg or 3.33 mg/m² orally daily, given in three divided doses. Other indications—417 μg (0.417 mg) to 1.67 mg/kg or 12.5 to 50 mg/m² orally daily, given in 3 or 4 divided doses.

sterile methylprednisolone acetate suspension (depMedalone, Depo-Medrol)

Adults. For intraarticular, intralesional, or soft tissue injections, administer 4 to 80 mg. May be repeated at 1- to 5-week intervals if necessary. Intramuscular, 40 to 120 mg. Repeat at 1- to 14-day intervals if needed. Acute exacerbation of multiple sclerosis—200 mg intramuscular daily for 7 days, then 80 mg every other day for 30 days.
Children. For adrenocortical insufficiency—117 μg (0.117 mg)/kg or 3.33 mg/m² intramuscular daily, given in 3 divided doses every third day; or 39 to 58.5 μg (0.039 to 0.0585 mg)/kg or 1.11 to 1.66 mg/m² daily. Other indications—139 to 835 μg (0.139 to 0.835 mg)/kg or 4.16 to 25 mg/m² intramuscular, every 12 to 24 hours.

methylprednisolone sodium succinate for injection (A-methaPred, Solu-Medrol)

Adults. Intramuscular or intravenous, 10 to 40 mg (base). May be repeated if needed. "Pulse" therapy, high dose—intravenous, 30 mg/kg given over a minimum of 30 minutes. Dose may be repeated every 4 to 6 hours if necessary. For acute exacerbation of multiple sclerosis—intramuscular or intravenous, 200 mg (base) daily for 7 days, then 80 mg (base) or by oral therapy, every other day for 1 month.
Children. For adrenocortical insufficiency—117 μg (0.117 mg) (base) per kg or 3.33 mg (base) per m² intramuscular daily, given in 3 divided doses every third day; or 39 to 58.5 μg (0.039 to 0.0585 mg) (base) per kg or 1.11 to 1.66 mg (base) per m² daily. Other indications—139 to 835 μg (0.139 to 0.835 mg) (base) per kg or 4.16 to 25 mg (base) per m² intramuscular, every 12 to 24 hours.

methylprednisolone acetate for enema (Medrol Enpak)

Adults. 40 mg rectally, three to seven times weekly for 2 or more weeks, as necessary.
Children. 500 μg (0.5 mg) to 1 mg/kg or 15 to 30 mg/m² rectally, every day or every second day, for 2 or more weeks.
Pregnancy safety. Not established

paramethasone acetate tablets (Haldrone)

Adults. 2 to 24 mg daily orally, as a single dose or in divided doses.
Children. 58 to 800 μg (0.058 to 0.8 mg)/kg or 1.67 to 25 mg/m² orally, as a single dose or in divided doses.
Pregnancy safety. Not established

prednisolone syrup (Prelone)
prednisolone tablets (Cortalone, Delta-Cortef)
prednisolone sodium phosphate oral solution
(Pediapred)

Adults. 5 to 60 mg orally, as a single dose or in divided doses. Maximum is 250 mg daily.

Children. For adrenocortical insufficiency—140 μg (0.14 mg)/kg or 4 mg/m² orally daily, in three divided doses. Other indications— 500 μg (0.5 mg) to 2 mg/kg or 15 to 60 mg/m² orally daily, in three or four divided doses.

sterile prednisolone acetate suspension (Articulose, Predate)

Adults. For intraarticular, intralesional, or soft tissue injection, administer 4 to 100 mg. May be repeated if necessary. Intramuscular use, 4 to 60 mg daily.

Children. For adrenocortical insufficiency—140 μg (0.14 mg)/kg or 4 mg/m² intramuscular daily, given in three divided doses every third day or 46 to 70 μg (0.046 to 0.07 mg)/kg or 1.33 to 2 mg/m² intramuscular daily. Other indications—166 μg (0.166 mg) to 1 mg/kg or 5 to 30 mg/m² intramuscular, every 12 to 24 hours.

sterile prednisolone acetate and prednisolone sodium phosphate suspension

Adults. For intraarticular, intramuscular, or intrasynovial, administer 20 to 80 mg of prednisolone acetate and 5 to 20 mg of prednisolone sodium phosphate. May repeat at 3- to 28-day intervals, if needed.

Children. Not established

prednisolone sodium phosphate injection (Codelsol, Hydeltrasol)

Adults. For intraarticular, intralesional, or soft-tissue injection, administer 2 to 30 mg of prednisolone phosphate. If necessary, the dose may be repeated at 3- to 21-day intervals. Other indications—166 μg (0.166 mg) to 1 mg/kg or 5 to 30 mg/m² intramuscular every 12 to 24 hours.

sterile prednisolone tebutate suspension (Hydeltra-TBA, Metalone TBA)

Adults. For intraarticular, intralesional, or soft-tissue injection, administer 4 to 40 mg. If necessary, dosage may be repeated in 2- to 3-week intervals.

Children. Not established
Pregnancy safety. Not established

prednisone oral solution
prednisone syrup (Liquid Pred)
prednisone tablets (Apo-Prednisone, Deltasone)

Adults. 5 to 60 mg orally daily, as a single dose or in divided doses. For acute exacerbation of multiple sclero-

sis—200 mg orally daily for 7 days, then 80 mg every other day for 30 days. For adrenogenital syndrome—5 to 10 mg orally daily. Maximum daily dose is 250 mg/day.

Children. For nephrosis—children less than 18 months old, not established. 18 months to 4 years old, 7.5 to 10 mg orally initially, four times daily. 4 to 10 years old, 15 mg orally initially, four times daily. 10 years or older, 20 mg orally initially four times daily. For rheumatic carditis, leukemia, tumors—500 μg (0.5 mg)/kg or 15 mg/m² orally four times a day for 14 to 21 days; then 375 μg (0.375 mg)/kg or 11.25/m² four times daily for 4 to 6 weeks. For tuberculosis, given with concurrent antitubercular therapy—500 μg (0.5 mg)/kg or 15 mg/m² orally four times daily for 2 months. For adrenogenital syndrome—5 mg/m² orally daily, given in two divided doses.

Pregnancy safety. Not established

triamcinolone tablets (Aristocort, Kenacort)
triamcinolone diacetate syrup (Aristocort, Kenacort)

Adults. For adrenocortical insufficiency—4 to 12 mg orally daily as single dose or in divided doses. Give with a mineralocorticoid. Other indications—4 to 48 mg orally daily or in divided doses.

Children. For adrenocortical insufficiency—117 μg (0.117 mg)/kg or 3.3 mg/m² orally daily, as a single dose or in divided doses; give with a mineralocorticoid. Other indications—416 μg (0.416 mg) to 1.7 mg/kg or 12.5 to 50 mg/m² orally daily, as a single dose or in divided doses.

sterile triamcinolone acetonide suspension (Cenocort A, Kenalog)

Adults. For intraarticular, intrabursal, or tendon-sheath injection, administer 2.5 to 15 mg. For intradermal or intralesional injection, administer up to 1 mg per site. May repeat at weekly (or less if necessary) intervals. Intramuscular, 40 to 80 mg. Repeat at 4-week intervals if necessary.

Children. Less than 6 years old—not recommended. 6 to 12 years old—intraarticular, intrabursal, or tendon-sheath injection, administer 2.5 to 15 mg. Repeat if necessary. Intramuscular, 40 mg, which may be repeated at 4-week intervals if needed, or 30 to 200 μg (0.03 to 0.2 mg)/kg or 1 to 6.25 mg/m². May repeat at 1- to 7-day intervals.

sterile triamcinolone diacetate suspension (Amcort, Aristocort Forte)

Adults. For intraarticular, intrasynovial, intralesional, sublesional, or soft-tissue injection, administer 3 to 48 mg. May repeat at 1- to 8-week intervals if necessary. Intramuscular, 40 mg weekly.

Children. Less than 6 years old—not recommended. 6 to 12 years old—intramuscular 40 mg weekly.

sterile triamcinolone hexacetonide suspension (Aristospan Intraarticular, Aristospan Intralesional)

Adults. Intraarticular, administer 2 to 20 mg. If necessary, may repeat at 3- or 4-week intervals. Intralesional or sublesional injection, administer up to 500 µg (0.5 mg) per square inch of affected skin. Repeat if necessary.

Children. Not established

Pregnancy safety. Not established

NURSING CONSIDERATIONS

Assessment. Use glucocorticoids cautiously in individuals with psychosis, peptic ulcer, tuberculosis, acute glomerulonephritis, vaccinia or varicella, herpes simplex of the eye, and infections uncontrolled by antibiotics.

Note that myasthenic crisis may be induced if these drugs are administered to patients with myasthenia gravis.

Use cautiously in pregnant women, since adrenal insufficiency in both mother and child is possible at delivery. Fetal abnormalities also can occur.

Carefully assess for severe fluid and electrolyte imbalances when hypertension is present, as well as with congestive heart failure, diabetes mellitus, thrombophlebitis, renal insufficiency, and osteoporosis.

Do not give glucocorticoids to clients with systemic fungal and amebiasis infections. These drugs can exacerbate the disease state.

Obtain baseline weight before therapy. Weigh daily; report any sudden increases, which would indicate fluid retention, to the prescriber. Monitor intake and output daily. Correlate with physical findings of edema.

Obtain baseline data for hematologic values, serum electrolytes, and serum and urine glucose. Check stool for occult blood. These determinations should be monitored during therapy.

Assess children for growth before and periodically during therapy.

Intervention. Note that an alternate-day regimen may be valuable when considering the long-term use of glucocorticoids in less severe disease processes, especially when an intermediate range–acting agent (methylprednisolone, prenisolone, prednisone) is used, since it diminishes hypothalamic-pituitary-adrenal (HPA) axis suppression. The alternate-day dose given every other morning before 9 AM is at least twice the daily dose equivalent. This therapy requires that a client possess a responsive pituitary axis and be stabilized initially on the alternate-day schedule.

Give glucocorticoids as a single daily dose in the morning before 9 AM if possible, with food or milk. They suppress adrenal activity the least when it is at its peak, which is early morning.

Administer IM injections of suspensions deep in the gluteal muscle to avert local tissue atrophy at the injection sites. Note that injections into the deltoid muscle can cause atrophy.

Note that clients taking cortisone who require surgery should receive a preoperative dose of a rapid-acting corticosteroid. The drug is continued postoperatively in decreasing doses for several days. Clients with atrophy of the adrenal gland may be unable to cope with the stress of surgery if cortisone treatment is interrupted.

Be prepared to do an HPA axis suppression test following high doses or long-term therapy to determine level of suppression.

Know that withdrawal should be carried out slowly and under close supervision to avoid adrenal insufficiency.

Note that the usual rate of withdrawal of systemic corticosteroids is the steroid equivalent of 2.5 mg prednisone every 4 days, when the client is under close and continuous medical supervision. When this is not possible, withdrawal of systemic corticosteroids is slower, approximately 2.5 mg prednisone (or equivalent corticosteroid dosage) every 10 days. When withdrawal symptoms such as weakness, lethargy, hypoglycemia, depression, anorexia, and nausea appear, the previous dose may be resumed for 7 days before continuing the decrease.

When the drug is to be discontinued, be aware that it usually is withdrawn gradually. If a medical-surgical emergency or stressful event occurs, the drug is given again to prevent the possibility of acute adrenal insufficiency

Education. After intraarticular injection, instruct the client not to overuse the injected joint.

Instruct clients to report any signs of infections, such as sore throat, fever, and poor wound healing. Corticosteroids can mask infection and increase its spread. The client should avoid individuals with known contagious illnesses.

Tell clients to avoid any immunizations while taking glucocorticoids, since they impair the antibody response.

Instruct clients to report any visual disturbances. Long-term glucocorticoid therapy can cause cataracts, glaucoma, or optic nerve damage.

Since these drugs can cause gastric distress, instruct clients to report any persistent symptoms and instruct them to take the drug with meals or milk in the morning. Antacids may be necessary to prevent or relieve gastric irritation.

Warn the client and family that changes in appearance (see box, p.791) and mood may develop following glucocorticoid use. The nurse should assist the client and family in dealing with the changes that occur, as well as reassure them that they will disappear when the drug is stopped.

ALTERATIONS IN BODY IMAGE THAT MAY OCCUR WITH GLUCOCORTICOID THERAPY

Alterations in body image may be a major problem in clients receiving glucocorticoid therapy. Among the body changes that may occur are the following:

Abdominal distention

Acneiform eruptions

Fat deposits on upper back ("buffalo hump")

Fluid retention

Hirsutism

Hyperpigmentation

Loss of muscle mass

Lupus erythematosus–like lesions

Nausea and vomiting

Round face ("moon face")

Petechiae and ecchymosis

Purpura

Straie

Thin fragile skin

Thinning of extremities with thickening of torso

Weight gain

Most clients receiving glucocorticoids should be on a high potassium, low sodium diet to counter the potassium-depleting and sodium-retaining effects of the drug. Clients should limit alcohol, caffeine, aspirin, and other gastric irritants to minimize peptic ulceration.

Inform female clients that they may experience menstrual irregularities while taking glucocorticoids.

Inform female clients that the following drugs are unsafe to take during pregnancy because of their effects on the fetus: metamethasone, cortisone, dexamethasone, hydrocortisone, methylprednisolone, and prednisolone.

Have clients carry a card describing their medical condition and drug therapy.

Remember that any client who has received a significant amount of cortisone or related glucocorticoids is likely to have some atrophy of the adrenal cortex. The amount of hormone that will produce atrophy is unknown, as is how long the atrophy will persist, but acute adrenal insufficiency may result from too rapid withdrawal of therapy. Instruct the client to report withdrawal symptoms including weakness, lethargy, malaise, restlessness, hypoglycemia, psychologic despondency, anorexia, and nausea.

Warn the client that changes in mental status (euphoria, mood swings, depression, insomnia), may occur during glucocorticoid therapy.

Caution the client to report to the physician any symptoms of abdominal pain, bone pain, tiredness, bruising, or tarry stools.

Evaluation. Assess for the following when excessive doses are given: CNS symptoms (anxiety, depression/stimulation) hyperglycemia, glycosuria, elevated blood pressure, and Cushing's syndrome.

Remember that not only the total daily dose, but also frequent individual doses during the day must be adjusted to meet the client's needs. Notify the physician of the client's varying responses to the drugs.

Assess children on glucocorticoid therapy for normal growth development, which these drugs can suppress.

Closely monitor the blood sugar of clients taking glucocorticoids, since these drugs can cause hyperglycemia. Diabetic clients may need changes in diet or insulin dosage to maintain blood sugar control.

MINERALOCORTICOIDS

The primary agents with mineralocorticoid effects are desoxycorticosterone and fludrocortisone. Desoxycorticosterone has mainly mineralocorticoid activity with no glucocorticoid effects, whereas fludrocortisone has high levels of mineralocorticoid activity with some moderate glucocorticoid effects. However, the latter is still used primarily for its mineralocorticoid effects.

Mechanism of action. The agents act on the renal distal tubule to reabsorb sodium and enhance excretion of potassium and hydrogen.

Indications. Treatment of Addison's disease (chronic primary adrenocortical insufficiency) and adrenogenital syndrome.

Pharmacokinetics. Desoxycorticosterone is administered parenterally. Fludrocortisone is available in oral dosage form.

Absorption. Fludrocortisone good orally. Half-life in plasma 30 minutes; biological half-life is 18 to 36 hours.

Duration of action. 24 to 48 hours

Metabolism. Liver, kidneys

Excretion. Kidneys, mainly as inactive metabolites

Side effects/adverse reactions. See Table 49-4.

Significant drug interactions. The following interactions may occur when mineralocorticoids are given concurrently with the drugs listed below.

Drug	Possible Effect and Management
amphotericin B parenteral	May produce severe hypokalemia. Monitor serum potassium and electrolyte levels closely. Also monitor cardiac function.

TABLE 49-4   Side Effects/Adverse Reactions of Mineralocorticoids

Drug	Side effects	Adverse reactions
desoxycorticosterone acetate (DOCA) desoxycorticosterone acetate pellets (Percorten) fludrocortisone acetate (Florinef)		Less frequent or rare: Severe or persistent headaches, hypertension, dizziness, edema of lower extremities, increase in weight, weakness in extremities (arms and legs)

Drug	Possible Effect and Management
digitalis glycosides	Hypokalemic effect may potentiate the risk for cardiac dysrhythmias or digitalis toxicity. Monitor closely.
diuretics	Effectiveness of diuretics may be decreased with these medications. Concurrent use of potassium-depleting diuretics may produce severe hypokalemia. Monitor serum potassium levels closely.
liver enzyme inducers	Increased metabolism of mineralocorticoids may result in a decrease in the effectiveness of these drugs.
potassium supplements	May decrease effectiveness of these drugs. Monitor serum potassium levels frequently.
sodium in food or medications	In type IV renal tubular acidosis, concurrent use of sodium with fludrocortisone may result in hypertension, hypernatremia, and edema. Monitor sodium intake closely and advise clients on safe consumption of foods and medications to avoid hypernatremia. Instruct patients to read labels on both foods and medication.

desoxycorticosterone acetate injection

Adults. For adrenocortical (mineralocorticoid) insufficiency—1 to 5 mg intramuscularly daily. To treat adrenogenital syndrome (salt losing)—Initially, up to 6 mg intramuscularly daily for 3 or 4 days. Then adjust dosage according to patient response and serum electrolyte levels. Maximum is usually 10 mg daily.

Children. 1 to 5 mg intramuscularly or 1.5 to 2 mg/m² intramuscularly.

deoxycorticosterone acetate pellets (Percorten)

Adults. Implant subcutaneously 1 pellet (125 mg) for each 500 µg (0.5 mg) of daily dose of the above injection. Repeat implantation at 8- to 12-month intervals.

Children. Not established

sterile desoxycorticosterone pivalate suspension (Percorten)

Adults. 25 mg for each 1 mg of daily maintenance dose of acetate injection, given intramuscularly. Repeat monthly.

Children. See adult dosage.

fludrocortisone acetate tablets (Florinef)

Adults. For treatment of chronic adrenocortical (mineralocorticoid) insufficiency—100 µg (0.1 mg) daily orally, given with a glucocorticoid. If transient hypertension occurs, decrease dose to 50 µg (0.05 mg). To treat adrenogenital syndrome (salt losing)—100 to 200 µg (0.1 to 0.2 mg) orally daily with a suitable glucocorticoid.

Children. 50 to 100 µg (0.05 to 0.1 mg) orally daily.

Pregnancy safety. Not established.

NURSING CONSIDERATIONS

Assessment. Determine that the client does not have hypertension, congestive heart failure, or cardiac disease for which these drugs are contraindicated.

Establish the client's baseline weight and blood pressure and report weight increases to the physician.

Periodically assess the client's blood pressure and check for evidence of edema. Monitor intake and output.

Intervention. Desoxycorticosterone comes as a sesame oil solution injection; it is not for intravenous use. Withdraw medication from the vial with a 19-gauge needle and administer with a 23-gauge needle.

Education. Advise the client to arrange periodic checking of the serum electrolyte levels, especially during prolonged therapy, and to implement dietary salt restrictions. Use of a potassium supplement may be necessary.

Instruct the client to take daily weight measurements and to report a sudden weight gain to the prescriber. Consult with the physician for specific weight-gain limitations for each individual client.

Evaluation. Monitor blood pressure, and if hypertension develops, adjust the dosage of the steroid and the salt intake.

Be aware that excessive loss of potassium can cause dysrhythmias and sudden weakness, palpitations, paresthesia, or nausea.

ANTIADRENALS (ADRENAL STEROID INHIBITORS)

Aminoglutethimide, metyrapone, and trilostane are examples of drugs that inhibit or suppress adrenal cortex function.

aminoglutethimide (Cytadren)

Mechanism of action. Aminoglutethimide inhibits the enzyme conversion of cholesterol to pregnenolone, thereby blocking the synthesis of adrenal steroids. It also may have other suppression effects in the synthesis and metabolism of the steroids.

By blocking the aromatase enzyme in the peripheral tissues, it inhibits estrogen production from androgens.

Indications. Treatment of Cushing's syndrome associated with adrenal carcinoma, ectopic adrenocorticotropic hormone tumors, or adrenal gland hyperplasia.

Pharmacokinetics

Absorption. Good

Half-life. 13 hours. After prolonged therapy of 2 to 32 weeks, the half-life decreases to 7 hours because of the increase in liver enzymes induced by aminoglutethimide. Time to peak concentration: 1.5 hours

Onset of action. Adrenal function is suppressed within 3 to 5 days of therapy.

Duration of action. Recovery of normal adrenal basal secretion and its response to stress usually occurs within 36 to 72 hours after aminoglutethimide and hydrocortisone are withdrawn. If client has taken these drugs for 1 year or longer, recovery may take longer.

Metabolism. Liver

Excretion. Kidneys

Side effects/adverse reactions. See Table 49-5.

Significant drug interactions. When aminoglutethimide is given concurrently with dexamethasone, it may reduce dexamethasone's half-life by one half. Therefore, if a glucocorticoid is necessary, hydrocortisone is the drug recommended, since it does not interact with aminoglutethimide.

Dosage and administration

Adults. Antiadrenal effect—Initially, 250 mg orally two or three times daily for approximately 14 days.

Maintenance, 250 mg orally every 6 hours (four times daily). In Cushing's syndrome, the prescribing limit for adults is usually 2 g/day.

Its antineoplastic use is still under investigational study.

Children. Not established

Pregnancy safety. FDA category D

NURSING CONSIDERATIONS

Because of the cortical hypofunction, use antiadrenals cautiously in clients undergoing stress such as surgery, trauma, and acute illness.

Do not give to pregnant women, since aminoglutethimide may harm the fetus.

Obtain baseline thyroid function studies. Monitor periodically during therapy.

Since this drug can cause blood dyscrasias and liver and electrolyte abnormalities, routinely monitor serum electrolytes and hematologic and liver function studies.

Because the client may experience orthostatic hypotension, advise the client to change position or to stand slowly to minimize this effect.

Alert the client to avoid activities that require alertness until response to the drug has been determined.

Since hypotension (weakness, dizziness) is caused by aldosterone suppression, monitor blood pressure.

metyrapone (Metopirone)

Mechanism of action. Metyrapone inhibits the synthesis of cortisol and corticosterone by inhibiting the 11 B-hydroxylation reaction that occurs in the adrenal cortex. This normally leads to an increase in ACTH production and secretion from the pituitary, which in turn produces

TABLE 49-5 Side Effects/Adverse Reactions of Antiadrenal Drugs

Drug	Side effects*	Adverse reactions†
aminoglutethimide (Cytadren)	Most frequent: Ataxia, dizziness, sedation, loss of energy, uncontrolled eye movements (CNS effects are usually dose-related. Effects may decline in 2-6 weeks of continuous therapy but if severe, drug may need to be stopped.) Anorexia, nausea, vomiting, measle-like rash on face and/or palms of hands Rare: Dark skin, depression, dizziness, headaches, pain in muscles	Rare: Increased temperature, chills, sore throat (caused by leukopenia or agranulocytosis), fever or jaundice of eyes and skin (hypersensitivity), increased bleeding episodes or unusual bruising (thrombocytopenia)
trilostane (Modrastane)	Most frequent: Diarrhea, abdominal distress Less frequent: Muscle aches, headache, increased temperature, flushing, increased salivation, nausea, dizziness, gas, burning sensation in mouth or nose, watery eyes	Rare: Dark skin, sedation, anorexia, vomiting, rash, depression

*If side effects continue, increase, or disturb the patient, the physician should be informed.
†If adverse reactions occur, contact the physician, since medical intervention may be necessary.

an increase in the precursors of the adrenal glucocorticoids. The result is an increase in the steroids 11-deoxycortisol and desoxycorticosterone in the plasma and of their metabolites in the urine. Metyrapone may also decrease the synthesis of aldosterone in the body.

Indications. To test the hypothalamic-pituitary ACTH function

Pharmacokinetics

Absorption. Good. Plasma concentration during treatment period is usually 0.5 to 1 μg/ml.

Peak steroid excretion. Within 24 hours of drug administration in normal individuals. See dosage and administration section for test interpretation.

Excretion half-life. 1 to 2.5 hours

Metabolism. Liver

Excretion. Kidneys

Side effects/adverse reactions. Nausea, stomach distress, dizziness, headache, drowsiness, rash

Significant drug interactions. When individuals are taking or have taken either cyproheptadine or phenytoin within the previous 2-week period, test results may be affected. Phenytoin accelerates the metabolism of metyrapone. Estrogens have also reportedly led to a subtherapeutic response with metyrapone.

Dosage and administration. All corticosteroid drugs should be discontinued before and during testing with this drug.

First day—Collect 24-hour urine to measure 17-hydroxycorticosteroids (17-OHCS) or 17-ketogenic steroids (17-KGS).

Second day—Administer ACTH test, that is, give 50 units of ACTH by intravenous infusion over 8 hours and measure the 24-hour steroids in the urine. If results are within normal limits, continue with test. (The normal 24-hour urinary excretion of 17-OHCS is 3 to 12 mg. After ACTH, this will increase to 15 to 45 mg/24 hours.)

Third and fourth day—Rest day

Fifth day—Administer the metyrapone. Adults: 750 mg orally, every 4 hours for 6 doses. Children: 15 mg/kg every 4 hours for 6 doses; minimum dose is 250 mg.

Sixth day—Collect and determine the 24-hour steroids in the urine. If the client has a normally functioning pituitary, metyrapone will increase the 17-OHCS by two-fold to fourfold or double the 17-KGS excretion.

A subnormal response indicates the possibility of an impaired pituitary function in patients with sufficient adrenal function (panhypopituitarism or partial hypopituitarism). The student is referred to the package insert or a suitable reference source for other interpretations of this test.

Pregnancy safety. FDA category C

NURSING CONSIDERATIONS

Measure the ability of the adrenal gland to respond to exogenous ACTH before the test, since acute adrenal insufficiency is precipitated in clients with reduced adrenal secretory capacity.

Note that metyrapone testing requires that all corticosteroid therapy be stopped before and during testing.

Explain to the client the purpose of and procedures for this test.

trilostane (Modrastane)

Mechanism of action. Suppresses synthesis of adrenal steroids by inhibiting enzyme in the adrenal cortex.

Indications. For the treatment of Cushing's syndrome

Pharmacokinetics

Metabolism. Liver

Half-life. 8 hours

Side effects/adverse reactions. See Table 49-5.

Significant drug interactions. None.

Dosage and administration

Adults. Initially, 30 mg orally, four times daily. May gradually increase the dosage every 3 or 4 days until the desired effect is noted. Maintenance—usually less than 360 mg in 24 hours orally daily, given in four divided doses. Maximum is 480 mg/day.

Children. Not established.

Pregnancy safety. FDA category X

NURSING CONSIDERATIONS

Trilostane is contraindicated in clients with adrenal insufficiency, severe renal disease, or hepatic disease.

Because trilostane may prevent physiologic responses to stress, it may be discontinued briefly before surgery or in times of physiologic stress.

Because orthostatic hypotension may occur with the drug, alert the client to change positions or come to a standing position slowly.

Monitor the blood pressure periodically and alert the prescriber if hypotension becomes a concern for the client.

KEY TERMS

antiallergenic, page 781
circadian rhythm, page 781
corticosteroid, page 780
glucocorticoid, page 780
immunosuppressant, page 781

BIBLIOGRAPHY

Alexander MR and others: Therapy of chronic obstructive airways disease, Drug Intell Clin Pharm 18(4):279, 1984.

American Hospital Formulary Service: AHFS Drug Information '88, Bethesda, Md, 1988, American Society of Hospital Pharmacists, Inc.

Balow JE: Steroids in immunologically mediated renal disease. Part 4, Hosp Pract 18(11):85, 1983.

Berg S: Dexamethasone's new use in cancer treatment, J Assoc Pediatr Oncol Nurses 2(2):46, 1985.

Blair GP and others: Treatment of chronic obstructive pulmonary disease with corticosteroids: comparison of daily vs alternate-day therapy, Chest 86(4):524, 1984.

Braunwald E and others, eds: Harrison's principles of internal medicine, ed 11, New York, 1987, McGraw-Hill Book Co.

Christy NP: HPA failure and glucocorticoid therapy—the hypothalamic-pituitary-adrenal axis. Part 12, Hosp Pract 19(7):77, 1984.

Claman HN: Glucocorticosteroids: anti-inflammatory mechanisms. Part 1, Hosp Pract 18(7):123, 1983.

Claman HN: Glucocorticosteroids: the clinical responses. Part 2, Hosp Pract 18(7):143, 1983.

Ellis EF: Corticosteroid regimens in pediatric practice, Hosp Pract 19(5):143, 1983.

Ellison GW: Corticosteroids in neurologic disease. Part 9, Hosp Pract 19(4):105, 1983.

Fauci AS: Corticosteroids in autoimmune disease. Part 3, Hosp Pract 18(10):99, 1983.

Fernandez E: Update on the pharmacologic approach to asthma: anticholinergics, corticosteroids, and cromolyn sodium. Part 2, Respir Ther 14(5):29, 1984.

Grammer LC: Corticosteroid therapy in allergic and pulmonary diseases, Hosp Pract 18(8):89, 1983.

Harris ED Jr: Wider options for rheumatoid arthritis, Emerg Med 18(19):74, 1986.

Herfindal ET and Hirschman JL: Clinical pharmacy and therapeutics ed 3, Baltimore, 1984, Williams & Wilkins.

Hoffman JR and others: Pharmacologic therapeutic modalities: corticosteroids—use in cerebral resuscitation, CCQ 5(4):52, 1983.

Kaplan FS: Glucocorticoid osteopenia, Orthop Nurs 4(3):35, 1985.

Kastrup EK, Ed: Facts and comparisons, St Louis, 1988, JB Lippincott.

Katzung BG: Basic and clinical pharmacology ed 3, Norwalk, Conn, 1987, Appleton & Lange.

Kent JM: Help for the stiff, sore shoulder, Patient Care 19(8):55, 1985.

Labson LH: Perennial problems: "Doctor, I can't stand this itching!" Patient Care 18(17):89, 1984.

Lippman ME: Steroids in malignant diseases: progress in patient selection. Part 11, Hosp Pract 19(6):93, 1984.

Miller K: Controversial corticosteroids—emergency prehospital care, Emergency 18(12):52, 1986.

Neuberger GB: The role of the nurse with arthritis patients on drug therapy, Nurs Clin North Am 19(4):593, 1984.

Peppercorn MA and others: Inflammatory bowel disease: medication for ulcerative colitis and Crohn's disease, Consultant 25(17):37, 1985.

Perry PJ and others: Prednisolone psychosis: clinical observations, Drug Intell Clin Pharm 18(7/8):603, 1984.

Post-White J: Glucocorticosteroid-induced depression in the patient with leukemia or lymphoma, Cancer Nurs 9(1):15, 1986.

Roberts AM and others: Corticosteroid therapy of ophthalmologic diseases. Part 7, Hosp Pract 19(2):181, 1983.

Ryan GM: Steroids as antiemetics, Cancer Nurs 6(2):147, 1983.

Sjogren E: Solu-Medrol (methyprednisolone sodium succinate, USP), Crit Care Nurse 3(5):26, 1983.

United States Pharmacopeial Convention: Drug information for the health care provider, ed 8, Rockville, Md, 1988, U.S. The Convention.

Wyngaarden JB and Smith LH: Cecil textbook of medicine, ed 18, Philadelphia, 1988, WB Saunders Co.

CHAPTER 50

Drugs Affecting the Pancreas

OBJECTIVES

After studying this chapter, the student will be able to:

1. Describe insulin dependent diabetes mellitus (type I) and non–insulin dependent diabetes mellitus (type II).

2. Compare and contrast the different insulin preparations.

3. Discuss oral hypoglycemic agents and related nursing considerations.

4. List hyperglycemic agents and their mechanism of action.

5. Apply appropriate nursing considerations to clients receiving agents affecting the pancreas.

Insulin and glucagon are the two primary hormones released by the pancreas. When serum blood glucose declines, glucagon is released from the pancreas. Glucagon, which is synthesized in the A cells of the pancreatic islets, facilitates the catabolism of stored glycogen in the liver. The result is an increase in blood glucose, or **gluconeogenesis.** The release of glucagon stimulates insulin secretion, which then inhibits the release of glucagon.

The most important disease involving the endocrine pancreas is diabetes mellitus. Diabetes mellitus is primarily a disorder of carbohydrate metabolism that involves an insulin deficiency or an insulin resistance or both. All causes of diabetes will lead to hyperglycemia (see Chapter 46, "Overview of the Endocrine System").

HYPERGLYCEMIA

The two general classifications for diabetes mellitus are **insulin dependent diabetes mellitus (type I)** and **non–insulin dependent diabetes mellitus (type II).** Clients with type I diabetes have very little or no endogenous insulin capacity. This type of diabetes usually occurs before early adulthood and so was previously called juvenile onset diabetes. The client with type I diabetes is ketosis prone and requires exogenous insulin therapy for survival.

Type II diabetes was previously known as maturity onset diabetes. Generally, clients with this type of diabetes have some insulin function, so they are not fully dependent on insulin for survival. At times insulin treatment may be necessary to control type II diabetes, but usually weight reduction through dietary treatment will help reduce the hyperglycemia in clients with type II diabetes. The vast majority of individuals with type II diabetes are obese, and ketosis is rare. Although insulin resistance may occasionally occur with type I diabetes, it is believed to be more common in type II diabetes because of receptor and postreceptor defects. See the box below for a comparison of the primary features of both types of diabetes.

INSULIN PREPARATIONS

Insulin, which is normally secreted by the beta cells of the pancreas, is composed of two amino acid chains, A (acidic) and B (basic). These chains are joined together by disulfide linkages. Insulin preparations are derived from animals (extracted from cattle or pig pancreas) or synthesized in the laboratory from either an alteration of pork insulin or recombinant DNA with strains of *E. coli* to form human insulin (a biosynthetic human insulin). The difference between the sources is that the beef insulin differs from human insulin by three amino acids, whereas the pork insulin differs from human insulin by only a single amino acid. The human insulin is identical to the insulin produced by the pancreas.

Usually, the beef-pork combination insulins are suitable for most clients. If the client has not developed insulin resistance, insulin allergies, or lipoatrophy at the insulin injection sites, the combination product is usually sufficient and also less expensive. The beef-only insulins are indicated mainly for clients who are allergic to pork or for use in clients who must avoid the use of pork for religious reasons. Pork insulin has been found to be useful for clients who have local or systemic allergies, insulin resistance, or lipoatrophy or for clients who have a short-term need for insulin. The pure pork insulin is closer to human insulin, and in many instances, its use has resulted in reduction of the insulin dose (in insulin resistance) and in the improvement of local allergy in approximately 80% of the clients with insulin allergies.

Human insulin can be substituted for the same reasons as pork insulin, and it has been used instead of pork insulin in clients who are allergic to pork. Human insulin is much less antigenic than the animal-based insulin. The physician will make the decision about which type of insulin is best for a specific client.

Mechanism of action. Insulin affects the storage and metabolism of carbohydrate, protein, and fat by attaching insulin molecules to receptor sites on cellular plasma membranes, especially in the liver, muscle, and adipose tissues.

Indications
1. For the treatment of diabetes mellitus, insulin dependent (type I, IDDM)
2. Treatment of non–insulin dependent diabetes mellitus during emergencies or in specific situations, such as when needed as a supplement to the low physiologic endogenous insulin in an individual, during high fevers, severe infection, ketoacidosis or significant ketosis, severe burns, after major surgery, following severe trauma or during pregnancy

Pharmacokinetics. See Table 50-1.
Side effects/adverse reactions. See Table 50-2.

FEATURES OF INSULIN DEPENDENT (IDDM) AND NON–INSULIN DEPENDENT (NIDDM) DIABETES

	IDDM	NIDDM
Synonym	Type I	Type II
Age of onset	Usually < 30	Usually > 40
Onset of symptoms	Sudden (symptomatic)	Gradual (usually asymptomatic)
Body weight	Usually nonobese	Obese (80%)
Incidence	10%	90%
Insulin dependent	Yes	Usually not required
Insulin resistance	No	Yes
Receptors	Normal	Usually decreased or defective
Plasma insulin	Decreased	Normal or increased
Complications	Frequent	Frequent
Ketoacidosis	Prone to	Usually resistant
Diet	Mandatory	Mandatory

TABLE 50-1   Characteristics of Insulin Preparations

Insulins*	Onset (hours)	Peak effect (hours)	Duration of action (hours)
RAPID ACTING			
regular crystalline insulin injection†	½-1	2-4	6-8
crystalline zinc insulin (Semilente)	1	2-6	10-12
INTERMEDIATE ACTING			
insulin zinc suspension (Lente Insulin)	1-3	8-12	18-28
isophane insulin suspension (NPH Insulin)	3-4	6-12	18-28
isophane insulin suspension (70%) plus insulin injection (30%) (Mixtard, Novolin 70/30)	½	4-8	24
LONG ACTING			
extended insulin zinc suspension (Ultralente)	4-6	18-24	36
protamine zinc insulin suspension (PZI)	4-6	14-24	36

*All above insulins, with the exception of Mixtard, Novolin combinations, are available in 40 unit and 100 unit strengths. Beef, pork, beef-pork, and human insulins are available in rapid-acting insulins and the three insulins listed under intermediate acting. The others are animal sources only.
†This is the only insulin for intravenous use. Intravenously, the onset of action is within ⅙ to ½ hour, peak effect within ¼ to ½ hour, and duration of action within ½ to 1 hour.

Significant drug interactions. The following interactions may occur when insulin is given concurrently with the drugs listed below.

Drug	Possible Effect and Management
adrenocorticoids, glucocorticoids	Adrenocorticoids and glucocorticoids may increase blood glucose levels. A dosage adjustment of one or both drugs may be necessary. Monitor closely.
alcohol	May increase the hypoglycemic effect of insulin. Monitor closely, since dosage adjustments may be necessary. If possible, avoid the concurrent use of alcohol.
antidiabetic agents, oral	These agents enhance hypoglycemic effects. Although a small number of carefully selected individuals may find the combination therapy more effective than single therapy, this type of treatment is not generally advocated.
beta adrenergic blocking agents (including eye preparations)	These agents may mask symptoms of hypoglycemia, such as increased pulse rate and decreased blood pressure. May also prolong hypoglycemia by blocking gluconeogenesis. Dosage adjustments of insulin may be necessary. Selective beta blockers in low dosages, such as metoprolol and atenolol, cause fewer problems than the other beta adrenergic blocking agents. Propranolol may cause hyperglycemia or hypoglycemia when given concurrently with insulin. Periodic blood glucose tests are recommended to monitor the combined effects and allow for adjustment of insulin dose, if necessary.

Dosage and administration. There is no average dose of insulin for the diabetic person; each client's needs must be determined individually. These needs are frequently determined by blood glucose monitoring, which has been simplified by the availability of both visual test strips and strips used in blood glucose meters or instruments. Such devices have allowed clients to monitor their diabetes and make the necessary adjustments with medication, diet, or exercise, as instructed by their physician or health care provider. The visual glucose testing strips are less expensive than the testing instruments, but the meter readings are much more precise (assuming they are properly calibrated). Thus clients with visual problems or a need for a more accurate blood glucose reading will benefit from using a blood glucose meter instrument.

Insulin dosage is expressed in units rather than in milliliters or minims. Insulin injection is standardized so that each milliliter contains 40 or 100 USP units. Insulin is classified according to its duration of action (short- or rapid-acting, intermediate-acting, and long-acting). Generally meals should occur at the same time that administered insulin reaches its peak effect. Insulin requirements can vary widely among individuals, so dosages must be adjusted to an individual's needs.

Clients with diabetes who become hyperglycemic, perhaps because of hospitalization or an infection (at home or in the hospital), may need insulin coverage in addition to their regular insulin. This is often referred to as sliding-scale insulin. The amount of insulin given will vary with the blood values or (in some instances), with the glucose in the urine, which roughly approximates blood glucose levels. The latter method is still used in many areas, but it is generally a poor way to monitor blood glucose. If at all possible, urine glucose tests should not be used to determine insulin dosages. There may be some variation between urine glucose tests; therefore, they should not be

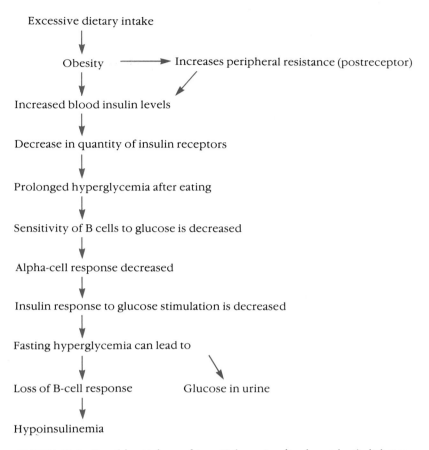

Excessive dietary intake

Obesity ⟶ Increases peripheral resistance (postreceptor)

Increased blood insulin levels

Decrease in quantity of insulin receptors

Prolonged hyperglycemia after eating

Sensitivity of B cells to glucose is decreased

Alpha-cell response decreased

Insulin response to glucose stimulation is decreased

Fasting hyperglycemia can lead to

Loss of B-cell response   Glucose in urine

Hypoinsulinemia

FIGURE 50-1   Possible etiology of type II (non–insulin dependent) diabetes.

TABLE 50-2   Symptoms of hypoglycemia and hyperglycemia

Persons administering insulin should be aware of the symptoms of hypoglycemia and hyperglycemia and know what action to take if they occur.

Hypoglycemia: Increased anxiety, blurred vision, chilly sensation, cold sweating, pallor, confusion, difficulty in concentrating, drowsiness, headache, nausea, increased pulse rate, shakiness, increased weakness, increased appetite	Hyperglycemia: Drowsiness; red, dry skin; fruity breath odor; anorexia; abdominal pain; nausea, vomiting; dry mouth; increased urination; rapid, deep breathing; unusual thirst; rapid weight loss

used interchangeably for urine glucose monitoring. (See box on urine tests.)

Dietary intake, physical activity, and the client's glucose tolerance are all taken into consideration when insulin doses are established. Insulin dosages should not be considered to be a fixed regimen; the dosage may need to be adjusted as a result of physical growth (child growing into adulthood), illness, stress, the development of antiinsulin antibodies, concomitant administration of certain medications, or changes in exercise and diet. Treatment programs need to be reviewed and adjusted as necessary, with the physician, nurse, and client working closely to manage the hyperglycemia and if possible, avoid its complications.

Insulin is given subcutaneously (or intravenously for regular insulin only). It cannot be given by mouth because it is destroyed by digestive enzymes. Regular insulin is usually given about 15 to 30 minutes before meals.

Insulin pumps and new devices. Portable insulin pumps have improved the metabolic state of some type I clients who did not have adequate diabetic control after intensive dietary restrictions and multiple daily injections of insulin. The insulin pump is a battery-operated pump connected to a small computer that is programmed to give small amounts of insulin per hour. It does not analyze the blood glucose level; however, it is programmed based on the individual's daily insulin needs, diet, and

GLUCOSE URINE TESTING

NAME OF TEST	PROCEDURE	COLOR RANGE	RESULTS
Chemstrip uG	Dip strip in urine, compare color to chart at 2 minutes.	Buff, green to dark blue	0, 1/10%, 1/4%, 1/2%, 1%, 2%, 3%, 5%
Clinistix	Dip strip in urine, compare color at 10 seconds.	Buff to dark purple	0, light (0.1%), medium, dark
Clinitest 2-Drop method	Add 2 drops of urine to 10 drops water in a test tube. Add a Clinitest tablet and watch reaction. Wait 15 seconds after boiling stops, shake tube and compare color to chart.	Blue, green, brown to orange	0, 1/2%, 1%, 2%, 3%, 5%
Clinitest 5-Drop method	Add 5 drops of urine to 10 drops of water in test tube. Add Clinitest tablet and watch reaction. Wait 15 seconds after boiling stops, shake tube and compare color to chart.	Blue, green, brown to orange	0, 1/4%, 1/2%, 3/4%, 1%, 2%
Diastix	Dip strip in urine, wait 60 seconds and compare color to chart.	Light blue, green to brown	0, 1/10%, 1/4%, 1/2%, 1%, 2%
Tes-Tape	Dip strip in urine, wait 60 seconds and compare color to chart.	Yellow to green	0, 1/10%, 1/4%, 1/2%, 2%

The urine glucose percentages are generally equivalent to the following; 1/10% = 100 mg/dl; 1/4% = 150 mg/dl; 1/2% = 500 mg/dl; 3/4% = 750 mg/dl; 1% = 1000 mg/dl; 2% = 2000 mg/dl; 3% = 3000 mg/dl; 5% = 5000 mg/dl.

Note that the above tests do not always report the same ranges of urinary glucose. For example, only Chemstrip uG and Clinitest 5-Drop report 3% and 5%, whereas Tes-Tape does not report 3/4% or 1% values. The only product that reports the 3/4% value is Clinitest-5 Drop. The nurse is therefore cautioned about substituting one test for another without being aware of the test limitations.

Urinary ketones (acetone, acetoacetic acid, and beta-hydroxybutyric acid) are found in the urine when fats are not properly metabolized in the body. Their presence is indicative of poorly controlled diabetes, ketonemia and diabetic acidosis (ketoacidosis) caused by a lack of available insulin. This is seen primarily in individuals with insulin dependent diabetes. The tests for urinary ketones include Acetest Tablets, Chemstrip K or uGK, Ketostix, and Keto-Diastix. Chemstrip uGK and Keto-Diastix measure both glucose and ketones by means of separate areas on the same strip.

Many drugs can cause urine discoloration thus interfering with the reading of the urine tests. Phenytoin (Dilantin), phenazopyridine (Pyridium), metronidazole (Flagyl), methyldopa (Aldomet), rifampin (Rifadin), and riboflavin are a few of the drugs that may cause test interference. Clients taking these medications will need to resort to blood testing as an alternative.

physical exercise. The client can also push a button that releases a bolus dose to cover each meal consumed. Although the pumps are effective and useful in clients who are properly trained, health care professionals need to be aware of several problems associated with them. Malfunction of the infusion of insulin may occur because of battery failure, and defects in the tubing may cause leakage of insulin solution or may block the infusion tub-ing. Therefore it is vitally important to teach the client to change the infusion set and battery. Clients must be highly motivated and educated in the handling of insulin pumps. The client should be capable of keeping records and following specific procedures, and should be willing to perform blood tests daily or more often. Also, these pumps are very expensive. Therefore insulin pumps currently are not recommended for every type I diabetic.

Needleless injectors, such as the Vitajet, Medi-jector, and Precijet 50 are also available. These devices are expensive and appear to have limited usefulness in practice. Many devices are also available for the visually impaired or blind client with diabetes. Information on injection aids for the blind may be obtained from state and national associations for the blind, such as the American Foundation for the Blind.

The future may hold some exciting new methods of insulin administration. Research is underway for a nasal spray insulin, insulin in a transdermal patch, and transplantation of the beta cells of the pancreas. Although periodic releases of information are available from time to time, these areas of exploration should be closely monitored.

Pregnancy safety. FDA category not established. Insulin is the drug of choice for control of diabetes in pregnancy. Insulin requirements may drop for 24 to 72 hours following delivery and slowly return to prepregnancy levels in about 6 weeks.

NURSING CONSIDERATIONS

Assessment. A comprehensive nursing history is necessary for the nurse to help the client manage his or her diabetic state. This is as essential for the newly diagnosed client with diabetes as it is for the client who is seeking reassurance that they are managing their diabetes appropriately or for readjustment of the therapeutic regimen because of stress, illness, change of life-style, or noncompliance.

Determine the client's daily exercise, dietary management and preferences, and understanding of diabetes and its control. Also note any physical impairments, such as decreased manual dexterity and limitations of vision, that would impede the self-administration of insulin. Because the cost of insulin, injection equipment, and blood and urine testing equipment can be considerable, assess the client's financial status and health insurance coverage and locate alternative resources if necessary. Clients with certain religious affiliations (such as Jewish or Islamic clients) prefer not to use pork insulin because their dietary codes involve the avoidance of pork.

Intervention. Note that all insulin preparations are stable as long as the vials are protected from heat or cold. Vials of insoluble preparations (all except regular insulin) should be rotated between the hands and inverted end-to-end several times before a dose is withdrawn. A vial should not be shaken vigorously or the suspension made to foam.

Use a properly calibrated syringe for insulin. For doses of less than 50 units of U-100, use a low-dose syringe (50 units of U-100/0.5 ml). The decreased diameter of the barrel of the syringe results in the calibrations being further apart, which enhances accuracy of measurement. Avoid bubbles in the solution because the displacement of a few units of insulin, particularly with U-100 insulin, can alter the actual dose that the client receives.

Administer the insulin subcutaneously, using a 25- or 26-gauge needle, with the length of the needle determined by the client's size. A ⅜ to ⅝ inch needle is usually used, and the injection is administered at 90 degree angle in a large fold of skin that has been gently pinched up. Alternately, the injection may be inserted at a 30 to 45 degree angle at the base of the fold of skin.

Understand that only the regular form of insulin may be injected by the intravenous route. Insulin adsorption onto plastic intravenous infusion administration sites removes up to 80% of an insulin dose; most often not less than 20% to 50% of a dose is removed by adsorption. The adsorption on the tubing surface occurs within 1 hour and requires individual client monitoring of insulin needs. Saturation of the adsorption sites on the tubing requires special care when changing the tubing for reexposure to the insulin and further monitoring of client needs. When insulin is administered as an infusion, use an intravenous pump for accurate administration.

Education. Teach clients about insulin administration and instruct them in urine and blood glucose monitoring so they can adjust insulin doses when their urine or blood levels are above normal limits. Instruct the client in the administration of insulin, including the type of insulin, the proper storage of insulin, the disposal of syringes, and rotation of the injection site.

Unopened vials of insulin should be stored under refrigeration. When a client is using a vial of insulin it is *not* necessary to store it in the refrigerator.

Be sure the patient understands that frequent urine testing and serum glucose monitoring are necessary to achieve insulin control. Stress compliance with the understanding that insulin helps to control hyperglycemia but is not a cure for diabetes.

Instruct clients about signs and symptoms of hypoglycemia that can occur secondary to insulin dosage. Dosage adjustment may be necessary to compensate for the hypoglycemia. The hypoglycemic individual should have a carbohydrate with a high sugar content (such as fruit juice) promptly, and the physician should be notified. If the patient is conscious, orange juice, candy, or a lump of sugar can be given. Early symptoms of hypoglycemia are fatigue, headache, drowsiness, lassitude, tremulousness, or nausea. Late symptoms are weakness, sweating, tremors, or nervousness. Observe the client at night for excessive restlessness and profuse sweating.

Teach clients to assess for signs of hyperglycemia: thirst, polyuria, drowsiness, flushed skin, fruity odor to breath, and unconsciousness. Instruct the family to have insulin available for administration and to observe the client closely after insulin has been given.

Discuss the following with the client and family to prevent recurrences of ketoacidosis:
- Use a regimented pattern of diabetic control.
- Never omit antidiabetic drugs, particularly when a secondary illness is manifested.
- Consume clear liquids and eat smaller meals when illness occurs.
- When ill, frequently test urine for ketones and sugar.

EFFECTS OF COMMONLY ABUSED DRUGS ON DIABETIC MANAGEMENT

Many drugs can increase or decrease blood glucose levels, but rarely are the commonly abused drugs reviewed in relation to diabetes. Because substance abuse by the client with diabetes can be very problematic, the most commonly abused drugs are reviewed here.

ALCOHOL

Alcohol promotes hypoglycemia; blocks the formation, storage, and release of glycogen. It also may interact with many other drugs, including oral hypoglycemic agents such as chlorpropamide. In alcoholics who have decreased their food intake, alcohol can cause a serious drop in blood glucose levels, leading to a need for acute intervention.

CNS STIMULANTS

Amphetamines, sympathomimetics, anorexics, cocaine, psychedelic drugs, and others may result in hyperglycemia and an increase in liver glycogen breakdown. Large amounts of caffeine in products such as coffee, tea, and cola drinks can also increase blood glucose levels.

MARIJUANA

Marijuana may increase appetite and food consumption. Heavy use may produce a glucose intolerance leading to hyperglycemia.

CIGARETTES

Nicotine in cigarettes is a potent vasoconstrictor. It can decrease the absorption of subcutaneous insulin or increase the person's insulin requirements by 15% to 20%. Cigarette smoking can cause a drop of 1 to 2 degrees in skin temperature. It also is a risk factor for the development of diabetic nephropathy.

ABUSE OF CNS-ACTING DRUGS

CNS-acting drugs (such as stimulants, depressants, sedative-hypnotics, opiates, marijuana, alcohol) can impair judgment and alter perceptions (time, place) and thus interfere with the individual's control of the diabetic state.

SUGAR-FREE PRESCRIPTION AND OVER-THE-COUNTER MEDICATIONS

Advise clients to always read the labels or check with their pharmacists before purchasing medications. The sugar contents of both prescription and over-the-counter medications are changed often by the manufacturer, so the best advice is to check the list of contents every time medication is purchased. The following is a selected listing of medications that are currently sugar-free:

ANTACIDS, ANTIFLATULENTS

Di-Gel Liquid	Alka-Seltzer	Maalox
Riopan-Plus	Maalox	Suspension
Pepto-Bismol	Therapeutic	Concentrate
Silain-Gel Liquid	Gelusil Liquid	Mylanta Liquid
	WinGel Liquid	Titralac

ANTIDEPRESSANTS, ANTIPSYCHOTICS

Aventyl HCl Liquid	Lithium Citrate Syrup
Sinequan Oral Concentrate	Mellaril Concentrate
Serentil Concentrate	Thorazine Concentrate

ANTIHISTAMINES, DECONGESTANTS

Bayhistine Elixir	Dimetapp Elixir
Bromophen Elixir	Novahistine Elixir

COUGH MEDICINES

Cerose DM Expectorant	Codimal DM Syrup
Conar Suspension	Hycomine Syrup
Tuss-Ornade Liquid	Tricodene Liquid

DRUGS COMMONLY REPORTED TO CAUSE HYPERGLYCEMIA

chlorthalidone (Hygroton)
corticosteroids
diazoxide (Proglycem, Hyperstat)
furosemide (Lasix)
Estrogens (birth control tablets, estrogen replacement)
epinephrine-type drugs (sympathomimetics or decongestants in cold preparations, diet pills)
nicotinic acid (in large doses)
phenytoin (Dilantin)
thyroid preparations
thiazide diuretics
caffeine (large quantities)
cyclophosphamide (Cytoxan)
ethacrynic acid (Edecrin)
asparaginase (Elspar)
morphine
nicotine (smoking)
lithium (Lithane)

ndx Selected Nursing Diagnoses for Clients Receiving Insulin

Nursing diagnosis	Outcome criteria	Nursing interventions
Knowledge deficit related to newly prescribed diabetic medication (insulin)	Client and family will: Demonstrate correctly appropriate storage, handling, and administration of insulin Be familiar with the signs and symptoms of insulin reaction/hypoglycemic reaction and appropriate response Understand the different insulin preparations and appropriate adjustment of drug therapy Be aware of possible side effects or adverse reactions to insulin	Administer insulin as prescribed. Teach the client and family: The function and importance of therapy Technique of blood (or urine) glucose monitoring and adjusting insulin appropriately Proper technique of administration Need for lifelong dietary and drug management The differences between the three forms of insulin How to correctly calculate dosages Proper storage and handling of insulin Importance of rotating sites to minimize adverse local reactions Signs and symptoms of insulin/hypoglycemic reaction and appropriate management Help client establish and maintain a monitoring record of blood (or urine) glucose and insulin administration. Advise client to wear or carry a medical identification tag, bracelet, or card. Provide client with a list of drugs and conditions that may alter insulin requirements.
Knowledge deficit related to newly diagnosed diabetes	Client and family will: Demonstrate an understanding of diabetes, its therapy and complications, and measures to minimize or prevent complications	Assess the understanding and level of intelligence of client and family. Determine educational needs and desires. Provide information regarding the pathophysiology of diabetes and the function of insulin. Explain methods and goals of diet and drug therapy. Explain function and purpose of tests. Answer questions and clarify misconceptions. Provide resources for further learning and support (American Diabetics Association [ADA], Juvenile Diabetics Foundation [JDF], and others).

Continued.

Selected Nursing Diagnoses for Clients Receiving Insulin—cont'd

Nursing diagnosis	Outcome criteria	Nursing interventions
Altered nutrition related to hyperglycemia or hypoglycemia or insulin administration	Client will: Achieve control of blood glucose and maintain desired nutritional intake Client and family will: Demonstrate knowledge of appropriate diabetic diet and modifications of dietary practices	Administer insulin as prescribed Teach client and family: Correct method of blood (or urine) glucose monitoring Signs, symptoms, and treatment for hyperglycemia and hypoglycemia Importance of balanced diabetic diet to control diabetes Provide dietary instruction and counseling in appropriate diet. Assist client and family in planning a sample diet.
Alteration in body image related to insulin dependence	Client and family will: Verbalize feelings and concerns Understand disease and measures of control Client will: Maintain, as much as possible, prediagnosis activities	Encourage client and family to express feelings and concerns. Determine assets and strengths. Determine, with client and family, strategies for managing areas of difficulty or concern. Provide resources for further learning and support (ADA, JDF, others). Be alert for signs of nonacceptance or difficulties such as noncompliance or denial.
Feelings of powerlessness related to perceived lack of personal control	Client and family will: Identify those areas of diabetes that are possible to control and participate in decision making related to diabetic management	Assess client and family coping patterns and support mechanisms. Assess client and family perceptions related to diagnosis. Allow and encourage expression of concerns and fears. Encourage client and family participation in therapy planning and implementation.

- Notify the physician of secondary illness, nausea and vomiting, fever, inability to eat, or inability to control blood glucose levels. Inform the family and client that the following factors may lead to diabetic ketoacidosis: insulin dependent diabetes mellitus, omission of insulin, infections, cerebrovascular accidents (stroke), myocardial infarction, pregnancy, trauma, surgery, and stress (especially emotional).

Teach the client the following about combining insulins and preparing syringes: When mixing insulins, draw regular insulin into the syringe first to avoid contamination of the regular insulin vial with the other insulin admixture. The interaction of regular and NPH insulin occurs within 15 minutes after mixing and then will remain at this stability for 30 days at room temperature and 90 days if refrigerated. Regular and lente mixtures require up to 24 hours for the interaction to reach a stable level of consistent response; if premixed in the same syringe, their activity is also 30 days at room temperature and 90 days under refrigeration. Clients stabilized on this premixed insulin will have a different response if they inject the insulin separately from each component. Dosage errors are avoided by not changing the injection order of mixing insulins or changing the model of needles, brands of syringes, or sources of insulins.

Instruct the client in the planned rotation of injection sites. Observe for **lipodystrophies,** abnormal accumulations of fat, and avoid such skin lesions.

Note that the abdomen is the area of rapid subcutaneous absorption patterns for insulin, followed by the upper arm, with intermediate absorption rate; the slowest rate is in the thigh. Physical activity in the client accelerates absorption, especially in the injected limb.

Teach the client that alternating the insulin injection

sites from the leg to the abdomen or arm has the effect of accelerating the absorption of insulin and diminishing the postprandial rise in plasma glucose. Varying the insulin injection sites within the same anatomic region rather than between different regions may diminish daily fluctuations or variations in insulin absorption and in metabolic control in insulin-dependent diabetic patients.

Inform the client that an important part of insulin control is diet therapy. The dietitian and the meal preparer must be included in the total care of the client with diabetes. Before clients are discharged, they must be able to verbalize and understand their diet therapy and be willing to participate in meal planning.

Caution clients against the ingestion of alcohol, since hypoglycemia could result. If alcohol is consumed, their insulin dosage may be reduced, since alcohol potentiates the hypoglycemic effect of insulin.

Emphasize that proper urine testing is important in determining correct insulin dosage. Whichever method is used, the client should test the second voided specimen. Urine should be tested before each meal.

At all times the client should carry a medical identification that describes the therapeutic regimen.

Evaluation. Monitor blood glucose levels frequently in the client with diabetes. Recently developed products, such as Chemstrip and Dextrostix, allow for blood glucose monitoring at home. The home glucose-monitoring devices are for clients with diabetes. They are much more reliable than urine glucose tests and facilitate tighter control of blood sugar levels.

Urine glucose testing is a much more commonly done assessment, although it is an indirect measurement of the client's glycemic status because of individual differences in the renal threshold for glucose. Usually glucose spillage into the urine occurs at blood levels of 160 to 180 mg/100 ml, but it may be higher in elderly clients or lower in children and pregnant women. Therefore it may not correlate well with serum glucose levels. See the box on p. 800 for various agents used for the testing of urine glucose levels. The maintenance of euglycemia (70 to 140 mg/100 ml) indicates the appropriate dosage of insulin for the client.

ORAL HYPOGLYCEMIC AGENTS

In the early days of insulin therapy, many attempts were made to obtain a preparation of insulin that remained active after oral administration. None were successful, and it is unlikely that any can be, since both polypeptides and proteins (which compose insulin) are susceptible to destruction in the gastrointestinal tract and are poorly absorbed in an intact state.

However, certain drugs have been found to have blood glucose-lowering or "insulin-like" action when given by mouth. They are principally the group of sulfonylureas. These compounds were originally discovered after observing that some of the antibacterial sulfonamides had hypoglycemic effects. Although these drugs are sometimes called "oral insulins," this definitely is incorrect, since chemically they are completely different from insulin. They also differ from insulin in origin and mode of action. Table 50-3 lists the agents that are available for clinical practice.

Mechanism of action. They enhance the release of insulin from the beta cells in the pancreas, decrease liver glycogenolysis and gluconeogenesis, and increase the sensitivity to insulin in body tissues. Therefore they reduce blood glucose concentration in persons with a functioning pancreas. Antidiuretic effect—chlorpropamide increases the effect of low levels of antidiuretic hormone present in persons with central diabetes insipidus.

Indications. For the treatment of non–insulin dependent diabetes mellitus (type II) in persons whose diabetes cannot be controlled by diet only.

Pharmacokinetics. See Table 50-4.

Side effects/adverse reactions. See Table 50-5.

Significant drug interactions. The following interactions may occur when the oral hypoglycemic agents are given with the drugs listed below.

Drug	Possible Effect and Management
alcohol	May result in a disulfiram-type reaction, especially with chlorpropamide. The reaction may include stomach pain, nausea, vomiting, flushing, lowered blood glucose levels, and headaches. Avoid concurrent administration if possible. This problem is reported less often with glipizide and glyburide.
anticoagulants, oral, coumarin or indandione	Initially increased serum levels of both drugs may be seen but with chronic therapy, a reduction in plasma levels and effectiveness of the anticoagulant is reported. An increased serum level of the oral hypoglycemic agent may result in increased effects and toxicity because of a decrease in liver metabolism. Monitor closely because one or both drugs may require a dosage adjustment.
chloramphenicol (Chloromycetin), guanethidine (Ismelin), insulin, monoamine oxidase (MAO) inhibitors, salicylates or sulfonamides	May result in an increase in hypoglycemic effect. Monitor closely, since dosage adjustments may be necessary.
beta adrenergic blocking agents (including ophthalmics)	Increases risk of hyperglycemia or hypoglycemia. See drug interaction for insulin for further information.

TABLE 50-3   Hypoglycemic Agents

Drug/trade name(s)	Remarks
FIRST GENERATION SULFONYLUREAS	
acetohexamide (Dymelor, Dimelor♣)	Intermediate-acting drug. Metabolized to active metabolite (hydroxyhexamide) in liver; a potent hypoglycemic agent. Use with caution in renal insufficiency.
chlorpropamide (Diabinese, Apo-Chlorpropamide♣)	Longest acting oral hypoglycemic. Generally more potent and more toxic than other drugs. Also indicated in treatment of polyuria of diabetes insipidus; may enhance effects of ADH. Usually given as single morning dose with food.
tolazamide (Tolinase, Ronase)	Intermediate-acting drug. Alternative drug for persons who do not respond to other sulfonylureas.
tolbutamide (Orinase, Mobenol♣)	Short-acting drug. Mildly goitrogenic at high doses and may reduce radioactive iodide uptake after prolonged administration without producing clinical hypothyroidism. It is rapidly metabolized to inactive metabolites. Useful in clients with kidney disease.
SECOND GENERATION SULFONUREAS	
glipizide (Glucotrol)	Highly protein bound. Metabolized by liver to inactive metabolites.
glyburide (DiaBeta, Euglucon♣, Micronase)	Highly protein bound (99%). Produces less active metabolites that are excreted by kidneys.
APPROXIMATELY EQUIVALENT THERAPEUTIC DOSES	
acetohexamide, 500 mg chlorpropamide, 250 mg glipizide, 5 mg glyburide, 5 mg tolazamide, 250 tolbutamide, 1000 mg	

TABLE 50-4   Pharmacokinetics of Oral Hypoglycemic Agents

Drug	Absorption orally	Half-life (hours)	Time to peak effect (hours)	Duration of action (hours)	Metabolism (in liver)	Excretion
acetohexamide	Good	6-8	1-3	12-24	To active metabolite	Kidneys (80%) bile (10%)
chlorpropamide	Good	25-60	3-6	24-48 or more	80% activity or metabolites unknown	Kidneys (6%-60% unchanged)
glipizide	Good	2-4	1-3	12-24	To inactive metabolites	Kidneys
glyburide	Good	10	4	24	To inactive metabolites	Kidneys (50%) bile (50%)
tolazamide	Fair (slow)	7	4-8	12-24	To slightly active metabolites	Kidneys (85%)
tolbutamide	Good	5	1-3	6-12	To inactive metabolite	Kidneys (85%) Bile (9%)

acetohexamide tablets (Dimelor, Dymelor)

Adults. Initially, 250 mg orally daily. Adjust dosage gradually until desired effect is achieved. Maximum daily dose is 1.5 g. (In persons requiring doses of 1 g or more, divided doses are recommended.) Usually administered before breakfast and evening meals. Elderly, undernourished, or debilitated clients or persons with impaired renal or liver function require a lower initial dose.

Children. Not effective in insulin dependent diabetes (type I)

Pregnancy safety. FDA category C.

chlorpropamide tablets (Apo-Chlorpropamide, Diabinese M Glucamide)

Adults. Initially 100 to 250 mg orally, once a day. May increase dose gradually by 50 to 125 mg every 7 days until diabetes is under control or the total daily dose reaches 750 mg. Antidiuretic effect—100 to 250 mg orally, once a day. Increase dosage at 2- to 3-day intervals if necessary, up to 500 mg daily. Although the maximum adult dose is 750 mg daily, generally clients who do not respond to 500 mg a day usually will not respond to 750 mg daily. In higher dosage range, divided doses (before breakfast and the evening meal) are recommended.

TABLE 50-5 Hypoglycemic Oral Agents: Side Effects/Adverse Reactions

Side effects*	Adverse reactions†
Most frequent: Diarrhea, dizziness, gas, anorexia, headache, nausea, vomiting, abdominal distress Less frequent/rare: Photosensitivity, rash	Less frequent: Chlorpropamide only—respiratory difficulties (CHF in persons with cardiac problems). Sedation; cramping of muscles; convulsions; edema of face, hands, or ankles; comatose, increased weakness (antidiuretic effect). Rare: Pruritus, jaundice, light colored stools, dark urine (impairment of liver function). Increased fatigue, sore throat, increased temperature, increased bleeding or bruising. Overdosage: Symptoms of hypoglycemia (see insulin side effects/adverse reactions)

*If side effects continue, increase, or disturb the client, the physician should be informed.
†If adverse reactions occur, contact the physician because medical intervention may be necessary.

Elderly. See comment under acetohexamide.
Children. See acetohexamide.
Pregnancy safety. FDA category C.

glipizide tablets (Glucatrol)

Adults. Initially, 5 mg orally daily. The dosage may be increased at 2.5 to 5 mg doses every 7 days until diabetic control is achieved, or the maximum total dose of 40 mg is reached.

Elderly persons or those with kidney or liver impairment should be started at on a daily dose of 2.5 mg. Persons receiving 15 mg daily or more should have the dosage divided in two, before breakfast and evening meals.
Children. Same as acetohexamide.
Pregnancy safety. FDA category C.

glyburide tablets (DiaBeta, Euglucon, Micronase)

Adults. Initially 2.5 to 5 mg orally daily. Increase dosage gradually at no more than 2.5 mg at 7-day intervals until diabetes is under control or the total daily dose reaches 20 mg.

Elderly clients or persons with kidney or liver impairment should start at 1.25 mg daily. Persons receiving 10 mg or more per day should receive a divided dosage, that is, before breakfast and evening meals.
Children. See acetohexamide.
Pregnancy safety. FDA category B

tolazamide tablets (Ronase, Tolinase)

Adults. Initially 100 to 250 mg orally daily in the morning. Dosage may be increased gradually until diabetes is under control or the total maximum daily dose of 1 g is reached. (When more than 500 mg/day is necessary, divide dose and administer before breakfast and evening meals.)
Elderly. See acetohexamide.

Children. See acetohexamide.
Pregnancy safety. FDA category C.

tolbutamide tablets (Apo-Tolbutamide, Mobenol, Oramide, Orinase)

Adults. Administer 500 mg orally once or twice a day. Adjust dosage gradually as necessary until diabetes is under control or the total maximum dose of 3 g per day is reached. Divided doses are recommended, usually before breakfast and evening meals.
Elderly. See acetohexamide.
Children. See acetohexamide.
Pregnancy safety. FDA category C.

NURSING CONSIDERATIONS

Assessment. Do not substitute these agents for insulin in clients with diabetic coma, ketoacidosis, significant ketosis or acidosis, severe burns, infection, or trauma or those undergoing major surgery. They are to be used with caution with clients with adrenal or pituitary insufficiency or renal or hepatic impairment. Consideration should be given to use of oral hypoglycemic agents other than chlorpropamide with clients with cardiac impairment because of chlorpropamide's antidiurectic effects.

Intervention. Remember that the client with diabetes requires close supervision, especially when an oral hypoglycemic agent is tried for the first time.

When converting from insulin to an oral hypoglycemic agent for control of the diabetic status, monitor the client's urine for sugar and acetone three times a day before meals. No transition period is usually required when changing from one hypoglycemic agent to another one, except with chlorpropamide. In the case of chlorpropamide caution should be exercised in the first week because of its prolonged half life, 25 to 60 hours.

Education. Recognize that the need for instruction stressing dietary restriction is even greater for clients receiving oral hypoglycemic agents than for those taking insulin. Remember that these clients should be taught testing for glycosuria and ketonuria, skin care, and signs and symptoms of hypoglycemia and hyperglycemia.

Caution clients about excessive alcohol intake (and medications containing alcohol) when oral sulfonylurea therapy is begun. Alcohol can increase the rate of metabolism of these drugs when there is long-term consumption of excessive quantities.

When clients are switched from insulin to oral sulfonylureas, advise them to perform urine testing frequently during this period.

Teach clients to carry or have access to forms of glucose at all times.

Have the client administer the initial dosage in the morning to decrease nocturnal hypoglycemia. Drugs given with food will decrease any gastric upset.

If the client is taking divided doses of oral sulfonylureas and omits a dose, advise him/her that it should be taken as soon as it is remembered. The missed dose should be administered near the time for the next dose, but they should not be taken together. Administration before meals will maximize postprandial insulin release.

Make the client aware that the administration of these agents has been associated with increased incidence of death from cardiovascular disease compared with treatment with diet alone or diet plus insulin.

Evaluation. Elderly persons tend to be more sensitive to the effects of the oral hypoglycemic agents. Because hypoglycemia may be more difficult to recognize in these clients, they require lower dosages and closer monitoring.

Observe for hypoglycemia in the client who has irregular meal patterns, exercises more than usual, or ingests significant amounts of alcohol; hypoglycemia is more likely in these clients. A moderate life-style is essential to diabetes management. Periods of physiologic or psychologic stress may necessitate a temporary use of insulin.

HYPERGLYCEMIC AGENTS

glucagon (glucagon for injection)

Mechanism of action. Glucagon is a polypeptide hormone secreted by the pancreatic islet alpha cells. Hepatic glycogenolysis is accelerated by glucagon through stimulation of synthesis of cyclic AMP (cAMP) and increasing phosphorylase kinase activity. The resulting blood glucose elevations are caused by both increased breakdown of glycogen to glucose and glycogen synthesis inhibition. Glucagon stimulates liver gluconeogenesis through promotion of amino acid uptake and then conversion of the amino acids to precursors of glucose. Hepatic and adipose tissue lipolysis is enhanced by activation of adenyl cyclase, producing free fatty acids and glycerol, which stimulate ketogenesis and gluconeogenesis.

Indications. Treatment of hypoglycemia in clients with diabetes or during insulin shock therapy. It is only effective if liver glycogen is available; thus it is ineffective in chronic states of hypoglycemia or starvation and adrenal insufficiency.

Used as an adjunct to barium in gastrointestinal radiography. It produces relaxation of the esophagus, stomach, duodenum, small bowel, and colon (hypotonicity).

Pharmacokinetics. Parenteral medication (intramuscular, intravenous or subcutaneous).

Half-life. 3 to 6 minutes.

Onset of action as diagnostic aid. Intravenous, 0.25 to 2 USP units, within 1 minute intramuscular, 1 USP unit, within 8 to 10 minutes; 2 USP units, within 4 to 7 minutes

Duration of effect as diagnostic aid. Intravenous, 0.25 to 0.5 USP units, 9 to 17 minutes; 2 USP units, between 22 and 25 minutes; intramuscular, 1 USP unit, between 12 and 27 minutes; 2 USP units, within 21 to 32 minutes.

Metabolism. Liver mainly; some by kidneys, in body tissues and plasma.

Excretion. Kidneys.

Side effects/adverse reactions. Not usually severe. Less frequent include rash, dizziness, respiratory distress (allergic reaction), nausea or vomiting.

Significant drug interactions. None.

Dosage and administration

Adults. For antihypoglycemic effects—Administer 0.5 to 1 USP units (0.5 to 1 mg) of glucagon, intramuscular, intravenous or subcutaneous. May repeat in 20 minutes if necessary.

Diagnostic aid—0.25 to 2 USP units (0.25 to 2 mg) of glucagon intramuscular or intravenous. Dosage depends on area to be examined, desired onset of action, and duration of effect. For example, to examine the colon, it is recommended that 2 USP units be given intramuscular approximately 10 minutes before the procedure.

Children. Antihypoglycemic effect—Administer 0.025 USP unit (0.025 mg) per kg up to a maximum dose of 1 USP unit (1 mg), intramuscular, intravenous, or subcutaneous; dose may be repeated in 20 minutes if needed.

Pregnancy safety. FDA category B.

NURSING CONSIDERATIONS

Assessment. It is important for the nurse to recognize the symptoms of hypoglycemia: anxiousness, irritability, nervousness, weakness, shakiness, inability to concentrate; perspiring, cool, pale skin; hunger, nausea, headache; and unconsciousness.

Intervention. Administer glucagon for hypoglycemia in the unconscious client. After administering, turn the individual on one side to prevent choking and/or aspiration. Inform the physician of the client's status. If the client has not regained consciousness in 5 to 20 minutes, give a second dose and transport the client to the hospital. Intravenous glucose will need to be started if the individual does not respond to the second dose of glucagon. Glucagon and glucose may be given at the same time.

If the client does regain consciousness and can swallow, offer some oral form of sugar followed by a more complex carbohydrate, such as crackers and cheese or a glass of milk. This will help prevent a recurrence of the hypoglycemia before the next meal. If the client is experiencing nausea and vomiting that prevent food intake for more than an hour after the administration of the glucagon, seek medical assistance.

Replace the client's supply of glucagon as soon as possible.

Education. Teach the family and the client how to mix the drug and how to inject properly before the need arises to use glucagon. Advise them to keep supplies on hand and check them frequently to be sure the expiration dates have not passed.

Instruct the client and family about the symptoms of hypoglycemia and the importance of the client ingesting some form of sugar when the symptoms first occur.

diazoxide (Proglycem)

Mechanism of action. Diazoxide administered orally produces a prompt, dose-related increase in blood glucose levels primarily by inhibition of insulin release from the pancreas and an extrapancreatic effect.

Indications. Treatment of hypoglycemia caused by hyperinsulinism, which is caused by an inoperable islet cell adenoma or carcinoma, an extrapancreatic malignancy, islet cell hyperplasia, adenomatosis and nesidioblastosis. It is not indicated for treatment in functional hypoglycemia.

Pharmacokinetics

Absorption. Very good.

Half-life. 21 to 36 hours in normal individual.

Onset of action. Within 1 hour.

Duration of effect. Not longer than 8 hours.

Protein binding. High (more than 90% bound to albumin).

Metabolism. Liver.

Excretion. Kidneys.

Side effects/adverse reactions. See Table 50-6.

Significant drug interactions. The following interactions may occur when diazoxide is given with the drugs listed below.

Drug	Possible Effect and Management
Anticonvulsants, hydantoin (phenytoin)	May decrease or nullify the action of both drugs. Avoid concurrent drug administration.
Medications that induce hypotension (alcohol, diuretics, calcium channel blocking agents, beta adrenergic blocking drugs) and peripheral vasodilators	Concurrent use may cause enhanced severe, hypotensive effect. Monitor closely, since dosage adjustments may be necessary.

Dosage and administration

diazoxide capsules/oral suspension (Proglycem)

Adults. Initially 1 mg/kg every 8 hours; adjust dosage as necessary. Maintenance—3 to 8 mg/kg orally daily; divide into 2 or 3 equal doses and administer every 12 or 8 hours, as indicated. Maximum dose is usually 15 mg/kg/day.

Children. Antihypoglycemic agent—neonates and infants, initially 3.3 mg/kg orally, every 8 hours; adjust dosage according to therapeutic response. Maintenance, 8 to 15 mg/kg orally daily; divide total dose into 2 or 3 equal doses and administer every 12 or 8 hours, as indicated. Children, see usual adult dosage.

Pregnancy safety. FDA category C.

TABLE 50-6   Side Effects/Adverse Reactions of Diazoxide

Side effects*	Adverse reactions†
Less frequent: Taste alterations, constipation, anorexia, nausea, vomiting, abdominal pain With chronic, long term use: Increased hair growth on arms, legs, back, and forehead (hypertrichosis); tremors of hands and fingers, stiffness (caused by extrapyramidal effects)	Most frequent: Decreased urination; edema of hands, feet, or lower extremities; weight gain (because of sodium and water retention) Less frequent: Fast or irregular heart rate Rare: Chest pain, confusion, increased temperature, rash, increased bleeding, bruising, hand numbness Overdose: signs of hyperglycemia—increased drowsiness, red, dry skin, fruity breath odor, anorexia, increased thirst and urination

*If side effects continue, increase, or disturb the client, the physician should be informed.
†If adverse reactions occur, contact the physician because medical intervention may be necessary.

NURSING CONSIDERATIONS

Assessment. Determine whether the client has a sensitivity to thiazide diuretics or other sulfonamide medication because he or she may also be sensitive to diazoxide.

Carefully consider the use of diazoxide in clients with cardiac problems because of its tendency to increase water and sodium retention. Observe clients for swelling of the feet and lower legs, increased weight gain, and decrease in urinary output as signs of fluid retention. Diuretics are sometimes given concurrently to avert these side effects.

Intervention. Since pain may occur at the site of injections, it is recommended that diazoxide be administered intravenously and then only into a peripheral vein by an established intravenous line. Avoid extravasation because it results in cellulitis and pain. Treat conservatively with cold packs if extravasation does occur. Keep the client recumbent during and at least 30 minutes after injection.

Education. Instruct clients in the importance of diet, testing of urine for glucose and ketones, regular visits to the physician, symptoms of hypoglycemia and hyperglycemia, and of not taking other medications unless discussed with the physician.

It is important to monitor the blood and urine glucose levels and check the urine for ketones.

glucose (Glutose, Insta-Glucose)

Mechanism of action. Glucose is a monosaccharide that is absorbed from the intestine and then used, distributed in the body, or stored in the tissues.

Indications. To treat or manage hypoglycemia.

Pharmacokinetics

Absorption. Rapid from gastrointestinal tract.

Distribution. Readily to tissues. Glucose provides 4 calories per gram.

Side effects/adverse reactions. No toxicity reported; some reports of nausea.

Significant drug interactions. None.

Dosage and administration

Adults. Approximately 10 to 20 grams administered orally; may repeat in 10 minutes if necessary. Glucose must be swallowed to produce an effect. It is not absorbed from the buccal cavity.

Children. Only under instructions of the physician.

KEY TERMS

gluconeogenesis, page 796
insulin dependent diabetes mellitus, page 796
lipodystrophies, page 804
non–insulin dependent diabetes mellitus, page 796
type I diabetes mellitus, page 796
type II diabetes mellitus, page 796

BIBLIOGRAPHY

Alexander CM: Intensive insulin therapy: multiple injections v pump, Consultant 25(6):25, 1985.

American Hospital Formulary Service: AHFS drug information '87, Bethesda, Md, 1987, American Society of Hospital Pharmacists, Inc.

Armstrong N: Coping with diabetes mellitus: a full-time job, Nurs Clin North Am 22(3):559, 1987.

Baker DE and others: The second generation sulfonylureas: glipizide and glyburide, Diabetes Educ 11(3):29, 1985.

Balik B and others: Diabetes and the school-aged child, MCN 11(5):324, 1986.

Beaser RS: Oral hypoglycemics: optimizing the benefits of new drugs and old, Consultant 24(10):82, 1984.

Billie DA: Tailoring your diabetic patient's care plan to fit his life-style, Nursing 16(2):54, 1986.

Bovington MM and others: Management of the patient with diabetes mellitus during surgery or illness, Nurs Clin North Am 18(4):661, 1983.

Bournemann M and others: Insulin-induced hypoglycemia in Type I diabetics, Diabetes Educ 10(3):13, 1984.

Branson HK: Defining diabetic emergencies, Emergency 9(7):16, 1987

Braunwald E and others, ed: Harrison's principles of internal medicine, ed 11, New York, 1987, McGraw-Hill Book Co.

Campbell RK: Blind diabetics, Am Pharm NS21(1):31, 1981.

Campbell RK: Diabetes and the pharmacist: a self-paced training program, ed 2, 1986, Ames Division, Miles Laboratories, Inc.

Campbell RK: The effect of temperature on insulin, Diabetes, Educ 12(1):80, 1986.

Campbell RK: Humulin BR, a new insulin for use in external insulin pumps, Diabetes 12(4):392, 1986.

Campbell RK: Understanding, monitoring, and preventing long-term complications of diabetes. Module 4 of Pharmaceutical services for patients with diabetes, 1986. American Pharmaceutical Association and Eli Lilly and Co.

Cassmeyer VL: Preventing, recognizing, and treating diabetic shock, Nursinglife 7(1):33, 1987.

Childs EP: Insulin infusion pumps, Nursing 83 (11):55, 1983.

Christman C and others: Diabetes: new names, new test, new diet, Nursing 17(1):34, 1987.

Crigler-Meringola ED: Making life sweet again for the elderly diabetic by gearing your teaching and interventions to his needs, Nursing 14(4):60, 1984.

Davidson DE: Handbook of nonprescription drugs, ed 8, Washington, DC 1986, American Pharmaceutical Association and The National Professional Society of Pharmacists.

Donohue-Porter P: Insulin-dependent diabetes mellitus . . . educating the diabetic person regarding diabetes and infections, Nurs Clin North Am 20(1):191, 1985.

Eisenbarth GS and others: Type I diabetes: clinical implications of autoimmunity, Hosp Pract 22(9):167, 1987.

Fain JA: Insulin administration in diabetic ketoacidosis, Focus Crit Care 13(6):47, 1986.

Feldman JM: Sulfonylureas: mechanisms of interactions; strategies to reduce them, Consultant 24(7):37, 1984.

Flavin K and others: The pharmacologic repertoire . . . drugs for diabetes, Am J Nurs 86(11):1244, 1986.

Francisco GE and others: Geriatric pharmacology: the use of oral hypoglycemics. Part 2, Hosp Formul 20(1):103, 1985.

Fredholm N and others: Insulin pumps: the patients' verdict, Am J Nurs 84(1):36, 1984.

Fuller E: Physicians ask about type II diabetes, Patient Care 18(18):18, 1984.

Fuller E: Glycemic emergencies: emergency handbook. Part 6, Patient Care 19(17):151, 1985.

Gever LN: Administering glucagon in an emergency, Nursing 15(1):66, 1985.

Gossel TA: Blood glucose self-testing products, US Pharmacist 11(3):91, 1986.

Graber AL: When you trade pills for insulin, Diabetes Forecast 40(1):40, 1987.

Gray DL: Elderly diabetics and urine testing, Geriatr Nurs. 6(6):332, 1985.

Haire-Joshu D and others: Contrasting Type I and Type II diabetes, Am J Nurs 86(11):1240, 1986.

Haire-Joshu D and others: Intensive conventional insulin therapy, Am J Nurs 86(11):1251, 1986.

Herfindal ET and Hirschman JL: Clinical pharmacy and therapeutics, ed 3, Baltimore, Md, 1984, Williams & Wilkins.

Hernandez CMG: Surgery and diabetes: minimizing the risks, Am J Nurs 87(6):788, 1987.

Huff PS: Second generation oral hypoglycemic agents, US Pharmacist 10(2):51, 1985.

Jeffries NR and others: Diabetes education and the older patient, Diabetes Educ 11(2):27, 1985.

Jenny JL: Differences in adaptation to diabetes between insulin-dependent and non-insulin-dependent patients: implications for patient education, Patient Educ Couns 8(1):39, 1986.

Jovanovic L: Utilizing high technology to achieve optimal insulin delivery for Type 1 diabetic patients, Caring 4(1):35, 1985.

Kastrup EK, ed: Facts and comparisons, St Louis, 1988, JB Lippincott Co.

Katzung BG: Basic and clinical pharmacology, ed 3, Norwalk, Conn, 1987, Appleton & Lange.

Knott SP and others: Teaching self-injection to diabetics: an easier and more effective way, Nursing 14(1):57, 1984.

Krosnick A: Diabetes treatment update: switching to biosynthetic human insulin, Consultant 27(7):78, 1987.

Levin PA and others: Diabetes mellitus: customizing management, Hosp Pract 19(10):137, 1984.

Morrisett WR: The role of sulfonylureas in managing type II diabetes, Physician Assist 8(8):33, 1984.

Pepper GA: What's news in insulin? Nurse Pract 11(1):62, 1986.

Popovich NG The new role of the pharmacist in the management of diabetes mellitus, W Lafayette, Ind, 1985, Purdue University.

Price MJ: Insulin and oral hypoglycemic agents, Nurs Clin North Am 18(4):687, 1983.

Samanta A and others: Management of the acutely ill diabetic patient, Intensive Care Nurs 1(4):194, 1986.

Schade DS: Choosing patients for insulin pump therapy, Hosp Ther 12(8):65, 1987.

Siperstein MD: Type II diabetes: some problems in diagnosis and treatment, Hosp Pract 20(3):55, 1985.

Skelly AH and others: Insulin allergy in clinical practice, Nurse Pract 12(4):16, 1987.

Stock PL: Action stat! Insulin shock, Nursing 15(4):53, 1985.

Thatcher G: Insulin injections: the case against random rotation, Am J Nurs 85(6):690, 1985.

United States Pharmacopeial Convention: Drug information for the health care provider, ed 8, Rockville, Md, 1988, The Convention.

Whitehouse FW: Diabetes mellitus: current concepts of proper management, Hosp Med 22(5):231, 1986.

Wyngaarden JB and Smith LH: Cecil textbook of medicine, ed 18, Philadelphia, WB Saunders Co.

Yarborough MC and Campbell RK: Developing a diabetes program for your pharmacy. Module 2 Pharmaceutical services for patients with diabetes, American Pharmaceutical Association and Eli Lilly and Co.

UNIT XIII

Drugs Affecting the Reproductive System

CHAPTER

51

Overview of the Female and Male Reproductive Systems

OBJECTIVES

After studying this chapter, the student will be able to:

1. Identify the anterior pituitary gland hormones that influence the female and male reproductive systems.

2. Describe hormonal influences on uterine function during the menstrual cycle.

3. Identify the primary male and female hormones.

4. Describe the effects of estrogen during the proliferative stage.

5. Trace the transport of sperm from production to ejaculation in the male body.

6. Discuss the role that vas deferens ducts play in male sterility.

REPRODUCTION

Reproduction is the sum of genetic and hormonal influences originating from the sexes of a species to perpetuate the species. In human beings, the reproductive process in both sexes is highly complex, involving **follicle-stimulating hormone** (FSH) and **luteinizing hormone** (LH) from the anterior pituitary gland, as well as the hormones from the reproductive systems of the male (**androgens**) and the female (**estrogens** and **progestogens**).

ENDOCRINE GLANDS

The reproductive system of the human female consists of the ovaries, fallopian tubes, uterus, and vagina. The male reproductive system consists of the testes, seminal vesicles, prostate gland, bulbourethral glands, and penis. The reproductive organs of both male and female are mainly under the control of the endocrine glands. The ovaries and testes, known as **gonads**, not only produce ova and sperm cells but also form endocrine secretions that initiate and maintain the secondary sexual characteristics in men and women. The structure and physiologic functions of the pituitary gland are reviewed in Chapter 46; the discussion of the pituitary gland in this chapter is limited to its effect on the female and male reproductive systems.

PITUITARY GONADOTROPIC HORMONES

The gonadotropins or pituitary hormones responsible for the development and maintenance of sexual gland functions are the following:

1. FSH, which stimulates the development of the ovarian (graafian) follicles up to the point of ovulation in

the female; in the male FSH stimulates the development of the seminiferous tubules and promotes spermatogenesis.

2. LH or **interstitial cell–stimulating hormone** (ICSH), which acts in the female to promote the growth of the interstitial cells in the follicle and the

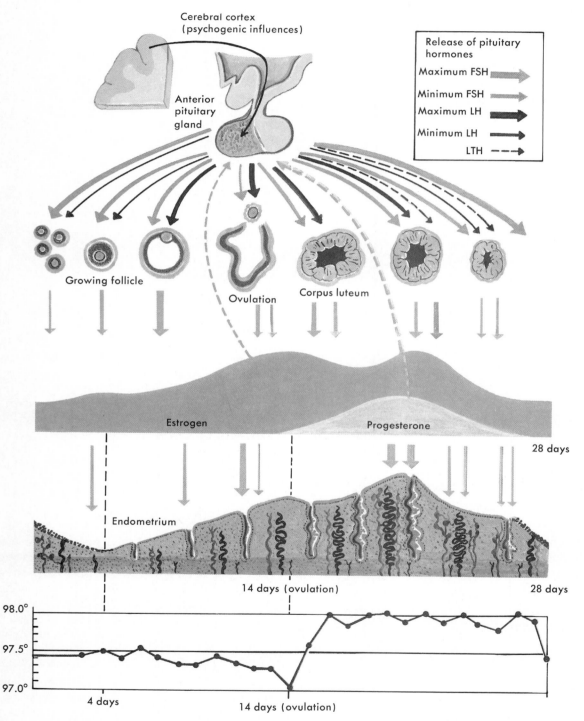

FIGURE 51-1   Effects of pituitary hormones and ovarian hormones on uterine functions during the menstrual cycle. Body temperature fluctuations are also demonstrated.

(From Anthony, C, and Thibodeau, G: Textbook of anatomy and physiology, ed 12, St Louis, 1987, Times Mirror/Mosby College Publishing.)

formation of the corpus luteum; in the male, ICSH stimulates the growth of interstitial cells in the testes and promotes the formation of the hormone androgen, testosterone.

3. **Luteotropic hormone** (LTH) or luteutropin, which is identical with the lactogenic hormone, or prolactin.

In the female, FSH initiates the cycle of events in the ovary. Under the influence of both FSH and LH the graafian follicle grows, matures, secretes estrogen, ovulates, and forms the corpus luteum. LTH promotes the secretory activity of the corpus luteum and the formation of **progesterone.** In the absence of LTH the corpus luteum undergoes regressive changes and fails to make progesterone.

FEMALE SYSTEM

Figure 51-1 illustrates the effects of the pituitary hormones, ovarian hormones, and uterine functions during the menstrual cycle. Body temperature fluctations are also included with this diagram.

Day 1 of the menstrual cycle is the onset of menses, and Day 5 usually signifies the end of menstruation. During this time, FSH is stimulating folicular growth in the ovary and also stimulating the ovary to produce estrogen, which is low at the beginning of the cycle. As estrogen levels increase, FSH levels decrease. The rising estrogen levels are preparing the uterus for a fertilized ovum, which is known as the proliferative stage of the uterus and results in the following:

1. Estrogen stimulates the growth of glandular surface of the **endometrium**, or inner lining of the uterus.

2. Estrogen affects the mucus glands of the cervix to produce a more plentiful, viscous mucus that contains nutrients that can be used by the sperm.

The increasing levels of estrogen also stimulate the pituitary gland to release LH. As FSH is decreasing, LH is increasing. At this time (day 14), **ovulation** occurs when the mature follicle ruptures and releases its ovum. The ovum travels through the fallopian tube to the uterus. Female pelvic organs are shown in Figure 51-2.

The increasing levels of LH will affect the ruptured fol-

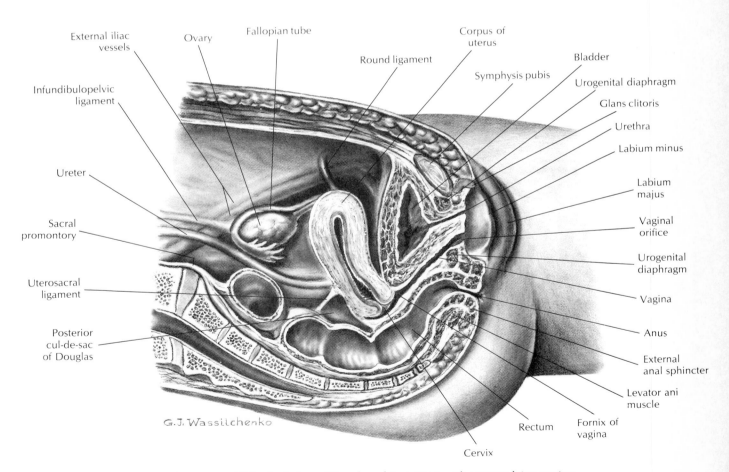

FIGURE 51-2 Midsagittal view of female pelvic organs, with woman lying supine.

(From Bobak and Jensen: Essentials of maternity nursing, ed 2, St Louis, 1987, The CV Mosby Co.)

licle by changing the follicle capsule into the corpus luteum. Under the influence of LH, the corpus luteum releases estrogen and progesterone. In the second phase, or secretory phase, both uterine hormones increase secretion of the glands of the endometrium. If the ovum is fertilized and reaches this area on approximately the eighteenth day of the cycle, it will be able to thrive on the nutrient secretions of the endometrium.

Progesterone has an additional effect: it inhibits the flow of cervical mucus and reduces the thickness of the vaginal lining. But if fertilization does not occur, the pituitary will respond to the increased levels of estrogen and progesterone by shutting off the release of FSH and LH. Without the central stimulation, the corpus luteum cannot produce estrogen or progesterone, so the surface layer of the endometrium will slough off, resulting in menstruation. Figure 51-3 depicts the feedback mechanism of FSH and LH and their main effects on the ovaries.

Most women demonstrate month-to-month variations in their menstrual cycles; therefore ovulation is not always predictable. The previous description of the menstrual cycle is based on a 28-day cycle, but ovulation varies and occurs on different days in different length cycles. Physiologically, this is the primary reason for the unreliability of the rhythm method of contraception, which depends on predicting the day of ovulation based on previous menstrual cycles.

FEMALE SEXUAL RESPONSE

For both males and females, psychic stimulation and local sexual stimulation are necessary for a satisfactory sexual experience. Psychic stimulation may be aided by an individual's erotic thoughts, although sexual desire is also affected by increasing levels of estrogen secretion, especially during the preovulatory period.

Local sexual stimulation causes similar responses in both sexes; that is, massage, increasing stimulation or irritation of the perineal region or sexual organs can result in an enhancement of sexual sensations. In the female, the clitoris is very sensitive, and its stimulation can initiate a sexual sensation. Erectile tissue is located in the **introitus** (vaginal opening) and clitoris areas. This tissue is under parasympathetic nerve control; therefore in early stimulation, the parasympathetic nerves dilate the arteries located in the erectile tissues. Blood collects in the erectile tissue in the area so that the introitus will tighten around the penis, which aids male satisfaction for sexual stimulation, thus leading to ejaculation.

The parasympathetic nerves also signal the Bartholin's glands situated near the labia minora resulting in an increase in mucus secretion inside the introitus. This secretion, in addition to mucus from the vaginal epithelium, serves as a lubricant during sexual intercourse.

The female climax, or orgasm, is reached when the local sexual stimulation reaches the maximum sensation or intensity. It is considered similar to emission and ejaculation in the male and may also help to promote fertilization of the ovum. It has been theorized that orgasm produces a rhythm in the female tract from spinal cord reflexes that increase both uterine and fallopian tube motility and may result in cervical canal dilation for up to 30 minutes. This will allow for easy sperm transport in the female.

The intense sexual sensations that develop during orgasms also result in an increase in muscle tension throughout the body. After the sexual act, this tension subsides into relaxation or feelings of satisfaction, sometimes referred to as resolution.

MALE SYSTEM

The effects of FSH and LH or ICSH in the male were described in the section on pituitary gonadotropic hormones. The effects of ICSH on secretion of testosterone are seen in Figure 51-4. **Testosterone**, an androgen, performs numerous functions, which are described below. FSH from the anterior pituitary gland stimulates the seminiferous tubules to increase production of spermatozoa, while ICSH stimulates the interstitial cells to increase secretion of testosterone. A high level of testosterone will inhibit the pituitary's release of FSH and ICSH.

Testosterone has many functions in the male. It aids in developing and maintaining the male secondary sex characteristics and male accessory organs, such as prostate, seminal vesicles, and bulbourethral glands. Testosterone promotes adult male sexual behavior, as well as regulating metabolism and protein anabolism, that is, growth of bone and skeletal muscles. This hormone affects fluid and electrolyte metabolism, by reabsorbing sodium and water and increasing excretion of potassium. FSH and ICSH secretion is also inhibited from the anterior pituitary by testosterone.

TRANSPORT OF SPERM IN THE MALE

Sperm produced in the testes mature by spending 1 to 3 weeks in the epididymis in the male. The sperm, or seminal fluid, then travels through the epididymis (ducts that lie around the top of the testes) to the vas deferens. The vas deferens, a duct extension of the epididymis, extends over the bladder surface (posteriorly) to the ampulla to form the ejaculatory duct. Sperm can be stored in the vas deferens in excess of one month without loss of fertility depending on sexual activity. Thus a vasectomy, or severing of the vas deferens will make a man sterile primarily because it interrupts the journey of sperm to the ejaculatory duct and urethra. Male pelvic organs and the anatomy of the ejaculatory ducts are shown in Figure 51-5.

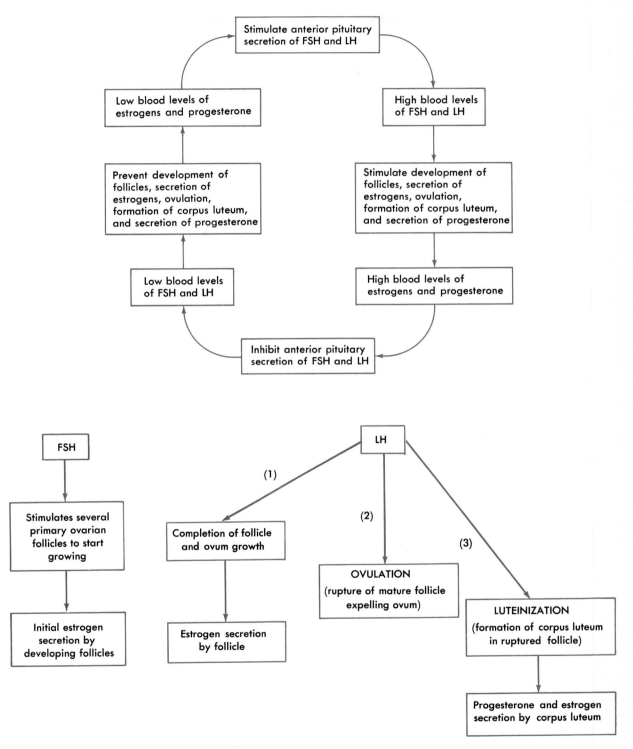

FIGURE 51-3 Feedback mechanism of FSH and LH and their main effects on the ovaries.

(From Anthony, C, and Thibodeau, G: Textbook of anatomy and physiology, ed 12, St Louis, 1987, Times Mirror/Mobsy College Publishing.)

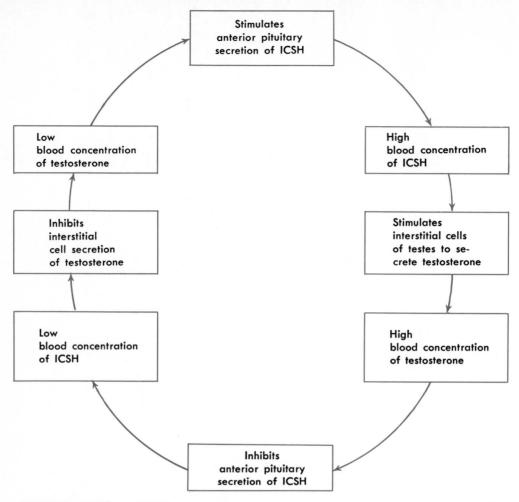

FIGURE 51-4   Effect of ICSH on testosterone.

(From Anthony, C, and Thibodeau, G: Textbook of anatomy and physiology, ed 12, St Louis, 1987, Times Mirror/Mosby College Publishing.)

MALE SEXUAL RESPONSE

Penile erection is a parasympathetic response that consists of dilation of the arteries and arterioles in the penis, which compresses the veins in this area. Thus more blood enters the penis than leaves, it becomes larger, and erection occurs. Emission and **ejaculation** of the sperm or semen is a reflex response. The stimulus that initiated erection will also help to move the sperm and secretions (**semen**) from the genital ducts to the prostatic urethra. Orgasm, the climax of the sexual act, moves the semen through the ejaculatory ducts. During coitus, the sperm can be transferred from male to female.

Later in life gonadal function ceases. Women undergo menopause or cessation of menses, and men have a decrease in sex hormone production, which is sometimes called the male climacteric.

KEY TERMS

androgen, page 815
ejaculation, page 820
endometrium, page 817
estrogens, page 815
follicle-stimulating hormone (FSH), page 815
gonads, page 815
interstitial cell-stimulating hormone (ICSH), page 816
introitus, page 818
luteinizing hormone (LH), page 815
luteotropic hormone (LTH), page 817
ovulation, page 817
progesterone, page 817
progestogens, page 815
semen, page 820
testosterone, page 818

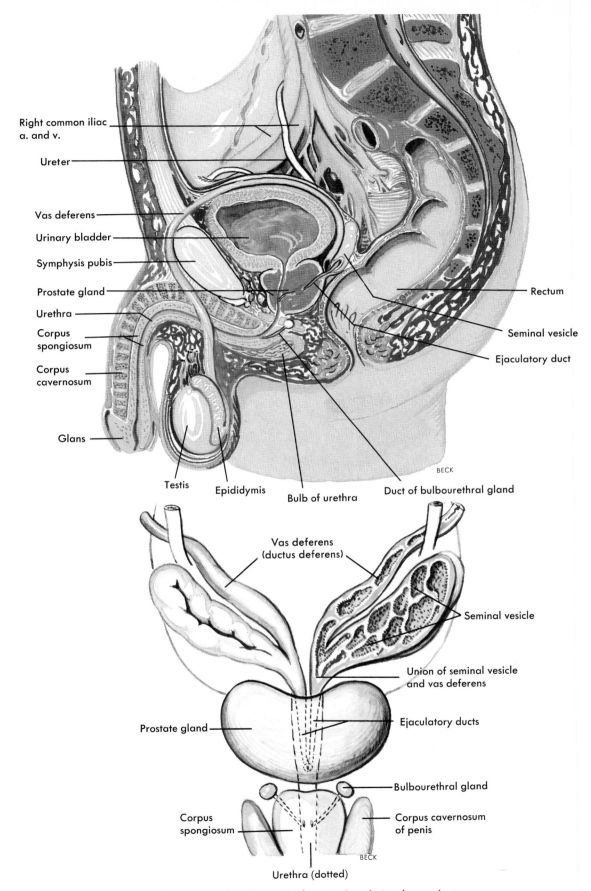

FIGURE 51-5 Male pelvic organs (median sagittal section) and ejaculatory ducts.

(From Anthony, C, and Thibodeau, G: Textbook of anatomy and physiology, ed 12, St Louis, 1987, Times Mirror/Mosby College Publishing.)

BIBLIOGRAPHY

Anthony CP and Thibodeau GA: Textbook of anatomy and physiology, ed 12, 1987, St Louis, Times Mirror/Mosby College Publishing.

Endacott J and others: Female and male climacteric, Nursing (Oxford) 2(14):399, 1983.

Guyton AC: Textbook of medical physiology, ed 7, Philadelphia, 1986, WB Saunders Co.

Maxwell M: Male reproductive physiology, Nurs Mirror 157(20):24, 1983.

Tyson JE: Reproductive endocrinology: new problems call for new solutions, Diagn Med 7(4):24, 1984.

CHAPTER 52

Drugs Affecting the Female Reproductive System

OBJECTIVES

After studying this chapter, the student will be able to:

1. List drugs affecting the female reproductive system.

2. Describe the source and action of chorionic gonadotropin.

3. Describe the function of the primary female sex hormones.

4. Describe side effects/adverse reactions of estrogens and progestins.

5. Compare and contrast monophasic, biphasic, and triphasic oral contraceptives.

6. Apply nursing considerations to the client receiving drugs affecting the female reproductive system.

Drugs affecting the female reproductive system include synthetic and natural substances, such as gonadotropin-releasing hormone, nonpituitary chorionic gonadotropin, menotropins, female sex hormones, oral contraceptives, and ovulatory stimulants and drugs used for infertility.

GONADOTROPIN-RELEASING HORMONE

Gonadotropin-releasing hormone or gonadorelin is a synthetic hormone used to diagnose **hypogonadism** in males and females. It is under investigation for use in the treatment of delayed puberty, amenorrhea, and infertility, alone and with other medications.

gonadorelin (Factrel and LHRH)

Mechanism of action. This synthetic hormone acts like LH/FSH-releasing hormone, that is, it stimulates the release of luteinizing hormone (LH) and follicle-stimulating hormone (FSH) from the anterior pituitary. It is used to detect a decreased response of LH/FSH caused by various medical conditions.

Indication. An aid to diagnosis of hypogonadism in the male or female.

Pharmacokinetics

Administration. Subcutaneous or intravenous

Distribution. Half-life is several minutes, and duration of action is 3 to 5 hours.

Excretion. Kidney in metabolite form
Side effects/adverse reactions. See Table 52-1.
Significant drug interactions. None
Dosage and administration
gonadorelin hydrochloride for injection
Adults. 100 µg (0.1 mg) subcutaneous or intravenous. Whenever possible, gonadorelin should be administered within the early follicular phase of the female's menstrual cycle.
Children (12 years or older). 100 µg (0.1 mg) subcutaneous or intravenous.
Pregnancy safety. FDA category B

NURSING CONSIDERATIONS

Education. The nurse should follow the manufacturer's insert for test procedures and explain procedures to the client. In general, baseline blood samples are drawn, an injection given, several blood samples are drawn at specific times and analyzed for serum LH concentrations.

Evaluation. A test result within the normal range indicates the presence of functional pituitary gonadotropins. A below normal or absent LH response following a test

TABLE 52-1   Side Effects/Adverse Reactions of Female Hormones/Drugs

Drug(s)	Side effects*	Adverse reactions
gonadorelin (Factrel and LHRH)	If given SC; pain and pruritus at site of injection	
gonodotropin, chorionic (A.P.L., Pregnyl, Follutein, Antuitrin✱)	Less frequent: headaches, increased anxiety, depression, edema of lower extremities, breast enlargement, increased weakness	More frequent; abdominal bloating, pain Less frequent in boys only: oily skin or acne, penis and testes enlargement, increase in height and growth of pubic hair
	Warning: may also see an increase in multiple births and, possibly, arterial thrombolism	
menotropins (Pergonal)	Less frequent for males: breast enlargement Warning: same as above	More frequent for females only; abdominal bloating or pain
estrogens (various manufacturers)	Most frequent: red or irritated skin with transdermal product Most frequent but can be reduced with continuous therapy: stomach cramps or gas, anorexia, nausea, enlarged and increased breast tenderness in both sexes Less frequent: brown skin spots, mild diarrhea, dizziness, increase in headaches or migraines, unable to tolerate contact lenses, vomiting, decrease in male sexual drive, increase in female sexual drive	In males, the large doses used to treat cancer increase the risk for a myocardial infarction, pulmonary embolism, and/or thrombophlebitis. Severe hypercalcemia reported in cancer patients with bone metastases treated with estrogens. Most frequent: edema of lower extremities Less frequent/rare: change in menstrual bleeding, spotting, break-through bleeding, excessive bleeding, and complete termination of bleeding have been reported; urinary incontinence, sudden ataxia, headaches (which may be severe), chest, groin or leg pain, sudden respiratory difficulties, slurred speech, visual changes, increased weakness in arms or legs, hypertension, chorea, breast lumps, jaundice, rash, abdominal or side pains
progesterone progestins (various manufacturers)	Most frequent: weight and appetite changes; redness or pain at site if injection; edema of lower extremities, increased weakness Less frequent/rare: oily skin (acne), brown skin spots, increase in body hair including facial hair, nausea, alopecia (some), increase in breast tenderness	Most frequent: changes in menstrual bleeding patterns Less frequent/rare: visual changes (double vision, bulging eyes, visual loss); sudden headaches or ataxia, severe headaches; pain in chest, leg (calf), or groin, slurred speech; depression; increased weakness or pain in extremities (blood clot); loss of breath, jaundice; lactation; rash; pruritus, abdominal or side pain

*If side effects continue, increase, or disturb the patient, the physician should be informed.
†If adverse reactions occur, contact the physician because medical intervention may be necessary.

TABLE 52-1   Side Effects/Adverse Reactions of Female Hormones/Drugs—cont'd

Drug(s)	Side effects*	Adverse reactions
contraceptives, oral	Most frequent (may decrease with chronic therapy): stomach cramps or gas, oily skin (acne) during first 3 months of therapy; anorexia, nausea, edema of lower extremities, weight gain, increased weakness Less frequent/rare: brown spots on skin, mild diarrhea, dizziness, increase in headaches or migraines, increase in hair on face and body, photosensitivity, unable to tolerate contact lenses, increased irritability, alopecia (some), significant increase or decline in sexual desire, vomiting	*Need immediate medical attention:* hemoptysis (coughing up blood); sudden, severe headaches or ataxia, sudden loss of breath, slurred speech or visual changes; pain in leg, chest, or groin, weakness or pain in extremities Less frequent/rare: visual changes (double vision, bulging eyes, visual loss), changes in menstrual bleeding patterns, faintness, increased frequency or painful urination, hypertension, chorea, lactation or breast lumps, depression, paresthesias, pain or cold fingers or toes, pain in abdomen or side, jaundice, rash, increased tenderness, swelling or pain in upper abdominal section (hepatoma), development of dark colored moles (malignant melanoma), increase in vaginal discharge (candidiasis)
clomiphene citrate (clomid, Serophene)	Most frequent: hot flashes Less frequent/rare: dizziness; headaches; nausea; vomiting, depression; increased anxiety; restlessness, weakness; breast feels uncomfortable in female, enlarged in males	Most frequent: abdominal pain or gas, visual disturbances (blurred vision) Rare: visual disturbances eyes sensitive to light, double vision, decline in vision (see light flashes), jaundice of eyes and skin

*If side effects continue, increase, or disturb the patient, the physician should be informed.
†If adverse reactions occur, contact the physician because medical intervention may be necessary.

dose frequently signifies a pituitary or hypothalamic dysfunction.

In men over 50 years, basal LH and FSH concentrations increase with age; LH response after gonadorelin administration is delayed and may be diminished in older males.

In menopausal and postmenopausal females, basal LH concentrations are elevated so the peak LH increases are exaggerated compared to concentrations in premenopausal women.

If side effects persist or increase in severity, the physician must be notified. No serious side effects have been reported; however, itching or pain may occur at the site of injection.

NONPITUITARY CHORIONIC GONADOTROPIN

Certain gonadotropic substances formed by the placenta during pregnancy are extracted from the urine of pregnant women. The action of human chorionic gonadotropin is nearly equivalent to the pituitary's luteinizing hormone (LH) with little or no follicle-stimulating effects. Although there is therapeutic use in both sexes, the discussion of nonpituitary chorionic gonadotropin and menotropins is in this chapter.

gonadotropin, chorionic (A.P.L, Pregnyl, Follutein, Antuitrin♣)

Mechanism of action. Used to make up for a deficiency in luteinizing hormone

Indications

1. Prepubertal cryptorchidism and hypogonadotropic hypogonadism: stimulates androgen production in the testes, which may enhance the descent of the testes and increase development of the secondary sex characteristics in the male
2. Diagnostic aid for hypogonadism
3. Corpus luteum insufficiency: stimulates progesterone production by the ovaries to promote the development and maintenance of the corpus luteum
4. Female infertility: substitute for LH in individuals with insufficient gonadotropin levels to cause ovulation in ovarian follicles that were prepared by FSH

Pharmacokinetics

Administration. Intramuscular

Distribution. Biphasic half-life is 5.6 and 24 hours. In females, ovulation usually occurs within 18 hours of administration.

Excretion. Kidneys, approximately 10% to 12% within 24 hours

Side effects/adverse reactions. See Table 52-1.

Significant drug interactions. None

Dosage and administration
chorionic gonadotropin for injection

Adults. Hypogonadotropic hypogonadism in males: 1000 to 4000 U intramuscular two to three times a week for several weeks to months. In some cases, it is administered indefinitely if a response occurs. Induction of ovulation: 5000 to 10,000 U intramuscular following last dose of menotropins or from 5 to 7 days after the last dose of clomiphene.

Children. Prepubertal cryptorchidism: 1000 to 5000 U intramuscular two to three times a week for up to several weeks (discontinued when desired response is achieved). Treatment for longer than 2 months is not recommended.

Pregnancy safety. FDA category C

NURSING CONSIDERATIONS

Assessment. It should be determined whether the client has a preexisting pituitary hypertrophy or tumor, because the medication will stimulate growth of the tumor. The drug should not be used with individuals with precocious puberty, prostatic cancer, abnormal vaginal bleeding, fibroids, ovarian cysts, or thrombophlebitis.

The drug should be used with careful monitoring in clients with asthma or those with cardiac disease and renal dysfunction, because of the possibility of fluid retention.

Intervention. Reconstitute with the 10 ml of sodium chloride provided by the manufacturer.

Education. Provide support for the client and spouse throughout their attempt to achieve fertility. Societal and familial pressures create stress for them as a couple and individually. They should be advised that gonadotropin-induced ovulation is expensive and may result in multiple births. Since success is difficult to achieve, the couple should be counseled on alternatives such as adoption.

If the physician has requested daily recording of woman's temperature, inform the client about the relationship of temperature to ovulation and its importance for the appropriate timing of intercourse to enhance the chance of pregnancy. Daily intercourse from the day before chorionic gonadotropin is given until ovulation occurs is advised. Ovulation usually occurs 18 hours after the medication is given.

Prepubertal males receiving chorionic gonadotropin should be prepared for an acceleration in sexual development and supported through self-image changes.

Evaluation. The client's progress should be assessed periodically. Although the regimen is lengthy and time consuming, the client should be supported and encouraged to cooperate.

To monitor the female client receiving the drug for induction of ovulation, an estrogen excretion determina-

tion should be done 1 week after the initiation of each course of the drug. Examinations of the cervical mucus will determine if there has been follicular maturation or ovulation.

Hyperstimulation of the ovaries may be indicated by stomach or pelvic pain and should be reported to the physician immediately. A pelvic examination may be done to evaluate ovarian size.

To monitor the male client for hypogonadism, serum testosterones may be measured periodically to assess progress. Sperm counts and determinations of sperm mobility should also be done.

MENOTROPINS

Menotropin is human pituitary gonadotropin, that is, a purified preparation of follicle-stimulating hormone (FSH) and luteinizing hormone (LH) obtained from the urine of postmenopausal women.

menotropins (Pergonal)

Mechanism of action. Action is equivalent to effects produced by FSH and LH. It stimulates the development of the ovarian follicle, causes ovulation, and may stimulate corpus luteum development. In males, it stimulates sperm production.

Indications

1. Treatment of female infertility, usually used in combination with chorionic gonadotropin. This is usually reserved for individuals that have not responded to other treatment modalities, such as clomiphene or bromocriptine.

2. Treatment of male infertility, used in combination with chorionic gonadotropin to stimulate spermatogenesis in primary or secondary hypogonadotropic hypogonadism.

Pharmacokinetics

Administration. Intramuscular

Distribution. Ovulation usually occurs 18 hours after administration.

Excretion. Kidneys

Side effects/adverse reactions. See Table 52-1.

Significant drug interactions. None

Dosage and administration

menotropins for injection

Adults. Induction of ovulation: 1 ampule (75 units of FSH and LH activity) intramuscular daily for 9 to 12 days. If necessary, dosage may be increased by 1 or 2 ampules every 4 to 5 days, up to a maximum of 6 ampules. When estrogen activity is equal to or greater than a normal individual, chorionic gonadotropin is administered a day after the last dose of menotropins. Hypogonadotropic hypogonadism in males: 1 ampule intramuscular three times weekly (in addition to chorionic gonadotropin twice a week) for a minimum of 4 months, following pretreatment with chorionic gonadotropin for 4 to 6 months. An increase in dose may be necessary if an increase in spermatogenesis does not occur within 4 months.

Pregnancy safety. Not established

NURSING CONSIDERATIONS

See chorionic gonadotropin.

FEMALE SEX HORMONES (OVARIAN HORMONES)

The ovaries, in addition to providing ova, manufacture and secrete steroid female hormones that control secondary sex characteristics, the reproductive cycle, and the growth and development of the accessory reproductive organs in the female. Two main types of hormones are secreted by the ovary: (1) the follicular or estrogenic hormones (estrogens) produced by the cells of the developing graafian follicle and (2) the luteal or progestational hormones (porgestogens) derived from the corpus luteum that is formed in the ovary from the ruptured follicle. The periodic cycling of the female sex hormones depends on an interaction between FSH and LH with the ovarian hormones estrogen and progesterone. This results in a menstrual cycle that normally continues throughout life, except for pregnancy, until menopause. While estrogens are primarily secreted by the ovarian follicles, some may also be secreted by the adrenals, corpus luteum, placenta, and testes.

ESTROGENS

Estrogens are available from natural sources (the urine of pregnant mares) and in conjugated dosage forms and have been synthetically formulated. Examples of natural steroidal estrogens include estradiol, estrone, and estriol; nonsteroidal estrogens include diethylstilbestrol (DES), dienestrol, and chlorotrianisene.

estrogen (various manufacturers)

Mechanism of action. Estrogen increases the synthesis of DNA, RNA, and protein in estrogen-responsive tissues. Elevated estrogen serum levels will inhibit the secretion of FSH and LH from the pituitary. This results in inhibition of lactation, ovulation, and the development of a proliferative endometrium.

Indications
1. Treatment of estrogen deficiency: estrogen replacement is recommended for atrophic vaginitis, female hypogonadism, insufficient primary ovarian function, abnormal uterine bleeding, and severe vasomotor symptoms in menopause.

2. Treatment of breast carcinoma: used in metastatic breast carcinomas in postmenopausal women with tumor estrogen-negative receptors; also in selected male breast carcinomas.
3. Treatment of advanced prostatic carcinomas
4. Prophylaxis of osteoporosis in postmenopausal women: may be effective in reducing or preventing bone mass loss and fractures in estrogen insufficiency.

Pharmacokinetics
Distribution. Protein bound
Metabolism. Liver
Excretion. Kidneys
Side effects/adverse reactions. See Table 52-1.
Significant drug interactions. The following interactions may occur when estrogens are given with the drugs listed below.

Drug	Possible Effect and Management
bromocriptine	Estrogens may result in amenorrhea, interfering with bromocriptine's therapeutic effect. Concurrent use is not recommended.
hepatotoxic drugs, especially dantrolene	Estrogens increase risk of inducing hepatotoxicity; females over 35 years old are at increased risk. Avoid concurrent drug administration if at all possible.
smoking tobacco	Tobacco smoking increases the risk of serious cardiac adverse reactions, such as cerebrovascular accident (CVA), transient ischemic attacks (TIAs), thrombophlebitis, and pulmonary embolism. The risk is higher in women over 35 years old who smoke; therefore, they should be advised against smoking while undergoing estrogen therapy.

Precautions
1. The risk of endometrial cancer increases with prolonged use of estrogens in postmenopausal women. However, low-dose estrogen given cyclically or the use of a progestin (concurrently or sequentially) may reduce the risk of inducing endometrial cancer.
2. Animal data indicate an increased risk of breast cancer with long-term estrogen administration. Estrogen should be used with caution in women with a family history of breast cancer, breast nodules, fibrocystic disease, or abnormal mammogram reports.
3. Males treated with estrogens should be checked regularly for the development of male breast carcinomas.
4. Estrogens should not be administered during pregnancy because studies indicate an increased risk of congenital malformations, especially with DES.
5. Estrogens are excreted in breast milk and will also inhibit lactation; therefore, administration of estrogens to nursing women is not recommended.

Dosage and administration

1. The lowest effective dose of estrogens should be administered for the shortest time period to reduce the possibility of serious adverse effects. When continuous therapy is required, the physician should reevaluate the client at least every 6 months.

2. To avoid overstimulation of estrogen-sensitive tissues, a cyclic dosing schedule of 3 weeks of estrogen administration and 1 week off or of adding progestin for the last 10 to 13 days of the cycle will most closely approximate the natural hormonal cycle. This is not the schedule for oophorectomized individuals or clients with cancer who are receiving hormonal therapy.

3. High-dosage or long-term therapy with estrogen should not be discontinued abruptly. It is recommended that medication be reduced over a 3- to 6-month period.

4. Estradiol and estrone are naturally occurring steroidal estrogens that are principal endogenous estrogens. Estradiol is available alone or synthetically as estradiol cypionate, estradiol valerate, ethinyl estradiol, and polyestradiol phosphate. The primary pharmacologic effects of all the estogens are similar.

5. Conjugated estrogens are a mixture of estrogenic substances, especially estrone and equilin. They are available in oral tablet, parenteral, and vaginal cream dosage formulations. Dosage must be individualized according to the diagnosis and the client's therapeutic response, for example, vasomotor symptoms associated with menopause. The usual oral adult dose is 0.3 to 1.25 mg orally daily for 21 days, followed by 7 days without estrogen. Some women may even require higher doses to achieve an adequate therapeutic response.

6. Diethylstilbestrol (DES) is a synthetic nonsteroidal estrogen that has the same indications primarily as the other estrogens. In addition, it has been used as a postcoital contraceptive after rape or incest to prevent pregnancy, although this use has not been approved in the United States. DES 25 mg orally twice a day for 5 days is given within 24 hours (at most 72 hours) following coitus. DES should not be administered to pregnant women since it will not terminate pregnancy but it can cause very serious fetal toxicities. Congenital defects plus an increased risk of developing a rare vaginal or cervical cancer in later life has been reported in females exposed in utero to DES. A higher incidence of genital tract abnormalities has also been reported in males exposed in utero to DES.

7. Transdermal estradiol (Estraderm) is also available in the United States. It is usually used to supply estrogen in conditions of estrogen deficiency. Applied topically to intact skin, 50 μg (0.05 mg) or 100 μg (0.1 mg) daily is released from the transdermal patch. It should be applied twice weekly for 3 weeks, followed by 1 week without medication; then the cycle is repeated.

Pregnancy safety. FDA category X

NURSING CONSIDERATIONS

Assessment. The drug is contraindicated if breast cancer is known or suspected, or if the client has abnormal or undiagnosed vaginal bleeding.

Estrogens are to be used with caution with the client who has hypercalcemia, active thrombophlebitis, or a history of thrombophlebitis secondary to estrogen use.

Intervention. Estrogens are usually administered on a cycle of 3 weeks on and 1 week off the medication, except for males.

Administer the intramuscular forms slowly to minimize client discomfort. Large muscles, such as the gluteus maximus, should be used to maximize absorption.

Administer intravenous estrogens slowly; vaginal burning occurs if administered too rapidly.

Vaginal forms should be administered at bedtime to enhance absorption. Sanitary napkins or panty shields may be used to protect clothing from stains.

Education. Assist the client in exploring her concerns about the risks of taking estrogens. Provide her with information regarding the occurrence of cardiovascular disease and cancer in relationship to her age, smoking habits, and other health characteristics. Encourage the client to read the patient package insert carefully and then discuss any concerns she might have.

Advise the client to have regular physical examinations, which should include a pelvic and breast examination and a Pap smear, every 6 to 12 months during treatment.

The client should be advised to stop the medication immediately and contact her physician if she suspects she is pregnant.

Caution the client that smoking increases the incidence of serious side effects of the drug, particularly in women over 35.

Instruct the client to notify her health provider in the instance of severe headache, blurred or lost vision (which may possible signal stroke), or symptoms of chest pain, shortness of breath, or leg pain, which may indicate thromboembolism elsewhere in the body. The physician should also be informed of severe abdominal pain or mass, jaundice, severe mental depression, or unusual bleeding. Instructions should be provided for monthly self-examination of the breasts and any lumps found should be reported to the physician. Mammograms should be done annually.

Nausea, frequently occurring at the beginning of therapy, usually ceases after 1 or 2 weeks. Seldom severe, it can be controlled by taking the medication with meals.

Advise the client to weigh one or two times weekly and report a sharp increase in weight or other signs of fluid retention, such as swollen ankles, puffy eyelids, and "tight" rings. A low-sodium diet and diuretic may be prescribed to control these symptoms.

Bleeding after estrogen withdrawal is expected. Explain to postmenopausal women that such bleeding does not indicate that a state of fertility has returned.

Instruct users with diabetes to report positive urine or blood sugar tests so the dosage of their antidiabetic medications can be adjusted.

Forewarn male clients of estrogen-induced feminization and impotence, which will disappear when therapy terminates. Advise clients of the increased risk of myocardial infarction, pulmonary embolism, and thrombophlebitis while undergoing estrogen therapy.

Instruct clients taking prescribed conjugated estrogens and esterified estrogens for osteoporosis prophylaxis to increase their intake of calcium and vitamin D and to engage in regular weight-bearing exercise such as walking.

When applying the transdermal form of the drug, the client should wash her hands before and after application of the patch. It should be applied to the abdomen on clean, dry, intact skin without hair. The sites on the abdomen should be rotated to prevent application to any site more frequently than every 7 days. The patch should not be applied to the breasts or to the waistline where clothing might cause the patch to become loose. The patch should be pressed into place for 10 seconds and then examined to ensure all the edges are tight. If the patch becomes loose, it may be reapplied or a new one may be applied.

Evaluation. Blood pressure should be monitored weekly. Hepatic function studies should be done every 6 to 12 months. Males treated with estrogens should be checked regularly for the development of breast carcinomas.

PROGESTERONE AND PROGESTINS

Progesterone is a naturally occurring progestin secreted from the corpus luteum mainly during the latter half of the menstrual cycle. The pituitary luteinizing hormone stimulates the synthesizing and secretion of progesterone from the **corpus luteum.** Progesterone may also be formed from steroid precursors available in the ovaries, testes, adrenal cortex, and placenta.

Progesterone and synthetic progestins have similar pharmacologic effects in the body. Progestins were developed because progesterone was not always satisfactory in therapeutic application. It often had to be administered in large oral dosages plus its injections were often painful and caused local reactions. The progestins provided many advantages for the client, as well as the physician. Their greater potency lowered the dose of progestins necessary to produce an equivalent response to progesterone; there is a longer duration of action and, with some products, an effective oral/sublingual dosage form.

progesterone/progestins (various manufacturers)

Mechanism of action. Progesterone and progestens cause induction of biochemical changes in the endometrium to prepare for the implantation and nourishment of the embryo. They supplement the action of estrogen in its effects on the uterus and mammary glands. They cause suppression of ovulation during pregnancy and relaxation of the uterine smooth muscles. They also increase the synthesis of DNA and RNA; large doses will inhibit the secretion of luteinizing hormone (LH) from the anterior pituitary.

Indications
1. Treatment of female hormonal imbalance of amenorrhea and dysmenorrhea
2. Treatment of endometriosis
3. Diagnosis for endogenous estrogen deficiency
4. Treatment of specific carcinomas
5. Prevention of pregnancy

Pharmacokinetics

Metabolism. Mainly by the liver

Excretion. Kidneys

Side effects/adverse reactions. See Table 52-1.

Significant drug interactions. Progestins may cause amenorrhea and/or excessive lactation, which will interfere with bromocriptine's therapeutic effect. Concurrent use is not recommended.

Precautions
1. Congenital anomalies have been reported with the use of progestins during the first 4 months of pregnancy. They should not be used as diagnostic tests for pregnancy.
2. Progestins are excreted in breast milk; therefore, they are not recommended for use by nursing women.

Dosage and administration

hydroxprogesterone caproate injection (Delalutin, Duralutin, Pro-Depo). Treatment of hormone imbalance, primary or secondary amenorrhea, or functional bleeding of the uterus: administer 375 mg intramuscular during the menstrual cycle. After 4 days of bleeding or, if no bleeding, 3 weeks (21 days) after the injection, start the cyclic therapy schedule. This cyclic schedule should be repeated every 28 days for four cycles with close monitoring of the client.*

*Cyclic schedule is 20 mg intramuscular estradiol valerate on first day of cycle, then 250 mg hy droxyprogesterone caproate injection and 5 mg estradiol valerate intramuscular on day 15 of the cycle.

For additional dosage schedules for other indications, the reader is referred to the current package insert or USP-DI.

medroxyprogesterone (Amen, Curretab, Provera)

For amenorrhea secondary to female hormone imbalance: Give 5 to 10 mg orally daily for 5 to 10 days. This dosage may be started anytime during the cycle.

To treat functional bleeding of the uterus: Give same dosage as stated above, but start therapy on day 16 or day 21 of the menstrual cycle. When therapy is discontinued, bleeding occurs within 3 to 7 days afterward.

Injectable dosage form, to treat renal or endometrial cancer: 400 mg to 1 g intramuscular initially. Repeat dose at 1-week intervals. Maintenance dosage: When improvement is noted or the disease state is stabilized, maintenance with a 400 mg/month dosage has been possible.

megestrol (Megace)

To treat breast cancer: 40 mg orally, four times daily

To treat endometrial cancer: 10 to 80 mg orally four times daily. Allow 2 months of therapy with megestrol before evaluating its effectiveness. Maximum daily dosage is 800 mg daily.

norethindrone (Micronor, Norlutim, Nor-Q.D.)

To treat amenorrhea or functional bleeding of the uterus caused by a female hormone imbalance: 5 to 20 mg orally from day 5 through day 25 of the menstrual cycle

To treat endometriosis: 10 mg orally daily for 14 days; then the daily dosage may be increased by 5 mg daily (every 2 weeks) up to a maximum of 30 mg/day. Continue this dosage for 6 to 9 months.

Contraceptive: 350μg (0.35 mg) orally daily, starting on first day of menstrual cycle

norethindrone acetate tablets (Aygestin, Norlutate)

For treatment of amenorrhea or functional bleeding of the uterus caused by female hormone imbalance: 2.5 to 10 mg orally from day 5 through day 25 of the menstrual cycle

To treat endometriosis: 5 mg daily for 2 weeks; then increase daily dosage by 2.5 mg every 2 weeks up to a maximum of 15 mg/day. Continue therapy for 6 to 9 months.

The potency of norethindrone acetate is double that of norethindrone, but the other features are the same.

norgestrel tablet (Ovrette). Contraceptive: 75 μg (0.75 mg) orally daily starting first day of menstrual cycle and continued daily thereafter

progesterone injection in oil (Gesterol, Femotrone in Oil, Progestaject). To treat amenorrhea caused by female hormone imbalance: 5 to 10 mg intramuscular daily for 6 to 8 days, usually starting 8 to 10 days before menses. Bleeding will usually occur within 2 to 3 days following the last injection; normal menstrual cycles may then follow. Discontinue injections if menstrual bleeding occurs during the series of injections.

Pregnancy safety. FDA category X

NURSING CONSIDERATIONS

Assessment. It should be determined that the client does not have preexisting cancer of the breast or reproductive tract, suspected pregnancy, abnormal and undiagnosed vaginal bleeding, a history of active thrombophlebitis, or hepatic dysfunction or conditions for which progestins are contraindicated.

Because of the tendency of progestins to cause fluid retention that might aggravate these conditions, these drugs should be used cautiously in clients with asthma, a history of active depression, epilepsy, cardiac insufficiency, or renal dysfunction. Clients with a history of ectopic pregnancy or diabetes should also be monitored carefully for any unusual symptoms.

Intervention. Give oil preparations deep intramuscular.

A low-sodium diet and diuretic may be prescribed to control symptoms of fluid retention, such as swollen ankles and puffy eyelids.

Education. Encourage the client to read the package insert carefully and then discuss with her health care provider any concerns she might have. Advise the client to have regular physical examinations, which should include a pelvic and breast examination and a Pap smear, every 6 to 12 months during treatment.

Instruct client to notify her health provider in the instance of severe headache, blurred or lost vision (which may possibly signal stroke), and symptoms of chest pain, shortness of breath, or leg pain, which may indicate thromboembolism elsewhere in the body. The physician should also be informed of severe abdominal pain or mass, jaundice, severe mental depression, or unusual bleeding. Instructions should be provided for monthly self-examination of the breasts, and any lumps found should be reported to the physician.

Instruct users with diabetes to report positive urine tests so that the dosage of their antidiabetic medications can be adjusted.

If progestins are used for contraceptive purposes, instruct the client to take the drug at same time of the day, every day of the year. The tablets need to be kept in their original containers. It is best to keep an extra month's supply, replacing it with the new container of tablets purchased each month. This will always ensure a fresh supply.

The client should be advised to discontinue the medication immediately and notify the physician if she suspects she is pregnant. Pregnancy should be avoided during the first month of administration of progestins and for at least 3 months after they have been discontinued. Contraceptives should be used during this time.

Evaluation. Since progestins may cause glucose intolerance, diabetic clients may need an adjustment in insulin or oral hypoglycemic dosage.

If fluid retention occurs, a low sodium diet may reduce edema.

Undesirable effects are usually mild or absent during short-term use. However, as the duration of progestion increases, the number and severity of adverse effects also increase. Evaluation for these effects must continue as long as therapy continues.

ORAL CONTRACEPTIVES

Oral contraception is the most effective form of birth control presently available. "The pill" is a fixed combination of estrogen and progestin that was approved for marketing by the FDA in 1960. Since then millions of women have used oral contraceptives, and through experience an enormous amount of information about effectiveness, estrogen-progestin combination, the relationship of risk factors to major side effects, and mortality have been collected. Performing a thorough history and physical examination, selecting an appropriate contraceptive method with the individual/couple, and instituting a client teaching and monitoring program are basic for the development of a good family planning program.

estrogens and progestins (oral contraceptives)
(various manufacturers)

Mechanism of action. Increased serum levels of estrogens and progestins inhibit the secretion of FSH and LH from the pituitary, resulting in suppression of ovulation. Changes in the endometrium result in failure of implantation of the ova, plus an increase in cervical mucus impedes sperm ingress.

Indications. Prevention of pregnancy; treatment of hypermenorrhea, endometriosis, and female hypogonadism

Pharmacokinetics

Distribution. Protein binding of estrogens is of a medium to high degree.

Metabolism. Estrogens and progestins, mainly by liver

Excretion. Estrogens and progestins, primarily by kidneys

Side effects/adverse reactions. See Table 52-1.

Significant drug interactions. The following interactions may occur when oral contraceptives are given with the drugs listed below.

Drug	Possible Effect and Management
inducers of hepatic enzymes	Barbiturates, anticonvulsants, griseofulvin, and rifampin are inducers of hepatic enzymes. Concurrent use with oral contraceptives may decrease the effectiveness of contraception.
anticoagulants, oral coumarin or indandione	Both increased and decreased anticoagulant effects have been reported. Monitor closely.
antidepressants, tricyclic	Antidepressant toxicity or a reduction in antidepressant therapeutic effects may be seen. These effects are probably dose-related. Low estrogen dosages have less effect on enzyme inhibition than larger dosages. Dosage adjustment of the antidepressant may be necessary; monitor closely for unusual effects.
bromocriptine	Concurrent use is not recommended. Oral contraceptives may cause amenorrhea and/or galactorrhea. Such effects interfere with the action of bromocriptine.
other hepatotoxic drugs, especially dantrolene	The risk of inducing hepatotoxicity is increased. Females over 35 years old are especially at risk. Avoid concurrent drug administration if possible; if not, monitor closely for hepatotoxicity.
smoking tobacco	Not recommended. An increase in cardiovascular risk such as CVA, transient ischemic attacks (TIAs), pulmonary embolism, and thrombophlebitis may result, especially in women over the age of 35. Avoid smoking if taking oral contraceptives.

Dosage and administration

1. Although the use of exogenous estrogenic substances alone will inhibit ovulation, undesirable bleeding frequently occurs during the latter phase of the cycle. If estrogen levels are increased to prevent this, severe nausea and breast tenderness occur. It is for these reasons that estrogens are combined with progestins in oral contraceptives.

2. Since naturally occurring progesterone is inactivated or extremely weak in its effect when taken orally and must be given by injection to be effective, the progestins (steroidal compounds related to progesterone) have been developed. The majority of the oral contraceptives contain a synthetic progestin, usually norethynodrel, norethindrone, or norgestrel.

3. Norethynodrel is a basic progestin, norethindrone is a more androgenic progestin, norgestrel is a synthetic progestogen similar to norethindrone. Norethindrone is sometimes recommended for patients

having excess side effects from estrogen, such as greater weight gain and amenorrhea. Norethynodrel is good for patients with oily skin, acne, hirsutism, and breakthrough bleeding.

4. Three methods of oral contraception are available: combination estrogen and progestin, low-dosage progestogens (minipill), and postcoital contraception with diethylstilbestrol. Table 52-2 lists the composition, doses, and brand names or oral contraceptives used in these three methods.

5. Combination estrogen and progestin contraceptives are divided into three types:

TABLE 52-2 Composition, Doses, and Brand Names of Oral Contraceptives

Estrogen	Progestin	Trade name
MONOPHASIC		
0.035 mg ethinyl estradiol	0.5 mg norethindrone	Brevicon 21-Day
0.035 mg ethinyl estradiol	0.5 mg norethindrone	Brevicon 28-Day (21 tablets active ingredients plus 7 tablets inert ingredients)
0.035 mg ethinyl estradiol	1 mg norethindrone	Norinyl 1 + 35 Tablet (21 tablets)
0.035 mg ethinyl estradiol	1 mg norethindrone	Norinyl 1 + 35 Tablet (28 tablets plus 7 tablets inert ingredients)
0.05 mg mestranol	1 mg norethindrone	Norinyl 1 + 50 Tablet (21 tablets)
0.05 mg mestranol	1 mg norethindrone	Norinyl 1 + 50 Table (28 tablets plus 7 tablets inert ingredients)
0.08 mg mestranol	1 mg norethindrone	Norinyl 1 + 80 Tablet (21 tablets)
0.08 mg mestranol	1 mg norethindrone	Norinyl 1 + 80 Tablet (28 tablets plus 7 tablets inert ingredients)
0.1 mg mestranol	2 mg norethindrone	Norinyl 2 mg Tablets
0.020 mg ethinyl estradiol	1 mg norethindrone	Loestrin 1/20 Tablets (21 tablets)
0.020 mg ethinyl estradiol	1 mg norethindrone	Loestrin FE 1/20 (contains 21 oral contraceptive tablets plus 7 tablets of ferrous fumarate [75 mg])
0.030 mg ethinyl estradiol	1.5 mg norethindrone	Loestrin FE 1.5/30 (contains 21 oral contraceptive tablets plus 7 tablets of ferrous fumarate [75 mg])
0.030 mg ethinyl estradiol	0.15 mg levonorgestrel	Nordette-21
0.030 mg ethinyl estradiol	0.15 mg levonorgestrel	Nordette-28 (21 tablets, plus 7 tablets inert ingredients)
0.030 mg ethinyl estradiol	0.3 mg norgestrel	Lo/Orval (21 tablets)
0.030 mg ethinyl estradiol	0.3 mg norgestrel	Lo/Ovral-28 (21 tablets plus 7 tablets inert ingredients)
0.035 mg ethinyl estradiol	0.4 mg norethindrone	Ovcon-35 (21 tablets)
0.050 mg ethinyl estradiol	1 mg norethindrone	Norlestrin 21 1/50 (21 tablets)
BIPHASIC		
0.035 mg ethinyl estradiol	0.5 mg norethindrone (10 tablets) 1 mg norethindrone (11 tablets)	Ortho-Novum 10/11-21 (21 tablets)
TRIPHASIC		
0.030 mg ethinyl estradiol	0.05 mg levonorgestrel (6 tablets)	Triphasil 21 (21 tablets)
0.040 mg ethinyl estradiol	0.075 mg levonorgestrel (5 tablets)	Triphasil 28 (21 tablets plus 7 tablets inert ingredients)
0.030 mg ethinyl estradiol	0.125 mg levonorgestrel	
0.035 mg ethinyl estradiol		Ortho-Novum 7/7/7-21 (21 tablets)
0.035 mg ethinyl estradiol	0.5 mg norethindrone (7 tablets)	
0.035 mg ethinyl estradiol	0.75 mg norethindrone (7 tablets)	
	1 mg norethindrone (7 tablets)	Ortho-Novum 7/7/7-28 (21 tablets plus 7 tablets inert ingredients)

a. **Monophasic** oral contraception is a fixed ratio of estrogen and progestin that is taken for 21 days of the normal menstrual cycle. Originally these preparations contained high doses of hormones and had increased reports of adverse side effects. Most of these preparations have been reformulated into lower dosage hormones, but the biphasic and triphasic oral contraceptives are more commonly used today.

b. **Biphasic** oral contraception supplies various amounts of hormone during the first and second halves of the menstrual cycle—that is, low levels of hormones in the follicular phase, which is increased during the luteal phase of the menstrual cycle.

c. **Triphasic** oral contraception is the newest form of oral contraception; it most closely simulates the normal estrogen and progesterone levels during the menstrual cycle. The dose of estrogen is kept at a low and constant level during the 21-day dosing period while the progestin is progressively increased to mimic the natural release of hormones in the female. Because the lowest dosages of hormones possible are used in this formulation, the incidence and severity of adverse reactions reported are considerably lower than with the monophasic or biphasic formulations.

6. Low-dosage progestogens (minipill) oral contraceptives do not contain any estrogen hormone. They are generally prescribed for 28 days of the menstrual cycle. These preparations are usually less effective than the combination products (approximately 97% protection from pregnancy), and they reportedly have a higher incidence of spotting and breakthrough bleeding. An advantage is that they generally do not cause the more serious adverse reactions associated with estrogen therapy.

7. For postcoital contraception with diethylstilbestrol, see the section on diethylstilbestrol on p. 828.

Pregnancy safety. FDA category X

NURSING CONSIDERATIONS

Assessment. See assessment in previous sections on estrogens and progestins.

Education. Instruct the client to take the medications as prescribed by the physician. The tablets should be taken at the same time each day, preferably in association with another daily routine, i.e., brushing of teeth, cleansing of face in the morning or at night. Nighttime administration may be preferable to decrease nausea. Nausea occurs in some clients during the first cycle but tends to subside after the third or fourth month. It may be prevented or reduced by taking the medication with food.

Caution clients never to let their tablet supply run out and to keep an extra month's supply on hand. The packages should be rotated by using the extra package after the pills currently being used and replacing the extra supply each month on a regular basis.

Instruct the client to use the pills in the same sequence that they appear in the container.

Instruct client beginning to use oral contraceptives to use a second method of birth control for the first cycle until the body adjusts to the medication. If she misses a dose of the medicine for 1 day of the 21-day schedule, she should take it as soon as she remembers. If she does not remember until the next day, tell her to take the missed tablet and the regularly scheduled one together. If she does not remember a dose for 2 days in a row, she should take 2 tablets a day for each of the next 2 days. In addition she may want to use a second method of birth control for full protection. If she misses 3 doses or more in a row, then she should stop taking the medicine and use another method of birth control until she menstruates or until it is determined she is not pregnant. Then she may restart the medication with the appropriate cycle.

If the client is using a 28-day schedule and misses any of the first 21 tablets, instruct her to follow the preceding instructions. If she misses any of the last 7 tablets, which are inactive, there is no hazard of pregnancy; however, the first tablet of the next month's series must be taken on the regularly scheduled day. Be sure to review the literature provided with the medication with the client to ensure understanding.

Assist the client in exploring her concerns about the risks of taking oral contraceptives. Provide her with information regarding the occurrence of cardiovascular disease and cancer in relationship to her age, smoking habits, and other health characteristics. Encourage the client to read the patient package insert carefully and then to discuss with her health care provider any concerns she might have.

Advise the client to have physical examinations, which should include a pelvic and breast examination and a Pap smear, every 6 to 12 months during treatment.

Instruct the client to notify her health provider immediately in the instance of severe headache, blurred or lost vision (which may possible signal stroke), and symptoms of chest pain, shortness of breath, or leg pain, which may indicate thromboembolism elsewhere in the body. The physician should also be informed of severe abdominal pain or mass, jaundice, severe mental depression, or unusual bleeding. Instructions should be provided for monthly self-examination of the breasts, and any lumps found should be reported to the physician.

Medical intervention is necessary for various changes in menstrual bleeding pattern, increased and painful urination, jaundice, abdominal cramping, ocular changes (double vision, partial or complete loss of vision, bulging eyes), increased blood pressure, breast alterations (lumps, secretions), depression, pain or numbness in fingers or toes.

Evaluation. Clients should be monitored for the development of side effects or adverse reactions. Among the more commonly seen reactions are salt and water retention, breakthough bleeding, thromboembolic disorders, hypertension, and nausea (see Table 52-2 for a more complete listing). If significant adverse reactions occur, a different birth control pill formula or alternate birth control method should be used.

Compliance with therapy is especially important if oral contraceptives are to be effective. Periodically review with the client the appropriate use and importance of taking the drug on a daily schedule. Ensure that the client knows the proper procedure to follow should one or more doses be missed.

OVULATORY STIMULANTS AND DRUGS USED FOR INFERTILITY

Anovulation, the absence of ovulation, is physiologic in women who are pregnant, breast feeding, or postmenopausal. It becomes a suspected pathologic condition in individuals with abnormal bleeding or infertility. The incidence of anovulation is unknown and cannot be ascertained, but diagnostic tests may determine its presence. Methods of ovulation induction include use of gonadotropins, thyroid preparations, cortisone preparations, estrogens, and synthetic agents.

clomiphene citrate (Clomid, Serophene)

Mechanism of action. Clomiphene has estrogen and antiestrogenic properties. Its exact mechanism of action is unknown, but it has been postulated that its completion with estrogen for receptor sites in the hypothalamus causes an increased secretion of FSH and LH. The result is ovarian stimulation, maturation of the ovarian follicle, and development of the corpus luteum.

Indication. Treatment of female infertility
Pharmacokinetics

Absorption. Freely absorbed from gastrointestinal tract. Also recirculated in enterohepatic system, which may account for its prolonged duration of action in the body.

Distribution. Half-life is 5 to 7 days in the plasma. Ovulation usually occurs between 4 to 10 days after the first day of treatment.

Metabolism. Hepatic
Excretion. Feces (biliary), for up to 6 weeks
Side effects/adverse reactions. See Table 52-1.
Significant drug interactions. None
Dosage and administration

Adults. For female infertility: 50 mg orally daily for 5 days, on the fifth day of the menstrual cycle if bleeding

occurs or start at any time in women who have no recent uterine bleeding. This cycle is repeated until conception occurs, up to three or four cycles. If ovulation does not occur, the dose is increased to 100 mg a day for 5 days, which may be repeated if necessary. Some clients may need larger doses to induce ovulation (up to 250 mg/day), but higher dosages are associated with a higher incidence of side effects.

Pregnancy safety. Not established

NURSING CONSIDERATIONS

Assessment. It should be determined whether the client has preexisting conditions for which clomiphene is contraindicated, such as abnormal and undiagnosed vaginal bleeding, fibroid tumors, mental depression, active or a history of hepatic dysfunction, or thrombophlebitis. If the client has ovarian cysts, clomiphrene may cause enlargement of them.

Education. Instruct the client to take basal body temperature daily and record on flow chart. This determines when ovulation occurs and assists in properly timing coitus so as to enhance fertilization. Easy to read oral thermometers are available that register 96° to 100° F; however, some physicians prefer rectal temperatures for accuracy. The temperature is taken from day 1 of the menstrual period and every morning upon awakening and before the client engages in any activity, such as drinking coffee, brushing teeth, smoking, and intercourse. The body temperature is low (approximately 97.5° F) and stable for 2 weeks after menstruation. At ovulation there is a slight decrease, followed the next day by an increase (approximately 98.5° F), which continues if progesterone levels are normal. The temperature decreases again just before menstruation. If this decrease does not occur, the client may be pregnant; the next series of the drug should be delayed until it is determined she is not pregnant, since clomiphene may have teratogenic effects. Coitus should occur every other day for 3 to 4 days before ovulation and for 2 to 3 days after ovulation to enhance fertilization.

Advise the client that taking the medication at the same time every day maintains drug levels and helps her remember the daily dose.

If the medication is to start on day 5, count the first day of the menstrual period as day 1.

If a dose is missed, advise client to take it as soon as possible. If the dose is not remembered until time for the next dose, both should be taken together. If more than one dose is missed, the physician should be consulted.

Inform the client and her spouse of the possibility of multiple births with this drug.

Advise the client that abdominal pain is an indication for immediate medical attention, since this may be symptomatic of ovarian cyst or enlargement.

Nursing Diagnoses Related to Hormone Therapy and Oral Contraceptive Use

Nursing diagnosis	Outcome criteria	Nursing interventions
Potential knowledge deficit related to female hormone therapy	Client will be able to verbalize action, use, dose, and side effects/adverse reactions of hormonal therapy. Client will demonstrate a reduction in symptoms without side effects/adverse reactions.	Instruct client to take medication as prescribed. Advise client taking dosage in vaginal cream form to administer at bedtime to increase absorption. Use a sanitary napkin, not tampons, to protect clothing. Advise client that the medication may be taken with food to minimize or prevent nausea. Alert client to stop taking her medication and consult with the physician if she suspects she is pregnant. Advise client to report to the prescriber any symptoms of thromboembolism (sudden, severe headache, sudden change in vision, sudden pain, weakness, or numbness); liver impairment (yellow eyes or skin, dark urine, pale stools); or mental depression. Alert client that cigarette smoking while on this medication increases the risk of thromboembolism (deep-vein thrombosis, pulmonary embolism, heart attack, stroke), particularly after age 35. Stress the importance of regular visits to the physician for follow-up care every 6–12 months.
Potential knowledge deficit related to oral contraceptive regimen	Client will demonstrate compliance with medication regimen (oral contraception) without side/adverse effects	Instruct client to take medication as prescribed. Advise client to use an additional method of birth control during the 3 weeks of the initial cycle. Encourage client to take the medication at the same time each day, not more than 24 hours apart. Alert client that although nausea may occur in the first few weeks of therapy, it is usually temporary and may be minimized by taking the dose with food. Advise client to always keep a month's supply on hand. Replace the extra supply each month. Provide specific information regarding appropriate action to be taken by the client when "missed" doses occur. Stress the importance of regular visits to the physician for follow-up care every 6 to 12 months. Advise client to alert other health care providers that she is taking oral contraceptives, since they may cause serious symptoms as well as interact with other drugs to lessen contraceptive effectiveness. Alert client to stop taking her medication and consult with the physician if she suspects she is pregnant. Advise client to report to the prescriber any symptoms of thromboembolism (sudden severe headache, sudden change in vision, sudden pain, weakness, or numbness); liver impairment (yellow eyes or skin, dark urine, pale stools); or mental depression. Alert client that cigarette smoking while on this medication increases the risk of thromboembolism (deep-vein thrombosis, pulmonary embolism, heart attack, stroke), particularly after age 35.

Counsel the client to report visual disturbances to the physician at once.

Advise the client to be cautious with tasks that require alertness, since clomiphrene may cause visual disturbances, vertigo, and light headedness.

Evaluation. If pregnancy does not occur, review the course of therapy with the client and her spouse to ensure understanding.

A pelvic examination to assess ovarian size should be completed before each course of the drug.

KEY TERMS

anovulation, page 834
biphasic, page 833
corpus luteum, page 829
hypogonadism, page 823
monophasic, page 833
oral contraception, page 831
triphasic, page 833

BIBLIOGRAPHY

American Hospital Formulary Service: AHFS drug information '88, Bethesda, Md, 1988, American Society of Hospital Pharmacists, Inc.

Atkinson LE and others: The next contraceptive revolution, Fam Plann Perspect 18(1):19, 1986.

Babington MA: Adolescent use of oral contraceptives, Pediatr Nurs 10(2):111, 1984.

Barrett-Connor E: Postmenopausal estrogen, cancer and other considerations, Women Health 11(3/4):179, 1986.

Block M and Rulin MC: Managing patients on oral contraceptives, Am Fam Physician 32(2):154, 1985.

Connell EB: Research on methods of fertility regulation, JOGN Nurs 13(2) (suppl):50s, 1984.

Cotter A: An ill for every pill? Nurs Times 79(46):12, 1983.

Coveney T: Osteoporosis and oestrogens, Nurs Mirror 158(19):19, 1984.

Cupit LG: Contraception: helping patients choose, JOGN Nurs 13(2) (suppl):23s, 1984.

Cutick R: Special needs of perimenopausal and menopausal women, JOGN Nurs 13(2)(suppl):68s, 1984.

D'Arcy PF: Drug interactions with oral contraceptives, Drug Intell Clin Pharm 20(5):353, 1986.

Dobson CL: Menopause: benefits of hormone replacement therapy, Consultant 25(7):242, 1985.

Emery MG and others: Nutritional consequences of oral contraceptives, Fam Community Health 6(3):23, 1983.

Fish S: Hormone replacement therapy, Nurs Mirror 157(6):Clinical Forum 7:i, 1983.

Flowers DS: Estraderm (Ciba-Geigy): a review of transdermal estrogen, Fla Pharm J 51(8):14, 1987.

Frazer J: The dilemma of the perimenopausal female: a sexual/physical health issue, Holistic Nurs Pract 1(4):67, 1987.

Fuller E: When your patient faces menopause, Patient Care 17(11):91, 1983.

Gambrell RD Jr: Banishing the shadow of menopause, Emerg Med 18(19):24, 1986.

Gilman AG and others: Goodman and Gillman's the pharmacological basis of therapeutics ed 7, New York, 1985, Macmillan Publishing Co.

Gleit CJ and others: The role of calcium and estrogen in osteoporosis, Orthop Nurs 4(3):13, 1985.

Goldzieher JW and others: Medical aspects of contraception, Hosp Pract 22(3):93, 1987.

Hadley A: Running a natural course... teaching women to understand their bodies' natural reproductive cycle, Nurs Mirror 156(21):Midwifery Forum 5:i, 1983.

Hammerslough CR: Characteristics of women who stop using contraceptives, Fam Plann Perspect 16(1):14, 1984.

Handy LC: Nursing management of the woman with osteoporosis, JOGN Nurs 14(2):107, 1985.

Johnson JH: Contraception—the morning after, Fam Plann Perspect 16(6):266, 1984.

Kanell RG: Oral contraceptives: the risks in perspective, Nurse Pract 9(9):25, 1984.

Kessler A and others: Contraception: fad and fashion, World Health, June 1984, p 24.

Klein L: Unintended pregnancy and the risks/safety of birth control methods, JOGN Nurs 13(5):287, 1984.

Klitsch M: Hormonal implants: the next wave of contraceptives... the NORPLANT system, Fam Plann Perspect 15(5):239, 1983.

Konicki AM: Physical and psychological effects of DES on exposed offspring, Cancer Nurs 8(4):233, 1985.

Ladewig PA: Protocol for estrogen replacement therapy in menopausal women, Nurs Pract 10(10):44, 1985.

Lehmann A: DES, a living legacy: what can nurses do about it? Can Nurse 79(11):34, 1983.

Lincoln R: The pill, breast and cervical cancer, and the role of progestogens in arterial disease, Fam Plann Perspect 16(2):55, 1984.

Lindsey AM and others: Endocrine mechanisms and obesity: influences in breast cancer, Oncol Nurs Forum 14(2):47, 1987.

Luy M: Primary osteoporosis: new thinking on an old problem, AD Nurse 2(3):15, 1987.

McKirdy, A. Community/outpatient nursing: smooth transition...women with menopausal problems...oestrogen is administered by implant, part 1, Nurs Mirror 160(1):29, 1985.

Milliliken SR: Oral contraceptives in the 1980s, Physician Assist 9(5):29, 1985.

Notelovitz M: The symptomatic menopausal patient, Hosp Med 21(1):21, 1985.

Orne R and others: Reexamining the oral contraceptive issues, JOGN Nurs 14(1):30, 1985.

Padilla SL and others: Anovulation: etiology, evaluation and management, Nurse Pract 10(12):28, 1985.

Piziak VK and others: Menopausal hormone replacement, Hosp Pract 20(2):82GG-II, 1985.

Polednak AP: Exogenous female sex hormones and birth defects, Public Health Rev 13(1/2):89, 1985.

Reid JS: Estrogen-depletion urethritis, Geriatr Nurs 6(1):42, 1985.

Riddick DH: Hormonal management of the climacteric, Physician Assist 7(4):37, 1983.

Sanders C: Concerns voiced on Depo Provera, RNAO News 42(3):15, 1986.

Sands CD and others: The oral contraceptive PPI: its effect on patient knowledge, feelings, and behavior... patient package insert, Drug Intell Clin Pharm 18(9):730, 1984.

Sasso SC: Biphasic oral contraceptives, MCN 9(2):101, 1984.

Skillman TG: Osteoporosis: management for all women, prevention for some, Consultant 24(2):153, 1984.

Spitz IM and others: Antiprogestins: prospects for a once-a-month pill, Fam Plann Perspect 17(6):260, 1985.

Standley CC and others: Contraception tomorrow, Int Nurs Rev 16(2):73, 1984.

Transdermal estrogen: a promising dosage form, Patient Care 21(2):25, 1987.

United States Pharmacopeial Convention. Drug information for the health care provider, ed 8, Rockville, Md, 1988. The Convention.

Veninga KS: Effects of oral contraceptives on vitamins B_6, B_{12}, C, and folacin, J Nurse Midwife 29(6):386, 1984.

Walter RM Jr: Osteoporosis: therapy that can make a difference, Consultant 27(3):115, 1987.

Wissing VS: The hormone factor: hormone manipulation in the treatment of breast cancer, Am J Nurs 84(9):1117, 1984.

CHAPTER
53

Drugs for Labor and Delivery

OBJECTIVES

After studying this chapter, the student will be able to:

1. Describe the altered pharmacokinetic pattern of drugs during labor and delivery.

2. Discuss the pharmacologic action of oxytocics on the uterus.

3. Identify the three primary indications of Pitocin.

4. Explain the two primary actions of ergonovine.

5. Discuss the mechanism of action and use of ritodrine.

6. Explain the action of the two lactation inhibitors.

Since many drugs are available for use during labor and delivery, it is important to consider the benefit versus risk to the fetus. The pharmacokinetics of drugs may be altered during labor and delivery. For example, during labor, gastric emptying is delayed and vomiting may result, which would alter drug absorption. Also, vomiting is often exacerbated by the use of opioid analgesics. Thus, because oral drug absorption is unpredictable at this time, parenteral routes should be used. Drug metabolism and excretion may be altered and prolonged during labor and, although clinical data are currently sparse, the potential for inducing adverse or undesirable effects is always a concern. If a drug, such as potent analgesics (opioid) and sedatives, may be potentially harmful to the fetus, then the smallest possible dose should be used if alternate methods are not available.

Complications in pregnancy may also dictate the use of additional medications, such as those to treat diabetes, hypertension, pre-eclampsia, eclampsia, and systemic infections. The medications and proper use of them are covered under the appropriate pharmacologic sections in this book. In this chapter, the discussion is limited to the drugs used to induce labor (oxytocics), avoid preterm labor, and suppress lactation.

DRUGS AFFECTING THE UTERUS

The uterus is a highly muscular organ that exhibits a number of characteristic properties and activities. The

837

smooth muscle fibers extend longitudinally, circularly, and obliquely in the organ. The uterus has a rich blood supply, but when the uterine muscle contracts, blood flow is diminished. Profound changes occur in the uterus during pregnancy: it increases in weight from about 50 g to approximately 1000 g, its capacity increases tenfold in length, and new muscle fibers may be formed. These changes are accompanied by changes in response to drugs.

Drugs that act on the uterus include (1) those that increase the motility of the uterus and (2) those that decrease uterine motility.

OXYTOCICS: DRUGS THAT INCREASE UTERINE MOTILITY

Oxytocics are drugs that exert a selective action on the smooth muscle of the uterus. The most commonly used oxytocics are alkaloids of synthetic oxytocin and ergot, although many other drugs may exhibit some effect on uterine motility.

Oxytocin is one of two hormones secreted by the posterior pituitary; the other hormone is vasopressin, or antidiuretic hormone (ADH). Oxytocin means "rapid birth," a term derived from its ability to contract the pregnant uterus. It also facilitates milk ejection during lactation.

The nonpregnant uterus is relatively insensitive to oxytocin, but during pregnancy, uterine sensitivity to oxytocin gradually increases, with the uterus being most sensitive at the termination of pregnancy. Oxytocin secretion may precede and possibly trigger delivery of the fetus. Large amounts of oxytocin have been detected in the blood during the expulsive phase of delivery. It is believed oxytocin is released in response to stretching of the uterine cervix and vagina. A positive feedback mechanism may be operant; that is, more forceful contractions of uterine muscle and greater stretching of the cervix and vagina result in more oxytocin release. Oxytocin acts directly on the myometrium, having a stronger effect on the fundus than on the cervix.

oxytocin (Pitocin, Syntocinon)

Mechanism of action. Oxytocin stimulates uterine smooth muscle contractions indirectly, which simulates normal contractions of a spontaneous labor and transiently reduces uterine blood flow. It also stimulates the mammary gland to increase milk excretion from the breast. (It does not increase the production of milk.)

Indications. Induction of labor, control of postpartum hemorrhage, and, stimulation of lactation.

Side effects/adverse reactions. See Table 53-1.

Pharmacokinetics

Administration. Available in nasal and parenteral dosage forms. Though rapidly absorbed nasally, absorption may be erratic by this route.

Distribution. Protein binding is low. Half-life is 1 to 6 minutes. Onset of action is as follows: nasal—within a couple of minutes, intramuscular—within 3 to 5 minutes, intravenous—immediate, although the uterine contractions will increase gradually over 15 to 60 minutes before it stabilizes. Duration of action is as follows: nasal—20 minutes, intramuscular—30 to 60 minutes, intravenous—20 minutes after the infusion is stopped.

Metabolism. Liver and kidneys

Excretion. Kidneys

Significant drug interactions. None.

Dosage and administration. Stimulation/induction of labor: 1 to 2 mU (0.001 to 0.002 units) per minute by intravenous infusion. The dose may be gradually increased by 1 to 2 mU per minute every 15 to 30 minutes until a contraction pattern is established that simulates normal labor (up to a maximum of 20 mU per minute).

Control of **postpartum uterine bleeding:** 10 units at a rate of 20 to 40 mU in a nonhydrating diluent infused intravenously, following birth of the infant. Nasal solution: 1 spray or 3 drops in one or both nostrils 2 or 3 minutes before nursing or pumping of breasts.

NURSING CONSIDERATIONS

Assessment. It should be ascertained that the client in labor does not have cord presentation or prolapse, **placenta previa** or vasa previa, fetal distress, hypertonic uterine patterns or uterine inertia, severe toxemia, or an obstetrical emergency requiring surgery.

Oxytocin should be used cautiously if the client in labor exhibits grand **multiparity** (several prior births), overdistention of the uterus, past history of trauma or major surgery on the cervix or uterus, invasive cervical carcinoma, partial placenta previa, prematurity of the fetus, or an unfavorable fetal position. Caution is also recommended in women over 35 years of age or those having an abortion using hypertonic saline.

It should be determined that there is pelvic adequacy of the client in labor and that there is fetal maturity.

Before administering the drug, record a baseline of data, including blood pressure and other vital signs, characteristics, frequency and duration of contractions, and fetal heart rate. During the infusion, assess the client for blood pressure and pulse and the fetus for heart rate at least every 15 minutes. Assess the myometrium for tonus during and between contractions and report hypertonic uterine contractions or a period of uterine relaxation. Discontinue oxytocin at the first sign of uterine hyperactivity.

Intervention. Administration should be only in a hospital setting and under the supervision of a physician.

Accurate administration by infusion pump is mandatory, as is using a Y connection so that the oxytocin solution

TABLE 53-1 Side Effects/Adverse Reactions of Labor and Delivery Drugs

Drug	Side effects*	Adverse reactions†
OXYTOCICS		
oxytocin (Pitocin, Syntocinon)	Rare or infrequent: With parenteral use only—nausea, vomiting, tachycardia, irregular heart rate	May occasionally cause nausea, vomiting, premature ventricular contractions, fetal bradycardia, dysrhythmias, neonatal jaundice, postpartum excessive bleeding Rarely: Hematoma in the pelvic area, increased loss of blood, and afibrinogenemia Allergic and anaphylactic reactions have also occurred. Expulsion of the placenta has also been reportedly inhibited on occasion, which may result in increased risk of bleeding and infections. Prolonged therapy may result in water intoxication and possibly, maternal death, because of its slight antidiuretic effects. Monitor clients closely during prolonged use, since hypertensive episodes and subarachnoid hemorrhage may result. When given in excessive dosages to hypersensitive patients, uterine spasms and tetania contractions can occur, which may lead to uterine rupture, abruptio placentae, reduction in blood flow to the uterus, amniotic fluid embolism, and trauma to the fetus (resulting in dysrhythmias, intracranial hemorrhage, and asphyxia)
ergonovine (Ergotrate)	Most frequent: Nausea or vomiting, seen mostly after IV administration Less frequent: Diarrhea, dizziness, tinnitus, increased sweating, confusion Dose-related effect: Abdominal cramping	Less frequent: Coronary vessel spasms resulting in chest pain Rare: Respiratory difficulties (allergic effect); hypertensive episode (patient complains of sudden, very severe headache); pruritus; pain in arms, legs, or lower back; cold hands or feet; leg weakness
methylergonovine maleate (Methergine)	Same as ergonovine	Same as ergonovine
PREMATURE LABOR INHIBITOR		
ritodrine (Yutopar)	With IV dosage form, nearly 80% to 100% of the clients have increased maternal heart rate and increased systolic and decreased diastolic maternal blood pressure. Oral dosage forms may cause small increases in maternal heart rate but do not affect maternal blood pressure or fetal heart rate.	
	Most frequent: Orally—trembling or tremors; IV—trembling or tremors, red colored skin, nausea, vomiting, headaches Less frequent: IV—increased anxiety or nervousness and restlessness; Orally—rash, jitteriness	Most frequent (10%–15% with oral dosage forms, 35% with IV administration): Tachycardia, irregular heartrate Rare (1% to 2% after IV use): Chest pain, respiratory difficulties Signs of excessive dosing: Severe nausea, vomiting, nervousness, trembling, shortness of breath, tachycardia or irregular heart rate With IV, monitor closely as some cases of maternal pulmonary edema resulting in death have occurred. Cause is unknown but contributing factors include concurrent corticosteroids, hypokalemia, twin gestations, a sustained rapid heartbeat of over 140 beats/minute and perhaps undiagnosed cardiac disease.

*If side effects continue, increase, or disturb the patient, the physician should be informed.
†If adverse reactions occur, contact the physician because medical intervention may be necessary.

may be discontinued while the vein is kept open. When preparing an infusion with oxytocin, distribute the drug throughout the solution by gently rotating the bottle.

When administered by nasal spray, instruct the patient to clear nasal passages. Then, holding the head vertically and the bottle upright, spray the solution into the patient's nostril.

Do not administer by more than one route simultaneously.

Evaluation. The maternal blood pressure and pulse should be monitored frequently, along with the frequency, duration, and force of the contractions. Continuous fetal monitoring should be done while the client is receiving oxytocin. Fluid intake and output determinations are needed as the drug has a slight antidiuretic effect, which, with prolonged intravenous, could result in severe water intoxication. Hypochloremia and hyponatremia may occur in the client because of water intoxication. Hyperbilirubinemia may occur in the neonate.

ergonovine (Ergotrate)

Mechanism of action. Direct stimulation of the smooth muscle of the uterine wall. Also has antiserotonin effects on the CNS and has been used as a diagnostic agent for coronary vasospasm (because it vasoconstricts the coronary arteries).

Indications. To prevent and treat postpartum hemorrhage.

Pharmacokinetics

Administration. Oral or parenteral.

Metabolism. Liver.

Onset of action. Uterus contraction—orally, within 6 to 15 minutes; intramuscular, within 2 to 5 minutes; intravenous, immediate effect.

Duration of action. Uterus contraction—orally, about 3 hours; intramuscularly, approximately 3 hours; intravenously, about 45 minutes but rhythmic contractions can persist for up to 3 hours

Excretion. Kidneys.

Side effects/adverse reactions. See Table 53-1.

Significant drug interactions. None.

Dosage and administration. Orally the dosage for ergonovine maleate tablets is 0.2 to 0.4 mg two to four times a day (on a schedule of every 6 to 12 hours) until the dangers associated with uterine atony and hemorrhage are over. The usual course is 48 hours. Parenterally, 0.2 mg is administered intramuscularly or intravenously and repeated in 2 to 4 hours if necessary, for up to five doses for use as a uterine stimulant. The intravenous route is usually only recommended in emergencies or when excessive uterine bleeding is present.

Injectable. Adult—200 μg (0.2 mg) intramuscular or intravenous, may repeat in 2 to 4 hours if needed, up to a maximum of five doses.

NURSING CONSIDERATIONS

Assessment. If the client does not tolerate other ergot derivatives, she may not tolerate ergonovine.

Ergonovine should be used with caution in clients with coronary artery disease because it causes coronary vasospasm. It may also increase blood pressure, thus its use should be limited in clients with hypertension, as well as in clients with toxemia of pregnancy. As with most drugs, it is to be administered with care to clients with hepatic or renal function impairment.

It is contraindicated before delivery of the placenta, since it may result in the entrapment of the placenta. It is not to be used for the induction of labor or in cases of threatened spontaneous abortion.

A baseline standard should be obtained for the pulse and blood pressure.

Intervention. When given intravenously, the drug should be administered slowly over a minimum of 1 minute.

Education. Clients should be instructed to avoid smoking, because the action of the drug is enhanced as nicotine constricts blood vessels. Caution the client about exposure to cold because the body's ability to respond may be diminished.

Evaluation. Blood pressure and pulse should be monitored, as well as uterine response; the character and amount of vaginal bleeding should also be assessed. If the client has chest pain, the physician should be notified immediately.

If the client does not respond to the drug, tests to determine serum calcium levels should be done. Correction of hypocalcemia with intravenous calcium salts will restore the oxytoxic action of the drug.

The client should be observed for signs of ergotism, such as headache, nausea and vomiting, peripheral ischemia, and paresthesia.

methylergonovine maleate (Methergine)

Mechanism of action. Direct stimulation of the smooth muscle of the uterine wall results in hemostasis. This drug has an antiserotonin effect in CNS.

Indications. To prevent and treat postpartum hemorrhage.

Pharmacokinetics

Absorption. Good orally.

Half-life. ½ to 2 hours.

Onset of action. Contraction of uterus—orally, within 6 to 15 minutes; intramuscularly, 2 to 5 minutes; intravenously, immediately.

Duration of action. Contraction of uterus—orally, about 3 hours; intramuscularly, approximately 3 hours; intravenously, 45 minutes although contraction can continue for up to 3 hours.

Metabolism. Liver.

Excretion. Kidneys.

Side effects/adverse reactions. See Table 53-1.

Significant drug interactions. None.

Dosage and administration

Oral tablets. 200 to 400 μg (0.2 to 0.4 mg) orally two to four times daily (spaced every 6 to 12 hours) until uterine bleeding and atony is under control. Usually oral dosing follows the administration of an initial parenteral dose.

NURSING CONSIDERATIONS

See discussion of nursing considerations for ergonovine.

PREMATURE LABOR INHIBITORS

Preterm labor, or labor that occurs before the thirty-seventh week of pregnancy, is a major problem in obstetrics. It occurs in approximately 10% to 15% of all pregnancies. Premature birth increases the possibility of neonatal morbidity and mortality.

ritodrine (Yutopar)

Mechanism of action. Ritodrine is a beta$_2$ adrenergic stimulant that relaxes the uterine muscle by inhibiting uterine contractions.

Indications. To prevent and treat premature labor in pregnancies of 20 weeks or more gestation.

Pharmacokinetics

Absorption. Approximately 30% available following oral administration.

Onset of action. Orally—within ½ to 1 hour. Intravenously—5 minutes.

Time to peak serum concentration. Orally—within ½ to 1 hour. Intravenously—within 1 hour.

Peak serum levels. Oral—5 to 15 nanograms/ml (following a 10 mg dose). Intravenous—42 to 52 nanograms/ml (following an infusion of 9 mg over 1 hour)

Half-life. Oral—two phases—1.3 and 12 hours. Intravenous—three phases—6 to 9 minutes, 1.7 to 2.6 hours, and 15 to 17 hours

Metabolism. Liver.

Excretion. Kidneys.

Side effects/adverse reactions. See Table 53-1.

Significant drug interactions. The following interactions may occur when ritodrine is given with the drugs listed below.

Drug	Possible Effect and Management
Corticosteroids, long acting (betamethasone, dexamethasone, paramethasone)	Pulmonary edema and death have been reported in pregnant women. If concurrent drug administration is absolutely necessary, monitor closely and
Beta adrenergic blocking agents (labetalol, nadolol, propranolol, and others)	discontinue both drugs at first sign of pulmonary edema. Usage is not recommended because the two drugs are antagonistic toward each other. Drugs with greater beta$_1$ selectivity may be less antagonistic.

Dosage and administration

Tablets. 10 mg orally initially ½ hour before the intravenous infusion is stopped; then 10 mg every 2 hours for 24 hours. Maintenance—10 to 20 mg orally every 4 to 6 hours until birth or as directed by the physician. Maximum recommended daily dosage is 120 mg.

Injectable. 50 to 100 μg (0.05 to 0.1 mg) intravenous/minute, increase every 10 minutes if necessary by increments of 50 μg (0.05 mg) to an effective dosage. Maintenance—150 to 350 μg (0.15 to 0.35 mg) intravenous/minute. Continue intravenous infusion for 12 to 24 hours after labor contractions have stopped, then institute oral therapy as described above.

Pregnancy safety. FDA category B.

NURSING CONSIDERATIONS

Assessment. Length of gestation should be determined, since ritodrine is not recommended for use before the twentieth week of pregnancy. Preterm labor should not have progressed more than 4 cm of cervical dilation or 80% effacement or the drug may not be effective.

Ritodrine is contraindicated when the client has cardiac disorders, hyperthyroidism, eclampsia, pulmonary hypertension, or intrauterine infection, hemorrhage, or fetal death. Caution is indicated if the client has diabetes or pre-eclampsia.

Intervention. A controlled infusion device should be used when administering ritodrine intravenously to better enable dosage titration. Avoid the use of sodium chloride for infusion because of the risk of pulmonary edema. The client is placed on her left side to reduce blood pressure changes. Intravenous administration is usually con-

---

TERBUTALINE

Terbutaline, a drug commonly used for bronchodilation, is used investigationally for the prevention and treatment of preterm labor. Terbutaline (oral and parenteral dosage forms) is a beta$_2$ adrenergic stimulant similar to ritodrine that is currently only marketed for its bronchodilator effects. Further research is necessary to find an agent more specific for the uterine beta$_2$ receptors.

tinued for 12 to 24 hours after contractions stop, and then followed by oral dosage.

Education. The client should be cautioned to notify the physician if her water breaks or if her contractions begin again. If the client's contractions do not recur, she may gradually resume ambulation and other activities of daily living after 36 to 48 hours.

Evaluation. The client's blood pressure, heart rate, and uterine activity should be monitored periodically, as well as the fetal heart rate. Increases in maternal heart rate and systolic blood pressure are common.

For those clients receiving prolonged intravenous therapy, blood glucose level and fluid and electrolyte balance should be monitored. Closely monitor fluids to prevent circulatory overload. Tachycardia and dyspnea may indicate impending pulmonary edema. Other side effects for which to observe are headache, nausea and vomiting, erythema, and trembling.

LACTATION INHIBITORS

Estrogens such as chlorotrianisene (Tace) and bromocriptine (Parlodel) have been used to treat postpartum breast engorgement and inhibition of lactation, respectively. The use of estrogens for breast engorgement has declined over the years, mainly because the incidence of painful engorgement is considered low and studies have indicated that analgesics or other supportive therapies are quite effective. Also, the physician must weigh the benefit of using estrogens for this purpose against the risk, especially the risk of possibly inducing a thromboembolism.

Bromocriptine directly inhibits the release of prolactin from the anterior pituitary gland, resulting in suppression of lactation. For further information on bromocriptine, see the drug monograph for dopamine agonist in Chapter 17.

KEY TERMS

multiparity, page 838
oxytocics, page 838
placenta previa, page 838
postpartum uterine bleeding, page 838
preterm labor, page 841

BIBLIOGRAPHY

American Hospital Formulary Service: AHFS Drug Information '87, Betheseda Md, 1987, American Society of Hospital Pharmacists, Inc.

Brengman SL and others: Ritodrine hydrochloride and preterm labor, Am J Nurs 83(4):537, 1983.

Dumoulin JG: Should we leave the third stage to nature? Midwife Health Visit Community Nurse, 22(1):12, 1986.

Fullerton JT and others: Outpatient co-management of the patient receiving oral ritodrine therapy, J Nurse Midwife 31(1):38, 1986.

Huston CJ: (1987) Action STAT, preterm labor, Nursing 17(3):33, 1987.

Inch S: Management of the third stage of labour—another cascade of intervention? Midwifery 1(2):114–22, 1985.

Lirette M and others: Management of the woman in preterm labor, Perinat Neonat 10(1):30, 1986.

Long, PJ: Management of the third stage of labor: a review, J Nurse Midwife 31(3):135, 1986.

Marshall C: The art of induction/augmentation of labor, JOGN Nurs 14(1):22, 1985.

Shortridge LA: Using ritodrine hydrochloride to inhibit preterm labor . . . (Yutopar), MCN 8(1):58, 1983.

Stephany T: Terbutaline sulfate for treating tetanic contractions, MCN 10(6):394, 1985.

Toofanian A and others: Preterm labor and its management, Perinat Neonat 9(1):19–20, 25–7, 1985.

United States Pharmacopeia Convention: drug information for the health care provider, ed 7, Rockville, Md, 1987, The Convention.

Warren C: Knowing when to leave well alone . . . induction of labour, Nurs Times 82(48):48, 1986.

CHAPTER
54

Drugs Affecting the Male Reproductive System

OBJECTIVES

After studying this chapter, the student will be able to:

1. Compare the pharmacokinetics of the three androgens.
2. Discuss the approved indications for androgen therapy.
3. List the side effects/adverse reactions of androgen therapy.
4. Use nursing considerations appropriately in managing the care of clients undergoing androgen therapy.

Normal development and maintenance of male sex characteristics depend on adequate amounts of the male sex hormones, the **androgens.** Testosterone and its derivatives plus synthetic agents are commonly used as replacement therapy for males who lack the hormone. In hypogonadism and eunuchoidism, the androgens produce marked changes in growth of the male sex organs, body contour, voice, and other secondary sex characteristics.

testosterone
methyltestosterone
fluoxymesterone

Testosterone, the natural hormone, is available in combination with esters to prolong the medication's duration of action. For example, testosterone propionate is formulated in an oily solution that produces hormonal effects for 2 or 3 days, whereas testosterone cypionate and testosterone enanthate in oil are much longer acting. They are usually administered once every 2 to 4 weeks. Testosterone pellets are available for subcutaneous implantation. This form will also provide an extended duration of action, depending on the number of pellets used it may extend from 2 to 6 months before replacement pellets are necessary.

Oral testosterone is absorbed but is mainly destroyed by the liver before it reaches systemic circulation. Admin-

843

istering methyltestosterone by the buccal route of administration increases its serum level and effectiveness. Fluoxymesterone is a synthetic androgen that is effective orally in tablet form.

Mechanism of action. As a natural hormone in normal males, testosterone stimulates the synthesis and activity of RNA, which results in an increased protein production. When androgens are converted to 5-alphadihydrotestosterone in the tissues, luteinizing hormone (LH) and follicle-stimulating hormone (FSH) will be suppressed by the negative feedback mechanism involving the hypothalamus–anterior pituitary gland.

Androgens are also potent **anabolic agents;** that is, they stimulate the formation and maintenance of muscular and skeletal protein. They bring about retention of nitrogen (essential to the formation of protein in the body) and enhance storage of inorganic phosphorus, sulfate, sodium, and potassium. Athletes have used androgens to increase weight, musculature, and muscle strength. Weight gains may be caused by fluid retention, a side effect of androgen therapy. The potential risk of developing the major serious adverse reactions from androgens far outweighs the advantages to be gained in athletic events. Many major sporting events disqualify athletes whose use of such products is documented. Chapter 9, on substance abuse, has additional information on the abuse of androgens.

Indications
1. Treatment of androgen deficiency, such as testicular failure caused by cryptorchidism, orchitis, orchidectomy, or pituitary-hypothalamic insufficiency
2. Treatment of delayed male puberty when not induced by a pathologic condition
3. Treatment of breast carcinoma: palliative or secondary treatment for inoperable metastatic breast cancer in postmenopausal women, although newer agents are generally available for this indication. Androgens have also been used in premenopausal women with breast cancer in association with an oophorectomy, if such tumors are believed to be responsive to the hormone.
4. Treatment of postpartum breast engorgement in nonnursing women
5. Anemia: androgens stimulate erythropoiesis in males and females

Pharmacokinetics
Half-life. Testosterone: between 10 and 100 minutes; fluoxymesterone: dose related—that is, a 2 mg dose is 13.7 hours, whereas a 10 mg dose is approximately 10 hours; methyltestosterone: between 2.5 and 3.5 hours

Time to peak concentration. Methyltestosterone: buccal tablet—within 1 hour; oral tablet—2 hours

Duration of action. Depends on the dose and the ester formulation administered. The longest duration of testos-

terone preparations is with enanthate, then cypionate, with the propionate form being the shortest.

Metabolism. Liver

Excretion. Kidneys; some in feces because of the enterohepatic circulation

Side effects/adverse reactions. See Table 54-1.

Significant drug interactions. When androgens are given with anticoagulants (oral coumarin or indanedione), anticoagulant effects may be enhanced. Monitor blood clotting levels closely, since dosage adjustments may be necessary.

Dosage and administration
1. Choice of dosage and length of therapy depend on the diagnosis, age, and sex, and the intensity of the side effects/adverse reactions.
2. Usually in delayed puberty and hypogonadal males, dosage regimens are started in the lower ranges and gradually increased according to the individual's needs and response. In delayed puberty, after 4 to 6 weeks of therapy, the androgens are discontinued for 1 to 3 months while x-rays are evaluated to determine the drug's effect on bone growth. The hypogonadal male will receive the androgens through puberty with dosage adjustments as required. Usually lower maintenance dosages are used after puberty.
3. Androgen antineoplastic therapy usually requires a 3-month period to evaluate effectiveness.
4. Temporary withdrawal of the drug is required if the male experiences **priapism.** This is an indication of excessive dosing of the androgen.
5. Women with metastatic breast cancer should receive a shorter-acting androgen, especially during the initial therapies. It has been reported that androgens occasionally increase the extension of breast cancer.

sterile testosterone suspension
Adults (intramuscular). Nonnursing female, to prevent postpartum breast pain or engorgement: 25 mg, one or two times a day for 3 to 4 days. Androgen replacement therapy: 25 to 50 mg two or three times a week. Antineoplastic therapy for metastatic breast carcinoma in females: 100 mg three times a week.

Children (intramuscular). Delayed puberty in males: 12.5 to 25 mg intramuscularly two or three times a week for approximately 4 to 6 months.

testosterone enanthate injection
Adults (intramuscular). Androgen replacement therapy: 50 to 400 mg every 2 to 4 weeks. Antineoplastic therapy for inoperable breast cancer in females: 200 to 400 mg every 2 to 4 weeks.

Children (intramuscular). Delayed puberty in males: 50 to 200 mg every 2 to 4 weeks for approximately 4 to 6 months.

TABLE 54-1   Side Effects/Adverse Reactions of Androgens

Drug(s)	Side effects*	Adverse reactions†
Androgens: testosterone, methyltestosterone, fluoxymesterone	Less frequent (occurs in both sexes): abdominal pain, insomnia, diarrhea or constipation, hives or redness at site of injection, increased salivation, mouth soreness, unusual increase or decrease in libido	Most frequent in females: increase in oily skin or acne, deep voice, increased hair growth or alopecia, enlarged clitoris, irregular menses (even when medication is stopped, the deep voice or hoarseness may not be reversed) Most frequent in males: urinary urgency, breast swelling or soreness, frequent or continuous erection Less frequent in both sexes: dizziness, increased weakness, red skin or changes in skin color, frequent headaches, confusion, respiratory difficulties, depression, nausea, vomiting, pruritus, allergic skin rash, edema of lower extremities, jaundice, increase in bleeding episodes In males only: difficult urination or an increase in urinary frequency; increase in sexual interests and desires Rare (long-term therapy in both sexes): constant stomach pain, black stools, vomiting of blood, breath odors, constant headaches (caused by hepatic necrosis); dark urine, hives, light colored stools, anorexia, purple-red spots on body or inside mouth or nose **(peliosis hepatis)**; pain or increased sensitivity in upper abdomen or liver section, swelling of stomach (hepatocellular tumors); sore throat and/or increased temperature (leukopenia)

*If side effects continue, increase, or disturb the patient, the physician should be informed.
†If adverse reactions occur, contact the physician, since medical intervention may be necessary.

methyltestosterone capsules

Adults (oral). Nonnursing female, to prevent postpartum breast pain or engorgement: 20 mg four times a day for 3 to 5 days. Replacement (hypogonadism, climacteric, or impotence): 10 to 50 mg daily. Postpubertal cryptorchidism: 10 mg three times a day. Antineoplastic therapy for metastatic breast carcinoma in females: 50 mg one to four times a day.

Children (oral). Delayed puberty in males: 5 to 25 mg per day for approximately 4 to 6 months.

methyltestosterone buccal tablets

Adults (buccal). Nonnursing female, to prevent postpartum breast pain or engorgement: 10 mg four times a day for 3 to 5 days. Replacement (hypogonadism, impotence, or climacteric): 5 to 25 mg daily. Postpubertal cryptorchidism: 5 mg three times a day. Antineoplastic therapy for metastatic breast carcinoma in females: 25 mg one to four times daily.

Children (buccal). Delayed puberty in males: 2.5 to 12.5 mg daily for approximately 4 to 6 months.

fluoxymesterone tablets

Adults (oral). Nonnursing female, to prevent postpartum breast pain or engorgement: 2.5 mg given shortly after delivery, then 5 to 10 mg daily in divided dosages for 4 to 5 days. Replacement therapy: 5 mg one to four times a day. Antineoplastic therapy for metastatic breast carcinoma in females: 2.5 to 10 mg four times a day. Antianemic agent (unapproved use): 10 mg orally twice daily, up to maximum of 40 mg daily.

Children (oral). Delayed puberty in males: 2.5 to 10 mg daily for approximately 4 to 6 months.

Pregnancy safety. FDA category X

NURSING CONSIDERATIONS

Assessment. Assess whether the male client has breast cancer or known or suspected prostatic cancer, since androgens are contraindicated in both conditions.

The drugs should be used with caution in clients with severe cardiorenal disease, prostatic hypertrophy, hepatic failure, hypercalcemia, and, because of their hypercholesterolemic effects, those with a history of myocardial infarction and coronary artery disease.

Intervention. Administer the oral preparations with food to minimize gastric distress. Administer intramuscular testosterone deep within the gluteal muscle. The nurse should be aware that testosterone cypionate and testosterone enanthate are not interchangeable with testosterone propionate and suspension forms of the drug because of the difference in duration of action. With testosterone cypionate, the preparation may be warmed and shaken to dissolve the crystals. It may also turn cloudy if a wet needle or syringe is used but this does not affect its potency.

The nurse should be sensitive to the emotional responses of patients taking androgens. Female clients may have changes in secondary sex characteristics such as unnatural hair growth or heightened libido, which will subside with the cessation of the drug. Other changes that may occur, such as enlarged clitoris or hoarseness or deepening of the voice, may not be reversible. Male clients may need support to deal with deepening of the voice and rapid changes in height, size of sex organs, and hair growth patterns. Frequent or continuing erection may be a concern.

Education. Work with the client and/or responsible family member to develop a diet high in protein, calories, vitamins, and minerals that is individualized to the client's food preferences.

Monitor the client with diabetes closely. Antidiabetic agents may require dosage adjustment with concurrent administration of androgens.

Instruct the client to weigh daily to monitor for fluid retention. Sodium restriction and/or diuretics may be required if edema occurs.

Advise the client to maintain regular visits to the physician for monitoring progress.

Evaluation. Monitor the client's serum calcium carefully. Promptly report indications of hypercalcemia: nausea and vomiting, lethargy, loss of muscle tone, polyuria, increased urine and serum calcium levels. Hypercalcemia in clients with metastic breast cancer usually indicates bone metastasis. The client should be encouraged to drink 3 to 4 L or more of fluids to ensure adequate urinary output to prevent urinary calculi. Active clients should be encouraged to include weight-bearing exercise, i.e., walking daily. Clients confined to bed should have range of motion exercises at least daily. This exercise inhibits mobilization of calcium from bone.

Serum cholesterol levels should be monitored to ascertain the client's risk of cardiovascular disease as the result of androgen administration.

Hepatic function should also be monitored; hemoglobin and hematocrit should be evaluated for polycythemia.

Bone age determinations should be done every 6 months to assess the rate of bone maturation in children and adolescents.

Tumor growth should be monitored by radiography.

Elderly men should be observed for increasing difficulty or frequency of urination, which may indicate enlargement of the prostate secondary to the drug.

KEY TERMS

anabolic agents, page 844
androgens, page 843
peliosis hepatis, page 845
priapism, page 844
testosterone, page 843

BIBLIOGRAPHY

American Hospital Formulary Service: AHFS drug information '87, Bethesda, Md, 1987, American Society of Hospital Pharmacists, Inc.

Burch WM: Impotence: serum testosterone levels can tell you a lot, Consultant 22(11):275, 1982.

Gilman AG and others: Goodman & Gillman's the pharmacological basis of therapeutics, ed 7, New York, 1985, Macmillan Publishing Co.

Haggerty BJ: Prevention and differential of scrotal cancer, Nurse Pract 8(10):45, 1983.

Maxwell M: Male reproductive physiology, Nurs Mirror 157(20):24, 1983.

Melamed AJ: Current concepts in the treatment of prostate cancer, Drug Intell Clin Pharm 21(3):247, 1987.

Sandella JA: Cancer prevention and detection: testicular cancer . . . programmed instruction, Cancer Nurs 6(6):468, 1983.

United States Pharmacopeial Convention: Drug information for the health care provider, ed 7, Rockville, Md, 1987, The Convention.

Drugs Affecting Human Sexual Behavior

Sexuality and sexual behavior have psychologic, social, and physiologic dimensions that reflect a complexity beyond drug-related effects. Contributing factors include self-esteem, general health, availability of a partner, appropriate environment, and perhaps, age. Since drugs can affect sexual activities or sexual identity, nurses must be sensitive to their clients' needs as sexual beings and alert to cues that reflect problems. Clients may present these cues, if given the chance—for example, confusion or embarrassment about lack of interest in sexual activities, about lack of arousal despite desire, or about other phenomena they consider unusual.

Certain drug therapies can produce one or more side effects or adverse reactions; among these are decreased levels of testosterone, which is normally present in both sexes and enhances **libido** or sexual drive; increased levels of estrogen; emotional depression that effectively limits interest or response to sexual stimuli; or autonomic nervous system blockade, which may interfere with tumescence, lubrication, erection, or ejaculation. The references at the end of this chapter and information in Chapter 51 provide a better understanding of the structure and function of the reproductive systems.

Many physiologic functions significant to sexual pleasure are controlled by the psyche and the autonomic nervous system (see also Chapter 18). This system comprises two parts—the sympathetic (adrenergic) and parasympathetic (cholinergic) systems—and its functional units are nerves, nerve plexuses, and ganglia. Although viewed as physiologic antagonists, the two systems often have synergistic effects on sexual functioning. The male and female sexual organs are composed of homologous tissues; although the shapes of the organs differ, they correspond, part for part, in structure, position, and embryologic origin. In the embryo the genital protruberance appears identical in both sexes. The embryo is characteristically female initially and does not differentiate until fetal androgens begin to masculinize tissues (seventh to twelfth weeks of pregnancy). Thus it is not surprising that the mature analogous organs function similarly.

In the male, sympathetic (adrenergic) impulses produce ejaculation by causing contraction of the prostate and seminal vesicles along with effects on the bulbocavernous and ischiocavernous muscles. Drugs that block adrenergic impulses may affect ejaculatory function through sympathetic blockade. Parasympathetic (cholinergic) stimulation controls penile erection. This response results from congestion of the vascular sinuses in the penile corpora caused by parasympathetic nerve action in the venous channels. Drugs that interfere with parasympathetic nerve transmitters (cholinergic nerves) can cause defects in erection. In addition, ganglionic blocking agents, which may block both sympathetic and parasympathetic nerve transmission, can cause complete impotence and impaired sexual functioning.

In the female, parasympathetic (cholinergic) impulses cause arterial dilation and venoconstriction, which produce clitoral erection and vasocongestion of the vulva, **transudation** (oozing of a fluid through pores) of lubricating secretions from the vaginal walls, and swelling of the **introitus** (vaginal opening). Continued stimulation of the clitoris and/or the **Graefenberg spot,** which is located on the anterior wall of the vagina, may then produce orgasm and, for some, a miniature facsimile of ejaculation from glands that surround the female urethra.

See Table 55-1 for drug effects on human sexual behavior.

DRUGS THAT IMPAIR LIBIDO AND SEXUAL GRATIFICATION
ANTIHYPERTENSIVES

Certain drugs successfully used to treat high blood pressure produce vasodilation through blockade of the sympathetic nervous system. This interferes with the response to sympathetic nervous stimulation. Such adrenergic inhibition, however, occasionally results in **impotence,** inability of a man to achieve or maintain an erection, and decreased sexual function. Guanethidine (Ismelin) and reserpine (Serpasil), which act partly by depleting the postganglionic adrenergic nerve transmitter norepinephrine (originating from nerve endings), or by

blocking release of this transmitter from the nerve terminal, may produce impotence by inactivating the nervous mechanisms responsible for sexual function. Experiments with guanethidine have shown that erectile potency, ability to ejaculate, and intensity of climax are all reduced significantly during use of this drug. Similar observations have been made with reserpine, which also has central nervous system effects that decrease libido and lead to male impotence. In women reserpine blocks ovulation, causes infertility and pseudopregnancy, and induces lactation. These actions can affect sexual function and behavior profoundly.

Anticholinergic drugs and especially those with ganglionic blocking activity may also produce impotence and other untoward effects on sexual function. Guanethidine falls into this category. Other agents include mecamylamine (Inversine) and trimethaphan (Arfonad), which are used as antihypertensive agents. Since these drugs may block both sympathetic and parasympathetic innervation of the sex organs, both erectile capability and ejaculatory function may be affected during their use.

Another drug used in treating hypertension is spironolactone (Aldactone), a diuretic. This drug displaces aldosterone in the kidneys, thus interfering with the normal resorption of sodium ions. Resultant sexual dysfunction in both men and women has been reported. Amenorrhea was observed in six women who took spironolactone for 9 months, with normal menses returning within 2 months after drug therapy was discontinued. Gynecomastia and impotence in men have also been observed during spironolactone therapy.

ANTIHISTAMINES

Histamine is a naturally occurring substance that possesses various physiologic properties, including smooth muscle stimulation, mediation of the inflammatory response, and cardiovascular effects. Antihistaminic drugs act as competitive inhibitors of histamine at physiologic receptor sites and prevent its action. Well-known examples of such drugs include diphenhydramine (Benadryl), promethazine (Phenergan), and chlorpheniramine (Chlor-Trimeton). These drugs are consumed by millions as antiemetics, as mild sedatives, and for the control of allergy symptoms. Most antihistamines display anticholinergic effects such as dryness of the mouth, urinary retention, and constipation. Continuous use of these drugs may interfere with sexual activity. This effect is presumably mediated by the blockade of parasympathetic nerve impulses to the sex glands and organs.

ANTISPASMODICS

Most antispasmodic drugs are quaternary ammonium compounds. Their primary effect is relaxation of the smooth muscle of the gastrointestinal tract, biliary tract,

TABLE 55-1 Drug Effects on Human Sexual Behavior

Drug or drug category	Principal effect	Probable action
ANTIDEPRESSANTS		
amitriptyline (Elavil) desipramine (Norpramin, Pertofrane) imipramine (Tofranil)	Adverse	Central depression; peripheral blockade of nervous innervation of sex glands
lithium nortriptyline (Aventyl) pargyline (Eutonyl) phenelzine sulfate (Nardil) protriptyline (Vivactil) tranylcypromine sulfate (Parnate)	Adverse	Impotence
ANTIHISTAMINES	Adverse	Blockade of parasympathetic nervous innervation of sex glands
chlorpheniramine (Chlor-Trimeton) diphenhydramine (Benadryl) promethazine (Phenergan)		
ANTIHYPERTENSIVES	Adverse	Peripheral blockade of nervous innervation of sex glands
guanethidine (Ismelin) mecamylamine (Inversine) methyldopa (Aldomet)	Adverse	Depression, decreased libido, breast enlargement, gynecomastia, galactorrhea, amenorrhea, impotence, failure to ejaculate
pargyline (Eutonyl)	Adverse	Impotence, delayed ejaculation
Rauwolfia alkaloids	Adverse	Decreased libido, impotence, breast engorgement, pseudolactation, gynecomastia
reserpine (Serpasil) spironolactone (Aldactone) trimethaphan (Arfonad)		
ANTISPASMODICS	Adverse	Ganglionic blockage of nervous innervation of sex glands
atropine (Lomotil) glycopyrrolate (Robinul) hexocyclium (Tral) methantheline (Banthine)	Adverse	Impotence
BARBITURATES	Adverse	Central depression; suppression of motor activity; hypnosis
DIURETICS		
chlorothiazide (Diuril) hydrochlorothiazide (HydroDIURIL)	Adverse	General fatigue; rarely, impotence
NARCOTICS AND PSYCHOACTIVE DRUGS	Eventually adverse	Central depression; decreased libido and impaired potency
amphetamines	Questionable	Release of inhibitions; increased suggestibility; relaxation
anorectic agents cocaine	Transiently positive	Impotence, gynecomastic, menstrual disorders
heroin LSD marijuana methadone morphine	Adverse	Suppression of secondary sex organ function in male, reduction of libido, impotence
NICOTINE	Adverse	Vasoconstriction may impair erection and lubrication
SEDATIVES AND TRANQUILIZERS	Adverse	Central sedation; blockade of autonomic innervation of sex glands; suppression of hypothalamic and pituitary function
haloperidol chlordiazepoxide (Librium) chlorpromazine (Thorazine) chlorprothixene (Taractan)		
diazepam (Valium)	Transiently positive	Tranquilization and relaxation

Modified from Woods JS: Drug effects on human sexual behavior. In Woods NF: Human sexuality in health and illness, ed 3, St Louis, 1984, The CV Mosby Co.
*Many effects are dosage-dependent and reversible on discontinuance of drug.
Continued.

TABLE 55-1   Drug Effects on Human Sexual Behavior—cont'd

Drug or drug category	Principal effect	Probable action
haloperidol (Haldol) mesoridazine (Serentil) phenoxybenzamine (Dibenzyline) prochlorperazine (Compazine) thioridazine (Mellaril)	Generally adverse	Impotence, gynecomastia, breast engorgement, lactation, menstrual irregularities
ETHYL ALCOHOL	Progressively adverse	Central depression; suppression of motor activity; diuresis; decreased testosterone
STEROID HORMONES AND DERIVATIVES	Adverse	Antiandrogenic effects on sexual function; loss of libido; decreased potency
cortisone cyproterone acetate methandrostenolone (Dianabol)	Adverse	Menstrual disorders, decreased libido caused by antiandrogenic effect
methyltestosterone nandrolone phenpropionate (Durabolin)	Mixed effects	Phallic enlargement, prolonged penile erections, testicular atrophy, impotence, decreased ejaculatory volume, oligospermia; menstrual disorders, hirsutism, clitoral enlargement, male pattern baldness
MISCELLANEOUS progesterone or estrogen	Adverse	Depression, decreased libido, breast tenderness, testicular atrophy
amyl nitrite	Questionable	Vasodilation of genitourinary tract; smooth muscle relaxation
cantharis (Spanish fly)	Adverse	Irritation and inflammation of genitourinary tract, systemic poisoning
L-dopa and p-chlorophenylalanine (PCPA)	Questionable	Improved feeling of well-being
histamine H_2 antagonist (cimetidine)	Adverse	Impotence, gynecomastia, alopecia or galactorrhea
vitamin E	Questionable	Supports fertility in laboratory animals
yohimbine	Questionable	Stimulation of lower spinal nerve centers

ureter, and uterus. Because these drugs may act as ganglionic blocking agents, postural hypotension and impotence can result from their use. Drugs in this category include glycopyrrolate (Robinul) and hexocyclium (Tral).

SEDATIVES AND TRANQUILIZERS

Many of the wide variety of sedatives and tranquilizers available in recent years affect sexual interest and capability both directly and indirectly. Two of the most frequently used classes of tranquilizers are the phenothiazines and the benzodiazepine compounds. Several minor categories of sedative drugs also affect sexual function.

Phenothiazines comprise one of the most widely used classes of drugs in medical practice today. More than 30 phenothiazines with a broad spectrum of action are currently available. Known as the major tranquilizers, phenothiazines are used primarily in the treatment of psychosis, but they are also used as antiemetics and analgesics. Examples are chlorpromazine (Thorazine), prochlorperazine (Compazine), thioridazine (Mellaril), and mesoridazine (Serentil). Although the precise workings of their

sedative effect are not fully understood, these drugs are thought to modify sensory input into the reticular formation of the brainstem. The sedative effect may partly account for decreased sexual interest of persons undergoing phenothiazine therapy.

In addition to their central nervous system effects, the peripheral effects of these drugs may contribute to inhibition of sexual function. Phenothiazines decrease skeletal muscle tone and block cholinergic synapses at both muscarinic and nicotinic receptors. Various adrenergic impulses may be inhibited as well. Impotence, decreased libido, ejaculation disorders, and prolonged amenorrhea have been reported in individuals taking phenothiazines. Failure to ejaculate has been reported in men treated with thioridazine, although erection and orgasm do not appear to be affected. Ejaculation problems have also been reported with the use of chlorprothixene (Taractan) and mesoridazine (Serentil).

Chlorpromazine may also influence sexual function by affecting the endocrine glands, possibly through acting on the hypothalamus. In animal studies phenothiazine derivatives have suppressed hypothalamic and pituitary function, resulting in decreased hormone secretion and affecting sex organ function in both males and females. Chlorpromazine has been shown to be **spermicidal** in dogs and to reduce the copulation rate of male rats. Regressive and atrophic changes in the testes of experimental animals receiving phenothiazines have also been reported. Chlorpromazine can reduce urinary levels of gonadotropins, as well as estrogens and progestins. Like reserpine, chlorpromazine blocks ovulation, suppresses estrus in animals, induces lactation, and maintains a decidual reaction. The release of pituitary gonadotropins by relatively small doses of chlorpromazine delays ovulation and menstruation in female patients.

Benzodiazepine compounds are the second most widely used class of tranquilizing drugs. The best known is diazepam (Valium). As a mild tranquilizer, this drug is used for anxiety, as a skeletal muscle relaxant, and in alcoholism. Sexual impairment has been associated with diazepam's effects on both cholinergic and adrenergic facets of the autonomic nervous system. The sedative and relaxing effects of this drug may account for the decreased interest in sexual activity also noted. Alternatively, the judicious use of these tranquilizers has been considered of value in the treatment of sexual impotence and other problems involving sexual performance when excessive anxiety was a factor in decreased sexual performance.

Several other types of drugs used in the treatment of psychologic problems depress sexual activity in human beings. Haloperidol, an antipsychotic, can adversely affect the libido in men. Failure to ejaculate without concomitant alteration of erection or orgasm has been reported in individuals treated with phenoxybenzamine (Dibenzyline), an alpha adrenergic blocking agent once used to supplement psychiatric therapy. Its potent adrenergic blocking effects have been advanced to account for the adverse reactions on sexual function. Lithium carbonate has also been associated with disturbed sexual function in clients treated for mania with this drug.

ANTIDEPRESSANTS

Increasingly, contemporary life, often fast-paced and frustrating, is associated with psychologic depression. Diminished sexual interest, drive, and activity are characteristic of such depression. (See also Chapter 16). The drugs used to treat this depression compound the negative effects on sexual function.

While antidepressants generally elevate mood and thus increase sexuality, they can cause impotence and influence sexual behavior adversely. Two groups of drugs commonly used as antidepressants are the tricyclic compounds and the monoamine oxidase (MAO) inhibitors. Adverse reactions on sexuality of the first group may be related to peripheral anticholinergic effects, such as those produced by some antihypertensives. Examples of these drugs include imipramine (Tofranil) and amitriptyline (Elavil). Although MAO inhibitors may also be used as antihypertensives and antidepressants, the impotence that can result may be caused by their tendency to block peripheral ganglionic nerve transmission.

ETHYL ALCOHOL

Ethyl alcohol is considered for its effects on human sexual function and behavior as a drug of individual and unique notoriety. Revered for centuries as a sexual stimulant and cure of all ills, alcohol is in fact a depressant and is recognized today to have far greater social than therapeutic value. Although a sedative, alcohol in moderate amounts may enhance sexual activity by relieving anxieties and loosening the inhibitions that often shroud sexual behavior. Beyond a certain limit, however, neither desire nor potency will overcome the depressed physical capability that occurs under its influence.

Studies on the pharmacologic action of alcohol show that the central nervous system is more affected by alcohol than any other system of the body. Electrophysiologic studies suggest that alcohol first depresses the part of the brain responsible for integrating the various activities of the nervous system. The result is that various processes related to thought and motor activities become disrupted. The first mental processes affected are related to sobriety and self-restraint, producing a less inhibited and less restrained approach to sexual behavior and other activities normally inhibited by previous training or experience. With continued consumption of alcohol, however, the brain becomes narcotized, reflexes become slowed, blood vessels are dilated, and the capacity for sexual function is diminished. In addition, alcohol produces a severe diuretic effect, which may also interfere with sexual function.

Alcohol overindulgence by males is a frequent cause of forcible sexual assault on females. One study assessed various types of sexual offenders for frequency of offense; drunk persons constituted 12% to 16% of reported incidents. Alcohol consumption had not reached the point of physical incapacitation but rather a stage of confusion, belligerence, and misinterpretation, resulting in violent antisocial acts. Thus, although it first lowers inhibitions, alcohol eventually decreases physical capability and enjoyment of sexual activities.

Typically, the male alcoholic experiences delayed ejaculation during intoxication and impotence after years of chronic alcoholism. Vascular changes, peripheral neuropathy, and lowered testosterone levels because of liver damages are thought to cause the impotence. Body image changes such as testicular atrophy and gynecomastia compound the problem. However, occasionally favorable effects have been reported after sex therapy, despite alcohol-induced organ damage. These effects may result from resolution of negative, sexually repressive feelings. Much remains to be learned about the effects of alcohol on sexuality.

Of the 10 million people who have a drinking problem, 2 million are women, many of them elderly. The effects on women are also mixed. But most women alcoholics lose interest in sex generally, and alcoholism adversely affects their sexual interactions.

BARBITURATES

Barbiturates, such as amobarbital (Amytal), pentobarbital (Nembutal), secobarbital (Seconal), and thiopental (Pentothal), are sedative-hypnotic drugs that have general depressant effects on all nervous tissues. As with alcohol, these drugs in prescribed dosage produce relaxation, hypnosis, and sleep with depression of various body functions, including sexual performance and ability. With prolonged use or overdose barbiturates can cause respiratory failure and death. Withdrawal after long-term heavy consumption of barbiturates may result in convulsions. There is no rationale for their use in altering sexual behavior in human beings.

STEROID HORMONES AND DERIVATIVES

Sex hormones act on the central nervous system and other body organs to influence sexual and aggressive behavior, as well as mood and emotional outlook. Thus variations in female hormones may produce the anxiety, irritability, and depression associated with **premenstrual tension** syndromes, whereas male hormones are associated with aggression and increased sexual interest. Evidence indicates that sexual drives may be influenced by sex hormone treatment.

Synthetic sex hormone preparations have also been shown to influence sexual behavior. The antiandrogen steroid cyproterone acetate decreases libido and potency and is used successfully in the treatment of male **hypersexuality** and investigatively in female polycystic ovary syndrome. Synthetic estrogens and progesterones are widely accepted as oral contraceptive agents. Another class of synthetic sex hormones are the anabolic steroids, derived from the male sex hormone testosterone. These drugs, which include methandrostenolne (Dianabol) and nandrolone phenpropionate (Durabolin), are used to promote nitrogen retention and weight gain in elderly or undernourished patients. The substances have also been the source of controversy over their use and misuse by athletes and other postpubertal persons to promote muscle growth and endurance. When used by normally developed, well-nourished individuals, the effects of these drugs on strength and development are questionable. Considerable evidence shows that sexual activity may be adversely affected because of the effects these drugs have on gonadal function.

METHADONE

Methadone, a drug widely used to treat the symptoms of heroin withdrawal and in narcotics maintenance programs, produces both serious fertility problems and impaired sexual performance in male users. Fertility changes are associated with greatly reduced size and secretory activity of the secondary sex organs, resulting in extremely low ejaculate volume and low sperm motility. Whether this condition is reversible after the drug is withdrawn is not known; animal studies suggest that normal secondary sex organ function returns after discontinuing methadone treatment.

DRUGS THAT ENHANCE LIBIDO AND SEXUAL GRATIFICATION

Substances to increase sexual potency or drive have been sought throughout history. Inscriptions in the ruins of ancient cultures have described the preparation of "erotic potions," and an endless number of "aphrodisiacs" have been described since then. In contemporary society many drugs and chemicals that modify mood and behavior are claimed to have aphrodisiac properties.

In reality, no known drugs specifically increase libido or sexual performance, and chemicals taken for this purpose without medical advice and especially in combination with other drugs pose the danger of drug interaction or overdose. However, many pharmacologically active agents temporarily modify both physiologic responsiveness and subjective perception to enhance the enjoyment, if not the fulfillment, of the sex act. Some of these agents are considered in this section.

cantharis

Cantharis (cantharidin, Spanish fly), a legendary sexual stimulant, is a powerful irritant and potent systemic poison. It is not an effective sexual stimulant. A powder made from dried beetles *(Cantharis vesicatoria)* found in southern Europe, cantharis can produce severe illness characterized by vomiting, diarrhea, abdominal pain, and shock. When taken internally, it causes irritation and inflammation of the genitourinary tract and dilation of the blood vessels of the penis and clitoris, sometimes producing prolonged erections (priapism) or engorgement, usually without increased sexual desire. Deaths have been reported from the promiscuous use of cantharis as an aphrodisiac. It is currently recognized that cantharis is not an effective sexual stimulant, and it is seldom used in modern medical practice.

yohimbine

Another natural substance with purported aphrodisiac properties is yohimbine, an alkaloid derived from the west African tree *Corynanthe yohimbe*. Yohimbine produces a competitive alpha adrenergic block of limited duration and antidiuresis, probably from the release of antidiuretic hormone. Although yohimbine stimulates the lower spinal nerve centers controlling erection, there is no convincing evidence that it acts as a sexual stimulant. It currently has no therapeutic uses.

narcotics and psychoactive agents

The use of drugs such as morphine, heroin, cocaine, marijuana, LSD, and amphetamines as aphrodisiacs has become widespread in contemporary society. These agents can, under certain circumstances, enhance the enjoyment of the sexual experience for some. More commonly, however, sexual behavior decreases. Responsiveness varies because these agents have no particular properties that specifically increase sexual potency, but rather they tend to affect the user according to expectations. Thus the user's state of mind and the amount consumed contribute considerably to the effect achieved. Like alcohol, these drugs act on the central nervous system to weaken inhibitions, which are often the cause of problems involving sexual behavior. Taken in excess or too often, however, these drugs have the opposite effect and inhibit sexual drive and function. Because of these variations, researchers are skeptical of their value.

Recent studies have shown that both morphine and heroin in sufficient doses produce markedly reduced sexual activity in men and women. In men **nonemissive erections** and impotence can result. Assessment of impotence among narcotics users is complicated by the multiplicity of drugs taken concurrently, the unknown composition and actual dosage strength of street drugs, and the addictive potential of narcotics.

Marijuana (cannabis), an extract of the *Cannabis sativa* plant, is considered by many to be a sexual stimulant. However, like alcohol, its effect results indirectly from relaxation and release of inhibitions surrounding sexual activity. The active ingredient in marijuana is tetrahydrocannabinol. The pharmacologic effects resulting from smoking marijuana depend on the expectations and personality of the user, the dose, and the prevailing circumstances. Usually the effects of marijuana are time distortion and enhanced suggestibility, producing the illusion that sexual climax is somewhat prolonged. Thus the expectation that marijuana is an aphrodisiac may enhance enjoyment of the sex act. Studies on the properties of marijuana for a specific effect on sexual behavior, however, have shown that it has no such properties. On the contrary, there is evidence that marijuana smokers have a higher incidence of decreased libido and impaired potency than nonusers. In addition, chronic intensive use of marijuana depresses plasma testosterone levels in healthy males and produces gynecomastia in some users. Chromosomal breaks have also occurred.

Lysergic acid diethylamide (LSD) is another drug that, although considered an aphrodisiac by some, has poten-

tially untoward effects on sexual function and behavior. Like marijuana, any alteration of sexual performance produced by LSD is principally subjective. This drug acts almost entirely on the central nervous system. Little response, if any, has been noted in other organ systems that can be attributed to a direct effect of LSD, and no biochemical or pharmacologic evidence supports the contention that LSD or similar drugs contain any sex-stimulating properties. On the other hand, the repeated use of LSD may produce serious psychologic problems, which could overall adversely affect sexual interest or activity. Users of LSD during pregnancy may have a higher rate of malformed babies or stillbirths than nonusers.

Amphetamines (Benzedrine and Dexedrine) have also been used to stimulate sexual function. These drugs have a powerful central stimulant action, in addition to peripheral alpha and beta sympathomimetic effects. The main results of an oral dose of 10 to 30 mg are wakefulness and alertness, mood elevation, increased motor and speech activity, and often elation and euphoria. Physical performance is usually improved, and fatigue can be prevented or reversed. The effects of amphetamines on sexual performance, however, are inconsistent. At moderate dosage levels there is seldom any effect on sexual behavior, aside from the accompanying mood elevation or reversal of fatigue. Doses in the range of 20 to 50 mg can alter sensations to enhance the orgasmic feeling. However, higher doses, such as 1 g taken intravenously, produce loss of interest and withdrawal from sexual activity.

Amphetamines, along with other psychoactive agents, do little to promote the enjoyment of sexual activity and over time may produce adverse psychologic and physical effects that reduce sexual interest and capability.

DRUGS THAT STIMULATE SEXUAL BEHAVIOR

Various clinically used or experimental drugs enhance sexual interest or potency as a side effect in both humans and laboratory animals.

L-dopa

Levodihydroxyphenylalanine (L-dopa) is a natural intermediate in the biosynthesis of catecholamines in the brain and peripheral adrenergic nerve terminals. In the biologic sequence of events it is converted to dopamine, which in turn serves as a substrate of the neurotransmitter norepinephrine. L-Dopa is used successfully in the treatment of Parkinson's syndrome, a disease characterized by dopamine deficiency. When L-dopa is administered to an individual with this syndrome, the symptoms are ameliorated, presumably because the drug is converted to dopamine, thereby counteracting the deficiency. Recently patients, especially elderly men, being treated with L-dopa have been observed to have a sexual rejuvenation. This effect has led to the belief that L-dopa stimulates sexual powers.

Consequently, studies with younger men complaining of decreased erectile ability have shown that L-dopa increases libido and incidence of penile erections. Overall, however, these effects have been short-lived and do not reflect continued satisfactory sexual function and potency. Thus L-dopa is not a true aphrodisiac, but the increased sexual activity experienced by parkinsonian clients treated with L-dopa reflects improved well-being and partial recovery of normal sexual functions impaired by Parkinson's disease.

p-chlorophenylalanine (PCPA)

PCPA, a drug chemically related to L-dopa, has been claimed to have potent aphrodisiac properties in laboratory animals. Considerable controversy characterizes the potential sex-stimulating powers of this drug, which is used experimentally as a selective blocker of serotonin biosynthesis in the brain. In one report PCPA, when used with the monoamine oxidase inhibitor phenelzine, significantly increased male sexual activity. The sexual improvement paralleled the amelioration of headaches and mood. Since PCPA has not yet come into clinical use, its direct effects on human libido or sexual ability are unknown.

amyl nitrite

Amyl nitrite, a drug used in the past to treat angina pectoris, is alleged to enhance sexual activity in humans. As a vasodilator and smooth muscle stimulant, amyl nitrite has been reported to intensify the orgasmic experience for men if inhaled at the moment of orgasm. This effect is probably the result of relaxation of smooth muscles and consequent vasodilation of the genitourinary tract. No effects of amyl nitrite on libido have been reported, but loss of erection or delayed ejaculation may result. Women generally experience negative effects on orgasm when taking this drug.

vitamin E

Much has been said about the positive effects of vitamin E (alpha-tocopherol) on sexual performance and ability in human beings. Unfortunately, little scientific rationale substantiates such claims. The primary reasons for attributing a positive role in sexual performance to vitamin E come from experiments on vitamin E deficiency in laboratory animals. In such experiments the principal manifestation of this deficiency is infertility, although the reasons for this condition differ in males and females. In female rats there is no loss in ability to produce apparently healthy ova or any defect in the placenta or uterus. However, fetal death occurs shortly after the first week of embryonic life, and fetuses are reabsorbed. This situation can be prevented if vitamin E is administered any time up to the fifth or sixth day of embryonic life. In the male rat the earliest observable effect of vitamin E deficiency is

immobility of spermatozoa, with subsequent degeneration of the germinal epithelium. However, secondary sex organs are not altered and sexual vigor is not diminished, although vigor may decrease if the deficiency continues. Because of experimental results such as these, vitamin E has been conjectured to restore potency, or preserve fertility, sexual interest, and endurance in humans. No evidence supports these contentions, but since sexual performance is often influenced by mental attitude, a person who believes vitamin E may improve sexual prowess may actually find improvement. The only established therapeutic use for vitamin E is for the prevention or treatment of vitamin E deficiency, a condition that is rare in humans.

THE NURSE'S ROLE IN HUMAN SEXUALITY

An appreciation of the serious effects of sexual dysfunction on people's lives can produce a special sensitivity to patients' concerns. People often find it easier to confide in and discuss such important personal information with a nurse, male or female, than with anyone else.

High-quality professional nursing therefore should be directed toward achieving the following goals:

- Gaining understanding and acceptance of feelings about one's own sexuality. It takes time and effort to be comfortable enough to be therapeutic with others who are having sexual problems.
- Being open to patients' discussions about sexual concerns.
- Allowing patients to hold any belief or sexual practice they choose that is not overtly harmful.
- Recognizing that it is probably impossible to be truly comfortable with all patients or all related topics. It may be necessary to refer some patients with questions to more adequately prepared personnel. This might be a clinical nurse specialist or a social worker with expertise in dealing with sexual issues.
- Keeping current with the constantly changing data about drugs with potential for causing sexual dysfunction. This becomes more complex with the discovery, for example, that certain drugs in combination elicit unusual sexual responses. Currently, some that are suspect include antihypertensives, antidepressants, antihistamines, antispasmodics, sedatives and tranquilizers, ethyl alcohol, barbiturates, steroid hormones and derivatives, narcotics and psychoactive drugs, and certain natural substances.
- Being able to identify and interpret patient cues about problems dealing with sexuality, such as unexplained noncompliance with medication instructions, certain subjective data from the nursing history, avoidance of the topic, or other subtle hints.
- Discussing patients' medication with them (casual use

of drugs and over-the-counter and prescribed drugs), including information about potential adverse reactions.

- Consulting with the prescriber when adverse reactions do appear and suggesting that alternate forms or dosages of drug therapy be sought, if feasible. Such changes may be the route to enhanced compliance.
- Listening with sensitivity to expressed feelings of frustration, anger, anxiety, or fear that may attend body image changes or perceptions of aging and waning sexual attractiveness, which may actually result from drug effects.

KEY TERMS

Graefenberg spot, page 848
hypersexuality, page 852
impotence, page 848
introitus, page 848
libido, page 847
nonemissive erection, page 853
premenstrual tension, page 852
spermicidal, page 851
transudation, page 848

BIBLIOGRAPHY

Bartscher, PW: Human sexuality and implications for nursing intervention: a format for teaching, JNE 22(3):123, 1983.

Caruso D: Helping your patients enjoy sex again, RN 50(5):69, 1987.

Chapman J and others: A model for sexual assessment and intervention, Health Care Women Int 8(1):87, 1987.

Durie B: Drugs and sexual function, Nurs Times 83(32):34, 1987.

Fisher SG: The psychosexual effects of cancer and cancer treatment, Oncol Nurs Forum 10(2):63, 1983.

Fuentes RJ and others: Sexual side effects . . . what to tell your patients, what not to say . . . commonly prescribed drugs, RN 46(2):34, 1983.

Koch JJ: Psychotherapeutic techniques and methods applied in teaching human sexuality, J Nurs Educ 24(8):346, 1985.

Korenman SG: Clinical assessment of drug-induced impairment of sexual function in men, Chest 83(2):391, 1983.

MacElveen-Hoehn P: Sexual assessment and counseling, Semin Oncol Nurs 1(1):69, 1985.

Mann KV and others: Sexual dysfunction with beta-blocker therapy: more common than we think? Sex Disabil 5(2):67, 1982.

Marks RG: Sexual side effects: how drugs can change fertility. Part 2, RN 46(3):61, 1983.

Melman A: Male sexual dysfunction: office evaluation that identifies the problem's source. Part 1, Consultant 26(12):72, 1986.

Melman A: Male sexual dysfunction: office management that leads to restored function. Part 2, Consultant 27(1):56, 1986.

Meredith L: Some thoughts on teaching student nurses human sexuality, Lamp, March 1984, p 21.

Osis M: Sexuality: an interactional perspective . . . drugs and healthy aging, Gerontion 1(1):6, 1986.

Rosenbaum J and others: A sexuality workshop: increasing sexual self-awareness, Can J Psychiatr Nurs 27(2):8, 1986.

Shuman NA and others: Nurses' attitudes towards sexual counseling, DCCN 6(2):75, 1987.

Turner DS and others: An analysis of alcoholism and its effects on sexual functioning, Sex Disabil 5(3):143, 1982.

Watts RJ: Sexual functioning, health beliefs, and compliance with high blood pressure medications, Nurs Res 31(5):278, 1982.

Webb C and others: Nurse' knowledge and attitudes about sexuality in health care: a review of the literature, Nurse Educ Today 7(2):75, 1987.

Welman C: Sexual health and the professional nurse, Curationis 6(4):37, 1983.

Williams LD: Strategies for sexual counseling: program to prepare staff members, Rehabil Nurs 11(5):21, 1986.

Woods NF: Human sexuality in health and illness, ed 3, St Louis, 1984, The CV Mosby Co.

UNIT XIV

Drugs Used in Neoplastic Diseases

CHAPTERS

56
Antineoplastic Chemotherapy

57
Antineoplastic Agents

chapter 56

Antineoplastic Chemotherapy

OBJECTIVES

After studying this chapter, the student will be able to:

1. Identify four major developmental stages of normal and malignant cells.

2. List common antineoplastic drugs and their effects on the cell cycle.

3. Describe the major principles of chemotherapy.

4. Describe the common toxicities of antineoplastic chemotherapy.

5. Discuss age-related considerations for cancer in the elderly and in the child.

6. Describe nursing considerations common to all antineoplastic drugs.

Cancer is a generic term that includes over 300 defined disease states. An estimated 25% of Americans face a cancer diagnosis during their lifetimes. Many people fear cancer, since it is difficult to accept that a small lump or mole that has the potential for rapid growth may lead to serious illness or death. Therefore education and early treatment are imperative to win the battle against cancer, which is second to cardiovascular disease as a cause of death.

Statistically, the chances of developing cancer and dying from cancer are greater now than ever before. However, more persons are cured of cancer today than ever before. In 1971 approximately 535,000 new cases of cancer were detected. In 1986, the number of new cases of cancer was estimated to be 930,000 persons. This is an increase of nearly 74% in the reported incidence of cancer. In 1971, 337,398 Americans died from cancer, whereas 1986 cancer-related deaths were estimated at 472,000. This is an approximate 40% increase in mortality. While the figures are still staggering, the fact that the rise in cancer deaths has not paralleled the rise in cancer incidence indicates that we have made some progress in the war against cancer.

This chapter discusses the principles of antineoplastic chemotherapy and the use of chemotherapeutic drugs in the treatment of cancer. However, to better understand the mechanisms and sites of action of the cancer chemotherapeutic agents, it is important to understand the kinetics of both normal cells and cancer cells.

CELL KINETICS

The reproductive cycles of normal and cancer cells are essentially the same (Figure 56-1). In the S-phase (DNA synthesis or replication stage) DNA doubles in preparation for cell division. The G_2 phase is the premitotic phase. At this time DNA synthesis ceases but RNA and protein synthesis continues to prepare the cell for **mitosis,** or spindle formation. During the M-phase the cells divide into two completely new cells that may leave the cell cycle for G_0 phase or continue in the cell cycle to G_1 phase. The G_0 phase involves the storage of nonreplicating cells that develop into mature, differentiated cells that will eventually die. During the G_1 phase enzyme, RNA, and protein synthesis may occur. The decision for cell replication or cell differentiation is determined during G_1 phase.

The four major developmental stages of normal and malignant cells are shown in Figure 56-2. Cancer chemotherapy is most effective in the first stage because the dividing cell is most vulnerable to the specific anticancer agents. Activity in the dividing cell stage occurs in the bone marrow, the hair follicles, and the gastrointestinal tract. These three areas are most affected by the toxicity of the anticancer drugs.

The anticancer agents have different sites of action on the dividing cell cycle. Agents that are most effective in one specific phase are referred to as cell cycle–specific agents. For example, methotrexate is more active in the S-phase of the cell cycle, so it is considered an S-phase cell cycle–specific agent. Antineoplastic agents that are active against both proliferating and resting cells are called cell cycle–nonspecific agents. An example of this group is the alkylating agents (see Table 57-1, p. 868). Antineoplastic classifications are an important consideration in selecting the appropriate drug(s) for the specific cancerous state. Methotrexate, an agent active predominantly in the S-phase of the cell cycle, would be much less effective in treating large tumor masses, which generally have slowly dividing cancer cells.

Normal cells grow and divide in an orderly fashion. The body process of cell adhesion inhibits the movement of the newly formed cells, and the body's homeostatic mechanisms control the entire cell growth process. Cancer cells may evolve from a hereditary or genetic predisposition plus contact with certain environmental conditions. Generally such neoplastic cells lack the cellular differentiation of the tissues in which they originate and therefore are unable to function like the normal cells around them. Cancer growth is enhanced by an increased rate of cell proliferation that lacks the normal body control system on cellular growth patterns. The cancer cells, because of the genetic differences, lack the cell adhesive property of normal cells, which may lead to metastasis, or spread of the cancer.

The growth of a cancer is usually rapid in the early stages, but as the tumor enlarges in size, it nearly outgrows its blood and nutrient supply, and the growth rate pattern decreases or reaches the plateau phase for the tumor. This is referred to as **Gompertzian growth kinetics** (see box on p. 861). A cell burden of 10^9 is usually the smallest tumor burden that is physically

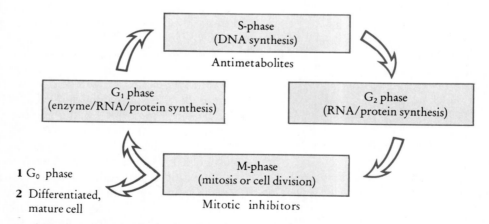

FIGURE 56-1   Reproductive cell cycle of normal and cancer cell with sites of action for antineoplastic drugs.

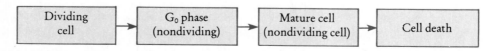

FIGURE 56-2   Overview of four major developmental stages of normal and malignant cells.

detectable. At this point the patient has approximately 1 billion cancer cells, which is equal to a tumor about the size of a small grape and weighing 1 g. This is the point at which clinical symptoms usually first appear.

The **Papanicolaou (Pap) smear** is a cytologic test capable of detecting carcinoma of the cervix and endometrium in the subclinical stages (10^2 to 10^6 cells). Early detection and treatment of small cancer lesions that are not detectable by visual examination have dramatically reduced the mortality of cancer of the cervix in the United States.

Animal studies have shown that chemotherapeutic drugs given in adequate doses for the host will kill a constant fraction of the cancer cells. For example, a drug or drug combination capable of killing 99.9% of the cells would only reduce a 10^{10} cell burden to 10^7 cancer cells. This reduction may produce a remission, but if further therapies are not instituted, the remaining cells may grow into another detectable tumor.

PRINCIPLES OF CHEMOTHERAPY

To obtain the maximal therapeutic effects with an antineoplastic agent or with combination cancer chemotherapies, the following principles should be considered:
1. Cancer chemotherapy is most effective against small tumors because they usually have an efficient blood supply and therefore drug delivery is increased. Also, small tumors generally have a higher percentage of proliferating cells so that a higher cell-kill factor is possible.
2. The removal of large, localized tumors by surgery reduces the tumor cell burden and thus contributes to the success of adjuvant chemotherapy. The major use of adjuvant chemotherapy is to help eradicate the **micrometastases** of cancer after surgery or radiation.
3. In general, combination cancer chemotherapeutic agents have a higher cancer cell-kill than treatment with a single drug agent.

COMBINATION CHEMOTHERAPY

In the 1960s combination chemotherapy was initiated for the treatment of acute lymphoblastic leukemia and Hodgkin's disease. When the complete response rates for single agents were compared with the response rates for combination drugs, the results were enlightening. The response rates for the MOPP treatment of advanced Hodgkin's disease are as follows:

	Drugs	Complete Response Rates
M	mustine (Mustargen)	20%
O	vincristine (Oncovin)	< 10%
P	procarbazine	< 10%
P	prednisone	< 5%
	MOPP combination	80%

The following considerations are used to select the drugs for combination chemotherapy:
1. Each drug when used alone should be active against the specific cancer.
2. Each drug should have a different site of action and act at a different point of the cell cycle (specificity).
3. Each drug should have a different organ toxicity or, if the toxic effect is similar, it should occur at different times after drug administration.

When the preceding principles are applied to the MOPP drug therapy, the concept of combination chemotherapy can be understood. First, the previous list illustrates the effectiveness of each of the drugs against Hodgkin's disease. Second, the sites of major activity for each antineoplastic agent are believed to be different.
1. Mustine (Mustargen) is an alkylating agent that can interfere with the replication, transcription, and translation of DNA.
2. Vincristine (Oncovin) inhibits mitosis by interfering with the mitotic spindle.
3. Procarbazine is a weak monoamine oxidase (MAO) inhibitor, and its antineoplastic action is believed to occur during the S-phase. It inhibits the synthesis of DNA, RNA, and protein.
4. Prednisone has lympholytic properties and may produce an antifibrotic effect that would be useful in treating cancer metastases surrounded by fibrous materials. It also improves appetite and general feelings of well-being.

The third principle, that of different organ toxicity or toxicities that occur at different times, has also been sub-

---

CANCER CELL GROWTH (GOMPERTZIAN)

	Number of cells present	
10^0	1	
10^1	10	
10^2	100	
10^3	1000	
10^4	10,000	Subclinical disease (undetectable by physical examination)
10^5	100,000	
10^6	1,000,000	
10^7	10,000,000	
10^8	100,000,000	
10^9	1,000,000,000	(1 g) Clinical symptoms appear
10^{10}	10,000,000,000	Regional spread
10^{11}	100,000,000,000	Metastases (regional-advanced)
10^{12}	1,000,000,000,000	
10^{13}	10,000,000,000,000	Possible lethal number of cancer cells

stantiated for the MOPP combination. The dose-limiting toxicity of bone marrow suppression is a property of both mustine and procarbazine, but the **nadir,** or the lowest depression point for this effect, occurs approximately 10 days after drug administration for mustine and 21 days after for procarbazine. Thus additive myelosuppressive effects from this combination are essentially avoided. Vincristine does not have bone marrow suppression effects but does exhibit a dose-limiting neurotoxicity. Prednisone does not demonstrate bone marrow suppression or neurotoxicity. Therefore the third principle of combination drug therapy is fulfilled.

Frequently the oncologist uses combination therapy in antineoplastic treatment. For other commonly prescribed drug combinations, see Table 56-1.

TOXICITY

Most of the currently available antineoplastic agents appear to act on similar metabolic pathways in both nor-

TABLE 56-1   Combination Chemotherapeutic Therapies

Cancer	Therapy	Drugs included*
Breast	CMF	cyclophosphamide (Cytoxan, Procytox♣)
		methotrexate
		5-fluorouracil
	Cooper's regimen (CVFMP)	cyclophosphamide (Cytoxan, Procytox♣)
		vincristine (Oncovin)
		5-Fluororacil
		methotrexate
		prednisone
Hodgkin's disease	ABVD	doxorubicin (Adriamycin)
		bleomycin (Blenoxane)
		vinblastine (Velban, Velbe♣)
		dacarbazine (DTIC)
	MOPP	mechlorethamine (Mustargen)
		vincristine (Oncovin)
		procarbazine (Matulane, Natulan♣)
		prednisone
Acute lymphocytic leukemia (ALL)	VP	vincristine (Oncovin)
		prednisone
	OAP	vincristine (Oncovin)
		cytarabine (Ara C, Cytosar-U, Cytosar♣)
		prednisone
Acute myelocytic leukemia (AML)	DA	daunorubicin (Cerubidine)
		cytarabine (Ara C, Cytosar-U, Cytosar♣)

*The underlined letters refer to the letters used in the combination therapy.

mal and malignant cells. A major limitation of cancer drugs is their lack of tumor specificity. Drug toxicities or side effects may be divided into (1) common side effects or adverse reactions and (2) specific dose-limiting drug effects.

The common toxic effects are hair loss **(alopecia),** nausea, vomiting, anorexia, diarrhea, and **stomatitis.** Leukopenia, thrombocytopenia, and anemia are common adverse effects that can lead to serious and even life-threatening infections. Bone marrow suppression is the major dose-limiting property most frequently encountered in cancer chemotherapy. Nursing assessment and monitoring are critical to improving patient care and will be reviewed in the nursing considerations section.

Specific dose-limiting effects are adverse reactions that occur only with certain drugs. For example, drugs that can produce liver disease include methotrexate, mercaptopurine, lomustine, dacarbazine, doxorubicin, and carmustine. Cyclophosphamide is associated with hemorrhagic cystitis. (Since dehydration increases the risk factor, adequate fluid intake is important when this agent is administered.) Methotrexate is associated with tubular necrosis, which can be prevented by **prehydrating** with normal saline and alkalinizing the urine to increase the elimination of the drug. Cisplatin is associated with tubular necrosis. Prehydration with 1 to 2 L of intravenous fluid and adequate fluids after drug administration help to reduce this adverse reaction. **Nephrotoxicity, ototoxicity,** and peripheral neuropathy have been reported with cisplatin.

Cardiac toxicity is reported with both doxorubicin and daunorubicin. **Cardiotoxicity** increases in patients who receive more than 550 mg/m^2 of body surface (total accumulated dosage given throughout therapy). Toxicity is also greater in geriatric patients and children under 2 years of age. Since this effect is cumulative if either drug is given, the amount of one drug already received by the patient must be considered when planning therapy with the other drug.

Neurologic toxicity may range from tingling of the hands and feet and loss of deep tendon reflexes to ataxia, footdrop, confusion, and personality changes. Drugs reported to produce neurologic effects include vincristine, vinblastine, and methotrexate.

AGE-RELATED CONSIDERATIONS
CANCER IN THE ELDERLY

Cancer is one of the most serious diseases of the elderly population, and its incidence increases sharply with age. Fifty percent of all cases of cancer in the United States occur in the oldest one eighth of the population. Sixty percent of all cancer deaths occur among persons 65 years of age or older. Compared with younger cancer victims, the elderly have more concurrent illnesses, which may decrease their ability to withstand the effects of cancer or the antineoplastic therapies. In addition, decreased pulmonary and renal function and decreased bone marrow cellularity may interfere with treatment. Other factors to be considered when managing regimens for elderly persons are the possibility of reduced income and loss of loved ones and family support. Often compromises in treatment are made because of a person's advanced age; however, data suggest that a dosage reduction of chemotherapy based on age alone is not indicated in clients with solid tumors. Clinical trials are needed to further examine the relationship between responsiveness to chemotherapy and the person's age.

CANCER IN CHILDREN

Cancer in children is relatively uncommon. In the United States only about 6000 pediatric cases are diagnosed annually; children represent approximately 3% of all cancer patients. Carcinomas are rare in children, with nearly 50% of pediatric carcinomas being leukemias and lymphomas and 20% nonepithelial tumors of the CNS. Since tumors in children grow rapidly, childhood cancer is generally more responsive to chemotherapy than is cancer in an adult. Children also tend to tolerate the acute side effects of chemotherapy better than adults. Fifty percent of children with cancer are long-term survivors or are actually cured.

THE NURSE'S ROLE IN ANTINEOPLASTIC CHEMOTHERAPY

Assessment. Nursing care for clients receiving drug therapy with antineoplastic agents is complex and inseparable from nursing care of the family. The client may be in any stage of the disease process and may even be facing impending death. In the assessment of the client and family, special considerations should be given to their coping abilities. The approach taken by the nurse should be sensitive and appropriate to the individual needs of the client and family. The client's degree of acceptance of chemotherapy should be assessed, and the nurse may need to help the patient deal with mixed emotions about the chemotherapy. The client's and family's knowledge of chemotherapy and their expectations should also be assessed. For specific nursing diagnoses related to the use of antineoplastic agents, see p. 865.

Intervention. The nurse has many responsibilities in dealing with the inevitable side effects of antineoplastic drugs. The potential for infection is increased because of bone marrow depression. Strict aseptic technique should be used during contact with the hospitalized patient, who should also be protected from persons harboring harmful microorganisms. Frequent blood counts are necessary, and the nurse is often responsible for ensuring that they are taken and the results monitored for early signs of bone marrow depression. A client with an absolute gran-

ulocyte count below 1000 cells/mm^3 is in danger of infection. Clients with granulocytopenia should maintain scrupulous oral hygiene and receive topical antibiotics for abrasions and scratches. Clients should be instructed to report to the physician any signs of infection, such as elevated temperature, sore throat, cough, mouth ulcerations, or burning on urination.

The potential for physical injury exists for clients with thrombocytopenia when platelet levels fall below 50,000 cells/mm^3. The nurse should avoid taking rectal temperatures and administering suppositories to such a client. Protective care for these clients might include the administration of stool softeners and the use of soft-bristled toothbrushes and electric razors. Soft tissue injury should be avoided, and the use of side rails on beds should be considered. Oral preparations of analgesics and other medications should be used to avoid the tissue damage resulting from intramuscular injections. Venipunctures should be done carefully by experienced personnel using strict sterile technique. The client should be instructed to report signs that indicate decreased platelets, such as petechiae, easy bruising, hemorrhage, bleeding from the gums, epistaxis, and blood in the stool and urine.

The kidneys are at risk of injury because of the effectiveness of the antineoplastic agents. Purines are released through cell destruction and converted to uric acid. The possibility of renal failure may result from the precipitation of uric acid crystals in the kidneys. The nurse should monitor the client's intake and output and serum uric acid and creatinine levels. Fluid intake should be 3 L daily. Cold, clear liquids such as tea, unsweetened apple juice or other juices, and soft drinks or carbonated beverages such as ginger ale may be well tolerated. Freezing a favorite beverage into ice cubes or popsicles is also recommended.

The client's body image may be disturbed as a result of alopecia. This side effect is extremely distressing to women, even when they have been prepared for it, have cosmetic aids available, and are aware that it is reversible. Clients, even those who have only thinning of the hair, need assurance that the hair will begin to grow back in about 6 to 8 weeks, although it may be a different texture or color. Treatment with hormones may necessitate support for the client in the event of such effects as masculinization in a female patient or feminization in a male patient. These clients need assistance in coping with body image problems.

Some clients lose their appetite or complain of a bitter or metallic taste in the mouth. Their desire for red meat or other protein foods may be reduced, since these foods are the most commonly perceived as bitter tasting. Because protein is essential for good nutrition, alternative methods of serving proteins should be pursued. Cold cooked turkey, fish, eggs, and dairy products may be suitable substitutes. The biggest meal of the day should be planned for the time the client is usually hungriest, even if that time is early morning or midnight.

Nausea and vomiting that accompany the use of antineoplastic drugs can be relieved by the administration of an antiemetic drug 1 to 3 hours before administration of the antineoplastic drugs. The antiemetic can then be continued afterward as necessary. Speeding the passage of food through the stomach is sometimes the solution to the problem of nausea, vomiting, and feelings of fullness. Some quantities of carbohydrates eaten at frequent intervals help achieve this effect. Liquids should not be drunk at mealtime but instead should be taken frequently throughout the day, up to 30 to 60 minutes before eating. Since hot foods have been reported to contribute to nausea, foods should be served at room temperature or cooler. Resting for 1 to 2 hours after eating is advised because activity can slow the digestive process.

Stomatitis, oral ulcerations, **xerostomia,** and other oral changes are common side effects of the potent antineoplastic agents and may interfere with the client's nutrition. Good oral hygiene is important to maintain a proper nutritional intake and decrease the possibility of oral infections becoming systemic. The kind of mouthwash solutions used depends on the status of the patient's lesions. Small, frequent servings of cold or room-temperature, bland, nonirritating foods are best tolerated by the client. This type of diet also decreases the diarrhea that is a common side effect of cancer chemotherapy.

Diarrhea, as a side effect of antineoplastic drugs, results from the death of the rapidly dividing cells of the bowel mucosa. The nurse should assess the client's bowel status, hydration, and electrolyte levels and record diarrhea as output. Fluid intake should be encouraged between meals, although intravenous therapy may be needed to replace lost fluids if the diarrhea is severe. Because of the client's frequent defecation, special attention should be given to skin care in the perianal area. Modification of the diet will prevent or decrease diarrhea. The client should be instructed to avoid foods that may cause gas and cramping, such as cabbage, beans, and highly spiced foods. Hot food should be avoided because it increases peristalsis that reduces nutrition absorption and may cause diarrhea. Reducing high-fiber foods in the diet, such as raw fruits and vegetables, bran, and whole grain cereals and bread, may help to control diarrhea. Foods that are high in potassium (to replace potassium loss through diarrhea) and that usually do not worsen diarrhea include bananas, apricot or pear nectar, red meat, saltwater fish, boiled or mashed potatoes, and orange juice.

Constipation may also be a problem with some clients. This may be an early symptom of CNS toxicity from the drug therapy or may result from eating mostly soft and liquid foods. High-fiber foods and prune juice have a laxative effect; 1 or 2 tablespoons of bran may be added to cooked cereals, casseroles, and homemade baked goods.

The client should be encouraged to drink plenty of fluids, preferably 8 to 10 glasses daily. Hot lemon water in the morning usually stimulates bowel activity. The physician may order a laxative or stool softener as needed.

Pain commonly occurs in clients receiving antineoplastic drugs. The treatment of pain associated with cancer, especially chronic pain, requires a careful assessment of the patient, consideration of appropriate nursing interventions, and skillful application of pharmacologic agents. Chronic pain may progress in a cycle to anxiety or depression, insomnia, fatigue, and increased pain. The following factors modify the pain threshold. (Analgesics are discussed in Chapter 11.)

Lower Threshold	Raise Threshold
Anger	Symptom relief
Fear	Adequate relief from pain
Discomfort	Rest
Fatigue	Diversion
Anxiety	Elevation of mood
Sadness	Understanding
Loneliness	Sympathy
Depression	
Isolation	

Nursing interventions may include physical activity to help prevent further deterioration resulting from inactivity. Deep breathing, turning the patient, and skin care are some of the actions that reduce complications. In addition to physical and pharmacologic interventions, the client may need psychosocial, intellectual, and spiritual support. The holistic approach of carefully assessing the client's current needs and anticipating and planning for continued care is important in the care of many illnesses but is crucial for a client dying of a progressive illness. A variety of home-care programs are available. In addition, hospice programs have been developed throughout the United States to help provide the supportive and palliative services necessary for clients with life-threatening illness and their families.

It must be remembered that anticancer drugs are potent drugs that are mutagenic and carcinogenic in animals and may be carcinogenic in humans. Nurses and pharmacists who prepare antineoplastic drugs should institute safety measures such as using good technique, wearing gloves, mask, and protective clothing, and whenever possible, preparing the solutions in a vertical laminar flow, biologically safe hood. All unused solutions, vials, needles, syringes, gloves, and materials used to clean up spills should be processed as hazardous materials; that is, the waste should be properly incinerated.

Although the development of cancer in professionals has not yet been directly related to handling of materials, a relationship between fetal loss and occupational exposure to antineoplastic drugs in nurses has been reported (Selevan 1988). Governmental regulatory agencies have indicated that it is unacceptable to allow exposure to

ndx Selected Nursing Diagnoses Relating to Antineoplastic Agents

Nursing diagnosis	Outcome criteria	Nursing interventions
Potential alteration in oral mucous membrane related to stomatitis	Client will: Demonstrate knowledge of oral hygiene Maintain adequate nutrition and hydration Maintain normal oral mucosa or have decreasing inflammation and/or ulceration	Instruct client to complete all dental work before beginning chemotherapy. Teach optimal oral hygiene to prevent stomatitis. Inspect oral cavity with a tongue blade and light twice daily and before each administration of the antineoplastic drug. Implement appropriate mouth care if inflammation is present. Encourage soothing foods: bland foods, cool liquids, cool foods (popsicles). Instruct client to avoid spicy or acidic foods, extremes in food temperature, and abrasive foods or foods that are difficult to chew. Consult with physician if oral pain relief solution is needed. Instruct client to report any ulcers in or around the mouth.
Potential for infection related to bone marrow depression	Client will: Remain free of infection	Instruct client in reading a thermometer. Teach client to take temperature daily in the afternoon and report any elevation over 101° F. Teach the client to avoid being immunized with live virus vaccines and having contact with people with infections. Instruct the client to report any signs of infection, such as cough, sore throat, and burning on urination.
Potential for injury related to bone marrow depression	Client will: Exhibit no signs of bleeding or excessive bruising	Avoid performing invasive procedures such as intramuscular injections and taking rectal temperatures. Inspect intravenous sites, skin, and mucous membranes for signs of bleeding and bruising. Instruct the client to report easy bruising, bloody urine, and bleeding from nose and gums. Test urine, emesis, and stool for occult blood. Instruct the client to exercise care in oral hygiene and in using safety razors and nail clippers. Teach the client to avoid constipation. Encourage the use of caution to prevent falls.
Potential for alterations in bowel elimination, diarrhea or constipation	Client will: Maintain a normal bowel pattern Have less constipation or diarrhea	Assess client's normal bowel pattern as baseline. If client is constipated, increase fluid intake and roughage in diet. If client has diarrhea, decrease roughage, increase fluids, and give small feedings. Consult with physician if stool softener, laxative, or antidiarrheal is needed. Assess client for fluid and electrolyte status. Monitor bowel movements; record diarrhea as output. Clean and dry the perianal area after each bowel movement.
Disturbance in self concept related to alopecia	Client will: Demonstrate progress toward coping with altered body image	Allow client to express apprehensions related to alopecia. Encourage client to obtain cap or hairpiece before treatment begins. Reassure client that hair growth should begin 8 weeks after therapy, but the new growth may be of a different color and texture.

potential carcinogens to continue until cancer actually occurs. Regulatory agencies should not wait for epidemiologic evidence before taking action to limit exposure to chemicals considered to be carcinogenic.

Education. Teaching the client about drug administration and drug effects may help to ease his or her anxiety. An assessment may reveal that expectations are unrealistic, and the client and the family may need assistance in accepting a more realistic view of the results of chemotherapy. Expectations of total cure may be unrealistic and should not be reinforced, whereas expectations of remission are often appropriate. One of the most important nursing interventions is emotional support to a client who

is receiving physically and psychologically distressing therapy. The long periods of therapy, with frequent interruptions and sporadic progress, may compound the client's anxieties.

A client receiving cancer chemotherapy should be cautioned *not* to take any over-the-counter medication before checking with the oncologist. Many over-the-counter preparations contain aspirin, alcohol, or other substances that could interfere with the antineoplastic agents or increase the risk for toxicity.

See above for specific areas of client instruction related to nursing diagnosis.

Evaluation. Evaluation of drug effects is an integral

nursing function in antineoplastic chemotherapy. Often no dosage schedule for antineoplastic agents is universally therapeutic, and the dosage is changed according to the client's response and the toxic effects of the drug. Thus the nurse's evaluation and communication of both drug toxicity and client response are essential. In evaluating toxic effects, the nurse should be vigilant for early signs, since progression of toxic effects may have severe and irreversible consequences.

KEY TERMS

BIBLIOGRAPHY

American Hospital Formulary Service, AHFS drug information 88, Bethesda, Md, 1988, American Society of Hospital Pharmacists, Inc.

American Cancer Society: Cancer facts and figures, New York, 1986, The Society.

Ballentine, R: Nursing implications of cancer chemotherapy, Nursing 83 13(7):56, 1983.

Baranovsky, A, and Myers, MH: Cancer incidence and survival in patients 65 years of age and older, CA 36(1):26, 1986.

Bersani, G, and Carl, W: Oral care for cancer patients, Am J Nurs 83:533, 1983.

Campbell, JB, and others: The leukemias: definition, treatment and nursing care, Nurs Clin North Am 18(3):523, 1983.

Chabner, BA: The volution of cancer chemotherapy, Hosp Practice 20(4):115, 1985.

Daeffler, R: Oral hygiene measures for patients with cancer. Part 2, Cancer Nurs 14:427, 1980.

Daeffler, R: Oral hygiene measures for patients with cancer. Part 3, Cancer Nurs, 1981, p 29.

Engelking, CH, and Steele, NE: A model for pretreatment nursing assessment of patients receiving cancer chemotherapy, Cancer Nurs 7(3):203, 1984.

Fuks, JZ, and Wiernik, PH: Adjuvant chemotherapy of cancer, Hosp Formulary, 17:1353, 1982.

Hemminki, K, and others: Spontaneous abortions and malformations in the offspring of nurses exposed to anaesthetic gases, cytostatic drugs, and other potential hazards in hospitals, based on registered information of outcome, J Epidemiol Community Health 39:141, 1985.

Holmes, S: Chemotherapy and the gastrointestinal tract, Nurs Times 80(8):28, 1984.

Holmes, W: SQ chemotherapy at home, Am J Nurs 85:168, 1985.

Hubbard, SM, and Seipp, CA: Administering cancer treatment: the role of the oncology nurse, Hosp Pract 20(7):167, 1985.

Katcher, BS, and others: Applied therapeutics, ed 3, San Francisco, 1983, Applied Therapeutics, Inc.

Klopovich, PM, and Trieworthy, RC: Adherence to chemotherapy regimens among children with cancer, Top Clin Nurs 7(1):19, 1985.

Longman, AJ, and Rogers, BP: Altered cell growth in cancer and the nursing implications, Cancer Nurs 7(5):405, 1984.

McCalla, JL: A multidisciplinary approach to identification and remedial intervention for adverse late effects of cancer therapy, Nurs Clin North Am 20(1):117, 1985.

Pelton, S: Easing the complications of chemotherapy, Nursing 84 14(2):58, 1984.

Pizzo, PA: Management of pediatric cancer, Hosp Pract 21(3):111, 1986.

Pratt, A, and others: Psychological parameters of chemotherapy-induced conditioned nausea and vomiting: a review, Cancer Nurs 7(6):483, 1984.

Ristuccia, AM: Hematologic effects of cancer chemotherapy, Nurs Clin North Am 20(1):235, 1985.

Rosenberg, SA: Combined-modality therapy of cancer (what is it and when does it work?), New Engl J Med 312(23):1512, 1985.

Selevan, SG, and others: A study of occupational exposure to antineoplastic drugs and fetal loss in nurses, New Engl J Med 313(19):1173, 1985.

Silverberg, E, and Lubera, J: Cancer statistics, 1986, CA 36(1):9, 1986.

Yasko, JM: Holistic management of nausea and vomiting caused by chemotherapy, Top Clin Nurs 7(1):18, 1985.

CHAPTER

57

Antineoplastic Agents

OBJECTIVES

After studying this chapter, the student will be able to:

1. Classify antineoplastic agents based on the major mechanism of action.

2. List common side effects/adverse reactions of antineoplastic drugs.

3. Describe the use of "leucovorin rescue" with methotrexate treatments.

4. Describe the indications and nursing considerations for the various classifications of antineoplastic agents.

5. Apply precautions in the preparation and administration of antineoplastic drugs.

CLASSIFICATION

The antineoplastic agents are divided into various classes based on their probable major mechanisms of action (Table 57-1).

These agents do not directly kill tumor cells; they act by interfering with cell reproduction or replication at some point in the cell cycle. For cells to proliferate, the genetic material DNA must be replicated once every cell cycle. DNA is the genetic substance in body cells that transfers information resulting in the production of RNA necessary to produce enzymes and protein synthesis (see Figure 57-1). The enzymes determine the structure, biochemical activity, growth rate, and functions of the cell.

The formation of the nucleic acids, DNA, and, ultimately, RNA, requires pyrimidines and purines (nitrogen compounds) as the basic building block materials. **Antimetabolites** have a structure similar to a necessary building block for the formation of DNA. This substance is accepted by the cell as the necessary ingredient for cell growth, but because it is an impostor, it interferes with the normal production of DNA. **Alkylating agents** are drugs that substitute an alkyl chemical structure for a hydrogen atom in DNA. This results in a cross-linking of each strand of DNA, thus preventing cell division.

Antibiotic antitumor agents interfere with DNA functioning by blocking the transcription of new DNA or RNA. Like the alkylating agents, they are used primarily to treat malignancies of the hematopoietic tissues, neuro-

TABLE 57-1   Antineoplastic Drugs and Cell-Cycle Effects

Drug and classification	Effect on cell cycle
ALKYLATING DRUGS	Cell cycle–nonspecific
busulfan (Myleran)	
carmustine (BCNU, BiCNU)	
chlorambucil (Leukeran)	
cisplatin (cis-platinum, Platinol)	
cyclophosphamide (Cytoxan)	
dacarbazine (DTIC-Dome)	
lomustine (CCNU, CeeNU)	
mechlorethamine hydrochloride (nitrogen mustard, Mustargen)	
melphalan (Alkeran)	
triethylenethiophosphoramide (Thiotepa)	
ANTIMETABOLITE DRUGS	Cell cycle–specific agents; main activity in S-phase
cytarabine (cytosine arabinoside, Cytosar-U)	
floxuridine (FUDR)	
fluorouracil (5-FU, Adrucil)	
hydroxyurea (Hydrea)	
mercaptopurine (Purinethol)	
methotrexate (Mexate)	
thioguanine	
ANTIBIOTIC ANTITUMOR DRUGS	Most agents in this classification believed to be cell cycle–nonspecific; doxorubicin believed to be cell cycle–specific for S-phase, whereas Mitomycin is most active in G- and S-phases
bleomycin sulfate (Blenoxane)	
dactinomycin (actinomycin D, Cosmegen)	
daunorubicin hydrochloride (Cerubidine)	
doxorubicin hydrochloride (Adriamycin)	
mithramycin (Mithracin)	
mitomycin (Mutamycin)	
MITOTIC INHIBITORS	Cell cycle–specific for M-phase; block mitosis in metaphase
vinblastine (Velban)	
vincristine (Oncovin)	
HORMONAL DRUGS	Primary effects in oncology reviewed in text; dexamethasone indicated for cerebral edema often associated with metastatic brain tumors
Adrenocorticosteroids	
dexamethasone (Decadron)	
prednisone	
Estrogens	Sex hormones used to offset tumor-stimulating effects of endogenous hormones; may inhibit tumor growth in specific tissues by altering hormonal environment
diethylstilbestrol (DES)	
estradiol (Estrace, Progynon)	
conjugated estrogens (Premarin)	
esterified estrogens	
ethinyl estradiol	
Androgens	
fluoxymesterone (Halotestin)	
methyltestosterone (Oreton-Methyl)	
testosterone	
Progestins	
hydroxyprogesterone caproate (Delalutin)	
medroxyprogesterone acetate (Provera, Depo-Provera)	
megestrol acetate (Megace)	
Antiestrogen	Blocks estrogen receptor sites in tumors that are estrogen dependent
tamoxifen citrate (Nolvadex)	
MISCELLANEOUS DRUGS	
asparaginase (L-asparaginase, Elspar)	Enzyme capable of breaking down asparagine, which is necessary for metabolism of malignant cells; cell cycle–specific for G_1-phase
mitotane (Lysodren)	Cytotoxic activity unknown but acts as adrenal gland suppressing agent; indicated for inoperable adrenocortical carcinomas
procarbazine (Matulane)	Cytotoxic activity unknown; weak MAO inhibitor; believed to have S-phase activity

Pyrimidines ----------------------> DNA -------------- RNA ----------------> Protein/enzymes

Purines ------------------/

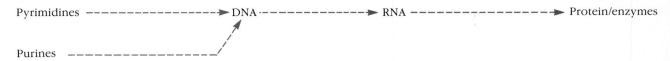

FIGURE 57-1   Protein synthesis.

blastoma, Ewing's and osteogenic sarcomas, and disseminated carcinomas of the lung, breast, ovary, and testis.

The **mitotic inhibitors,** vinblastine and vincristine, are plant alkaloids that block cell division in metaphase. They probably have other major sites of action because vinblastine differs from vincristine pharmacologically and in therapeutic application. Vinblastine has been used in the treatment of various lymphomas and carcinoma of the breast and testis. Vincristine is frequently used to treat acute leukemias and Hodgkin's disease.

Hormonal agents are used in the treatment of neoplasms that are sensitive to hormonal growth controls in the body. Their exact mechanism of action against neoplasms is unknown, but apparently they interfere with growth-stimulating receptor proteins at the cellular membrane. Estrogens are used to treat androgen-sensitive prostatic carcinomas or in postmenopausal women with breast cancer, and progestins are used for endometrial tumors and renal carcinomas. Androgens are used in the treatment of menopausal women with breast cancer and in prostatic cancer, and antiestrogens (tamoxifen citrate) are used to treat breast cancer and endometrial cancer.

Since corticosteroids retard lymphocytic proliferations, their greatest value lies in the treatment of lymphocytic leukemias and lymphomas. They are also used in conjunction with radiation therapy to decrease the occurrence of radiation edema in such critical areas as the superior mediastinum, brain, and spinal cord. Individual drugs belonging to this category are discussed in Chapter 49.

Alkylator-like drugs are chemically different agents that are believed to have an action similar to the alkylating agents.

Miscellaneous agents are those that cannot be classified by their mechanism of action into any of the groups previously mentioned. L-Asparaginase is capable of reducing asparagine to aspartic acid. Certain cancer cells depend on a circulating supply of asparaginase within the blood. When the available asparaginase is reduced, the cancer cells will eventually die. Normal body cells are capable of synthesizing adequate supplies of asparaginase and therefore are not affected by an asparaginase deficiency. L-Asparaginase has been used in the treatment of acute lymphocytic leukemia.

Mitotane is an adrenal gland suppressing agent whose exact mechanism of cytotoxic activity is unknown. Its primary indication is in the treatment of an inoperable carcinoma of the adrenal cortex.

The exact mechanism of action of procarbazine is unknown, but it is believed to interfere with DNA structure and thus has an effect similar to the alkylating agents. It is also a weak MAO inhibitor and may have activity in the S-phase of the cell cycle. It is commonly prescribed for the treatment of Hodgkin's disease.

ANTIMETABOLITE DRUGS

fluorouracil (Adrucil, 5-fluorouracil, 5-FU)

Mechanism of action. Fluorouracil is a pyrimidine antagonist that interferes with the synthesis of DNA and RNA. It is a cell cycle–specific agent that produces its effect in the S-phase of cell division.

Indications

1. Palliative treatment of carcinomas of the colon, rectum, breast, stomach, and pancreas
2. Administered by intracavitary route for malignant effusions and intraarterially for liver, head, and neck tumors

Pharmacokinetics

Metabolism. Metabolized rapidly (within 1 hour) in the tissues to active metabolite floxuridine monophospate. Final metabolic degradation occurs in the liver.

Distribution. Distributed throughout the body and also crosses the blood-brain barrier; half-life for alpha phase is 10 to 20 min; beta phase is prolonged owing to tissue storage of metabolites and it may extend to 20 hours.

Excretion. Depends on catabolic degradation to inactive metabolites in the liver; primary excretion route is respiratory as carbon dioxide (60% to 80%); balance is excreted by way of the kidneys (up to 15% unchanged).

Side effects/adverse reactions. See Table 57-2.

Significant drug interactions. When fluorouracil is given with other bone marrow depressant drugs or radiation, increased bone marrow depression may occur. A decrease in drug dosage is usually indicated.

Dosage and administration (adults only)

Intravenous injection. 7 to 12 mg/kg body weight per day for 4 days; if no toxicity occurs during following 3 days, a dose of 7 to 10 mg/kg body weight is administered every 3 to 4 days for 2 weeks, or 12 mg/kg body weight daily for 5 days. If no toxicity occurs after another day, 6 mg/kg body weight is administered on alternate days for an additional 4 or 5 doses. Total course for therapy is 2 weeks.

Maintenance dosage. 7 to 12 mg/kg body weight intravenously every 7 to 10 days or 300 to 500 mg/m^2 body surface daily for 4 or 5 days, repeated on a monthly cycle.

TABLE 57-2   Side Effects/Adverse Reactions of Antineoplastic Agents

Drug(s)	Side effects*	Adverse reactions†
fluorouracil (Adrucil, 5-fluorouracil, 5-FU)	More frequent: Anorexia, alopecia, nausea, vomiting, rash, pruritus, lethargy	Diarrhea, chills, elevated temperature, sore throat, stomatitis, heartburn, abdominal distress, dark stools, increased frequency of bleeding and bruising
methotrexate (Mexate, Folex)	More frequent: Anorexia, nausea, vomiting Less frequent: Alopecia, pale skin, rash, pruritus, acne, boils High-dose therapy: Erythematous (red) skin	Black stools, diarrhea, abdominal distress, blood in vomitus, elevated temperature, chills, sore throat, stomatitis, increased frequency of bleeding and bruising Intrathecal: Seizures, headaches, lethargy, visual disturbances, dizziness, disorientation
mechlorethamine (Mustargen)	More frequent: Nausea and vomiting Less frequent: Anorexia, diarrhea, headache, alopecia, metallic taste in mouth, drowsiness	Elevated temperature, chills or sore throat, increased bleeding or bruising, painful rash, amenorrhea, abdominal distress, joint pain, edema of lower extremities With high-dose therapy or regional perfusion: Tinnitus, hearing loss, and dizziness
leucovorin (citrovorum factor, folinic acid, Wellcovorin, calcium folinate♣)	None reported	Allergic reaction: Rash, hives, pruritus, or difficulty in breathing
cyclophosphamide (Cytoxan, Beisar, Procytox♣)	More frequent: Dark discoloration of skin and fingernails, alopecia, anorexia, nausea, vomiting Less frequent: Facial flushing, headache, rash, pruritus, increased perspiration, swollen lips	Elevated temperature, chills, sore throat, irregular menstrual cycle, increased bleeding High dose or long-term therapy: Lethargy, disorientation, blood in urine, pain on urination, cough, shortness of breath, tachycardia, edema of lower extremities, painful joints, abdominal distress
cisplatin (Platinol)	More frequent: Nausea, vomiting Less frequent: Anorexia	Tinnitus, impaired hearing, elevated temperature, chills, sore throat, increased bleeding episodes, anemia, abdominal distress, painful joints, edema of lower extremities, impairment of taste perception, blurred vision, peripheral neuropathy, facial edema, difficulty in breathing
doxorubicin (Adriamycin)	More frequent: Alopecia, nausea, vomiting Less frequent: Diarrhea; dark discoloration of soles, palms, or nails, which is reported most often in blacks and children	Elevated temperature, chills, sore throat, stomatitis, inflammation of esophageal lining, red skin rash, abdominal distress, painful joints, edema of lower extremities, tachycardia, difficulty in breathing, increased bleeding or bruising
vinca alkaloids vincristine (Oncovin)	More frequent: Alopecia Less frequent: Nausea, vomiting, rash, weight loss, gas	Neurotoxicity that includes diplopia or blurred vision, paresthesias of hands and feet, ataxia, loss of deep tendon reflexes, ptosis, headache, jaw pain, abdominal distress, constipation, edema of lower extremities, disorientation, seizures, depression, insomnia
vinblastine (Velban, Velbe♣)	More frequent: Alopecia Less frequent: Nausea, vomiting, muscular pains	Elevated temperature, chills, sore throat, abdominal distress, edema of lower extremities, increased bleeding or bruising; neurotoxic side effects are considered rare

*If side effects continue, increase, or disturb the patient, the physician should be informed.
†If adverse reactions occur, contact the physician because medical intervention may be necessary.

Maximum dosage for adults is 800 mg/day or 400 mg/day for the high-risk patient. Investigational protocols may employ higher dosages than stated in the product's package insert. Review Chapter 2 for legal implications.

Topical. For treatment of skin cancer (basal cell carcinomas) and precancerous skin lesions.

Pregnancy safety. Not established

NURSING CONSIDERATIONS

Assessment. Carefully consider use of fluorouracil when the patient is pregnant or breast-feeding or has renal or hepatic function impairment, infection, bone marrow depression, or tumor cell infiltration of the bone

Intervention. Dosages are determined by the patient's weight. In obese patients or those with edema or ascites, estimated lean body mass is used.

Administer antiemetics to reduce nausea and vomiting.

Fluorouracil may be administered intraarterially by an infusion pump to ensure a consistent rate of infusion. The nurse should be knowledgeable about and skillful with the specific equipment being used.

Take precautions against intravenous infiltration. If extravasation occurs, administration should be stopped immediately and the remaining dose injected into another vein. Cold compresses may reduce local tissue damage.

Safety precautions should be taken if the platelet count is low. The precautions include avoidance of invasive procedures or use of extreme care in such procedures; regular examination of skin, mucous membranes, and injection sites for bruising or bleeding; testing of emesis, urine, and stool for signs of occult bleeding; care in the use of grooming implements, toothbrushes, toothpicks, razors, and nail clippers; prevention of constipation; and prevention of physical injury. Protective isolation should be instituted if WBC falls below 3500/mm^3. Broad-spectrum antibiotics may be administered pending appropriate cultures.

The client's mouth should be examined for ulcerations before each dose is administered, since stomatitis is a sign of toxicity. Therapy should be discontinued but may be reinstated at a lower dosage when the side effects have subsided.

Gastrointestinal disturbances usually occur about the fourth day of therapy and subside 2 or 3 days after the medication is withdrawn. Weakness occurs immediately after the dose is administered and lasts for 12 to 36 hours or longer.

Watch for signs of toxicity and indications for discontinuing the drug, including intractable vomiting, diarrhea, severe stomatitis, WBC below 3500/mm^3, thrombocytopenia (below 10,000/mm^3), and gastrointestinal bleeding.

Education. Be aware that skin and ocular sensitivity to the sun may occur. Sunglasses and sun-blocking lotions may be advised.

Clients should be instructed to avoid excessive alcohol and any aspirin intake because of the risk of gastrointestinal bleeding.

The client should be cautioned against being immunized with live virus vaccines during fluorouracil therapy, since it may cause rather than prevent the disease. Vaccination is also contraindicated in family members and other persons in close contact with the client. The client should avoid being exposed to infections.

Inform the patient that alopecia may occur but is reversible.

Evaluation. Monitor CBC and hematocrit and watch patient for signs of bruising and bleeding, particularly gastrointestinal bleeding. Lowest levels of leukocyte and platelet counts generally occur 21 to 25 days after the first day of fluorouracil therapy and recover by 30 days.

Monitor BUN, creatinine clearance, and serum uric acid level. A decrease in creatinine clearance and an increase in the other test values may indicate nephrotoxicity. Fluid intake should be 3000 ml daily.

Monitor temperature and observe for signs of infection, fever, chills, or sore throat.

methotrexate (Mexate, Folex)

Mechanism of action. Methotrexate is an antimetabolite that is cell cycle–specific for the S-phase. To synthesize DNA, folic acid must be reduced to tetrahydrofolic acid by the enzyme folic acid reductase. Methotrexate binds with folic acid reductase, thus inhibiting the synthesis of DNA and RNA. Since malignant cellular growth is usually greater than cell growth of normal tissues, cancer growth may be impaired by methotrexate.

Indications

1. Gestational choriocarcinoma, advanced lymphosarcoma, acute lymphocytic leukemia, meningeal leukemia, lung and breast cancers, epidermoid cancers of the head and neck, and mycosis fungoides
2. Severe, disabling psoriasis that is unresponsive to standard therapies

Pharmacokinetics

Absorption. Administered orally, intramuscularly, intravenously, and intrathecally. Oral formulation is usually rapidly absorbed with peak serum levels reached in 1 to 2 hours. Oral doses below 30 mg are completely absorbed, whereas doses above 30 mg are only partially absorbed.

Distribution. Limited amounts of methotrexate can cross the blood-brain barrier, but significant quantities pass into the systemic circulation following intrathecal drug administration. Systemically, approximately 50% of the drug is protein bound.

PRECAUTIONS FOR HANDLING ANTINEOPLASTIC DRUGS

DRUG PREPARATION AND ADMINISTRATION

Wear vinyl gloves when handling drugs.

Wear a face mask and eye protection when preparing powdered medications.

Use areas for the preparation of drugs only for that purpose. Limit access to that area.

Remove only the required amount of the drug into the syringe. If more is withdrawn accidently, inject the excess back into the vial and dispose of it properly.

Vent vials with a 20-gauge needle to avoid the creation of aerosol particles.

Nurses should not prepare intravenous chemotherapy if they are pregnant because of suspected risk to the fetus from these agents.

DISPOSAL OF ANTINEOPLASTIC DRUGS AND EQUIPMENT

All antineoplastic drugs and all vials, needles, syringes, tubing, and equipment used in their administration need to be discarded with caution. Special leak-proof, puncture-proof double bagged containers should be used and labeled BIOHAZARD for disposal by incineration.

Needles and syringes should not be broken and/or separated before disposal because it might cause leakage of the medication.

SPILLAGE OF ANTINEOPLASTIC DRUGS

Wear two pairs of gloves when cleaning up an antineoplastic drug spill. Wash hands before and after.

Wear a mask and eye protection if the medication is powdered.

Place the spilled substance in a plastic bag. Wipe up the remainder with a damp cloth and also place in the plastic bag.

Seal the bag and place it inside of a second bag, and seal the second bag. Label it BIOHAZARD and send it for disposal by incineration.

Wash the area with soap and water.

DISPOSAL OF PATIENT EXCRETA

Urine, vomitus, and other body fluids from patients receiving antineoplastic drugs should be handled with caution. Flush excreta down the toilet; wear gloves to avoid contact. Wash containers thoroughly.

Metabolism. Intracellular and hepatic.

Excretion. Unchanged drug is primarily excreted renally with a small percentage excreted in the bile (feces). Individuals vary in their excretion of this drug. Small amounts have remained in body tissues for periods of weeks to months.

Side effects/adverse reactions. See Table 57-2.

Significant drug interactions. The following interactions may occur when methotrexate is given with the drugs listed below.

Drug	Possible Effect and Management
alcohol and hepatotoxic drugs	Increases risk of hepatotoxicity. Avoid combination or if absolutely necessary, monitor closely.
acyclovir injection	Neurologic complications may occur with use of intrathecal methotrexate.
probenecid or sulfinpyrazone	Hyperuricemia and gout may occur. To manage, the physician may adjust the antigout medications or prescribe allopurinol. The latter is often preferred to prevent drug induced hyperuricemia.
asparaginase	Cell replication is inhibited by asparaginase, thus impairing the therapeutic effects of methotrexate. If asparaginase is administered 9 to 10 days before or within 24 hours after methotrexate, this effect in not reported. The major side effects of methotrexate—gastrointestinal and hematologic (blood components suppression)—are usually reduced with this drug administration schedule.
bone marrow depressants or radiation	Bone marrow depressant effects increase. A decrease in drug dosage is usually indicated.
NSAIAs (nonsteroidal antiinflammatory agents)	Concurrent administration may result in severe methotrexate toxicity. Refer to manufacturer's recommendations on individual NSAIAs to reduce this possibility.
probenecid or salicylates	May interfere with excretion of methotrexate, which results in elevated serum levels. Salicylates may also displace methotrexate from its protein-binding sites, also resulting in increased, and possibly toxic, serum levels. If necessary to use in combination, monitor serum methotrexate levels closely. Methotrexate dosage level should be decreased and the patient closely monitored for signs of toxicity.
vaccines, live oral	May result in a decrease in antibody response along with an increase in side effects/adverse reactions. Avoid if possible, or, if necessary, monitor closely for adverse effects and patient response.

Dosage and administration

Antineoplastic

Adults. Dosage 15 to 50 mg/m² of body surface given orally, intramuscularly, or intravenously, once or twice a week.

Children. 20 to 30 mg/m² of body surface orally or intramuscularly, once a week.

Meningeal leukemia

Adults. Use methotrexate sodium for injection without preservative. Dosage 12 to 15 mg/m² of body surface at specific intervals that vary according to purpose (induction treatment or prophylaxis) by the intrathecal route.

Children. Children over 2 years old, administer 12 mg/m^2 of body surface intrathecally, every 3 to 5 days until cerebrospinal fluid cell count returns to normal.

Other uses for an adult

Mycosis fungoides. Orally, 2.5 to 5 mg daily for weeks or if necessary, for extended periods. Intramuscularly, either 25 mg twice weekly or 50 mg once a week.

Psoriasis. Oral initial dosages (for 70 kg person) may vary from 2.5 to 6.25 mg daily for 5 days, followed by at least 2 drug-free days. Other dosage regimens also total up to a range of 30 to 50 mg in a 7-day period. See package insert for detailed information. The recommended intramuscular or intravenous methotrexate dosage is a single 10 to 25 mg dose weekly, up to a maximum of 50 mg.

Rheumatoid arthritis. Administer 2.5 to 25 mg (usually 7.5 mg) per week, orally.

Pregnancy safety. FDA category D

NURSING CONSIDERATIONS

Assessment. Carefully consider use of methotrexate when the patient is pregnant or breast-feeding or has bone marrow depression, infection, oral mucositis, peptic ulcer, renal function impairment, ulcerative colitis, or a history of gout, urate renal stones, or previous cytoxic drug therapy or radiation therapy. Caution should be used with debilitated, very young, or elderly patients.

Intervention. Administer leucovorin calcium within the first 36 to 42 hours of starting methotrexate (or earlier) to block the systemic toxic effects of high-dosage methotrexate (known as "leucovorin rescue"). Leucovorin should be immediately available for administration or high-dosage methotrexate administration should not be initiated.

Reconstitute with sterile, preservative-free sodium chloride for injection for intrathecal use.

Safety precautions should be taken if the platelet count is low. Precautions include avoidance of invasive procedures or use of extreme care in such procedures; regular examination of skin, mucous membranes, and injection sites for bruising or bleeding; testing of emesis, urine, and stool for signs of occult bleeding; care in the use of grooming implements, toothbrushes, toothpicks, razors, and nail clippers; prevention of constipation; and prevention of physical injury.

Education. Caution the client against being immunized with live virus vaccines during methotrexate therapy, since it may cause the disease rather than prevent it. It is also contraindicated in family members and other persons in close contact with the client. The client should avoid being exposed to infections.

Instruct the client in the importance of continuing the medication despite gastric distress.

Alcohol ingestion should be avoided, since it increases the hepatotoxicity associated with the drug.

The client should be aware that skin sensitivity and photophobia may occur. Sun-blocking lotions and sunglasses may be advised.

Inform the client that alopecia may occur but is reversible.

Evaluation. Monitor serum uric acid levels and intake and output to ensure that the patient is adequately hydrated to prevent hyperuricemia and uric acid nephropathy. Alkalinization of urine will also help prevent renal toxicity.

Monitor SGOT and SGPT and observe the patient for signs of hepatotoxicity (yellowing of eyes and skin and dark urine).

Monitor CBC and watch the patient for signs of bruising and bleeding, particularly gastrointestinal bleeding. The nadir of the platelet count occurs after 7 to 10 days, with recovery about 7 days later.

Monitor temperature and observe for signs of infection, fever, chills, or sore throat. The nadir of the leucocyte count occurs after 7 to 10 days, with recovery about 7 days later.

The client's mouth should be examined for ulcerations before the administration of each dose, since stomatitis is a sign of toxicity. Therapy should be discontinued, but may be reinstated at a lower dosage when the side effects have subsided.

---

leucovorin (citrovorum factor, folinic acid, Wellcovorin, calcium folinate✤)

Mechanism of action. Leucovorin or folinic acid is a form of folic acid that does not require dihydrofolate reductase to produce folic acid. Therefore it is used to prevent or treat toxicity induced by folic acid antagonists.

Indications

1. Use as an antidote for folic acid antagonists, such as methotrexate, pyrimethamine, and trimethoprim. **Leucovorin rescue** is a term used to describe high-dose methotrexate treatments that use leucovorin to reduce the time that sensitive (normal) cells are exposed to the toxic effects of methotrexate. It has been useful in the treatment of osteogenic sarcoma, carcinomas of the head and neck, refractory acute leukemia, and lung carcinomas.
2. Treat megaloblastic anemia caused by nutritional deficiencies, sprue, in infants and whenever oral folic acid therapy is not appropriate.

Pharmacokinetics

Absorption. Orally, rapid absorption.

Distribution and metabolism. It is rapidly converted in the intestinal mucous membrane and liver primarily, to

5-methyl tetrahydrofolate, an active metabolite. This substance is transported and stored in the body, mainly in the liver (50%). It can also cross the blood-brain barrier.

Onset of action. Orally, in 20 to 30 minutes. Intramuscularly, in 10 to 20 minutes. Intravenously, less than 5 minutes.

Duration of action. 3 to 6 hours by all methods of administration

Excretion. Kidneys mainly (80% to 90%) and feces (5% to 8%).

Side effects/adverse reactions. See Table 57-2.

Significant drug interactions. None reported.

Dosage and administration

Folic acid antagonist

Adults. Orally, intramuscularly, or intravenously, administer a dose equivalent to or greater than the dose of methotrexate (i.e., 15 to 50 mg/m^2 of body surface). It is usually given within 24 to 42 hours of starting the high-dose methotrexate therapy.

Leucovorin is given together with pyrimethamine or trimethoprim (in high doses to avoid the induction of megaloblastic anemia). Oral or intramuscular doses range from 0.4 mg to 5 mg per dose. Treatment of the anemia requires an oral or intramuscular dose of 5 to 15 mg daily.

In antianemia dosage for megaloblastic anemia caused by folic acid deficiency, oral or intramuscular dose is up to 1 mg daily.

Children. See usual adult recommended dosage schedule.

Pregnancy safety. FDA category C.

NURSING CONSIDERATIONS

Leucovorin is administered after methotrexate rather than simultaneously with methotrexate. The first dose is usually administered within 24 to 42 hours of beginning high-dose methotrexate therapy. Such high-dose therapy should not be initiated unless leucovorin is immediately available for administration since rescue is critical. All nursing considerations for methotrexate administration should be observed.

ALKYLATING DRUGS

Alkylating drugs are frequently used as anticancer agents and are believed to be the first class of medications applied clinically in the modern era of antineoplastic drug therapy. Although research was conducted during World War I with sulfur and nitrogen mustards, this information was kept classified because mustard gas was used by the military. Not until 1942 was nitrogen mustard used to treat a lymphosarcoma patient who had become resistant to

radiation therapy. Since then a variety of alkylating agents have been tested and used in the treatment of various cancerous states.

mechlorethamine (Mustargen)

Mechanism of action. Mechlorethamine is an alkylating agent capable of cross-linking DNA and interfering with DNA and RNA, thus preventing cell division and protein synthesis. It is cell cycle–nonspecific.

Indications. Intravenously or by **intracavitary** route (such as intrapleurally or intraperitoneally) for treatment of Hodgkin's disease, lymphomas, chronic leukemia, malignant effusions, mycosis fungoides, lymphosarcoma, metastatic carcinomas, and polycythemia vera.

Pharmacokinetics

Absorption. Given intravenously or by intracavitary route.

Distribution and metabolism. When given intravenously, rapidly converted to reactive ion that usually is not detectable in the blood after approximately 10 minutes; rapidly inactivated in body fluids.

Excretion. Probably by way of the kidneys, although only a minute amount of unchanged drug is excreted in the urine.

Side effects/adverse reactions. See Table 57-2.

Significant drug interactions. The following interactions may occur when mechlorethamine is given with the drugs listed below.

Drug	Possible Effect and Management
bone marrow depressants or radiation	Increased bone marrow depression may occur. A decrease in drug dosage is usually indicated.
probenecid or sulfinpyrazone	Hyperuricemia and gout may occur. The physician may adjust the antigout medications or prescribe allopurinol. The latter is often preferred to prevent drug-induced hyperuricemia.
vaccines, live viral	See methotrexate drug interactions

Dosage and administration

Adults. Intravenously, total dosage of 0.4 mg/kg ideal body weight in divided doses (2 to 4 daily doses) or in a single dose. If patients have previously received drug chemotherapy or radiation, this dosage should not exceed 0.2 to 0.3 mg/kg body weight. Intracavitary, 0.4 mg/kg of body weight. Intrapericardial, 0.2 mg/kg of body weight. Topically, for mycosis fungoides, available in ointment (0.01% to 0.04%) and topical solution (approximately 10 mg/50 ml). Medication is applied topically to skin surface daily until a complete response is achieved. With ointment and solution dosage forms, maintenance usually requires application one or more times per week for approximately 3 years.

Children. See recommended adult dosages.

Pregnancy safety. Not established.

NURSING CONSIDERATIONS

Assessment. Carefully consider use of mechlorethamine when the patient is pregnant or breast-feeding or has bone marrow depression, infection, or a history of gout, urate renal stones, or previous cytotoxic drug therapy or radiation therapy.

Caution should be taken against intravenous infiltration. If extravasation occurs, promptly infiltrate the area with sterile isotonic sodium thiosulfate or 1% lidocaine and apply ice compresses for 6 to 12 hours.

Intervention. Do not use if droplets of water appear in the vial before reconstitution. Reconstitute with sterile water for injection or sodium chloride injection fluid only.

Reconstitute immediately before or less than 15 minutes before each dose. Discard any unused solution after neutralizing.

Avoid contact with the solution by wearing gloves while preparing and administering it. If contact with the skin, mucous membranes, or eye occurs, irrigate the affected area immediately with large amounts of water for 15 minutes; follow with 2% thiosulfate solution. Neutralize all equipment used in the administration of the drug by soaking for 45 minutes in a solution of equal parts of 5% sodium thiosulfate and 5% sodium bicarbonate.

When mechlorethamine is given by the intracavitary route, change the patient's position (prone to supine to right side to left side) every 10 minutes for an hour to distribute the drug. Removal of fluid before intracavitary administration of mechlorethamine improves contact of the medication with the cavity lining. Fluid is usually removed from the cavity again 24 to 36 hours after therapy.

Safety precautions should be taken regarding invasive procedures and infection avoidance as mentioned previously with antimetabolite drugs.

When applying mechlorethamine topically, follow the specific instructions for application for that client. Usually the client showers, rinses, and dries thoroughly before each treatment and does not shower until treatment the next day. Use plastic gloves to apply mechlorethamine, avoiding contact with the eyes, nose, and mouth. The treatment may be continued for months or even years.

Nausea and vomiting occur in about 90% of patients, generally within 1 to 3 hours of the dose. Although the vomiting usually lasts only 8 hours, nausea may persist 24 hours. These symptoms may be decreased by the administration of antiemetics before mechlorethamine dosing. However, if the use of sedatives is also required to control the nausea and vomiting, the mechlorethamine may be administered at night for the convenience of the patient.

Avoid invasive procedures such as intramuscular injections when the platelet count is low. The nadir of thrombocytopenia usually occurs within 6 to 8 days, with recovery in 10 days to 3 weeks.

Education. The client should be instructed not to be immunized with live virus vaccines during mechlorethamine therapy and to avoid contact with others receiving immunization during that time.

The female client should be alerted that menstrual periods may become irregular.

Hair loss may occur in clients but they should be told that this effect is usually temporary.

The client should be instructed in the importance of adequate hydration in the prevention of complications.

Alert the client to the frequency of nausea and vomiting with the administration of this drug, but stress the importance of continuing the medication despite these symptoms.

Evaluation. Monitor serum uric acid and BUN levels. Adequate hydration will help prevent renal complications, although alkalinization of the urine may be necessary if serum uric acid levels begin to increase.

Monitor the client's CBC and monitor for the presence of fever, chills, and sore throat. Within 24 hours of the first dose, lymphocytopenia occurs. Granulocytopenia occurs 6 to 8 days after the dose and lasts 10 days to 3 weeks.

---

cyclophosphamide (Cytoxan, Neosar, Procytox✤)

Mechanism of action. Cyclophosphamide is a cell cycle–nonspecific agent that cross links DNA and RNA strands and also inhibits the synthesis of protein.

Indications

1. Acute and chronic leukemias, carcinomas of the ovary and breast, neuroblastomas, retinoblastomas, Hodgkin's and non-Hodgkin's lymphomas, multiple myeloma, sarcomas, and mycosis fungoides
2. As an immunosuppressant in drug-resistant nephrotic syndrome, rheumatoid arthritis, and other autoimmune disease states

Pharmacokinetics

Absorption. The drug is well absorbed from the gastrointestinal tract with distribution across the blood-brain barrier.

Metabolism. Cyclophosphamide undergoes hepatic metabolism to active and inactive metabolites. There is little binding, but active metabolites are approximately 50% protein bound. Serum half-life is approximately 4 to 6½ hours, but drug or drug metabolites have been detected for up to 72 hours in the plasma.

Excretion. Excretion is primarily by way of the kidneys.

Side effects/adverse reactions. See Table 57-2.

Significant drug interactions. The following interactions may occur when cyclophosphamide is given with the drugs listed below.

Drug	Possible Effect and Management
bone marrow depressants or radiation	Increased bone marrow depression may occur. A decrease in drug dosage is usually indicated.
probenecid or sulfinpyrazone	Hyperuricemia and gout may occur. The physician may adjust the antigout medications. Allopurinol is not indicated, since it may increase the bone marrow toxicity of cyclophosphamide. If drugs are given concurrently, monitor closely for toxicity.
immunosuppressant agents including adrenocorticoids, azathioprine, chlorambucil, cyclosporine, and mercaptopurine	Increased risk of infections and further development of neoplasms
vaccines, live viral	See methotrexate drug interactions

Dosage and administration
Antineoplastic

Adults. Orally, 1 to 5 mg/kg body weight daily. Induction dose is given intravenously, 40 to 50 mg/kg body weight in divided dosages given over 2 to 5 days. Maintenance dose is given intravenously, 10 to 15 mg/kg body weight every 7 to 10 days or 3 to 5 mg/kg body weight twice a week or 1.5 to 3 mg/kg body weight daily.

Children. Induction dose is given orally or intravenously, 2 to 8 mg/kg body weight or 60 to 250 mg/m^2 in divided dosages daily, given over 6 to 7 days. Maintenance dose is given orally, 2 to 5 mg/kg body weight or 50 to 150 mg/m^2 of body surface area, twice weekly. Intravenously, 10 to 15 mg/kg body weight 7 to 10 days or 30 mg/kg body weight at 21- to 28-day intervals, following bone marrow recovery.

Other uses

Immunosuppressant, adults. Rheumatoid arthritis, orally 1.5 to 2 mg/kg body weight daily, up to a maximum of 3 mg/kg body weight daily.

Nephrotic syndrome, children. Orally 2 to 2.5 mg/kg body weight daily.

Pregnancy safety. FDA category C.

NURSING CONSIDERATIONS

Assessment. Carefully consider use of cyclophosphamide when the patient is pregnant or breast-feeding or has renal or hepatic function impairment, infection, bone marrow depression, or tumor cell infiltration of the bone marrow.

Intervention. Reconstituted solutions may be stored for 24 hours at room temperature or 6 days if refrigerated. Antiemetics may be administered concurrently to reduce nausea and vomiting.

Education. Alopecia may occur but is reversible; however, the new hair may be different in color and texture.

As with antineoplastic agents, previously discussed, instruct the client not to be immunized with live virus vaccines during the course of therapy.

Advise the client that nausea and vomiting frequently occur with cyclophosphamide therapy, but stress that the medication needs to be taken despite these symptoms.

Evaluation. Monitor BUN, creatinine clearance, and serum uric acid level determinations. A decrease in creatinine clearance and an increase in the other test values may indicate nephrotoxicity. Intake should be 3000 ml daily for adequate hydration to prevent uric acid nephropathy. Alkalinization of urine or allopurinol administration may also be used to prevent uric acid nephropathy.

Observe the patient for reduced urinary output, weight gain over several days, edema of the feet and lower legs, flank pain, pruritus, urine odor on breath, anorexia, nausea, and vomiting.

Monitor for myelosuppression as evidenced by anemia and leukopenia. Monitor hematocrit, platelet count, and total and differential leukocyte counts. Lowest levels of leukopenia generally occur 7 to 12 days after the first dose. The leukocyte count recovers 17 to 21 days after the last dose. Observe the patient for fever of unknown origin, chills, sore throat, unusual bleeding, or bruising.

Monitor urinalysis for microscopic hematuria and the client for painful urination as indications of hemorrhagic cystitis.

ALKYLATOR-LIKE DRUGS
cisplatin (Platinol)

Mechanism of action. The mechanism of action of cisplatin is unknown, but it is believed to be a cell cycle–nonspecific agent that has an action similar to the alkylating agents.

Indications. Bladder, testicular, and ovarian carcinomas.

Pharmacokinetics

Distribution. When administered intravenously, cisplatin locates in the liver, small and large intestines, and kidney, but it does not significantly cross the blood-brain barrier. Half-life is biphasic; alpha or initial half-life is 25 to 49 minutes, and beta or later phase is 58 to 73 hours.

Metabolism. Metabolized to inactive metabolites that are highly protein bound (greater than 90%); partially renally excreted (27% to 43%) after 5 days, although platinum has been detected in body tissues for 4 months or longer.

Side effects/adverse reactions. See Table 57-2.

Significant drug interactions. The following interactions may occur when cisplatin is given with the drugs listed below.

Drug	Possible Effect and Management
bone marrow depressants or radiation	Increased bone marrow depression may occur. A decrease in drug dosage is usually indicated.
probenecid or sulfinpyrazone	Hyperuricemia and gout may occur. The physician may adjust the antigout medications or prescribe allopurinol. The latter is often preferred to prevent drug-induced hyperuricemia.
nephrotoxic or ototoxic drugs	Concurrent or sequential administration is not recommended. The risk for nephrotoxicity and ototoxicity is increased, especially in patients with renal impairment.
vaccines, live viral	See methotrexate drug interactions

Dosage and administration (adults only). Dosage varies according to site of cancerous growth; for example, for advanced bladder cancer intravenous dosage is 50 to 70 mg/m^2 of body surface area every 3 to 4 weeks. For metastatic ovarian tumors or testicular tumors, cisplatin and other antineoplastic agents are given in combination or by sequential drug administration. Recommended dosages vary according to protocol and also whether therapy is initial or maintenance. Current recommendations should be reviewed to determine indications, dosages, dosage schedules, or different drug combinations for specific cancers.

Pregnancy safety. Not established.

NURSING CONSIDERATIONS

Assessment. Carefully consider use of cisplatin when the patient is pregnant or breast-feeding or has renal function impairment, infection, healing impairment, bone marrow depression, or a history of gout, urate renal stones, or previous cytotoxic drug or radiation therapy.

Intervention. Hydrate patient with 1 to 2 L of intravenous infusion fluid, and dilute cisplatin in 2 L of 5% dextrose in one-half or one-third normal saline containing 37.5 g of mannitol. This infusion should be administered over 6 to 8 hours. To reduce nephrotoxicity, adequate hydration of 3000 ml daily should be maintained. Urinary output should be closely monitored. Alkalinization of urine and allopurinol administration may also be used to prevent uric acid nephropathy.

Reduce nausea and vomiting by administering a parenteral antiemetic ½ hour before cisplatin is given. These symptoms usually begin 1 to 4 hours after a dose. Therefore the antiemetic therapy is continued on a schedule as long as necessary. If the nausea and vomiting are severe, cisplatin may be discontinued.

As with antineoplastic agents previously discussed (p. 872), observe safety precautions regarding invasive procedures.

Do not use aluminum needles or other equipment containing aluminum. Cisplatin is incompatible with aluminum, which causes a black precipitate and a potency loss.

Education. As with other antineoplastic agents previously discussed, caution the client against being immunized with live virus vaccines.

Evaluation. Evaluate for nephrotoxicity, hyperuricemia, and uric acid nephropathy. Nephrotoxicity is cumulative, and the effects may be irreversible with repeated or high dosages. Symptoms are reduced urinary output, weight gain over several days, edema of the feet and lower legs, flank pain, pruritus, urine odor on breath, anorexia, nausea, and vomiting. Metoclopramide is indicated for cisplatin-induced emesis.

Monitor BUN, creatinine clearance, and serum uric acid level. A decrease in creatinine clearance and an increase in the other test values may indicate nephrotoxicity.

Test hearing status before the initial dose and each subsequent dose. Ringing in the ears and difficulty in hearing high frequencies may indicate ototoxicity. Hearing loss is cumulative and may be unilateral.

Monitor for myelosuppression as evidenced by anemia, leukopenia, and thrombocytopenia. Hematocrit, platelet count, and total and differential leukocyte counts should also be monitored. The lowest leukocyte and platelet counts generally occur 18 to 23 days after a dose and recover by 39 days. The patient should be observed for fever of unknown origin, chills, sore throat, unusual bleeding, or bruising.

Discontinue administration of cisplatin at the first indication of peripheral neuropathy because it may be irreversible. Symptoms to watch for are numbness or tingling in the fingers, toes, or face and loss of taste.

Do not administer subsequent doses of cisplatin until platelet levels are over 100,000 cells/mm^3, WBC is over 4000 cells/mm^3, creatinine concentration is under 1.5%, or BUN is under 25 mg/100 ml.

ANTIBIOTIC ANTITUMOR DRUGS
doxorubicin (Adriamycin)

Mechanism of action. Doxorubicin is an antineoplastic and antibiotic agent that is specific for the S-phase of cell division. It binds DNA and inhibits RNA synthesis. It is a cell cycle–nonspecific agent.

Indications. Acute leukemia, Wilms' tumor, neuroblastoma, soft tissue and bone sarcomas, Hodgkins' disease, lymphomas, breast and various other carcinomas

Pharmacokinetics

Absorption. Given intravenously.

Distribution. Does not cross the blood-brain barrier; rapidly cleared from the blood and highly tissue bound

Metabolism. Metabolized in the liver to both active metabolite (adriamycinol) and inactive metabolites.

Excretion. Mainly by way of bile (50% unchanged drug and 23% active metabolite); kidney excretion is approximately 10%

Side effects/adverse reactions. See Table 57-2.

Significant drug interactions. For interactions with bone marrow depressant drugs or radiation, probenecid or sulfinpyrazone, and live virus vaccines, see comments regarding mechlorethamine drug interactions (p. 874).

Dosage and administration

Adults. Give 60 to 75 mg/m² body surface intravenously and repeat every 3 weeks, or 25 to 30 mg/m² daily on 2 or 3 successive days. Repeat in 21 to 28 days. An intravenous weekly schedule is 20 mg/m² once a week. Maximum dosage is 550 mg/m² or 450/m² in clients who have had chest radiation or medications that cause cardiotoxicity.

Children. Intravenously, 30 mg/m² daily on 3 successive days every 28 days.

Pregnancy safety. Not established.

NURSING CONSIDERATIONS

Assessment. Carefully consider use of doxorubicin when the patient is pregnant or breast-feeding or has bone marrow depression, heart disease, hepatic function impairment, or a history of gout, urate kidney stones, or cytotoxic drug or radiation therapy. Caution should be used with elderly patients because of their decreased bone marrow reserves.

Intervention. Reconstitute with sterile sodium chloride for injection.

Avoid contact with the solution by wearing gloves while preparing and administering it. If contact with the skin or mucous membranes occurs, wash thoroughly with soap and water.

Use reconstituted solutions within 24 hours if stored at room temperature or within 48 hours if stored between 2° and 8° C (36° and 46° F) and protected from light.

Take precautions against intravenous extravasation. If extravasation occurs, the intravenous line should be moved to another site for completion of the dose. Local infiltration of sodium bicarbonate and steroids may be used to reduce the local inflammation. If inflammation is extensive, surgical excision of the area may be required.

Do not give intramuscularly or subcutaneously because it will cause tissue necrosis.

As with other antineoplastic agents previously discussed (p. 872), observe safety precautions for invasive procedures.

Education. The client's urine may become reddish for 1 or 2 days after administration of doxorubicin, but it generally clears in 48 hours.

As with previously discussed antineoplastic agents, discuss with the client the importance of adequate hydration, the possibility of alopecia, the contraindication of being immunized with live virus vaccines during therapy, and the importance of taking medications despite gastric distress.

Evaluation. Monitor serum uric acid levels and intake and output to ensure that the patient is adequately hydrated to prevent hyperuricemia.

Monitor CBC and watch the patient for signs of bruising and bleeding, particularly gastrointestinal bleeding.

Monitor the electrocardiogram and observe the patient for swelling of the feet and lower legs and shortness of breath, which indicate cardiotoxicity. Cardiotoxicity is more common in elderly persons over 70 years of age and in children under 2 years of age. It usually occurs within 1 to 6 months after therapy is begun. Cardiotoxicity may develop suddenly and may be irreversible; it is critical that cardiotoxicity be detected early, when it usually responds to therapy.

Monitor temperature and observe for signs of infection, fever, chills, or sore throat. The lowest leukocyte count usually occurs 10 to 14 days after dosage and recovers within 21 days.

Examine the client's mouth for ulcerations before the administration of each dose since stomatitis is a sign of toxicity.

MITOTIC INHIBITORS
vincristine (Oncovin)

Mechanism of action. Vincristine is a cell cycle–specific agent that inhibits mitosis during M-phase.

Indications. Acute lymphoblastic leukemia, Hodgkin's disease, lymphosarcoma, rhabdomyosarcoma, neuroblastoma, Wilms' tumor, carcinomas of lung and breast.

Pharmacokinetics

Absorption. Given intravenously; does not cross blood-brain barrier

Metabolism. Highly tissue bound; metabolized by liver

Excretion. Mainly through bile metabolized by liver

Side effects/adverse reactions. See Table 57-2.

Significant drug interactions. The following interactions may occur when vincristine is given with the drugs listed below.

Drug	Possible Effect and Management
probenecid or sulfinpyrazone	Hyperuricemia and gout may occur. The physician may adjust the antigout medications or prescribe allopurinol. The latter is often preferred to prevent drug-induced hyperuricemia.

Drug	Possible Effect and Management
asparaginase	When given concurrently with vincristine, an increase in neurotoxicity may result. To reduce the possibility of this interaction, asparaginase should be given only after vincristine is administered, not concurrently or before vincristine.
doxorubicin	If administered with vincristine and prednisone, an increase in bone marrow depressant effects may occur. This combination should be avoided.
vaccines, live viral	See methotrexate drug interactions

Dosage and administration

Adults. Intravenously, 0.01 to 0.03 mg/kg body weight or 0.4 mg to 1.4 mg/m² of body surface as a single dose, weekly.

Children. Intravenously, 1.5 to 2 mg/m² body surface as a single dose, weekly.

Combination therapies may employ various dosage regimens, according to the patient's condition and the cancer under treatment.

Pregnancy safety. FDA category D

• • •

Vinblastine (Velban, Velbe♣) is also a vinca alkaloid. Although similar to vincristine in mechanism of action and metabolism, it differs in its tumor specificity and toxic effects. It is indicated for the treatment of Kaposi's sarcoma, carcinoma of the breast and testes, and choriocarcinoma. Its major undesirable effect is bone marrow suppression. Neurotoxicity is the major dose-limiting side effect of vincristine.

NURSING CONSIDERATIONS

Assessment. Carefully consider use of vincristine when the patient is pregnant or breast-feeding or has hepatic function impairment, infection, leukopenia, neuromuscular disease or a history of gout, urate kidney stones, or cytotoxic drug or radiation therapy.

Intervention. Reconstitute with bacteriostatic sodium chloride injection provided by the manufacturer, sterile water for injection, or sodium chloride injection. Store reconstituted solutions up to 14 days if refrigerated.

Take precautions against intravenous infiltration. If extravasation occurs, stop administration immediately and inject remaining dose into another vein. To alleviate discomfort and inflammation, inject hyaluronidase locally and apply heat, or apply cold compresses, or inject hydrocortisone locally.

Administer by intravenous push or inject into the tubing of a running intravenous infusion for 1 minute.

Administer only intravenously; to administer intramuscularly or subcutaneously will cause tissue necrosis; intrathecal administration will cause death.

As with other antineoplastic agents previously discussed (p. 872), observe safety precautions for invasive procedures and avoidance of infections.

Education. As with previously discussed antineoplastic agents (p. 875), stress the importance of adequate hydration, the possibility of alopecia, the contraindication of being immunized with live virus vaccines during therapy, and the importance of taking medications despite gastric distress with the client.

Evaluation. Monitor the patient's bowel status for early signs of autonomic toxicity, such as constipation. Use of a laxative or stool softener will help prevent upper colon impaction.

Monitor serum uric acid levels and the patient's intake and output to ensure adequate hydration for the prevention of uric acid nephropathy. Intake should be 3000 ml daily. Urine may be alkalinized if serum uric acid levels increase.

Monitor CBC and observe client for fever, chills, sore throat, bleeding, and bruising to assess potential for infection or physical injury. The lowest level of leukocytes occurs 5 to 10 days after the last day of administration, and recovery occurs within another 7 to 14 days.

Monitor the patient's neuromuscular status. Watch for ataxia, numbness, tingling or pain in the fingers or toes, headache, double vision, and other early signs of neurotoxicity.

ADDITIONAL ANTINEOPLASTIC AGENTS

Prednisone and dexamethasone are corticosteroids that are often prescribed for patients with cancer. Predni-

---

AIDS AND CANCER

Acquired immune deficiency syndrome (AIDS) is a disease without a known cure. It has been postulated that the AIDS virus originated in Africa (Poirier, 1986). In Zaire, Africa, Karposi's sarcoma is common. Karposi's sarcoma is also one of the most common opportunistic diseases seen in AIDS patients (Popkin, 1983).

Anti-AIDS drugs under current investigational use include:

Suramin—antiviral agent
Ribavirin—antiviral agent
Alpha-interferon—immune system modifier
HPA-23—antiviral agent
Zidovudine (Azidothymidine, AZT)—antiviral agent

THE DOUBLE SYRINGE METHOD FOR ADMINISTERING VESICANT ANTINEOPLASTIC DRUGS

Some antineoplastic agents have **vesicant** properties (cause blisters) and require careful handling. The following are common vesicant agents:

dactinomycin	mithramycin
carmustine (BiCNU)	mitomycin C
daunorubicin	vinblastine
doxorubicin	vincristine
mechlorethamine	

These agents should be administered by the double-syringe technique as follows:
1. Select site for administration according to following order of preference: forearm, dorsum of hand, wrist, or antecubital fossa.
2. Use 20- or 21-gauge "butterfly" needle for drug administration. Administer 5 ml normal saline solution and withdraw small amount of blood into tubing to test vein patency. If blood return is poor, select site other than distal location.
3. Administer vesicant agent for at least 3 minutes, drawing blood back into tubing after every 2 to 3 ml solution.
4. Flush with 3 to 5 ml saline solution after administration.
5. If patient has pain at site of injection or an unusual sensation during drug administration, extravasation may have occurred, and a new site for drug injection should be selected.

PROGESTERONE RECEPTORS IN BREAST CANCER

Progesterone receptors (PR) are important factors in predicting patient response and length of survival in both newly diagnosed and advanced stage breast cancer patients. Estrogen receptors (ER)–positive women generally are reported to have significantly longer survival times than ER–negative patients. The risk of earlier recurrence of cancer is also more prevalent in the ER–negative patient. It is predicted that PR analysis will be an important biologic variable that can provide quantitative assay data that are more significant for survival prognosis than the presence of estrogen receptors. The further development of this test will allow for improved treatment planning for the patient with breast cancer (McGuire, 1986).

sone has demonstrated a lympholytic and antiinflammatory effect that is useful in the treatment of leukemias, lymphomas, and breast carcinomas. Steroids, especially dexamethasone, are useful in reducing cerebral edema induced by the increasing growth of a brain tumor or from radiation therapy.

Mitotane (Lysodren) is a cytotoxic agent with a high affinity for the adrenal cortex. It is indicated for inoperable adrenal cortex carcinomas. Side effects include adrenal gland insufficiency, skin rash or darkening of the skin, depression, and lethargy.

Estramustine phosphate (Emcyt) is indicated for the palliative treatment of prostatic carcinoma, especially in clients resistant to estrogen. This product combines nitrogen mustard with estradiol; thus cytotoxic effects are combined with hormonal therapy.

Tamoxifen (Nolvadex, Nolvadex-D✿) is a synthetic (nonsteroidal) antiestrogen agent indicated for the treatment of breast cancer. It blocks the uptake of estradiol, thus it is effective for tumors that contain high concentrations of estrogen receptors. Common side effects include nausea, vomiting, weight gain, and hot flashes. A flare-up of bone pain or erythema is sometimes reported by patients, but such effects are usually transient and are not related to the disease process. Some physicians believe such effects are positive indicators of patient response to the drug.

Interferon alfa-2a, recombinant (Roferon-A), and interferon alfa-2b, recombinant (Intron A), were approved in 1986 for the treatment of hairy cell leukemia. Both interferon products induce partial or complete remissions in larger numbers of hairy cell leukemia cases than reported with previous therapies. Interferons are natural body proteins formed in response to viral infections and stimulation of the immune system and by certain chemical substances. Natural interferon is very scarce and expensive; however, recombinant interferon is a synthetic agent that is produced in a laboratory, so it is more plentiful and less expensive.

Although the exact mechanism of action is unknown, in some types of cancer, interferon appears to have a dual effect of both cytotoxic and immune stimulation. Some patients demonstrate an increase in the hematologic factors, that is, granulocytes, platelets, and hemoglobin serum levels. Toxicities reported include a flulike syndrome that includes fever, chills, muscle pain, loss of appetite, and lethargy. At higher doses, myelosuppression, nausea, vomiting, neurotoxicity (changes in personality, disorientation, paranoid behavior), and various cardiotoxic signs may occur.

Interferon is not the "cure-all" it was promoted to be in the 1970s. Research studies are being performed to assess the gamma form of interferon, which seems to affect different receptor sites than the alpha and beta forms. Many questions remain to be answered: Is immune modification or growth inhibition more important? Should interferon be used as the primary treatment, or as an adjunct to other modalities, such as chemotherapy or radiation? Will various combinations of interferons, such as alpha and gamma, be safer and more effective than the single agents? Such questions must be answered to determine the future role of interferon in neoplastic disease.

KEY TERMS

BIBLIOGRAPHY

American Hospital Formulary Service: AHFS drug information 88, Bethesda, Md, 1988, American Society of Hospital Pharmacists, Inc.

Anderson RW and others: Risk of handling injectable antineoplastic agents Am J Hosp Pharm 39:1881, 1982.

ASHP technical assistance bulletin on handling cytotoxic drugs in hospitals, Am J Hosp Pharm 42:131, 1985.

Bingham E: Hazards to health workers from antineoplastic drugs, New Engl J Med 313(19):1220, 1985.

Black DJ: Breast cancer, Differential Insights 4:4, 1983. Cancer chemotherapy: continuous cancer chemotherapy infusions. II. Types of continuous infusions, US Pharmacist, April, 1985, p H-6.

Chabner BA and others: Investigational trials of anticancer drugs: establishing safeguards for experimentation, Public Health 99(4):355, 1984.

D'Arcy PF: Reactions and interactions in handling anticancer drugs, Drug Intell Clin Pharm 17:532, 1983.

Goldstein D and Laszlo J: The role of interferon in cancer therapy, Hosp Formul 21:932, 1986.

Gullatte MM and Foltz A: Hepatic chemotherapy via implantable pump, Amer J Nurs 83:1674, 1983.

Gurwell A: Protect yourself from the hazards of anticancer drugs, RN, 46(10):66, 1983.

Hughes CB: Giving cancer drugs IV: Some guidelines, Amer J Nurs 86:34, 1986.

Kraha EM: You can't be too careful with cytotoxic drugs, RN 48(2):71, 1985.

Krakoff IH: Cancer chemotherapeutic agents, American Cancer Society Professional Education Pub no 3078-PE 6/78, New York, 1978, The Society.

Lynn J: Choices of curative and palliative care. CA 36(2):100, 1986.

Mattia MA and Blake SL: Hospital hazards: cancer drugs, Am J Nurs 83:759, 1983.

McGuire WL and Clark GM: Role of progesterone receptors in breast cancer, CA 36(5):302, 1986.

Miakowski C: Potential and actual impairments in skin integrity related to cancer and cancer treatment, Top Clin Nurs 5(2):64, 1983.

OSHA develops guidelines for handling cytotoxic drugs, Am J Hosp Pharm 43:1116, 1986.

Poirier T: AIDS: where do we stand today? US Pharmacist, 11:52, 1986.

Popkin B and others: Caring for the AIDS patient—fearlessly, Nursing '83, 13(9): 50, 1983.

Rahr V: Giving intrathecal drugs Am J Nurs 86:829, 1986.

Reich SD: Pharmaceutics: old regulations, new enforcement, Cancer Nursing 6(6):229, 1983.

Schaffner A: Safety precautions in home chemotherapy, Am J Nurs 84:346, 1984.

Speciala JL and Kaalaas J: Infuse-a-port, new path for I.V. chemotherapy, Nursing 85 15(10):40, 1985.

United States Pharmacopeial Convention: Drug information for the health care provider, ed 8, Rockville, Md, 1988, The Convention.

INVESTIGATIONAL DRUGS

Investigational drugs are agents that have not been released for marketing by the Food and Drug Administration. While responsibility for regulating drugs rests with the FDA, the National Cancer Institute (NCI) is the largest developer of antineoplastic agents in the United States. The NCI has established stringent regulations to monitor the receipt, use, and disposal of investigational drugs. It also requires that investigators report adverse reactions on an established time schedule. For example, anaphylactic reactions to an investigational drug must be reported by phoning a specific branch office that is available on a 24-hour basis. This call must be followed up with a written report within 10 working days.

Investigational drugs are divided into three groups:

	Drug Group	Purpose
Phase I	A	To determine maximum tolerated dosage
		To detect toxicities associated with various dosage schedules
		To determine pharmacokinetics and optimum dosing schedule
Phase II	B	To identify antineoplastic activity in specific cancers affecting humans
		To determine patient's response to various drug dosages and schedules
Phase III	C	New agent is now compared with previously marketed drugs to ascertain effectiveness, effect on quality of life, mortality, and morbidity

UNIT XV

Drugs Used in Infectious Diseases and Inflammation

CHAPTER 58

Overview of Infections, Inflammation, and Fever

INFECTIONS

Infectious diseases comprise a wide spectrum of illnesses caused by pathogenic microorganisms. Some common pathogens and their most likely sites of infection in the body are listed in Table 58-1. These pathogens cause pneumonia, urinary tract infections, upper respiratory tract infections, venereal disease, vaginitis, tuberculosis, and candidiasis.

Infections are classified primarily as either local or systemic. A localized infection, which may involve the skin or internal organs, may progress to a systemic infection. A systemic infection involves the whole body rather than a localized area of the body. Several terms describe the degree of local or systemic infection. **Colonization** is the localized presence of microorganisms in body tissues or organs. These microorganisms can be pathogenic or part of the normal flora. Colonization alone does not denote infection but rather signifies the potential for infection resulting from the multiplication of the resident organisms or the alteration in host defense mechanisms of the individual. When flora at its normal colonization site is altered (e.g., by the administration of an antibiotic that affects pathogens and some but not all normal microorganisms), unaffected microorganisms within that environment may grow uninhibited and cause a secondary infection.

TABLE 58-1   Primary Organisms Causing Infectious Diseases and their Common Sites of Infection

Organism	Infection site
GRAM-POSITIVE COCCI	
Staphylococcus aureus	Burns, skin infections, decubital and surgical wounds, paranasal
Non–penicillinase producing	and middle ear (chronic sinusitis and otitis), lungs, lung
Penicillinase producing	abscess, pleura, endocardium, bone (osteomyelitis), and
Staphylococcus epidermidis	joints
Non–penicillinase producing	
Penicillinase producing	
Methicillin resistant	
Streptococcus pneumoniae	Paranasal and middle ear, lungs, pleura
Streptococcus pyogenes (group A β-hemolytic)	Burns, skin infections, decubitus and surgical wounds, paranasal and middle ear, throat, bone (osteomyelitis), and joints
Streptococcus, viridans group	Endocardium
GRAM-POSITIVE BACILLI	
Clostridium tetani (anaerobe)	Puncture wounds, lacerations, and crush injuries; toxins affecting nervous system
Corynebacterium diphtheriae	Throat, upper part of the respiratory tract
GRAM-NEGATIVE COCCI	
Neisseria gonorrhoeae	Urethra, prostate, epididymis and testes, joints
Neisseria meningitidis	Meninges
ENTERIC GRAM-NEGATIVE BACILLI	
As a group (Bacteroides, Enterobacter, Escherichia coli, Klebsiella pneumoniae, Proteus mirabilis, other Proteus, Salmonella, Serratia, Shigella)	Peritoneum, biliary tract, kidney and bladder, prostate, decubital and surgical wounds, bone
Bacteroides	Brain abscess, lung abscess, throat, peritoneum
Enterobacter	Peritoneum, biliary tract, kidney and bladder, endocardium
Escherichia coli	Peritoneum, biliary tract, kidney and bladder
Klebsiella pneumoniae	Lungs, lung abscess
OTHER GRAM-NEGATIVE BACILLI	
Haemophilus influenzae	Meninges, paranasal and middle ear, lungs, pleura
Pseudomonas aeruginosa	Burns, paranasal and middle ear (chronic otitis media), decubital and surgical wounds, lungs, joints
ACID-FAST BACILLI	
Mycobacterium tuberculosis	Lungs, pleura, peritoneum, meninges, kidney and bladder, testes,
Mycobacterium avium	bone, joints
MYCOPLASMAS	
Mycoplasma pneumoniae	Lungs
SPIROCHETES	
Treponema pallidum (syphilis)	Any tissue or vascular organ of the body
FUNGI	
Aspergillus	Paranasal and middle ear, lungs
Candida species	Skin infections, throat, lungs, endocardium, kidney and bladder,
Cryptococcus	vagina
VIRUSES	
Herpes virus or varicella-zoster virus	Skin infections (herpes simplex or zoster)
Enterovirus, mumps virus, and others	Meninges, epididymis, and testes
Respiratory viruses (including Epstein-Barr virus)	Throat, lungs
ANAEROBES	
Gram-positive	Deep wounds
Clostridium difficile	
Clostridium perfringens	
Peptococcus species	
Peptostreptococcus species	
Gram-negative	
Bacteroides fragilis	
Fusobacterium species	

Inflammation is a defense mechanism of body tissues in response to invasion or toxins produced by colonizing microorganisms. This reaction consists of cytologic and histologic tissue responses for the localization of phagocytic activity and destruction or removal of injurious material leading to repair and healing. **Bacteremia** is the presence of viable bacteria in the circulatory system. **Septicemia** refers to a systemic infection caused by the multiplication of microorganisms in the circulation. Although bacteremia may lead to septicemia in the immunocompromised host, it is (depending on the pathogen) usually a short-lived, self-limited process. In the immunocompromised host, bacteremia may rapidly produce an overwhelming systemic disease. **Sepsis** is a syndrome involving multiple system organ involvement that is a result of microorganisms or their toxins circulating in the blood.

For nonpathogenic organisms colonizing humans or causing transient bacteremias without tissue invasion, antibiotic therapy is rarely required in the immunocompetent host, whereas prophylactic antibiotic therapy may be required in immunocompromised hosts. In most cases of localized inflammation, such as wound infections, pneumonia, or urinary tract infections, antimicrobials reduce the number of viable pathogens. This permits the immune system to eliminate microorganisms. Antimicrobials are also an essential part of the treatment of septicemia and sepsis.

Microorganisms are divided into several groups: bacteria, mycoplasmas, spirochetes, fungi, and viruses. Bacteria are classified according to shape, such as bacilli, spirilla, and cocci, and their capacity to be stained. Specific identification of bacteria requires a Gram stain and culture with chemical testing. Gram stain is a sequential procedure that involves crystal violet and iodine solutions followed by alcohol. Gram stain allows the rapid identification of organisms into groups, such as gram-positive or gram-negative rods or cocci. The culture procedures identify specific organisms, but they require 24 to 48 hours for completion. Often the initial or empiric antibiotic selection is based on the physician's clinical impression plus the Gram-stain procedure; the antibiotic may be changed once culture and sensitivity results are available.

INFLAMMATION

Inflammation is the reaction of body tissues to injury, such as physical trauma, foreign bodies, chemical substances, surgery, radiation, and electricity. The area affected will undergo a series of changes as the body processes attempt to wall off, heal, and/or replace the injured tissue. For example, after an injury occurs, the body will release chemical substances into the tissue that form a wall (called a **chemotactic gradient**). Fluids and cells will begin to move toward this area.

Blood vessels dilate within 30 minutes of the insult. This will provide for an increase in blood flow and an increase in exudation of fluid from the blood vessels into the injured tissues. The exudate includes protein-rich fluids high in fibrinogen that will attract other substances to the area, such as complement, antibodies, and leukocytes. Fluids collecting in this area will result in edema or swelling. Generally, this occurs within 4 hours of the injury.

During the cellular phase, granulocytes will migrate to the area from the dilated blood vessels at the site. The granulocytes will migrate toward the chemotactic site, accumulate in the area of injury, and if the injury is a foreign substance or bacteria, will engulf and destroy the foreign material (phagocytosis). Neutrophils, monocytes (macrophages), and lymphocytes (which arrive later) are the granulocytes that affect the injured area. The phagocytosis process tends to localize or wall off the foreign material, to prevent its spread through the tissues. Large numbers of phagocytes lead to pus accumulation and the eventual destruction and removal of the foreign material.

Some pathogens are resistant to destruction and are only walled off, such as tuberculosis bacilli. Thus they can live for many years within the confined cells in the body. Others may transform from a local infection into a systemic infection, thus requiring antimicrobial or antibiotic treatment.

MEDIATORS OF THE INFLAMMATORY SYSTEM

The complement system is composed of complement components (18 distinct proteins and their cleavage products) present in the blood in the form of inactive proteins called **zymogens.** Complement is essential in reacting to an acute inflammatory reaction caused by bacteria, some viruses, and immune complex diseases. Complement enhances chemotaxis, increases blood vessel permeability, and eventually causes cell lysis.

Histamine, prostaglandins, arachidonic acid, and leukotrienes are other mediators capable of producing local reactions, smooth muscle contraction, increased chemotaxis, blood vessel vasodilation, and other inflammatory effects. When the foreign agent is destroyed, the resulting debris will be removed by the macrophages and neutrophils, thus resolving the inflammatory reaction.

FEVER

Fever, or elevated body temperature, is a sign of inflammation. It may be caused by the release of endogenous pyrogens from the macrophages. These **pyrogens,** or fever-producing substances, will interfere with the temperature-regulating centers located in the hypothalamus, raising the thermostat set point. The body may respond to the pyrogens by releasing arachidonic acid and prostaglandin (PGE1) that also affect the central control, further increasing the hypothalamic set point. The body will react by conserving heat through vasoconstriction, piloerection (goose flesh), and shivering—all factors that increase the body temperature.

The normal body temperature is 98.6° F (37° C), and the normal range is 97° F to approximately 99° F when measured orally. Rectally, a person's body temperature is 1° F higher than oral. Hyperthermia occurs when the body's temperature rises above normal. When the body temperature reaches 106° F, convulsions may result. If the body's thermoregulatory mechanisms have trouble returning the body temperature to a normal setting, body metabolism may increase so rapidly that the body cannot regulate its own heat production. At 108° F tissue damage occurs and cells begin to die, resulting in irreversible brain damage.

Several types of fever are known. For example, a **constant fever** that rises or falls only a few degrees above or below a specified point, is seen with typhoid fever. An **intermittent fever** may return to normal once or several times in 24 hours. This type of fever is associated with pyogenic infections, abscesses, lymphomas, tuberculosis, and drug reactions. A **remittent fever** fluctuates but does not usually return to normal; this occurs in many viral and bacterial infections. **Relapsing fever** consists of afebrile episodes of 1 or more days between fevers, such as in malaria and Hodgkin's disease. **Fever of unknown origin (FUO)** has been described as a temperature greater than 103° F recorded daily for more than 2 weeks in a patient with an uncertain diagnosis, following a week's evaluation in a hospital setting. Most patients with FUO are later found to have an infection, neoplasm, or connective tissue disease.

Body temperature is regulated by nervous system feedback mechanisms through a temperature-regulating center in the hypothalamus. When the hypothalamus is no longer in contact with the pyrogens, it will reset the temperature to the normal set point. Experimental studies indicate that prostaglandins of the E series are produced in response to endogenous pyrogens. The E prostaglandins act on the anterior hypothalamus to increase the set point, thus resulting in fever. Drugs that inhibit the synthesis of E prostaglandins have antipyretic activity (acetaminophen, salicylates). For example, salicylates reduce raised body temperatures by causing the hypothalmic center to reestablish a normal set point. Heat production will not be inhibited, although heat loss will be increased by an increase in cutaneous blood flow and sweating, caused by the lowered thermostat (see Figure 58-1). Antibiotics indirectly reduce temperature by destroying the bacteria causing the fever.

ANTIMICROBIAL THERAPY

The treatment of an infectious disease caused by a microorganism depends on the group to which the microorganism belongs; different groups of antimicrobial agents are used for treating different groups of microorganisms. Table 58-2 lists some antimicrobial agents used in the treatment of infectious diseases. Antimicrobial drugs can help cure or control most infections caused by microorganisms. However, antimicrobials alone do not necessarily produce the cure. They are adjuncts to methods such as surgical incision and drainage, pulmonary toilet, and wound debridement for removal of nonviable, infected tissue.

The first major antimicrobial agents were the sulfonamides. The second group of antimicrobials were the true antibiotics, such as penicillin. They were substances derived from certain organisms used against infections caused by other organisms. As a result of research, there are now many synthetic and semisynthetic antibiotics. Other antimicrobial agents include the urinary tract antiseptics and the antimycobacterial, antifungal, and antiviral agents.

MECHANISM OF ACTION

The goal of antimicrobial therapy is to destroy or to suppress the growth of infecting microorganisms so that normal host defense and other supporting mechanisms can control the infection, resulting in its cure. To exert their effects, antimicrobial agents must first gain access to target sites. Usually this can be accomplished by absorption and distribution of the drug into and by way of the circulatory system. More specific antibiotics or antimicrobial agents are capable of penetrating to the site, distributing, and having an affinity for the bacterial target proteins. Sometimes, as in the case of infections of the skin and eyes, local application to the infected area may be necessary. Once the drug has reached its site of action, it can have bactericidal or bacteriostatic effects, depending on its mechanisms of action.

Bacteriostatic agents inhibit bacterial growth, allowing host defense mechanisms additional time to remove the invading microorganisms. **Bactericidal agents,** on the other hand, cause bacterial cell death and lysis, superimposing the killing effect of the drug on the effects of host defenses. Antimicrobial agents may be divided into bacteriostatic and bactericidal categories, with the sulfonamides as an example of the former and the penicillins exemplifying the latter. Such categorization is not always valid or reliable, however, because the same antimicrobial agent may have either effect depending on the dose administered and the concentration achieved at its site of action. Tetracycline, for example, is generally bacteriostatic but may be bactericidal in high concentrations. Chloramphenicol, which is often listed as a bacteriostatic drug, has bactericidal effects against *S. pneumoniae* and *H. influenzae* in the cerebrospinal fluid.

Antimicrobial agents may exert their bacteriostatic or bactericidal effects in one of four major ways:

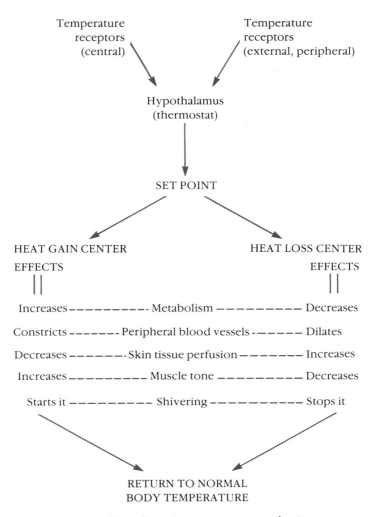

FIGURE 58-1 Set point temperature mechanism.

1. Inhibition of cell wall synthesis in bacteria. Unlike host cells, bacteria are not isotonic with body fluids. Their contents are under high osmotic pressure and their viability depends on the integrity of the cell walls. Any compound that inhibits any step in the synthesis of this cell wall causes it to be weakened and the cell to lyse. Antimicrobial agents having this mechanism of action are bactericidal.
2. Disruption or alteration of membrane permeability, resulting in leakage of essential bacterial metabolic substrates. Agents causing these effects can be either bacteriostatic or bactericidal.
3. Inhibition of protein synthesis. Antimicrobial agents may induce the formation of defective protein molecules; such agents are bactericidal in their action. Antimicrobial agents that inhibit specific steps in protein synthesis are bacteriostatic.
4. Inhibition of synthesis of essential metabolites. Antimicrobial agents that work in this manner structurally resemble physiologic compounds and act as competitive inhibitors in a metabolic pathway. Generally, they are bacteriostatic agents. (See the box on p. 891.)

GENERAL ADVERSE REACTIONS TO ANTIMICROBIAL DRUGS

Although the development of antimicrobial agents represents one of the most important advances in drug therapy, these drugs can have adverse and toxic effects. The list of side effects and toxic effects of each specific drug group is long and varied. Table 58–3 identifies some of the major allergic and toxic effects of a few antimicrobial agents. All antimicrobial agents, however, are capable of producing two general types of adverse reactions of which the nurse must be aware.

Allergic or Hypersensitivity Reactions

Allergic or hypersensitivity reactions occur in response to all available antimicrobial agents. Such reactions in-

TABLE 58-2   Antimicrobial Drugs of Choice

Organism	Drug(s)
GRAM-POSITIVE COCCI	
Staphylococcus aureus	
Non–penicillinase producing	penicillin G or V, first generation cephalosporins, vancomycin
Penicillinase producing	first generation cephalosporins, cloxacillin, dicloxacillin, methicillin
Methicillin resistant	ciprofloxacin, vancomycin
Streptococcus pneumoniae	penicillin G or V
Streptococcus pyogenes (group A)	penicillin G or V
Streptococcus (group B)	penicillin G or V, ampicillin, amoxicillin
Streptococcus viridans	penicillin G or V
GRAM-POSITIVE BACILLI	
Bacillus anthracis	penicillin G or V
Corynebacterium diphtheriae	erythromycin
Corynebacterium, JK strain	erythromycin, vancomycin
Listeria monocytogenes	amikacin, gentamicin, tobramycin, netilmicin
GRAM-NEGATIVE COCCI	
Neisseria gonorrhoeae	penicillin G or V, ampicillin, amoxacillin, azlocillin, piperacillin, cefoxitin, and most third generation cephalosporins
Neisseria meningitidis	penicillin G or V
GRAM-NEGATIVE ENTERIC BACILLI	
Escherichia coli	amikacin, gentamicin, tobramycin, cefamandole, cefotetan, third generation cephalosporins, ciprofloxacin
Klebsiella pneumoniae	same as E. coli
Proteus mirabilis	same as E. coli
Salmonella sp	ampicillin, amoxocillin, ciprofloxacin
OTHER BACILLI	
Pseudomonas aeruginosa	azlocillin, amikacin, gentamicin, piperacillin, ceftazidime, ciprofloxacin
ANAEROBES	
Gram-positive	
Clostridium difficile	tetracyclines
Clostridium perfringens	penicillin G or V
Clostridium tetani	penicillin G or V
Peptococcus sp	penicillin G or V
Peptostreptococcus sp	penicillin G or V
Gram-negative	
Bacteroides fragilis	clindamycin, metronidazole
MYCOPLASMAS	
Mycoplasma pneumoniae	clindamycin, erythromycin, tetracyclines
SPIROCHETES	
Treponema pallidum (syphilis)	penicillin G or V
FUNGI	
Asperigillus, candida sp	amphotericin B
VIRUSES	
Herpes simplex	vidarabine, acyclovir

clude rash, fever, urticaria with pruritis, chills, a generalized erythema, anaphylaxis, and the Stevens-Johnson syndrome. **Stevens-Johnson syndrome** is a form of toxic epidermal necrolysis in which the epidermis separates from the dermis, leaving the patient with a skin loss similar to a second degree burn.

A minor rash may be easily tolerated, but an individual with a generalized rash or erythema accompanied by chills and fever needs medical intervention. For example, an allergic response to a rapid infusion of vancomycin can result in a generalized red skin reaction, fever and chills; to mitigate this reaction, antihistamines would need to be given. Some rashes fade with continued treatment, as with some individuals receiving ampicillin, whereas other symptoms may become more severe, necessitating discontinuing the medication. Respiratory distress (wheezing) or anaphylaxis is a medical emergency requiring immediate attention to prevent a fatal outcome.

Sensitization has occurred through indirect exposure to a drug, such as drinking milk from cows treated with antibiotics or eating poultry or beef from livestock treated with antimicrobials. Also, previous topical application of antimicrobials may cause sensitization.

Treatment of allergic reactions includes the use of antihistamines and epinephrine, which block or counteract the effects of the vasoactive mediators of allergy, and the use of corticosteroids, which may reduce tissue injury and edema in the inflammatory response. The use of steroids is controversial in the face of systemic infection because of their prolonged inhibition of normal host defense responses.

Superinfection

Superinfection is an infection that occurs during the course of antimicrobial therapy delivered for either therapeutic or prophylactic reasons. Most antibiotics reduce or eradicate the normal microbial flora of the body, which is then replaced by resistant exogeneous or endogenous bacteria. If the number of these replacement organisms is large and the host conditions favorable, clinical superinfection can occur. Approximately 2% of persons treated with antibiotics get superinfections. The risk is greater when large doses of antibiotics are used, when more than one antibiotic is administered concurrently, and when broad-spectrum drugs are employed. The administration of some specific antimicrobials are more commonly associated with superinfection than others. For example, *Pseudomonas* organisms frequently colonize in and infect individuals taking cephalosporins. In a similar manner, clients taking tetracyclines may become infected with *Candida albicans*. Generally, superinfections are caused by microorganisms that are resistant to the drug the client is receiving. In the past, penicillinase-producing staphylococci were the most common cause of superinfection. *S. aureus* and *S. epidermidis* superinfections especially with methicillin-resistant strains, are again on the rise. Also, gram-negative enteric bacilli and fungi are the most common offenders. The proper management of superinfections includes (1) discontinuation of the drug being given or replacement of it by another drug to which the organism is sensitive, (2) culture of the suspected infected area, and (3) possible administration of an antimicrobial agent effective against the new offending organism.

GENERAL GUIDELINES FOR USE

Several important principles guide the judicious and optimal use of the antimicrobial agents. Causes of adverse

---

CLASSIFICATION OF ANTIMICROBIAL DRUGS BY MECHANISM OF ACTION

Inhibit cell wall synthesis
  penicillins
  cephalosporins
  vancomycin
  bacitracin
  cycloserine
  ristocetin
Alter membrane permeability
amphotericin B
nystatin
polymyxin
colistin
Inhibit protein synthesis
Impede replication of genetic information
  nalidixic acid
  griseofulvin
  novobiocin
  rifampin
  pyrimethamine
Impair translation of genetic information
  chloramphenicol
  tetracycline
  erythromycin
  aminoglycosides
  lincomycins
Antimetabolites
  sulfonamides
  sulfones
  PAS
  INH
  ethambutol

Modified from Kagan BM, ed: Antimicrobial therapy, ed 2, Philadelphia, 1980, WB Saunders Co.

TABLE 58-3 Summary of Some Major Allergic and Toxic Effects of Antimicrobial Drugs

Effect	Drug
Anaphylaxis	penicillin
Hematologic effects	chloramphenicol (low incidence but high mortality) sulfonamides (low incidence)
Nephrotoxicity	polymyxins aminoglycosides sulfonamides (low incidence with newer drugs)
Potential for neuromuscular blockade	polymyxins aminoglycosides
Injury to eighth cranial nerve	aminoglycosides

reactions to antimicrobial agents and of therapeutic failures are often related to lack of adherence to the following principles of antimicrobial therapy.

Identification of Infecting Organism

Because most antimicrobial agents have a specific effect on a limited range of microorganisms, the physician must formulate a specific diagnosis about the potential pathogens or organisms most likely causing a given infectious process. The drug most likely to be specifically effective against the suspected microorganism can then be selected. This objective is most validly and reliably accomplished by obtaining specimens from the infected area if possible (e.g., urine, sputum, wound drainage) or by obtaining venous blood specimens and sending them to the laboratory for culture and identification of the causative organism. The recovery of a specific microorganism from appropriate specimens is a significant factor in the determination of antimicrobial therapy. When a significant microorganism has been isolated, laboratory tests for antimicrobial susceptibility (sensitivity) to various antimicrobial agents are completed.

It is desirable to receive culture and sensitivity reports before initiating antimicrobial therapy. In some situations, however, it is not practical to wait for these laboratory results. For example, antimicrobial therapy must be initiated without delay in acute, life-threatening situations, such as peritonitis, septicemia, or pneumonia. In such situations the choice of antimicrobial agent for initial use must be based on tentative identification of the pathogen and Gram stain. It is known, for example, that microorganisms commonly isolated in acute adult infections of the lung include pneumococci, Haemophilus strain streptococci, and staphylococci. Antimicrobial agents specifically toxic to those organisms may be administered temporarily. The drugs can then be changed, if necessary, after laboratory reports have been received. When even tentative identification is difficult, *broad-spectrum* antibiotics, which are effective against a wide range of microorganisms, can be prescribed or several antimicrobial agents may be prescribed for simultaneous administration.

Some infections are most effectively treated with the use of only one antibiotic. In other situations *combined antimicrobial drug therapy* may be indicated. Indications for the simultaneous use of two or more antimicrobial agents include (1) treatment of mixed infections, in which each drug may act on a separate portion of a complex microbial flora; (2) need to delay the rapid emergence of bacteria resistant to one drug; and (3) need to reduce the incidence or intensity of adverse reactions by decreasing the dose of a potentially toxic drug. Indiscriminate use of combined antimicrobial drug therapy should be avoided because of expense, toxicity, and higher incidence of superinfections and resistance.

Sensitivity and Resistance of Microorganisms

Sensitivity testing measures the ability of a specific antibiotic to limit the growth or kill microorganisms in vitro. Two accepted methods of testing sensitivity of microorganisms to selected antibiotics are the disk method and the tube dilution method. The disk method, which is rapid and inexpensive, gives an index to microbial susceptibility. Tube dilution testing is required when bactericidal activity is essential, as in bacterial endocarditis. By this method the minimum inhibitory concentration (MIC) and the minimum bactericidal concentration (MBC) of an antibiotic agent against a particular organism are measured.

Frequently, a discrepancy exists between the in vitro testing and the activity of the drug within the body. This depends on a number of variables such as affinity for antibiotic active sites and penetration into the bacteria, pH, temperature, and ability of the drug to reach the site of an infection. For example, in the case of meningitis it would be inappropriate to use a drug that does not cross the blood-brain barrier even though the organism tested may be sensitive to the drug.

Resistance refers to the ability of a particular microorganism to resist the effects of a specific antibiotic. Resistance occurs in one of three ways: (1) the antibiotic is unable to reach the potential target site of its action—some organisms, such as *Pseudomonas,* elaborate a protective membrane (a glycocalyx or slime) that prevents the antibiotic from reaching the cell wall; (2) the microorganism may produce an enzyme that acts to reduce or eliminate the toxic effect of the antibiotic to the cell wall. Examples of these enzymes are the beta lactamases that cleave the beta-lactam ring on penicillins and cephalosporins, forming inactive compounds; acylases that acetylate chloramphenicol to yield inactive derivatives and enzymes that inactivate aminoglycosides by phosphorylation, adenylation, and acetylation; and (3) the microorganism may also be altered in the individual through several biochemical changes. The changes occur in such a way that the target site for the antibiotic no longer accommodates the drug. In this case a specific organism is said to have "become resistant" to a previously susceptible antibiotic. As a rule, microorganisms resistant to a certain drug will tend to be resistant to other chemically related antimicrobial agents, a phenomenon known as cross-resistance. For example, bacteria unresponsive to tetracycline will also be resistant to oxytetracycline and chlortetracycline.

Role of Host Defense Mechanisms

No antimicrobial agent will effect the cure of an infectious process if host defense mechanisms are inadequate. Such drugs act only on the causative organisms of infectious disease and have no effect on the defense mechanisms of the body, which need to be assessed and supported. Many infections do not require drug therapy and are adequately combated by individual defense mechanisms, including antibody production, phagocytosis, interferon production, fibrosis, or gastrointestinal rejection (vomiting, diarrhea). However, host defense mechanisms may be diminished, as in, for example, diabetes mellitus, neoplastic disease, and immunologic suppression. In addition, the very ill client may require supportive care to ensure adequate oxygenation, fluid and electrolyte balance, and optimal nutrition for antimicrobial therapy to be effective. In some situations surgical intervention is also necessary. In general, in the presence of a substantial amount of pus, necrotic tissue, or a foreign body, the most effective treatment is a combination of an antimicrobial agent and an appropriate surgical procedure.

The status of the host's defense mechanisms will also influence choice of therapy, route of administration, and dosage. If an infection is fulminating, for example, parenteral (preferably intravenous) administration of a bactericidal drug will be selected rather than oral administration of a bacteriostatic drug. Large "loading" doses of antimicrobial agents are often administered at the beginning of treatment of severe infections, to achieve maximum blood concentrations rapidly. However, factors influencing drug dosage are also related to the status of a client's renal function. Because many antimicrobial agents are metabolized and/or excreted by the kidneys, a major management problem exists in regard to individuals with compromised renal function. Drug doses are then generally reduced in parallel with the client's creatinine clearance levels. Hemodialysis may further alter the therapeutic regimen. In some disease states (such as burns) antibiotic dosage may need to be increased to achieve therapeutic levels.

In short, the administration of an antimicrobial agent specifically toxic to the isolated microorganism is not the only important measure in antimicrobial therapy. An additional and very important determinant of the effectiveness of an antimicrobial agent is the functional state of the host's defense mechanisms.

Proper Dosage and Duration of Therapy

Administering antimicrobial drugs for therapeutic purposes in adequate dosage and for long enough periods of time is an important principle of infectious disease therapy. Fortunately, serum levels of some of the more potent antibiotics can be monitored to avoid or reduce the potential for toxicity, for example, aminoglycosides. The nurse should assess for alterations in renal and hepatic functions, since they both can affect drug dosage, dosing interval, and/or drug toxicity.

Failures in antimicrobial therapy are frequently the result of drug doses being too small or being given for too short a period of time. Generally, antimicrobial therapy should not be discontinued until the patient has been afebrile and clinically well for 48 to 72 hours. Follow-up cultures should be obtained to assess the effectiveness of therapy.

Inadequate drug therapy may lead to remissions and exacerbations of the infectious process and may contribute to the development of resistance. When antibiotics are used prophylactically, they usually are given for short periods of time to enhance host defense mechanisms. For example, with perioperative antibiotics a loading dose is given immediately before surgery and continued for 48 hours following surgery.

Antimicrobial agents currently being used will be discussed as chemically related groups of drugs. The nurse should be familiar with the general characteristics of each drug group or category and with one or two prototype drugs in each group. Because the dosage for any given antibiotic varies with the type of infection, the site of infection, and the age of the patient, only general dosages are given in this text. It is recommended that the manufacturer's package insert or a formulary be consulted for specific dosages.

THE NURSE'S ROLE IN ANTIMICROBIAL THERAPY

Antimicrobial agents destroy or inhibit the growth of microorganisms. Some of these agents are derived from living organisms; others are synthetic and semisynthetic chemical compounds. The goal of antimicrobial therapy for infectious diseases is to destroy or suppress the growth of infecting microorganisms so that normal host defense mechanisms can gain control and eliminate the infecting organisms. Among the microorganisms that can be controlled by these drugs today are most bacteria, many fungi, and a few viruses. For the nurse to safely and effectively manage clients taking antimicrobials, knowledge of host defenses and antimicrobial drugs is necessary.

The primary defense mechanisms against infection in the body are intact skin and mucous membranes, the chemical composition and pH of specific body secretions, phagocytic cells, mechanical movements of certain cells or tissues such as cilia action, coughing, peristalsis, and the inflammatory process. Many factors can impair host defenses and thereby increase the risk for the development of infection by virulent organisms.

Any disruption in the integrity of skin or mucous membranes becomes a portal of entry for disease-producing organisms. In very ill, hospitalized clients or in those who are immunoincompetent (e.g., individuals with acquired immune deficiency syndrome [AIDS] or receiving immunosuppressive therapies), relatively minor breaks in the skin or mucosa can lead to fatal infections. Vigorous teeth cleaning, tube insertions, and injections should be avoided, if possible. Environmental hazards such as furniture obstructions, wet flooring, or the presence of irritating agents should be corrected so that injury is prevented. An impairment of blood supply to body tissues will also reduce host defenses by reducing the overall resistance of the tissues to injury and by preventing the migration of inflammatory cells to the area of injury. Other factors that impair the body's defenses against infection include neutropenia, anemia, protein malnutrition, and autoimmune and antiinflammatory agents such as antineoplastic agents and corticosteroids. Persons with chronic preexisting cardiopulmonary, renal, or metabolic disease and those at the extremes of age are more susceptible to the development of infection because of altered organ function. Poor personal hygiene and the suppression of the normal bacterial flora by antibiotics create conditions whereby normal defenses are overwhelmed, resulting in pathogen overgrowth (superinfection).

To exert their effects, antimicrobial agents must first gain access to target sites, usually by absorption of the drug into and distribution through the circulatory system. Then they have bacteriostatic or bactericidal effects, depending on the mechanism of action. Bacteriostatic agents such as sulfonamides inhibit bacterial growth, allowing host defense mechanisms additional time to remove the invading microorganisms. Bactericidal agents, such as the penicillins, cause bacterial cell death and lysis, superimposing this effect on the effects of host defenses. Antimicrobial agents may exert their bacteriostatic or bactericidal effects by inhibition of cell wall synthesis in bacteria, disruption or alteration of membrane permeability, inhibition of protein synthesis, or inhibition of synthesis of essential metabolites.

Hundreds of antimicrobial agents are marketed currently, and it is impossible for the nurse to be infinitely knowledgeable about each drug. However, in spite of the numerous and varied drugs available, there are still only a few drug categories to remember. Knowledge of general characteristics of each drug category and of general principles of antimicrobial drug therapy should enable the nurse to function effectively.

In addition to the antibiotics, which include penicillins, cephalosporins, macrolides, lincomycins, vancomycin, aminoglycosides, tetracyclines, chloramphenicol, and polymyxins, major groups of antiinfective drugs include sulfonamides, urinary tract antiseptics, and antimycobacterial, antifungal, and antiviral agents. Table 58–3 gives a brief summary of some major allergic and toxic effects of antimicrobial agents.

Nursing interventions in antimicrobial drug therapy generally relate to (1) assisting in the identification of the infecting organism, (2) actual administration of the drug, (3) assessment of the client's response to the drug, (4) client education, and (5) prevention and treatment of adverse reactions, including pharmacologic and chemical drug interactions.

Assisting in identification of infecting organism. Obtaining cultures to determine the source and type of infection is frequently the nurse's responsibility. In the event that orders for an antimicrobial agent are given before establishment of an infective source, the nurse should obtain cultures before administering the first dose of the drug ordered. Specimens obtained for culture should be taken directly to the laboratory and not allowed to stand. Delay may cause the death of fastidious organisms and allow contaminating organisms to overgrow the pathogen. Subsequent culture specimens obtained while the patient is receiving antimicrobials should be sent to the laboratory with information regarding the drug(s) being administered. The appropriate selection of laboratory tests for the identification of offending organisms often depends on this knowledge.

Administration of antimicrobial drugs. Because the constant and consistent administration of an antimicrobial drug at prescribed dosage intervals is necessary for maintaining therapeutic blood levels of the drug, the nurse should administer such a drug according to prescribed times as accurately as possible. This may mean awakening sleeping patients and ensuring that tests or therapies do not interrupt this schedule.

When antimicrobial agents are administered intravenously, the nurse must observe additional precautions: (1) the drugs should be diluted in neutral solutions (pH 7.0 to 7.2) of isotonic sodium chloride (0.9%) or 5% dextrose in water; (2) the drugs should be administered without the admixture of any other drug, to avoid chemical or physical incompatibilities; (3) the drugs should be administered by intermittent intravenous infusions to avoid inactivation (e.g., by temperature) and prolonged vein irritation from high drug concentration; (4) the infusion site must be changed every 48 hours to reduce the risk of chemical phlebitis; and (5) intramuscular antimicrobials should be injected deeply into large muscle masses (such as gluteal), and injection sites should be rotated to prevent tissue irritation.

Assessment of client's response to drug. Assessment of the client for therapeutic responses to antimicrobial agents is also a primary nursing responsibility. A decrease in the severity or a disappearance of the clinical and laboratory manifestations of infection indicates a positive response to antimicrobial therapy. With local infections redness, heat, edema, and pain should decrease. In the case of a systemic infection, temperature, heart rate, respiratory rate, and white blood cell count should return to normal, and appetite and a sense of well-being should improve. Purulent drainage, if present, should decrease in amount and change to a more normal appearance and consistency. In patients who are seriously ill, an improvement in organ function should accompany other signs of resolution of infection. Serum antibiotic concentrations can be monitored through the course of therapy to assess for therapeutic and toxic levels of individual antimicrobials.

In addition to monitoring therapeutic effects of antimicrobials, nurses must monitor the client for the development of common side effects of individual drugs. Fluid and electrolyte imbalances can occur during the course of administering many antibiotics, either from the drug itself, the mode of administration, or side effects such as diarrhea. For example, extracellular volume excess may result from administering multiple intravenous drugs, each of which is diluted in 100 ml of saline. Edema, pulmonary congestion with subsequent shortness of breath, and an increase in body weight all indicate the presence of an extracellular volume excess. Hypokalemia, resulting from severe diarrhea or the administration of antibiotic containing large quantities of sodium, produces no obvious clinical signs or symptoms until the potassium deficit is significant. At this point, widespread muscular weakness and cardiac conduction abnormalities appear. In the client whose cardiac function is being monitored, the appearance of U waves may be an earlier indication of low serum potassium. Laboratory demonstration of hypokalemia is frequently the only way to detect this disorder. Hypernatremia, another commonly seen disorder in clients receiving antimicrobial therapy, is also associated with few early clinical signs or symptoms, with the exception of a high serum sodium value, which occurs frequently because many antimicrobials have a sodium base. In general, when individuals must take prolonged courses of antimicrobials that can cause fluid and electrolyte imbalances, it may be necessary to periodically obtain serum electrolyte studies.

Education. Clients should be taught principles of antimicrobial therapy clearly enough to understand that these drugs should never be taken without medical supervision and should be taken in strict accordance with physicians' prescriptions. This is especially important because many individuals receiving antimicrobial drugs are not hospitalized and are responsible for self-medication. Clients should be taught, for example, not to take "leftover" antimicrobial drugs for new illnesses, even if symptoms appear similar; not to stop taking these drugs as soon as symptoms abate; and not to share these drugs with family and friends. Clients who are allergic to an antimicrobial agent should be taught how to protect themselves from future treatment with the drug in question such as by medical alert wallet cards or tags.

Expected effects, side effects, and adverse reactions of individual antimicrobials could be appropriately described on "drug sheets" for clients to refer to at home while taking antimicrobial therapy. A telephone number to call when questions arise could also be written on the drug sheets and would convey the message that it was expected and desirable for clients to discuss their concerns about their medications with health care workers.

Occasionally, antimicrobials will interfere with the results of home laboratory testing kits and patients using these must be cautioned. For example, the cephalosporins may produce a false positive reading when individuals with diabetes use commercial chemical testing strips to monitor their urine glucose.

Prevention and Management of Adverse Responses

Allergic response. Assessment of a client's previous reactions to drugs and to antimicrobial agents in particular is especially important in avoiding allergic reactions to drugs. Careful questioning of the individual regarding drugs previously taken and exact clinical responses to them is an important part of the client's history. Some clients equate common side effects such as nausea and diarrhea with drug allergy. Although these drug responses are important, knowledge of their appearance may not be as sufficient a reason to withhold a specific antibiotic as would a true allergy. Once drug allergy is known, warnings should be prominently displayed on the client's record or hospital chart. As additional precautions, the nurse should (1) ask the client if he or she has drug allergies before administering any medications; (2) tell the client what drug he is receiving; (3) observe the client for at least half an hour after administration of the drug (penicillin in particular), especially if it is administered parenterally and the client has never taken the drug previously; and (4) know what drugs are used for the treatment of allergic responses and where they are kept.

Anaphylaxis. The most serious allergic reaction to antimicrobials is an acute anaphylaxis. This reaction can occur anywhere from a few seconds to 30 minutes after an antibiotic injection. The syndrome associated with this reaction usually begins with diffuse flushing, itching, and a feeling of warmth. Hives may appear on the patient's face, neck, and chest. As the syndrome progresses, generalized body edema develops. Massive facial edema signals the possibility of upper airway edema, with impending obstruction and respiratory difficulty from pulmonary involvement. These problems are manifested as a choking sensation, stridor, chest tightness and pain, wheezing, shortness of breath, and restlessness.

The initial step in the emergent management of anaphylaxis is to immediately stop the antibiotic if it is still being infused. If the individual is not in a medical facility, immediate transport to one should be arranged, preferably by a vehicle staffed by paramedics who could establish an artificial airway in the event the patient's airway becomes totally obstructed. Reversal of anaphylaxis is accomplished by drug therapy. The antihistamine diphenhydramine HCl (Benadryl) is administered parenterally or orally. Epinephrine 1:1000 can be injected subcutaneously and will reverse the vascular effects of anaphylaxis.

Aminophylline or theophylline is administered if bronchospasm persists. If the individual is in anaphylactic shock, vasopressors may be necessary concomitantly with the administration of intravenous fluids for short-term management of hypotension. Corticosteroids (methylprednisolone) may be administered for prevention of protracted symptoms in severe reactions.

Superinfection. The emergence of superinfection may be suspected in the presence of diarrhea or recurrent fever in the patient taking antimicrobial drugs. Stomatitis is indicated by the presence of a sore mouth or white patches on the oral mucosa. Monilial vaginitis may produce a vaginal discharge or perineal rash. Localized superinfections may be heralded by increasing redness, heat, edema, pain, and possibly drainage. Children, elderly persons and others whose normal host defense mechanisms may be weakened should be especially observed for signs of superinfection. In the course of prolonged antimicrobial drug therapy, periodic cultures of the upper respiratory tract and of feces may be indicated to determine changes in bacterial flora that subsequently may be responsible for secondary infection. The nurse should be careful not to introduce new microorganisms and should emphasize asepsis in contacts with clients receiving antimicrobial therapy.

Stop and renewal orders. The establishment of automatic stop and renewal orders in many hospitals is another precaution against adverse reactions. Such orders restrict the administration of a prescribed antimicrobial agent to a definite time period (e.g., 7 days); its continued use past that time requires a new prescription from the physician.

Drug interactions. Because the administration of more than one drug to a client is the rule rather than the exception in current hospital practice, the possibility of drug interactions must be taken into account if antimicrobial therapy is to be optimally effective. The nurse should be alert to drugs that interact biologically with antimicrobial agents, as well as chemical incompatibilities between antimicrobial drugs and other agents when they are mixed for intravenous administration. The hospital formulary on each unit provides accurate and current information about these interactions.

Nursing interventions in antimicrobial drug therapy are essential to the safe and effective use of such agents.

KEY TERMS

bacteremia, page 887
bactericidal agents, page 888
bacteriostatic agents, page 888
chemotactic gradient, page 887
colonization, page 885
constant fever, page 888
fever of unknown origin (FUO), page 888
inflammation, page 887
intermittent fever, page 888
pyrogens, page 887
relapsing fever, page 888
remittent fever, page 888
sepsis, page 887
septicemia, page 887
Stevens-Johnson syndrome, page 890
zymogens, page 887

BIBLIOGRAPHY

Babcock JB and others: Effective antibiotic use in the hospital, J Med Technol 3(4):218, 1986.

Baron KA and White RL: Antibiotic efficacy review, Pharmacy Practice News 14(9):19, 1987.

Braunwald E and others, eds: Harrison's principles of internal medicine, ed 11, New York, 1987, McGraw-Hill Book Co.

Bullock BL and Rosendahl PP: Pathophysiology, adaptations and alterations in function, ed 2, Glenview, Ill, 1988, Scott, Foresman and Co.

Carlson KR: I.V. antibiotics: nursing considerations in the administration of the initial dose, NITA 9(1):62, 1986.

Saxon A (moderator) and others: Immediate hypersensitivity reactions to beta-lactam antibiotics, Ann Intern Med 107:204, 1987.

Tideiksaar R: Infections in the elderly: antibiotic selection. Part 2, Physician Assist 11(3):70, 1987.

Wyngaarden JB and Smith LH: Cecil textbook of medicine, ed 18, Philadelphia, 1988, WB Saunders Co.

Zenk KE: Special delivery: administering I.V. antibiotics to children, Nursing 16(12):50, 1986.

CHAPTER 59

Antibiotics

OBJECTIVES

After studying this chapter, the student will be able to:

1. Discuss the nurse's role in antibiotic therapy.

2. Differentiate between peak, trough, and mean serum levels.

3. List four major classifications of antibiotics.

4. Differentiate between different antibiotics within the same general classification.

5. Apply nursing considerations to the client receiving antibiotic therapy.

Antibiotics are chemical substances that kill or suppress the growth of microorganisms. The many available antibiotics vary in antibacterial spectrum, mechanism of action, potency, toxicity, and pharmacokinetic properties. An understanding of the general principles of antibiotic therapy, as discussed in Chapter 58, is essential for the nurse. In addition, before administering antibiotics, nurses must familiarize themselves with particular drugs, their actions, and effects.

THE NURSE'S ROLE IN ANTIBIOTIC THERAPY

Assessment. When an infection is suspected, the nursing assessment is particularly important. Detailed information regarding client's general health, as well as symptoms indicating an infection, such as elevated temperature, chills, sweats, redness, pain or swelling in an area previously unaffected, fatigue, anorexia, weight loss, cough, change in character or amount of sputum, increased white blood cell count, amount and quality of pus or drainage, should be obtained.

Whenever possible, the infecting organism should be identified before drug therapy begins. The collection of specimens (blood, urine, sputum, wound drainage and discharge) and cultures should be completed before antibiotic therapy starts. Specimens should be carefully obtained following institutional and agency guidelines to ensure test accuracy and to protect personnel from exposure to infectious organisms. Prompt treatment is imper-

897

ative in serious infections, and antimicrobial drugs should not be withheld pending laboratory study and culture results.

Antibiotics, particularly penicillins, have been associated with serious hypersensitivity and allergic reactions. A complete drug history of the client and family helps identify possible hypersensitivity or cross-sensitivity administration of the drugs. Information regarding possible contraindications, cautions, potential drug interactions and drug-taking patterns is also obtained.

Intervention. Dosage and routes of administration are highly individualized and are based on the organism or infection being treated, as well as a variety of individual client factors such as age, weight, general health, and preexisting diseases or organ or system dysfunction. Antibiotics are available in various dosage forms for topical, oral, or parenteral use. Dosage adjustments between different forms or routes of administration are necessary because of differences in absorption, distribution, metabolism, or excretion. For example, an oral dose of penicillin G requires five times the parenteral dose to achieve the same serum levels of the drug.

Special attention must be paid to interactions of oral antibiotics with food or other drugs. Some antibiotics should not be administered with food. For example, tetracycline forms a nonabsorbable complex with dairy products, whereas other antibiotics are administered with food to minimize gastric irritation.

Cross-sensitivity often exists between drugs of the same class (e.g., penicillins). Clients intolerant of one antibiotic may be intolerant of similar antibiotics.

The time of antibiotic administration should be spaced as evenly as possible over a 24-hour period to ensure stable and consistent serum levels. Antibiotics ordered four times a day (q.i.d.) should be administered every 6 hours. Three times a day (t.i.d.) means every 8 hours. It is important to administer antibiotics at the scheduled time to maintain a consistent blood level. Allowable variation differs with specific drugs and institutional policy. As a general rule, antibiotics should be administered within 15 minutes of the scheduled time.

Serum levels of many antibiotics are monitored to determine if the concentration is at the correct, or **therapeutic, level,** a high **(toxic level)** or low **(subtherapeutic level).** Timing of serum determinations is also important. To determine the lowest, or **trough, level,** the blood is drawn immediately before administering a dose. Mean serum levels are determined at some point between doses, and the highest serum level, or **peak level,** is determined shortly after dose administration. The desired serum concentration may vary with different drugs and the infecting organism. The exact timing of peak, mean, or trough serum level determinations is determined by each particular drug and route of administration.

Education. Clients should be fully informed about the nature of their condition and the treatment plan. They should understand the medication regimen, including the name of medication (generic as well as trade name), general action, its purpose, proper handling, dosage, and correct administration. Provide the client with a list of adverse drug effects, drug-drug interactions, and food-drug interactions, and advise the client of the proper response if these interactions occur.

Clients should be instructed to take the medication exactly as prescribed, at evenly spaced intervals, for the full length of time prescribed or until all the drug is gone. Even if the client feels well, the infection may return if the full course of therapy is not completed. Any leftover medication should be appropriately discarded.

A rash, itching, hives, fever, chills, joint pain or swelling, difficulty breathing, or wheezing are signs of an adverse reaction. The drug should be stopped and the health care provider contacted immediately.

Evaluation. When an antibiotic is adminstered for prophylaxis, the client should be monitored for signs indicating the absence or development of infection. When a specific infection is treated, a therapeutic response will be indicated by a decrease in specific signs of infection identified in the initial assessment (fever, malaise, WBC count, redness, inflammation, pain, cultures). Evaluation of the therapeutic response is important, since antibiotic therapy may be ineffective for several reasons, including incorrect route of administration, inadequate drainage of abscesses, poor antibiotic penetration of infected tissues, subtherapeutic serum levels, or bacterial resistance to the antibiotic.

Reducing or eliminating normal flora by antibiotic therapy provides an environment conducive to growth of undesirable bacteria, fungus, or yeasts, a condition known as **superinfection.** Examples commonly seen include diarrhea from altered intestinal flora or vaginal yeast infections resulting from a reduction in normal vaginal flora, which suppresses yeast growth.

Adverse effects vary widely, depending on drug, dose, route of administration, and client-related factors. Refer to nursing considerations of specific antibiotics for side effects or adverse reactions and specific nursing evaluation related to those drugs.

Allergic reactions are always possible following the first or successive doses. In general it is important to monitor for allergic reactions such as anaphylaxis, skin rashes, urticaria, and bronchospasm. Administration should immediately stop at the first sign of an allergic reaction, and the prescriber should be notified.

PENICILLINS

Penicillins are antibiotics derived from a number of strains of *Penicillium notatum* and *P. chrysogenum,* common molds often seen on bread or fruit (Figure 59-1).

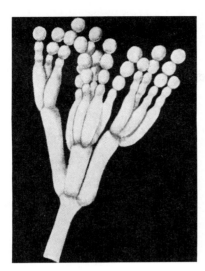

FIGURE 59-1 Typical penicillus of *Penicillium notatum;* Fleming's strain.

(From Raper, K.B., and Alexander, D.F.: J. Elisha Mitchell Sc. Soc. 61:74, 1945.)

Introduced into clinical practice in 1941, the penicillins constitute a large group of antimicrobial agents that remain the most effective and least toxic of all available antimicrobial drugs. Table 59-1 lists the penicillins used in current therapeutic practice and their route of administration. Penicillins encompass true antibiotics, as well as many newer, semisynthetic compounds that share a common structural nucleus and a common mechanism of action.

Mechanism of action. The penicillins specifically inhibit synthesis of bacterial cell walls, probably by interfering with the biosynthesis of mucopeptides and preventing linkage of structural components of the cell wall. They are bactericidal for a wide variety of gram-positive and some gram-negative organisms. Bacterial species considered highly susceptible to the penicillins include *streptococcus pneumoniae,* group A beta hemolytic streptococci, *Neisseria meningitidis, N. gonorrhoeae,* non-penicillinase-producing *Staphylococcus aureus, Clostridium tetani, Clostridium perfringens, Corynebacterium diphtheriae, Actinomyces,* and *Treponema pallidum* and other spirochetes. Most pencillins are much more active against gram-positive than gram-negative bacteria. There are exceptions, however. Gram-negative gonococci, for example, are penicillin susceptible. Generally, gram-negative bacteria have thinner cell walls and a lipopolysaccharide coat; *Neisseria* and *Haemophilus* species have much thicker cell walls and more permeable lipopolysaccharide coats than other gram-negative pathogens and thus are more penicillin sensitive.

Indications. Antibacterial agents are used to treat microorganisms or infections that are susceptible to their individual effects. The penicillins are not useful in the presence of bacteria-producing enzymes capable of de-

stroying penicillins, such as penicillinase-producing strains of the beta-lactamase enzymes produced by these strains (via chromosomal and plasmid-mediated enzymes) with strains of *S. aureus, E. coli,* indole-positive *Proteus* or *P. aeruginosa.* However, in some instances, synthetic penicillins are effective in treating infections caused by these organisms.

TABLE 59-1 Penicillins

Generic name (brand name)	Routes of administration
amdinocillin, sterile (Coactin)	IM, IV
amoxicillin (Amoxil, Apo-Amoxi♣)	PO
amoxicillin and clavulanate potassium (Augmentin, Clavulin♣)	PO
ampicillin (Amcill, Apo-Ampi♣)	PO
ampicillin sodium (Ampicin♣, Omnipen-N, Polycillin-N)	IM, IV
azlocillin sodium (Azlin)	IV
bacampicillin hydrochloride (Spectrobid, Penglobe♣)	PO
carbenicillin indanyl sodium (Geocillin, Geopen Oral)	PO
carbenicillin disodium (Geopen, Pyopen)	IM, IV
cloxacillin sodium (Apo-Cloxi♣, Cloxapen)	PO
cyclacillin (Cyclapen-W)	PO
dicloxacillin sodium (Dynapen, Pathocil)	PO
methicillin sodium (Staphcillin)	IM, IV
mezlocillin sodium (Baypen, Mezlin)	IM, IV
nafcillin sodium (Unipen)	PO
oxacillin sodium (Bactocill, Prostaphlin)	IM, IV
penicillin G benzathine (Bicillin)	PO, IM
penicillin G potassium (P-50♣, Pentids, Megacillin♣)	PO
penicillin G procaine suspension (Ayercillin♣, Crysticillin)	IM
penicillin V potassium (Apo-Pen-VK♣, Beepen-VK, Pen Vee K, PVF K♣)	PO
piperacillin sodium (Pipracil)	IM, IV
ticarcillin disodium (Ticar)	IM, IV, IV infusion
ticarcillin disodium and clavulanate potassium (Timentin)	IV infusion

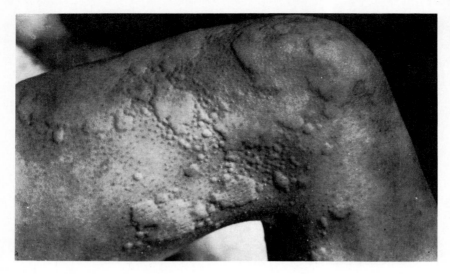

FIGURE 59-2   Urticaria such as those seen in patients sensitive to penicillin.

Studies of the prophylactic use of penicillin have shown it to be of value in (1) treating persons exposed to group A *S. pyogenes,* (2) preventing rheumatic fever recurrences, (3) treating persons exposed to gonorrhea and syphilis, and (4) preventing subacute bacterial endocarditis in patients with valvular heart disease who must undergo surgical or dental procedures.

Pharmacokinetics. See Table 59-2.

Side effects/reactions. See Table 59-3.

Significant drug interactions. When penicillins are given with the following drugs, the following interactions may occur.

Drug	**Possible Effect and Management**
anticoagulants, oral coumarin or indandione, heparin or thrombolytic agents	Increased risk of bleeding when given with high doses of parenteral carbenicillin or ticarcillin; these drugs inhibit platelet aggregation. Monitor closely for signs of bleeding. Concurrent use of these penicillins with thrombolytic agents also increases the risk for severe bleeding; thus, concurrent drug administration is not recommended.
anti-inflammatory nonsteroidal analgesics, platelet aggregation inhibitors (such as salicylates, dextran, dipyridamole, valproic acid) and sulfinpyrazone	With high dosages of carbenicillin or ticarcillin (parenteral dosage forms), an increased risk for bleeding or hemorrhage exists. These drugs inhibit platelet function and large doses of salicylates may induce hypoprothrombinemia and also gastrointestinal ulcers (from NSAIDs, salicylates, or sulfinpyra-

Drug	**Possible Effect and Management**
	zone), all adding to the potential risk of hemorrhage.
captopril or potassium-sparing diuretics, or Enalapril or potassium-containing drugs or potassium supplements	If given concurrently with parenteral penicillin G potassium, serum potassium levels may increase, causing hyperkalemia. Monitor closely, as dosage adjustments may be necessary.
cholestyramine or colestipol	May decrease absorption of oral penicillin G if given concurrently. Advise clients to take antibiotic first and other medications 3 hours later.
probenecid	Decreases renal tubular secretion of penicillins, resulting in elevated serum levels and an increase in half-life. It may also increase toxicity. Several combinations of penicillin and probenecid are marketed to take advantage of this effect.
estrogen-containing contraceptives	When used concurrently with ampicillin, bacampicillin, or penicillin V, the effectiveness of the oral contraceptives may be decreased due to increase in estrogen metabolism or reduction in enterohepatic circulation of estrogens. Advise clients to use an alternate method of contraception while taking these antibiotics.

TABLE 59-2   Pharmacokinetics of Penicillins

Drugs	Oral absorption (%)	Time to peak serum levels (hr)	Half-life (hr) Normal renal function	Neonate	Liver metabolism (%)	Kidney excretion (% unchanged)
amdinocillin	None	IM, ½	0.9	—	Very low	70 in 6 hr
amoxicillin	75-90	P.O., 2	1-1.3	—	28-50	68
amoxicillin and clavulanate	Very good	P.O., 1-2	1.3 (amoxicillin) 1 (clavulanate)	—	28-50 (amoxicillin)	50-70 (amoxicillin)
ampicillin	35-50	P.O., 1.5-2 IM, 1	1-1.5	1.7-4	12-50	25-60 (P.O.) 50-85 (IM)
azlocillin	—	—	1	—	<10	50-70 in 24 hr.
bacampicillin	Very good (98)	P.O., ½-1 (young children) P.O., 0.9-1 (adults)	0.7-1.1	—	Mostly liver	75 within 8 hr.
carbenicillin disodium	None	IM, 1	1-1.5	2.7-4	2	60-90
carbenicillin indanyl sodium	30-50	P.O., 1-3	1-1.5	2.7-4	2	60-90
cloxacillin	50	P.O., 1-2	0.5-1.1	—	9-22	30-45
cyclacillin	Very good	P.O., 0.5-1	0.5-0.7	—	15-17	85
dicloxacillin	37-50	P.O., 0.5-1	0.5-1	Not recommended	9-10	60
methicillin	None	IM, 0.5-1	0.4-0.8	—	8	80
mezlocillin	Very little	IM, 0.75	0.8-1	1.8-2.1	45	55-60 in 6 hr
nafcillin	Poor to variable	P.O., 1-2 IM, 1-2	0.5-1	—	60	10-30
oxacillin	30-33	P.O., 0.5 (solution) 1 (capsule) IM, 0.5	0.5-0.7	1.2-1.6	49	40
penicillin G	Poor to variable (15-30)	P.O., 1-2	0.5-0.7	1.4-3	19	20 (P.O.)
benzathine	Poor	IM, 24	—	—		
potassium	30	IM, 0.25-0.5	—	—		60 (pen GK)
procaine	—	IM, 1-4	—	—		60-90 (pen G procaine)
penicillin V	60	P.O., 0.5-1	1	—	56	20-40
piperacillin	None	IM, 0.5	0.6-1.2	—	None	60-90 in 24 hr
ticarcillin	None	IM, 0.5-1	1-1.2	5	Minimal	86
ticarcillin and clavulanate	None	—	1-1.2 (ticarcillin)	—	Minimal	60-70 (ticarcillin)

Dosage and administration
amdinocillin, sterile (Coactin)

Adults. 10 mg/kg intramuscularly or intravenously every 4 hours. If given with another beta-lactam antibiotic, the time should be extended to every 6 hours.

In renal impairment (<30 ml/min), 10 mg/kg every 6 to 8 hours.

Children. Infants and children up to 12 years old: not established. Children 12 years and older: see adult dosage.

TABLE 59-3   Penicillins: Side Effects and Adverse Reactions

Side effects*	Adverse reactions†
Most frequent: mild diarrhea (ampicillin, amoxicillin with clavulanate, carbenicillin, penicillin G, penicillin V, ticarcillin); taste alterations (carbenicillin); nausea or vomiting (amoxicillin with clavulanate ampicillin, carbenicillin, penicillin G, penicillin V, ticarcillin); sore mouth or tongue (bacampicillin); dark or discolored tongue (penicillin G, penicillin V) Less frequent: alterations in taste and smell (azlocillin, ticarcillin and clavulanate); mild diarrhea (amdinocillin, amoxicillin, azlocillin, bacampicillin, cloxacillin, dicloxacillin, methicillin, mezlocillin, nafcillin, oxacillin, piperacillin); sore mouth (azlocillin, ticarcillin and clavulanate); sore mouth or tongue (amoxicillin, amoxicillin and clavulanate, ampicillin); abdominal distress (amoxicillin and clavulanate, bacampicillin); taste alterations (mezlocillin); dark or discolored tongue (amoxicillin, amoxicillin and clavulanate, ampicillin, bacampicillin)	Most frequent: pseudomembranous colitis—stomach pain, gas, severe diarrhea, fever, increased thirst, weight loss, nausea or vomiting, increased weakness (amoxicillin, amoxicillin and clavulanate, ampicillin, bacampicillin); bloody urine, edema of face and ankles, respiratory difficulties due to intersitial nephritis (parenteral methicillin); convulsions with high injectable doses, especially in renal impairment (penicillin G); rash, hives, pruritis, wheezing—hypersensitivity reaction (See Fig. 59-2) amoxicillin, amoxicillin and clavulanate, ampicillin, bacampicillin, cloxacillin, cyclacillin, dicloxacillin, methicillin, mezlocillin, nafcillin, oxacillin, penicillin G and penicillin V); increased bleeding episodes and bruising (carbenicillin, ticarcillin, ticarcillin and clavulanatin)

*If side effects continue, increase, or disturb the client, inform the physician.
†If adverse reactions occur, contact physician because medical intervention may be necessary.
All penicillins except amdinocillin can cause pseudomembranous colitis after the medication is discontinued. Medical intervention is necessary.

amoxicillin capsules/oral suspension (Amoxil, Apo-Amoxi✼, Novamoxin✼)

Adults. 250 to 500 mg (anhydrous base) orally every 8 hours. Maximum daily dose is 4.5 g (anhydrous base). For gonorrhea, 3 g orally and 1 g of probenecid simultaneously as one dose.

Children. Infants up to 6 kg of body weight, 25 to 50 mg orally (anhydrous base) every 8 hours. Infants, 6 to 8 kg, 50 to 100 mg orally (anhydrous base) every 8 hours.

Infants and children, 8 to 20 kg, 6.7 to 13.3 mg/kg (anhydrous base) orally every 8 hours; 20 kg and over, see adult dose.

If dosage for infants and children calculates to a larger dose than for an adult on the weight basis, the total daily adult dose should not be exceeded in the pediatric client.

For gonorrhea, 50 mg/kg orally (anhydrous base) and 25 mg/kg of probenecid concurrently as a single dose in a prepubertal child. Probenecid is not recommended for children under 2 years old.

amoxicillin tablets (chewable) (Amoxil). See above for dosage.

amoxicillin and clavulanate potassium for oral suspension/tablets (Augmentin, Clavulin)

Adults. Pneumonia, other severe infections: 500 mg anhydrous amoxicillin and 125 mg clavulanic acid orally every 8 hours. For other severe infections, 250 mg anhydrous amoxicillin and 125 mg (clavulanic acid) orally every 8 hours.

Children. Infants or children up to 40 kg: for severe infections such as acute otitis media, sinusitis, or pneumonia, 13.3 mg/kg (anhydrous base) orally every 8 hours. For other infections, 6.7 mg/kg (anhydrous amoxicillin) orally every 8 hours. Children 40 kg and over, see adult dose.

ampicillin capsules/oral suspension (Amcil, Apo-Ampi✼, Polycillin)

Adults. 250 to 500 mg (anhydrous base) orally every 6 hours. Maximum daily dose is 6 g. For gonorrhea, 3.5 g (anhydrous base) and 1 g of probenecid concurrently orally as a single dose.

Children. Infants and children up to 20 kg, 12.5 to 25 mg/kg (anhydrous base) orally every 6 hours or 16.7 to 33.3 mg/kg orally every 8 hours. Children 20 kg and over, see adult dosage. Some infants and children may need up to 200 mg/kg (anhydrous base) daily in divided doses, depending on type and severity of infection.

sterile ampicillin sodium (Ampicin✼, Omnipen-N, Polycillin-N)

Adults. 250 to 500 mg (base) intramuscularly or intravenously every 6 hours. Maximum daily dose is up to 300 mg/kg (base) or 16 g daily.

For bacterial meningitis (septicemia), 1 to 2 g (base IM or IV every 3 to 4 hours; 18.75 to 25 mg/kg every 3 hours or 25 to 33.3 mg/kg every 4 hours).

For gonorrhea, 500 mg (base) intramuscularly or intravenously every 8 to 12 hours for 2 doses. If necessary, dosage may be repeated.

Children. Infants up to 20 kg, 6.25 to 25 mg/kg intramuscularly or intravenously every 6 hours or 8.3 to 33.3 mg/kg every 8 hours. Infants and children, 20 kg and over, see adult dose.

For bacterial meningitis (septicemia), 18.75 to 25 mg/kg (base) intramuscularly or intravenously every 3 hours or 25 to 33.3 mg/kg every 4 hours.

Some infants and children may need up to 400 mg/kg given in divided doses daily, depending on type and severity of infection.

sterile azlocillin sodium (Azlin)

Adults. 33.3 to 50 mg/kg (base) intravenously every 4 hours, 50 to 75 mg/kg every 6 hours; 3 g every 4 hours, or 4 g every 6 hours.

For urinary tract infections (complicated), 37.5 to 50 mg/kg (base) intravenously every 6 hours or 3 g every 6 hours.

For urinary tract infections (uncomplicated), 25 to 31.25 mg/kg (base) intravenously every 6 hours or 2 g every 6 hours.

Clients with impaired renal function need a reduced dosage; check package insert for dosage instructions.

Maximum daily dose is 350 mg/kg (base) or 24 g daily, in life-threatening infections.

Children. Newborn infants, not established. Children with acute pulmonary exacerbation of cystic fibrosis, 75 mg/kg (base) intravenously every 4 hours. Maximum daily dose should not exceed 24 g (base).

bacampicillin hydrochloride tablets/oral suspension (Spectrobid, Penglobe♣)

Adults. 560 mg (ampicillin) orally every 12 hours. Maximum daily dose is 2.24 g (ampicillin).

For skin, soft tissue infections, acute otitis media, pharyngitis, sinusitis, and urinary tract infections, 280 to 560 mg (ampicillin) every 12 hours.

For gonorrhea, acute, uncomplicated urogenital infections in males and females, 1.12 g (ampicillin) and 1 g of probenecid orally, concurrently, as a single dose.

Children. For pneumonia: infants and children up to 25 kg, 17.5 mg/kg (ampicillin) orally every 12 hours; children 25 kg and over, see adult dose.

For skin and soft tissue infections, acute otitis media, pharyngitis, sinusitis, and urinary tract infections: infants and children up to 25 kg, 8.75 to 17.5 mg/kg (ampicillin) orally every 12 hours; children 25 kg and over, see adult dose.

Dosage not established for acute gonorrhea in pediatric patients; however, 125 mg of bacampicillin hydrochloride is equivalent to 87.5 mg of ampicillin.

Tablet dosage form is not recommended for pediatric clients.

carbenicillin indanyl sodium tablets (Geocillin, Geopen Oral)

Adults. 382 to 764 mg (base) orally every 6 hours.
Children. Not established.

sterile carbenicillin disodium (Geopen, Pyopen)
Adults

For skin and soft tissue infections, septicemia, meningitis, pneumonia: 50 to 83.3 mg/kg (base) intramuscularly or intravenously every 4 hours.

For urinary tract infections, 1 to 2 g (base) intramuscularly or intravenously every 6 hours or up to 50 mg/kg, every 6 hours.

For gonorrhea, 4 g (base) intramuscularly, divided into two injection sites, and 1 g of probenecid orally, which should be given 30 minutes before the carbenicillin.

Clients with impaired renal function (creatinine clearance less than 5 ml/min), 2 g (base) intravenously every 8 to 12 hours.

Children

For septicemia, meningitis, pneumonia or skin and soft tissue infections: neonates to 2 kg, 100 mg/kg (base) intramuscularly or intravenously initially, then 75 mg/kg every 8 hours during the first 7 days of life, then 100 mg/kg every 6 hours.

Neonates 2 kg and over, 100 mg/kg (base) intramuscularly or intravenously initially, then 75 mg/kg every 6 hours during the first 3 days of life, then 100 mg/kg every 6 hours thereafter.

Older infants and children, see adult dose.

For urinary tract infections, 12.5 to 50 mg/kg (base) intramuscularly or intravenously every 6 hours or 8.3 to 33.3 mg/kg every 4 hours. Dosage is not established for pediatric clients with renal impairment. Dosages of 600 to 800 mg/kg daily in divided doses has been used in very young infants with life-threatening infections (1.1 g of carbenicillin disodium is equivalent to approximately 1 g of the base).

cloxacillin sodium capsules/oral solution (Apo-Cloxi♣, Cloxapen)

Adults. 250 to 500 mg (base) orally every 6 hours. Maximum daily dose is up to 6 g (base) per day.

Children. Infants and children up to 20 kg, 12.5 to 25 mg/kg (base) orally every 6 hours; children 20 kg and over, see adult dosage. (1.05 g of cloxacillin sodium is approximately equivalent to 1 g of base).

cyclacillin tablets/oral suspension (Cyclapen-W)

Adults. 250 to 500 mg orally every 6 hours. Maximum daily dose is 8 g/day. Clients with renal impairment need a dosage adjustment; see package insert for dosages.

Children

For acute otitis media: 16.7 to 33.3 mg/kg orally every 8 hours.

For pharyngitis, including tonsillitis: infants and children up to 20 kg, 125 mg orally every 8 hours; children 20 kg and over, 250 mg orally every 8 hours.

For other infections: 12.5 to 25 mg/kg orally every 6 hours.

This drug is not recommended for infants under 2 months old. Maximum daily dose is 2 g.

dicloxacillin sodium capsules/oral suspension (Dynapen, Pathocil)

Adults. 125 to 250 mg (base) orally every 6 hours. Maximum daily dose is 6 g (base) daily.

Children. Infants and children up to 40 kg, 3.125 to 6.25 mg/kg (base) orally every 6 hours; children 40 kg and over, see adult dose. No dosage schedule has been established for neonates. (1.05 g of dicloxacillin sodium is approximately equivalent to 1 g of base.)

methicillin sodium for injection (Staphcillin)

Adults. 1 g intramuscularly every 4 to 6 hours or 1 to 2 intravenously every 4 hours. Maximum daily dose is 24 g.

Children. Intramuscularly, 25 mg/kg every 6 hours; intravenously, 16.7 to 33.3 mg/kg every 4 hours, or 25 to 50 mg/kg every 6 hours. Neonates should receive lower doses of this drug. Some infants and children may need up to 200 or 300 mg/kg daily in divided doses, depending on infection type and severity. (1 g of methicillin sodium is approximately equal to 900 mg of base.)

sterile mezlocillin sodium (Baypen, Mezlin)

Adults. Intramuscularly or intravenously, 33.3 to 58.3 mg/kg every 4 hours; 50 to 87.5 mg/kg every 6 hours; or 3 to 4 g every 4 to 6 hours.

For acute, uncomplicated gonococcal urethritis infection, intramuscularly or intravenously, 1 to 2 g (base) as single dose plus 1 g of probenecid orally, the latter given ½ hour before or concurrently with mezlocillin.

For complicated urinary tract infection, intravenously, 37.5 to 50 mg/kg (base) every 6 hours, or 3 g every 6 hours.

For uncomplicated urinary tract infection, intramuscularly or intravenously, 25 to 31.25 mg/kg (base) every 6 hours, or 1.5 to 2 g every 6 hours.

Persons with impaired renal function will require a dosage adjustment; check a current package insert for dosage instructions.

Maximum daily dosage is 24 g/day (base). Dosages up to 500 mg/kg/day have been used.

Children. Intravenously or intramuscularly, infants up to 7 days old, 75 mg/kg (base) every 12 hours; infants 8 to 30 days old, 75 mg/kg (base) every 6 to 8 hours; infants over 1 month old and up to 12 years old, 50 mg/kg (base) every 4 hours.

nafcillin sodium capsules/tablets/oral solution (Unipen)

Adults. 250 mg to 1 g (base) orally every 4 to 6 hours. Maximum daily dose is 6 g/day (base).

Children. Neonates, 10 mg/kg (base) orally every 6 to 8 hours; older infants and children, 6.25 to 12.5 mg/kg (base) orally every 6 hours.

For streptococcal pharyngitis, 250 mg (base) orally every 8 hours. (1.1 g of nafcillin sodium is approximately equivalent to 1 g of base.)

nafcillin sodium for injection (Nafcil, Nallpen, Unipen)

Adults. Intramuscularly, 500 mg (base) every 4 to 6 hours; intravenously, 500 mg to 1.5 g (base) every 4 hours. Daily maximum dose: Intramuscularly, 12 g/day (base); intravenously 20 g/day (base).

Children. Neonates, intramuscularly, 10 to 20 mg/kg (base), every 12 hours; intravenously, 10 to 20 mg/kg (base) every 4 hours, or 20 to 40 mg/kg every 8 hours. Older infants and children, intramuscularly, 25 mg/kg (base) every 12 hours; intravenously, 10 to 20 mg/kg (base) every 4 hours or 20 to 40 mg/kg every 8 hours. Some neonates, infants and children may need up to 200 mg/kg/day (base) in divided dosages, depending on infection type and severity.

oxacillin sodium capsules/oral solution (Bactocill, Prostaphlin)

Adults. 500 mg to 1 g (base) orally every 4 to 6 hours. Maximum daily dose is 6 g/day.

Children. Children up to 40 kg, 12.5 to 25 mg/kg (base) orally every 6 hours; children 40 kg and over, see adult dosage. Maximum daily dosage is 4 to 6 g (base).

oxacillin sodium for injection (Bactocill, Prostaphlin)

Adults. Intravenously or intramuscularly, 1 to 2 g (base) every 4 hours. Maximum daily dose is 20 g/day (base) in severe septicemia and meningitis.

Children. Intravenously or intramuscularly, children up to 40 kg, 12.5 to 25 mg/kg (base) every 6 hours or 16.7 mg/kg every 4 hours; children 40 kg and over, see adult dosage.

In some premature infants and neonates, doses of 25 mg/kg (base) daily may provide adequate serum concentrations.

Neonates 2 kg and under may receive 25 mg/kg (base) every 12 hours (from 1 to 14 days old) or 25 mg/kg every 8 hours (from 15 to 30 days old). Neonates over 2 kg may receive 25 mg/kg every 6 hours (15 to 30 days old).

Depending on type and severity of the infection, some children may need up to 300 mg/kg (base) daily, in divided doses. (1.05 g of oxacillin sodium is approximately equivalent to 1 g of base.)

penicillin G benzathine tablets (Bicillin)

Adults. 400,000 to 600,000 units (base) orally every 4 to 6 hours.

To prevent streptococcal infection in individuals with a history of rheumatic heart disease, 200,000 units (base), orally every 12 hours. Maximum daily dose is up to 12 million units/day (base).

Children. Infants and children up to 12 years old, 4167 to 15,000 units/kg (base) orally every 4 hours, or 6250 to 22,500 units/kg every 6 hours or 8333 to 30,000 units/kg every 8 hours; children 12 years and older, see adult dosage.

sterile penicillin G benzathine suspension (Bicillin L-A, Permapen)

Adults

For group A streptococcal pharyngitis, 1.2 million units (base) intramuscularly as a single dose.

To prevent a streptococcal infection in persons with a history of rheumatic heart disease, intramuscularly

1.2 million units (base) month, or 600,000 units every 2 weeks.

Syphilis (primary, secondary, or latent), intramuscularly 2.4 million units (base) as single dose.

Syphilis (tertiary and neurosyphilis), intramuscularly, 2 million units (base) weekly for 3 weeks, or 3 million units once a week for 2 or 3 weeks.

Maximum daily dose is up to 2.4 million units.

Children

For congenital syphilis: infants and children up to 2 years old, 50,000 units/kg (base) intramuscularly as single dose; 2 to 12 years old, adult dose based on usual dose for syphilis.

For group A streptococcal pharyngitis: infants and children up to 27.3 kg, 300,000 to 600,000 units (base) intramuscularly as single dose; children 27.3 kg and over, 900,000 units (base) intramuscularly as a single dose.

penicillin G potassium for oral solution/tablets (P-50♣, Pentids, Megacillin♣)

Adults. 200,000 to 500,000 units (125 to 312 mg base) orally every 6 to 8 hours.

To prevent rheumatic heart disease in persons requiring prophylaxis from streptococcal infection, 200,000 to 250,000 units (125 to 156 mg base) orally every 12 hours.

Maximum daily dose is up to 12 million units/day (7.5 g base).

Children. Infants and children up to 12 years old, 4167 to 15,000 units/kg (2.5 to 9.3 mg base) orally every 4 hours; 6250 to 22,500 units/kg (3.75 to 14 mg) every 6 hours; or 8333 to 30,000 units/kg (5 to 18.7 mg) every 8 hours. Children 12 and over, see adult dosage.

penicillin G potassium for injection (Pfizerpen)
sterile penicillin G potassium
penicillin G sodium for injection (Crystapen)

Adults. 1 million to 5 million units (base) intramuscularly or intravenously, every 4 to 6 hours.

For the following specific infections:

Antinomycosis, intravenous infusion of 10 million to 20 million units (base) daily.

Clostridial infections, 20 million units (base) daily.

Erysipeloid endocarditis, 10 million to 20 million units (base) daily.

Gingivostomatitis, necrotizing ulcerative, 10 million to 20 million units (base) daily.

Gonococcal endocarditis and arthritis, 10 million to 20 million units (base) daily.

Meningococcal meningitis 1 million to 2 million units (base) every 2 hours or by intravenous infusion, 20 million to 30 million units daily.

Rat-bite fever, 10,000 to 20 million units (base) daily.

Maximum daily dose is up to 100 million units/day (base) per day.

Children. Premature and full-term neonates, intramuscularly or intravenously, 30,000 units/kg (base) every 12

hours. Older infants and children, 4167 to 16,667 units/kg (base) intramuscularly or intravenously every 4 hours, or 6250 to 25,000 units/kg every 6 hours. Depending on infection type and severity, some pediatric clients have needed up to 400,000 units/kg/day (base) in divided doses. Neonates: *Listeria* infections, 500,000 to 1 million units/day (base).

sterile penicillin G procaine suspension (Ayercillin♣, Crysticillin, Duracillin A.S.)

Adults. Intramuscularly, 600,000 to 1.2 million units (base)/day.

For diphtheria, administer 300,000 to 600,000 units (base)/day intramuscularly, along with diphtheria antitoxin.

For gonorrhea, 4.8 million units (base) intramuscularly divided into two injection sites with 1 g of probenecid orally (given ½ hour before or with the penicillin) as a single dose.

For syphilis, intramuscularly, 600,000 units (base) daily for 8 days (primary, secondary, and latent) or for 10 to 15 days (tertiary, neurosyphilis).

Maximum daily dose is up to 4.8 million units (base)/day.

Children

For congenital syphilis, infants and children up to 32 kg, 50,000 units (base)/kg intramuscularly daily for 10 days.

For syphilis (primary, secondary, and latent) in children over 12 years old, see adult dose for syphilis.

Depending on infection type and severity, some pediatric patients may need up to 100,000 units (base)/kg daily in divided doses.

penicillin V potassium tablets (Apo-Pen-VK♣, Beepen-VK, Pen Vee K, V-Cillin K, Veetids, PVF K♣)
penicillin V potassium for oral solution (Beepen-VK, Ledercillin VK, Pen Vee K, VC-K♣)

Adults. 125 to 500 mg (200,000 to 800,000 units; base) orally every 6 to 8 hours. Maximum daily dose is 7.2 g (11,520,000 units, base; daily).

To prevent streptococcal infections in persons with a history of rheumatic heart disease, administer 125 to 250 mg (200,000 to 400,000 units base) every 12 hours.

Children. Infants and children up to 12 years old, 2.5 to 9.3 mg (4167 to 15,000 units, base)/kg orally every 4 hours; 3.75 to 14 mg (6250 to 22,500 units)/kg orally every 6 hours; or 5 to 18.7 mg (8333 to 30,000 units)/kg every 8 hours. Children 12 years and older, see adult dose.

sterile piperacillin sodium (Pipracil)

Adults. 3 to 4 g (base) intramuscularly or intravenously every 4 to 6 hours.

For uncomplicated gonorrhea, 2 g (base) intramuscularly as a single dose and 1 g of probenecid orally, given ½ hour before injection.

Perioperative prophylaxis in:

Clients undergoing abdominal hysterectomy surgery, 2 g (base) intravenously, ½ to 1 hour before surgery 2 g on return to recovery room, and 2 g 6 hours later.

Client undergoing cesarean-section, 2 g (base) intravenously when umbilical cord is clamped, then 2 g intravenously at 4 hours and 8 hours after the first dose.

Intraabdominal procedures, 2 g (base) intravenously ½ to 1 hour before surgery, 2 g during surgery, and 2 g every 6 hours after surgery for up to 24 hours.

Clients undergoing vaginal hysterectomy, 2 g (base) intravenously ½ to 1 hour before surgery and 2 g intravenously at 6 and 12 hours after the first dose.

Septicemia, nosocomial pneumonia, intraabdominal or genitourinary tract infections, skin and soft tissue infection: 2 to 3 g (base) intravenously every 4 hours; 3 to 4 g every 6 hours; 33.3 to 50 mg/kg every 4 hours; or 50 to 75 mg/kg every 6 hours.

For complicated urinary tract infections: 3 to 4 g (base) intravenously every 6 to 8 hours; 31.25 to 50 mg/kg every 6 hours; or 41.7 to 66.7 mg/kg every 8 hours.

For uncomplicated urinary tract infections and community-acquired pneumonia: intramuscularly or intravenously 1.5 to 2 g (base) every 6 hours; 3 to 4 g every 12 hours; 25 to 31.25 mg/kg every 6 hours; or 50 to 62.5 mg/kg every 12 hours.

Persons with impaired renal function require a dosage reduction; see package insert for exact dosages recommended.

Maximum daily dose is 24 g (base)/day. In selected situations, dosages up to 500 mg/kg have been given.

Children. Infants and children under 12 years old, not established. 12 years and over, see adult dose.

sterile ticarcillin disodium (Ticar)

Adults

For septicemia, pneumonia, skin and soft tissue infections, intraabdominal infections, and genitourinary tract infections: intravenous infusion, administer 3 g (base) every 3 to 6 hours, or 25 to 37.5 mg/kg every 3 hours, or 33.3 to 50 mg/kg every 4 hours, or 50 to 75 mg/kg every 6 hours.

For complicated urinary tract infections, intravenous infusion, 3 g (base) every 4 to 6 hours; 25 to 33.3 mg/kg every 4 hours; or 37.5 to 50 mg/kg every 6 hours.

For uncomplicated urinary tract infections, intramuscularly or intravenously, 1 g (base) every 4 to 6 hours.

For clients with impaired renal function, refer to the package insert for specific dosing schedules.

Children. Neonates up to 2 kg with septicemia, pneumonia, skin or soft tissue infections, intraabdominal infections or genitourinary tract infections: intramuscularly or intravenously, 100 mg (base)/kg initially, then 75 mg/kg every 8 hours during first week of life, followed by 100 mg/kg every 4 hours thereafter. Neonates 2 kg and over for same infections, administer intramuscularly or intravenously, 100 mg (base)/kg initially, then 75 mg/kg every 4 to 6 hours during the first 14 days of life, then 100 mg/kg every 4 hours thereafter. Children up to 40 kg, for same infections as noted previously, intravenous infusion, 33.3 to 50 mg (base)/kg every 4 hours or 50 to 75 mg/kg every 6 hours.

For complicated bacterial urinary tract infections: intravenous infusion, 25 to 33.3 mg (base)/kg every 4 hours, or 37.5 to 50 mg/kg every 6 hours.

For uncomplicated urinary tract infections (bacterial): intramuscularly or intravenously 12.5 to 25 mg (base)/kg every 6 hours, or 16.7 to 33.3 mg/kg every 8 hours; for children 40 kg and over, see adult dose. (1.1 g of ticarcillin disodium is approximately equivalent to 1 g of base.)

sterile ticarcillin disodium and clavulanate potassium (Timentin)

Adults. For systemic and urinary tract infections: adults under 60 kg, intravenous infusion of 33.3 to 50 mg/kg (ticarcillin) every 4 hours or 50 to 75 mg/kg every 6 hours; adults over 60 kg, intravenous infusion, 3 g (ticarcillin) and 100 mg (clavulanic acid) every 4 to 6 hours.

For persons with impaired renal function, check current package insert for dosing instructions.

Children. Infants and children up to 12 years old, not established. Children 12 years and older, see adult dosage.

Combinations. Amoxicillin and ticarcillin have been combined with a beta-lactamase inhibitor, clavulanic acid, and marketed as Augmentin and Timentin, respectively. In recent years, the usefulness of ampicillin has been limited because of an increase in bacterial resistance resulting mainly from the enzymatic inactivation of ampicillin by bacteria beta-lactamases. In 1987, the third combination of a beta-lactam antibiotic and beta-lactamase inhibitor was released: ampicillin and sulbactam (Unasyn). The sulbactam binds with beta-lactamase-producing bacteria, thus preventing the inactivation of ampicillin.

The pharmacokinetics of ampicillin are not affected by the concurrent administration of sulbactam (see pharmacokinetics of ampicillin). The antibacterial in vitro activity of ampicillin has been extended to include bacterial strains that produce beta-lactamase, such as *Proteus, Klebsiella, E. coli, H. influenza, Staphylococcus aureus,* and many anaerobes. Therefore this combination may be effective in urinary tract, skin, intraabdominal, and gynecologic infections that usually have a mixture of aerobic and anaerobic organisms.

The side effects and adverse reactions are similar to those of ampicillin alone. Unasyn should be avoided in individuals with mononucleosis, since a high incidence of skin rash is reported with its usage. Several other concerns include the following:

1. The drug may produce a false-positive reaction for glucose with Clinitest; therefore diabetics should use Clinistix or Ketodiastix for monitoring when using this drug.
2. The sodium content of Unasyn is 5 mEq/1.5 g. At the maximum dosage of 12 g/day, over 900 mg of sodium will be administered. Clients with cardiac disease on sodium-restricted diets should be monitored.
3. Dosage is by the intravenous or intramuscular route. The usual dose is 1.5 g (1 g of ampicillin/0.5 g sulbactam) to 3 g (2 g ampicillin/1 g sulbactam) every 6 hours. In clients with impaired renal function, check package insert or current USP DI for dosing instructions.

NURSING CONSIDERATIONS

Assessment. Obtain cultures to assess sensitivity before administering the first dose of penicillin, but begin therapy before obtaining the results.

Intervention. In addition to performing nursing measures common to all types of antimicrobial drug therapy, as discussed in the previous chapter, the nurse must be especially cognizant of several factors when penicillins are prescribed.

In administering penicillins, the nurse should remember that oral penicillins are bound to food and that they are poorly absorbed in acid media. Their administration, therefore, should not be preceded or followed by food for at least 1 hour, to minimize binding. Penicillins should not be taken with acidic fruit juices, since juices may facilitate decomposition of penicillins.

In administering penicillins intravenously, the nurse should note that most penicillins in clinical use are sodium or potassium salts. Significant amounts of cation can be administered when these drugs are given intravenously in massive dosage. For example, 20 million units of potassium penicillin G contains 33 mEq of potassium ion. Fatalities have occurred because of the toxic effect of potassium on the heart following administration of such large doses in the presence of renal insufficiency. Carbenicillin contains 4.7 mEq of sodium per gram and may be administered in doses of 30 to 40 g daily. Signs and symptoms of hyperkalemia and hypernatremia should be duly noted and reported.

When administering penicillins intravenously, do so intermittently to prevent blood vessel irritation. The intravenous site should be changed at least every 48 hours.

Education. Instruct the client to take the full course of medication, even though feeling better and symptom free. Emphasize the importance of taking evenly spaced doses to maintain therapeutic blood levels. Prescriptions for antibiotics should never be shared with others or saved and taken for a different episode of illness.

Ampicillin, carbenicillin, cloxacillin, cyclacillin, dicloxacillin, naficillin, oxacillin, penicillin G, and the liquid form of bacampicillin should be taken when the stomach is empty. Amoxicillin, penicillin G, and the tablet form of bacampicillin, however, may be taken with food to decrease gastrointestinal distress.

Women taking ampicillin, bacampicillin, and penicillin V should be cautioned to use an alternate form of contraception if they are using estrogen-containing contraceptives.

Clients with diabetes mellitus using copper sulfate urine glucose tests (Clinitest) may have false-positive

---

PENICILLINS: FDA PREGNANCY SAFETY CATEGORIES

Category B	amdinocillin
	amoxicillin
	amoxicillin and clavulanate
	ampicillin
	azlocillin
	bacampicillin
	mezlocillin
	piperacillin
	ticarcillin and clavulanate
Not established	all others

EFFECT OF FOOD ON ORAL PENICILLIN ABSORPTION*

DRUG	FOOD EFFECT
amoxicillin	None
amoxicillin and clavulanate	None
ampicillin	Decreased slightly
bacampicillin	None
carbenicillin indanyl sodium	Increased
cloxacillin	Decreased
dicloxacillin	Decreased
nafcillin	Decreased
oxacillin	Decreased
penicillin G benzathine	Decreased very slightly
penicillin V potassium	Decreased very slightly

*Penicillins whose absorption decreases after food intake are generally acid labile; therefore, administer with a full glass of water on an empty stomach one hour before or 2 hours after meals.

results while taking amoxicillin, ampicillin, bacampicillin, and penicillin G. Have the client use glucose-enzymatic tests, such as Clinistix or Ketodiastix.

Instruct clients to report failure of their condition to improve in a few days or the development of rash, fever, or chills, which may indicate a delayed sensitivity reaction.

Evaluation. Because allergic reactions are a significant problem in the use of penicillins, the nurse must meticulously assess the patient's previous drug experiences with special attention to the development of prior drug-related rashes. For infants less than 3 months old, a history of penicillin allergy in the mother should be sought. If at all possible, no penicillin preparation of any kind should be prescribed for or administered to a patient with a history of allergic reaction to the drug. Because of possible cross-sensitization, it also seems wise to avoid the use of cephalosporins in patients with severe or immediate allergic reactions to penicillins.

Drug interactions with penicillins can increase or decrease the effectiveness of the penicillins and should be monitored. Gentamicin acts synergistically with penicillins against enterococci, as well against *Staphylococcus aureus,* when used with nafcillin or methicillin. Probenecid, by decreasing the rate of renal excretion of penicillins, increases and prolongs therapeutic blood levels. On the other hand, acidifying agents such as ammonium chloride, ascorbic acid, methenamine, methionine, and citrus juice destroy oral penicillins, making them less effective. Tetracyclines slow bacterial multiplication and thereby inhibit the penicillins that act against rapidly multiplying bacteria. Erythromycin inhibits the bacteriocidal activity of penicillins against most organisms.

Because of the possibility of bacterial and fungal superinfection (see page 898), elderly and debilitated clients should be observed carefully for unusual weight loss (pseudomembraneous colitis), abdominal cramps and diarrhea, darkened or discolored tongue, and sore mouth.

CEPHALOSPORINS

Cephalosporin antimicrobial agents are chemical modifications of the penicillin structure. These modifications created compounds with different microbiologic and pharmacologic activities. To classify the differences in antimicrobial activity, cephalosporins are divided into generations. At present, there are three generations of cephalosporins. Table 59-4 lists the cephalosporin generations and generic and trade names.

Cephalosporins also inhibit cell wall synthesis and are bactericidal. They are effective in numerous situations, but until the third-generation cephalosporins were marketed, the majority were not considered to be drugs of

TABLE 59-4   Cephalosporins

Parenterals	Oral preparations
FIRST GENERATION	
cefazolin (Ancef, Kefzol)	cephalexin (Ceporex✿, Keflex)
cephalothin (Keflin)	cephradine (Anspor, Velosef)
cephapirin (Cefadyl)	cefadroxil (Duricef, Ultra-cef)
SECOND GENERATION	
cefamandole (Mandol)	cefaclor (Ceclor)
cefonicid (Monocid)	
ceforanide (Precef)	
cefotetan (Cefotan)	
cefoxitin (Mefoxin)	
cefuroxime (Zinacef)	
THIRD GENERATION	
cefoperazone (Cefobid)	
cefotaxime (Claforan)	
ceftazidime (Fortaz, Tazicef)	
ceftizoxime (Cefizox)	
ceftriaxone (Rocephin)	
moxalactam (Moxam)	

choice for any serious infection. Initially their advantage over penicillins was their resistance to enzymatic degradation by the penicillinases (beta-lactamase). Now, however, drug resistance has been reported to drugs from all three generations, possibly through four mechanisms: (1) a microorganism lacking an outer cell membrane permeability; (2) bacteria lacking a receptor for the drug; (3) bacteria producing a beta-lactamase enzyme that can split the beta-lactam ring in the cephalosporins (many such enzymes have been isolated); or (4) development of a type of bacteria tolerance, that is, bacterial strains that are inhibited but not killed by the cephalosporins. The reason for this effect is the lack of, or deficiency in, autolytic enzymes in the bacterial cell wall (Katzung, 1987). Unfortunately, this class of drugs has been overused, and reports of bacterial resistance are increasing.

Physicians often prescribe cephalosporin antibiotics, even for clients allergic to penicillins. The possibility of a cross-reaction is approximately 5% to 10%; however, if the individual reports a serious reaction or anaphylaxis to penicillin, cephalosporins should not be used.

Mechanism of action. Inhibits cell wall synthesis, cell division, and growth. Rapidly dividing bacteria respond best to the cephalosporins.

Indications. Treatment of a variety of infections and as presurgery prophylactic agents. Used in combination with aminoglycosides and third-generation cephalosporins to treat synergistically *P. aeruginosa, S. marcescens,* and other susceptible organisms.

Pharmacokinetics. See Table 59-5.

Side effects/adverse reactions. See Table 59-6.

Significant drug interactions. When cephalosporins are given with the following drugs, the following interactions may occur.

Drug	Possible Effect and Management
alcohol	Not recommended with cefamandole, cefoperazone, cefotetan, or moxalactam. An increase in acetaldehyde in the blood may result, producing a disulfiram (Antabuse)-type reaction such as stomach pain, nausea, vomiting, headaches, low blood pressure, tachycardia, respiratory difficulties, increased sweating, or flushing of the face. Avoid drinking alcohol-containing beverages, medications containing alcohol, or using intravenous alcohol solutions during the administration of these drugs and for 3 days afterward.
anticoagulants, oral coumarin or indandione, heparin, or thrombolytic agents	Increased risk of bleeding and hemorrhage when given concurrently with cefamandole, cefoperazone, cefotetan or moxalactam. These cephalosporins interfere with vitamin K metabolism in the liver, resulting in hypoprothrombinemia. Also, moxalactam causes irreversible platelet damage. Dosage adjustments of the anticoagulants may be necessary during and after administration of these drugs. Avoid concurrent use of these drugs with thrombolytic agents because of the increased risk of serious bleeding and hemorrhage.
Nonsteroidal antiinflammatory drugs (NSAIDs), especially aspirin, platelet aggregation inhibitors, and sulfinpyrazone	When given with high doses of moxalactam or, less commonly, with cefamandole, cefoperazone, or cefotetan, an increased risk of hemorrhage exists because of the additive effect on platelet inhibition. Also, high dosages of salicylates and/or the specified antibiotics may induce hypoprothrombinemia, and the GI potential for ulcers or hemorrhage with NSAIDs, salicylates, or sulfinpyrazone may increase when used with the previous mentioned cephalosporins. Monitor closely.
probenecid	Probenecid decreases renal tubular secretion of the cephalosporins that are excreted by this mechanism, which can result in increased serum levels, extended half-life, and increased potential for toxicity. Probenecid does not affect the secretion of ceforanide, ceftazidime, or ceftriaxone. Cephalosporins and probenecid are also used concurrently to treat specific infections such as sexually transmitted diseases, in which a high serum level and prolonged effect is desirable.

Dosage and administration

cefaclor capsules/oral suspension (Ceclor)

Adults. 250 to 500 mg orally (anhydrous base) every 8 hours. Maximum daily dose is up to 4 g daily.

Children. Not recommended in infants under 1 month old. Infants 1 month and over, 6.7 to 13.4 mg/kg (anhydrous base) orally every 8 hours. Although doses up to 60 mg/kg have been used, it is recommended that the maximum daily dose not exceed 2 g.

cefadroxil capsules/oral suspension/tablets (Duricef, Ultracef)

Adults

For tonsillitis and beta-hemolytic streptococcal pharyngitis, administer 500 mg (anhydrous base) every 12 hours for 10 days.

For skin and soft tissue infections, 500 mg (anhydrous base) orally every 12 hours or 1 g once a day.

For urinary tract infections, 500 mg to 1 g (anhydrous base) every 12 hours or 1 to 2 g once daily.

In persons with impaired renal function, check a current package insert for dosage recommendations.

Maximum daily dose is 6 gs (anhydrous base) daily.

Children. 15 mg (anhydrous base)/kg orally every 12 hours.

cefamandole nafate for injection (Mandol)

Adults

Pneumonia, uncomplicated, and soft tissue infections, 500 mg (base) intramuscularly or intravenously every 6 hours.

For urinary tract infections, 500 mg to 1 g intramuscularly or intravenously every 8 hours.

For other infections, 500 mg to 2 g (base) intramuscularly or intravenously every 4 to 6 hours.

For preoperative prophylaxis, 1 to 2 g (base) intramuscularly or intravenously, ½ to 1 hour before surgery; 1 to 2 g every 6 hours after surgery for up to 24 hours.

For persons with impaired renal function, check a current package insert for dosing recommendations.

Maximum adult daily dose is up to 12 g (base) daily. (Dosages of up to 16 g/day have been used.)

Children. Premature infants and infants up to 1 month old, not recommended. Infants 1 month and older, 8.3 to 16.7 mg/kg (base) intramuscularly or intravenously every 4 hours; 12.5 to 25 mg/kg every 6 hours; or 16.7 to 33.3 mg/kg every 8 hours. For preoperative prophylaxis children 3 months and older, 12.5 to 25 mg/kg (base) intramuscularly or intravenously, ½ to 1 hour before surgery and 12.5 to 25 mg/kg every 6 hours after surgery. Maximum daily dose is 150 mg/kg (base) or the maximum daily adult dose. Do not exceed these dosages.

cefazolin sodium injection (Ancef)

Adults. 250 mg to 1 g (base) by intravenous infusion every 6 to 8 hours.

For preoperative prophylaxis, 1 g (base) by intravenous infusion ½ to 1 hour before surgery; 500 mg to 1 g during surgery, and 500 mg to 1 g every 6 to 8 hours after surgery for up to 24 hours.

For pneumococcal pneumonia, 500 mg (base) by intravenous infusion every 12 hours.

For urinary tract infections, acute (uncomplicated) 1 g (base) by intravenous infusion every 12 hours.

For persons with impaired renal function, see current package insert for dosing recommendations.

TABLE 59-5 Pharmacokinetics of the Cephalosporins

Drug	Absorption	Half-life (hr)	Time to peak level (hr)	Peak serum level μg/ml	Peak serum level Dose	Peak urine level μg/ml	Peak urine level Dose	Liver and kidney metabolism of the drug	Kidney excretion* (%/hr)
cefaclor		0.6-0.9	0.5-1					No	60-85/8
PO	Very good			7	250 mg	600	250 mg		
				13	500 mg	900	500 mg		
cefadroxil		1.2-1.5	1.5-2					No	70/6, 93/24
PO	Very good			16	500 mg	1800	500 mg		
				28	1 g				
cefamandole		0.5-1.2						No	65-85/8
IM			1-2	17	250 mg	2400	500 mg		
			0.1	38	500 mg	4000	1 g		
				64	1 g				
IV				188	1 g				
cefazolin		1.4-1.8						No	60-90/6
IM			1-2	17	250 mg	2400	500 mg		
				38	500 mg	4000	1 g		
				64	1 g				
IV			0.1	188	1 g				
cefonicid		4.5						No	99/24
IM			1	99	1 g	385	500 mg		
IV			0.1	220	1 g				
cefoperazone								No	15-30/6
PO	Fair-poor	1.6-2.6							
IM			1 (1 g)	65	1 g	1000	2 g		
			2-3 (2 g)	95	2 g				
IV			At end of infusion	155	1 g				
				250	2 g				
				340	3 g				
				510	4 g				
ceforanide		2.9						No	80-95/12
IM			1	40	500 mg	1250	500 mg		
				75	1 g	2900	1 g		
IV				125	1 g	2550	1 g		
				240	2 g	5130	2 g		
cefotaxime		1						Yes (50%)	20-36/6
IM			0.5	21	1 g				
IV				102	1 g				
				214	2 g				
cefotetan		3-4.6						—	50-80/24
IM			1 (1 g)	71	1 g				
			2-3 (2 g)	91	2 g				
IV			0.5	158	1 g	1700	1 g		
				237	2 g	3500	2 g		
cefoxitin		0.7-1.1						Slight	85/6
IM			0.3-0.5	24	1 g	>3000	1 g		
IV			0.1	110	1 g				
ceftazidime								No	80-90/24
IM		2	1	17	500 mg				
				40	1 g				
IV		1.9	0.5	42	500 mg				
				70	1 g				
				170	2 g				
ceftizoxine		1.7						No	—
IM			1	14	500 mg				
				39	1 g				

*The percent excreted unchanged/hours.

TABLE 59-5   Pharmacokinetics of the Cephalosporins—cont'd

Drug	Absorption	Half-life (hr)	Time to peak level (hr)	Peak serum level μg/ml	Peak serum level Dose	Peak urine level μg/ml	Peak urine level Dose	Liver and kidney metabolism of the drug	Kidney excretion (%/hr)
			0.1	60	1 g	>6000			
				132	2 g	1 g			
				220	3 g				
ceftriaxone								Yes	33-67/?
IM		5.8-8.7	2	43	500 mg	425	500 mg		
IM				75	1 g	630	1 g		
IV		4.3-4.6	0.5	80	500 mg	525	500 mg		
				150	1 g	995	1 g		
				260	2 g	2690	2 g		
cefuroxime		1-3						—	90/8
IM			0.75	27	750	1300	750 mg		
IV			0.25	50	750 mg	1150	750 mg		
				100	1.5 g	2500	1.5 g		
cephalexin								No	80/6, 90/8
PO		0.9-1.2	1	9	250 mg	1000	250 mg		
				18	500 mg	2200	500 mg		
				32	1 g	5000	1 g		
cephalothin		0.5-1						Yes (33%)	60-70/6
IM			0.5	10	500 mg	800	500 mg		
				20	1 g	2500	1 g		
IV			0.25-0.5	30	1 g				
				80-100	2 g				
cephapirin		0.5-0.6						Yes (40%)	50-70/6
IM			0.5-1	9	500 mg	900	500 mg		
IM				16	1 g				
IV			0.1	35	500 mg				
				67	1 g				
cephradine		0.8-1.3						No	60-90/6
PO	Very good		1	9	250	1600	250 mg		
				17	500	3200	500 mg		
				24	1 g	4000	1 g		
IM			0.8-2	6	500 mg				
				14	1 g				
IV			0.1	86	1 g				
moxalactam								No	55-65/24
IM		2.1-2.3	1-2	10	250 mg				
				15	500 mg				
				25	1 g				
IV		1.7-3.5	At end of infusion	50	500 mg	170	250 mg		
				100	1 g	445	500 mg		
				200	2 g	1800	1 g		
				260	3 g	4200	2 g		
				440	4 g				

Maximum adult daily dose is up to 12 g (base)/day.

Children. Premature infants and infants under 1 month old, not recommended; infants and children 1 month and older, 6.25 to 25 mg/kg (base) by intravenous infusion every 6 hours or 8.3 to 33.3 mg/kg every 8 hours.

sterile cefazolin sodium (Ancef, Kefzol)

Adults. 250 mg to 1 g (base) intramuscularly or intravenously every 6 to 8 hours.

For preoperative prophylaxis, 1 g (base) intramuscularly or intravenously ½ to 1 hour before surgery; 500 mg to 1 g during surgery; and 500 mg to 1 g every 6 to 8 hours after surgery for up to 24 hours.

For urinary tract infections, acute (uncomplicated), 1 g (base) intramuscularly or intravenously every 12 hours.

For persons with impaired renal function, check the

TABLE 59-6   Cephalosporins: Side Effects and Adverse Reactions

Side effects*	Adverse reactions†
Most frequent: the following can be less frequent with some of the cephalosporins: diarrhea, mild (less with cefoxitin); abdominal cramps or distress (rare with cefoxitin); mouth soreness, tongue soreness (due to fungal overgrowth); rash, pruritis, redness, or edema (hypersensitivity reaction) Less frequent: pruritis in rectal or genital area	All cephalosporins: Rare: stomach pain, gas, distress, severe, watery diarrhea, bloody diarrhea, elevated temperature, thirst, nausea or vomiting, increased weakness, weight loss (pseudomembranous colitis) For cefamandole, cefoperazone, cefotetan, and moxalactam only: Rare: increased bleeding episodes, increased bruising (hypothrombinemia) For moxalactam only: Rare: if given in high doses to patients with renal impairment: convulsions.

*If side effects continue, increase, or disturb the client, inform the physician.
†If adverse reactions occur, contact physician because medical intervention may be necessary.

most current package insert for dosing recommendations.

Maximum daily dose is 12 gs (base)/day.

Children. Premature infants and infants up to 1 month old, not recommended; infants and children 1 month and older, 6.25 to 25 mg/kg (base) intramuscularly or intravenously every 6 hours or 8.3 to 33.3 mg/kg every 8 hours.

sterile cefonicid sodium (Monocid)

Adults. 500 mg to 2 g (base) intramuscularly or intravenously every 24 hours.

For preoperative prophylaxis:

Clients with cesarean-section surgery, 1 g (base) intravenously when umbilical cord is clamped.

Preoperative prophylaxis for other surgical patients, 1 g (base) intravenously 1 hour before surgery.

For persons with impaired renal function, check the current package insert for dosing recommendations.

Children. Not established.

cefoperazone sodium injection (Cefobid)

Adults. Intravenous infusion:

In mild to moderate infections, 1 to 2 g (base) every 12 hours.

Severe infections, 1.5 to 3 g (base) every 6 hours, 2 to 4 g every 8 hours, or 3 to 6 g every 12 hours.

Persons with impaired liver function and/or biliary obstruction should not receive more than 4 g/day without serum levels being drawn.

Persons with both liver and kidney function impairment should not receive more than 1 to 2 g/day without serum levels being drawn.

Maximum daily dose is 12 g daily. (Doses up to 16 g/day given by continuous intravenous infusion in severely immunocompromised persons have been reported without adverse effects.)

Children. Not established.

sterile cefoperazone sodium (Cefobid, Cefobine)

Adults. Intramuscular or intravenous infusion:

For mild to moderate infections, 1 to 3 g every 12 hours.

For severe infections, same dose as cefoperazone sodium injection.

For persons with impaired liver function and/or biliary obstruction or combined liver and kidney function impairment, same dose as cefoperazone sodium injection.

Maximum daily dose, same as cefoperazone sodium injection.

Children. Not established.

ceforanide for injection (Precef)

Adults. 500 mg to 1 g intramuscularly or intravenously every 12 hours.

For preoperative prophylaxis, intramuscularly or intravenously, 500 mg to 1 g 1 hour before surgery.

For persons with impaired renal function, check current package insert for dosing recommendations.

Children. Infants and children up to 1 year old not established; children 1 year and older, intramuscularly or intravenously, 10 to 20 mg/kg every 12 hours.

cefotaxime sodium injection (Claforan)

Adults. Intravenous infusion, 1 to 2 g every 4 to 8 hours.

For preoperative prophylaxis:

Clients with cesarean section surgery, intravenous infusion, 1 g when umbilical cord is clamped and 1 g 6 to 12 hours after the initial dose.

Preoperative prophylaxis for other surgical patients, intravenous infusion, 1 g, ½ to 1½ hours before surgery.

Infections (uncomplicated), intravenous infusion, 1 g every 12 hours.

For adults with impaired renal function, (creatinine clearance < 20 ml/min/1.73 m^2), give one-half the usual adult dose.

Maximum daily dose is 12 g daily.

Children. Neonates up to 7 days old, intravenous infusion, 50 mg/kg every 12 hours; neonates 1 to 4 weeks old intravenous infusion, 50 mg/kg every 8 hours; infants and children up to 50 kg; intravenous infusion, 8.3 to 30 mg/kg every 4 hours or 12.5 to 45 mg/kg every 6 hours; children over 50 kg, see usual adult dose. Maximum daily dose in infants and children should not be more than 12 g.

sterile cefotaxime sodium (Claforan)

Adults. Intramuscularly or intravenously, 1 to 2 g every 4 to 8 hours.

For gonorrhea, 1 g intramuscularly, as a single dose.

Preoperative prophylaxis for clients with cesarean section surgery, 1 g intravenously when umbilical cord is clamped and 1 g intramuscularly or intravenously 6 and 12 hours after initial dose.

Preoperative prophylaxis for other surgical patients, 1 g intramuscularly or intravenously, 0.5 to 1.5 hours before surgery.

Infections, uncomplicated, 1 g intramuscularly or intravenously every 12 hours.

Adults with impaired renal function, same as cefotaxime sodium injection.

Children. Same as cefotaxime sodium injection.

sterile cefotenan disodium (Cefotan)

Adults

For mild to moderate infections, 1 to 2 g intramuscularly or intravenously every 12 hours for 5 to 10 days.

For severe infections, 2 g intravenously every 12 hours.

For life-threatening infections, 3 g intravenously every 12 hours.

For preoperative prophylaxis:

Clients with cesarean section, 1 to 2 g intravenously when umbilical cord is clamped.

Preoperative prophylaxis for other patients, 1 to 2 g intravenously 0.5 to 1 hour before surgery.

Urinary tract infections, 500 mg to 2 g intramuscularly or intravenously every 12 hours, or 1 to 2 g every 24 hours.

Persons with impaired renal function, check current package insert for dosing recommendations.

Maximum daily dose is 6 g/day.

Children. Not established.

cefoxitin sodium injection (Mefoxin)

Adults. Intravenously, 1 to 2 g every 4 to 8 hours.

Preoperative prophylaxis:

Client with cesarean section, 2 g intravenously when umbilical cord is clamped; 2 g 4 and 8 hours after initial dose and 2 g every 6 hours for up to 24 hours.

Clients with transurethral prostatectomy surgery, 1 g intravenously immediately following surgery and 1 g every 8 hours up to 24 hours.

Other surgical clients, 2 g intravenously 0.5 to 1 hour before surgery and 2 g every 6 hours after surgery for up to 24 hours.

For persons with renal function impairment, check a current package insert for dosing recommendations.

Maximum daily dose is up to 12 g/day.

Children. Infants and children up to 3 months old, not recommended; infants and children 3 months and older, 13.3 to 26.7 mg/kg intravenously every 4 hours or 20 to 40 mg/kg every 6 hours.

For preoperative prophylaxis, infants and children 3 months and older, intravenously, 30 to 40 mg/kg 0.5 to 1 hour before surgery and 30 to 40 mg/kg every 6 hours after surgery for up to 24 hours. Total daily dose in infants and children is up to 12 g.

sterile cefoxitin sodium (Mefoxin)

Adults. Intravenously, 1 to 2 g every 4 to 8 hours.

For gonorrhea (uncomplicated), 2 g intramuscularly, and 1 g of probenecid orally, given 30 minutes before or with cefoxitin.

Preoperative prophylaxis for clients with cesarean section, same as cefoxitin sodium injection.

For clients with transurethral prostatectomy, same as cefoxitin sodium injection.

For other surgical patients, intramuscularly or intravenously, same dosage as cefoxitin sodium injection.

For impaired renal function, same as cefoxitin sodium injection.

Children. Infants and children up to 3 months old, not recommended; infants and children 3 months and older, intramuscularly or intravenously, same dosage as cefoxitin sodium injection.

For preoperative prophylaxis, infants and children 3 months and older, intramuscularly or intravenously, same dosage as cefoxitin sodium injection.

ceftazidime injection (Fortaz)

Adults. Intravenous infusion, 1-2 g every 8-12 hours.

For urinary tract infections, uncomplicated, intravenous infusion 250 mg every 12 hours.

For urinary tract infections, complicated, intravenous infusion, 500 mg every 8 to 12 hours.

For persons with renal impairment, check current package insert for dosing recommendations.

Children. Neonates up to 4 weeks old, intravenous infusion, 30 mg/kg every 12 hours. Infants and children 1 month to 12 years old, intravenous infusion, 30 to 50 mg/kg every 8 hours. Maximum daily dose in infants and children is up to 6 g/day.

ceftazidime for injection (Fortaz, Magnacef✣, Tazicef, Tazidime)

Adults. 1 to 2 g intramuscularly or intravenously every 8 to 12 hours. For urinary tract infections, complicated and uncomplicated, intramuscularly or intravenously, same dose as ceftazidime injection.

Children. Same as ceftazidime injection.

ceftizoxime sodium injection (Cefizox)

Adults. 1 to 4 g intravenously every 8 to 12 hours.

For urinary tract infections, uncomplicated, 500 mg intravenously every 12 hours.

For persons with impaired renal function, see current package insert for dosing recommendations.

Children. Infants and children up to 6 months old, not established; children 6 months and over, 50 mg/kg intravenously every 6 to 8 hours. The maximum daily dose in children should not exceed 200 mg/kg or the maximum total daily adult dose.

sterile ceftizoxime sodium (Cefizox)

Adults. 1 to 4 g intramuscularly or intravenously every 8 to 12 hours.

For gonorrhea, uncomplicated, 1 g intramuscularly as a single dose.

For urinary tract infections, uncomplicated, 500 mg intramuscularly or intravenously every 12 hours.

For persons with impaired renal function, check current package insert for dosing recommendations.

Children. Infants and children up to 6 months old, not established; children 6 months and over, 50 mg/kg intramuscularly or intravenously every 6 to 8 hours. Maximum total daily dose is the same as for ceftizoxime sodium injection.

sterile ceftriaxone sodium (Rocephin)

Adults. 1 to 2 g intramuscularly or intravenously every 24 hours or 500 mg to 1 g every 12 hours.

For gonococcal infections, uncomplicated, 250 mg intramuscularly as single dose.

For preoperative prophylaxis, 1 g intravenously 0.5 to 2 hours before surgery.

Maximum daily dose is 4 g/day.

Children. 25 to 37.5 mg/kg intramuscularly or intravenously every 12 hours.

For meningitis, 50 mg/kg intravenously every 12 hours. Therapy can be started with or without a loading dose of 75 mg/kg.

Maximum daily dose is 4 g for meningitis or 2 g for other infections.

cefuroxime sodium injection (Zinacef)

Adults. 750 mg to 1.5 g intravenously every 6 to 8 hours.

For meningitis, bacterial, up to 3 g intravenously every 8 hours.

Preoperative prophylaxis:

For clients with open-heart surgical procedures, 1.5 g intravenously at start of anesthesia and every 12 hours for up to 24 hours.

For other surgical clients, 1.5 g intravenously 0.5 to 1 hour before surgery and 750 mg intravenously every 8 hours, if surgery is prolonged, for up to 24 hours.

For persons with impaired renal function, check current package insert for dosing recommendations.

Children. Infants and children up to 3 months old, 10 to 33.3 mg/kg intravenously every 8 hours or 15 to 50 mg/kg every 12 hours; infants and children 3 months and over, 12.5 to 25 mg/kg intravenously every 6 hours or 16.7 to 33.3 mg/kg every 8 hours.

For bone infections, 50 mg/kg intravenously every 8 hours.

For meningitis, bacterial, 50 to 60 mg/kg intravenously every 6 hours or 66.7 to 80 mg/kg every 8 hours.

sterile cefuroxime sodium (Kefurox, Zinacef)

Adults. 750 to 1.5 g intramuscularly or intravenously every 6 to 8 hours.

For gonococcal infections, uncomplicated, 1.5 g intramuscularly divided into two separate injection sites, and 1 g probenecid orally, given concurrently as a single dose.

For meningitis, bacterial, same as for cefuroxime sodium injection.

For clients with open heart surgical procedures, same as cefuroxime sodium injection.

For other surgery patients, same as cefuroxime sodium injection.

Children. Infants and children up to 3 months old, 10 to 33.3 mg/kg intramuscularly or intravenously every 8 hours or 15 to 50 mg/kg every 12 hours. Infants and children 3 months and older, 12.5 to 25 mg/kg intramuscularly or intravenously every 6 hours or 16.7 to 33.3 mg/kg every 8 hours.

For bone infections, same as for cefuroxime sodium injection.

For meningitis, bacterial, same as for cefuroxime sodium injection.

cephalexin capsules/oral suspension (Ceporex❀, Keflex, Novolexin❀)

Adults. 250 to 500 mg orally every 6 hours.

For cystitis, uncomplicated, skin and soft tissue infections, and streptococcal pharyngitis: 500 mg orally every 12 hours.

Maximum daily dose is 4 g or more per day.

Children. 6.25 to 25 mg/kg orally every 6 hours.

For otitis media, 18.75 to 25 mg/kg orally every 6 hours.

For skin and soft tissue infections and streptococcal pharyngitis, 12.5 to 50 mg/kg orally every 12 hours.

cephalothin sodium injection

Adults. Intravenous infusion, 1 to 2 g every 4 to 6 hours.

For preoperative prophylaxis, intravenous infusion, 1 to 2 g 0.5 to 1 hour before surgery; 1 to 2 g during surgery; and 1 to 2 g every 6 hours after surgery for up to 24 hours.

For pneumonia, uncomplicated, furunculosis (with cellulitis) and urinary tract infections, intravenous infusion, 500 mg every 6 hours.

For persons with impaired renal function, check current package insert for dosing recommendations.

Maximum daily dose is 12 g/day.

Children. Intravenous infusion, 13.3 to 26.6 mg/kg every 4 hours or 20 to 40 mg/kg every 6 hours. For preoperative prophylaxis, intravenous infusion, 20 to 30 mg/kg 0.5 to 1 hour before surgery; 20 to 30 mg/kg during surgery; and 20 to 30 mg/kg every 6 hours after surgery for up to 24 hours.

NURSING CONSIDERATIONS

Assessment. Determine whether the client is hypersensitive to other cephalosporins. In some clients the use of cephalosporins is contraindicated. If the client has a history of sensitivity to penicillin, cephalosporins should be used with caution, since cross-sensitivity is possible.

Cultures for sensitivity of the organism should be obtained before the first dose of cephalosporin is administered; however, therapy should begin before the results are obtained.

Intervention. In addition to performing nursing measures common to all types of antimicrobial drug therapy as discussed in the previous chapter, the nurse must be aware of other factors when cephalosporins are prescribed.

Intramuscular cephalosporins, because they are irritating to tissues and can cause pain, induration, and sterile abscesses following injection, should be given deeply into a large muscle mass.

Education. Instruct client to take the full course of medication, even though feeling better and symptom free. Stress the importance of taking evenly spaced doses to maintain therapeutic blood levels.

Cephalosporins may be taken with food if gastric irritation develops.

Clients with diabetes mellitus who are using copper sulfate urine glucose tests (Clinitest) may have false-positive results while taking cephalosporins. Have the client use glucose-enzymatic tests such as Clinistix or Ketodiastix.

The client should be cautioned not to drink alcoholic beverages or to take alcohol-containing medications because abdominal cramps, nausea, and vomiting; hypotension, tachycardia, and shortness of breath; and sweating and facial flushing may occur.

Instruct clients to read labels, because many cough remedies contain alcohol.

Evaluation. Because of the possibility of superinfection, observe clients, particularly the elderly and debilitated, for symptoms of bacterial and fungal overgrowth.

Precautions with cephalosporins should include monitoring those drugs that increase the effects of cephalosporins (loop diuretics, gentamicin, and probenecid) and those that decrease the effects (tetracyclines). Loop diuretics and aminoglycosides can lead to acute renal failure, which subsequently impairs renal excretion of the cephalosporins. Proberecid decreases renal excretion of the cephalosporins and thereby increases blood levels. Tetracyclines slow the rate of bacterial reproduction and thus, when given concurrently with the cephalosporins, which act against rapidly multiplying bacteria, inhibit the effectiveness of the cephalosporins.

For clients taking cefamandole, cefoperazone, and moxalactam, bleeding time and prothombin time should be monitored, as hypoprothrombinemia has occurred with these drugs.

CEPHALOSPORINS: FDA PREGNANCY SAFETY CATEGORIES

Category B	cefadroxil
	cefamandole
	cefazolin
	cefonicid
	ceforanide
	cefotaxime
	cefotetan
	ceftazidime
	ceftizoxime
	ceftriaxone
	cefuroxime
	cephalexin
	cephalothin
	cephapirin
	cephradine
Category C	moxalactam
Not established	all others

MACROLIDE ANTIBIOTICS

The macrolide antibiotics constitute a large group of substances that were introduced in the early 1950s. They are bacteriostatic, since they inhibit protein synthesis, but in high concentrations with selected organisms, they may also be bactericidal.

The most important macrolide antimicrobial agent is erythromycin. Troleandomycin (TAO) is a macrolide antibiotic similar to erythromycin. Troleandomycin has limited usefulness in clinical practice; therefore only erythromycin is reviewed in this section.

erythromycin delayed-release capsules (Eryc, Eryc Sprinkle✿)

erythromycin tablets (Erythromic✿, Novorythro✿)

erythromycin delayed-release tablets (E-Mycin, Ery-Tab, Ilotycin, and others)

erythromycin estolate capsules/oral suspension (Ilosone, Novorythro✿)

erythromycin estolate tablets and chewable tablets (Ilosone)

erythromycin ethylsuccinate oral suspension (E.E.S., E-Mycin E, Pediamycin)

erythromycin ethylsuccinate tablets and chewable tablets (E.E.S.)

erythromycin stearate tablets (Apo-Erythro-S✿; Erypar, Novorythro✿)

sterile erythromycin gluceptate (Ilotycin)

erythromycin lactobionate for injection (Erythrocin)

Mechanism of action. Inhibits protein synthesis by penetrating the bacterial cell membrane and binding ribosomes of susceptible bacteria.

Indications

Treatment of susceptible bacterial infections such as chlamydial conjunctivitis, genitourinary tract and systemic infections caused by *Chlamydia trachomatis, Corynebacterium diphtheriae, Neisseria gonorrhoeae,* Legionnaires' disease, *Listeria monocytogenes, Haemophilus influenzae, Bordetella pertussis, Streptococcus epidemicus, Staphylococcus aureus,* and others.

Prevention of bacterial endocarditis in individuals who are allergic to penicillin.

Pharmacokinetics. Oral preparations.

Absorption. On empty stomach, very good. When taken with food, absorption of the base tablets and stearate form decreases.

Distribution. To most fluids in the body, except cerebrospinal fluid. Highest levels are noted in the liver, bile, and spleen, with sufficient concentrations in the pleural and ascitic fluids.

Protein binding. High to very high.

Metabolism. Partial, in the liver. Erythromycin ethylsuccinate is hydrolyzed to free drug in the gastrointestinal tract and the blood. Erythromycin stearate is reduced to free drug in the gastrointestinal tract. Erythromycin estolate is reduced to propanoate ester in the gastrointestinal tract, absorbed, and then hydrolyzed to free drug in the blood.

Half-life. Between 1.4 and 2 hours. Renal function impairment may extend the half-life to 4.8 to 6 hours.

Time to peak level. 1 to 4 hours.

Excretion. Via the liver and bile primarily.

Side effects/adverse reactions. See Table 59-7.

Significant drug interactions. When erythromycin is given with the following drugs, the following interactions may occur.

Drug	Possible Effect and Management
alfentanil (Alfenta)	May increase plasma levels and action of alfentanil. Monitor closely if given in combination.
carbamazepine (Tegretol)	Carbamazepine metabolism may be inhibited, leading to elevated serum levels and, possibly, toxicity. This is reported more often with troleandomycin than erythromycin, but similar precautions and monitoring are indicated for both drugs.
chloramphenicol or lincomycins	May antagonize the therapeutic effects of chloramphenicol and lincomycin. Avoid concurrent administration.
hepatotoxic medications	Increased possibility for liver toxicity; monitor closely if given concurrently.
warfarin (coumarin, coumadin)	May result in decreased warfarin metabolism and excretion leading to an increased risk of bleeding or hemorrhage. Dosage adjustments of coumarin may be necessary during and after treatment with erythromycin. Monitor prothrombin times closely.
xanthines, such as aminophylline, caffeine, oxtriphylline, and theophylline (exception dyphylline)	An increase in theophylline levels and/or toxicity is reported with this combination of drugs. This effect is usually seen at approximately the sixth day of erythromycin therapy, as it appears to be related to the peak erythromycin serum level. Monitor closely, as dosage adjustments of the xanthines may be necessary during and after erythromycin therapy.

Dosage and administration

erythromycin tablets, delayed-release capsules/tablets

Adults

For systemic bacterial infections, 250 mg orally every 6 hours or 333 mg every 8 hours.

For disseminated gonorrhea, 500 mg orally every 6 hours for 1 week.

For Legionnaires' disease, 500 mg to 1 g orally every 6 hours.

To prevent streptococcal infections in individuals with a history of rheumatic heart disease, 250 mg orally twice daily (every 12 hours).

Maximum is 4 g (or more, in some circumstances) orally, daily.

Children. For systemic infections, 7.5 to 25 mg/kg orally every 6 hours or 15 to 50 mg/kg every 12 hours.

erythromycin estolate tablets/capsules/oral suspension/chewable. See preceding section.

TABLE 59-7 Antibiotics: Side Effects and Adverse Reactions

Drug(s)	Side effects*	Adverse reactions†
erythromycin	Less frequent: diarrhea, nausea or vomiting, soreness of tongue and mouth, abdominal distress	Rare (except for erythromycin estolate—more frequent): yellow eyes or skin, severe abdominal pain, increased weakness, pale stools, or dark, orange urine (due to cholestatic jaundice); if clients have renal impairment and receive high drug doses, hearing loss may occur but is usually reversible
lincomycins (clindamycin and lincomycin)	Most frequent: mild diarrhea, skin rash Less frequent: pruritus of skin, rectum, or genital areas (due to fungal infection)	Most frequent: severe abdominal cramps, pain or gas; severe watery and perhaps bloody diarrhea; increased temperature; thirst; weight loss, increased weakness (from pseudomembranous colitis) The above symptoms may occur after drug is discontinued.
vancomycin	Oral dosage form, most frequent: nausea, vomiting or taste alterations Parenteral: none	Parenteral: Less frequent: hearing loss, ringing or buzzing in ears (ototoxicity), respiratory difficulties, hematuria, sedation, increased frequency of urination, thirst, anorexia, nausea, vomiting, weakness (nephrotoxicity) Rare (usually with bolus or rapid injection of drug): "red-neck syndrome"—chills; fever; tachycardia; pruritus; nausea; vomiting; rash or red face; rash of neck, upper body, back, and arms; paresthesia (due to histamine release) Ototoxicity and nephrotoxicity may occur after the medication is stopped. Medical attention is necessary.
aminoglycosides (amikacin, gentamicin, kanamycin, neomycin, netilmicin, streptomycin, tobramycin)		Most frequent: hearing loss, ringing or buzzing in ears (ototoxicity); bloody urine, thirst, anorexia, increased or decreased urination (nephrotoxicity); ataxia, dizziness (ototoxicity, vestibular); nausea, vomiting, paresthesias (usually only from streptomycin); numbness, tingling, muscle twitching, convulsions (neurotoxicity) Less frequent: visual loss, skin rash, pruritus, edema (hypersensitivity with gentamicin or steptomycin, less often with others) Rare: respiratory difficulties, weakness, sedation (neuromuscular blocking effects, nephrotoxicity) If signs and symptoms of ototoxicity or nephrotoxicity occur after drug is discontinued, contact physician. Also, after local irrigation or topical application of aminoglycosides during surgery, neuromuscular blockade, respiratory paralysis, ototoxicity and nephrotoxicity have been reported.

*If side effects continue, increase, or disturb the patient, inform the physician.
†If adverse reactions occur, contact physician, as medical intervention may be necessary.

Continued.

TABLE 59-7   Antibiotics: Side Effects and Adverse Reactions—cont'd

Drug(s)	Side effects*	Adverse reactions†
tetracyclines	Most frequent: stomach cramps, diarrhea, pruritus of rectum or genitals, sore mouth or tongue (fungal overgrowth), nausea, vomiting Photosensitivity to sunlight reported with all tetracyclines except minocycline (rare) Ataxia, dizziness or CNS toxicity reported with minocycline only	With aminoglycosides given concurrently by parenteral and intrathecal routes, leg cramps, skin rash, elevated temperature, and convulsions have been reported. Most frequent: discoloration of teeth in infants and children Low frequency: demeclocycline may increase thirst, frequency of urination, or weakness (nephrogenic diabetes insipidus); minocycline may cause skin and mucous membrane discoloration (pigmentation)
chloramphenicol (Chloromycetin, Mychel, Novochlorocap✦)	Less frequent: diarrhea, nausea, or vomiting	Less frequent: pale skin, elevated temperature, sore throat, increase in bleeding episodes or bruises, increased weakness (blood dyscrasias) Rare: gas, bloated stomach, sedation, gray skin, hypothermia, respiratory difficulties (Gary syndrome) Visual disturbances or loss (optic neuritis); numbness, burning sensation, tingling or weakness in hands or feet (peripheral neuritis) Bone marrow depression can occur during or after the drug is discontinued; if sore throat, fever, unusual bleeding episodes, or tiredness occur, contact a physician immediately
quinolones (ciprofloxacin, norfloxacin)	Most frequent: nausea, diarrhea, vomiting, headache, skin rash, stomach upset, restlessness	Rare: nephritis, increased urination, urinary retention, impaired renal function, seizures, depersonalization, cardiac toxicity (atrial flutter, ventricular ectopy, angina pectoris, syncope); most of these effects occur with ciprofloxacin.
metronidazole (flagyl, flagyl I.V., Neo-Metric✦)	Most frequent: diarrhea, dizziness, headache, anorexia, nausea, vomiting, abdominal pain, or cramping Less frequent/rare: constipation, taste alterations, dry mouth, metallic taste in mouth, increased weakness Dark urine reported—no need for medical intervention.	Most frequent: hand or feet pain, tingling, weakness or numbness (peripheral neuropathy) Less frequent: vaginal discharge or irritation (treatment failure or fungus infection); rash, hives, pruritus, sore throat, elevated temperature. CNS effects—ataxia, mood changes, convulsions (with high doses)

erythromycin ethylsuccinate tablets/oral suspension

Adults

For systemic infections, 400 mg orally every 6 hours.

For disseminated gonorrhea, 800 mg orally every 6 hours for 1 week.

For Legionnaires' disease, 400 mg to 1 g orally every 6 hours.

To prevent streptococcal infections in individuals with a history of rheumatic heart disease, 400 mg orally, twice daily (every 12 hours).

Maximum daily dose is 4 g, although dosages up to 8 g/day have been well tolerated.

Children. For systemic infections, 7.5 to 25 mg/kg orally every 6 hours or 15 to 50 mg/kg every 12 hours.

Note: 1.17 g of erythromycin ethylsuccinate is approximately equivalent to 1 g of erythromycin. The recommended dose is 60% greater than the dose suggested for erythromycin base.

erythromycin stearate. See erythromycin.

erythromycin gluceptate parenteral
erythromycin lactobionate for injection

Adults. For systemic infection, 250 to 500 mg by intravenous infusion every 6 hours or 3.75 to 5 mg/kg every 6 hours. Maximum daily dose is 4 g.

Children. For systemic infections, 3.75 to 5 mg/kg by intravenous infusion every 6 hours.

Note: 1.3 g of erythromycin gluceptate or 1.5 g of erythromycin lactobionate is approximately equivalent to 1 g of erythromycin.

NURSING CONSIDERATIONS

Assessment. If the client has hepatic impairment, use erythromycin with caution. Periodic hepatic function studies may be required for those clients receiving high-dose or prolonged intravenous erythromycin gluceptate therapy. Observe clients for symptoms of hepatic dysfunction.

Intervention. General nursing considerations related to antimicrobial therapy discussed earlier also apply to the client receiving erythromycin.

Erythromycins should be administered with a full glass of water on an empty stomach (1 hour before or 2 hours after meals) to obtain maximum effect. Enteric-coated tablets, delayed-release capsules, and estolate and ethylsuccinate preparations may be taken with meals and may be used with clients who have a gastrointestinal intolerance to other forms of oral erythromycin. When administering oral suspensions, ensure that they have been refrigerated, shaken well, and that the calibrated liquid-measuring device has been used for accurate dosing.

Continuous infusion is preferable to intermittent; however, if intermittent infusion is considered, it should be diluted in 100 to 250 ml of 0.9% sodium chloride injection or 5% dextrose injection and administered over 20 to 60 minutes.

Education. The importance of complying with a full course of therapy, even though the patient feels better or is symptom-free, should be stressed with the client. This course of therapy should continue at least 10 days in group A beta-hemolytic streptococcal infections to prevent the occurrence of acute rheumatic fever.

Evaluation. Observe the client for symptoms of superinfection.

LINCOMYCINS

clindamycin hydrochloride capsules/oral
solution/injectable (Cleocin, Dalacin C✦)
lincomycin hydrochloride capsules/injection
(Lincocin)

Lincomycin is primarily bacteriostatic, although it may be bactericidal in high doses with selected organisms. Clindamycin, which is a semisynthetic derivative of linco-

mycin, is more effective and causes fewer untoward effects.

Clindamycin and lincomycin are effective against most aerobic gram-positive cocci, including staphylococci, streptococci, and pneumococci. Both antibiotics are also active against several anaerobic and microaerophilic gram-negative and gram-positive organisms.

Because clindamycin is more effective in general than lincomycin, most clinicians believe that there are no recommended uses for lincomycin. Clindamycin has also been used in combination with aminoglycosides to treat mixed aerobic-anaerobic bacterial infections.

Mechanism of action. Inhibit protein synthesis in bacteria by binding ribosomes of susceptible bacteria.

Indications. Treatment of chronic bone infections, genitourinary tract infections, intraabdominal infections, anaerobic pneumonia, septicemia caused by streptococci and staphylococci, and serious skin and soft tissue infections when caused by susceptible bacteria.

Pharmocokinetics

Absorption. Oral. Clindamycin: very good (90% absorption before meals). Absorption is not affected by meals. Lincomycin: fair absorption (20% to 30%). Absorption decreases if drug is given with meals.

Distribution. Rapidly to most body fluids and tissues, except for cerebrospinal fluid. Highest concentrations noted in bone, bile, and urine and, following parenteral therapy with lincomycin, in the eye.

Half-life
Clindamycin: between 2 and 2.5 hours (pediatric clients); 2.4 to 3 hours (adults).
Lincomycin: between 4 and 5.4 hours.
With impaired renal function:
  Clindamycin, 3 to 5 hours (children); 10 to 13 hours (adults).
  Lincomycin, 10 to 13 hours.
With impaired liver function:
  Lincomycin: 9 hours.

Time to peak blood levels. Clindamycin: orally, ¾ to 1 hour; intramuscularly, 1 hour (pediatric); 3 hours (adults); intravenously at the end of the infusion. Lincomycin: orally, 2 to 4 hours; intramuscularly, ½ hour; intravenously at the end of infusion.

Metabolism. Liver. Rate of metabolism is increased in pediatric clients. Clindamycin palmitate and phosphate are inactive. They are hydrolyzed in the body to active clindamycin.

Excretion. Kidneys, bile and intestine.

Side effects/adverse reactions. See Table 59-7.

Significant drug interactions. When lincomycins are given with the following drugs the following interactions may occur.

Drug	Possible Effect and Management
Anesthetics, such as chloroform, cyclopropane, enflurane, halothane, isoflurane, methoxyflurane, trichloroethylene, or the neuromuscular blocking agents	May result in enhanced neuromuscular blockade, skeletal muscle weakness, respiratory depression, or paralysis. Use extreme caution if this combination is used during or immediately after surgery. Monitor closely and, if necessary, treat with calcium salts or anticholinesterase agents if blockade occurs.
Antidiarrheals, adsorbent type (kaolins, attapulgite)	Decreases absorption of oral lincomycins. Avoid concurrent usage or advise client to take the antidiarrheal 2 hours before or 3 to 4 hours after the oral lincomycins.
chloramphenicol or erythromycins	May antagonize the therapeutic effect of lincomycins. Avoid concurrent administration.

Dosage and administration

clindamycin hydrochloride capsules/oral solution
Adults. 150 to 450 mg orally every 6 hours.
Children. Oral solution. Infants under 30 days old, use cautiously. 1 month and over, 2 to 6.3 mg/kg every 6 hours or 2.7 to 8.3 mg/kg every 8 hours. If child weighs 10 kg or under, the minimum dose recommended is 37.5 mg every 8 hours. (1.09 g of clindamycin hydrochloride is approximately equivalent to 1 g of clindamycin.)

clindamycin phosphate injection
Adults. 300 to 600 mg intramuscularly or intravenously every 6 to 8 hours. Maximum is 2.4 g daily.
Children. Infants up to 30 days old, use cautiously. 1 month and older, intramuscularly or intravenously 3.75 to 10 mg/kg or 87.5 to 112.5 mg/m² every 6 hours or 5 to 13.3 mg/kg or 116.7 to 150 mg/m² every 8 hours. Regardless of body weight, in severe infections, the minimum recommended dose is 300 mg/day. For bone infections, intramuscularly or intravenously, 7.5 mg/kg every 6 hours.

lincomycin hydrochloride capsules
Adults. 500 mg orally every 6 to 8 hours.
Children. Infants under 30 days old, not recommended. 1 month and older, 7.5 to 15 mg/kg orally every 6 hours or 10 to 20 mg/kg every 8 hours. (1.13 g of lincomycin hydrochloride is approximately equivalent to 1 g of lincomycin).

lincomycin hydrochloride injection
Adults. Intramuscularly 600 mg every 12 to 24 hours. Intravenously, 600 mg to 1 g every 8 to 12 hours. Subconjunctivally, 75 mg. Maximum adult dose is 8.4 g/day.
Children. Infants under 30 days old, not recommended. 1 month and older, intramuscularly, 10 mg/kg every 12 to 24 hours or more often if needed; intravenously, 3.3 to 6.7 mg/kg every 8 hours or 5 to 10 mg/kg every 12 hours.

NURSING CONSIDERATIONS

Assessment. Determine whether the client has a history of gastrointestinal disease, particularly colitis or enteritis, because pseudomembranous colitis may occur with lincomycin therapy.

Intervention. Administer clindamycin capsules with a full glass of water or with meals to prevent esophageal ulceration. Administer lincomycin on an empty stomach.

Education. Stress the importance of complying with a full course of the medication, even though the patient feels well and is symptom-free. Ten days is considered a minimal course of therapy for streptococcal infections.

Instruct the client to take the medication at evenly spaced times to ensure maintenance of serum levels.

Evaluation. During therapy, observe the client for abdominal cramps, diarrhea, weight loss, or weakness, which might be indications of pseudomembraneous colitis.

VANCOMYCIN

Vancomycin is derived from *Streptomyces orientalis* cultures. It is bactericidal for many organisms and bacteriostatic for enterococci.

Mechanism of action. Inhibits bacterial cell walls, resulting in lysis by a mechanism that differs from that in penicillin or cephalosporins. Also inhibits RNA synthesis.

Indications. Treatment of antibiotic-induced pseudomembranous colitis (*Clostridium difficile*). Treatment of staphylococcal enterocolitis.

Pharmacokinetics
Absorption. Poor from intestinal tract.
Peak serum levels. Less than 1 µg/ml. Higher in some clients.
Concentration in feces. Between 180 and 530 µg/g after a dose of 500 mg daily; between 2000 to 5000 µg/g after a 2-g dose.
Excretion. Feces.
Side effects/adverse reactions. See Table 59-7.
Significant drug interactions. When vancomycin is given with the following drugs, the following interactions may occur.

Drug	Possible Effect and Management
aminoglycosides, amphotericin B parenteral, aspirin, bacitracin parenteral, bumetanide	Increases potential for ototoxicity and/or nephrotoxicity. In clients with pseudomem-

Drug

parenteral, capreomycin, cis-platin, cyclosporine, ethacrynic acid parenteral, furosemide parenteral, paromomycin, polymyxins, or streptozocin

cholestyramine or colestipol

Possible Effect and Management

branous colitis or severe kidney impairment, the serum levels of vancomycin may be increased, thus leading to an increased potential for toxicity. Monitor closely.

When given concurrently, a reduction in vancomycin antibacterial activity is reported. Avoid this combination if possible. If not, dose oral vancomycin several hours apart from the other medications.

Dosage and administration
vancomycin hydrochloride capsules/oral solution

Adults. Treatment of pseudomembranous (antibiotic-induced) colitis in *C. difficile* or staphylococcal enterocolitis: 125 to 500 mg orally every 6 hours or 167 to 667 mg every 8 hours for 5 to 10 days. If necessary, this regimen may be repeated. Maximum dosage is 4 g/day.

Children. Treatment of pseudomembranous (antibiotic-induced) colitis in *C. difficile* or staphylococcal enterocolitis: 11 mg/kg every 6 hours for 5 to 10 days. (Some experts have suggested dosages up to 50 mg/kg/day.) Dosage may be repeated if necessary.

sterile vancomycin hydrochloride (Diatracin✿, Vancocin I.V.)

Adults

For prophylaxis of endocarditis in penicillin-allergic clients with prosthetic heart valves or valvular heart disease who are undergoing dental surgery or upper respiratory tract procedures: 1 g by intravenous infusion; start 1 hour before the procedure and repeat in 8 hours.

For gastrointestinal and genitourinary tract procedures, 1 g by intravenous infusion; start 1 hour before the procedure and give with gentamicin (1.5 mg/kg) intramuscularly or intravenously or streptomycin, 1 g intramuscularly, ½ to 1 hour before the procedure. Repeat both drugs in 8 hours.

For the treatment of enteric infections such as pseudomembranous colitis (antibiotic-induced by *C. difficile*) or systemic infections, 7.5 mg/kg or 500 mg every 6 hours or 15 mg/kg or 1 g every 12 hours by intravenous infusion. In patients with impaired renal function, reduce the dosage according to creatinine clearance or serum concentrations of the drug.

Maximum daily dose is up to 3 to 4 g daily intravenously for short periods in very serious infections.

Children

For prevention of endocarditis in penicillin-allergic cli-

ents with prosthetic heart valves or valvular heart disease who are undergoing dental, surgical, or upper respiratory tract procedures, 20 mg/kg by intravenous infusion administered 1 hour before the procedure. Repeat in 8 hours.

For gastrointestinal and genitourinary tract procedures, intravenous infusion, 20 mg/kg 1 hour before procedure and concurrently give gentamicin, 2 mg/kg (IM or IV) or streptomycin, 20 mg/kg intramuscularly, ½ to 1 hour before procedure. Repeat both drugs in 8 hours.

For treatment of enteric infections (antibiotic-induced pseudomembranous colitis caused by *C. difficile*) or systemic infections: by intravenous infusion, 11 mg/kg every 6 hours or 22 mg/kg every 12 hours. Dosages of up to 60 mg/kg/day have been used in very serious infections such as staphylococcal infections of the central nervous system.

NURSING CONSIDERATIONS

Assessment. Assess the client for hearing loss, since vancomycin has ototoxic properties. Assess elderly clients for hearing loss over the course of therapy, as they excrete vancomycin more slowly.

Intervention. The general nursing considerations for the administration of antimicrobial therapy should be applied to vancomycin administration.

Administer the oral liquid using the calibrated liquid-measuring device provided by the manufacturer. If the intravenous form is used for oral administration, each vial should be dissolved in 30 ml of water or juice. It may be administered straight or through a nasogastric tube to minimize the unpleasant taste.

Parenteral vancomycin is only to be administered intravenously because it is so irritating to the tissues. Care must be taken to avoid extravasation. To avoid side effects such as hypotension, thrombophlebitis, and "red-neck syndrome," do not administer as a bolus injection. Vancomycin may be administered intermittently in at least 100 ml of 0.9% sodium chloride injection or 5% dextrose injection over 60 minutes. Rotation of the venous sites will help prevent local irritation.

Education. Alert the client to possible side effects or adverse reactions. Instruct the client to take the medication as prescribed and for the full course of therapy.

Evaluation. Urinalysis and renal function studies may be needed before and periodically during high-dose or prolonged therapy. Vancomycin serum concentration determinations may be necessary in clients with renal impairment or in clients over 60.

AMINOGLYCOSIDES

amikacin sulfate injection (Amikin)
gentamicin sulfate injection (Apogen, Cidomycin♣, Garamycin)
kanamycin sulfate injection (Kantrex, Klebcil)
neomycin sulfate (Neo-IM, Mycifradin♣)*
netilmicin sulfate injection (Netromycin)
streptomycin sulfate injection
tobramycin sulfate injection (Nebcin)

Aminoglycosides are potent bactericidal antibiotics that are usually reserved for serious or life-threatening infections. They are very effective against many bacteria (gram-positive and gram-negative) but are generally reserved for gram-negative infections. Safer and less toxic agents are available to treat the majority of gram-positive infections.

Mechanism of action. Irreversibly binds ribosomes of susceptible bacteria, thus inhibiting protein synthesis and leading to eventual cell death. Bactericidal effects.

Indications

Treatment of serious or life-threatening infections when other agents are ineffective or contraindicated.

Used with penicillins, cephalosporins, or vancomycin for their synergistic effects.

Especially useful for the treatment of gram-negative infections such as those caused by *Pseudomonas* spp., *E. coli, Proteus* spp., *Klebsiella* spp., *Serratia* spp., and others.

Pharmacokinetics

Absorption. Orally, poor from an intact gastrointestinal tract. Intramuscularly, rapid absorption. Topically, local topical application or irrigation may lead to absorption from most areas of the body except for the urinary bladder.

Distribution

amikacin. Mainly in extracellular fluid. The cerebrospinal fluid of normal infants is approximately 10% to 20% of the plasma drug level, but if the meninges are inflamed, these levels may increase to 50% of the blood concentration. High and therapeutic concentrations are also reached in the synovial fluid and the urine.

gentamicin. Mainly in extracellular fluid. High concentrations are reported in the urine.

kanamycin. Mainly to extracellular fluid. The cerebrospinal fluid of normal infants is approximately 10% to 20% of the plasma drug level, but if the meninges are inflamed, these levels may increase to 50% of the blood concentration. High concentrations also reported in urine and synovial fluids.

netilmicin. Rapidly distributed to body tissues (liver, gallbladder, stomach, appendix, renal cortex) and body fluids (urine, blood, bile, sputum, peritoneal, synovial, pleural, pericardial, and blister fluids).

streptomycin. Mainly to extracellular fluids; to most body tissues except the brain. High levels found in urine. Also found in pleural, bile, and ascitic fluids and tuberculous tissues and/or abscesses.

tobramycin. Mainly to extracellular fluid. High concentrations in urine and synovial fluids.

Metabolism. Not metabolized.

Time to peak bile concentration. Kanamycin, intramuscular, in approximately 6 hours.

Plasma levels

amikacin. Intramuscularly, peak serum levels (mean) of 12, 16, and 21 μg/ml is achieved in 1 hour after a single dose of 250, 375, and 500 mg, respectively. Intravenously, peak serum levels (mean) of 38 μg/ml is noted at the end of a 30-minute infusion of a single 500 mg dose.

gentamicin

Adults: Intramuscularly, up to four times the single intramuscular dose in mg/kg. Intravenously, 4 to 6 μg/ml within ½ to 1 hour after infusion.

Infants: 3 to 5 μg/ml after a dose of 2.5 mg/kg. Clients with high fevers or extensive burns usually have decreased serum levels.

kanamycin. Intramuscularly or intravenously, peak serum level (mean) of 22 μg/ml after a dose of 7.5 mg/kg. Clients with high fever or severe burns usually have decreased serum levels.

netilmicin. Intramuscularly, 3 to 3.5 times the single intramuscular dose in mg/kg. Intravenously, given over 1 hour by infusion, similar to intramuscular levels.

streptomycin. Intramuscularly, 25 to 50 μg/ml after a 1-g intramuscular dose.

tobramycin. Intramuscularly, 4 μg/ml after an intramuscular dose of 1 mg/kg. Intravenously, similar to levels after an intravenous infusion given over 1 hour. Clients with high fever or severe burns usually have decreased serum levels.

Bile concentration. Netilmicin is usually 10% of the serum level. If patient has liver impairment, this value may increase to up to 25%.

Urine concentrations

amikacin. The average urine concentration is approximately 560, 700, and 830 μg/ml, respectively, recorded 6 hours after an intramuscular dose of 250, 375, and 500 mg, respectively.

gentamicin. Urine concentration may be in excess of 100 μg/ml.

kanamycin. Urine concentration is 10 to 20 times greater than the serum levels.

netilmicin. Urine concentration is up to 800 μg/ml.

tobramycin. Urine concentration is 75 to 100 μg/ml following a single intramuscular dose of 1 mg/kg. Also see box.

Side effects/adverse reactions. See Table 59-7.

---

*Safer drugs are available; therefore the systemic use of this drug is not recommended.

Significant drug interactions. When aminoglycosides are given concurrently with the following drugs, the following interactions may occur.

Drug

other aminoglycosides (two or more concurrently) or capreomycin

Possible Effect and Management

Potential for ototoxicity, nephrotoxicity, and neuromuscular blockade is enhanced. Hearing loss may progress to deafness even after the drug is stopped. In some cases, hearing loss may be reversed.

Administration of two or more aminoglycosides may reduce uptake of both drugs, possibly resulting in reduced effectiveness.

An increased potential for neuromuscular blockade. Treat with an anticholinesterase agent or calcium salts to prevent or reverse this effect.

The administration of topical and systemic aminoglycosides is not recommended. Hypersensitivity effects are reported more frequently with this combination.

amphotericin B, parenteral; aspirin; bacitracin, parenteral; bumetanide, parenteral; cephalothin; cisplatin; cyclosporine; ethacrynic acid, parenteral; furosemide, parenteral; paromomycin; streptozocin or vancomycin

Increased potential for ototoxicity and/or nephrotoxicity. Hearing loss may be permanent. If drugs are given concurrently, serial audiometric hearing determinations are suggested.

Vancomycin and aminoglycosides may be ordered to prevent bacterial endocarditis or to treat specific infections such as endocarditis caused by organisms such as streptococci and corynebacteria. In such instances, frequent determinations of drug serum levels and renal

Drug

anesthetics (halogenated hydrocarbon) or citrate-anticoagulated blood by massive transfusions or neuromuscular blocking agents

indomethacin, intravenous

methoxyflurane or polymyxins, parenteral

Possible Effect and Management

function is recommended, as dosage adjustments or other interventions may be necessary.

May increase neuromuscular blockade. Monitor closely as interventions may be necessary.

May reduce excretion of aminoglycosides, leading to elevated serum levels and possible aminoglycoside toxicity. Monitor closely, as dosage adjustments may be indicated. Aminoglycoside toxicity is usually reported in the premature neonate, but it may also occur in the adult.

Increased possibility for nephrotoxicity and/or neuromuscular blockade. If used concurrently, monitor closely.

Dosage and administration
amikacin sulfate injection (Amikin)
Adults. Intramuscular or intravenous infusion, 5 mg/kg every 8 hours or 7.5 mg/kg every 12 hours for 6 to 10 days.

For uncomplicated urinary tract infections, intramuscular or intravenous infusion, 250 mg every 12 hours.

If client is receiving hemodialysis, after the dialysis, give a supplemental dose of 3 to 5 mg/kg.

Maximum dose is 15 mg/kg/day. Do not exceed 1.5 gs daily for more than 10 days.

Children. Intramuscular or intravenous infusion: Neo-

AMINOGLYCOSIDE PHARMACOKINETICS

| DRUG | HALF-LIFE | | KIDNEY EXCRETION (% unchanged/hr) |
	NORMAL RENAL FUNCTION (hr)	IMPAIRED RENAL FUNCTION (hr)	
amikacin	2-2.5	Up to 150	84-92/9
	1-1.5*	(anuric)	94-98/24
gentamicin	2-3	40-50	50-93/24
kanamycin	2-4	27-80	50/4
			80-90/24
netilmicin	2-3.4	>30	75-90/24
streptomycin	2.4-2.7	50-100	80-98/24
tobramycin	1.9-2.2	53-56	60-85/6
			85-93/24

*Young clients and burn patients.

nates, 10 mg/kg initially, then 7.5 mg/kg every 12 hours; older infants and children; see adult dose.

Maintenance dosages have also been calculated as follows:

$$\text{Maintenance dose (q 12 hr)} = \frac{\text{Patient's creatinine clearance (ml/min)}}{\text{Normal creatinine clearance (ml/min)}} \times 7.5\text{ mg/kg}$$

Burn patients may need a 5 to 7.5 mg/kg dose every 4 to 6 hours.

gentamicin sulfate injection (Apogen, Garamycin)

Adults. Intramuscular or intravenous infusion, 1 to 1.7 mg/kg every 8 hours or 750 μg to 1.25 mg/kg every 6 hours for 7 to 10 days.

For uncomplicated urinary tract infections, intramuscular or intravenous infusion:

Adults under 60 kg, 3 mg/kg daily or 1.5 mg/kg every 12 hours.

Adults 60 kg and over, 160 mg daily or 80 mg every 12 hours.

After hemodialysis, a supplemental dose of 1 to 1.7 mg/kg may be administered.

Intralumbar or intraventricular, 4 to 8 mg daily.

Maximum daily dose is 8 mg/kg in serious, life-threatening situations.

Children. Intramuscular or intravenous infusion:

Premature or neonates up to 7 days old, 2.5 mg/kg every 12 hours for 7 to 10 days (more if necessary).

Older neonates and infants, 2.5 mg/kg every 8 hours for 7 to 10 days (more if necessary).

Children, 2 to 2.5 mg/kg every 8 hours for 7 to 10 days (more if necessary).

Intralumbar or intraventricular, infants up to 3 months old, dose not established; infants and children 3 months and older, 1 to 2 mg daily. Dosages of up to 8 mg/day have been used in infants that have a functioning ventricular shunt.

gentamicin in sodium chloride injection (Garamycin). Same as preceding.

kanamycin sulfate injection (Kantrex, Klebcil)

Adults

Inhalation: 250 mg every 6 to 12 hours.

Intramuscular: 3.75 mg/kg every 6 hours; 5 mg/kg every 8 hours; or 7.5 mg/kg every 12 hours for 7 to 10 days.

Intraperitoneal: 500 mg.

Intravenous infusion: 5 mg/kg every 8 hours or 7.5 mg/kg every 12 hours for 7 to 10 days.

Maximum daily dose is 15 mg/kg, not exceeding 1.5 g daily.

Children. Intramuscular or intravenous infusion, see adult dosage.

netilmicin sulfate injection (Netromycin)

Adults. Intramuscularly or intravenously:

For systemic (severe) infections, 1.3 to 2.2 mg/kg every 8 hours or 2 to 3.25 mg/kg every 12 hours for 7 to 14 days.

For complicated urinary tract infections, 1.5 to 2 mg/kg every 12 hours for 1 to 2 weeks.

After hemodialysis, a dose of 1 mg/kg may be given.

Maximum daily dose is up to 7.5 mg/kg. (In cystic fibrosis patients, doses up to 12 mg/kg/day have been used.)

Children. Intramuscularly or intravenously: Neonates up to 6 weeks old, 2 to 3.25 mg/kg every 12 hours for 1 to 2 weeks. Infants and children 6 weeks to 12 years old, 1.83 to 2.67 mg/kg every 8 hours or 2.75 to 4 mg/kg every 12 hours for 1 to 2 weeks.

tobramycin sulfate injection (Nebcin)

Adults. Intramuscular or intravenous infusion, 750 μg to 1.25 mg/kg every 6 hours or 1 to 1.7 mg/kg every 8 hours for 7 to 10 days (or more if necessary). Maximum daily dose is 8 mg/kg/day in serious, life-threatening infections. Total daily dosages greater than 3 to 5 mg/kg should be reduced as soon as clinically possible.

Children. Intramuscular or intravenous infusion: premature or full-term neonates 1 week old or less, up to 2.5 mg/kg every 12 hours. Older infants and children, 1.5 to 1.9 mg/kg every 6 hours or 2 to 2.5 mg/kg every 8 hours.

sterile tobramycin sulfate (Nebcin). For intravenous infusion only; see dosage in preceding discussion.

tobramycin in dextrose injection. See dosage in discussion of tobramycin sulfate injection.

NURSING CONSIDERATIONS

Assessment. Elderly clients are at greater risk of nephrotoxicity and ototoxicity because of reduced renal function, and they generally require smaller daily doses. Loss of hearing however, may occur in clients with normal renal function. Audiograms, renal function studies, and vestibular function studies should be done before and periodically during high-dose therapy or therapy over 10 days. Intake and output should be monitored.

Intervention. For intravenous administration, dilute appropriately and administer slowly over a 30- to 60-minute period to prevent neuromuscular blockade for toxic serum levels.

Clients should be well hydrated while taking these medications to minimize chemical irritation of the urinary tubules.

Education. Instruct the client to report any loss of hearing or any ringing or buzzing in the ears that would indicate ototoxicity; any change in urinary pattern or blood in the urine that would indicate nephrotoxicity; dizziness that would indicate vestibular toxicity; or numbness, tingling or twitching that would indicate neurotoxicity.

Stress the importance of taking the full course of medication as prescribed.

Evaluation. Monitor peak and trough drug levels routinely, since evidence suggests that the incidence of ototoxicity and nephrotoxicity with aminoglycosides correlates with slight elevations of either drug level but particularly with trough levels. The trough concentration is believed to be a more sensitive indicator of renal function than the serum creatinine.

TETRACYCLINES

The tetracyclines, the first broad-spectrum antibiotics, were introduced in 1948. They include a large group of drugs that have a common basic structure and similar chemical activity.

demeclocycline (Declomycin)
doxycycline (Doxychel, Vibramycin, Vibra-Tabs)
methacycline (Rondomycin)
minocycline (Minocin)
oxytetracycline (Terramycin)
tetracycline (Achromycin V, Novotetra✷, Sumycin)

Mechanism of action. Tetracyclines block the binding of transfer RNA complex to the ribosome. No amino acid is available to the messenger RNA to produce polypeptides; therefore protein synthesis is prevented. These agents are bacteriostatic for many gram-negative and gram-positive organisms. The tetracyclines exhibit cross-sensitivity and cross-resistance.

Indications. Treatment of acne vulgaris, actinomycosis, anthrax, bacterial urinary tract infections, and systemic bacterial infections sensitive to the tetracyclines.

Pharmacokinetics

Absorption. Orally, fair to very well absorbed (from 59% for oxytetracycline to 90% to 100% for doxycycline or minocycline).

Distribution. All tetracyclines distribute well to most body fluids (bile, sinus secretions, synovial, pleural, ascitic). Cerebrospinal fluid levels vary and may range from 10% to 25% of the plasma drug concentration after parenteral administration. Tetracyclines localize in teeth, liver, spleen, tumors, and bone. Doxycycline can reach clinical concentrations in the eye. Prostatic levels are approximately 60% of the serum level. High levels of minocycline are reported in saliva, sputum, and tears.

Metabolism. Doxyxline and minocycline are inactivated by the liver. For half-life and excretion routes, see box, "Tetracycline Half-Lives and Excretion."

Onset of action. In treatment syndrome of unappro-

priate ADH secretion with demeclocycline, within 1 to 2 days.

Time to peak serum level. Tetracycline, 2 to 3 days; other tetracyclines, orally within 2 to 4 hours.

Side effects/adverse reactions. See Table 59-7.

Significant drug interactions. When tetracyclines are given concurrently with the following drugs, the following interactions may occur.

Drug	Possible Effect and Management
aminosalicylate calcium; antacids; calcium supplements (such as calcium lactate, calcium gluconate); choline and magnesium salicylates; iron supplements; magnesium salicylate or magnesium-containing laxatives; foods containing milk and milk products	May result in nonabsorbable complex, thus reducing the absorption and serum levels of the antibiotic. Also, antacids may increase gastric pH, which decreases the absorption of tetracyclines. If given concurrently, advise clients to separate medications by 1 to 3 hours of the oral tetracycline.
colestipol	Decreases absorption of tetracyclines. Avoid concurrent usage.
methoxyflurane	Except for doxycycline, this combination may increase the risk for nephrotoxicity.
penicillins	Bacteriostatic drugs may block the effect of bactericidal antibiotics in meningitis or other infections in which a rapid bactericidal action is needed. Avoid concurrent therapy.
sodium bicarbonate	May decrease absorption of oral tetracyclines. Advise clients to separate medications by at least 1 to 2 hours.

Dosage and administration

demeclocycline hydrochloride capsules/tablets (Declomycin)

Adults

To treat a systemic protozoal infection, 150 mg orally every 6 hours or 300 mg every 12 hours.

AMINOGLYCOSIDES: FDA PREGNANCY SAFETY CATEGORIES

Category C	amikacin
	gentamicin
Category D	netilmicin
	tobramicin
Not established	kanamycin

TETRACYCLINE HALF-LIVES AND EXCRETION

DRUG	HALF-LIFE (hr)	ROUTE OF EXCRETION*
demeclocycline (Declomycin)	10-17	Kidneys/bile (42%)
doxycycline (Vibramycin, others)	12-22	Bile/kidneys (35%)
methacycline (Rondomycin)	14-17	Kidneys/bile (50%)
minocycline (Minocin)	11-23	Bile/kidneys (5-10%)
oxytetracycline (Terramycin)	6-10	Kidneys/bile (70%)
tetracycline	6-11	Kidneys/bile (60%)

*Major route of excretion/secondary route of excretion (percentage of drug excreted unchanged or unmetabolized).

Treatment of the syndrome of inappropriate ADH secretion (diuretic effect), 3.25 to 3.75 mg/kg orally every 6 hours.

Maximum daily dose to treat antiprotozoal infection is 2.4 g.

Maximum dose to treat syndrome of inappropriate ADH secretion is 300 mg to 1.2 g daily.

Children. To treat a systemic protozoal infection, 1.65 to 3.3 mg/kg orally every 6 hours or 3.3 to 6.6 mg/kg every 12 hours. *Do not administer tetracyclines to infants and children up to 8 years old, because these drugs can cause permanent discoloration of the teeth, enamel hypoplasia, and a decrease in linear skeletal growth rate (premature infants).*

doxycycline for oral suspension (Doxychel, Vibramycin)
doxycycline calcium oral suspension (Vibramycin)
doxcycline capsules (Doxy-Caps, Vibramycin)
doxycycline delayed-release capsules (Doryx)
tablets (Doxy-Tabs, Vibra-Tabs)
Adults

Treatment of protozoal infections, 100 mg orally every 12 hours the first 24 hours, then 100 to 200 mg daily or 50 to 100 mg every 12 hours.

To prevent traveler's diarrhea, doxycycline 100 mg orally daily for 3 weeks.

Maximum daily dose is 300 mg. Dosages up to 600 mg/day for 5 days have been used in acute gonococcal infections.

Children. Treatment of protozoal infections: children 45 kg and under, 2.2 mg/kg orally every 12 hours the first 24 hours, then 2.2 to 4.4 mg/kg daily or 1.1 to 2.2 mg/kg every 12 hours. For children over 45 kg, see adult dose.

The precaution listed for infants and children up to 8 years old applies to all tetracyclines.

doxycycline hyclate for injection (Doxy, Doxychel, Vibramycin)

Adults. 200 mg daily or 100 mg every 12 hours by intraveous infusion the first 24 hours, then 100 to 200 mg daily or 50 to 100 mg every 12 hours. Maximum daily dose is up to 300 mg.

Children. Intravenous infusion: children 45 kg and under, 4.4 mg/kg daily of 2.2 mg/kg every 12 hours the first 24 hours, then 2.2 to 4.4 mg/kg daily or 1.1 to 2.2 mg/kg every 12 hours. For children over 45 kg, see adult dose. See precaution for children up to 8 years old.

methacycline hydrochloride capsules (Rondomycin)

Adults. For treatment of protozoal infections, 150 mg orally every 6 hours or 300 mg every 12 hours. For pneumonia (*Mycoplasma pneumoniae,* Eaton agent), 450 mg orally every 12 hours for 6 days. Maximum daily dose is 2.4 g.

Children. Children 8 years and older, 1.65 to 3.3 mg/kg orally every 6 hours or 3.3 to 6.6 mg/kg every 12 hours.

minocycline hydrochloride capsules/oral suspension/tablets (Minocin)
Adults

For treatment of protozoal infections, orally, 200 mg initially, then 100 mg every 12 hours or 100 to 200 mg initially, then 50 mg every 6 hours.

For *Mycobacterium marinum* infections, 100 mg orally every 12 hours for 6 to 8 weeks.

For *Neisseria meningitidis* carriers that are asymptomatic, 100 mg orally every 12 hours for 5 days.

Maximum daily dosage is 350 mg the first day, 200 mg/day thereafter.

Children. Children 8 years and older, 4 mg/kg orally initially, then 2 mg/kg every 12 hours.

sterile minocycline hydrochloride (Minocin)

Adults. Intravenous infusion, 200 mg initially, then 100 mg every 12 hours. Maximum daily dose is 400 mg.

Children. Intravenous infusion, children 8 years and older, 4 mg/kg initially, then 2 mg/kg every 12 hours.

oxytetracycline tablets/capsules (Terramycin)

Adults. For treatment of protozoal infections, 250 to 500 mg orally every 6 hours. Maximum daily dose is up to 4.

Children. For children 8 years and older, 6.25 to 12.5 mg/kg orally every 6 hours.

oxytetracycline injection (Terramycin)

Adults. Intramuscularly, 100 mg every 8 hours, 150 mg every 12 hours, or 250 mg once daily. Maximum daily dosage is 500 mg.

Children. Children 8 years and older, 5 to 8.3 mg/kg intramuscularly every 8 hours or 7.5 to 12.5 mg/kg every 12 hours. Maximum daily dose is 250 mg.

oxytetracycline hydrochloride for injection (Terramycin)

Adults. Intravenous infusion, 250 to 500 mg every 12 hours. Maximum daily dose is 2 g/day.

Children. Children 8 years and older, intravenous infusion, 5 to 10 mg/kg every 12 hours.

tetracycline oral suspension (Achromycin V, Novotetra✿, Panmycin)
tetracycline hydrochloride capsules (Achromycin V, Bristacycline, Medicycline✿)
tetracycline hydrochloride tablets (Cefracycline✿, Novotetra✿, Panmycin)
tetracycline phosphate complex capsules (Tetrex)

Adults

For treatment of protozoal infections, 250 to 500 mg orally every 6 hours or 500 mg to 1 g every 12 hours.

As antiacne agent, 500 mg to 2 g orally daily, in divided doses initially. When improvement is noted, usually after 21 days of therapy, the dosage should be reduced gradually to a maintenance dose of 125 to 1000 mg/day. Some persons respond to alternate-day or intermittent drug therapy.

To treat gonorrhea, 500 mg orally every 6 hours for 5 days.

To treat syphilis, 500 mg orally every 6 hours for 15 days for early syphilis or 30 days for late syphilis. Maximum daily dose is 4 g.

Children. To treat protozoal infections in children 8 years and older, 6.25 to 12.5 mg/kg orally every 6 hours or 12.5 to 25 mg/kg every 12 hours.

tetracycline hydrochloride for injection, intramuscular (Achromycin)

Adults. 100 mg every 8 hours intramuscularly 150 mg every 12 hours, or 250 mg daily. Maximum daily dose is 1 g.

Children. Children 8 years and older, 5 to 8.3 mg/kg intramuscularly every 8 hours or 7.5 to 12.5 mg/kg every 12 hours. Maximum dose is 250 mg/day.

tetracycline hydrochloride for injection (intravenous) (Achromycin)

Adults. 250 to 500 mg intravenously every 12 hours. Maximum daily dose is 2 g.

Children. Children 8 years and older, 5 to 10 mg/kg intravenously every 12 hours.

NURSING CONSIDERATIONS

In addition to nursing measures common to all types of antimicrobial drug therapy, the nurse should observe the following measures when patients are receiving drugs of the tetracycline family.

Assessment. Tetracyclines are contraindicated in pregnant women and children under 8 years of age because they cause permanent mottling and discoloration of the teeth and a decrease in linear skeletal growth rate.

Clients with a hypersensitivity to one tetracycline may be hypersensitive to the others as well. In addition, clients with hypersensitivities to "caine-type" drugs, such as lidocaine or procaine, may be intolerant of the lidocaine in oxytetracycline injection or the procaine in the tetracycline intramuscular injection.

Use of tetracyclines in clients with renal impairment is not recommended (except for doxycycline and minocycline).

Intervention. Tetracyclines should be taken with a full glass of water to prevent esophageal erosion and gastrointestinal irritation. Except for doxycycline and minocycline, they should be taken on an empty stomach (1 hour before or 2 hours after meals) for maximum effectiveness. Avoid administering antacids and laxatives containing aluminum, calcium, or magnesium; iron products; and food, milk, or other dairy products for 1 hour before and 2 hours after tetracycline administration, as they form nonabsorbable complexes with tetracyclines.

Administer the oral suspension using the calibrated liquid-measuring device provided by the manufacturer.

Education. Stress the importance of taking the full course of the medication and of taking the medication in evenly spaced doses to maintain serum levels.

Photosensitivity may occur and persist for some time after discontinuance of the drug. Instruct the client to avoid direct sunlight and ultraviolet light. If exposure is unavoidable, a sun screen may help prevent a reaction.

Instruct the client to discard outdated tetracyclines (show client where date is found), since they become toxic as they decompose.

Evaluation. Because the potential for superinfections is greater in tetracycline therapy than in therapy with other antimicrobial agents, observe clients carefully for signs and symptoms of secondary infections, especially monilial infections. Meticulous oral and perineal hygiene is helpful in preventing monilial superinfections.

CHLORAMPHENICOL

Chloramphenical (Chloromycetin), discovered in 1949, is a potent inhibitor of protein synthesis. It is a bacteriostatic agent for a wide variety of gram-negative and gram-positive organisms, but because it is potentially seriously toxic to bone marrow (aplasia leading to aplastic anemia and possibly death), its approved indications are limited.

Mechanism of action. Usually bacteriostatic but in high doses with highly susceptible organisms, it may be bactericidal. It penetrates bacteria cell membranes and reversibly prevents peptide bond formation, thus inhibiting protein synthesis.

Indications. For the treatment of meningitis *(Haemophilus influenzae),* paratyphoid fever, Q fever, rickettsialpox, Rocky Mountain spotted fever, typhoid fever *(Salmonella typhi),* typhus infections, and bacterial septicemia.

Pharmacokinetics

Absorption. Rapid from gastrointestinal tract.

Distribution. High concentrations in liver, kidneys, eyes, urine, and other body fluids.

Metabolism. Primarily liver. Chloramphenicol palmitate is hydrolyzed in the gastrointestinal tract to free drug before absorption. Chloramphenicaol sodium succinate is hydrolyzed to free drug in the liver, lungs, blood, and kidneys.

Half-life

Adults. For persons with normal kidney and liver function, between 1.5 and 3.5 hours. For persons with impaired kidney function, between 3 and 4 hours. In persons with more severe kidney dysfunction, half-life is prolonged.

Infants. If 1 to 2 days old (24 hours or longer), variable; 10 to 16 days old, 10 hours.

Time to peak blood levels. Orally, within 1 to 3 hours.

Excretion. Kidneys (5% to 10% by glomerular filtration in 24 hours; 80% by tubular secretion as inactive metabolites.)

Side effects/adverse reactions. See Table 59-7.

Significant drug interactions. When chloramphenicol is given concurrently with the following drugs, the following interactions may occur.

Drug	Possible Effect and Management
alfentanil	May result in increased alfentanil blood levels, prolonging its effect. Monitor closely.
anticonvulsants, hydantoin, bone marrow depressants, radiation therapy	May result in enhanced bone marrow depressant effects. Dosage reduction may be necessary.
	Decreased hydantoin metabolism may result in increased serum levels and toxicity. Monitor closely, as dosage adjustments may be needed.
antidiabetic oral agents	May displace the antidiabetic drug from protein binding, leading to hypoglycemia. Dosage adjustment may be necessary. Monitor closely.
erythromycins or lincomycins	Therapeutic action of chloramphenical and these drugs may be antagonized. Avoid this drug combination.

Dosage and administration

chloramphenicol capsules (Chloromycetin, Mychel)
chloramphenicol palmitate oral suspension (Chloromycetin)

Adults. 12.5 mg/kg orally every 6 hours. Maximum daily dose is 4 g.

Children. Premature and full-term infants up to 14 days old, 6.25 mg/kg orally every 6 hours; infants 2 weeks and older, 12.5 mg/kg orally every 6 hours or 25 mg/kg every 12 hours. In serious infections, doses up to 75 to 100 mg/kg daily may be used.

sterile chloramphenicol sodium succinate (Chloromycetin, Mychel-S)

Adults. 12.5 mg/kg intravenously every 6 hours. Maximum daily dose is 4 g.

Children. See preceding recommendations.

Pregnancy safety. Not established.

NURSING CONSIDERATIONS

Assessment. Consider carefully before using chloramphenicol in clients with hepatic and renal impairment.

Intervention. Administer chloramphenicol with a full glass of water on an empty stomach (1 hour before meals or 2 hours after) to maximize effectiveness. When administering the oral suspension, use the calibrated liquid-measuring device provided by the manufacturer.

If administered intravenously, the drug should be infused over at least a 1-minute period. Check the intravenous site daily for local irritation.

Education. Because the bone marrow depressant effects of chloramphenicol may increase gingival bleeding and delay healing, instruct the client to delay dental work until blood counts return to normal. Instruct all clients in proper oral hygiene, with cautious use of toothbrushes, dental floss, and toothpicks.

Advise the client to report to the physician immediately any symptoms of blood dyscrasias, such as sore throat, fever, extreme fatigue, or unusual bleeding or bruising.

Caution clients who test their urine with copper sulfate glucose tests (Clinitest tablets) that they may get false-positive reactions. For the course of the antibiotic therapy, recommend the use of Clinistix or Keto-diastix.

Evaluation. Perform complete blood counts periodically to monitor for dose-related reversible bone marrow depression.

QUINOLONES

The quinolone antibiotics (also referred to as 4-quinolone or fluoroquinolone), are recent synthetic chemical additions to the antimicrobial classification. Two members of this class, ciprofloxacin and norfloxacin, are reviewed.

ciprofloxacin (Cipro)

Mechanism of action. Alters bacterial DNA by interfering with DNA gyrase and possibly by direct interaction with DNA itself. May also inhibit bacterial RNA synthesis, especially at high concentrations. It is bactericidal.

Indications. To treat susceptible strains of bacteria (gram-negative and gram-positive) affecting the lower respiratory tract, bone and joint infections, infectious diarrhea, urinary tract infections, and skin infections.

Pharmacokinetics

Absorption. Good (approximately 70%).

Maximum serum concentration. Within 1 to 2 hours after oral dose.

Half-life. 4 hours.

Metabolism/excretion. Approximately 40% to 50% of the dose excreted in the urine as unchanged drug. Also approximately four less active metabolites have been identified in the urine.

Side effects/adverse reactions. See Table 59-7.

Significant drug interactions. When ciprofloxacin is given concurrently with the following drugs, the following interactions may occur.

Drug	Possible Effect and Management
antacids, especially magnesium hydroxide or aluminum hydroxide	May decrease absorption of ciprofloxacin, reducing drug effectiveness. Avoid concurrent drug administration.
probenecid	Blocks renal tubular secretion of

Drug	Possible Effect and Management
	ciprofloxacin, resulting in elevated serum levels.
theophylline	May result in increased plasma levels of theophylline and increased risk of toxicity. Monitor plasma levels closely, as dosage adjustments may be necessary. Monitor closely.

Dosage and administration

To treat urinary tract infections, 250 mg orally every 12 hours.

For respiratory tract infections, skin, bone and joint infections, 500 mg orally every 12 hours.

For more serious or complicated infections, 750 mg every 12 hours.

For infectious diarrhea, 500 mg orally every 12 hours.

In patients with impaired renal function, check current package insert or USP DI for dosing instructions.

Pregnancy safety. FDA category C.

norfloxacin (Noroxin)

Mechanism of action. Inhibits bacterial DNA synthesis, bactericidal.

Indications. To treat urinary tract infections (complicated or uncomplicated) caused by susceptible strains of bacteria such as *E. coli, K. pneumoniae, Enterobacter cloacae, Proteus mirabilis, Pseudomonas aeruginosa, Staphylococcus aureus,* group D streptococci, and others. It is effective against many gram-negative and gram-positive organisms.

Pharmacokinetics

Absorption. Fair (approximately 30% to 40% of an oral dose is absorbed on an empty stomach).

Peak plasma level. Within 1 hour.

Half-life. 3 to 4 hours.

Metabolism/excretion. Bile and kidney excretion.

Side effects/adverse reactions. See Table 59-7.

Significant drug interactions. When norfloxacin is given with the following drugs, the following interactions may occur.

Drug	Possible Effect and Management
antacids	Decreases absorption of norfloxacin. Avoid concurrent drug administration.
probenecid	Decreases urinary excretion of norfloxacin. Monitor closely to avoid toxicity.
nitrofurantoin	Avoid concurrent drug administration. Norfloxacin's effectiveness may be antagonized.

Dosage and administration
Adults

For treatment of urinary tract infections, individuals with normal renal function and uncomplicated urinary tract infection, administer 400 mg orally twice a day for 7 to 10 days.

For complicated infections, 400 mg twice a day for 10 to 21 days.

For clients with impaired renal function, check a current package insert or USP DI for prescribing information.

Pregnancy safety. FDA Category C.

NURSING CONSIDERATIONS

Assessment. Since norfloxacin adminstration may result in CNS toxicity, another drug should be used if possible for clients with a history of seizures.

Intervention. Administer norfloxacin with a full glass of water on an empty stomach.

Hydrate the client to maintain a urinary output of at least 1200 to 1500 ml daily for adults, as crystalluria has been reported.

Education. Stress the importance of taking a full course of therapy, taking all doses as prescribed at evenly spaced intervals to maintain therapeutic serum levels.

Caution the client that the drug may decrease salivation and that dry mouth may result. This may be relieved by sugar-free candies or gum, ice cubes, or frequent mouth rinses. If the therapy is long-term, caries and gum disease may result and the client should be advised to have regular dental checkups.

Advise the client to report dizziness, lightheadedness, or depression, as these signs indicate CNS toxicity. Visual disturbances such as blurred or double vision and increased light sensitivity should be reported for the same reason.

Avoid taking antacids and norfloxacin within 2 hours of each other.

Advise the client that photophobia is a possible effect of this drug. Avoiding bright lights and wearing sunglasses may assist the client with this symptom.

Because visual disturbances, dizziness, lightheadedness, or drowsiness may occur, advise the client to limit activities that require alertness and dexterity until the response to the drug has been determined.

MISCELLANEOUS ANTIBIOTICS

Except for metronidagole hydrochloride and spectinomycin, the other antibiotics in current use are topical agents and will be discussed in Chapter 67.

metronidazole hydrochloride (Flagyl, Flagyl I.V., Neo-Metric✤)

Mechanism of action. Metronidazole is reduced intracelluarly to a short-acting, cytotoxic agent that interacts with DNA, thus inhibiting bacteria synthesis and resulting in cell death (microbicidal). It is active against many anaerobic bacteria and protozoa.

Indications. For the treatment of amebiasis (intestinal and extraintestinal), bone infections, brain abscesses, CNS infections, bacterial endocarditis, genitourinary tract infections, liver abscess (amebic), septicemia, trichomoniasis, *Bacteroides* pneumonia and other infections due to organisms susceptible to metronidazole's action.

Pharmacokinetics

Absorption. Very good orally.

Distribution. To many body fluids and areas such as saliva, bile, bone, liver, lungs, seminal fluid, and others.

Half-life. 6 to 12 hours (mean is 8 hours).

Time to peak serum level. Within 1 to 2 hours (orally). Peak serum levels after a 250-mg, 500-mg, and 2-g oral dose are 6, 12, and 40 µg/ml respectively. With intravenous dosage form at recommended doses, the peak steady-state serum level is approximately 25 µg/ml; trough levels are approximately 18 µg/ml.

Metabolism. Liver.

Excretion. Kidneys (60% to 80%), feces.

Side effects/adverse reactions. See Table 59-7.

Significant drug interactions. When metronidazole is given concurrently with the following drugs, the following interactions may occur.

Drug	Possible Effect and Management
alcohol	Metronidazole interferes with the metabolism of alcohol, leading to an accumulation of acetaldehyde. This may result in disulfiram-type effects, that is, flushing, headaches, nausea, vomiting, and abdominal distress. Avoid concurrent drug administration.
anticoagulants (coumarin or indandione)	May enhance anticoagulant effects by inhibiting their metabolism. Monitor closely with prothrombin tests if given concurrently. Dosage adjustments may be necessary.
disulfiram	Avoid concurrent administration with metronidazole. Adverse effects, including confusion and psychosis, have been reported.

Dosage and administration
Tablet form
Adults

To treat systemic anaerobic bacterial infections, 7 mg/kg orally to a maximum of 1 g every 6 hours for 7 days or more, if necessary.

Antiprotozoal, 500 to 750 mg orally three times daily for 5 to 10 days.

Trichomoniasis, 2 g orally as single dose or 1 g twice a day for 7 day or 250 mg three times a day for 1 week.

Maximum daily dose is 4 g.

Children. Systemic anaerobic antibacterial use not established.

Antiprotozoal:

Amebiasis, 11.6 to 16.7 mg/kg orally, three times daily for 10 days.

Trichomoniasis, 5 mg/kg orally, three times daily for 7 days.

Parenteral form

Adults

To treat systemic anaerobic bacterial infections, intrave-

ndx Selected Nursing Diagnoses Related to Antibiotic Therapy

Nursing diagnosis	Outcome criteria	Nursing interventions
Knowledge deficit related to antimicrobial drug therapy	Client will: Express understanding of the purpose, function, and side effects/adverse reactions of drug therapy Demonstrate understanding of proper handling and administration	Assess client's level of knowledge and understanding. Determine education needs of client. Provide information related to: Specific problem being treated with the antimicrobial agent Purpose and function of drug therapy Side effects/adverse reactions of the drug Methods of reducing side effects Answer questions and clarify misconceptions. If drug is to be self-administered, instruct the client in: Proper route and method for administration Proper storage and handling Importance of taking all of the prescribed drug Alert client to possible drug interactions. Instruct the client not to take additional medications without first checking with the prescriber.
Altered nutrition related to gastrointestinal effects of antimicrobrial drugs	Client will maintain desired nutritional status.	Assess client's normal dietary patterns and intake. Assess normal pattern of bowel function. Emphasize the importance of adequate nutrition. Instruct client to report any gastrointestinal changes (nausea, vomiting, cramping, gas, diarrhea, constipation). Administer in relation to meals and food to minimize side effects (with meals, before or after, depending on specific drug) yet maintain effectiveness of therapy. Encourage intake of yogurt, buttermilk, or lactin to maintain or restore intestinal flora. Report adverse effects to prescriber.

nous infusion, 15 mg/kg initially, then 7.5 mg/kg up to a maximum or 1 g every 6 hours for 7 days or more, if necessary.

To prevent perioperative infections of the colon, intravenous infusion, 15 mg/kg 1 hour before surgery and 7.5 mg/kg 6 and 12 hours after the first dose.

Maximum daily dose is 4 g.

Children. Not established.

Pregnancy safety. Not established.

NURSING CONSIDERATIONS

Assessment. Because metronidazole may cause CNS toxicity, any individual with preexisting CNS disease should be carefully evaluated before treatment with the drug.

Intervention. Administer oral forms with meals to minimize gastrointestinal irritation.

Parenteral metronidazole is to be administered by slow intravenous infusion. It may be administered continuously or intermittently over 1-hour period.

The sodium content of the parenteral forms of the drug should be considered in the sodium intake for clients on sodium restriction.

Education. Advise the client that the drug may cause an unpleasant taste in the mouth, diminished taste sensation, and a dry mouth. The use of sugar-free candies, ice cubes, and frequent mouth rinses may bring some relief to the client. If therapy is long-term, dry mouth may contribute to dental caries and gum disease, and the client should receive regular dental checkups.

Stress the importance of completing a full course of therapy, even though the client may be feeling well and be symptom free. The doses should be evenly spaced to ensure therapeutic serum levels are maintained.

Advise the client not to ingest alcoholic beverages while taking metronidazole, as a disulfiramlike effect may result (flushing, nausea and vomiting, and abdominal cramping).

If metronidazole is being prescribed for trichomoniasis, the client will need to prevent reinfection from her male partner. He will need concurrent drug therapy and to use a condom until the infection is resolved in both partners.

Advise the client that the urine may turn a darker color, but this change is not medically significant.

Evaluation. Assess clients periodically for symptoms of peripheral neuropathy such as numbness and tingling of the hands or feet. Mood changes and irritability also indicate of CNS toxicity.

Monitor complete blood counts frequently for blood dyscrasias and instruct the client to report immediately to the physician any symptoms of sore throat, unusual tiredness or weakness, or unusual bleeding or bruising.

spectinomycin (Trobicin)

Spectinomycin was marketed in 1971, but its sole therapeutic indication is the treatment of infections caused by *Neisseria gonorrhoeae*. It inhibits protein synthesis in the bacteria cell. It is for intramuscular use only and generally is recommended for individuals with gonorrhea who are allergic to penicillin, cephalosporins, or probenecid and who cannot tolerate tetracyclines. It also has been recommended for gonorrhea treatment in geographic locations where high antibiotic resistance has been reported. It is not effective for treating syphilis and should not be used for mixed infections (gonorrhea and syphilis), as it can mask the symptoms of syphilis.

KEY TERMS

peak level, page 898
subtherapeutic level, page 898
superinfection, page 898
therapeutic level, page 898
toxic level, page 898
trough level, page 898

BIBLIOGRAPHY

Abramowicz, M ed: Ampicillin/sulbactam (Unasyn). In The Medical Letter 29(747):79, 1987.

American Hospital Formulary Service: AHFS Drug Information'88, Bethesda, Md., 1988, American Society of Hospital Pharmacists, Inc.

Anderson, PO: Rational antibiotic use, US Pharmacist, 10(5): H-2-13, 1985.

Baron, KA, and White, RL: Antibiotic efficacy review, Pharmacy Practice News, 14(9):19-20, 29, 1987.

Barriere, SL: Economic impact of oral quinolones, Hosp. Formulary 22 (suppl A):21, 1987.

Braunwald, E, and others, eds: Harrison's Principles of internal medicine, ed 11, New York, 1987, McGraw-Hill Book Co.

Cobb, DK: Mechanisms of resistance to extended-spectrum cephalosporins, Hosp Pract 21(1):100, 1986.

Cohen, MS: Antibiotic therapy 1985: what are the challenges?, Hosp Formul 20(12):1247, 1985.

Davidson, DE: Handbook of nonprescription drugs, ed 8, Washington, DC, 1986, American Pharmaceutical Association and The National Professional Society of Pharmacists.

Fass, RJ: Efficacy and safety of oral ciprofloxacin, Hosp. Formulary 22 (suppl), 1987.

Fazio, VW: Surgical conferences: penicillins vs. cephalosporins on the surgical service, M01076, 1987, Miles Pharmaceuticals.

Gilman, AG, and others: Goodman and Gilman's the pharmacological basis of therapeutics, ed 7, New York, 1985, Macmillan Publishing Co.

Glatt, AE: Third-generation cephalosporins, Physician Assist 10(1):73, 1986.

Glatt, AE: Second-generation cephalosporins, Hosp Pract 21(3):158, 1986.

Gleckman, RA, and Bergman, MM: When to turn to the newer cephalosporins, part 2, J Resp Dis, p 51, Dec. 1986.

Gleckman, RA, and others: Selected newer uses of some older antibiotics, Hosp Formul 21(8):844, 1986.

Guay, DRP, Peterson, PK, and Breitenbucher, R: Pharmacy: oral fluoroquinolone antimicrobial therapy in the geriatric patient, TNH, p:38, March 1988.

Herfindal, ET, and others, eds: Clinical pharmacy and therapeutics, ed 4, Baltimore, 1988, Williams & Wilkins.

Kastrup, EK, ed: Facts and comparisons, St Louis, 1988, JB Lippincott Co.

Marble, DA, and others: Norfloxacin: a quinoline antibiotic, Drug Intell Clin Pharmacol 20(4):261, 1986.

Nahata, MC, and others: Ceftriaxone: a third-generation cephalosporin, Drug Intell Clin Pharmacol 19(12):900, 1985.

Neu, HC: Oral quinolones: the potential role of ciprofloxacin in modern antibiotic therapy, Infections in Med (suppl), Miles Pharmaceuticals, pp 1-27, 1987.

New Drugs, Formulary Review: Cipro, new oral quinolone, Hosp Ther, 12(12): 85, 1987.

Norris, SM: Clinical pharmacology of antibiotics: the cephalosporin antibiotic agents—third-generation cephalosporins part 3, Infect Control 6(2):78, 1985.

Rapp, RP: Pharmacologic and microbiologic activity of the carbapenems, Symposia Reporter 10(2):1, 1986.

Rewers, RF: Unasyn (ampicillin sodium/sulbactam sodium), Saint Margaret Hosp Drug Infor Bull, 13(10):32, 1987.

Rocklin, RE: Penicillin reactions—desensitize or discontinue? Hosp Pract, p 75, Jan. 1986.

Rubinstein, E, Segev, S, and Lev, B: The 4-quinolones: a promising new class of antibiotics. I. Antibacterial spectrum and pharmacokinetics, Hosp Ther, 11(8):39, 1986.

Rubinstein, E, Segev, S, and Lev, B: The 4-quinolones: a promising new class of antibiotics. II. Clinical efficacy, Hosp Ther 11(8):53, 1986.

Saxon, A, moderator: Immediate hypersensitivity reaction to beta-lactam antibiotics, Ann Intern Med, 107(2):204, 1987.

Sheng, F.C., and Busuttil, R.W.: Vascular infections: the role of antibiotics in surgical prophylaxis and primary treatment, Hosp Form 21(7):770, 1986.

Scherer, P: New drugs of 1985: in theory and in practice, Am J Nurs 86(4):406, 1985.

Shibl, AM, and others: New cephalosporin antibiotics: selection and uses, Hosp Formul 20(7):802, 1985.

Squires, E, and Cleeland, R: Microbiology and pharmacokinetics of parenteral cephaloporins, Rep No 18-02-7300-064-057, Rutherford, NJ, Roche Laboratories.

Tabor, PA: Antibiotic-related bleeding disorders, Focus Crit Care 12(3):31, 1985.

United States Pharmacopeial Convention: Drug information for the health care provider, ed 8, Rockville, Md, 1988, United States Pharmacopeial Convention, Inc.

Weintraub, M, et al: Amdinocillin: application of new knowledge about beta-lactam antibiotics, Hosp Formul 20(1):26, 1985.

Weintraub, M, and others: Norfloxacin: an emerging quinolone for use in treating serious and uncomplicated UTI, Hosp Formul 21(11):1102, 1986.

Wyngaarden, JB, and Smith, LH: Cecil's textbook of medicine, ed 18, Philadelphia, 1988, WB Saunders Co.

chapter 60

Antifungal and Antiviral Drugs

OBJECTIVES

After studying this chapter, the student will be able to:

1. List commonly used antifungal agents.

2. Describe side effects/adverse reactions of antifungal agents.

3. Discuss nursing considerations for the client receiving antifungal agents.

4. Give two reasons why effective antiviral drug therapy is more limited than antibacterial and antifungal therapy.

5. List commonly used systemic antiviral agents.

6. Discuss nursing considerations for the client receiving antiviral agents.

ANTIFUNGAL DRUGS

Infection of humans by **fungi** (plantlike, parasitic microorganisms) can be caused by 1 of about 50 species. These infections, termed **mycoses**, can range from mild and superficial to severe and life threatening. Infecting organisms can be ingested orally or become implanted under the skin after injury; air-borne fungal spores can be inhaled. One species of fungi, *Candida albicans*, is usually part of the normal flora of the skin, mouth, intestines, and vagina. Overgrowth and systemic infection from *C. albicans* can occur with antibiotic, antineoplastic, and corticosteroid drug therapy. Oral **candidiasis** (thrush) is common in newborn infants, whereas vaginal candidiasis is common in pregnant women with diabetes mellitus or in women who take oral contraceptives.

Antifungal chemotherapy has not developed to the same degree as antibacterial chemotherapy. Most fungi are completely resistant to the action of chemicals at concentrations that can be tolerated by the human host, and only a few antifungal compounds are available for use internally. As a result most antifungal drugs are used topically. Table 60-1 lists the antifungal agents most commonly used in clinical medicine. All topical preparations will be discussed in Chapter 67. The following discussions include only those agents that are taken by oral or parenteral routes.

TABLE 60-1 Systemic Antifungal Agents

Drug	Trade names
amphotericin B	Fungizone
flucytosine	Ancobon, Ancotil✦
griseofulvin	Grisactin
griseofulvin (microsize)	Grifulvin V, Grisovin-FP✦
griseofulvin (ultrami-crosize)	Fulvicin P/G, Grisactin Ultra
ketoconazole	Nizoral
miconazole	Monistat IV
nystatin	Mycostatin

amphotericin B (Fungizone)

Mechanism of action. Amphotericin can be fungistatic or fungicidal, depending on the concentrations achieved clinically. It does not affect bacteria or viruses. It is believed to bind to sterols in the fungus cell membrane, thereby increasing permeability and removing potassium and other elements from the cell.

Indications. It is effective for treating aspergillosis; blastomycosis; candidiasis (moniliasis); coccidioidomycosis; cryptococcosis; histoplasmosis; leishmaniasis; and American mucocutaneous, disseminated sporotrichosis.

Pharmacokinetics. Parenteral drug.

Distribution. To lungs, liver, kidneys, adrenal glands, muscle, spleen, and other body tissues.

Protein binding. Very high.

Half-life. Initially 24 to 48 hours; terminal or elimination half-life is approximately 15 days.

Peak plasma level. Between 2 and 4 μg/ml after an initial infusion of 1 to 5 mg daily.

Metabolism. Unknown.

Excretion. Kidneys. Very slow excretion; approximately 40% excreted over 7 days but can still be found in the urine for at least 7 weeks after stopping the drug.

Side effects/adverse reactions. See Table 60-2.

Significant drug interactions. When amphotericin B is given concurrently with the following drugs, the following interactions may occur.

Drug	Possible Effect and Management
adrenocorticoids, glucocorticoids, mineralocorticoids, corticotropin (ACTH)	May result in severe hypokalemia; if given concurrently, frequent serum potassium determinations should be performed. May decrease adrenal cortex response to corticotropin (ACTH).
bone marrow depressants, radiation therapy	May produce increase bone marrow depressant effects; monitor closely, as dosage adjustments may be necessary.

Drug	Possible Effect and Management
	If given with flucytosine, the antifungal effects of both drugs may be increased. Also, amphotericin B may increase the uptake of flucytosine into cells and impair its renal excretion, thus possibly increasing toxicity with flucytosine.
digitalis glycosides	Amphotericin B–induced hypokalemia may increase the potential for digitalis toxicity. Monitor closely for arrythmias, anorexia, nausea, vomiting or other indications of possible toxicity.
nephrotoxic medications	Increase potential for nephrotoxicity; monitor closely, as dosage adjustments may be necessary.

Dosage and administration

Adults. For systemic fungus infections, 25 to 100 μg (0.025 to 0.1 mg) initially every 48 to 72 hours; increase the dose gradually to 500 μg (0.5 mg), as tolerated by the individual, up to a maximum of 15 mg.

Intravenous infusion: initially, test dose 1 mg in 5% dextrose injection given over 2 to 4 hours. Dose may then be increased by 5- to 10-mg increments or more, depending on individual tolerance and the severity of the infection. Maximum dose is 50 mg daily.

Children. For systemic fungus infections, initially administer by intravenous infusion, 250 μg (0.25 mg)/kg daily in 5% dextrose injection over a 6-hour period. Gradually increase the dose (usually by 250 μg/kg increments every other day), depending on individual tolerance, up to a maximum of 1 mg/kg or 30 mg/m^2.

Pregnancy safety. Not established.

NURSING CONSIDERATIONS

Assessment. The renal function status of the client should be ascertained and amphotericin B used with caution if renal impairment exists.

Intervention. Amphotericin B should not be used if there is any evidence of precipitate or foreign matter in the vial. The package inserts should be read before administration of the drug for major points of safe delivery. It should not be mixed with any other drug unless absolutely necessary.

Reconstitute only with the diluents recommended; others will cause the drug to precipitate. If in-line intravenous filters are used, they should have at least a 1-μm mean pore diameter, or they may filter out clinically sig-

TABLE 60-2   Antifungal Drugs: Side Effects/Adverse Reactions

Drug	Side effects*	Adverse reactions†
amphotericin B	*With IV infusion.* Most frequent: weight loss, headaches, nausea, vomiting, diarrhea, gas, anorexia. *With intrathecal injection.* Pain in back, leg, or stomach; dizziness; headache; nausea; or vomiting	With IV infusion: Most frequent: chills, fever, muscle pain, increased weakness, irregular heart rate, (hypokalemia) Less frequent/rare: visual disturbances, increased or decreased urination, tinnitus, convulsions, hand or feet numbness, pain, respiratory difficulties, skin rash, (hypersensitivity), sore throat, fever (leukopenia), bleeding episodes (thrombocytopenia) With intrathecal injection: Less frequent: hands or feet numbness, tingling, weakness or pain; urinary difficulties Rare: visual disturbances
flucytosine	Most frequent: diarrhea, nausea, or vomiting Less frequent: headache, sluggishness, dizziness	Most frequent: rash, sore throat, elevated temperature, increased bleeding episodes, increased weakness Less frequent: confusion, hallucinations
griseofulvin	Most frequent: headaches Less frequent: diarrhea, dizziness, nausea or vomiting, abdominal pain, insomnia, increased weakness	Less frequent: confusion, photosensitivity, rash, hives, pruritus, sore mouth or tongue Rare (occurs more often with chronic use and/or high dosages): hand or feet numbness, pain, tingling, or weakness; sore throat and elevated temperature
ketoconazole	Most frequent: nausea or vomiting Less frequent: rash, pruritus, insomnia, diarrhea, dizziness, sluggishness, photosensitivity, sexual impairment in males	Rare: dark urine, pale stools, abdominal pain, increased weakness, jaundice of eyes or skin; in males, breast enlargement (gynecomastia)
miconazole	Most frequent: nausea or vomiting Less frequent: diarrhea, sluggishness, red flushing of skin (face), anorexia.	Most frequent: chills, elevated temperature, pain at injection site, rash, pruritus Less frequent: increase in bleeding episodes, increased weakness, respiratory difficulties

*If side effects continue, increase, or disturb the client, inform the physician.
†If adverse reactions occur, contact physician because medical intervention may be necessary.

nificant amounts of the drug. Gloves should be worn while preparing the drug. Every half hour during administration, shake the hanging solution to keep it in suspension.

Administering the drug on alternate days and over a 6-hour period may reduce the incidence of side effects. If therapy is interrupted for more than 7 days, the dosage should be restarted at the lowest level and increased to the appropriate therapeutic level. The duration of the course of amphotericin B should be sufficient to prevent a relapse.

Febrile reactions to drug administration may be minimized if the physician orders a small dose of intravenous adrenocorticoid to be given just before the infusion of amphotericin B. Nephrotoxicity may also be minimized by sodium bicarbonate diuresis or salt loading just before administration of amphotericin B.

Heparin may be added to the intravenous infusion of amphotericin B to help prevent thrombophlebitis at the intravenous site. Sites should be changed with each dose to minimize thrombophlebitis.

If the client experiences gastrointestinal symptoms with the administration of amphotericin B, a pleasant and relaxed atmosphere for mealtimes should be provided, small, frequent feedings of high-protein, high-calorie foods of the client's choice should be encouraged, and good oral hygiene maintained. Palliative medication may be necessary if the client is experiencing indigestion, vomiting, or diarrhea.

Education. The client should be advised to complete essential dental work before starting therapy with amphotericin B or to delay it until completing the course of the drug because the bone marrow depressant effects may cause gingival bleeding and delay healing. Appropriate oral hygiene should be taught, including gentle use of toothbrushes and floss and avoidance of toothpicks.

Advise the client to alert the nursing staff at the first indication of pain at the intravenous site.

Evaluation. Blood urea nitrogen (BUN) and serum creatinine values should be determined every other day as the dosage is increased to optimal level, and then weekly until the drug is discontinued. If BUN levels exceed 40 mg/dl or serum creatinine increases to 3 mg/ml, dosage should be decreased or discontinued until renal function improves. Serum potassium levels should be monitored twice a week. Blood counts should be monitored in anticipation of bone marrow depression.

Monitor vital signs and observe the client carefully during the test dose (1 mg in 50 to 150 ml of dextrose 5% in water and administered over 20 to 30 minutes) and the first 1 to 2 hours of each dose for shortness of breath, fever, chills, nausea, and vomiting. Febrile response usually lasts for less than 4 hours after the end of the infusion.

Pain at the site of infusion may indicate extravasation. Be cautious, as the drug causes local tissue irritation and thrombophlebitis.

Clients receiving the drug intravenously should be assessed for gastrointestinal disturbances such as anorexia, indigestion, nausea and vomiting, and diarrhea. Daily monitoring of weights will determine if these symptoms are associated with weight loss.

Monitor fluid intake and output to determine renal status. Observe for signs of hypokalemia such as muscle cramps, irregular pulse, and weakness or lethargy.

Monitor for symptoms of bone marrow depression (fever, sore throat, and unusual bleeding or bruising) and report them to the physician.

flucytosine capsules (Ancobon, Ancotil✿)

Mechanism of action. Flucytosine enters fungus cells, where it is converted to fluorouracil, an antimetabolite. It interferes with pyrimidine metabolism, thus preventing nucleic acid and protein synthesis. It has selective toxicity against susceptible strains of fungi because the body cells do not convert significant quantities of this drug into fluorouracil.

Indications. Fungal endocarditis (usually caused by *Candida* spp.) fungal meningitis (*Cryptococcus* spp.), fungal pneumonia, fungal septicemia, and fungal urinary tract infections.

Pharmacokinetics

Absorption. Very good orally.

Distribution. Widely distributed in the body. Even cerebrospinal fluid (CSF) concentrations are approximately 60% to 90% of serum concentrations.

Metabolism. Not significantly metabolized.

Half-life. With normal renal function, 0.5 to 2 hours; with impaired renal function, may range from 4 to 6 hours.

Time to peak serum concentration. 4 to 6 hours.

Excretion. Kidneys (80% to 90% as unchanged drug).

Side effects/adverse reactions. See Table 60-2.

Significant drug interactions. Administration of flucytosine concurrently with bone marrow depressants or radiation therapy may enhance bone marrow suppressant effects; monitor closely, since dosage adjustments may be necessary.

Dosage and administration

Adults. 12.5 to 37.5 mg/kg orally, every 6 hours.

Children. 12.5 to 37.5 mg/kg orally or 375 to 562.5 mg/m² every 6 hours.

Pregnancy safety. Not established.

NURSING CONSIDERATIONS

Assessment. Use with caution if a client has preexisting bone marrow depression or hepatic or renal function impairment. Renal impairment necessitates a dosage adjustment. Monitor fluid intake and output. Perform blood counts and renal function studies before and frequently during the course of therapy. Periodically perform hepatic studies such as SGOT, SGPT, and serum alkaline phosphatase during therapy.

Intervention. As with antibiotics, obtain specimens for culture and sensitivity before starting therapy. However, the initial dose is administered as soon as adequate specimens are obtained.

Administer multiple-dosage units, prescribed as a single dose, over 15 minutes to help prevent nausea and vomiting. Treat palliatively with antiemetics if these symptoms occur.

Education. Encourage the client to comply with the full course of therapy, even if feeling better. Progress should be monitored by regular visits to the health care provider.

Advise the client to report any syncope, dizziness, or drowsiness to the physician.

As with amphotericin B, advise the client to complete dental work prior to, or delay it until after, a course of flucytosine. Recommend the gentle use of toothbrushes and dental floss and avoiding toothpicks because of the risk of gingival bleeding.

Evaluation. The serum level of flucytosine may be measured to ascertain whether it is being maintained in the therapeutic range, 25 to 120 μg/ml. Monitor the client for signs of bone marrow depression such as sore throat and fever and signs of unusual bleeding, bruising, weakness, or tiredness.

griseofulvin capsules (Grisactin)
griseofulvin oral suspension, microsize (Grifulvin V)
griseofulvin tablets, microsize (Fulvicin-U/F,
Grifulvin V, Grisovin-FP✳)
griseofulvin tablets, ultramicrosize (Fulvicin P/G,
Grisactin Ultra, Gris-PED)

Mechanism of action. Inhibits fungus cell mitosis during metaphase. Also deposited in the keratin precursor cells in skin, hair, and nails, thus inhibiting fungal invasion of the keratin. When infested keratin is shed, healthy keratin will replace it.

Indications. Treatment of strains of organisms susceptible to griseofulvin; onychomycosis, tinea barbae, tinea capitis, tinea corporis, tinea cruris, and tinea pedis.

Pharmacokinetics

Absorption. Microsize oral absorption varies from 25% to 70%; ultramicrosize is nearly completely absorbed. If administered with or after a fatty meal, absorption is enhanced.

Distribution. Keratin layers in skin, hair, and nails. Little of the drug is distributed in body tissues and fluid.

Half-life. 24 hours.

Time to peak serum level. In approximately 24 hours after a single dose of the ultramicrosize griseofulvin (250 mg) or microsize griseofulvin (500 mg).

Metabolism. Liver.

Excretion. Kidneys.

Side effects/adverse reactions. See Table 60-2.

Significant drug interactions. When griseofulvin is given concurrently with the following drugs, the following interactions may occur.

Drug	Possible Effect and Management
anticoagulants, oral: coumarin or indandione	Decreased anticoagulant effect may be noted; monitor prothrombin times closely until a stable serum level is achieved. Dosage adjustments may be required during and after griseofulvin administration.
contraceptives, estrogen-containing oral	Chronic, long-term use of griseofulvin may decrease the effectiveness of oral contraceptives. May see intercycle menstrual bleeding, amenorrhea, or pregnancy. Advise client to use an alternate method of contraception when taking griseofulvin.
other photosensitizing medications	May result in additive photosensitive effects; monitor closely if given concurrently.

Dosage and administration

griseofulvin capsules/tablets (microsize)
griseofulvin oral suspension (microsize)
Adults
To treat tinea corporis, tinea cruris, or tinea capitis: 500 mg orally daily as single dose or in two divided doses.
To treat tinea pedis or onychomycosis: 1 g orally in two divided doses.

Children. 10 mg/kg orally or 300 mg/m² daily in single dose or in two divided doses; children 14 to 23 kg, 125 to 250 mg orally daily as single dose or in two divided doses; children 23 kg and over; 250 to 500 mg orally daily as a single dose or in two divided doses.

griseofulvin tablets (ultramicrosize)
Adults
To treat tinea corporis, tinea cruris, or tinea capitis: 250 to 330 mg orally daily as a single dose or in two divided doses.
To treat tinea pedis or onychomycosis: 500 to 660 mg orally daily in two divided doses.
Children. 5.5 to 7.3 mg/kg orally daily as a single dose or in two divided doses; children 14 to 23 kg, 62.5 to 165 mg orally daily as a single dose or in two divided doses; children 23 kg and over, 125 to 330 mg orally daily as a single dose or in two divided doses.

Pregnancy safety. Not established.

NURSING CONSIDERATIONS

Assessment. If the client has preexisting porphyria, lupus erythematosus, or hepatic function impairment, administer the drug with caution.

Intervention. Administer with meals to help prevent gastrointestinal distress and to enhance absorption. Therapy is even more effective if the meal is fatty. If the client is on a low-fat diet, consult the physician.

Administer the oral suspension using the calibrated measuring device provided by the manufacturer.

Education. Encourage the client to comply with the full course of therapy, even if feeling better. Regular visits to the physician are necessary to check progress. Therapy is continued until a clinical or laboratory examination indicates the causative organism is eradicated.

Frequent shampoos and clipping of the hair and nails will support the therapeutic effect of the drug, as will keeping affected skin areas clean and dry.

Advise the client that skin may be more sensitive to sunlight and recommend avoiding direct sunlight and using sun screens.

Advise the client to report any symptoms of fever and sore throat to the health care provider, as they may indicate blood dyscrasias.

Because the drug may cause dizziness, the client should avoid tasks that require mental alertness until the response to the drug can be ascertained.

Instruct the client about good oral hygiene and to report any soreness or irritation of the mouth, which might indicate a fungal overgrowth.

Instruct female clients taking estrogen-containing oral contraceptives to use an alternative or additional form of contraception while taking griseofulvin.

Advise the client not to ingest alcoholic beverages

while taking griseofulvin, because it may potentiate the effects of alcohol, causing tachycardia and flushing.

Evaluation. Monitor blood counts and hepatic and renal function studies periodically during therapy.

ketoconazole (Nizoral)

Mechanism of action. Depending on concentration, ketoconazole may be fungistatic or fungicidal. It alters the biosynthesis of fungal cell wall sterols, thus altering cell permeability and causing loss of essential intracellular substances. It also inhibits the synthesis of triglycerides and phospholipids by fungus and inhibits oxidative and peroxidative enzyme activity, which leads to an intracellular accumulation of toxic concentrations of hydrogen peroxide, which subsequently causes cellular deterioration and death. In *Candida albicans,* it interferes with the conversion of blastospores into the invasive mycelial form.

Indications. Treatment of blastomycosis, disseminated candidiasis, mucocutaneous candidiasis, oropharyngeal candidiasis, candiduria, chromomycosis, coccidioidomycosis, histoplasmosis, paracoccidioidomycosis, and tinea corporis, tinea cruris, tinea pedis, and tinea versicolor by strains of organisms susceptible to this drug.

Pharmacokinetics

Absorption. Requires acid media for dissolution and absorption. Usually very well absorbed in otherwise healthy clients.

Distribution. Widely distributed in humans to inflamed joint fluid, saliva, bile, urine, sebum, feces, tendons, skin, or soft tissues.

Protein binding. High, primarily to albumin.

Half-life. Alpha phase: between 1.4 and 3.3 hours during first 10 hours; beta phase: 8 hours afterward.

Time to peak serum level. Within 1 to 4 hours.

Metabolism. Liver.

Excretion. Bile, primary route; kidneys, 13%.

Side effects/adverse reactions. See Table 60-2.

Significant drug interactions. When ketoconazole is given concurrently with the following drugs, the following interactions may occur.

Drug	Possible Effect and Management
alcohol or other hepatotoxic drugs	Increases risk for hepatotoxicity. If possible, avoid other hepatotoxic medications. Monitor closely.
cyclosporine	May increase serum levels of cyclosporine and increase potential for nephrotoxicity. If given together, monitor closely. Serum levels of cyclosporine should be obtained and monitored.
histamine H_2-receptor blocking agents (cimetidine, famotidine, ranitidine)	Usually increases GI pH, which can reduce absorption of ketoconazole. Advise clients to take these drugs approximately 2 hours after ketoconazole.
isoniazid or rifampin	When both isoniazid and rifampin are given with ketoconazole, a decrease in serum levels of ketoconazole or rifampin is noted. In some cases, serum levels are not detectable. If necessary to use this combination, monitor very closely.

Dosage and administration. Oral suspension/tablets.

Adults. For systemic antifungal effects, 200 to 400 mg orally daily. Tinea versicolor, 200 mg orally once daily for 5 to 10 days. Maximum daily dose is 1 g.

Children. For systemic antifungal effects in infants and children up to 2 years old, not established. For children 2 years and older, 3.3 to 6.6 mg/kg orally, once daily.

Pregnancy safety. FDA category C.

NURSING CONSIDERATIONS

Assessment. Ascertain whether the client has a history of alcoholism or liver function impairment. If so, ketoconazole should be used with caution, as the drug is hepatotoxic.

Intervention. Take culture specimens before beginning drug therapy. Once adequate specimens are obtained, therapy should not be delayed.

For clients with aclorhydria, absorption may decrease. To minimize this effect, dissolve each tablet in 4 ml of 0.2N hydrochloric acid. The solution may be further diluted with a small amount of water and administered through a plastic or glass straw to prevent contact with the teeth. Have the client rinse his or her mouth with water and swallow the solution. If antacids, anticholinergics, or H_2 blockers are needed, give at least 2 hours after administering ketoconazole, since these drugs may decrease absorption.

Education. Recommend that the client take ketoconazole with meals or food to decrease the risk of gastrointestinal distress. Therapy is usually long term; at times it lasts months or years. Encourage the client to continue to take the medication for the full course of therapy even if feeling better. Taking the drug at the same time every day increases compliance.

Advise the client to visit the health care provider regularly to monitor progress. Infected areas should be evaluated periodically.

Caution the client to avoid alcoholic beverages while on this course of therapy.

Advise the client to avoid exposure to bright light or to wear sunglasses because of the drug's photophobic effects.

Because ketoconazole causes drowsiness, caution the client to avoid activities that require mental alertness until the response to the drug has been determined.

Evaluation. Perform hepatic function studies before and periodically during the course of therapy. Observe the client for clinical symptoms such as nausea, lethargy, yellowing of the eyes or skin, skin rash, dark urine, or clay-colored stools.

Men may experience enlargement of the breasts and decreased sexual ability because the drug decreases testosterone and adrenal steroid levels.

miconazole injection (Monistat IV)

Mechanism of action. Depending on its concentration, miconazole may be fungistatic or fungicidal. It alters the biosynthesis of fungal cell wall sterols, thus altering cell permeability, which results in the loss of essential intracellular substances. It also inhibits the synthesis of triglycerides and phospholipids by fungus; inhibits oxidative and peroxidative enzyme activity, which leads to an intracellular accumulation of toxic concentrations of hydrogen peroxide and subsequent cellular deterioration and death. In *Candida albicans,* it interferes with the conversion of blastospores into invasive mycelial form.

Indications. Susceptible strains of fungus in disseminated candidiasis, mucocutaneous (chronic) candidiasis, coccidioidomycosis, cryptococcosis, fungal meningitis, paracoccidioidomycosis, petriellidiosis, and fungal urinary bladder infections. This drug is reserved as a second-line drug (after systemic amphotericin B and ketoconazole) for the treatment of severe systemic fungal infections. It is more toxic and often not as effective as the previously mentioned drugs.

Side effects/adverse reactions. See Table 60-2.

Significant drug interactions. None.

Dosage and administration. Parenteral dosage form.

Adults. 200 mg to 1.2 g by intravenous infusion. See package insert or current USP-DI for specific recommended doses for fungal infections.

Children. Children up to 1 year old, doses are not established. For children 1 year and older, 20 to 40 mg/kg daily by intravenous infusion. Do not exceed 15 mg/kg.

Pregnancy safety. Not established.

NURSING CONSIDERATIONS

Assessment. As with other antifungal agents, obtain culture specimens before beginning drug therapy. However, start therapy as soon as adequate specimens are obtained rather than waiting for the culture results.

Intervention. Administer intravenous infusions of miconazole over 30 to 60 minutes to prevent dysrhythmias or increases in heart rate that may result from rapid administration.

Minimize nausea and vomiting secondary to the administration of miconazole by reducing the dosage, slowing the infusion rate, or administering an antiemetic before beginning the infusion. Infusions of the drug should not be administered at mealtimes to also help prevent gastrointestinal effects.

Dilute each dose of miconazole in at least 200 ml of 0.9% sodium chloride solution or 5% dextrose injection for intravenous infusion. This solution will be stable at room temperature for 24 hours. If the solution darkens, it should be discarded, as it has deteriorated. Do not mix with other medications.

Education. Instruct the client to alert the nurse if he or she has trouble breathing, skin rash, or fever and chills, which are signs of hypersensitivity.

Evaluation. Monitor the client's infection throughout the course of therapy. The intravenous site should be monitored periodically for pain and inflammation, which would indicate phlebitis. Monitor hematocrit and hemoglobin values for adverse effects of anemia. Serum electrolytes and lipids should be monitored periodically.

nystatin lozenges (Mycostatin)
nystatin oral suspension (Mycostatin, Nadostine✽)
nystatin for oral suspension (Nilstat)
nystatin tablets (Mycostatin, Nadostine✽, Nilstat)

Nystatin, an antibiotic obtained from *Streptomyces noursei,* is primarily used to treat oropharyngeal infections caused by the monilial organism *Candida albicans.* Although not an approved indication, oropharyngeal candidiasis is often treated with nystatin vaginal tablets in lozenge form, mainly because they dissolve slowly.

Mechanism of action. Adheres to sterols in the fungal cell membrane, leading to a loss of essential intercellular contents.

Indications. Candidiasis-induced oropharyngeal infections.

Pharmacokinetics

Absorption. Not absorbed from gastrointestinal tract.

Excretion. Feces.

Side effects/adverse reactions. Infrequent. In high dosages, may cause diarrhea, nausea, vomiting, or abdominal distress.

Significant drug interactions. None.

Dosage and administration

nystatin lozenges

Adults. Oral: dissolve lozenge completely in mouth (200,000 to 400,000 units) four or five times daily for up to 2 weeks.

Children. See adult dosage.

nystatin oral suspension

Adults. Orally, 400,000 to 600,000 units four times daily.

Children. Premature and low-birth-weight infants: 100,000 units orally four times daily; older infants: 200,000 units orally four times daily; children, see adult dose.

nystatin tablets

Adults. Orally, 500,000 to 1 million units three times daily.

Children. Premature and low-birth-weight infants and older infants: see nystatin oral suspension; children, orally, 500,000 units four times daily.

Pregnancy safety. Not established.

NURSING CONSIDERATIONS

Intervention. Shake oral suspensions thoroughly before measuring dosages. With the prepared oral suspension, use the calibrated dosage-measuring device provided by the manufacturer. When mixing dry powdered nystatin, add the dose to 120 to 240 ml of water; administer immediately as it contains no preservatives. Vaginal tablets may be used as lozenges to treat oral candidiasis because they are slow to dissolve and are in contact longer with the buccal mucous membrane.

Education. Instruct the client to perform oral hygiene before taking each dose of nystatin. Half the dosage is placed in each side of the mouth. The medication is swished and then held in the mouth for as long as possible. Vaginal tablets are to be dissolved slowly in the mouth as with throat lozenges.

Caution the client to complete the full course of therapy even if feeling better. It should be continued for at least 48 hours after normal culture results are obtained and symptoms have disappeared.

Alert the client to report to the health care provider symptoms of nausea, vomiting, diarrhea, or increased irritation at the site of infection.

Evaluation. Nystatin is virtually nontoxic and well tolerated by all age groups. Monitor the client's infection throughout the course of therapy.

ANTIVIRAL DRUGS

Chemotherapy for viral diseases has been more limited than chemotherapy for bacterial diseases because development and clinical application of antiviral drugs are difficult. In many viral infections, the replication of the virus in the body reaches its peak before any clinical symptoms appear. By the time signs and symptoms of illness appear, the multiplication of the virus is ending, and the subsequent course of the illness has been determined. To be clinically effective, therefore, antiviral drugs must be administered in a **chemoprophylactic** manner—that is, before disease appears. A second factor limiting the development of antiviral drugs is that viruses are true parasites; they replicate within the mammalian cell and utilize the host cells' enzyme systems. Thus drugs that would inhibit virus replication would also disturb the host cells and

therefore would be too toxic for use.

Table 60-3 lists common systemic antiviral agents.

acyclovir capsules/tablets (Zovirax)

Mechanism of action. Acyclovir is selectively taken up by herpes simplex virus (HSV)–infected cells and converted to an active triphosphate form, which is then incorporated into growing DNA chains produced by the virus, thus terminating chain development.

Indications. Herpes genitalis infections; the oral form is used to treat and manage herpes genitalis infections in immunocompromised and uncompromised clients. Injectable acyclovir is used to treat severe initial herpes genitalis infections in nonimmunocompromised clients.

Pharmacokinetics

Absorption. Oral dosage form is poorly (15% to 30%) absorbed, but serum levels achieved are therapeutic.

Distribution. Widely disseminated to various body fluids and tissues such as brain, kidneys, lungs, muscle, spleen, uterus, vaginal mucosa and secretions, cerebrospinal fluid (CSF), and herpetic vesicular fluid. CSF levels are approximately 50% of the serum concentration.

Half-life. Normal creatinine clearance is approximately 2.5 hours.

Mean peak serum level at steady state

Oral. Approximately 0.6 μg/ml after a 200 mg dose every 4 hours for 5 days; approximately 1.2 μg/ml after a 400 mg dose every 4 hours for 5 days.

Parenteral. Approximately 10 μg/ml after a 5 mg/kg dose every 8 hours (administer over 1 hour).

Metabolism. Liver.

Excretion. Kidneys.

Side effects/adverse reactions. See Table 60-4.

Significant drug interactions. When acyclovir is given concurrently with the following drugs, the following interactions may occur.

Drug	Possible Effect and Management
Interferon or methotrexate, intrathecal	When given with parenteral acyclovir, monitor closely for neurologic abnormalities, such as lethargy, obtundation, tremors, confusion, hallucinations, agitation, seizures, or coma.

TABLE 60-3 Systemic Antiviral Agents

Drug	Trade names
acyclovir	Zovirax
amantadine HCl	Symadine, Symmetrel
ribavirin	Virazole, Vilona✦, Viramid✦
vidarabine	Vira-A
zidovudine	Retrovir

TABLE 60-4 Antiviral Drugs: Side Effects/Adverse Reactions

Drug	Side effects*	Adverse reactions†
acyclovir	*Oral* Most frequent with chronic usage: diarrhea, dizziness, headache, pain in joints, nausea or vomiting. Less frequent with chronic use: acne, anorexia, insomnia. *Injectable form* Dizziness. Less frequent: headache, sweating.	*Oral* Less frequent with chronic usage: menstrual irregularities, rash. *Injectable form* More frequent: rash or hives. Less frequent: bloody urine, confusion, hallucinations, tremors. Rare (usually with bolus injection): stomach pain, respiratory difficulties, decreased urination, thirst, anorexia, nausea or vomiting, increased weakness, convulsions.
amantadine	Most frequent: anorexia, nausea, anxiety, red-purple skin spots, increased irritability, dizziness, insomnia, difficulty concentrating, nightmares. Less frequent/rare: visual disturbances, dry mouth, nose, and throat, headache, rash, vomiting, constipation, increased weakness.	Most frequent: mood changes, hallucinations, confusion (especially in elderly). Less frequent: difficulty in urination, hypotension. Rare: slurred speech, oculogyric crisis, sore throat, fever. With chronic dosing: edema of feet or lower legs, shortness of breath, weight gain. Overdosage: severe confusion, serious mood alterations, convulsions, severe insomnia or nightmares.
ribavirin	Less frequent: dizziness, blurred vision, increased weakness, lightheadedness (hypotensive effect), visual alterations (feeling of particles in eye; photosensitivity, edema, pruritus, or red eyes).	None reported.
vidarabine	Frequency not reported: increased lacrimation, feeling of particles in eye.	Frequency not reported: photosensitivity, eye irritation (pruritus, redness, edema, pain, burning.)
zidovudine	Most frequent: taste alterations, nervousness, diarrhea, dizziness, headaches, anorexia, nausea, rash. Less frequent: stomach distress or pain, pruritus, mouth sores, edema of lips or tongue, insomnia, vomiting, faintness, confusion, anxiety, agitation.	Most frequent: chills, sore throat, elevated temperature, pale skin, increase in bleeding tendencies, increased weakness. Bone marrow depression may occur when drug is stopped: pale skin, chills, sore throat, elevated temperature, increase in bleeding episodes, increased weakness (agranulocytopenia and anemia).

*If side effects continue, increase, or disturb the client, inform the physician.
†If adverse reactions occur, contact the physician because medical intervention may be necessary.

Drug	Possible Effect and Management
other nephrotoxic drugs	May increase the potential for nephrotoxicity, especially if client already has renal impairment. Monitor renal function closely.

Dosage and administration
acyclovir capsules/tablets (Zovirax)

Adults. Herpes genitalis infections: initially, 200 mg orally every 4 hours during waking hours (five times daily) for 10 days. Intermittent therapy, 200 mg orally every 4 hours during waking hours (five times daily) for 5 days. As a chronic suppressant agent for recurrent infections, 200 mg orally every 8 hours for up to 6 months. (If necessary, may be increased up to 200 mg five times daily for up to 6 months.)

Note: adults with renal impairment will require a dosage adjustment. Check current package insert or USP DI for dosing instructions.

Children. Not established.

sterile acyclovir sodium (Zovirax)
Adults

For serious herpes genitalis infections: initially, 5 mg (base)/kg by intravenous infusion every 8 hours for 5 days. Administer at a constant rate over a minimum of 1 hour.

For herpes simplex (HSV-1 and HSV-2) mucocutaneous infections in immunocompromised individuals: 5 to 10 mg/kg by intravenous infusion every 8 hours for 7 to 10 days. Administer at a constant rate for a minimum of 1 hour.

For renal impairment: see current package insert or USP-DI for dosing instructions.

Maximum daily dose is up to 30 mg/kg or 1.5 g/m². Children

For serious herpes genitalis infections: initially for infants and children up to 12 years old, 250 mg (base)/m² every 8 hours for 5 days. Give at a constant rate for a minimum of 1 hour. Children 12 years and older, see adult dose.

For herpes simplex (HSV-1 and HSV-2) mucocutaneous infections in immunocompromised individuals: infants and children up to 12 years old, 250 mg (base)/m² every 8 hours for 1 week. Give at a constant rate for a minimum of 1 hour; children 12 years and older: see adult dose.

Pregnancy safety. FDA category C.

NURSING CONSIDERATIONS

Assessment. If the client has preexisting dehydration or renal function impairment, use acyclovir with caution, as these clients are at greater risk for nephrotoxicity. A history of neurologic abnormalities or a previous neurologic reaction to cytotoxic agents may indicate a tendency for such responses to acyclovir.

Assess lesions before administering the drug and daily throughout therapy.

Intervention. The capsules may be administered with meals to minimize gastrointestinal distress. Intravenous acyclovir should be administered via infusion pump at a constant rate for at least 1 hour to prevent precipitation of drug crystals in the renal tubules. The client should also be hydrated during the infusion to prevent this effect. Avoid rapid or bolus injection of the drug. Rotate infusion sites to prevent phlebitis. The intravenous solution is not to be used topically, orally, or administered intramuscularly or subcutaneously.

Education. The client will need accurate information about herpes. Because herpes genitalis is sexually transmitted, misinformation about it abounds. The client should avoid sexual activity if either or any participant has symptoms of herpes. Condom use may help prevent the spread of the infection, but spermicidal jellies or diaphragms probably will not. Acyclovir will not prevent the transmission of the disease or cure it.

The full course of therapy should be taken; however, caution the client not to take the drug longer than prescribed. Six months is generally the limit of long-term therapy. Report to the health care provider if symptoms do not ease.

Medication should be initiated as soon as possible after symptoms appear. The client should be instructed to begin the medication as soon as itching, tingling, or pain develop at the site to minimize the episode of herpes.

Instruct the client regarding comfort measures such as wearing loose-fitting clothing to minimize irritation of the lesions. The infected areas should be kept clean and dry.

Caution female clients to obtain a Pap smear at least annually, as women with genital herpes are at higher risk for cervical cancer than women without genital herpes.

As dizziness is an adverse effect of this agent, the client should be cautioned against performing tasks that require mental alertness, such as driving, until the response to the drug has been ascertained.

The client should be encouraged to maintain good dental hygiene and visit the dentist regularly for teeth cleaning and to monitor for the development of gingival hyperplasia.

Evaluation. Renal function studies should be done before and during therapy to monitor for the drug's nephrotoxic effects. Fluid intake and output should be monitored, particularly if the client is receiving bolus injections of acyclovir.

---

amantadine hydrochloride capsules (Symadine, Symmetrel)
amantadine hydrochloride syrup (Symmetrel)

Mechanism of action. Although its mechanism of action is not fully understood, amantadine is believed to prevent influenza A virus from penetrating respiratory epithelial cells, to uncoat the virus, and thus release viral nucleic acid into host cells.

Indications. Influenza A (prevention and treatment) parkinsonism, and extrapyramidal reactions (drug-induced).

Pharmacokinetics

Absorption. Very good.

Distribution. To nasal secretions and saliva.

Metabolism. None.

Half-life. Normally, within 11 to 15 hours. In renal failure, within 24 hours (7 to 10 days in chronic dialysis clients).

Onset of action. For drug-induced extrapyramidal reactions, approximately 48 hours.

Time to peak serum level. Within 2 to 4 hours (range is 1 to 8 hours). Steady-state is reached in 2 to 3 days of daily drug administration.

Peak serum level. Approximately 0.3 µg/ml; steady-state levels are 0.2 to 0.9 µg/ml. Toxicity is seen when serum levels exceed 1.5 to 2 µg/ml.

Excretion. Kidneys.

Side effects/adverse reactions. See Table 60-4.

Significant drug interactions. When amantadine is given concurrently with the following drugs, the following interactions may occur.

Drug	Possible Effect and Management
alcohol	Not recommended; increased risk for CNS side effects such as dizziness, fainting episodes, confusion, or circulatory problems reported.

Drug
CNS-stimulating agents

Possible Effect and Management
May cause increased CNS stimulation, resulting in insomnia, increased irritability and nervousness. Cardiac arrhythmias and convulsions may also occur. Avoid if possible. If given concurrently, be sure to monitor closely.

Dosage and administration. Oral.

Adults. As antiviral agent: 200 mg orally daily or 100 mg every 12 hours. Antidyskinetic: 100 mg orally once or twice a day. Clients with renal impairment should check the current PDR or USP DI for dosing instructions. Maximum daily dosage: antiviral, 200 mg/day; antidyskinetic, 400 mg/day.

Children. Neonates and infants up to a year old, not established; Children 1 to 9 years old, 1.5 to 3 mg/kg orally every 8 hours or 2.2 to 4.4 mg/kg orally every 12 hours; maximum dose is 200 mg daily; children 9 to 12 years old, 100 mg orally every 12 hours; children 12 years old and older, see adult dosage.

Pregnancy safety. FDA category C.

NURSING CONSIDERATIONS

Assessment. When the client's health assessment is done before drug therapy, the following health problems should indicate cautious use of amantadine: congestive heart failure and/or peripheral edema, as the drug may worsen the condition; epilepsy, as the drug may increase seizure activity; and renal impairment, as accumulation of the drug increases CNS adverse effects.

Elderly clients are more prone to experience confusion and difficulty in urination as frequent effects of amantadine because of its antimuscarinic activity.

Intervention. Syncope, insomnia, and nausea may be minimized by changing from a once-daily dosage to a twice-daily schedule. Administering the last daily dose several hours before bedtime helps to minimize insomnia.

When administering the syrup form of the drug, use the calibrated measuring device provided by the manufacturer.

Education. Caution the client to avoid alcoholic beverages while taking amantadine, as alcohol increases the risk of CNS effects such as dizziness, syncope, and confusion.

If the client is taking amantadine as an antiviral medication, its course should be started before, or as soon as possible after, exposure. Client should complete the full course of therapy and should notify the health care provider if symptoms do not decrease within a few days.

Clients taking the drug as an antidyskinetic medication,

should complete the course of therapy as prescribed and not take more than the prescribed dosage. The client should be advised that it may require 2 or more weeks to obtain full benefit from the drug. Counsel the client to gradually resume physical activities. The drug dosage should be discontinued gradually.

Mental confusion, hallucinations, and difficulty sleeping are indications of CNS toxicity and should be reported to the physician promptly.

Advise clients to change positions from lying to sitting or standing and from sitting to standing with caution because of the orthostatic effects of amantadine.

Clients may decrease the discomfort of mouth dryness with ice, sugarless gum, or candy.

Alert the client to the possible occurrence of a purplish, red rash, which disappears 2 to 12 weeks after the medication is discontinued.

Because amantadine may cause drowsiness or dizziness, caution the client to avoid tasks such as driving until the response to the drug has been determined.

Evaluation. Closely monitor clients receiving dosages over 200 mg/day for side effects or adverse reactions. Blood pressure and TPR monitoring is indicated, particularly for the first few days after a dosage increase.

If the client is taking amantadine for parkinsonism, dyskinetic symptoms such as tremors, rigidity, and disturbances of gait should be monitored throughout the course of therapy.

ribavirin for inhalation aerosol (Virazole, Vilona❋, Viramid❋)

Mechanism of action. Unknown. The drug is believed to reduce intracellular guanosine triphosphate (GTP) storage and impair viral RNA and protein synthesis, thus inhibiting viral duplication, spread to other cells, or both.

Indications. Serious viral pneumonia caused by respiratory syncytial virus (RSV).

Pharmacokinetics

Absorption. Well absorbed after oral inhalation; orally, rapidly absorbed from gastrointestinal tract.

Distribution. To plasma, secretions in respiratory tract, and erythrocytes. High levels are found in respiratory tract secretions.

Half-life. Elimination half-life: inhalation, 9.5 hours; orally, approximately 24 hours; in erythrocytes (RBCs), 40 days.

Time to peak serum level. Orally, within 1 to 1.5 hours.

Mean peak serum level. Approximately 0.2 μg/ml (0.8 μmol) in children who receive ribavirin aerosol by face mask for 2.5 hours daily over 3 days; approximately 1.7 μg/ml (6.8 μmol) in children who receive ribavirin aerosol by face mask or mist tent for 20 hr/day for 5 days.

Metabolism. Liver.

Excretion. Kidneys (between 30% and 55% in urine in 72 to 80 hours).

Side effects/adverse reactions. See Table 60-4.

Significant drug interactions. None.

Dosage and administration

ribavirin for inhalation aerosol

Adults. Not established.

Children. For viral pneumonia, oral inhalation via a Viratek small-particle aerosol generator, using a 20-mg/ml ribavirin concentration in the reservoir. Administer over 12 to 18 hr/day for 3 to 7 days.

Pregnancy safety. FDA category X.

NURSING CONSIDERATIONS

Intervention. Therapy with ribavirin may begin before the diagnosis is determined by diagnostic tests; however, treatment should not continue if the presence of the respiratory syncytial virus (RSV) is not confirmed.

Ribavirin aerosol is to be administered only with the Viratek SPAG Model SPAG-2. See the SPAG-2 manual for exceptions.

To prepare the solution for inhalation, add a measured quantity of sterile water for injection or for inhalation, which is adequate to dissolve the drug, to each 6-g vial. Do not use bacteriostatic water. Transfer the solution to a clean, sterilized SPAG-2 reservoir. Dilute the solution with sterile water to a total volume of 300 ml. Ensure that the final solution is free of particulate matter. Always discard the remaining solution as its level gets low and add freshly reconstituted solution to the reservoir. The solution retains its potency at room temperature for 24 hours. Do not administer concurrently with any other medication by aerosolization.

Evaluation. If administered to clients receiving ventilation assistance, observe for increased positive-end expiratory pressure and increased positive inspiratory pressure, which occur if ribavirin precipitates within the ventilator apparatus. The equipment should be checked at least every half hour to prevent fluid accumulation in the tubing.

vidarabine (Adenine Arabinoside, Ara-A) (Vira-A)

Mechanism of action. Unknown, although in cells it is converted to a triphosphate that is a selective competitive inhibitor of DNA polymerase. It may also penetrate the viral DNA molecule at different positions, thus terminating the chain.

Indication. Herpes simplex encephalitis virus.

Pharmacokinetics

Parenteral dosage form

Distribution. Well distributed to body tissues; con-

verted to Ara-Hx, which has about 10% of the antiviral activity of vidarabine.

Metabolism. Half-life (mean) for Ara-A is 1 hour; for Ara-Hx, OS 3.3 hours.

Excretion. Kidneys.

Side effects/adverse reactions. See Table 60-4.

Significant drug interactions. None reported. Monitor when client is given allopurinol, as it may interfere with vidarabine metabolism.

Dosage and administration

Adults. For slow intravenous infusion only. Administer 15 mg/kg for 19 days. Infuse the total daily dose very slowly over 12 to 24 hours. Closely follow manufacturer's instructions for preparation.

Pregnancy safety. FDA category C.

NURSING CONSIDERATIONS

Intervention. Parenteral vidarabine is for intravenous use only. It is poorly absorbed from intramuscular or subcutaneous sites.

For intravenous administration, dilute to a concentration of less than 0.5 mg/ml with any intravenous solution except for blood products or protein solutions. For ease of dissolution, warm the intravenous solution to 35° to 40° C (95° to 100° F). Shake until the solution is completely clear. Administer using an in-line filter (0.45-μm pore size or smaller). Use an infusion pump for accurate rate flow.

Evaluation. When vidarabine is administered for herpes simplex virus (HSV) encephalitis, monitor the level of consciousness and neurologic status throughout therapy.

Monitor blood studies, including hemoglobin, hematocrit, and blood cell counts, periodically during therapy.

zidovudine capsules (Retrovir)

Mechanism of action. May be virustatic. Converted in the virus to triphosphate, which competes with natural thymidine triphosphate for incorporation in growing chains of viral DNA. Once in the DNA chain, it inhibits viral replication. It has a greater affinity for retroviral reverse transcriptase than for the human alpha-DNA polymerase; thus it selectively inhibits viral replication.

Indications. Acquired immune deficiency syndrome (AIDS) or treatment of AIDS-related complex (ARC).

Pharmacokinetics

Absorption. Very good from gastrointestinal tract. It has a first-pass metabolism in the liver that reduces the average bioavailability to 65%.

Distribution. To plasma and cerebrospinal fluid (CSF). CSF concentration is between 50% to 60% of serum levels 4 hours after dosing.

Half-life. Zidovudine: orally, about 1 hour (range, 0.8 to 1.9 hours). Major metabolite, or GAZT: 1 hour (range, 0.6 to 1.7 hours). Intravenous, about 1.1 hours (range 0.5 to 2.9 hours).

Time to peak plasma level. Between 0.5 to 1.5 hours

Peak serum level. Between 1.5 and 2 μmol/l after a 1 hour intravenous infusion of 1 mg/kg or an oral dose of 2 mg/kg. Between 4 and 6 μmol/l after a 1-hour intravenous infusion of 2.5 mg/kg or an oral dose of 5 mg/kg. Between 6 and 10 μmol/l after a 1-hour intravenous infusion of 5 mg/kg or an oral dose of 10 mg/kg.

Metabolism. Liver.

Excretion. Kidneys.

Side effects/adverse reactions. See Table 60-4.

Signficant drug interactions. When zidovudine is given concurrently with the following drugs, the following interactions may occur.

Drug	Possible Effect and Management
acetaminophen, aspirin, benzodiazepines, cimetidine, indomethacin, morphine, or sulfonamides	May inhibit hepatic metabolism and decrease excretion of zidovudine. Avoid concurrent usage to avoid toxicity.
bone marrow depressants, radiation therapy	May exacerbate bone marrow depression and toxicity. Dosage reductions may be necessary. Monitor closely.

Dosage and administration

Adults. 200 mg orally every 4 hours around the clock. Maximum daily dose is up to 60 mg/kg.

Children. Not established.

Pregnancy safety. FDA category C.

NURSING CONSIDERATIONS

Assessment. Assess the client's health before initiating zidovudine therapy. The following health problems indicate that the drug is to be used with caution: bone marrow depression, which may result in blood dyscrasias; hepatic and renal function impairment, which may affect elimination of the drug and cause toxicity; and folic acid or vitamin B$_{12}$ deficiency, which may result in increased sensitivity to hematotoxicity.

Intervention. The client may experience changes in taste, swelling of the lips and tongue, and mouth ulcers. These symptoms may affect the client's desire or ability to eat. The client must receive good oral hygiene to prevent infection and promote comfort. Food and fluid intake should be monitored to ensure adequate nutrition. Encourage the client to take small but frequent high-protein meals. Serve meals attractively and cater to the client's food preferences. Bland and smooth textured foods may be better tolerated.

Education. Advise the client to take the medication exactly as prescribed and not to take more in the hope that it will be more effective or to discontinue the medication without medical advice in despair that it is not effective. Other medications should not be taken concurrently without the approval of the physician. The client should take the medication every 4 hours around the clock. Setting an alarm clock to interrupt sleep and maintain this schedule can ensure therapeutic blood levels.

The client should be advised of the importance of regular supervision by the health care provider to check blood counts.

Alert the client that dizziness and syncope are effects of zidovudine and that hazardous activities requiring mental alertness should be avoided until the response to the drug has been determined.

Advise the client to avoid sexual contact, to use condoms to prevent transmission of the AIDS virus to sexual partners, and not to share needles with others.

Advise the client to complete essential dental work before starting therapy with zidovudine or to delay it until completing the course of the drug because bone marrow depressant effects may result in gingival bleeding and delayed healing. Teach appropriate oral hygiene, including gentle use of toothbrushes and floss and avoiding toothpicks.

Evaluation. Perform CBCs at least every 2 weeks during therapy. Observe the client for fever, sore throat, unusual bleeding or bruising, or unusual tiredness, all of which are symptoms of bone marrow depression. These symptoms may occur even after the medication is discontinued and should be reported to the health care provider.

KEY TERMS

candidiasis, page 934
chemoprophylactic, page 941
fungi, page 934
mycoses, page 934

BIBLIOGRAPHY

American Hospital Formulary Service: AHFS drug information '87, Bethesda, 1987, American Society of Hospital Pharmacists, Inc.

Braunwald, E, and others, eds. Harrison's principles of internal medicine, ed 11, New York, 1987, McGraw-Hill Book Co.

Casto, DT: Amantadine hydrochloride: an agent for the prevention and treatment of influenza A infection, J Pediatr Health Care 1(1):51, 1987.

Collins, PJ: Fighting back against AIDS, Patient Care 19(19):131, 1985.

Crawshaw, JP: New options for genital herpes Dx/Rx, Patient Care 20(7):20, 1986.

DeQuesne, T: Drugs for viral infections, Midwife Health Visit Community Nurse 22(1):32, 1986.

Eggleston, M: Therapy of ocular herpes simplex infections, Infect Control 8(7):294, 1987.

Einstein, HE: Update on treatment of systemic fungal disease, Respir Ther 15(6):75, 1985.

Editorial: A sharper focus on flu control . . . emphasis on amantadine, Emerg Med 17(15):105, 1985.

Editorial: Acyclovir: antiviral agent, Aust Nurses J 15(9):57, 1986.

Hall, JE, and others: Amphotericin B dosage for disseminated candidiasis in premature infants, J Perinat 7(3):195, 1987.

Halpern, JS: Amantadine: antiviral agent for influenza A, JEN 11(3):158, 1985.

Hawkins, CC, and others: Fungal infections: opportunistic organisms in the immunocompromised, Consultant 25(8):93, 1985.

Job, ML, Matthews, HW, and Shulman, EM: Your guide to therapy of systemic fungal infections, US Pharmacist 11(7):41, 1986.

Kastrup, EK, ed: Facts and comparisons, St Louis, 1988, JB Lippincott Co.

Lamb, C: Fighting viral infections: a survey of new agents, Patient Care 20(19):65, 1986.

Lamb, C: Fungal infections from head to toe, Patient Care 21(11):62, 1987.

Lewis, MR: Tinea versicolor, Nurse Pract 11(2):30, 1986.

Masur, H: Fungal infections in AIDS patients. II. Optimal treatment regimens, Hosp Ther 12(9):47, 1987.

Mathewson, HS: Antiviral drugs for acute respiratory infections, Respir Care 31(1):46, 1986.

Pepper, GA: Oral acyclovir (Zovirax): major or minor miracle? Nurse Pract 10(12):50, 1985.

Rimar, JM: Ribavirin for treatment of RSV infection, MCN 11(6):413, 1986.

Ruben, FL: Influenza: when and how to use drug therapy . . . amantadine, Consultant 25(5):60, 1985.

Schoeneck, CLE: Acyclovir: a recently developed anti-herpes agent, Crit Care Nurse 5(4):8, 1985.

Schwarz, RH: Neonatal herpes: detection, treatment and prevention, Med Aspects Human Sexuality 19(3):36, 1985.

Sethi, ML: Viral diseases and drug therapy, US Pharmacist 10(11):42, 1985.

United States Pharmacopeial Convention: Drug information for the health care provider, ed 8, Rockville, Md, 1988, United States Pharmacopeial Convention, Inc.

Weintraub, M, and others: Ciclopirox: a chemically unique antifungal agent, Hosp Formul 20(5):575, 1985.

Weintraub, M, and others: Rimantadine: a new agent for the prophylaxis and treatment of influenza A, Hosp Formul 21(4):431, 1986.

Zabrosky, CA, and others: Acyclovir, Infect Control 7(4):228, 1986.

CHAPTER 61

Other Antimicrobial Drugs and Antiparasitic Drugs

Antimicrobial and antiparasitic agents include antimalarial, antituberculous, amebicidal, anthelmintic, and leprostatic medications. Sulfonamides are reviewed in Chapter 34, "Antimicrobials for Urinary Tract Infections."

MALARIA

Malaria is a prevalent disease in spite of efforts to control the causative parasite and insect vector. Malaria is generally limited to the tropics and subtropic areas, but cases are also imported into the United States and Canada. Four species of the genus *Plasmodium* are responsible for human malaria: *Plasmodium vivax, P. malariae, P. ovale,* and *P. falciparum. P. ovale,* which is found in West Africa, is considered rare. *P. falciparum* malaria is the most lethal form of malaria and is usually resistant to chloroquine.

Malaria is transmitted to humans by the bite of an infected female *Anopheles* mosquito, as well as by blood transfusions, congenitally, or contaminated needles commonly used by drug abusers. For clinical differences between the four species of malaria, see Table 61-1.

LIFE CYCLE OF MALARIAL PARASITE

To understand the chemotherapy of malaria, it is essential to review the life cycle of the malarial parasite, the

TABLE 61-1   Clinical Differences Between the Four Species Causing Malaria

Species	Presentation	Asexual cycle	Relapse
P. falciparum	Parasitemia (elevated), anemia (severe), renal impairment, possible brain tissue infestation, pulmonary edema, death	2 days	No; usually resistant to chloroquine
P. vivax	Rupture of spleen, anemia	2 days	Yes
P. ovale	—	2 days	Yes
P. malariae	Infection of red blood cells that persists for years; nephritis	3 days	No

plasmodium. Figure 61-1 presents the cycle in seven basic steps.

Plasmodia have two interdependent life cycles: the sexual cycle, which takes place in the mosquito, and the asexual cycle, which occurs in the human body.

Sexual cycle. The sexual cycle is noted in step 7 of Figure 61-1. The female *Anopheles* mosquito becomes the carrier of the parasite by drawing blood containing male and female forms from an infected person. These sexual forms of the parasite are known as *gametocytes.* In the stomach of the mosquito the female gametocytes are fertilized by the males; zygotes form, which result in numerous cell divisions that develop into sporozoites. The formation of sporozoites in the mosquito completes the sexual cycle. Sporozoites then migrate to the salivary glands of the infected mosquito and are injected into the bloodstream of the human by the bite of the female insect (step 1, Figure 61-1).

Asexual cycle. In the human the asexual cycle of the plasmodium consists of the *exoerythrocytic phase* and the *erythrocytic phase.*

Exoerythrocytic phase. Shortly after the introduction of the sporozoites into the circulation of the human, they leave the blood and enter fixed tissue cells (reticuloendothelial cells) of the liver, where multiplication and maturation take place (step 2). For a period of time (8 to 42 days), which varies with different plasmodia, the patient exhibits no symptoms, no parasites are found in erythrocytes, and the blood is noninfective. This phase is known as the *preerythrocytic* stage. The parasites are called primary tissue schizonts, or preerythrocytic forms. After the preerythrocytic stage, the young parasites burst from the liver cells as merozoites.

Erythrocytic phase. When merozoites enter the bloodstream, they penetrate the erythrocytes and begin the erythrocytic phase of their existence (step 3a). In the case of *P. vivax* (but not *P. falciparum*) some of the merozoites invade other tissue cells to form secondary exoerythrocytic forms (step 3b). The relapses in vivax and other forms of malaria are believed to be caused by the successive formations of merozoites produced by various secondary exoerythrocytic forms of the parasite. *Drugs affecting malarial parasites in the bloodstream do not always destroy those in the exoerythrocytic, or tissue, stage.*

After the merozoites bore into the red blood cells, they again multiply, but this time asexually, and erythrocytic schizonts are formed. The erythrocytic phase is completed when the parasitized red blood cells rupture, setting free many more merozoites that are formed from the schizonts. Pyrogenic substances are also liberated, causing a rapid rise in body temperature (step 4). Some of the merozoites may be destroyed in the plasma of the blood by leukocytes and other agents, but some enter other erythrocytes to repeat the cycle (step 5). The recurring chills, fever, and prostration that are prominent clinical symptoms of malaria occur when the red blood cells rupture and release the young parasites with foreign protein and cell products. The erythrocytic phase lasts 48 to 72 hours, depending on the plasmodium involved. After a few cycles, some of the asexual forms of the malarial parasites develop into sexual forms called gametocytes (step 6). When the mosquito bites a person infected with malarial parasites and ingests the sexual forms, the cycle begins again.

Persons who harbor the sexual forms of plasmodia are called *carriers,* since it is from carriers that mosquitoes receive the forms of the parasite that perpetuate the disease. The asexual forms cause the clinical symptoms of malaria. Carriers should avoid giving blood, since it is possible that the recipient of this blood will contract malaria or become a carrier. An increasing number of malaria cases (some fatal) have occurred from transfusions of infected blood. Some of these infected individuals who donated blood may have once lived in a malarious area. Any person who has had malaria or has been exposed to the disease by visiting a region where it is prevalent must be disqualified as a blood donor.

ANTIMALARIAL MEDICATIONS

The choice of a drug for treatment of malaria is based on the particular malarial strain involved and the stage of the *Plasmodium* life cycle. The drugs, therefore, are clas-

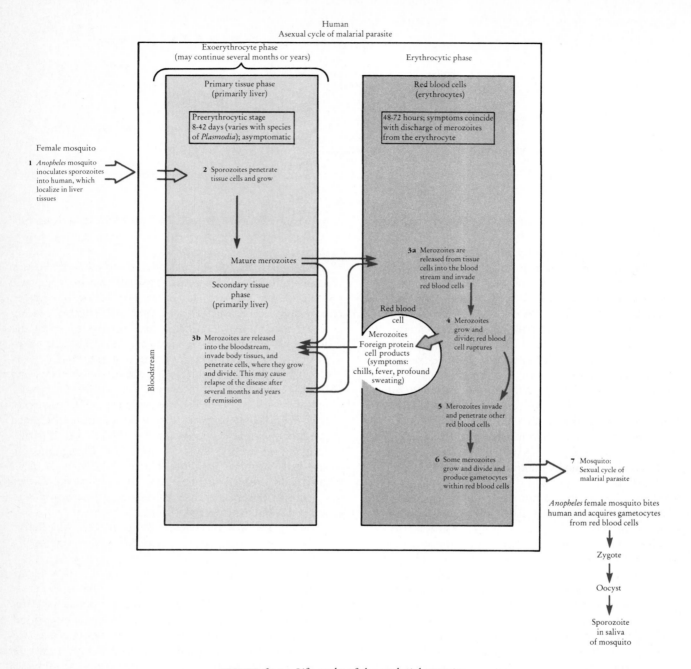

FIGURE 61-1   Life cycle of the malarial parasite.

sified according to the type of therapy they provide, which is as follows:

1. Prophylaxis is achieved in the preerythrocytic stage with drugs that are called *primary tissue schizonticides*. They destroy erythrocytic forms of the parasite, thereby preventing invasion of red blood cells. As a consequence, the drug prevents a malarial infection after the host is bitten by an infected mosquito. Pyrimethamine exerts an effective prophylactic effect on *P. falciparum*. However, these drugs are usually so toxic that their prophylactic use is avoided.

2. Suppressive treatment of clinical symptoms involves drugs that *inhibit* the erythrocytic stage of parasite development. Thus the infected individual is free of the clinical symptoms manifested by the disease. However, the exoerythrocytic forms continue to exist in the liver. The drugs administered for suppressive treatment are chloroquine, hydroxychloroquine, and pyrimethamine. *P. falciparum* infection is usually cured by this treatment. In other forms of malaria, relapses occur when therapy is discontinued.

3. Clinical cure of an acute attack occurs when multiplication of the parasites within the erythrocyte is *interrupted,* thereby

terminating the malarial symptoms of the attack. These drugs are called *blood schizonticides* and include the 4-aminoquinolines. Pyrimethamine is also used but has a slower action than the other drugs. Infections with *P. vivax and P. falciparum* respond well. If relapse occurs, therapy should be repeated with other agents such as quinine as combination therapy.

4. Radical cure requires drugs (secondary tissue schizonticides) that destroy both the exoerythrocytic and erythrocytic parasites to prevent relapsing malaria. This is generally reserved for individuals with vivax malaria. The only drug available is primaquine. It is usually given with chloroquine, which suppresses the erythrocytic cycle to effect a radical cure.

The emergence of drug-resistant strains of malaria, particularly that caused by *P. falciparum,* poses a major public health problem throughout the world. Despite the combined efforts of many countries to eradicate malaria, it remains the most devastating infectious disease in the world because of the many lives lost and the economic burdens it imposes. Fortunately, in the United States, endemic malaria has been completely eradicated.

It is essential that travelers contemplating a trip to malarious areas of the world be aware of the need to obtain information from their physician about measures for reducing exposure to the disease. Malaria exists in Haiti, Mexico, Central America, South America, the Middle East, India, Africa, Southeast Asia, Korea, and Indonesia. To reduce exposure to mosquitoes, the individual should stay indoors in well-screened areas after sundown, sleep under mosquito netting, wear adequate clothing, and use mosquito repellents over exposed areas of the body.

Antimalarial products include quinine sulfate, quinacrine HCl, 4-aminoquinoline compounds (chloroquine phosphate, chloroquine HCl, and hydroxychloroquine sulfate), 8-aminoquinoline compounds (primaquine phosphate), folic acid antagonist (pyrimethamine), and combinations (chloroquine phosphate with primaquine phosphate; sulfadoxine and pyrimethamine).

quinine sulfate capsules (Strema)
quinine sulfate tablets (Quinamm, Quinite)

Mechanism of action. Antiprotozoal: unknown, but it is believed to bind to and alter DNA properties. Action is schizonticidal. Drug concentrates in parasitized erythrocytes, which may be why it has selective toxicity during the erythrocytic stages of plasmodial infections. Antimyotonic: increases refractory period of skeletal muscle and decreases the excitability of the motor end-plate, thus reducing response to nerve stimulation.

Indications. Treatment of malaria, especially chloroquine-resistant malaria, by *P. falciparum;* prevention and treatment of leg muscle cramps.

Pharmacokinetics
Absorption. Very good orally.
Protein binding. High.

Half-life. About 8.5 hours.
Time to peak serum level. Within 1 to 3 hours after a single dose.
Mean serum level. Approximately 7 μg/ml after chronic administration of 1 g total daily dose.
Metabolism. Liver.
Excretion. Kidneys.
Side effects/adverse reactions. see Table 61-2.
Significant drug interactions. When quinine is given concurrently with alfentanil, alfentanil may accumulate, and its duration of action may increase.

Dosage and administration
Adults
Antiprotozoal: 200 mg to 1 g orally three times daily for 6 to 12 days.
For *P. falciparum* (chloroquine-resistant) malaria: 650 mg orally every 8 hours for a minimum of 3 days in most areas of world (7 days in southeast Asia), with pyrimethamine twice daily for the first 3 days and 2 g of sulfadiazine daily for the first 5 days; 650 mg every 8 hours for a minimum of 3 days in most areas (7 days in southeast Asia), with 250 mg of tetracycline every 6 hours for 10 days; or 650 mg every 8 hours for a minimum of 3 days with 1.5 g of sulfadoxine and 75 mg of pyrimethamine as a single dose.
Antimyotonic: for night-time leg cramps, 260 mg orally at bedtime. An extra dose of 260 mg may be taken after supper.

Children
Antiprotozoal: for *P. falciparum* (chloroquine-resistant) malaria, 8.3 mg/kg orally every 8 hours for a minimum of 3 days in most areas of world (7 days in southeast Asia). Antimyotonic: not established.
Pregnancy safety. Not established.

NURSING CONSIDERATIONS

Assessment. Quinine is contraindicated for use in clients with glucose-6-phosphate dehydrogenase (G-6-PD) deficiency, rhinitis, optic neuritis, myasthenia gravis, and pregnancy. Use with caution in patients with cardiac disease, particularly cardiac dysrhythmia that is treated with quinidine. Note quinine has quinidinelike activity.

Intervention. Since quinine irritates the gastrointestinal mucosa, the capsule should be administered intact with food. Except for its use in chloroquine-resistant falciparum malaria, quinine, which has been the traditional antimalarial remedy, has been replaced by more effective and less toxic drugs.

Education. Instruct the client to remain compliant to the antimalarial medication regimen for the full course of the prescription.

Instruct patient to report to the physician if any side/adverse effects appear.

Evaluation. Observe for symptoms of cinchonism (tin-

TABLE 61-2   Antimalarial Drugs: Side Effects/Adverse Reactions

Drug	Side effects*	Adverse reactions†
quinine sulfate	Most frequent: diarrhea, nausea, vomiting, abdominal pain or discomfort	Most frequent: visual disturbances, dizziness, severe headaches, tinnitus, hearing loss Less frequent: rash, pruritus, hives, respiratory difficulties, wheezing Rare: sore throat, elevated temperature, increased bleeding episodes, increased weakness
quinacrine HCl	Most frequent: transient headaches, dizziness, GI distress, diarrhea, nausea; temporary yellow skin and urine coloration—not jaundice	Chronic therapy: hepatitis, skin eruptions, aplastic anemia, corneal deposits/edema, visual disturbances, seizures (after high doses), psychosis. Less frequent: anxiety, mood changes, nightmares
4-aminoquinolines: chloroquine phosphate or hydrochloride; and hydroxychloroquine	Most frequent: diarrhea, headaches, anorexia, nausea, vomiting, abdominal distress Less frequent: alopecia or bleaching of hair; dark discoloration of skin, nails, or inside of mouth; dizziness, increased anxiety, rash, pruritus	Less frequent: visual disturbances Rare: mood alterations, tinnitus, convulsions, sore throat, fever, increased bleeding episodes Overdosage: sedation, lightheadedness, severe respiratory difficulties
8-aminoquinoline: primaquine phosphate	Most frequent: nausea, vomiting, abdominal distress Less frequent: headaches, pruritus	Most frequent: dark discoloration of urine (hemolytic anemia due to G-6-PD deficiency) Less frequent: dizziness, respiratory difficulties, increased weakness Rare: sore throat, elevated temperature
folic acid antagonist: pyrimethamine	Most frequent with high dosages: anorexia, vomiting	Most frequent with high dosages: taste alterations; sore, red, swelling or burning of tongue; diarrhea; throat pain; swallowing difficulties; sores, ulceration or white spots in mouth; sore throat; fever; increased bleeding; increased weakness Rare: rash Overdose: ataxia, tremors, convulsions

*If side effects continue, increase, or disturb the client, inform the physician.
†If adverse reactions occur, contact physician because medical intervention may be necessary.

nitus, dizziness, altered auditory acuity, visual disturbances, headache, gastrointestinal distress, nausea, and diarrhea). These symptoms disappear when the drug is discontinued.

quinacrine HCl (Atabrine HCl)

Mechanism of action. Combines with DNA, interfering with its ability to replicate or even to serve in transcription of RNA; therefore, protein synthesis decreases. It suppresses and destroys erythrocytic asexual forms of *P. falciparum* and *P. vivax* and sexual forms (gametocytes) of *P. vivax.* It is not effective against *P. falciparum* gametocytes and sporozoites of all species of malaria-causing pathogens.

Indications. Treatment and suppression of malaria (see preceding); treatment of giardiasis and cestodiasis.

Pharmacokinetics

Absorption. Good.

Maximum plasma level. Within 1 to 3 hours.

Biologic half-life. Approximately 5 days.

Metabolism. Unknown.

Excretion. Kidneys.

Side effects/adverse reactions. See Table 61-2.

Significant drug interactions. When quinacrine HCl is given concurrently with the following drugs, the following interactions may occur.

Drug	Possible Effect and Management
alcohol	Quinacrine may interfere with the metabolism of alcohol, resulting in a mild disulfiram-type reaction.
primaquine	Primaquine toxicity may be increased; concurrent usage is contraindicated.

Dosage and administration

For treatment:

Adults and children 8 years and older, 200 mg with 1 g of sodium bicarbonate orally every 6 hours for 5 doses, then 100 mg three times a day for 6 days (total dose is 2.8 g in 1 week).

Children 4 to 8 years old, 200 mg orally three times a day for 24 hours, then 100 mg every 12 hours for 6 days.

Children 1 to 4 years old, 100 mg orally three times daily for 24 hours, then 100 mg daily for 6 days.

For suppression, continue therapy for 1 to 3 months. Adults take 100 mg a day; children 50 mg a day.

Pregnancy safety. Not established.

NURSING CONSIDERATIONS

Assessment. Observe caution in clients with psychosis, glucose-6-phosphate dehydrogenase (G-6-PD) deficiency, renal or cardiac disease, hepatic disease, and alcoholism. Cautious use is also indicated in pregnant women, children, and individuals over age 60. Use in patients with porphyria or psoriasis may exacerbate these conditions; therefore, the benefit must outweigh the risk.

Intervention. Administer drug after meals with a large glass of water or other fluid (tea or fruit juice) to minimize gastric irritation. The bitter taste may be masked by jam or honey.

Education. Advise client that the drug imparts a reversible yellow coloration to urine and skin (not jaundice). It also causes a cyanotic coloration (gray-blue tinge) to fingernail beds, ears, and nasal cartilage.

Instruct client to report to the physician any skin eruptions, psychotic behavior (may last up to 2 weeks after discontinuation of drug), or visual disturbances (blurred vision, halos of light, or difficulty in focusing).

Evaluation. Perform compete blood counts and ophthalmoscopic examinations periodically, particularly in clients on prolonged therapy. Drug may need to be discontinued if there are significant abnormalities.

4-Aminoquinoline Compounds

chloroquine phosphate tablets (Aralen)
chloroquine HCl injection (Aralen)
hydroxychloroquine sulfate tablets (Plaquenil)

Mechanism of action. Antiprotozoal: for treatment of malaria, unknown; perhaps due to ability to bind or alter DNA properties. During suppressive therapy, they inhibit the erythrocytic stage of development of plasmodia. In acute malarial attacks, they interfere with erythrocytic schizogony of parasites. These drugs selectively accumulate in parasitized erythrocytes, which may be the reason for their selective toxicity in the erythrocytic stages of plasmodial infestation.

Indications

Prevention and treatment of acute attacks of malaria caused by the four *Plasmodium* species. To cure *P. vivax* and *P. ovale* malaria, 8-aminoquinoline compounds should be given concurrently with or subsequently to a 4-aminoquinolone compound.

Treatment of extraintestinal (primarily hepatic) amebiasis. Chloroquine is usually used in combination with an effective intestinal amebicide.

Treatment of acute and chronic rheumatoid arthritis. Both drugs are used in clients who do not respond to other less toxic drugs.

Treatment of systemic erythematosus: hydroxychloroquine is used as a suppressant for chronic discoid and systemic lupus erythematosus.

Pharmacokinetics

Absorption. Rapid and complete.

Distribution. Throughout body tissues, especially eyes, liver, lungs, and kidneys.

Metabolism. Liver.

Time to peak level. 1 to 2 hours.

Excretion. Kidneys.

Side effects/adverse reactions. See Table 61-2.

Significant drug interactions. When 4-aminoquinolines are given concurrently with alcohol or other hepatotoxic agents, the potential for inducing hepatotoxicity increases. Monitor very closely.

Dosage and administration

chloroquine

Adults

Malaria:

Suppressant effect: 500 mg orally once a week. If therapy was not started at least 2 weeks before exposure to malaria, an initial loading dose of 1 g (given in two divided doses, 6 hours apart) is recommended.

Therapeutic: 1 g orally, followed by 500 mg in 6 to 8 hours, then 500 mg daily on the second and third days.

For extraintestinal amebiasis: give with other antiprotozoals that are toxic to tissue, 250 mg orally four times daily for 48 hours, then 250 mg twice daily for 14 to 21 days.

Dosage schedules may be increased or decreased if necessary. Therapy may also be repeated.

Antirheumatic: 250 mg orally daily; may increase to 750 mg daily if necessary.

Lupus erythematosus: 250 mg orally twice daily for 14 days, then 250 mg daily.

Children

Malaria:

Suppressant effect: 8.3 mg/kg orally; do not exceed adult dosage. Administer once weekly. If therapy not started at least 2 weeks before exposure to malaria, administer a loading dose of 16.7 mg/kg in two divided doses (6 hours apart).

Therapeutic: 41.7 mg/kg orally given over 3 days as follows: 16.7 mg/kg (do not exceed a single dose of 1 gm); 8.3 mg/kg (do not exceed a single dose of 500 mg) given at 6, 24, and 48 hours after the first dose.

To treat extraintestinal amebiasis: 10 mg/kg orally (up to maximum of 600 mg) per day for 3 weeks.

chloroquine HCl injection (Aralen)
Adults
Malaria: 200 to 250 mg intramuscularly; repeat in 6 hours if needed. Do not exceed 1 g in first 24 hours.
For extraintestinal amebiasis: 200 to 250 mg intramuscularly per day for 10 to 12 days.
Children
Malaria: 6.25 mg/kg intramuscularly; repeat in 6 hours if needed. Do not exceed a total dose of 12.5 mg/kg in 24 hours.
For extraintestinal amebiasis: 7.5 mg/kg intramuscularly, daily for 10 to 12 days.
Note: do not exceed 6.25 mg/kg in children. Severe reactions and even death have occurred after injectable administration of this drug.

hydroxychloroquine sulfate tablets (Plaquenil)
Adults. Antiprotozoal, malaria:
Suppressant therapy: 400 mg orally, once weekly. If therapy was not started at least 2 weeks before malaria exposure, administer an initial loading dose of 800 mg in two divided doses (6 hours apart).
Therapeutic: initially 800 mg orally, then 400 mg in 6 to 8 hours, then 400 mg daily on the second and third days.
Antirheumatic: 200 mg initially orally two or three times daily; take with meals or a glass of milk. For maintenance, 200 mg orally, once or twice a day, with a glass of milk or with meals.
To suppress lupus erythematosus: initially, 400 mg orally once or twice a day. For maintenance, 200 to 400 mg orally daily.
Children. Antiprotozoal, malaria:
Suppressant: 6.4 mg/kg orally, weekly. Do not exceed adult dosage. If therapy not started 2 weeks before malaria exposure, give a loading dose of 12.9 mg/kg orally in two divided doses (6 hours apart).
Therapeutic: 32 mg/kg orally over 3 days as follows: 12.9 mg/kg, not to exceed an 800-mg single dose; then 6.4 mg/kg, not to exceed a 400-mg single dose at 6, 24, and 48 hours after the initial dose.
Pregnancy safety. Not established.

NURSING CONSIDERATIONS

Assessment. Perform baseline ophthalmoscopic and audiometric examinations.
These drugs are contraindicated in the presence of hypersensitivity to 4-aminoquinolines, retinal or visual field changes, and pregnancy (to prevent retinal damage in the fetus). Long-term therapy in children is also contraindicated.
Intervention. Administer oral drugs with milk or meals to minimize gastric irritation. If client is on parenteral therapy, substitute oral administration as soon as possible.
Hydroxychloroquine tablets may be crushed and placed in gelatin capsules or mixed with jam or jello to make them easier to swallow.
Initiate suppressive therapy 2 weeks before exposure and continue medication while staying in malarious area. Maintain drug regimen for 6 to 8 weeks after leaving the region.
Education. Instruct client to take drug for the full course of treatment even if feeling better. This will ensure that the infection is completely eradicated, and the symptoms will not return. To obtain the full effect of the drug, inform the client to follow a regular schedule by taking it the same day each week. Keep drug out of reach of children. Fatalities in children have occurred following ingestion of three or four tablets.
Instruct the client to keep regularly scheduled visits for ophthalmoscopic and audiometric examinations and report to the physician any signs of visual and auditory disturbances. This is to prevent irreversible retinopathy, which may occur even after discontinuation of therapy.
Explain to client that the drug may cause a red or brown discoloration of the urine.
When drug is administered for rheumatoid arthritis, inform the client that therapeutic benefits usually do not occur until 6 to 12 months after therapy has been initiated.
Caution the client to avoid alcoholic beverages while taking this drug.
In addition to taking this medication to avoid contracting malaria, the client should also be instructed to sleep under mosquito netting at night, to wear trousers and long-sleeved shirts, and to use mosquito repellent on exposed skin surfaces.
Since the medication may cause dizziness, advise the client to avoid tasks that require mental alertness until the response to the medication has been determined.
Evaluation. Obtain a baseline and periodic complete blood count and test for glucose-6-phosphate dehydrogenase (G-6-PD) deficiency to avoid the occurrence of hemolytic anemia. Signs of blood dyscrasia are fever, sore throat, fatigue, and easy bruising.
Perform periodic tests of muscle strength and reflexes, particularly in patients on long-term therapy. Discontinue therapy if positive signs occur.
Observe client for drug resistance to 4-aminoquinolines. Failure to prevent or cure clinical malaria may require treatment with quinine if the person is infected with a resistant strain of the parasite. Avoid the use of these drugs in individuals with psoriasis or porphyria, since these conditions may become exacerbated. Discontinue drugs at first sign of retinal changes and/or visual disturbances and continue to observe client for possible progression even after therapy has been discontinued.

Use with caution in individuals with liver disease or alcoholism, individuals with G-6-PD deficiency hematologic disorders, and in children.

8-Aminoquinoline Compound
primaquine phosphate tablet

Mechanism of action. Unknown, but primaquine binds and alters DNA properties. It is very effective in the exoerythrocytic stages of *P. vivax* and *P. ovale* malaria and against the primary phase (exoerythrocytic stage) of *P. falciparum* malaria. It is also effective against the sexual forms (gametocytes) of plasmodia (especially *P. falciparum*).

Indications. Treatment of malaria and prevention of relapses of malaria caused by *P. vivax* and *P. ovale;* also effective against gametocytes of *P. falciparum.*

Pharmacokinetics
Absorption. Good.
Peak serum level. Within 2 to 3 hours.
Half-life. Approximately 7 hours.
Metabolism. Rapidly metabolized, site unspecified.
Excretion. Kidneys (1% unchanged).
Side effects/adverse reactions. See Table 61-2.
Significant drug interactions. When primaquine is given concurrently with the following drugs, the following interactions may occur.

Drug	Possible Effect and Management
other hemolytic agents	May increase risk for toxicity; monitor closely.
quinacrine	Not recommended; an increase in primaquine toxicity is reported.

Dosage and administration
Adults. 26.3 mg (15 mg of base) orally daily for 14 days. To cure some strains of *P. vivax* malaria (especially the strain from southeast Asia), a dose of 52.6 mg (30 mg of base) daily for 14 days may be necessary. To eradicate gametocytes of *P. falciparum,* administer a single dose of 78.9 mg (45 mg of base).
Children. 667 μg (0.667 mg) (390 μg, or 0.39 mg of base) per kg orally, daily for 14 days.
Pregnancy safety. Not established.

NURSING CONSIDERATIONS

Assessment. Persons with active forms of rheumatoid arthritis or lupus erythematosus have a tendency to develop granulocytopenia. Avoid the use of primaquine in these individuals.
Intervention. Gastric irritation can be minimized by administering drug with meals.

Education. Encourage the client to comply with the full course of medication.
Evaluation. Emphasize the importance of periodic complete blood counts and hemoglobin determinations to the client. The signs of hemolytic anemia are fever, chills, precordial pain, darkened urine, and a sudden decrease in hemoglobin.

Discontinue medication if a sudden decrease in hemoglobin concentration, erythrocyte count, or leukocyte count occurs.

The more serious adverse effects of primaquine involve individuals with a genetically determined glucose-6-phosphate dehydrogenase (G-6-PD) deficiency, which can cause a lethal hemolysis of red blood cells. This disorder occurs in about 8% of black males and other dark-skinned individuals such as Asians and some Mediterranean peoples. However, there is evidence that the enzyme G-6-PD in the red blood cells is essential for metabolism in the plasmodia; hence persons with a genetic deficiency of G-6-PD in their red blood cells are believed to have some natural immunity to malaria.

Folic Acid Antagonist
pyrimethamine tablets (Daraprim)

Mechanism of action. Blocks protozoal enzyme dihydrofolate reductase, thus inhibiting the conversion of dihydrofolic acid to tetrahydrofolic acid. The depletion of folate reduces protozoal nucleic acid and protein production. Effective against asexual erythrocytic forms of malaria, and it has a lesser effect against the tissue forms of *P. falciparum.* It arrests sporogony in the mosquito but it does not destroy gametocytes.

Indications. For preventing and treating malaria caused by *Plasmodium* spp. Used in combination with sulfadoxine to suppress chloroquine-resistant, *P. falciparum* malaria. Also combined with quinine and a sulfapyrimidine sulfonamide (sulfadiazine, trisulfapyrimidines) to treat uncomplicated attacks of chloroquine-resistant *P. falciparum* malaria. For treating toxoplasmosis, drug is combined with a sulfapyrimidine sulfonamide to treat toxoplasmosis caused by *Toxoplasma gondii.*

Pharmacokinetics
Absorption. Very good orally.
Distribution. Concentrated mainly in red and white blood cells, kidneys, liver, lungs, and spleen. Can cross the placenta.
Protein binding. Highly bound.
Half-life. 96 hours.
Time to peak plasma levels. Within 2 to 4 hours.
Metabolism. Liver.
Excretion. Kidneys.
Side effects/adverse reactions. See Table 61-2.
Significant drug interactions. None reported.

Dosage and administration

Adults

For chloroquine-resistant, *P. falciparum* malaria: for an acute attack, combine with other antimalarials, 25 mg orally, twice daily for 3 days.

For suppressant effect or chemoprophylaxis: 25 mg orally daily for 7 days.

For toxoplasmosis, give with a sulfapyrimidine sulfonamide: orally, 50 to 100 mg daily for 1 to 3 days, then 25 mg daily for 4 to 6 weeks.

Maximum daily dose for chloroquine-resistant *P. falciparum* malaria: acute attack, up to 75 mg/day; for suppressive cure, up to 75 mg weekly.

Children. To treat chloroquine-resistant *P. falciparum* malaria: acute attack, give with other antimalarials, 300 μg (0.3 mg)/kg orally three times daily for 3 days; for suppressant cure or chemoprophylaxis, 900 μg (0.9 mg)/kg orally once weekly. Do not exceed the recommended adult dose.

Pregnancy safety. Not established.

NURSING CONSIDERATIONS

Assessment. Since the drug crosses the placenta, its use is not recommended in pregnancy. In animal studies defects have occurred in the fetus. Moreover, risk-benefit must be considered in nursing mothers because pyrimethamine may disrupt the folic acid metabolism in the nursing infant. The drug also can cause hemolytic anemia in glucose-6-phosphate dehydrogenase (G-6-PD)–deficient infant.

To prevent possible central nervous system toxicity in individuals with convulsive disorders, use a small initial dose for treatment of toxoplasmosis.

Do not use for treatment of resistant form of parasite.

Intervention. Administer medication with milk or food to minimize gastric irritation. For children, tablets may be crushed to prepare 1% solution in normal saline. Use within 24 hours at room temperature. If mixed with cherry syrup NF, use immediately after preparation.

If taken to prevent malaria, the medication should be taken 2 weeks before entering a malarious area and be continued for 6 weeks after leaving it. Besides building tissue stores of the drug, early administration will allow assessment of the client's tolerance of the drug.

Education. Advise the client to have semiweekly blood counts and platelet counts during therapy.

If taken as a malaria suppressant, instruct the client to follow the dosage schedule as prescribed by taking the drug the same day each week.

Advise the individual to sleep under mosquito netting to avoid being bitten by malaria-carrying mosquitoes while in the endemic areas. Advise the wearing of proper clothing so that arms and legs are covered, especially at dawn and during evening hours, when mosquitoes are out. The use of mosquito repellent on uncovered areas of the skin may help to protect the individual from the bites of infected mosquitoes.

Instruct the client to report to physician any signs of possible blood dyscrasia (fever, sore throat, unusual bleeding or bruising, extreme weakness and fatigue).

Fansidar (pyrimethamine with sulfadoxine) should only be used when the traveler is going to areas where chloroquine-resistant malaria is prevalent and is planning to stay longer than 3 weeks because of the risk of severe skin reactions. The drug should be discontinued and a health care provider notified at the first sign of a rash.

Evaluation. The high dosage required for treating toxoplasmosis could approach the toxic level. If folic acid deficiency develops, dosage may be reduced. Clinical symptoms of folic acid deficiency are soreness, redness, or burning of the tongue; pharyngitis; ulcers in the mouth; or diarrhea. Folinic acid (leucovorin) restores the depressed platelet or white blood counts to normal levels.

Combination Therapy for Malaria

Chloroquine phosphate with primaquine phosphate tablets is used for malaria prophylaxis in all areas where the disease is prevalent, regardless of the causative organism. The tablets are available as 500 mg of chloroquine phosphate (300 mg of base) and 79 mg primaquine phosphate (45 mg base). Adult dose is one tablet before entering the area, then one tablet weekly on the same day each week. Continue this dosage for 2 months after leaving the endemic area. For further information on this product, see previous section describing the individual drugs.

Sulfadoxine and pyrimethamine tablets (Fansidar) are used to treat *P. falciparum* malaria (chloroquine resistant). They are also used to prevent malaria in travelers in areas where this malaria strain is prevalent. For additional information on the ingredients in this product, see previous section and sulfonamides in Chapter 37. Refer to a current package insert or a current *Facts and Comparisons Drug Information* (Kastrup, E.K., ed.) reference for detailed dosing and additional information on this product.

TUBERCULOSIS

Tuberculosis (TB) in native-born Americans increased in 1986 for the first time since 1953. Nationwide, nearly 23,000 cases of TB were reported in 1986 (Hayden, 1987). Approximately 12 million Americans are infected with this disease, and nearly 10% will develop tuberculosis. This increase is largely attributed to the increasing numbers of individuals with AIDS, to street living or homelessness, drug abusers, undernourished or malnourished persons, or those taking immunosuppressant drugs or suffering from cancer. With the antituberculosis chemotherapy and chemoprophylaxis available today, great progress has been made in treating this disease state.

Mycobacterium tuberculosis is the bacteria that causes tuberculosis. The most common infection site is the lungs, but other body areas can also be infected, such as bones, joints, skin, meninges, or genitourinary tract. This bacteria is an aerobic bacillus that needs a highly oxygenated organ site for growth; thus the lungs, growing ends of bones, and cerebral cortex are ideal sites. Tubercle bacilli may be transmitted by airborne droplets but *cannot be transmitted on objects such as dishes, clothing, or sheets and bedding.* Sharing an enclosed environment with an infected person creates a high risk of developing this infection (Health Information for International Travelers, 1988).

Fortunately, though, the transmission of the bacilli is blocked by good room ventilation, ultraviolet light, and specific chemotherapy. Many clients are treated as outpatients, assuming they are not public health hazards (that is, highly infectious) and do not have severe symptoms of disease. Usually after 2 weeks of appropriate chemotherapy, most clients are no longer infectious to their family or contacts (Herfindal and others, 1988). When sputum cultures are negative, many persons return to their work setting.

PATHOGENESIS

Tubercle bacilli droplets are transmitted by coughing or sneezing by an infected person. Persons producing sputum generally have many bacilli and are more infectious than the infected person that does not cough. Nevertheless, an uninfected person must be exposed to an infectious case of tuberculosis for many weeks before the infection can be transferred (Glassroth, 1981). Three types of tubercle bacilli are pathogenic to humans: human to human, bovine to human, and avian to human. Avian TB is rare in the United States and with the pasteurization of milk and testing of cows, bovine TB is much less prevalent. Thus the primary source of transmission is human to human.

When the tubercle bacilli enters the lungs, infection can spread from there to other body organs through the blood and lymphatic system. Usually, however, the infection becomes dormant and is walled off by calcified and fibrous tissues. The bacilli become inactive, perhaps for the lifetime of the host. If host defenses break down, however, or if the host receives an immunosuppressive drug, the bacilli may be reactivated. The ensuing disease may be chronic tuberculosis or miliary tuberculosis. Chronic tuberculosis may occur in any body organ but, as previously stated, it occurs most frequently in areas with the greatest oxygen tension. Miliary tuberculosis refers to the spread of many bacilli in the body; it is most often seen in children under 4 years old and can rapidly lead to death of the individual (Herfindal and others, 1988).

DRUG TREATMENT REGIMENS

Effective drug regimens are available to treat tuberculosis. Drug selection is based on toxicity and also on the development of drug-resistant organisms. General guidelines include:

1. For clients with tuberculosis, administer two or more sensitive drugs for the specific TB bacilli. One drug alone will increase the risk of organisms developing drug resistance. Isoniazid is recommended for newly infected persons without existing disease, which is determined by the individual's delayed hypersensitivity reaction to an intradermal injection of purified protein derivative (PPD).

2. Two or more drugs are combined to treat the disease because they will provide additive antituberculous action and also because one drug will help to prevent or delay the development of resistance to the other drug.

3. Avoid combinations with additive toxicities, such as nephrotoxic or ototoxic effects.

4. Monitor the prescribed therapy regimen closely to avoid client noncompliance, to detect side effects or adverse reactions, and to register progress of the treatment program (Roffman, 1981).

Although in the past tuberculosis treatment required 1 to 2 years of therapy, today 9 to 12 months of combined isoniazid and rifampin therapy is reported to be effective. Short-course drug regimens are also used, especially in areas where client noncompliance has led to the development of drug-resistant organisms. Various drug protocols range from daily drug administration to twice-weekly administration (Braunwald and others, 1987). See Table 61-3 for typical drug treatment regimens for tuberculosis.

THE NURSE'S ROLE IN THE ADMINISTRATION OF ANTITUBERCULOUS AGENTS

These general nursing considerations for antituberculous agents are supplemented by specific considerations for each agent.

Assessment. Cultures for *Mycobacterium* and tests for the organism's susceptibility to the antitubercular drugs should be obtained before and periodically during the course of drug therapy.

Intervention. The nurse should attempt to administer

TABLE 61-3 Selected Drug Treatment Regimens for Tuberculosis

Drug regimen (adult dosage)	Comments
isoniazid (INH)(300 mg) and rifampin 600 mg daily for 9 to 12 months	Common regimen for initial treatment of TB; if drug resistance is possible, ethambutol 15 mg/kg is added
INH 300 mg and ethambutol (15 mg/kg) daily for 12 to 18 months	Least toxic protocol; used for individuals with minimal disease state; also used for pregnant women
INH (300 mg), rifampin (600 mg), pyrazinamide (2 g), and streptomycin (1 g) or ethambutol (15 mg/kg) daily for 2 months, followed by one of the following regimens: 1. INH, 300 mg, and rifampin, 600 mg, daily for 4 months 2. INH, 300 mg, rifampin, 600 mg, and streptomycin, 1 g, twice weekly for 6 months	Typical short, intensive course of therapy; these regimens need close client supervision; the regimens have been reported to be effective

these drugs with consideration for the client's comfort. For example, gastrointestinal disturbances following administration can be reduced by concurrent administration of food or antacids.

Education. The client must take prescribed medications regularly and without interruption for maximum therapeutic effectiveness. A person who is responsible for self-medication should be instructed about the necessity to take these drugs according to the prescribed regimen and not to discontinue them when feeling better.

Instruct clients responsible for self-medication about the necessity for periodic medical evaluations to evaluate the effectiveness of therapy.

Because of the long-term nature of drug therapy in tuberculosis, clients may need support in maintaining the therapeutic regimen and in managing side effects of the tuberculosis drugs.

When peripheral neuritis appears as a side effect of the antitubercular drugs, teach clients precautionary strategies to avoid injury from burning agents and sharp objects until the alteration in sensation is remedied.

Teach clients measures that minimize disease transmission, such as covering the mouth when coughing and sneezing. The disease may also be transmitted through unpasteurized milk or milk products.

Evaluation. Monitor the client for symptoms that indicate resolution of the infection: diminished cough and sputum production; decreased fever and night sweats; reduction of cavitation on x-ray; reduction of anorexia with concomitant weight gain; and decreased acid-fast bacteria (AFB) in sputum specimens. If the drug is taken to prevent tuberculosis, the absence of the disease demonstrates its effectiveness.

ANTITUBERCULOUS AGENTS
aminosalicylates, systemic
aminosalicylate calcium tablets
aminosalicylate sodium for oral solution (Teebacin)
aminosalicylate sodium tablets (Nemasol♣, PAS, Teebacin)
aminosalicylic acid tablets

Mechanism of action. Bacteriostatic agent. Inhibits bacterial resistance to streptomycin and isoniazid. It is closely related to aminobenzoic acid (PABA) and competitively inhibits folic acid formation in *tuberculosis,* thus suppressing growth and reproduction.

Indications. Treatment of tuberculosis, pulmonary and extrapulmonary, caused by *M. tuberculosis.*

Pharmacokinetics

Absorption. Very good orally. Sodium dosage form is more rapidly absorbed than other dosage forms.

Distribution. To various body fluids, with high levels accumulating in pleural fluids, kidney, lungs, and liver tissues.

Half-life. With normal renal function, within 45 to 60 minutes; with impaired renal function, up to 23 hours.

Time to peak serum level. Within 1 to 2 hours but persisting for nearly 4 hours.

Metabolism. Liver.

Excretion. Kidneys.

Side effects/adverse reactions. See Table 61-4.

Significant drug interactions. When aminosalicylates are given concurrently with the following drugs, the following interactions may occur.

Drug	Possible Effect and Management
aminobenzoic acid (PABA)	May antagonize the bacteriostatic effect of aminosalicylates; do not administer concurrently.
cellulose sodium phosphate or tetracyclines, oral	Decreases effect of cellulose sodium phosphate in preventing hypercalciuria; monitor closely or avoid this combination. Nonabsorbable complexes are formed with the oral tetracyclines. Advise clients to separate intake of tetracyclines from aminosalicylate calcium by at least 2 to 3 hours.

Dosage and administration

aminosalicylate calcium tablets. Not available in United States

TABLE 61-4   Antituberculous Agents: Side Effects/Adverse Reactions

Drug	Side effects*	Adverse reactions†
aminosalicylates	Most frequent: diarrhea, abdominal distress	Most frequent: chills, rash, sore throat, increased temperature, increased weakness, confusion, constipation, sedation, increased thirst and frequency of urination, anorexia, depression, nausea, vomiting, pruritus, low back pain, pain on urination Less frequent: bloody urine, menstrual changes, decreased libido, dry skin, weight gain, edema in throat (goiter), headaches, photosensitivity, jaundice of eyes/skin
capreomycin	Less frequent: rash, pruritus, swelling, increased temperature, pain, bleeding, hardness at site of injection	Most frequent: bloody urine, increased thirst and frequency of urination, anorexia (hypokalemia), Less frequent: hearing loss, tinnitus, ataxia, dizziness, increased weakness, irregular heart rate, mood alterations, muscle pain or cramps, abdominal distress, weak pulse, nausea, vomiting
cycloserine	Most frequent: headaches Less frequent: pale skin, more frequent bleeding episodes, weakness	Most frequent: increased anxiety, confusion, dizziness, sedation, increased irritability, restlessness, depression, muscle tremors, nightmares, mood alterations, speech difficulties, suicidal tendencies Less frequent: visual disturbances, photosensitivity, tingling, pain, numbness in hands or feet, jaundice of eyes or skin Rare: convulsions
ethambutol	Less frequent: lightheadedness, abdominal distress, rash, pruritus	Less frequent: chills, joint pain or swelling, (especially big toe, ankle, or knee), hot skin over affected joints Rare: visual disturbances, pain, burning, tingling, or numbness of hands or feet
ethionamide	Most frequent: diarrhea, drooling, anorexia, metal mouth taste, nausea, vomiting, mouth soreness, abdominal distress, hypotension, sedation, tiredness Less frequent/rare: acne, breast enlargement in men, alopecia, photosensitivity, rash	Most frequent: depression Less frequent: ataxia, confusion, mood alterations, jaundice of eyes or skin Rare: menstrual irregularities, decreased libido, dry skin, goiter, joint swelling and pain
isoniazid (INH)	Most frequent: lightheadedness, abdominal distress, tingling, Less frequent: breast enlargement in males	Most frequent: hands and feet pain, burning dark urine, jaundice of eyes or skin, anorexia, nausea, increased weakness Rare: visual disturbances
pyrazinamide	Less frequent: nausea, vomiting, urination difficulties Rare: pruritus, rash, photosensitivity	Most frequent: anorexia, increased temperature, increased weakness, jaundice of eyes or skin Less frequent: joint pain and swelling, especially of big toe, ankle, and knee; feeling of heat over affected joint
rifampin	Most frequent: anorexia, discoloration of body fluids (urine, saliva, feces, tears, sweat—red orange to brown), abdominal distress Less frequent: pruritus, rash, mouth or tongue soreness	Less frequent: chills, respiratory difficulties, lightheadedness, shivers, increased temperature, headaches, fever, bone and muscle pain Rare: bloody urine, decreased urination, anorexia, nausea, vomiting, increased weakness, sore throat, increased bleeding episodes, jaundice of eyes or skin

*If side effects continue, increase, or disturb the client, inform the physician.
†If adverse reactions occur, contact physician because medical intervention may be necessary.

aminosalicylate sodium for oral solution/tablets

Adults. Given in combination with other antitubercular drugs, 3.3 to 4 g orally (aminosalicylic acid) every 8 hours or 5 to 6 g every 12 hours. Maximum is 20 g day.

Children. Given with other antitubercular drugs, 50 to 75 mg/kg (aminosalicylic acid) orally every 6 hours or 66.7 to 100 mg/kg every 8 hours.

Pregnancy safety. Not established.

NURSING CONSIDERATIONS

Assessment. Aminosalicylates should be used with caution if the client has the following preexisting conditions: gastric ulcer, as gastric irritation may increase; G-6-PD deficiency because there is a risk of hemolytic anemia; severe renal or hepatic function impairment. Avoid the administration of aminosalicylate calcium in conditions in which there might be increased calcium levels, such as adrenal insufficiency, hyperparathyroidism, and carcinoma. Congestive heart failure should preclude the use of aminosalicylate sodium because of the risk of fluid accumulation.

Intervention. Administer with meals or antacids to minimize gastrointestinal distress.

When administering the dry powder form of the drug, mix thoroughly with diluent and ensure that the client takes all of liquid to obtain the full dose.

Do not administer aminosalicylates within 6 hours of rifampin or aminosalicylate calcium within 2 or 3 hours of oral tetracyclines.

Education. Clients with diabetes who test their urine with copper sulfate urine glucose tests may have false-positive test results. Clients should instead use Clinistix or Ketodiastix.

Evaluation. Serum electrolytes and urinalyses should be monitored periodically during drug therapy.

capreomycin sulfate, sterile (Capastat)

Mechanism of action. Unknown.

Indications. Treatment of pulmonary tuberculosis caused by *M. tuberculosis* after primary medications (streptomycin, isoniazid, rifampin, and ethambutol) fail or when these medications cannot be used because of resistant bacilli or drug toxicity.

Pharmacokinetics. The following apply to parenteral drug administration.

Distribution. High concentration in urine; does not enter the cerebrospinal fluid.

Half-life. With normal renal function, within 3 to 6 hours; with impaired renal function, delayed and prolonged.

Time to peak serum level. Within 1 to 2 hours of intramuscular administration.

Peak serum level. Average 28 to 32 μg/ml (range is 20 to 47 μg/ml).

Urine concentration. 1680 μg/ml following a 1-g dose.

Excretion. Kidneys.

Side effects/adverse reactions. See Table 61-4.

Significant drug interactions. When capreomycin is given concurrently with the following drugs, the following interactions may occur.

Drug	Possible Effect and Management
aminoglycosides	Avoid concurrent drug administration. The risk for developing ototoxicity, nephrotoxicity and neuromuscular blockade is increased. Hearing loss may progress to deafness, even after the drug is stopped. This can be a very dangerous combination. *Avoid.*
amphotericin B, parenteral; bacitracin, parenteral; bumetanide, parenteral; cisplatin, cyclosporine, ethacrynic acid, parenteral; furosemide, parenteral; paromomycin, streptomycin; or vancomycin	Concurrent or even sequential use of capreomycin with any of these drugs can increase the risk for ototoxicity and/or nephrotoxicity. Hearing loss may occur and progress to deafness—even if drugs are stopped. *Avoid if at all possible.*
anesthetics, halogenated hydrocarbon inhalation, or citrate anticoagulated blood in massive transfusions or neuromuscular blocking agents	May result in increased neuromuscular blocking effects, resulting in respiratory depression or paralysis. Monitor closely, especially during surgery or in the postoperative period. If possible, avoid this combination. If not, closely monitor and keep anticholinesterase agents or calcium salts on hand to reverse the blockade.
methoxyflurane or polymyxins, parenteral	*Avoid concurrent or sequential drug administration.* The potential for nephrotoxicity and/or neuromuscular blockade is increased, which may lead to respiratory depression or paralysis.

Dosage and administration. Parenteral dosage form.

Adults. Given with other antitubercular drugs 1 g (base) intramuscularly daily for 2 to 4 months, followed by 1 g two or three times a week. Maximum is 20 mg/kg (base) daily.

Children. Not established.

Pregnancy safety. Not established.

NURSING CONSIDERATIONS

Assessment. The health assessment should determine if the client has the following preexisting conditions: dehydration, which increases the risk of toxicity due to increased serum levels of the drug; myasthenia gravis and parkinsonism, in which the neuromuscular deficits may increase; impairment of the eighth cranial nerve, because the drug may cause increased auditory and vestibular toxicity; and renal impairment, which may increase because of the nephrotoxic effects of the drug.

Because of these effects, audiograms and vestibular and renal function determinations should be monitored before and periodically during therapy. If the BUN is above 30 mg/dl, the medication should be stopped. Fluid intake and output should be monitored throughout therapy. In addition, liver function studies should be done periodically, as well as serum potassium levels.

With prolonged therapy, the client should be monitored for an overgrowth of nonsusceptible organisms.

Intervention. To prepare for intramuscular administration, add 2 ml of 0.9% sodium chloride injection or sterile water for injection to the vial. Allow 2 to 3 minutes for dissolution to occur. Reconstituted solutions may darken, but this does not affect their potency. They are stable for 48 hours at room temperature or 14 days if refrigerated.

Administer intramuscularly deep into a large muscle mass to minimize pain and the risk of sterile abscesses.

Education. The client should maintain regular contact with the health care provider to monitor his or her condition. Symptoms of tinnitus, hearing deficit, and/or vertigo should be reported to the physician.

cycloserine capsules (Seromycin)

Mechanism of action. This is a broad-spectrum antibiotic that can be bacteriostatic or bactericidal, depending on drug concentration at infection site and organism susceptibility. It interferes with bacterial cell wall synthesis.

Indications. Treatment of active pulmonary and extrapulmonary tuberculosis after failure of the primary antitubercular medications; treatment of urinary tract infections.

Pharmacokinetics

Absorption. Very good orally.

Distribution. To most body tissues and fluids, including cerebrospinal fluid (CSF); lungs; ascitic, pleural and synovial fluids. Urine concentrations very high, up to 50 µg/ml.

Half-life. With normal renal function, 10 hours; with impaired renal function, delayed and prolonged.

Time to peak serum level. Within 3 to 4 hours.

Metabolism. Up to 35%.

Excretion. Kidneys.

Side effects/adverse reactions. See Table 61-4.

Significant drug interactions. When cycloserine is given concurrently with the following drugs, the following interactions may occur.

Drug	Possible Effect and Management
alcohol	In chronic alcohol abusers, it may increase the risk of seizures. *Avoid concurrent usage.*
ethionamide	May increase CNS side effects such as seizures. Monitor closely, as dosage adjustments may be necessary.

Dosage and administration

Adults

For tuberculosis (with other antitubercular agents), 250 mg orally every 12 hours for 14 days, then increase as necessary and as tolerated by the patient—up to 250 mg every 6 to 8 hours. Monitor by serum level testing.

For urinary tract infections, 250 mg orally every 12 hours.

Maximum is 1 g daily, although doses of up to 1.5 g daily have been used.

Children

For tuberculosis (with other antitubercular agents), 5 to 20 mg/kg daily in divided doses.

For urinary tract infections: infants up to 2 years old, 62.5 mg orally every 12 hours; 2 to 10 years old, 125 mg orally every 12 hours; over 10 years old, see adult dosage.

Pregnancy safety. Not established.

NURSING CONSIDERATIONS

Caution the client to avoid alcohol while taking this medication, as it increases risks of CNS toxicity such as dizziness, mental disturbances, and seizures.

Advise the client to report immediately to the physician any signs of dizziness, drowsiness, vision disturbances, or thoughts of suicide.

ethambutol hydrochloride tablets (Etibi✿, Myambutol)

Mechanism of action. A bacteriostatic agent that is believed to diffuse into the mycobacteria bacilli and suppress RNA synthesis. It is only effective against actively dividing mycobacteria.

Indications. Treatment of tuberculosis.

Pharmacokinetics

Absorption. Very good orally.

Distribution. Very good to most body tissues and fluids, except for cerebrospinal fluid. High concentrations found in kidneys, lungs, saliva, urine, and erythrocytes.

Half-life. With normal renal function, within 3 to 4 hours; with impaired renal function, up to 8 hours.

Time to peak serum level. Within 2 to 4 hours.

Metabolism. Liver.

Excretion. Kidneys.

Side effects/adverse reactions. See Table 61-4.

Significant drug interactions. None.

Dosage and administration

Adults

For tuberculosis (with other antitubercular agents), 15 mg/kg initially daily.

For retreatment, 25 mg/kg orally daily for 2 to 3 months, then 15 mg/kg daily.

Maximum daily dose in tuberculosis is initial treatment, from 500 to 1.5 g day; retreatment, from 900 mg to 2.5 g day.

Children. Children up to 13 years old, not established; 13 years and older, see adult dosage.

Pregnancy safety. Not established.

NURSING CONSIDERATIONS

Assessment. When the client has preexisting optic neuritis and/or renal impairment, use ethambutol with caution. It may also increase uric acid concentrations, so care must be taken with clients with gout. Uric acid determinations are required periodically during the course of therapy.

Intervention. Administer with food to minimize gastrointestinal distress.

Administer ethambutol in a single daily dose, as divided doses may not result in therapeutic serum levels. It is administered concurrently with other antitubercular agents because of the tendency for bacterial resistance to occur when it is used alone.

Education. Encourage the client to visit the health care provider regularly to monitor progress. If no improvement occurs in 2 to 3 weeks, this should be reported to the physician.

Report promptly signs of optic neuritis (blurred vision, any loss of vision or red-green perception, or eye pain) or peripheral neuritis (numbness, tingling, or weakness in the hands and feet).

Evaluation. Ethambutol is known to decrease visual acuity and the ability to see red and green. This presents a safety hazard, especially in driving motor vehicles, and patients should be tested for these visual disturbances fre-

quently during drug therapy. Discontinuation of the drug is usually indicated when visual acuity is disturbed.

ethionamide tablets (Trecator-SC)

Mechanism of action. Unknown, but believed to inhibit peptide synthesis. Depending on concentration at site of infection and susceptibility of the organism, ethionamide may be bacteriostatic or bactericidal.

Indications. Treatment of tuberculosis after failure of the primary antitubercular agents (streptomycin, isoniazid, rifampin, and ethambutol)

Pharmacokinetics

Absorption. Very good orally.

Distribution. To most body tissues and fluids, including cerebrospinal fluid.

Half-life. 3 hours to peak serum level.

Metabolism. Possibly liver.

Excretion. Kidneys.

Side effects/adverse reactions. See Table 61-4.

Significant drug interactions. When ethionamide is given with cycloserine, an increase in CNS side effects (especially convulsions) may result. Monitor closely, as dosage adjustments may be necessary.

Dosage and administration

Adults. For tuberculosis, in combination with other antitubercular agents, 250 mg orally, every 8 to 12 hours. Maximum is 1 g daily.

Children. For tuberculosis, in combination with other antitubercular agents, 4 to 5 mg/kg orally every 8 hours. The maximum daily dose should not exceed 750 mg/day.

Pregnancy safety. Not established.

NURSING CONSIDERATIONS

Assessment. Carefully weigh risks and benefits for clients with diabetes mellitus or severe hepatic dysfunction before prescribing a course of ethionamide.

To monitor for hepatotoxic effects, AST (SGOT) and ALT (SGPT) should be done before and at least monthly during the course of therapy. Observe the client for jaundice.

Cultures and sensitivity testing should be done before and periodically throughout therapy to monitor progress.

Intervention. Administer with meals to minimize gastrointestinal distress. If gastrointestinal upset occurs, it may be minimized by a divided dosage schedule or by administration with a rectal suppository. In both cases, however, serum concentrations may not be adequate.

Pyridoxine may be prescribed concurrently to prevent peripheral neuritis.

Education. Advise the client about the importance of complying with the medication regimen, particularly when such a course may be continued for 1 or 2 years or more.

Regular visits to the physician are necessary to monitor progress and for periodic eye exams. Any symptoms related to changes in vision should be promptly reported to the physician.

Advise the client that because ethionamide may cause dizziness, drowsiness, or weakness, hazardous activities requiring mental alertness such as driving should be avoided until the response to the medication has been ascertained.

Alert the client to other potential side effects, such as mental depression or mood changes.

Evaluation. Although its incidence is rare, optic neuritis (blurred vision, vision loss, and/or eye pain) does occur. The client should have a thorough ophthalmologic exam before starting the drug and at the first indication of symptoms related to vision changes. Symptoms of CNS toxicity such as mental depression, mood changes, and weakness may be observed.

isoniazid syrup (Isotamine✸, Laniazid, PMS Isoniazid✸)
isoniazid tablets (DOW-Isoniazid, Isotamine✸, Rimifon✸)
isoniazid injection (Nydrazid)

Mechanism of action. A bactericidal agent that affects mycobacteria in the division phase. Exact mechanism of action is unknown but is believed to inhibit mycolic acid synthesis and cause cell wall disruption in susceptible organisms.

Indications. For preventing all forms of tuberculosis. In combination with other agents, treatment of all forms of tuberculosis.

Pharmacokinetics
Absorption. Very good orally.

Distribution. To all body tissues, fluids, and cerebrospinal fluid.

Half-life. For fast acetylators, within 0.5 to 1.6 hours; for slow acetylators, within 2 to 5 hours; with impaired liver or kidney function, delayed and prolonged.

Time to peak serum levels. 1 to 2 hours or 4 to 6 hours, depending on whether the client is a fast or slow acetylator.

Metabolism. Liver, primarily by acetylation to inactive metabolites, some of which may be hepatotoxic. The rate of acetylation by the liver is genetically determined, that is, slow acetylators have a decrease in hepatic N-acetyl transferase.

Excretion. Kidneys.

Side effects/adverse reactions. See Table 61-4.

Significant drug interactions. When isoniazid is given concurrently with the following drugs, the following interactions may occur.

Drug	Possible Effect and Management
alcohol	Daily use of alcohol may result in increased isoniazid metabolism and increased risk of hepatotoxicity. Monitor clients closely, as dosage adjustment may be necessary.
alfentanil	Isoniazid inhibits liver metabolism. This effect may decrease the metabolism of alfentanil, leading to increased serum levels and duration of action. Monitor closely.
disulfiram	May increase incidence of CNS side effects such as ataxia, irritability, dizziness, or insomnia. Monitor closely, as dosage reduction or even discontinuation of disulfiram may be required.
hepatotoxic drugs	May increase potential for hepatotoxicity. Avoid concurrent drug administration.
ketoconazole, miconazole (parenteral), or rifampin	Isoniazid with ketoconazole may increase serum levels of ketoconazole; if both isoniazid and rifampin are given with ketoconazole, the serum levels of ketoconazole or rifampin have been reported to be undetectable. Therefore, combining isoniazid or rifampin together or singly with ketoconazole, with ketoconazole or parenteral miconazole is not recommended. Rifampin with isoniazid may increase the potential for hepatotoxicity, especially in clients with liver impairment and/or in fast acetylators of isoniazid. Monitor closely for hepatotoxicity, especially during the first 90 days of therapy.
phenytoin	May result in impaired phenytoin metabolism, leading to increased serum levels and toxicity. Phenytoin dose may need to be adjusted. Monitor closely.

Dosage and administration
Oral dosage forms

Adults. Tuberculosis: prophylaxis, 300 mg orally daily, treatment with other antitubercular agents, 300 mg orally daily; maximum daily dose is 300 mg.

Children. Tuberculosis: prophylaxis, 10 mg/kg orally; maximum, 300 mg daily. Treatment with other antitubercular agents, 10 to 20 mg/kg orally; maximum, 300 mg daily. (Some children with severe tuberculosis—tubercular meningitis—have required doses up to 30 mg/kg—maximum 500 mg—per day.)

isoniazid injection

Adults. Tuberculosis: prophylaxis, 300 mg intramuscularly daily. Treatment with other antitubercular agents, 5 mg/kg up to 300 mg intramuscularly daily.

Children. Tuberculosis: prophylaxis, 10 mg/kg intramuscularly, to maximum of 300 mg daily. Treatment with other antitubercular agents, 10 to 20 mg/kg, to 500 mg intramuscularly daily.

isoniazid combinations. Isoniazid is combined with vitamin B_6 (because of the increased need for vitamin B_6 (pyridoxine) induced by isoniazid). Preparations containing this combination are Teebaconin and Vitamin B_6 and P-I-N- Forte. Another combination is 150 mg of isoniazid with 300 mg of rifampin (Rifamate) or 300 mg isoniazid tablets with 300 mg rifampin capsules (Rimactane/INH Dual Pack).

Pregnancy safety. Not established.

NURSING CONSIDERATIONS

Assessment. Mycobacterial cultures and sensitivities should be done before and periodically throughout therapy to monitor progress.

As isoniazid is metabolized in the liver, this drug should be administered cautiously to clients with a history of alcoholism and/or hepatic function impairment.

Intervention. Administer with meals to minimize gastrointestinal distress.

Pyridoxine may be prescribed concurrently to prevent peripheral neuritis. This may not be required for children if their dietary intake of vitamins is adequate.

Education. Encourage the client's compliance with the full course of isoniazid therapy.

Regular visits to the physician are necessary to monitor progress and for periodic eye exams. Any symptoms related to changes in vision should be promptly reported to the physician.

Since alcohol and oral antacids decrease the effects of isoniazid, they should not be used in combination with it. Alcohol increases ioniazid metabolism, and antacids decrease its absorption from the gastrointestinal tract.

Clients with diabetes who test their urine with copper sulfate tests (Clinitest) may obtain false-positive test re-

sults. Other tests (Clinistix, Tes-Tape) for urine glucose are unaffected.

Evaluation. To monitor for hepatotoxic effects, AST (SGOT) and ALT (SGPT) should be done before and at least monthly during the course of therapy. The client should be observed for symptoms of jaundice.

Although its incidence is rare, optic neuritis (blurred vision, vision loss, and/or eye pain) does occur. The client should have an ophthalmologic exam before and at the first indication of symptoms related to vision changes.

pyrazinamide tablets (PMS Pyrazinamide✿, Tebrazid✿)

Mechanism of action. Unknown. Depending on concentration at site of action and susceptibility of the mycobacteria, it can be bacteriostatic or bactericidal.

Indications. Treatment of tuberculosis after failure of primary medications (streptomycin, isoniazid, rifampin, and ethambutol).

Pharmacokinetics

Absorption. Good orally.

Distribution. To most body fluids and tissues, including cerebrospinal fluid.

Half-life. With normal renal or hepatic functions, within 9 to 10 hours; with impaired kidney or liver function, increased.

Time to peak serum level. 2 hours.

Time to peak urine concentration. 2 hours.

Metabolism. Liver primarily, also stomach and bladder.

Excretion. Kidneys.

Side effects/adverse reactions. See Table 61-4.

Significant drug interactions. None.

Dosage and administration

Adults. Tuberculosis: combined with other antitubercular agents, 5 to 8.75 mg/kg orally every 6 hours or 6.7 to 11.7 mg/kg every 8 hours. Maximum is 3 g/day. (In isoniazid-resistant infections, dosages up to 60 mg/kg have been used.)

Children. Not recommended.

Pregnancy safety. Not established.

NURSING CONSIDERATIONS

Assessment. Mycobacterial cultures and sensitivity testing should be done before and periodically throughout therapy to monitor progress. Clients with impaired hepatic function should not receive pyrazinamide unless absolutely essential.

Intervention. Reduced dosages may be required for clients with impaired renal function.

Education. Encourage the client to remain compliant with the full course of therapy, which may take years.

Regular visits to the health care provider are essential for monitoring progress.

Clients testing their urine with sodium nitroprusside urine ketone tests may have color interference and should use another test for urine ketones.

Teach clients measures to prevent gout, such as maintaining a fluid intake of 2500 ml daily, adjusting to optimum weight, and limiting intake of alcohol and foods high in purines, such as organ meats (liver, kidneys, hearts, sweetbreads), shellfish, and sardines.

Evaluation. In addition to the hepatic function studies required before and intermittently during therapy with other antitubercular drugs, serum uric acid determinations should be monitored to ensure that an acute episode of gout may be prevented. Observe clients for jaundice and symptoms of acute gouty arthralgia (pain and swelling of joints such as the big toe, knee, and ankle).

rifampin capsules (Rifadin, Rimactane, Rofact✳)

Mechanism of action. Broad-spectrum bactericidal antibiotic. Blocks RNA transcription.

Indications

Treatment of tuberculosis in combination with other antitubercular agents.

To prevent meningococcal meningitis (drug eliminates *Neisseria meningitidis* from the nasopharynx in carriers of meningococcal infections; asymptomatic clients only—not recommended for treatment of meningococcal infections.)

Pharmacokinetics

Absorption. Very good orally.

Distribution. To most body fluids and tissues, including cerebrospinal fluid.

Protein binding. Very high.

Half-life. 1.5 to 5 hours. High after a single dose; decreases after chronic dosing.

Time to peak serum level. 1.5 to 4 hours.

Metabolism. Liver.

Excretion. Feces primarily.

Side effects/adverse reactions. See Table 61-4.

Significant drug interactions. When rifampin is given concurrently with the following drugs, the following interactions may occur.

Drug	Possible Effect and Management
alcohol	Daily usage of alcohol may increase the risk of rifampin-induced hepatotoxicity and increase rate of rifampin metabolism. Monitor closely, as dosage adjustments may be necessary.
adrenocorticoids, glucocorticoids, and mineralocorticoids, anticoagulants, oral coumarin or indandione, corticotropin, digitalis glycosides, disopyramide, or quinidine	Rifampin increases levels of liver-metabolizing enzymes and therefore may decrease the effectiveness of these medications, which are metabolized by liver. Monitor closely, as dosage adjustments may be needed. (Except for digoxin—a cardiac glycoside—because liver plays small role in its metabolism.)
estrogen-containing oral contraceptives, estramustine, or estrogens	Decreases effectiveness due to increased liver metabolism of estrogen. May result in menstrual irregularities, spotting, and unplanned pregnancies. Advise clients of the possible effects when these drugs are combined and advise alternative contraception.
isoniazid or ketoconazole (oral) or miconazole (parenteral)	Increased risk for hepatotoxicity. See comments under isoniazid.
methadone	May decrease the effectiveness of methadone, which may induce methadone withdrawal in dependent clients. Monitor closely, as dosage adjustments may be necessary during and after rifampin therapy.

Dosage and administration

Adults. Tuberculosis: given in combination with other antitubercular agents, 600 mg orally daily. To treat asymptomatic *N. meningitidis* carriers, 600 mg orally daily for 4 days.

Children. Children under 5 years old not established.

To treat tuberculosis in children 5 years old and older, 10 to 20 mg/kg orally daily in combination with other antitubercular agents.

To treat asymptomatic *N. meningitidis* carriers, 10 mg/kg orally every 12 hours for 4 doses.

To prevent *Haemophilus influenzae* infection in carriers, 20 mg/kg orally daily for 4 days.

Maximum daily dose is 600 mg.

Elderly. 10 mg/kg orally daily. Maximum daily dose is up to 600 mg.

Pregnancy safety. Not established.

NURSING CONSIDERATIONS

Assessment. Mycobacterial cultures and sensitivity testing should be done before and periodically throughout therapy to monitor progress. Clients with impaired hepatic function should not receive rifampin unless absolutely essential.

Intervention. Reduced dosages may be required for clients with impaired renal function.

Education. Encourage the client to complete the full course of therapy, which may take years. Clients testing their urine with sodium nitroprusside urine ketone tests may have color interference and should use another test for urine ketones saliva to become reddish. Clients should be reassured that this effect is not hazardous. However, clients that wear soft contact lens should be alerted that this same effect may permanently color the lens.

Women taking oral contraceptives who are also receiving rifampin should be cautioned to use an alternate form of contraception.

Clients should be advised to avoid alcoholic beverages while taking rifampin because it increases the risk of hepatotoxicity.

Caution the client, too, that rifampin may cause drowsiness and to avoid hazardous tasks involving mental alertness until the response to the drug has been ascertained.

Evaluation. In addition to the hepatic function studies required before and intermittently during therapy with other antitubercular drugs, serum uric acid determinations should be monitored to ensure that an acute episode of gout may be prevented. Clients should be observed for jaundice as well as symptoms of acute gouty arthralgia (pain and swelling of joints such as the big toe, knee, and ankle).

Regular visits to the health care provider are essential for monitoring progress.

streptomycin sulfate injection

Streptomycin is a aminoglycoside antibiotic that is poorly absorbed from the gastrointestinal tract; therefore, it is given intramuscularly. It was one of the first effective agents used in the late 1940s to treat tuberculosis, and it still is an important agent in managing severe tuberculosis. Like the other aminoglycosides, its major toxicities include ototoxicity and nephrotoxicity, especially when given to clients with impaired renal function or with other medications with the same toxicities. See Chapter 59 for detailed information on the aminoglycosides.

Dosage and administration

Adults. For tuberculosis, given with other antitubercular agents, 1 g (base) intramuscularly daily. As soon as possible, reduce the dosage to 1 g (base) to two or three times a week.

Children. For tuberculosis, given in combination with other antitubercular agents, 20 mg/kg intramuscularly daily. Maximum daily dose is 1 g. For other infections in combination with other antibacterials, 5 to 10 mg/kg intra-

muscularly every 6 hours or 10 to 20 mg/kg every 12 hours.

Elderly. Reduce dosage to 500 to 750 mg intramuscularly daily.

For other infections, in combination with other antibiotics or antibacterials, 250 mg to 1 g (base) intramuscularly every 6 hours or 500 mg to 2 g every 12 hours.

For plague, 500 mg to 1 g intramuscularly every 6 hours or 1 to 2 g every 12 hours.

For tularemia, 250 to 500 mg intramuscularly every 6 hours or 500 mg to 1 g every 12 hours for 7 to 10 days.

Maximum daily dosage: tuberculosis, 1 g twice a week to 2 g daily; other infections up to 4 g daily.

AMEBIASIS

Amebiasis is an infection of the large intestine produced by a protozoan parasite, *Entamoeba histolytica.* This infestation is found worldwide but is prevalent and severe in tropical areas. It also has been detected in poorly sanitized areas, including some rural communities, Indian reservations, and migrant farm camps. Transmission is usually through ingestion of cysts (fecal to oral route) from contaminated food or water or from person-to-person contact. Poor personal hygiene can increase the spread of this parasite.

LIFE CYCLE OF AMEBA

The protozoan has two stages in its life cycle: (1) the trophozoite (vegetative ameba), which is the active, motile form, and (2) the cyst, or inactive, drug-resistant form that appears in intestinal excretion. The *trophozoite stage* is capable of ameboid motion and sexual activity. Because of its susceptibility to injury, it generally succumbs to an unfavorable environment. However, under certain circumstances, the trophozoite protects itself by entering the *cystic stage.* During this phase the protozoan becomes inactive by surrounding itself with a resistant cell wall within which it can survive for a long time, even in an unsuitable environment.

The complete life cycle of the ameba occurs in humans, the main host. It begins by ingestion of cysts that are present on hands, food, or water contaminated by feces. On reaching the stomach the hydrochloric acid does not destroy the swallowed cysts, but instead they pass unharmed into the small intestine. The digestive juices penetrate the cystic walls, and the trophozoites are released. The motile amebae later pass into the colon, where they live and multiply for a time, feeding on the bacterial flora of the gut. The presence of bacteria is essential for their survival. Finally, before excretion, the trophozoites move toward the terminal end of the bowel and again become encysted. After the cysts are eliminated in the feces, they remain viable and infective. Unfortunately, the cycle may begin again when the cysts appearing in fecal excretion are ingested through contamination of food or water.

The parasite causing amebiasis replicates in three major locations: (1) the lumen of the bowel, (2) the intestinal mucosa, and (3) extraintestinal sites. Thus, amebiasis is classified according to its primary site of action: intestinal amebasis, where amebic activity is restricted to the bowel lumen or intestinal mucosa, or extraintestinal amebiasis, where parasitic invasion occurs outside the intestine.

Intestinal amebiasis. Intestinal amebiasis may be manifested as an asymptomatic intestinal infection or a symptomatic intestinal infection that may be mild, moderate, or severe.

Asymptomatic intestinal amebiasis. In asymptomatic intestinal amebiasis the action of the parasite is restricted to the lumen of the bowel. The individual is asymptomatic but becomes a carrier of the disease by passing mature cysts of the parasite in formed stools. Outside the body the cysts can live for several weeks, surviving dry, freezing, or high temperature conditions. By this means the infection is transmitted from person to person by flies or contaminated food or water. Ordinary concentrations of chlorine in water purification do not destroy the cysts. If the carrier fails to follow any drug treatment, serious gastrointestinal pathologic problems eventually develop. Occasionally mild symptoms exist; they include vague abdominal pain, nausea, flatulence, fatigue, and nervousness.

Symptomatic intestinal amebiasis. Symptomatic amebiasis occurs when the trophozoites in the lumen of the bowel penetrate the mucosal lining of the colon. After they multiply and thrive on bacterial flora, a large infestation occurs, producing diarrhea and abdominal pain. The increased loss of fluid may cause prostration. In addition, ulcerative colitis may result. This state of the disease is called intestinal amebiasis and is usually diagnosed as mild, moderate, or severe according to the intensity of the symptoms and the extent of the disease.

Extraintestinal amebiasis. The term "extraintestinal amebiasis" means that the parasites have migrated to other parts of the body, such as the liver or occasionally the spleen, lungs, or brain. When the parasites are in the liver, necrotic foci develop because of the parasites' destructive effect on tissues. When there is liver involvement, the terms "liver abscess" and "hepatic amebiasis" are usually used.

ANTIAMEBIASIS AGENTS

Drugs for the treatment of amebiasis are classified according to the site of the previously described amebic action. Luminal amebicides act primarily in the bowel lumen and are generally ineffective against parasites in the bowel wall or tissues. Tissue amebicides are drugs that act primarily in the bowel wall, liver, and other extraintestinal tissues. See Table 61-5 for the more commonly used drugs in each classification. No single drug is effective for both types of amebiasis; therefore a luminal and extraluminal (tissue) amebicide or combination therapy is often prescribed.

Luminal Amebicides
carbarsone (Carbarsone Pulvules)

Mechanism of action. An arsenical (contains 29% arsenic), is believed to combine with thiol (SH) groups in the parasite's essential enzyme systems, thus producing a direct amebicidal effect.

Indications. Treatment of intestinal amebiasis and the trophozoites of *E. histolytica* in the lumen of the colon.

Pharmacokinetics

Absorption. Very good after oral administration.

Excretion. Slowly in urine; also in bile.

Side effects/adverse reactions. See Table 61-5.

Significant drug interactions. None.

Dosage and administration

Adults. 250 mg orally two or three times a day for 10 days. If additional courses are necessary, wait 10 to 14 days before resuming therapy.

Children. Specific instructions are given in the recent package insert or in *1988 Facts and Comparisons Drug Information Book.* Generally, the average total dose is 75 mg/kg given in divided doses three times a day.

Pregnancy safety. FDA category C.

NURSING CONSIDERATIONS

Assessment. Administer with caution to clients with hepatic function impairment or to clients with a history of

---

GENERAL RECOMMENDATIONS FOR AMEBICIDES

INTESTINAL AMEBIASIS
carbarsone
emetine HCl
iodoquinol
metronidazole
paromomycin

EXTRAINTESTINAL AMEBIASIS
chloroquine
emetine HCl
metronidazole

TABLE 61-5   Amebicides: Side Effects/Adverse Reactions

Drug	Side effect*	Adverse reactions†
carbarsone		Intolerance or toxic signs: GI distress, nausea, vomiting, cramps, skin lesions, edema, sore throat, hepatitis, neuritis, visual problems, splenomegaly Overdose: diarrhea, nausea, vomiting, stomach pain, shock, coma, seizures, kidney problems, mucous membrane ulcers
iodoquinol	Most frequent: diarrhea, nausea, vomiting, abdominal pain Less frequent: dizziness, headaches, pruritus of rectum	Less frequent: chills, increased temperature, rash, hives, pruritus, neck swelling Chronic use of high doses: visual disturbances, ataxia, increased tiredness, muscle pain Children with chronic, high-dose therapy: eye pain, decreased visual acuity; pain, tingling, or weakness in hands or feet
paromomycin	Nausea, vomiting diarrhea	Stomach cramps, hearing loss, dizziness, tinnitus
emetine	Muscle aching, stiffness, nausea, vomiting, headache, diarrhea, dizziness	Toxic reactions may occur at any dose. Cardiotoxic effects, increased heart rate, precordial pain, ECG disturbances, congestive heart failure, gallop rhythm, severe hypotension, extreme weakness

*If side effects continue, increase, or disturb the client, inform the physician.
†If adverse reactions occur, contact physicians because medical intervention may be necessary.

sensitivity to arsenical agents. Hepatic function studies should be completed before and periodically during therapy. Observe the client for signs of hepatotoxcity such as dark urine, light-colored stools, and yellowing of the skin and sclera of the eyes. Document frequency and character of stools.

Intervention. For ease of administration with clients that have difficulty swallowing, the contents of the capsule may be diluted with applesauce or jelly or in 120 ml of fruit juice. Cleansing enemas may be prescribed to be given before a carbarsone enema.

Education. The client must take the medication as prescribed. Toxicity may occur if the prescribed dose is exceeded. Discontinue at the first indication of toxicity. Notify the physician immediately of skin lesions occur; severe exfoliative dermatitis may result.

Teach clients proper hygiene to prevent reinfestation.

Evaluation. The effectiveness of carbarsone is evaluated by an improvement in the client's condition, an increased sense of well-being, weight gain, a decrease in abdominal discomfort, and return to normal bowel patterns, and a decrease of the parasites in the stool.

Monitor fresh, warm stool specimens periodically for amebic cysts, which indicate a need for continued treatment.

When the course of carbarsone is completed, examine stools for amebic cysts at the end of the first week and monthly thereafter to confirm that the client no longer carries the ameba.

emetine hydrochloride

Mechanism of action. Emetine is a potent amebicide that is highly effective against the trophozoites (vegetative) forms of *E. histolytica*. Emetine blocks protein synthesis by inhibiting attachment of tRNA to the ribosomes. The drug acts primarily on the intestinal and extraintestinal parasites.

Indications

Treatment of acute amebic dysentery or acute intestinal amebiasis.

Treatment of extraintestinal amebiasis, amebic abscesses, and amebic hepatitis.

Also used in other parasite infections such as balantidiasis, fascioliasis, and paragonimiasis.

Pharmacokinetics

Absorption. Administered parenterally. Rapidly absorbed from subcutaneous and intramuscular injection.

Distribution. Liver, lungs, spleen, and kidney. High concentrations in the liver with insignificant levels in the gastrointestinal tract may account for the greater success in treaitng hepatic than in intestinal amebiasis.

Excretion. Some of the drug is excreted in the urine in 20 to 40 minutes; the remainder is eliminated very slowly, with some of it remaining in the tissues for 40 to 60 days after administration. For this reason, the potential for cumulative toxic reactions is a constant danger.

Side effects/adverse reactions. See Table 61-5.

Significant drug interactions. None.

Dosage and administration. Do not give this drug

intravenously, as this route is dangerous and contraindicated.

Adults. Deep subcutaneous injection is preferred; it may also be given intramuscularly. Some authorities recommend a dose of 1 mg/kg/day, not to exceed 65 mg/day or 10 days of therapy (total dose of 650 mg). If therapy needs to be repeated, wait at less 6 weeks before starting another course of therapy.

Children. Use *only* in very severe dysentery that cannot be controlled by other amebicides. Under 8 years old, do not exceed 10 mg/day; over 8 years old; do not exceed 20 mg/day. For amebic hepatitis or abscesses, administer for 10 days.

Pregnancy safety. FDA category X.

NURSING CONSIDERATIONS

Assessment. Emetine is containdicated in individuals with cardiac or renal disease, except those with amebic hepatitis or abscess not controlled by chloroquine. It should not be used during pregnancy or in children except those with severe dysentery not responsive to other amebicidal agents. Do not repeat therapy in clients who have received a course of treatment less than 6 to 8 weeks previously.

Use emetine with caution in elderly or debilitated clients. Discontinue medication if tachycardia, hypotension, muscular weakness, or dyspnea occurs.

Intervention. Emetine is administered in a hospital, and bed rest is indicated for the course of therapy and for several days after emetine is discontinued. Treatment is usually limited to 10 days. If necessary, a course of therapy may be repeated only after a 6- to 8-week rest period.

Administer medication by deep subcutaneous or intramuscular injection. Aspirate syringe before injecting drug to avoid inadvertent intravenous administration, which can result in dangerous toxic effects. Rotate injection site to prevent local irritation and swelling.

When preparing emetine for parenteral use, avoid contact with eyes or mucous membranes, as the drug is irritating.

Monitor pulse and blood pressure several times a day. Perform ECG before administering emetine to use as a baseline; repeat after the fifth dose, on completion of therapy, and 1 week later. ECG pattern resembles that of myocardial infarction (e.g., ST elevation, T-wave inversion, Q-T interval prolongation). These changes occur about 7 days following drug administration and are reversible, with complete return to normal in about 6 weeks. If tachycardia occurs, anticipate the appearance of ECG abnormalities.

Education. Because the drug is cardiotoxic, advise client to avoid strenuous exercise for several weeks following termination of therapy.

Teach client meticulous personal hygiene to avoid reinfection. Stress the importance of handwashing and of sanitary disposal of feces. Family members should also observe proper hygiene.

Evaluation. Observe client for unusual symptoms such as muscle stiffness, restlessness, fatigue, or pain in the neck or upper extremities. Report these signs to the physician, for the drug may need to be discontinued.

Monitor intake and output. Report oliguria or any other change in renal function. Keep a record of the character of stools: number, consistency, unusual odor, presence of mucus or other abnormal matter.

Deliver still-warm stool specimen to the laboratory so that ameba can be identified. Inform client that stool specimens must be examined periodically for up to 3 months following therapy to ensure continued elimination of ameba. Because clients with acute amebic dysentery frequently become asymptomatic carriers, it is essential to check family members and other contacts.

iodoquinol (Diiodohydroxyquin, Yodoxin, Moebiquin)

Mechanism of action. Iodoquinol is an amebicidal agent that destroys both the trophozoites and cysts of *EG histolytica.* Since the drug is poorly absorbed from the tract, its amebicidal activity is mostly limited to the intestinal site. It is ineffective in amebic abscess and amebic hepatitis.

Indications. Treatment of acute and chronic intestinal amebiasis.

Pharmacokinetics

Absorption. Poor from gastrointestinal tract.

Excretion. Feces.

Side effects/adverse reactions. See Table 61-5.

Significant drug interactions. May increase the blood levels of protein-bound iodine, thus interfering with certain thyroid function tests. This effect may last up to 6 months after the drug is stopped.

Dosage and administration

Adults. 650 mg orally two or three times a day; after meals for 20 days.

Children. 40 mg/kg orally in three divided doses for 20 days.

Pregnancy safety. Not established.

NURSING CONSIDERATIONS

Assessment. Intake and output should be documented, as well as frequency and character of stools. Fresh, warm stools should be monitored for the presence of amebae. Diarrhea may occur the first few days of therapy with iodoquinol. Alert the physician if it continues for more than 3 days.

Clients should have an ophthalmologic exam before and periodically during therapy.

Intervention. Administer drug with meals to minimize gastrointestinal irritation. The course of therapy may be repeated if necessary only after a 2- to 3-week rest period.

For ease of administration to children and for clients that may have difficulty swallowing, tablets may be crushed and mixed with applesauce, Jello, or ice cream.

Education. Clients should be instructed in proper hygiene to prevent reinfection. Inform the client that any results of thyroid function studies completed within 6 months of the discontinuance of iodoquinol may be distorted.

Evaluation. The development of a neurologic disorder such as myelooptic neuropathy has been implicated in treatment with prolonged high doses. This is characterized by the presence of blurred vision, optic atrophy, optic neuritis, and peripheral neuropathy (numbness, pain, or weakness in hands or feet).

Iodoquinol can cause thyroid enlargement, and it interferes with certain thyroid function tests by increasing protein-bound serum iodine levels. The drug contains approximately 64% iodine.

In children, the administration of iodoquinol for chronic diarrhea has been responsible for causing optic atrophy and permanent loss of vision. Thus administration of this drug is not advocated for treatment or prophylaxis of "traveler's diarrhea" or for use in chronic nonspecific diarrhea.

Contraindicated for use in patients who have liver disease or who are hypersensitive to iodine.

paromomycin (Humatin)

Mechanism of action. Paromomycin is both an amebicidal and an antibacterial agent. The drug is a broadspectrum aminoglycoside antibiotic that is produced from cultures of *Streptomyces rimosus*. Its antibacterial properties are similar to those of kanamycin and neomycin. Paromomycin acts directly on intestinal amebae and on bacteria such as *Salmonella* and *Shigella*. Because the drug is poorly absorbed from the gastrointestinal tract, it exerts no effect on systemic infections such as extraintestinal amebiasis.

Indications. Treatment of acute and chronic intestinal amebiasis, adjunct therapy in management of hepatic coma.

Pharmacokinetics

Absorption. Poor from gastrointestinal tract.

Excretion. Feces.

Side effects/adverse reactions. See Table 61-5.

Significant drug interactions. None.

Dosage and administration. For intestinal amebiasis: adults and children, 25 to 35 mg/kg orally daily, given in three divided doses with meals for 5 to 10 days. For management of hepatic coma, adults, 4 g orally daily in divided doses at regular intervals for 5 to 6 days.

Pregnancy safety. Not established.

NURSING CONSIDERATIONS

Assessment. Paromomycin is contraindicated for use in intestinal obstruction and in ulcerative bowel lesions because of possible systemic absorption. Notify the physician if ringing of the ears or dizziness occurs.

Intervention. Administer after meals to minimize gastrointestinal distress.

Education. Teach the client proper personal hygiene to prevent reinfection.

Evaluation. Examine fresh, warm stools for the presence of amebae at weekly intervals for 6 weeks after the end of therapy and monthly for 2 years to indicate that the client is not harboring the parasite.

Other Drugs

Chloroquine phosphate and chloroquine hydrochloride are also used to treat extraintestinal amebiasis. See drug monograph for further information on these drugs. Dehydroemetine (Mebadin) and diloxanide furoate (Furamide) are also antiinfective agents used to treat amebiasis but are only available from the Centers for Disease Control (Parasitic Disease Drug Service, Division of Host Factors, Center for Infectious Disease, Atlanta, GA 30333), as they are considered investigational agents.

OTHER PROTOZOAN DISEASES

Several other protozoan diseases are widespread throughout the world and may be encountered in medical practice in the United States. In this section each disease and the primary antiprotozoan agent used in its treatment will be described.

BALANTIDIASIS

Balantidium coli, which causes **balantidiasis,** is the largest of the protozoa that infest the lumen of the large intestine. The organism performs ciliated movement and reproduces asexually and sexually. It feeds on intestinal bacteria and can also invade the intestinal wall by penetrating the mucosa. The organism is capable of producing lesions similar to those caused by *E. histolytica.* The symptoms are nausea, vomiting, abdominal pain, and diarrhea. The organism also forms cysts, which are eliminated with the feces. Some individuals become asymptomatic carriers. The pharmacologic treatment of the disease is emetine and iodoquinol.

GIARDIASIS

The distribution of **giardiasis,** caused by *Giardia lamblia,* is worldwide. The parasite is similar to *E. hisolytica* in that it appears in two forms. The motile trophozoites exist and multiply in the upper small intestine, the duodenum, jejunum, and occasionally the biliary tract of the human. The cysts develop in the gastrointestinal tract and are usually expelled with the feces.

G. lamblia is transmitted by ingesting water or food contaminated with fecal matter that contains cysts. The incubation period is 1 month. Symptoms include anorexia, nausea, diarrhea, and foul-smelling, bulky stools. However, the disease is not life-threatening. Sporadic outbreaks of the disease have developed in various parts of the United States. Old overworked filtration systems allow the organisms to enter the water supply. Giardiasis is treated with metronidazole.

PNEUMOCYSTOSIS

Pneumocystosis is a disease found commonly in individuals who have impaired immune systems caused by malignancies, collagen vascular diseases, AIDS, or immunosuppressive therapy. It is caused by the parasite *Pneumocystis carinii.* Characteristically the disease's symptoms initially are vague and generalized and include a dry cough, dyspnea or tachypnea or both, chest discomfort, and marked pallor. Cyanosis is the most common and consistent finding. If untreated, the disease progresses into interstitial plasma cell pneumonia, where its infiltration into the lungs and lung tissue causes a honeycombed appearance. Fatality is 50% or more of individuals who do not receive treatment at this advanced stage of the disease. Children are more susceptible to pneumocystosis than are adults. The drug of choice for treatment is trimethoprim/sulfamethoxazole. Clients who do not respond to this drug or who have a severe adverse reaction to it are often given pentamidine.

TRYPANOSOMIASIS

Trypanosomiasis is not commonly found in the United States but is found extensively in other parts of the world. There are two types of trypanosomiasis, the African variety and the South American variety.

African trypanosomiasis (sleeping sickness) is caused by *Trypanosoma gambiense* or *T. rhodesiense.* These protozoans are transmitted from host to host by the bite of the tsetse fly. The organism then invades the lymphatic system and causes intermittent attacks of fever, lymphadenopathy, hepatosplenomegaly, dyspnea, and tachycardia. This is called the hemolytic stage of the disease and is treated with suramin sodium, the drug of choice.

As the disease progresses into the central nervous system, the victim experiences headaches, disturbances in coordination, mental dullness, apathy, and eventually constant sleep, resulting in emaciation and death. This latter state, with involvement of the central nervous system, has been treated effectively with melarsoprol, an investigational drug available from the Centers for Disease Control.

The South American variety of trypanosomiasis is often referred to as Chagas' disease. It is caused by the protozoan *T. cruzi* and is transmitted by the bite of reduviid bugs infected with these parasites. The disease may be asymptomatic or symptomatic, varying from region to region. Early symptoms may be local swelling (chagoma) at the site of the insect bite, rash, fever, and edema of eyelids and face. The chronic form of the disease may result in visceromegaly, cardiopathy, or meningoencephalitis resulting in death, or the individual may remain asymptomatic. *T. cruzi* seems to have an affinity for cardiac parenchymal cells and nerve cells in the mesenteric plexus.

Chagas' disease is resistant to most forms of therapy. The drug nifurtimox has shown activity against both extracellular and intracellular parasites that no other drug has demonstrated.

All the agents now used in treating both African and South American trypanosomiasis are severely toxic. As a result, their usefulness in treating these diseases has been limited. All three agents used in treating trypanosomiasis are available from the U.S. Centers for Disease Control.

TOXOPLASMOSIS

Toxoplasmosis is caused by an intracellular parasite, *Toxoplasma gondii.* This parasite is found worldwide and infests a variety of animals, including humans. It is often harbored in the host with no evidence of the disease. Toxoplasmosis is contracted by ingesting cysts found in inadequately cooked raw meat or by accidentally ingesting cysts from cat feces.

The most common form of the disease in the United States is usually subclinical. Symptomatically the individual may experience lymphadenopathy, fever, and occasionally a rash on the palms and soles. The most serious complication of toxoplasmosis is meningoencephalitis. Toxoplasmosis is treated with a combination of sulfadiazine and pyrimethamine, both of which alter the folic acid cycle of the *Toxoplasma* organism, resulting in its death. The oral dosage of pyrimethamine is 25 mg/day for 3 to 4 weeks; the dosage of sulfadiazine is 4 g/day for 3 to 4 weeks.

TRICHOMONIASIS

Trichomoniasis is a disease of the vagina caused by *Trichomonas vaginalis.* Its characteristic presentation consists of a wet, inflamed vagina, a "strawberry" cervix, and a thin, yellow, frothy malodorous discharge. Usually both sexual partners are infected by this organism, which can be identified microscopically from semen, prostatic fluid, or exudate from the vagina. Infections often recur, which indicates that the protozoans persist in extravaginal foci, male urethra, or the periurethral glands and ducts of both sexes. Metronidazole is the drug of choice, and treatment must be given simultaneously to both partners involved for cure. Two other agents—tinidazole and nimorazole—are being used successfully in its treatment in other countries.

HELMINTHIASIS

The disease-producing **helminths** are classified as metazoa, or multicellular animal parasites. Unlike the protozoa, they are large organisms that have a complex cellular structure and that feed on host tissue. They may be present in the gastrointestinal tract, but several types also penetrate the tissues, and some undergo developmental changes during which they wander extensively in the host. Because most anthelmintics used today are highly effective against specific parasites, the organism must be accurately identified before treatment is started, usually by finding the parasite ova or larvae in the feces, urine, blood sputum, or tissues of the host.

Parasitic infestations do not necessarily cause clinical manifestations, although they may be injurious for a number of reasons.

1. Worms may cause mechanical injury to the tissues and organs. Roundworms in large numbers may cause obstruction in the intestine; filariae may block lymphatic channels and cause massive edema; and hookworms often cause extensive damage to the wall of the intestine and considerable loss of blood.
2. Toxic substances produced by the parasite may be absorbed by the host.
3. The tissues of the host may be traumatized by the presence of the parasite and made more susceptible to bacterial infections.
4. Heavy infestation with worms will rob the host of food. This is particularly significant in children.

Helminths that are parasitic to humans are classified as (1) Platyhelminthes (flatworms), which include two subclasses: cestodes (tapeworms) and trematodes (flukes), and (2) Nematoda (roundworms).

PLATYHELMINTHS (FLATWORMS)

Cestodes. Cestodes are tapeworms, of which there are four varieties: (1) *Taenia saginata* (beef tapeworm), (2) *T. solium* (pork tapeworm), (3) *Diphyllobothrium latum* (fish tapeworm), and (4) *Hymenolepis nana* (dwarf tapeworm). As indicated by the name of the worm, the para-

site enters the intestine by way of improperly cooked beef, pork, or fish or from contaminated food, as in the case of the dwarf tapeworm.

The cestodes are segmented flatworms with a head or scolex, which has hooks or suckers that are used to attach to tissues, and a number of segments, or proglottids, which in some cases may extend for 20 to 30 feet in the bowel. Drugs affecting the scolex allow expulsion of the organisms from the intestine. Each of the proglottids contains both male and female reproductive units. When filled with fertilized eggs, they are expelled from the worm into the environment. Upon ingestion, the infected larvae develop into adults in the small intestine of the human. The larvae may travel to extraintestinal sites and enter other tissues such as the liver, muscle, and eye. The tapeworms, with the exception of the dwarf tapeworm, spend part of their life cycle in a host other than humans—pigs, fish, or cattle. The dwarf tapeworm does not require an intermediate host.

The tapeworm has no digestive tract and, therefore, it depends on the nutrients that are intended for the host. Subsequently, the victim suffers by eventually developing nutritional deficiency.

Trematodes. Trematodes, or flukes, are flat, nonsegmented parasites with suckers that attach to and feed on host tissue. The life cycle begins with the egg, which is passed into fresh water following fecal excretion from the body of the human host. The egg containing the embryo forms into a ciliated organism, the *miracidium.* In the presence of water the miracidium escapes from the egg and enters the intermediate host, the freshwater snail, which exists extensively in rice paddies and irrigation ditches. After entry, the fluke forms a cyst in the lungs of the snail. In the cyst, many organisms develop. They can penetrate other parts of the snail and grow into worms called *cercariae.* Eventually, the cercariae are released from the snail into the water, attaching themselves to blades of grass to encyst. Humans, the final host, then becomes infected by the parasite.

When encysted organisms in snails or even fish and crabs are swallowed by humans, they develop into adult flukes in different structures of the body. The flukes, therefore, are classified according to the type of tissues they invade. Following ingestion, the eggs of *Schistosoma haematobium* appear in the urinary bladder and cause inflammation of the urogenital system. This can result in chronic cystitis and hematuria. Infestations with *S. japonicum* and *S. mansoni* produce intestinal disturbance with resultant ulceration and necrosis of the rectum. *S. japonicum* is more concentrated in the veins of the small intestine. If the liver and spleen become infected, the disease is usually fatal. *S. mansoni* prefers the portal veins that drain the large intestine, particularly the sigmoid colon and rectum. Unlike the other parasites, the cercariae of *S. mansoni* are not ingested but burrow through the skin, especially between the toes of the human host who is standing in contaminated water. They then make their way to the portal system, where they mature into adult flukes.

Schistosomiasis (bilharziasis) occurs endemically in Africa, Asia, South America, and the Caribbean islands. The disease can be controlled largely by eliminating the intermediate host, the snail. Travelers to these areas must avoid contact with contaminated water for drinking, bathing, or swimming. Unfortunately, the disease has been introduced in the United States by immigrants or individuals who have traveled to the endemic areas.

NEMATODA (ROUNDWORMS)

Nematoda are nonsegmented, cylindrical worms that consist of a mouth and complete digestive tract. The adults reside in the human intestinal tract; there is no intermediate host. Two types of nematode infection exist in the human: the egg form and the larval form.

Egg infective form. Ascaris lumbricoides is a large nematode (about 30 cm in length) and is known as the "roundworm of humans." The adult *Ascaris* usually resides in the upper end of the small intestine of the human, where it feeds on semidigested foods. The fertilized egg, when excreted with feces, can survive in the soil for a long time. When inadvertently ingested by another host, the embryos escape from the eggs and mature into adults in the host. To prevent the disease, proper sanitary conditions and meticulous personal habits must be observed.

Infection with *Enterobius vermicularis,* or pinworm, is highly prevalent among children and adults in the U.S. Adult pinworms reside in the large intestine. However, the female migrates to the anus, depositing her eggs around the skin of the anal region. This causes intense itching and can be noted especially in children. Diagnosis is made with the Graham sticky tape method. Ingestion of excreted eggs can infect an individual. In addition, eggs that contaminate clothing, bedding, furniture, and other items may be responsible for continuing the reinfection of an individual and initiating the infection of others.

Larval infective form. Necator americanus (New World) or *Ancylostoma duodenale* (Old World) hookworms are somewhat similar in action. They reside in the small intestine of humans. When the eggs are excreted in the feces, the larvae hatch in the soil. The larvae can penetrate the skin of humans, particularly through the soles of the feet, producing dermatitis (ground itch). On entry into the small intestine, they develop into adult worms. During the process they extravasate blood from the intestinal vessels and cause a profound anemia in the victim. The presence of eggs in the feces indicates a positive test for hookworm disease. This infection can be avoided by wearing shoes.

Trichinella spiralis is a small pork roundworm that causes trichinosis. In humans the disease begins by ingestion of insufficiently cooked pork or bear meat. On entry of encysted meat into the small intestine, the larvae are released from the cysts. Following maturation, the females develop eggs that later form into larvae. They then migrate by the bloodstream and the lymphatic system to the skeletal muscles and encyst. Encapsulation and eventually calcification of the cysts occur. Diagnosis of trichinosis is made by muscle biopsy, whereby microscopic examination reveals the presence of larvae. The disease is prevented by thoroughly cooking pork and bear meat before eating.

ANTHELMINTIC AGENTS

Anthelmintic drugs are used to rid the body of worms (helminths). Anthelmintics (*anti,* against; Gr. *helmins,* worm) are among the most primitive types of chemotherapy. It has been estimated that one third of the world's population is infested with these parasites.

diethylcarbamazine citrate (Hertazan)*

Mechanism of action. Synthetic organic compound that is specific for certain common parasites; see Table 61-6.

Indications. Treatment of Bancroft's filariasis, onchocerciasis, ascariasis, tropical eosinophilia, and loiasis.

Pharmacokinetics. Not available.

Side effects/adverse reactions

In *Wuchereria bancrofti* infestations, the most common reactions are headache, tiredness, or weakness. Less frequent effects include nausea, vomiting, and skin rash. Therapy is only discontinued when a severe allergic reaction is noted.

In onchocerciasis, the most frequent reactions are facial edema, especially around the eyes, and pruritus. When the infestation is intense, a severe reaction may occur after only one dose. Monitor closely.

In ascariasis, nausea, vomiting, giddiness, and tiredness occur most often, especially in undernourished or debilitated children.

Significant drug interactions. None.

Dosage and administration

Adults

For Bancroft's filariasis, onchocerciasis, and loiasis: usually 2 mg/kg orally after meals, three times a day. In acute stage, the treatment may be given for 3 to 4 weeks.

For ascariasis: clients are treated in the community health facilities with a dose of 13 mg/kg orally daily for 1 week, which should reduce the number of worms by 85% to 100%; no posttreatment purging is

*Drug is available free from Lederle Laboratories. For address and phone number, see *Facts and Comparisons Drug Information* (Kastrup, EK, ed) reference.

TABLE 61-6   Drugs Used in Treatment of Helminthiasis

Disease	Organism	Drug of choice	Alternate choice
CESTODES (TAPEWORMS)			
Diphyllobothriasis	*Diphyllobothrium latum* (fish tapeworm)	Niclosamide*	Paromomycin
Hymenolepiasis	*Hymenolepis nana* (dwarf tapeworm)	Niclosamide*	Paromyomycin
Taeniasis	*Taenia saginata* (beef tapeworm)	Niclosamide*	Paromomycin
Taeniasis	*Taenia solium* (pork tapeworm)	Niclosamide,* Quinacrine	Paromomycin
TREMATODES (FLUKES)			
Fascioliasis	*Fasciola hepatica* (liver fluke)	Bithionol*	None
Fasciolopsiasis	*Fasciolopsis buski* (intestinal fluke)	Hexylresorcinol†	None
Paragonimiasis	*Paragonimus westermani* (lung fluke)	Bithionol*	None
Schistosomiasis *(Bilharziasis):*	*Schistosoma* (blood fluke):		
Urinary *Bilharziasis*	*S. haematobium*	Metrifonate*	Niridazole*
Oriental schiztosomiasis	*S. japonicum*	Niridazole*	Antimony sodium dimercapto-succinate*
Intestinal or hepatosplenic *Bilharziasis*	*S. mansoni*	Niridazole* or oxamniquine	Antimony sodium dimercapto-succinate*
NEMATODES (ROUNDWORMS)	Intestinal roundworms:		
Ascariasis	*Ascaris lumbricoides* (giant roundworm)	Pyrantel pamoate or Mebendazole	Piperazine citrate
Enterobiasis	*Enterobius vermicularis* (pinworm)	Pyrantel pamoate or Mebendazole	Piperazine citrate
Uncinariasis	*Necator americanus* (hookworm)	Pyrantel pamoate or Mebendazole	Thiabendazole
Strongyloidiasis	*Strongyloides stercolaris* (threadworm)	Thiabendazole	
Trichuriasis	*Trichuris trichiura* (whipworm)	Mebendazole	None
TISSUE ROUNDWORMS			
Cutaneous larva migrans (creeping eruptions)	*Ancylostoma braziliense*	Thiabendazole	
Dracunculoida	*Dracunculus medinensis* (guinea worm)	Niridazole*	Metronidazole
FILARIAL NEMATODES			
Filariasis	*Brugia (W.) malayi*	Diethylcarbamazine	None
No common name	*Dipetalonema perstans*	Diethylcarbamazine	
Loiasis	*Loa loa*	Diethylcarbamazine	
Filariasis	*Wuchereria bancrofti*	Diethylcarbamazine	
Tropical eosinophilia	Tropical pulmonary eosinophilia	Diethylcarbamazine	
Onchocerciasis	*Onchocerca volvulus*	Diethylcarbamazine plus Suramin*	
Trichinosis	*Trichinella spiralis* (pork roundworm)	Thiabendazole plus steroids for severe symptoms	Mebendazole

*Drug is available for use only from the Parasitic Disease Service Centers for Disease Control, Atlanta, GA 30333.
†Not available in the United States.

necessary. The ascarids are excreted within 1 to 2 days after therapy is started.

Children. Give 6 to 10 mg orally three times a day for 7 to 10 days. At times, an additional course of therapy is necessary.

NURSING CONSIDERATIONS

Assessment. Use with caution in children under 2 years of age.

Drug should not be used during pregnancy. Fetal damage in laboratory animals has been demonstrated. Do not use in individuals who are hypersensitive to mebendazole.

Intervention. For ease of administration, the tablet may be chewed, swallowed whole, or crushed and mixed with food. No dietary restrictions, laxatives, or posttreatment purging are required. A second course of therapy will be required if the patient is not cured in 3 weeks.

Anticipate expulsion of roundworms in 1 to 2 days following initial therapy.

An individual with a recent history of malaria should be given an antimalarial agent before initiating diethylcarbamazine therapy. This prevents recurrence of a malarial attack.

In pinworm infestation, treat all family members because it is readily transmitted from person to person.

Collect stool specimen in clean, dry, and properly labeled container and send to laboratory. Do not contaminate specimen with water, urine, or chemicals because parasite may be destroyed. Collect *pinworm specimen:* wrap a transparent strip of cellophane (sticky side out) around a tongue blade and press against perianal area. Then place sticky side of tape on a glass slide and send to laboratory. Female worm emerges from the rectum during the night to lay eggs in the perianal area. This causes the client to become restless during sleep. The emerging worms can be seen at night with a flashlight.

Education. Emphasize the importance of following meticulous hygiene: washing hands before eating and after going to toilet; keeping hands or objects from mouth. Avoid walking barefoot to prevent hookworm. The larvae hatch in the soil and penetrate through the skin. Instruct client to take frequent showers rather than baths, to change underclothes, nightclothes, bedclothes, and towels daily, and to disinfect toilet facilities daily.

For treatment of filiaris, stress the importance of remaining under physician's care. Failure to follow drug regimen eventually can obstruct lymph flow, thereby producing hydrocele, elephantiasis of limbs, enlarged scrotum or breasts, and chyluria (milk-like urine).

Evaluation. If allergic reactions occur (swelling and itching of skin, fine papular rash, tenderness of lymph nodes, headache, fever, tachycardia, conjunctivitis, uveitus), report to physician. Antihistamine therapy or corticosteroids are usually prescribed to relieve these symptoms. Ophthalmoscopic examinations are performed on clients treated for onchocerciasis. Report immediately any signs of itching or swelling of eyes. Corticosteroid eye drops may be administered for treatment of this condition.

mebendazole (Vermox)

Mechanism of action. Blocks glucose uptake by the helminths, which depletes glycogen stores necessary for survival and reproduction of the infestation.

Indications. Treatment of *Trichuris trichiura* (whipworm), *Enterobius vermicularis* (pinworm), *Ascaris lumbricoides* (roundworm), *Ancylostoma duodenale* (common hookworm), or *Necator americanus* (American hookworm), singly or in mixed infestations.

Pharmacokinetics

Absorption. Poor orally (5% to 10%).

Peak plasma levels. Within 2 to 4 hours.

Excretion. Feces.

Side effects/adverse reactions. Some transient stomach pain and diarrhea.

Significant drug interactions. None.

Dosage and administration

Adults and children. Trichuriasis, ascariasis, and hookworm infestations: one tablet morning and evening for 3 consecutive days. If not cured, a second treatment may be administered. Enterobiasis: one tablet only.

Pregnancy safety. FDA categeory C.

NURSING CONSIDERATIONS

Intervention. For ease of administration, tablets may be crushed and mixed with applesauce or other food. No dietary restrictions, laxatives, or posttreatment enemas are necessary.

Education. Stress the importance of handwashing and of sanitary disposal of feces. Instruct the client to wash the perianal area daily to prevent reinfestation. Underwear and bed linens should be changed daily. All family members should be treated at the same time.

niclosamide (Niclocide)

Mechanism of action. Niclosamide affects the mitochondria of the cestode, inhibiting aerobic metabolism. It also impedes anaerobic metabolism, on which many cestodes depend for survival. Contact with the drug results in destruction of the scolex and proximal segments of the organism, the proglottids. The scolex, when loosened from the intestinal wall, is usually digested in the intestine. Consequently, identification of the worm in the feces cannot be made.

Indications. Treatment of *Taenia saginata* (beef tapeworm), *Diphyllobothrium latum* (fish tapeworm), and *Hymenolepis nana* (dwarf tapeworm) infestations.

Pharmacokinetics

Absorption. Poor. This means the drug can exert its effect at the intended site of action, namely the intestine, for a prolonged period of time.

Excretion. Feces.

Side effects/adverse reactions. See Table 61-7.

Significant drug interactions. None.

Dosage and administration

Adults. Thoroughly chew, then swallow the tablets with a little water.

For *T. saginata* and *D. latum* (beef and fish tapeworms): four tablets (2 g) as single dose; for *H. nana* (dwarf tapeworm), four tablets (2 g) daily for 1 week.

Children. For young children, tablets may be crushed to a fine powder and a paste made with water. Take after a light meal such as breakfast.

For *T. saginata* and *D. latum* (beef and fish tapeworms): child over 75 pounds, three tablets (1.5 g) as single dose; child from 25 to 75 pounds, two tablets (1 g) as single dose.

For *Hymenolepis nana* (dwarf tapeworm): child over 75 pounds, three tablets (1.5 g) on first day, then two tablets (1 g) daily for 6 days; between 25 and 75 pounds, two tablets (1 g) the first day, then one tablet (0.5 g) daily for next 6 days.

Pregnancy safety. FDA category B.

NURSING CONSIDERATIONS

Assessment. The safety for use in pregnancy has not been established. The drug should be used only if the potential benefit outweighs the risk to the fetus. It is not known whether niclosamide is excreted in breast milk. Since it is not absorbed in significant amounts from the gastrointestinal tract, the drug is unlikely to be excreted through this route.

Niclosamide should not be administered to clients who are hypersensitive to the drug.

Intervention. Treatment may be administered on an outpatient basis.

TABLE 61-7   Selected Anthelmintic Agents: Side Effects/Adverse Reactions

Drug	Side effects*	Adverse reactions†
niclosamide		Most frequent: stomach pain or distress, anorexia, nausea, vomiting Less frequent/rare: diarrhea, dizziness, sedation, pruritus of rectum, rash, bad taste in mouth
pyrantel	Less frequent: stomach cramps or distress, diarrhea, dizziness, sedation, headaches, insomnia, anorexia, nausea, vomiting	Less frequent: skin rash Overdose: muscle tremors or weakness, respiratory difficulties, lightheadedness, collapse
thiabendazole	Most frequent: lightheadedness, anorexia, nausea, vomiting Less frequent/rare: diarrhea, sedation, headache, bed wetting, back pain (lower), pain on urination, abdominal distress	Less frequent: chills, elevated temperature, muscle or joint aches, rash, pruritus, skin redness, blistering or peeling, edema, increased weakness Rare: yellow or blurred vision, visual disturbances, tinnitus, tingling or numbness of hands or feet

*If side effects continue, increase, or disturb the client, inform the physician.

†If adverse reactions occur, contact physician because medical intervention may be necessary.

Administer the drug after a light meal such as breakfast.

No dietary restrictions are required before or after treatment. Instruct client to chew tablet thoroughly and swallow with a small amount of water. For children crush the tablet to a fine powder and mix with a small amount of water to form paste. If the patient is constipated, a mild laxative should be prescribed to ensure a normal bowel movement.

Education. Advise client to take the drug for the full course of therapy to prevent return of infection. Stress the importance of reporting progress to the physician. If there is no improvement, a second course of therapy may be required. Niclosamide destroys the tapeworm on contact while in the intestine. The killed worms (including the scolex) are passed in the stool and may not be seen. In the treatment of *T. solium* (pork tapeworm), a saline purge such as magnesium sulfate should be given 1 or 2 hours after the administration of niclosamide to prevent the development of cysticercosis in the intestinal tract. Moreover, the procedure provides a good possibility of expulsion of an intact scolex. Note that niclosamide has no effect on cysticercosis.

Because the drug may cause dizziness, warn individual about driving a motor vehicle or operating dangerous machinery.

Instruct client to observe strict hygiene (both personal and environmental) to prevent reinfection. This observance applies particularly to *H. nana* (dwarf tapeworm).

Evaluation. Stress the importance of followup studies; the client is considered cured only if stool examination results are negative for a minimum of 3 months. Stool examination is required 1 month and 3 months following drug regimen.

oxaminiquine (Vansil)

Mechanism of action. Although male schistosomes are more susceptible to this drug than female, after treatment the female schistosomes stops laying eggs, which may be one reason for the drug's effectiveness.

Indications. Treatment of all stages of *Schistosoma mansoni* infections, including those with hepatosplenic involvement.

Pharmacokinetics
Absorption. Good.
Peak serum levels. In 1 to 1.5 hours.
Half-life. 1 to 2.5 hours.
Metabolism. Extensive.
Excretion. Kidneys.
Side effects/adverse reactions. Usually well tolerated. Some transitory dizziness, sedation, nausea, vomiting, stomach pain, anorexia, and headaches reported.

Significant drug interactions. None.
Dosage and administration
Adults. 12 to 15 mg/kg as single dose or recommended dosage schedule as follows;
   30 to 40 kg, 500-mg dose
   41 to 60 kg, 750-mg dose
   61 to 80 kg, 1000-mg dose
   81 to 100 kg, 1250-mg dose.
Children. Under 30 kg, 20 mg/kg in two divided doses, with 2 to 8 hours separating each dose.
Pregnancy safety. FDA category C.

NURSING CONSIDERATIONS

Assessment. Use oxaminiquine with caution in individuals with a history of convulsive disorders.

Intervention. Administer after meals to minimize side effects such as dizziness, drowsiness, and gastrointestinal distress. Oxaminiquine therapy does not require special preparation such as fasting, dietary restrictions, or enemas.

Education. Caution the client to avoid hazardous tasks requiring mental alertness, such as driving, until the response to the drug has been ascertained.

Advise the client that oxaminiquine causes a reddish orange discoloration of the urine that is harmless.

Encourage the client to complete the full course of therapy and to check with the health care provider if there is no improvement after completing a full course of therapy.

piperazine (Vermizine)

Mechanism of action. Piperazine affects the musculature of the helminth, possibly by blocking the stimulating effects of acetylcholine at the myoneural junction. Accordingly, muscle paralysis of the roundworms makes them unable to maintain their position in the host. The paralyzed worms are then dislodged and expelled as a result of normal peristalsis.

Indications. Treatment of enterobiasis (pinworms) and ascariasis (roundworm).

Pharmacokinetics
Absorption. Readily absorbed from gastrointestinal tract.
Metabolism. Approximately 25%.
Excretion. Primarily by kidneys within 24 hours.
Side effects/adverse reactions. Adverse effects include gastrointestinal (nausea, vomiting, stomach cramps, diarrhea); central nervous system (headaches, dizziness, ataxia, trembling, muscle weakness, paresthesia, convulsions, memory defect); ocular (blurred vision, nystagmus, and other visual disturbances); hypersensitivity (rash, hives,

fever, cough, bronchospasm, lacrimation). If gastrointestinal or hypersensitivity responses are severe, the drug should be discontinued.

Significant drug interactions. When piperazine is given with chlorpromazine, the extrapyramidal side effects of chlorpromazine may be increased. Also, fatal seizures have been reported. Avoid concurrent administration.

Dosage and administration

Adults. For ascariasis (roundworm): 3.5 g as single dose daily for two consecutive days.

Children. 75 mg/kg as single dose daily for 2 consecutive days. Maximum daily dose is 3.5 g.

Adults and children. For enterobiasis (pinworm): single daily dose of 65 mg/kg (maximum daily dose is 2.5 g) for 7 consecutive days. For severe infections, dose may be repeated after a 1-week interval.

NURSING CONSIDERATIONS

Assessment. Observe individuals with renal insufficiency for signs of neurologic symptoms.

The drug is contraindicated for use in renal or hepatic impairment and in convulsive disorders.

Intervention. The drug may be taken with food. Some physicians prefer single-dose therapy with mebendazole or pyrantel pamoate. No dietary restrictions, laxatives, or enemas are required with piperazine.

Education. Stress the importance of handwashing and of sanitary disposal of feces. Instruct the client to wash the perianal area daily to prevent reinfection. Underwear and bed linens should be changed daily to prevent reinfection. All family members should be treated at the same time.

praziquantel (Biltricide)

Mechanism of action. Penetrates cell membranes and increases cell permeability in susceptible worms. This results in an increased loss of intracellular calcium, contractions, and muscle paralysis of the worm. Drug also disintegrates the schistosome tegument (covering). Subsequently, phagocytes are attracted to the worm and kill it.

Indications. Treatment of *Schistosoma mekongi, S. japonicum, S. mansoni,* and *S. haematobium* infestations.

Pharmacokinetics

Absorption. Good orally.

Peak serum level. Within 1 to 3 hours. Cerebrospinal fluid levels are between 14% and 20% of plasma levels.

Half-life (elimination). 0.8 to 1.5 hours; metabolites, 4 to 5 hours.

Excretion. Kidneys.

Side effects/adverse reactions. Generally well tolerated. Side effects are mild, transient, and are only more severe in clients with a large worm infestation. Headache, lightheadedness, stomach distress, weakness, fever, rash.

Significant drug interactions. None.

Dosage and administration

Adults and children. Three doses of 30 mg/kg as a 1-day treatment. The interval between the doses should be 4 to 8 hours.

Children. Under 4 years old, dosage not established.

Pregnancy safety. FDA category B.

NURSING CONSIDERATIONS

Assessment. Praziquantel is contraindicated in clients with ocular cysticercosis, as destruction of the parasites in the eye by the medication may cause severe ocular damage.

Intervention. No special preparations such as fasting, dietary restrictions, or laxatives are necessary for the administration of praziquantel. However, the tablets should be taken with meals and swallowed whole with a small amount of fluid to avoid the extremely bitter taste. Chewing the tablets may cause gagging and vomiting.

Education. The client should be encouraged to comply with the medication regimen and to visit the health care provider regularly to monitor progress. Because of praziquantel's side effects of dizziness and drowsiness, caution the client to avoid hazardous activities such as driving until the response to the medication has been ascertained.

Evaluation. To monitor the effectiveness of praziquantel, stool examinations are completed at specific intervals, depending on the parasite:

- Intestinal, liver, and blood flukes: 1 week and 1, 6, and 12 months following treatment
- Lung flukes: 1 month following treatment.
- Tapeworms: 1 and 3 months following treatment

For *Schistosoma haematobium* and *S. mekongi,* urine examinations are required at 1, 3, and 6 months to determine proof of cure. A client is not considered cured unless examination results have been negative for several months.

pyrantel pamoate oral suspension (Antiminth, Aut✿, Combantrin✿)
pyrantel pamoate tablets (Combantrin✿)

Mechanism of action. A depolarizing neuromuscular blocking agent, that is, it causes contraction then paralysis of the helminth muscles. The helminths are dislodged and then expelled from the body by persistalsis.

Indications. Treatment of ascariasis, enterobiasis, and helminth infestations.

Pharmacokinetics

Absorption. Poor and incomplete orally.

Time to peak serum level. Within 1 to 3 hours.

Peak serum level. 0.05 to 0.13 μg/ml.

Excretion. Feces.

Side effects/adverse reactions. See Table 61-7.

Significant drug interactions. When pyrantel is given concurrently with piperazine, it may reduce or antagonize pyrantel's antihelmintic action. Avoid concurrent administration.

Dosage and administration

Adults. For ascariasis, 11 mg/kg (base) orally as a single dose. If necessary, may repeat in 2 to 3 weeks. For enterobiasis, 11 mg/kg (base) orally as single dose. Repeat in 2 to 3 weeks. Maximum daily dose is 1 g.

Children. Infants and children up to 2 years old, not established; 2 years and over, see adult dose or check a recent package insert or USP DI for current dosing recommendations.

Pregnancy safety. Not established.

NURSING CONSIDERATIONS

Assessment. Use cautiously in individuals with hepatic impairment.

Intervention. The administration of pyrantel does not require special preparation such as fasting, dietary restrictions, laxatives, or enemas. It may be taken with or without food or at any time of day. Shake well and use the calibrated measuring device provided to accurately measure the dosage.

Education. Encourage the client to take the full course of therapy and visit the health care provider on a regular basis to monitor progress.

Alert the client to avoid hazardous tasks requiring mental alertness such as driving until the response has been determined.

For pinworm infestation, it is important to wash, without shaking, all the bed linens and nightclothes to prevent reinfestation. All household members should be treated simultaneously.

Stress proper hygiene, both personal and environmental, with the client.

Evaluation. For pinworms, perianal examinations using cellophane tape swabs should be completed before and 1 week following pyrantel therapy. Negative examination results for 7 consecutive days indicative cure. Swab tests are taken in the morning before bathing or defecation. For roundworms, stool examination results should be negative for ova, larvae, or worms 2 to 3 weeks after completion of therapy.

quinacrine HCl (Atabrine)

Mechanism of action. Unknown.

Indications. Treatment of giardiasis and cestodiasis.

Pharmacokinetics. Not available.

Side effects/adverse reactions. If visual disturbances occur, notify physician. Transient psychosis (especially in elderly) and a yellow color to skin or urine may occur.

Significant drug interactions. None.

Dosage and administration

Dwarf tapeworm infestations

Adults. Give 1 tablespoon of sodium sulfate in water the night before administering this medication. On first day, administer 900 mg on an empty stomach in three portions approximately 20 minutes apart; 90 minutes later give a sodium sulfate purge. For the next 3 days, administer 100 mg three times a day.

Children. Administer ½ tablespoon of sodium sulfate the night before the medication. Then:

4- to 8-year-olds, give initial dose of 200 mg followed by 100 mg after breakfast for 3 days.

8- to 10-year-olds, give initial dose of 300 mg followed by 100 mg twice a day for 3 days.

11- to 14-year olds, give initial dose of 400 mg, followed by 100 mg three times daily for 3 days.

Tapeworm (beef, pork, and fish) infestation. Start clients on a bland, semisolid, nonfat or milk diet the day before administering the medication. The client should fast after supper. A saline purge and cleansing enema may be administered before treatment and be followed by a saline purge 1 to 2 hours later.

Adults. Four doses of 200 mg (total 800 mg) administered 10 minutes apart. Give sodium bicarbonate, 600 mg, with each dose to reduce nausea or vomiting.

Children. Give following doses in three to four divided doses, 10 minutes apart with 300 mg of sodium bicarbonate with each dose, if tolerated: 5- to 10-year-olds, 400 mg total dose; 11- to 14-year olds, 600 mg total dose. The expelled worm will be stained yellow, which will help in identifying the scolex.

Giardiasis

Adults. 100 mg three times a day for 5 to 7 days.

Children. 7 mg/kg in three divided doses (to maximum of 300 mg/day) after meals for 5 days. Check stools 2 weeks later and, if necessary, repeat treatment course.

Pregnancy safety. Not established.

NURSING CONSIDERATIONS

Assessment. Observe caution in clients with psychosis, G-6-PD deficiency, renal or cardiac disease, hepatic disease, and alcoholism. Cautious use is also indicated in pregnant women, children, and individuals over age 60. Use in individuals with porphyria or psoriasis may exacerbate these conditions; therefore, the benefit must outweigh the risk.

Quinacrine should not be used concomitantly with primaquine because the former increases toxicity of the latter. In pregnant women with tapeworm infestation or giardiasis, treatment should be postponed until after delivery because quinacrine crosses the placenta.

Intervention. Administer drug after meals with a large glass of water or other fluid (tea or fruit juice) to minimize gastric irritation. The bitter taste may be masked by jam or honey.

The client generally requires hospitalization. Give a bland, semisolid, nonfat diet for 1 to 2 days before drug therapy. Individual should fast after evening meal the night before and on morning of drug therapy.

Give a saline or cleansing enema in the evening and 1 or 2 hours before medication. This will decrease the amount of stool required to examine for scoleces after the drug is given. Repeat saline enema 1 or 2 hours after quinacrine is administered to dispel worms. Sodium bicarbonate is given concurrently with the drug to prevent nausea and vomiting. Vomiting may cause the worms to move toward the stomach, where the ova can pass through the stomach wall and cause cycticercosis, or invasion of tissue. Vomiting is also prevented by administering the drug through a duodenal tube, particularly for treatment of pork tapeworm.

Education. Instruct the client to report to the physician any skin eruptions, psychotic behavior (may last up to 2 weeks after discontinuation of drug), or visual disturbances (blurred vision, halos of light, or difficulty in focusing).

Tell the client that the drug imparts a temporary reversible yellow coloration to urine and skin (not jaundice). It also causes a cyanotic temporary coloration (gray-blue tinge) to fingernail beds, ears, and nasal cartilage.

Evaluation. Collect entire stool specimen after treatment (usually for 48 hours); do not put toilet paper in bedpan. The search for scoleces in the laboratory is done by using ultraviolet light: the worm fluoresces on absorption of quinacrine. Scoleces must be found to be certain of a cure; otherwise the tapeworm will grow again.

Perform complete blood counts and ophthalmoscopic examinations periodically, particularly in clients on prolonged therapy. Drug may need to be discontinued if there are significant abnormalities.

thiabendazole oral suspension/tablets (Foldan✿, Mintezol, Triasox✿)

Mechanism of action. Unknown, but thiabendazole inhibits specific enzymes in the helminth (fumarate reductase). Vermicidal.

Indications. Treatment of cutaneous larva migrans, strongyloidiasis, toxocariasis, and trichinosis.

Pharmacokinetics
Absorption. Very good orally.
Half-life. Thiabendazole, in normal and anephric clients, 1.2 hours (0.9 to 2 hours).
Time to peak serum level. 1 to 2 hours.
Peak serum level. Metabolites, between 6.5 and 10 μg/ml.
Metabolism. Liver.
Excretion. Kidneys.
Side effects/adverse reactions. See Table 61-7.
Significant drug interactions. None.
Dosage and administration
Adults
For capillariasis, 25 mg/kg orally, once daily for 20 to 30 days.
For larva migrans, cutaneous, 25 mg/kg orally, twice a day for 2 to 5 days. May be repeated 2 days after treatment is completed if active lesions are present.
For strongyloidiasis, uncomplicated infections, 25 mg/kg orally twice a day for 2 days or 50 mg/kg as a single dose.
For hyperinfection syndrome, 25 mg/kg orally twice a day for 5 to 7 days. If necessary, may be repeated.
For toxocariasis, 25 mg/kg orally twice a day for 5 to 10 days. May repeat in 1 month if needed.
For trichinosis, 25 mg/kg orally twice daily for 2 to 7 days.
For trichostrongyliasis, 25 mg/kg orally twice daily for 2 to 3 days.
Maximum daily dose is 3 g.
Children. See adult dose. For children up to 13.6 kg, the clinical experience of this drug with ascariasis, strongyloidiasis, trichinosis, trichuriasis, and uncinariasis is limited.
Pregnancy safety. FDA category C.

NURSING CONSIDERATIONS

Assessment. The drug should be used with caution in patients with hepatic or renal dysfunction, severe malnutrition, or anemia.

Intervention. Thiabendazole should be administered after meals; no dietary restrictions, laxatives, or enemas are required with this drug.

For the oral suspension form, shake well and use the calibrated measuring device provided to ensure accurate dosage. Chew or crush tablet form before swallowing.

Education. Encourage the client to comply with the full course of treatment and to visit the health care provider to monitor progress.

Because of the side effects of dizziness and drowsiness, caution the client to avoid hazardous activities such as driving that require alertness.

Teach proper hygiene, personal and environmental.

Evaluation. Observe client for hypersensitivity reaction to prevent severe erythema multiforme (Stevens-Johnson syndrome).

Sputum and stool examinations are required to monitor progress of the roundworm infection.

LEPROSY

Leprosy, or **Hansen's disease,** is caused by *Mycobacterium leprae* in humans. Although estimates indicate that nearly 15 million people have leprosy worldwide, in the United States it is more frequently found in Hawaii and areas of Texas, Louisiana, and Florida. Leprosy has also been seen in foreign-born clients, especially those from the Philippines, Mexico, and Vietnam.

Although the precise mode of transmission is unknown, the incubation period for leprosy is a few months to decades. Large numbers of leprosy bacilli are generally shed from skin ulcers, nasal secretions, the gastrointestinal tract and, perhaps, biting insects. It is more prevalent in males than females (3 to 1) in some areas.

M. leprae is a bacillus that in humans first presents as a skin lesion—a large plaque or macule that is erythematous or hypopigmented in the center. More numerous lesions, peripheral nerve trunk involvement, and the common complications of plantar ulceration of the feet, footdrop, loss of hand function, and corneal abrasions may follow.

Most cases can be arrested, if not cured, by appropriate therapy and management. The drugs of choice are dapsone, rifampin, and clofazimine.

dapsone (DDS; Avlosulfon✦)

This drug is not currently marketed in the United States but may be obtained by contacting the National Hansen's Disease Center, Carville, LA 70721.

Mechanism of action. Dapsone is a bacteriostatic agent with an action that is probably similar to that of the sulfonamides. It is effective against *M. leprae*.

Indications. Treatment of all forms of leprosy, except for cases that are dapsone resistant; treatment of dermatitis herpetiformis.

Pharmacokinetics

Absorption. Very good orally.

Peak serum levels. 1 to 3 hours or up to 4 to 8 hours.

Protein binding. High (70% to 90%). Main metabolite, monoacetyl dapsone (MADDS) is 99% bound. To achieve a plateau serum level of 0.5 to 0.7 μm/ml, this drug must be administered daily in 100-mg doses for a minimum of 8 days.

Metabolism. Liver.

Half-life. 10 to 50 hours (average 28).

Excretion. Kidneys.

Side effects/adverse reactions. See Table 61-8.

Significant drug interactions. When dapsone is given concurrently with the following drugs, the following interactions may occur.

Drug	**Possible Effect and Management**
aminobenzoic acid (PABA)	May reduce effect of dapsone by interfering with its mechanism of action. Avoid concurrent usage.
hemolytic agents	Increase the potential for serious adverse effects; avoid if possible.

Dosage and administration

Adults

Antileprosy agent: 100 mg orally daily or 1.4 mg/kg daily.

Dermatitis herpetiformis suppressant initially 50 mg orally daily. Dosage may be increased until symptoms are controlled (up to 300 mg or higher in some cases). Reduce daily dose to the lowest effective maintenance dose as soon as possible.

Maximum daily dose in antileprosy applications, 200 mg daily; as dermatitis herpetiformis suppressant, from 50 to 500 mg/day.

Children. Antileprosy agent: 1.4 mg/kg orally daily.

Pregnancy safety. FDA category A.

NURSING CONSIDERATIONS

Assessment. Administer dapsone cautiously in clients with anemia, deficiencies of G-6-PD and methemoglobin reductase, or hepatic or renal impairment.

CBC should be completed prior to dapsone therapy for a baseline assessment.

Education. Encourage the client to comply with the dapsone regimen and stress that use of the drug is long-term or indefinite. Taking the medication at the same time each day will assist compliance.

Stress the importance of regular visits to the health care provider to monitor progress.

Caution the client that dapsone may cause dizziness and drowsiness; hazardous activities requiring mental alertness such as driving should be avoided until the response to the drug has been determined.

Evaluation. Once therapy has started, a complete blood count should be determined weekly for the first month, monthly for 6 months, and then semiannually for the remainder of dapsone therapy. The dosage may be reduced or suspended if CBC values are diminished: RBCs, below 2.5 million/mm^3; hemoglobin, below 9 g/dl; WBCs, below 5000/mm^3. In addition, the client should be observed for the development of hemolytic anemia; symptoms are pale skin, fever, and unusual tiredness and weakness.

Hepatic function studies should be done if the client develops anorexia, nausea, vomiting, or jaundice.

Peripheral neuritis (numbness and tingling of the hands and feet) and exfoliative dermatitis (itching and scaling of the skin and loss of hair) are also indications for dosage interruption.

clofazimine (Lamprene)

Mechanism of action. Unknown. May have a slow bactericidal effect on *M. leprae.* It inhibits the growth and tends to bind preferentially to mycobacterial DNA.

Indications. A secondary agent for the treatment of leprosy, especially dapsone-resistant leprosy caused by *M. leprae.*

Pharmacokinetics

Absorption. Fair to good (45% to 62%) orally.

Distribution. Very lipophilic.

Half-life. 70 days after chronic dosing.

Mean serum level. 0.7 and 1 μg/ml after daily dosages of 100 and 300 mg, respectively.

Peak serum level. 1.8 to 3.5 μg/ml after a daily dose of 300 mg for 60 days or more.

Excretion. Kidneys.

Side effects/adverse reactions. See Table 61-8.

Significant drug interactions. None.

Dosage and administration

Adults. For dapsone-resistant leprosy, given in combination with one or more antileprosy agents, 50 to 100 mg orally daily. Maximum daily dosages above 300 mg are not recommended in the treatment of leprosy.

Children. Not established.

Pregnancy safety. FDA category C.

NURSING CONSIDERATIONS

See discussion of dapsone.

Alternate Drug Therapy

Rifampin has been used investigationally in the treatment of leprosy, but leprosy is not yet an approved indication for this drug. In the treatment of multibacillary leprosy, the World Health Organization (WHO) has recommended a three-drug combination of dapsone, clofazimine, and rifampin. (For further information on dosing schedules and alternate treatment modalities, see Wyngaarden and Smith, 1988.)

KEY TERMS

amebiasis, page 966
balantidiasis, page 970
giardiasis, page 971
Hansen's disease, page 981
helminths, page 972
leprosy, page 981
malaria, page 948
pneumocystosis, page 971
toxoplasmosis, page 971
trichomoniasis, page 971
trypanosomiasis, page 971
tuberculosis, page 956

BIBLIOGRAPHY

Baciewicz, AM, and others: Update on rifampin drug interactions, Arch Intern Med 147(3):565, 1987.

TABLE 61-8　Leprostatic Agents: Side Effects/Adverse Reactions

Drug	Side effects*	Adverse reactions†
dapsone	Rare: dizziness, headaches, nausea, vomiting	Most frequent: pain in abdomen, legs, or back; anorexia; pale skin, elevated temperature; rash; increased weakness Rare: jaundice; sore throat; hand or feet pain; tingling, or burning sensations; blue nails, lips, or skin; respiratory difficulties; pruritus; dry, red, or scaling of skin; alopecia; mood alterations In high doses, more peripheral motor (muscle) weakness is seen
clofazimine	Most frequent: dry, scaly skin Less frequent/rare: anorexia, rash, taste alterations, dizziness, sedation, dryness, burning, irritation, itching, or photosensitivity of eyes	Most frequent: stomach colic or pain, diarrhea, nausea, vomiting, red to brown or black skin discoloration Rare: visual loss, jaundice, depression, red or black tarry stools (GI bleeding)

*If side effects continue, increase, or disturb the client, inform the physician.

†If adverse effects occur, contact physician because medical intervention may be necessary.

Bailey, WC: Treatment of atypical mycobacterial disease, Chest 84(5):625, 1983.

Braunwald, E, and others, eds: Harrison's Principles of internal medicine, ed 11, New York, 1987, McGraw-Hill Book Co.

Beausoleil, EG: Malaria and drug resistance . . . chloroquine, World Health p. 7, Aug.-Sept, 1986.

Bonner, A., and others: Giardia lamblia: day care diarrhea, Am J Nurs 86(7):818, 1986.

CDC amends its malaria prophylaxis recommendation . . . no longer recommends the use of amodiaquine, Nurses Drug Alert 10(6):42, 1986.

Standard therapy for tuberculosis, 1985, Chest (Suppl) 87(2):117s

Crompton DWT, and others: Malnutrition's insidious partner . . . intestinal parasitic disease (pictorial), World Health p. 18, March 1984.

Eggleston, M: Metronidazone, Infect. Control 7(10):514, 1986.

Fernex, M: Mefloquine and its allies, World Health p 6, May 1985.

Garcia, LS, and others: Parasitic infection and the compromised host Diagnost Med 7(7):22, 1984.

Gever, LN: Pentamidine: treatment for A.I.D.S. complications, Nursing 16(9):92, 1986.

Gilman, AG, and others: Goodman & Gilman's The pharmacological basis of therapeutics, ed 7, New York, 1985, Macmillan Publishing Co.

Glassroth, J: Tuberculosis: a review for clinicians. In Clinical notes on respiratory diseases, American Thoracic Society 20:25, 1981.

Harding, SM, and others: Tuberculosis: 1986 (pictorial), Hosp Med 22(9):147, 1986.

Harter L, and others: Giardiasis in an infant and toddler swim class, Am J Public Health 74(2):155, 1984.

Hayden, C (Tuberculosis Surveillance Officer, Centers for Disease Control, Atlanta, Ga.): Miami Herald, p 12A, March 25, 1987.

Health Information for International Travelers, Washington, DC, 1988, US Dept of Health and Human Services.

Herfindal, ET, and others, eds: Clinical pharmacy and therapeutics, ed 4, Baltimore, 1988, Williams & Wilkins.

In the matter of tuberculosis, Emerg Med 18(2):57, 1986.

Isom, VV: Preventive health care to Peace Corps Volunteers in a third world country, Occup Health Nurs 32(8):421, 1984.

Kastrup, EK, ed: Facts and comparisons, St Louis, 1988, JB Lippincott Co.

Krupp, MA, Schroeder, SA, and Tierney, LM, Jr: Current medical diagnosis and treatment, Norwalk, Conn, 1987, Appleton & Lange.

Loken, S: Giardiasis: diagnosis and treatment, Nurse Pract 11(12):20, 1986.

Montonye, JM: Isoniazid poisoning, JEN 11(2):66, 1985.

No shortcut to treating vaginitis, Emerg Med 18(3):95, 1986.

Preventive treatment of tuberculosis . . . with isoniazid, Chest 87(2)(Suppl.):128s, 1985.

Roffman, DS: Tuberculosis: differential insights. A continuing education publication for the hospital pharmacist, Bristol Lab 2(5):2, 1981.

Sanford, JP: Guide to antimicrobial therapy, West Bethesda, Md, 1987, Merck Sharp & Dohme.

Sheahan SL, and others: Management of common parasitic infections encountered in primary care, Nurse Pract 12(8): 19, 1987.

Summers, L: Tuberculosis: a persistent health care problem, J Nurse Midwife 32(2):68, 1987.

United States Pharmacopeial Convention: Drug information for the health care provider, ed 8, Rockville, Md, 1988, U.S. Pharmacopeial Convention, Inc.

Wyngaarden, JB, and Smith, LH: Cecil's Textbook of medicine, ed 18, Philadelphia, 1988 WB Saunders.

CHAPTER 62

Nonsteroidal Antiinflammatory Drugs

GENERAL CHARACTERISTICS

Aspirin and other selected agents are used to treat the signs and symptoms of inflammation, fever, and pain. The gastric irritation and undesirable side effects induced by moderate to large doses of aspirin led to a search for alternate medications. With the discovery of ibuprofen in the mid-1970s, the era of aspirin-like drugs or nonsteroidal antiinflammatory drugs (NSAIDs) was introduced. Although aspirin is also a NSAID, this term most commonly refers to the newer aspirin substitutes on the market.

All of these products have anytipyretic, analgesic, and antiinflammatory effects, but the indications for the individual products may vary according to specific testing and clinical data submitted to the FDA for approval. In this chapter the specific drugs are divided by their chemical groups: fenamates, indoles, oxicams, and derivatives of propionic acid, pyrroleacetic acid, and salicylic acid.

Mechanism of action. Although the exact mechanism of action is unknown, the inhibition of the biosynthesis of **prostaglandin** may be responsible for the therapeutic effects and some of the adverse effects of this drug classification. See Figure 62-1 for prostanglandin synthesis and NSAID effects. It is quite possible that other actions (currently unknown) may also contribute to the therapeutic effects of these medications. Possible effects include the following:

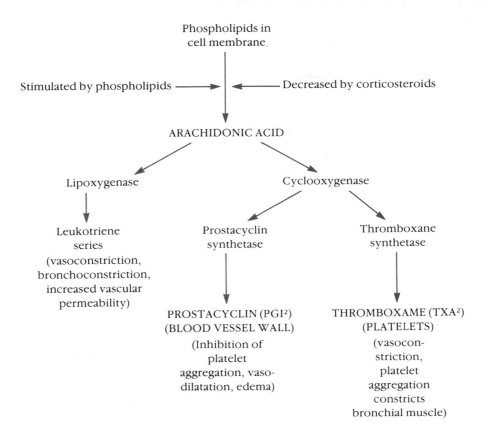

During cell injury, phospholipids will be converted to prostaglandins. Some prostaglandins are vasodilators that enhance blood vessel permeability, resulting in edema.

FIGURE 62-1 Prostaglandin synthesis and NSAID effects in inflammation.

1. Analgesic effect—decreases the biosynthesis of prostaglandins peripherally, and the generation of pain impulses may be blocked. It is also possible that the synthesis of other substances is also reduced, such as substances (mechanical or chemical) that generally sensitize the pain receptors to stimulation.

2. Antigout effect—may be due to the analgesic and antiinflammatory effects of the agents. They do not affect hyperuricemia.

3. Antiinflammatory effect—not fully understood. It has been hypothesized that NSAIDs act in peripheral, inflamed areas by inhibiting the synthesis and perhaps reducing the action of prostaglandins in the area. They may also affect the synthesis and/or effects of other local inflammatory substances. They also inhibit leukocyte migration and lysosomal enzyme release and activity and, perhaps, provide additional inhibition effects on both cellular and connective tissues.

4. Antipyretic effect—may reduce prostaglandin effects centrally in the hypothalamus, resulting in peripheral vasodilation, an increase in blood flow through the skin, and an increase in sweating and heat loss.

5. Antidysmenorrheal effect—prevents the synthesis and action of intrauterine prostanglandins, which may be responsible for the pain and symptoms of primary dysmenorrhea. NSAIDs may also decrease uterine contractions and increase blood perfusion to the uterus, which relieves ischemia and spasmodic pains.

6. Vascular headaches—may be prevented. Specific types of headaches that are believed to be caused by prostaglandin-induced dilation or constriction of cerebral blood vessels may be suppressed. The action may be caused by the reduction of prostaglandin activity or by a direct effect centrally.

7. Platelet inhibition—exerted by NSAIDs but to a lesser degree than by aspirin. The usual doses of

meclofenamate or mefenamic acid do not usually significantly alter platelet aggregation. Additional information on platelet inhibition, gastrointestinal sides effects, and renal toxicity will be noted in the section on side effects/adverse reactions.

Indications

The treatment of acute or chronic rheumatoid arthritis, osteoarthritis, ankylosing spondylitis, and other rheumatic diseases as listed in the package inserts of the individual drugs

The treatment of mild to moderate pain, especially when the antiinflammatory effect is also desirable (such as after dental procedures, obstetric and orthopedic surgery, and soft tissue athletic injuries)

The treatment of gouty arthritis (naproxen, sulindac), fever (ibuprofen), nonrheumatic inflammation (naproxen, sulindac), and dysmenorrhea (ibuprofen, mefenamic acid, naproxen). The reader is referred to a current package insert or USP-DI for a listing of approved and investigational NSAIDs use.

Pharmacokinetics. The following are general pharmacokinetics; pharmacokinetics for specific drugs are noted later.

Absorption. Very good orally. Although food may delay absorption, it has not been proven to significantly change the total amount absorbed. To decrease the gastrointestinal side effects, it is recommended that indomethacin, sulindac, and mefenamic acid be administered with antacids or meals.

Protein binding. Very high (greater than 90%)

Metabolism. Sulindac is an inactive substance (prodrug) that is converted by the liver to an active sulfide metabolite. Most of the agents are metabolized by the liver.

Excretion. Kidneys

Side effects/adverse reactions. See Table 62-1.

Significant drug interactions. The following interactions may occur when NSAIDs are given concurrently with the drugs listed below.

Drug	Possible Effect and Management
anticoagulants, oral (coumarin or indanedione, heparin, streptokinase, or urokinase)	May increase the risk of gastrointestinal ulcers or hemorrhage. Monitor closely for signs of these effects. Coumarin or indanedione anticoagulants may be displaced from protein-binding sites, resulting in an increased risk of bleeding episodes. Monitor closely with laboratory coagulation tests. Platelet inhibition by fenoprofen, ibuprofen, naproxen, piroxicam, sulindac, tolmetin, or diflunisal (in higher than recommended dosages) may be dangerous for the individual receiving anticoagulant or thrombolytic agents. Avoid concurrent drug

Drug	Possible Effect and Management
	administration if possible. If not, monitor closely for potential serious side effects.
cefamandole, cefoperazone, moxalactam, or plicamycin	These drugs may cause a decrease in prothrombin blood levels, an inhibition of platelet aggregation, and with moxalactam, irreversible platelet damage. Concurrent administration with a NSAID may increase the risk for bleeding episodes, gastrointestinal ulceration, and hemorrhage. Avoid concurrent administration if possible. If not, monitor closely for side effects.
indomethacin	When given with diflunisal, the renal excretion of indomethacin is decreased, which may result in increased serum levels, increased risk of toxicity, and even fatal gastrointestinal hemorrhage. Avoid concurrent drug administration.
probenecid	May result in an increase in serum levels of the NSAIDs and an increased risk of toxicity. Monitor closely, since a decrease in NSAID dosage may be indicated.

THE NURSE'S ROLE IN NSAID THERAPY

Assessment. The nurse should establish the client's allergies before administering these drugs. In individuals with a documented history of allergy or hypersensitivity to aspirin, the anaphylactoid reaction is life threatening. Clients with the triad of aspirin allergy, nasal polyps, and bronchospastic disease experience bronchospasm leading to respiratory failure with the use of the NSAIDs. The NSAIDs are contraindicated in these individuals when the drugs have caused asthmatic symptoms, rhinitis, urticaria, nasal polyps, angioedema, or bronchospastic events.

NSAIDs are to be used with caution in elderly clients, who are more prone to upper gastrointestinal, hepatic, or renal effects of these agents.

These drugs should be used cautiously in individuals with preexisting hepatic impairment. Prudent long-term management for clients should include liver enzyme monitoring and determinations of the baseline level.

Cautious use in individuals with impaired renal function is required; creatinine clearance should be closely monitored in these clients. A reduced dosage should be employed in clients with diminished renal function to prevent drug accumulation.

Intervention. The doses may be taken 30 to 60 minutes before meals or 2 hours postprandially to reach a blood level more readily. Administration with a meal, however, followed by a full glass of water, will aid in preventing gastric upset.

Education. The woman who is pregnant or intends to

TABLE 62-1 NSAIDs: Side Effects/Adverse Reactions

Drug(s)	Side effects*	Adverse reactions†
diflunisal, fenoprofen, ibuprofen, meclofenamate, mefenamic acid, naproxen, piroxicam, sulindac, tolmetin	Most frequent: stomach distress (all except fenoprofen); constipation (fenoprofen, naproxen, sulindac); diarrhea (diflunisal, meclofenamate, mefenamic acid, sulindac, tolmetin); dizzy spells (all except diflunisal and piroxicam); sedation (fenoprofen, mefenamic acid, naproxen); headaches (all except diflunisal, fenoprofen, piroxicam); nausea or vomiting (all); anxiety, (fenoprofen); tachycardia (fenoprofen). Less frequent: gas or mild stomach distress (diflunisal, fenoprofen, ibuprofen, piroxicam, sulindac); constipation (diflunisal, ibuprofen, meclofenamate, piroxicam, tolmetin); anorexia (fenoprofen, ibuprofen, sulindac, piroxicam, meclofenamate; diarrhea (fenoprofen, ibuprofen, naproxen, piroxicam); dizziness (diflunisal, piroxicam); sedation (diflunisal, piroxicam, tolmetin); increased sweating (fenoprofen, naproxen); sore, dry mouth (fenoprofen, meclofenamate, naproxen); tremors (fenoprofen); insomnia (diflunisal, fenoprofen, tolmetin); nervousness (ibuprofen, sulindac, tolmetin).	Most frequent: itching (ibuprofen, naproxen); edema and increased blood pressure (naproxen, tolmetin); tinnitus (naproxen); respiratory difficulties (naproxen); allergic skin rash (all); sedation (diflunisal, ibuprofen, meclofenamate, sulindac); increased bleeding episodes (naproxen); weakness (fenoprofen, tolmetin). Less frequent: weakness (diflunisal) (piroxicam-anexmia), increased thirst (naproxen); edema (ibuprofen, meclofenamate, piroxicam, white areas or sores in mouth (meclofenamate, naproxen, piroxicam); skin rash (fenoprofen, mefenamic acid, naproxen, piroxicam, tolmetin); tinnitus (diflunisal, fenoprofen, ibuprofen, tolmetin, sulindac, meclofenamate, piroxicam); elevated blood pressure (ibuprofen, meclofenamate, piroxicam, sulindac); pruritis (ibuprofen, meclofenamate, piroxicam, sulindac, tolmetin); hives (fenoprofen, meclofenamate); visual changes (fenoprofen, tolmetin); gastrointestinal ulcers or perforation (meclofenamate, tolmetin).
indomethacin	Incidence of 3% to 9%—stomach distress, dizzy spells, gas, nausea or vomiting. Between 1% and 3%—constipation, diarrhea, sedation, ill feeling.	Greater than 10%—morning headaches. About 1%—black or bloody stools; mental disturbances; memory lapses; depression; tinnitus; edema of face, feet, or lower extremities; weight gain; rectal irritation (suppository dosage form). Incidence of approximately 1%—severe stomach pain or cramps; severe and, perhaps, bloody diarrhea; vomiting of blood; bleeding sores on lips; blood in urine; pain in chest; seizures; hearing loss; elevated blood pressure; hallucinations; fainting episodes; muscle weakness; skin peeling; respiratory difficulties; allergic skin reaction; white mouth sores; sore throat, fever, chills; increased bleeding episodes; weakness; decreased urine output; nosebleeds; unexplained vaginal bleeding; jaundice. With chronic therapy: visual disturbances, eye pain
ketoprofen	Greater than 3% incidence—gas, indigestion, nausea, abdominal distress, pain, itching in rectum, constipation, diarrhea, headache, anxiety, insomnia. Between 1% and 3% incidence—dizzy spells, anorexia, vomiting, ill feeling. About 1%—decreased libido; dry nose or throat; tachycardia; photosensitivity; sore tongue, gums, or mouth; paresthesia of hands/feet; alopecia; increased thirst.	Greater than 3% incidence—rectal bleeding from suppository form; edema in feet or lower legs; weight gain. Between 1% and 3% incidence—severe stomach pain, visual disturbances, urinary problems, increased urinary frequency, depression, tinnitus, mouth sores or ulcers, allergic skin reaction. About 1% incidence—black or bloody stools, vomiting of blood, blood in urine, decreased urine output, edema of face, hives, chills, itching skin, runny nose, memory loss, confusion, hearing loss, red eyes, fever, severe headaches, loose fingernails, red and scaly skin, respiratory difficulties, sore throat and fever, increased bleeding episodes, weakness, nosebleeds, jaundice.

*If side effects continue, increase, or disturb the client, the physician should be informed.
†If adverse reactions occur, the physician should be contacted, since medical intervention may be necessary.

become pregnant while using a NSAID should notify her physician, since these drugs may interfere with maternal and infant blood clotting and prolong the duration of pregnancy and parturition. There is an increase in the incidence of stillbirths and neonatal deaths in humans. If the mother intends to breastfeed, she should be made aware of the fact that salicylates are detected in the breast milk and are cleared from the body more slowly by infants.

The client with a clinical problem such as errosive gastritis, ulcers, bleeding disorders, mild diabetes, or gout or those individuals receiving anticoagulant drugs should be warned to discuss this new change with their physician before commencing therapy again with a NSAID. Large doses of salicylates are to be avoided in clients with carditis. The effect of edema caused by these agents should be considered in individuals with diseases such as congestive heart failure and hypertension.

To reduce the risk of esophageal irritation caused by tablets lodging against the lining of the esophagus, the client should be instructed to take the medication with a full glass of water and to remain upright for 15 to 30 minutes after taking the medication.

The client who omits a scheduled dose should not double the next dose but resume the usual dosing interval.

Alcoholic beverages produce a synergistic effect with the NSAID and aspirin in causing gastrointestinal bleeding. Aspirin used chronically has caused iron deficiency anemia.

The nurse should discuss with the client the most common side effects and adverse reactions, which, however, are not always an indication of excessive dosage and should be reported to the physician. Clients should be told that if a skin rash, itching, visual disturbances, edema, persistent headache, or dark stools occur, they should immediately notify their prescribing physician, and a therapeutic alternative may be reevaluated.

Some individuals have drowsiness and dizziness and should be cautioned about performing tasks with which the drug would interfere. The problem of morning stiffness in affected joints may be overcome by taking the last dose as late as possible in the evening.

The client should be cautioned not to use any over the counter analgesics concurrently with the NSAID unless the physician specifically prescribes them.

Evaluation. Clients should be made aware of the need for periodic determinations of WBCs, hemoglobin, and/or hematocrit. They require close prothrombin time monitoring in clients receiving concomitant anticoagulant therapy and those with other intrinsic hemostatic coagulation defects.

Precipitation of acute renal failure may occur in clients with preexisting diminished sodium excretion, congestive heart failure, cirrhosis, hypertension, or renal disease.

The surfacing of eye problems during therapy should be handled by an ophthalmologic examination and discontinuation of the drug therapy until evaluation has ruled out the drug therapy as a causal agent.

FENAMATES

meclofenamate sodium capsules (Meclomen)

Dosage and administration

Adults. 200 to 400 mg orally daily, in three or four divided doses. Maximum is 400 mg/day.

Children. Children less than 14 years old: not established.

Pregnancy safety. Not established

NURSING CONSIDERATIONS

In addition to the following points, see the general nursing considerations for NSAIDs on p. 986.

Improvement in the client's condition may occur within a few days; however, 2 to 3 weeks may be necessary for maximum effect.

A client with a history of upper gastrointestinal tract disease requires close supervision, since peptic ulceration and sometimes severe gastrointestinal bleeding are reported to have occurred with this drug.

If the client is undergoing long-term meclofenamate therapy, CBC and renal and hepatic functions should be evaluated periodically. Decreases in hemoglobin and/or hematocrit levels may occur, and these values need determination if anemia is suspected.

If gastrointestinal side effects occur with meclofenamate, it may be necessary to reduce the dose or discontinue the drug.

mefenamic acid capsules (Ponstan✳, Ponstel)

Dosage and administration

Adults. 500 mg orally initially, then 250 mg every 6 hours when needed.

Children. For children less than 14 years old: not established.

Pregnancy safety. FDA category C

NURSING CONSIDERATIONS

In addition to the following points, see the general nursing considerations for NSAIDs on p. 986.

Monitor the client for diarrhea or skin rash. Both are indications to discontinue the drug immediately. If diarrhea develops, the client will be unable to tolerate mefenamic acid in the future. Mefenamic acid is not administered for more than 7 days.

Use with caution in individuals with a history of renal disease, hepatic dysfunction, blood dyscrasias, or asthma and in those with diabetes or gastrointestinal disorders.

Mefenamic acid is more likely to cause gastrointestinal symptoms, dizziness, and drowsiness than other NSAIDs.

Caution client to avoid driving or operating machinery in early stages of therapy because of drowsiness and dizziness.

INDOLES

Indomethacin is an indoleacetic acid derivative. Sulindac and tolmetin are chemically related to indomethacin, but since they are pyrroleacetic acid derivatives, they will be listed in that section.

indomethacin capsules (Indocin, Imbrilon♣, Indocid♣)
indomethacin extended-release capsules (Indocid R♣, Indocid SR♣, Indocin SR, Indolar SR♣)
indomethacin oral suspension (Indocid♣, Indocin)

Pharmacokinetics
Absorption
Capsule or oral suspension—very good; usually 90% is absorbed within 4 hours.
Extended release capsule is designed to release 25 mg initially, then 50 mg over the following 12 hours. 90% of a dose is absorbed within 12 hours.
A suppository may be absorbed more rapidly than a capsule. It needs to be retained at least 1 full hour in the rectum to obtain the maximum absorption and effect.
Protein binding. Very high to albumin (approximately 99%)
Half-life. Biphasic
Distribution. Within 1 hour
Elimination. Approximately 4.5 hours, but the range is from 2.6 to 11.2 hours. Individual times can vary greatly.
Onset of action
Antirheumatic: usually within 1 week, but some individuals have required up to 2 weeks, depending on the severity of their condition.
Antigout: within 2 to 4 hours
Time to peak serum levels
Capsules: within ½ to 2 hours after a 25-mg dose
Extended-release capsules: within 2 to 4.25 hours
Peak serum level
Capsules: 25-mg dose, 0.8 to 2.5 μg/ml; 50-mg dose, 2.5 to 4 μg/ml
Extended-release capsules: 1.5 to 3 μg/ml
Oral suspension: 50-mg dose, 2.5 to 4 μg/ml
Time to peak effect
Antirheumatic effect: up to 4 weeks, depending on individual and severity of condition
Antigout: 24 to 36 hours for heat and tenderness; 3 to 5 days for swelling

Metabolism. Liver
Excretion. Kidneys (approximately 60%); 33% is excreted via the bile
Side effects/adverse reactions. See Table 62-1.
Significant drug interactions. See interactions for NSAIDs. In addition, the following are potentially significant interactions.

Drug	Possible Effect and Management
triamterene	The antihypertensive and diuretic effect may be decreased because of inhibition of prostaglandin synthesis.
	May increase the serum levels of potassium when used with potassium-sparing diuretics. Monitor potassium levels closely since dosage adjustments may be necessary.
	May block the increase in plasma renin activity induced by bumetanide, furosemide, or indapamide.
	Renal function impairment has been reported with the concurrent administration of triamterene and indomethacin. Concurrent drug administration is not recommended.
lithium	Indomethacin may decrease lithium excretion, resulting in increased serum levels and toxicity. Monitor for signs of lithium toxicity and monitor serum lithium levels, since a dosage adjustment may be necessary.
methotrexate	The renal excretion of methotrexate may be decreased, leading to increased serum levels and an increased risk of renal and systemic toxicity. It is recommended that indomethacin therapy be stopped for 24 to 48 hours before and for at least 12 hours after medium- or high-dose methotrexate infusion therapy. Closely monitor methotrexate serum levels.

Dosage and administration
indomethacin capsules/oral suspension
Adults
Antirheumatic effects: 25 or 50 mg orally two to four times a day. If necessary and tolerated, the dose per day may be increased by 25 or 50 mg/week until a satisfactory response is obtained. Maximum is 200 mg/day.
For arthritic patients with persistent night pain and/or morning stiffness, up to 100 mg of the total daily dose can be administered at bedtime.
Generally, a dose of 150 to 200 mg/day or more may result in an increased risk of adverse effects without the advantage of additional therapeutic effects.
Antigout effects: 100 mg orally initially, then 50 mg three times daily until pain has subsided. The dosage is then reduced until the medication is discontinued.
Antiinflammatory effect: 75 to 100 mg orally daily, in 3 or 4 divided doses. When used for acute bursitis or tendonitis, discontinue drug when inflammation symptoms have been controlled for several days. Therapy length is usually 7 to 14 days. Adult maximum daily dose is 200 mg.

Children. Antirheumatic effect: 1.5 to 2.5 mg/kg orally daily, divided into 3 or 4 doses, up to a maximum of 4 mg/kg/day, or 150 to 200 mg/day, the lesser amount.

indomethacin extended-release capsules
Adults. 75 mg orally, once daily (in morning or at bedtime); may be increased to 75 mg twice daily, if needed

Children. Not established

indomethacin suppositories
Adults. 50 mg rectally up to four times daily

Children. See dosage information for indomethacin capsules.

Pregnancy safety. Not established.

NURSING CONSIDERATIONS

In addition to those listed below, see the general nursing considerations for NSAIDs on pp. 986 and 988.

Indomethacin should be used with caution in individuals with mental depression or other psychiatric problems. Evaluate the client periodically for confusion, mood changes, and hallucinations.

Although the capsules may be taken with antacids or after meals to minimize gastrointestinal distress, the oral suspension should not be mixed with antacids or other liquids for administration.

When administering the suppository form of the drug, ensure that it remains in the rectum for at least 1 hour to maximize effectiveness.

Administer sterile indomethacin sodium intravenously for 5 to 10 seconds. Avoid extravasation because the drug is irritating to the tissues. Fluid restriction usually accompanies intravenous use of the drug.

Dosages in the elderly may begin as low as half the usual adult dose.

Encourage long-term compliance as it may take 2 weeks for a noticeable effect or up to a month for maximum effectiveness.

OXICAMS
piroxicam capsules (Apo-Piroxicam✣, Feldene)

Dosage and administration
Adults. 20 mg orally daily or 10 mg orally twice a day

Children. Not established
Pregnancy safety. Not established.

NURSING CONSIDERATIONS

In addition to those listed below, see the general nursing considerations for NSAIDs on pp. 986 and 988.

The effectiveness of piroxicam therapy may not be determined for 2 weeks because therapeutic plasma concentrations are not reached until 7 to 12 days after administration of the drug has begun.

PROPIONIC ACID DERIVATIVES

Propionic acid derivatives include fenoprofen, ibuprofen, ketoprofen, and naproxen derivatives.

fenoprofen calcium capsules (Nalfon)
fenoprofen calcium tablets (Fenopron✣, Nalfon, Progesic✣)

Dosage and administration
Adults
Antirheumatic effect: 300 to 600 mg orally of fenoprofen (base) three or four times daily. The higher doses are usually needed in rheumatoid arthritis.

Analgesic effect (mild to moderate pain) or as an antidysmenorrheal agent: 200 mg orally of fenoprofen (base) every 4 to 6 hours when necessary

Usual maximum daily amount is 3.2 g of fenoprofen (base).

Children. Not established
Pregnancy safety. Not established

NURSING CONSIDERATIONS

In addition to those listed below, see the general nursing considerations for NSAIDs on pp. 986 and 988.

The nurse should be aware that headache and drowsiness occur in about 15% of individuals taking fenoprofen.

Advise the client with arthritis that although improvement may be noticeable in a few days, maximum effectiveness may not occur until fenoprofen has been taken regularly for 2 to 3 weeks.

ibuprofen capsules (Amersol✣)
ibuprofen tablets (Advil, Apo-Ibuprofen✣, Motrin, Brufen✣)

Dosage and administration
Adults
Antirheumatic effect: 300 to 600 mg orally three or four times daily. Higher dosages are usually necessary for rheumatoid arthritis.

Analgesic (mild to moderate pain), antipyretic, or antidysmenorrheal effect: 200 to 400 mg orally, every 4 to 6 hours as necessary

Maximum daily dose: 3.2 g (although some physicians have prescribed up to 3.6 g/day) For over-the-counter use (200-mg tablets): dosage is up to 6 tablets in 24 hours

Children. Not established; therefore dosage schedule must be determined by the physician

Pregnancy safety. Not established

NURSING CONSIDERATIONS

In addition to those listed below, see the general nursing considerations for NSAIDs on pp. 986 and 988.

Gastrointestinal side effects and dizziness are more common with ibuprofen than with other NSAIDs.

Advise the client with arthritis that although improvement may be noticeable in the first few days of ibuprofen therapy, it may be 1 to 2 weeks before maximum effectiveness is reached.

Because photosensitivity occurs with ibuprofen, advise the client to avoid the use of sun lamps and prolonged exposure to the sunlight.

Ibuprofen is available without prescription in the 200 mg strength for self-medication. Clients using ibuprofen as an over-the-counter medication should be instructed to report to their health care provider if their symptoms do not improve, if fever persists for more than 3 days, or if swelling or redness occur in the painful area.

ketoprofen capsules (Orudis, Alrheumat✱, Profenid✱)
ketoprofen enteric-coated tablets (Orudis-E✱)
ketoprofen suppositories (Orudis✱)

Indications. Treatment of rheumatoid arthritis, osteoarthritis, pain, and dysmenorrhea

Pharmacokinetics

Absorption. Very good orally

Enteric coated: takes approximately 1.5 hours longer than noncoated tablets

Rectally: approximately 73% to 93% of oral tablet absorption

Protein binding. Very high

Half-life. Biphasic

Distribution. Within 21.4 minutes

Elimination. Within 1.5 to 4 hours or an average of 3 hours. In elderly clients, this may be increased to 5 hours. In clients with impaired renal function, it is approximately 3.5 hours.

Onset of action for rheumatoid arthritis. Within 7 days

Time to peak serum level

Oral, following a 50-mg dose:

Capsules—within 0.5 to 2 hours; or 1.1 hours on an empty stomach or 2 hours if taken with meals

Enteric-coated tablets—within 1.5 to 4 hours

Rectally—within 0.5 to 2 hours

Time to steady-state plasma levels. Within one day

Time to peak synovial fluid levels. Within 2 hours after a single 50-mg dose

Peak serum level. Orally, 4.1 μg/ml after a single 50-mg dose taken on an empty stomach. May decrease to 2.4 μg/ml if taken with meals. Serum levels may be elevated in elderly.

Peak synovial fluid level. 0.7 to 0.9 μg/ml after a single 50-mg or 100-mg dose

Metabolism. Liver

Excretion. Kidneys

Side effects/adverse reactions. See Table 62-1.

Significant drug interactions. See previous comments on cefamandole, cefoperazone, moxalactam, plicamycin, methotrexate, and probenicid.

Dosage and administration

ketoprofen capsules/enteric-coated tablets

Adults

Antirheumatic effects: 75 mg orally three times daily or 50 mg four times a day initially, then increased or decreased according to patient response

Analgesic or antidysmenorrheal effects: 50 mg orally every 6 to 8 hours when needed

In clients with impaired renal function: reduce dosage by 33% to 50% of recommended dosage.

Elderly clients: reduce initial dosage up to 50% of usual recommended dosage. Adjust dosage as necessary according to individual response.

Maximum daily dose: 300 mg orally, given in 3 or 4 divided doses.

Children. Not established.

ketoprofen suppositories (not available in the United States)

Adults. 100 mg rectally twice a day, morning and night. Maximum daily dose for oral and rectal combined is 200 mg/day.

Pregnancy safety. FDA category B

NURSING CONSIDERATIONS

In addition to those listed below, see the general nursing considerations for NSAIDs on pp. 986 and 988.

Advise the client that the maximum effectiveness of ketoprofen therapy may not occur for 2 to 4 weeks.

Use caution in elderly clients or in clients with impaired renal function.

naproxen oral suspension (Naprosyn)
naproxen tablets (Apo-Naproxen✱, Naprosyn, Naxen✱)
naproxen sodium tablets (Anaprox, Synflex✱)
naproxen suppositories (Naprosyn✱)

Dosage and administration
naproxen suspension/tablets
Adults

For antirheumatic effects: 250, 375, or 500 mg orally twice daily, morning and night. Dosages above 1000 mg/day have not been evaluated.

For analgesic effect (mild to moderate pain): 500 mg orally initially, then 250 mg every 6 to 8 hours when necessary

As antigout agent: 750 mg initially orally, then 250 mg every 8 hours until attack is under control

Antidysmenorrheal effect: 500 mg orally initially, then 250 mg every 6 to 8 hours when necessary

Maximum daily dose for mild to moderate pain and dysmenorrhea: 1.25 g/day

Children. Antirheumatic effect: 10 mg/kg orally daily; administer in two divided doses

naproxen sodium tablets
Adults

For antirheumatic effects: 275 mg orally twice a day, (morning and night) or 275 mg in the morning and 550 mg at night. Doses above 1.1 g have not been evaluated.

Analgesic effect (mild to moderate pain): 550 mg orally initially, then 275 mg every 6 to 8 hours when necessary

Antigout effects: 825 mg orally initially, then 275 mg every 8 hours until attack is under control

Antidysmenorrheal effects: 550 mg orally initially, then 275 mg every 6 to 8 hours when necessary

Maximum daily dose: 1.375 g for pain and dysmenorrhea

Children. Not established

naproxen suppositories (not available in the United States)

Adults. 500 mg rectally at bedtime.
Maximum daily dose of both oral and rectal dosage form cannot exceed 1 g/day.

Children. Not established.
Pregnancy safety. FDA category B

NURSING CONSIDERATIONS

In addition to the ones listed below, see the general nursing considerations for NSAIDs on pp. 986 and 988.

Caution should be used in elderly clients and those with hepatic and renal impairment.

Monitor fluid intake and output because of the fluid-retaining effects of naproxen. Observe the client for clinical signs of fluid retention (unusual weight gain; swelling of the face, feet, and lower extremities; and shortness of breath).

Advise the client that it may be as long as 2 to 4 weeks before the maximum therapeutic effect of naproxen is achieved.

Carprofen

Carprofen (Rimadyl) is a new NSAID, released in early 1988. It is currently reserved for individuals who are unresponsive to or cannot tolerate the other agents on the market. Although experience with this product is limited, it appears to cause more skin rashes, and, perhaps, a higher rate of lower urinary tract symptoms than the previously discussed drugs. More clinical experience is needed to assess the benefits and side effects of this drug to properly compare it with the earlier marketed agents.

PYRROLEACETIC ACID DERIVATIVES

This chemical class includes sulindac and tolmetin.

sulindac tablets (Clinoril)

Dosage and administration
Adults

For antirheumatic effects: 150 to 200 mg orally twice daily. Adjust dosage as necessary according to client response.

For antigout effects: 200 mg orally twice daily. Adjust dosage as necessary according to client response.

For antiinflammatory effects (e.g., for an acute painful shoulder): 200 mg orally twice daily. Adjust dosage as necessary.

Children. Not established.
Pregnancy safety. Not established

NURSING CONSIDERATIONS

In addition to those listed below, see the general nursing considerations for NSAIDs on pp. 986 and 988.

Advise the client with arthritis that although improvement may be felt within a week of the initiation of sulindac therapy, continuous use for 2 to 3 weeks may be necessary before the maximum effect occurs.

tolmetin sodium tablets (Tolectin)
tolmetin sodium capsules (Tolectin DS)

Dosage and administration
Adults. 400 mg (base) orally initially, three times daily. (Administer doses to include one in the morning and one at bedtime.) Maintenance:

For rheumatoid arthritis: 600 mg to 1.8 g orally (base) in 3 or 4 divided doses daily

For osteoarthritis: 600 mg to 1.6 g orally (base) in 3 or 4 divided doses daily

Maximum daily dose is 2 g base per day for rheumatoid arthritis or 1.6 g base per day for osteoarthritis.

Children. Less then 2 years old: not established. Two years old and older:

Initial: 20 mg (base) per kg orally daily in divided doses

Maintenance: 15 to 30 mg (base) per kg daily in divided doses

Pregnancy safety. FDA category C

NURSING CONSIDERATIONS

In addition to those listed below, see the general nursing considerations for NSAIDs on pp. 986 and 988.

Tolmetin is not to be used in individuals with a history of upper gastrointestinal tract disease unless there is close supervision for signs of ulcer perforation or severe gastrointestinal bleeding.

Advise the client that although improvement of the condition occurs within the first days, the maximum effect of tolmetin may not occur until 1 to 2 weeks after the initiation of therapy.

Monitor the fluid intake and output because of the fluid-retaining properties of tolmetin. Observe the client for increase in weight, increase in blood pressure, and headache.

SALICYLIC ACID DERIVATIVE

Diflunisal is the only product listed under this category; however, it is not metabolized to salicylic acid in humans.

diflunisal tablets (Dolobid)

Dosage and administration

Adults

Antirheumatic effects: 250 to 500 mg orally twice daily; adjust dosage as necessary according to client's response

Analgesic: 500 mg to 1 g orally initially, then 250 to 500 mg every 8 to 12 hours as necessary

Maximum daily dose: 1.5 g

Children. Not established.

Pregnancy safety. FDA category C

NURSING CONSIDERATIONS

In addition to the ones listed below, see the general nursing considerations for NSAIDs on pp. 986 and 988.

Tablets are to be swallowed whole and not crushed.

Administration of a loading dose is recommended to initiate diflunisal therapy. Otherwise, a delay of 2 to 3 days may occur in reaching a therapeutic level and in evaluating alterations of the medication regimen.

Because of the possibility of photosensitivity with diflunisal, alert the client to avoid the use of sunlamps and prolonged exposure to sunlight.

PROSTACYLCIN (PGI$_2$) AND THROMBOXANE (TXA$_2$)

Thromboxane A$_2$ is a potent vasoconstrictor that stimulates additional platelet aggregation. Therefore inhibiting the formation of thromboxane A$_2$ will decrease platelet aggregation. NSAIDs inhibit synthetase, thereby preventing prostaglandin formation. Aspirin irreversibly blocks prostaglandin synthetase, whereas the other NSAIDs are primarily reversible inhibitors.

Prostacyclin is a vasodilator and an inhibitor of platelet aggregation; therefore inhibiting its effects might increase the potential of a thrombus formation. Studies have indicated that very high blood levels of aspirin (perhaps equivalent to 100 mg to 200 mg/kg dosage) are needed to inhibit prostacyclin, resulting in these effects. Studies of individuals with rheumatoid arthritis receiving high doses of aspirin did not reveal an increased risk of atherosclerotic thrombotic episodes. Thus this is a potential problem that is not frequently detected clinically (Quandt and others, 1987).

OTHER DRUGS

Several other products, such as the antimalarial agents (Chapter 61), gold salts, and penicillamine, are also used to treat inflammation in clients who have not responded to or cannot tolerate salicylates or the other NSAIDs.

Although in use for over 50 years in the treatment of rheumatoid arthritis, gold compounds are generally much slower acting and more toxic than the other products. Therefore they are reserved for individuals who demonstrate continued or increased disease activity while receiving conservative therapy.

auranofin capsules (Ridaura)
aurothioglucose suspension, sterile (Solganal)
gold sodium thiomalate injection (Myochrysine, Myocrisin✿)

Mechanism of action. The mechanism of action is unknown, but they appear to suppress the synovitis of the acute stage of rheumatoid disease. Proposed mechanisms of action include inhibition of prostaglandin synthesis, inhibition of various enzyme systems; suppression of phagocytic action of macrophages and leukocytes; and alteration of immune response.

Indications. Treatment of juvenile arthritis and rheumatoid arthritis. These agents may induce remission or suppression of rheumatoid arthritis in patients not responding to other therapies. In chronic disease states, they may help avoid further joint damage.

Pharmacokinetics

Absorption. Approximately 25% orally

Protein binding

auranofin: 60% bound to plasma proteins, remainder in RBCs

Aurothioglucose and gold sodium thiomalate: very high to plasma proteins only

Half-life (elimination)

Oral:
  Blood—3 to 4 weeks with an average of 26 days
  Body tissues—42 to 128 days (average, 80 days)

Parenteral: dependent on dose and duration of treatment

Onset of action

Oral: within 3 to 4 months usually, but in some clients up to 6 months

Parenteral: in 6 to 8 weeks

Time to steady-state serum level. Auranofin: in 3 months

Steady-state serum level. Auranofin: approximately 68 μg/ml with daily drug administration of 6 mg

Metabolism

Auranofin: so rapid that the original drug is not detected in the bloodstream

Aurothioglucose and gold sodium thiomalate: unknown

Excretion

Oral: kidneys (60%), remainder in feces

Parenteral: kidneys (60% to 90%), very slowly excreted; biliary and feces excretion, 10% to 40%

Side effects/adverse reactions. See Table 62-2.

Significant drug interactions. When gold compounds are given concurrently with penicillamine, the risk for very serious kidney and/or blood adverse reactions is increased. AVOID this combination.

Dosage and administration

auranofin

Adults. 6 mg daily or 3 mg twice daily orally. If after 6 months an adequate client response is not noted, the daily dose may be increased to 9 mg given in three divided doses. If an adequate client response is not noted after 90 days of treatment with the higher dose, discontinue therapy. Maximum daily dose is 9 mg.

Children. Not established.

aurothioglucose

Adults

Initially: 10 mg intramuscularly first week, 25 mg intra-

TABLE 62-2   Side Effects/Adverse Reactions of Gold and Penicillamine

Drug(s)	Side effects*	Adverse reactions†
gold products: auranofin aurothioglucose gold sodium thiomalate	Most frequent: abdominal distress or pain, gas, diarrhea, nausea, vomiting. (GI irritation is a delayed effect occuring with all 3 drugs.) Anorexia (auranofin). Less frequent: usually occurs after injection. Hypotension, faintness, red face, nausea, vomiting, tiredness (not reported with auraxofin). Constipation and taste alterations reported (auranofin).	Most frequent: sore, irritated tongue or gums (all but auranofin); allergic skin reaction or pruritis; mouth ulcers or fungus in mouth (all three drugs). Metallic taste in mouth (all but auranofin); protein in urine (auranofin); eye redness (auranofin). Less frequent: blood in urine; hives, glossitis, increase in bleeding tendencies (auranofin). Protein in urine reported with all drugs except auranofin.
penicillamine	Most frequent: diarrhea, decrease in taste, anorexia, nausea, vomiting, mild abdominal distress.	Most frequent: elevated temperature, rash, hives, pruritis, joint pain, swollen lymph glands, mouth ulcers or white spots. Less frequent: blood in urine; edema of face, feet, or lower extremities; weight gain, sore throat, chills, fever, increased bleeding episodes, weakness. Rare: stomach pain (severe because of peptic ulcer reactivation), skin blisters, chest pain, dark urine, pruritis, jaundice or pale stools, respiratory difficulties, increased weakness, difficulty talking or swallowing, diplopia, muscle weakness, visual disturbances, red or irritated skin or eyes, tinnitus.

*If side effects continue, increase, or disturb the client, the physician should be informed.

†If adverse reactions occur, the physician should be contacted, since medical intervention may be necessary.

muscularly for second and third weeks, then 25 to 50 mg weekly until 800 to 1000 mg total has been administered

Maintenance: 25 to 50 mg intramuscularly every 2 weeks for 2 to 20 weeks, then 25 to 50 mg every 3 or 4 weeks

Maximum dose: 50 mg weekly.

Children.

Up to 6 years old: not established

6 to 12 years old: 2.5 mg intramuscularly the first week, 6.25 mg the second and third weeks, then 12.5 mg weekly until 200 to 250 mg total dose has been administered. Afterward, administer 6.25 to 12.5 mg every 3 to 4 weeks.

gold sodium thiomalate injection

Adults

Initially: 10 mg intramuscularly the first week, 25 mg the second week, then 25 to 50 mg weekly until a clinical response is achieved or toxicity occurs. Maximum total dose is 1000 mg.

Maintenance: 25 to 50 mg intramuscularly every 2 weeks for 2 to 20 weeks, then 25 to 50 mg every 3 or 4 weeks

Children. 10 mg intramuscularly the first week, then 1 mg/kg (do not exceed 50 mg per dose)

Pregnancy safety. FDA category C

NURSING CONSIDERATIONS

Assessment. Clients should be assessed for a sensitivity to gold and other heavy metals, since they may also be intolerant to gold salts.

Gold therapy is contraindicated in renal or hepatic dysfunctions, uncontrolled severe diabetes, debilitation, marked hypertension, congestive heart failure, systemic lupus erythematosus, urticaria, eczema, colitis, hematologic disorders, and following radiation therapy.

Intervention. To administer the intramuscular injection, the nurse must first shake the vial vigorously and warm it to body temperature to ease drawing the suspension into the syringe. An 18-gauge, 1½-inch needle should be used to deposit the gold deep into the muscular tissue of the upper quandrant of the gluteal region. A 2-inch needle may be used for obese patients.

Adverse responses such as anaphylaxis, angioedema, and syncope may result after an injection. Have emergency equipment available.

Education. Advise clients that dental work should not be undertaken if the administration of gold compounds has had a leukopenic and/or thrombocytopenic effect. In addition, instruction should be provided by the nurse regarding appropriate oral hygiene, including gentle toothbrushing and flossing and the avoidance of the use of toothpicks.

Caution the client that exposure to sunlight may aggravate gold-induced dermatitis and/or cause a rash.

Encourage compliance; relief from symptoms may not occur for 3 to 6 months. Regular visits to the health care provider are necessary to monitor progress.

With parenteral forms of the medication, there is the possibility of a nitritoid reaction following the injection and joint pain for 1 to 2 days following an injection.

Alert the client that side effects may occur even after the discontinuation of gold compounds.

Evaluation. Platelet counts, WBCs, and urinalyses should be completed before and periodically during therapy (urinalysis before every injection and platelets and WBCs before every second injection). All three should be accomplished monthly with auranofin therapy. Also with auranofin therapy, renal and hepatic function studies are required before and periodically during the course of therapy.

Glossitis, gingivitis, and stomatitis may result from gold compound therapy. Since these conditions may cause a lack of appetite, monitor the client's food intake.

Skin symptoms such as itching and rash are quite common with auranofin. Gastrointestinal symptoms such as abdominal cramps and diarrhea are quite common. Both should be reported promptly to the physician.

---

penicillamine capsules (Cuprimine)
penicillamine tablets (Depen, Distamine✳,
Pendramine✳)

Mechanism of action

Chelating agent for heavy metals, such as mercury, lead, copper, iron and others. The metals are made more soluble so that they can be readily excreted by the kidneys.

Antirheumatic agent, action unknown. It has been proposed that it may improve lymphocyte function. This product also reduces IgM rheumatoid factor and immune complexes located in the serum and synovial fluids, but overall it does not significantly decrease the absolute levels of serum immunoglobulins. The relationship of these effects to rheumatoid arthritis is unknown.

Indications

Prophylaxis and treatment of **Wilson's disease**

Treatment of rheumatoid arthritis, especially with individuals with severe arthritis that has not responded to other therapies

Prophylaxis of cystine renal calculi (recurrence) and treatment of **cystinuria**

Side effects/adverse reactions. See Table 62-2.

Significant drug interactions. When penicillamine is given concurrently with gold compounds or immunosuppressants (with exception of glucocorticoids), an increased potential for serious adverse reactions is noted;

these reactions include severe hematologic and/or kidney disease effects. *Avoid concurrent drug administration.*

Dosage and administration

Adults

Chelating agent: 250 mg orally four times daily

Antirheumatic agent: initially 125 or 250 mg orally daily. Increase dose if necessary at 2- to 3-month intervals by 125 or 250 mg/day. Maximum dose recommended is 1.5 g/day.

Antiurolithic agent: 500 mg orally four times daily

Elderly clients: initially 125 mg orally daily. Increase dose if necessary by 125 mg/day at 2- to 3-month intervals. Maximum daily dose: 750 mg.

Children

Chelating agent: Infants and children over 6 months old (young children)—250 mg orally in fruit juice, as a single dose; older children—see adult dose.

Antirheumatic agent: not established

Antiurolithic agent: 7.5 mg/kg orally, four times daily

Pregnancy safety. Not established

NURSING CONSIDERATIONS

In addition to the following discussion, see the general nursing considerations for NSAIDs on pp. 986 and 988.

Assessment. Use with caution in clients with hepatic or renal dysfunctions.

Twenty-four-hour urinary copper analyses are recommended for clients with Wilson's disease to determine optimum penicillamine dosages.

Intervention. Administer drug on empty stomach at least 1 hour apart from any other drug, food, antacid, or milk.

If the course of therapy is interrupted, it needs to be restarted at a low dosage and gradually increased to the appropriate dosage.

Penicillamine dosage should be reduced to 250 mg if the client is going to have surgery because of the drug's effects on collagen and elastin, which results in increased skin friability. Return to the usual dosage should be delayed until wound healing is complete.

If administered for cystinuria, the client should be on high fluid intake, especially at night when the urine is more acidic and concentrated; 500 ml at bedtime and 500 ml once in the middle of the night is adequate. The greater the fluid intake, the lower the therapeutic dose of penicillamine.

Education. The client should be encouraged to comply with the medication regimen, since an interruption in the medication for even a few days may cause a sensitivity

reaction when it is restarted. Long-term compliance may be especially difficult for clients with rheumatoid arthritis because an improvement in the status of their illness may require 2 to 3 months of therapy.

If administered for Wilson's disease, the dosage is calculated on the basis of the urinary copper excretion; the objective is to maintain a negative copper balance. The client should be advised that a low copper diet may be necessary. This means omitting mushrooms, chocolate, nuts, shellfish, liver, molasses, and broccoli.

Alert the client that taste may be impaired. The ability to taste may be enhanced by administering 5 to 10 mg of copper daily, except for individuals with Wilson's disease in which copper intake is restricted.

Evaluation. Take urinalyses and complete blood and platelet counts twice a month for the first 6 months and each month thereafter to monitor for toxicity.

Hepatic function studies should be completed every 6 months for the first 18 months of therapy to monitor for toxic hepatitis.

For clients with cystinuria, x-ray examinations for renal calculi should be done on an annual basis.

KEY TERMS

chelating agent, page 995
cystinuria, page 995
prostaglandin, page 984
Wilson's disease, page 995

BIBLIOGRAPHY

Beard, K, Walker, AM, and others: Nonsteroidal antiinflammatory drugs and hospitalization for gastroesophageal bleeding in the elderly, Arch Intern Med 147(9): 1621, 1987.

Braunwald, E, and others, eds: Harrison's principles of internal medicine, ed 11, New York, 1987, McGraw-Hill Book Co.

Carson, JL, Strom, BL, and others: The relative gastrointestinal toxicity of the nonsteroidal antiinflammatory drugs, Arch Intern Med 147(6): 1054, 1987.

Kastrup, EK, ed: Facts and comparisons, St Louis, 1988, JB Lippincott Co.

Katzung, BG: Basic and clinical pharmacology, ed 3, Norwalk, Conn, 1987, Appleton & Lange.

Quandt, CM, Talbert, RL, and De Los Reyes, RA: Current concepts in clinical therapeutics: ischemic cerebrovascular disease, Clin Pharm 6(4): 292, 1987.

United States Pharmacopeial Convention: Drug information for the health care provider, ed 8, Rockville, Md, 1988, The Convention.

Wyngaarden, JB, and Smith, LH: Cecil's textbook of medicine, ed 18, Philadelphia, 1988, WB Saunders Co.

CHAPTER 63

Uricosuric Drugs

OBJECTIVES

After studying this chapter, the student will be able to:

1. Recall the process of production of uric acid in the body.

2. Describe the classic symptoms of gout and the objectives for the treatment of gout.

3. Identify other diseases in which a secondary hyperuricemia may occur and common drugs that may increase or decrease a client's uric acid level.

4. List the common side effects/adverse reactions and the significant drug interactions for uricosuric drugs.

5. Formulate an appropriate plan of care for an individual client receiving an uricosuric drug.

Gout is a metabolic disease of unknown origin. Heredity may have a bearing on the incidence of this disease, since it occurs more often in relatives of persons with gout than in the general population. The hallmark of gout is **hyperuricemia.**

Countries with an increase in protein cosumption appear to have the highest reported incidences. For example, gout previously was rare in Japan, but it is much more common now because of the increase in protein consumption in that country (Wyngaarden, 1988).

Gout occurs most often in adult men, with only about 5% of the diagnosed cases occurring in women. It is characterized by a defective purine metabolism and manifests itself by attacks of acute pain, swelling, and tenderness of joints, such as those of the big toe, ankle, instep, knee, and elbow. The amount of uric acid in the blood becomes elevated, and **tophi,** which are deposits of uric acid or urates, form in the cartilage of various parts of the body. These deposits tend to increase in size. They are seen most often along the edge of the ear. Chronic arthritis, nephritis, and premature sclerosis of blood vessels may develop if gout is uncontrolled.

Treatment goals for gout are (1) to end the acute gouty attack as soon as possible, (2) to prevent a recurrence of acute gouty arthritis, (3) to prevent the formation of uric acid stones in the kidneys, and (4) to reduce or prevent disease complications that result from sodium urate deposits in joints and kidneys.

The drugs used to treat an acute gout attack include

colchicine, nonsteroidal antiinflammatory drugs (NSAIDs), and corticosteroids. Colchicine, specifically used to treat gout, will be reviewed in this chapter. To treat chronic gouty arthritis or to prevent gout attacks, allopurinol, probenecid, sulfinpyrazone, and salicylates have all been used. Salicylates require very high daily dosages, such as 4 to 6 g/day. Since few individuals can tolerate this high dose on a long-term basis, it is not commonly prescribed for gout.

The reader should be aware that a secondary hyperuricemia may occur from neoplastic diseases or cancer, psoriasis, Paget's disease, and other common and rare disease states. Many drugs have also been reported to cause an increase or a decrease in uric acid levels (see Table 63-1). It is preferable for the physician to identify the cause of the hyperuricemia and then to make the decision whether or not to treat it. Asymptomatic hyperuricemia in an elderly person may or may not be drug induced and often is not treated by the physician because of the adverse reactions and the cost of the medications. But if symptoms are present or a treatable disease state is identified, then specific treatments would be indicated.

colchicine tablets
colchicine injection

Mechanism of action

Antigout activity: unknown. It has been reported to decrease the motility of leukocytes, phagocytosis, and production of lactic acid, which results in a decrease in deposits of urate crystals and the inflammatory reaction. This drug does not correct for hyperuricemia.

Antiosteolytic: appears to inhibit mitosis of osteoprogenitor cells and the action of pre-existing osteoclasts.

Colchicine also constricts blood vessels and effects central vasomotor stimulation (resulting in hypertension), depresses the respiratory center, and causes a decline in body temperature.

TABLE 63-1 Medications Affecting Uric Acid Serum Levels

Increase levels	Decrease levels
alcohol	acetohexamide
cancer chemotherapeutic agents	ACTH hormone
	allopurinol
diuretics	glyceryl guaiacolate
levodopa	mannitol
ethambutol	tetracycline (outdated)
salicylates (less than 2 g/day)	probenecid
	radiopaque dyes
epinephrine (adrenalin)	salicylates (more than 3 g/day)
norepinephrine	

Indications. Treatment of prophylaxis of acute gouty arthritis, treatment of chronic gouty arthritis

Pharmacokinetics

Absorption. Good orally

Half-life. Biphasic; 20 minutes for distribution and approximately 1 hour of elimination after a 2-mg intravenous dose is administered

Onset of action. In acute gouty arthritis after the first dose of the drug:
Intravenous: within 6 to 12 hours
Oral: approximately 12 hours

Time to peak serum level. Oral, within 0.5 to 2 hours

Peak serum level. 2.2 nanograms/ml after an oral dose of 2 mg

Time to peak effect in acute gouty arthritis. For antiinflammatory effect and pain relief, 24 to 48 hours after the first oral dose, for reduction of swelling or relief, usually 3 days or more

Metabolism. Liver

Excretion. Mainly biliary, with only 10% to 20% by way of the kidneys. Because of tissue take-up of this drug, excretion of this drug may take 10 days or more after the drug is discontinued.

Side effects/adverse reactions. See Table 63-2.

Significant drug interactions. When colchicine is given concurrently with radiation therapy or drugs that induce blood dyscrasia or bone marrow depression, the risk of inducing bone marrow depressant effects or other serious toxic, hematologic effects may be increased.

Dosage and administration

Oral dosage form

Adults. Antigout effect:
Prophylactic effect: 500 to 650 μg (0.5 to 0.65 mg) orally, one to three times daily; if client has planned surgery, orally 500 to 650 μg (0.5 to 0.65 mg) three times daily for 3 days before and 3 days after surgery

Therapeutic application (for relief of acute attacks): 500 μg (0.5 mg) to 1.3 mg orally; then 500 to 650 μg (0.5 to 0.65 mg) every 1 or 2 hours or 1 to 1.3 mg every 2 hours until pain subsides, or until nausea, vomiting, or diarrhea occurs, or until the maximum dose of 10 mg is reached

Children. Not established

Injection

Adults. Antigout effect:
Prophylactic action: 500 μg (0.5 mg) to 1 mg intravenously once or twice daily

Therapeutic effect to relieve an acute attack: 2 mg initially intravenously, then 500 μg (0.5 mg) every 6 hours until the desired clinical response is noted

Maximum adult daily dose: 4 mg/day

Children. Not established.

Pregnancy safety. FDA category D

TABLE 63-2 Side Effects/Adverse Reactions of Uricosuric Drugs

Drug	Side effects*	Adverse reactions†
colchicine	Most frequent (with oral): diarrhea, nausea, vomiting, abdominal pain. Less frequent: anorexia. With chronic therapy or after a serious toxicity: alopecia.	Rare: redness, edema, or pain at site of injection. With chronic drug administration: pain, tingling, feelings of numbness or weakness in hands or feet, skin rash, sore throat, elevated temperature, chills, increased bleeding episodes, weakness. Serious overdose may occur 24 to 72 hours after administration: blood in urine, decreased urine output, seizures, severe or bloody diarrhea, mood alterations, severe muscle weakness, respiratory difficulties, burning sensations in stomach, throat, or on skin; severe vomiting (which can lead to profound dehydration and hypotension).
allopurinol	Less frequent/rare: diarrhea, sedation, abdominal pain, gas, headaches, nausea, vomiting, alopecia.	Most frequent: rash, hives, pruritis, allergic-type reaction. Rare: bloody urine or bleeding from sores on the lips; painful urination; pain in lower back area; chills; elevated temperature; sore throat, muscle pain or muscle aches, nausea, vomiting, decrease in quantity of urine, edema of face, or lower extremities, nosebleed, jaundice; red, itching, or peeling skin; red eyes; scaly skin; mouth or lip sores; ulcers or white spots; increased weakness.
probenecid	Most frequent: headaches, anorexia, mild nausea or vomiting. Less frequent: lightheadedness, red face, increased need to urinate, sore gums.	Less frequent: blood in urine, lower back pain, pain on urination. Rare: respiratory difficulties, elevated temperature, pruritus, rash, allergic reaction, increased bleeding episodes, weakness, decrease in urine output, weight gain, edema of face or lower extremities, jaundice. Acute overdose: seizures, CNS stimulation, serious vomiting.
sulfinpyrazone	Most frequent: nausea, vomiting, abdominal pain.	Less frequent: rash or allergic reaction. Rare: black or bloody stools, blood in urine, lower back pain, elevated temperature, sore throat, increased bleeding episodes, weakness, difficulty or pain on urination. Overdose: ataxia, seizures, diarrhea; severe, persistent nausea or vomiting; abdominal pain; respiratory difficulties.

*If side effects continue, increase, or disturb the client, the physician should be informed.
†If adverse reactions occur, the physician should be contacted because medical intervention may be necessary.

NURSING CONSIDERATIONS

Assessment. Caution should be used when this drug is given to elderly persons and to those with cardiac, renal, or gastrointestinal disease.

Intervention. Oral colchicine may be administered with food to prevent gastrointestinal distress.

The drug should not be administered for 3 days after the dosage for the acute episode to avoid toxic effects from accumulation.

When given intravenously, it is highly irritating if injected outside a vein (necrosis and extravasation) and therefore cannot be given subcutaneously or intramuscularly. Change the needle before administration. Administer the intravenous injection over an interval of 2 to 5 minutes.

To be effective, colchicine must be given properly at the first indication of an oncoming attack, and dosage must be adequate. Once the dose that will cause diarrhea has been determined, it is often possible to reduce subsequent doses to prevent diarrhea and still achieve satisfactory relief of pain.

Colchicine is incompatible with and will precipitate if mixed with or injected into intravenous tubing containing 5% dextrose solution, solutions which contain a bacteriostatic agent, or any solution that would change the pH of the colchicine solution. To dilute, use 0.9% sodium chloride injection or sterile water for injection.

Fluids need to be encouraged to ensure a urinary output of at least 2000 ml daily.

Education. Advise the client to maintain regular visits to the health care provider to monitor progress.

Caution the client not to drink alcoholic beverages while taking colchicine, since it increases the risk of gastrointestinal toxicity and decreases the effectiveness of the medication by increasing uric acid levels. With clients who are chronic alcoholics, the intravenous route of administration may be preferred to avoid the risk of gastrointestinal symptoms.

Since colchicine has such a narrow margin of safety, alert the client to report to the physician as soon as possible any signs of nausea, vomiting, diarrhea, sore throat, unusual bleeding or bruising, or unusual tiredness.

Caution the client to tell any health care providers that colchicine is being taken before any surgery or dental procedures are done.

Evaluation. The nurse should monitor the client's involved joints for range of motion, pain, and swelling. The drug should be discontinued as soon as the pain of the acute gout episode is relieved, if gastrointestinal symptoms occur, or if the maximum dosage is reached.

Monitor fluid intake and output to assess adequacy of urinary output.

CBCs should be monitored for clients on long-term therapy because the drug's effects on bone marrow may result in blood dyscrasias.

allopurinol tablets (Zyloprim, Alloprin✿, Aluline✿)

Mechanism of action. Decreases the production of uric acid by inhibiting **xanthine oxidase,** the enzyme necessary to convert hypoxanthine to xanthine and xanthine to uric acid (see Figure 63-1). It also increases the reutilization of both hypoxanthine and xanthine for nucleic acid synthesis, thus resulting in a feedback inhibition of de novo purine synthesis. The result is a decrease of uric acid in both the serum and urine.

This decrease of uric acid will prevent or decrease urate deposits, thus avoiding or reducing both gouty arthritis and **urate nephropathy.** The reductions in urine urate levels prevents the formation of uric acid or calcium oxalate calculi stones.

Indications

Treatment of chronic gouty arthritis
Prevention and treatment of hyperuricemia and uric acid nephropathy
Prevention of uric acid calculi in the kidneys.
Prevention of calcium oxalate calculi (recurrence) in the kidneys

Pharmacokinetics

Absorption. Very good orally (approximately 80% to 90%)

Half-life

Allopurinol within 1 to 3 hours
Oxipurinol (metabolite): between 12 and 30 hours (average 15 hours). In clients with renal impairment, this time can be prolonged.

Onset of action. Serum uric acid is reduced significantly within 48 to 72 hours.

Time to peak serum level

Allopurinol: within 0.5 to 2 hours after a single 300-mg dose
Oxipurinol: between 4.5 and 5 hours

Peak serum level (after a single 300-mg dose)

Allopurinol: approximately 2 to 3 µg/ml. In clients with renal impairment, this can increase to 30 to 50 µg/ml.

Time to peak effect. Reducing serum uric acid to normal range may take from 1 to 3 weeks. Reducing the number of acute gout attacks may take several months of drug therapy.

Duration of action. After drug is stopped, the serum uric acid levels usually will increase to pretreatment levels within 1 to 2 weeks.

Metabolism. Mainly liver. Nearly 70% of the drug is metabolized to oxipurinol, an active metabolite.

Excretion. Mostly liver, then kidneys. Approximately 10% of a drug dose is excreted as allopurinol, and nearly 70% is excreted as oxipurinol.

Side effects/adverse reactions. See Table 63-2.

Significant drug interactions. The following interactions may occur when allopurinol is given concurrently with the drugs listed below.

Drug	Possible Effect and Management
anticoagulants, oral (coumarin or indanedione)	Allopurinol may inhibit metabolism of the oral anticoagulant resulting in an increase in serum levels, activity and, perhaps, toxicity. Monitor prothrombin levels closely, since dosage adjustment may be necessary.
azathioprine or mercaptopurine	allopurinol's effect of inhibiting xanthine oxidase may result in decreased metabolism of these medications, leading to an increased potential for therpetic and/or toxic effects (especially bone marrow depression). Monitor closely since interventions or dosage adjustments may be necessary.

Dosage and administration

Adults

For hyperuricemia:

Antigout effect: initially, 100 mg orally daily. Increase by 100 mg/day at 7-day intervals if necessary. Do not exceed 800 mg/day. Maintenance, 100 to 200 mg orally two or three times a day or 300 mg daily in a single dose. (Maintenance dose for mild gout is 200 to 300 mg daily. For moderate to severe gout [tophaceous], maintenance dose is 400 to 600 mg daily.)

Treatment of hyperuricemia in neoplastic disease: initially, 600 to 800 mg orally daily, beginning 2 to 3 days before beginning of chemotherapy or radiation therapy. Maintenance therapy, adjust dosage according to serum uric acid levels that are analyzed about 2 days after the initiation of allopurinol and periodically thereafter. Discontinue the allopurinol during the period of tumor regression.

To treat uric acid calculi **(antiurolithic)**: 100 to 200 mg orally one to four times daily or 300 mg daily as a single dose

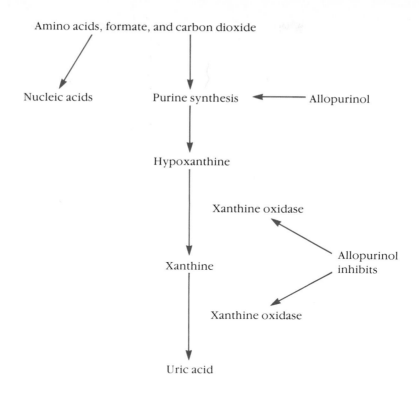

Amino acids, formate, and carbon dioxide

Nucleic acids   Purine synthesis ←—— Allopurinol

Hypoxanthine

Xanthine oxidase

Xanthine   Allopurinol
                  inhibits

Xanthine oxidase

Uric acid

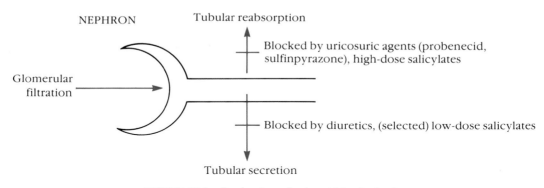

NEPHRON   Tubular reabsorption

Glomerular
filtration

Blocked by uricosuric agents (probenecid,
sulfinpyrazone), high-dose salicylates

Blocked by diuretics, (selected) low-dose salicylates

Tubular secretion

FIGURE 63-1   Production of uric acid in the body.

To treat calcium oxalate calculi (antiurolithic): 200 to 300 mg orally daily as a single dose or in divided doses

For clients with renal impairment: check a current package insert or USP-DI for prescribing information.

Maximum daily dose: 300 mg/dose or up to 800 mg/day

Children. Antihyperuricemic in neoplastic disease states:

Children less than 6 years old: 50 mg orally three times daily

Children 6 to 10 years old: 100 mg orally three times daily or 300 mg daily as a single dose

Dosage adjustments, if needed, should be made after approximately 2 days of therapy.

Pregnancy safety. FDA category C

NURSING CONSIDERATIONS

Assessment. If the client has impaired renal function, a reduction in dosage may be necessary.

Intervention. Administer with food to minimize gastrointestinal distress. For ease of administration for clients with difficulty swallowing, the tablets may be crushed and mixed with a small amount of applesauce or jelly.

A high fluid intake (80 to 96 ounces daily to produce 2 L of urine) and alkalinization of the urine are necessary to lessen the risk of stone formation and sludging of the tubules with urates.

Any single dose of allopurinol should not exceed 300 mg; it may be given in divided doses.

Education. Encourage the client to comply with the medication regimen. The client should be advised that allopurinol helps prevent, but does not relieve, acute gout episodes.

Regular visits to the physician are necessary to monitor progress through periodic blood testing and assessment for side effects/adverse reactions.

Caution the client not to drink alcoholic beverages because alcohol increases uric acid concentrations.

Alert the client that drowsiness may occur and that hazardous activities requiring mental alertness, such as driving, need to be avoided until the response to the medication has been determined.

Stress the importance of the large amount of fluid intake necessary to ensure adequacy of fluid output.

To minimize the formation of calcium oxalate stones, the client should maintain a diet that enhances the alkalinity of the urine. Large doses of vitamin C should be avoided.

The client should be advised to report to the physician immediately any signs of a skin rash or other adverse reactions. Skin rash usually precedes severe hypersensitivity reactions.

Evaluation. For proper dosing, serum uric acid levels should be monitored. CBCs and renal and hepatic function studies are recommended at periodic intervals during therapy, particularly in the first few months.

Monitor fluid intake and output to ensure the adequacy of fluid intake.

probenecid tablets (Benemid, Benuryl✤, Probalan)

Mechanism of action. Used in the treatment of hyperuricemia or to prevent gout, probenecid competitively inhibits the reabsorption of urate at the proximal renal tubule, thus increasing the urinary excretion of uric acid, which effectively lowers the serum urate levels. It has no antiinflammatory action or analgesic effects.

As an adjunct to antibiotic therapy, probenecid competitively inhibits the secretion of weak organic acids, such as penicillin and some of the cephalosporin antibiotics, at both the proximal and distal renal tubules in the kidneys. The result is an increase in blood concentrations and duration of action of these antibiotics. Probenecid may also block the renal and/or biliary transport and the transport of many other substances and drugs in or out of the cerebrospinal fluid (CSF).

Indications. Treatment of chronic gouty arthritis and hyperuricemia, adjunct therapy for selected antibiotics for the treatment of sexually transmitted diseases, such as gonorrhea, acute pelvic inflammatory disease (PID), and neurosyphillis

Pharmacokinetics

Absorption. Very good

Protein binding. High to very high with albumen

Half-life. Dose dependent, i.e., 3 to 8 hours after a 500-mg dose is administered, or 6 to 12 hours after a 2-g dose is given

Time to peak levels

Adults. 2 to 4 hours after a 1-g dose; 4 hours after a 2-g dose

Children. 3 to 9 hours after a dose of 25 mg/kg

Peak serum levels. Greater than 30 µg/ml after a single 1-g dose; 150 to 200 µg/ml after a single 2-g dose

Therapeutic serum levels. Uricosuric action: 100 to 200 µg/ml; suppression of penicillin excretion: 40 to 60 µg/ml

Time to peak effect. Uricosuric effect within 30 minutes; suppression of penicillin excretion, appproximately 2 hours

Duration of effect. Penicillin serum levels will persist for approximately 8 hours after a single dose.

Metabolism. Liver; several metabolites may be active

Excretion. Kidneys, mainly as metabolites

Side effects/adverse reactions. See Table 63-2.

Significant drug interactions. The following interactions may occur when probenecid is given concurrently with the drugs listed below.

Drug	Possible Effect and Management
indomethacin, ketoprofen	Probenecid decreases the renal excretion of ketoprofen by 66%, protein binding by 28%, and the formation of ketoprofen conjugates. This leads to an increase in ketoprofen serum levels and, possibly, toxicity. Avoid this combination.
antineoplastic drugs, rapidly cytolytic	Do not administer with probenecid because of potential toxicity of uric acid nephropathy. Also, the rapidly acting antineoplastic drugs may increase plasma uric acid levels and interfere with any control of the previous hyperuricemia and gout.
aspirin or salicylates	Not recommended because salicylates in moderate to high doses given chronically will inhibit the effectiveness of probenecid. Also, if high doses of salicylates are being given for their uricosuric effects, probenecid may lower the excretion of salicylates, which may result in elevated serum salicylate levels and toxicity.
cephalosporins, penicillins	Probenecid decreases the renal tubular secretion of penicillin and selected cephalosporins, which may result in an increased serum level and pro-

Drug	Possible Effect and Management
	longed duration of action of the antibiotic. An increased risk of toxicity may also be present. Monitor serum levels closely if given concurrently. Two cephalosporins not affected by probenecid are ceforanide and ceftazidime.
heparin	The anticoagulant effects of heparin may be enhanced and prolonged. Avoid concurrent administration if possible; if not, monitor laboratory tests closely.
methotrexate	Probenecid may decrease the renal excretion of methotrexate, which may increase the risk of serious toxicity with methotrexate. If used concurrently, administer a lower dose of methotrexate and monitor closely for toxicity or monitor methotrexate serum levels.
nitrofurantoin	Probenecid may decrease the renal tubular secretion of nitrofurantoin, resulting in an increase in serum levels and, possibly, toxicity. This may reduce the urinary levels and effectiveness of nitrofurantoin. A reduction in probenecid dosage may be necessary to use nitrofurantoin in urinary tract infections. Monitor effectiveness closely.

Dosage and administration
Adults
Antigout effect or antihyperuricemic: 250 mg orally twice daily for 7 days, then 500 mg twice a day

Adjunct to antibiotic therapy (penicillin or selected cephalosporins): 500 mg orally four times daily

Treatment of sexually transmitted disease: 1 g orally, given with the appropriate antibiotic regimen. (E.g., to treat neurosyphilis, 500 mg orally of probenecid four times daily is given with 1 dose of 2.4 million units of penicillin G procaine daily for 10 days.)

Children
Antihyperuricemia: not established

Adjunct to antibiotic therapy (penicillin or selected cephalosporins):

Children less than 2 years old: not recommended

Children 2 to 14 years old or weighing up to 50 kg: initially 25 mg/kg orally or 700 mg/M^2, then 10 mg/kg or 300 mg/M^2, four times daily

Children over 50 kg: see adult dose

To treat gonorrhea: Postpubertal children or those who weigh over 45 kg—25 mg/kg orally up to a maximum of 1 g as a single dose given with the appropriate antibiotics

Pregnancy safety. Not established

NURSING CONSIDERATIONS

Assessment. Probenecid is well tolerated by most pa-

tients (except those with peptic ulcer disease, glucose-6-phosphate dehydrogenase deficiency, acute intermittent porphyria, blood dyscrasias, and a history of uric acid kidney stones).

Intervention. Probenecid may be administered with an antacid or food to minimize gastrointestinal distress.

A high fluid intake (10 glasses of water daily) to produce copious volumes of urine is recommended to minimize formation of uric acid stones and occurrence of renal colic and hematuria.

Alkalinization of the urine may be required to minimize the formation of kidney stones. Sodium bicarbonate, potassium citrate, and acetazolamide are agents recommended for the alkalinization of urine. Diet therapy is also recommended.

Education. Encourage the client to comply with the medication regimen. Variations in the dosages may precipitate an acute episode of gout. It is important for the client to understand that this drug is to help prevent attacks, but it does not relieve acute gout episodes. Regular visits to the physician are necessary to monitor progress.

Stress the importance of maintaining adequate fluid intake.

Alert clients with diabetes who test urine for glucose with copper sulfate tests (Clinitest) that a false positive result may result while taking this medication. Enzymatic tests (Ketodiastix, Tes-Tape) should be used to assess urine glucose levels.

Caution the client not to drink alcohol because it increases uric acid levels. Aspirin and other salicylates should be avoided because they decrease the effectiveness of probenecid and may precipitate a gout attack.

The client should be cautioned to report to the physician any symptoms of hypersensitivity (skin rash), renal stones (hematuria, dysuria, low back pain), or blood dyscrasias (sore throat, fever, unusual bleeding or bruising, unusual fatigue).

Evaluation. The nurse should monitor the client's involved joints for range of motion, pain, and swelling during the course of medication.

Fluid intake and output are monitored to ensure adequacy of urinary output (2000 to 3000 ml) to minimize urate stone formation.

CBCs, uric acid determinations, and renal function studies should be evaluated periodically during probenecid therapy.

---

sulfinpyrazone capsules (Anturane, Aprazone)
sulfinpyrazone tablets (Antazone♣, Anturan♣, Anturane)

Mechanism of action. Same as probenecid

Indications. Treatment of chronic gouty arthritis and hyperuricemia

Pharmacokinetics

Absorption. Very good

Protein binding. Very high

Half-life

Sulfinpyrazone: between 1 and 5 hours (usually 3 hours)

Para-hydroxy-sulfinpyrazone: nearly 1 hour

Sulfide metabolite: up to 13 hours

Time to peak serum levels

Sulfinpyrazone: within 1 to 2 hours

Sulfide metabolite: between 9 and 15 hours after a single dose; with multiple dosing, about 7 hours.

Peak serum levels. Sulfinpyrazone:

200-mg dose: 14 to 23 μg/ml

400-mg dose: approximately 30 μg/ml

Long-term drug administration of 800 mg daily: up to 160 μg/ml

Duration of action. Uricosuric effect lasts approximately 4 to 6 hours, but in some persons it can last up to 10 hours.

Metabolism. Liver. One active metabolite, para-hydroxy-sulfinpyrazone is approximately one half as potent as sulfinpyrazone.

Side effects/adverse reactions. See Table 63-2.

Significant drug interactions. The following interactions may occur when sulfinpyrazone is given concurrently with the drugs listed below.

Drug	Possible Effect and Management
Anticoagulants, (coumarin or indanedione, heparin, streptokinase or urokinase)	Sulfinpyrazone may increase the anticoagulant effect by displacing coumarin or indanedione from their protein-binding sites and by inhibiting their metabolism. Monitor prothrombin time closely, since dosage adjustments may be necessary. An increase in bleeding episodes or hemorrhage may result from concurrent administration of sulfinpyrazone and anticoagulant or thrombolytic therapy. The potential for this reaction is caused by the platelet aggregation inhibition effect of sulfinpyrazone and its possibility of causing gastrointestinal ulceration or hemorrhage.
azlocillin; carbenicillin, parenteral; dextran; dipyridamole; divalproex; mezlocillin; piperacillin; ticarcillin or valproic acid	These drugs inhibit platelet aggregation; therefore concurrent drug administration may increase the potential of bleeding episodes. Monitor closely.
antineoplastic agents, rapidly cytolytic	Do not give concurrently with sulfinpyrazone. Increased risk of inducing uric acid nephropathy or losing control of uric acid serum levels (pre-existing levels) and gout is possible.
aspirin or salicylates	Concurrent use is not recommended. When salicylates are given long term in moderate to high doses, the uricosuric effect of sulfinpyrazone may be inhibited. See comments about probenecid.
cefamandole, defoperazone, moxalactam, or plicamycin	These drugs can cause platelet function inhibition and hypoprothrombinemia. (Moxalactam can cause irreversible platelet damage and inhibition of platelet aggregation by sulfinpyrazone.) Monitor closely.
nitrofurantoin	Sulfinpyrazone may decrease kidney excretion of nitrofurantoin, which may increase the risk of nitrofurantoin toxicity and reduce the effectiveness of nitrofurantoin as a urinary tract antiinfective agent. Avoid this combination.

Dosage and administration

Adults. Antigout effect: Initially, 100 mg to 200 mg orally twice daily. Increase dosage gradually, if needed, over a 1-week period to a dosage sufficient to control the elevated serum uric acid levels (usually 400 to 800 mg/day).

Maintenance. 100 to 400 mg orally twice daily.

Children. Not established.

Pregnancy safety. Not established

NURSING CONSIDERATIONS

Assessment. Sulfinpyrazone is used with caution in clients with a history of blood dycrasias, peptic ulcer, renal stones, or renal function impairment.

Intervention. Sulfinpyrazone may be administered with an antacid or food to minimize gastrointestinal distress.

Clients should maintain adequate fluid intake (8 ounces 10 to 12 times daily) and urinary alkalinzation if necessary, since sulfinpyrazone is a potent uricosuric agent that may cause urolithiasis and renal colic, especially in the initial stages of therapy.

Education. Encourage the client to comply with therapy. This is essential since optimal effectiveness of the drug may not be reached for several months. Advise the client that sulfinpyrazone helps prevent gout attacks but does not relieve an acute episode. Regular visits to the health care provider should be maintained to monitor progress.

Stress the importance of adequate fluid intake in the prevention of the formation of stones.

Caution the client not to use alcohol because it increases uric acid levels. Aspirin and other salicylates should be avoided because they decrease the effectiveness of sulfinpyrazone and may precipitate a gout attack.

Evaluation. CBCs, uric acid determinations, and renal function studies should be completed at intervals during therapy.

Monitor fluid intake and output to ensure that intake is adequate for sufficient urinary output (2 to 3 L/day) to help prevent urinary stones.

KEY TERMS

antiurolithic, page 1000
gout, page 997
hyperuricemia, page 997
tophi, page 997
urate nephropathy, page 1000
xanthine oxidase, page 1000

BIBLIOGRAPHY

Braunwald, E, and others, eds: Harrison's principles of internal medicine, ed 11, New York, 1987, McGraw-Hill Book Co.

Kastrup, EK, ed: Facts and comparisons, St Louis, 1988, JB Lippincott Co.

United States Pharmacopeial Convention: Drug information for the health care provider, ed 8, Rockville, Md, 1988, The Convention.

Wyngaarden, JB, and Smith, LH: Cecil's textbook of medicine, ed 18, Philadelphia, 1988, WB Saunders.Co.

UNIT XVI

Drugs Affecting the Immunologic System

Overview of the Immunologic System

The immunologic system is composed of cells and organs that defend the body against invasion of foreign biologic and/or chemical substances. The immunocompetent cells in the body have an inherent ability to identify foreign protein substances from their own body cells. This chapter will review the organs and tissues of the immune system, the immunocompetent cells, and the types of immunity.

OBJECTIVES

After studying this chapter, the student will be able to:

1. Identify the lymphoid organs of the immune system.

2. Describe the role of each of the lymphoid organs in the defense of the body against foreign biologic and/or chemical substances.

3. Identify the immunocompetent cells involved in the immune response.

4. Compare and contrast the function of the three major groups of T cells.

5. Describe the action of B cells in response to foreign antigens.

6. Identify the five classes of antibodies and their function.

7. Compare and contrast humoral and cell-mediated immunity.

8. Describe the various types of immunity: active and passive immunity; natural immunity and natural acquired immunity; and active artificially acquired immunity and passive artificially acquired immunity.

ORGANS AND TISSUES OF THE IMMUNE SYSTEM

The spleen, tonsils, lymph nodes, and thymus are the lymphoid organs located in the body. The lymphoid tissues are mainly lymphocytes and plasma cells, which travel freely throughout the human system. The two major classes of lymphocytes are T cell and B cell lymphocytes, which are discussed in the section "Immunocompetent Cells." Figure 64-1 identifies the organs and tissues of the immune system.

SPLEEN

The spleen, the largest lymphatic organ in the body, performs two main functions: (1) a storage site or reservoir for blood and (2) a processing station for red blood cells, i.e., the RBCs near the end of their life cycle will break down in the spleen.

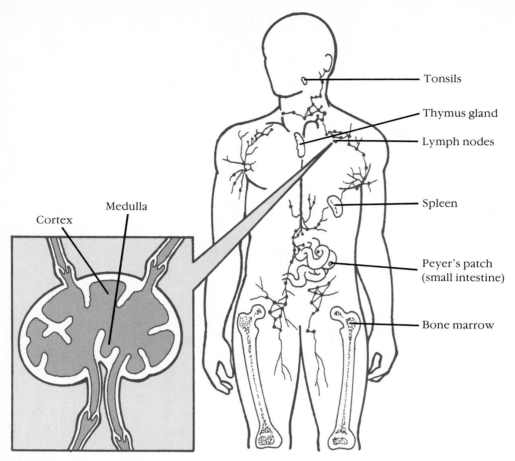

FIGURE 64-1   Location of organs and tissues of the immune system; inset shows cross-section of lymph node.

Macrophages lining the pulp and sinuses of the spleen remove cellular debris and process hemoglobin in the red pulp area of the spleen.

The white pulp area of the spleen contains lymphocytes and plasma cells that are involved in the immune process. The spleen intercepts foreign matter or antigens that have reached the bloodstream.

TONSILS

The tonsils are an accumulation of lymphoid tissue, named according to their location; lingual, palatine, and pharyngeal tonsils. They intercept foreign bodies or antigens that enter the body by way of the respiratory tract. Similar lymphoid tissue is located in the submucosal areas of the gastrointestinal tract (Peyer's patches) to intercept antigens (bacteria and viruses) entering from the gut. Other lymphoid tissues are located in the bone marrow (help to intercept antigens in the blood) and in the lymph nodes.

LYMPH NODES

The lymph nodes are capsulated organs located throughout the body that are involved with lymph circulation. The outer portion of the lymph node is the cortex, and the inner portion is the medulla. The thymus-dependent zone exists in the deep area or middle cortex. This area contains mainly T lymphocytes; that is, lymphocytes formed or seeded from the thymus gland.

Lymph nodes are essentially a row of in-line filters that screen the lymph flowing through it. Many lymphocytes and macrophages are located throughout the lymph nodes, especially in the cortical, paracortical, and medullary areas. T lymphocytes are located mainly in the paracortical region, whereas plasma cells are found in the medullary sinuses.

THYMUS GLAND

The thymus gland is located in the mediastinal area. It processes lymphocytes, and in the early years up to puberty, it rapidly produces lymphocytes. The immune system is developed when immature lymphocytes from the bone marrow are processed in the thymus gland and then sent to the spleen, the lymphatic system, and other tissues and organs in the body to mature. The lymphocytes are active against some bacteria and viruses, allergens, fungus infections, and foriegn tissue.

At birth, the thymus gland is larger than in an adult. By the time a person reaches puberty, the thymus has grown to nearly six times its original size. After puberty, this gland undergoes involution, and in the elderly, it is usually a small mass of reticular fibers with some lymphocytes and connective tissue. Although its importance was largely discounted over the years, today it is one of the most important areas for medical research. Scientists are searching for answers to the many questions about the thymus gland and its relationship to the other tissues and organs in the immune system.

IMMUNOCOMPETENT CELLS

Mononuclear T and B cells and the polymorphonuclear leukocytes (PMLs) are involved in the immune response, although only the mononuclear T cells and B cells are **immunocompetent cells.** The PMLs are nonspecific cells that interact with lymphocytes to produce an inflammatory response, whereas the B cells and T cells are capable of recognizing specific antigens and initiating the immune response.

In humans, stem cells from the bone marrow are transformed to T cells or **T lymphocytes** in the thymus gland and B cells or **B lymphocytes** elsewhere in the body. The T lymphocytes then migrate to lymphoid tissue and organs as reviewed in the previous section. When in contact with an antigen, T lymphocytes will form specialized cells to provide cellular immunity. The B lymphocytes form antibodies to provide humoral immunity.

T LYMPHOCYTES (T CELLS)

T cells are generally long-lived. When they are not in their special areas, they circulate continuously through the body by way of the bloodstream and lymphatic system. They are involved with the B lymphocytes (B cells) in that they can cooperate with them (helper T cells) or inhibit them (suppressor T cells). The B cells do not interact with the thymus. Clones are groups of lymphocytes capable of forming one specific antibody (B cell or T cell) to respond to a specific type of antigen. Only the specific antigen can activate the specialized clones.

When the T cells first contact an antigen, the lymphocytes that recognize the foreign substance will proliferate, thus giving rise to larger numbers of cells that have the capacity to recognize and respond to this antigen. Some of the cells will go on to produce antibody or cell-mediated immune-type responses, whereas others will increase the population of antigen-sensitive memory cells. This is called acquired immunity. The second exposure to this antigen will provoke a more powerful response by the specific T cells.

Three major groups of T cells have been identified in the past few years: (1) cytotoxic T cells, (2) helper T-cells, and (3) suppressor T cells.

Cytotoxic T cells. This type of cell can bind tightly to organisms or cells that contain their binding-specific antigen. Then the T-cells release cytotoxic (probably lysosomal) enzymes directly into the cell. Cytotoxic T cells are capable of killing microorganisms, cancer cells, viruses, heart transplant cells, and other cells that are foreign to the person's body. Body tissues that contain viruses or foreign cells may also be attacked by the killer cells.

Helper T cells. These compose the majority of the T cells and help the immune system in many ways.

They increase the activation of B cells, cytotoxic T cells, and suppressor T cells by antigens. Helper T cells clones are activated by very small amounts of antigens, quantities that may not activate the previously mentioned three cells. Once the helper T cells are activated, they secrete **lymphokines** that will increase the response of the three lymphoid cells to the antigen.

Helper T cells may also secrete interleukin-2 (a lymphokine), that is capable of stimulating the action of other T cells (cytotoxic T cells, some suppressor T cells).

Helper T cells also secrete macrophage migration inhibition factor, another lymphokine. This slows or stops the migration of macrophages into the affected area and will also activate the macrophages present to be more effective phagocytotic agents. The activated macrophages can attack and destroy a vastly increased number of the invading organisms.

Suppressor T cells. Less is known about these cells than the others, but it is known that they can suppress the function of both cytotoxic and helper T cells. This suppression may be useful in preventing excessive immune reactions that can cause severe body damage. These cells are often called the regulatory T cells.

B LYMPHOCYTES (B CELLS)

B lymphocytes clones are dormant in lymphoid tissue until a foreign antigen appears. The macrophages in the lymphoid tissue phagocytize the foreign substance and the adjacent B lymphocytes and perhaps the T cells are activated. B cells specific for the antigen will enlarge, and some will differentiate to form plasmablasts, a plasma cell precursor, and memory cells. The plasmablasts proliferate and divide, so that in 4 days, approximately 500 plasma cells will be present for each original plasmablast. The plasma cells rapidly produce gamma globulin antibodies that are secreted into the lymph and transported by the blood.

Cells similar to those in the original clone are called memory cells. A second exposure to the same antigen will cause a more rapid and potent antibody response. The first response to an antigen may be slow, weak, and of short duration. The second response will be much more rapid, far more potent and prolonged, and antibodies will be formed for months rather than only for a few weeks. This is the reason why vaccination using several doses given at periods of weeks or months apart is so effective.

ANTIBODIES

Antibodies are gamma globulins (a type of protein), called immunoglobulins, that are specific for particular antigens. At the present time, five clases of antibodies have been identified: IgG, IgM, IgA, IgD, and IgE. (The "Ig" stands for immunoglobulin, and the other letters designate the classes.)

IgG is the major immunoglobulin in the blood (about 75% to 80% of the total antibodies in the normal person) and is capable of entering tissue spaces, coating microorganisms, activating the complement system and thus accelerating phagocytosis. It is the only immunoglobulin capable of crossing the placenta to provide the fetus with passive immunity until the infant can produce its own immune defense system.

IgM is the first immunoglobulin produced during an immune response. It is located primarily in the bloodstream and develops in response to an invasion of bacteria or viruses. IgM activates complement and can destroy foreign invaders during the initial antigen exposure. Its level decreases in approximately 1 week, while IgG levels are progressively increasing.

IgA is located primarily in external body secretions— that is, saliva, sweat, tears, mucus, bile, and colostrum— and it is found in respiratory tract mucosa and in plasma. It helps to provide a defense against antigens on exposed surfaces and antigens that enter the respiratory and gastrointestinal tracts. The plasma cells in the intestinal area secrete IgA and secretory component to defend the body against bacteria and viruses.

The function of IgD is unknown. It is in the plasma and has been located on lymphocyte surfaces together with IgM, so it may be associated with binding antigens to the cell surface. Although levels of IgD are increased in chronic infections, IgD does not appear to have a particular affinity for specialized antigens.

IgE binds to histamine-containing mast cells and basophils. It can mediate the release of histamine in immune response to parasites (helminths) and in some allergic conditions. It is often called the reaginic antibody because of its involvement in immediate hypersensitivity reactions. Concentrations of it are low in the serum because the antibody is firmly fixed on tissue surfaces. Once activated by an antigen, it will trigger the release of the mast cell granules, resulting in the signs and symptoms of allergy and anaphylaxis.

IMMUNITY

Links in the chain of the infectious disease may be broken at many points. One link can be broken by attacking the pathogen (human disease-causing organism) with antimicrobial or antiinfective therapy. Another can be broken by augmenting human resistance by using biologic agents such as vaccines and serums, which artificially supply antibodies or catalyze the ability of the immune system to produce its own. An immunologic reaction that destroys or resists foreign cells or their products (antigens) is termed **immunity.** The most successful antigens, or immunogens, are protein or polysaccharide macromolecules that are usually bacterial, viral, fungal, or rickettsial in origin.

The primary types of immunity are humoral immunity and cell-mediated immunity.

HUMORAL IMMUNITY

Antigens may be recognized by T helper cells that activate specific B cells, by a strong B cell response to the invasion of certain antigens (such as large polymers, *E. coli,* dextrans), or by a macrophage intermediary. Macrophage interactions often enhance the antigen recognition by both T and B cells in the body. Humoral response is described as primary or secondary immune response.

Primary response. The foreign antigen in the body will bind to specific B cells to produce specialized antibody-producing plasma cells. Usually within 6 days, antibodies that are specific to the antigen can be found in the blood. Initially the immunoglobulin is IgM, which increases in quantity for up to 2 weeks; then production declines so that very little IgM is present in a few weeks.

After the initial IgM evaluation, IgG antibodies start to appear at approximately day 10, peak in several weeks, and maintain high levels for a much longer time period.

Secondary response. This response is often called the memory response, because the immune system responds so much faster to the second exposure to the same antigen. Both T and B memory cells are involved in beginning immediate production of antibodies in large amounts.

The second part of humoral immunity is activation of the **complement system,** a series of approximately 20 proteins that circulate in the blood in an inactive form. When an antigen-antibody complex triggers complement, each component in the cascade is activated in precise order. (See Figure 64-2.) This reaction causes the mast

CELL SURFACE ◄────── Site of antigen-antibody reaction

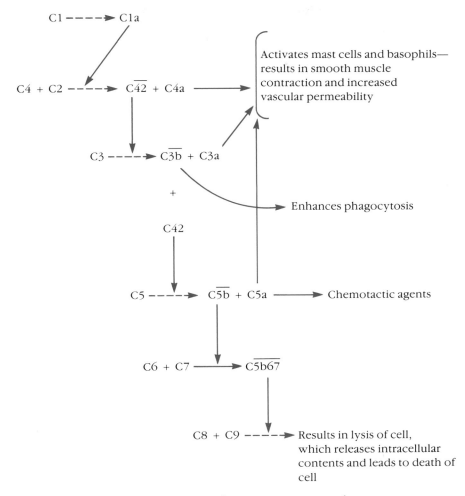

FIGURE 64-2 Complement system or cascade.

cell release of substances that produces redness, increased heat, and edema of inflammation. It may also cause bacteria cell death and damage to normal tissue that surrounds the affected area.

CELL-MEDIATED IMMUNITY

Cell-mediated immunity is the result of contact between T cells and antigens. Receptors on the T cell surface are capable of recognizing foreign antigens and antigen destruction may occur through one of two processes: (1) directly, by injecting chemical compounds into the target cell membrane (killer activity by cytotoxic T cells) or (2) by secreting lymphokines. The lymphokines can enhance or suppress the action of other lymphocytes, or they can create a chemotactic gradient in the area that will attract macrophages (and eosinophils, basophils, neutrophils) to

the site. Cell-mediated immunity (delayed hypersensitivity) involves only the direct action of T cells without humoral assistance.

NATURAL AND ACQUIRED IMMUNITY

The body has certain inherited and innate abilities to resist encounters with antigens. This ability is known as **natural resistance** (or natural immunity, which is not to be confused with naturally acquired immunity). Some general defenses inherent to natural resistance come from factors familiar to the focus of nursing: for example, adequate rest, nutrition, exercise, and freedom from undue stress. Physiologic factors, which discourage proliferation of microbes, include the acidity of gastric secretions, respiratory tract cilia, and bactericidal lysozymes in tears. During a lifetime an individual may also acquire further immune capabilities through both natural and artificial means. This type of **acquired immunity** is conferred by either active or passive action (see Figure 64-3).

Unbroken skin is extremely effective in barring entry to microorganisms, but a barrage of defenses is mounted by the inflammatory response if invasion does succeed. The immune system identifies the threatening antigens or allergens and creates specific gamma globulins destructive to the particular species of antigen. These gamma globulins, or antibodies or immunoglobulins (Ig), are proteins that are chemically complementary and specially configured to lock into the foreign antigen, inactivating it. Antibodies also activate cellular defenses to phagocytize the invading microorganisms. Custom-made gamma globulins, or antibodies, provide acquired immunity to the specific type of antigen for varying lengths of time. Those antibodies will then gradually disappear from the serum, but the potential for their rapid replication in response to a repeat challenge by that specific antigen continues to exist after the initial exposure. Consequently, the result is known as *naturally acquired immunity,* which is a process of *naturally acquired active immunity* because of the body's active involvement in creating the antibodies. Naturally acquired immunity can also result from a process of **passive immunity** when antibodies made by the mother's body are passively transferred by means of the placenta or by breast milk (especially colostrum, the breast milk produced shortly after delivery) to the fetus or infant.

On the other hand, artificial induction of the immune state, *artificially acquired immunity,* is initiated purposefully for protection of the susceptible individual. It may also be either induced actively or passively. Artificially acquired *active* immunity is evoked by the deliberate administration of antigens, either live partially modified organisms, killed organisms, or their toxins. The parenteral route is the predominant mode of administration. Periodic reactivation of actively acquired artificial immunity against certain organisms (by booster doses, e.g., tetanus) is sometimes necessary. Artificially acquired passive immunity is conferred by the parenteral administration of antibody-containing immune serum from immune humans or animals (Figure 64-3).

Artificially acquired active immunity generally secures protection for a longer duration than any kind of passive immunity and is usually the prophylactic treatment of choice for populations at potential risk. Side effects may include local pain at the injection site and headache with mild to moderate fever. Because of the agents used, *active* immunity results in fewer adverse effects than passive immunity. Artificially acquired *passive* immunity is often chosen for susceptible individuals following a known exposure. A combination of active and passive approaches is also occasionally used. A number of products used in artificial passive immunization have caused adverse reactions because of individual hypersensitivities to animal products, especially horse serum or eggs, to the preservative used in a medication, or to an antibiotic. The

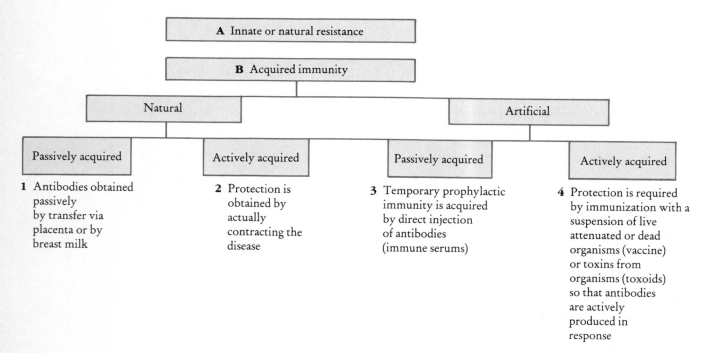

FIGURE 64-3   Immunity.

TABLE 64-1 Comparison of Active and Passive Immunity

	Active immunity	Passive immunity
Source	Self	Another human or animal
Effectiveness	High	Moderate to low

Method	Contracting disease itself (clinical or sublinical case)
	Immunization
	   Vaccines (killed or attenuated)
	   Toxoids
		Administration of antibody itself by:
		   Injection
		   Maternal transplacental transfer
		   Breast milk

Time taken to develop	5-14 days	Immediate effect
Duration	Relatively long (up to years)	Relatively short (few days or weeks)
Ease of reactivation	Easy, by booster dose	May be dangerous; possible anaphylaxis, especially if animal antiserum used
Purpose	Prophylactic	Prophylactic and therapeutic

Modified from Barrett JT: Textbook of immunology, ed 3, St Louis, 1978, The CV Mosby Co.

products of bacterial metabolism are the agents responsible for other adverse reactions. Presence of a mild to moderate upper respiratory tract infection or pregnancy does not always prohibit immunization; however, an immunosuppressed state (as a result of cancer chemotherapy or disease) may. Current manufacturers' instructions should always be consulted. Table 64-1 makes a direct comparison of the capabilities and effects of active and passive immunities.

KEY TERMS

acquired immunity, page 1014
antibodies, page 1012
B lymphocytes (B cells), page 1011
complement system, page 1012
immunity, page 1012
immunocompetent cells, page 1011
lymphokines, page 1011
natural resistance, page 1013
passive immunity, page 1014
T lymphocytes (T cells), page 1011

BIBLIOGRAPHY

Abernathy, E: Immunology: how the immune system works, Am J Nurs 87(4):456, 1987.

Barrett, JT: Textbook of immunology: an introduction to immunochemistry and immunobiology, ed 4, St Louis, 1984, The CV Mosby Co.

Bullock, BL, and Rosendahl, PP: Pathophysiology, adaptations and alterations in function, ed 2. Glenview, Ill, 1988, Scott, Foresman and Co.

Dale, MM, and Foreman, JC, eds: Textbook of immunopharmacology, Oxford, UK, 1984, Blackwell Scientific Publications.

Gurevich, I: The competent internal immune system, Nurs Clin North Am 20(1):151, 1985.

Guyton, AC: Human physiology and mechanisms of disease, ed 4, Philadelphia, 1987, WB Saunders Co.

Guyton, AC: Textbook of medical physiology, ed 7, Philadelphia, 1986, WB Saunders Co.

Kemp, D: Development of the immune system, CCQ 9(1):1, 1986.

Reckling, JB, and others: Understanding immune system dysfunction, Nursing 17(9):34, 1987.

Smith, SL: Physiology of the immune system, CCQ 9(1):7, 1986.

CHAPTER 65

Serums, Vaccines, and Other Immunizing Agents

OBJECTIVES

After studying this chapter, the student will be able to:

1. Discuss the present status and anticipated future developments of immunization.

2. State the appropriate immunization schedule for children until the age of two years.

3. Identify immunizations recommended for adults.

4. Describe the recommended use of tetanus toxoid and tetanus immune globulin in wound management.

5. Discuss the role of the nurse in the administration of immunizations.

6. List side effect/adverse reactions of immunizations and correlate with client education necessary for the management of those effects.

7. Compare the advantages and disadvantages of live attentuated and inactivated biologic products.

THE PRESENT

The critical age period for immunization is 2 months of age through grade school entry and during the school years (several states now require maintenance of immunizations as a criterion for retention in the school system). Certain groups are found to be at high risk: adolescents, new parents (unimmunized or with waning immunity, exposed to childhood illness or vaccines), and health care providers. Other groups such as migrant workers and recent immigrants to the United States are predictably at high risk for infectious diseases.

International political and economic upheavals and the Indochinese and Cuban refugee influx to the United States all have pointed up the major problems these people encounter: diphtheria, measles deaths, hepatitis B, and malaria carrier status. Screening has proved to be the easier problem, preventing outbreaks during the refugee relocation holding period the more difficult. Immunization programs that are taken for granted in the United States and other countries are virtually unheard of in many others. As a group adolescents also seem to be at high risk for preventable infections. Typically, they may lack immunization because of their life-style or their emphasis on present rather than future goals. Of these, certain subgroups may be particularly in need of immunization, such as athletes, heavy drug users, runaways, foreign travelers, and those isolated from or rejecting traditional health care.

Several million children are not immunized against measles, polio, rubella (German measles), mumps, diphtheria, pertussis (whooping cough), and tetanus.

Newspapers and television news coverage have reported the adverse reactions associated with pertussis vaccine and some of the other vaccines, which have served to bias some viewers against vaccination. It is important to stress that the vaccines are not without some risks, but the serious risks associated with not being vaccinated and actually contracting the disease are greater still. Diphtheria, tetanus, polio, and the other diseases can cause crippling and death, and most are very contagious. Schedules for immunizations of these diseases have been developed as guidelines for the practitioner and for parents to ensure adequate protection for their children (Table 65-1).

A valid history of clinical disease or obtaining an **antibody titer** for some of these diseases is useful in determining disease exposure and immunity. However, proven exposure to the disease does not always guarantee immunity. Therefore timely immunizations are even more important if the potential for development of the disease is imminent or increased, as it is for persons traveling to foreign countries where some diseases are **endemic.** Required and recommended immunizations for foreign travel are constantly changing and are best obtained before travel from the local department of health.

Special assessments must be made when exposure, for example, to measles or tetanus has occurred. Measles can be prevented if exposure is followed within 72 hours by administration of the live measles vaccine. However, people who were vaccinated with the *killed*-virus measles vaccine between 1963 and 1967 and who have never had the disease have now been found to be at considerable risk. They are not protected from measles, and they are at serious risk of developing an atypical type of measles with fever spiking to 104° F (40° C), cough with abnormal infiltrates as seen on roentgenograms, a rash progressing paradoxically from the periphery, and occasionally cardiomegaly and a mild drop in the platelet count. Nurses should advise all individuals over 12 years of age who have not had the live measles vaccine or the disease itself to get immunized with the *live* measles vaccine. Other special immunizations recommended for adults 18 years and older are listed in Table 65-2.

Any time a traumatic wound (especially a puncture wound) is encountered, the individual's tetanus immunization status must be assessed. If the person has not been fully immunized within the past 10 years, or if the wound is contaminated and an immunization is more than 5 years old, a booster dose of tetanus toxoid may be in order (Table 65-3).

Predictions for the future are that vaccines will be available for most of the common bacterial and viral infectious diseases and that measles will be eradicated in the United States (a goal of the Centers for Disease Control). Renewing and reinforcing the public's trust in immunotherapy will be a necessary corollary to this goal. Most new parents today are too young to remember the fear engendered by the very mention of childhood illnesses a few decades ago. If parents are not convinced, outbreaks of diseases (e.g., poliomyelitis) may make the argument for us.

Complacency about childhood illnesses and their current and potential threats must be shaken. The initial effects of childhood illnesses can be very serious, and more potential future hazards are currently being discovered (e.g., the possible association of mumps with eventual diabetes and of chickenpox with shingles).

During the National League for Nursing–supported Department of Health, Education and Welfare immunization campaign at the end of the 1970s, it was reported that: "Immunization is one of the easiest health services to deliver and to measure. Yet in 1977 nearly 40% of the 52

TABLE 65-1 Recommended Schedule for Active Immunization of Normal Infants and Children

Age	Vaccines	Special comments
2 months	DPT-1,* OPV-1	If necessary, may be given earlier if endemic to the area.
4 months	DPT-2, OPV-2	
6 months	DPT-3	A third dose of OPV is optional in areas of high endemicity of poliomyelitis.
15 months	MMR, DPT-4, OPV-3	May be given simultaneously.
25 months	Hemophilus B poly-saccharide vaccine	May be given between 18 to 23 months for infants at increased risk, i.e., those that attend daycare centers.
4-6 years	DPT-5, OPV-4	Given before or when entering the school system.
14-16 years	Td	Repeat every 10 years during lifetime.

From Immunization Practices Advisory Committee, Centers for Disease Control, MMWR, 1986.
*DPT, Diphtheria, tetanus toxoid, and pertussis vaccine; *OPV*, oral, attenuated poliovirus vaccine containing poliovirus types 1, 2, and 3; *MMR*, live measles, mumps, and rubella viruses; *Td*, adult tetanus toxoid and diphtheria toxoid in combination; this contains the same dose of tetanus toxoid as DPT or DT, but it has a reduced dose of diphtheria toxoid.

TABLE 65-2 Immunizations Recommended for Adults (18 and older)

Immunizing agent	Indication(s)/dosage schedule
For all adults routinely:	
Tetanus toxoid	Management of wounds. IM* dose every 10 years.
Diphtheria toxoid	As a preventive or to help in management of contacts with persons with diphtheria. IM dose every 10 years.
For selected persons:	
Influenza vaccine	Elderly persons or persons with chronic disease states. Adults living in high-risk situations: nursing home residents, medical personnel, or healthy persons 65 years and older. SC annually.
Pneumococcal vaccine	High-risk persons, such as those with underlying health problems and healthy elderly persons 65 years and older. SC once only.
For adolescents and young persons:	
Measles vaccine	For persons born after 1956 who have not had measles or have not previously received a live virus vaccine. SC once.
Mumps vaccine	For prepuberty and adolescent males who have not had the vaccine or mumps. SC once.
Rubella vaccine	For hospital workers, adolescent and adult females who are not immunized and have no laboratory evidence of immunity. SC once.
Hepatitis B vaccine	For persons at high risk of hepatitis exposure, such as health care personnel, hemodialysis patients, drug abusers, those exposed to a family member with hepatitis, and travelers. Three doses are the usual dosage schedule.

Modified from Williams, WW Hickson, and others, 1988; Wyngaarden and Smith, 1988.
*IM, Intramuscularly; SC, subcutaneously

million children under 15 were not protected against one or more of the vaccine-preventable diseases. This represents a major national problem."* The campaign focused on vigorous enforcement of state school entry laws and a

*From National League for Nursing News 26:(6), July-Aug. 1978.

one-time assessment of all children at *all* grade levels. It sought to allay school officials' fear of a reaction to tougher enforcement with a concerted show of community support. The Centers for Disease Control (CDC), U.S. Public Health Service, is an excellent source of information for nurses directing or implementing vaccination programs. Free publications are available to health care professionals.†

Requests for exemption from required immunizations for school entry or for continued attendance on medical grounds can be obtained from the child's physician. A model form for exemption on religious grounds can be obtained from the Christian Science Committee on Publications. However, it is *theoretically* possible that the right to exempt certain children could interfere with "herd immunity" by sustaining a continued pool of susceptibles, thereby maintaining a hazard that would be unacceptable to other parents who might apply legal and other pressures.

Community health nurses, school nurse-teachers, local public health departments, the Department of Health and Human Services, and the World Health Organization need to work together to share expertise in educating the public, in casefinding and reporting, in screening, and in mass immunization programs.

CURRENT AND FUTURE DEVELOPMENTS

The overall picture of immunization shows that currently there is renewed evaluation of the effects and effectiveness of the "vaccine era" during which morbidity and mortality rates of infectious diseases (especially childhood illness, with the exception of pertussis) were significantly reduced by artificially acquired means. Refinements and developments in clinical immunology are advancing even as still more dilemmas arise.

1. Live vaccine–related diseases have surfaced as problems. During the 1970s, in approximately 1 case in 11 million live poliovirus vaccinations, the vaccinee developed the disease itself. About 1 in 4 million of the vaccinees' contacts was found to develop polio of the vaccine type (versus the wild poliovirus type). This was thought to be an outstandingly safe record by comparison with some countries (e.g., the Soviet Union) and a deplorable record by comparison with others. Studies indicate the possibility that mutant strains of neurovirulent polioviruses (especially Type 3 virus) may be excreted in vaccinees' feces. There was some consideration of the renewed use of the inactivated poliovirus vaccine (IPV) of the 1950s or a new one being developed to avoid this eventuality. This approach must be weighed according to feasibility and

†Public Inquiries, Centers for Disease Control, Atlanta, GA 30333; this address may also be used to request subscriptions to *Morbidity & Mortality Weekly Report* (MMWR), containing up-to-date statistics, findings, and instructions about infectious diseases and immunizations worldwide.

TABLE 65-3   Guide to Tetanus Prophylaxis in Wound Management

History of tetanus immunization (doses)	Clean, minor wounds		All other wounds†	
	Td*	TIG	Td	TIG
Uncertain or less than 3	Yes	No	Yes	Yes
3 or more‡	No§	No	No″	No

From the 1988 Report of the Committee on Infectious Diseases, ed 21. Published by the American Academy of Pediatrics, Elk Grove Village, Ill.
*Td = adult type tetanus and diphtheria toxoids. If the patient is less than 7 years old, DT or DTP is given (see text). TIG = tetanus immune globulin.
†Including but not limited to wounds contaminated with dirt, feces, soil, saliva, etc.; puncture wounds, avulsions; and wounds resulting from missiles, crushing, burns, and frostbite.
‡If only three doses of *fluid* toxoid have been received, a fourth dose of toxoid, preferably an adsorbed toxoid, should be given.
§Yes, if more than 10 years since the last dose.
″Yes, if more than 5 years since the last dose.

risk versus benefits: the probability of a family returning for the necessary booster doses of IPV must be balanced against the probability of their contracting poliovirus as a result of vaccination with trivalent oral poliovirus vaccine (TOPV). Intensive campaigns to immunize infants and small children have since significantly reduced the number of susceptible individuals.

The whole question of vaccine safety seems to loom large in the decision-making process of the public. When questioned, only about half the parents interviewed at the close of the 1970s thought vaccines were *very* safe, and only one third thought they were moderately safe. This belief may partly account for the statistics that, at the same time, only about 68% of 10- to 14-year olds were found to be adequately protected against the common infectious diseases. The other reason may be that childhood diseases are just not seen as significant anymore.

2. Immunization with the killed-virus measles vaccine given from 1963 to 1967 apparently left the vaccinee more vulnerable to an atypical measles virus with severe side effects. Increasingly a college-age person or parent is the subject of a relatively virulent form of some childhood disease for which he or she was much earlier immunized or whose antibody titers are waning.

3. Other secondary effects are surfacing: some booster injections (e.g., tetanus) seem to increase sensitivity to the antigen, resulting in severe reactions. Following the swine flu vaccination program, there were significant reports of apparently vaccine-related cases of Guillain-Barré syndrome. Since increasing numbers of liability claims against vaccine producers can be anticipated among our more astute population, children's health care practitioners can increasingly anticipate being objects of a lawsuit or being called as expert witnesses.

4. Poultry allergy is less of a potential threat than originally supposed, since only minute quantities of potential allergens are found in the vaccines and then only in those grown in egg embryo culture. Reactions to antibiotics and thimerosal allergy must still be dealt with, however.

5. Evidence is building that desired antibody formation from vaccines is subject to interference from concurrent passive transfer by way of immune serum or antitoxin, or by way of maternal transplacental or breast milk transfer of maternal antibodies, or interference when one single-virus vaccine is injected simultaneously with another virus vaccine. Such coincidences must be avoided through immunization schedules.

ADMINISTRATION

Before an immunization is given, an interview with the client and family should take place. The individual's age, current physical condition and general resistance to disease, history of exposure to infectious disease (both past and potential), and previous immunizations should be assessed. A list of the general contraindications to immunization follows:

1. Current acute or febrile illness
2. Immunosuppressive therapy in progress or immunodeficient state
3. Recent immune serum globulin (ISG), plasma, or blood transfusions
4. Pregnancy—"live" vaccines especially may prove to be teratogenic or may cause infection in the fetus and therefore need to be avoided or given with caution (see Table 65-4)
5. Certain malignancies that leave the individual infection-susceptible (e.g., leukemias, lymphomas)
6. Simultaneous administration of another *single* live virus, unless proved safe
7. Prior unusual or allergic reaction to the same or similar vaccine
8. Allergy to antibiotics in vaccine, thimerosal as a preservative, or other constituents

Minor afebrile infections such as the common cold are not usually contraindications to immunization.

Perceptions and misconceptions concerning immuni-

TABLE 65-4   Vaccination During Pregnancy

	Vaccine	Indications for vaccination during pregnancy
LIVE VIRUS VACCINES		
Measles	Live-attenuated	Contraindicated.
Mumps		
Rubella		
Yellow fever	Live-attenuated	Contraindicated except if exposure is unavoidable.
Poliomyelitis	Trivalent live-attenuated (OPV)	Persons at substantial risk of exposure may receive live-attenuated virus vaccine.
INACTIVATED VIRUS VACCINES		
Hepatitis B	Plasma derived, purified hepatitis B surface antigen	Pregnancy is not a contraindication.
Influenza	Inactivated type A and type B virus vaccines	Usually recommended only for patients with serious underlying disease. It is prudent to avoid vaccination during the first trimester. Consult health authorities for current recommendations.
Poliomyelitis	Killed virus (IPV)	OPV, not IPV, is indicated when immediate protection of pregnant females is needed.
Rabies	Killed virus Rabies IG	Substantial risk of exposure
INACTIVATED BACTERIAL VACCINES		
Cholera	Killed bacterial	Should reflect actual risks of disease and probable benefits of vaccine.
Typhoid		
Plague	Killed bacterial	Selective vaccination of exposed persons.
Meningococcal	Polysaccharide	Only in unusual outbreak situations.
Pneumococcal	Polysaccharide	Only for high-risk persons.
TOXOIDS		
Tetanus-diphtheria (Td)	Combined tetanus-diptheria toxoids, adult formulation	Lack of primary series, or no booster within past 10 years.
IMMUNE GLOBULINS, POOLED OR HYPERIMMUNE	Immune globulin or specific globulin preparations	Exposure or anticipated unavoidable exposure to measles, hepatitis A, hepatitis B, rabies, or tetanus.

From Health Information for International Travel, Atlanta, 1988, US Department of Health and Human Services, Centers for Disease Control.

zation must be clarified. The relative safety and merits of immunization versus risks of the disease process itself (both short- and long-range) should be discussed, using statistics where appropriate. The client and/or family should be told that a repeat immunization, if records are unclear, is usually not contraindicated; the risk is usually minimal, and future protection is ensured. Unimmunized parents should be identified and probably immunized before their children, especially when TOPV is administered.

Noncompletion of an immunization series may occasionally be prevented if vaccinees or their parents know that interruption of the series or a prolonged period between phases of immunization makes no difference to eventual antibody levels. A copy of the immunization schedule given to the patient or family also enhances compliance with the immunization series.

Complete, written, and accurate documentation of immunizations with dates is rare even in office records. Nonetheless, having access to these data is important. Therefore teaching parents or vaccinees to keep careful written records for each vaccination, especially in view of the high mobility of our population, is crucial. Simple blank forms are available for this purpose and should be given to parents or the vaccinee with an explanation and advice to keep them updated and in a safe place (e.g., with health record files at home or in the family Bible) and to bring them to each child's appointment.

Almost all immunotherapy is parenteral and must be given by the specified route and with the specified diluent to avoid either local reactions (especially seen when the intracutaneous route is used) or possible anaphylaxis (especially when the intravenous route is used). All needles should be changed after withdrawing the vaccine from the vial, if possible. Aspiration after insertion is, of course, also necessary to prevent the danger of depositing the dose into the bloodstream.

SIDE EFFECTS/ADVERSE REACTIONS

As important as protection from debilitating infectious disease is, even immunization is not without some risk. Side effects (i.e., slight fever, sore injection site, or minor rash) are usually mild and transient; occasionally more serious effects (i.e., encephalitis and convulsions) are reported. Although serious, the incidence of these effects, when weighed against effects of diseases preventable through immunization, usually tips the balance in favor of immunization, particularly for those at high risk.

Joint pains and malaise may also be seen, especially after certain live and inactivated vaccines. Rarely allergy to the egg protein providing the culture medium for the organism involved, to antiserums or antitoxins, to the mercury preservative, or to contained antibiotics causes a reaction that is usually controllable by antihistamines. When any unusual or severe reaction occurs, the nurse should contact the practitioner and an informational form should be sent to the Centers for Disease Control. Vaccinees should be given a contact's name in case they become sick and visit a physician, hospital, or clinic within 4 weeks after immunization. Adverse reaction monitoring is part of a surveillance system to detect uncommon, severe, previously unrecognized, and rare reactions to vaccination. Past examples are the Guillain-Barré syndrome accompanying a small percentage of influenza vaccinations, encephalitis following measles vaccine, and peripheral neuropathy after rubella vaccinations; these are all *very* rare occurrences. Even though uncommon, a large number of benign, expected reactions could indicate a "hot" lot of vaccine. Data are collected by the Centers for Disease Control for comparison with national data and are published in the *Quarterly Adverse Reaction Report.*

Minor expected reactions can be treated with acetaminophen and rest. Severe fevers (more than 103°F) can be treated with acetaminophen and sponge baths to reduce the temperature; occasionally a convulsion may accompany a high temperature, and parents need to be advised. Serum sickness sometimes occurs after repeated serum injections; it consists of rash, urticaria, arthritis, adenopathy, and fever starting hours or even days after the injection. Treatment consists of analgesics, antihistamines, ephedrine, or corticosteroids. Rare but serious anaphylactic reactions can cause urticaria, dyspnea, cyanosis, shock, or unconsciousness that occurs within minutes of injection. This is not normal; it is an emergency situation. Therefore a nurse or someone responsible should observe any recipient of immunotherapy for up to half an hour after therapy. Treatment for anaphylaxis may involve epinephrine 1:1000 (0.01 ml/kg) in a 1:10 dilution subcutaneously or intramuscularly immediately, administered slowly in a physiologic saline solution. This may possibly be repeated and followed by intravenous administration of epinephrine. Vasopressors and intermittent positive pressure breathing (IPPB) oxygen, antihistamines, and corticosteroids may help. Immunization therapy may cautiously be resumed after all signs of anaphylaxis are gone.

Nurses often find themselves in charge of vaccination programs and clinics. Since nurses are often the first to be consulted by clients, keeping current about the changes in immunizations is important. A description of biologic agents (active and passive) used for immunization and their secondary effects may be found in Table 65-5 and 65-6.

The Nurse's Role in Immunotherapy

Assessment. Passive immunization or **immunoprophylaxis** should always be administered as soon as possible after exposure to the agent.

Routinely assess individuals (especially children) for immune status. High-risk groups include adolescents, new parents, individuals not vaccinated with the live measles vaccine, migrant workers, or recent immigrants. Elderly individuals, especially those in nursing homes, as well as those with chronic health problems, are at particular risk for respiratory infections and should be encouraged to obtain annual influenza virus vaccinations. Individuals who have been exposed or are at risk of exposure to one of the childhood diseases or serious communicable diseases or who have incurred a traumatic wound are also candidates for immunization.

Contraindications to immunization are found under "administration." Be aware that a history of hypersensitivity reactions to the biologic agent or to any contained antibiotics or preservatives are contraindications to immunotherapy. Pregnancy may or may not be a contraindication, depending on clinical judgment and manufacturers' instructions.

Always assess client's allergy history carefully and test for hypersensitivity before administering animal sera.

Intervention. Immune antisera and globulin are administered intramuscularly unless otherwise noted.

Be aware that a crying, wriggling baby or child presents a challenging moving target for injection and must be temporarily restrained. This can often be accomplished just as effectively in the warmth and security of another's arms (the mother's, if feasible) rather than on a hard table surface. Taking out the needle and syringe and explaining that "this may hurt for only a minute" *just before* the actual injection will lessen fear of pain.

Record the dates of immunization at the time of administration, and give a copy to the recipient or parents for permanent safekeeping. Explain that this record may be invaluable later when these dates may be required on applications to school, summer camp, or college.

Be aware that most products will lose potency at temperatures higher than 2° to 8° C (35.6° to 46.4° F) except for TOPV, which must be frozen. Most immunization

Text continued on p. 1030.

TABLE 65-5 Biological Agents for Active Immunization

Active immunization uses either inactivated (K or killed) material or live (L) attenuated agents.
Advantages: Usually higher levels of antibody are induced and it is not necessary to repeat the procedure frequently.
Disadvantages: Adverse effects may occur, such as allergic reactions, that are not usually seen with passive immunization. See box on p. 65-16 for advantages and disadvantages of live attenuated and inactivated biologic products.

Product	Route of administration	Primary immunization schedule	Comments	Nursing considerations
Cholera vaccine	(K) bacteria SC, IM	Two doses, 1-4 wk apart	Provides 50% protection for about 6 mo.	*Assessment.* Contraindications: acute illness; severe reaction or allergic response to previous dose; pregnancy evaluated individually Precautions: review of hypersensitivity history Side effects: redness, induration, pain at site; occasionally—malaise, headache, mild to moderate temperature elevations *Implementation.* Administer IM in the deltoid muscle to adults and children over 3. Have epinephrine 1:1000 on hand.
Diphtheria toxoid	IM	Three doses, 4 or more wk apart; follow schedule in Table 66-1.	If seizures occur, use Td.*	*Assessment.* Contraindications: acute infection; reaction to initial dose, such as high fever, seizure, shock, purpura; preexisting neurologic disorder; immunosuppression; febrile states. Side effects: usual—local redness and possible tenderness; possible abscess; mild to moderate fever
Hemophilus b polysaccharide vaccine (Hib)	SC	One dose to children 18-24 mo.	Efficacy improved if given to child over 2 years old. Should be given to high-risk infants at age 18 mo.	*Assessment.* Contraindicated in immunosuppression, acute illnesses, and febrile states. *Implementation.* Shake vial well. Store in medical refrigerator. 　May be given at the same time as DPT but at different sites. 　Reconstitute with diluent provided. Record date on vial. Refrigerate; stable 30 days. 　Have epinephrine 1:1000 available.
Hepatitis B	(K)-IM	Three doses. First two doses 1 mo apart, third at 6 mo. In immunocompromized persons give double dosage.	Provides >90% protection.	*Assessment.* Contraindications/precautions: hypersensitivity. Safety and efficacy not yet established for children under 3 mo of age and in pregnant or breast-feeding women. Clinical judgment would probably weigh the risk of the disease higher then the potential risks caused by the vaccine's secondary effects. Delay giving vaccine in serious active infection or in presence of severely compromised cardiopulmonary status. Frequent handwashing, gloving (especially if any breaks in skin), and isolation modalities are essential for nurses in particular.

*Td, Combination of tetanus toxoid and diphtheria toxoid. Less diphtheria toxoid is contained in Td as compared with diphtheria toxoid.

TABLE 65-5 Biological Agents for Active Immunization—cont'd

Product	Route of administration	Primary immunization schedule	Comments	Nursing considerations
				Side effects: 50% report various degrees of temporary injection site soreness; occasionally—101° F fevers are reported; infrequently—malaise, headache, nausea, myalgias, arthralgias *Implementation.* Shake before drawing up suspension; inspect for particles; do not dilute. Store opened and unopened vials in the refrigerator.
Influenza	(K)-IM	One dose. Split doses used in persons under 13 years old (lower incidence of side effects).	Give annually by November.	*Assessment.* Contraindications: hypersensitivity to egg products; individuals who are immunosuppressed; acute febrile illness; do not inject intravenously Precautions: pregnancy; keep epinephrine on hand; not effective against all possible strains of influenza virus; resterilize jet injection apparatus if contaminated with blood; complete immunizations by November. Toxic drug reactions may occur (especially with phenytoin, warfarin, or theophylline) following viral infection or vaccination Side effects: local tenderness, redness, induration; fever, malaise, myaglia; rare—allergic skin and respiratory reactions and Guillian-Barré syndrome; very rare—encephalopathy *Implementation.* Inject IM into deltoid or lateral mid-thigh or gluteus. Refrigerate. Have epinephrine 1:1000 available.
Measles virus vaccine	(L)-SC	One dose at 15 mo; earlier if epidemic occurs.	If given before 15 mo, may reimmunize. Also may prevent disease if given within 48 hr of exposure to measles.	*Assessment.* Contraindications: neomycin or chicken product hypersensitivity; active febrile infection; active untreated TB; immunosuppression or immunodeficiency; bone marrow or lymphatic deficiencies; pregnancy (pregnancy should also be avoided for 3 mo after vaccination) Precautions: give no sooner than 3 mo after transfusion of blood/plasma/human ISG of more than 0.02 ml/lb body weight. Give with or after TB skin test. Do not give within 1 mo of immunization by other live virus vaccines except one of the M-M-R type or combination. Side effects: moderate fever to 102° F, rash (in 5-12 days); rare—fever more than 103° F with convulsions; 1 per million occurrences—encephalitis or subacute sclerosing panencephalitis; previous recipients of *killed* virus vaccine—local swelling, redness, vesiculation. *Implementation.* A 25-gauge ⅝-inch needle is recommended. Refrigerate before reconstitution and afterward. Use within 8 hr; avoid light at all times. Inject 0.5 ml reconstituted vaccine subcutaneously. Solution may be pink or yellow but must be clear. Discard cloudy solutions. Have epinephrine 1:1000 available.

Continued.

TABLE 65-5   Biological Agents for Active Immunization—cont'd

Product	Route of administration	Primary immunization schedule	Comments	Nursing considerations
Meningococcal meningitis vaccine	SC	One dose. If a household disease, antibiotic prophylaxis (rifampin) should be given for several days, since antibody response requires at least 5 days.	Used in epidemics.	*Assessment.* Obtain immunization and allergy history. Contraindications: immunosuppression; acute illness. Precautions: pregnancy. Side effects: mild, local erythema. *Implementation.* Administer in a single parenteral dose. Do not give IV. Have epinephrine 1:1000 available.
Mumps vaccine	(L)-SC	One dose	If administered before 1 year old, reimmunization may be necessary.	*Assessment.* Contraindications and precautions: same as for measles vaccine with following exceptions in side effects. Side effects: mild fever (uncommonly more than 103° F); low incidence of parotitis, orchitis, purpura, allergic reactions (urticaria); very rare—encephalitis and other nervous system reactions. *Implementation.* Same as measles vaccine.
Pertussis (in DPT and pertussis vaccine alone)	(K)-IM	As per DPT (see Table 65-1)	Not usually given after age 6.	*Assessment.* Contraindications: acute infection; previous reactions to an initial dose (all 3 antigens or only pertussis may be omitted then) such as fever greater than 103° F (39° C), convulsion, altered consciousness, focal neurologic signs, "screaming fits," shock/collapse, purpura; preexisting neurologic disorder; immunosuppression; older than 6 yr (give Td instead). Precautions: reactions to DPT call for reevaluation and possibly administration of Td only. Side effects: usual—local redness, induration, and possible tenderness; possible abscess; mild to moderate fever. *Implementation.* Administer IM into deltoid or thigh, varying site each time. Shake before using. Refrigerate. Have epinephrine 1:1000 available.
Pneumococci polysaccharide vaccine	SC, IM	0.5 ml	Not used in children under 2 yr old.	*Implementation.* Keep refrigerated. Inject into deltoid or midlateral thigh. Have epinephrine 1:1000 available. *Assessment.* Contraindications: hypersensitivity, revaccination, pregnancy, intradermal administration, and IV administration. Will not protect against specific antigens not included. Within 10 days of start of chemotherapy for Hodgkin's disease, vaccine is contraindicated. Precautions: active infection; under 2 yr of age; immunosuppression; severely compromised cardiac or pulmonary function; history of pneumococcal infection. Keep epinephrine on hand. Side effects: local redness and soreness, induration, fever greater than 100.9° F; rare—anaphylactoid reactions

TABLE 65-5 Biological Agents for Active Immunization—cont'd

Product	Route of administration	Primary immunization schedule	Comments	Nursing considerations
Poliomyelitis vaccine	(L)-Oral	Two doses, 6-8 wk apart (see Table 66-1).		*Assessment.* Contraindications: never administered parenterally or in acute illness; advanced, debilitated condition; persistent vomiting or diarrhea; immunodeficient or immunosuppressed states. Precautions: will not modify/prevent existing or incubating disease. Side effects: rarely—paralytic disease after vaccination or after contact with vaccinee (advise unimmunized close contacts of vaccinee to seek immunization as needed. *Implementation.* Store frozen, thaw before use, and agitate before giving 2 drops orally, in chlorine-free water, simple syrup, or milk, or on bread, cake, or cube sugar (using dropper supplied). See package insert for specific storage advice. Change of color from pink to yellow is not remarkable.
Rabies vaccine	(K)-IM	Preexposure: two doses a week apart followed by a third dose in 14-21 days in endemic areas. Postexposure: five doses on days 1, 3, 7, 14, and 28. Give rabies immune globulin concurrently.		*Assessment.* History of hypersensitivity dictates cautious use of rabies vaccine. *Implementation.* Flush and cleanse wound; possible initial prophylaxis with tetanus and antibiotic therapy. Have epinephrine 1:1000 available. Discontinue corticosteroids during immunization.
Rubella	(L)-SC	One dose.	Give after client 15 mo old. Do not give during pregnancy. Women must not become pregnant for 3 mo after injection. Contraceptive counseling may be needed.	*Assessment.* Contraindications and precautions as for Attenuvax with the following exceptions Contraindications: postpubertal females with rubella titers of more than 1:8; pregnancy (pregnancy also to be avoided for 3 mo after vaccine) Precautions: theoretical possibility of live virus transmission from nose/throat of vaccinees Side effects: occasionally—mild symptoms of naturally acquired rubella (lymphadenopathy, urticaria, rash, malaise, sore throat, fever, headache, polyneuritis, arthralgias, local pain, swelling, redness; fever rarely more than 103°F); very rarely—encephalitis *Implementation.* Same as for measles vaccine.
Smallpox vaccine	(L)-intradermal	One dose.	Today this vaccine is only indicated for the military and laboratory personnel who work with poxviruses.	*Assessment.* Contraindications: not to be used for treatment of warts or recurrent herpes simplex infections; infants with "failure to thrive" syndrome; anyone with disturbed skin integrity; immunosuppression or immunodeficiency; pregnancy. Precautions: blot off excess vaccine; vaccination equipment should be burned, boiled, or autoclaved before disposal.

Continued.

TABLE 65-5 Biological Agents for Active Immunization—cont'd

Product	Route of administration	Primary immunization schedule	Comments	Nursing considerations
			No longer required for travel; production for local use was discontinued in 1983.	Side effects: severe neurologic disorders; generalized rashes; local pyrogenic infections (see package insert for details). *Implementation.* Injection is by needle punctures through a drop of vaccine on the skin; site should be inspected for presence of desired vesicle after 6-8 days. Store dry but refrigerated.
Tetanus toxoid	IM	Two doses 1 mo apart. Third dose 6-12 months after second dose. Included in DPT (see Table 65-1).	School children and adults receive fourth dose 6-12 mo after initial series. Duration of effect, 10 yr.	*Assessment.* Contraindications; not for *treatment* of an actual tetanus infection; any acute infection; immunosuppression Precautions: hypersensitivity; keep epinephrine on hand; history of cerebral damage, neurologic disorders, or febrile convulsions should be evaluated individually Side effects: occasionally—Arthus-type response to high levels of tetanus antibody (antitoxin) in those receiving regular or frequent tetanus toxoid boosters (thus the recommended 10-yr interval between Td booster). Response may include significant local symptoms of redness, edema resembling a giant "hive," axillary lymphadenopathy; systemic symptoms can include low fever, malaise, aches and pains, general urticaria, tachycardia, and hypotension. Prolonged intervals between primary immunizing doses has no effect on eventual immunity status. *Implementation.* Shake well and give deep IM, avoiding blood vessels. Refrigerate, but do not freeze. Have epinephrine 1:1000 available.
Tuberculosis BCG vaccine	(L)-SC or intradermal	One dose.	Because of questionable efficacy, this product is not commonly used in the U.S.	*Assessment.* Contraindications: altered immune states Precautions: pregnancy; postvaccination sensitivity may mimic positive reaction to tuberculin following a skin test for TB. Full, lasting protection from TB cannot be ensured postvaccination (great variance in efficacy among BCG products). Side effects (can occur up to 1 yr later): severe local ulceration, lymphadenitis; very rare—osteomyelitis, lupoid reactions, disseminated BCG infection, death. *Implementation.* Reconstitute, do not shake, protect from light, and use within 8 hr. Halve dose on label for those under 28 days old and revaccinate with full dose after 1 yr old (intracutaneous route or follow label). Strains and efficacy vary among different preparations.

TABLE 65-5   Biological Agents for Active Immunization—cont'd

Product	Route of administration	Primary immunization schedule	Comments	Nursing considerations
Typhoid vaccine	(K)-SC or intradermal	Two doses 1 mo or more apart.	Approximately 70% protective. Only recommended for travel, epidemics, or identified household carriers.	*Assessment.* Contraindications: acute infection; allergic reaction to previous dose. Precautions: get history of possible hypersensitivity. Keep current regarding recent literature. Side effects: local redness, induration, tenderness; malaise, headache, myalgia, elevated temperature. *Implementation.* Shake vial well before use. Keep refrigerated. Have epinephrine 1:1000 available.
Yellow fever vaccine	(L)-SC	One dose.	Only for persons living in or traveling to Africa and South America.	*Assessment.* Contraindications: pregnancy; altered immune states; hypersensitivity to eggs and certain contained antibiotics Precautions: administer at least 1 mo apart from other live virus vaccines. Side effects: mild—headache, myalgia, fever; extremely rare—encephalitis. *Implementation.* Keep frozen. Reconstitute with sodium chloride without preservatives. Rotate vial; do not shake. Use within 1 hr; discard the rest. Have epinephrine 1:1000 available.

TABLE 65-6   Biological Agents For Passive Immunization

Passive immunization is a transfer of antibodies from animal or human sources to a person incapable of forming antibodies OR to prevent disease when time does not allow for active immunization OR to treat a disease that is normally prevented by immunization OR for situations where active immunization is not available, such as snake bites.

Product	Dosage	Comments	Nursing considerations
Black widow spider antivenin, equine	One vial of 6000 units, IM or IV	Use is limited to children >15 kg.	*Assessment.* Do not proceed without hypersensitivity history, hypersensitivity skin test (0.02-0.03 ml of a 1:10 dilution of horse serum or antivenin intracutaneously) with a control injection of sodium chloride in opposite extremity. Give serum based on above results and individual evaluation of risks and benefits (see package insert for detailed instructions). Do not pack wound in ice; discontinue vaccine if there are any systemic reactions. *Implementation.* Mix to reconstitute by swirling (to avoid foaming); have available epinephrine, oxygen, resuscitation equipment (airway, tourniquet, injectable antihistamines, corti-

Continued.

TABLE 65-6   Biological Agents For Passive Immunization—cont'd

Product	Dosage	Comments	Nursing considerations
			costeroids, and injectable pressor amines); give first 5-10 ml of infusion slowly over a 3-5 min period and observe for reactions; if given by IM route, give into large muscle mass (e.g., gluteal); consider possible tetanus prophylaxis and antibiotics if local tissue damage is evident; treat shock with blood, plasma expanders; give aspirin or codeine as needed for pain; give sedative or tranquilizer as needed.
Botulism antitoxin	One vial IV and 1 vial IM. Repeat in 2-4 hr if client's symptoms get worse.	Available from CDC.*	*Implementation:* Follow directions closely on administration. Given only to asymptomatic individuals with unequivocal exposure. *Assessment.* Observe contacts carefully; if symptoms occur, then administer antitoxin.
Diphtheria antitoxin	20,000 to 120,000 units IM. Same dose for adults children.	Available from CDC.	*Implementation.* Active immunization and erythromycin prophylaxis preferred rather than antitoxin administration for nonimmune contacts of active cases.
Hepatitis B immune globulin	0.06 ml/kg IM after exposure, preferably within 1 wk. A second injection should be given 25-30 days after first exposure except if this vaccine was given with HBIG.		*Assessment.* Contraindications: hypersensitivity to this product or thimerosal. *Implementation.* Deltoid and buttocks are preferred injection sites. All exposures should be treated as if confirmed, and appropriate isolation procedures should be instituted.
Hepatitis non-A, non-B immune globulin Hypogammaglobulinemia immune globulin	0.06 ml/kg IM immediately after exposure. 0.6 ml/kg IM every 21-28 days.	Should give double dose at onset of therapy.	*Assessment.* Contraindications: do not give IV; IgA deficiency (may develop possible anaphylactic reactions to blood products); coagulation disorder; allergy to thimerosal; do not give Gamastan to those with clinical signs of hepatitis A or if exposure within past 2 weeks; vaccination for measles, mumps, polio, or rubella within 3 mo after IG Side effects: local pain, urticaria, angioedema; rare—anaphylaxis *Implementation.* Given to individuals with sera exposure to

*CDC, Centers for Disease Control. Central number (404) 329-3311; (404) 329-2888 for nights, weekends, and holidays for emergencies only.

TABLE 65-6   Biological Agents For Passive Immunization—cont'd

Product	Dosage	Comments	Nursing considerations
			clients with hepatitis. IM route (gluteal is preferred site) in several muscle sites as needed. Do not inject more than 3 ml per site. Refrigerate; do not freeze; use before expiration date. Have epinephrine 1:1000 available.
Measles immune globulin	0.25 ml/kg IM immediately after exposure.		*Implementation.* Live vaccine usually prevents measles if given within 2 days of exposure. If immunoglobulin is given, do not administer the live vaccine for 3 mo.
Pertussis immune globulin	1.25 ml/IM (child).		Its effectiveness is questionable.
Poliomyelitis globulin	0.15 ml/kg IM.		*Implementation.* Use only for exposed, nonimmunized persons. After 2 to 3 months, immunize with live or inactivated vaccine.
Rabies immune globulin	20 IU/kg, up to ½ infiltrated locally at wound site and remainder of dose given IM.	Give immediately after bite or at scratches caused by bats, skunks, foxes, coyotes, raccoons, or other carnivores.	*Assessment.* Obtain specific history of animal bite. Do not give to anyone previously adequately immunized with rabies vaccine. Side effects: local soreness, slight fever; rare—angioneurotic edema, nephrotic syndrome, or anaphylaxis. *Implementation.* Administer 5 ml or less at each site; use different sites. Give intramuscularly only and never intravenously. Repeated doses may interfere with full development of active immunity. Flush and cleanse wound; possible initial prophylaxis with tetanus and antibiotic therapy.
Rho (D) immune globulin	Treat Rho-negative woman; 1 dose IM within 3 days of abortion, delivery, or amniocentesis of Rho-positive infant, or transfusion Rh-positive blood.	For nonimmune women only. May administer after 3 days if necessary.	*Assessment.* Contraindicated in Rho (D)-positive or D^u positive individuals. *Implementation.* Keep refrigerated.
Rubella immune globulin	20-40 ml IM at exposure.	Not recommended for pregnant women because it will protect the mother but not the fetus.	
Coral snake antivenin, equine	Minimum of 3-5 vials IV.	Use dosage sufficient to reverse symptoms of snakebite.	See nursing considerations for black widow spider antivenin, equine.

Continued.

TABLE 65-6   Biological Agents For Passive Immunization—cont'd

Product	Dosage	Comments	Nursing considerations
Tetanus immune globulin	Preventive: 250-500 units IM. Therapeutic: 3000-6000 units IM.	Given along with Td immunization, but administer in separate syringe at different IM sites. Use only for major or dirty wounds if the wound is more than 24 hours old and the person received less than 2 doses of toxoid in the past.	*Assessment.* Side effects: occasionally—local tenderness, stiffness, allergic or anaphylatic systemic reactions. *Implementation.* Do not give intravenously; avoid blood vessels. Have epinephrine available.
Vaccinia immune globulin	Preventive: 0.3 ml/kg IM. Therapeutic: 0.6 ml/kg IM. May repeat if necessary for treatment; in 1-week intervals for prophylaxis.	Available from CDC.	
Varicella-zoster	125 units/10 kg for persons up to 50 kg. 625 unit maximum for patients >50 kg. Give IM within 4 days of exposure.	For immunosuppressed or immunoincompetent children under 15 years old.	*Assessment.* Modifies the natural disease but may not prevent the development of the illness. (Costly; approximately $400 to treat one adult.)

ADVANTAGES AND DISADVANTAGES OF LIVE ATTENUATED AND INACTIVATED BIOLOGIC PRODUCTS

TYPE OF IMMUNIZATION	ADVANTAGES	DISADVANTAGES
Attenuated (live)	Immunity long lasting. Can simulate resistance as produced by natural disease.	Increased risk of inducing disease. Mild disease needed usually to induce immunity. Higher risk of containing contaminants than inactivated product. Usually more labile and requires special storage.
Inactivated (killed)	Easy to ship and store. Usually highly purified. Little risk of inducing a disease from infection.	Provides a short-acting immunity. Often need re-immunization. May not stimulate protective type factors. May not prevent a reinfection without disease or a carrier state.

---

agents should therefore be stored in a medical refrigerator, where a thermometer is placed nearby, and replaced immediately after use. They should not be stored near a radiator, on a window sill, or on a refrigerator door shelf because of unpredictable temperatures.

Education. Teach clients or their parents how to recognize and differentiate between anticipated side effects and serious adverse reactions. (See Tables 65-5 and 65-6). After any immunization, ask clients to remain in the area for up to half an hour for observation of any developing adverse reactions. Keep epinephrine on hand to counter any potentially dangerous event (such as anaphylaxis). Antipyretics may be taken for the not uncommon aches, local pain and swelling, or mild temperature elevations, which may occur within 24 hours. Recipients of immunotherapy should understand whom they are to contact if complications occur later.

Apply and explain appropriate isolation precautions when caring for individuals with known or suspected exposure to the communicable diseases. Assuming that someone else will take this responsibility at the outset is unwise.

Evaluation. Because of the risk of anaphylaxis, clients should be observed for up to half an hour after administration.

Sources of information on immunization include primarily the Public Health Service Advisory Committee on Immunization Practices (ACIP), which advises the public health agencies, and the Committee on Control of Infectious Diseases (the Red Book Committee), which is drawn from the members of the American Academy of Pediatrics and advises the private health sector. The ACIP can be contacted through the Centers for Disease Control in Atlanta. Since the two groups maintain a slightly different perspective, minor inconsequential variations in recommendations may occasionally be noted. Other sources include local public health departments and printed package inserts included with the vaccine or serum. Biologic preparations and accompanying inserts are regulated by the Bureau of Biologics of the FDA. The state of the art of immunotherapy is in rapid flux. The only constant in immunization practice is change itself. To read, attend seminars, and consult with experts is to keep pace.

KEY TERMS

active immunization, page 1022
antibody titer, page 1017
endemic, page 1017
immunoprophylaxis, page 1021
passive immunization, page 1027

BIBLIOGRAPHY

Bruni, PJ: Pertussis vaccine: assets and liabilities, Patient Care 18(15):173, 1984.

Fedson, DS: Adult immunization: protocols and problems, Hosp Pract 21(7):143, 1986.

Few, BJ: Pertussis vaccine, MCN 12(4):243, 1987.

Frank, T, and others: Pertussis immunizations? Pediatr Nurs 10(5):360, 1984.

Giangrasso, J, and others: Misuse of tetanus immunoprophylaxis in wound care, Ann Emerg Med 14(6):573, 1985.

Halpern, JS: Rabies vaccine: reduced risks and fears, JEN 10(2):101, 1984.

Hinman, AR: The pertussis vaccine controversy, Public Health Rep 99(3):255, 1984.

Katz, SL: The campaign against pertussis vaccination, Perinat Neonat 8(1):72, 1984.

Kastrup, EK, ed: Facts and comparisons, St Louis, 1988, JB Lippincott Co.

Katzung, BG: Basic and clinical pharmacology, ed 3, Norwalk, Conn, 1987, Appleton & Lange.

Kent, JM: The new flu and pneumococcal vaccines, Patient Care 18(14):62, 1984.

Kynes, P: The hepatitis B vaccine, J Enterostom Ther 12(4):144, 1985.

Lelyveld, S: An update of immunization practices for the emergency physician, Top Emerg Med 8(1):76, 1986.

Longyear, LA, and others: Keeping children safe: the *Haemophilus influenzae* type b immunization, J Pediatr Health Care 1(2):73, 1987.

Pajares, KF, and others: Rubella vaccination, Pediatr Nurs 10(1):72, 1984.

Poland, V: What high-risk personnel need to know about the hepatitis B vaccine, AORN J 40(3):372, 1984.

Poser, CM: Vaccine, infection complications: neurologic syndromes that arise unpredictably, Consultant 27(1):45, 1987.

Rimar, JM: *Haemophilus influenzae* type b polysaccharide vaccine, MCN 11(1):57, 1986.

Thompson, CE, and others: Tetanus and the aged, Nurse Pract 10(6):28, 1985.

Todd, B: Preventing influenza and pneumonia, Geriatr Nurs 5(8):399, 1984.

True, L, and others: Routine pertussis immunization, Drug Intell Clin Pharm 19(10):729, 1985.

Veatch, RM: The ethics of promoting herd immunity, Fam Community Health 10(1):44, 1987.

Wiedermann, G, and others: Risks and benefits of vaccinations, Infect Control 5(9):438, 1984.

Williams, WW, Hickson, MA, and others: Immunization policies and vaccine coverage among adults: the risk for missed opportunities, Ann Intern Med 108(4):616, 1988.

Windom, RE: Adult vaccination should be routine, too, Public Health Rep 102(3):245, 1987.

Wyngaarden, JB, and Smith, LH: Cecil textbook of medicine, ed 18, Philadelphia, 1988, WB Saunders Co.

UNIT XVII

Drugs Affecting the Integumentary System

CHAPTER
66

Overview of the Integumentary System

OBJECTIVES

After studying this chapter, the student will be able to:

1. Describe the two layers of the skin.
2. Differentiate between the three types of exocrine glands.
3. Explain five major functions of the skin.
4. Name three appendages of the skin.

The skin (or integument) has been described as the largest organ in the body. In most disease states, medications are administered at a site that is distant from the target organ, but in dermatology, medications can be directly applied to the target site. Since skin functions are vital to an individual's survival and also quite diverse, this chapter reviews the structure of the skin, functions of the skin, and skin appendages. (See Figure 66-1.)

STRUCTURE OF THE SKIN

The skin is made up of two layers, the epidermis and dermis.

The **epidermis,** or outer skin layer, consists of four strata or layers:

1. Stratum corneum (horny layer)—outer dead cells that have been converted to keratin, a water-repellent protein. This layer forms a protective cover for the body; it will desquamate or shed and be replaced by new cells from the bottom layers.
2. Stratum lucidum or clear layer—this area contains translucent flat cells; keratin is formed here.
3. Stratum granulosum or granular layer—granules are located in the cytoplasm of these cells. Cells die in this layer of skin.
4. Stratum germinativum—this has been divided into two layers in some references; the top layer is the

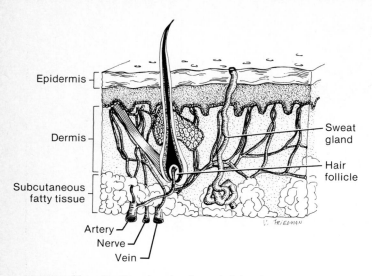

FIGURE 66-1   Section showing layers of the skin.
(From Potter, PA: Pocket nurse guide to physical assessment, St. Louis, 1986, The CV Mosby Co.)

stratum spinosum, and the innermost layer is the stratum basale. The latter two names were devised to describe the cellular structure of the two layers; stratum spinosum contains spinelike cells, whereas stratum basale has column-shaped cells. The cells in the latter area germinate—that is, undergo cellular mitosis to generate new cells for the skin.

Melanocytes, which are responsible for synthesizing **melanin,** a skin color pigment, are also located deep in the stratum germinativum. The more melanin that is present, the deeper the brown skin color. Melanin also is a protective agent; it blocks ultraviolet rays, thus preventing injury to underlying dermis and tissues.

The epidermis has no direct blood supply of its own; it is nourished only by diffusion.

The **dermis** lies between the epidermis and subcutaneous fat. It is approximately 40 times thicker than the epidermis, and it contains and provides skin support from its blood vessels, nerves, lymphatic tissue, and elastic and connective tissues.

The two main divisions of the dermis are the papillary dermis and the reticular dermis. Sweat glands, sebaceous glands, and hair follicles originate in the reticular dermis, and their structures branch out in the papillary dermis.

Below the dermis layer is the hypodermis, which contributes flexibility to the skin. Subcutaneous fat tissue is an area for thermal insulation, nutrition, and cushioning or padding.

The skin contains three types of **exocrine glands**— sebaceous, eccrine, and apocrine. **Sebaceous glands** are large, lipid-containing cells that produce sebum, the oil or film layer that covers the epidermis. This protects and lubricates the skin, so it is not only water repellent but also has some antiseptic effects.

The sebaceous fluid travels by way of a short duct (sebaceous duct) to the hair follicles in the upper dermis. Thus hair, which is located everywhere on the skin except the palms, soles, and mucous membrane tissues, is lubricated.

The **eccrine glands,** or sweat glands, are also widely distributed on the skin surface, including the soles and palms. These glands help regulate body temperature and also help prevent excessive skin dryness.

The **apocrine glands** are located mainly in the axillae, genital organs, and breast areas. They are odoriferous and are believed to represent scent or sex glands.

Normal skin pH is 4.5 to 5.5, which is weakly acidic. This acid mantle is a protective mechanism because microorganisms grow best at pH 6 to 7.5. Infected skin areas usually have a higher skin pH.

FUNCTIONS OF THE SKIN

The skin serves many functions in the body. Some of the major functions are listed here:

1. Protective function—The skin forms a protective covering for the entire body. It protects the internal organs and their environment from external forces. Thus it is a barrier against microorganism and chemical body invasion.

2. Organ of sensation—Nerve endings permit the transfer of stimuli sensations, such as heat, cold, pressure, and pain.

3. Body temperature regulator—It maintains a body temperature homeostasis by regulating heat loss or heat conservation. Blood vessels in the dermis area can dilate, and perspiration increases when the body temperature is elevated. If the body temperature is below normal, the skin blood vessels constrict and perspiration is decreased to conserve body heat.

4. Skin excretes fluid and electrolytes (sweat glands), stores fat, synthesizes vitamin D (when skin is exposed to sunlight or ultraviolet rays, the steroid 7-dehydrocholesterol that is normally present in the skin is converted to vitamin D_3), and provides a site for drug absorption. Fat soluble vitamins (A, D, and K), estrogens, corticoid hormones, and some chemicals can be absorbed through skin.

5. Skin contributes to the concept of body image and a feeling of well-being. A disfiguring skin condition can lead to emotional problems, and a chronic skin condition may also lead to depression.

APPENDAGES OF THE SKIN

The appendages of the skin are hair, nails, and skin glands. These areas are discussed when drug therapy is specific for these sites.

Skin injuries, lesions, and disorders result in a variety of dermatologic problems for the individual and nursing care issues for the health care provider. In the next chapter, major skin problems are discussed.

KEY TERMS

apocrine glands, page 1036
dermis, page 1036
eccrine glands, page 1036
epidermis, page 1035
exocrine glands, page 1036
melanin, page 1036
sebaceous glands, page 1036

BIBLIOGRAPHY

Cahn, RL, and Longe, RL: The skin assessment, Washington, D.C., 1986, Syntex Laboratories, Inc. and The American Pharmaceutical Association.

Dossey, L: The skin: what is it? . . . the potency of touch, Top Clin Nurs 5(2):1, 1983.

Gilchrest, BA, ed: The aging skin, Dermatologic Clinics 4(3):345.

Marks, RM, Barton, SP, and Edwards, C: The physical nature of the skin, Norwell, Mass, 1988, MTP Press.

Shroot, B, and Schaefer, H, eds: Skin pharmacokinetics, New York, 1988, Karger.

Thibodeau, GA: Anatomy and physiology, St Louis, 1987, Times Mirror/Mosby College Publishing.

Wooldridge, W: Aging skin: medical, cosmetic, and aesthetic considerations, Consultant 26(2):186, 1986.

Dermatologic Drugs

Many dermatologic preparations are available and used to treat the numerous skin disorders common in the United States and Canada. Often particular ointments, creams, powders, or specific vehicles provide a desired effect without the addition of an active ingredient. For example, for the person with dry, scaly skin found in psoriasis or dry eczema, an ointment that has an occlusive emollient effect is desired, such as an emulsifying ointment, lanolin, or a synthetic base. The person with a moist or dry skin condition may receive a cooling emollient-type preparation that is also moisturizing, such as a cream formulation.

The individual with an acute inflammation that is weeping or oozing would need a drying and soothing lotion, such as a saline solution, aluminum acetate solution, or calamine lotion. A lichenified oozing skin problem (an example being eczema) may need a protective and drying agent, such as coal tar paste, Lassar's paste, or zinc compound paste. If the skin problem is located on an elbow or knee and the site is sore and wet, then a dusting powder may be appropriate to reduce friction and help dry the area. Talcum or starch-type preparations may be used.

SKIN DISORDERS

Reactions or disorders of the skin are manifested by symptoms such as itching, pain, or tingling and by signs such as swelling, redness, papules, pustules, blisters, and hives. Some common dermatologic disorders in the United States and Canada are:

Acne vulgaris (cystic acne and acne scars)
Atopic dermatitis
Dyshidrotic eczema
Folliculitis
Fungus infections (tinea pedis, tinea unguium, tinea versicolor, tinea cruris)
Hand eczema
Herpes simplex
Lichen simplex chronicus
Psoriasis
Seborrheic dermatitis
Verruca vulgaris
Vitiligo

A reaction of the skin that makes the individual uncomfortable or unsightly may be attributed to or related to sensitivity to drugs, allergy, infection, emotional conflict, hormonal imbalance, or degenerative disease. Sometimes the cause of the skin disorder is unknown and the treatment may be empiric in the hope that the right remedy will be found.

Dermatologic diagnosis includes physical inspection, personal and family medical history, and laboratory tests including blood and urine tests, cytodiagnosis, and biopsy. The physical examination of the skin sometimes includes the use of Wood's light. This instrument provides long-wave ultraviolet light, which is helpful in detecting hair and skin infected with fungi that fluoresce and in aiding in differentiation of hypopigmented areas and depigmented areas of the skin. The potassium hydroxide 10% (KOH) test aids in diagnosis of mycotic infection. The solution will disintegrate keratin, disclosing, under microscopic examination, mycelia (vegetative part as filaments), fungal elements, and hyphae (which acquire food). Other tests include the Tzanck test for epidermal giant cells (seen in herpes zoster viral infections, usually with inclusion bodies, and in pemphigus vulgaris without bodies), biopsy, and patch tests. The dermatophyte test medium is a fast-acting medium that creates a marked color change when a dermatophyte is grown in it.

When the nature of the lesion has been established, its characteristics should be defined according to size, shape, surface, and color. See the box on p. 1042 for different types of lesions and some of the conditions associated with them.

The next step is to discover the distribution of the condition. In some diseases the diagnosis can be made from the distribution alone, and in others, it provides some assistance. The inference should not be drawn, however, that because a disease is not found in its common pattern of distribution that it can be excluded. For example, psoriasis is commonly found on the extensors, but occasionally it will be seen as a solitary lesion in the external ear. A basal cell carcinoma is most common on the face, but occasionally it occurs on the trunk. On the other hand, rosacea only attacks those areas of the face that flush.

The regional distribution of common conditions is shown in the box on p. 1043 (several diseases may overlap or occur simultaneously but in different areas).

The box on pp. 1044 to 1047 is a summary of the vast number of dermatologic reactions from drugs and their characteristic lesions and sequelae. Some may even be life-threatening. See Table 67-1 for the most common drugs involved. The nurse always needs to be cognizant of a client's drug history and current therapy to relate such lesions and sequelae to the appropriate cause; this often saves the client many unnecessary and uncomfortable diagnostic examinations and lessens the anxiety of the client and of the medical team. Simply discontinuing a particular drug often resolves a complicated dermatologic problem or sequelae of unknown origin.

Eczema and dermatitis are noninfectious inflammatory dermatoses. Contact dermatitis has clinical features that include skin rash with eczema (a red, thick, crusty, fissured, suppurating area) in various stages. The causes may be from contact with a primary irritant (acids, oils, soaps) in the environment, home, or work place or from a delayed allergic reaction (as seen with poison ivy contact).

Atopic dermatitis appears as a general eczema dermatitis frequently on the flexor body surfaces having genetic associations such as hay fever or asthma.

Seborrheic dermatitis often appears on the scalp, eyebrows, ears, or sternum as a brown to red scaly rash.

Text continued on p. 1047

PRINCIPLES OF SKIN ABSORPTION

Keratin in the outer skin layer provides a waterproof barrier. To enhance drug absorption, the epidermis, or keratin skin layer, needs to be hydrated. Therefore some medications are placed under an occlusive dressing (such as plastic wrap) or administered in an occlusive-type ointment (petroleum jelly) because both will trap and prevent water loss (sweat) from the skin, thus increasing epidermis hydration.

Fat or lipid soluble drugs are better absorbed through skin than water soluble drugs.

In specific body areas, the skin is very thin (eyelids, scrotum area, or the skin of a child) or very thick. The palms of the hands or soles of feet are nearly impenetrable by topical agents.

Products with ETOH content may be administered for drying effects.

Steroid products thin the skin and many are contraindicated for the face.

TABLE 67-1   Life-Threatening Drug-Induced Skin Eruptions

Drug eruptions	Drug involved	Reported sequelae
Exfoliative dermatitis	antidiabetics, oral	
	arsenicals	
	barbiturates	
	carbamazepine (Tegretol)	
	demeclocycline (Declomyein)	
	diphtheria and tetanus toxoids and pertussis vaccine, absorbed and Salk poliomyelitis vaccine	Death; probably caused by penicillin in the poliovirus vaccine
	furosemide (Lasix)	
	gold	
	griseofulvin (Grifulvin)	Lymphadenopathy
	hydroflumethiazide (Saluron)	
	isorbide (Isordil)	
	measles virus vaccine	
	mercury	
	methotrimeprazine (Levoprome)	
	nitrofurans	
	nitroglycerin	
	oral antidiabetics	
	para-aminosalicylic acid (PAS)	Hepatitis, hemolytic anemia
	penicillin	
	phenothiazines	
	phenylbutazone (Butazolidin)	
	phenytoin (Dilantin)	Atypical lymphocytes, hypoproteinemia, hepatosplenomegaly
	streptomycin	
	sulfasalazine (Azulfidine)	
	sulfonamides	
	tetracyclines	
Stevens-Johnson syndrome (erythema multiforme)	aminophenazone	
	ampicillin	
	antipyrine	
	arsenicals	
	barbiturates	
	carbamazepine (Tegretol)	
	chloramphenicol	
	chlorpropamide (Diabinese)	
	clindamycin	
	codeine	
	cold preparation 666	
	mephenytoin (Mesantoin)	
	novobiocin	
	paramethadione	
	penicillin	
	phenophthalein	
	phenylbutazone (Butazolidin)	
	phenytoin (Dilantin)	Death
	phenytoin and trimethadione	Lupus erythematosus occurred simultaneously
	rifampin (Rifadine, Rimactane)	
	salicylates	
	sulfasalazine (Azulfidine)	
	thiazides	
	thiouracil	
	trimethadione (Tridione) and phenobarbital	Lupus erythematosus with subsequent medication
	triple sulfas (trisulfapyrimidines, multiple sulfonamides)	
	tetracycline	

Modified from Martin EW: Hazards of medication, ed 2, Philadelphia, 1978, JB Lippincott Co.

TABLE 67-1 Life-Threatening Drug-Induced Skin Eruptions—cont'd

Drug eruptions	Drug involved	Reported sequelae
Toxic epidermal necrolysis (Lyell's syndrome)	acelaziamide (Diamox)	
	antihistamines	
	antipyrine	
	barbiturates	
	chenopodium oii	Death
	dapsone	
	diallylbarbituric acid	
	diphtheria	
	ethylmorphine HCI (Didial)	
	gold salts	
	ipecac	
	methyl salicylate	
	neomycin sulfate	
	nitrofurantoin (Furadantin)	Death; cause questionable
	opium powder	
	PABA	
	penicillin	
	pentazocine (Talwin)	
	phenobarbital	
	phenolphthalein	
	phenylbutazone (butazolidin)	Death; 1 out of 4 cases
	phenytoin (Dilantin)	Death
	procaine penicillin, aqueous injection and oral mixed sulfonamide preparation	
	sulfasalazine (Azulfidine)	Death
	sulfathiazole	
	sulfonamides	
	tetracycline	
Lupus erythematosus	chlorpromazine (Thorazine)	
	chlortetracycline (Aureomycin)	
	corticosteroid withdrawal	
	digitalis (long term)	
	ethosuximide (Zarontin)	
	gold compounds (long term)	
	griseofulvin	
	hydantoin anticonvulsants	
	hydralazine (Apresoline)	
	isoniazid (Nydrazid)	
	isoquinazepon	
	mephenytoin (Mesantoin)	
	methyldopa (Aldomet)	
	methysergide	
	methylthiouracil	
	oral contraceptives (mestranol?)	
	para-aminosalicylic acid (PAS)	
	penicillamine	
	penicillin	
	phenobarbital (long term)	
	phenylbutazone (Butazolidin)	
	phenytoin (Dilantin)	
	practolol	
	primidone (Mysoline)	
	procainamide (Pronestyl)	
	propylthiouracil	
	reserpine (long term)	
	rifampin (Rifadin, Rimactane, rifampicin)	
	streptomycin	
	sulfadiazine	
	sulfasalazine (Azulfidine)	
	sulfonamides (long acting)	
	tetracycline	
	thiazides (long term)	
	trimethadione (Tridione, Troxidone)	

DIFFERENT TYPES OF LESIONS AND SOME OF THE CONDITIONS ASSOCIATED WITH THEM

ATROPHY

Senile skin
Lupus erythematosus

BULLAE

Contact dermatitis (poison ivy)
Dermatitis herpetiformis
Drug eruptions (sulfonamides, barbiturates)
Erythema multiforme
Herpes zoster
Impetigo
Insect bites
Pemphigoid
Pemphigus

CRUSTS

Any ulcerating disease
Any vesicular or bullous dermatitis

DEPIGMENTATION

Albinism
Vitiligo

HYPERKERATOSIS

Corns
Ichthyosis

HYPERPIGMENTATION

Addison's disease
Chloasma
Cushing's disease
Freckles
Hemochromatosis
Neurofibromatosis
Pregnancy

MACULES

Addison's disease
Drug eruptions
Freckles
Measles
Nevus flammeus
Neurofibromatosis (café-au-lait spots)
Vitiligo

NODULES

Basal cell carcinoma
Chilblains
Erythema induratum
Erythema nodosum
Hemangiomas
Keratoacanthoma
Lipomas
Molluscum contagiosum
Neurofibromas
Syphilis
Warts

PAPULES

Acne
Basal cell carcinoma (rodent ulcer)
Granuloma pyogenicum
Melanoma
Molluscum contagiosum
Pigmented nevi
Tuberculids
Warts
Xanthomas

PLAQUES

Atopic dermatitis
Lichen planus
Lupus erythematosus
Paget's disease of the nipple
Psoriasis
Seborrheic dermatitis

PUSTULES

Acne
Chickenpox
Folliculitis
Herpes simplex
Herpes zoster
Rosacea
Smallpox

SCALY MACULES

Pityriasis rosea
Pityriasis versicolor
Seborrheic dermatitis
Tinea corporis

SCALY PAPULES

Atopic dermatitis
Contact dermatitis
Lichen planus
Localized neurodermatitis
Psoriasis
Syphilis

SCARS

Any ulcerating disease

ULCERS

Basal cell carcinoma
Bedsores
Self-inflicted conditions, e.g., dermatitis artefacta
Squamous cell carcinoma
Syphilitic gummas
Trauma
Tuberculosis
Venous stasis

VEGETATIVE

Condylomas
Squamous cell carcinoma
Warts

VESICLES

Atopic dermatitis
Burns
Chickenpox
Contact dermatitis
Dermatitis herpetiformis
Herpes simplex
Herpes zoster
Insect bites
Scabies

WHEALS

Insect bites
Urticaria

From Solomons, B: Lecture notes on dermatology, ed 4, Oxford, London, 1977, Blackwell Scientific Publications, Ltd.

REGIONAL DISTRIBUTION OF COMMON DERMATOLOGIC CONDITIONS

ABDOMEN

Candidiasis
Drug eruptions
Pityriasis rosea
Psoriasis
Scabies
Seborrheic warts
Urticaria

ANOGENITAL AREA

Candidiasis
Contact dermatitis
Herpes simplex
Intertrigo
Lichen planus
Pediculosis pubis
Pruritus
Psoriasis
Scabies
Seborrheic dermatitis
Syphilis
Tinea cruris (in males)
Warts

ARMS

Contact dermatitis
Lichen planus
Psoriasis

AXILLAE

Boils
Candidiasis
Contact dermatitis
Pediculosis
Seborrheic dermatitis
Tinea

BACK

Acne
Pityriasis rosea
Psoriasis
Seborrheic dermatitis
Seborrheic warts

CHEST

Acne
Pityriasis rosea
Pityriasis versicolor
Psoriasis
Seborrheic dermatitis
Seborrheic warts

EARS

Contact dermatitis
Lupus erythematosus
Neoplasm
Otitis externa
Psoriasis
Seborrheic dermatitis

EYELIDS

Contact dermatitis
Neoplasms
Warts
Xanthelasma

FACE

Acne
Contact dermatitis
Impetigo
Infantile eczema
Lupus erythematosus
Neoplasms
Rosacea
Sebaceous cysts
Seborrheic dermatitis
Seborrheic warts

FEET

Atopic dermatitis
Contact dermatitis
Corns
Dyshidrosis
Psoriasis
Tinea
Warts

HANDS

Atopic dermatitis
Contact dermatitis
Dyshidrosis
Hyperhidrosis
Scabies
Warts

LEGS

Contact dermatitis
Erythema nodosum
Insect bites
Lichen planus
Neurodermatitis
Psoriasis
Purpura
Varicose dermatitis

LIPS

Cheilitis
Contact dermatitis
Herpes simplex
Leukoplakia
Neoplasms

MOUTH

Aphthous stomatitis
Leukoplakia
Lichen planus
Neoplasms
Pemphigus

SCALP

Alopecia
Pediculosis
Psoriasis
Sebaceous cysts
Seborrheic dermatitis
Tinea

Modified from Solomons B: Lecture notes on dermatology, ed 4, Oxford, London, 1977, Blackwell Scientific Publications, Ltd.

DRUG-INDUCED COMMON DERMATOLOGIC CONDITIONS

DRUGS CAUSING AN ACNEFORM REACTION

ACTH
androgenic hormones
bromides
corticosteroids
cyanocobalamin
hydrantoins
iodides
methandrostenolone (Dianabol)
methyltestosterone (Metandren)
oral contraceptives

DRUGS CAUSING PURPURA

ACTH
allopurinol (Zyloprim)
amitriptyline (Elavil, Endep)
anticoagulants
barbiturates
carbamides
chloral hydrate
chlorothiazide (Diuril)
chlorpropamide (Diabinese)
chlorpromazine (Thorazine)
corticosteroids
digitalis
fluoxymesterone
gold salts
griseofulvin (Grifulvin)
iodides
mepesulfate
meprobamate
penicillin
phenylbutazone (Butazolidin)
quinidine
rifampin (Rifadin, Rimactane, rifampicin)
sulfonamides
thiazides
trifluoperazine

DRUGS CAUSING URTICARIA

ACTH
amitriptyline
barbiturates
bromides
chloramphenicol (Chloromycetin)
dextran
enzymes
erythromycin (Erythrocin, Ilotycin)
griseofulvin (Grifulvin)
hydantoins (Dilantin)
insulin
iodides
iodopyracet (Diodrast)
meperidine (Demerol)
meprobamate (Equanil, Miltown)
mercurials
nitrofurantoin (Furadantin)
novobiocin
opiates
penicillin
penicillinase
pentazocine (Talwin)
phenolphthalein
phenothiazines
propoxyphene (Darvon)
rifampin (Rifadin, Rimactane, rifampicin)
salicylates
serums
streptomycin
sulfonamides
tetracyclines
thiouracil

DRUGS CAUSING ALOPECIA

alkylating agents
anticoagulants
antimetabolites
bleomycin (Blenoxane)
mephenytoin (Mesantoin)
methimazole
methotrexate
norethindrone acetate (Norinyl, Noriestrine, Ortho-Novum)
quinacrine
oral contraceptives
sodium warfarin (Coumadin)
trimethadione (Tridione)

DRUGS CAUSING MORBILLIFORM REACTIONS

anticonvulsants
anticholinergics
antihistamines
barbiturates
chloral hydrate
chlordiazepoxide (Librium)
chlorothiazide (Diuril)
chlorpromazine (Thorazine)
gold salts
griseofulvin (Grifulvin)
hydantoins (Dilantin)
insulin
meprobamate
mercurials
methaminodiazepoxide
novobiocin
organic extracts
para-aminosalicylic acid
penicillin
phenothiazines
phenylbutazone (Butazolidin)
quinacrine (Atabrine)
salicylates
serums
streptomycin
sulfonamides
sulfones
tetracyclines
thiouracil

DRUGS CAUSING LICHENOID REACTIONS

amiphenazole (Daptazole)
chloroquine
gold salts compounds
organic arsenicals
para-aminosalicylic acid
quinacrine (Atabrine, mepacrine)
quinidine
thiazides

DRUGS CAUSING FIXED ERUPTIONS

acetanilid
acetarsone
acetophenetidin
acetylsalicylic acid
aconite
acriflavine
aminopyrine
amobarbital
amodiaquine
amphetamine sulfate
anthralin
antimony potassium tartrate
antipyrine
arsphenamine
barbital
barbiturates
belladonna
bismuth salts
bromides
chloral hydrate
chlorguanide
chloroquine
chlorothiazide and sun
chlorpromazine
chlortetracycline
cinchophen
copaiba
dextroamphetamine
diacetyldiphenotisatin
diallybarbituric acid
diethylstilbestrol
digilanid
digitalis
dimenhydrinate (Dramamine)
dimethylamine acetarsone
diphenhydramine (Benadryl)

disulfiram and alcohol
eosin
ephedrine
epinephrine
ergot alkaloids
erythrocin
eucalyptus oil
formalin
frangula
gold compounds
griseofulvin (Grifulvin)
iodine
ipecac
ipomea
2-isopropyl-4-pentenoyl urea
   (Sedormid)
karaya gum
magnesium hydroxide
meprobamate
mercury salts
methenamine
neoarsphenamine
opium alkaloids
oxophenarsine
oxytetracycline (Terramycin)
para-aminosalicylic acid
penicillin
phenacetin
phenazone
phenobarbital
phenolphthalein
phenylbutazone (Butazolidin)
5-phenylethylhydantoin
phenylhydantoin
phenytoin (Dilantin)
phosphorus

potassium chlorate
pyramidine derivatives
quinacrine
quinidine
quinine
reserpine
salicylates
santonin
saccharin
scopolamine
sodium salicylate
sterculia gum
stramonium
streptomycin
strychnine
sulfadiazine
sulfaguanidine
sulfamerazine
sulfamethazine
sulfamethoxypyridazine (Kynex)
sulfapyridine
sulfarsphenamine
sulfathiazole
sulfisoxazole (Gantrisin)
sulfobromophthalein sodium
sulfonamides
tetracyclines
thiambutosine
thiram and alcohol
thonzylamine HCl (Neohetramine)
tripelennamine (Pyribenzamine)
trisodium arsphenamine sulfate
tryparsamide
urease
urginin
vaccines and immunizing agents

DRUGS CAUSING CONTACT DERMATITIS

acriflavine
amethocaine
antazoline
antazoline and phenocide
antazoline and pyribenzamine
antihistamine
arsphenamine
atabrine
bacitracin (occupational)
benzocaine
benzoyl peroxide and chlor-
   hydroxyquinoline
bleomycin (Blenoxane)
cetrimide
chloramphenicol
chlorcyclizine

chlorhexidine
chlorhydroxyquinaline and
   benzoyl peroxide
chlorxylenol
chlorphenesin
chlorpromazine
colophony
crotamiton
cyclomethycaine
diphenhydramine
domiphen
ephedrine
formaldehyde
halogenated phenolic compounds
hedaquinium chloride

iodine
iodochlorhydroxyquinoline
isoniazid (occupational)
lanolin
meprobamate
mypyramine (Pyrilamine)
mercurials
mercury
neomycin
nitrofurazone
novobiocin
para-aminosalicylic acid
parabens
penicillin
peru balsam
phenindamine

Continued.

DRUGS CAUSING CONTACT DERMATITIS—cont'd

phenocide and antazoline
phenol
potassium hydroxyquinoline sulfate
procaine and other anesthetics
promethazine
propamidine
pyribenzamine and antazoline

quinacrine (Atabrine)
quinine
resorcin
spiramycin (occupational)
streptomycin

sulfonamides
sulfur and salicylic acid ointment
tetracyclines
thiamine
thimerosal (Merthiolate)

PHOTOSENSITIZERS

acetohexamide (Dymelor)
acridine preparations (slight)
agave lechuguilla (amaryllis)
agrimony
9-aminoacridine
aminobenzoic acid
amitriptyline (Elavil)
anesthetics (procaine group)
angelica
anthracene
antimalarials
arsenicals
barbiturates
bavachi (corylifolia)
benzene
benzopyrine
bergamot (perfume)
bithionol (Actamer, Lorothidol)
blankophores (sulfa derivatives)
bulosemide (Jadit)
bromchlorsacylanilid
4-butyl-4-chlorosalicylanilide
carbamazepine (Tegretol)
carbinoxamine d-form (Twiston R-A)
carbutamide (Nadisan)
carrots, wild
cedar oil
celery
chlorophyll
chlorothiazide (Diuril)
chlorpromazine (Thorazine)
chlorpropamide (Diabinese)
chlortetracycline (Aureomycin)
citron oil
citrus fruits
clover
coal tar
contraceptives, oral
corticosteroids, topical
cyproheptadine

demeclocycline (Declomycin, deme-
  thylchlortetracycline)
desipramine (Norpramin, Pertofrane)
dibenzopyran derivatives
dicyanine-A
diethylstilbestrol
digalloyl trioleate (sunscreen)
dill
diphenhydramine hydrochloride
  (Benadryl)
disopyramide
doxycycline
dyes (methylene blue, toluidine blue)
eosin (slight)
estrone
fennel
fluorescein dyes
5-fluorouracil
furocoumarins (bergamot oil)
glyceryl p-aminobenzoate (sunscreen)
gold salts
grass (meadow)
griseofulvin (Fulvicin)
haloperidol
hematoporphyrin
hexachlorophene (rare)
hydrochlorothiazide (Esidrix,
  HydroDiuril)
imipramine HCI (Tofranil)
isothipencyl (Theruhistin)
isothipendyl (Theruhistin)
lady's thumb (tea)
lantinin
lavender oil
lime oil
meclothiazide (Enduron)
mepazine (Pacatal)

9-mercaptopurine
methotrimeprazine (Levoprome)
methoxsalen (Meloxine, Oxsoralen)
5-methoxypsoralen
8-methoxypsoralen
monoglycerol para-aminobenzoate
mustards
nalidixic acid (NegGram)
naphthalene
neuroleptics
nortriptyline (Aventyl)
oral contraceptives
oxytetracycline (Terramycin)
para-dimethylaminoazobenzene
paraphenylenediamine
parsley
parsnips
penicillin derivates (Griseofulvin)
perloline
perphenazine (Trilafon)
phenanthrene
phenazine dyes
phenolic compounds
phenothiazines
phenoxazines
phenylbutazone (Butazolidin)
phenytoin (Dilantin)
pitch and pitch fumes
porphyrins
prochlorperazine (Compazine)
promazine hydrochloride (Sparine)
profriptyline (Vivactil)
promethazine hydrochloride (Phenergan)
psoralens (perfume)
pyrathiazine hydrochloride (Pyrrolazote)
pyrazinamide
pyridine

PHOTOSENSITIZERS—cont'd

quinethazone (Hydromox)	sulfamerazine	trichlormethiazide (Metahydrin)
quinidine	sulfamethazine	tricyclic antidepressants
quinine	sulfapyridine	tridione
rose bengal perfume (slight)	sulfathiazole	triethylene melamine (TEM)
rue	sulfonamides	triflupromazine hydrochloride (Vesprin)
salicylanilides	sulfisomidine (Elkosin)	trimeprazine tartrate (Temaril)
salicylates	sulfonylureas (antidiabetics, oral	trimethadione (Tridione)
sandalwood oil (perfume)	hypoglycemics)	tripyrathiazine
silver salts	tetrachlorasalicylanilide (TCSA)	trypaflavine
smartweed (tea)	tetracyclines	trypan blue
stilbamidine isethionate	thiazides (Diuril, HydroDiuril)	vanillin oils
sulfacetamide	thiophene	water ash
sulfadiazine	thiopropazate dihydrochloride (Dartal)	xylene
sulfadimethoxine	tolbutamide (Orinase)	yarrow
sulfaguanidine	toluene	
sulfanilamide (slight)	tribromosalicylanilide (TBS)	
	(deodorant soaps)	

Stasis dermatitis often preceding a decubitus is found on the lower legs secondary to venous stasis and poor vascularity and is a brown eczematous area in appearance.

Erythemato-papular-squamous eruptions are noninfectious inflammatory dermatoses that include urticaria (hives), psoriasis, pityriasis rosea, lichen planus, and exfoliative dermatitis. The nurse will see acute urticaria as an incidious-appearing, itchy erythematous wheal (which is a release mediated from complement of histamine from mast cells and basophils) resulting from an allergen. Chronic urticaria appears as a large hive without the sensation of itch or pruritis and is often accompanied by angioneurotic edema resulting from a genetic predisposition to diminished protease inhibitors (esterase).

Psoriasis often appears as erythematous plaques and orange-red-brown papules covered with silvery scales. Psoriasis is often found on the scalp and extensor surfaces of the limbs and neck. Often thick irregular nails are present. These erythemato-papular-squamous eruptions may bleed easily.

Pityriasis rosea is a self-limited oval salmon-colored patch that follows the axis of skin cleavage lines. The major patches appear on the trunk, and smaller scales appear on the peripheral areas.

Infectious inflammatory dermatoses include viral diseases (**verruca** [wart], herpes simplex, varicella-zoster-chicken pox), bacterial diseases (impetigo, folliculitis, **furuncle** [boil]) and fungal diseases (**tinea** [dermatophytosis], mucocutaneous candidiasis).

The verruca or wart is of various types, including the following: verruca vulgaris (commonly found on the hands and fingers); verruca plantaris (inward wart growth on the sole of the foot that may be covered with a callus or hyperkeratosis); verruca plana (found on the dorsa of the hands and face as a flat wart); condyloma acuminatum or venereal wart (cauliflower-like growth in the anogenital area often with hyperkeratosis).

Herpes simplex and infectious inflammatory dermatoses appear as vesicles with an inflamed base and have an incubation period of up to 2 weeks in the primary infection. Late antibody development occurs. The herpes virus Type 1 affects skin and the oral cavity, and the herpes virus Type 2 affects the skin of neonates and genital mucosa. The recurrent infection is a reactivation of the older infection or new infection; antibodies appear early.

Fungal diseases, which include tinea or dermatophytosis, appear in the following various clinical classifications: tinea capitis (caused by either a *Trichophyton* or *microsporum* fungal infection as nonfluorescent or fluorescent in children and in adults tinea barbae); tinea corporis (or *Microsporum* in children and *Trichophyton* in adults); tinea cruris (*Epidermophyton* or *Trichophyton*); and tinea pedis; onychomycosis (*Trichophyton*); and tinea versicolor (*Malassezia furfur*). Tinea or dermatophytosis often appear as a scaly erythematous circular lesion. Tinea versicolor appears as a brown discoloration. Breaking of the hair is seen in tinea capitis or barbae, and with onychomycosis the patient has thick discolored nails.

• • •

As previously stated, dermatologic products are so vast in number it would be difficult to cover them all in this chapter. For the sake of simplicity, this chapter will discuss three major groups of dermatologic products: general, prophylactic agents, and therapeutic agents. Some general dermatologic products include those previously discussed plus solutions, baths, soaps, wet dressings, and soaks. Prophylactic agents include sunscreens, protectives, and antiseptics and disinfectants. Therapeutic agents include the antiinfectives, and antiinflammatory corticosteroids, keratolytic agents, acne products, stimulants and irritants, topical anesthetics, burn products for second- and third-degree burns, antiaging products, and ectoparasiticidal topical drugs.

GENERAL DERMATOLOGIC PREPARATIONS

This section refers to single and combination formulations used as bath preparations, cleansers, soaps, solutions and lotions, emollients, skin protectants, wet dressings and soaks, and rubs and liniments.

BATHS

Baths may be employed to cleanse the skin, to medicate it, or to reduce temperature. The usual method of cleansing the skin is by the use of soap and water, but this may not be tolerated in skin diseases. In some cases even water is not tolerated and inert oils must be substituted. Persons with dry skin should bathe less frequently than those with oily skin. It is possible to keep the skin clean without a daily bath. Nurses are sometimes accused of overbathing hospital patients, causing the client's skin to become dry and itchy. An oily lotion is preferable to alcohol (isopropyl or ethyl) for dry skin.

To render baths soothing in irritative conditions, bran, starch, or gelatin may be added in the proportion of about 1 to 2 ounces per gallon of water. Oils such as Alpha-Keri, Lubath, and oilated oatmeal in a proportion of 1 ounce to the tub of water decrease the drying effect of water and thus help to relieve the itching of a sensitive, xerotic skin.

SOAPS

Ordinary soap is the sodium salt of palmitic, oleic, or stearic acids or mixtures of these. Soaps are prepared by saponifying fats or oils with the alkalies. The fats or oils used vary considerably. The oil used for castile soap is supposed to be olive oil. Some soaps are made with coconut oil to which the skin of some persons is sensitive. Soaps contain glycerin unless it has been removed from the preparation. The consistency of the soap depends on the predominating acid and alkali used.

Although all soaps are relatively alkaline, the presence of an excess of free alkali or acid will constitute a potential source of skin irritation.

Medicated soaps contain antiseptics and other added substances, such as cresol, thymol, and sulfur, but soaps per se are antiseptic only insofar as they mechanically clean the skin.

Many people believe that soap and water are bad for the complexion. This is erroneous for the most part. A clean skin helps to promote a healthy skin. The soap used in maintaining a clean skin should be mild and contain a minimum of irritating materials. Soaps may be harmful if skin is extra sensitive to soap products, the soap is not adequately rinsed off the skin, if it stimulates excess production of natural skin oils, or if it excessively dries the skin.

Soaps are irritating to mucous membranes, and they are used in enemas mainly because of this action. They are also used in the manufacture of liniments and tooth powders. One of the mildest soaps is shaving soap.

SOLUTIONS AND LOTIONS

Soothing preparations may also be liquids that carry an insoluble powder or suspension, or they may be mild acid or alkaline solutions, such as boric acid solution, limewater, or aluminum subacetate used as wet dressings and soaks. The bismuth salts (the subcarbonate or subnitrate) and starch are also commonly used for their soothing effect.

Aluminum acetate solution (Burow's solution, modified Burow's solution). This mild protein precipitant astrigent coagulates bacterial and serum protein and contains 545 ml aluminum subacetate solution and 15 ml glacial acetic acid in 1000 ml aqueous medium. It is diluted with 10 to 40 parts of water before application. This may be prepared from Domeboro or Bluboro products.

Aluminum subacetate solution. This preparation contains 145 g aluminum sulfate, 160 ml acetic acid, and 70 g precipitated calcium carbonate in 1000 ml aqueous medium. It is applied topically after dilution with 20 to 40 parts of water as a wet dressing.

Calamine lotion. Prepared calamine, zinc oxide, bentonite magma, glycerine, and calcium hydroxide solutions are included in this lotion. It is a soothing lotion used for the dermatitis caused by poison ivy, insect bites, prickly heat, and so on. It is patted on the involved skin area and is available with an antihistamine, diphenhydramine, as Caladryl lotion.

CLEANSERS

Cleansers are usually soap free or modified soap products that are recommended for persons with sensitive, dry, or irritated skin or who may have had a previous reaction to soap product. These cleansers are less irritating, may contain an emollient substance, and may also have been adjusted to a slightly acidic or neutral pH. Included in this category are Aveeno Cleansing Bar, Lowila Cake, Keri Facial Cleanser, pHisoDerm, Spectro-Jel, and Lobana Body Shampoo.

GENERAL GOALS OF THERAPY

Identify and remove the cause of the skin disorder, if possible.

Institute measures to restore and maintain the structure and normal function of the skin.

Relieve symptoms that are produced by the disorder, such as itching, dryness, pain, and infection.

EMOLLIENTS

Emollients are fatty or oily substances that may be used to soften or soothe irritated skin and mucous membrane. An emollient is often used as a vehicle for other medicinal substances. Examples of emollients include lanolin, petroleum jelly (vaseline), vitamin A and D ointment, vitamin E, and cold cream. Examples of emollient products on the market include Panthoderm; vitamin E oil, cream, ointment, or liquid; Aquacare; Nutraplus; vitamin A and D creams and ointments; Moisturel Lotion; Allercream Skin; Lubriderm; Dermassage; Nivea Skin; and many more.

SKIN PROTECTANTS

Skin protectants are used to coat minor skin irritations or to protect the person's skin from chemical irritants. Some commercially available products include AeroZoin, Benzoin, Kerodex, Hydropel, Covicone, and Benzoin Compound.

WET DRESSINGS AND SOAKS

Wet dressings and soaks include some of the preparations previously discussed under solutions and lotions. These liquids are either a wet dressing or an astringent-type wet dressing used to treat inflammatory skin conditions, such as insect bites, poison ivy, bruises, and edema. Aluminum acetate solution (Burow's or modified Burow's solution), Bluboro powder, Domeboro Powder, and Pedi-Boro Soak Paks are available for this use.

A lime sulfur solution (Viem-Dome, Vlemasque, Vleminckx') is often used as a soak or dressing for cystic acne, seborrheic dermatoses, and various types of pustular infections.

RUBS AND LINIMENTS

Rubs and liniments are indicated for pain relief when the skin is intact. Pain caused by muscle aches, neuralgia, rheumatism, arthritis, and sprains are the types of pain that usually respond to these products. The ingredients in the preparations may include a counterirritant (e.g., cajuput oil, camphor, oil of cloves, methyl salicylate), an antiseptic (chloroxylenol, eugenol, thymol), local anesthetic (benzocain), or analgesics (salicylate-containing substances). The formulations are usually gels, creams, lotions, liniments, aerosols, or ointments. Examples from this category include Aspercreme, Myoflex Creme, infra-RUB Cream, Musterole Deep Strength Rub, Ben-Gay Ointment, Counterpain Rub, Vicks VapoRub, Doan's Backache Spray, Panalgesic Liniment, Banalg Liniment, and Sloan's Liniment.

PROPHYLACTIC AGENTS
PROTECTIVES

Protectives are soothing, cooling preparations that form a film on the skin. Protectives, to be useful, must not macerate the skin, must prevent drying of the tissues, and must keep out light, air, and dust. Nonabsorbable powders are usually listed as protectives, but they are not particularly useful because they stick to wet surfaces and have to be scraped off and do not stick to dry surfaces at all.

Collodion. Collodion is a 5% solution of pyroxylin, or guncotton, in a mixture of ether and alcohol. When collodion is applied to the skin, the ether and alcohol evaporate, leaving a transparent film that adheres to the skin and protects it.

Flexible collodion. Flexible collodion is a mixture of collodion with 2% camphor and 3% castor oil. The addition of the latter makes the resulting film elastic and more tenacious. Styptic collodion contains 20% tannic acid and therefore is astringent, as well as protective.

Nonabsorbable powders. Nonabsorbable powders include zinc stearate, zinc oxide, certain bismuth preparations, talcum powder, and aluminum silicate. The disadvantages associated with their use have been mentioned previously.

Although it is safe to say that no substances known at present can stimulate healing at a more rapid rate than is normal under optimal conditions, preparations that act as bland protectives may help by preventing crusting and trauma. In some instances they may reduce offensive odors.

SUNBURN PREPARATIONS

Sunburn is an acute erythema caused by too long an exposure to the rays of the sun. In some cases, especially if a large area is involved, it may be serious, and the skin surface should be treated as in any serious burn. Exposure to the sun should be done gradually, a few minutes each day, when a general tan is desired. As would be true for any minor partial-thickness burn, when the epithelium is intact and remains so, ordinary protective demulcents or emollients are sufficient to allay irritation.

The use of chemical sunscreens such as para-aminobenzoic acid (PABA) and its esters, benzophenones and cinnamates, can minimize the absorption of ultraviolet (UV) rays by the skin, which causes sunburn. These preparations, however, are only of value in preventing sunburn if they are applied before intense sun exposure.

Physical sunscreens such as zinc oxide, red petrolatum, or titanium dioxide are the most effective in preventing a sunburn, but cosmetically they are not appealing to most people.

Chemical sunscreen agents absorb the sun's burning and tanning UV rays that are in the medium wavelength (UV-B range 290 to 320 nm). The UV rays of the long wavelength (UV-A range 320 to 400 nm) produce tanning and photosensitivity reactions secondary to drug and cosmetic use. Both the UV-B and UV-A range are absorbed by the benzophenone products (e.g., Sundown Sunblock Ultraprotection, Total Eclipse Sunscreen), and their usefulness extends to both protection from direct UV ray exposure and from drug-induced photosensitivity.

Physical sunscreen agents may also prevent drug- or cosmetic-induced photosensitivity reactions, tanning, and burning. These opaque substances reflect the UV rays in a range of 290 to 770 nm; however, they tend to lack the cosmetic appeal of chemical sunscreens (zinc oxide and others).

Routine application of these products prevents sunburn and premature skin aging secondary to UV light overexposure; they may reduce actinic-induced skin cancer incidence. The nurse should advise the use of these agents to individuals who become exposed to photosensitizing agents and to those clients with medical conditions sensitive to UV light exposure such as systemic lupus erythematosus (SLE), porphyria, and solar urticaria.

Individuals allergic to analine dyes, benzocaine, sulfonamides, or thiazides may experience cross-allergic reactions to PABA and its esters. PABA topical products will stain clothing a yellow color. PABA and its esters (glyceryl PABA), benzophenones and cinnamates, may cause a dermatitis on application of these products. Sunscreen vehicles containing alcohol should not be used on eczematous or inflamed skin.

The nurse will frequently see a **sun protection factor** (SPF) rating statement on suntanning products (SPF ranges from 2 to 15). A high SPF number rating denotes more protection or increased resistance to burning and tanning. An individual who requires burn protection because he or she always burns on sunlight exposure or who uses photosensitive drugs requires maximum protection with an SPF rating number from 8 to 15. A person who burns moderately but gradually tans would require an SPF number of 4 to 5. A person who seldom burns and tans readily requires an SPF number of 2 to 3. The FDA has stated that SPFs over 15 are not recommended. However, this has not been finalized by a ruling, so products are available with SPFs over 15.

Two additional formulas are available: waterproof formulas indicate the person using this product can maintain sunburn protection even after being in the water for up to 80 minutes, wheras water-resistant formulas maintain the sunburn protection after being in the water for up to 40 minutes. See Table 67-2 for examples of sunscreen agents including their SPF and waterproof or water-resistant label, if appropriate.

THERAPEUTIC AGENTS
TOPICAL ANTIINFECTIVES

Antiinfectives include topical antibiotics, antiviral agents (for use with minor skin abrasions and superficial infected wounds), and antifungal agents.

Antibiotics

The most frequent causative organisms of skin infections (**exodermas**) are *Streptococcus pyogenes* and *Staphylococcus aureus.* Folliculitis, impetigo, furuncles, carbuncles, and cellulitis often result from these organisms. These common skin disorders are infections for which topical prophylaxis antibiotics may be applied. Only some of the agents follow; other topical antibiotics will be discussed in sections on acne products, antifungals, and antivirals.

Bacitracin. Bacitracin is very useful in the local treatment of infectious lesions. Bacitracin is most often used in an ointment (Baciguent, over the counter), although it can be used to moisten wet dressings or as a dusting powder. It is odorless and nonstaining, and its use seldom results in sensitizing; however, allergic contact dermatitis has occurred.

Neomycin. Neomycin has been used successfully in the treatment of infections of skin and mucous membrane. It is applied topically (Myciguent, over the counter). It occasionally irritates the skin, and allergic contact dermatitis is reported especially when used on stasis ulcers. An ointment (Mycitracin, over the counter), which combines *neomycin, bacitracin, and polymyxin B,* may be more efficacious in mixed infections than when these agents are used singly.

In conditions where absorption of neomycin may occur (including burns and trophic ulceration), there is the potential of nephrotoxicity, ototoxicity, and neomycin hypersensitivity reactions. This risk is seen more frequently in persons with compromised renal function, in clients with extensive burns (over 20% of area), and in clients using other aminoglycoside antibiotics. Sensitization may occur to any of the antibiotic ingredients, and prolonged use may produce suprainfection as an overgrowth of nonsuspective organisms such as fungi. Photo-

TABLE 67-2   Sunscreen Formulations

Commercial name	SPF	Waterproof/water resistant
Hawaiian Tropic Baby Faces Sunblock	22	Water resistant
Sundown 15 Ultra Protection	20	Waterproof
Hawaiian Tropic Swim 'N' Sun	20	Water resistant
Coppertone Sunblock w/ Vitamin E and Aloe	15	—
Ray Block	15	—
Block Out by Sea & Ski	15	Waterproof
Block Out Clear by Sea & Ski	15	Waterproof
TI-Screen	15	Water resistant
Coppertone Shade Plus	8	Water resistant
PreSun 8 Creamy	8	Waterproof
Shade Sunscreen	6	Waterproof
PreSun 4 Creamy	4	Waterproof
Coppertan Suntan	4	—
Coppertone Dark Tanning	2	—
Hawaiian Tropic Professional "Light" Tanning	2	—
LIP BALM PROTECTANTS		
PreSun 15 Lip Protector	15	
Chapstick Sunblock 15	15	
Lipkote by Coppertone	15	
Blistik	10	

TABLE 67-3   Spectrum of Antimicrobial Activity of Topical Antibiotics*

Antibiotic	Spectrum of activity		
	Gram+	Gram−	Broad spectrum
bacitracin ointment		X	
chlortetracycline ointment			X
chloramphenicol cream			X
erythromycin liquid or ointment	X		
gentamicin cream and ointment			X
neomycin cream and ointment			X

Topical preparations and antibiotic combinations available over the counter include all the above with the exception of chloramphenicol, erythromycin, and gentamicin.

The over-the-counter products must be labeled as first aid products to help prevent infection in minor cuts, burns, or injuries. They cannot be recommended to treat known infections.

Prescription antibiotic ointments are generally indicated for the treatment of minor or surface bacteria infections.

Antivirals

acyclovir (Acycloguanosine, Zovirax Ointment 5%)

Mechanism of action. Acyclovir inhibits the viral enzymes necessary for DNA synthesis.

Indications. Used in the management of active initial infections of genital herpes genitalis and in limited, non–life threatening mucocutaneous herpes simplex infections (primarily herpes labialis) in immunocompromised patients.

Side effects/adverse reactions
GU. Vulvitis
Skin. Mild pain, transient burning, stinging, pruritis, rash

Dosage and administration. Adequate covering with ointment of the lesions every 3 hours six times daily for 7 days.

Pregnancy safety. FDA category C

NURSING CONSIDERATIONS

Assessment. A thorough assessment of the lesion provides a baseline for monitoring effectiveness and response to therapy.

Intervention. Dose per application will vary depending

sensitivity is reported with topical gentamicin.

The possibility of hypersensitivity occurs with chloramphenicol when used topically as does the additional risk of bone marrow hypoplasia, blood dyscrasias, itching, burning, angioneurotic edema, urticaria, and vesicular and maculopapular dermatitis. Tetracyclines may stain clothing and cause erythema, irritation, and swelling locally. See Table 67-3 for list of topical antibiotics and their spectrum of activity.

Although erythromycin generally has activity against gram positive organisms, in the United States it is approved only for treatment of acne vulgaris caused by an anaerobe, *Propionibacterium acnes (Corynebacterium acnes).*

on lesion area; a 1/2-inch ribbon of ointment covers approximately 4 inches of surface area.

Store ointment at 15° C to 25° C (59° F to 78° F).

Education. Instruct the client to use a finger cot or rubber glove when applying the ointment to prevent autoinoculation to other sites and transmissions to other patients. Avoid contact with eyes.

Advise annual or more frequent Pap smears because women with herpes genitalis are more likely to develop cervical cancer.

Recommend the wearing of loose clothing and keeping affected areas clean and dry to prevent further irritation.

Advise the client to avoid sexual activity if lesions are active for either partner. Even if partner is asymptomatic, the disease may still be sexually transmitted; use of a condom probably will help prevent transmission of herpes.

Antifungals

There are few fungi that produce keratinolytic enzymes to provide for their existence on skin. There are three infectious fungi that can cause local fungal infections without systemic effects: *Microsporum, Trichophyton,* and *Epidermophyton.* The possibility of a mixed infection with these fungi must never be overlooked.

Fungi exist in a moist, warm environment, preferably in dark areas (such as shoes and socks). Tinea pedis (athlete's foot, ringworm of the foot) is commonly encountered. Immunologic mechanisms may have an important role in fungal control. The triad for suspicion for fungal infections is an immunologic deficit, a specific fungi involvement, and the skin condition.

The stratum corneum is a layer of dead desquamated cells that are shed normally or are dissolved in sebum. The fungi invade this layer and cause inflammation and induce sensitivity when they penetrate the epidermis and dermis. Since the stratum corneum is shed daily, the ability to spread or transmit the fungi is by contact.

Most commonly reported side effects/adverse reactions include local irritation, pruritus, burning sensation, and scaling. Erythema, blistering, stinging, peeling, urticaria, pruritus, and general irritation may occur with products like clotrimazole.

Pregnancy safety has been noted only for the following antifungal agents: econazole nitrate (FDA category C), ciclopirox olamine (FDA category B), clotrimazole (FDA category B), haloprogin (FDA category B), and ketoconazole (FDA category C).

The primary topical antifungal agents include undecylenic acid products, iodochlorhydroxyquin, miconazole nitrate, econazole nitrate, ciclopirox olamine, clotrimazole, triacetin, haloprogin, tolnaftate, nystatin, amphotericin B, gentian violet, ketoconazole, and a variety of antifungal combination ointments, powders and liquids. See Table 67-4 for the generic, trade name, status (over-the-counter or prescription), and comments about the products.

NURSING CONSIDERATIONS

Assessment. Carefully note skin characteristics, symptoms, and predisposing factors such as trauma, suppressed immunity, general health, hygiene practices, or exposure to infecting agent.

If laboratory tests are to be obtained, such as cultures of exudate or tissue, they should be obtained before application of topical agent.

Intervention. Topical substances for antifungal purposes should be applied liberally to a clean, dry, affected skin area. An occlusive dressing should not be applied unless directed by the physician.

Avoid contact of these substances with the eyes.

Store below 85° F (30° C) but without freezing.

Education. Encourage compliance with the full course of therapy. Fungal infections generally require prolonged therapy.

The nurse may encourage the client with a superficial fungal infection to practice adequate hygienic principles to discourage growth. Some of the principles are the following: (1) the affected area should be dry and aerated, and clothing that is warm or that causes an occlusive environment of moisture should be avoided; (2) the body areas may be kept dry by using powders (with or without antifungal ingredients) to prevent maceration; (3) before applying the antifungal medication, the patient should wash the area with mild soap and water and dry; (4) friction or trauma of the area may be avoided by not wearing tight-fitting clothing, which causes friction; clothing should be laundered daily. For infants with anogenital lesions, avoid tight diapers, disposable diapers, and plastic pants. For clients with foot infections, advise well-ventilated shoes or sandals.

Evaluation. Use of these agents may lead to skin sensitization and result in symptoms of hypersensitization, increasing redness and swelling, weeping, and itching and burning not present at the beginning of therapy. If no improvement is seen within 4 weeks, the client needs to be reevaluated.

CORTICOSTEROIDS

Topical corticosteroids are generally indicated for relief of inflammatory and pruritic dermatoses. They also offer the benefit of lessening systemic corticosteroid side effects and allowing direct contact with the localized lesion. Table 67-5 lists some of the most commonly used corticosteroids in current practice.

The effectiveness of the topical corticosteroids is a result of their antiinflammatory, antipruritic, and vasocon-

TABLE 67-4   Topical Antifungal Agents

Name	Prescription drug	Over-the-counter	Special comments
amphotericin B (Fungizone)	X		Equivalent to nystatin against *Candida albicans* (Monilia) infections.
ciclopirox olamine (Loprox)	X		Broad spectrum antifungal. Used for tinea pedis, tinea cruris, tinea corporis, candidiasis caused by *C. albicans* and tinea versicolor caused by *M. furfur*.
clotrimazole (Lotrimin, Mycelex)	X		Broad spectrum antifungal agent.
econazole nitrate (Spectrazole)	X		Broad spectrum antifungal agent.
gentian violet (Crystal Violet)		X	Antibacterial and antifungal dye. Bactericidal to gram + organisms. Because of its staining properties, it has been replaced by newer agents.
haloprogin (Halotex)	X		Synthetic antifungal agent. Broad spectrum.
iodochlorhydroxyquin (Vioform)		X	Antibacterial and antifungal. Used for athletes foot, eczema, and other fungal infections. May cause staining of clothes, skin, or hair.
ketoconazole (Nixoral)	X		Broad spectrum synthetic antifungal agent. Resistance to drug not yet reported.
miconazole (Micatin)		X	Used for tinea pedis (athlete's foot), tinea cruris, tinea corporis, and tinea versicolor. Available in cream, powder, and spray.
(Monistat-Derm)	X		Lotion preferred for intertriginous areas.
nystatin (Mycostatin, Nilstat)	X		Antifungal antibiotic with both fungicidal and fungistatic effects. Indicated for wide variety of yeast or yeastlike fungi.
tolnaftate (Tinactin, Aftate)		X	Available as cream, powder, spray, and liquid. Used for topical fungus skin infections.
triacetin (Enzactin)		X	To treat athlete's foot (tinea pedis) and other topical fungus infections.
undecylenic acid (Desenex, Caldesene)		X	Antifungal and antibacterial for athlete's foot and ringworm, with exception of nails and hairy sites. Also used for diaper rash, prickly heat, minor skin irritations, jock itch, excessive perspiration, and skin irritation in the groin area.

strictor actions. Topical corticosteroids may also stabilize epidermal lysosomes in the skin, and flourinated steroids are antiproliferative. By decreasing the cell proliferation, the flourinated topical corticosteroids are used in treating dermatologic disorders with rapid cellular turnover (psoriasis). A correlation exists between the potency and the therapeutic efficacy of corticosteroids (see the box on p. 1055). The vehicle (aerosol, cream, gel, lotion, ointment, solution, or tape) in which the corticosteroid is placed also alters the vasoconstrictor property and the therapeutic efficacy. Corticosteroid skin penetration is enhanced by the following vehicles in decreasing order of effectiveness: ointments, gels, creams, and lotions.

Ointment bases and propylene glycol both enhance the penetration of the corticosteroid and its vasoconstrictor effects. Ointments, as a result of their occlusive nature, hydrate the stratum corneum, permitting granular steroid penetration. The lotion form is well suited for hairy areas or a lesion that is oozing and wet. Creams and ointments are well suited for dry, scaling, thickened, and pruritic areas. Sprays, lotions, and gels are suited for the scalp or hairy areas. Sprays are esthetically suitable for acute weeping lesions, are cooling, and have antipruritic effects. All these vehicles influence absorption and therapeutic effect.

The rate of percutaneous penetration (through the epidermal stratum corneum) after application also influences therapeutic efficacy. Steroid percutaneous penetration increases with its vehicle base solubility. It is limited by three factors: rate of dissolution, rate of passive diffusion, and drug penetration rate (the skin itself is a barrier, and the stratum corneum is a rate-limiting membrane). The skin is selectively permeable by regional variations in absorptive capacity. Since most topical corticosteroids are

TABLE 67-5 Topical Corticosteroids

Generic name	Trade name
amcinonide	Cyclocort Cream and Ointment
betamethasone benzoate	Benisone Cream, Gel, and Ointment Uticort Cream, Lotion, and Gel
betamethasone dipropionate	Alphatrex Ointment, Cream, and Lotion Diprolene Ointment and Cream Diprosone Ointment, Cream, Lotion, and Aerosol
betamethasone valerate	Betatrex Ointment, Cream, and Lotion Valisone Ointment, Cream, and Lotion
clobetasol propionate	Temovate Ointment and Cream
clocortolone pivalate	Cloderm Cream
desonide	Tridesilon Ointment and Cream DesOwen Cream
desoximetasone	Topicort Ointment, Cream, and Gel Topicort LP Cream
dexamethasone	Decaderm Gel Aeroseb-Dex Aerosol Decaspray Aerosol
dexamethasone sodium phosphate	Decadron Phosphate Cream
diflorasone diacetate	Florone Ointment and Cream Maxiflor Ointment and Cream
fluocinolone acetonide	Fluonid Ointment, Cream, and Solution Synalar Ointment, Cream, and Solution
fluocinonide	Lidex Ointment, Cream, Solution, and Gel
flurandrenolide	Cordran Ointment, Lotion, and Tape Cordran SP Cream
halcinonide	Halog Ointment, Cream, and Solution
hydrocortisone	Cortril Ointment Hytone Ointment, Cream, and Lotion Cort-Dome Cream and Lotion HC-Jel Cortaid Spray
triamcinolone acetonide	Aristocort Ointment and Cream Kenalog Ointment, Cream, Lotion, and Aerosol

in suspension vehicles (ointments, creams, lotions), the addition of a solvent (propylene glycol) to the product can enhance drug dissolution, which may improve absorption. The sebum, enzymes, and perspiration of the skin convert topical suspensions to solutions only partially, needing the inclusion of a solvent, surfactant, or emulsifier in the vehicle to increase the rate of dissolution and distribution and to overcome the barrier to penetration (the dissolution barrier). Inflamed skin absorbs topical steroids to a greater degree than thick or lichenified skin.

Side effects/adverse reactions

Skin. Acneiform eruptions, allergic contact dermatitis, burning sensations, dryness, itching, hypopigmentation, bruising, hirsutism (usually face), folliculitis, round and swollen face, alopecia (usually scalp)

Other. Overgrowth of bacteria, fungus, and virus; immunosuppression

Dosage and administration

Adults. Once or twice daily as directed

Children. Once or twice daily with steroids in potent or less potent drug category. Application frequency depends on infection site, response of the cutaneous eruption to medication, and application technique.

Pregnancy safety. FDA category C

NURSING CONSIDERATIONS

Assessment. The age of the skin affects absorption of the potent fluorinated corticosteroids; the very young and the very old have skin that is more permeable. If prolonged treatment is required, it is prudent for the physician to clinically monitor plasma cortisol levels monthly until the steroid is discontinued. Most side effects are temporary and are resolved when the topical steroid is discontinued. Do not stop therapy suddenly.

Education. To enhance client compliance the reasons for the occlusive dressing procedure should be described to the patient. This technique intensifies percutaneous penetration of the topical steroid and concentrates the medication in the area where it is most needed.

Evaluation. Occlusive dressings may cause folliculitis from bacterial or candidal infection, hyperthermia from heat retention, or systemic effects related to increased drug absorption.

KERATOLYTICS

Keratolytics (keratin dissolvers) are drugs that soften scales and loosen the outer horny layer of the skin. Salicylic acid and resorcinol are drugs of choice. Their action makes possible the penetration of other medicinal substances by cleaning the lesions involved. Salicylic acid is particularly important for its keratolytic effect in local treatment of scalp conditions, warts, corns, fungous infections, acne, and chronic types of dermatitis. It is used up to 20% in ointments, plasters, or collodion for this purpose.

ACNE PRODUCTS

Acne vulgaris involves an intrafollicular hyperkeratinization that leads to the formation of a keratin plug at the base of the pilosebaceous follicle; it afflicts 30% to 85% of adolescents. The reduction and removal of sebum and bacteria, specifically *Propionibacterium acnes,* are the target of acne vulgaris therapy. Treatment of acne therapy may include (1) removal of keratin plugs, (2) decreasing the amount of *P. acnes,* (3) lowering the amounts of free fatty acid and formation, (4) decreasing the sebum production, and (5) effectively improving the appearance of the individual for psychosocial benefits.

Grades of acne have been classified as follows. Grade I includes primarily sparse comedones; grade II has comedones, papules, and occasionally pustules; grade III has a predominance of papules and pustules with small cysts; grade IV has overt signs of cystic acne. Treatment varies with the needs of each grade.

Of the many treatment modalities in acne therapy, only the topical forms of benzoyle peroxide, tetracycline, erythromycin, clindamycin, and tretinoin will be discussed here.

benzoyl peroxide

Mechanism of action. Benzoyl peroxide slowly and continuously liberates active oxygen, producing antibacterial, antiseptic, drying, and keratolytic actions. The release of oxygen into the pilosebaceous and comedome area creates unfavorable growth conditions for *P. acnes* and reduces the release of the fatty acids from sebum. Additionally, the drying vehicle aids in shrinking the papules or pustules but does not have an effect on comedones or cysts.

Indication. Treatment of acne vulgaris

Pharmacokinetics

Absorption. Absorbed by the skin

Metabolism. In skin to benzoic acid

Onset of action. Within 4 to 6 weeks improvement is usually noted.

Excretion. Kidneys

Side effects/adverse reactions

Occur infrequently and are rarely a problem: dry or peeling skin, red skin, or sensation of warmth of skin

Adverse effects that require medical intervention: severe redness, pruritus, blisters, burning, or swelling of skin caused by an allergic reaction

Significant drug interactions. None

Dosage and administration. Usually applied topically

POTENCIES OF TOPICAL STEROID PRODUCTS

The following drug list compares the relative potency of the topical corticosteroid products. The fluorinated products (fluocinonide, betamethasone, halcinonide, triamcinolone, clobetasol, and others) are the most potent drugs and are less likely to cause sodium retention.

MOST POTENT

betamethasone dipropionate (Diprosone cream, ointment, 0.05%)

clobetasol propionate (Temovate cream, ointment, 0.05%)

VERY POTENT

amcinocide (Cyclocort cream, ointment, 0.1%)

betamethasone dipropionate (Diprosone lotion 0.05%)

desoximetasone (Topicort cream, ointment, 0.25%)

diflorasone diacetate (Florone cream, ointment, 0.05%)

fluocinolone (Synalar HP cream, 0.2%; Lidex and Lidex-E cream, gel, ointment, 0.05%)

halcinonide (Halog cream, ointment solution, 0.1%)

triamcinolone acetonide (Aristocort A), or Kenalog cream, ointment, 0.5%)

POTENT

betamethasone (Benisone cream, gel, ointment, lotion, 0.025%)

betamethasone valerate (Valisone cream, ointment, lotion, 0.1%)

desoximetasone (Topicort LP; Topicort Gel, 0.05%)

flucinolone acetonide (Fluonid cream, ointment, 0.025%)

flurandrenolide (Cordran, Dordran SP cream, ointment, lotion, 0.025%)

halcinonide (Halog cream, 0.025%)

triamcinolone acetonide (Aristocort or Kenalog cream, ointment, lotion, 0.1%)

LESS POTENT

betamethasone valerate (Valisone, reduced strength cream, 0.01%)

clocortolone (Cloderm cream, 0.1%)

desonide (Tridesiloncream, 0.05%)

fluocinolone acetonide (Synalar cream, 0.01%)

flurandrenolide (Cordran, Cordran SP cream, ointment, 0. 025%)

hydrocortisone valerate (Westcort cream, ointment,) 0.2%

triamcinolone acetonide (Aristocort, Aristocort A, Kenalog cream, ointment, lotion, 0.025%)

LEAST POTENT

dexamethasone (Decadron cream, 0.1%)

Hydrocortisone (Cortef; Cort-Dome and others, cream, ointment, 2.5%)

methylprednisolone (Medrol ointment, 0.25%; 1%)

Data from Katcher BS Young, LY, and Koda-Kimble, MA: Applied therapeutics: the clinical use of drugs, ed 4, San Francisco, 1988, Applied Therapeutics, Inc, pp. 1404-1405.

to skin once daily for the first few days; then dosage is increased or decreased as therapeutic response indicates.

Pregnancy safety. FDA category C.

tretinoin (retinoic acid, vitamin A acid, Retin-A)

Mechanism of action. Tretinoin is an irritant that stimulates epidermal cell turnover, which causes skin peeling; this reduces the free fatty acids and horny cell adherence within the comedone.

Indications. Used in the treatment of acne vulgaris in which comedones, pustules, and papules predominate

Side effects/adverse reactions

Skin. Excessively red and edematous blisters, crusted skin, temporary alterations in pigmentation

Significant drug interactions. Concomitant topical use with drying or peeling agents such as benzoyl peroxide, resorcinol, salicylic acid, and sulfur results in excessive keratolytic and peeling effects.

Dosage and administration. Applied each night by covering the area lightly before the person retires. Some clients require less frequent applications or use a lower percentage strength, and others may respond to the higher percentage dosage forms.

Pregnancy safety. FDA category B

NURSING CONSIDERATIONS

Clients with sunburned skin, skin sensitive to ultraviolet light, or skin exposed to weather extremes must exercise caution and avoid tretinoin until the skin has recovered.

The client must avoid medicated or abrasive cleansers, astringents, soaps, and cosmetics that have a drying effect and a high alcohol concentration.

The client will be excessively sensitive to sun and should wear SPF sunscreens during therapy.

Irritation and desquamation are most likely during the first 1 to 3 weeks of treatment.

isotretinoin

Isotretinoin (Accutane) is an oral product indicated for the treatment of severe recalcitrant cystic acne. Women who are pregnant or are planning to become pregnant should not use this preparation. Many spontaneous abortions have been reported in pregnant women, as well as major abnormalities in the fetus at birth. Hydrocephalus, microcephalus, external ear abnormalities, facial dysmorphia, cleft palate, and cardiovascular problems have all been documented. This product is listed as contraindicated in pregnancy (FDA category X.)

Investigations are in progress to determine the status of this product. It will either have stronger restrictions placed on its use, or it may be removed from the market.

If this product is available and ordered, the nurse is urged to read the current package insert or current reference guides *(Facts and Comparisons, USP-DI, ASHP Formulary,)* carefully before drug administration.

TOPICAL ANTIBIOTICS

Topical antibiotics used in the treatment of acne (clindamycin, erythromycin, tetracycline, meclocycline) have unknown mechanisms of action. Therefore the postulated mechanisms of action of these antibiotics are antiinflammatory or inhibitory or suppressive of acne-causing bacteria and the reduction of short-chain free fatty acids of the surface lipids.

clindamycin phosphate (Cleocin T topical solution)

Topical clindamycin efficacy in the treatment of acne is reported to be equal to or better than oral tetracycline therapy and superior to topical erythromycin or topical tetracycline therapy. Skin phosphatases, by hydrolysis, convert the clindamycin phosphate to the antibacterial active clindamycin base.

Approximately 10% of a dose penetrates and is absorbed in the stratum corneum layer. Clindamycin has appeared in the urine without detectable activity in the plasma and with detectable activity in comedonal extracts. After topical application, there is an inhibition of acne-causing bacteria and reduction of free fatty acids on the skin surface.

Indications. This is one of the most widely used topical antibiotics indicated in the treatment of acne vulgaris.

Side effects/adverse reactions. The following side effects infrequently occur and rarely require physician intervention: mild diarrhea; dry, scaly and/or peeling of skin; a stinging or burning sensation. Medical intervention is necessary if the following adverse effects occur: hypersensitivity skin reaction; severe stomach distress and pain; severe watery and, perhaps, bloody diarrhea; elevated temperature; increased thirst; nausea; vomiting; increased weakness; and unintentional weight loss.

The signs and symptoms of pseudomembranous colitis occurring after the medication is discontinued require immediate physician intervention.

Dosage and administration

Adults. Apply a thin film twice daily to affected area.

Children. See usual adult dosage.

Pregnancy safety. FDA category B

NURSING CONSIDERATIONS

Cross-resistance exists with lincomycin and antagonism with erythromycin. Contraindications demonstrated by hypersensitivity to any form of clindamycin or lincomycin may apply to the topical preparation. During the client interviews the nurse should inquire about any previous sensitivity not only to clindamycin but also to other antibiotics or allergens and a history of regional enteritis. Atopic patients should be questioned since some absorption may possibly occur through the skin.

erythromycin topical solution (A/T/S, Eryderm, Staticin, Erymax)

Indications. Erythromycin topical solution is indicated for the treatment of acne vulgaris.

Side effects/adverse reactions. With this product, suprainfection and an overgrowth of antibiotic-resistant organisms may occur. Skin reactions may be erythema, desquamation, tenderness, dryness, pruritus, burning, oiliness, and acne.

Dosage and administration. Erythromycin topical solution is applied with the fingertips and hands each morning and evening to the affected areas. These areas are to be washed and rinsed and patted dry; after application, the hands and fingers should be washed.

NURSING CONSIDERATIONS

Hypersensitivity to erythromycin or the other components of the solution (alcohol, propylene glycol, or acetone) is a containdication to its use. Its safe use in pregnancy and lactation has not been established. A cumulative irritant effect may occur with concomitant use of peeling, desquamating, or abrasive agents.

Caution the client that erythromycin solution should not be used near the eyes, nose, mouth, and other mucous membranes.

meclocycline sulfosalicylate (Meclan) cream

Indications. Meclocycline sulfosalicylate is a topical oxytetracycline derivative that is indicated in the treatment of acne vulgaris.

Side effects/adverse reactions. Acute contact dermatitis and skin irritation may occur. Excessive application may result in temporary follicular staining and fabric staining.

Dosage and administration. This nonalcoholic vanishing cream is applied in the morning and evening or less often depending on client response. The cream contains formaldehyde and may cause allergic reactions.

NURSING CONSIDERATIONS

The percutaneous absorption resulting from prolonged use of this tetracycline derivative necessitates cautious monitoring of clients with hepatic or renal dysfunctions. No adequate well-controlled studies have been made in pregnant women or nursing mothers.

tetracycline topical solution (Topicycline)

Mechanism of action. Topical tetracycline is directly applied to the pilosebaceous unit (hair follicle and sebaceous gland), which is most numerous on the face, back, chest, and upper arms. Systemic tetracycline decreases the amount of free fatty acids present in acne lesions, but the mechanism by which topical tetracycline therapy improves acne is unknown.

Indications. Acne vulgaris

Side effects/adverse reactions. Topical tetracycline by percutaneous absorption produces serum levels of 0.1 μg/ml, which is less than 7% of that produced by a 500 mg/day oral dose. Liver damage in clients with renal impairment using topical tetracycline is unlikely, but it should be considered in those with hepatorenal dysfunction. No data are available regarding the use of topical tetracyclines in pregnant women, and no established data are available concerning its use during lactation.

Transient stinging or burning may often occur. The slight yellow superficial coloring of the skin of light-complected clients may be washed off. Under a source of ultraviolet light (sun, sunlamp), the treated areas will fluoresce.

Dosage and administration. Tetracycline is generously applied twice daily (morning and evening) to affected areas until the skin is wet. Because of the 40% ethanol and other components, the eyes, nose, mouth, and mucous membrane areas should be avoided. Normal use of cosmetics is permitted. (See Chapter 59 for a more complete discussion.)

BURN PRODUCTS

Approximately 6000 or more people die each year of thermal injury in the United States alone. The chief cause of death is shock, a fact of considerable significance in any effective plan of treatment.

Burns cause lesions of the skin accompanied by pain. The burn may be caused by heat (thermal burn), chemical cauterizing agents (chemical burns), or electricity (electrical burns). Sources may be friction, lightning, or electromagnetic energy sources (ultraviolet light, x-rays, lasers, or atomic explosion). The types of burns that result from various sources are relatively specific and diagnostic.

Consideration of what takes place in the damaged tissues clarifies many points of treatment. At first there is an altered capillary permeability in the local injured area. That is, the permeability is increased, resulting in a loss of plasma and weeping of the surface tissues. If the burn is at all extensive, considerable amounts of plasma fluid may be lost in a relatively short time. This depletes the blood volume and causes a decreased cardiac output and diminished blood flow. Unless the situation is rapidly brought under control, irreparable damage may result from the rapidly developing tissue anoxia. Lack of sufficient oxygen and the accumulation of waste products from inadequate oxidation result in loss of tone in the minute blood vessels, and the increased capillary permeability then extends to tissues remote from those suffering the initial injury. Thus a generalized edema often develops, and the vicious cycle once established tends to be self-perpetuating. One of the aims in the treatment of burns is therefore to stop the loss of plasma insofar as it is possible and replenish that which is lost as quickly as possible.

Partial- or full-thickness burns must be thought of as open wounds with the accompanying danger of infection. The infection must be prevented or treated. The treatment, however, must be such that it will not bring any further destruction of tissue or of the small islands of remaining epithelium from which growth and regeneration can take place.

When burns are divided into three degrees, they are classified by the depth of skin involved within a geographic designation. First-degree burns involve only the epidermis, causing erythema with characteristic dry, painful reddening and edema without blistering or vesiculation (e.g., overexposure to sun or flash burn). Second-degree burns involve the epidermis extending into the dermis and may be superficial or involve deep dermal necrosis. Epithelial regeneration may extend from the deep skin appendages such as hair follicles and sebaceous glands that penetrate the dermis. This burn is characterized by a moist, blistered, very painful surface (e.g., flash or scald burns from nonviscous liquids). Third-degree burns involve destruction of the entire dermis and epidermis characterized by white, lustrous, or opaque skin; dry, leathery skin; or coagulated, charred skin without sensation as a result of the destruction of nerve endings (e.g., flame burns or hot viscous liquids). Deep third-degree burns extend into subcutaneous fat, muscle, or bone; they cause scarring and may require skin grafting (see box).

The severity of electrical burns depends on the amount of voltage received, the condition of the skin (e.g., cuts, abrasions, and moisture, which lower resistance), and contraction of flexor muscles, which inhibits release from the power source. This may result in cardiac systole, ventricular fibrillation, or nervous system paralysis, which can lead to respiratory arrest. Electrical burns develop necrosis of more tissue than thermal burns. Electrical burns are of three types. In Type I, the electrical current causes effects on blood vessels such as occlusion, thrombosis, or tissue destruction. In Type II, electrical burns from high-tension currents (e.g., an electrical arc) produce a crater in the skin. Type III electrical burns are similar to flame burns because the arc flame ignites the person's clothes.

Chemical burns occur after contact with acid or alkali; the initial treatment is water irrigation of the affected area followed by neutralization. Chemical burns may occur in the mouth and appear as a white slough owing to necrosis of the epithelium and underlying connective tissues.

BURNS

DEGREE	DESCRIPTION
First	Superficial injury involving only the epidermis. Characterized by pain, red skin without blistering, and perhaps, swelling. This is a mild partial thickness burn that will heal without scarring.
Second	Burn extends from epidermis into the dermis area. Pain is intense, skin surface will be red, blistered, and may have a mottled appearance. This type burn usually has edema and blistering for 2 days after the initial burn injury. This is a partial thickness burn that generally leaves minimal scarring, if properly treated.
Third	This burn involves destruction of the epidermis and dermis and may extend into fat, muscle, or tissues. Some areas will be charred black, person will complain of severe pain or no pain at all if nerves have been destroyed. This is a full-thickness burn that may require skin grafting. Healing results in significant scarring.

First aid treatment of burns. An important first aid treatment for minor and major burns regardless of cause (chemical, electric, thermal) is to immediately cool the wound to remove irritants, decrease inflammation, and constrict blood vessels; this reduces the permeability of the blood vessels and checks edema formation. Cold tap water can be used to thoroughly flush the wound and to cool hot clothing. The more quickly the wound is cooled, the less tissue damage there is likely to be, and the more rapid will be the recovery. No greasy ointments, lard, butter, or dressings should be applied, since these agents will inhibit loss of heat from the burn, which will increase both discomfort and tissue damage. The burn may be left exposed to the air or cold wet compresses may be applied until the person can be transported for medical attention.

Burn victims treated in an emergency room or burn unit will be stabilized with intravenous fluids, given analgesics for pain, and sedated, if necessary. Such individuals are immunized with tetanus toxoid and/or tetanus immunoglobulin, depending on their immunization status. Catheterization may be necessary to measure urinary output, depending on client's status. Following stabilization, the burn wound is cleaned in a whirlpool (Hubbard) tank if available. Povidone iodine (Betadine whirlpool concentrate) is usually added to the tank. Hair around the wound is shaved, loose skin is removed. Following the bath, topical antibiotic therapy is started.

silver sulfadiazine (Silvadene)

Silver sulfadiazine is an antiinfective agent with broad antimicrobial activity against many gram-negative and gram-positive bacteria and yeast. It is particularly effective against *Pseudomonas* organisms. It is produced by the reaction of silver nitrate with sulfadiazine. Silver sulfadiazine acts only on the cell membrane and cell wall to produce its bactericidal effect.

Silver sulfadiazine is used in second- and third-degree burns for the prevention and treatment of sepsis. Control of infection may prevent the conversion of infected second-degree burns resulting in necrosis. Since silver sulfadiazine is not a carbonic anhydrase inhibitor, it does not alter acid-base balance; neither does it alter electrolyte balance nor stain tissues, linen, or dressings. Silver sulfadiazine softens eschar, facilitating eschar removal and preparation of the wound for grafting.

Silver sulfadiazine is available as a 1% cream to be applied topically to cleansed, debrided burn wounds once or twice daily. It should be applied with a sterile gloved hand to a thickness of about $\frac{1}{16}$ inch. Burn wounds should be continuously covered with the cream. If the cream is removed by activity, it should be reapplied. Daily bathing and debriding are important. Dressings may or may not be used.

Therapy is usually continued until satisfactory healing has occurred or the wound is ready for grafting. Since silver sulfadiazine inhibits bacterial growth, delayed eschar separation may occur, necessitating escharotomy to prevent contractures.

Pain, burning, and itching occur infrequently following application of the silver sulfadiazine cream.

Silver sulfadiazine may cause a hypersensitivity reaction; if this occurs, the drug should be discontinued. Hemolysis may occur in persons with glucose-6-phosphate dehydrogenase deficiency.

When applied to extensive areas of the body, significant amounts of the drug may be absorbed, reaching therapeutic serum levels, producing adverse reactions characteristic of the sulfonamides. Renal function in these patients should be monitored and the urine examined for sulfa crystals.

Silver sulfadiazine may cause kernicterus. Although it is not recommended for pregnant women at term, premature neonates, or infants under 6 months, it is useful in pediatric burn clients. Proteolytic enzymes may be inactivated by this silver salt.

For nursing considerations, consult Chapter 72.

silver nitrate

An aqueous solution of silver nitrate 0.5% has been used extensively in some burn centers during the past few years. As a 0.5% solution it is a relatively safe antiseptic agent for gram-negative bacteria. Dressings soaked in silver nitrate 0.5% are applied early to the burn; the dressings must be kept moist and must not be allowed to dry, which would cause precipitation of silver salts into the wound and irritation. Concentrations of silver nitrate above 1% produce tissue necrosis; concentrations below 0.5% are not antiseptic. Silver nitrate stains anything with which it comes in contact. The brown or black tissue discoloration is usually not permanent. Silver nitrate solution 0.5% is a hypotonic solution, and when it is used on extensive burns or for extensive periods of time it may cause electrolyte imbalance. Serum electrolytes should be frequently determined and clients observed for symptoms of sodium or potassium depletion (such as change in behavior and confusion); blood sample color (brownish) is indicative of methemoglobinemia.

For nursing considerations, consult Chapter 72.

mafenide acetate (Sulfamylon)

One of the most important therapeutic agents developed to combat burn infection in avascular tissue has been the discovery of mafenide acetate. Mafenide (a sulfonamide) is a water-soluble ointment (bacteriostatic to gram-negative and gram-positive organisms, including *Pseudomonas aeruginosa*) that is applied topically to the complete burn wound area with sterile gloves following wound cleansing and debridement. The exposure method of therapy is preferred, although occasionally thin-layer dressings may be applied; however, this may result in tissue maceration. Environmental pus, serum, or acidity do not affect the activity of this agent.

The ointment (applied with a sterile gloved hand) should always form a protective coating over the burn. It rapidly diffuses through partial (second-degree) and full-thickness (third-degree) burns and has proved to be one of the most effective means for preventing and retarding bacterial invasion in burn wounds. It has decreased deaths resulting from septicemia and decreased extension of the wound from infection. It has decreased the number of burn cases requiring plastic surgery or skin grafting. However, eschar separation is delayed.

Mafenide acetate is relatively nontoxic but has reported allergic reactions. It is rapidly metabolized to a metabolite and eliminated by way of the kidneys. Since this drug and metabolite are strong carbonic anhydrase inhibitors, acidosis (metabolic) may occur, usually compensated by hyperventilation. The client should be carefully observed for any signs resulting in respiratory alkalosis. If rapid or labored respirations occur, the ointment should be washed off the wound. Therapy can be interrupted for 2 to 3 days without impairing the bacterial control of the wound while continuing fluid therapy and acid-base restoration.

Mafenide may cause some discomfort when first applied (in $\frac{1}{16}$-inch layer once or twice daily)—a burning or pain sensation may occur that lasts from a few minutes to as long as an hour.

This is a highly stable drug. It remains active for several years and does not need to be refrigerated except in tropical countries.

gentamicin sulfate

Gentamicin sulfate (Garamycin) topical has been used to treat burns in some areas of the country. Many burn units have discontinued its use though, because of the development of bacterial resistance, especially *Pseudomonas* organisms. Silver sulfadiazine (Silvadene) is usually the preferred agent in many burn centers, although the other topical agents (Povidone iodine, mafenide acetate) are also commonly used.

TOPICAL ANTIPRURITICS

Antipruritics are drugs given to allay itching of skin and mucous membranes. There is less need for these preparations as the constitutional treatment of persons with skin disorders is better understood. Dilute solutions containing phenol, as well as tars, have been widely used. They may be applied as lotions, pastes, or ointments. Dressings wet with potassium permanganate 1:4000, aluminum subacetate 1:16, boric acid, or physiologic saline solution may cool and soothe and thus prevent itching. Lotions such as calamine or calamine with phenol (phenolated calamine) and cornstarch or oatmeal baths may also be used to relieve itching.

Local anesthetics such as dibucaine and benzocaine may decrease pruritus, but their use is not recommended because of their high sensitizing and irritating effects. The application of hydrocortisone in a lotion or ointment in a strength of 0.5% to 1% has proved to be one of the best methods of relieving pruritus and decreasing inflammation. It has the additional advantage of possessing a low sensitizing index.

TOPICAL ECTOPARASITICIDAL DRUGS

Ectoparasites are arthropods (insects) that live on the outer surface of the body. Ectoparasiticides are drugs used against those animal parasites. For human use these drugs are more frequently referred to as pediculicides and scabicides (miticides), reflecting the parasite treated with each group.

Pediculosis is a parasite infestation of lice on the skin of a human. Lice infestations have been increasing in North America and western Europe. It was once thought that pediculosis could be attributed to crowded dwellings and poor hygiene, but recently this assumption has proved not to be true. The lice are transmitted from one person to the next by close contact with infested persons, clothing, combs, and towels. There are three different varieties of the infestations: (1) pediculosis pubis, caused by *Phthirus pubis* (pubic louse, or "crabs"), (2) pediculosis corporis, caused by *Pediculus humanus* var. *corporis* (body louse), and (3) pediculosis capitis, caused by *P. humanus* var. *capitis* (head louse). See Figure 67-1.

Common findings in a person who is infested include pruritis, nits (eggs of louse) on hair shafts, lice on skin or clothes, and, when there are pubic lice, occasionally sky-blue macules on the inner thighs or lower abdomen. The drug of choice is the pediculicide lindane (gamma-benzene hexachloride).

A characteristic finding of pediculosis corporis, except in heavily infested individuals, is that the parasite is absent from the body but inhabits seams of clothing that come in contact with the axillae or that are in the beltline or collar.

Scabies is a parasitic infestation caused by the itch mite, *Sarcoptes scabiei.* It is transmitted from one person to the next by close contact, such as sleeping with an infested individual. It bores into the horny layers of the skin in cracks and folds, causing irritation and pruritus. Itching occurs almost exclusively at night. The infestation is usually generalized over the body except the head and neck regions. The drug of choice is the scabicide, crotamiton.

The first approach to the treatment of both pediculosis and scabies is identification of the source of infestation. Next, decontamination of clothing and personal articles used by the infested person is necessary. This can be done by washing clothing and bedding with hot, soapy water or by having items that cannot be washed dry-cleaned. Usually all persons involved, such as the whole family, are treated to prevent reinfestation. Table 67-6 summarizes

Pubic louse   Body louse

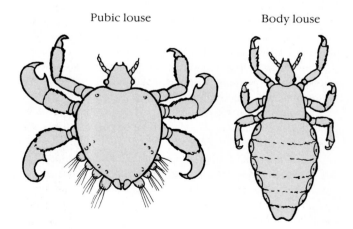

FIGURE 67-1   Pubic louse *(Phthirus pubis), left,* and body louse *(Pediculus humanus), right.* Notice the first pair of legs on the pubic louse are thinner than the second and third pairs. Also, the abdomen is shorter. On the body louse, all legs are approximately the same length, and the abdomen is longer.

TABLE 67-6   Drugs Used in the Treatment of Ectoparasitic Diseases

Disease	Drug
Pediculosis (lice infestation)	
Pediculus humanus var. *capitis* (head louse)	lindane (gamma-benzene hexachloride)
	malathion (0.5% Prioderm)
Pediculus humanus var. *corporis* (body louse)	pyrethrins with piperonylbutoxide
Phthirus pubis (pubic louse)	copper oleate, 0.03%
Scabies (mite infestation)	crotamiton
Sarcoptes scabiei	lindane (gamma-benzene hexachloride)
	benzyl benzoate, 12%-25%
	sulfur in petrolatum

the various topical pediculicides and scabicides used in the treatment of these parasitic infestations.

lindane (gamma-benzene hexachloride; Kwell)

Lindane is considered both a scabicide and a pediculicide because it is effective in the treatment of both lice and mite infestations. It is available in a 1% cream, lotion, and shampoo. For the treatment of pediculosis pubis and infestations of *Pediculus humanus* var. *capitis,* the cream or lotion is applied in a sufficient quantity to cover the skin and hair of the infected and surrounding areas. It is left on for 12 hours and then thoroughly washed. It seldom needs to be applied more than once. The shampoo is worked into the hair and left on for 4 minutes. Then the hair is rinsed and dried, and nits (eggs) are combed from the hair shafts. Retreatment is usually not necessary.

For the treatment of scabies, only the cream or lotion is used. If crusted lesions are present, a warm bath preceding the application of lindane is recommended. Lindane is applied over the entire body from the neck down. Again, it is left on for 8 to 12 hours and then washed off. Usually one application is sufficient. It is common to have pruritus after application, but this does not indicate a need for reapplication unless living mites can be demonstrated.

Lindane occasionally will cause an eczematous skin rash. It penetrates human skin and has a potential for central nervous system toxicity, especially in children. Rarely do convulsions or aplastic anemia occur with use of this drug.

malathion (0.5% Prioderm)

The FDA has recently approved the use of malathion for the treatment of head lice and ova. In addition, the drug has been shown to destroy lindane-resistant lice. Re-

search studies reveal that this agent is effective in lice-infested individuals within 24 hours after use. Also, the drug is well tolerated and no central nervous system toxicity has been reported. Malathion is a lotion that is rubbed into the scalp and left to air dry. Because the drug is flammable, the individual must be warned to avoid open flames and not to use a hairdryer. The hair should be shampooed 8 to 12 hours after application; dead lice are combed out. If necessary, a second application may be tried 7 to 9 days later. Malathion is available only as a prescription in 2-ounce bottles.

crotamiton (Eurax)

Crotamiton has scabicidal and antipruritic actions. It is massaged into the skin from the chin down, particularly in the folds and creases of the body. It is reapplied in 24 hours, and 48 hours after the second application it is washed from the body surface.

Two applications of crotamiton usually eradicate most mite infestations. In resistant cases it may be applied again 1 week later.

Crotamiton is available as a 10% cream or lotion. Occasionally a skin rash may occur with its application. Rarely allergic or irritant contact dermatitis occur.

KEY TERMS

ectoparasites, page 1060
exodermas, page 1050
furuncle, page 1047
keratin, page 1039
keratolytics, page 1054
pediculosis, page 1060
scabies, page 1060
SPF (sun protection factor), page 1050
tinea, page 1047
verruca, page 1047

BIBLIOGRAPHY

Braunwald, E, and others, eds: Harrison's principles of internal medicine, ed 11, New York, 1987, McGraw-Hill Book Co.

Coody, D: There is no such thing as a good tan, J Pediatr Health 1(3):125, 1987.

Cooper, D and others: The burn injury: incidence, initial assessment, and management, Emerg Care Q 1(3):1, 1985.

Davis, SK, and Bennett, RW: Topical treatment of burn wounds, US Pharmacist 9(1):39, 1984.

Davidson, DE: Handbook of nonprescription drugs, ed 8, Washington, DC; 1986, American Pharmaceutical Association and The National Professional Society of Pharmacists.

Does topical Trentinoin prevent cutaneous aging? Lancet 8592(1):977, 1988.

Gossel, TA: Topical antibiotics, US Pharmacist 10(7):22, 1985.

Herfindal, ET, and Hirschman, JL: Clinical pharmacy and therapeutics, ed 3, Baltimore, 1984, Williams & Wilkins.

Kastrup, EK, ed: Facts and comparisons, St. Louis, 1988, JB Lippincott Co.

Knoben, JE, and Anderson, PO: Handbook of clinical drug data, ed 5, Hamilton, Ill, 1986, Drug Intelligence Publications, Inc.

Rasmussen, JE: The management of acne, Physician Assist 10(5):179, 1986. United States Pharmacopeial Convention: Drug information for the health care provider, ed 8, Rockville Md, 1988, The Convention.

Weiss, SS, Ellis, CN, Headington, SS, Tinoff, T, Hamilton, TA, and Voorhees, JJ: Topical trentinoin improves phot aged skin, JAMA 259(4):977, 1988.

Weston, WL: Topical corticosteroids in dermatologic disorders. Part 6, Hosp Pract 19(1):149, 1984.

Debriding Agents

The **decubitus ulcer** (bedsore or pressure sore) is a break in the skin and underlying subcutaneous and muscle tissue caused by abnormal and sustained pressure or friction being exerted over the bony prominences of the body by the object on which the body part rests. It results in vascular insufficiency and ischemic necrosis, and it most frequently affects debilitated, comatose, immobilized, or paralyzed patients.

There are many contributing causes to this condition that must be treated. Among the local and systemic are the following: obesity or malnutrition; debilitation; a pressure and shearing force on the lower body if the head of the bed is raised more than 30 inches; a loss of sensation of pressure or pain; muscle atrophy and motor paralysis, as a result of a reduction in the amount of adipose tissue between skin and underlying bone; emaciation and dehydration; poor nutrition because of vitamins, minerals, and trace elements (such as copper and zinc); friction; local anatomic defects; trauma; incontinence; edema; infections; heat and moisture (maceration); hypertension; septicemia; and local circulatory interference.

The bacterial flora of a decubitus ulcer are both gram-negative and gram-positive organisms, which include *Staphylococcus aureus*, streptococcus A and D, *Escherichia coli*, *Clostridium tetani*, and *Bacteroides, Proteus, Pseudomonas, Klebsiella*, and *Citrobacter* organisms. Parenteral antibiotics (adequate levels in granulating wounds are not reached) may be needed in difficult-to-treat infected decubitus ulcers as an adjunct to surgical management just before and at time of surgery.

An individual with a full thickness loss of skin may be a candidate for surgical intervention either to cover the ulcer area or to stabilize the wound. Surgical decisions include the underlying disease, the ability of the client to withstand surgery, and the ulcer condition or prognosis (especially those in which all soft tissue is destroyed, exposing bone).

NURSING MANAGEMENT OF DECUBITUS ULCERS

Prevention and treatment of decubitus ulcers are centered around treatment of underlying causes, providing a well-balanced nutritional state, and minimizing or eliminating the pressure or friction causing vascular stasis and tissue damage. The following are some preventive and treatment measures that the nurse may use to reduce the occurrence of decubitus ulcers.

1. Change the client's position frequently (every 1 to 2 hours day and night) for pressure relief.
2. Maintain a clean, dry, and wrinkle-free bed. Bedclothes should be smooth rather than coarse and should be changed frequently.
3. Provide active and passive exercise to increase muscle and skin tone and to improve vascularity, or use a whirlpool for hydrotherapy.
4. Position the client with pillows and pads, not exceeding a 30-inch elevation of the head.
5. Use sheepskin, hydrofloat devices, silica gel pads, polystyrene, and foam rubber pads and heel protectors to relieve pressure. Place them on a mattress in direct contact with the client's skin. The mattress should be free of surface bulges and indentations and have a uniform, flat surface to prevent friction or wrinkles. Reduced pressure on skin is below capillary pressure in the skin (59 to 60 mm Hg).
6. Use an alternating pressure mattress pad covered with one layer of sheet to promote circulation and reduce the occurrence of tissue ischemia.
7. Massage the client's back with nonalcoholic skin lotion, covering and checking the bony prominences of the ankles, coccyx, elbows, heels, hips, knees, shoulders, and other areas having thin layers of subcutaneous tissue.
8. Provide meticulous skin hygiene with frequent inspections for abnormal alterations. Wash gently with warm water and, if needed, mild nondetergent soap, rinse, and blot dry with a soft towel. An emollient lubricating lotion may be used following washing to keep the skin soft.
9. Keep the skin of incontinent client's dry and clear of urine and fecal contamination, since maceration from moisture promotes tissue breakdown and predisposes patients to infection. Trimmed nails prevent self-inflicted injury caused by scratching of the skin.
10. Maintain nutritional support for a positive nitrogen balance, tissue turgor, and adequate fluid intake with 3800 to 4600 cal/24 hours, a diet high in protein, vitamins, minerals, and trace elements. The client's hemoglobin level should be 12 g/100 ml or more and the serum protein above 6 mg/100 ml.
11. Necrotic decubitus ulcers often require debridement by surgical or drug methods and meticulous wound care.
12. Treatment regimens are based on the extent of skin involvement.
13. Assess the decubitus ulcer on a daily basis for gradual reduction in size, redness, and swelling; presence of granulation tissue; and signs and symptoms of infection (warmth, edema, and unusual drainage from site).

The preventive measures should be taught to clients, family members, or other caregivers of bedridden or other clients who are at risk for developing decubiti.

DRUG MANAGEMENT OF DECUBITUS ULCERS

The treatment of decubitus ulcers depends on the stage of the ulcer. In early stages, topical steroids (fluorinated) may be used to hasten healing. Topical antibiotics are only used when an infection is documented by a culture of the decubitus wound to identify the specific type of microorganisms present. Inflammation of the area, pus, or odor may indicate the need for a laboratory culture.

Decubitus or pressure sores have been classified into five grades or stages:

Grade I—A red area that overlies a bony or tendinous (tendons) site that remains even when the pressure is relieved (blanching erythema)

Grade II—A superficial ulceration (skin blister or break) into the dermis area (nonblanching erythema)

Grade III—Skin ulcer extends into exposed subcutaneous tissue; presence of blister and eschar formation

Grade IV—Deep skin ulcer that exposes muscle and bone; usually the body enzymes separate the eschar, sloughing of tissue results in an ulcer; generally, noninfectious

Grade V—Ulcer has extended into bursae, or joints, or into body cavities; or ulcer is the same as Grade IV with the addition of an infection

In addition to the nursing management previously reviewed, numerous treatment protocols have been applied. Decubitus ulcers are problem areas that generally do not have widely accepted, standard treatment programs. Therefore, depending on the physician and local practice, the treatment approach can vary considerably. Table 68-1 is a recommended treatment protocol based on the previous staging system.

TABLE 68-1   Recommended Treatment Protocol for Decubitus Ulcers

Staging	Typical treatment modalities
Grade I or II	Corn starch, silicone spray
Grade III	Wet to dry dressings (antiseptics) Collagenase or enzyme ointments Surgical debridement
Grade IV and V	Dextranomer beads Enzyme ointments Wet to dry dressings (antiseptics) Surgical debridement

PROTEOLYTIC ENZYME PREPARATIONS

In grade IV or V, debriding agents are often used to remove sloughing tissue and to help facilitate granulation of the wound. The debridement can be performed with a wet-to-dry dressing method, usually using normal saline or hypertonic saline solution or one-fourth to one-half strength betadine or one-half strength Dakin's solution as antiseptics. Chemical debridement is performed with proteolytic enzymes. In very serious ulceration, or if complications are present (osteomyelitis), surgical debridement may be required. The focus of this section will be limited to the use of proteolytic enzymes.

Proteolytic enzymes digest or liquefy necrotic tissue and purulent exudate without affecting fat, keratin, fibrin, or granulation tissues. The drawback with these preparations is that 2 or 3 days are usually needed to get rid of an eschar, and some physicians believe this should be done more quickly. Sutilains (Travase) debrides a new or fresh burn effectively, but enzymes that debride an ischemic decubitus ulcer are lacking, according to some specialists (Sawyer, PN and others, 1980).

Most enzymes contain the suffix "ase" in their name plus the name of the substrate on which they act. For example, collagenase acts on and degrades collagen; hyaluronidase acts on hyaluronic acid, a ground substance of connective tissue. Enzymes are also grouped according to the reactions they catalyze. For example, **proteolytic enzymes** hasten the hydrolysis of proteins.

Since enzymes are proteins, they may be antigenic and cause toxic reactions of an immunologic type.

The enzymes discussed in this chapter are used topically for *medical* or *chemical* **debridement**—i.e., the removal, by enzymatic digestion, of necrotic and injured tissue, clotted blood, purulent exudates, or fibrinous accumulations in wounds. This action cleans the wounds and facilitates healing. Systemic antibiotic therapy and topical antibiotic or antiseptic therapy may be used in conjunction with enzymatic debridement to control or inhibit infection.

The Nurse's Role in Proteolytic Enzyme Therapy

The following are aspects of care for clients being treated with topically applied enzymatic drugs (not the nonenzymatic agents). These are in addition to the previously discussed nursing management. Before topical aseptic application of enzymes, the wound should be thoroughly cleansed (flushing away necrotic debris and fibrinous exudates) with a solution that does not inactivate the enzyme (e.g., physiologic saline or sterile distilled water). Solutions containing metal or acidic ions should be avoided to prevent inactivation of the enzymes. As much necrotic tissue should be removed with forceps and scissors as can be readily removed. All previously applied ointment should be removed before new ointment is applied to the substrate.

- Dense, dry, and thick eschar should be crosshatched by the physician with a No. 10 or 11 blade for adequate contact of enzyme to the substrate of necrotic debris.
- Ointment should be applied directly to the wound with a tongue depressor or spatula and then covered with sterile petrolatum gauze or sterile gauze (or other nonadhering dressing), or it can be applied with a sterile gauze pad that is then placed over the wound. A bandage and/or tape should then be used to hold the dressing in place.
- Ointment or jelly preparations should be confined to the wound. The surrounding healthy tissue (or skin) should be protected from the enzyme (e.g., zinc oxide paste can be used).
- The treated lesion should be kept moist and protected from drying.
- The enzyme must be in direct contact with the wound for a sufficient length of time, usually about 4 days.
- To avoid delayed healing, the enzyme should be discontinued when the wound is cleaned and debrided.
- Secondary skin closure or grafting may follow optimal debridement.
- Debilitated clients should be carefully monitored, since debriding enzymes increase the risk of bacterial infection.
- Client's should be observed for allergic or sensitivity reactions, e.g., dermatitis and febrile reactions.

collagenase (Santyl, Biozyme-C)

Mechanism of action. Collagenase is an enzymatic debriding agent derived from *Clostridium histolyticum*. It is capable of degrading both denatured and undenatured collagen. Other proteolytic enzymes act only on denatured collagen. Thus it is claimed that collagenase produces more effective debridement by acting on collagen at the wound edges, where necrotic slough is anchored. These actions promote the formation of granulation tissue and the epithelization of dermal ulcers and burned tissue.

Side effects/adverse reactions. This ointment should be applied only within the area of the lesion, since a transient erythema has been reported as a cutaneous reaction on the wound surface or the area adjacent to the lesion. This reaction may be prevented by applying a protectant (for example, zinc oxide paste) around the lesion.

Topical enzymes used for debriding may increase the risk of bacteremia in the debilitated individual; this may necessitate monitoring of these clients for systemic bacterial infections.

Significant drug interactions

1. Collagenase can be inactivated by irrigating the lesion with an acidic solution such as Burow's solution (pH 3.6 to 4.4). The optimal pH range for collagenase is 6 to 8; a local pH alteration outside this range will decrease the enzymes' activity.
2. The activity is adversely affected by detergents, soaps, cleansing agents, hexachlorophene, heavy metal ions (as found in antiseptics, iodine, thimerosal, mercury compounds silver sulfadiazine and silver nitrate), boric acid, and soaks such as Burow's solution (which has a low pH and contains an interacting metal ion).

Dosage and administration. Collagenase should be applied once daily. If the wound is deep, collagenase should be applied directly with a wooden tongue depressor or spatula. The application should be repeated if the dressing area is soiled (e.g., because of incontinence).

NURSING CONSIDERATIONS

See p. 1064 for nursing management of decubitus ulcer.

Before collagenase is applied, the area is cleansed of debris by gentle rubbing with a gauze pad saturated with hydrogen peroxide, Dakin's solution, or sterile normal saline. The ulcer should be patted dry with a clean gauze pad. If infection is present, a topical antibacterial agent (for example, neomycinbacitracin-polymyxin B solution or powder) is applied directly to the ulcer surface before collagenase.

The average time for complete debridement of dermal ulcers and decubiti with collagenase is about 11 days. This time permits debridement of necrotic tissue and establishment of granulation tissue.

The ointment does not have to be refrigerated; it is stored at room temperature.

fibrinolysin and desoxyribonuclease ointment (Elase)

Mechanism of action. The proteolytic enzymes fibrinolysin and desoxyribonuclease are derived from bovine

plasma and pancreas, respectively. Purulent exudates consist of fibrinous material and nucleoprotein. Desoxyribonuclease attacks deoxyribonucleic acid, and fibrinolysin (plasmin) acts on fibrin of blood clots and fibrinous exudates. The mechanism of action is fibrinolytic activity on denatured proteins (devitalized tissue); protein elements of living cells are unaffected.

An ointment product that contains the two enzymes in combination with chloromycetin is also available. The added bacteriostatic properties inhibit bacterial protein synthesis by interfering with transfer of activated amino acids from soluble ribonucleic acid to ribosomes in infected lesions. Systemic antibiotics are also indicated.

Indications

1. Used to debride inflamed and infected lesions, including surgical wounds, ulcerative lesions (trophic, decubitus, stasis, arteriosclerotic), second- and third-degree burns, and wounds resulting from circumcision or episiotomy. The combination product with antibiotic is preferred for infected lesions.
2. Used for treatment of vaginitis and cervicitis (intravaginal use) and irrigation of infected wounds and superficial hematomas not adjacent to or near fatty tissue.

Side effects/adverse reactions. Allergic reactions have been observed in persons who are sensitive to bovine source materials, mercury compounds (thimerosal, a mercury derivative, is used as a preservative in the ointment base of Elase), or chloromycetin.

Dosage and administration. The topical solution (use within 24 hours following reconstitution) may be used in a spray or a wet dressing. Elase is also available as a dry powder in vials. Dressing should be changed at least once a day or preferably, two or three times daily. After 24 hours, this product is practically inactive.

sutilains (Travase)

Mechanism of action. Sutilains is a sterile preparation of proteolytic enzymes isolated from culture filtrates of *Bacillus subtilis.* It digests necrotic soft tissues and purulent exudates.

Indications. Aids in the selective removal of only nonviable or undenatured protein in necrotic soft tissue and purulent exudate from open wounds and ulcers (which may impair granulation tissue formation and wound healing) resulting from second- and third-degree burns, decubiti, peripheral vascular disease, and wounds (incisions, trauma, pyogens).

Side effects/adverse reactions. Side effects are mild; they include mild, transient pain (managed with a mild analgesic), local paresthesia, bleeding, and transient dermatitis.

Significant drug interactions

1 The use of detergents and antiseptics (benzalkonium chloride, hexachlorophene, iodine, nitrofura-

zone) concomitantly should be avoided because of possible inactivation of enzyme activity.

2 Compounds containing metallic ions, such as silver sulfadiazine, silver nitrate, or thimerosal, interfere adversely with the action of the enzyme.

Dosage and administration. First thoroughly clean the area with normal saline or water solutions. Moisten wound area by bathing or with wet soaks. Apply a thin layer of the ointment to the necrotic tissue extending ¼ to ½ inch beyond the desired area to be debrided. Cover with a loose moist dressing. This procedure is usually repeated three or four times daily.

NURSING CONSIDERATIONS

See also the general nursing considerations for topical enzymatic agents on p. 1065.

Assessment. Sutilains should not be applied to wounds communicating with major body cavities, wounds with exposed major nerves or nerve tissue, neoplastic ulcers, or wounds in women of childbearing age.

Intervention. Sutilains is prepared as an ointment containing 82,000 casein units/g ointment base (15-g tubes). It must be refrigerated at a temperature between 2° C and 10° C.

A wound should be thoroughly cleansed (including removal of antiseptics) with water or isotonic sodium chloride solution and left moist or wet before a thin layer of sutilains ointment is applied up to ½ inch beyond the area needing debriding. The area should then be covered with loose, wet dressings.

This procedure should be repeated three or four times daily. A moist environment is necessary for this agent's enzymatic activity.

This drug must be kept away from the eyes; if contact occurs, the eyes should be rinsed with copious amount of sterile water.

Evaluation. If dissolution does not occur in 24 to 48 hours, the drug should be discontinued.

If bleeding or dermatitis occurs, the drug should be discontinued.

Although systemic allergic reactions have not been reported, the drug is capable of causing an antibody response.

Topical Enzyme Combination Products

Trypsin and papain (proteolytic enzymes), balsam Peru (mild antibacterial agent that aids in improving circulation in the wound area by stimulating the capillary bed), castor oil (protective covering, improves epithelialization), urea (emollient and keratolytic), and chlorophyll derivatives (aid in controling wound odor and healing) have been formulated into various combinations and marketed. For example, Granulex contains trypsin, bal-

sam Peru, and castor oil, whereas Panafil contains papain, urea and chlorophyll derivatives.

Such products may be ordered for administration once or twice daily. The wound area should be cleaned by flushing with physiologic saline before application each time. Be aware that hydrogen peroxide solution can inactivate papain activity.

NONENZYMATIC AGENTS

dextranomer (Debrisan)

Mechanism of action. Dextranomer is a hydrophilic dextran polymer in the form of small beads (0.1 to 0.3 mm in diameter); it is used for cleansing only a wet or secreting wound (not dry wounds). Each gram of beads absorbs about 4 ml of fluid (swelling to four times in size) from a secreting lesion or wounds. This rapid action continues until all the beads are saturated. The assumption of a grayish yellow color by the beads indicates that they are saturated and ready for removal. The spaces between the beads produce a powerful dehydrating suction force and capillary action in the area. Low-molecular-weight substances (bacteria and bacterial forms) in the secretions of wound exudates (e.g., toxins, peptides) are drawn up (absorbed) within the beads. The higher molecular weight substances (plasma, protein, fibrinogen, fibrin, split products) are absorbed in the spaces between adjacent swollen beads, and this removal retards eschar formation.

Indications

1. Application of dextranomer to the surface of a secreting wound removes exudates and particles that impede tissue repair and increase wound healing time and reduces edema and inflammation.

2. Secreting or exudative wounds for which dextranomer can be used include (clean wet ulcer) venous stasis ulcers, decubitus ulcers, infected traumatic and surgical wounds, and infected burns.

Dosage and administration. Dextranomer is available in 4-g packages and 60- and 120-g containers and a paste form. To initially prepare the wound, it should be irrigated with sterile water or saline and the area should be left moist. The beads should cover the wound surface to a depth of 3 mm to 6 mm (⅛ to ¼ inch) (e.g., 4 g of beads covers a wound or ulcer 1½ × 1½ inches). A paste mixture is often used for areas that are either irregular body surfaces or are difficult to reach. If the premade paste dosage form is not available (10-g foil packets) then the nurse may mix the beads with glycerin (only glycerin) and dress the wound in the usual manner. The beads or paste must be reapplied every 12 hours or more often while reducing the number of applications as the exudate diminishes.

NURSING CONSIDERATIONS

The contents of each container should be used for only one person to limit cross-contamination. If the wound is a cratered decubitus ulcer, the nurse should allow for expansion of the beads by not packing the wound tightly. During the first few days, as the edema is reduced, the wound itself may appear larger in size than it did before treatment. Therapy should be discontinued when healthy granulation is established. Treatment of an underlying pathologic condition (such as venous or arterial flow or pressure) is concurrent. Diabetic and immunosuppressed patients may be susceptible to severe infections.

The wound should be lightly bandaged on all four sides to hold the beads in place and prevent maceration from occlusion. The degree of wound secretion determines the number of dressing changes (usually one or two daily profuse secretions may necessitate three or four dressing changes). Changes are done before encrustation or full saturation of the beads (grayish yellow color) to prevent drying and to facilitate bead removal by irrigation (e.g., sterile water, saline). A client occasionally may have some minor pain during dressing changes. The nurse should be aware that if the beads are spilled on the floor, the floor becomes slippery, creating a work hazard. Dextranomer should be used only in body areas where complete removal is possible (not deep fistulas or sinus tracts).

flexible hydroactive dressings and granules (Duo-Derm)

Mechanism of action. These moisture-reactive dressings for pressure sores and leg ulcers remain in place for 1 to 7 days, and by interacting with the available skin moisture, a bond is created that keeps them in place. While in place over the wound, the moisture-reactive particles imbedded in a polymer base interact with the wound fluid exudate creating a soft moist gel over the wound, which eases dressing removal with minimal damage to newly formed regenerating tissues. The control of wound fluid exudate absorption is a function of the rate at which the dressing interacts with the exudate.

Indications. For necrotic wounds only after the thick eschar at the wound margin is removed. Local management of venous stasis ulcers, ulcers secondary to arterial insufficiency, diabetes mellitus, trauma, pressure sores, and superficial wounds. The granule form is for local management of exudating dermal ulcers in association with the dressings.

Dosage and administration. Clean the wound site before applying this product. Follow the specific instructions outlined in the package labeling.

NURSING CONSIDERATIONS

Assessment. Use in the following dermal conditions should be avoided: tissue of muscle, tendon, or bone, ulcers with infection (tuberculosis, syphilis, or deep fungal infections), active vasculitis (periarteritis nodosa, systemic lupus erythematosus, and cryoglobulinemia).

Intervention. The liquefied material left in the wound (seen when the dressing is removed) has the appearance of pus and should be washed away before further wound evaluation proceeds.

The characteristic disagreeable dermal ulcer odor, apparent when the dressing is removed or from wound leakage, may be diminished with the use of the granule dosage form during excess exudation periods.

Evaluation. During the initial phase of treatment, the wound increases in size and depth because of the cleaning away of the necrotic debris.

During periods of infection, the dressings or granules should be discontinued and antibiotic treatment started until infection is completely treated.

Excessive exudate, when present, may necessitate the granule dosage form application into the wound to prevent leakage and allow the dressing to remain in place longer and reduce dressing changes.

KEY TERMS

BIBLIOGRAPHY

Alteresen, V: Debriding enzymes, J Enterostom Ther 11(3):122, 1984.

Barnes, SH: Patient/family education for the patient with a pressure necrosis, Nurs Clin North Am 22(2):463, 1987.

Becker, L, and others: Treating pressure sores with or without antacid, Am J Nurs 84(3):351, 1984.

Bergtoom, N: A clinical trial of the braden scale for predicting pressure sore risk, Nurs Clin North Am 22(2):417, 1987.

Blom, MF: Dramatic decrease in decubitus ulcers. . . VA quality assurance program stimulated changes, Geriatr Nurs 6(2):84, 1985.

Bobel, LM: Nutritional implications in the patient with pressure sores, Nurs Clin North Am 22(2):379, 1987.

Boykin, A, and others: Pressure sores: nursing management, J Gerontol Nurs 12(12):17, 1986.

Brockenshire, A: Pressure sores: dressings for success, Perspectives, 10(3):4, 1986.

Burg, FD, Johnson, J, and Ellis, N: Managing decubitus ulcers: a case history, Hospital Therapy, 12(12):67, 1987.

Byrne, N, and others: Overcoming the red menace: preventing and treating decubitus ulcers, Nursing 14(4):55, 1984.

David, J: Pressure sore care: float like a butterfly. . . range of aids which can help prevent them, Community Outlook, May 1986, p 19.

Fellin, R: Managing decubitus ulcers: cost savings by substituting hydrocolloid for gauze dressings, Nurs Manage 15(2):29, 1984.

Fowler, E: Comparison of the wet-to-dry dressing and a copolymer starch in the management for bebrided pressure sores, J Enterostom Ther 11(1):22, 1984.

Fowler, EM: Equipment and products used in management and treatment of pressure ulcers, Nurs Clin North Am 22(2):449, 1987.

Frye, BA: A coat of many colors: a program to reduce the incidence of hospital-originated pressure sores, Rehabil Nurs 11(1):24, 1986.

Gesnell, DJ: Assessment and evaluation of pressure sores, Nurs Clin North Am 22(2):399, 1987.

Gould, D: Pressure sore prevention and treatment: an example of nurses' failure to implement research findings, J Adv Nurs 11(4):389, 1986.

Hamilton, L: A pressure sore monitoring program: just the beginning, Perspectives 11(1):6, 1987.

Jones, J: An investigation of the diagnostic skills of nurses on an acute medical unit relating to the identification of risk of pressure sore development in patients, Nurs Pract 1(4):257, 1986.

Kastrup, EK, ed: Facts and comparisons, St Louis, 1988, JB Lippincott Co.

Kendrick, VM, and others: Nursing research at a VNA. . . a transparent, semi-permeable adhesive waterproof dressing. . . in the home, Home Healthcare Nurse 2(5):44, 1984.

Kynes, PM: An integrated approach to risk assessment. . . pressure sores, J Enterostom Ther 13(5):173, 1986.

Lingner, C, and others: Clinical trial of a moisture vapor-permeable dressing on superficial pressure sores, J Enterostom Ther 11(4):147, 1984.

Maklebust, J: Pressure ulcers: etiology and prevention, Nurs Clin North Am 22(2):359, 1987.

Osborne, S: A quality circle investegation. . . reducing the incidence of pressure sores, Nurs Times 83(7):73, 1987.

Preston, KM: Dermal ulcers: simplifying a complex problem, Rehabil Nurs 12(1):17, 1987.

Pritchard, V: Pressure sores: calculating the risk, Nurs Times 82(8):59, 1986.

Robnett, MK: The incidence of skin breakdown in a surgical intensive care unit, J Nurs Qual Assur 1(1):77, 1986.

Ryan, B: Updating skin care for the orthopeadic patient, CONA J k(4):10, 1986.

Sawyer, PN (moderator; a Modern Medicine Forum): Treatment alternatives for pressure sores, Modern Medicine, November 15-30, 1980, p. 49.

Shannon, ML: Five famous fallacies about pressure sores, Nursing 14(10):34, 1984.

Stoneberg, C, and others: Pressure sores in the homebound: one solution. . . alternating pressure pads (APPs), Am J Nurs 86(4):426, 1986.

United States Pharmacopeial Convention: Drug information for the health care provider, ed 8. Rockville, Md, 1988, The Convention.

VanDuyn, OM and Stanaszek, WF: Decubitus ulcers: case studies in pharmacy practice, US Pharmacist 6(3):28, 1981.

Wright, D, and others: Pressure to act. . .pressure sore survey applied to everyday clinical practice, Senior Nurse 5(1):12, 1986.

Yankony, GM, and others: Pressure sore management: efficacy of a moisture reactive occlusive dressing, Arch Phys Med Rehabil 65(10):597, 1984.

UNIT XVIII

Intravenous and Nutritional Therapy

Vitamins and Minerals

OBJECTIVES

After studying this chapter, the student will be able to:

1. Review the recommended daily allowances of vitamins and minerals.

2. Discuss factors that might contribute to inadequate intake of vitamins and minerals.

3. Describe the difference between fat-soluble and water-soluble vitamins.

4. Cite the results of a deficiency or excess of each vitamin.

5. Identify the nursing considerations essential to the administration of vitamins in general and for each vitamin specifically.

6. Compare the contents of OTC vitamin and mineral preparations with the recommended daily allowances.

Under usual circumstances, nutritional needs are best met by adequate oral ingestion of fluids and regular, balanced meals. Breast milk or formula meets the normal nutrition needs of the infant; strained and chopped table foods are added to the diet as tolerated by the growing child. Throughout life, challenges to nutrition status can occur that necessitate nutrient, vitamin, mineral, electrolyte, and fluid replacement or supplementation.

Debilitation from nutritional deprivation may impair wound healing; reduce collagen, hormone, and enzyme synthesis; and decrease essential protein production, reducing circulating albumin, fibrinogen, and hemoglobin. Malnutrition or mild to moderate starvation produces serious cellular biochemical changes, including diminished liver glycogen stores starting the first day of deprivation. Diminished protein stores are supplemented via **gluconeogenesis,** since amino acids are converted into glucose as an energy source. Tissue proteins are depleted and short-lived in the intestinal mucous membranes, liver, pancreas, and kidney tubular epithelia. Muscle proteins are converted to provide energy, and adipose tissues are metabolized to produce free fatty acids for energy substrates. The byproducts of fatty acid oxidation (ketones) are used as energy for the brain if starvation is prolonged.

Unusual or abnormal circumstances necessitating administration of the various nutritional modalities such as vitamin replacement and enteral or parenteral feedings are discussed in the following sections.

VITAMINS

Adequate vitamin intake is of critical biochemical importance because vitamins help maintain normal metabolic functions, growth, and repair of tissue. Mechanisms of action, specific indications for use, and pharmacokinetics are not well understood for all vitamins, nor have dosages been established for all vitamins. However, vitamin supplement therapy may be essential during periods of nutrition challenge, typically during rapid growth, pregnancy, lactation, or convalescence. Other challenges to nutrition occur with inadequate nutrient ingestion or absorption and inordinate nutrient drain caused by neoplastic disorders; cancer thus has been called the "nitrogen trap."

Insufficient dietary intake of vitamins and other essential nutrients occasionally may be traced to impoverished diets resulting from cultural, religious, or personal beliefs; fad diets; alcoholism; poverty; ignorance; or lack of available foodstuffs. Mild forms of **avitaminosis,** however, are more common in the United States and Canada (often as a result of alcoholism) than the pronounced deficiency states of beriberi, pellagra, rickets, or scurvy. The potential for iatrogenic starvation, however, exists because of ignorance or oversight on the part of health care personnel who routinely fail to assess their clients'

nutrition status or do not know how to correct it when necessary. Many medical procedures also may potentiate client malnutrition. In addition, clients often are kept from oral intake or on a restricted diet for too long.

The ubiquitous IV D5W infusion only delivers 170 calories/L—and purely in the form of a carbohydrate. Multiple cleansing enemas or prolonged gastrointestinal suction rob the body of essential electrolytes. Only perfunctory medical assessment may be made of the effects of intraoperative blood losses or of wound drainage on nutrition needs, and surgery always is accompanied by increased nitrogen excretion. Also, common nursing problems that result when the client does not, cannot, or will not eat are often not given adequate medical attention to enable satisfactory nursing care. Vitamin preparations and other, more aggressive supportive nutrition therapies are needed for the hospitalized patient more often than recognized.

Few vitamins are synthesized by the body. Vitamin K is formed by bacteria in the gut; vitamin D is produced when skin is exposed to sunlight; and small, insufficient amounts of vitamin B also are made in the gut. Thus most vitamins must either be ingested in food or taken as dietary supplements. Although the average American diet contains adequate vitamins, vitamin sales in the United

TABLE 69-1   Recommended Daily Dietary Allowances (Designed for the Maintenance of Good Nutrition of Practically All Healthy People in the United States)*

| | Age (years) | Weight | | Height | | Protein (g) | Fat-Soluble Vitamins | | |
		kg	lb	cm	in		Vitamin A (µg RE)†	Vitamin D (µg)‡	Vitamin E (mg α TE)§
Infants	0-0.5	6	13	60	24	kg × 2.2	420	10	3
	0.5-1.0	9	20	71	28	kg × 2	400	10	4
Children	1-3	13	29	90	35	23	400	10	5
	4-6	20	44	112	44	30	500	10	6
	7-10	28	62	132	52	34	700	10	7
Males	11-14	45	99	157	62	45	1000	10	8
	15-18	66	145	176	69	56	1000	10	10
	19-22	70	154	177	70	56	1000	7.5	10
	23-50	70	154	178	70	56	1000	5	10
	51+	70	154	178	70	56	1000	5	10
Females	11-14	46	101	157	62	46	800	10	8
	15-18	55	120	163	64	46	800	10	8
	19-22	55	120	163	64	44	800	7.5	8
	23-50	55	120	163	64	44	800	5	8
	51+	55	120	163	64	44	800	5	8
Pregnant						+30	+200	+5	+2
Lactating						+20	+400	+5	+3

From Food and Nutrition Board, National Academy of Sciences–National Research Council, Washington, DC, 1980.
*The allowances are intended to provide for individual variations among most normal persons as they live in the United States under usual environmental stresses. Diets should be based on a variety of common foods in order to provide other nutrients for which human requirements have been less well defined.
†Retinol equivalents. 1 Retinol equivalent = 1 µg retinol or 6 µg β carotene.
‡As cholecalciferol, 10 µg cholecalciferol = 400 IU vitamin D.
§α-Tocopherol equivalents. 1 mg d-α-tocopherol = 1 α TE.

States constitute a multimillion-dollar industry, largely because of advertising. Widespread vitamin use is often an unjustified effort to improve on normal health. **Hypervitaminosis** is an occasional result.

Tables 69-1 and 69-2 list recommended daily dietary allowances (RDAs) for various vitamins and minerals.

The Food and Drug Administration issues a vitamin dosage listing known as the "U.S. Recommended Daily Allowance" (U.S. RDA) for labeling purposes. This listing is the common reference used in pharmacist-client teaching. Also the latter values are usually higher than the RDA values. See Table 69-3.

Vitamins are classified as being fat soluble or water soluble. **Fat-soluble vitamins** are A, D, E, and K. They are stored in the liver and fatty tissue in large amounts, and a deficiency in these vitamins occurs only after long deprivation from an adequate supply or disorders preventing their absorption. **Water-soluble vitamins** include the B-complex group and C. These vitamins are not stored in the body in large amounts, and short periods of inadequate intake can lead to a deficiency. Vitamins are important components of enzyme systems that catalyze the reactions for protein, fat, and carbohydrate metabolism.

The FDA proposes regulations dividing vitamin mineral products into three categories:

1. *Supplement*—all ingredients are within established limits
2. *Over-the-counter proprietary*—vitamin-mineral contents exceed the limits established for supplement use, but not excessively
3. *Prescription status*—contents exceed the upper limit for over-the-counter proprietary products

Many multivitamin capsules and tablets vary in their contents. Some contain ingredients such as biotin and pantothenic acid, for which evidence about their essential role in human nutrition is inconclusive.

"Optional vitamins" (E, B_6, folic acid, pantothenic acid, and B_{12}) may or may not be included as ingredients in over-the-counter multivitamin preparations. However, the most popular over-the-counter multivitamin preparations contain all vitamins needed by human beings. Most over-the-counter vitamin preparations are designed to fulfill daily body needs completely without regard for the amounts of various vitamins contained in the daily diet.

THE NURSE'S ROLE IN VITAMIN USE

Good nutrition is essential for good health. The nurse's participation in health promotion includes the provision of information regarding all aspects of nutrition. With the

Water-soluble vitamins							Minerals					
Vitamin C (mg)	Thiamin (mg)	Riboflavin (mg)	Niacin (mg NE)‖	Vitamin B_6 (mg)	Folacin¶ (µg)	Vitamin B_{12}# (µg)	Calcium (mg)	Phosphorus (mg)	Magnesium (mg)	Iron (mg)	Zinc (mg)	Iodine (µg)
35	0.3	0.4	6	0.3	30	0.5	360	240	50	10	3	40
35	0.5	0.6	8	0.6	45	1.5	540	360	70	15	5	50
45	0.7	0.8	9	0.9	100	2.0	800	800	150	15	10	70
45	0.9	1.0	11	1.3	200	2.5	800	800	200	10	10	90
45	1.2	1.4	16	1.6	300	3.0	800	800	250	10	10	120
50	1.4	1.6	18	1.8	400	3.0	1200	1200	350	18	15	150
60	1.4	1.7	18	2	400	3.0	1200	1200	400	18	15	150
60	1.5	1.7	19	2.2	400	3.0	800	800	350	10	15	150
60	1.4	1.6	18	2.2	400	3.0	800	800	350	10	15	150
60	1.2	1.4	16	2.2	400	3.0	800	800	350	10	15	150
50	1.1	1.3	15	1.8	400	3.0	1200	1200	300	18	15	150
60	1.1	1.3	14	2	400	3.0	1200	1200	300	18	15	150
60	1.1	1.3	14	2	400	3.0	800	800	300	18	15	150
60	1.0	1.2	13	2	400	3.0	800	800	300	18	15	150
60	1.0	1.2	13	2	400	3.0	800††	800	300	10	15	150
+20	+0.4	+0.3	+2	+0.6	+400	+1.0	+400	+400	+150	**	+5	+25
+40	+0.5	+0.5	+5	+0.5	+100	+1.0	+400	+400	+150	**	+10	+50

‖NE (niacin equivalent) is equal to 1 mg of niacin or 60 mg of dietary tryptophan.

¶The folacin allowances refer to dietary sources as determined by *Lactobacillus casei* assay after treatment with enzymes ("conjugates") to make polyglutamyl forms of the vitamin available for the test organism.

#The RDA for vitamin B_{12} in infants is based on average concentration of the vitamin in human milk. The allowances after weaning are based on energy intake (as recommended by the American Academy of Pediatrics) and consideration of other factors such as intestinal absorption.

**The increased requirement during pregnancy cannot be met by the iron content of habitual American diets nor by the existing iron stores of many women; therefore the use of 30-60 mg of supplemental iron is recommended. Iron needs during lactation are not substantially different from those of nonpregnant women, but continued supplementation of the mother for 2-3 months after parturition is advisable to replenish stores depleted by pregnancy.

††New recommendations may be adopted to prevent postmenopausal osteoporosis in this age-group.

TABLE 69-2   Estimated Safe and Adequate Daily Intakes of Additional Selected Vitamins and Minerals*

	Age (years)	Vitamins			Trace elements†	
		Vitamin K (μg)	Biotin (μg)	Pantothenic acid (mg)	Copper (mg)	Manganese (mg)
Infants	0-0.5	12	35	2	0.5-0.7	0.5-0.7
	0.5-1	10-20	50	3	0.7-1	0.7-1
Children	1-3	15-30	65	3	1-1.5	1.0-1.5
	4-6	20-40	85	3-4	1.5-2	1.5-2
	7-10	30-60	120	4-5	2-2.5	2.0-3
Adolescents	11 +	50-100	100-200	4-7	2-3	2.5-5
Adults		70-140	100-200	4-7	2-3	2.5-5

From Recommended dietary allowances, Food and Nutrition Board, National Academy of Sciences–National Research Council, Washington, DC, 1980.
*Because there is less information on which to base allowances, these figures are not given in the main tables of the RDA and are provided here in the form of ranges of recommended intakes.
†Since the toxic levels for many trace elements may be only several times usual intakes, the upper levels for the trace elements given in this table should not be habitually exceeded.

TABLE 69-3   U.S. Recommended Daily Allowances for Labeling Purposes

Vitamins, minerals	Infants	Children under 4	Adults and children 4 years and older	Pregnant† lactating women
vitamin A	1500 IU	2500 IU	5,000 IU	8,000 IU
vitamin D	400 IU	400 IU	400 IU	400 IU
vitamin E	5 IU	10 IU	30 IU	30 IU
vitamin C	35 mg	40 mg	60 mg	60 mg
folacin*	0.1 mg	0.2 mg	0.4 mg	0.8 mg
thiamine	0.5 mg	0.7 mg	1.5 mg	1.7 mg
riboflavin	0.6 mg	0.8 mg	1.7 mg	2.0 mg
niacin	8 mg	9 mg	20 mg	20 mg
pyridoxine	0.4 mg	0.7 mg	2 mg	2.5 mg
cyanocobalamin	2 ug	3 ug	6 ug	8 ug
pantothenic acid	3 mg	5 mg	10 mg	10 mg
calcium	0.6 Gram	0.8 Gram	1 Gram	1.3 Gram
phosphorus	0.5 Gram	0.8 Gram	1 Gram	1.3 Gram
iodine	45 ug	70 ug	150 ug	150 ug
iron	15 mg	10 mg	18 mg	18 mg
magnesium	70 mg	200 mg	400 mg	450 mg
manganese†	0.5 mg	1 mg	4 mg	4 mg
copper	0.6 mg	1 mg	2 mg	2 mg
zinc	5 mg	8 mg	15 mg	15 mg

*Folacin refers to all folic acid derivatives that have vitamin activity.
†Proposed U.S. RDA values. (Davidson, 1986)

many misconceptions regarding vitamins and their function in health and the prevention of illness prevalent today, the nurse has an important role in the provision of accurate dietary counseling with regard to vitamins.

Assessment. A dietary history for the client will provide the nurse with insights into the client's eating patterns, i.e., the last 24-hour period. This will enable the nurse to be more specific with the client regarding his or her dietary needs.

Assess for signs of the specific vitamin deficiency throughout therapy.

Intervention. Use the calibrated measuring devise provided by the manufacturer for accurate dosing. Chewable tablets should be thoroughly chewed or crushed before swallowing.

Caution is to be used in administering fat-soluble vitamins to children, since they are more sensitive to high doses.

Education. Discussions with the client regarding vitamins should cover their function in the body, signs of vitamin deficiency, and unproven uses.

Diet is the treatment of choice in vitamin deficiencies;

Trace elements†				Electrolytes		
Fluoride (mg)	Chromium (mg)	Selenium (mg)	Molybdenum (mg)	Sodium (mg)	Potassium (mg)	Chloride (mg)
0.1-0.5	0.001-0.04	0.01-0.04	0.03-0.06	115-350	350-925	295-700
0.2-1	0.02-0.06	0.02-0.06	0.04-0.08	250-750	425-1275	400-1200
0.5-1.5	0.02-0.08	0.02-0.08	0.05-0.1	325-975	550-1650	500-1500
1-2.5	0.03-0.12	0.03-0.12	0.06-0.15	450-1350	775-2325	700-2100
1.5-2.5	0.05-0.2	0.05-0.2	0.1-0.3	600-1800	1000-3000	925-2775
1.5-2.5	0.05-0.2	0.05-0.2	0.15-0.5	900-2700	1525-4575	1400-4200
1.5-4	0.05-0.2	0.05-0.2	0.15-0.5	1100-3300	1875-5625	1700-5100

vitamins are not a substitute for a balanced diet. Instruct the client in the four basic food groups and, in particular, specific foods that supply the vitamin in which he or she is deficient. Supplements are only needed if the dietary intake is insufficient to meet body requirements. Megadoses are not recommended, and there is the risk of toxicity with chronic overdoses. The RDA should not be exceeded.

FAT-SOLUBLE VITAMINS

vitamin A:
vitamin A capsules (Alphalin, Aquasol A)
vitamin A oral solution (Aquasol A)

Vitamin A, the fat-soluble, growth-promoting vitamin, is essential for growth in the younger age-groups for maintenance of health at all ages. The chemistry of this vitamin is related to the carotenoid pigments of plants, especially carotene; the term *vitamin A* may be applied to vitamin A, α-carotene, β-carotene, γ-carotene, and cryptoxanthin. The last four factors are formed in plants and are precursors of vitamin A in the body; β-carotene is hydrolyzed in the body to form two molecules of vitamin A.

Vitamin A may be found in spinach. Plant carotene also supplies the provitamin from which the body tissues prepare vitamin A. The amount of chlorophyll in the plant is a rough indication of the amount of carotene present. Animal fats, such as those found in butter, milk, eggs, and fish liver, are sources of the carotenoids that were originally derived from plants and stored in animal tissues.

Mechanism of action. Vitamin A is essential in promoting normal growth and development of bones and teeth and maintaining the health of epithelial tissues of the body. Its function in relation to normal vision and the prevention of night blindness has been studied carefully. Vitamin A actually is part of one of the major retinal pigments, rhodopsin, and thus is required for normal "rod vision" in the retina of human beings and many animals.

Vitamin A also has a function in the conversion processes resulting in corticosterone and cholesterol.

Indications
1. Used to treat or relieve symptoms associated with a deficiency of vitamin A, such as night blindness (**nyctalopia**), **hyperkeratosis,** retarded growth, **xerophthalmia, keratomalacia,** weakness, and increased susceptibility of mucous membranes to infection.
2. Certain analogs are used to treat acne (see Chapter 67).
3. The diet low in vitamin A should be corrected with foods rather than with drugs. It appears that large doses of vitamin A may cause neurologic and skin damage in adults, and excessive doses are known to produce highly toxic effects in rats and in young children.
4. At times vitamin A concentrates have a legitimate use as dietary supplements. Increased need occurs during pregnancy and lactation, in infancy, and in conditions characterized by lack of normal absorption and storage of vitamin A.

Pharmacokinetics. Vitamin A and carotene are readily absorbed from the normal gastrointestinal tract. Efficient absorption depends on fat absorption and therefore on the presence of adequate bile salts in the intestine. Certain conditions, such as obstructive jaundice, some infectious diseases, and the presence of mineral oil in the intestine, may result in vitamin A deficiency in spite of the amount ingested being normal.

Vitamin A is stored to a greater extent in the liver than elsewhere. The liver also functions in changing carotene to vitamin A; this function is inhibited in liver diseases and in diabetes. The amount of vitamin A stored depends on the dietary intake. When intake is high or excessive, the stores formed in the liver may be sufficient to last a long time.

Metabolism. Liver
Excretion. Feces/kidneys
Side effects/adverse reactions. See Table 69-4.
Significant drug interactions. When vitamin A is given concurrently with isotretinoin, an additive increase in side effects may result. Avoid concurrent administration if possible. If not, monitor closely.

TABLE 69-4   Vitamins: Significant Side Effects/Adverse Reactions

Vitamin	Side effects	Adverse reactions
vitamin A	—	Acute overdose: Diplopia, severe headaches, increased agitation, skin peeling on lips and palms, severe vomiting, gum bleeding, mouth soreness, confusion or enhanced excitability, diarrhea, sedation, dizziness, convulsions. In babies, may see a bulging spot on the head and hydrocephalus. Older children and adults may have an increase in intracranial pressure. Toxicity appears approximately 6 hours after an overdose. Reversible if vitamin ingestion is discontinued. Chronic overdose: May result in pain in bones and joints, elevated temperature, feeling of weakness, headaches, anorexia, alopecia, abdominal pain, vomiting, increased irritability, increased frequency of urination (especially at night), skin photosensitivity, yellow-orange color discoloration on soles of feet, palms of hands or skin near nose and lips. May also see hepatotoxicity, intracranial and portal hypertension, anemia, hemolysis, and papilledema. Toxicity is slowly reversible on discontinuing vitamin A.
vitamin D	—	Early signs of toxicity associated with hypercalcemia: Diarrhea, constipation seen more often in children and adolescents, dry mouth, continuous headaches, thirst, anorexia, metallic taste in mouth, nausea or vomiting—more often seen in children and adolescents. Increased weakness. Later signs of vitamin D toxicity associated with hypercalcemia: bone pain, elevated blood pressure, pruritus, increased urinary frequency (especially at night), eye irritation or increased sensitivity of eyes to lights, cloudy urine, mood alterations, nausea or vomiting, severe abdominal pain, convulsions, weight loss, irregular heart rate. Severe toxicity is manifested by vascular and soft tissue calcification that may result in hypertension or renal failure. Growth in children may be arrested. Death can occur because of renal or heart failure.
vitamin E	Large doses: Visual disturbances, diarrhea, headaches, flu symptoms, nausea, abdominal cramps, severe weakness, lightheadedness, breast enlargement in both sexes	Very large doses, that is, over 800 units/day for long time periods—altered hormone metabolism such as thyroid, adrenal and pituitary, altered immunity, increased bleeding problems in vitamin K deficient persons.
niacin	Less frequent with niacin only: Feeling flush or warm, red skin especially in face and neck areas, headaches. Large doses: Diarrhea, lightheadedness, dry skin, nausea or vomiting, abdominal pain	Less frequent with niacin only: rash, pruritus or wheezing (with IV administration). Large doses may also result in elevated serum levels of glucose and uric acid, liver toxicity, and cardiac arrhythmias.
ascorbic acid	Less frequent/rare: Lightheadedness (with IV injection). With high doses: Diarrhea (in oral daily doses of more than 1 g), red, flushing of skin, headaches, nausea or vomiting, increased urination in doses more than 600 mg/day, abdominal cramps	Dose-related effects: Side or back (lower) pain because of oxalate stones in urinary tract.

Dosage and administration

Recommended daily dietary allowance (RDA). Studies have established conclusively that the vitamin A daily requirement is rather large if optimal conditions of nutrition are to be maintained. Vitamin A RDAs are 400 to 420 μg RE (retinol equivalents) for infants, 400 to 700 μg RE for children, and 800 to 1000 μg RE for adults. During pregnancy and lactation, requirements increase by 200 and 400 μg RE, respectively. Therapeutic dosages may be 3 times these amounts. Although larger doses have been used in experimental studies, no evidence justifies the use of more than 25,000 μg RE/day. Excessive dosage over the daily requirements has not been shown to help in the prevention of colds, influenza, and so on. When the vitamin A requirement is met in the form of carotene or the provitamin A, twice as many units of the carotene are required to produce the same effect.

vitamin D:
calcifediol capsules (Calderol)
calcitriol capsules (Rocaltrol)
calcitriol injection (Calcijex)
dihydrotachysterol capsules (Hytakerol)
dihydrotachysterol oral solution (DHT, DHT Intensol, Hytakerol)
dihydrotachysterol tablets (DHT)
ergocalciferol capsules (Deltalin, Drisdol, Ostoforte✻, Radiostol✻)
ergocalciferol tablets (Calciferol)
ergocalciferol infection (Calciferol)

The term *vitamin D* is applied to two or more substances that affect the proper utilization of calcium and phosphorus in the body. Two forms of naturally occurring vitamin D have been isolated. One is obtained as a product of irradiated ergosterol and is known as vitamin D_2 or ergocalciferol. Ergosterol has therefore been shown to be a precursor of vitamin D. Further investigation has shown that several precursors can be changed by irradiation into compounds that have vitamin D activity. Irradiation of 7-dehydrocholesterol results in the formation of vitamin D_3 (cholecalciferol), which is stored in the body. It also is formed in skin exposed to sunlight. Irradiated ergosterol (calciferol) is the active constituent in various vitamin preparations, such as viosterol and irradiated yeast.

Vitamins D_2 and D_3, as well as other products of irradiated ergosterol, are capable of antirachitic activity (see "mechanism of action").

Although an essential vitamin, vitamin D is contained in only a few foods (milk, bread, cereals, animal livers) of the average American diet. Small amounts are present in herring, sardines, salmon, tuna fish, eggs, and butter. Vitamin D is found in high concentrations in a number of fish oils (cod, halibut).

At present, milk is the chief commercial food product fortified by the addition of vitamin D concentrate. By federal regulation, milk products are standardized at 400 IUg of vitamin D/quart, which represents a day's requirement.

Mechanism of action. The exact mechanism by which vitamin D functions in the metabolism of calcium and phosphorus is not known. Evidence suggests that a complex relationship exists between vitamin D and parathyroid hormone, but this is not yet conclusive. The vitamin seems to be involved directly with the absorption of calcium and phosphorus from the intestinal tract and their deposition in bone and teeth. In the absence of vitamin D, the amount of these substances absorbed from the bowel is diminished to such an extent that even though the calcium and phosphate intake is adequate, rickets results in the child and osteomalacia in the adult.

When skin is exposed to the ultraviolet rays in sunlight, cholecalciferol (vitamin D_3) is formed. Ergocalciferol (calciferol, vitamin D_2) is usually found in vitamin preparations, and cholecalciferol is added to vitamin D–fortified milk. Both cholecalciferol and ergocalciferol are metabolized in the liver to calcifediol (25-hydroxycholecalciferol), which is then transported to the kidney where it is converted to calcitriol (1,25-dihydroxycholecalciferol, which is believed to be the most active analog). Dihydrotachysterol is a synthetic product of ergocalciferol that has only weak **antirachitic** activity; it is activated metabolically in the liver. Calcifediol appears to have intrinsic vitamin D activity in addition to its conversion to the active metabolite.

Calcitriol, which appears to bind to a receptor in the intestinal mucosa, is incorporated into the cell nucleus, resulting in the formation of a calcium-binding protein that increases calcium absorption from the intestine. Parathyroid hormone and calcitriol both act to control the transfer of calcium ions from bones into the extracellular fluid; therefore they maintain a calcium homeostasis effect in the extracellular fluid.

Indications

For the prevention and treatment of rickets. The incidence of rickets is low in the United States but it can occur in young children who are restricted to vegetarian diets without milk supplementation or in infants who are breast fed by mothers who did not take prenatal vitamins nor drink milk. It is primarily caused by a vitamin D deficiency that results in an inadequate intake and perhaps, an excessive loss of calcium from the body. Rickets results in soft bones, deformed joints, and bone deformities.

For the treatment of chronic hypocalcemia, hypophosphatemia, and osteodystrophy.

For the prevention and treatment of vitamin D deficiency states caused by improper nutrition or intestinal malabsorption conditions.

For the prevention and treatment of tetany. (Dihydrotachysterol is the preferred product for acute, chronic, or latent types of postsurgical tetany and idiopathic tetany.)

For the treatment of osteomalacia in adults.

Pharmacokinetics

Absorption. Absorption best from the small intestine. Cholecalciferol is absorbed better than ergocalciferol because the latter requires the presence of bile salts for absorption.

Protein binding. Transported by specific alpha globulins

Storage. Mostly in liver and fat depots

Metabolism. See discussion in Mechanism of Action. Both cholecalciferol and ergocalciferol require two steps for metabolic activation, that is the liver and kidneys. Calcifediol is activated by the kidneys, whereas dihydrotachysterol is activated in the liver. Calcitriol does not require any special metabolic activation. The kidneys are also responsible in part for degradation of these substances.

Serum half-life. Calcifediol: 10 to 22 days (usually 16 days); calcitriol: within 3 to 8 hours; ergocalciferol: within 19 to 48 hours, but it can be stored in fat sites for longer time periods

Onset of action. Hypercalcemic effect: calcitriol—orally within 2 to 6 hours; dihydrotachysterol—within hours, although maximum effect is seen in 7 to 14 days; ergocalciferol—within 12 to 24 hours, although therapeutic response may not be seen until 10 to 14 days later

Time to peak serum concentration. Calcifediol: in about 4 hours; calcitriol: orally in approximately 2 hours

Duration of effect following oral administration. Calcifediol: 15 to 20 days (in renal failure this can be increased 2 or 3 times); calcitriol: in 24 to 48 hours; dihydrotachysterol: up to 9 weeks; ergocalciferol: up to 6 months

Excretion. Bile, kidneys

Side effects/adverse reactions. See Table 69-4.

Significant drug interactions. The following interactions may occur when vitamin D products are given concurrently with the drugs listed below.

Drug	Possible Effect and Management
antacids containing magnesium	If given with calcifediol or calcitriol, hypermagnesemia may result, especially in clients with chronic renal failure. Avoid concurrent administration if possible; if not, monitor closely.
vitamin D, other products	Not recommended because of additive effects resulting in an increased risk of toxicity.

Dosage and administration

calcifediol capsules (Calderol)

Adults. 0.3 to 0.35 mg orally initially weekly on a daily or alternate day schedule. Dosage may be increased if necessary, at monthly intervals.

Children

Less than 2 years old: 0.02 to 0.05 mg (20 to 50 μg) orally daily

2 to 10 years old: 0.05 mg (50 μg) orally daily

10 years and over: see adult dosage

calcitriol capsules (Rocaltrol)

Adults. 0.25 μg (0.00025 mg) orally initially daily. Dosage may be increased by 0.25 μg every 2 to 4 weeks if necessary up to the following:

Hypocalcemia in chronic dialysis clients: orally, 0.5 to 3 μg or more daily

Hypoparathyroidism: 0.25 to 2.7 μg orally daily

Renal osteodystrophy: 0.25 μg orally every other day up to 3 μg or more daily

Divided doses daily may be the preferred way of giving this drug.

Children. 0.25 μg orally daily. Dosage may be increased by 0.25 μg every 2 to 4 weeks if necessary up to following:

Hypocalcemia in chronic dialysis: 0.25 to 2 μg orally daily.

Hypoparathyroidism: 0.04 to 0.08 μg/kg orally daily.

Renal osteodystrophy: 0.014 to 0.041 μg/kg orally daily.

calcitriol injection (Calcijex)

Adults. As antihypocalcemic agent:

Initially: 0.5 to 0.01 μg/kg by rapid intravenous injection, three times per week. Dosage may be increased by 0.25 to 0.5 μg every 2 to 4 weeks if necessary.

Maintenance: 0.5 to 0.3 μg or 0.01 to 0.05 μg/kg by rapid intravenous injection, three times per week

Children. Not established

dihydrotachysterol capsules (Hytakerol)/oral solution (DHT, DHT Intensol, Hytakerol)/tablets (DHT)

Adults. Usually 0.125 mg (125 μg) to 2 mg daily. Hypocalcemic tetany:

Initially:

Acute—750 μg (0.75 mg) to 2.5 mg orally daily for 3 days

Less acute situation—250 to 500 μg (0.25 to 0.5 mg) orally daily for 3 days

Maintenance: 250 μg (0.25 mg) orally per week to 1 mg/day, as needed

Hypoparathyroidism:

Initially: 750 μg (0.75 mg) to 2.5 mg orally daily for several days

Maintenance: 200 μg (0.2 mg) to 1 mg orally daily

Children. Hypoparathyroidism:

Initially, 1 to 5 mg orally daily for 4 days; then either continue or decrease to one-fourth the dose

Maintenance: 500 μg (0.5 mg) to 1.5 mg orally daily

ergocalciferol capsules (Deltalin, Drisdol, Ostoforte, Radiostol)/oral solution (Calciferol, Drisdol, Radiostol, Radiostol Forte)/tablets (Calciferol)

Adults

Vitamin D deficiency: 1000 to 2000 units orally daily. Reduce dosage to 400 units/day as soon as possible (when appropriate).

Vitamin D–resistant rickets: 12,000 to 500,000 units orally per day

Osteomalacia resulting from chronic administration of anticonvulsants: 1000 to 4000 units orally daily

Familial hypophosphatemia: 50,000 to 100,000 units orally daily

Hypoparathyroidism: 50,000 to 150,000 units orally daily

Children

Vitamin D deficiency: 1000 to 4000 units orally daily. Reduce dose to 400 units daily when appropriate.

Osteomalacia caused by chronic administration of anticonvulsants: 1000 units orally daily

Hypoparathyroidism: 50,000 to 200,000 units orally daily

ergocalciferol injection (Calciferol)

Adults. Malabsorption: administer 10,000 units intramuscularly daily

Children. See adult dose.

Pregnancy safety. No documented problems in humans with intake of normal daily requirements. In animals, doses of calcitriol, dihydrotachysterol, and calcifediol in excess of recommended daily dose (4 to 15 times more), have been found to be teratogenic. Thus, pregnancy safety is FDA category C.

NURSING CONSIDERATIONS

See also the nurse's role in vitamin therapy.

Assessment. The administration of vitamin D is contraindicated in clients with hypercalcemia and hypervitaminosis D. The nurse's assessment should rule out these conditions before initiation of vitamin D therapy. Other conditions for which caution should be used in the administration of vitamin D are arteriosclerosis, hyperphosphatemia, hypersensitivity to vitamin D, and renal or cardiac impairment.

Along with periodic evaluations of renal function, serum calcium levels should be monitored, particularly in the early weeks of therapy, to assist in the determination of the appropriate dosage levels. Serum calcium values should be in the 8 to 9 mg/100 ml range and the calcium times phosphorus product (Ca x P in milligrams per 100 ml) should not be greater than 58. Other examinations may be required according to the client's response to therapy.

Children should have their growth measurements monitored over the course of therapy. Growth may be inhibited by prolonged administration of the drug.

Assess for signs of toxicity: constipation; anorexia, nausea, and vomiting; metallic taste and dryness in the mouth; and headache.

Education. Stress the importance of regular visits to the health care provider to monitor progress.

Review with the client any instructions for a special diet or for a calcium supplement, if prescribed. Foods high in vitamin D include fish and fish liver oils, as well as vitamin D–fortified milk.

The client should be cautioned not to use any over-the-counter products that contain calcium, phosphorus, or vitamin D unless approved by the physician. Clients taking calcifediol or calcitriol should avoid the use of antacids containing magnesium.

vitamin E (tocopherol):
vitamin E capsules (Aquasol E; E-Ferol; Eprolin; Epsilan-M)
vitamin E solution (Aquasol E)
vitamin E tablets (Pheryl-E)
vitamin E chewable tablets (Chew-E)
vitamin E injection in oil (E-Ferol)

Vitamin E is a fat-soluble vitamin, the richest source of which is wheat germ oil. Vitamin E also occurs in other vegetable oils, such as cottonseed oil and peanut oil, and is found in green, leafy vegetables.

Several compounds have been found that exhibit vitamin E activity. The most active of these are the tocopherols, of which three are naturally occurring compounds known as α-, β-, and γ-tocopherol. The most biologically potent of these compounds is α-tocopherol.

A vitamin E deficiency was seen in the late 1960s, induced in premature infants that were fed a formula that lacked vitamin E. The symptoms exhibited were hemolysis of erythrocytes, thrombocytosis, and edema that cleared up with administration of vitamin E. Since infant formulations now are supplemented with this vitamin, a vitamin E deficiency in infants is probably remote.

In adults, neuropathies in clients with biliary disease and cystic fibrosis have reportedly responded to vitamin E therapy. Interestingly, animals suffer severe symptoms (muscular dystrophy, sterility, cardiac lesions, and others) from a deficiency in this vitamin that are not recorded in human beings. The reason for this is unknown.

Mechanism of action. Vitamin E is an essential nutrient, but its exact function is unknown. It has antioxidant properties; i.e., when combined with dietary selenium, vitamin E will prevent the effects of peroxidase on unsaturated bonds in the cell membranes and will also protect red blood cells from hemolysis. It is also known to be a cofactor for several enzyme systems in the body.

Indications. For the prevention and treatment of vitamin E deficiency

Pharmacokinetics

Absorption. Orally from 20% to 80% of a dose is absorbed from the duodenum. Absorption requires the presence of bile salts and dietary fat.

Protein binding. Binds to beta lipoproteins in the blood

Storage. In all body tissues but especially fat depots, which contain up to a 4-year requirement of this vitamin

Metabolism. Liver

Excretion. Bile, kidneys

Side effects/adverse reactions. See Table 69-4.

Significant drug interactions. When Vitamin E is given

concurrently with iron supplements, iron's therapeutic effect for iron deficiency anemia may be impaired. Also, large daily doses of iron may result in an increased requirement for vitamin E. If given concurrently, monitor closely to determine an appropriate intervention.

Dosage and administration

vitamin E capsules/oral solution/tablets/chewable tablets

Adults. To prevent vitamin E deficiency, 30 units orally daily. To treat a vitamin E deficiency, 60 to 75 units orally per day.

Children. Treatment of deficiency: 1 unit/kg orally daily or four to five times the RDA orally daily. If premature infants are receiving formulas that are high in polyunsaturated fatty acids, then add 15 to 25 units per day of vitamin E (or 7 units per liter of formula). In normal-birth-weight infants, add 5 units per liter of formula.

vitamin E injection in oil

Adults. Treatment of vitamin E deficiency: administer 60 to 75 units intramuscularly per day.

Children. Treatment of deficiency: administer 1 unit/kg daily, intramuscularly.

NURSING CONSIDERATIONS

See also the nurse's role in vitamin therapy.

Assessment. Before the initiation of vitamin E therapy, it should be ascertained whether the client has hypoprothrombinemia as a result of vitamin K deficiency or iron deficiency anemia because vitamin E will aggravate the former and interfere with the hematologic response to iron therapy in the latter.

Intervention. Water-miscible forms are more readily absorbed from the gastrointestinal tract, but parenteral administration may be necessary if the malabsorption syndrome is severe.

The client taking large doses of vitamin E for prolonged periods of time should be assessed for signs of toxicity: dizziness and drowsiness; impaired vision; breast enlargement; and flulike symptoms.

Education. Although vitamin E deficiency is infrequent, dietary instruction for clients may be necessary. Foods high in vitamin E are vegetable oils, wheat germ, whole-grain cereals, egg yolk, and liver.

vitamin K

Vitamin K is a fat-soluble vitamin. (See Chapter 29 for drug monograph.)

WATER-SOLUBLE VITAMINS

The vitamin B complex refers to a group of vitamins that often are found together in food, although they are chemically dissimilar and have different metabolic functions. Grouping them together is based largely on the historic basis of their having been discovered in sequential order. They have little in common other than their sources and their water solubility. A sensible and increasingly popular trend promotes discarding such names as vitamin B_1 and B_2 and referring to these vitamins as thiamine and riboflavin. The vitamin B complex includes thiamin, riboflavin, nicotinic acid, pyridoxine, folic acid, pantothenic acid, biotin, choline, inositol, and vitamin B_{12} (cyanocobalamin).

This discussion will be limited to the B vitamins that are associated with deficiency states and for which information on therapeutic application is available: thiamine hydrochloride (vitamin B_1), riboflavin (vitamin B_2), niacin (nicotinic acid), pyridoxine hydrochloride (vitamin B_6), vitamin B_{12} (cyanocobalamin), and folic acid.

thiamine (vitamin B_1):
thiamine hydrochloride elixir/tablets (Betalin S, Bewon) thiamine hydrochloride injection (Betalin S, Betaxin✤)

Mechanism of action. Thiamine combines with adenosine triphosphate (ATP) to form thiamine pyrophosphate coenzyme. This is necessary for carbohydrate metabolism.

Indication. To prevent and treat thiamine deficiency, which can result in beriberi or Wernicke's encephalopathy

Pharmacokinetics

Absorption. Very good from duodenum except in malabsorption syndrome

Metabolism. Liver

Excretion. Kidneys

Side effects/adverse reactions. Usually rare. Skin rash, pruritus, or respiratory difficulties (wheezing) may occur rarely after a large intravenous dose is administered (anaphylactic reaction).

Significant drug interactions. Alcohol will inhibit the absorption of thiamine from the gastrointestinal tract.

Dosage and administration

thiamine hydrochloride elixir/tablets

Adults. As nutritional supplement:

Beriberi: 5 to 10 mg orally three times daily in a multivitamin formulation

Treatment of deficiency: 5 to 10 mg orally three times daily until client improves; then reduce to RDA dose

Neuritis in pregnancy caused by thiamine deficiency: 5 to 10 mg daily

Alcohol induced deficiency: 40 mg orally daily

Dietary supplement: 1 to 2 mg orally daily

Children

Infants with mild beriberi: 10 mg orally daily

Treatment of thiamine deficiency: 10 to 50 mg orally daily in divided doses

Dietary supplement:

   Infants—300 to 500 μg (0.3 to 0.5 mg) orally daily
   Other children—500 μg (0.5 mg) orally daily

thiamine hydrochloride injection

Adults. Nutritional supplement–for severe beriberi: 5 to 100 mg intramuscular or by slow intravenous, three times daily followed by oral maintenance

Children. For severe beriberi: 10 to 25 mg by intramuscular or slow intravenous injection

Pregnancy safety. FDA category A

NURSING CONSIDERATIONS

Also see the nurse's role in vitamin therapy.

Assessment. Thiamine rarely causes toxicity in individuals with normal renal function. Skin rash or wheezing may occur as signs of hypersensitivity.

Since it is infrequent that a deficiency of a single B vitamin would occur, the client needs to be assessed for multiple deficiencies.

Intervention. In most instances the vitamin is administered in an oral preparation; however, if this is not acceptable or possible, parenteral forms are available.

Education. Instruction for the client should include sources that are high in thiamine, such as whole grain or enriched cereals and meats, particularly pork.

riboflavin (vitamin B$_2$): riboflavin tablets

Mechanism of action. In the body riboflavin is converted into two coenzymes—flavin mononucleotide (FMN) and flavin adenine dinucleotide (FAD)—that are necessary to normal tissue respiration. Riboflavin is also necessary for pyridoxine activation and may also be connected to maintenance of erythrocyte integrity.

Indications. For the prevention and treatment of riboflavin deficiency; usually does not occur in healthy persons but may be detected as a result of malnutrition or intestinal malabsorption

Pharmacokinetics

Absorption. Very good from gastrointestinal tract, except for malabsorption states

Protein binding. Moderate

Metabolism. Liver

Excretion. Kidneys

Side effects/adverse reactions. Relatively nontoxic. Large doses may cause yellow discoloration of the urine.

Significant drug interactions. Alcohol impairs the absorption of riboflavin.

Dosage and administration

riboflavin tablets

Adults. To treat riboflavin deficiency: 5 to 30 mg orally daily in divided doses for several days; then 1 to 4 mg daily orally

Children. To treat riboflavin deficiency in children 12 years and older: 3 to 10 mg orally for several days; then 600 μg (0.6 mg)/1000 calories consumed orally daily

Pregnancy safety. Not established

NURSING CONSIDERATIONS

Also see the nurse's role in vitamin therapy.

Assessment. Vitamins that are water-soluble rarely cause toxicity in individuals with normal kidney function.

Education. Alert the client that large doses of riboflavin may cause the urine to become yellow in color.

The best food sources of riboflavin are milk and dairy products, meats, and green, leafy vegetables.

niacin (nicotinic acid):
niacin capsules
niacin extended-release capsules (Diacin, Niac, Nico-400, Nicobid, Tr-B3✿)
niacin oral solution (Nicotinex)
niacin tablets (Nicolar)
niacin extended-release tablets (Span-Niacin)
niacinamide capsules/tablets
niacinamide injection

Mechanism of action. Niacin is converted to niacinamide in the body; then it is a part of two coenzymes, nicotinamide adenine dinucleotide (NAD) and nicotinamide adenine dinucleotide phosphate (NADP), which are necessary for glycogenolysis, tissue respiration, and lipid or fat metabolism.

As an antihyperlipid agent, niacin lowers serum cholesterol and triglyceride levels. Niacinamide does not possess these effects.

Indications. For the prevention and treatment of vitamin B$_3$ deficiency conditions. Niacin deficiency may result in pellagra. Niacin only is a treatment adjunct for hyperlipidemia. It's usefulness may be limited by its side effects, especially its vasodilating effects.

Pharmacokinetics

Absorption. Very good from gastrointestinal tract

Metabolism. Liver. Dietary tryptophan is metabolized by intestinal bacteria to niacin and niacinamide (approximately 60 mg of tryptophan is equivalent to 1 mg of niacin). Niacin is also changed to niacinamide as necessary.

Half-life. 45 minutes

Onset of action

To reduce cholesterol levels: Within several days following oral administration

To reduce triglyceride levels: Within several hours after oral administration

Time to peak serum level. Orally within 45 minutes

Excretion. Kidneys

Side effects/adverse reactions. See Table 69-4.

Significant drug interactions. None

Dosage and administration

niacin oral dosage forms

Adults

Vitamin usage to treat pellagra: 50 mg orally 3 to 10 times daily

Dietary supplement: 10 to 20 mg orally daily

In Hartnup disease: 50 to 200 mg orally daily

Antilipidemic effects: 100 mg orally intially, three times daily: increase dosage by 300 mg/day every 4 to 7 days as necessary

Maintenance: 1 to 2 grams orally three times daily (Maximum is 6 g/day.)

Children

To treat pellagra: 100 to 300 mg orally daily in divided dosages

As dietary supplement: 50 to 200 mg orally daily

niacin injection

Adults. Vitamin to treat pellagra: intramuscularly, 50 to 100 mg given five or more times daily; or 25 to 100 mg by slow IV, twice daily, or more often if necessary

Children. Vitamin to treat pellagra: give a dose lower than the oral dose by slow IV.

niacinamide oral

Adults

Vitamin to treat pellagra: 50 mg orally 3 to 10 times daily

As dietary supplement: 10 to 20 mg orally daily

In Hartnup disease: 50 to 200 mg orally daily

Children

Vitamin to treat pellagra: 100 to 300 mg orally in divided dosages

As dietary supplement: 50 to 200 mg daily

niacinamide injection

Adults. Vitamin to treat pellagra: 50 to 100 mg intramuscularly, five or more times daily, as necessary, or 25 to 100 mg by slow IV twice daily or more often, if necessary

Children. Vitamin to treat pellagra: give a dose lower than the oral dose by slow IV.

Pregnancy safety. FDA category C

NURSING CONSIDERATIONS

Also consult the nurse's role in vitamin therapy.

Assessment. Before large doses, it should be determined if the client has arterial bleeding, diabetes mellitus (niacin only), peptic ulcer, or hepatic disease, since all these conditions will be aggravated by niacin and niacinamide.

Intervention. Administer with milk or food to help prevent gastrointestinal distress.

Oral administration of niacin is preferred. Parenteral niacin is used only when the oral route is not acceptable or possible. If administered intravenously, do not exceed a rate of 2 mg/min.

If individuals are receiving large doses of niacin or niacinamide for prolonged periods, blood glucose and hepatic function should be monitored.

Education. Alert the client that for the first 2 weeks of therapy to expect a feeling of warmth, a flushing of the skin of the face and neck shortly after taking the tablets. This sensation may be reduced by starting with a low dosage and gradually increasing to the therapeutic dose. Niacinamide is preferred because it lacks this blushing effect.

Stress the importance of regular visits to the health care provider to monitor the effective of the medication and the client's progress.

Since one of the adverse effects is dizziness, caution the client to avoid hazardous tasks that require mental alertness until the response to the medication has been determined.

The best food sources of niacin are meats, eggs, milk, and other dairy products.

pyridoxine (vitamin B_6):

pyridoxine hydrochloride tablets (Hexa-Betalin)

pyridoxine hydrochloride extended-release capsules (Rodex, TexSix T-R)

pyridoxine hydrochloride injection (Beesix, Hexa-Betalin, Pyroxine)

Mechanism of action. Pyridoxine is taken up by erythrocytes and converted into pyridoxal phosphate. This is a coenzyme necessary for many metabolic functions that affect proteins, carbohydrates, and lipid utilization in the body. Pyridoxine is also involved with the conversion of tryptophan to niacin or serotonin.

Indications. To prevent or treat pyridoxine deficiency. A deficiency state can lead to sideroblastic anemia, neurologic disturbances, seborrheic dermatitis, cheilosis, and xanthurenic aciduria.

Pharmacokinetics

Absorption. Very good from gastrointestinal tract; mainly absorbed from the jejunum

Protein binding. Pyridoxine is not bound to plasma proteins but pyridoxal phosphate is highly bound to plasma proteins.

Metabolism. Liver

Half life. 15 to 20 days

Excretion. Kidneys

Side effects/adverse reactions. Very rare. Side effects are seen only when dosages of 200 mg/day are given for more than a month, resulting in a dependency-type syndrome. Megadoses also can cause severe sensory neuropathy such as ataxia, numb feet, clumsiness. It is reversible when pyridoxine is stopped.

Significant drug interactions. When pyridoxine is given with levodopa, the antiparkinsonian effects of levodopa may be reduced or reversed. This effect is not reported with the carbidopa-levodopa combination.

Dosage and administration
oral dosage forms
Adults
As a nutritional supplement for a pyridoxine dependency syndrome: 30 to 600 mg orally daily initially. Maintenance is 50 mg daily orally for life.
As a dietary supplement: 10 to 20 mg orally daily for 21 days, followed by 2 to 5 mg daily (usually given in a multivitamin formulation) for several weeks
In congenital metabolic dysfunctions (hyperoxaluria, homocystinuria, xanthurenic aciduria): 100 to 500 mg orally daily
For drug-induced deficiency:
Prevention of deficiency—10 to 50 mg orally daily for penicillamine or 100 to 300 mg daily for cycloserine, hydralazine, or isoniazid (INH)
To treat deficiency that is drug induced—50 to 200 mg orally daily for 21 days, followed by 25 to 100 mg daily as required to prevent a relapse
In alcoholism: 50 mg orally daily for 14 to 28 days. If anemia responds, continue pyridoxine indefinitely.
Hereditary sideroblastic anemia: 200 to 600 mg orally daily for 30 to 60 days; then 30 to 50 mg daily for life if drug is effective.
Children.
Nutritional supplement for pyridoxine dependency syndrome:
Infants—maintenance, 2 to 10 mg orally daily for life
Other children—see adult dosage
Dietary supplement: 2.5 to 10 mg orally daily for 21 days, followed by 2 to 5 mg/day (in multivitamin formulation) for several more weeks
pyridoxine hydrochloride injection
Adults
Nutritional supplement for pyridoxine dependency syndrome: 30 to 600 mg intramuscular or intravenous daily initially
To treat a drug-induced deficiency: 50 to 200 mg intramuscular or intravenous daily for 21 days, followed by 25 to 100 mg daily as necessary
Children. Nutritional supplement for pyridoxine dependency syndrome in infants with convulsions: 10 to 100 intramuscular or intravenous initially
Pregnancy safety. Not established

NURSING CONSIDERATIONS

Also consult the nurse's role in vitamin therapy.
Assessment. Initial assessment should determine whether the client has Parkinson's disease, which is treated with levodopa. Pyridoxine reverses the antiparkin-

sonian effects of levodopa.
Education. Large doses of pyridoxine for a period of several months may result in sensory neuropathy affecting gait and numbness of the hands and feet.
Best food sources of pyridoxine are meats, bananas, potatoes, lima beans, and whole grain cereals.

cyanocobalamin (vitamin B_{12}):
cyanocobalamin tablets
cyanocobalamin soluble tablets (Kaybovite)
cyanocobalamin injection (Amacobin✱, Bedoz✱, Betalin 12, Rubramin✱)
hydroxocobalamin:
hydroxocobalamin injection (Acti-B 12✱, alphaREDISOL)

Mechanism of action. A coenzyme for a variety of metabolic functions that include fat and carbohydrate metabolism and protein synthesis. Also needed for growth, cell replication, hematopoiesis, and nucleoprotein and myelin synthesis.
Indications. To treat pernicious anemia (caused by lack of intrinsic factor) or to prevent and treat vitamin B_{12} deficiency caused by malabsorption or strict vegetarianism. Vitamin B_{12} deficiency can lead to megaloblastic anemia and irreversible neurologic damage.
Pharmacokinetics
Absorption. Well absorbed from the lower half of the ileum. Intrinsic factor (IF) must be present in the GI tract for oral absorption to occur.
Protein binding. Very high to transcobalamins. Hydroxocobalamin is higher than cyanocobalamin.
Storage. Liver (90%), some in kidneys
Metabolism. Liver
Half-life. Approximately 6 days, but in liver up to 400 days
Time to peak serum level. Orally within 8 to 12 hours
Excretion. Bile; excess above needs of the body by way of the kidneys
Side effects/adverse reactions. Rare. After parenteral injection, anaphylactic reactions are rarely seen. Less frequently seen are diarrhea and pruritus.
Significant drug interactions. None
Dosage and administration
cyanocobalamin
Oral dosage forms
Adults (dietary supplement): 1 μg (0.01 mg) orally daily or up to 25 μg (0.025 mg) daily if necessary
Children. (dietary supplement):
Up to 1 year old: 0.3 μg (0.0003 mg) orally daily
1 year and older: 1 μg (0.001 mg) orally daily
Parenteral dosage form
Adults:
To treat a deficiency state—100 μg (0.1 mg) intra-

muscular or deep subcutaneously, daily for 6 or 7 days, then 100 μg (0.1 mg) every other day for 7 doses. If clinically improved and a reticulocyte response occurs, then 100 μg (0.1 mg) every 3 or 4 days for another 2 to 3 weeks.

Maintenance—100 to 200 μg (0.1 to 0.2 mg) intramuscular monthly in pernicious anemia and after a total gastrectomy or extensive ileal resection; this is continued for life.

Children:

To treat a deficiency state:—initially, 30 to 50 μg (0.03 to 0.05 mg) intramuscular or deep subcutaneous daily for 2 or more weeks (Total dose is 1 to 5 mg.)

Maintenance—100 μg (0.1 mg) intramuscular or deep subcutaneous monthly as needed. In pernicious anemia and after a total gastrectomy or extensive ileal resection, administer it for life.

hydroxocobalamin. Although the indications for cyanocobalamin and hydroxocobalamin are the same, hydroxocobalamin is often preferred to treat vitamin B_{12} deficiency states because the optic neuropathies reported may degenerate with the administration of cyanocobalamin.

Parenteral dosage form

Adults:

To treat B_{12} deficiency—30 to 50 μg (0.03 to 0.05 mg) intramuscular or deep subcutaneous daily. If the megaloblastic anemia is severe, administer 100 mg (0.1 mg) daily for 5 to 10 days.

Maintenance—100 to 200 mg intramuscular (0.1 to 0.2 mg) monthly for life for pernicious anemia, following a total gastrectomy and extensive ileal resection.

Children:

To treat a vitamin B_{12} deficiency—30 to 50 mg (0.03 to 0.05 mg) intramuscular or deep subcutaneous daily for 2 or more weeks (Total dose is 1 to 5 mg.)

Maintenance—100 mg (0.1 mg) intramuscular or deep subcutaneous monthly as needed. For life administration, see the listing for adults.

Pregnancy safety. FDA category C

NURSING CONSIDERATIONS

See also the nurse's role in vitamin therapy.

Assessment. The administration of cyanocobalamin is contraindicated in Leber's disease because the levels of the substance are already elevated.

Caution should be used if the client has a history of gout.

Plasma vitamin B_{12} levels should be determined before therapy begins and on about the sixth day of therapy. Diagnosis of vitamin B_{12} deficiency should be confirmed by the lab or the initiation of B_{12} therapy will mask a folic acid deficiency.

During the first 48 hours of therapy, serum potassium should be monitored closely for the possibility of severe hypokalemia.

Hypersensitivity, which occurs rarely, is demonstrated by skin rash and, after parenteral administration, wheezing.

Education. Stress compliance with the medication regimen if the client is on life-long therapy following a gastrectomy or ileal resection, or for pernicious anemia. For these conditions the drug is administered intramuscularly.

Best food sources for vitamin B_{12} are meats, seafood, egg yolk, milk, and fermented cheeses.

folic acid (vitamin B_9):
folic acid tablets (Apo-Folic✤, Folvite, Novofolacid✤)
folic acid injection (Folvite)

Mechanism of action. Folic acid is converted to tetrahydrofolic acid in the body, which is then utilized for normal erythropoiesis and nucleoprotein synthesis.

Indications. To prevent and treat folic acid deficiency. Folic acid should not be administered until pernicious anemia has been ruled out as a potential diagnosis. Folic acid will correct the hemotologic changes and mask pernicious anemia while the underlying neurologic damage progresses.

A folic acid deficiency may result in megaloblastic and macrocytic anemias and glossitis.

Pharmacokinetics

Absorption. Absorbed well in gastrointestinal tract. Mostly absorbed from the upper duodenum, even in the presence of malabsorption (tropical sprue). But food folate absorption would be impaired in malabsorption syndromes.

Protein binding. High to plasma proteins

Storage. Liver

Metabolism. Liver. Folic acid in the presence of vitamin C (ascorbic acid) is converted in the liver and serum to its active form, tetrahydrofolic acid, by dihydrofolate reductase.

Excretion. Kidneys

Side effects/adverse reactions. Rare. Allergic reaction (elevated temperature and rash) or yellow discoloration of urine reported.

Significant drug interactions. None

Dosage and administration

Oral dosage forms

Adults

As a dietary supplement: 100 μg (0.1 mg) orally daily (up to 1 mg daily in pregnancy). The dose may be increased to 500 μg (0.5 mg) to 1 mg if necessary. In tropical sprue, a dose of 3 to 15 mg daily is used.

To treat folic acid deficiency: 250 μg (0.25 mg) to 1 mg orally daily until a hematologic effect is noted

Maintenance: 400 μg (0.4 mg) orally daily; 800 μg (0.8 mg) orally in pregnancy and lactation

Children.

As a dietary supplement: 100 μg (0.1 mg) orally daily; increase to 500 μg (0.5 mg) to 1 mg daily if necessary. Infants fed goat milk formulas should receive 50 μg (0.05 mg) daily.

To treat folic acid deficiency: 250 μg (0.25 mg) to 1 mg orally daily until a hematologic effect is noted

Maintenance:

Infants—100 μg (0.1 mg) orally daily

Children less than 4 years old—up to 300 μg (0.3 mg) orally daily 4 years and older—400 μg (0.4 mg) orally daily

Parenteral dosage form

Adults. For vitamin supplement to treat a folic acid deficiency, 250 μg (0.25 mg) to 1 mg daily, intramuscularly, intravenously, or deep secretory component until a hematologic effect is noted.

Children. See adult dose.

Pregnancy safety. Not classified

NURSING CONSIDERATIONS

See also the nurse's role in vitamin therapy.

Assessment. It should be determined if the client has pernicious anemia because folic acid will reverse hematologic abnormalities, but the neurologic aspects of the disease will continue to progress.

The only side effect reported with folic acid, even with large doses, is allergic rash and fever.

Education. Alert the client that large doses of folic acid may turn the urine yellow.

The best food sources of folic acid are vegetables, fruits, and organ meats.

ascorbic acid (vitamin C):
ascorbic acid tablets (Apo-C✤, Cevalin)
ascorbic acid chewable tablets (Flavorcee)
ascorbic acid effervescent tablets (Redoxon)
ascorbic acid oral solution (Cecon, Ce-Vi-Sol)
ascorbic acid extended-release capsules (Ascorbicap, Cetane)
ascorbic acid extended-release tablets (Arco-Cee, Cemill)
ascorbic acid and sodium ascorbate chewable tablets (Apo-C)
ascorbic acid injection (Cetane, Cevalin)
sodium ascorbate injection (Cenolate, Cetane, Redoxon✤)

The well-known effects of lemon and orange juices in curing scurvy led to the discovery of vitamin C or ascorbic acid. Scurvy only occurs in humans and a few other species because ascorbic acid cannot be produced in the body. Today it is a very rare disease in the United States, only seen when all ascorbic acid intake is discontinued for 3 to 5 months.

Mechanism of action. Although less is known about its function when compared to other water-soluble vitamins, ascorbic acid is involved in the formation of collagen in all fibrous tissue, including bone, and in the development of teeth, blood vessels, and blood cells. It also plays a role in carbohydrate metabolism. It is believed to stimulate the fibroblasts of connective tissue and thus promote tissue repair and the healing of wounds. It is thought to help maintain the integrity of the intercellular substance in the walls of blood vessels, and the capillary fragility associated with scurvy is explained on this basis. It is also involved in phenylalanine, tyrosine, folic acid, and iron metabolism.

When given as an adjunct to deferoxamine for a chronic iron overdose, it may serve to improve the chelating effect of deferoxamine, thus increasing the amount of iron excreted from the body (an unapproved indication).

The effectiveness of ascorbic acid in preventing or relieving cold symptoms is also an unapproved indication. Many studies have been performed over the years that have not substantiated the claims that megadoses of vitamin C reduce or eliminate cold symptoms (Davidson, 1986).

Indications. To prevent and treat vitamin C deficiency

Pharmacokinetics

Absorption. Absorbed well in jejunum. May be reduced if large doses are given.

Protein binding. Low

Storage. In plasma and cells; highest concentration is found in glandular sites

Metabolism. Liver

Excretion. Kidneys

Side effects/adverse reactions. See Table 69-4.

Significant drug interactions. None noted

Dosage and administration

oral dosage forms

Adults. As a dietary supplement, 50 to 100 mg orally daily. In clients undergoing chronic dialysis, 100 to 200 mg orally daily. To treat a vitamin C deficiency, 100 to 250 mg orally, one to three times daily.

Children. As a dietary supplement, infants and children under 4 years old, 20 to 50 mg daily orally. To treat a vitamin C deficiency, 100 to 300 mg orally daily, given in divided doses.

Ascorbic acid and sodium ascorbate chewable tablets are not available in the United States. Dosage is usually one tablet daily.

ascorbic acid injection

Adults. To treat a vitamin C deficiency, 100 to 250 mg intramuscularly or intravenously, from one to three times daily

Children. To treat a vitamin C deficiency, 100 to 300 mg intramuscularly or intravenously daily, in divided doses
sodium ascorbate injection. Adults and children: same as ascorbic acid injection
Pregnancy safety. FDA category C

NURSING CONSIDERATIONS

See also the nurse's role in vitamin therapy.

Assessment. Because of the risk of the formation of urinary stones when large doses of vitamin C are given to persons with the following conditions, it should be determined that the client does not have cystinuria, oxalosis, or a history of gout or urate renal stones.

Large doses may also precipitate a crisis in sickle cell anemia. Clients with diabetes mellitus may find interference with glucose testing with large doses of vitamin C.

If the purpose of administering vitamin C is to acidify the urine, urinary pHs will need to be monitored to determine effectiveness of the drug.

Education. Clients taking more than 600 mg daily may have a small increase in urination; more than 1 g daily, diarrhea; and more than 2 to 3 g daily of prolonged therapy, withdrawal scurvy.

The best food sources of vitamin C are citrus fruits, tomatoes, strawberries, cantaloupe, and raw peppers.

MULTIPLE-VITAMIN PREPARATIONS

Numerous multivitamin preparations are available in the United States and Canada. Supplemental preparations should provide 100% of the U.S. RDA to meet the needs of the vast majority of clients. Extra-potency or high-potency vitamins are rarely necessary for routine supplementation. In addition, the nurse should be aware that many preparations contain chemicals that are not yet known to be associated with any known deficiency states.

MINERALS

Oral sources of minerals are available commercially either as single sources or in combination with other minerals or multiple-vitamin preparations. The U.S. RDA is noted in Table 69-3 (p. 1076).

IRON

Iron is an essential mineral for the proper functioning of all biological systems in the body. It functions as an oxygen carrier in hemoglobin and myoglobin, for tissue respiration, and for many enzyme reactions in the body. It is also stored in various body sites, such as the liver, spleen and bone marrow. Iron deficiency is the most common nutritional deficiency in the United States resulting in anemia. Young children and women, especially pregnant women, are most frequently affected.

Iron is supplied through diet (meats and certain vegetables and grains) and iron supplements. Ingested iron is converted to the ferrous state by gastric juices which are then more readily absorbed in the body. The absorption of iron is affected by many substances, though; for example, ascorbic acid (vitamin C), orange juice, veal, and fish all potentiate iron absorption. Eggs, corn, beans, and many cereal products (containing phytates) inhibit iron absorption.

Mechanism of action. See previous section.

Indications. Iron deficiency anemia.

Pharmacokinetics

Oral dosage forms

Absorption: Mainly in the duodenum and proximal jejunum. In iron deficiency, between 20% to 30% of iron is absorbed. In normal individuals, 3% to 10% is usually

TABLE 69-5   Iron Supplements: Significant Side Effects and Adverse Reactions

	Side effects	Adverse reactions
iron salts: ferrous fumarate, ferrous fluconate, ferrous sulfate, iron-polysaccharide	Most frequent: nausea, vomiting. Less frequent: dark urine, constipation, diarrhea, teeth staining with liquid dosage formulations.	Most frequent: stomach cramps, pain. Less frequent/rare: pain on swallowing, bloody stools. *Iron toxicity:* *Early signs of* *acute toxicity:* Diarrhea which may contain blood, elevated temperature, severe abdominal cramps or pain, vomiting. *Late signs:* Pale, cold skin, convulsions, increased weakness, sedation, blue lips, fingernails, palms of hands, irregular heart rate (weak and tachycardic).

absorbed. The quantity absorbed is approximately equivalent to the deficiency. Ferrous iron is better absorbed than the ferric dosage form.

Protein binding. High, approximately 90%.

Excretion. Not eliminated physiologically by the body. Excess iron intake can result in accumulation and iron toxicity. Small amounts are lost daily in shedding of skin, nails, hair, breast milk, urine, and menstrual blood. In healthy adults, the daily iron loss is approximately 1 mg per day for males and postmenopausal females and 1.5 mg per day in premenopausal females.

Side effects/adverse reactions. See Table 69-5.

Significant drug interactions. When iron salts are given concurrently with

Drug	Possible Effect and Management
calcium supplements, milk or dairy products, coffee, fiber or selected food products (see previous section)	Decreased iron absorption may result. Schedule iron supplements at least 1 hour prior or 2 hours after administration of these substances.
tetracyclines, oral administration	Decreases absorption of tetracycline which may result in reduced antibiotic effectiveness. Avoid concurrent Vitamin E May impair the hematologic effectiveness of the iron supplement. Avoid concurrent administration.

Dosage and administration. See Table 69-6.

NURSING CONSIDERATIONS

Assessment. Complete a thorough dietary history and assess the client's nutritional status to ascertain the possible causes of the anemia and the need for client education.

Iron should be administered for iron deficiency anemias specifically rather than all anemias in general. Some anemic conditions such as thalassemia may actually result in excess deposits of iron in the body.

It should be determined that the client does not have a disorder of iron metabolism such as hemochromatosis, which causes an excess depotism of iron in the tissues, skin pigmentation, cirrhosis of the liver, and decreased carbohydrate tolerance; or hemosiderosis, an increase in tissue iron stores without associated tissue damage.

Some elderly clients may need larger doses of iron than the usual daily adult dose for iron deficiency anemia, for the reduction of gastric secretions and achlorhydria as a consequence of aging inhibits the ability to absorb iron.

Intervention. The ferrous rather than ferric preparation of iron provides for the most efficient absorption of iron. Iron is best administered on an empty stomach. When taken with food, its absorption may be decreased by as much as a half to a third. Administer with a full glass of water to prevent staining of the teeth with liquid iron preparations. A drinking straw or a dropper may be used

TABLE 69-6   Iron Supplements

Drug	Dosage and administration*	Percent
ferrous fumarate (Feostat, Palafer†, Fem-iron, Ircon)	Adults: 200 mg orally 3-4 times daily. Children: 3 mg/kg 3 times daily. May be increased to 6 mg/kg if necessary.	33
ferrous gluconate (Fergon, Simron)	Adults: 325 mg orally, 4 times daily. May be increased to 650 mg 4 times daily if necessary. Children (2 yrs and over): 16 mg/kg orally 3 times daily.	11.6
ferrous sulfate (Feosol, Fer-In-Sol, Mol-Iron)	Adults: 300 mg orally 2 times daily. May be increased to 4 times daily, if necessary. Children: 10 mg/kg orally 3 times daily.	20
extended release tablets (Fero-Grad, Fero-Gradument)	Adults: 160 to 525 mg orally 1 or 2 times daily. Children: 160 mg orally daily.	
iron polysaccharide† (Hytinic, Nu-Iron)	Adults: 150 mg orally 2 times daily. May be increased to 150 mg 4 times daily, if necessary. Children: therapeutic dosage not available.	Ferric, percentage depends on product.

*Dosages are therapeutic recommendations, that is, for the treatment of iron deficiency anemia.

†Contains a water soluble complex of elemental ferric ion.

to place the dose well back on the tongue to prevent contact with the teeth.

Oral preparations of iron should be discontinued before parenteral iron therapy begins.

Anaphylaxis has been known to occur up to 24 hours after parenteral administration. Epinephrine should be available during injection of iron dextran, particularly in clients with asthma and known allergies. A test dose of 25 mg should be administered, intramuscularly or intravenously, to all clients at least one hour or longer before their first therapeutic parenteral dose.

For intravenous administration of iron dextran, do not mix with other medications or add it to parenteral nutrition solutions. It should be administered undiluted and at a rate of not more than 1 mL per minute. Flush the intravenous line with normal saline for injection. Maintain the client in a recumbent position for 30 minutes in case orthostatic hypotension should occur.

It is recommended that iron dextran be administered by the Z-track technique (see Chapter 6), using a 2-3 inch, 19 or 20 gauge needle, into the muscle mass of the upper outer quadrant of the buttock. It is never to be injected into the upper arm or any other exposed area because of the possibility of the preparation staining the skin dark brown. To minimize staining use a separate needle to withdraw the drug from the vial.

Education. The client should be alerted that iron preparations cause black stools which are medically insignificant. However, if the client experiences other symptoms of internal blood loss, such as bloody streaks in the stool, abdominal tenderness, cramping, or pain, the physician should be notified.

Instruct the client to maintain a diet rich in sources of iron, such as liver, green leafy vegetables, potatoes, dried peas and beans, dried fruit, and enriched flour, bread, and cereals.

Evaluation. The hemoglobin, hematocrit, reticulocyte count, and plasma iron values should be monitored at three weekly intervals during the first two months of oral iron therapy or a few days after the initiation of parenteral therapy. It usually takes 1-2 months for the hemoglobin concentration of a person with iron deficiency anemia to reach normal levels on oral therapy.

KEY TERMS

antirachitic, page 1079
avitaminosis, page 1074
fat-soluble vitamins, page 1075
gluconeogenesis, page 1073
hyperkeratosis, page 1077
hypervitaminosis, page 1075
keratomalacia, page 1077

nyctalopia, page 1077
water-soluble vitamins, page 1075
xerophthalmia, page 1077

BIBLIOGRAPHY

American Hospital Formulary Service: AHFS drug information '88, Bethesda, Md, 1988, American Society of Hospital Pharmacists.

Austen, C: Vitamin chart no. 10: biotin, Nutr Support Serv 6(8):28, 1986.

Bailey, LB: Vitamin chart no. 8: vitamin B_6, Nutr Support Serv 6(6):28, 1986.

Baumgartner, TS, and others: Vitamin chart no. 11: folic acid. Part 1, Nutr Support Serv 6(9):33, 1986.

Baumgartner, TS, and others: Vitamin chart no. 11: folic acid. Part 2, Nutr Support Serv 6(10):25, 1986.

Blair, KA: Vitamin supplementation and mega doses, Nurse Pract 11(7):19, 1986.

Bowman, BB: Vitamin chart no. 5: vitamin B_1, Nutr Support Serv 6(2):52, 1986.

Bowman, BB: Vitamin chart no. 7: niacin, Nutr Support Serv 6(6):38, 1986.

Davidson, DE, ed: Handbook of nonprescription drugs, ed 8, Washington, DC, 1986, American Pharmaceutical Association and The National Professional Society of Pharmacists.

Dawson-Hughes, B: Vitamin chart no. 2: vitamin D, Nutr Support Serv 5(10):51, 1986.

DeMaeyer, EM: Vitamin and mineral deficiencies, World Health, Oct 1984, p. 25.

Flink, EB: Magnesium deficiency: causes and effects, Hosp Pract 22(2):116A, 1987.

Gardner, SS: Vitamin B_{12} deficiency anemia, SGA J 9(3):126, 1987.

Gums, JG: Clinical significance of magnesium: a review, Drug Intell Clin Pharm 21(3):240, 1987.

Hardin, SR: Rocaltrol (calcitriol/Roche): potent form of vitamin D, Crit Care Nurs 5(3):66, 1985.

Holmes, P: The value of vitamins, Nurs Times 83(16):31, 1987.

Katzung, BG: Basic and clinical pharmacology, ed 3, Norwalk, Conn, 1987, Appleton & Lange.

Krasinski, SD: Vitamin chart no. 4: vitamin K, Nutr Support Serv 6(1):46, 1986.

Loescher, LJ, and others: Vitamin therapy for advanced cancers, Oncol Nurs Forum 11(6):38, 1984.

Luke, B: Megavitamins and pregnancy: a dangerous combination, MCN 10(1):18, 1985.

Moss, BK: Using vitamin and mineral supplements, Patient Care 18(16):81, 1984.

Moss, BK: Who really needs nutrition supplements? Patient Care 18(10):86, 1984.

Rolig, EC: Vitamins: physiology and deficiency states, Nurse Pract 11(7):38, 1986.

Rubin, MB: Vitamins and wound healing, Plast Surg Nurs 4(1):16, 1984.

Sitren, HS: Vitamin chart, Nutr Support Serv 6(7):30, 1986.

Shamberger, RJ: The subtle signs of chronic vitamin undernutrition: fat-soluble vitamins. Part 1, Diagn Med 7(3):75, 1984.

Shamberger, RJ: The subtle signs of chronic vitamin undernutrition: water-soluble vitamin. Part 2, Diagn Med 7(4):61, 1984.

Smith, S: How drugs act: vitamins. Part 7, Nurs Times 81(3):35, 1985.

Solomons, N: Vitamin chart no. 6: vitamin B_2, Nutr Support Serv 6(3):30, 1986.

Solomons, NW: Nutrient chart no. 13: adverse and toxic effects of excessive intakes of mineral nutrients, Nutr Support Serv 5(6):39, 1985.

Thibodeau, GA: Anatomy and physiology, St Louis, 1987, Times Mirror/Mosby College Publishing.

Travis, HR: Vitamin C and the common cold revisited, Health Educ 15(1):13, 1984.

United States Pharmacopeial Convention: USP DI-88 drug information for the health care provider, ed 8, Rockville, Md, 1988, The Convention.

Yen, PK: Vitamin C - a miracle cure? Geriatr Nurs 7(5):276, 1986.

chapter 70

Fluids and Electrolytes

Injecting substances, including blood, into the bloodstream of animals or humans has been the subject of experiments since the seventeenth century. Although a few successes were recorded, the majority of cases resulted in complications, infections, and/or death.

In the early 1900s, it was discovered that all human blood was not the same and that sodium citrate could be safely added to blood to prevent it from clotting. From this point on, rapid advances were made in blood administration.

The administration of parenteral fluids intravenously has become more prevalent during the past 50 years. The problems associated with the use of unsafe solutions because of pyrogens had to first be resolved. This was first recognized in 1923; throughout the years advances in scientific knowledge and pharmaceutical technology have resulted in products that have significantly improved patient safety. See the box "Intravenous Therapy: 1930s to Today," which outlines nursing progress in intravenous therapy since the early 1930s.

CURRENT OVERVIEW OF INTRAVENOUS THERAPY

Approximately 25% of all clients in hospitals today receive some type of intravascular therapy. New, sophisticated delivery systems have been developed and different methods of application are constantly being conceived. Intravenous solutions are infused for various therapeutic reasons; some examples are listed here:

To replace fluids and electrolytes
To correct acid-base imbalance

To administer medications

To maintain ready access to the venous system if any of the first three measures is anticipated

To measure changes in venous pressure

To measure the kidneys' excretory capabilities by diagnostic test

To administer essential nutrients

Blood and its components are transfused intravenously to (1) replace blood volume or plasma fractions; (2) restore the blood's capabilities for oxygen carrying, clotting, or oncotic pressure; or (3) cleanse the plasma of harmful constituents by exchanges.

Intravenous hyperalimentation or parenteral nutrition solutions are infused to complement or supplement individuals in deprived nutrition states.

FLUIDS

Water comprises from 45% to 75% of the total human body weight, depending on the amount of adipose tissue present. Infants and young children have more water per unit of body weight than adults, and female adults have less water content than male adults. The greatest amount of body water (up to 45% of body weight) is to be found in the **intracellular fluid,** i.e., the fluid inside the cells. In this fluid the chemical reactions of all metabolism so essential to life occur. The remainder of body water is located in the **extracellular fluid,** that is, the fluid surrounding the cells. This extracellular fluid consists of plasma, interstitial fluid, and lymph, as well as extracellular portions of dense connective tissue, cartilage, and bone. The volume of fluid in the two body fluid compartments varies with age and differs in the sexes. In this fluid metabolic exchanges between cells and tissues and the external environment occur.

The importance of body water is highlighted by two facts: (1) it is the medium in which all metabolic reactions occur, and (2) precise regulation of volume and composition of body fluid is essential to health. In the healthy individual, body water remains remarkably constant, maintained by a balance between intake and excretion—the water gained each day is equal to the water lost. If the water gained exceeds the water lost, **water excess,** or **overhydration,** and edema will occur. If the water lost exceeds the water gained, **water deficit,** or **dehydration,** will occur. If 20% to 25% of body water is lost, death usually occurs.

Water is an excellent solvent that permits many substances to be dispersed through it. It also has a high dielectric constant, which permits ionization of electrolytes. These electrolytes are important in maintaining body fluid volume and distribution. They include the cations sodium (Na^+) for extracellular fluid, and potassium (K^+) and magnesium (Mg^{++}) for intracellular fluid; and the anions chloride (Cl^-) and bicarbonate (HCO_3^-) for extracellular fluid, and phosphate (PO_4^{--}) and protein for intracellular fluid. Intracellular ions also occur in the extracellular fluid but in smaller amounts.

Water is also an excellent lubricant between membranes, and it functions well as a heat insulator and heat exchanger.

Daily intake of water in some form is essential to maintain water balance. During starvation, human beings can go several weeks without food but can survive only a few days without water. The average volumes of water consumed daily are as follows: 120 to 150 ml/kg body weight in neonates and infants, 120 to 130 ml/kg in children, and 30 ml/kg in adults.

Thirst, the subjective desire to ingest water, helps maintain water balance. Although thirst is complex and not well understood, a decrease in saliva and dryness of the mouth and throat induces it. Dehydration of thirst receptors may lead to their stimulation.

INTRAVENOUS THERAPY: 1930s TO TODAY

EARLY 1930s

Intravenous injections were reserved for only seriously ill clients.

Only a physician could perform the venipuncture.

1940s

Massachusetts General Hospital became one of the first hospitals to assign a nurse to intravenous therapy.

The job description included administering intravenous solutions and blood transfusions, cleaning the infusion sets for reuse, and cleaning and sharpening needles for reuse.

Primary responsibility was of a technical nature: administering and maintaining the infusions and keeping the equipment clean and functional.

1950s TO 1990s

Improvements and innovations in equipment, needles (Intracaths, and so forth), tubing, development of plastic and disposable equipment, and an increased variety of commercially prepared intravenous fluids increase the safety of intravenous therapy.

The development of intravenous filters prevent particulate matter, bacteria, or fungus from entering the bloodstream.

Intravenous route is used to administer many medications and hyperalimentation fluids, in addition to intravenous fluids.

The development of intravenous nurse specialists, intravenous departments or teams in the hospital, standards for client care, and professional organizations to promote intravenous therapy as a speciality area in nursing.

Water intake occurs primarily by (1) drinking fluids, (2) ingesting food containing moisture (most foods contain a high percentage of water), and (3) absorbing water formed by the oxidation of hydrogen in the food during metabolic processes, which produces about 0.5 L of water per day.

Water is lost from the body in five principal ways: (1) by way of the kidneys as urine, (2) through the skin as insensible perspiration and sweat, (3) through expired air as water vapor, (4) through feces, and (5) through the excretion of tears and saliva. Urine excretion accounts for 50% to 60% of the total daily water loss. Urine output, of course, varies with the amount of water ingested.

Water loss by the kidney varies with the solute load and the antidiuretic hormone (ADH) level. The kidney excretes sufficient urine to transport the solutes into the bladder if an increase in solute load occurs, as in diabetes mellitus or following ingestion of excessive amounts of food. The reabsorption of water in the distal convoluted tubules is controlled by ADH. An increase in ADH levels will lead to an increase in water reabsorption, which produces a more concentrated urine. ADH (vasopressin) is secreted by the posterior pituitary gland. This secretion is regulated by osmoreceptors located in the supraoptic nucleus. ADH has an action on specific vasopressin receptors on the medullary tubular cell to stimulate cyclic AMP (cAMP) production in this cell. The cAMP activates an enzyme that alters protein structure in the cell membrane to increase tubular cell permeability to water. This will increase water resorption and increase urine osmolality.

WATER TRANSPORT IN THE BODY

Water travels from less concentrated areas to areas with higher concentrations of solutes or dissolved substances **(osmosis).** The solutes may be electrolytes, such as potassium chloride or sodium chloride, which, when dissolved in water, yield potassium cations and chloride anions (a chemical balance that is maintained) or nonelectrolytes, such as dextrose, urea, or creatinine. Each fluid compartment in the body, i.e., intracellular and extracellular compartments, has its own electrolyte composition. (See Table 70-1 for electrolyte composition in body compartments.) Disturbances in electrolyte composition can be reflected in clinical symptoms in the client.

Osmolality refers to the total solute concentration usually expressed per liter of serum. The osmotic pressure is decided by the number of solutes in solution. For example, if the extracellular fluid contained a large amount of dissolved particles and the intracellular fluid had a small amount of dissolved particles, then the osmotic pressure from the intracellular fluid would force water to pass from the less concentrated area to the more con-

centrated area. This would occur until both concentrations were equal. Therefore deciding on the appropriate intravenous therapy for a client would necessitate knowing the electrolyte values. The level of sodium, the principal electrolyte in the extracellular fluid is essential to know, although potassium levels are also important, along with serum osmolality, current disease state or illnesses, specific laboratory values if appropriate, and the initial signs and symptoms.

PARENTERAL SOLUTIONS

Parenteral solutions generally may be divided into four categories: (1) hydrating solutions, (2) isotonic solutions, (3) maintenance solutions, and (4) hypertonic solutions. See Table 70-2 for examples of the four categories of parenteral solutions.

Hydrating solutions include dextrose 2.5%, 5%, or higher in water or in 0.2% to 0.5% normal saline. (Hypotonic saline—note that full strength normal saline is not included in this category.) Hydrating solutions are used to hydrate or to prevent dehydration. They are often used to assess kidney status before specific electrolytes are ordered as replacement and maintenance therapy and also to help increase diuresis in dehydrated individuals.

Dextrose is a source of calories (one liter of 5% dextrose = approximately 170 calories) and is rapidly metabolized in the body. Therefore, although considered isotonic or more than isotonic in the bottle, in the body dextrose is metabolized, leaving water that decreases the osmotic pressure of the plasma and easily transfers to body cells, providing water immediately to dehydrated tissues.

Isotonic solutions are usually prescribed to replace extracellular fluid losses that occur from blood loss, severe vomiting episodes, or any situation in which the chloride loss is equal to or greater than the sodium loss. Isotonic or normal saline is also used before and after a blood transfusion. The reason is that hemolysis of red

TABLE 70-1 Normal Body Electrolyte Distribution*

Electrolytes	Extracellular (mEq/L)		Intracellular (mEq/L)
	Plasma	Interstitial	
sodium (Na$^+$)	142	146	15
potassium (K$^+$)	5	5	150
calcium (Ca^{++})	5	3	2
magnesium (Mg^{++})	2	1	27
chloride (Cl$^-$)	103	114	1
bicarbonate (HCO$_3^-$)	27	30	10

*In addition, phosphates, sulfates, and other substances are located in the extracellular and intracellular fluids.

TABLE 70-2 Four Categories of Selected Parenteral Solutions*

	Na$^+$	K$^+$	Mg^{++}	Ca^{++}	Cl$^-$	Osmolarity$^+$
HYDRATING SOLUTIONS						
dextrose 2.5%, 5%, 10%						
dextrose 2.5% in 0.45% NaCl injection†	56				56	280
dextrose 5% in 0.45% NaCl injection‡	7				77	405
ISOTONIC SOLUTIONS						
normal saline or sodium chloride injection (0.9% NaCl)	154				154	310
Ringer's injection	147	4		4	155	310
lactated Ringer's injection§	130	4		3	109	275
MAINTENANCE SOLUTIONS						
Plasmalyte 56	40	13	3		40	111
Plasmalyte 148 (or Normosol-R, Isolyte S)	140	5		3	98	295
HYPERTONIC SOLUTIONS						
sodium chloride, 3% injection	513				513	1025
sodium chloride, 5% injection	855				855	1710

*Normal plasma contains Na$^+$ (136-145), K$^+$ (3.5-5), Mg^{++} (1.5-2.5), Ca^{++} (4.3-5.3), Cl$^-$ (100-106), HCO$_3$ (27); osmolarity (280-300 m0sm).

+ electrolytes given as mEq/L; osmolarity as m0sm/L.

†Dextrose 2.5% = 25 g dextrose/L or 85 calories. 0.33% NaCl is also referred to as half-strength normal saline (NS).

‡Dextrose 5% = 50 g dextrose/L or 170 calories.

§Note a major difference between Ringer's injection and lactated Ringer's injection is the 28 mEq of lactate, a precursor of bicarbonate, in the lactated injection. Thus lactated Ringer's is preferred for patients with metabolic acidosis perhaps caused by burns or infections. Ringer's injection, however, has more chloride ions; thus it is more useful in treating dehydration from reduced water intake, vomiting, or diarrhea or for patients with hypochloremia.

blood cells, which occurs with dextrose in water, is avoided by utilizing this product.

Isotonic sodium chloride is also used to treat metabolic alkalosis, especially when it occurs in the presence of fluid loss. The increased administration of chloride ions will help to decrease the number of bicarbonate ions in the individual. Other solutions considered isotonic preparations include Ringers injection and lactated Ringers injection.

Maintenance solutions or multiple electrolyte solutions have been formulated to replace daily electrolyte and extracellular needs and water. Such solutions may also be indicated to replace electrolytes and water loss from severe vomiting or diarrhea. With these preparations, the extracellular replacement is usually achieved within 2 days (usually 1 to 3 liters/day is administered) and this should be closely monitored by laboratory tests. If maintenance solutions are continued after the client's deficits have been corrected, the excess sodium may lead to circulatory overload, pulmonary edema, and heart failure.

Examples of maintenance solutions include Plasma-Lyte and Normosol.

Hypertonic solutions are used to treat hypotonic expansion (water intoxication) when the increased body fluid volume is caused by water only. This can happen under several different circumstances; e.g., (1) hospitalized patients that receive large amounts of dextrose 5% in water or electrolyte-free solutions to replace fluid and electrolytes lost from vomiting, diarrhea, diuresis, or gastric suction, or (2) it is most apt to occur in elderly clients during the postoperative period when water is retained in response to stress (endocrine response to stress).

When behavorial changes, such as lethargy, confusion, and perhaps, disorientation occur postoperatively in the elderly person, overhydration or hypotonic expansion should be considered. Central nervous system signs and symptoms such as increased tiredness, muscle twitching, headaches, nausea, vomiting, and even seizures have been noted. Weight gain is always present and the blood pressure may be normal or elevated.

In milder cases, the treatment usually includes withholding all fluids until excess fluids are excreted. In severe cases of hyponatremia, small quantities of hypertonic sodium chloride are administered to (1) increase the osmotic pressure, (2) increase the water flow from body cells to the extracellular compartment, and (3) to enhance excretion of the fluids by the kidneys.

The typical hypertonic saline is a 3% or 5% solution that when ordered, must be administered slowly with close supervision, (to prevent pulmonary edema) and requires close monitoring of laboratory tests for electrolytes.

ABNORMAL STATES OF FLUID-ELECTROLYTE BALANCE

A dynamic relationship exists in the human body between water and sodium, and abnormal states of hydration can be classified as (1) dehydration (volume depletion), (2) overhydration (**hypervolemia** or volume excess), (3) loss of water in excess of sodium (hypernatremia), and (4) loss of sodium in excess of water (hyponatremia).

The second abnormal state, or overhydration or volume excess, was reviewed previously, under the description of hypertonic solutions on p. 1095. The other three abnormal states may be classified as various types of dehydration.

DEHYDRATION

Table 70-3 illustrates the differences between the three types of dehydration. Note that the causes of the three dehydration states are different, as are the effects on fluid compartments in the body and some of the initial signs and laboratory values, especially sodium concentration. This is very important information because it will aid the physician not only in diagnosing the initial condition but also in choosing an appropriate intravenous therapy for the individual client.

Hypertonic dehydration caused by heat exhaustion resulting from water depletion can occur on land or sea. Many cases of boaters lost at sea running out of water or refugees fleeing their countries in the Caribbean (Haiti, Cuba) and running out of water for days before being rescued or reaching land have been reported. Such persons require intensive care for their dehydration, and others may die from this deprivation. See Table 70-4 for the symptoms of hypertonic dehydration by clinical grading.

ELECTROLYTES

The major electrolytes in the body are sodium, potassium, calcium, and magnesium. This section will review the normal requirements, sources, specific functions, and problems associated with an excess or deficiency of the electrolyte.

SODIUM

Sodium is the major electrolyte in the extracellular fluid; the normal range is from 136 to 145 mEq/L of plasma. The sodium content in the body is regulated by sodium consumption (dietary) and sodium excretion by the kidneys. In the average person with normal renal function, sodium excretion will closely match sodium intake. This aids in keeping sodium content in body at a constant, even if sodium intake is somewhat varied (Braunwald, 1987).

The major dietary sources of sodium are table salt (sodium chloride), catsup, mustard, cured meats and fish,

TABLE 70-3 Differences Between the Three Types of Dehydration

	Hypotonic	Isotonic	Hypertonic
Cause	Loss of salt (NaC1)	Blood loss	Water loss or lack of sufficient fluid intake
Effect on ICF and ECF compartments	Volume ICF ↑ Volume ECF ↓	Decrease in ECF volume	Decrease in ICF and ECF volume
Significant signs:			
Rate of water elimination	Increased	Decreased	Decreased
Thirst	—	—	Early warning, because of cell dehydration
Pulse rate	Increased, weak, thready	Regular	Regular in early stages
Behavioral signs	May see vomiting, abdominal cramps	—	Confusion, irritability, agitation
Late stages	Skin turgor Weak pulse, lethargy, confusion, death owing to circulatory failure	Shock, weak Weak, thready	Skin turgor Dry, furrowed tongue; death
Clinical lab results:			
Hematocrit	Increased	Increased	Increased
Hemoglobin	Increased	Increased	Increased
Sodium levels	Decreased	—	Increased

TABLE 70-4   Symptoms of Hypertonic Dehydration by Clinical Grading

Clinical grading	Symptoms
Mild or early	Increased thirst. Usually a 2% body weight loss.
Moderate to severe	Very dry mouth, difficulty in swallowing, scant urine output (highly concentrated urine), increased pulse rate and body temperature, poor skin turgor; an approximate 6% body weight loss.
Extreme or very severe	All previous symptoms plus impaired mental and physical capabilities, rectal temperature very high, respiratory difficulties (hyperventilation that may lead to tetany), cyanosis, severe oliguria or anuria, circulatory failure, loss of more than 7% in body weight. Usually coma and death occur when approximately 15% of body weight is lost.

cheese, peanut butter, pickles, olives, potato chips, and popcorn. The recommended dietary allowance for sodium is from 1100 mg (women, 23 to 50 years old) to 3300 mg (men 23 to 50 years old). Sodium is necessary for control of body water; for the electrophysiology of nerve, muscle, and gland cells; and for the regulation of pH and isotonicity.

Hyponatremia

Hyponatremia may be detected when the serum level falls below 135 mEq/L. It is induced by excessive sweating with replacement of only the water; infusion of large quantities of nonelectrolyte parenteral fluids; adrenal insufficiency or gastrointestinal suctioning with replacement fluids limited to water by mouth.

Symptoms include lethargy, hypotension, stomach cramps, vomiting, diarrhea, and possibly, seizures. Deficiency states are usually treated with Ringer's solution or normal saline injection.

Hypernatremia

Hypernatremia is seen when the serum sodium levels are higher than normal. This excess may be induced by excessive use of saline infusions, inadequate water consumption (as described previously), or excess fluid loss without a corresponding loss of sodium.

Signs and symptoms include edema; hypertonicity; red, flushed skin; dry, sticky mucous membranes; increase in thirst; temperature elevation; and a decrease in or absence of urination. Treatment includes reducing salt intake and using dextrose in water intravenously to promote diuresis and increase the excretion of both excess salt and water from the blood.

POTASSIUM

Potassium is the major electrolyte in the intracellular fluids. The amount of potassium in the intracellular fluid is approximately 150 mEq/L, whereas the amount in the plasma is between 3.5 and 5 mEq/L. Even though this plasma amount appears to be low, it is of great importance, since serum potassium must be maintained between 3.5 and 5 mEq/L for survival. The diet of most individuals contains from 35 to 100 mEq of potassium daily. Normally, any excess potassium is excreted by the kidney in the urine. Potassium plays an important part of (1) muscle contraction, (2) conduction of nerve impulses, (3) enzyme action, and (4) cell membrane function.

Hypokalemia

Hypokalemia or potassium deficit may be caused by chronic administration of intravenous solutions containing little or no potassium; diuretic therapy with potassium-depleting medications; reduced dietary intake as in persons on "starvation diets"; poor absorption because of steatorrhea, regional enteritis, or short bowel syndrome; loss of gastrointestinal secretions, which are very rich in potassium, because of vomiting, diarrhea, gastrointestinal suction or fistula drainage; extensive burn conditions, and in the presence of excessive amounts of adrenocortical hormone.

Unlike sodium, which is reabsorbed when the serum sodium level is low, potassium ions continue to be excreted in the urine when the serum potassium level is low. As potassium loss continues, the individual's condition deteriorates unless potassium intake is increased and normal levels are reestablished.

With hypokalemia, impaired muscle function occurs. Impairment of skeletal muscle function may cause profound weakness or paralysis, including paralysis of the respiratory muscles. Impaired smooth muscle function may result in ileus.

Cardiac effects of hypokalemia include increased sensitivity to digitalis with potential toxicity and ECG changes such as ST segment depression, U waves, and T wave flattening, depression, or inversion. For example, early potassium deficiency may be detected by the use of the electrocardiogram. The T wave tends to flatten when serum potassium levels are below 3.5 mEq/L. The T wave tends to elongate vertically when the serum potassium level is 5.8 mEq/L or higher. Atrioventricular block and cardiac arrest may occur.

Hypokalemia also causes movement of Na^+ and H^+ from extracellular fluid and the excretion of H^+. This elevates the plasma pH, which results in **metabolic alkalosis.** Other effects are decreased water reabsorption in the renal tubule, resulting in polyuria, and hypochloremia.

Hypokalemia is treated by replacing potassium orally or parenterally. A hazard of parenteral correction of potassium deficit is the production of potassium poisoning, or hyperkalemia.

Parenteral or intravenous administration of potassium. The dosage of potassium supplements depends on the individual requirements of the client, and it requires close monitoring of laboratory values. Intravenous potassium solutions must always be *diluted* and administered slowly. Potassium generally is only given to individuals with a documented adequate urine flow. In dehydrated clients, it is best to give a potassium-free fluid first to hydrate the client and determine urinary output.

It has been generally recommended (AHFS, 1988) that parenteral fluids should not contain more than 40 mEq/L of potassium and the rate of administration should not be more than 20 mEq/hour. Whenever possible, the oral preparations or consumption of foods high in potassium should replace the intravenous potassium solutions.

The parenteral potassium salts are available as potassium chloride, potassium acetate, and potassium phosphate. Generally, the potassium chloride is the preferred preparation, since the chloride ion is present also to correct the hypochloremia that often is seen with hypokalemia. The alkalinizing potassium salts may be necessary to treat hypokalemia associated with metabolic acidosis (a rare situation).

Oral dosage forms of potassium. Potassium acetate, potassium bicarbonate, potassium chloride, potassium citrate, and potassium gluconate are available alone or in combinations for oral administration. Liquid preparations are generally preferred for oral therapy and most contain 10, 20, or 40 mEq of potassium/15 ml. These preparations must be diluted with fruit juice or water before ingestion and taken after meals with a full glass of water to minimize the gastrointestinal irritation. For powder preparations, closely follow the manufacturer's instructions. See Table 70-5 for a listing of oral potassium preparations.

The uncoated and enteric-coated dosage forms of potassium have caused intestinal and gastric ulcers with bleeding episodes. Although still available, they are rarely used medically. Instead, liquid, effervescent preparations, powders, and extended-release dosage forms (wax matrix, microencapsulated) are the currently available preferred products. The nurse should be aware that ulceration has also been reported with the extended-release products (although much less frequently than with the other products), and these preparations should be reserved for clients that cannot or will not take the liquid or effervescent potassium.

If the client complains of stomach pain, swelling, or severe vomiting, or gastrointestinal bleeding is noted, the extended-release potassium should be stopped immediately and the physician should be contacted. Potassium supplements are contraindicated in clients with severe renal impairment, untreated chronic adrenocortical insufficiency (Addison's disease), hyperkalemia, and severe burn conditions or acute dehydration. Solid dosage forms of potassium should not be administered to clients with esophageal compression caused by an enlarged left atrium or other anatomic variation resulting in increased compression in this area. In such cases, ingestion of potassium-rich foods may also be helpful.

Approximately 45 mEq of potassium may be added to the diet by consuming 2 medium-sized bananas and 8 ounces of orange juice; 40 mEq of potassium may be derived from eating 20 large dried apricots, and a cup of dates will yield 36 mEq. A salt substitute (KCl) may provide 60 mEq of potassium/level teaspoon.

The dosage of potassium supplements depends on individual requirements. The approximate daily allowance for adults is 40 to 50 mEq; for infants, about 2 to 3 mEq/kg body weight daily. Oral dosage usually is increased gradually over a 3- to 7-day period to avoid producing hyperkalemia.

Hyperkalemia

Hyperkalemia, or potassium excess, can be caused by acute or chronic renal failure; the release of large amounts of intracellular potassium in burns, crush injuries or severe infections; overtreatment with potassium salts; or in metabolic acidosis, which causes a shift of potassium from the cells into the extracellular fluids.

Hyperkalemia causes interference with neuromuscular function, which can produce weakness and paralysis. Abdominal distention and diarrhea also occur. Cardiac effects caused by hyperkalemia result from impaired conduction. The ECG shows widening and slurring of the QRS complexes, peaked T waves, depressed ST segments, and possibly disappearance of P waves. Ventricular fibrillation and cardiac arrest may occur.

The treatment of hyperkalemia depends on the serum level of potassium and the electrocardiogram (EKG) patterns. If the serum level is below 6.5 mEq/L and the EKG changes are limited to peaking of the T waves, then this may be considered mild hyperkalemia. If the serum level of potassium is between 6.5 and 8 mEq/L with EKG changes limited to peaking of the T waves, then this is moderate hyperkalemia. Severe hyperkalemia is described as a serum level of potassium above 8 mEq/L with an EKG pattern of absent P waves, widened QRS complex or ventricular dysrhythmias.

For *mild* hypokalemia treatment includes removing or treating the cause. For example, if the client is receiving potassium supplements or diuretics with a potassium-sparing property, stop the medications. If metabolic acidosis is present, then treat this condition.

Moderate to severe hyperkalemia may require more aggressive therapy. Infusing hypertonic dextrose solutions will help shift potassium into the cells. Insulin has been used, especially in diabetic clients with hyperkalemia; it also reduces potassium serum levels by 1 to 2 mEq/L

TABLE 70-5 Oral Potassium Preparations

Products	Strength	Additional information
LIQUIDS		
potassium chloride	10 mEq/15 ml	(5% KC1 solution)
Potassine	15 mEq/15 ml	Contains saccharin
potassium chloride	20 mEq/15 ml	
Cena-K		Contains saccharin
Kaochlor 10%		Contains 5% alcohol, tartrazine, and saccharin
Kaochlor S-F		Contains 5% alcohol and saccharin
Kay Ciel		Contains 4% alcohol and saccharin
Klorvess		Contains 0.75% alcohol, saccharin; cherry flavor
Potachlor 10%		Contains 5% alcohol; cherry and orange flavors
Potachlor 10%		Unit dose, 15 and 30 ml. 3.8% alcohol, tartrazine, and lemon flavor
potassium chloride	30 mEq/15 ml	
Rum-K		Alcohol free; butter rum flavor
potassium chloride	40 mEq/15 ml	
Kaon-C1 20%		Contains 5% alcohol and saccharin
Klor-Con		Contains tartrazine
Potachlor 20%		Alcohol free; cherry flavor
potassium gluconate	20 mEq/15 ml	
Kaon		Contains 5% alcohol, saccharin; grape flavor
Kaylixir		Contains 5% alcohol, saccharin
K-G Elixir		Contains 5% alcohol
My-K Elixir		Contains 5% alcohol, saccharin; grape flavor
Trikates	45 mEq/15 ml K (from K acetate, K bicarbonate, K citrate)	Contains saccharin
Tri-K		Contains saccharin; orange flavor
Bi-K	20 mEq/15 ml K (from K gluconate and K citrate)	Contains sorbitol, saccharin
Twin-K		Contains sorbitol, saccharin
Twin-K-C1	15 mEq/K and 4 mEq C1/15 ml (K gluconate, K citrate and ammonium chloride)	Contains sorbitol, saccharin
Duo-K	20 mEq/K and 3.4 mEq C1/15 ml (from K gluconate and KC1)	
Kolyum		Contains sorbitol, saccharin; cherry flavor
POWDERS		
K-Lor	15 mEq KC1/pkt	Saccharin; fruit flavor
Kay Ciel	20 mEq KC1/pkt	4% alcohol, saccharin
K-Lor		Saccharin; fruit flavor
Klor-Con		Saccharin; fruit flavor
Potage		Beef or chicken flavor
Klor-Con/25	25 mEq KC1/pkt	Contains saccharin; fruit flavor
K-Lyte/C1	25 mEq KC1	Contains fruit punch flavor
Klorvess Effervescent Granules	20 mEq each K and C1 (from potassium chloride, bicarbonate, citrate, and lysine HC1)/pkt	Sodium free; saccharin
Kolyum	20 mEq K and 3.4 mEqC1 (from potassium gluconate and chloride)/pkt	Contains sorbitol, saccharin; cherry flavor
EFFERVESCENT TABLETS (must be dissolved in water)		
Kaochlor-Eff	20 mEq KC1 (from potassium chloride, citrate, bicarbonate, and betaine HC1)	Contains tartrazine, saccharin; citrus fruit flavor

Continued.

TABLE 70-5   Oral Potassium Preparations—cont'd

Products	Strength	Additional information
Klorvess	20 mEq KC1 (from potassium chloride, bicarbonate, lysine HC1)	Sodium free; contains saccharin
K-Lyte/C1	25 mEq KC1 (from potassium chloride and bicarbonate, 1-lysine monohydrochloride and citric acid)	Contains saccharin; fruit punch or citrus flavor
K-Lyte/C1 50	50 mEq K (same as above)	
Effer-K	25 mEq K (bicarbonate and citrate)	Saccharin; orange flavor
Klor-Con/EF		Orange flavor
K-Lyte		Contains saccharin; orange or lime flavor
K-Lyte DS	50 mEq K (as bicarbonate and citrate)	Contains saccharin; orange or lime flavor
CAPSULES AND TABLETS		
potassium chloride tablets	1.33 mEq, 8 mEq, 10 mEq	
Kaon-C1	Controlled-release tablets 6.7 mEq (500 mg) KC1 in wax matrix	Contains tartrazine
Klor-Con 8; Slow-K	Controlled-release tablets, 8 mEq (600 mg) KC1 in wax matrix	
Kaon C1-10; Klor-Con-10	Controlled-release tablets, 10 mEq (750) KC1 in wax matrix	
Klotrix	Same as previous	
K-Tab	Same as previous	
K-Dur 10; Ten-K	Controlled-release tablets, microcrystalloids; 10 mEq (750 mg) KC1	
K-Dur 20	Controlled-release tablets, microcrystalloids; 20 mEq (1500 mg) KC1	
Micro-K Extencaps	Controlled-release capsules, 8 mEq (600 mg) KCL; microencapsulated particles	
K-Norm; Micro-K 10	Controlled-release capsules, 10 mEq (750 mg) KC1; microencapsulated particles	
Kaon	Tablets, 5 mEq (1.17 g) potassium gluconate	
K-Forte Regular	Chewable tablets, 1 mEq (39 mg) K (from gluconate, chloride and citrate) and 10 mg vitamin C	Orange flavor
K-Forte Maximum Strength	Chewable tablets, 2.5 mEq (99 mg) potassium (from gluconate, chloride, and citrate) plus 25 mg vitamin C	Contains 0.52 mg sodium; orange flavor

for hours. Sodium bicarbonate parenterally will also help shift serum potassium into the cells. Calcium gluconate intravenously is administered under constant EKG monitoring for the client that has severe cardiac toxicity. The calcium helps counteract the adverse effects of potassium on the neuromuscular membranes, so this is a temporary measure only. Lowering of the potassium levels is critical to reversing this situation.

All of the above-described methods do not remove potassium from the body. Sodium polystyrene sulfonate (Kayexalate) is a cation exhange resin that can be given orally or rectally to reduce potassium serum levels. A single enema can reduce the serum level of potassium by 0.5 to 2 mEq/L within 1 hour. Additional enemas can be given if necessary.

The potassium is eliminated with feces or enema. Lax-atives must be used when the drug is given orally. Since its action is considered slow, the previously discussed treatments are indicated if EKG changes indicate severe potassium intoxication. Administration should be discontinued when the serum potassium levels falls to 4 or 5 mEq/L.

Side effects of sodium polystyrene sulfonate treatment include anorexia, nausea, vomiting, constipation, hypokalemia, and hypocalcemia. Fecal impaction has also been reported; it can be prevented with the use of laxatives.

The oral dose of sodium polystyrene sulfonate for adults is 15 g, one to four times daily in 20 to 100 ml of water or syrup. Add sorbitol to reduce the possibility of constipation. The rectal dose for adults is 25 to 100 g of the resin suspended in 100 ml of sorbitol or 10% dextrose in water. This dose may be administered every 6 hours.

The solution should be retained rectally for several hours, if possible. Then, to remove the resin, administer a cleansing enema.

CALCIUM

Calcium (Ca^{++}) is essential for growth and bone ossification, neuromuscular transmission, cell membrane permeability, the maintenance of excitability in nerve fibers, hormone secretion and action, muscle contraction, maintenance of cardiac and vascular tone, many enzyme activities, and the normal coagulation of blood.

Almost all of the 1000 to 1200 g calcium in the normal adult is in the skeletal tissue, and only about 1% of the total body calcium is in solution in body fluids. About half the calcium in plasma is bound to serum proteins; a small portion is bound to complex organic anions (e.g., bicarbonate and phosphate). Almost all unbound serum calcium is ionized. Normal serum calcium concentration is 4.5 to 5.5 mEq/L or 9 to 11 mg/100 ml.

The recommended dietary allowance of calcium for adults is 800 to 1200 mg daily. Pregnant or lactating women need 1.2 g; children 6 to 18 years of age need 0.8 to 1.2 g. The intake of calcium in a balanced diet is sufficient for normal body needs. Absorption of calcium depends on how well it is kept in solution in the digestive tract. An acid medium favors calcium solubility; thus calcium is absorbed mainly in the upper intestinal tract. Absorption is decreased by the presence of alkalis and large amounts of fatty acids, with which the calcium forms insoluble soaps. Adequate intake of vitamin D appears to promote calcium absorption. Calcium is excreted in the urine and feces, as well as in perspiration. Estrogen deficiency promotes calcium loss.

Maintenance of normal concentration of serum calcium depends on the interactions of three agents: parathyroid hormone, vitamin D, and calcitonin. Parathyroid hormone and vitamin D mobilize the removal of calcium from bone, the principal source of calcium for extracellular fluids. Parathyroid hormone also promotes renal tubular reabsorption of calcium and a slight increase in intestinal absorption of calcium. Calcitonin is synthesized in the thyroid gland; it moderates or decreases the rate of removal of calcium from the bone.

Hypocalcemia

Hypocalcemia, a decrease in serum calcium, results from (1) hypoparathyroidism, (2) chronic renal insufficiency, (3) rickets and osteomalacia, (4) malabsorption syndrome, and (5) deficiency of vitamin D. Hypoparathyroidism may follow thyroidectomy, since several parathyroid glands frequently are removed with this surgery. If the function of the remaining gland(s) is impaired, the result is depressed parathyroid activity.

Individuals who are bedridden tend to develop a negative calcium balance because the ion is lost from bones and is excreted. This effect is likely to be serious when long immobilization of the patient is necessary.

Hypocalcemia causes increased excitability of the nerves and neuromuscular junction, which leads to muscle cramps, muscle twitching, and tetany. Numbness and tingling of the fingers, toes, and lips occur. The hypertonicity of muscle may cause tonic contractions of the hands and feet (carpopedal spasm). The increased neural excitability may cause convulsions, abnormal behavior, and personality changes. In children, prolonged hypocalcemia has resulted in mental retardation. Other effects of hypocalcemia include dyspnea, laryngeal spasm, diplopia, abdominal cramps, and urinary frequency. Diminished cardiac contractility may occur. The ECG shows a prolonged QT interval and an inverted T wave. In prolonged hypocalcemia, defects can occur in the nails, skin, and teeth; cataracts may appear; and calcification of the basal ganglia may occur.

Regardless of the underlying cause, severe hypocalcemia is treated initially with intravenous administration of rapidly available calcium ions. For latent tetany, mild symptoms of hypocalcemia, and maintenance therapy, a calcium salt is given orally. Vitamin D may be given. Parathyroid injection is now considered obsolete and is not used for therapy; its biologic activity is uncertain. Overdosage of calcium may cause hypercalcemia, which results in anorexia, nausea, vomiting, weakness, depression, polyuria, and polydipsia. Calcium must be administered cautiously to clients on digitalis therapy, since calcium potentiates the effect of digitalis and may precipitate dysrhythmias. ECG monitoring of the client is recommended when parenteral calcium is administered.

Calcium salts are used as a nutritional supplement, particularly during pregnancy and lactation. They are specific in the treatment of hypocalcemic tetany. They have also been used for their antispasmodic effects in cases of abdominal pain, tenesmus, and colic resulting from disease of the gallbladder or painful contractions of the ureters. The basic salts of calcium are also used as antacids. Although controversial, approximately 1 to 1.5 g calcium per day has been recommended to prevent postmenopausal bone loss or osteoporosis.

The most widely used calcium salt is calcium carbonate. It requires an acid medium to form soluble calcium salts, since it is nearly insoluble in water. Calcium phosphate and calcium sulfate are also pH dependent, whereas calcium lactate, calcium citrate, and calcium gluconate are considered pH independent. In elderly persons and postmenopausal women, an impaired stomach acid production is noted. The higher stomach pH or achlorhydria state will result in a decreased solubility of the pH-dependent calcium salts.

Since the different calcium salts have different amounts of calcium present, many professionals choose the calcium salt with the highest percentage of calcium per gram present because it would then require a smaller quantity of drug to be administered. For example, if the recommended daily dose of calcium is 1000 mg/day, then it would be necessary to administer nearly 10 g calcium gluconate to reach this amount; whereas only 2.5 g/calcium carbonate per day would be required. This would require the consumption of smaller quantities of tablets to obtain the same amount of calcium. This, of course, is assuming all the present calcium is soluble under the conditions present in the client. (See Table 70-6.)

To improve the solubility of calcium carbonate tablets, especially in individuals that might be achlorhydric, it is recommended that the tablets be taken with meals, when acid secretion is highest. Avoid taking the tablets on an empty stomach or at night because these are times when acid secretions are at a minimal point. Calcium phosphates and tricalcium phosphate have little usefulness in possible achlorhydric states and perhaps, even in the normal person. Both products have a very poor dissolution rate or pattern, thus reducing the possibility of calcium absorption. Perhaps in clients with known achlorhydric states, the soluble calcium salts (lactate or citrate) might be the appropriate form to use even though it will be necessary to use more tablets to provide sufficient quantities of calcium.

Selected food consumption is another source for calcium. See Table 70-7 for foods with a high calcium content.

Hypercalcemia

Hypercalcemia, or elevated serum calcium levels, may be caused by neoplasms with or without bone metastases. Carcinoma of the ovary, kidney, or lung can synthesize and secrete a parathyroid-like hormone, causing hypercalcemia. Other common causes are hyperparathyroidism, thiazide or diuretic therapy, multiple myeloma, sarcoidosis, and vitamin D intoxication.

Clinical manifestations of hypercalcemia are highly variable and involve many organ systems. Calcium may be deposited in various body tissues.

Gastrointestinal symptoms are anorexia, nausea and vomiting, constipation, and abdominal pain.

Central nervous system symptoms include apathy, depression, amnesia, headaches, and drowsiness. In severe cases, disorientation, syncope, hallucinations, and coma may occur.

Renal symptoms include polyuria and polydipsia, which occur from loss of renal-concentrating ability. Kidney stones may be formed. Nephrocalcinosis may occur, seriously impairing renal function. This may lead to edema, uremia, and hypertension, which may be irreversible.

In the *neuromuscular* system, neural excitability is diminished, causing weakness and muscle flaccidity.

Cardiovascular symptoms include elevated serum calcium, which causes increased cardiac contractility, ventricular extrasystoles, and heart block. ECG changes in-

TABLE 70-6　Calcium Content in Various Calcium Salts

Salt	% Calcium	Amount (g) needed for 1 g Calcium
calcium ascorbate	10.3	9.75
calcium carbonate	40.0	2.50
calcium citrate	24.1	4.20
calcium gluconate	9.3	10.75
calcium lactate	18.4	5.40
calcium sulfate	36.1	2.80
dibasic calcium phosphate	29.5	3.40
tribasic calcium phosphate	38.8	2.60

TABLE 70-7　Selected Foods with High Calcium Content

Food	Calcium content
Yogurt, low fat (1 cup)	400 mg
Skim milk (1 cup)	300 mg
Cheese, Swiss (1 ounce)	250 mg
Cheese, cottage (1 cup)	215 mg
Cheese, cheddar (1 ounce)	200 mg
Broccoli, raw	100 mg
Ice cream (½ cup)	100 mg

clude a short QT segment and characteristic signs of heart block. In severe calcium toxicity, cardiac arrest in systole may occur.

Treatment is variable and aimed at controlling the underlying disease. If hypercalcemia is caused by thiazide diuretic therapy, the diuretic is discontinued; the serum calcium returns to normal levels in about 1 month.

Renal excretion of calcium can be promoted with several drugs. Infusions of sodium chloride may be given to increase sodium excretion, which in turn increases calcium excretion. Natriuretic drugs, such as furosemide (Lasix) or ethacrynic acid (Edecrin), may be used. Chelating (binding) agents, such as disodium edetate, increase renal excretion of calcium by forming soluble complexes with the calcium that are not reabsorbed by the renal tubules. Inorganic phosphates may be given orally or intravenously to foster deposition of calcium in bone, thereby decreasing serum levels. An antineoplastic drug, mithramycin, also reduces serum calcium levels.

MAGNESIUM

Magnesium (Mg^{++}) is an important ion for the function of many enzyme systems.

Hypomagnesemia

Hypomagnesemia, a deficit of magnesium, may be encountered in chronic alcoholism, severe malabsorption, starvation, diarrhea, prolonged gastrointestinal suction, vigorous diuresis, diseases causing hypocalcemia and hypokalemia, acute pancreatitis, and primary aldosteronism.

Hypomagnesemia is characterized by increased irritability of the nervous system, which may lead to disorientation and convulsions. Increased neuromuscular irritability and contractility also occur. Coarse tremor, muscle spasm, delirium, athetoid movements, and nystagmus may appear. Tetany may occur. Hypomagnesemia also causes tachycardia, hypertension, and vasomotor changes. The use of intravenous fluids containing from 3 to 5 mEq magnesium/L may avert magnesium deficiency that arises from prolonged administration of intravenous solutions that do not contain magnesium.

Hypomagnesemia is treated with intravenous fluids containing magnesium, 10 to 40 mEq/day for severe deficit, followed by 10 mEq/day for maintenance.

Hypermagnesemia

Hypermagnesemia occurs primarily in patients with chronic renal insufficiency. An excess of magnesium causes depression of the central nervous system, which leads to sedation and confusion. Blockade of the myoneural junction occurs by inhibiting acetylcholine release and diminishing muscle cell excitability. This causes muscle weakness. Respiratory muscle paralysis may occur, causing death. Hypermagnesemia also causes blockade of sympathetic ganglia and has a direct vasodilating effect that causes decreased blood pressure.

Excess magnesium has a cardiac inhibitory effect. Conduction time is increased, and the ECG shows a lengthened PR segment and a prolonged QRS complex. If the Mg^{++} concentration continues to increase, cardiac arrest in diastole may occur. Third-degree atrioventricular block may also occur.

An excess of Mg^{++} may require dialysis. Since calcium acts as an antagonist to Mg^{++}, calcium salts may be given parenterally. Normal serum concentration is 1.5 to 2.5 mEq/L, with one third bound to protein and two thirds as free cation. A toxic blood level is greater than 4 mEq/L. About 50% of the total body magnesium exists in an insoluble state in bone, 45% is intracellular cation, and 5% extracellular cation. The normal dietary intake of magnesium has a range of approximately 8 to 24 mEq/24 hours in the adult (recommended dietary allowance is 300 to 400 mg daily). Magnesium is excreted by way of the kidney. Magnesium has physiologic effects on the nervous system similar to those of calcium.

ADDITIONAL SINGLE-SALT SOLUTIONS

In addition to the previously discussed salt preparations, ammonium chloride injection and sodium lactate injection are also available for use.

Ammonium chloride injection is indicated to treat hypochloremia and metabolic alkalois (not associated with severe liver disease) to prevent tetany or renal damage. Most cases will respond to sodium chloride solution, but for the rare, nonresponsive situation, ammonium chloride is available.

This product is most often required for infants that have severe, protracted vomiting caused by pyloric obstruction. It is available as a 2.14% solution (0.4 mEq/ml) and must be infused slowly to allow for metabolism of the ammonium ions by the liver to avoid ammonia toxicity.

Sodium lactate injection is available as a ⅙ molar solution containing 167 mEq/L each of sodium and lactate ions. It is used to treat metabolic acidosis when no evidence of an elevated lactic acid level exists. Sodium lactate is converted to sodium bicarbonate in the liver. In persons with lactic acidosis or impaired liver function, sodium bicarbonate should be administered.

THE NURSE'S ROLE IN INTRAVENOUS THERAPY

With the increasing prevalence of clients receiving some type of intravascular therapy in hospitals, as well as in home settings, the role of the nurse in intravenous therapy has also grown and developed.

Assessment. Begin assessment by understanding the purpose of the particular client's intravenous therapy and his or her potential risks. Every individual with an intravenous infusion runs the risk of circulatory overload, iatrogenic starvation or dehydration, infiltration, phlebitis, air embolism, infection of the site, or sepsis. Those who are debilitated, have a renal or cardiovascular problem, are prone to infection, or have badly sclerosed veins are particularly at risk. Continued reassessments of laboratory data reports are essential for patients receiving electrolyte replacement therapy. Serum electrolytes should not exceed the following accepted ranges during intravenous therapy:

Sodium	135 to 145 mEq/L
Chlorides	95 to 108 mEq/L
Potassium	3.5 to 5 mEq/L
Calcium	4.5 to 5.8 mEq/L
Magnesium	1.5 to 2.5 mEq/L

Note that fluctuations in potassium, calcium, and magnesium must be watched carefully during intravenous electrolyte therapy, since even a small deviation in these creates a much greater risk than in those electrolytes with a wider range of normal values. Understanding that milliequivalents (mEq) are not related to milligrams also is important; "mEq" does not reflect a measure of weight. Milliequivalents measure the number of chemically active ions in solution, which is a more precise measure of the relative potency of an electrolyte solution than weight-by-volume measurements. (See Chapter 6 for equipment and technical aspects of intravenous therapy.)

Remember that ongoing assessment of client response is essential to preventing complications from intravenous therapy. Such assessments are made frequently in some critical care units. Calculating the need for hourly changes in intravenous flow rates based on patient fluid output may be your responsibility. You may titrate infusion fluid intake according to the amount of hourly urine, gastric, or other outputs over specified periods.

Complications. The ongoing assessment of the client receiving intravenous therapy should include observations for the following complications:

Infiltration. Infiltration occurs when the needle is dislodged from the vein, permitting the solution to enter the surrounding tissues, which causes pain and edema. Clients or family members should be informed to notify the nurse if pain or swelling occurs at the infusion site. In addition, nurses should check the infusion site frequently for signs of infiltration and stop the infusion if infiltration occurs. Restarting intravenous therapy usually requires a new infusion site.

Thrombosis. An intravascular blood clot occurs when platelets agglutinate and fibrin strands and red and white blood cells adhere to the platelet mass. A thrombus may form any time a blood vessel is injured, including injury by venipuncture. A thrombus may form in or around the needle or catheter, plugging the lumen; if this occurs, the infusion stops. The infusion should be restarted at a new site with a new needle or catheter. Attempts to unplug the needle by forcing a bolus of solution in a syringe through the needle into the vein is unwise and unsafe. The thrombus may become an embolus and lodge in a vital organ, causing more serious complications such as pulmonary embolus.

Thrombophlebitis. Blood clot formation and inflammation of the vein may result from several factors: prolonged duration of infusion, use of contaminated equipment or contaminated solutions, irritation from drugs in the infusion, toxicity and pH of the solution, the use of leg vein as site of administration, and infection. Thrombophlebitis is manifested by pain, heat, swelling, redness along the vein's course, and loss of motion of the affected part. When this occurs, the infusion should be stopped, the needle withdrawn, and the condition reported and recorded immediately. Treatment usually consists of applying moist heat to the affected area and resting the body part; anticoagulant therapy also may be ordered.

Nurses should take the necessary precautions to prevent thrombophlebitis by doing the following:

- Using sterile aseptic technique with proper cleansing of skin before insertion of the needle
- Being certain equipment is not contaminated
- Checking solutions for precipitation, debris, sedi-

ment, or change in color before and during intravenous therapy
- Ascertaining that no intravenous bottle or tubing is left in place for more than 24 hours, since some organisms proliferate at room temperature in intravenous fluids
- Changing the intravenous setup every 24 hours to reduce the possibility of sepsis
- Administering irritating drugs slowly
- Avoiding intravenous needle infusion into leg veins or small veins

Pain at administrative site. Pain occurs when (1) the needle touches the venous wall, (2) too much tension is put on the needle or tubing, and (3) irritating drugs are administered too rapidly. Adjusting the needle, relieving the tension by readjusting the needle support or relaxing the pull on the tubing, and administering irritating drugs at a slow rate may alleviate the pain and discomfort.

Necrosis. Death and sloughing of tissue can occur when irritating drugs or solutions, such as epinephrine or levarterenol, infiltrate into the tissues. The infusion should be stopped *immediately.* If the infiltration contains levarterenol, the antidote phentolamine (Regitine) may be injected subcutaneously in minute amounts immediately at many sites in the edematous area.

Pulmonary edema. Pulmonary edema occurs when the circulatory system is overloaded with fluids. Central venous pressure monitoring, particularly in clients with cardiac disease, can help to prevent this hazardous complication.

Pyrogenic reactions. Pyrogenic reactions occur when pyrogens, or fever-producing substances, are introduced into the circulatory system. Bacterial pyrogens are filtrable, thermostable products of bacterial origin and activity that may accumulate and tend to cause a severe rigor when injected into the body. Pyrogenic reactions are characterized by fever and chills, malaise, headache, nausea, and vomiting. The infusion should be stopped *at once.* The solution should not be discarded but instead sent to the pharmacist. Pyrogenic reactions must be reported and recorded. The stock number should be noted, since an entire batch of solutions may be contaminated.

•   •   •

Note that the recommended system for surveillance and reporting of problems with large-volume parenteral solutions in hospitals has been delegated to the National Coordinating Committee on Large-Volume Parenterals. The Committee is composed of legally recognized standards-setting bodies, enforcement agencies, and national groups with a major influence over the manufacture and use of large-volume parenteral solutions. Organizations represented on the committee are the American Hospital Association, American Medical Association, American Nurses' Association, American Society of Hospital Pharmacists, Centers for Disease Control, Food and Drug Administration, Joint Commission of Accreditation of Hospitals, National Association of Boards of Pharmacy, National Association for Practical Nurse Education and Service, Parenteral Drug Association, The United States Pharmacopeial Convention, and major large-volume parenteral manufacturers (Abbott, Cutter, McGraw, Travenol). The committee's mission is to find workable solutions to those large-volume parenteral problems judged to have the greatest clinical significance. The National Intravenous Therapy Association is composed largely of intravenous team nurses who make procedure and policy recommendations. The recommendations relate to problems with large-volume parenteral solutions in health care facilities, methods for compounding intravenous admixtures in hospitals, labeling of large-volume parenteral solutions, and procedures for in-use testing for contamination or adverse reactions and for filter selection.

Intervention. Be aware that intravenous fluid and dextrose or electrolyte replacement by infusion continues to be the most common application of intravascular therapy. Although the dosage and choice of solution is tailored to the client's needs by the physician according to his or her disorder and body surface area, monitoring the therapy is the nurse's responsibility. A member of the therapy team, the nurse, or the physician may be responsible for initiating therapy by inserting the necessary needle or catheter.

Consider intravascular therapy a closed-system, sterile procedure. It is invasive, and its effects are relatively irreversible. Therefore take care to perform and maintain it precisely. Maintain a steady, even flow at the rate ordered; do not speed up rates to make up for lost time (watch the literature, however, for a resolution of the question about slowed rates being more compatible with basal metabolic rates during the before-dawn hours). Use every aid to facilitate therapy, such as calculating drops to be infused per minute and then time-taping the container. Do not allow containers to empty completely, since air in the tubing could be driven into the vein when another full container is attached. Throughout all client activities keep containers about 3 feet above the site. If too high, the solution will infuse too rapidly; if too low, blood may find its way into the needle or tubing and clot there. Consult agency infusion specialists such as members of the intravenous therapy team, when available, if you encounter difficulties.

Be aware of the options available in selecting a filter for the intravenous infusion. Several different intravenous filter products are designed for different filtration needs. Filters are available in a range of sizes and in an add-on or in-line form:

- A 5 μm filter removes *particulate* material and is designed to filter gross particulate matter. The smallest particle visible to the unaided eye is approximately 30 μm across.

- A 0.5 μm filter is considered a *bacteria-retention* filter, which is designed to prevent passage of most particulate matter and certain fungi and bacteria. A yeast cell is approximately 3 μm in diameter.

- The 0.22 μm filter is called a *sterilizing* filter, since it is designed to prevent passage of virtually all particulate matter and most bacteria for at least 24 hours. Bacteria range in size from 0.2 to 2 μm in diameter. Travenol Laboratories and other manufacturers provide these filters for use with the add-on or in-line systems. Select a 0.22 μm filter for parenteral nutrition solutions.

Education. If your client is a child, keep in mind that intravenous therapy may be a frightening experience. Interesting, nonthreatening coloring booklet pages at the back of the *Nursing Photobook, Managing Intravenous Therapy* (see Bibliography) may be copied and provided to make the child more at ease.

Instruct the client receiving intravenous therapy to report to the nurse any symptoms of the complications previously mentioned.

KEY TERMS

BIBLIOGRAPHY

Abramowicz, M, ed: Prevention and treatment of postmenopausal osteoporosis, The Medical Letter 29:746, 1987.

American Hospital Formulary Service: AHFS drug information '88, Bethesda, Md, 1988, American Society of Hospital Pharmacists, Inc.

Barrus, DH, and others: Should you irrigate an occluded I.V. line? Nursing 17(3):63, 1987.

Beckwith, N: Fundamentals of fluid resuscitation, Nursinglife 7(3):49, 1987.

Braunwald, E, and others, eds: Harrison's principles of internal medicine, ed 11, New York, 1987, McGraw-Hill Book Co.

Bryan, CS: "CDC says . . .": the case of intravenous tubing replacement, Infect Control 8(6):255, 1987.

Buckalew, VM, Jr: Hyponatremia: pathogenesis and management, Hosp Pract 21(11):49, 1986.

Coward, DD: Cancer-induced hypercalcemia, Cancer Nurs 9(3):125, 1986.

Davidson, ED: Handbook of nonprescription drugs, ed 8, Washington, DC, 1986, American Pharmaceutical Association and The National Professional Society of Pharmacists.

DeRubertis, FR: Hypercalcemia and hypocalcemia, Top Emerg Med 5(4):64, 1984.

Diseases, Nurse's Reference Library, Horsham, Pa, 1981, Intermed Communications.

Flink, EB: Magnesium deficiency: causes and effects, Hosp Pract 22(2):116A, 1987.

Gilman, AG, and others: Goodman and Gilman's the pharmacological basis of therapeutics, ed 7, New York, 1985, Macmillan Publishing Co.

Kastrup, EK, ed: Facts and comparisons, St Louis, 1988, JB Lippincott Co.

Metheny and Snively: Nurses' handbook of fluid balance, ed 2, Philadelphia, 1974, JB Lippincott Co.

Nursing photobook: managing intravenous therapy, Horsham, Penn, 1980, Intermed Communications.

Otrakji, J: Disorders of potassium metabolism, Top Emerg Med 5(2):53, 1983.

Persons, CB: Preventing infection from intravascular devices, Nursing 17(4):75, 1987.

Plumer, AL: Principles and practice of intravenous therapy, ed 2, Boston, 1975, Little, Brown & Co.

Poe, CM, and others: The challenge of hypercalcemia in cancer, Oncol Nurs Forum 12(6):29, 1985.

Rice, V: Magnesium, calcium, and phosphate imbalances: their clinical significance (home study program), Crit Care Nurse 3(3):90, 1983.

Rice, V: Shock management: fluid volume replacement, Crit Care Nurse 4(6):69, 1984.

Shangraw, RF: Factors affecting dissolution and absorption of calcium supplements, Fla Pharm J 51(1):10, 1987.

Stanaszek, WF, and others: Current approaches to the management of potassium deficiency, Drug Intell Clin Pharm 19(3):176, 1985.

Stark, JL: Water regulation in health and renal disease: a review, NITA 8(6):497, 1985.

Thomas, AG: Disorders of sodium metabolism, Top Emerg Med 5(2):46, 1983.

Verbalis, JG, and others: Hypernatremia and hyponatremia, Top Emerg Med 5(4):79, 1984.

Walter, RM, Jr: Hypercalcemia: therapy that addresses the causal mechanism, Consultant 26(9):91, 1986.

CHAPTER
71

Enteral and Parenteral Nutrition

OBJECTIVES

After studying this chapter, the student will be able to:

1. Identify the consequences of malnutrition on the hospitalized or elderly client.

2. Describe common techniques used for the delivery of enteral feedings.

3. Distinguish between elemental, polymeric, modular, and altered amino acid formulations for enteral feedings.

4. Identify common commercial enteral formulations according to their formulation category.

5. Identify major drug-food interactions to be aware of when enteral nutrient formulations are being administered.

6. Develop a nursing care plan for a client receiving enteral formulations.

7. Differentiate between partial parenteral nutrition and total parenteral nutrition.

8. Describe central hyperalimentation and the indications for its use.

9. Identify the components of total parenteral solutions and the function of each element in the attainment of the body's requirement.

10. Cite the complications possible during parenteral nutrition; correlate with the clinical manifestations, nursing assessments and nursing interventions.

Pioneers in parenteral hyperalimentation in the late 1960s to the 1970s were Drs. Stanley Dudrick and Jonathan Rhoads. As surgeons and researchers, they were concerned about the tremendous weight loss in acutely ill patients, so they performed animal studies, and later human studies, to prove their theory that a positive nitrogen balance could be achieved by providing nutrients intravenously.

Since then, many advances have been recorded in the fields of both enteral and parenteral nutrition. Clinical nutrition is now a recognized and active entity for improving health care in all settings, including the client's home, long-term care facilities, and hospitals. Today nutritional programs or specific products have even been developed for individuals with specific disease states or illnesses. In this chapter, enteral and parenteral nutrition will be reviewed, along with selected disease states and criteria for use of the specific nutritional system.

ENTERAL NUTRITION

ENTERAL FEEDINGS (LIQUID ORAL AND TUBE FEEDINGS)

The high incidence of reported malnutrition among hospitalized persons and nursing home residents is associated with such complications as muscle atrophy, slow wound healing, impaired immunocompetence, sepsis, and death. Other signs include peripheral edema caused by reduced plasma proteins, dry and flaky skin, and hair loss. Nearly half of hospitalized patients have some degree of malnutrition; 5% to 10% have severe protein-calorie deficiencies. Malnutrition is reflected in reduced total lymphocyte count, serum albumin, and transferrin levels, or iron-binding capacity; increased 24-hour urine urea nitrogen concentration reflects protein catabolism.

Stress in reaction to hospitalization may alter a client's usual eating habits. Unfamiliar foods and general malaise resulting from illness cause patients to lose their appetites. Oral intake may be inadequate or be impossible because of oropharyngeal surgery, trauma, neoplasm, paralysis, or esophageal fistula. Fasting before surgery or for diagnostic workup also may be depleting. When sepsis, trauma, major surgery, inflammation or infection, or severe burns supervene, energy needs may be doubled. If the gastrointestinal tract is functional, however, enteral or tube feedings may effectively supply essential nutrition. The cost per person for tube feedings is about equal to a regular hospital diet and provides more complete control and assessment of intake. Tube feedings also may be used to supplement parenteral nutrition as it is being tapered. Enteral feedings generally are contraindicated in individuals who are capable of oral intake or who have adynamic ileus, intestinal obstruction, intractable vomiting, or esophageal fistulas.

Enteral feedings may be administered either by bolus doses, typically 250 to 400 ml of formula every 4 to 6 hours; by intermittent feedings by means of a 20 to 30 minute drip; or by continuous gravity or enteral pumps. The continuous method, for 16 to 24 hours, has had more success because it helps prevent complications such as the dumping syndrome (nausea, vomiting, cramping, diarrhea, and malabsorption caused by sudden influxes of undigested feedings of high osmolality into the small intestine) and obviates the need for frequent tube irrigations. Enteral feedings can be administered by the following routes: nasogastric, nasoduodenal, esophagostomy, gastrostomy, and jejunostomy. The last three are more invasive, requiring surgically created stomas, and thus are less preferred routes. Nasogastric, esophagostomy, and gastrostomy feedings allow for more natural digestion in the stomach and preclude the risk of the dumping syndrome. Aspiration, however, is more likely because gastric reflux can occur, since only the gastroesophageal sphincter is operant. Although feedings administered directly into the small intestine avoid this problem, hypoglycemia and the dumping syndrome may develop because of the sudden influx. Skin excoriation and infection are potential risks in gastrostomies and jejunostomies because the surgical opening penetrates the peritoneum. These complications are avoided in the cervical esophagostomy, a surgically created, skin-lined canal tunneled from the lower neck border and extending to below the cervical esophagus.

The selection of tube feeding formula depends on the client's nutrition needs, organ or metabolic disorders, lactose intolerance, gastrointestinal competence, convenience, feasibility, and cost. Nutritional assessment may be based on anthropometric parameters, biochemical data, and physical findings, as well as on medical, diet,

drug, and socioeconomic histories. Ideal weight can be obtained from tables or by estimation:

Men: 106 pounds (48 kg) for the first 5 feet (150 cm) plus 6 pounds (2.7 kg) per inch (2.5 cm) over 5 feet (plus or minus 10%)

Women: 100 pounds (45 kg) for the first 5 feet plus 5 pounds (2.2 kg) per inch over 5 feet (plus or minus 10%)

ENTERAL FORMULATIONS

Over 80 enteral formulations are available in the United States. These products can be divided into elemental (monomeric), polymeric, modular, and altered amino acid formulations.

1. Elemental formulations contain dipeptides and tripeptides and/or crystalline amino acids, glucose oligosaccharides, and vegetable oil or the medium-chain triglycerides. This formula requires minimum digestion from the client. The residue is also minimal.

   Elemental formulations are indicated for persons with partial bowel obstruction, inflammatory bowel disease, radiation enteritis, bowel fistulas, and short bowel syndrome.

2. Polymeric formulations contain complex nutrients: protein (e.g., casein and soy protein); carbohydrate (e.g., corn syrup solid, maltodextrins); and fat (vegetable oil or milk fat).

   Polymeric formulas are preferred to elemental formulations for patients with a fully functional gastrointestinal tract who have few or no specialized nutrient requirements. These formulas are preferred because the hyperosmolarity of the elemental formulas causes more gastrointestinal problems than the polymeric formulations. It should not be used in clients with a malabsorption problem.

3. Modular formulations are single nutrient formulas, i.e., protein, carbohydrate, or fat. This formula can be added to a monomeric or polymeric formulation to provide a more individual specialized nutrient formulation.

4. Altered amino acid formulations are indicated for clients with genetic errors of metabolism (e.g., phenylketonuria, homocystinuria, maple syrup urine disease), for clients with acquired disorders of nitrogen accumulation (e.g., cirrhosis or chronic renal failure), and in clients who are catabolic because of injuries or infection. (For selected examples of the four categories, see Table 71-1.)

DRUG-FOOD (NUTRIENT) INTERACTIONS

A number of drug-food interactions have been identified, but this is often overlooked when enteral nutrient formulations are being administered. Since the interac-

TABLE 71-1   Selected Commercial Enteral Formulations

	Comments
ELEMENTAL FORMULATIONS*	
Flexical	Approximately 30% of the calories are from fat. Proteins are short-chain peptides. Lactose free.
Vital	Proteins are short-chain peptides. Lower osmolality than others. Lactose free.
Vivonex	Proteins are amino acids. Lactose free.
Vivonex HN	Less fat content than Vivonex. Its higher osmolality necessitates dilution and slower infusion to avoid complaints of cramping. Lactose free.
POLYMERIC FORMULATIONS	
Compleat-B	For tube feedings only. Contains lactose.
Ensure	Lactose free.
Ensure-Plus	Higher caloric formula. Lactose free.
Isocal	For tube feedings only. Lactose free. Low osmolality.
Magnacal	Good for clients with sodium or water restrictions. Has a high caloric formula (2 calories/ml).
Meritene	High protein formula. Contains lactose.
Osmolite	An isotonic formula. Lactose free.
Portagen	Used in malabsorption syndromes because the fat content is from MCT oil. Lactose free.
Precision LR	Lactose free. Low in fat and residue.
Sustacal	Contains a high protein content and lactose.
MODULAR FORMULATIONS	
Carbohydrate	
Controlyte	A carbohydrate supplement. Has low sodium; no vitamins, minerals, or lactose.
Polycose	Unflavored carbohydrate supplement. 2 calories/ml.
Fat	
MCT Oil	Fat supplement. Used in malabsorption, GI alterations, and pancreatitis. Contains 94% medium-chain triglyceride.
Microlipid	Fat supplement. Is a concentrated source for calories, i.e., it contains 4.5 calories/ml.
Proteins	
Amin-aid	Contains a high biologic protein and has high caloric formula (1.9 calories/ml). Used for clients with renal failure (acute and chronic).
Casec	A protein supplement for use in severe burns or trauma, fistulas, and complicated surgery. Contains milk but no vitamins, minerals, or lactose.
Hepatic-Aid Instant Drink Powder, Hepatic-Aid II Instant Drink Powder	Contains high concentrations of branched-chain amino acids and low concentrations of aromatic amino acids to correct for the abnormal serum amino acid profiles. Use in chronic liver disease.
Travasorb Renal Powder	Contains amino acids, glucose, and sucrose and MCT (medium-chain triglycerides). 1.35 calories/ml. For renal failure.
Traum-Aid HBC Powder	Contains amino acids (high BCAA), carbohydrates, and fats (MCT, soybean oil. For trauma and sepsis clients.

*All these elemental formulations contain vitamins and trace elements. They also have 1 calorie/ml.

Continued.

TABLE 71-1   Selected Commercial Enteral Formulations—cont'd

	Comments
Stresstein Powder	Amino acids (BCAA), carbohydrates (maltodextrins), and fats (MCT, soybean oil). Indicated for severe trauma and stress.

ALTERED AMINO ACID FORMULATIONS

For chronic renal failure: see Amin-aid above.
For pre-eclampsia, congestive heart failure:

Lonalac	Protein supplement used for low sodium requirements. It has vitamins, trace elements, and lactose.

For genetic disorders:

Phenylketonuria: diet prescribed is low in phenylalanine. Tyrosine may need to be supplemented.

Homocystinuria: diet low in methionine and cystine

Maple syrup urine disease: diet low in leucine, isoleucine, and valine

tions can be clinically significant, the major ones are listed in Table 71-2.

THE NURSE'S ROLE IN ENTERAL NUTRITION

Assessment. Assess periodically for residual gastric volume and tube placement, particularly before each feeding or before administering a dose of a medication into the feeding tube. For continuous feedings, simply stop the feeding and measure the residual by aspirating the stomach contents with a bulb syringe. It is not necessary to clamp off the tube and wait for an interval of time because these feedings should move through the system continuously. If the residual is greater than 50% of an hour's

TABLE 71-2   Drug-Food Interactions

Drug(s)	Food or nutrient	Possible effect/management
ampicillin	Decrease in serum levels by food.	Administer on an empty stomach.
aspirin	Absorption prolonged by food.	Administer with milk or crackers; avoid giving on a full stomach.
cephalosporins (cefamandole, cefaperazone, moxalactam)	Absorption prolonged by food. May produce disulfiram reaction if alcohol is present.	Administer on schedule. Avoid alcohol-containing medications, beverages, sauces and topical preparations.
doxycycline	Iron will reduce serum levels of antibiotic.	Schedule iron preparations and doxycycline about 3 hr apart.
oxacillin	Absorption prolonged and serum levels decreased.	Administer on an empty stomach.
tetracyclines (with exception of doxycycline and minocycline)	Milk, dairy items, eggs, cereals, and divalent and trivalent cautions.	Administer on an empty stomach.
digoxin	Absorption prolonged or delayed if given with food.	Be consistent; give digoxin with or without food. This will reduce problems with bioavailability.
griseofulvin	Absorption is increased in presence of fats.	If client appears to have an inadequate absorption, consider giving the drug with a high fat meal.
levodopa	High protein diets will delay and prolong absorption.	Schedule apart from a high protein meal.
metoprolol, propranolol, phenytoin	Food will increase absorption and bioavailability.	Be consistent; give medication with or without food. This will reduce problems of fluctation in bioavailability.
warfarin	Foods with high vitamin K will reduce the anticoagulant action.	Avoid excessive consumption of foods with high vitamin K content (broccoli, spinach, and other green, leafy vegetables).

volume, return the aspirate and notify the physician. For cyclic administration, measure residual volume halfway between feedings. If the residual is more than 50% of the volume of the previous feeding, return the aspirate and consult with the physician. In both of these instances, a reduction in the volume of the feeding may be necessary.

Monitor bowel sounds to ensure that the client has good bowel function. Fluid intake and output should be carefully documented. If the client develops diarrhea, the physician needs to be consulted.

Many types of enteral formulas are lactose-free (nonmilk proteins are the base) for patients who lack sufficient lactase in intestinal brush bodies for lactose absorption. Blacks, Orientals, American Indians, and Jews are particularly prone to lactase deficiency. Lactose ingestion causes varying degrees of diarrhea, abdominal cramps, bloating, and flatulence. Isotonic formulas may be useful to prevent the dumping syndrome.

Intervention. Although the gastrointestinal tract is the optimal route for nutrient administration, in many ill clients the normal ingestion of food is difficult, if not nearly impossible, to achieve. The availability of many enteral nutrient preparations was designed for such persons. These formulations may be given by the nasoenteral route through thin, flexible tubing that is generally well tolerated by the client. These feeding tubes are now made from silicone or polyurethane compounds and have much smaller lumen sizes, No. 5 through 10 French. These are much preferred to the older, thicker rubber or polyvinyl chloride types (Salem pump, Levin tube) that stiffen in contact with digestive juices. Aspiration for residual gastrointestinal contents and irrigation of these small-lumen tubes, however, may be more difficult than with the older, larger types.

Small-diameter feeding tubes also get clogged more easily. To prevent this formula residue buildup, some suggest flushing tubes every 4 hours (and each time feeding is interrupted) with 20 ml of cranberry juice followed by 10 ml of water. Acidity of the juice breaks up the formula residue, and the water prevents sugar from crystallizing.

Transnasal tube placement in the intestine requires the use of longer, mercury- or tungsten-weighted feeding tubes that gradually are passed by peristalsis. This takes about 24 hours, and radiographic confirmation of tube placement must be made.

If tube feedings must be administered for long time periods, then the surgical placement of a gastrostomy (G) tube or a jejunostomy (J) tube can surgically be instituted. This will help reduce the need for the frequent flushing and replacement of the nasoenteral tube. A newer procedure in use today is the placement of a G tube percutaneously by using endoscopic guidance; this is known as the percutaneous endoscopic gastrostomy (PEG).

Initially, the infusion of enteral formulas are begun at half-strength concentrations and given at a rate of 50 ml/hour. This rate and strength can then be titrated according to the client's tolerance to the formulation. For example, the rate may be increased 25 ml/hour and the concentration increased to three-quarter strength, which eventually will be increased to the full-strength formulation. The desired calories and total volume ordered will then be administered, assuming the client can tolerate the full-strength preparation. To avoid inducing vomiting or diarrhea, the increases in rate and fluid concentration should not be made simultaneously. The more rapid the feeding, the more likely is hyperglycemia or the dumping syndrome. However, nursing efforts should be maintained to encourage intake because the milk-based formulas, for example, contain 1 kcal/ml, and the client must take 1000 to 2000 ml of formula to obtain all the RDAs for the vitamins and minerals.

The enteral preparation may be given continuously or by cyclic administration. Cyclic feedings are similar to a person's normal feeding cycle and is the preferred method in some settings. If the client cannot or does not drink additional water while on the formulations, it is suggested that additional water be added to the enteral formulations. In general, enteral formulations that have 1 kcal/ml usually contain approximately 80% water, whereas the formulations with more concentrated kcal per ml have less than 70% water.

In the case of accidental aspiration after a tube feeding into the stomach, the tube may be advanced through the pyloric sphincter to prevent future regurgitation. Resultant hyperosmolality, however, potentiates hyperglycemia or the dumping syndrome. Physiologic osmolality is approximately 280 mOsm/L, but some preparations are greater than 400 mOsm/L.

The state of the art of enteral feedings is in rapid evolution. One source for current information is Ross Laboratories, 625 Clinton Ave, Columbus, OH 43216.

Education. Tube feedings self-administered at home are now possible with the advent of smaller tubes and infusion instrumentation that incorporates improved human engineering features. Necessary preparation of the client and another family member should begin 5 to 7 days before discharge. Individualized instruction with return demonstrations of learning take about 3 to 6 hours, perhaps more if it includes learning insertion and removal of the tube for nocturnal administration. Incorrect tube placement is signified by coughing, choking, difficulty in speaking, or cyanosis. Written and verbal instructions related to possible complications are also necessary (see Table 71-3). Resumption of daily activities at home is more inconvenient for the tube-fed ostomy patient who must loosen clothing or undress for each feeding.

Patients receiving tube feedings are deprived of the usual personal and social gratifications of the eating act.

TABLE 71-3   Most Common Secondary Effects of Tube Feedings

Condition	Cause	Action
Aspiration	Impaired gag reflex	Stop; suction trachea; inflate cuff before feedings
	Uncuffed tracheostomy tube	Put head of bed at 30-60 degrees for feedings and for 1 hour after
	Decreased gastric motility	Check for residual of feedings and tube placement
	Misplaced tube	Check taping of tube Advance tube through pyloric sphincter
Obstructed tube	Plugged tube end-ports	Flush tubing before and after feedings or instillation of medications Shake or mix formula well
Hyperglycemia, dumping syndrome: nausea, vomiting, diaphoresis, cramping	Osmotic intolerance to hyperosmolar load of feeding, rapid rate, or high concentration; ice-cold feeding	Change volume or rate of delivery and dilute feeding temporarily Allow feedings to warm slightly

They may feel "different" and alienated from others. To some, it may be symbolic of a rapidly deteriorating state of health and a last resort for survival. They especially need to understand the procedure, its rationale, and what to expect from it. Once given the opportunity to discuss its meaning, many can go on to participate actively in their own feedings and to express greater satisfaction.

PARENTERAL NUTRITION

Parenteral nutrition is the treatment of choice for selected clients who cannot eat, will not eat, should not eat, or cannot eat enough. Often called *hyperalimentation* or **total parenteral nutrition (TPN),** it is the intravenous approach to complete nutrition. TPN can supply all the calories, dextrose, amino acids, fats, trace elements, and other essential nutrients needed for growth, weight gain, wound healing, convalescence, immunocompetence, and other health-sustaining functions, and TPN provides these components in the ratio of a regular diet. It promotes anabolism by supplying all necessary nutrients in excess of those needed for energy expenditure, and it may be infused through a central vein, a peripheral vein, or both, simultaneously. Although related nomenclature has not yet been standardized, **partial parenteral nutrition** has come to denote parenteral nutrition therapy by intravenous solutions that are lacking some essential elements, notably fats, of the regular diet. Insulin and heparin have been added to parenteral nutrition preparations, but many other medications are avoided as admixtures because they may present potential incompatibilities with the nutrients in the solution. The three major parenteral systems for nutritional support are these:

1. Protein-sparing nutrition
2. Peripheral-vein total parenteral nutrition (PTPN)
3. Central-line venous hyperalimentation

PROTEIN-SPARING NUTRITION

This type of nutrition is usually reserved for the client who has minimal protein deficiencies and sufficient fat stores. A 3% to 5% isotonic amino acid is mixed with carbohydrate-free fluids, vitamins, minerals, and electrolytes that are administered by peripheral vein. The solution will provide approximately 400 to 600 calories/day. The individual will meet many energy requirements by using the free fatty acids and ketones derived from their endogenous adipose tissue, thereby preserving their protein compartment in the body. This type usually is used for short-term periods for clients who are not nutritionally compromised and are not in a hypermetabolic state.

PERIPHERAL-VEIN TOTAL PARENTERAL NUTRITION

Peripheral-vein total parenteral nutrition (PTPN) is ordered for clients needing nutritional support, but at the time, insertion of a central venous line for total parenteral nutrition may not be possible or necessary. The individual may be nutritionally healthy or have slight to moderate nutritional deficits without being in a hypermetabolic state. Their current medical situation indicates that a nutritional deficit will probably occur if nutritional therapy is not instituted.

It is considered a temporary measure, an attempt to provide an approximate nitrogen balance in clients who have mild deficits or in NPO clients who have a slightly elevated metabolic rate. It may be prescribed to precede a procedure that imposes restrictions on oral feedings; or for gastrointestinal illnesses that prevent oral food ingestion; or for anorexia caused by radiation or chemotherapy in cancer treatment programs; or following surgery, if the individual's nutritional deficits are minimal but oral food consumption will not be instituted for 5 or more days. It is not indicated for nutritionally depleted clients with a hypermetabolic state. If used in such persons, it should be a temporary measure until central vein hyperalimentation can be initiated.

The solution is composed of a 3% to 5% isotonic amino acid, which is mixed with a carbohydrate solution, vitamins, minerals, and electrolytes for administration through a peripheral vein. The solution will provide between 500 and 700 calories/day. The major advancement in this therapy is the use of a lipid as a nonprotein source of calories. Dextrose, when administered peripherally, must be limited to a 10% solution to avoid sclerosing of the veins. Peripherally administered lipid preparations or intravenous fat emulsions (Liposyn, Travamulsion, Intralipid, and Soyacal) are a source of additional calories for the individual.

CENTRAL HYPERALIMENTATION

A catheter is placed in a central vein, the subclavian vein most commonly, in order to administer solutions that contain hypertonic glucose and amino acids. Because of its blood flow, the central vein can accept the high-osmolar concentrated solutions. Central hyperalimentation or total parenteral nutrition (TPN) is usually composed of the three major nutrients—dextrose, crystalline amino acids, and lipid emulsions—plus vitamins, minerals, trace elements, electrolytes, and water. The solutions may vary according to the individual's requirements and, in general, according to the supplier of the basic amino acid solution. Special preparations of amino acids are also available for the client with a specific disease state.

The primary indications for central hyperalimentation are the following:

1. Malnutrition or a weight loss of more than 10% of body weight is present in a person before or after surgery.
2. Individuals with conditions of short bowel syndrome; acute pancreatitis; enteric or enterocutaneous fistulas; gastrointestinal tract obstructions; major trauma or burns when enteral feedings are not possible; clients with cancer, who are undergoing treatment and cannot maintain an adequate nutrition; comatose clients or persons with neurologic illnesses that interfere with eating (pseudobulbar palsy); or in selected persons with renal, cardiac, or liver failure.

COMPONENTS OF SOLUTIONS
Amino Acids

Amino acids are necessary to promote the production of proteins (anabolism), to reduce protein breakdown (catabolism), and to help promote healing of wounds. A healthy adult usually requires approximately 0.9 g protein/kg, whereas an infant or child needs from 1.4 to 2.2 g/kg. In undernourished or traumatized persons, this requirement can increase substantially.

The protein must be of high biologic value. This requirement is significantly increased (almost six times) in a traumatized or a seriously ill individual, since this patient's daily need is approximately 3 g/kg body weight. A nonprotein source of calories must be provided with the amino acids to offset their use as an energy source.

Protein is composed of amino acids, which are identified as essential and nonessential (see Table 71-4). The term **essential** indicates that the amino acid cannot be synthesized by the body. **Nonessential** amino acids can be synthesized from a nitrogen source (amino acids, ammonium salts, urea). All natural amino acids are needed for growth and development and must be present concurrently in the proper amounts for protein synthesis to occur. The adult can synthesize all but eight of these amino acids; these eight therefore are considered essential in adults. To the extent that oral intake of amino acids is limited, protein synthesis depends on an exogenous source. The **semiessential** amino acids (histidine, arginine) are not synthesized in adequate amounts during growth periods; thus 10 amino acids are considered essential in infants.

> amino acids, crystalline (Aminosyn 3.5%, 5%, 10%; FreeAmine III 8.5%, 10%; Novamine; Travasol 5.5%, 8.5%, 10%). Also available with electrolytes.

Amino acid crystalline solutions contain synthetic amino acids but not peptides. This is the preferred form of amino acid because most persons are able to tolerate this formulation.

TABLE 71-4 Classification of Amino Acids

Essential	Nonessential	Semiessential
isoleucine	alanine	arginine
leucine	aspartic acid	histidine
lysine	cysteine	
methionine	glutamic acid	
phenylalanine	glycine	
threonine	proline	
tryptophan	serine	
valine	tyrosine	

Dextrose usually is administered with these solutions because of the protein-sparing action of carbohydrates. If the protein is administered without adequate calories in the form of carbohydrate, the protein will be used for the body's caloric need rather than for repair and regeneration of tissue.

Carbohydrates

Generally, dextrose is the primary source of carbohydrate in nutritional preparations. Both carbohydrate and lipids are used as sources of calories. One gram of d-glucose provides 3.4 calories, whereas fat supplies 9 calories/g and protein supplies 4 calories/g. Concentrations of dextrose solutions above 10% are hyperosmolar and too irritating to be given continuously peripherally, thus they should be administered through central venous catheters. Centrally, the concentration of dextrose solutions infused is usually between 25% and 35%.

When dextrose is administered without lipids as the primary source of calories, then hyperglycemia may occur. As dextrose requires insulin for utilization, using a combination of caloric sources, dextrose and lipids, will help decrease the potential for hyperglycemia and extra need for insulin in some individuals. Also, dextrose alone increases the rate of metabolism and production of carbon dioxide, which may increase the person's respiratory demands. Administering a combination caloric preparation of dextrose and lipids will reduce the increase in ventilatory demands.

Other sources of calories available, although not as prevalent in usage, include alcohol in dextrose solution, fructose (Levulose) in water, and invert sugar in water. Fructose is a carbohydrate normally found in the blood that does not require insulin for peripheral utilization. But fructose administration has resulted in elevated lactic acid levels, and deaths have occurred in persons with hereditary fructose intolerance.

The dextrose used in formulations is derived from corn sugar; however, a very small portion of the population may be sensitive to corn derivatives. For such persons, invert sugar derived from cane or beet sugar is an alternative.

Alcohol is another substrate providing 7 kcal/g, and it does not require insulin for peripheral utilization. Providing enough calories would necessitate a quantity of alcohol that would produce a potential for intoxication and hepatotoxicity. Since dextrose is inexpensive and readily available, it is often the preferred product for administration.

Fat

lipid emulsions (Intralipid 10%, 20%; Liposyn 10%, 20%; Liposyn II 10%, 20%; Travamulsion 10%, 20%; Soyacal 10%, 20%)

Fat constitutes 40% to 50% of the total calories supplied in the average North American diet. Fat emulsions are derived from either soybean or safflower oil, which provides a mixture of neutral triglycerides and unsaturated fatty acids. The two functions of intravenous fat emulsions in parenteral nutrition are to supply essential fatty acids and to be a source of energy or calories (9 calories/g).

Linoleic, linolenic, and arachidonic acids are essential in humans. Linoleic acid cannot be synthesized in the body, and it is the precursor to both linolenic and arachidonic acid (a tetraene). If it is not available or if a deficiency of linoleic acid is present, then the enzyme system will act on oleic acid to synthesize eicosatrienoic acid (a triene), which is incapable of functioning like arachidonic acid. Essential fatty acid deficiency (EFAD) with clinical signs of hair loss, scaly dermatitis, retardation of growth, reduced wound healing, decreased platelets and fatty liver is noted when the triene-to-tetraene ratio is greater than 0.4. This necessitates the intravenous administration of a fat emulsion to correct the biochemical alteration.

The fat emulsions may be administered peripherally or by central veins. Fat emulsions break down when mixed with amino acid and dextrose solutions, but they may be coinfused from separate containers that flow into the same vein as the dextrose and amino acid solutions, by means of a Y connector positioned just in front of the infusion site. The lipid infusion line should be higher than the dextrose–amino acid line because the lipid emulsion has a lower specific gravity. If it is not administered in this order, the lipid emulsion may retract into the amino-dextrose line.

The fat emulsions currently available are either safflower oil (Liposyn) or soybean oil (Intralipid) or a combination of both (Liposyn II).

Daily intake may be 2 L (which provides 1980 calories) or 2.5 L (which provides 2475 calories). Or if administered with 500 ml Liposyn 10%, the 2 L fluid plus the Liposyn equals 2530 calories; if given with the 2.5 L fluid, it will provide 3025 calories. Larger amounts of liposyn may be administered, which in turn will increase caloric intake.

The formula is modified according to the client's condition and individual needs (Central Vein, 1982).

Fat emulsion particles are thought to be metabolized from the bloodstream in a manner similar to that of the chylomicrons, which appear in the blood postprandially. No more than 60% of the total daily caloric needs of the individual should be provided by fat emulsions. The fat emulsions may prevent hyperglycemia, hyperinsulinemia, and hyperosmolar syndrome, which often occurs in clients given dextrose as the only source of parenteral caloric nutrition. Fat emulsions pose some dangers for persons with severe liver disease, pulmonary disease, anemia, or blood coagulation disorders and for acutely ill patients with elevated serum concentrations of C-reactive protein. Fat emboli and accumulation of intravascular fat may occur in lungs of premature, preterm, or low-birth-weight infants (infusion rate not to exceed 1 g/kg in 4 hours). A normal diet should be 40% fat, 40% protein, and 20% carbohydrate.

Trace Elements (Minerals) and Electrolytes

Although some of the commercial parenteral nutrition solutions contain trace elements, persons placed on long-term administration should be evaluated for trace element deficiencies. Trace element solutions are available individually (zinc, copper, manganese, molybdenum, chromium, selenium, and iodine) and in combination formulations (M.T.E. 4, 5, or 6 Concentrated and others). Several trace metal formulations are also available in combination with electrolytes (Tracelyte, Tracelyte with Double Electrolytes, and others).

Examples of the signs and symptoms of trace element deficiency, normal serum levels, and primary excretion sites are noted in Table 71-5. It is also critical to monitor electrolyte serum levels, especially the cations sodium, potassium, calcium, and magnesium and the anions of chloride, phosphate, bicarbonate, and acetate. Combination of electrolyte concentrates are available for administration to large volume parenteral solutions, such as Hyperlyte, Lypholyte, TPN Electrolytes, and others. Such preparations are usually used only in compounding of preparations in the pharmacy.

If iron replacement is necessary, it can be given by intramuscular injection by way of the Z track technique or injection or by intravenous injection or infusion. Do not mix iron with other drugs or add it to parenteral nutrition solutions. For additional information on iron (Iron Dextran), the reader is referred to a current package insert or current reference book.

Vitamins

The client receiving parenteral feedings will need additional vitamins. Usually a combination of multivitamin infusion (MVI) and, perhaps, additional vitamins will be given on alternate days to meet the client's needs for vitamins A and D and the water-soluble vitamins (B and C). Such preparations can be added to the parenteral nutrition solution. Vitamin K and vitamin B_{12} may be given at 3-week intervals, whereas folate (folic acid) is usually given on a weekly basis. The specific dose and frequency for vitamin regimens depend primarily on the individual client's needs and the usual protocols of the prescribing physician. See Table 71-6 for a typical daily total parenteral nutrition formulation for adults without any cardiac, liver, or kidney complications.

SPECIAL FORMULATIONS

Specially formulated amino acid preparations are available for clients in renal failure, those with high metabolic stress, and those in liver failure or encephalopathy.

Aminosyn-RF, NephrAmine, and ReNamin	Contains essential amino acids and hypertonic dextrose to promote protein synthesis. These preparations decrease the rise of urea nitrogen in the blood, allowing it to be recycled to glutamate (a precursor for the synthesis of nonessential amino acids). The latter aids in reducing many azotemic symptoms. Indicated for persons in renal failure. Since NephrAmine does not contain arginine, its use in infants would increase the risk of developing hyperammonemia. The other two preparations contain arginine.
FreAmine HBC	A mixture of essential and nonessential amino acids with a high concentration of branched-chain amino acids (BCAA). It is used to prevent nitrogen loss or to treat a negative nitrogen balance in adults when (a) the gastrointestinal tract cannot or should not be used to obtain an adequate protein intake, (b) the absorption of protein by the gastrointestinal tract is impaired, or (c) in severe trauma or sepsis, the nitrogen balance is significantly impaired. This formulation provides approximately 1.5 g/kg of amino acids for adults. This is a high metabolic stress formulation.
HepatAmine	This is a mixture of essential and nonessential amino acids with a high concentration of BCAA. It is indicated to treat hepatic failure and encephalopathy. In studies the BCAA reversed the abnormal plasma–amino acid levels in liver failure. The shift to normalization of amino acids was reflected by an improved mental status and EEG tests. Nitrogen balance was improved and mortality decreased in the reports.

THE NURSE'S ROLE IN PARENTERAL NUTRITION

Assessment. Close, ongoing reassessment of clients' responses to this complex therapy is essential. In particular, developing circulatory overload of fluids or electrolytes should be monitored by assessments of vital signs and fluid intake and output. A uniform infusion rate should be maintained at all times. Infusion instrumentation does not eliminate the need for alert nursing care, since it has the same potential for malfunction as all equipment does.

Some level of glucosuria may occur, particularly at initiation of therapy, since insulin response is challenged by the glucose load. The urine should be tested for glucosuria, and blood glucose may be tested at 6-hour intervals. The patient's daily weight must be taken accurately and recorded. Blood urea nitrogen (BUN) is tested daily for 3 to 5 days, then every other day as needed. A sequential multichannel antoanalyzer (SMA) 12/60 procedure should be done weekly with tests for protein, partial thromboplastin time (PTT), and complete blood count (CBC). Serum electrolytes should be monitored daily.

Daily recording of the data and communication of atypical values to the attending physician are critical. These data include blood glucose in excess of 200 mg/100 ml; weight loss; urine glucose in excess of 1+ (glucosuria); an increase in pulse and blood pressure and sweating; elevated temperature; swelling and edema over the punc-

TABLE 71-5   Trace Elements

Elements	Normal serum levels	Excretion sites	Deficiency symptoms
copper	80-163 µg/dl	Bile (80%), intestinal wall (16%)	Decrease in red and white blood cells, hair and skeletal abnormalities, defective tissue growth
chromium	1-5 µg/L	Kidneys, bile	Neuropathy, confusion, impaired glucose tolerance, ataxia
iodine	0.5-1.5 µg/dl	Kidneys, bile	Goiter, cretinism, impaired thyroid functioning
manganese	6-12 µg/L	Bile	Defective growth, nausea, vomiting, weight loss, skin rash, CNS alterations (ataxia, seizures)
molybdenum	—	Mainly kidneys, some bile	Increased heart rate, tachypnea, headache, nausea, vomiting, edema, malaise, disorientation, coma; also may see hypouricemia, hypouricosuria, and hypermethioninemia
selenium	10-37 µg/dl	Kidneys, feces	Muscle aches, pain, or tenderness, cardiomyopathy, kwashiorkor
zinc	100±12 µg/dl	Stool (90%), kidneys, sweat	Nausea, vomiting, diarrhea, weakness, anorexia, growth retardation, anemia, hepatosplenomegaly, hypogeusia, rash, depression, defective wound healing, eye lesions

TABLE 71-6   Typical Daily TPN Formulation for Adults without Heart, Liver, or Kidney Compromise

Calories	dextrose	60%-80% of total energy needs
	lipids	20%-40% of total energy needs
Protein	amino acids, crystalline	100% of individual's requirement

An example of a typical formulation is (per unit or bottle):
  amino acids (Aminosyn 7%)—500 ml
  dextrose 50%—500 ml
  TPN electrolytes—20 ml
  multivitamins, including vitamin A, D, and E—10 ml
  trace metals—5 ml
  potassium phosphate (3 mM P/ml)—4 ml (12 mM P)

This formulation would provide the following per bottle or unit:
  water—1039 ml
  calories—990 kcal
  nitrogen—5.5 g
  protein equivalent—35 g
  sodium—35 mEq
  potassium—40 mEq
  chloride—35 mEq
  magnesium—5 mEq
  calcium—4.5 mEq
  phosphorus—12 nM
  acetate—82 mEq

ture site or on the head, neck, or face; low serum electrolytes; distended veins in the neck, arms, and hands; convulsions; coma; or other radical changes in the client's condition.

Complications of parenteral nutrition therapy include infection; hyperglycemia/hypoglycemia; dehydration; hypervolemia; depressed levels of the electrolytes potassium, phosphate, calcium, or magnesium; EFAD, caused by prolonged fat-free hyperalimentation therapy, and trace element deficiencies (see the box on p. 1117). Because these balanced nutritional solutions provide an excellent medium for growth of microorganisms, strict asepsis

---

COMPLICATIONS OF PARENTERAL NUTRITION

COMPLICATIONS ARISING FROM INFECTION AND SEPSIS

Catheter seeding from bloodborne or distant infection
Contamination of catheter entrance site during insertion or long-term catheter placement
Solution contamination

COMPLICATIONS THAT ARE METABOLIC IN ORIGIN

Azotemia
Cholelithiasis (children under 15 years)
Dehydration from osmotic diuresis
Electrolyte imbalance
Hyperammonemia
Hyperosmolar, hyperglycemic, nonketotic coma (HHNC)
Hyperphosphatemia and hypophosphatemia
Hypocalcemia
Hypomagnesemia
Rebound hypoglycemia on sudden cessation of parenteral nutrition
Trace element deficiencies

COMPLICATIONS ARISING FROM SUBCLAVIAN CATHETERIZATION

Air embolism
Arteriovenous fistula
Brachial plexus injury
Cardiac perforation, tamponade
Catheter embolism
Catheter misplacement
Central vein thrombophlebitis
Endocarditis
Hemothorax
Hydromediastinum
Hydrothorax
Pneumothorax
Subclavian artery injury
Subclavian hematoma
Subcutaneous emphysema
Tension pneumothorax
Thoracic duct injury

---

must be employed when preparing solutions (usually done by pharmacists, ideally under a laminar flow hood) and when handling solutions or the insertion site.

Starvation among the general population usually is associated with poverty. Alert nursing assessments of all patients' nutrition states is the key to avoiding the need for any of the complex regimens discussed. Nutrition by natural means is always more successful. If necessary, oral or tube feedings should be the first choice; parenteral nutrition should be employed when these are impossible or ineffective.

Intervention. Hickman or Broviac catheters are two central venous catheters that can be used for intermittent infusions of drugs, parenteral feedings, and other adjunctive therapies. These catheters are designed so that the ends may be capped between infusions. Heparinized saline is instilled at the completion of infusions, and the tube is recapped. Except during lipid infusions, in-line filters may be used to trap air and bacteria. Parenteral lines are reserved for feedings.

Parenteral nutrition intake may begin at a rate less than 1 L/12 hours for the first 2 days. If tolerated, the rate may be increased gradually during the first 5 days to 3 L/day. Ideally, the rate of parenteral nutrition solutions should be regulated by infusion pump for steady flow with no oscillations.

Do not shake lipid emulsion infusions that have separated in solution to mix them; instead discard them. Fats in these lipid emulsions have been found to leach out the plasticizer DEHP in polyvinyl chloride tubing. Since the toxic potential of DEHP is not known, it is wise to use the administration sets provided by the manufacturer for use with fat emulsions in parenteral nutrition therapy. As noted, the fat emulsion arm of the Y connector must be 6 inches higher than the other arm; otherwise the lower density of the fat emulsion will cause it to run up into the other arm of the tubing.

Dressings should be changed if they become wet or dislodged; they are designed to be air-occlusive. Protocols for dressing changes can be found in selected references; usually staff nurses who are part of a specially trained team should do dressing changes. If a client's temperature becomes elevated, it must be reported immediately. Cultures (fungal, bacterial) should be taken of the insertion site, tubing, and parenteral solutions. Peripheral vein sites should be changed routinely every 10 to 12 hours.

Air embolism is a potential hazard with central venous lines because of the low pressure in the venous system. Tubing connections must be kept taped to prevent their separation. When necessary, tubing should be changed quickly with the client in a supine position and executing Valsalva's maneuver (forced exhalation against a closed glottis). Insertions should be accomplished in Trendelenburg's position.

Education. Parenteral nutrition can now be continued at home for indefinite periods for those who need ongoing nutritional support and who meet the criteria. Education of the patient and family is essential with regard to the purposes and techniques of the following: preventing infection, care of the solution and flow rate regulation, daily weights, recording of intake and output, and the need for close contact with community health nurses and other personnel. The patient must understand infusion pump monitoring before taking on full responsibility for this technology. Every attempt should be made to resume the usual activities of daily living and to integrate this therapy in the patient's life-style.

KEY TERMS

essential amino acids, page 1113
nonessential amino acids, page 1113
partial parenteral nutrition, page 1112
peripheral-vein total parenteral nutrition (PTPN), page 1112
semiessential amino acids, page 1113
total parenteral nutrition (TPN), page 1112

BIBLIOGRAPHY

American Hospital Formulary Service: AHFS drug information '88, Bethesda, Md, 1988, American Society of Hospital Pharmacists, Inc.

Barrocas, A: Advances in nutritional support, Nutr Support Serv 5(5):6, 1985.

Birdsall, C: Do total nutritional admixtures benefit your patients? Amer J Nurs 87(1):14, 1987.

Birdsall, C: How do I administer medication by NG? Amer J Nurs 84(10):1259, 1984.

Birdsall, C: Clinical savvy: when is TPN safe? Amer J Nurs 85(1):73, 1985.

Bradley, J: Principles of enteral nutrition, Hosp Pharm 23(2):197, 1988.

Braunwald, E, and others, eds: Harrison's principles of internal medicine, ed 11, New York, 1987, McGraw-Hill Book Co.

Brendel, V: Catheters utilized in delivering total parenteral nutrition, NITA 8(3):488, 1984.

Central vein, Contemporary parenteral nutrition, Abbott Laboratories, Hospital Products Division, 97-1357/R1-10-June '84, 1982.

Drescher, MR: Advances in peripheral vein nutrition, NITA 8(6):533, 1985.

Flynn, KT, and others: Enteral tube feeding: indications, practices and outcomes, Image J Nurs Sch 19(1):16, 1987.

Ford, R: History and organization of the Seattle Area Hickman Catheter Committee, NITA 8(3):123, 1985.

Fox, B, and others: Take precautions now . . . patients receiving total parenteral nutrition, Nursing 15(5):48, 1985.

Guthrie, P, and others: Peripheral and central nutritional support, NITA 9(5):393, 1986.

Haynes-Johnson, V: Tube feeding complications: causes, prevention, and therapy, Nutr Support Serv 6(3):17, 1986.

Heymsfield, ST, Horowitz, J, and Lawson, DH: Enteral hyperalimentation developments. In Berk, JE, ed: Digestive Diseases, Philadelphia, 1980, Lea & Febiger.

Horbal-Shuster, M, and others: Keeping enteral nutrition on track, Amer J Nurs 87(4):523, 1987.

Kastrup, EK, ed: Facts and comparisons, St Louis, 1988, JB Lippincott Co.

LaFranco, M: Drug-food interactions, Parenterals 6(1):6, 1988.

Leider, Z, and others: Intermittent tube feedings: pros and cons, Nutr Support Serv 6(2):47, 1986.

Lipman, TO, and Murphy, L: Types of parenteral nutrition: a comparison, Drug Ther Hosp 6(3):61, 1981.

Lyman, B, and others: The role of the nutritional support team in preventing and identifying complications of parenteral and enteral nutrition, QRB 13(7):232, 1987.

Matthews, L: Enteral nutrition in the geriatric stroke patient, Nutr Support Serv 6(11):22, 1986.

Miller, LS, and others: Enteral and parenteral nutrition in the critically ill patient, Hosp Formul 21(6):672, 1986.

Munro-Black, J: The ABCs of total parenteral nutrition, Nursing 14(2):50, 1984.

Nursing photobook: managing IV therapy, Horsham, Penn, 1980, Intermed Communications.

Olson, GB, and others: Balanced parenteral nutrition, Nutr Support Serv 5(6):16, 1985.

Peripheral Vein TPN, Contemporary parenteral nutrition, Abbott Laboratories, Hospital Products Division, 97-1035/R4-10-May '85, 1981.

Rutherford, C: Peripheral parenteral nutrition, NITA 9(3):232, 1986.

Strommer, RS: Nursing care of parenteral nutrition patients, Hosp Formul 18(11):1083, 1983.

Wilhelm, L: Helping your patient "settle in " with TPN, Nursing 15(4):60, 1985.

Wyngaarden, JB, and Smith, LH: Cecil textbook of medicine, ed 18, Philadelphia, 1988, WB Saunders Co.

UNIT XIX

Miscellaneous Agents

CHAPTER
72

Antiseptics, Disinfectants, and Sterilant Agents

OBJECTIVES

After studying this chapter, the student will be able to:

1. Compare and contrast nosocomial infections and community- or home-acquired infections.

2. Differentiate between medical and surgical asepsis.

3. Describe the characteristics of an ideal antiseptic/disinfectant.

4. Describe the mechanism of action of antiseptics and disinfectants.

5. List the indications for use of common antiseptics and disinfectants.

6. Identify the uses and limitations of silver nitrate and silver sulfadiazine.

7. Describe the effectiveness of iodine compounds and iodophors.

8. Explain the mechanism of action of oxidizing agents.

9. Describe the current uses of sterilants.

10. Identify nursing considerations for the safe and effective use of antiseptics, disinfectants, and sterilants.

INFECTIONS AND INFECTIOUS DISEASES

Infections and infectious diseases, although differing in type and character, occur in people in all settings—hospitals, institutions, the community at large, and the home.

Community- or home-acquired infections are usually fairly benign and relatively responsive to treatment. Characteristic examples are appendicitis, animal bites, lacerations, and foreign bodies.

Nosocomial infections are those that are acquired in a hospital. Between 2 to 4 million of the 40 million persons hospitalized yearly in the United States develop an infection that was not present or incubating upon admission to the hospital. Such nosocomial infections are responsible for an estimated 30,000 to 60,000 deaths. They also lead to extra hospitalization, resulting in approximately a $5 billion economic burden. Nosocomial infections have been called one of the most significant current ecologic problems in the United States. They are occasionally caused by virulent microorganisms resistant to antibiotics.

The emergence of antibiotic-resistant bacteria has become an increasingly important problem, especially in health care agencies. Relative virulence of strains of these bacteria tends to change over time. Before 1940 and the introduction of antibiotics, group A streptococci represented the major microbial problem. By the mid-1950s, when antibiotics were beginning to proliferate, coagulase-positive *Staphylococcus aureus* predominated. Sub-

1121

sequently, the problem became more complex, with the frequent appearance of aerobic gram-negative bacilli (such as *Pseudomonas*), fungi or yeast such as *Candida albicans*, and herpesvirus hominis. *Serratia marcescens* has also rather quickly become a challenge. Anerobic organisms such as *Clostridia, Bacteroides,* and *Peptostreptococcus* are increasingly common, but the organisms now most frequently responsible for hospital-acquired infections include *Staphylococcus aureus, Escherichia coli, Klebsiella, Enterobacter, Pseudomonas, Proteus, Serratia, Providencia, Actinetobacter,* and species of *Flavobacterium*. All are common, can survive at room temperature or under refrigeration, and have potential to develop resistance to antibiotics.

Urinary tract infections and postoperative wound infections account for the majority (approximately 70% or more) of the nosocomial infections detected in a hospital setting. The high-risk areas, such as critical care units, burn units, and dialysis units, usually have the highest incidence of infection outbreaks and of antibiotic resistance in the hospital. Nurses must be aware of the problem and of methods used to reduce the incidence of nosocomial infections in their practice.

MEDICAL AND SURGICAL ASEPSIS

Medical and surgical asepsis are used in health care to reduce the number and spread of organisms. These approaches presume the presence of pathogens (organisms capable of inducing disease or infection in human beings) or potential pathogens in the immediate environment and seek to limit their transmission (Figure 72-1). Methods in surgical asepsis destroy *all* microorganisms including spores; in medical asepsis, only *pathogens* are destroyed or inhibited. The focus in surgical asepsis is to keep *all* organisms out of a designated area (e.g., fresh wound), but in medical asepsis it is to remove or destroy the pathogens in the area and to contain the remaining nonpathogens there by conscious efforts. The former uses "sterile technique" (use of sterile equipment or sterile fields) and the latter uses "clean technique" (such as hygienic measures, cleaning agents, antiseptics, disinfectants, and barrier fields). Which is applied in any given situation depends largely on the susceptibility of the host, the organism's virulence, and other factors in the infectious cycle.

STERILIZATION

An object is "sterile" if it is free of *all* forms and types of life. **Sterilization** is a process that destroys all forms of life on an instrument or utensil, in a liquid, or within a substance. Living tissue (of clients, nurses, or surgeons) cannot be sterilized by any known means without damage to that tissue; therefore the process known as sterilization

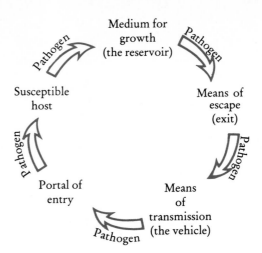

FIGURE 72-1 A theoretical model of the process of any infection. The infectious process is vulnerable to interruption at any or all of these steps. Antiseptics, disinfectants, sterilants, and other medical and surgical aseptic techniques are used by nurses to impede the process. These practices prevent escape, transmission, or entry of the pathogen into a host. Immunization techniques increase the host's resistance.

is only applied to objects. It is also important to grasp the concept put forth by the Council on Pharmacy and Chemistry that use of the terms "sterile," "sterilizer," and "sterilization" can be used only in the absolute sense; there is no acceptable concept of *relative* sterility. However, just because a piece of equipment is labeled "sterilizer" does not mean that is totally and permanently effective for sterilizing. Nor does the term "sterilized" testify to an item's current condition of purity.

Several acceptable and practicable sterilization methods now exist. Steam under pressure (autoclaving) is preferred as the most effective. Ethylene oxide is a gas sterilant used for heat-labile materials, for sharp-edged instruments that could be dulled by steam, for electrical and anesthesia equipment, and for bedding. Hot air ovens are used to sterilize glassware. Chemical sterilants are also employed when necessary.

ANTISEPTICS AND DISINFECTANTS

Antiseptics and disinfectants are agents, usually chemical, used to kill many of the pathogens within a given population of microorganisms. Their mechanisms of action are generally not very effective against spores of bacteria and fungi, many viruses, and some very resistant bacterial strains. As a group, the effects of disinfectants and antiseptics differ from sterilization largely in the degree and type of organisms destroyed. Disinfectants and antiseptics kill only pathogens, but sterilizing kills all types of organisms.

Although some of the literature uses the terms "disinfectant" and "antiseptic" interchangeably, this is erroneous and confusing. Disinfectants differ from antiseptics in the matter on which they are used and in their degree of ability to destroy organisms. Disinfectants are used only on nonliving objects; they are toxic to living tissue. Antiseptics are chemicals typically applied only to living tissue, so they must be less potent or made more dilute to prevent cell damage. Such lessening of potency, although crucial to viable tissue, decreases effectiveness accordingly. Some definitions of antiseptics emphasize their inhibiting rather than destructive effects. The narrow range of tolerance by tissues to antiinfective topical preparations tends to limit the variety and number of acceptable antiseptic agents available. Therefore antiseptics may differ markedly from disinfectants in chemical composition or may simply be a dilute version of a disinfectant for use on intact tissue. Thus some chemical substances may be used either as an antiseptic or as a disinfectant, depending on concentration gradients.

Antiseptics and disinfectants are further categorized as **bacteriostatic** or **bactericidal** in character. Antiseptics are most often bacteriostatic; that is, they act to retard only the growth and replication of bacteria but do not kill off the entire bacteria population. Disinfectants, as bactericides, actually kill bacteria but perhaps not all types (depending on the disinfectant, its specificity, and so on) and often not fungi, viruses, or spores. Other disinfectants—*fungicides, virucides,* and *sporicides*—act specifically on these organisms. **Germicides** is an all-encompassing term for agents that work against many types of "germs"—bacteria, fungi, viruses, and spores.

Organisms vary in sensitivity to disinfectants and antiseptics in general (see box). However, factors such as the dormant and impervious spore forms of some bacteria, the waxy envelopes of the tubercle bacilli, certain properties of some types of gram-positive bacteria (staphylococci and enterococci), some gram-negative ones (*Salmonella* and *Pseudomonas* species), and hepatitis viruses make them highly refractory to many forms of disinfectants or antiseptics.

Ideal antiseptic/disinfectant. The ideal all-around antiseptic/disinfectant does not yet exist. Such an ideal agent would have to do the following:

1. Be destructive to all forms of microorganisms without being toxic to human cells
2. Have a low incidence of hypersensitivity
3. Be active in the presence of organic matter and soaps
4. Be stable, noncorrosive, nonstaining, and inexpensive

The current criteria for an *effective* disinfectant, however, includes the ability to destroy within 10 minutes all vegetative bacteria (but not spores) and fungi, tubercle bacilli, animal parasites, and viruses (but not hepatitis viruses). Many variables affect the relative efficiency of a product. These include the ingredients' abilities to dissolve, mix, work in the presence of organic matter such as blood or other exudate, and penetrate into recesses. Other properties include chemical composition, concentration, pH, ionization, surface tension, temperature, and length of time required for action. Thus in actual clinical use, there may be extreme variability in the effectiveness of any given product, depending on the specific application and the situation. Although several standard tests for efficacy of these products are available, the results are subject to the same variables and, in several cases, are unwieldy to administer.

Currently, there are few established guidelines for specific approved use of any particular disinfectant: a disinfectant is considered a disinfectant whether it is to be used on corridor floors or on surgical instruments. This method of classifying permits widespread practices such as the common use of iodophor solutions as disinfectants when they have earned FDA approval as antiseptics. Antiseptics are not required to be as potent as disinfectants. Relative usefulness of various antiseptics can be compared based on their therapeutic index. This index is the relationship between the specific antiseptic concentration that is proved effective against microorganisms without irritating tissues or interfering with healing. Other decisive factors are the potential for causing hypersensitivity reactions or systemic absorption. *Thorough handwashing*

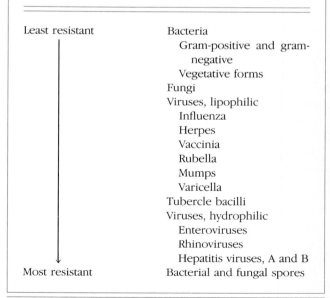

GENERAL RANKING OF ORGANISM TYPES ACCORDING TO THEIR RELATIVE SENSITIVITY TO DISINFECTANTS AND ANTISEPTICS*

Least resistant | Bacteria
Gram-positive and gram-negative
Vegetative forms
Fungi
Viruses, lipophilic
Influenza
Herpes
Vaccinia
Rubella
Mumps
Varicella
Tubercle bacilli
Viruses, hydrophilic
Enteroviruses
Rhinoviruses
Hepatitis viruses, A and B
Most resistant | Bacterial and fungal spores

*May vary with concentration of compound and other factors.

still predominates as the most effective measure for controlling the spread of infection.

To place the concepts of sterilization, disinfection, and antisepsis in perspective, it should be clear that these processes differ in the degree to which they destroy organisms. Thus anything that is sterile can also be considered both disinfected and antiseptic. (The converse is, of course, not true.) All of these processes correctly begin with handwashing, even when gloves are worn. It has been repeatedly demonstrated that clean, washed hands are crucial deterrents to microorganism growth, reproduction, and transmission in any environment.

Mechanism of action. Antiseptics and disinfectants may act in three ways.

1. They may bring about a change in the structure of the protein of the microbial cell (denaturation), which often proceeds to coagulation of protein with increased concentration of the chemical agent.
2. They may lower the surface tension of the aqueous medium of the parasitic cell. This increases the permeability of the plasma membrane, and the cellular constituents are destroyed by lysis. The cell is unable to maintain its equilibrium in its environment. (The surface-active agents are thought to act this way.)
3. They may interfere with some metabolic processes of the microbial cells in such ways as to interfere with the cell's ability to survive and multiply.

Table 72-1 is an overview of typical indications of selected disinfectants, antiseptics, and sterilants. In practice, applications may vary depending on the concentration of the solution and its purpose.

PHENOLIC COMPOUNDS

cresol, carbolic acid, Lysol

A 50% solution of cresol in vegetable oil (saponified, a milky emulsion) in 2% to 5% strength is known as Lysol.

Mechanism of action. Phenols denature microbial protein structures and, in high concentrations, will precipitate cellular proteins. The actions of these compounds are relatively unaffected by the presence of organic matter or heavy bacterial inocula.

Indications. Cresol is used for disinfecting excreta, sinks, bedpans, toilets, and equipment.

Dosage and administration. Solutions of phenol are antiseptic, bactericidal, or escharotic, depending on the strength of the concentration used. In aqueous solutions, from 1% to 2% of carbolic acid kills all but the hepatitis virus and bacterial or fungal spores within 20 minutes; it destroys even spores after 12 hours of contact. Cresol is two to five times as effective as phenol but no more toxic. Although it is only slightly soluble in water, it is soluble in liquid soaps.

Side effects/adverse reactions. All phenols are deadly poisons if taken internally or applied topically to abraded skin. They are also corrosive to equipment.

NURSING CONSIDERATIONS

Carbolic acid, cresol, and Lysol are intended for disinfectant use only. These phenolic compounds should not be applied to the skin in concentrations stronger than 2%; they should never be applied to broken skin. If accidental skin contact is made or if a burning sensation is noted, the area should be washed with copious amounts of water.

hexachlorophene (pHisoHex, pHiso Scrub, Septisol)

Hexachlorophene is a bacteriostatic agent that was incorporated into detergent creams, soaps, lotions, shampoos, and other topical products to reduce the incidence of pathogenic bacteria on the skin. Because of its toxicity, especially in infants, it is currently available only by prescription for surgical scrub purposes and as a bacteriostatic skin cleanser.

Mechanism of action. Hexachlorophene is a bacteriostatic agent effective against staphylococci and other gram-positive bacteria.

Indications. A surgical scrub and bacteriostatic skin cleansing agent, hexachlorophene is used to control gram-positive infection outbreaks when other methods have been unsuccessful.

This product is a cumulative antibacterial agent, especially with repeated use. It is also reported to be resistant to removal by many soaps and detergents, sometimes for several days.

Side effects/adverse reactions. This is a topical agent that is toxic if taken orally; ingestion results in gastric symptoms and central nervous system signs because of increased intracranial pressure. It is less toxic to tissues than phenol, but concentrations of 3% or more have a narrow margin of safety.

Daily topical use on newborns or application several times daily to the skin or vagina in adults has resulted in confusion, diplopia, lethargy, convulsions, respiratory arrest, and death. It is usually not routinely used or recommended for bathing infants. It also should not be used on mucous membranes or burned or denuded skin or for any prolonged skin contact without rinsing. Dermatitis and photosensitivity are also reported.

Dosage and administration

For surgical hand scrubs

Without a brush. A preliminary wash of 20 to 30 seconds, adding only a small amount of water is followed by a sudsy 2 to 4 minute scrub and a thorough rinsing.

With a brush. A first scrub is followed by a scrub of varying length (see manufacturer's instructions), depending on the frequency of previous pHisoHex hand scrubs.

TABLE 72-1 Typical Indications: Selected Disinfectants, Antiseptics, and Sterilants

Agent	Sterilant	Disinfectant	Antiseptic
PHENOLIC COMPOUNDS			
Cresol, Lysol, carbolic acid		√	
Hexachlorophene			√
Resorcinol			√
Hexylresorcinol			√
DYES			
Gentian violet			√
Carbol-fuchsin solution			√
HEAVY METALS			
Mercurials			
Ammoniated mercury ointment			√
Merbromin (Mercurochrome)			√
Nitromersol (Metaphen)			√
Thimerosal (Merthiolate)			√
Silver compounds			
Silver nitrate, silver sulfadiazine			√
HALOGENS			
Chlorine compounds			
Sodium hypochlorite		√	√
Chloramines			
Halazone		√	
IODINE COMPOUNDS			
Tincture of iodine		√	√
Aqueous iodine solution		√	√
Iodophors			√
OXIDIZING AGENTS			
Hydrogen peroxide		?*	√
Zinc peroxide			√
Benzoyl peroxide			√
BIGUANIDES			
Chlorhexidine gluconate			
Hibiclens, Hibitane			√
SURFACE-ACTIVE AGENTS			
Benzalkonium chloride			
Zephiran chloride			?
NITROFURAZONE			
Furacin			√
ALCOHOLS			
Ethanol		√	√
Isopropranol		√	√
ALDEHYDES			
Formaldehyde	√	√	
Glutaraldehyde	√	√	
ACIDS			
Acetic		√	√
Benzoic			√
Lactic			√
Boric			?
ETHYLENE OXIDE	√		

*?, This property of compound is questionable.

Assessment. Observe clients with prolonged exposure for signs of CNS toxicity: change in sensorium, double vision, lethargy, and seizures.

Intervention. These products are highly toxic if ingested and easily absorbed even through intact skin if not thoroughly rinsed. Do not leave in contact with skin or mucous membranes, as in occlusive dressings, wet packs, lotions, or vaginal packs. Avoid contact with the eyes. Most authoritative sources recommend against the use of pHisoHex for bathing infants or in pregnant or hypersensitive persons. Use should be discontinued if gastric or central nervous signs appear.

pHisoHex is most effective for handwashing when no other antiseptic or solvent follows the rinse, since its antibacterial effects are progressive and cumulative with repeated use. If used for a preoperative preparation, scrub the operative site and surrounding areas every day for 3 days for optimal effectiveness.

pHisoHex may burn brown when exposed to light, but this does not affect its action.

Dispensers should be cleaned every 1 to 2 weeks.

resorcinol

Resorcinol is bactericidal and fungicidal and is about one third as effective as phenol.

Mechanism of action. It is a protein precipitant and is keratolytic.

Indications. Resorcinol is used for treatment of acne, ringworm, eczema, psoriasis, seborrheic dermatitis, and similar skin lesions. Its efficacy is said to be variable or erratic in these disorders.

Side effects/adverse reactions. If systemically absorbed, this topical agent has a toxicity similar to phenol except that there is no prominent CNS stimulation.

Dosage and administration. Usually marketed as an ointment, cream, or lotion in 1% to 10% concentrations.

Assessment. Observe the application site for erythema, swelling, and peeling. Discontinue applications and notify the health care provider.

Intervention. Treatment on alternate days is suggested when used concomitantly with tretinoin for acne vulgaris to avoid excessive skin dryness or irritation.

hexylresorcinol

Hexylresorcinol is a stainless and odorless antiseptic. Although quite irritating to body tissues, diluted solutions of hexylresorcinol are used to cleanse skin wounds and are also used in mouthwashes or pharyngeal antiseptic preparations.

Side effects/adverse reactions. Occasionally a marked hypersensitivity reaction may occur.

Dosage and administration. A 1:1000 solution of hexylresorcinol in glycerin and water is marketed for use as a mouthwash and gargle.

Watch for and advise discontinuation of this product if there are signs of inflammation or irritation, which may indicate hypersensitivity rather than simple dermal irritation.

DYES

Rosaniline dyes are a group of basic dyes only used occasionally today as antiseptic or antiprotozoal agents. This group includes crystal violet, gentian violet, methyl violet, brilliant green, and fuchsin (red). Very few of these dyes continue to be used with any frequency, mainly because of their cosmetic effects (staining of skin, tissues, and clothing). Even gentian violet has largely been replaced by newer topical agents.

gentian violet

Mechanism of action. Gentian violet is bactericidal to gram-positive organisms and bacteriostatic to *Monilia, Epidermophyton,* and *Trichophyton.* It is an antibacterial and antifungal dye.

Indication. Topical antiinfective

Side effects/adverse reactions. Permanent purple staining may result if gentian violet solution is applied to granulation tissue. These agents are not intended for oral ingestion.

Dosage and administration. Gentian violet solutions are available as 1% and 2% preparations. It also is available as gentian violet tampons, 5 mg, for intravaginal use in vulvitis.

Assessment. Assessment of the rate and quality of healing lesions may be difficult because of discoloration of the involved skin areas.

Although healing may be slow and require repeated treatments, these agents produce fewer adverse effects than some other antiseptic agents, which is a distinct advantage in the treatment of some complex dermatologic conditions.

Intervention. Question an order to apply to facial wounds or other frequently exposed body areas, since permanent staining may result. Suggest another topical antiseptic as a substitute.

Use nonocclusive dressings.

Do not apply to granulation tissue, since permanent discoloration or tattooing may occur.

Education. Alert clients that permanent staining of treated areas may occur. Advise clients to avoid use of occlusive dressing.

Caution parents that children are attracted to these colorful solutions and will drink them if they are accessible.

HEAVY METALS

Mercury Compounds

> ammoniated mercury ointment/lotion; merbromin (Mercurochrome); thimerosal (Merthiolate)

The therapeutic effectiveness of mercurial antiseptics is quite low. These antiseptics are primarily bacteriostatic agents whose individual effectiveness in some cases is surpassed by the accompanying vehicle in the particular compound. Inorganic mercury compounds such as ammoniated mercury ointment may owe their effectiveness primarily to the vehicles in the compounds, which permit sustained action of the agent. Organic mercurial agents (e.g., thimerosal) are more bacteriostatic, less irritating, and less toxic than the inorganic mercurials, yet they also have a relatively low therapeutic index. Merbromin is the least effective of the common mercurial antiseptics.

Mechanism of action. The mercurial antiseptics probably act by inhibiting bacterial sulfhydryl enzymes. However, they inhibit tissue enzymes as well, which reduces their usefulness.

Mercurial antiseptics are relatively slow acting, and organisms may revive if they come into contact with open wounds or body fluids. Bacterial spores will resume activity even after prolonged application of a mercurial antiseptic. Tissue and fluid proteins may compete for the mercury, leaving less free mercury for activity against microorganisms.

Indications

> *ammoniated mercury.* Used for psoriasis, seborrheic dermatitis, impetigo contagiosa, dermatomycoses, pediculosis pubis, and superficial pyodermas. Since resistance to mercury has been demonstrated and more effective, less toxic preparations are available, the use of this product is not often recommended.
>
> *merbromin (25% mercury and 20% bromine; Mercurochrome).* An antiseptic and first aid product
>
>> *thimerosal (Merthiolate)*
>> Aerosol pump: used to treat contaminated wounds after cleansing; for antisepsis of intact skin, pustular topical dermatoses, and dermatomycoses; also for preoperative and postoperative use

> Glycerite: used for local application to vagina and cervix area and also to irrigate open wounds
> Solution: used whenever the tincture is contraindicated; a 1:5000 dilution is used in the eye, nose, throat, or genitourinary tract
> Tincture: for skin antisepsis before surgery, for first aid treatment in contaminated wounds, and as an antifungal agent in athlete's foot infections

Side effects/adverse reactions. Skin irritations. For ammoniated mercury, prolonged use may lead to mercury poisoning. This product should not be used in infants or young children. Hypersensitivity reactions or allergic reactions have been reported with ammoniated mercury and thimerosal.

Dosage and administration

> *ammoniated mercury ointment.* Apply once or twice daily.
>
> *merbromin (Mercurochrome).* Clean injury first with soap and water; then apply freely until injury is healed.
>
> *thimerosal (merthiolate).* Apply topically one to three times daily.

NURSING CONSIDERATIONS

Assessment. Before using, assess if client has a history of hypersensitivity to mercury compounds. Observe site of application for contact allergy dermatitis.

Intervention. Cleanse wound thoroughly before applying agent. Let dry before dressing wound. Thimerosal will sting when applied.

Do not apply to large areas of abrasions, since the mercury may be absorbed systemically and cause toxicity.

Education. Make consumers aware of the very limited value of these products as antiseptics and disinfectants in comparison to their potential risks as poisons and allergens. There may be unwarranted reliance on them in the home, since they are relatively inexpensive. Children especially seem to like the pretty red stain left on the skin as evidence of germicidal effectiveness. These products should be stored out of reach of children.

Silver Compounds

> silver nitrate; silver acetate (Healthbreak); silver protein, mild; silver sulfadiazine (Silvadene)

Locally applied, many inorganic silver compounds have antiseptic qualities. Those silver salts that are highly ionizable and soluble produce astringent or caustic actions.

Mechanism of action. Release of free silver ions precipitates bacterial cellular proteins, resulting in bactericidal effects because of disruption of cell walls and plasma membranes.

Effectiveness of these agents is directly proportional to

their concentration and duration of contact time. There is an immediate bactericidal effect when silver solutions are applied to tissue. The silver proteinate that is formed slowly liberates small amounts of ionic silver, which provides continued bacteriostatic action. An unexplained strongly bactericidal quality resides in distilled water when it is in contact with metallic silver. Silver nitrate reacts with soluble chloride, iodides, and bromides to form insoluble salts, stopping the action of silver nitrate. Thus its action can be halted if necessary to irrigation of the area by sodium chloride solutions. This chemical characteristic explains why solutions of silver salts penetrate tissues slowly; apparently chlorides there precipitate the silver ions and inactivate them.

Indications

silver nitrate 1% solution. To prevent gonorrheal ophthalmia neonatorum

10% ointment. Used in podiatry to treat neurovascular helomas, to cauterize and seal small nerve endings and blood vessels, and as a protective cover after corns and calluses have been removed

10% solution. Used to treat impetigo vulgaris and pruritus and in podiatry

25% solution. Used to treat pruritus; in podiatry, used to treat plantar warts

50% solution. Used primarily in podiatry for plantar warts, papillomatous growths, and other selected problems

silver acetate (Healthbreak Chewing Gum). Temporary aid to help break the cigarette habit. At the present time, the FDA over-the-counter advisory panel has stated this product is safe, but its effectiveness is not yet established.

silver protein, mild (Argyrol S.S. 10%). To treat local mild inflammation in the eye, ear, nose, throat, rectum, urethra, and vagina

silver sulfadiazine (Silvadene). Bactericidal for many gram-positive and gram-negative organisms and yeast. It also inhibits bacteria that is resistant to other agents and is considered superior to sulfadiazine alone. It is used to prevent and treat infections in second and third degree burns.

Side effects/adverse reactions

silver nitrate 1% solution. Eye redness or irritation

Other silver nitrate preparations. Skin irritation. With long-term use, it can cause permanent discoloration of the skin because of the deposit of reduced silver (argyria).

In higher concentrations it is limited to podiatric supervision because it is a strong caustic and escharotic agent, so tissues and membranes can be affected or damaged.

silver acetate (Healthbreak Gum). Prolonged use of this product may cause a local argyria, a permanent blue staining of the oral mucous membranes. This effect is not harmful, just not cosmetically acceptable; therefore clients should not use this product for more than 21 days.

silver protein, mild. Prolonged use can result in permanent skin discoloration and conjunctival argyria.

silver sulfadiazine (Silvadene). Allergic skin reaction. Other adverse effects are difficult to attribute directly to this product, since other therapeutic drugs are usually being administered concurrently. Leukopenia and perhaps systemic sulfonamide adverse reactions may occur.

Dosage and administration

silver nitrate 1% solution. Following birth, the eyelids of infants are cleaned with sterile water and sterile cotton or gauze. Then 2 drops of this solution is instilled and allowed to remain in the eyes for no longer than 30 seconds. (In some hospitals, topical erythromycin or tetracycline preparations are used.)

Other silver nitrate preparations. 10% ointment: applied to lesion or affected area as needed, for up to 5 days. 10% solution: applied by cotton applicator to affected area or lesion two or three times a week for 2 to 3 weeks, as necessary. Stronger preparations: podiatric use only.

silver acetate. One tablet is chewed slowly (from 10 to 15 minutes) every 4 hours. Maximum is 6 tablets in 24 hours. Do not use for more than 21 days.

silver protein, mild (Argyrol S.S.). For infections, instill 1 to 3 drops in eye(s) every 3 to 4 hours for several days.

For preoperative use, place 2 or 3 drops in eye(s), then rinse with a sterile irrigating solution.

silver sulfadiazine (Silvadene). Apply with a sterile gloved hand once or twice daily to a 1/16-inch thickness. Keep burn areas covered with this product at all times.

Pregnancy safety. FDA category C

NURSING CONSIDERATIONS

Assessment. Question client about hypersensitivity to silver (or sulfonamides in Silvadene Cream) or a glucose-6-phosphate dehydrogenase deficiency; these preclude treatment with these compounds. The effects in children and in pregnant or breast-feeding women are not known.

Intervention. Store silver nitrate solutions at temperatures between 15° and 30° C (59° to 86° F) and protected from light. Do not use Silvadene Cream if its white color has darkened.

Use only the appropriate concentrations of antiseptic solutions for antiseptic purposes to avoid irritations and burns to tissue. Sodium chloride can be used to flood the area should this occur accidentally.

Store silver nitrate solutions out of reach of children and never take internally. Since sulfadiazine may be absorbed from Silvadene Cream, clients should increase their fluid intake to prevent crystalluria.

Although application of silver sulfadiazine is not painful, application of silver nitrate in solution may be quite painful, especially when applied to burns. Therefore give clients analgesics before dressing changes.

Cleanse wounds before treatment to remove exudate, debris, and blood; this will prevent premature inactivation of these products.

Dressings are not necessary over silver sulfadiazine.

Take care with silver solutions to keep spills and stains to a minimum. Gloves are advised when working with silver solutions. Most tissue stains caused by Silvadene gradually disappear. Stains may be removed from linens, clothing, and shoes by applying household chlorine bleach.

Evaluation. Evaluate affected skin areas daily and note any changes.

Perform ongoing evaluation of clients treated with these compounds to limit adverse effects related to hypersensitivities, crystalluria, or electrolyte imbalances because of absorbed drug components. If silver sulfadiazine is used in the treatment of extensive burns, monitor clients for serum sulfa concentrations, crystalluria, and renal function.

HALOGENS

Chlorine Compounds

chlorine

Chlorine, a nonmetallic element, is a greenish yellow gas with an intensely disagreeable odor. It is corrosive in all forms and acts as a bleaching agent. One part of chlorine in 10,000 parts of air causes respiratory tract irritation progressing to laryngospasm, unconsciousness, and, after 5 minutes, death.

Mechanism of action. Although chlorine can be bactericidal (though it is ineffective against acid-fast bacteria), sporicidal, viricidal, and amebicidal, the elemental form of chlorine itself has limited usefulness as a disinfectant because the gas is difficult to handle. The antibacterial action of chlorine is said to be caused by the formation of hypochlorous acid, which results when chlorine reacts with water. Hypochlorous acid is rapidly antibacterial, depending on the amount of organic matter, the size of the inoculum, the acidity of the medium, and the warmth of the solution's temperature. Prepared solutions decompose fairly rapidly and in a short time become markedly less microbicidal.

Indications. Several chlorine compounds act by slowly yielding hypochlorous acid when combined in various concentrations with water.

1. *Sodium hypochlorite solutions* in common use include the 5% solution, which is limited to the disinfection of utensils, walls, furniture, floors, and swimming pools, and to Dakin's solution, which is a 0.5% concentration used as an antiseptic for fungous infections (e.g., athlete's foot). These solutions are of

limited usefulness for wound irrigations, except for debridement purposes, because they are irritating to the skin and delay the clotting process. Common household bleaches are usually 5.25% solutions of sodium hypochlorite. Therapeutic solutions are unstable and must be freshly prepared before use.

2. *Chloramines* are compounds in which chlorine in water is linked chemically with nitrogen to release hypochlorous acid. Chloramines are more stable, less irritating, slower and more prolonged in action, and less readily affected by organic matter than hypochlorite solutions. Halazone is the only important chloramine used in the United States. It is available in tablet form for sanitizing drinking water. All pathogens usually found in water will be killed in 30 to 60 minutes by adding 1 or 2 tablets per liter of water.

Side effects/adverse reactions. Chlorine compounds are toxic if taken internally and are harmful to delicate tissues and mucous membranes. Over a period of time they are corrosive to equipment.

NURSING CONSIDERATIONS

Store chlorine products in marked containers out of the reach of children. If a chlorine agent is swallowed, a poison control center should be contacted and emergency treatment sought. Small amounts of fluids may be given, but not so much that vomiting occurs.

Store these products away from light and in airtight containers, if possible. Therapeutic solutions should be prepared just before use. Avoid spills on skin or delicate tissues because it will cause irritation. Avoid spills on clothing or contact with hair because of its bleaching properties. Rinse thoroughly with clear water if a spill occurs.

Iodine compounds and iodophors

iodine tincture, povidone-iodine solution (Betadine)

Iodine is a heavy, bluish black, crystalline solid that has a metallic luster and a characteristic odor. It is slightly soluble in water but is soluble in alcohol and in aqueous solutions of sodium and potassium iodide. Iodine is volatile, and solutions should not be exposed to air except during use. In its elemental form, iodine is very rapidly bactericidal, viricidal, fungicidal, and lethal to protozoa; it is less effective against spores. It is one of the most efficient chemical disinfectants and antiseptics currently in use. Some of the iodine compounds are believed to be superior to other antiseptics, including hexachlorophene scrubs. This is controversial in view of the short life of topical iodine's effectiveness in comparison to that of hexachlorophene. All types of bacteria are destroyed at a single concentration of iodine. It is effective over a wide range of pH.

Mechanism of action. Organic matter interferes with the potency of iodine only when it is first applied; later, effectiveness increases because of diffusion as the iodine complexes dissociate. This initial delayed effect in the presence of organic material may also be offset by the increased strengths of the solution concentrations now on the market.

Indications. Iodine compounds are used chiefly for treatment of minor wounds, abrasions, infected wounds, indwelling urethral catheter care, skin preparation before invasive procedures, Hickman catheter and parenteral nutrition dressing changes, and intravenous needle insertions. They are also used for disinfecting indwelling catheters for peritoneal dialysis and for sanitizing water and air. An aqueous solution of 5% iodine and 10% potassium iodide (Lugol's solution) can also be given orally in the treatment of goiter. Various iodine compounds are marketed for antisepsis and disinfection.

iodine topical solution (2% iodine), iodine tincture (2% iodine in alcohol solution), strong iodine solution (5% iodine in water), strong iodine tincture (7% iodine in alcohol). These are used preoperatively to disinfect the skin. They are applied topically for antimicrobial effects against bacteria, fungi, viruses, protozoa, and yeasts.

povidone-iodine (Betadine, Operand, Pharmadine). This water-soluble iodine combined with povidone releases approximately 10% free iodine. It has the same germicidal action of iodine without producing irritation to skin and mucous membranes. Povidone-iodines (Betadine, Isodine) are available in many formulations, such as 10% applicator solution, 2% scrub, spray, foam, vaginal gel, ointment, mouthwash, perineal wash, or whirlpool concentrate. With iodine tincture, the area cannot be bandaged. Povidone-iodine areas may be bandaged if necessary.

tincture of iodine. Iodine tincture, the most commonly used iodine antiseptic, contains 2% iodine and 2.4% sodium iodide in 46% ethyl alcohol. This is frequently employed for cutaneous infections caused by bacteria and fungi. Even a 1% tincture will kill almost an entire bacterial population in 1½ minutes. Three drops of iodine tincture added to a quart of drinking water will reduce ameba and bacterial counts in 15 minutes without impairing palatability.

aqueous iodine solution. This aqueous solution contains 2% iodine and 2.4% sodium iodide in water. Aqueous solutions are thought to be as effective as tincture of iodine for similar therapeutic purposes. They are also less irritating and therefore are used for abraded skin areas.

solution of iodine (2%) in glycerin. This solution is the treatment of choice for application to mucous membranes.

iodophors (Betadine, Prepodyne). Iodophors have become widely used as *antiseptics.* This is the only purpose for which they have been approved by the FDA, although in practice they continue to be used for disinfection of certain equipment. Iodophors are a group of iodine compounds that are combined with a carrier or agent, which increases the water solubility of iodine and provides a sustained-release pool of iodine. Studies show that *as a group* the iodophors are approximately equivalent in germicidal effectiveness but less effective than iodine tinctures or solutions because of their lower concentrations. However, iodophors have been shown to be more effective than chlorhexidine when hands are contaminated with gram-negative organisms.

Poloxamer-iodines (Prepodyne, Septodyne) are available as solutions containing 0.75% and 1% of available iodine, among other forms. Iodophors may also be combined with a detergent (e.g., Wescodyne), adding the power of a surface-acting agent. It is said that Wescodyne kills tubercle bacilli, as well as iodine's usual repertoire of organisms. However, detergents in iodophors for surgical scrubs have been associated with increased toxicity; povidone-iodine by itself is relatively low in tissue toxicity. Iodophor solutions have also been found to be susceptible to contamination within the container according to two reports circulated by the Centers for Disease Control (CDC).

Side effects/adverse reactions. Iodine is toxic if taken internally. It is locally corrosive to gastrointestinal tissues but is inactivated by gastrointestinal contents. Iodine tinctures may be transiently quite painful when applied to open skin areas, but the aqueous solution form stings only slightly. Neonates have developed hypothyroidism following topical application of povidone-iodine. Marked hypersensitivity reactions do occur occasionally even with topical application. These are manifested by severe systemic reactions of fever and generalized skin eruptions.

Dosage and administration. See Indications section.

NURSING CONSIDERATIONS

Assessment. Before iodine compounds and iodophors are applied, ask clients about any past allergic reactions to iodine, shellfish, or iodine-containing diagnostic agents. If there is doubt substitute another product. If irritation develops, wash the skin.

Do not use povidone-iodine as vaginal douche during pregnancy.

Intervention. These products are exceptionally valuable because of their efficiency, low toxicity, and low cost.

Do not bandage or tape areas treated with tincture of iodine; if treated with povidone-iodine, a cover dressing may be applied.

Iodophors will stain only starched linen or clothing. Tinctures and solutions of iodine may stain more freely.

Soap and water cleansing of fingertips before skin puncture for blood glucose monitoring by some reagent strips is recommended. Artificially elevated blood glucose determinations have been noted when povidone-iodine swabs were used for skin preparation.

If appropriate, give the client medication for pain before iodine tinctures are applied.

Education. Advise the client to purchase iodine preparations in very small quantities and discard routinely after a short time, since evaporation of the solvent or vehicle will leave a concentrated iodine preparation that may burn tissues on application.

OXIDIZING AGENTS

hydrogen peroxide

Hydrogen peroxide is a colorless, odorless antiseptic that deteriorates readily to form water and oxygen.

Mechanism of action. When hydrogen peroxide comes into contact with organic matter such as tissues, enzymatic reactions cause decomposition of hydrogen peroxide and rapid formation of oxygen bubbles. Solutions have a high surface tension. Because of this and the resulting effervescence, there is limited penetrability.

Although the antiseptic action of hydrogen peroxide is fairly fast acting, it is short lived. It acts as an antibacterial only as long as the bubbling action continues.

Indications. Oxygen that is released is particularly suited for destroying anerobic microorganisms, but effects vary depending on the type of organism. Several products containing hydrogen peroxide are marketed.

hydrogen peroxide topical solution. This is a 3% solution of hydrogen peroxide in water, which is used to irrigate suppurating wounds and some extensive traumatic wounds. It should not be instilled into closed body spaces because of its effervescence. It is also used for wound cleansing, before Hickman catheter dressing changes, for surgical repair of cleft lip, as irrigations following some radical head and neck surgeries, for some oral lesions, for oral cleansing (Peroxyl mouthrinse), and for removal of collections of mucus from the inner cannula of tracheostomy tubes. It is used with caution, if at all, for ear irrigations to remove excess cerumen because of damage to the tympanic membrane.

The official solution should be further diluted with water into a half-strength or 1:4 strength for most applications.

medicinal zinc peroxide. This peroxide, a combination of zinc and hydrogen peroxide, yields hydrogen peroxide. The residue of zinc oxide is mildly astringent. It is used topically for antisepsis and deodorizing of wounds, especially those infected with anerobes.

benzoyl peroxide. Benzoyl peroxide is used as a topical antiseptic, keratolytic, antiseborrheic, and mild irritant to treat acne. (See Chapter 67.)

Side effects/adverse reactions. If small amounts of dilute solutions are swallowed, rapid decomposition of the substances in the stomach into relatively harmless molecular oxygen and water occurs. Repeated use as a mouthwash may cause hypertrophied papillae of the tongue ("hairy tongue"), a reversible condition. Some products may cause contact dermatitis and bleaching of clothing.

NURSING CONSIDERATIONS

To delay deterioration of the contents, store solutions in tightly capped, amber containers to protect from light and air. Solutions in containers should be discarded frequently, and fresh solutions should be used. The rapidity and vigor with which bubbling occurs may be used as a general guide to the freshness of the solution.

The bubbling action makes hydrogen peroxide useful for removing mucous secretions from equipment (i.e., inner cannulae of tracheostomy tubes).

Do not leave paper cups containing hydrogen peroxide where clients can reach them. Because the solution looks like water, patients have mistakenly drunk it despite the unusual taste. Although very small amounts will not be harmful, large amounts in the stomach could be harmful because of resultant effervescence in the stomach, a closed cavity. These compounds, like all medications, should be kept secured and out of children's reach.

BIGUANIDES

chlorhexidine gluconate (Hibiclens, Hibitane Tincture)

Chlorhexidine gluconate is a biguanide with antiseptic activity. It is effective against both gram-positive and gram-negative bacteria.

Mechanism of action. Chlorhexidine acts by disrupting the bacterial cell's plasma membrane.

Indication. Hibiclens is a bactericidal skin cleansing solution containing chlorhexidine gluconate. It is useful as a surgical scrub, a handwashing agent for personnel, and a skin wound cleanser. It is also used for the treatment of aphthous ulcers in the mouth and the prevention of dental caries.

Side effects/adverse reactions. Orally ingested, chlorhexidine is believed to have low toxicity; however, low concentrations in the bloodstream can cause hemolysis. There have been reports of deafness occurring when these products came into contact with the middle ear through a perforated eardrum. Rare secondary effects include dermatitis, photosensitivity, and irritation of mucosal tissue. Physiochemical properties of these agents suggest that absorption through the skin is minimal.

Dosage and administration. The action of chlorhexidine is not affected by the presence of blood or exudate, but effectiveness may be directly related to the concentration of the solution. Hibiclens (the 4% solution) is more effective than Hibitane (1% aqueous solution), according to studies. Studies comparing Hibiclens and povidone-iodine produced equivocal results. As a handwash, Hibiclens is applied, water added, and friction applied for 15 seconds. Skin wounds should be washed gently with Hibiclens and rinsed. For surgical scrubs hands and forearms are scrubbed with approximately 5 ml Hibiclens for 3 minutes without water, while using a brush or sponge. After hands and forearms are rinsed, washing is repeated for 3 more minutes. Hibitane Tincture should be applied liberally to the surgical site, swabbed for 2 minutes or more, and the area then air-dried. Pooled Hibitane has caused skin burns during electrocautery. The tinctures are said to have a persistent bactericidal effect against many gram-positive and gram-negative bacteria (some of the latter are completely resistant to chlorhexidine, however). Furthermore, there have been a few reports of epidemic infections caused by *Pseudomonas maltophilia* and *P. cepacia* that were traced to diluted solutions in 0.05% to 0.2%.

NURSING CONSIDERATIONS

Intervention. Since this product has been used outside the United States for about 20 years and only briefly in the United States, data regarding secondary effects may be incomplete.

Use judgment when diluting these agents, since their effectiveness may be greatly reduced in proportion to the dilution. Certain solutions less than 4% may actually support bacterial growth. Chlorhexidine-treated areas should not be wiped with alcohol, which will neutralize the intended residual action.

Do not use chlorhexidine on delicate tissues such as eyes and mucous membranes. The area should be rinsed promptly if this occurs.

Education. Advise clients not to swallow chlorhexidine compounds (especially when used for mouth care).

SURFACE-ACTIVE AGENTS

benzalkonium chloride (Zephiran Chloride)

As wetting agents, emulsifiers, or detergents, surface-acting agents are considered superior to soaps because they can be used in hard water, are stable in acid or alkaline solutions, decrease surface tension more effectively, and are less irritating to the skin. Benzalkonium chloride is a cationic (bearing a positive electric charge on the active portion of the agent) quaternary ammonium compound used in solution as a topical antiseptic or as a disinfectant. It is generally believed that benzalkonium chloride is not very reliable in either role.

Mechanism of action. The mechanism of action is not known for certain, but it is thought that this agent and others like it act by inactivating enzymes, precipitating proteins, and causing increased permeability of bacterial cell membranes.

Indications

1. Used in an aqueous solution as an antiseptic for skin, mucous membranes, wounds, and preoperative skin preparation of personnel and patients.
2. Used to immersion-store sterile instruments and equipment. However, its documented ability to support the growth of contaminants has caused the CDC to recommend the substitution of other agents, such as iodophors and alcohols.

Side effects/adverse reactions. Chemical burns may occur if benzalkonium chloride is allowed to stay in contact with tissues, as in wet packs or occlusive dressings. The tincture and the spray formulations are flammable. Delicate tissues may be injured if specified dilution recommendations are not used. Ingestion only rarely causes toxicity. Hypersensitivity reactions can occur.

Dosage and administration. This agent is slow acting in comparison to iodine. Therapeutic effects are thought to be in direct relation to the concentration of the solution used. Depending of the purpose and tissues or equipment to be treated, recommended dilutions range from 1:750 to 1:5000 or 1:10,000. A variety of gram-positive and gram-negative organisms and many fungi and viruses (not hepatitis) are said to be susceptible. Bacterial spores and *Pseudomonas cepacia* are resistant, and *Mycobacterium tuberculosis* is relatively resistant to Zephiran chloride. Organic materials inactivate benzalkonium chloride. Tap water that contains metallic ions, organic matter, or resindeionized water may reduce its effectiveness. Many materials, soaps, and anionic detergents may absorb the active ingredient, rendering it weak for many purposes.

NURSING CONSIDERATIONS

Assessment. If any of these compounds have been used, continue to monitor the area or utensil critically for contamination.

Intervention. In view of the highly questionable efficacy of surface-active agents, especially benzalkonium chloride, question an order or a suggestion to use them as antiseptics or disinfectants. Suggest the substitution of an iodophor, alcohol, or other compound. Use only the concentration recommended for each specified area. Do not use with occlusive dressings.

Do not apply these compounds to areas previously treated with soaps or anionic agents.

Do not apply to delicate tissues. Flood the area with water if these agents are accidentally introduced.

Do not reuse solutions after soaking cotton balls, dressings, or instruments.

Avoid using Zephiran to disinfect thermometers. If it must be used, use not less than the recommended 1:750 concentration.

Do not use the tincture or spray formulations near an open flame.

MISCELLANEOUS AGENTS

nitrofurazone (Furacin)

Mechanism of action. Nitrofurazone is a broad antibacterial agent active against many bacteria that cause local infections, including *Staphylococcus aureus, Streptococcus, E. coli,* and others.

Indications

1. Used mainly as adjunct therapy to clients with second and third degree burns when bacterial resistance to other agents is a problem.
2. Also used during skin grafting when bacterial contamination may result in graft rejection or a donor site infection.

Side effects/adverse reactions. Rash, itching, local edema (dermatitis), and allergic reactions have been reported. Hypersensitivity occurs early in the treatment of a few individuals. Furacin is not absorbed significantly through mucosal or burned tissues, and systemic toxicity is rare. However, its propylethylene glycol base may be absorbed and challenge the client with renal dysfunction. Bacterial and fungal suprainfections may occur. Clients with glucose-6-phosphate dehydrogenase deficiency should avoid the use of nitrofurazone if possible.

Significant drug interactions. Nitrofurazone may inhibit the effectiveness of the enzyme sutilains (Travase).

Dosage and administration. The 0.2% powder, cream, ointment, soluble dressing, or topical solution may be applied directly on the area or to a gauze dressing for application. The soluble dressing form is useful as an preparatory antiseptic for skin graft areas. The solution is bacteriostatic in concentrations of 1:100,000 to 1:200,000 and bactericidal at twice these concentrations. Efficacy is reduced in the presence of heavy microbial contamination, plasma, or blood. Resistance seldom develops.

Pregnancy safety. FDA category C

NURSING CONSIDERATIONS

Assessment. Watch for dermatitis or other manifestations of hypersensitivity to this product. Severe skin reactions may require topically applied steroids. Pregnant women should avoid use of this product until it has been proved safe; persons with glucose-6-phosphate dehydrogenase deficiency are likewise cautioned to avoid Furacin. Judgment should be used in treating individuals who have renal disorders with preparations that include polyethylene glycol. Clients should be alerted to these adverse reactions.

Intervention. Cleanse the affected area before each dressing change.

Treatment by Furacin may be suggested in instances of burn or wound infections resistant to other medications.

Treatment for a developing secondary infection may become necessary. Meticulous sterile technique is essential during dressing changes and when opening and withdrawing Furacin-saturated dressings from their sterile packets.

Evaluation. Evaluate affected areas daily. Areas that do not seem to be responding to treatment by Furacin or any areas becoming inflamed because of hypersensitivity should continue to be assessed for discontinuance.

ALCOHOLS

ethanol (ethyl alcohol); isopropanol (isopropyl alcohol)

Mechanism of action. Alcohols may precipitate cellular proteins.

Indications

1. Alcohols are variably effective in topical application for the destruction of gram-positive and gram-negative bacteria, fungi, lipophilic viruses, and tubercle bacilli.
2. In topical application alcohols are commonly used to prepare skin for minor invasive procedures (using commercially packaged skin wipes), such as before parenteral injections, in combination with iodine for the same purpose, or for disinfection of vial tops and thermometers.
3. Alcohols are also used for disinfection of heat-labile instruments, polyethylene tubing, catheters, implants, prostheses, smooth hard-surfaced objects, hinged instruments, and inhalation and anesthesia equipment.
4. Because of their rapid evaporation rate, dilute solutions of alcohols are still occasionally used as sponge baths to reduce fever, although systemic absorption may be especially harmful to neonates and children.
5. Alcohols are also used as preservatives in solutions, used as diluents or to dissolve other drugs, and in combination with many other drugs for over-the-counter purchase (often without rationale).
6. Ethyl alcohol is also ingested purposefully as an intoxicating beverage.

Side effects/adverse reactions. Essentially, all of the alcohols are poisonous drugs when taken internally, depending on the dose. Isopropyl alcohol is inherently highly poisonous; ethyl alcohol, pure alcohol made from vegetables, fruits, canes, and grains, is the alcohol of alcoholic beverages. The degree to which fractional distillation is carried out determines the resultant concentration. When continuously inhaled or absorbed through the skin, alcohols can cause intoxication. Ethyl alcohol is irritating if left in contact with skin for prolonged periods. If ethyl alcohol is applied to open skin, a film that can harbor microorganisms develops. Isopropyl alcohol causes subcutaneous vaodilation, which can cause needle sites and incisions to bleed somewhat more freely.

Dosage and administration. Ethyl alcohol is slightly less effective as an antiseptic than isopropyl alcohol. Efficacy may depend highly on the concentration used and the amount of mechanical friction applied. The most effective solutions of ethyl alcohol are concentrations of 50% to 70%; stronger solutions are less effective. At concentrations of 70%, almost 90% of the bacteria on skin are killed within 2 minutes if the wet surface is allowed to dry naturally. Inadequate disinfection may occasionally result even if friction is conscientiously applied to surfaces.

Isopropyl alcohol is employed in aqueous solutions of 70% concentration or undiluted as 99% concentration (isopropyl rubbing alcohol). It may be combined with other disinfectants such as iodine and formaldehyde to improve efficiency.

NURSING CONSIDERATIONS

Intervention. Leave on the skin for at least 2 minutes. Allow to dry without fanning. Do not use with open wounds.

Cleanse thermometers before placing them to soak in an alcohol solution, because any adherent organic matter will inhibit the solution's action. Alcohol solutions themselves *may harbor organisms* and *may rust instruments;* therefore, they are often not the best solution for disinfecting or for sterile storage of equipment.

When alcohol is used as a disinfectant or antiseptic, its effectiveness is heightened when friction in applied and when it is allowed to dry naturally (without fanning with the hand or other object) before proceeding. Nonetheless, studies (see Bibliography) show that the sterility of tops of freshly uncapped vials is maintained whether or not alcohol swabs are applied to the tops, *unless* the alcohol itself is contaminated. Sterile tops of medication containers such as vials should not be wiped with a disinfectant before using, unless they have become contaminated or have remained uncovered too long.

Be prepared to apply more pressure and possibly a small pressure dressing after giving an injection or discontinuing an intravenous infusion if alcohol has been applied to the site. If the individual is also receiving anticoagulant therapy, the bleeding may be extensive.

Education. Make personnel, clients, and parents aware that all alcohols are inherently or potentially poisonous and that intoxication or dangerous poisoning can occur as a result of their absorption, inhalation, or ingestion. Keep alcohols secured and out of the reach of children.

ACIDS

acetic acid (vinegar); benzoic acid; lactic acid; boric acid

Various acids have been used as antiseptics or cauterizing agents. Of these, vinegar is the most commonly used, especially in community health nursing, because of its practicality, availability, and low cost. Other acids that are employed as antiseptics include benzoic acid (0.1%), which prevents bacterial and fungous growth; lactic acid, which is used primarily as a component of spermatocides in the United States (and as a topical antiseptic elsewhere); and boric acid, which is so mild that it is used in eye and ear preparations. Of these other acids, most have lost credibility as effective antiseptics. Specifically, boric acid has been implicated in cases of serious systemic intoxication by absorption.

Mechanism of action. Vinegar (acetic acid) provides an acid medium that inhibits the growth of organisms dependent on a neutral or alkaline medium.

Indications. In a 5% concentration, acetic acid is germicidal to many organisms. It is bacteriostatic at lower concentrations. A mild vinegar solution is often recommended as a vaginal douche for antisepsis in the prevention or suppression of vaginal infections caused by *Trichomonas, Candida,* and *Gardenella vaginalis* organisms and for spermatocidal purposes. Acetic acid may also be used as a mild antiseptic-deodorant for many other applications, such as for instillation into the collection container of indwelling urinary drainage catheters, bladder irrigation (0.25% concentration), and diaper soaks. The 1% concentration may be used as a topical antiseptic for certain surgical wounds and burns since it is particularly effective against *Pseudomonas aeruginosa.* When applied to skin graft donor sites, a 0.25% acetic acid solution does not interfere with healing.

Side effects/adverse reactions. The residual pungent odor of acetic acid may be a deterrent to its use. Ingestion may produce laryngospasm. Preservatives that are incorporated in vinegar may be responsible for some hypersensitivity reactions.

Dosage and administration. See Indications.

A mildly effective, soothing vaginal douche can be prepared by adding 1 to 2 tablespoons of white household vinegar (5%) to 1 quart of warm water. Stronger concentrations are no more effective and may irritate mucosal tissues.

Antiseptics instilled in urinary collection bags should be of concentrations that are not injurious to bladder mucosa in case the bag is inadvertently raised so that contents reflux into the bladder.

STERILANTS

ALDEHYDES

formaldehyde solution

Formaldehyde solution is a 37% concentration of formalin (by weight). It is a clear, colorless disinfectant liquid that, on exposure to air, liberates a pungent, irritating gas. It is effective against bacteria, fungi, and viruses.

Mechanism of action. Proteins are precipitated by strong formaldehyde concentrations.

Indications

1. When formaldehyde is combined with isopropyl alcohol or hexachlorophene, it is probably the most potent germicidal solution currently available.
2. Preparations that combine formaldehyde solution, isopropyl alcohol, and antirust agents for the disinfection of instruments and heat-labile articles are used for "cold sterilization." Hemodialysis equipment is often cleaned with formaldehyde solutions. The solution may be applied as a strong astringent.
3. It is also used as a preservative for sputum and other types of specimens and in certain medicinals and biologicals, such as toxoid vaccines.
4. It is also used commercially to make clothing crease-resistant.

Side effects/adverse reactions. Personnel who are in frequent contact with formaldehyde compounds are at great risk. In the past only the adverse reactions of itchy and watery eyes, runny noses, coughing, dermatitis, and browning and blistering of hands were noted. Increasing attention is being paid to formaldehyde's confirmed mutagenicity and possible carcinogenicity. Studies show that formaldehyde may not only inhibit the repair of DNA that has been damaged by x-rays but also actually potentiate this damage. Investigations may also show that aldehydes, which are produced by nitrosamine degradation in the body, may contribute to the mutagenicity and carcinogenicity associated with nitrosamines. When hydrogen chloride fumes and formaldehyde fumes combine in moist air, the product may be associated with increased risk of lung cancer.

A report from the National Institute for Occupational Safety and Health (NIOSH) states that formaldehyde should be considered and handled as a potential occupational carcinogen and recommends that appropriate controls be developed and implemented accordingly. Currently, standards set by the Occupational Safety and Health Administration (OSHA) limit an 8-hour concentration limit to 3 parts per million (ppm), along with other specific limitations related to air concentration. In view of its latest findings, NIOSH recommends that exposure be limited to a concentration no more than 1 ppm for any 30-minute period.

Dosage and administration. The action of formaldehyde is slow. It is usually employed in 2% to 8% solutions as a disinfectant. Even at 8% concentrations, formaldehyde takes 18 hours to destroy bacterial spores.

Help disseminate important information to other workers about the dangers of exposure to formaldehyde. Wear gloves when handling formaldehyde. All who work with formaldehyde should see that adequate ventilation is maintained in work areas and that goggles and filter masks are available and in good condition for use whenever fumes are strong enough to cause respiratory and eye irritations. Always dilute the 37% solution.

glutaraldehyde (Cidex)

Glutaraldehyde is considered to be a more effective disinfectant sterilant than formaldehyde. Glutaraldehyde is less volatile than formaldehyde; therefore it is less musty, and fewer irritating fumes generally occur.

Mechanism of action. At a pH of 7.5 to 8.5, glutaraldehyde is a very effective antibacterial agent with potent bactericidal, tuberculocidal, fungicidal, sporicidal, and virucidal action. This effectiveness is recorded even in the presence of organic material (blood, tissue, mucus).

Indications. Glutaraldehyde is a germicidal agent used to disinfect and sterilize plastic and rubber equipment (respiratory, anesthesia), surgical and dental instruments, catheters, thermometers, and other hard-surfaced, heat-labile equipment.

Side effects/adverse reactions. Glutaraldehyde is irritating to skin or mucous membranes. It is also a severe eye irritant, and fumes may irritate the respiratory tract. It should be used cautiously in a well-ventilated area.

Dosage and administration

Disinfection of instruments: Immerse instruments in glutaraldehyde solution for 10 minutes. Rinse equipment before use.

Sterilization: Immerse equipment or instruments for a minimum of 10 hours to destroy pathogenic spores.

Use sterile technique in removing the items from the solution and rinse thoroughly with sterile water. Flush all lumens and cannulas and dry the items before use.

NURSING CONSIDERATIONS

Do not use this disinfectant-sterilant on living tissue. If accidentally exposed, thoroughly rinse the area.

When feasible, consider steam under pressure, gas, or heat in preference to sterilization by glutaraldehyde.

To prepare a glutaraldehyde solution, add the specified activator powder, which contains a rust inhibitor.

Completely cover articles with the solution for the entire prescribed time. (The time necessary depends on the purpose for which the solution is used—for disinfection or for chemical sterilization.) During the immersion period, cap the container to prevent escape of fumes. Remove articles from the immersion fluid with sterile forceps and thoroughly airdry.

Post instructions for use in full view of personnel. Also instruct them in the use of glutaraldehyde. Ongoing inservice education should be maintained.

ETHYLENE OXIDE

Ethylene oxide is a colorless gas at ordinary temperatures. Its use is more dangerous, more complex, more expensive, and less reliable than steam under pressure. It is highly toxic, flammable, and thought to be mutagenic and carcinogenic as well. Carboxide is a combination of 10% ethylene oxide and 90% carbon dioxide; other combinations include gases such as Freon (to reduce flammability and explosive hazards). External exhaust systems are recommended when ethylene oxide is used.

Mechanism of action. Ethylene oxide is an alkylating agent, which allows it to unite chemically with living cells, thereby interfering with cellular metabolism and destroying the cells.

Indications

1. Used for gaseous sterilization of materials that cannot be subjected to intense heat or pressure, such as plastic machinery parts, optical instruments, or prosthetic devices (i.e., artificial hip replacements and pacemakers).
2. It is highly penetrating and is destructive to all types of microorganisms, including viruses, tubercle bacilli, and spores.
3. Articles removed from gas sterilizers should be allowed adequate time for residual gases to be diffused from internal parts before they are removed and used.

Side effects/adverse reactions. Careful studies by the National Institute for Occupational Safety and the Ameri-

can Hospital Supply Corporation have correlated ethylene oxide exposure with chromosomal defects, low sperm counts, spontaneous abortion, and leukemia and other cancers in factory workers. Other toxic effects include respiratory, eye, and skin irritation, anemia, vomiting, and diarrhea. Studies recommend that "ethylene oxide be regarded in the workplace as a potential occupational carcinogen, and that appropriate controls be used to reduce worker exposure."* It has now been ruled that current minimal standards relating to exposure be changed so that workers are exposed to no more than 1 ppm in the air as an 8-hour time-weighted average and that those who work with ethylene oxide be provided with ongoing medical surveillance. The Occupational Safety and Health Administration has jurisdiction over standard setting. It was found that white blood cells of hospital workers who had been exposed to currently allowable levels of ethylene oxide for as little as 4 minutes/day for 6 months showed the same anomalous chromatid breaks and rejoinings that are used as criteria for determining genetic risk for mutagenesis and carcinogenesis.

NURSING CONSIDERATIONS

Assessment. If badges to monitor ambient air concentrations of ethylene oxide are issued, employees and nurses should wear them. Monthly EtO level checks by facility engineers are recommended.

All who are frequently exposed (central supply room workers, operating room nurses, employees of manufacturers, and other users) should have routine follow-up examinations. Nurses and nurse practitioners may want to include questions related to industrial exposure in taking health histories of those with repeated respiratory tract conditions.

Those in their childbearing years should avoid prolonged exposure, especially early in pregnancy.

Intervention. Substitute other forms of sterilization for ethylene oxide, if feasible. There may be no other acceptable forms of sterilization for the specific applications, however. Implementation of recommended standards may compromise patient care and possibly place an inordinate financial burden on hospitals not now suitably equipped.

If ethylene oxide sterilization is frequently employed, hospital workers should be actively working with the hospital administration to have steps taken to monitor the ambient air levels of ethylene oxide during the use of gas sterilizers and to install air-exhaust systems that vent to the outside.

Post instructions for the preparation and use of ethyl-

*See Coene, RF: Bulletin No. 35, Washington, DC, 1981, Government Printing Office.

ene oxide and gas sterilizers where they are used and where they are manufactured. Risks are incurred when articles are transferred from the ethylene oxide sterilizer to the aerator, when aeration time guidelines are not followed, or when the aerator malfunctions.

Monitor court proceedings, which will probably result in new standards for exposure, and disseminate findings to those in the occupational nursing field.

KEY TERMS

bacteriocidal, page 1123
bacteriostatic, page 1123
community- or home-acquired infections, page 1121
germicides, page 1123
nosocomial infections, page 1121
sterilization, page 1122

BIBLIOGRAPHY

Block, SS: Disinfection, sterilization, and preservation, ed 2, Philadelphia, 1977, Lea & Febiger.

Coene, RF: Formaldehyde: evidence of carcinogenicity, Current Intelligence Bulletin No. 34, DDHS (NIOSH), Washington, DC, 1981, Government Printing Office.

Coene, RF: Ethylene oxide (EtO): evidence of carcinogenicity, Current Intelligence Bulletin No. 35, DDHS (NIOSH), Washington, DC, 1981, Government Printing Office.

Contaminated povidone-iodine solution (Northeastern U.S.), Morbid Mortal Week Rep 29(46):553, 1980.

Do disinfectants need tests for effectiveness? Hosp Infect Control 10(3):29, 1982.

Feingold, KR, and others: Iodine-induced artifacts in home blood glucose measurements (letter), Diabetes Care 6(3):317, 1983.

Formaldehyde limits a cell's DNA repair, Sci News 123:231, April 1983.

Gilman, AG and others, eds: The pharmacologic basis of therapeutics, ed 7, New York, 1980, Macmillan, Inc.

Hamilton, HK: Procedures, Nursing '83 Books, Springhous, Pa, 1983, Intermed Communications.

Hargiss, CO, and Larson, E: Guidelines for prevention of hospital acquired infections, Am J Nurs 11:2175, 1981.

Herfindal, ET and Hirschman JL: Clinical pharmacy and therapeutics, ed 3, Baltimore, 1984, Williams & Wilkins.

Kastrup, EK, ed: Facts and comparisons, St Louis, 1988, JB Lippincott Co.

Katzung, BG: Basic and clinical pharmacology, ed 3, Norwalk, Conn, 1987, Appleton & Lange.

Kimbrough, RD: Review of evidence of toxic effects of hexachlorophene, Pediatrics 51:391, 1973.

Malizia, WF, and others: Benzalkonium chloride as a source of infection, New Engl J Med 263:800, 1960.

Mattia, MA: Hazards in the environment, the sterilants: ethylene oxide and formaldehyde, Am J Nurs 13:240.

Morrison, RT and others: Organic chemistry, ed 3, Boston, 1978, Allyn & Bacon, Inc.

Osol, A, ed: Remington's pharmaceutical sciences, ed 16, Easton, Pa, 1980, Mack Publishing Co.

Perkins, J: Principles and methods of sterilization in the hospital, ed 3, Springfield, Ill, 1982, Charles C Thomas, Publisher.

Pseudomonas aeruginosa peritonitis attributed to a contaminated iodophor solution (Georgia) Morbid Mortal Week Rep 31(15):197, 1982.

Reddish, GF, ed: Antiseptics, disinfectants, fungicides, and chemical and physical sterilization, Philadelphia, 1978, Lea & Febiger.

Reducing the risks from ethylene oxide, Am J Nurs 83:1643, 1983.

Sobel, J and others: Nosocomial Pseudomonas cepacia infection associated with chlorhexidine contamination, Am J Med 73:183, 1982.

Spaulding, EH: Role of chemical disinfection in the prevention of nosocomial infections, Proceedings of the International Conference on Nosocomial Infections. Atlanta, 1970, Centers for Disease Control.

Speight, TM, ed: Avery's drug treatment, ed 3, Baltimore, 1987, Williams & Wilkins.

United States Pharmacopeial Convention: Drug information for the health care provider, ed 8, Rockville, Md, 1988, The Convention.

US Occupational Safety and Health Administration: General industry: OSHA safety and health standards (29 CFR, part 1910), rev ed, 1976, Washington, DC: US Government Printing Office.

CHAPTER 73

Diagnostic Agents

OBJECTIVES

After studying this chapter, the student will be able to:

1. Describe the mechanism of action of radiopaque contrast medium.

2. State the method of absorption, metabolism, and excretion of barium sulfate and iodinated contrast media.

3. Identify the nursing assessments necessary to detect side effects/adverse reactions from the administration of iodinated contrast medium and the appropriate nursing interventions to manage the initial symptoms.

4. Describe the pharmacokinetics of diagnostic agents used as radioactive tracers and imaging agents.

5. Describe the indications, secondary effects, and nursing considerations of common nonradioactive agents used for visualization of organ function and challenging glandular response.

6. Identify common tests used for screening selected health conditions.

Diagnostic agents are considered drugs in the sense that they are chemical substances used to diagnose or monitor a condition or disease. As diagnostic agents, certain secondary chemical characteristics are used to confirm a diagnosis or prognosis or to guide therapy. For example, one type of diagnostic agent may interact with a bodily fluid specimen as a reagent to produce one or another color as an indicant, or it may induce an inflammatory response or an enhancement of a particular gland's functioning. Other agents act by contrasting and enhancing visibility on x-ray film of the lumens or cavities of internal body structures. Some, because of a special affinity and uptake by certain organs, permit critical assessment of organ function. Diagnostic agents may also have side effects and adverse reactions, just like any drug. Thus it is necessary that the nurse know the agent used, its mechanism of action, and indications. Secondary effects are equally important, since many agents have a somewhat narrow range of safety. In some instances, nurses are responsible for correctly collecting and testing specimens and interpreting the results. Specialized training and professional education are necessary to administer some kinds of agents; others are packaged in simple kit form for over-the-counter sale. Because the field of diagnostics and its products is burgeoning, manufacturers' instructions should always be consulted to be assured of current information.

Products used for diagnostic testing are categorized in various ways. Here they are organized by their diagnostic applications and presented (not all-inclusively) in chart form wherever feasible:

- For assessment of the size, location, and integrity of structures, such as those of the gastrointestinal tract, gallbladder, kidneys, blood vessels, spleen, and joints, or as an adjunct to computed tomography examinations.
- For functional assessment of organ systems, for example, the heart, pancreas, stomach, liver, pituitary, adrenal cortex, thyroid, or gallbladder.
- For assessment of sensitivities to specific substances, as in allergy states, tuberculosis, mumps, coccidioidomycosis, blastomycosis, or histoplasmosis.
- For assessment of glandular responsivity to provocative challenge by certain agents.
- For screening assessments or monitoring of indicative components in urine, blood, or feces.

RADIOPAQUE AGENTS FOR VISUALIZING ORGAN STRUCTURE

Mechanism of action. When injected or instilled, radiopaque contrast agents make the body cavity or compartment more radiographically dense or opaque than neighboring anatomic structures. They are used when the structural integrity of a soft-tissue organ system is under study. Ordinary x-ray examinations are useful only for studies of dense materials such as bone. Radiopaque contrast media may also permit visualization of organs' functional dynamics as part of associated diagnostic tests. (See table 73-1.)

Many of these agents contain molecular iodine in the radiopaque contrast medium to provide the opacity necessary for outlining internal organ cavities, lumens, or ducts that would otherwise be invisible by x-ray examination or fluoroscopy. The high atomic weight of iodine provides the characteristic radiodensity. Visual contrast is directly proportional to the iodine concentration of the medium.

Barium contrast media do not contain iodine compounds. Instead, they consist of barium sulfate powder and a vehicle such as hydrosol gum for mixing with prescribed volumes of water to provide a suspension for oral or rectal administration. Additives may include compounds for coloring and flavoring. Iodinated radiopaque agents consist of substituted, triiodinated, benzoic acid derivatives or water-soluble, triiodinated, benzoic acid salts. Manufacturers' instructions should always be reviewed.

The physician should be consulted when a client reports a history of idiosyncratic response or hypersensitivity to iodine, shellfish, or contrast media, or a history of multiple radiographic or radionuclide studies. The most common radiopaque contrast agents are barium sulfate suspensions and iodinated contrast materials.

Indications

1. Barium-containing preparations are typically used to opacify the gastrointestinal tract. Radiographic techniques of upper gastrointestinal tract and colon examinations are generally performed when ulcers, inflammatory bowel disease, or cancer is suspected. One of the most common uses of barium contrast media is in "double-contrast" studies for gastrointestinal tract evaluation.

2. The most frequent clinical uses of iodinated contrast media include intravenous urography and angiography. Iodinated contrast media are often used during computed tomography (CT) of the head and body to visualize vascular structures and to detect tumors. See Table 73-1 for details.

Pharmacokinetics. Radiopaque agents may be administered by the oral, vaginal, rectal, intravenous, or intraarterial routes. They may also be instilled into other body cavities.

Absorption. Orally administered iodinated agents for visualization of the gallbladder are absorbed across the gastrointestinal mucosa and enter the systemic circulation through the portal venous system. Orally or rectally administered iodinated media for delineation of the gastrointestinal tract are absorbed only minimally, but enough so that the renal tract may also be visualized. Barium sulfate preparations are not absorbed.

Metabolism. Liver, gallbladder

Excretion. Urine

Side effects/adverse reactions. These products are not without risk. Effects are diverse, are mild to moderate in severity, and usually occur within 1 to 3 minutes. However, delayed reactions may occur up to 1 hour after injection. Secondary effects are increased by dysfunctional excretory routes. Intravenous cholangiography has caused the highest number of reactions and has therefore been largely replaced by radionuclide diagnostics and retrograde duodenal examination. Excretory urography is performed frequently with only rare serious reactions. Milder reactions result from administration of oral cholecystographic agents. Certain agents are more likely to cause secondary effects than others; manufacturers' information should be consulted.

A history of allergy puts the client at twice the risk of reaction to contrast media, although, paradoxically, these are not true hypersensitivity reactions. Those with a previous reaction to contrast media are at three times the risk. Certain individualized reactions may occasionally have serious results. Death occurs in less than 0.01% of patients, and most of these are attributable to cardiac arrest associated with predisposing cardiovascular disease. The dosage and the injection rate influence hemodynamics and thus perfused organ damage, if any. Barium sulfate preparations, since they are not absorbed internally, are only potentially hazardous when administered to

TABLE 73-1   Common Diagnostic Tests Using Common Radiopaque Agents: Barium Sulfate and Iodinated Contrast Media

| | Cholangiography/ Cholecystography | | Computerized tomographic enhancement | Angiography | Myelography | Lymphography | Arthrography | Discography | Urography | | Hysterosalpingography | GI Radiography | FDA pregnancy category |
	Oral	IV							IV	Retrograde			
ORAL CHOLECYSTOGRAPHICS													
iocetamic acid (Cholebrine)	✔												B
iopanoic acid (Telepaque)	✔												C
ipodate salts (Oragrafin sodium)	✔												U†
tyropanoate sodium (Bilopaque)	✔												C
INTRAVENOUS AGENTS													
diatrizoate salts (Hypaque Sodium 50%, Urovist Sod. 300)		✔	✔	✔			✔		✔		✔		C
iodamide meglumine (Renovue)			✔						✔				U
iodamide meglumine (Cholegrafin)		✔								✔			U
iothalamate salts (Conray)		✔	✔	✔									B
metrizamide (Amipaque)			✔	✔	✔								B
ORAL GASTROINTESTINAL AGENTS													
diatrizoate salts (Hypaque sodium)												✔	B
barium sulfate (Barotrast)												✔	U
MISCELLANEOUS AGENTS													
diatrizoate salts (Hypaque 20%)										✔			C
iothalamate salts (Cysta-Conray)										✔			B
ethiodized oil (Ethiodol)						✔					✔		U

Modified from Facts and Comparisons, St Louis, 1988, JB Lippincott Co.
*When combined with diatrizoate.
†U, unclassified.

persons with bowel perforations or fistulas. If allowed to remain in the colon, barium sulfate may cause constipation. Hospitalization and close observation during the procedures are recommended for persons who have high potential for reactions or complications.

Isosulfan blue (for lymphography) should be administered *only subcutaneously.* Certain iothalamate, meglumine, or diatrizoate sodium compounds *are not for injection;* they are for instillation only.

Potential side effects/adverse reactions of iodinated contrast media. Cardiovascular reactions commonly include reports of "feeling warm" and vasodilation. Howev-er, most clients have no sensation or discomfort. The most common reactions are nausea or flushing, with feelings of warmth over the abdomen and chest. Severely dehydrated patients, the elderly, infants, and the seriously ill tolerate these hemodynamic and hyperosmolar changes less well than others do. Rare adverse reactions include cerebral hematomas, hemodynamic alterations, sinus bradycardia, transient ECG changes, ventricular fibrillation, and petechiae. Individuals with pheochromocytoma may have hypertensive crises. Circulatory load is temporarily increased and may challenge myocardial competence in clients with congestive heart failure if agents are administered intravascularly. If hypertonic solutions are given by the enteral route, intraluminal osmolarity may increase and cause hypovolemia and shocklike states.

Gastrointestinal effects may include nausea, vomiting, and parotid gland and submaxillary gland swellings.

Central nervous system symptoms may include paresthesias, dizziness, convulsions, paralysis, shock, or coma.

Skin lesions may result: urticaria, necrosis, or pain at the injection site (especially in urography).

Hematologic signs may include thrombocytopenia, leukopenia, or anemia. Diazoate salts inhibit all stages of coagulation. Platelet aggregation is inhibited by several of the agents. Exacerbations of sickle cell disease may attend intravascular injections of contrast media.

Renal system involvement may be manifested by nephrosis of proximal tubular cells in excretory urography, which may proceed to renal failure.

Respiratory signs may include rhinitis, cough, dyspnea, bronchospasm, asthma, laryngeal or pulmonary edema, and subclinical pulmonary emboli. Overt signs of pulmonary emboli and infarction may attend lymphography with ethiodized oil.

Special senses may be impaired: distorted taste sensations; irritated, itching, tearing eyes, or conjunctivitis.

Hypersensitivity reactions and others may include anaphylaxis. Incidence of paradoxic reactions is highest in the 20- to 40-year-old group. History of allergy predisposes to reactions to contrast media. Almost 20% of those who had had a previous reaction to some characteristic of contrast media (not iodine) again experienced a reaction. Although these reactions (primarily urticaria) may be similar to hypersensitivity reactions, they do not seem to be associated with allergy to iodine compounds. The cause is not known. Almost 13% of the remaining group had an iodine allergy history. About 25% of the rest of those with allergy histories had reactions to contrast media.

Significant drug interactions. The following interactions may occur when the oral cholecystographic agents are given with the drugs listed below.

Drug	Possible Effect and Management
cholestyramine (Cuemid, Questran)	The cholestyramine will adsorb the cholecystographic agents, thus interfering with the test. Avoid concurrent administration for at least 8 hours or more when these tests are scheduled.
iodipamide meglumine IV	Prior administration of the oral agents may block liver metabolism and excretion of this drug. Administration of both drugs, within 24 hours is not recommended.
urographic agents	Renal toxicity has been reported in clients with abnormal liver function when these tests were given following the oral agents. Avoid concurrent administration.

The following interactions may occur when the radiopaque parenteral agents are given with the drugs listed below.

Drug	Possible Effect and Management
aspirin, nonsteroidal antiinflammatory drugs, and other antiplatelet agents	May enhance the antiplatelet effect, since high levels of iodipamide meglumine, diatrizoate sodium, and diatrixoate meglumine all inhibit platelet aggregation. Monitor closely.
inotropic agents	May result in a paradoxic cardiac depressant effect, which is dangerous if client has an ischemic myocardium. Monitor closely if agents must be administered concurrently.

Dosage and administration. Manufacturers' instructions for dose preparation and administration should be followed.

Iodinated radiopaque agents may be variously administered orally (tablets, paste, granules, or suspensions), rectally (enema), parenterally or instilled. Four to six of the tablet formulations may be taken over a short interval the morning before the test, with nothing else but water after that. Barium sulfate compounds are noniodinated, and most are prepared from powders for suspensions to be taken orally or rectally. The volume of orally administered reconstituted agents is about 8 ounces; the enema volume may range from 500 ml to 3 pints. Intravenous injection volumes vary according to the agent, from 20 to 300 ml. Direct injection of certain high concentrations of iothalamate solutions should never be made into carotid or vertebral arteries. Elderly patients should be hydrated before barium tests.

NURSING CONSIDERATIONS

Assessment. Radiographic examinations are not without hazard to the client or to personnel. Risk/benefit ratios must be established on an individual basis. Reactions may arise from either physical or chemical properties of the compounds used. Almost any organ system may be affected. (See side effects/adverse reactions.) Take an allergy history with particular attention to previous reactions to contrast media or iodine-containing foods, such as shellfish or iodized table salt. Pretreatment with prednisone, diphenhydramine, and ephedrine for clients with a history of iodine hypersensitivity and those with a generally positive allergy history may minimize but not prevent hypersensitivity reactions. This pretreatment regimen reduced the incidence of adverse reactions in 1 study from 35% to 3%. Do not mix these medications for concurrent administration with the contrast media; they are incompatible.

Maintain radiologic histories. Apprise clients and all those working in an environment of ionizing radiation that there may be current and long-term effects of radiation and of the fact that these effects are cumulative. Since there is no established safe dosage, single or cumulative, keep exposure to a minimum. The risks to benefits of each procedure should be weighed carefully by the clinician and the informed client.

It is recommended that radiography, fluoroscopy, or computed tomography not be performed if the woman is pregnant or after the first 10 days after menses.

Nurses should ask for lead shielding devices and client-supporting devices before participating in radiographic examinations. If frequently involved, monitor the individual cumulative exposure by wearing a film badge that is checked monthly or quarterly. Wear it outside any shields; obtain reports.

Take a careful history related to kidney, thyroid, or liver disease. Instruct the client, as appropriate, to prepare by taking the agent with water the night before the procedure or to administer effective enemas or to ingest nothing but water until the test is completed. Explain as appropriate that the procedure may include the administration of about 8 ounces of a fairly thick oral suspension or a retention enema and that position changes may be necessary during the procedure. Prepare the examination platform for unexpected bowel evacuation. Transport as necessary along with the client to the department a bedpan, an emesis basin, tissues, and a warm blanket (room temperatures and equipment in radiologic units are often noted to be cold).

Assist in making the decision to administer anesthesia to restless or agitated clients, especially children. Closely monitor the condition of anesthetized patients; they are at higher risk for adverse reactions than unanesthetized patients.

Intervention. Prepare clients appropriately for their examinations using protocols from the radiology department. If visualization is sufficiently impaired because of inadequate bowel preparation or because tablets were not taken as directed, or because foods and fluids other than water were not withheld, it may necessitate a repeat preparation and examination.

Have drugs, equipment, and medical assistance readily available in case of an emergency such as cardiac arrest. Monitor levels of consciousness and vital signs during the procedure as feasible and afterward for at least 1 hour.

Education. Obtain an order for clear enemas or laxatives as necessary after the procedure or similarly instruct the client.

AGENTS FOR EVALUATING ORGAN FUNCTION

Some diagnostic agents can be used to track and visualize the functional processes of organ systems. Inferences can be made about organ function by measurement of the degree or rate at which the agent is distributed, taken up, sequestered, secreted, or excreted from the target organ system or by measurement of the volumes or flow rates. Some of these diagnostic agents are radionuclides (a species of radioactive atom characterized by higher atomic number than bodily tissues) whose gamma-ray emissions can be tracked or whose residues can be sampled. Other nonradioactive agents are dyes, polysaccharides, or other substances whose dissemination may be traced by color changes or chemical analysis.

RADIOACTIVE AGENTS

See Table 73-2.

Mechanism of action. A **radionuclide** is an unstable form of a chemical element. Radiopharmaceutical agents are those in which one of the nonradioactive atoms has been replaced by a radioactive atom. They are either of natural origin or are produced by particle accelerators or generators. The process of neutron activation used in nuclear medicine to produce radionuclides describes the

TABLE 73-2   Common Diagnostic Tests Using Approved Radioactive Tracer and Imaging Agents

Indications	Agent
Addison's disease, intestinal absorption	cyanocobalamin Co 57, Co 58, Co 60, oral/injectable (Raco-balamin-57 kit, Rubatrope-57)
Blood iron studies	ferrous citrate (Fe 59), injectable
Blood plasma volume determinations or blood pool imaging	radioiodinated (I 125) serum albumin (RISA-125-H, Albumotope I 125), radioiodinated (I 131) serum albumin (RISA-131-H, Albumotope I 131), sodium pertechnetate Tc 99m solution (Pertscan-99m), pertechnetate sodium Tc 99m (Technetium Tc 99m Generator Solution) (see above)
Brain imaging	chlormerodrin Hg 197 injection chlormerodrin Hg 203 injection Sodium pertechnetate Tc 99m solution (Pertscan-99m) Ytterbium (Yb) pentetate sodium (for cisternography); previously called DTPA (penetetic acid)

TABLE 73-2 Common Diagnostic Tests Using Approved Radioactive Tracer and Imaging Agents—cont'd

Indications	Agent
Brain, thyroid, and salivary gland imaging; placental localization; blood pool imaging	pertechnetate sodium Tc 99m (Technetium Tc 99m Generator Solution, Elutek, Mektec 99, Minitec, ScintiCheck, Technetope)
Bone imaging	flourine F 18 injection strontium Sr 87m generator solution strontium nitrate Sr 85, injection (Strotope, Stronscan-85) technetium Tc 99m etidronate sodium kit (osteoscan, Hedspa) technetium Tc 99m stannous pyrophosphate kit (TechneScan PYP kit, Phosphotec, Pyrolite)
Cardiac abnormalities, cerebral blood flow, pulmonary function, muscle blood flow studies	xenon Xe 133 injection (Xeneisol Xe 133 Injection) xenon Xe 133 gas (not used for diagnosis of cardiac abnormalities)
Deep vein thrombosis	radio-iodinated I 125 fibrinogen injection (Ibrin)
Fats, fatty acid absorption (estimations)	triolein I 131, oral/injection oleic acid I 125, oral
Gastrointestinal protein loss, hypoproteinemia	chromium (Cr 51) serum albumin (human), injection (Chromalbin)
Heart blood pool, pericardial effusion, ventricular aneurysms	technetium Tc 99m serum albumin kit
Intestinal absorption	cyanocobalamin (see Addison's disease, above), oral/injection
Hodgkin's disease, lymphomas, bronchogenic carcinoma	gallium citrate Ga 67
Liver function and liver imaging	sodium rose bengal I 125 injection (Robengatope) sodium rose bengal I 131 injection technetium Tc 99m sulfur colloid kit (Tesuloid, Techne-Coll) technetium Tc 99m sulfur colloid injection
Ocular or cerebral tumors (localization)	sodium phosphate P 32, oral/injection (Phosphotope) (Also used in the treatment of polycythemia vera and chronic leukemia)
Pancreatic imaging	selenomethionine Se 75 injection (Sethotope)
Placental localization	chromated (Cr 51) serum albumin (human) (Chromalbin) technetium Tc 99m (see above for brand names)
Pulmonary emboli, pulmonary carcinoma, pneumonitis, emphysema, tuberculosis; congenital heart disease, pulmonary vascular obliteration, pulmonary emboli, diffuse pulmonary disorders	iodinated I 131 aggregated albumin (Macroscan-131, MAA I 131) (Albumotope L-S, used for diagnosing disorders following the semicolon) technetium Tc 99m aggregated albumin kit (Macrotec, TechneScan MAA, MAA kit, Pulmolite: Technetated Albumin Lungaggregate, Instant Microspheres)
Red blood cell volume, mass, or survival times; evaluation of blood loss	sodium chromate Cr 51 injection (Rachromate-51, Chromitope Sodium)
Reduction of Tc 99m accumulation in choroid plexus and in salivary and thyroid glands	potassium perchlorate, oral (Perchloracap)
Renal and urinary tract function	chlormerodrin Hg 197 injection sodium ortho-iodohippurate, iodohippurate sodium, I 131 injection (Hippuran-131, Hipputope) sodium iothalamate I 125 (Glofil-125) technetium Tc 99m pertechnetate sodium kit (Renotec; previously called DTPA)
Thyroid function and imaging	sodium iodide I 125 (MPI Iodine 123) sodium iodide I 125 oral solution, sodium iodide I 131 oral solution (Iodotope) (latter also used for treatment of hyperthyroidism or selected thyroid carcinomas) sodium pertechnetate Tc 99m (Pertscan-99m) technetium Tc 99m (see also thyroid above)

capture of a slow neutron into a stable nucleus with the subsequent emission of a gamma ray. Transmutation is a similar operation, using instead a fast neutron. After injection or ingestion of the resultant nuclide, its pharmacokinesis can be followed by a gamma-ray detector combined with either a rectilinear scanner, scintillation camera, Bender-Blau camera, or other radiation-display device. For nonemitters (such as glucose ^{14}C), air, blood, lymph, spinal fluids, urine, or biopsy specimens may be collected and the residual radioactivity analyzed or counted as it is excreted. These data are used to make inferences about organ disorders and the body's ability to absorb, metabolize, or excrete substances.

Ionizing radiation. Much can be learned through the use of radiation that could not otherwise be discovered or diagnosed. Like any other diagnostic technique, a risk-benefit ratio must be determined.

Ionizing radiation has the ability to knock electrons out of atoms, creating electrically charged ions. It may be defined as electromagnetic radiation (x-rays and gamma rays) or particulate radiation (electrons, occasionally beta particles, protons, neutrons, or atomic nuclei with kinetic energy).

Impact by emitted radiation energy may disrupt bonds between atoms in such crucial biologic molecules as DNA. Disruption can lead to cell death, mutations, or defective mitosis. Energy that is absorbed by tissues can lead to acute effects (as in radiotherapy or radiation accidents) or chronic effects (as from multiple low radiation doses). Effects may appear only after long periods (like cataracts) or in subsequent generations.

The amount of radiation absorbed by tissues during radiologic tests is determined by the dose administered, the half-life of the radionuclide, the energy, the mode of decay, and the length of time the agent dwells within the body. There is no known safe dosage of ionizing radiation despite limits set by the Nuclear Regulatory Commission and the National Council on Radiation, Protection and Measurements.

Estimations of the amount of radiation emitted, the effect, and the dose absorbed may be denoted by the following terms:

A **roentgen** is the amount of gamma or x radiation that creates 1 electrostatic unit of ions in 1 ml of air at o'c.

A **rem** is the predicted effect on the human body of a 1-roentgen dose.

A **rad** is equivalent to the absorption of ionizing radiation energy. One rad = 100 ergs of radiation energy per gram of matter.

Although arbitrary, annual limits for the general population and for any single gestational period have been set at 0.5 rem (for x rays, 1 rem is equal to 1 rad) and for closely monitored occupational workers at about 3 rem/year. Most nurses, physicians, and other health personnel are not routinely monitored for radiation exposure unless assigned to an area with high potential for exposure. Their risk for cumulative exposure is nonetheless higher than that of the general population.

Very little is known about the full effects of radiation. Certain increased risks are associated, however, as follows: infertility, birth defects, potential for certain malignant neoplasms, and manifestations of aging. Exposure to low-level ionizing radiation, such as that from radiographic examinations, and agents containing radionuclides add to the individual's total radiation history. Effects may be insidious, perhaps manifesting themselves in crucial enzyme defects many years after exposure. There is some evidence of the body's ability to repair chromosomal damage, but the scope of this ability is unknown.

"Excessive radiation exposure" is any unnecessary exposure above natural background levels. Although natural background radiation adds to the cumulative risk, medical and dental therapies account for the largest proportion of artificially generated exposure.

Indications. Most radionuclides in use today in radiology are for imaging of organs, evaluating organ function, or detecting or treating cancer. The role of nuclear imaging is gradually diminishing because there is increased reliance on computed tomography, ultrasound, and magnetic resonance imaging. Radionuclides are used as tracers to evaluate physiologic and biochemical functioning of organ systems. Extremely sensitive radioactivity sensing devices make it possible to detect, count, and visualize by imaging methods and to analyze minute amounts of radionuclides. Uniquely useful applications of nuclear imagery include the following (see Table 73-2 for specifics):

1. Thyroid enlargement or disease. Agents currently used include ^{131}I, ^{125}I, and ^{123}I. All are isotopes of iodine that emit a type of radiation that can be mapped externally. Usually a 24-hour uptake study is employed to determine the extent and areas of thyroid activity. A scan is then performed to evaluate any thyroid mass or enlargement. "Cold" tumors have a 20% to 25% probability of representing a thyroid cancer. Tumors that localize the radionuclide well are usually benign.

2. Screening individuals with diagnosed malignancies for metastases. Many clients treated for breast cancer, colon cancer, malignant melanoma, lymphoma, prostate cancer, and lung cancer, among others, are often successfully evaluated periodically by scintigrams of the liver, spleen, and skeletal system. The risk-benefit ratio is very high, and information about new or recurrent disease can help the oncologist make crucial decisions about goals, management, prognosis, and so forth.

3. Evaluation of heart disease. This is a primary application of nuclear imagery. Computers are used to analyze data from the images to detect the extent of

myocardial damage and wall motion abnormalities and to estimate the ejection fraction of the ventricles. Underlying coronary artery disease can also be estimated before catheterization or other invasive procedures by the use of radionuclides.

4. Tracking physiologic substances and assessment of the status of an organ (e.g., renal function and—more recently by new products—biliary excretion).

In addition to diagnostic uses, some radiopharmaceuticals may be administered therapeutically to deliver radiation to internal body tissues (e.g., iodine 131 for destruction of thyroid tissue in hyperthyroidism). Radioactive tracer substances may also be incorporated into a nonradioactive drug to track the second drug's pharmacokinetics for research purposes.

Computed tomography (CT) scans body parts in a series of contiguous slices with pencil-thin x-ray beams, which, after passing through the body, produce data from detectors positioned diametrically across from the beam source. Huge amounts of collected data are integrated and displayed by computer as a video image. CT presents a series of two-dimensional images representing a reconstructed "slice" in the axial plane. By viewing a series of these images, one can perceive the anatomy in a three-dimensional sense. CT therefore often conveys more information than other modalities about lesion density, location, and size. CT has largely replaced older techniques such as pneumoencephalography and angiography in the diagnosis of intracranial disease, though angiography is still used in this application. CT may eliminate the need for other x-ray examinations, but it is not considered a first-line, or screening, technique. Radionuclide scans continue to be used for initial diagnostic screening and for specific tests where their results are more fruitful. Radiation exposure from CT varies depending on the equipment used and the frequency of testing, but it said to be equal to or sometimes considerably higher than with ordinary x-ray techniques or radionuclides. Although CT is considered to be a noninvasive procedure, intravenous contrast material is frequently injected to enhance structures for differential diagnosis (Figure 73-1).

Ultrasound is a nonradioactive diagnostic tool with cardiovascular, abdominal, obstetric, and other applications. It is used with anatomic and physiologic information obtained by other nuclear medicine techniques. Ultrasound examinations yield data about organ contours and tissue consistency or, in the case of Doppler scanning, blood flow patterns. Results can be distorted in the presence of bone or gases in the body. The secondary effects

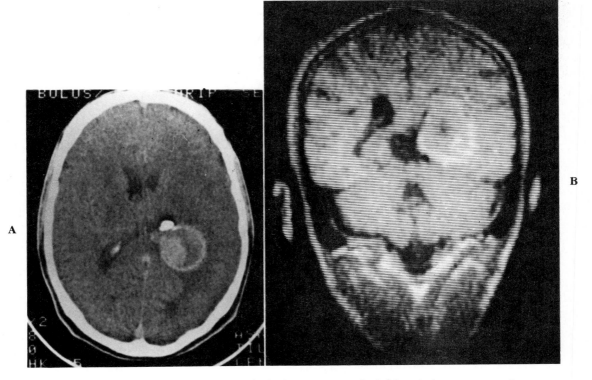

FIGURE 73-1 A, This CT scan shows a high-density mass in the left hemisphere, representing a hematoma. **B,** Coronal NMR saturation-recovery scan shows a high-density mass with a high-intensity rim and low-intensity center, representing the hematoma. (From Alfidi RJ and others: Radiology 143:175-181, 1982.)

of high-frequency sound waves on cellular structures and functions are not fully known, though such tests are considered to be noninvasive and innocuous by many in the field.

Nuclear magnetic resonance imaging (MRI) is a diagnostic modality that uses radio waves and a magnet, not radiation, drugs, biopsy specimens, or body fluids (Figure 73-2). Like CT, MRI provides sectioned imagery but gives more than the gross anatomic information gained by CT scanning. MRI supplies extremely detailed images of internal heart and brain structures, for example, and is capable of imaging areas of the spine, abdomen, and extremities. It can differentiate between lesions and normal tissue. MRI is now FDA approved and is rapidly becoming integrated into the radiologist's armamentarium. Those ineligible for diagnostics by MRI include pregnant women, children under 2 years of age, and those with metal prostheses or pacemakers.

Pharmacokinetics. Each type of radionuclide emits alpha or beta particles or gamma rays, or a combination of these. This spontaneous emission of charged particles is termed radioactive decay and eventually results in disintegration of the nucleus. The time it takes for the original radioactivity to decay to one half its original value is known as the physical or radioactive *half-life* of the particular radionuclide. Like a drug, the rate at which a tracer substance is excreted from the body also influences its effects, both valuable and undesirable.

Dosage and administration. Manufacturers' current directions should be reviewed. Dosages are not detailed here because they vary with individual needs.

The major considerations in radionuclide dosing are the amount of radioactivity that is administered to produce effective readings and the secondary effects of that radioactivity. While the radioactive material is in the body, it is irradiating even after the study has been completed, whereas x-rays irradiate from an external source and do so only while the body is exposed during the examination. The radionuclide dosage unit for imaging or nonimaging doses of radionuclides is a **microcurie** (one millionth of a curie). A **curie** is a specified measure of radioactivity associated with a specific amount of a radioactive substance, e.g., a radionuclide. Recommended dosages are spelled out in manufacturers' literature. The patient's absorbed dose of each radionuclide has been predicted for each procedure with the following three factors being taken into account:

1. The biologic parameters that describe the uptake, distribution, retention, and release of the radiopharmaceutical in the body
2. The energy released by the radionuclide and whether it is penetrating or nonpenetrating
3. The fraction of the emitted energy that is absorbed by the target

The ultimate radiation dose to both the target organ and the whole body is somewhat less in radionuclide

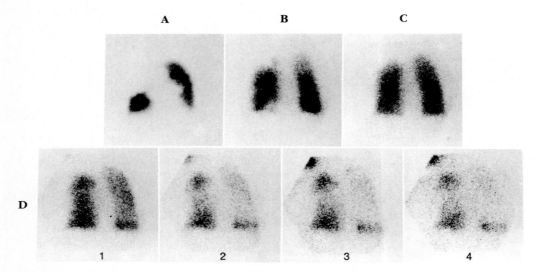

FIGURE 73-2 Patient, 74 years of age, with moderately severe COPD (emphysema) and history of acute chest pain, increasing shortness of breath. **A,** Posterior perfusion (Tc 99m MAA) lung image reveals absent perfusion in left upper lobe and superior left lower lobe, as well as in mediastinal region of right lung. **B,** Xe 133 ventilation study (posterior position). Inhalation phase—note ventilation of left lung and mediastinal portion of right lung. **C,** Xe 133 equilibrium phase. Even distribution of Xe 133 throughout both lung fields. **D,** Washout phase. Note delayed washout of Xe 133 from areas of increased dead air space (emphysema). Combined studies infer that patient has pulmonary embolization superimposed on COPD. (From Early PJ and Sodee DB: Principles and practice of nuclear medicine, St Louis, 1985, The CV Mosby Co.)

nonimaging procedures than in imaging procedures. It is considerably more in radiation therapy (not discussed here).

Shielding is a practical method to prevent or reduce excess radiation exposure of staff or patients during certain diagnostic examinations. Shielding acts to reduce radiation intensity to acceptable limits in body areas not intended for exposure during the radiologic examination. Alpha and beta radiation require very little shielding. An alpha particle can be blocked by the thickness of a sheet of paper, a beta particle by an inch of wood, but several feet of concrete or several inches of lead are necessary to stop gamma or x radiation. Half-value layer is the term describing the thickness of any material required to reduce the intensity of an x-ray or gamma-ray beam to half its original value. Because of its characteristic density, lead is the material typically used in radiation shielding equipment and coverings such as aprons and gloves.

NURSING CONSIDERATIONS

Assessment. As in the nursing considerations for individuals receiving radiopaque contrast media, assessments should include appropriate histories related to allergies to iodine or iodine-containing foods, previous exposures to ionizing radiation, and menstrual histories.

Intervention. The basic principles of radiation exposure safety are relative to the source of radiation: *time* spent in the radioactive field, *distance* from the source, and *shielding.* The amount of radiation absorbed is directly proportional to the time spent in a radioactive field and inversely related to the distance from the source of radioactive emission. Thus quality nursing care requires careful planning so that sensible limitations on time spent in the radioactive field do not reduce the quality of client care.

Wear rubber or plastic gloves when handling bedpans, urine specimens, or continuous drainage bags of clients within a day or two after nuclear medicine procedures. Wherever radionuclides are used, one person, designated the radiation safety officer, has the responsibility for safety in case of spills or accidents with radioactive materials. This officer should be consulted if there is a break in safety procedures or if, for example, linen has been contaminated by vomitus or excreta within 24 hours of administration of a radiopharmaceutical. Although it may be determined that unusual precautions are not needed, it is wise to seek consultation as needed.

Follow instructions by radiopharmaceutical manufacturers about radionuclide storage (some require refrigeration), dosage, and technique. Errors in technique must not be tolerated, especially with regard to the handling of radiopharmaceuticals, disposal of contaminated equipment, and proper shielding of all present for radiologic

and imaging procedures. Monitoring badges should be issued and worn by those regularly participating in these procedures. Protection should be assured for those who are unfamiliar with these procedures. Women of childbearing age who are more than 10 days after menses or who are pregnant should not assist. (*Radiation therapy* requires other precautions.)

Education. Clients' anxieties may be heightened by the uncertainty of unknown diagnosis, fear of radiation, and cold or unfamiliar surroundings. Clients may be introduced to the personnel, surroundings, and the large equipment some time before scheduled examinations and given opportunity for questions and explanations. They should know that there may be some discomfort at the site of injection, taste alterations, or a feeling of warmth or discomfort in various parts of the body if the administered agent contains an iodine preparation. If a counter or rectilinear scanner is used, clients should be advised that it may typically emit irregular clicks as it collects data; it does not emit radiation. Since clients may be required to maintain a single position on a hard surface for extended periods or may be briefly restrained, supply foam wedge supports and coverings as necessary. Explain that personnel may wear strange-looking gray or green apparel to shield them from excess radiation and that clients too will be protected by protocols that have been established. Then adhere to them.

Give clients written instructions, especially about the specific time they should return for the examination after the nuclide dose. Explain that the test must be performed at a very specific time after the medication is administered (at the point of a specific half-life).

NONRADIOACTIVE AGENTS

Nonradioactive Agents for Evaluating Organ Function via Volumes and Flows

These relatively biologically inert and nonradioactive substances are commonly used to measure flow rates, fluid volumes, diffusion, concentration ability, and organ function. These compounds are mostly dyes, polysaccharides, or other substances that can be assayed chemically or detected by characteristic colors after administration. Many of the dye tests determine the rate of plasma clearance of the dye by the organ under study. The ability to measure certain parameters against known normal values at defined points in the procedure makes these compounds useful as diagnostic aids. They are used variously for evaluation of cardiac output, liver or kidney function or blood flows, circulation time, intestinal absorption, and so forth (see box, "Selected Multiple Urine Tests").

Pharmacokinetics. These compounds are administered primarily by the intravenous or intramuscular routes. They are rapidly absorbed by the organ system under examination and are usually excreted by that system.

Side effects/adverse reactions. These drugs are relatively pharmacologically inert and are used to permit measurement of specific physiologic functions without themselves significantly altering those functions (Table 73-3).

Nonradioactive Agents for Challenging Glandular Response

Mechanism of action. Certain compounds are used diagnostically to challenge a particular system, often glandular, to produce measurable responses. Secretory responses indicate whether there is functional integrity within the secreting gland or system. Many of these agents are protein substances that mimic the action of naturally occurring bodily chemicals such as secretagogues for exocrine gland response and stimulants for endocrine secretion.

Pharmacokinetics. Since most are administered intramuscularly or intravenously, these agents move rapidly to the site of action. Degradation of these agents is equally rapid.

Indications. Nonradioactive agents are used to evaluate or enhance capabilities such as hypothalamic-pituitary function, thyroid secretion, gallbladder contraction, insulin response, gastric acid secretory function, alkalinity of pancreatic juice, or titrated responses to angiotensin II.

Side effects/adverse reactions. These compounds act on the targeted gland or site as releasing factors. Thus secondary effects may be as widespread and disruptive to bodily chemical balance as a large dose of the secretion or hormone itself (Table 73-4). Epinephrine, antihistamines, corticoids, and a tourniquet should be readily available for all tests in case of severe reactions. Analgesics, nasogastric suction equipment, vasodilators (for histamine agents), intravenous glucose solutions (for tolbu-

TABLE 73-3 Common Nonradioactive Compounds for Visualization of Organ Function

Compound	Indications	Secondary effects	Nursing considerations
aminohippurate sodium (PAH)	Renal function tests, especially of renal plasma flow	Considered safe; some reports of feelings of warmth and nausea High-protein diet, penicillin, salicylates, phenolsulfonphthalein, and diuretics inhibit PAH secretion in the tubules Procaine and sulfonamides may interfere with laboratory test results	Give intravenously at constant rate Handle blood samples carefully without agitating Observe site for hematoma or phlebitis
indocyanine green (Cardio-Green)	Liver function tests; blood flow, uptake, storage, and excretion Renal blood flow in anuric patients Cardiac output studies by the indicator dilution method	No reported toxicities Half-life decreased by phenytoin, phenobarbitol, haloperidol, and other drugs; check Package Insert	The dye is unstable and must be dissolved and used within 10 hours
inulin (Alantin)	Glomerular filtration rate	Renal clearance may be altered in pregnancy	Intravenous injections
mannitol (Osmitrol)	Glomerular filtration rate Used also for treatment of oliguria, cerebral edema, chemical poisoning, congestive glaucoma	Dry mouth, thirst, headache, acidosis, dehydration Contraindicated in congestive heart failure, pulmonary edema, persistent renal disease after initial dose Edetate may increase absorption of mannitol	Intravenous infusion Monitor vital signs and urinary output closely
sodium indigotindisulfonate (Indigo Carmine)	Renal function tests and for locating urethral orifices during cystoscopy		Intramuscular or intravenous use Replaced by more specific agents

TABLE 73-4 Common Nonradioactive Agents for Challenging Grandular Response

Compound	Indications and secondary effects	Nursing considerations
corticotropin (ACTH)	Adrenocortical functioning Contraindications: scleroderma, osteoporosis, systemic fungal infections, ocular herpes simplex, postoperative status, congestive heart failure, hypertension, allergy to pork Secondary effects: fluid-electrolyte imbalances, muscle weakness, GI ulceration, hypertension, increased intracranial pressure, infections, hypersensitivity	Withhold food and restrict activity for 12 hr before test Low-carbohydrate diet for 2 days before test (usually); rest for 30 min before test Withhold medications; corticosteroids, estrogens, calcium gluconate, amphetamines, spironolactone, ethanol, lithium (as feasible) Test results may be altered by radioactive scanning examinations administered within the week before test
edrophonium chloride (Tensilon)	Differential diagnosis of myasthenia gravis Contraindications: hypersensitivity, mechanical obstructions of the intestinal or urinary tracts Secondary effects: severe cholinergic reactions—bradycardia or cardiac standstill; dysrhythmias; cholinergic reactions of the eye, CNS, respiratory, GI, or muscular systems	A placebo may be administered first as if it were the test dose to evaluate baseline muscular capabilities Withhold medications: procainamide, muscle relaxants, prednisone, quinidine, and anticholinergics (for at least 8 hr) Observe for developing signs of adverse effects Keep available a syringe containing 1 mg atropine sulfate for IV use to reverse severe cholinergic reactions
gonadorelin (Factrel)	Anterior pituitary function; differential diagnosis of anterior pituitary from hypothalamic dysfunction; induction or inhibition of ovulation (investigational use) Secondary effects: hypersensitivity, headache, lightheadedness, nausea; pain, pruritus, or rash at injection site	Withhold medications affecting pituitary secretion of gonadotrophins: androgens, estrogens, progestins, and glucocorticoids Avoid interacting drugs: spironolactone, levodopa, digoxin, phenothiazines, and dopamine antagonists
histamine phosphate	Ability of gastric mucosa to produce hydrochloric acid and to diagnose pheochromocytoma Contraindications: asthma and allergies; hypotension; severe cardiac, pulmonary, or renal disease Secondary effects: flushing, dizziness, headache, dyspnea, asthma, urticaria, hypotension or hypertension, tachycardia, GI distress, or convulsions	Withhold food for 12 hr and fluids and smoking for 8 hr before test Withhold medications: antacids, anticholinergics, alcohol, cimetidine, reserpine, adrenergic blockers, corticosteroids Instruct client to expectorate excess saliva to prevent mixing it with specimen Keep epinephrine available for severe hypotension
pentagastrin (Peptavlon)	Gastric acid secretory function in pernicious anemia, atrophic gastritis, gastric carcinoma, duodenal ulcers, Zollinger-Ellison tumors and to evaluate effectiveness of acid-reducing surgery Secondary effects: hypersensitivity, stimulation of pancreatic secretion, GI distress or bleeding; effects less likely than with histamine or betazole	Withhold food, liquids, and smoking after midnight before test Inform client that a nasogastric tube will be passed Withhold medications: antacids, anticholinergics, adrenergic blockers, cimetidine, reserpine After test, observe for GI distress Usual diet and medications may be resumed
protirelin (Thypinone)	Thyroid function response to therapy; pituitary or hypothalamic dysfunction Secondary effects are usually transitory and minor but occur in 50%: blood pressure swings, breast engorgement in lactating women, nausea, urinary urgency, light-headedness, flushing, bad taste, headache, mouth dryness	Measure blood pressure every 15 min during test, especially for increases of up to 20 to 30 mm Hg Administered by IV bolus over 15 to 30 sec with the patient supine
secretin (Secretin-Kabi)	Diagnosis of pancreatic exocrine disorders; gastrinoma; as an aid in collecting pancreatic cells for microscopic examination Contraindications: acute pancreatitis attack, pregnancy	Withhold food overnight before test (12 to 15 hr) Prepare patient for discomfort of double-lumen oral tube

Continued.

TABLE 73-4 Common Nonradioactive Agents for Challenging Grandular Response—cont'd

Compound	Indications and secondary effects	Nursing considerations
	Hypersensitivity reactions may occur	
sincalide (Kinevac)	For gallbladder contraction to make possible aspiration of bile from the duodenum for assessment of cholesterol saturation Used also as adjunct to secretin for pancreatic evaluation Secondary effects: hypersensitivity, GI symptoms (not necessarily indicating biliary tract abnormality), dizziness, or flushing	Use solution within 24 hr
thyrotropin, TSH (Thytropar)	Differential diagnosis of source of myxedema: thyroid or pituitary; monitoring of drug therapy Given with ^{131}I to enhance uptake of ^{131}I Secondary effects: hypersensitivity, coronary thrombosis, exacerbation of Addison's disease, headache, hypotension, menstrual irregularities, fever, nausea, vomiting, urticaria, cardiac dysrhythmias	Used for 1-3 days to determine thyroid status; to diagnose thyroid cancer after surgery, usually given for 3-7 days Blood may be drawn between 6 and 8 AM Withhold all steroids and thyroid hormones for 2 days before test
Tolbutamide sodium (Orinase Diagnostic)	Diagnosis of islet cell adenomas differentiated from functional hypoglycemia Secondary effect: severe hypoglycemia; may be falsely positive or unsafe for pregnant woman, for fetus, or for children Containdications: severe renal or liver disease Rarely: burning sensations in shoulder or arm; thrombophlebitis	Instruct patients to adhere to a 150-300 g/day carbohydrate diet for 3 days before test and to fast overnight Avoid smoking during the fast and the test Withhold medications: dicumarol, salicylates, sulfonamides, oxyphenbutazone, phenylbutazone, probenecid, MAO inhibitors, beta blockers, and chloramphenicol for 3 days before test Use drug solution within 1 hr after preparation If severe hypoglycemia occurs, obtain a blood sample, stop the test, and prepare an IV glucose solution

tamide sodium), and atropine (for edrophonium chloride) should also be kept available.

Dosage and administration. Manufacturers' instructions should be followed very closely because almost all these compounds are administered parenterally and in very small dosages.

AGENTS FOR SCREENING AND MONITORING DISORDERS AND IMMUNE STATUS

See also Chapter 65.

Various screening and monitoring agents may be extracts of common allergens (ragweed, grasses, trees, molds, animal dander, and foods), purified derivatives or concentrates of microbial antigens, hormones, or animal cellular antigens, or they may be chemical reagents. Many chemical reagents for common diagnostic purposes are packaged in simple kit form for over-the-counter or prescribed purchase; they may also be used routinely in institutions and physicians' offices.

Mechanism of action; pharmacokinetics. Antigens applied topically or intradermally cause antigen-antibody reactions, which may be manifested by a local inflammatory response at the test site. The test site is assessed after a prescribed time interval. A positive response is indicated by the presence of erythema, the typical "wheal and flare" response, and induration (a firm lump under the skin). In the case of microbial antigen challenge, this positive response may merely indicate a previous exposure to the microbe or its products, but not necessarily the presence of an active disease process. False negative results may also occur, and further investigation may be necessary. The size of the erythematous area or induration may be measured to estimate the degree of the person's sensitivity or immune response. These responses may be short lived or of lifelong duration. (See Chapter 65.) Persons who are in an immunosuppressed state because of cancer chemotherapy or radiation treatments, malnutrition, debilitation, or congenital or acquired immune deficiency syndrome (AIDS) may demonstrate no response when tested with a prescribed battery of antigen challenges. These persons are extremely vulnerable to infection and may need metabolic support and precautions to avoid infection. Test results may not be reliable in those who have viral infections, are febrile or uremic, or have recently received live viral vaccinations. In vitro tests of body fluids and the like are usually performed by addition of antigens, reagents, or agglutinating substances to

SELECTED MULTIPLE URINE TESTS AVAILABLE ON THE MARKET

Measures	Chemstrip GP	Combistix	HemaCombistix	Uristix-4	Keto-Diastix	Chemstrip 5L	Labstix	BiliLabstix	Multistix SG*	Multistix 7	Multistix 10 SG*	Chemstrip 9	Multistix 9	Chemstrip LN	Multistix 2
glucose	X	X	X	X	X	X	X	X	X	X	X	X	X		
protein	X	X	X	X		X	X	X	X	X	X	X	X		
pH		X	X			X	X	X	X	X	X	X	X		
blood		X				X	X	X	X	X	X	X	X		
ketones					X	X	X	X	X	X	X	X	X		
bilirubin								X	X		X	X	X		
urobilinogen									X		X	X	X		
nitrite				X						X	X	X	X	X	X
leukocytes				X		X				X	9	X	X	X	X

Modified and adapted from Facts and comparisons, St Louis, 1988, JB Lippincott.
*Also measures specific gravity.

the specimen and by interpretation of results based on established phenomena such as the presence or absence of agglutination.

Indications. Some diagnostic agents measure a person's physiologic response or hypersensitivity to the agent as a specific chemical challenge. They are typically used in simple baseline screening procedures as part of the initial diagnostic workup. Some are used in skin tests by patch, prick, scratch, or intradermal injection for assessment of hypersensitivity (allergy), anergy (congenital or acquired inability to develop a cell-mediated reaction), cellular immunity, or antibody response. (See Table 73-5.) Others are used as reagents in specimens of blood, urine, and bodily discharges for detection of the levels of certain components to facilitate diagnosis or to monitor known conditions. (See Table 73-6.)

Side effects/adverse reactions. Local reactions to skin tests do not usually cause discomfort. Occasionally a highly positive reaction will result in vesiculation and necrosis of overlying skin; corticosteroids may be ordered. Transient tachycardia, malaise, or low-grade fever may occur separately. Occasionally, a person may report systemic allergic reactions of urticaria, sneezing, or dyspnea. Rarely, an overwhelming antigen-antibody response may occur, an anaphylactic response, calling for emergency measures such as the administration of epinephrine and respiratory and circulatory support. All these secondary effects are more likely if hyposensitization therapy is begun, since this includes a well-controlled program of increasing dosages of the allergen in question.

Dosage and administration. For certain standardized tests as coccidioidomycosis, the dosage is fixed (0.1 ml of a 1:100 dilution). Dosages for allergy testing are also very small (0.02 to 0.05 ml) but may be individualized. Manufacturers' instructions for all these diagnostic agents should be followed carefully.

NURSING CONSIDERATIONS

Intervention. Inspect the liquid extract for clarity; do not use it if particles are seen. As appropriate, use one of the following methods for administering these diagnostic test agents:

A sterile needle or other instrument may be used to prick or scratch the skin after a drop of the extract is placed on the skin. Depending on the approach used, the results may be read directly or after the testing patch has been removed.

Intradermal injections are commonly made into the ventral surface of the forearm. Use a tuberculin syringe with a 25- to 27-gauge needle. Inject intradermally with the needle nearly parallel to the skin surface, making certain that the needle does not penetrate deeper, into sub-

TABLE 73-5   Biologic Agents for Diagnostic Tests

Biologic product	Purpose, preparation, and storage	Alerts
BIOLOGIC DIAGNOSTIC TESTS		
Tuberculin, old; tine test	Multiple-puncture, disposable test device for the detection of tuberculin reactivity; especially useful in mass screening; initial test should be done at or before rubeola immunization, thereafter annually or biannually or as indicated by individual risk of exposure (repeated testing may increase the size of reaction but will not sensitize to tuberculin). Apply the disk with its 4 coated prongs quickly and firmly to the volar surface of the forearm so that puncture sites and disk impression are seen. Reaction read 48-72 hr (criteria for positive reaction—extent of induration or vesiculation as per enclosed ruler in package—2 mm or greater). Store unrefrigerated below 30° C (86° F)	Precautions: test with caution those with active tuberculosis (possible activation of quiescent lesions); hypersensitivity to acacia gum; immunosuppression or recent vaccination with live virus vaccines may suppress reactivity; doubtful or positive reaction—further test using Mantoux, chest roentgenogram, sputum culture Side effects: local vesicles, ulceration, or necrosis in highly sensitive persons; pain or pruritus may be relieved by cold packs
Tuberculin purified protein derivatives—PPD test (Mantoux) (Aplitest, multipuncture)	Solution obtained from human strain of *Mycobacterium tuberculosis* for more conclusive results than the tine test. Given intradermally 0.1 ml strength either 1 US unit (for those who are highly sensitized), 5 US units, or 250 US units (for those failing to react), which should never be used as initial dose. Given intracutaneously. Positive reaction when read 48-72 hr later: an induration 10 mm or more; 5-9 mm is "doubtful" reaction except in case of known exposure. Positive reaction only indicates previous exposure to tuberculosis, not necessarily active disease; further testing for diagnosis is thus required. Store at 2°-8° C.	Contraindications: never inject a 250 US unit/0.1 ml dose as initial test Precautions: immunosuppression or concurrent or recent immunization with certain virus vaccines or recent viral infection (may cause suppressed reactivity). Those over 55 year may need second testing Side effects: see package insert for details
ALLERGENIC EXTRACTS	Several hundred individual purified fluid allergens for diagnosis and hyposensitization for specific allergies: pollens, poison ivy/oak, foods, dusts, skin contactants, insects, fungi, yeasts, autogenous bacteria, based on intracutaneous skin test responses. Treatment is periodic subcutaneous injection of gradually increasing potency of dilutions of specific allergen(s); schedule and dosages highly individualized	Contraindications: severe anaphylaxis Precautions: severe anaphylaxis (reduce dose); keep on hand epinephrine, antihistamines, oxygen, etc. Side effects (grass allergens most reactive of all): local—edema, redness, pain (reduce dose); systemic—urticaria, sneezing, dyspnea (give epinephrine, antihistamines, steroids; reduce dose)

TABLE 73-6   Common Tests for Screening Selected Conditions

Preparation	Condition monitored or detected	Procedure
Acetone tests (Acetest, Chemstrip K, Ketostix)	Tests of urine or blood for ketones, in diabetes mellitus	Tablets, papers, or strips
Albumin (Albustix)	Protein detection in urine	Strips
Bacteria in urine tests (Microstix-Nitrite; Microstix-3 Strips, Uricult)	Tests for nitrite to detect bacteria in urine	Strips
Bilirubin test (Ictotest)	Tests for bilirubin in urine	Tablets
Blood urea nitrogen test (Azostix)	Tests for urea nitrogen in blood	Strips
C-reactive protein (LAtest-CRP)	Serum test for acute inflammation	Kit
Chlamydia trachomatis Test (Micro Trak *Chlamydia trachomatis* Direct Specimen Test)	Tests of tissue specimens for *Chlamydia trachomatis*	Slide test
Gastrointestinal tests (Entero-Test, Entero-Test Pediatric)	Upper gastrointestinal fluid used to test for bleeding, parasites, pH differences, achlorhydria, and esophageal reflux	Capsules

TABLE 73-6   Common Tests for Screening Selected Conditions—cont'd

Preparation	Condition monitored or detected	Procedure
Gastro-Test	Test for stomach pH to help locate/diagnose gastrointestinal bleeding	
Glucose blood tests (Chemstrip bG, Dextrostix, Glucostix, Visidex II)	Measure of blood glucose	Strips
Glucose urine tests (Clinitest, Chemstrip uG, Clinistix, Diastix, Tes-Tape)	Detection of urine glucose	Tablets, strips
Gonorrhea tests (Gonodecten, Biocult-GC)	Screen of discharges or swabs of urethral, rectal, pharyngeal, and endocervical areas for *Neisseria gonorrhoeae*	Kit
Mononucleosis tests (Mono-Chek, Mono-Diff, Monospot, Monosticon, Monosticon Dri-Dot, Mono-Sure, Mono-Test)	Physician office use, tests for antibodies to diagnose infectious mononucleosis	Kits
Occult blood screening CS-T, Early Detector, EZ-Detect, Fleet Detecatest	Home testing for blood in feces	Tests
Hemoccult II	Fecal sample from home sent to laboratory for check	Kit
Gastroccult	Tests of gastric content for blood	Kit
Coloscreen, Coloscreen/VPI, Hema-Chek, Hematest, Hemoccult, Hemastix	Tests of feces for blood	Tablets, slides, strips
Ovulation tests	Prediction of ovulation	Test, kit
(Clearplan, OvuStick)	Home tests	
(First Response Ovulation Predictor, Fortel Ovulation, OvuSTICK Urine hLH)	Immunoassay test for hLH in urine	
Pregnancy tests—home kits (Advance Test, Answer, Answer 2, Answer Plus, Answer Plus 2, Clearblue, Daisy 2, e.p.t. Plus, e.p.t. Stick test, Fact)	Urine testing	Kits
Pregnancy tests—for professional use only (Pregnate Clone Slide, Pregnosis, Pregnosticon Dri-Dot, UCG Slide Test, Nimbus, Pregnospia)	Tests of urine for chorionic gonadotropins	Test
Rheumatoid factor test (LAtest-RF kit, Rheumanosticon Dri-Dot)	Test of blood for rheumatoid factor	Kit
Sickle cell test—for professional use only		
Sickledex Test	Detection of hemoglobin S	Test
Streptococci tests—for professional use only (Culturette 10 minute Group A Strep ID, Insta Kit, Rapid Test Strep)	A latex slide agglutination test for Group A streptococci	
Taste function		
Accusens T	Measure of taste function and dysfunction	Kit
Virus tests		
Abbott HTLV III EIA	Tests for antibody to human T-lymphotrepic virus type III in blood	Kit
Micro Trak HSV 1/HSV 2 culture/typing	Identification of herpes simplex in tissue cultures	Kit
Rotalex Test	Detection of rotavirus in feces	Kit
Rubacell II	Detection of antibody to rubella virus in serum	Test

cutaneous tissue. This will increase the precision with which the results may be interpreted; in tuberculin tests it will also prevent febrile reactions. A correctly administered intradermal injection will immediately raise a small, colorless bleb or lump. Stop inserting the needle as soon as the tip of the needle, bevel up, has entered the skin but is still visible. Then inject the antigen with steady pressure.

Be prepared for major allergic manifestations such as angioedema, urticaria, serum sickness, or anaphylactic shock, which can occur. Have the person wait for 30 minutes to observe for development of an allergic reaction. Have available medications for emergency administration: antihistamines such as diphenhydramine four and epinephrine, 0.2 ml for subcutaneous use. Equipment for full circulatory and respiratory support should also be available.

Assessment. Administer these preparations with care because of their propensity to trigger allergic reactions.

Question the client regarding any previous reactions to skin testing. Dilute test doses of less than one tenth the usual concentration may then be administered.

After the injection, there is a prescribed wait, often 20 minutes or several days (depending on the antigen), before the local reaction should be assessed for erythema and induration. A positive reaction to some antigens is determined by the presence of induration alone; erythema is not always a criterion. **Erythema** is categorized as follows:

"tr" (trace)	Faint discoloration
+ (one plus)	Pink
++	Red
+++	Purplish red
++++	Vesiculation or necrosis

Measure the single largest induration or the largest coalesced induration. Induration can be measured with precision in the following way: Placing your index, middle, and ring fingers together, stroke the test site to determine the presence of induration. To delimit the indurated area, using a ball-point pen, draw a line *toward* the indurated area in all four directions. Edges of the induration can easily be perceived as the ball-point tip touches them. Stop each marking when the edge is perceived. Then measure the diameter of the remaining unmarked indurated area in millimeters. Or use the following criteria for indurations:

"tr" (trace)	Barely palpable
+	Palpable, but not visible
++	Easily palpable and visible; indurated area buckles when squeezed gently
+++	Easily palpable and visible; does not buckle when squeezed gently
++++	Vesiculation or necrosis

Criteria used to categorize Mantoux tuberculin test results according to induration diameter are as follows.

- Less than 5 mm is a negative result.
- 5 to 9 mm is a questionable result; retesting by another method may be necessary.
- More than 9 mm is a positive result.

Indurations resulting from multiple puncture tuberculin testing devices are interpreted as positive if more than 2 mm in diameter. Results are considered less reliable than results of Mantoux tests.

KEY TERMS

computed tomography (CT), page 1145
curie, page 1146
erythema, page 1154
microcurie, page 1146
nuclear magnetic resonance imaging (MRI), page 1146
rad, page 1144
radionuclide, page 1142
rem, page 1144
roentgen, page 1144
ultrasound, page 1145

BIBLIOGRAPHY

American Hospital Formulary Service: AHFS drug information 88, Bethesda, Md, 1988, American Society of Hospital Pharmacists, Inc.

Berger, ME., and Hubner, KF: Hospital hazards: diagnostic radiation, *Am J Nurs 83:*1155, 1983.

Chest x-ray screening statements, FDA Drug Bull 13(2):13, 1983.

Early, PJ., and Sodee, DB: Principles and practice of nuclear medicine, St. Louis, 1985, The CV Mosby Co.

Haaga, JR., and Alfidi, RJ: Computed tomography of the brain, head, and neck, St. Louis, 1985, The CV Mosby Co.

Herrmann, CS: Performing intradermal skin tests the right way, Nursing '83 13(10):50, 1983.

Kastrup, EK, ed: Facts and comparisons, St. Louis, 1988, JB Lippincott Co.

Leahy, IM, St Germain, JM, and Varricchio, CG: The nurse and radiotherapy, St. Louis, 1979, The CV Mosby Co.

Radiation safety (address at NEHW/NY Program), Nurses' Environmental Health Watch Quarterly 6(1):2, 1985.

Rhodes BA, and Croft, BY: Basics of radiopharmacy, St. Louis, 1978, The CV Mosby Co.

Poisons and Antidotes

Alphonse Poklis

POISONING

Although incidents of poisoning are common in the United States, only an estimated 10% are reported. About 2 million cases occur each year, with about 5000 fatalities. Carbon monoxide is the most common cause of death by poison. Most poisonings are accidental and caused by drug intoxication; some are suicide attempts. **Criminal poisonings** are rare, possibly because of the sophisticated poison detection capabilities of police toxicologic laboratories. **Industrial poisonings** may be more widespread than previously suspected, since both the sources of toxic agents in the environment and their effects can be insidious. Individuals or groups may be exposed over a lifetime to toxic by-products or toxic waste because of modern technologies. Common sources include chemical waste disposal sites (e.g., dioxin) or transport systems (e.g., radioactive substances), exhaust gases, insecticides, and fumigants.

Two thirds of accidental poisonings occur in children under age 5. According to the National Clearinghouse for Poison Control, ingestions of toxic substances by these children generally are deemed accidental; ingestions by older children are more likely to be true suicide attempts. Poisonings in children under 1 year of age are usually accidental medication overdoses by parents; from 1 to 5 years, the curious, experimenting, or hungry child is usually the initiator. Denatonium saccharide, the most vile-tasting substance ever known, is in the process of being patented, with plans to add this white, crystalline powder to household products to prevent accidental ingestion by children.

Morbidity and mortality from accidental poisonings in children under age 5 have dropped partly because of public awareness of the potential hazards in children's environments, the effectiveness of poison control centers, and childproof containers. Unfortunately this encouraging trend is not reproduced in other age-groups — a cause for continuing concern.

Currently the most frequent adult poison is a medication, most often a tranquilizer or sedative. Children most often ingest plants, household cleaners, antihistamines or medications for colds, perfumes, or vitamins and minerals. However, they suffer the most toxic effects from the nonprescription medications they ingest. Although aspirin poisonings in children have decreased, poisonings by acetaminophen products are increasing. Package tampering of this and other over-the-counter products increases their toxic potential, even though the pharmaceutical industry has created new protective packaging in response. This trend warrants particular attention, since an acute acetaminophen overdose can cause centrilobular hepatic necrosis, especially in adults.

An unusual type of poisoning has resulted from the proliferation of battery-operated games, cameras, hearing aids, calculators, and watches. An estimated 500 to 600 miniature button or disk batteries are swallowed each year by persons of all ages. Their major component is aqueous potassium hydroxide, which also is used to unclog pipes. Children can mistake the batteries for candy; adults may mistake them for medication tablets. Batteries that lodge in the esophagus, cecum, or other areas of the gastrointestinal tract present two problems: (1) they are locally corrosive to mucosa, causing ulceration or perforation in 1 to 2 hours; and (2) they may cause mercury poisoning when certain battery contents leak. Current recommendations suggest the battery be located by x-ray film, with daily serial x-ray films following its transit through the tract. If it is stalled in the stomach, a qualified endoscopist may choose to remove the battery immediately; vomiting usually is not effective. Endoscopic or surgical removal is necessary if the battery remains in the stomach for more than 24 hours, if gastric or peritoneal irritation develops, if radiologic evidence shows the battery lodging or leaking in the gastrointestinal tract, or if the particular type of battery is prone to leakage. A quicker method for removal employs a magnet wedged into an orogastric tube and a Foley catheter with an intact balloon, which the patient swallows.

Evidence indicates that a swallowed battery should be suspected if anorexia and vomiting follow a child's visit to a home of a person wearing a hearing aid, especially if the person habitually takes out the aid and leaves it accessible. Persons who wear hearing aids should be advised to dispose of worn-out disk or button batteries so they will not be mistaken for candy or medication tablets.

DETECTION OF POISONS

Toxicology is the study of poisons, their action and effects, methods of their detection, and diagnosis and treatment of poisoning. A poison can be defined as any substance that in relatively small amounts can cause death or serious bodily harm by chemical action. All drugs are potential poisons when used improperly or in excess dosage. Poisoning may be acute or chronic. In **acute poisoning** the effects are immediate. In **chronic poisoning** the effects are insidious because of cumulative effects of small amounts of poison absorbed over a prolonged period. Chronic poisoning causes chronic illness, which may or may not be reversible.

Nurses may be confronted with a suspected poisoning in many ways. A mother may call, upset that her small child has taken one of her contraceptive pills; a patient may accidentally drink the glass of peroxide mixture intended as a mouthwash; or a teenager who cannot be aroused may be brought into the emergency room. Often the nurse is alone in the situation, but speedy detection and treatment are essential.

Cues that typically point to poisoning include sudden, violent symtpoms of severe nausea, vomiting, diarrhea, collapse, or convulsions. If possible, it is important to find out what poison has been taken and how much. Additional information that might prove helpful to the physician in making a diagnosis includes answers to questions or reports of observed phenomena, with the nurse noting the following:

1. Any reports of poison contact by the victim
2. Poisoning in the "at-risk" age-group of children 1 to 5 years old
3. Report of a history of previous poisonings or ingestion of foreign substances
4. Diverse symptoms or signs referable to multiple organ system involvement that defy diagnosis
5. A history of suicidal intent or thought
6. Symptoms appearing suddenly in an otherwise healthy individual or a number of persons becoming ill about the same time, as might occur in food poisoning
7. Anything unusual about the person, the clothing, or the surroundings; evidence of burns about the lips and mouth; discolored gums; needle (hypodermic) pricks, pustules, or scars on the exposed and accessible surface of the body or dilated or constricted pupils, as may be seen in drug addicts; any skin rash or discoloration
8. The odor of the breath, the rate of respiration, any difficulty in respiration, and cyanosis
9. The quality and rate of the pulse
10. Appearance and odor of vomitus, if any, as well as accompanying diarrhea or abdominal pain
11. Any abnormalities of stool and urine; any change in color or the presence of blood
12. For signs of involvement of the nervous system, the

presence of excitement, muscular twitching, delirium, difficulty in speech, stupor, coma, constriction or dilation of the pupils, and elevated or subnormal temperature

Coma caused by drug overdose is characterized by the following categories:

Grade I — patient asleep but easily aroused, reacts to painful stimuli, deep tendon reflexes present, pupils normal and reactive, ocular movements present, and vital signs stable

Grade II — pain response absent, deep tendon reflexes depressed, pupils slightly dilated but reactive, and vital signs stable

Grade III — deep tendon and pupillary reflexes absent and vital signs stable

Grade IV — respiration and circulation depressed

Table 74-1 further assists in differentiating the signs of coma of toxic origin from those of coma resulting from structural neurologic damage. The nurse should *refrigerate in a covered container all specimens* of vomitus, urine, or stool in case the physician wishes to examine them and turn them over to the proper authority for analysis. This is of particular importance not only in making or confirming a diagnosis, but also in the event that the case has medicolegal significance.

Any of the signs listed earlier should be noted carefully for report to the poison control center or physician in charge. However, full reliance on signs and symptoms for clear-cut diagnosis and poison identification is fraught with danger, since these incidents may occur concurrently with an episode of acute disease, especially in children (e.g., aspirin intoxication), and symptoms may be similar or otherwise confusing. Also, more than one substance may be responsible for the signs of poisoning observed. Onset may vary, depending on the amount of substance taken, when it was taken (in relation to meals), and in what form it was taken (solutions will act faster than solid toxins).

Estimating the amount of poison ingested is one of the guideposts to treatment. In drug overdoses five times the average therapeutic dose is considered a reasonable predictor of toxicity. A single tablet of medication, even in adult dosage, ingested by a child will not be significantly toxic. One exception is the opiates, such as diphenoxylate hydrochloride (Lomotil). The volume of a liquid ingested can be estimated by the following rule of thumb: the volume of one swallow of a liquid by a child up to 5 years old is about 5 ml; in the adult, about 15 ml.

Another clue in determining whether a toxic amount of any substance could have been ingested can be found in the type of packaging. Spray aerosol containers, pump containers, and squeeze tubes rarely cause poisoning. The label also provides clues. The content can be assumed to be extremely toxic in amounts up to a teaspoon if the label states, "Call physician immediately" or "Danger — Poison," or if it gives any antidote information. If the label notes, "Warning" or "Caution," it is automatically assumed to have toxic potential. The label "Keep Out of Reach of Children," however, if unaccompanied by any of the other warnings, usually implies only minimal toxicity except under unusual conditions.

Not all substances commonly ingested accidentally are toxic if small amounts are taken only once. Poison control centers define a small amount as the quantity of a substance contained in "a taste," "one bite," or "a small piece," as opposed to "a mouthful." Although subjective, this is typical of data received when taking a poisoning history. A list of some frequently ingested products* that are *usually systemically nontoxic* if taken in small amounts follows:

Abrasives, bleaches (sodium hypochlorite, less than 5%)
Chalk
Cigarettes, cigarette ash, cigars
Cosmetics, perfume, cologne, deodorants
Crayons (if labelled C.P., A.P., or C.S., -130-46)
Glues, rubber cement
Hydrogen peroxide (medicinal, 3%)
Indelible pen or magic markers
Ink in a full cartridge of a ballpoint pen
Paint (latex)
Pencil (graphite or coloring)

*From Mofenson HC, Greensher J, and Carraccio T: Emergency Clin North Am 2:10, Feb. 1984.

TABLE 74-1 Signs of Coma of Toxic Origin Differentiated from Signs of Coma Resulting from Structural Neurologic Damage (to be Used as Corroborating Guide Only)

Signs	Structural neurologic damage	Toxic neurologic effects
Motor activity	Spasticity	Flaccidity
Pupillary reactions	Absent or variable	Present
Toe-to-head progression of signs	Yes	No
Blood pressure	May increase early; may decrease later	Usually decreases

Adapted with permission from Howard C Mofenson: Poison control manual, 1979, unpublished data.

Play-Doh

Saccharin and cyclamates

Safety matches (ingestion of less than 20 books of matches)

Soaps, liquid shampoos, household detergents (except dishwasher detergents)

Toothpaste (unless heavy ingestion of fluorides)

Vitamins (in amounts usually available for a single overdose, unless containing iron)

Ingestion of small amounts of these nonedible substances may produce mild gastric irritation but not systemic poisoning. Just knowing this can eliminate many panicky trips to the physician and has reduced unnecessary emergency room visits by about 5% in some health facilities. However, contact with a poison control center or physician is important (essential, if symptoms exist), since no product or drug is entirely safe for ingestion, and hypersensitivity reactions can occur.

In assisting with poisoning diagnosis and toxic substance identification, nurses (especially emergency room nurses and nurse practitioners) should familiarize themselves with certain clusters of signs associated with common drug poisonings or overdoses. These have been called "toxidromes" and are listed in Table 74-2. Other common single signs and their associated causative toxins are listed in Table 74-3.

Certain presumptive laboratory screening tests may be performed to help establish a more definitive diagnosis or for medicolegal reasons, but treatment should not be based solely on these tests, nor should treatment be delayed awaiting test results. Specimens of urine, blood, stool, or emesis; the results of the first lavage; and/or the suspect substance may need to be tested. Therefore all such products should be saved under refrigeration in closed containers for analysis. X-ray films of the abdomen may identify the presence of radiopaque substances such as certain medications, lead in paint chips, or other heavy metals such as arsenic, bismuth, iron, or thallium. Challenge doses of specific antidotes may be given to test for reversal of symptoms. However, the typical nursing situation in poisoning incidents calls for immediately contacting the nearest poison control center.

POISON CONTROL CENTERS*

There are about 600 poison control centers in the continental United States, Hawaii, Alaska, the Virgin Islands,

*The address of the coordinating agency for all poison control centers is the National Clearinghouse for Poison Control Centers, US Department of Health and Human Services, Food and Drug Administration, 5660 Fishers Lane, Room 1345, Rockville, MD 20857.

TABLE 74-2   Toxidromes That May Suggest Certain Drug Poisonings or Overdoses

Signs	Inference	Signs	Inference
Agitation, panic, depression Beet-red skin color Dilated pupils Dry skin with fever Hallucinations	atropine scopolamine	Ataxia Drowiness } Slurred } Without alcohol odor to breath speech	barbiturates sedative-hypnotics tranquilizers
Argumentativeness Dysrhythmias Diarrhea Dilated pupils Dry mouth with fetid odor	amphetamines	Dysrhythmias Coma Convulsions	tricyclic antidepressants: imipramine (Tofranil), amitriptyline (Elavil)
Headache Hyperactivity Sweating Tachycardia Tremors		Fever Hyperpnea Vomiting Ataxia	salicylates phenothiazines
Euphoria or coma Pinpoint pupils Slow respirations	opiates	Oculogyric crisis (coordinated deviation of eyes, usually upward) Torsion head and neck syndrome (torticollis)	
Involuntary defecation Involuntary urination Lacrimation Miosis Pulmonary congestion	organophosphates mushrooms (particularly genus *Amanita* or *Galerina*)		

Adapted with permission from Howard C Mofenson: Poison control manual, 1979, unpublished data.

TABLE 74-3   Single Signs That Suggest Presence of Certain Toxins

Sign	Inference	Sign	Inference
Abdominal colic	black widow spider bite heavy metals withdrawal from narcotic depressant	Pulse rate changes Increased	alcohol amphetamines atropine ephedrine
Ataxia	alcohol barbiturates bromides carbon monoxide hallucinogens heavy metals organic solvents phenytoin (Dilantin) tranquilizers	Slowed Pupillary changes Dilated	digitalis lily-of-the-valley narcotic depressants amphetamines antihistamines atropine barbiturates (when combined with coma)
Coma and drowsiness	alcohol (ethyl) antihistamines barbiturates, other hypnotics carbon monoxide opiates salicylates tranquilizers		cocaine ephedrine LSD (occasionally) methanol withdrawal from narcotic depressants (occasionally)
Convulsions or muscle twitching	alcohol amphetamines antihistamines boric acid camphor chlorinated hydrocarbon insecticides (DDT) cyanide lead organophosphate insecticides plants (azalea, iris, lily-of-the-valley, water hemlock) salicylates strychnine withdrawal from drugs: barbiturates, benzodiazepines (Valium, Librium), meprobamate	Nystagmus on lateral gaze Pinpoint pupils Respiratory alterations Increased	barbiturates minor tranquilizers (meprobamate, benzodiazepines), phenytoin (Dilantin) mushrooms (muscarinic) opiates organophosphate insecticides amphetamines barbiturates (early sign) carbon monoxide methanol petroleum distillates salicylates
Paralysis	botulism heavy metals plants (poison hemlock, etc.) triorthocresyl phosphate (plasticizer)	Paralysis Slowed or depressed	botulism organophosphate insecticides alcohol (late sign) barbiturates (late sign) opiates tranquilizers
Oliguria/anuria	carbon tetrachloride ethylene glycol (antifreeze) heavy metals hemolysis caused by naphthalene, plants, and so on methanol mushrooms oxylates petroleum distillates solvents	Wheezing/pulmonary edema Skin color changes Jaundice	mushrooms (muscarinic) opiates organophosphate insecticides petroleum distilates aniline dyes/coal tar colors arsenic carbon tetrachloride castor bean fava bean

Oral signs
  Breath odors
    Acetone
	acetone
	alcohol (methyl or isopropyl)
	phenol
	salicylates
			mushroom
			naphthalene (moth repellent/insecticide)
			yellow phosphorus

Continued.

TABLE 74-3   Single Signs That Suggest Presence of Certain Toxins—cont'd

Sign	Inference	Sign	Inference
Oral signs—cont'd		Red flush	alcohol
			antihistamines
			atropine
Alcohol	ethyl alcohol		boric acid
Bitter almonds	cyanide		carbon monoxide
Coal gas	carbon monoxide		nitrites
Garlic	arsenic		tricyclic antidepressants
	dimethyl sulfoxide (DMSO)	Cyanosis	aniline dyes
	phosphorus		carbon monoxide
	organophosphate insecticides		cyanide
	thallium		nitrites
Oil of winter-	methyl salicylate		strychnine
green		Violent emesis (with	aminophylline
Petroleum	petroleum distillates	or without hema-	bacterial food poisoning
Violets	turpentine	temesis)	boric acid
Dryness	amphetamines		corrosives
	antihistamines		fluoride
	atropine		heavy metals
	narcotic depressants		phenol
	tricyclic antidepressants		salicylates
Salivation	arsenic		
	corrosive substances		
	mercury		
	mushrooms		
	organophosphate insecticides		
	thallium		

Guam, Puerto Rico, the Canal Zone, and the District of Columbia. Most are located near hospitals or in emergency rooms of large community hospitals. Their telephone numbers are listed in the local telephone book or may be obtained from a pharmacist. Many are open 24 hours every day and are staffed to (1) answer specific questions from the public or from professionals about identification of ingredients in trade-named products, (2) estimate their toxicity, and (3) suggest specific treatment for poisonings. They also handle calls about drug abuse, suicide, food poisoning, dog bites, insect bites, snake bites, drugs and breast-feeding, and teratogenic drugs.

Poison control centers can be highly instrumental in reducing the number of poisonings (aside from treatment). They provide annual nationwide statistical analyses of poisonings by category, which help clarify the magnitude of the problem. Poison control centers also make available a wide selection of pamphlets, resources, and presentations to educate the public and professionsals on the ubiquity of poisons in the environment and on procedures to follow in dealing with poisons.

Other sources of information include the *Poisindex,* a microfiche data base of computer-generated information describing nearly all known substances, including product ingredients. It is updated every 3 months. Another source is *Drugdex,* a compendium of information specifically about drugs that includes their ranges of toxicity. It is well referenced for efficient use.

CLASSIFICATION AND MECHANISMS OF ACTION OF POISONS

The classification of poisons is as broad as the classification of drugs, since any drug is a potential poison when used in excess.

Poisons may be classified in various ways. They may be grouped according to chemical classifications as organic and inorganic poisons; as alkaloids, glycosides, and resins; or as acids, alkalis, heavy metals, oxidizing agents, halogenated hydrocarbons, and so on.

They also may be grouped by locale of exposure—poisons found in the home, encountered in industry, encountered while camping, and so on.

Poisons also may be classified according to the organ or tissue of the body in which the most damaging effects are produced. Some poisons injure all cells they contact. Such chemical substances are sometimes called protoplasmic poisons or cytotoxins. Others have more effect on the kidney (**nephrotoxins**), the liver (**hepatotoxins**), or the blood-forming organs.

Poisons that affect chiefly the nervous system are called neurotoxins or neurotropic poisons. They must be studied separately because different symptoms characterize each one. Symptoms of toxicity are mentioned with each of these drugs in previous chapters. Although symptoms of this group of poisons are to some extent specific, certain symptoms are encountered repeatedly and are associated with many poisons. Drowsiness, dizziness, headache, delirium, coma, and convulsive seizures always indicate central nervous system involvement. On the other hand, dry mouth, dilated pupils, and difficult swallowing are associated with overdosage of atropine or one of the atropine-like drugs; ringing in the ears, excessive perspiration, and gastric upset are associated with salicylate overdosage.

Many of the central nervous system depressants cause death by producing excessive depression of respiration and respiratory failure. The general anesthetics, barbiturates, chloral hydrate, and paraldehyde are examples of such drugs.

Many times the precise mechanism of action is not known; death may be caused by respiratory failure, but exactly what happens to cause depression of the respiratory center may not be known.

Central nervous system stimulants such as pentylenetetrazol and strychnine in toxic amounts cause convulsive seizures, exhaustion, and depression of vital centers.

The human body depends on a constant supply of oxygen if various physiologic functions are to proceed satisfactorily. Anything that interferes with the use of oxygen by the cells or with the transportation of oxygen will produce damaging effects faster in some cells than in others. Carbon monoxide from automobile engines and unvented gas heaters is one of the most widely distributed toxic agents. It poisons by producing hypoxia and finally asphyxia. Carbon monoxide has a great affinity for hemoglobin and forms carboxyhemoglobin. Thus the production of oxyhemoglobin and the free transport of oxygen is interfered with; oxygen deficiency soon develops in the cells. Unless exposure to the carbon monoxide is terminated before 40% of hemoglobin has been changed to carboxyhemoglobin, anoxia may produce serious brain damage. Death occurs when 60% of the hemoglobin has been changed to carboxyhemoglobin.

The cyanides act somewhat similarly in that they bring about cellular anoxia, but they do so differently. They inactivate certain tissue enzymes so that cells are unable to utilize oxygen. Death may occur very rapidly.

Curare and the curariform drugs in toxic amounts bring about paralysis of the diaphragm, and again the victim dies from lack of oxygen.

Certain drugs have a direct effect on muscle tissue from the body, such as that of the myocardium, or the smooth muscle of the blood vessels. Death results from the failure of circulation or cardiac arrest. The nitrites, potassium salts, and digitalis drugs may exert such toxic effects.

Arsenic is an example of a protoplasmic poison or cytotoxin. Compounds of arsenic inhibit many enzyme systems of cells, especially those that depend on the activity of their free sulfhydryl (SH) groups. The arsenic combines with these SH groups and makes them ineffective. Thus extensive tissue damage in the body occurs.

Methyl alcohol owes its toxic effect to an intermediate product of metabolism—formic acid. This produces a severe acidosis, lowered pH of the blood, reduced cerebral blood flow, and decreased consumption of oxygen by the brain. A selective action also affects the retinal cells of the eye, but the exact cause of this injury is unknown.

Benzene is an example of a poison that acts by inhibiting the formation of all types of blood cells. In some instances the precursor of one type of blood cell is injured more than another. Depression of the formation of any of the blood cells can cause death.

Strong acids and alkalis denature and destroy cellular proteins. Examples of corrosive acids are hydrochloric, nitric, and sulfuric. Sodium, potassium, and ammonium hydroxides are examples of strong or caustic alkalis. Locally, these substances cause destruction of tissue, and death may result from hemorrhage, perforation, or shock. Corrosive poisons may also cause death by altering the pH of the blood or other body fluids, or they may produce marked degenerative changes on vital organs such as the liver or kidney.

SPECIFIC POISONS, WITH SYMPTOMS AND SUGGESTED EMERGENCY TREATMENT

Since the emphasis is on *prompt* treatment, health care may be best served by quick action by informed bystanders at the scene who apply first-aid measures while help is sought from the poison control center and while transportation to a hospital, clinic, or physician's office is arranged. A first-aid chart that offers instruction for various poisoning emergencies is included in the box on p. 1162 as an example to delineate specific actions for different poisonings.

The caller to the poison control center should have the following information, if available:
1. Physical appearance of the substance
2. Odor, color, and texture; distinguishing characteristics of the substance
3. Trade name or chemical name, if known
4. Purpose or how the substance was meant to be used
5. Label statements relating to "poison" content or flammability

After the events of the suspected poisoning have been assessed thoroughly and problems analyzed, including the identification of the substance if possible, prompt nursing actions must be instituted. Nursing management will be guided by four major goals:
1. Vital functions (respirations, circulation, and others) will be maintained, supported, or restored.
2. The toxic substance will be removed or eliminated from the system as soon as possible.
3. The action of certain specific poisons may be counteracted, reversed, or antagonized by specific antidotes.
4. Recurrences will be reduced or prevented.

Based on the priority of nursing problems in each poisoning episode, these goals may best be implemented simultaneously or in order of need. Prompt removal of the poison or supportive care may be all the treatment needed.

Support of vital functions. Basic to the treatment of poisoning is intensive supportive therapy, good nursing care, and minimal dangerous invasive interventions. Nursing care of the poisoned patient should focus on restoration, support, and maintenance of such vital functions as ventilation, circulation, and acid-base and fluid-electrolyte balance. Emotional support for the patient and others involved in this crisis is crucial.

A general assessment and history should be performed quickly and competently to determine the extent of any impairments of body systems or particular susceptibilities. Expert nursing care is essential to observe the following for information indicating impending complications:

1. Level of consciousness
2. Vital signs. Temperature may be elevated with certain central nervous system (CNS) stimulants and salicylates and depressed with others. Transient cardiac dysrhythmias may occur; anticipate obtaining an electrocardiogram. Pulmonary congestion, airway obstruction, or apnea is common; aspiration of vomitus can occur.

Implemented plans may include:

1. Turning, deep breathing, coughing, and suctioning
2. Auscultation to demonstrate a need for chest x-ray examination, suctioning, tracheostomy, endotracheal intubation, blood gas determinations, supplemental oxygen and a respirator/ventilator, and so on
3. Initiation of intravenous infusion
4. Placement of a central venous pressure line or a Swan-Ganz catheter if hypotension persists

It is also essential that the victim be positioned to prevent aspiration of vomitus and that mouth care be attended to promptly after emesis. Moderate amounts of plain water by mouth (if a gag or swallow reflex is present) may be all that is needed to dilute or effectively inactivate many ingested poisons.

Close attention to developing problems and responsive intervention can often fend off the need for more aggressive medical therapies that tax the already tenuous condition of the poisoned patient.

Removal or elimination of poison. Careful evaluation of the patient who has been affected by a toxic substance is essential to determine which of the foregoing steps take priority and by which route the poison should be removed or eliminated, if necessary. The route is largely determined by the manner of the poisoning. Removal of ingested substances can be attempted in several ways: (1) by directly removing it from the stomach, if the poisoning is discovered early; (2) by increasing the

---

FIRST AID FOR POSSIBLE POISONING

REMEMBER: ANY NONFOOD SUBSTANCE MAY BE POISONOUS.

1. Keep all potential poisons—household products and medicines—out of children's reach.
2. Use "safety caps" (child-resistant containers) to avoid accidents.
3. Have 1 ounce of ipecac syrup in your home and in your first-aid kit for camping, travel, and so on.
4. Keep your poison center's and your physician's phone number handy.

IF YOU THINK AN ACCIDENTAL INGESTION HAS OCCURRED:

1. Keep calm. Do not wait for symptoms—call for help promptly.
2. Find out if the substance is toxic; your poison control center or your physician can tell you if a risk exists and what you should do.
3. Have the product's container or label with you at the phone.
   a. If a poison is on the skin:
   Immediately remove affected clothing.
   Flood involved parts of body with water, wash with soap or detergent, and rinse thoroughly.
   b. If a poison is in the eye:
   Immediately flush the eye with water for up to 20 minutes.
   c. If a poison is inhaled:
   Immediately get the victim to fresh air. Give mouth-to-mouth resuscitation if necessary.
   d. If vomiting has been recommended:
   Give 1 tablespoon of ipecac syrup followed by at least one glass (8 ounces) of clear liquid (water, juices, carbonated beverage). If the patient does not vomit within 15 to 20 minutes, give 1 more tablespoon of ipecac and more water. Do *not* use salt water.

NEVER INDUCE VOMITING IF:

1. The victim is in a *coma* (unconscious).
2. The victim is *convulsing* (having a seizure).
3. The victim has swallowed a *caustic* or *corrosive* (e.g., lye).

FOR REEMPHASIS:

1. Always call to be certain of possible toxicity before undertaking treatment.
2. Never induce vomiting until you are instructed to do so.
3. Do not rely on the label's antidote information, since it may be out of date. Call instead.
4. If you have to go to an emergency room, take the tablets, capsules, container, and/or label with you.
5. Do not hesitate to call your poison center or your physician a second time if the victim seems to be getting worse.

Adapted from American Association of Poison Control Centers, William O Robertson, MD, Secretary. Copyright © Physician's desk reference for nonprescription drugs, 1981 edition. Published by Medical Economics Co., Inc., Oradell, NJ 07649.

rate of transit of the poison through the colon, even though little or no absorption occurs there and thus may not be effective; or (3) if the substance has probably already been assimilated into the system or was injected, by attempting to remove or filter it from the bloodstream. Contact poisons may be flushed from the skin, eyes, and other external areas by copious volumes of plain, flowing water from a pitcher or other container. Soapy warm water is needed to remove organic solvents and tenacious oils. Inhaled toxins are treated by removing the patient to fresh air and administering artificial respiration or oxygen and other supportive measures as necessary.

Various methods exist for the removal or elimination of poisons from the gastrointestinal tract or systemic circulation: emesis, gastric lavage, cathartics, diuretics, dialysis, or occasionally blood exchange transfusions or hemoperfusion through charcoal or exchange resins. There are numerous approaches to treatment of the poisoning emergency; each must be tailored by clinical judgment to individual patient needs.

Generally, if more than 4 hours have elapsed since a poison ingestion, emptying the stomach will be ineffective. Exceptions are poisonings by anticholinergic drugs, which slow gastric motility, and by salicylates, which promote pyloric spasm. Some drugs, such as ethanol, are absorbed too rapidly to be recovered after 1 hour. However, when situations have warranted emptying the stomach, whole tablets have occasionally been recovered even a day later. Because of this, some recommend emptying the stomach even after a delay.

The most effective method for removing ingested toxins is usually the most natural one — emesis, done as soon as possible. In some instances, however, emesis is contraindicated (see box).

If vomiting does not or cannot occur naturally, either ipecac syrup or apomorphine is usually administered. However, neither emetic may be effective if the ingested substance is a sedative-hypnotic, a phenothiazine, or a tricyclic antidepressant, all of which have antiemetic properties.

The most commonly used emetic is ipecac syrup. (Fluid extract of ipecac, which is about 14 times more concentrated and has caused a number of deaths, should never be used.) Ipecac syrup tastes bitter-sweet. It probably acts both centrally and locally by directly stimulating the vomiting center, and by irritating the gastric mucosa. The usual dose for adults is 15 to 30 ml, followed by 200 to 300 ml of water, milk, or fruit juice or as much fluid as the patient can drink. For children under 1 year of age, a 7.5-ml dose is given; children 1 to 5 years old, a 15-ml dose; and those over 5 years, a 30-ml dose.

Vomiting usually occurs in 15 to 30 minutes. The dose may be repeated once after 20 minutes if the first dose is not effective. If vomiting does not occur within 30 minutes, gastric lavage should be performed, since ipecac

---

> ## CONTRAINDICATIONS FOR INDUCED EMESIS IN POISONINGS
>
> Infants up to 1 year of age
> Comatose or convulsing patient
> Absent gag and cough reflexes
> Ingestion of:
> Convulsion-inducing substances
> Sharp objects (e.g., glass, nails) along with toxic substance
> Central nervous system (CNS) poisons (e.g., camphor, strychnine), which must be removed more quickly by lavage
> Acids, alkalis, or petroleum distillates
> When risk of aspiration outweighs benefits: ingestion of less than 1 mg/kg body weight of a petroleum distillate that does not contain toxic components such as pesticides, heavy metals, and so on
> Patients who have already vomited copiously
> During pregnancy (decision may depend on clinical judgment)

Modified with permission from Howard C Mofenson: Poison control manual, 1979, unpublished material.

is a cardiotoxic if absorbed and may cause conduction disturbances, atrial fibrillation, or myocarditis.

Ipecac syrup is available without a prescription in 1-ounce (30-ml) bottles bearing the following instructions:

1. For emergency use to cause vomiting in poisoning. Before using, call physician, poison control center, or hospital emergency room immediately for advice.
2. Warning — Keep out of reach of children. Do not use if strychnine, corrosives such as alkalis (lye) and strong acids, or petroleum distillates such as kerosene, gasoline, fuel oil, coal oil, paint thinner, or cleaning fluid have been ingested.

Apomorphine, although more dangerous to use, may be used to induce vomiting when more rapid emesis is necessary; it is effective within 1 to 15 minutes after administration. Apomorphine is a narcotic emetic that causes a reflex action of the vomiting center in the brainstem. It can cause severe, protracted emesis and should be used with extreme caution. Naloxone hydrochloride (Narcan) should be on hand to counteract any respiratory depression. The single dose, which may *not* be repeated, is 0.1 ml/kg body weight, resulting in a dose range of 2 to 10 mg. Adults are usually given 5 to 6 mg; children between 1 and 2 years of age are usually given 1 to 2 mg. Since apomorphine comes in a 6 mg tablet that requires crushing and diluting with 3 ml of sterile water for subcutaneous injection, some awkwardness, delay, and questionable accuracy or potency of the produced solution may occur. (The crushed powder will account for some of the resultant volume, so one cannot be certain that 1 ml of solution contains an evenly distributed 2 mg of this potent CNS depressant.)

If the patient is conscious, drug-induced vomiting is usually preferable to gastric lavage, particularly in children, since aspiration of vomitus is less likely to occur. Nurses should employ the necessary measures to reduce the likelihood of aspiration of vomitus (e.g., proper positioning of patient). Occasionally, induction of vomiting may be facilitated by stimulating the pharynx, but time should not be wasted in repeated futile attempts.

If emesis cannot be induced, **gastric lavage** should be begun *except* under most of the same contraindicating conditions (e.g., untreated convulsions, absent reflexes, corrosives). Lavage *may* be preferred treatment for pregnant women and for patients who have ingested more than 2 ml/kg body weight of a petroleum distillate and who should have endotracheal intubation to protect the airway. Lavage may be contraindicated in the presence of cardiac dysrhythmias.

An Ewald orogastric tube, no. 16 to 30 French, may be used to lavage children; tube sizes for adult lavage range from no. 34 to 42. The newer, clear-plastic Lavacuator tube also may be used. A standard nasogastric tube is too narrow for extraction of particulate matter such as intact tablets (Figure 74-1). Stomach contents should be aspirated first and saved for toxicologic analysis if necessary. Several liters of half-strength saline solution may be used

in increments of 50 to 100 ml for children and 150 to 200 ml for adults during repeated lavages until return flows are clear. (Remember that dead space in the tube itself accounts for 20 to 25 ml of the fluid instilled.) Neither emesis nor lavage is guaranteed to empty the stomach completely.

Following emesis or lavage, activated charcoal may be instilled or swallowed to act as an adsorbent. Activated charcoal should be given as soon after poison ingestion as feasible, but not after ipecac and emesis, since it will adsorb the ipecac. Activated charcoal adsorbs many substances, both simple and complex. It is used as an adjunct in the treatment of oral poisonings with heavy metals, mercuric chloride, strychnine, phenol, atropine, phenolphthalein, oxalic acid, poisonous mushrooms, aspirin, and most drugs. It is not effective for poisoning with cyanide, DDT, ethanol, methanol, caustic alkalis, ferrous sulfate, boric acid, organophosphates, or carbonate. The charcoal mixture need not be removed from the stomach afterward because no known adverse effects exist. Activated charcoal can also serve as a stool marker to indicate when further gastrointestinal absorption of the ingested poison has ended.

For emergency treatment of adults or children, 5 to 50 g of the charcoal powder is mixed with tap water to form a slurry with the consistency of thick soup; this is taken orally by the patient or passed through a lavage tube. A dose of 50 g is used routinely by some emergency cen-

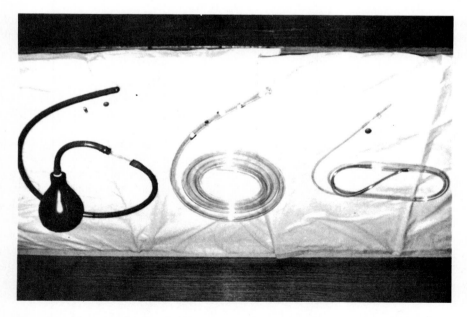

FIGURE 74-1   The two tubes on the left are used in various lavage techniques. The Ewald tube (left) has a single lumen. The orogastric hose, or Lavacuator (middle), has numerous openings up the side of the distal end and a double lumen. Note the sizes of the tablets in comparison to the nearby tubes. Standard nasogastric tubes (right) have no role in lavage of the poisoned patient since the tube is too narrow to enable evacuation of whole drug forms or even large particles.

(From Goldfrank L: Toxicologic emergencies, ed 2, New York, 1982, Appleton-Century-Crofts.)

ters; the dose may be as high as 120 g. In general the dose should be 10 times the estimated weight of the ingested substance. To improve palatability, a small amount of a flavoring agent (e.g., cherry), concentrated fruit juice, or chocolate powder may be added to the slurry; ice cream or sherbet should not be used, since these substances decrease the adsorptive capacity of the charcoal. Tablets or capsules of charcoal should not be used for treatment of poisoning, since they are less effective than the powder.

Administration of activated charcoal and ion exchange resins such as cholestyramine and colestipol, if given within 1 hour, may prevent intestinal reabsorption of some drugs that normally undergo recycling through the liver and thus may facilitate intestinal elimination. Digitoxin and phenprocoumon toxicity has been effectively treated this way. Paraquat, which is a lethal weed killer used on some marijuana plants and which is extremely rapidly absorbed from the gastrointestinal tract, is known to bind strongly to Fuller's earth and bentonite, but these adsorbents must be given too early to be practical. Cholestyramine binds to acidic drugs such as acetaminophen, but again, it must be given almost immediately.

Other ways used to block or eliminate toxins from the system include forced diuresis, cathartics and enemas, dialysis, hemoperfusion, and exchange transfusions. These methods should be reserved as treatment under certain conditions and for specific poisons; they are not universally effective and are much less commonly used than emesis or lavage.

Diuresis may be effective if the poison is one in which the total body clearance of active substance depends largely on renal clearance. For example, if only 1% of a drug dose is normally excreted in the urine, even a 20-fold increase in renal clearance will not be clinically significant. When performed, diuresis may be forced by infusing 1 to 2 L of fluid per hour or by the administration of mannitol, an osmotic diuretic. Hazards related to fluid overload in conditions of heart failure, organ edema, renal failure, or acid-base imbalances are clear.

In addition, changing the pH of the urine may enhance excretion of certain drugs. Alkalinization by administering sodium bicarbonate or other bases is particularly effective in salicylate overdoses and probably in phenobarbital and 2,4-dichlorophenoxyacetic acid (weed killer, 2,4-D). It is reported to be questionably effective for some barbiturates and amitriptyline. Forced acid diuresis is probably more potentially hazardous but is often recommended for poisoning with amphetamines, quinine, and fenfluramine (Pondimin), despite lack of full documentation of efficacy.

Cathartics and enemas are sometimes used to enhance toxin elimination and to reduce potential for absorption from the gastrointestinal tract. However, this is not very effective, since absorption is usually rapid and occurs in the upper small intestine. Castor oil or cathartics such as sodium sulfate or magnesium sulfate (Epsom salt) are used in overdoses of glutethimide (Doriden), a nonbarbiturate hypnotic, or short-acting barbiturates, among others. Efficacy has not been established.

Clearance of poisons directly from the bloodstream by peritoneal dialysis or hemodialysis, hemoperfusion, or transfusion is occasionally done to augment other measures previously discussed. These more complex methods may be ineffective, overly taxing to the poisoned patient, unnecessary, or even harmful in some instances. Not enough well-controlled studies have been done to prove efficacy. The degree to which they may be useful depends in part on the properties of the substance (i.e., whether it freely circulates or whether it is bound to plasma proteins or to tissues). Various lists of substances amenable to dialysis exist; some substances for which dialysis has *not* proved useful are as follows*:

amitriptyline (Elavil)
anticholinergics
antidepressants
antihisitamines
atropine
chlordiazepoxide (Librium)
desipramine hydrochloride (Pertofrane)
diazepam (Valium)
digitalis
diphenoxylate hydrochloride (Lomotil)
glutethimide (Doriden)
hallucinogens
imipramine (Tofranil)
methaqualone (Quaalude)
methyprylon (Noludar)
narcotic opiate depressants (e.g., heroin)
nortriptyline (Aventyl)
oxazepam (Serak)
phenelzine sulfate (Nardil)
propoxyphene (Darvon)

The following are some common criteria for considering dialysis:

1. Presence of potentially lethal levels of a dialyzable substance
2. Presence of high levels of a substance that breaks down into dialyzable poisons
3. When usual supportive or corrective measures will not suffice to prevent further damage (e.g., coma, apnea, shock, hyperthermia)
4. When major degradation or excretion routes are damaged, blocked, or otherwise dysfunctional (e.g., renal or liver failure)
5. Often when the patient is pregnant (hemodialysis)

*Modified from Krupp MA and Chatton MJ: Current medical diagnosis and treatment, 1979, Los Altos, Calif, 1979, Lange Medical Publications.

Although hemodialysis is more efficient for short-term dialysis, peritoneal dialysis may be less hazardous and may be continued over a longer period. Hemoperfusion is a more promising technique. Studies seem to show that more efficient removal of drugs occurs when heparinized blood can be passed through a column packed with adsorbents such as activated charcoal or, better yet, newer exchange resins such as polacrilin (Amberlite). Possible complications include embolism; loss of white cells, platelets, and fibrinogen; and hemorrhage.

Table 74-4 lists some specific poisons, with associated symptoms and the appropriate emergency treatment.

PREVENTION OF POISONING

The focus of nursing on primary care and its corollary, prevention, applies readily to poisonings. Prevention has always been emphasized by the nursing profession, and now other disciplines are beginning to take part. Combined efforts with drug information centers and other health professionals and creative approaches have already had an impact on the frequency of certain categories of drug poisoning, notably aspirin poisoning.

Various creative graphic symbols appear on labels of poisonous substances to alert the adult and/or nonreading child to the potential hazard contained therein. "Mr Yuk," an ugly, green-faced, scowling image, is one of these. Tricky-to-open caps appear to delay if not totally prevent children's indiscriminate use of medicines. Others who have no need for these caps can request medication in the familiar easy-to-open caps.

There is much to learn about toxins in our environment, both apparent and potential, and therefore much to do in the way of poison prevention, but concerted, thoughtful efforts have already had a positive effect on statistics.

ANTIDOTES

The number of antidotes for specific toxins is minimal (Table 74-5); no widely accepted "universal antidote" exists. Delaying nursing care while specific substance identification is made and the antidote sought may be more injurious in the long run. Antidotes can be as toxic as the original poison if not used appropriately.

Antidotes are more effective after the stomach is empty. The correct dose to reverse toxicity depends on the specific drug involved, its half-life, and the severity of toxicity shown. Antidotes work by any of the following mechanisms: (1) antagonizing or stimulating receptor sites that have been rendered hyperfunctional or dysfunctional by the poison; (2) interfering with enzyme inhibition; (3) administering the product of metabolism that has been interfered with; (4) inhibiting the biotransformation of a substance to a poisonous metabolite; (5) giving an agent that inactivates the toxic product; (6) chelation (forming highly stable complexes, tying up the substance — usually a heavy metal such as iron); (7) producing immunotherapy — the use of antidrug antibodies to bind and inactivate drugs (for example, there is a report of severe digoxin poisoning reversed with sheep digoxin–specific antibodies); and (8) reducing compounds that have bound tightly to oxygen in the bloodstream.

THE NURSE'S ROLE IN CARE OF THE CLIENT WITH POISONING

Assessment. An assessment should be done quickly to determine what substance is involved so that immediate action can be taken to prevent or minimize its effects. Symptoms may include, depending on the causative agent, nausea and vomiting, abdominal cramping, convulsions, change in the level of consciousness, and a decreased rate of pulse and respiration.

To assist in the determination of the agent, the lips and mouth are checked for excessive salivation, burns, or difficulty swallowing. The breath should be assessed for its odor. Some petroleum and cleaning products have distinctive smells which can be identified. The pupils should be checked for dilation or constriction, which may also help to indicate the substance.

If the patient is conscious, he should be questioned as to what substance and what quantity was taken. With the unconscious person, identification of the substance is facilitated by clues in the environment. Empty containers, open bottles or medication containers, or syringes should be gathered and taken to the hospital with the patient. Often the containers will list the ingredients of the substance to assist the medical staff in the choice of treatment or antidote.

Intervention. Immediate action is required in the case of poisoning to prevent the absorption of the substance. If the person is unconscious, he should be transported as soon as possible to a hospital. If the individual is conscious, a physician and/or the poison control center should be contacted immediately. The telephone number of the nearest poison control center is usually listed in the front of the telephone directory with other emergency numbers for the community.

If the poison has been inhaled, such as a toxic gas or carbon monoxide, the individual should be removed from the source to the fresh air and oxygen administered if available. Cardiopulmonary resuscitation should be started if indicated. The victim will need to be transported to the hospital.

If the substance is a contact poison, absorbed through the skin and mucous membranes, the individual should be rinsed off immediately with copious amounts of water.

TABLE 74-4   Some Specific Poisons, with Symptoms and Suggested Emergency Treatment*

Poison	Symptoms†	Treatment‡
alcohol (ethanol)	*Acute:* CNS depression with decreased inhibitions and higher mental processes, gastric irritation with nausea and vomiting, hypoglycemia with seizures, hypothermia, jaw spasms, extensor rigidity, positive Babinski's sign, ketoacidosis, convulsions, fever, cerebral edema with severe headache, coma. *Chronic:* vitamin and mineral deficiencies, polyneuropathy, myopathy, chronic gastritis, cirrhosis, pancreatitis, anemias, thrombocyte and granulocyte deficiencies.	Gastric lavage with tap water, or emesis. Give 4 g sodium bicarbonate. Maintain airway; support respirations; get blood gas, alcohol, and glucose levels. Oral or intravenous 50% glucose is given as needed for hypoglycemia/ketoacidosis. Diazepam is given as needed for hyperexcitability or vomiting. Treatment varies, especially for children.
amphetamines, psychedelic drugs—methamphetamine (Desoxyn), phentermine (Fastin, Ionamin), phenylpropanolamine (in diet pills), cocaine, LSD, mescaline, and so on.§	CNS stimulation, paranoia, visual hallucinations, but oriented to time and place. Mydriasis, increased blood pressure and pulse, hyperreflexia, tremor, piloerection, muscular weakness, fever, and occasionally drowsiness, nausea, and decreased urine output.	Provide secure environment, presence of familiar persons; "talking down" the patient. Sedative barbiturates and diazepam may be helpful. Give follow-up for symptoms, depression. Provide conservative, supportive measures.
arsenic (found in weed killers, insecticides, sheepdip, rodenticides, and so on.	Rapidity of onset of symptoms related to whether or not poison is taken with food. Odor of garlic on breath and stools. Faintness, nausea, difficulty in swallowing, extreme thirst, severe vomiting, gastric and mouth pain, "rice water" stools, oliguria, hematuria, albuminuria, cold clammy skin, skeletal muscle cramps Collapse and death.	Induce emesis with ipecac syrup. Give 0.5-10 g of activated charcoal in glass of water followed by repeated lavage with warm water or weak sodium bicarbonate solution or by an emetic (warm water) repeated until vomiting occurs. Give intravenous fluids. Allow sedation, analgesics. Dimercaprol (BAL) is the antidote of choice; penicillamine is an alternative. Keep patient warm. Relieve pain and diarrhea.
barbiturates (sleep inducers, anticonvulsants, sedatives)—amobarbital (Amytal), pentobarbital (Nembutal), phenobarbital (Luminal), secobarbital (Seconal), thiopental (Phentothal), and others	Similar to alcohol intoxication. Deep sleep or stupor occasionally preceded by confusion, excitement. Later, coma, with sluggish or absent reflexes. Extremes in respiratory rate. Shock with decreased blood pressure, pinpoint pupils, weak and thready pulse. Death from respiratory failure, hypostatic pneumonia, or pulmonary edema. Very early, sluggishness in actions, thinking, and speech; poor memory; faulty judgment; narrow attention; emotional lability; untidy grooming; suicidal tendencies. Also, nystagmus, strabismus, diplopia, vertigo, positive Romberg's sign, superficial reflexes, skin rashes. Concurrent use of amphetamines is common.	Gradual withdrawal for the chronic user. General supportive care for all: Keep warm; turn; see to hydration, nutrition, and so on. For acute poisoning, emesis or lavage with sodium bicarbonate after passing endotracheal tube if less than 2 hr since ingestion; hemodialysis may be effective. Pressor agents and use of ventilators may be necessary.

*Treatment may vary with individual situation and clinical judgment.
†Symptoms will vary with concentration of poison in body.
‡See text for specific antidote therapies.
§Toxicity usually involves more than a single substance.

Continued.

TABLE 74-4 Some Specific Poisons, with Symptoms and Suggested Emergency Treatment*—cont'd

Poison	Symptoms†	Treatment‡
caustics/corrosives **Acids** Contact or ingested acids—carbolic or crude creosol (disinfectants), hydrochloric‖ (metal cleaners, soldering), nitric‖ and oxalic (cleaning solutions), sulfuric (auto batteries) acids	Parts in contact with acid are first white, later brown or yellow. Coagulation necrosis with somewhat superficial tissue damage. Pain; thirst, difficulty breathing, speaking, swallowing; circulatory collapse; death from asphyxia.	Avoid stomach tube, emesis (danger of perforation), or sodium bicarbonate (danger of gaseous distention/rupture). Give copious amounts of water. Relieve pain and treat shock. Corticosteroid therapy possibly effective. Keep patient warm and quiet.
Inhaled, volatile acids—bromine, chlorine, fluorine, iodine	Cough, dyspnea, pulmonary edema.	Remove from area. Inspect skin and clothing. Treat pulmonary edema.
alkalis (identifiable by "soapy" or slippery texture)	Deep penetrating tissue destruction (e.g., esophageal perforation) with possibly severe scarring and stricture formation. Symptoms similar to acid ingestion; additionally, bloody vomitus and stools. Mucous membranes white and swollen; mouth, throat, and lips swollen.	If liquid agent, prepare for possible esophagoscopy and/or surgery. Avoid stomach tube and emesis and acids (e.g., fruit juices, vinegar). Give large amounts of water. Corticosteroid therapy possibly effective in presence of burns. Relieve pain and treat shock.
Contact or ingested alkalis—ammonia, automatic dishwater detergent, caustic soda (soapmaking), Clinitest tablets, lime (building construction), potash (lye, drain chemicals‖), potassium hydroxide, sodium hydroxide	Skin cold and clammy, hypotension, rapid pulse, violent vomiting, great anxiety.	
CNS or autonomic nervous system stimulant/depressant (depends on dosage)—phencyclidine (PCP, Sernylan, "angel dust")	Giddy euphoria at low doses may be accompanied (dose-related) by nystagmus, analgesia, paresthesias, pupillary constriction, ptosis, hypertension, muscle rigidity, blank stare, stupor without respiratory depression, confusion. Higher doses: coma, seizures, hypotension, cardiac dysrhythmias.	"Talking down" patient may not be effective. Gastric lavage for oral doses. Intravenous diazepam for seizures; intravenous diazoxide, 300 mg, rapidly, for severe hypertension; ammonium chloride, 0.5-1 g every 6 hr, titrate to decrease urine pH to 5.5-6.
hydrocarbons or petroleum distillates (present in kerosene, gasoline, naphtha, cleaning fluids, paint thinner, charcoal lighter fluid, benzene—most dangerous effect in blood-forming tissue)	*Ingestion* (more hazardous because of potential for aspiration to occur during ingestion and treatment): symptoms of intoxication similar to those of alcohol; burning sensation in mouth, esophagus, and stomach. Vomiting, dizziness, tremor, muscle cramps, confusion, fever, dullness. Cold, clammy skin; weak, irregular pulse; thirst; convulsions; unconsciousness; coma. Pulmonary symptoms include cough, cyanosis, bloody sputum, rales, edema, pneumonia. Death from respiratory failure. *Inhalation:* visual difficulties, transient euphoria, headache, nausea. Death from respiratory failure.	Avoid emetics and lavage. Use emesis if more than 1 ml/kg body weight ingested or if dangerous additives are involved; lavage after endotracheal intubation if more than 1 ml/kg ingested *and* loss of gag reflex, convulsions, or dyspnea occurs. Emesis is precluded in ingestion of (1) high-viscosity, low-volatility products such as oils in home fuel, lubrication, machine oil (unless it contains triorthoresyl phosphate); (2) tar, asphalt, glues, greases, petroleum jelly, mineral oil. Measures supportive to the maintenance of normal temperature, respirations, blood pressure, and fluid-electrolyte balance.

‖Most common examples.

TABLE 74-4   Some Specific Poisons, with Symptoms and Suggested Emergency Treatment* — cont'd

Poison	Symptoms†	Treatment‡
MAO inhibitors — phenelzine (Nardil), tranylcypromine (Parnate)	*Acute:* agitation, hallucinations, hyperreflexia, fever, and convulsions may appear later. *Chronic:* mostly excess CNS stimulation, convulsions, and orthostatic hypotension.	Measures supportive to the maintenance of normal temperature, respirations, blood pressure, and fluid-electrolyte balance.
nonbarbiturate sedatives — chloral hydrate, ethchlorvynol (Placidyl),¶ glutethimide (Doriden — toxic near 2.5-4 mg/day),¶ methaqualone (Quaalude),¶ methyprylon (Noludar),¶ paraldehyde. Benzodiazepines in large doses: chlordiazepoxide (Librium), diazepam (Valium — toxicity increased in intramuscular or intravenous doses or in combination with other drugs/ethanol), flurazepam (Dalmane), oxazepam (Serax), and so on	*As a group:* extinction of inhibitions, ataxia, clumsiness, nystagmus, excess sedation, possible coma and death. Drug dependency and withdrawal symptoms. *Glutethimide:* occasionally sudden apnea on being touched, hypotension, dilated pupils, no gag or corneal reflexes, coma. *Diazepam:* respiratory or circulatory insufficiency.	*Glutethimide:* intubate first, then lavage and give intravenous fluids. Recommended medications are intramuscular ephedrine, Neo-Synephrine, intravenous Benzedrine, intramuscular sodium benzoate. Provide respiratory system support and urinary catheterization as needed. Hemodialysis may be considered. Admit for close surveillance. *Diazepam:* lavage may be too late to prevent absorption. Supportive care may be sufficient even with large doses (300-400 mg).
opiates, opioids (having morphinelike pharmacologic actions) — codeine, heroin, hydromorphone hydrochloride (Dilaudid), meperidine hydrochloride (Demerol), methadone (Methadon, Dolophine), morphine sulfate and hydrochloride, oxycodone (Percodan), pentazocine (Talwin), powdered opium (Pantopon), propoxyphene (Darvon), and so on	Depending on the drug, dosage, and duration of use, varied symptoms may be seen. The typical triad may be present: (1) depressed respirations, (2) pinpoint pupils (dilated if severely hypoxic), (3) coma. Respiratory rate may be 2-4 min and irregular; cyanosis. Hypotension directly related to decreased respiratory exchange. Urine output and body temperature are decreased. Pulmonary edema, shock can occur. Frank convulsions and death usually attributable to respiratory failure.	Gradually reduce dosage if chronic user, or substitute methadone and so on for opiates. Maintain vital functions, especially airway, and provide ventilation. Give naloxone as antagonist. Position to prevent pneumonia and complications of shock, coma.
plants House and garden, various plant parts (seeds often contain a compound that releases cyanide when eaten)	Varied, including irritation and swelling of the mouth, tongue, throat; nausea, vomiting, diarrhea; irregular pulse; hypotension; convulsions; occasionally kidney damage.	Varied depending on plant and part ingested; emesis or lavage, then supportive and symptomatic care as needed. For example, give atropine, 2 mg subcutaneously for decreased blood pressure; phentolamine for increased blood pressure; alkalinize urine with sodium bicarbonate, 5-15 g every 4 hr to prevent precipitation of hemoglobin in the kidneys, as needed. Control convulsions as needed.
mushrooms (genus *Amanita*, causal agent most frequently fatal)	Confusion, excitement, thirst, nausea, vomiting, diarrhea, wheezing, salivation, bradycardia, small pupils, (muscarinic effects) or dilated pupils, tremors, collapse or death.	Treatment may vary with species involved. Induction of emesis or lavage; possible catharsis. For muscarinic symptoms give atropine sulfate, 1-2 mg subcutaneously, every 30 min as needed. Give sedatives for excitement. Increase oral and intravenous fluids. Treat shock.

¶Highly addictive with narrow margin of safety, especially in combination with ethanol.

Continued.

TABLE 74-4   Some Specific Poisons, with Symptoms and Suggested Emergency Treatment*—cont'd

Poison	Symptoms†	Treatment‡
psychopharmacologic agents (antipsychotics, mood stabilizers, antidepressants, sedatives—make up the single most frequently encountered group of toxins treated by poison control centers according to the latest accounting)—butyrophenones (haloperidol [Haldol]—also used in Tourette's syndrome); phenothiazines; chlorpromazine (Thorazine), thioridazine (Mellaril), trifluoperazine (Stelazine), triflupromazine (Vesprin)	Excess sedation, hypotention. Extrapyramidal effects: parkinsonian syndrome, akathisia (constant walking, no agitation), acute dystonic reactions (facial grimacing, seen at start of therapy), tardive dyskinesia (involuntary mouth movements and choreiform movements of extremities). Symptoms pronounced in elderly clients.	Phenothiazines: gastric lavage; admit to intensive care unit for at least 3 days; monitor vital signs, cardiac signs. Given diazepam for seizures. Treat hypertension very cautiously. Give sponge baths for fever. Give lidocaine for dysrhythmias. Physostigmine intramuscularly or intravenously slowly has been effective in reversing anticholinergic central nervous system effects.
salicylates—acetylsalicylic acid: aspirin	*Adults:* initial event is vomiting (denotes toxicity above 40 mg %). *Children* (less than 5 years old): respiratory alkalosis appears first, then metabolic acidosis, hyperpnea, flushed face, tinnitus, hyperthermia (above 70 mg %), abdominal pain, vomiting, dehydration, bleeding (rare), tremors/convulsions, pulmonary edema, shock (above 80 mg %), and coma.	Induce emesis or aspirate stomach without fluids, then lavage with 2-4 L of 5% sodium bicarbonate solution. Add activated charcoal. Give 5%-10% D5W solution with 75 mEq/L chloride intravenously and 25 mEq sodium bicarbonate (up to 40-80 mEq/L, according to level of acidosis). Give 40-80 mEq potassium chloride/L in D5W solution according to potassium deficit, after renal flow is established. Furosemide, 1 mg/kg body weight, to keep diuresis at 3-6 ml/kg/hr. Intravenous fluids should be titrated with serum electrolyte levels. Phytonadione, 0.1 mg/kg body weight, may be given once intramuscularly to correct prothrombin levels. Transfuse for low platelet counts. Dialysis may be considered. Give sponge baths for hyperthermia.
tricyclic antidepressants—amitriptyline (Elavil), imipramine (Tofranil)	*Acute:* fever, hypertension, seizures, coma. In children cardiac dysrhythmias may occasionally be seen.	Induce emesis or perform a gastric lavage. Control convulsions with intravenous diazepam, 0.2 mg/kg. Give physostigmine salicylate, 2 mg intramuscularly or intravenously. (See text.) Maintain respirations.

The clothing should then be removed and the skin rinsed again. A shower would be the best method of removal of the agent from the skin.

If the poison is ingested, the objective is to prevent absorption of the substance either by inducing vomiting or by lavage to remove the agent or by administering an agent to inactivate the poisonous substance. The most recommended method of inducing vomiting is to have the patient take 15 ml of syrup of ipecac followed by a full glass of water. This procedure may be repeated in 20 minutes if necessary. If lavage is attempted and the patient is unconscious, it should be done while a cuffed endotracheal tube is in place to prevent aspiration. Vomiting or lavage should not be attempted with the ingestion of caustic substances or hydrocarbons, found in petroleum products. Care for the ingestion of these substances is to give nothing by mouth and urgently seek medical assistance.

The poisonous substance may be inactivated by admin-

TABLE 74-5 Antidotes for Specific Drugs and Poisons

Poison	Specific antidote
Acetaminophen (Tylenol, Datril, over-the-counter cold preparations)	N-acetylcysteine (Mucomyst)*
Alcohol (methanol) and ethylene glycol (antifreeze)	Alcohol (ethanol)
Anticholinergics (atropine)	Physostigmine salicylate
Carbon monoxide	Oxygen administered under high pressure
Coumarin anticoagulants	Vitamin K, clotting factors
Cyanide	Amyl nitrite, sodium nitrite, sodium thiosulfate
Heavy metals: Arsenic	Dimercaprol (BAL)
Copper	Penicillamine (Cuprimine)
Iron	Deferoxamine (Desferal)
Lead	Dimercaprol, penicillamine, calcium disodium edetate (CaEDTA)
Mercury	Dimercaprol, deferoxamine
Narcotics	Naloxone
Nitrates and nitrites	Methylene blue
Opiates	Naloxone (Narcan)
Organophosphates (insecticides)	Atropine sulfate, pralidoxime (2-PAM)
Tricyclic antidepressants	Physostigmine salicylate

Adapted with permission from Howard C Mofenson, Poison control manual, 1979, unpublished data.
*Not yet FDA approved (see text).

istering activated charcoal, minimally 50 grams of the powdered preparation in 60-90 ml of water as an aqueous slurry, after the ipecac. The activated charcoal adsorbs the substance and prevents it from being absorbed by the body. Saline laxatives are then administered to remove the adsorbed poison from the body.

If the substance has a known antidote, it will be administered by the physician.

Other nursing interventions relate to the supportive care of the acutely ill client. Monitor vital signs and report changes immediately. If respirations are depressed, administer oxygen and suction. Maintain intravenous fluids as ordered. Observe the patient for nausea, vomiting, diarrhea, and abdominal cramping. The patient's vomitus, stool, and urine should be observed for abnormalities such as the presence of blood. Keep the patient warm and turn frequently to promote drainage from the respiratory tract.

If the poisoning was intentional, as a suicide attempt, safety precautions should be instituted to protect the client from further self-destructive behavior and a psychiatric referral should be considered.

Education. All medications should be clearly labeled as to type, dosage, and storage requirements and the client's ability to safely self-medicate should be assessed before there is an expectation for self-medication.

In interactions with clients, nurses should be alert to the presence of anger, depression, withdrawal, and faulty judgment that might precede intentional or unintentional poisoning.

Clients should be cautioned that toxic substances are not to be stored in food containers, containers that are not properly labeled, or stored in a place that is accessible to children. Medication should not be stored beyond the date of expiration. Poisonous plants should not be kept in households where there are small children.

Syrup of ipecac is a necessary ingredient in a household first aid container, as well as the appropriate directions for its use.

Evaluation. To prevent accidental poisoning, families should be assisted to evaluate environmental hazards in the home.

Clients should be monitored as with other life-threatening illnesses and specific interventions taken. Regression of the symptoms would indicate the successful elimination and inactivation of the poison.

COMMON POISONS

Some of the most commonly encountered poisons and their appropriate antidotal therapies are presented in Table 74-4.

acetaminophen

Acetaminophen is an analgesic-antipyretic ingredient in over 200 prescription and nonprescription drug formulations used therapeutically in adults and children. The drug is sold as a "safe substitute" for aspirin. However, when taken in massive overdose (greater than 15 gms, the equivalent of 15 to 20 "extra-strength" capsules), acetaminophen can produce acute hepatic damage. When overdosage is promptly diagnosed and treated with a specific antidote, patients readily recover with no permanent ill effects. However, if not treated, hepatic coma and death may occur. Acute acetaminophen intoxication has four stages. Initial symptoms in patients with potentially hepatotoxic blood concentrations include nausea, vomiting, anorexia, and diaphoresis, accompanied by overwhelming malaise, which begins 4 to 14 hours after ingestion. The second stage begins 24 to 72 hours after ingestion. During this time the patient seems to improve and have a feeling of well-being. However indices of impaired liver

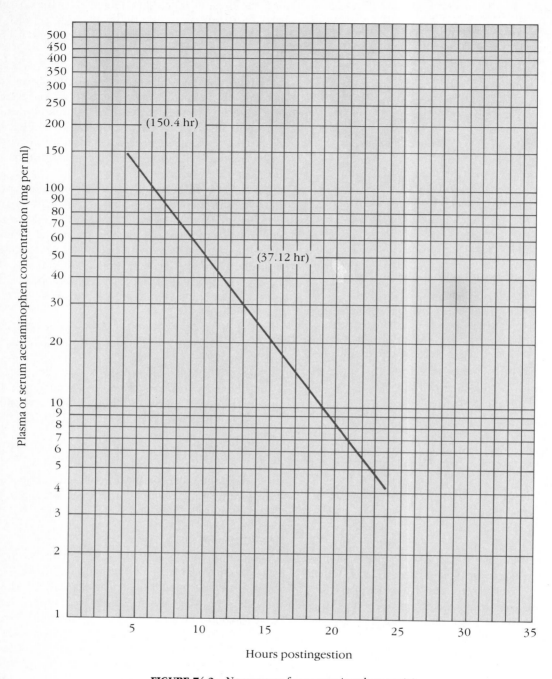

FIGURE 74-2   Nomogram for acetaminophen toxicity.
(Redrawn from Rumack, BH, and Matthew, H: Acetaminophen poisoning and toxicity. Pediatrics 55(6):871-878, 1975. Reproduced by permission of Pediatrics.)

function begin to occur including increased serum hepatic enzymes (SGOT, SGPT) and bilirubin, and prolongation of prothrombin time. The right upper quadrant abdominal area becomes tender to palpation. Stage 3 begins 3 to 7 days after ingestion with signs of hepatic necrosis characterized by abdominal discomfort, jaundice, dramatically increased prothrombin times, hypoglycemia, hepatic encephalopathy, and death. Should the

patient survive, stage 4 is the return of normal liver function within several weeks.

The initial symptoms of acetaminophen poisoning are nonspecific (vomiting, general malaise), but this diagnostic dilemma can be easily avoided by the laboratory analysis of plasma for acetaminophen. The severity of the ingestions is evaluated by use of a nomogram for toxicity developed by Rumack and Matthew (Figure 74-2). Plasma

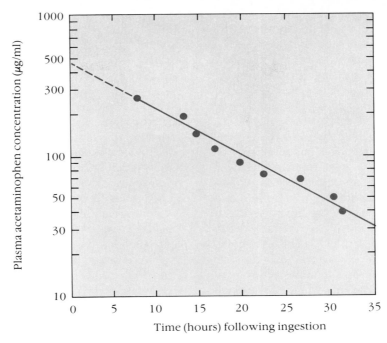

FIGURE 74-3 Decrease in patient plasma acetaminophen concentration during treatment of acetaminophen overdose ($t\frac{1}{2}$ = 9 hr).

(Redrawn from Melethil, S, Poklis, A, and Schwartz, HS: Vet Hum Toxicol 23(6):422, 1981.)

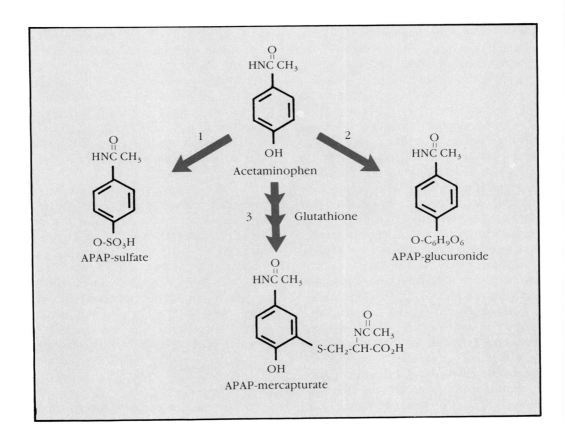

FIGURE 74-4 Hepatic metabolism of acetaminophen.

concentrations are correlated with the time after ingestion. Plasma concentrations above the line indicate hepatotoxicity may develop and antidotal treatment should be initiated. The nomogram begins 4 hours after ingestion; concentrations drawn before this time may be misleading, since peak plasma concentrations may not occur before 4 hours after ingestion. Additionally, the delayed symptoms of hepatotoxicity (elevation of serum SGOT, SGPT, and bilirubin concentrations and increased prothrombin time at 24 to 36 hours after ingestion) may be predicted by multiple plasma acetaminophen determinations between 4 and 8 to 12 hours after ingestion. At therapeutic doses, the plasma half-life (t½, time required to eliminate half of the amount of drug present in plasma) is 2 to 4 hours. In overdoses in which hepatotoxicity develops, half-life increases to 6 to 10 hours. Half-lives of greater than 10 hours indicate severe damage and possible hepatic coma. Figure 74-3 presents multiple plasma concentrations determined in a patient with acetaminophen hepatotoxicity (SGOT, 4040 units/ml, 24 hrs, postingestion) and a plasma half-life of 9 hours.

The development of potentially fatal liver damage in cases of acetaminophen overdose is caused by alterations in the drug's biotransformation (Chapter 4). At therapeutic doses, 98% of ingested acetaminophen is biotransformed by three different metabolic pathways (Figure 74-4). Normally the sulfate and glucuronide conjugates resulting from pathways 1 and 2, respectively, in Figure 74-4, represent 70% to 90% of excreted acetaminophen. Less than 10% of the dose is handled by the cytochrome P-450 (a drug-metabolizing enzyme) pathway, which combines glutathione with acetaminophen to produce mecapturic acid (pathway 3 in Figure 74-4). With the usual oral adult dose of acetaminophen (300 to 500 mg, which may be repeated every 4 hours but should not exceed 2.6 mg daily), toxicity does not occur.

When a massive overdose of acetaminophen is ingested, the enzymes controlling pathways 1 and 2 become saturated such that only a fixed amount of acetaminophen is converted to sulfate or glucuronide metabolites per unit time. This requires the glutathione pathway (3) to handle the excess acetaminophen no longer biotransformed by pathways 1 and 2. In overdoses the demands on pathway 3 soon deplete available liver stores of glutathione. When no glutathione is available, the acetaminophen product of pathway 3 binds to cellular constituents of the hepatocyte. These include enzymes or structural proteins necessary for normal function, and their complexion with acetaminophen leads to their inactivation and results in cellular injury and death. This mechanism also explains why patients taking chronic dosages of acetaminophen, even in moderate excess, rarely develop toxicity. Glutathione is continuously regenerated in the liver, and its rate of synthesis exceeds the demand for acetamin-

ophen biotransformation at therapeutic doses. Only when the dose exceeds the capacities of pathway 1 and 2 and depletes glutathione in pathway 3 does hepatic damage occur.

Antidotal therapy for acetaminophen poisoning is based on the administration of sulfur-containing compounds to replace the sulfur-containing glutathione as a receptor for the toxic product of acetaminophen biotransformation by pathway 3. Glutathione itself is not an effective antidote because it is readily broken down in plasma, and although normally synthesized in the liver cells, it is not taken up by the cells from external sources. In the United States the oral administration of N-acetyl-L-cysteine (Mucomyst) at a loading dose of 140 mg/kg followed by 70 mg/kg every 4 hours for a total of 17 doses, is the recommended antidote. It is administered orally in orange juice or soft drinks. The antidote must be administered within 24 hours after ingestion. As previously discussed, use of the nomogram in Figure 74-2 indicates the appropriateness of antidotal therapy.

NURSING CONSIDERATIONS

Assessment. Determine if acetylcysteine has been approved by the Food and Drug Administration (FDA) for use as an antidote for acetaminophen overdoses.

If not approved, obtain informed consent, since this is an experimental and investigational use of N-acetylcysteine. Make sure accepted protocol is the most current one, and follow it precisely.

Perform all procedures usually associated with treatment for ingested poisons before administering this antidote: assess patient condition and vital signs, institute emesis or lavage, and so forth.

Intervention. Avoid spilling this agent on materials such as iron, copper, and rubber because a reaction will occur.

Note that prolonged, chronic contact with this agent may result in dermal eruptions, which may indicate a hypersensitivity reaction. Nursing staff are probably at higher risk than patients and should take appropriate precautions.

Consider an occasional light purple coloration of the solution in an opened vial a harmless chemical reaction in its approved application. However, since no antimicrobial agent exists in the solution, refrigerate and discard opened containers if not used within 96 hours. Store unopened vials at controlled room temperature.

alcohols

The low molecular weight alcohols (methanol, isopropanol, and ethylene glycol) are relatively weak poisons themselves, but their metabolites are lethal. Lethal doses of these alcohols are relatively large. Unfortunately, these alcohols are as tasteless as vodka, as pleasant to sniff as cognac, and as drinkable as cold beer. Although they share many physical and chemical properties with ethanol (Chapter 9), and low molecular weight, small molecular size, and miscibility with water, they are not euphorigenic, and severe intoxication is usually life threatening. They do share a dehydrogenase to their corresponding aldehyde or ketone. The resultant aldehydes are rapidly converted by aldehyde dehydrogenase to their respective acids. However, unlike ethanol, which gives rise to acetic acid that may be utilized in normal metabolic processes, the other alcohols produce toxic acids. Fortunately, this metabolic interrelationship may be used for the management of their intoxication. Ethanol is the antidote for isopropanol, methanol, and ethylene glycol poisoning. Ethanol will compete with the other alcohols for alcohol dehydrogenase, thereby blocking or significantly slowing their conversion to their respective aldehydes and ultimately their toxic acids.

The alcoholic patient is particularly susceptible to exposure to these other alcohols for a variety of reasons. Either deliberately or accidentally, the alcoholic may ingest methanol, isopropanol, or ethylene glycol to alter his mental status. It is not unusual for derelict ("skid row") alcoholics to resort to drinking inexpensive products such as rubbing alcohol (isopropanol) when ethanol is not available. The early stages of poisonings from these agents produces a clinical picture much like ethanol intoxication: nausea, vomiting, motor incoordination, and impaired mental function. A history of ingestion of these other alcohols is often not obtained, either because the patient conceals it or is too intoxicated to be interviewed or is in coma. In such instances a misdiagnosis of ethanol intoxication may be made. Laboratory testing for both ethanol and serum chemistries may clarify this picture. Each of these common toxic alcohols will be discussed in turn.

NURSING CONSIDERATIONS

Assessment. Make baseline assessment of level of consciousness initially; reassess frequently.

Note that emesis or lavage may be unsuccessful because these toxins leave the stomach very rapidly.

Intervention. Perform continuous assessment of vital signs and emergency supportive measures.

Do frequent monitoring of blood glucose levels to assess for hypoglycemia or ketoacidosis.

Monitor intravenous infusion flow rates carefully to keep blood ethanol levels at approximately 100 mg 100 ml.

Education. Keep patients and concerned others in-formed about the progress of recovery and treatment measures.

carbon monoxide

Carbon monoxide (CO) is an odorless, colorless, tasteless gas produced by the incomplete combustion of carbon or carbonaceous materials. Any flame or combustion device is likely to emit CO. Sources of the gas include improperly maintained heating systems, improperly ventilated charcoal cookers or fire places, and industrial furnaces such as those in steel mills. Automobile exhaust contains 3% to 7% CO.

No other poison causes as many deaths in the United States as does CO. Inhalation of automobile exhaust is a common method of suicide. Accidental home and industrial exposure to CO is much more common than generally appreciated.

Poisoning by CO results from pulmonary absorption of the gas. CO readily combines with hemoglobin to form carboxyhemoglobin. CO combines with hemoglobin 200 to 300 times more strongly than oxygen. From 1 to 4 molecules of CO combine with 1 hemoglobin molecule, displacing the 1 to 4 oxygen molecules present. Not only does CO replace oxygen in hemoglobin, thus lowering available oxygen carried by the blood to the body tissues, but with the addition of each CO molecule the oxygen molecules remaining on the hemoglobin become so tightly bound that they are not readily released to the oxygen starved tissues. CO is measured in blood as the percent carboxyhemoglobin (%HbCO). The %HbCO is closely dependent on the concentration of CO in the inspired air, the time of exposure, and the state of activity of the person exposed. Additionally, CO gas dissolved in blood but not bound to hemoglobin diffuses into the body tissues and poisons cytochrome enzymes necessary for cellular utilization of oxygen.

The symptoms of CO poisoning are generally related to %HbCO. Clinically, only mild if any symptoms occur at 10% HbCO. Cigarette smokers may have CO up to this level. The initial signs of poisoning usually occur at 10% to 30% HbCO; these signs include throbbing headache, nausea, vomiting, dizziness, weakness, and visual disturbances. These early symptoms of intoxication are nonspecific and may be attributed to a number of other causes unless a history of CO is available or laboratory tests demonstrate elevated %HbCO. At 40% to 50% HbCO, syncope, tachycardia, tightness in the chest, and tachypnea occur. HbCO has a cherry pink color rather than the red color of oxyhemoglobin; therefore the patient may have a cherry pink coloration of the skin. Percent HbCO in excess of 50% causes life-threatening convulsions, coma, dangerously compromised cardiopulmonary function, and possible death. Fatalities from suicide or victims of fires often have %HbCO of 60% to 80%.

Treatment for CO poisoning is based on the patient's symptoms and %HbCO. Hyperbaric oxygen is the antidote of choice as oxygen under pressure is capable of replacing CO from hemoglobin and the iron containing respiratory cytochrome enzymes in the tissues. Ninety-five percent of absorbed CO is excreted by the lungs; however, once removed from the source of exposure, the half-life (t 1/2) of CO in normal ambient air is 4 hours. If 100% oxygen is administered, the half-life decreases to 40 minutes. Hyperbasic oxygen at 3 atm decreases the t 1/2 of CO to only 23 minutes. In severe poisoning, cardiopulmonary support is maintained throughout therapy. Additional drug therapy to control dysrhythmias, cerebral edema, and convulsions may be indicated.

NURSING CONSIDERATIONS

See the general nursing considerations for poisoning on p. 1166.

cyanide

Few poisons are as lethal as cyanide; large doses can produce death in minutes. Numerous industrial processes, including electroplating, chemical and dye syntheses, and extraction of precious metals, utilize cyanide or its salts. Cyanide is also commonly used as a fumigant-rodenticide in grain elevators, railway cars, and ship holds. It is available to the general public in photographic supplies, pesticides, and metal polishes. Certain seeds, particularly of the *genus Prunus* (wild cherry, bitter almonds, and others) contain cyanide-liberating glycosides. Sodium cyanide (NaCN), potassium cyanide (KCN), and calcium cyanide (Ca[CN]$_2$) are its common salts. Hydrogen cyanide (HCN) is a gas liberated when any acid reacts with a cyanide salt. HCN has a characteristic odor of bitter almond or peach pits.

Cyanide salts are often used as homicidal or suicidal agents. Numerous accidental poisonings arise from use of cyanide compounds in agriculture and industry. The popularity of the supposed antineoplastic agent **laetrile** has been responsible for a number of acute and subacute cyanide poisonings. Laetrile is usually amygdalin, a cyanide-containing glycoside that releases cyanide when metabolized by the body. Cigarette smoke contains HCN, and smokers have a significantly higher blood concentration of cyanide than nonsmokers. Much national attention was focused on cyanide poisoning during the Tylenol tampering incident in Chicago in 1982 when cyanide salts were feloniously added to headache capsules and placed on the shelves of retail stores.

Cyanide salts are readily absorbed from the alimentary tract and hydrogen cyanide from the respiratory tract. In the stomach large ingested doses also produce a corrosive necrosis. Liquid HCN is rapidly absorbed through the skin, but the gas is absorbed slowly. Cyanide is biotransformed in the body to cyanate and thiocyanate and excreted in the urine. This conversion of cyanide is rapid enough to permit the continuous inhalation of low concentrations (less than 30 ppm) of HCN for 8 hours.

After absorption, the cyanide radical (CN$^-$) rapidly binds to and inactivates certain oxidative enzymes of all tissues. CN has a particular affinity for compounds containing oxidized iron (Fe^{+3}). Cytochrome oxidase and other respiratory enzymes containing oxidized iron are commonly inactivated. One part CN per 100 million parts of solution blocks all cytochrome oxidase activity. This inhibition prevents tissue utilization of oxygen, and rapid death follows. Another deadly effect of CN is the reflex stimulation of respiration by action of the sensory nerves ending in the cortoid body. When cyanide vapor is inhaled, the carotid body and medullary stimulation cause a deep breath to be taken, thus allowing greater quantities of the poison to be inhaled.

Following ingestion or inhalation the onset of symptoms of cyanide poisoning is rapid and dramatic. Cyanide poisoning initially causes headache, sweating, ataxia, and varying degrees of mental confusion, which may quickly progress to coma. Cyanosis or, as with carbon monoxide poisoning, a cherry pink coloration of the skin may be noted. Vomiting frequently occurs, and the pupils are dilated. Depending on the degree of poisoning, convulsions and involuntary micturition and defecation may occur. Circulatory function may be strong or weak; the pulse is often decreased initially, then becomes rapid. Death resulting from asphyxia may occur with minutes of exposure; either circulation or respiration may fail first. The average fatal dose of sodium or potassium cyanide is 0.25 g; however, as little as 0.06 g has caused death. HCN is twice as toxic as its salts. Generally, death ensues when only a small fraction of an ingested dose is absorbed.

The classical treatment of cyanide poisoning is the administration of sodium nitrite and sodium thiosulfate (Figure 74-5). Sodium nitrite is given to convert the reduced iron (ferrous, Fe^{+2}) in hemoglobin to the oxidized (ferric, Fe^{+3}) state thus forming methemoglobin. Because of cyanide's great affinity for iron in the ferric state, cyanide combines immediately with methemoglobin to form cyanomethemoglobin, thus competing with respiratory enzymes such as cythochrome oxidase for CN and restoring normal cellular function. As much as 40% of the blood hemoglobin may be converted to methemoglobin without hindering normal oxygen transport and body respiration by the remaining normal hemoglobin. As mentioned above, cyanide is normally detoxified in the body to thiocyanate (SCN), which is excreted in the urine.

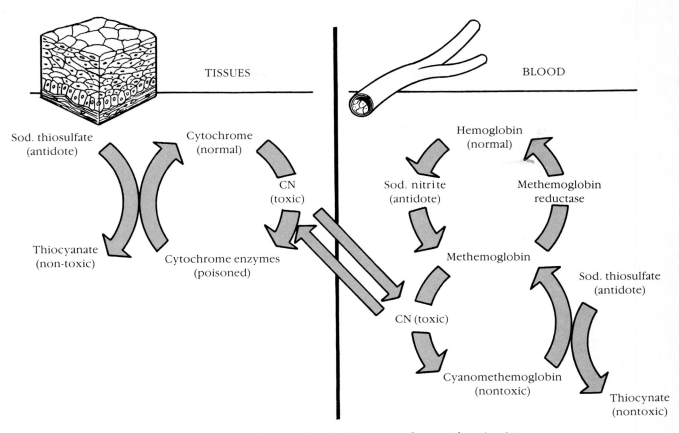

FIGURE 74-5 Mechanism of antidotal treatment for cyanide poisoning.

This metabolic conversion requires thiosulfate (or reducing sulfur) as a sulfur donor. In overdose situations the normal body stores of reducing sulfur are exhausted by the excess cyanide, thereby limiting the amount cyanide that can be detoxified. Sodium thiosulfate is administered to provide a source of reducing sulfur for the enzyme transsulfurase (rhodanese) to convert cyanomethemoglobin to thiocyanate, which is subsequently excreted in the urine. The remaining methemoglobin is then reconverted to hemoglobin by the enzyme system, methemoglobin reductase, which is present in the red blood cells.

Amyl nitrite is immediately administered by inhalation from several "pearls" or capsules broken into gauze, followed by 300 mg of sodium nitrite intravenous Amyl nitrite converts 5% of hemoglobin to methemoglobin, whereas the sodium nitrite converts 25% to 30%. Sodium thiosulfate, 12.5 mg, is then slowly administered intravenously. Excessive methemoglobineurea with this dose is rare in adults; however, children develop severe or even fatal methemoglobineurea if adult doses are given. For children weighing less than 60 lbs (25 kg), sodium nitrite doses should be based on blood hemoglobin; however, if

hemoglobin values are not readily available, 10 mg/kg may be initially administered. The concurrent administration of oxygen with nitrite-thiosulfate therapy enhances the antidotal effects of the combination.

NURSING CONSIDERATIONS.

Assessment. Do not delay initiating treatment; rapid, competent care is essential in cyanide poisoning.

Perform a baseline assessment of (1) vital signs, with particular attention to quality, rate, and rhythm of apical pulse, and (2) blood pressure; measure these parameters repeatedly throughout treatment.

Intervention. Initiate removal of ingested cyanide from stomach immediately by using rapid-acting emetic or lavage.

If poison has been inhaled, patient must be moved to fresh air and may be given oxygen.

Be prepared to have blood drawn and to record the time and results; determinations of hemoglobin level and methemoglobinemia probably will be needed repeatedly to titrate antidote dosages. Advise against administration of methylene blue for excessive methemoglobinemia resulting from this therapy. Blood products should be ordered and available in case a transfusion is necessary.

Note that the patient will be uncomfortable, with headache, feelings of chest constriction, and dyspnea.

ethylene glycol

Ethylene glycol ($HOCH_2CH_2OH$) is a colorless, odorless, water soluble liquid. It is an important starting material in many chemical processes and is widely used as a solvent. It is readily available as antifreeze or windshield de-icer solution. Although poisoning with ethylene glycol occurs more sporadically than with methanol or isopropanol, it is one of the most serious and dramatic intoxications encountered in clinical toxicology. As with other alcohols, alcoholics are often the victims; however, the compound is often used for suicide. Additionally, children attracted to the bright colors of adulterants added to antifreeze are often victims of accidental ingestions. The first reports of ethylene glycol poisoning were the result of a spectacular epidemic in which 76 people died after use of an elixir of sulfanilimide (an antibiotic) that contained diethylene glycol as a solubilizing agent. At the time, in the 1930s, the poisonous nature of ethylene glycol was unknown. In adults, 100 ml is the accepted lethal dose, though recovery has been reported following ingestions of up to 970 ml.

Absorption of ethylene glycol from the gastrointestinal tract is rapid with initial symptoms of intoxication occurring as early as 30 minutes after ingestion. It is evenly distributed throughout the body water, with only about 20% of the dose being excreted by the kidneys. The remaining 80% is converted in the liver by way of the alcohol dehydrogenase pathway to various aldehyde and acid metabolites (Figure 74-6). The major toxicity of ethylene glycol results from the accumulation of these metabolites.

The clinical effects of ethylene glycol poisoning in untreated patients follow three stages: (1) metabolic and central nervous system effects, (2) cardiopulmonary effects, and (3) renal effects. The first stage occurs within 12 hours after ingestion; it involves gastritis and abdominal pain with nausea and vomiting. The victim may experience transient exhilaration, but central nervous system depression soon sets in with motor incoordination, stupor, and finally coma. Convulsions may also occur. Like methanol, the production of acid metabolites, particularly glycolic acid, causes a profound metabolic acidosis. An anion gap and metabolic acidosis with accompanying central nervous system depression are characteristic of both methanol and ethylene glycol poisoning. Oxalic acid, another acid metabolite, chelates calcium salting in hypocalcemia, tetanic muscle contractions, and cardiac disturbances. Calcium oxalate is poorly soluble at physiologic pH, and microcrystals of the salt precipitate throughout the body tissues, causing cellular damage, particularly in the kidney. The presence of calcium oxalate crystals in urine strongly suggests ethylene glycol poisoning. The second stage is characterized by cardiopulmonary dysfunction at 12 to 36 hours after ingestion. Tachypnea, cyanosis, and pulmonary edema occur, and the possibility of the patient dying within 1 to 3 days is imminent. Death is the result of central nervous system depression or pulmonary edema. If the patient survives the first two stages, he then undergoes the third, or renal, stage of intoxication. A common symptom is flank pain, and the effects of kidney damage are present—oliguria, proteinurea, and anuria. Kidney damage is caused by precipitation of calcium oxalate crystals in the renal tubular lumina and distribution of normal cellular metabolism by other acid metabolics (glycoaldehyde, glycolic acid, and glyoxylic acid) (Figure 74-

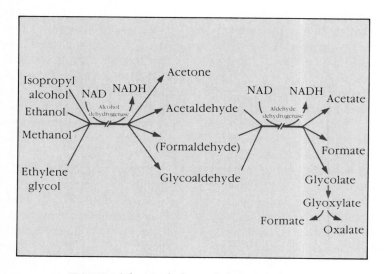

FIGURE 74-6   Metabolism of alcohols: summary.

6). Signs of renal damage predominate 2 to 3 days after ingestion. Should anuria persist, death from uremia may occur. Recovery from renal damage may take up to 4 months.

Treatment for ethylene glycol poisoning is similar to that for methanol intoxication. Sodium bicarbonate is given intravenously to neutralize metabolic acidosis. Ethanol is administered immediately to inhibit the production of toxic metabolites (see discussion of methanol). If serum ethylene glycol concentrations exceed 50 mg/dl or severe uremia develops, hemodialysis is indicated.

NURSING CONSIDERATIONS

See the general nursing considerations for poisoning on page 1166.

iron

Iron deficiency is a primary cause of anemia in both infants and adults. Thus iron is often added to infant formulas and foods and is available in over 100 commercial products for adults, including multiple and prenatal vitamins. Available products use a number of forms of iron, various salts and chelates. The toxic effects of iron are caused by its elemental form; therefore the relative toxicity of iron salts is related to the percent of elemental iron. For example, ferrous fumerate (33% iron) is more toxic on a weight basis than ferrous gluconate (12% iron). The accidental ingestion of iron preparations is a common form of pediatric poisoning, and suicidal ingestion of iron salts by adults is not uncommon. Though rarely fatal, iron overdose can result in profound mental retardation. Taken in overdose, iron produces both local and systemic deleterious effects.

Once ingested, large amounts of iron cause local corrosive actions on the gastric and duodenal mucosa and upper gastrointestinal tract. Thus initial symptoms of iron poisoning include nausea, vomiting, upper abdominal pain, and bloody diarrhea. The corrosive action destroys the normal mucosal barrier to iron absorption, allowing rapid absorption of large amounts of iron into the general circulation. These overdose concentrations of iron exceed the binding capacity of transferrin, the iron-carrying protein of the blood. The excess free iron readily diffuses into various tissues and binds to the sulfhydryl (SH) radicals of numerous enzymes and structural proteins. This binding of iron to compounds necessary for normal cellular function poisons the tissue cells. Thus 6 to 24 hours after ingestion symptoms of systemic intoxication — cyanosis, pulmonary edema, and possible cardiovascular collapse — start to occur. Within a few days, coagulation defects, hepatic necrosis, and renal failure may develop. As with adults, the initial symptoms of pediatric iron poisoning are characterized by repeated vomiting, abdominal pain, and diarrhea. However, frequently a latent phase occurs when the initial symptoms abate and the child appears well for a 6- to 12-hour period, which is followed by rapid illness and the development of shock. The determination of serum iron will indicate the severity of the intoxication and prevent the possible dangerous misinterpretation of this latency period. Additionally, serum iron values will indicate the necessity of the initiation of antidotal therapy. Serum iron concentrations of 350 μg/dl or less are rarely associated with clinical illness. Concentrations between 350 and 500 μg/dl call for observation of the patient for the development of clinical signs of intoxication. For concentrations above 500 μg/dl, deferoxamine (an iron chelating agent) therapy is recommended. The prognosis of patients with serum iron of 500-2000 μg/dl is reasonably good; however, concentrations exceeding 10,000 μg/dl are indicative of severe hepatic and renal damage. Heroic measures are required in such instances.

The treatment for iron poisoning includes not only general supportive measures, blood transfusion for hemorrhage, and intravenous bicarbonate to correct metabolic acidosis, but also specific antidotes to precipitate or chelate the ingested iron. Emesis may be induced to expel unabsorbed iron tablets in the stomach; also, sodium bicarbonate lavage is indicated, since bicarbonate converts ferrous iron to ferrous carbonate, which is poorly absorbed. After lavage, 200 to 300 ml of the bicarbonate solution should be left in the stomach. When indicated by toxic serum iron concentrations (+500 mg/dl), deferoxime, a chelating agent produced by *Streptomyces pilosus,* should be administered. Deferoxamine is a specific chelator that binds free serum iron and iron associated with hepatic and splenic stores. Deferoxamine does not bind with zinc, copper, or other trace metals. The deferoxamine-iron complex is nontoxic and freely excreted by the kidneys. Should the patient develop renal failure, the complex is readily dialyzable. If the patient is normotensive, 50 to 100 mg/kg up to 2 g, may be given intramuscularly every 4 to 8 hours to a maximum of 6 g/24 hr. However, if the patient is hypotensive, the intravenous administration is preferred, usually an infusion of 1 g at a rate no greater than 15 mg/kg/hr, repeated every 4 to 6 hours. Experience with the treatment of pregnant women who have overdosed on iron is limited. Generally, antidotal treatment is withheld; however, the highly polar nature of deferoxamine may reduce its fetal entry and thereby be useful.

NURSING CONSIDERATIONS

Assessment. Take careful history to elicit possibility of pregnancy.

Advise against the use of deferoxamine is patient is pregnant, or may have severe renal impairment.

Perform baseline assessments, including attention to vital signs, especially blood pressure and apical pulse.

Intervention. Institute emesis or gastric lavage as soon as possible.

Initiate supportive measures, including maintenance of clear airway and interventions related to presence of shock and to acidosis.

Administer deferoxamine using long needle and Z-track method; may add 0.2 to 0.3 ml of air to medication in syringe to prevent pain and induration at site of injections. Carefully controlled, slow intravenous infusion rates may be equally effective in preventing such pain.

Education. Tell patients to expect reddish brown coloration of urine and stools.

isopropanol

Isopropanol ($CH_3CHOHCH_3$) is a colorless, volatile, and flammable liquid present in numerous household products including disinfectants, cosmetics, solvents, linaments, and cleaning solutions. Most commonly, it is available in a 70% solution as rubbing alcohol. Isopropanol poisoning is more common than generally recognized. It is often ingested by debilitated alcoholics because it is cheaper than alcohol. Accidental ingestion by children is also common. Isopropanol is approximately twice as toxic as ethanol but less toxic than methanol. The lethal dose in adults is considered to be 240 ml; however, as little as 20 ml has caused intoxication.

Isopropanol is rapidly absorbed from the alimentary tract and the lungs. Percutaneous absorption is minimal. Following absorption, like other alcohols, it is evenly distributed in the body water. Most of an absorbed dose is slowly excreted by the kidneys and lungs. Only about 15% is oxidized to acetone by alcohol dehydrogenase (Figure 74-6). Acetone itself is very slowly excreted. This accounts for the prolonged effects of isopropanol poisoning and the characteristic acetone odor of the patient's breath. Although isopropanol and ethanol share the same metabolic pathway, ethanol has proved clinically ineffective as an antidote, since only a small fraction of isopropanol is converted to acetone.

The signs and symptoms of isopropanol poisoning are similar to those of ethanol; however, because of its slower metabolism and excretion, the symptoms of isopropanol intoxication persist two to four times longer than those of ethanol. Following ingestion, nausea, vomiting, gastritis, and severe abdominal pain may occur. Absorption is rapid, and dizziness, headache, lack of coordination, mental confusion, and stupor progressing to central nervous system depression and coma may occur within a few hours of ingestion. Cardiac dysrhythmia and severe hypotension progressing to cardiopulmonary collapse may occur. Dehydration and hemorrhagic gastritis are common features of isopropanol intoxication. Isopropanol poisoning may be differentiated from that of other alcohols by the presence of metabolic ketosis and a serum anion gap without metabolic acidosis. The determination of serum isopropanol and acetone concentration confirms the diagnosis. Serum values in excess of 150 mg/dl are usually associated with coma.

Treatment for isopropanol intoxication involves supportive therapy. If serum values are elevated, hemodialysis is indicated.

NURSING CONSIDERATIONS

See the general nursing considerations on p. 1166.

methanol (methyl alcohol)

Methanol (CH_3OH) is a colorless liquid prepared either by the destructive distillation of wood or by chemical synthesis. The two products are chemically and physiologically identical. Methanol is widely used in commercial and industrial processes and is found in numerous home and garage products such as varnish and paint solvent, windshield wiper solution, and gas line de-icer. It is also used as a canned fuel (Sterno) and as an adulterant to make ethanol unfit to drink when sold as a cleaning disinfectant (denatured alcohol).

Most cases of acute methanol poisoning are associated with the accidental or deliberate ingestion of adulterated ethanolic beverages. During World War II, 6% of all cases of blindness in the U.S. armed forces were caused by ingestion of methanol itself or in adulterated ethanol. Many ethanol poisonings have occurred as the result of methanol-contaminated illicit whiskey. In Georgia in 1951, 323 people were poisoned, 41 fatally, over a single week, because of a supply of adulterated "moonshine" whiskey. Similarly, in a single week 372 people were poisoned, 18 fatally, from an illicit beverage containing 82% methanol-isopropanol distributed in Papua, New Guinea. Suicidal ingestion of windshield washer solution (up to 95% methanol) also accounts for many acute poisonings. The inhalation of methanol vapors in a closed area will also induce intoxication. As little as 15 ml of methanol has proven fatal in some patients; however, 80 ml is generally considered a fatal dose.

Methanol is absorbed from the alimentary tract and the lungs. Once absorbed, it is evenly distributed in the body water. Only small amounts of methanol are excreted by the kidney; as little as 3% is found unchanged in the urine. As described above, methanol is primarily biotransformed by alcohol dehydrogenase to formaldehyde and ultimately to formic acid (Figure 74-6).

The most common presentation of methanol poisoning consists of a triad of symptoms relating to the gastrointestinal tract, the eyes, and metabolic acidosis. The onset of symptoms after ingestion ranges from 30 minutes to 72 hours. This great variance probably results from individual variation in alcohol dehydrogenase activity, as well as the coingestion of ethanol. Like other aliphatic alcohols, methanol is a central nervous system depressant, but depression is rarely fatal. In equal doses, ethanol produces a greater depression. Gastrointestinal irritation is much greater with methanol than ethanol; vomiting, gastrointestinal bleeding, and severe abdominal pain are common symptoms. Following gastric symptoms, weakness, lethargy, and a general malaise, not unlike symptoms of an ethanol hangover, occur. These conditions may rapidly proceed to mental confusion, convulsions, coma, and death.

Two primary features of methanol poisoning are caused by its metabolite, formic acid. The conversion of methanol to formic acid in the liver causes a profound metabolic acidosis, which may cause the patient to become short of breath and tachypneic and in severe cases result in shock, multisystem failure, and death. Accumulation of formic acid in the retinal nerve fibers and their ganglion cells results in optic disc swelling. This swelling apparently inhibits the neural axoplamic flow, which results in demylination of the optic nerve. Ocular symptoms generally may develop as early as 2 minutes or as late as 3 days after methanol ingestion; they include blurred vision, photophobia, constructed visual fields, "spots before the eyes," "snow vision," and blindness. Good visual recovery slowly unfolds following mild intoxications; however, complete recovery from optic neuritis is rare.

Laboratory tests are critical in establishing a correct diagnosis and in guiding therapy. As small water-soluble molecules, methanol and its metabolites produce metabolic acidosis and serum anion and osmolal gaps. These findings in the presence of visual disturbances and gastric distress lead to the immediate consideration of methanol poisoning. Serum methanol analysis can confirm this diagnosis. If the patient has ingested methanol within the previous 4 hours, the stomach should be emptied by administration of syrup of ipecac or gastric lavage. To block the conversion of methanol to toxic metabolites, an intravenous injection of a 10% ethanol solution in a loading dose of 10 ml/kg, followed by an infusion of 1.5 ml/kg/h, is administered. Should serum methanol concentrations exceed 50 mg/dl, hemodialysis, in addition to ethanol therapy, is indicated. In such cases, a maintenance infusion of 3.0 ml/kg/h ethanol is necessary during hemodialysis. Both ethanol and methanol serum concentrations should be frequently monitored. These regimens will result in blood ethanol concentrations of 100 to 130 mg/dl, which appears optimal for inhibition of alcohol dehydrogenase. The affinity of ethanol for the enzyme is at least seven times greater than that of methanol. A serum profile of a patient successfully treated for methanol poisoning by both ethanol infusion and hemodialysis is presented in Figure 74-7.

To correct metabolic acidosis, sodium bicarbonate is given intravenously; however, although bicarbonate may neutralize serum formic acid, it may not prevent optic nerve damage. Severe acidosis may require hemodialysis to remove methanol and formic acid. While experience is limited in man, recent studies in primates have demonstrated that infusion of sodium folate protects against methanol-induced blindness. Normally, small, single carbon molecules such as formic acid are metabolized to carbon dioxide and water by enzymes associated with tetrahydrofolic acid. When large concentrations of formic acid are present, the tetrahydrofolic acid becomes depleted. The administration of sodium folate replaces the depleted folic acid and accelerates the normal conversion of formic acid to carbon dioxide and water, thus preventing optic neuritis and blindness. The optimum dosage of sodium folate in man is yet to be determined; however, presently 50 mg intravenously every 4 hours is recommended. This antidote is sufficiently safe to warrant its use in all methanol-intoxicated patients. If sodium folate is unavailable, leucovorin, an active form of folate, may be substituted.

NURSING CONSIDERATIONS

See the general nursing considerations for poisoning on p. 1166.

organophosphate insecticides

Organophosphate compounds are highly effective insecticides. Their chemical structure is unstable, resulting in their disintegration into nontoxic radicals within days after their application. Therefore they do not persist or accumulate in the environment or animal tissues as do the chlorinated insecticides such as DDT. This accounts for their addition to numerous commercial products from flea collars, bug bombs, and flypapers to most home and commercial insect sprays. This popularity accounts for the high potential for accidental poisoning by organophosphates. Popular organophosphate insecticides and their relative toxicity are presented in Table 74-6.

Organophosphate compounds are powerful inhibitors of the enzyme acetylcholinesterase (ACHE), which breaks down the neurohumeral transmitter acetylcholine (ACh) (Chapter 18). Organophosphates were developed during World War II as nerve gases, and much of our knowledge of their actions and effects is related to work on the poison gases sarin, tabun, and soman. They are rapidly absorbed into the body by all routes, respiratory, dermal, gastrointestinal, and ocular. However, individual organophosphates display wide variation in their ability to penetrate the skin, in their oral absorption, and thus in their

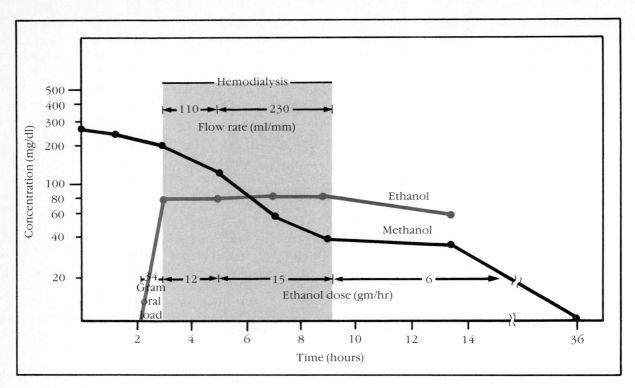

FIGURE 74-7   Blood methanol (black line) and blood ethanol (colored line) concentrations before, during, and after hemodialysis. Methanol elimination was enhanced during hemodialysis (shaded area).

(Redrawn from McCoy, HG, Cipolle, RJ, Ehlers, SM, and others: Severe methanol poisoning, Am J Med 67:806, 1979.)

toxicity. For example, malathion does not penetrate the skin well and its oral toxicity is low, making it a popular insecticide for use in home products (Table 74-6).

The signs and symptoms of organophosphate insecticide poisoning are related to inhibition of AChE, which results in an accumulation of ACh in the parasympathetic nervous system. Hence, all organs acted on by ACh are overstimulated. Table 18-2 (p. 361) indicates the expected results of organophosphate poisoning: bradycardia, hypotension, dyspnea, wheezing, miosis, blurred vision, convulsions, muscular fasciculations, and profuse sweating. A common mnemonic for symptoms of organophosphate intoxication is **SLUDGE:** *s*alivation, *l*acrimation, *u*rination, *d*efecation, *g*astrointestinal distress, and *e*mesis. The usual mode of death is respiratory arrest caused by bronchospasm, decreased pulmonary muscle strength, and finally depression of central nervous system control of respiration. The sequence in which specific systems develop is related to the route of exposure. Respiratory tract effects appear first after inhalation, whereas gastrointestinal effects appear initially after ingestion. Skin absorption results in immediate profuse sweating and muscle weakness. Both red blood cell cholinesterase and serum pseudocholinesterase activities are determined to aid in the diagnosis and assessment of the severity of organophos-

phate poisoning. A reduction in erythrocyte cholinesterase by 50% or more signifies a serious degree of poisoning.

Therapy for organophosphate poisoning involves the support of cardiopulmonary function, clearance of respiratory tract secretions to maintain a clear airway, and the use of appropriate antidotes, atropine and 2-PAM (Pralidoxamine, Protopam). Atropine competitively antagonizes the action of ACh at muscarinic receptors on organs innervated by postganglionic parasympathetic nerves and cholinergic sympathetic nerves (Chapter 19). An initial dose of 2 to 4 mg is given every 3 to 8 minutes to increase heart rate and decrease secretions. If these effects do not occur, an insufficient dose has been given. Patients poisoned with organophosphates may be particularly resistant to atropine. Therefore repeated larger doses may be necessary. Doses of 50 mg/24 hrs up to 2 to 4 g over a week have been safely administered in severe poisoning. The dangers of prolonged organophosphate intoxication exceed the risk of atropine overdose.

Atropine is effective in blocking muscarinic symptoms of bradycardia, bronchoconstriction, and excess secretions; however, muscular fasciculations are refractory to this antidote. These involuntary contractions and twitchings and respiratory paralysis are best treated with 2-PAM,

TABLE 74-6 The Relative Toxicity of Organophosphates

Organophosphate	Relative toxicity Oral LD$_{50}$ (mg/kg rates)
TEPP	1.5
Paraoxon (metabolite of parathion)	2.5
Parathion	6
EPN	40
Leptophos	46
Dichlorvos (DDVP)	80
Diazinon	200
Dichlofenthion	270
Malaoxon (metabolite of malathion)	308
Malathion	1375

Reprinted with permission from Eto M: Organophosphorous pesticides: organic and biological chemistry, Cleveland, 1974, CRC Press, pp 234-297. Copyright CRC Press, Inc., Boca Raton, Fla.

a cholinesterase reactivator that removes organophosphates bound to AChE. This then frees AChE to break down the accumulated ACh, thereby resuming normal activity at the neuromuscular junction. 2-PAM also directly detoxifies certain organophosphates. The initial dose of 2-PAM is 1 to 2 g intravenously in 100 ml of saline over 15 to 30 minutes. For children the dose is 20 to 40 mg/kg. Doses are repeated every 3 to 8 hours if muscle weakness persists. Side effects of 2-PAM include dizziness, nausea, headache, and tachycardia.

NURSING CONSIDERATIONS

Assessment. Remember that full assessment of vital signs is crucial.

Intervention. If there is cyanosis, establish and maintain an airway first. Copious secretions may necessitate nearly continuous suctioning at first; anticipate supplemental oxygen therapy.

Induce vomiting or perform gastric lavage if poison was ingested.

Cleanse skin of any insecticide contaminant if present.

Closely monitor both respiratory status and secretion production, since doses of atropine may be predicted on this information.

If signs of excessive atropinization appear, plan for treatment with physostigmine to antagonize atropine.

Anticipate need to administer pralidoxime (Protopam) if poisoning is severe.

Plan to monitor patient's status closely for 72 hours.

KEY TERMS

acute poisoning, page 1156
apomorphine, page 1163
chronic poisoning, page 1156
criminal poisoning, page 1155
gastric lavage, page 1164
hepatotoxins, page 1160
industrial poisoning, page 1155
laetrile, page 1176
nephrotoxins, page 1160
SLUDGE, page 1182

BIBLIOGRAPHY

1. Acetaminophen, Poison Information Bull 4(3):1, 1982.
2. Aronow R and others: Phencyclidine overdose: an emerging concept of management, Am Coll Emergency Physicians 7(2):56, 1978.
3. As bitter as they come, Science News 125:9, Jan 7, 1984.
4. Avery GS: Drug treatment, Sydney, 1980, Adis Press.
5. Bailey BO: Acetaminophen hepatotoxicity and overdose, Am Fam Physician 22:83, 1980.
6. Bean J: Use of bethanechol to treat anticholinergic side effects of tricyclic antidepressants and phenothiazines, Hosp Pharm 15(6):317, 1980.
7. The bio-science handbook of clinical and industrial toxicology, Van Nuys, Calif, 1979, Bio-Science Laboratories.
8. Bulletin, National Clearinghouse for Poison Control Centers, US Department of Health and Human Services, 25(6), 1981.
9. Calesnick B: Tricyclic antidepressant toxicity, Am Fam Physician 21(6):104, 1980.
10. Clark JF, Queener SF, and Karb VB: Pharmacological basis of nursing practice, St Louis, 1986, The CV Mosby Co.
11. Driesbach RH: Handbook of poisoning: diagnosis and treatment, ed 8, Los Altos, Calif, 1980, Lange Medical Publications.
12. Gellis SS and Kagan BM, eds: Accident and emergencies. In Current pediatric therapy, vol 6, Philadelphia, 1980, WB Saunders Co.
13. Gilman AG, Goodman LS, and Gilman A, eds: The pharmacological basis of therapeutics, ed 6, New York, 1980, Macmillan Publishing Co, Inc.
14. Goldfrank LR: Toxicologic emergencies, ed 2, New York, 1982, Appleton-Century-Crofts.
15. Greensher J and others: Activated charcoal updated, J Am Coll Emergency Physicians 8:7, 1979.
16. Haddad LM and Winchester JF, eds: Clinical management of poisoning and drug overdose, Philadelphia, 1983, WB Saunders Co.
17. Kastrup EK, ed: Facts and comparisons, St Louis, 1988, JB Lippincott Co.
18. Krogh C: Toxicities in perspective—acetylsalicylic acid and acetaminophen, Can Pharmaceutical J 113:169, 1980.
19. Long Island Regional Poison Control Center: The poisoned patient: emergency toxicology, Nassau County Medical Center Symposium, April 9, 1983.
20. Lovejoy F: Priorities in poisoning, Emergency Med 11:265, 1979.

21. Mofenson HC and Caraccio TR: First aid treatment of common ingestions, unpublished material, 1983.

22. Mofenson HC and Caraccio TR: Hydrocarbon intoxications, unpublished material, 1983.

23. Mofenson HC, Caraccio TR, and Brody GM: Carbon monoxide poisoning, unpublished material, 1983.

24. Mofenson HC, Caraccio TR, and Brody GM: Clinical toxicology of tricyclic antidepressants and cyclic antidepressants, unpublished material, 1983.

25. Mofenson HC, Caraccio TR, and Greensher J: Salicylate intoxication, unpublished material, 1983.

26. Mofenson HC and Greensher J: Poisoning — an update, Clin Pediatr 18(3):144, 1979.

27. Mofenson HC, Greensher J, and Caraccio TR: Ingestions considered nontoxic, Emergency Clin North Am 2:10, 1984.

28. Mofenson HC and others: Ingestion of small flat disc batteries, Ann Emergency Med 12(2):88, 1983.

29. Mofenson HC and others: Poison control formulary: common antidotes, unpublished material, May 1983.

30. Moore RA and others: Nalaxone, J Dis Child 134(2):156, 1980.

31. News. In Pediatr Pharmacol/Toxicol Newsletter 2(12):4, 1983.

32 1988 drug information for the health care provider: U.S.P.D.I., vol. 1, Rockville, Md., The US Pharmacopeial Convention, Inc.

33. Osman M: Reduction in oral penicillamine absorption by food, antacid, and ferrous sulfate, Clin Pharmacol Ther 33:465, 1983.

34. Page LB: Mushroom poisoning, West J Med 132(1):66, 1980 (editorial).

35. Parkhouse J, Pleuvry BJ, and Rees JMH: Analgesic drugs, Oxford, 1979, Blackwell Scientific Publications.

36. Poison prevention materials list. In Directory of United States Poison Control Centers and Services, US Department of Health and Human Services, 1988.

37. Shirkey H and others, eds: Pediatric therapy, ed 6, St Louis, 1980, The CV Mosby Co.

38. Special report: button batteries, Pittsburgh, 1983, National Poison Center Network.

Appendixes

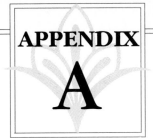

Commonly Used Medications: Generic to Trade Name Listing

The following is an alphabetical listing, by generic name, of selected prescription and over-the-counter medications.

Generic Name	Trade Name
acetaminophen	Tylenol, Datril, Anacin-3
acetazolamide	Diamox, Diamox Sequels
acetohexamide	Dymelor
acetylcysteine	Mucomyst
acetylsalicylic acid (ASA)	aspirin
acyclovir	Zovirax
albuterol	Proventil, Ventolin
allopurinol	Zyloprim
alprazolam	Xanax
aluminum hydroxide gel	Amphogel
aluminum-magnesium suspension	Maalox, Mylanta, Gelusil
amikacin	Amikin
amiloride	Midamor
aminoglutethimide	Cytadren
amitriptyline	Elavil, Endep
amobarbital	Amytal
amoxicillin	Amoxil, Larotid, Polymox
amphotericin B	Fungizone
ampicillin	Amcil, Omnipen, Polycillin
ascorbic acid	vitamin C
aspirin, buffered	Bufferin
aspirin, enteric coated	Ecotrin
atenolol	Tenormin
baclofen	Lioresal

Generic Name	Trade Name
beclomethasone	Vanceril, Beclovent
belladonna alkaloids and phenobarbital	Donnatal
benzocaine	Americaine, Hurricaine
benzquinamide	Emeta-Con
benztropine	Cogentin
betamethasone	Celestone, Valisone
bethanechol chloride	Urecholine
biperiden	Akineton
bisacodyl	Dulcolax
bleomycin	Blenoxane
bretylium tosylate	Bretylol
bromocriptine	Parlodel
brompheniramine	Dimetane
bumetanide	Bumex
busulfan	Myleran
butabarbital	Butisol
butorphanol	Stadol
calcitonin	Calcimar
calcium carbonate	Tums, Titralac, Alka-2
camphorated tincture of opium	Paregoric
captopril	Capoten
caramiphen and phenylpropanolamine	Tuss-Ornade
carbamazepine	Tegretol
carbenicillin	Geocillin, Geopen, Pyopen
carbidopa	Lodosyn
carbidopa and levodopa	Sinemet

Generic Name	Trade Name	Generic Name	Trade Name
carmustine	BiCNU	diethylstilbestrol	Stilbestrol, DES
cefaclor	Ceclor	diflunisal	Dolobid
cefamandol	Mandol	digitoxin	Crystodigin
cefapirin	Cefatrex	digoxin	Lanoxin
cefazolin	Ancef, Kefzol	dimenhydrinate	Dramamine
cefoperazone	Cefobid	dioctyl calcium sulfosuccinate (DOCS)	Surfak
cefoxitin	Mefoxin		
ceftizoxime	Cefizox	dioctyl sodium sulfosuccinate (DSS)	Colace
cephalexin	Keflex		
cephalothin	Keflin	dioctyl sodium sulfosuccinate with casanthranol	Pericolace
cephapirin	Cefadyl		
cephazolin	Ancef, Kefzol	diphenhydramine	Benadryl
cephradine	Anspor, Velosef	diphenoxylate HCL with atropine	Lomotil
chloral hydrate	Noctec		
chlorambucil	Leukeran	dipyridamole	Persantine
chloramphenicol	Chloromycetin, Chloroptic	disopyramide	Norpace
chlorazepate, dipotassium	Tranxene	disulfiram	Antabuse
chlorazepate, monopotassium	Azene	dobutamine	Dobutrex
chlordiazepoxide	Librium, Libritab	docusate calcium	Surfak
chlordiazepoxide and amitriptyline	Limbitrol	docusate sodium (DSS)	Colace
		dopamine	Intropin
chlordiazepoxide and clidinium	Limbrax	doxapram	Dopram
		doxepin HCl	Adapin, Sinequan
chloroquine	Aralen	doxorubicin HCl	Adriamycin
chlorothiazide	Diuril	doxycycline	Vibramycin
chlorotrianisene	Tace	dyphylline	Lufyllin
chlorpheniramine	Chlortrimeton	edrophonium	Tensilon
chlorpromazine	Thorazine	ephedrine	Vaponefrin
chlorpropamide	Diabinese	epinephrine	Adrenalin, Sus-Phrine
chlorprothixene	Taractan	ergoloid mesylates	Hydergine
chlorthalidone	Hygroton	ergonovine	Ergotrate
cholestyramine	Questran	ergotamine	Ergomar, Ergostat
cimetidine	Tagamet	erythromycin	Erythrocin, Ilotycin
cinoxacin	Cinobac	erythromycin estolate	Ilosone
cisplatin	Platinol	estrogens, conjugated	Premarin
clemastine	Tavist	ethacrynic acid	Edecrin
clidinium	Quarzan	ethchlorvynol	Placidyl
clindamycin	Cleocin-T	fentanyl	Sublimaze
clofibrate	Atromid-S	ferrous fumarate	Femiron
clonazepam	Clonopin	ferrous gluconate	Fergon
clonidine	Catapres	ferrous sulfate	Moliron, Feosol
colestipol	Colestid	flucytosine	Ancobon
conjugated estrogens	Premarin	fludrocortisone	Florinef
corticotropin	ACTH, Acthar	fluocinolone acetonide	Synalar
cortisone acetate	Cortone	fluocinonide	Lidex
cromolyn	Intal	fluphenazine HCl	Prolixin
cyclizine	Marezine	flurazepam	Dalmane
cyclophosphamide	Cytoxan	folic acid	Folvite
cyproheptadine	Periactin	folinic acid	Leucovorin calcium
dactinomycin	Cosmegen	furosemide	Lasix
dantrolene sodium	Dantrium	gemfibrozil	Lopid
demeclocycline	Declomycin	gentamicin	Garamycin
desipramine	Norpramin, Pertofrane	glycopyrrolate	Robinul
deslanoside	Cedilanid-D	griseofulvin	Fulvicin P/G
dexamethasone	Decadron, Hexadrol	guaifenesin (glyceryl guaiacolate)	Robitussin
diazepam	Valium		
diazoxide	Hyperstat, Proglycem	guanabenz	Wytensin
dibucaine	Nupercaine, Nupercainal	guanethidine	Ismelin
dicyclomine	Bentyl	haloperidol	Haldol

Generic Name	Trade Name	Generic Name	Trade Name
haloprogin	Halotex	meclizine HCl	Antivert, Bonine
halothane	Fluothane	melphalan	Alkeran
heparin	Lipo-Hepin, Liquaemin	menadiol	Synkayvite, vitamin K
hetacillin	Versapen	meperidine	Demerol
hyaluronidase	Wydase	mephenytoin	Mesantoin
hydralazine	Apresoline	mephobarbital	Mebaral
hydrochlorothiazide	HydroDiuril, Esidrex	meprobamate	Miltown, Equanil
hydrochlorothiazide and spironolactone	Aldactazide	mesoridazine	Serentil
		metaproterenol	Alupent
hydrochlorothiazide and timolol	Timolide	metaraminol	Aramine
		methadone	Dolophine
hydrochlorothiazide and triamterene	Dyazide	methandrostenolone	Dianabol
		methenamine hippurate	Hiprex, Urex
hydrocodone	Dicodid	methenamine mandelate	Mandelamine
hydrocodone and homatropine	Hycodan	methicillin	Staphcillin
		methimazole	Tapazole
hydrocortisone	Solu-Cortef	methocarbamol	Robaxin
hydromorphone	Dilaudid	methoxyflurane	Penthrane
hydromorphone and guaifenesin	Dilaudin cough syrup	methyldopa	Aldomet
		methylphenidate	Ritalin
hydroxyzine HCl	Atarax	metoclopramide	Reglan
hydroxyzine pamoate	Vistaril	metolazone	Zaroxolyn
ibuprofen	Advil, Motrin, Rufen	metoprolol	Lopressor
idoxuridine	Stoxil, Herplex	metronidazole	Flagyl
imipramine	Tofranil	miconazole	Monistat
indomethacin	Indocin	milk of magnesia (MOM)	magnesium hydroxide
INH (isoniazid)	Nydrazid	mineral oil emulsion	Kondremul
iron dextran	Imferon	minocycline	Minocin
isoetharine HCl	Bronkosol	minoxidil	Loniten
isoproterenol	Isuprel	mithramycin	Mithracin
isosorbide dintrate	Isordil, Sorbitrate	mitotane	Lysodren
isotretinoin	Accutane	molindone HCl	Moban
isoxsuprine HCl	Vasodilan	moxalactam	Moxam
kanamycin	Kantrex	nadolol	Corgard
kaolin-pectin	Kaopectate	nalbuphine	Nubain
ketoconazole	Nizoral	nalidixic acid	Neg Gram
labetalol	Normodyne, Trandate	naloxone	Narcan
lactulose syrup	Chronulac	naproxen	Naproxyn
lanatoside C	Cedilanid	naproxen sodium	Anaprox
levarterenol	Levophed	neostigmine	Prostigmin
levodopa	Dopar, Larodopa	niacin (nicotinic acid)	Nicobid, Nicolar
levorphanol	Levo-Dromoran	nifedipine	Procardia
levothyroxine	Synthroid	nitrofurantoin	Furadantin
lidocaine	Xylocaine	nitrogen mustard	Mustargen
lindane	Kwell	nitroglycerin	Nitrobid, Nitrospan, Nitrostat
liothyronine	Cytomel	nitroprusside	Nipride
liotrix	Euthroid, Thyrolar	norepinephrine	Levophed
lithium carbonate	Lithane, Lithobid	norethindrone	Norlutin
lomustine	Cee Nu	norethindrone acetate	Norlutate
loperamide HCl	Imodium	nortriptyline	Aventyl, Pamelor
lorazepam	Ativan	nylidrin	Arlidin
loxapine succinate	Loxitane	nystatin	Mycostatin, Nilstat
magaldrate	Riopan	orphendrine	Norflex
magnesium sulfate	Epsom salt	oxacillin	Prostaphlin
maprotiline	Ludiomil	oxazepam	Serax
mazindol	Sanorex	oxtriphylline	Choledyl
mebendazole	Vermox	oxycodone, ASA	Percodan
mecamylamine	Inversine	oxycodone, acetaminophen	Percocet
mechlorethamine	Mustargen, nitrogen mustard	oxymetazoline, nasal	Afrin, Dristan Long Lasting

Generic Name	Trade Name	Generic Name	Trade Name
oxyphenbutazone	Tandearil	pyridostigmine	Mestinon
oxytetracycline	Terramycin	pyrvinium pamoate	Povan
oxytocin	Pitocin	quinacrine	Atabrine
pancrelipase	Cotazym, Viokase	quinidine gluconate	Quinaglute
pancuronium	Pavulon	quinidine sulfate	Quinora
papaverine	Pavabid, Cerespan	quinine sulfate	Auinamm
paraldehyde	Paral	racepinephrine	Vaponefrin, Asthmanefrin
pargyline	Eutonyl	ranitidine	Zantac
pemoline	Cylert	rauwolfia serpentina	Raudixin
penicillamine	Cuprimine	reserpine	Serpasil
penicillin and benzathine	Bicillin	rifampin	Rimactane, Rifadin
penicillin G potassium	Pfizepen, Pentid	ritodrine	Yutopar
penicillin procaine	Duracillin, crysticillin, Wycillin	salsalate	Disalcid
		scopolamine	Transderm-Scop
penicillin V potassium	Pen-Vee K, V-cillin K	secobarbital	Seconal
pentaerythritol tetranitrate	Peritrate	selenium sulfide	Selsun Blue, Selsun
pentazocine	Talwin	senna	Senokot
pentobarbital	Nembutal	silver sulfadiazine	Silvadene
perphenazine	Trilafon	simethicone	Mylicon
phenazopyridine HCl	Pyridium	sodium polystyrene sulfonate	Kayexalate
phenazopyridine and sulfisoxazole	Azo-Gantrisin	spironolactone	Aldactone
		streptokinase	Streptase
phenelzine sulfate	Nardil	succinylcholine	Anectine
pentoxifylline	Trental	sucralfate	Carafate
phenmetrazine	Preludin	sulfamethoxazole	Gantanol
phenobarbital	Luminal	sulfamethoxazole and trimethoprim	Bactrim, Septra
phenolphthalein	Ex-Lax, Feen-A-Mint		
phenoxymethyl penicillin	V-Cillin, Penicillin VK	sulfasalazine	Azulfidine
phenylbutazone	Butazolidin, Azolid-A	sulfisoxazole	Gantrisin
phenylephrine	Neosynephrine	sulfisoxazole and phenazopyridine	Azo-Gantrisin
phenytoin	Dilantin		
phosphate enema	Fleet enema	sulindac	Clinoril
phosphated carbohydrate solution	Emetrol	tamoxifen	Nolvadex
		temazepam	Restoril
physostigmine	Antilirium	terbutaline	Brethine, Bricanyl
phytonadione (vitamin K_1)	Mephyton, Aquamephyton	tetanus immune globulin	Hyper-tet
pilocarpine	Isoptocarpine	tetracaine	Pontocaine
piroxicam	Feldene	tetracycline	Achromycin, Sumycin
potassium chloride	KLor, Kaon, Cl, Slow K, Micro K, Klorvess	theophylline	Elixophyllin, Theo-Dur
		thioridazine	Mellaril
potassium gluconate	Kaon	thiothixene	Navane
povidone-iodine	Betadine	thyroglobulin	Proloid
prazosin	Minipress	ticarcillin disodium	Ticar
prednisolone	Meticortelone, Delta Cortef	timolol maleate	Biocadren, Timoptic
primidone	Mysoline	tobramycin	Nebcin, Tobrex
probenecid	Benemid	tocainide	Tonocard
procainamide	Pronestyl	tolazamide	Tolinase
procaine	Novocain	tolbutamide	Orinase
procarbazine	Matulane	tranylcypromine sulfate	Parnate
prochlorperazine	Compazine	trazodone	Desyrel
procyclidine	Kemadrin	triamcinolone	Kenacort, Aristocort
promazine	Sparine	triamterene	Dyrenium
promethazine	Phenergan	triamterene and hydrochlorothiazide	Dyazide, Maxzide
propantheline	Probanthine		
propoxyphene	Darvon	triazolam	Halcion
propoxyphene, napsylate, acetaminophen	Davocet-N	trifluoperazine	Stelazine
		trihexyphenidyl HCl	Artane, Tremin
propranolol	Inderal	trimethadione	Tridione
psyllium hydrocolloid	Effersyllium	trimethaphan	Arfonad

Generic Name	Trade Name
trimethobenzamide	Tigan
trimethoprim	Proloprim. Trimpex
undecylenic acid	Desenex
urokinase	Breokinase
valproic acid	Depakene
vancomycin	Vancocin
vasopressin	Pitressin
verapamil	Calan, Isoptin
vidarabine	Vira-A
vinblastine	Velban
vincristine	Oncovin
vitamin B_6	Pyridoxine, Hexabetalin
vitamin B_{12}	cyanocobalamin, Redisol
vitamin C	ascorbic acid
vitamin D	Deltalin
vitamin K_1	phytonadione
warfarin	Coumadin

Drug Interferences with Laboratory Tests

Drugs may modify the results of laboratory tests by:

1. Changing the color of urine or stool, which may result in masking other abnormal circumstances, interfering with specific laboratory tests (colorimetric, photometric, and others), or causing undue concern for the uninformed client.
2. Direct chemical interference with the testing procedure.
3. Specific damage to a body organ, such as the liver or kidneys, or by specific metabolic alterations within the body. Often the reason for the laboratory test interference is unknown. The following sections will note the drugs that may cause test alterations, the type of changes induced (increased or decreased) and specific drug-test interferences when applicable.

CHANGING THE COLOR OF URINE OR STOOL

Medications That May Alter Urine Color

Drug	Possible color changes
amitriptyline (Elavil)	Blue-green
anticoagulants (coumarin and others)	Pink, red, or dark brown (indicative of systemic bleeding)
cascara	In acid urine, brown; basic urine, yellow to pink; on standing, black
iron salts, dextran, and others	Brown to black
laxatives (danthron, senna)	Pink to red or brown
laxatives (phenolphthalein)	Pink to red
levodopa (Laradopa, Dopar) methyldopa (Aldomet, Dopamet✤)	May cause dark urine and sweat; Pink, amber to dark urine
metronidazole (Flagyl)	Dark urine
nitrofurantoins (Furadantin, Macrodantin, Novofuran✤)	Yellow to rusty brown urine
phenazopyridine (Pyridium, Phenazo✤, and others)	Orange red urine; may stain clothing
phenytoin (Dilantin)	Red-brown or darkening of urine
phenothiazines (chlorpromazine, or Thorazine, and others)	Pink, red, or orange urine
rifampin (Rifadin, Rofact✤, and others)	Red, orange, or brown urine, stool, saliva, sweat, and tears

Medications That May Alter Color of Stools

Drug	Possible color changes
antacids with aluminum salts (Maalox, Mylanta, and others)	White specks or discoloration of stools
anticoagulants (coumarin and others)	Red, orange, to black because of internal bleeding
bismuth or iron salts	Black
laxative (phenolphthalein)	Red
laxative (senna)	Yellow, orange to brown
phenazopyridine (Pyridium and others)	Orange, red

DIRECT CHEMICAL INTERFERENCE WITH THE LABORATORY PROCEDURE

Selected Drug Examples of Direct Chemical Interference with Laboratory Tests*

Test	Testing method	Possible result
IN THE PRESENCE OF ACETAMINOPHEN (TYLENOL AND OTHERS)		
Blood glucose	Glucose oxidase/peroxidase method	False decrease
Pancreatic function testing	Bentiromide	False increase
Serum uric acid	Phosphotungstate uric acid test	False increase
IN THE PRESENCE OF ANTICONVULSANTS, SUCH AS PHENYTOIN (DILANTIN), ETHOTOIN (PEGANONE), MEPHENYTOIN (MESANTOIN)		
Thyroid test	Protein-bound iodine (PBI)	False decrease
IN THE PRESENCE OF ANTIHISTAMINES		
Skin testing	Allergen extracts	False negative
IN THE PRESENCE OF NONSTEROIDAL ANTIINFLAMMATORY AGENTS (NSAIDs)		
Urinary bile	Diazo tablets	False positive with mefenamic acid (Ponstel)
Urinary 5-hydroxyindoleacetic acid (5-HIAA) and urinary steroid determinations	Various assays -m-dinitrobenzene	False increase
IN THE PRESENCE OF THE ANTIMUSCARINIC, ATROPINE		
Urine test	phenolsulfonphthalein (PSP) excretion test	False decrease
IN THE PRESENCE OF MEGADOSING WITH ASCORBIC ACID (VITAMIN C)		
Occult blood in stool		False negative
Liver tests, LDH and serum transaminases	Auto-analyzer	Interference
Urine glucose	Glucose oxidase test (Tes-tape)	False decrease
IN THE PRESENCE OF COFFEE, TEA, COLA DRINKS, CHOCOLATE, AND ACETAMINOPHEN		
Theophylline test (clients receiving aminophylline, oxtriphylline, and theophylline)	Spectrophotometric	False increase
IN THE PRESENCE OF CEPHALOSPORIN ANTIBIOTIC		
Blood glucose	Ferricyanide test	False negative with cefuroxime
Antiglobulin test	Combs test, direct	False positive in neonates when mother received cephalosporins or cephamycins before delivery
Urine glucose	Copper sulfate tests (Benedict's or Fehling's)	False positive or increase
Bleeding time (coagulation)	Prothrombin time (PT)	Increased or prolonged with cefamandole, cefoperazone, and cefotetan; May require therapeutic intervention with vitamin K
IN THE PRESENCE OF HEPARIN		
Thyroid test	Resin T$_3$ uptake and, possibly, other thyroid test	Increase in serum thyroxine

*For additional drug-test interferences, see appendix bibliography.

SPECIFIC DAMAGE TO A BODY ORGAN

Following are examples of drugs altering laboratory tests because of unwanted or adverse effects on the liver or kidneys. For each section, generic names or general drug categories are listed. (Examples of registered trade names that are usually available in the United States or trade names generally available in Canada [✽] follow most of the entries.)

DRUGS THAT ARE HEPATOTOXIC

acetaminophen (Tylenol and others) with chronic, high-dose therapy or in an acute overdose situation

4-aminoquinolines or chloroquine (Aralen), hydroxychloroquine (Plaquenil)

amiodarone (Cordarone)

anabolic steroid agents such as dromostanolone (Drolban), ethylestrenol (Maxibolin), nandrolone (Anabolin IM, Durabolin), and others

antithyroid agents (Tapazole)

asparaginase (Elspar)

azlocillin (Azlin)

carbamazepine (Tegretol, Mazepine♣)

carmustine (BCNU)

contraceptives, estrogen containing, oral

dantrolene (Dantrium)

daunorubicin (Cerubidine)

disulfiram (Antabuse)

divalproex (Depakote, Epival♣)

erythromycin (most often with estolate form, Ilosone)

estrogens (DES, conjugated estrogens and others)

etretinate (Tegison)

gold compounds (Ridaura and others)

halothane (Fluothane, Somnothane)

isoniazid (INH, Nydrazid, Rimifon♣)

ketoconazole, oral (Nizoral)

mercaptopurine (Purinethol)

methotrexate (Mexate, Folex)

methyldopa (Aldomet)

mezlocillin (Mezlin, Baypen♣)

naltrexone, chronic high-dose therapy (Trexan)

nitrofurans (Furadantin, Macrodantin, Novofuran♣)

phenothiazines (Thorazine, Largactil♣, and others)

phenytoin (Dilantin)

pipercillin (Pipracil)

plicamycin (Mithracin)

rifampin (Rifadin, Rimactane, Rofact♣)

sulfonamides, systemic (Gantrisin, Gantanol, and others)

tetracycline, intravenous, high-dose therapy, especially in pregnant women.

valproic acid (Depakene, Depakote, Epival♣)

DRUGS THAT ARE NEPHROTOXIC

acyclovir, parenteral (Zovirax)

aminoglycosides antibiotics (Garamycin, Nebcin, and others)

amphotericin B, parenteral (Fungizone)

analgesic combinations with acetaminophen and aspirin or salicylates used chronically in high-dose therapy (Excedrin, Trigesic, and others.)

antiinflammatory analgesics, nonsteroidal (NSAID)

capreomycin (Capastat)

captopril (Capoten)

cisplatin (Platinol)

cyclosporine (Sandimmune)

demeclocycline (Declomycin)

edetate calcium disodium, high doses (Calcium Disodium Versenate)

enalapril (Vasotec)

gold compounds (Ridaura and others)

lithium (Eskalith, Lithane, and others)

methotrexate, high doses (Mexate, Folex)

methoxyflurane (Penthrane)

neomycin, oral (Mycifradin)

penicillamine (Cuprimine, Distamine♣)

pentamidine (Pentam, Lomidine♣)

plicamycin (Mithracin)

rifampin (Rifadin, Rofact♣)

streptozocin (Zanosar)

sulfonamides, systemic (Gantrisin, Gantanol, and others)

tetracyclines (with exception of doxycycline and minocycline)

vancomycin, parenteral (Vancocin I.V., Diatracin♣)

sulfonamides, systemic (Gantrisin, Gantanol, and others)

tetracyclines (with exception of doxycycline and minocycline)

vancomycin, parenteral (Vancocin I.V., Diatracin♣)

SELECTED DRUG EFFECTS ON SPECIFIC BLOOD SUBSTANCES*

Drugs	Glucose	K⁺	Na⁺	PT	SGOT/SGPT	Uric acid	BUN	Bilirubin
aminoglycosides (garamycin, and others)		(−)	(−)		(+)		(+)	(+)
anticonvulsants (phenytoin, mephenytoin)	(+)							
antidepressants, tricyclic (amitriptyline, and others)	(+/−)							
antiinflammatory analgesics, nonsteroidal (NSAID) (ibuprofen/piroxicam)	(−)							
mefenamic acid				(+)				
diflunisal						(−)		
all agents					(+)			

Drugs	Glucose	K⁺	Na⁺	PT	SGOT/ SGPT	Uric acid	BUN	Bilirubin
Beta adrenergic blocking agents (propranolol and others)		(+)			(+) esp. with labetalol	(+)	(+)	
carbamazepine (Tegretol)					(+)		(+)	(+)
carbidopa/levodopa (Sinemet)					(+)		(+)	(+)
cephalosporins (cefamandole, cefoperazone, cefoxitin, moxalactam)				(+)				
majority of cephalosporins					(+)			
cinoxacin (Cinobac)					(+)		(+)	
cisplatin (Platinol)		(−)				(+)	(+)	
diuretics, loop (bumetanide, furosemide, ethacrynic acid)	(+)	(−)	(−)			(+)	(+)	
diuretics, thiazides (hydrochlorothiazide and others).	(+)	(−)	(−)			(+)		(+)
diuretics, potassium-sparing (amiloride, spironolactone, triamterene)	(+)	(+)	(−)			(+)	(+)	
methyldopa (Aldomet)		(+)	(+)		(+)	(+)	(+)	(+)
norfloxacin (Noroxin)					(+)		(+)	
propoxyphene (Darvon and others)					(+)			(+)
Penicillin G-K		(+)						
injectable azlocillin, carbenicillin, mezlocillin, piperacillin, or ticarcillin			(+)					
azlocillin, ticarcillin						(−)		
azlocillin, mezlocillin, piperacillin, ticarcillin								(+)
majority of penicillins					(+) except methicillin, nafcillin, penicillin G-V			
prazosin (Minipress)			(+)					
rifampin (Rifadin and others)					(+)	(+)	(+)	(+)
trimethoprim (Proloprim)					(+)		(+)	(+)
tetracyclines (Terramycin, and others)					(+)		(+) except doxycycline minocycline	(+)
valproic acid (Depakene, Depakote)					(+)			(+)

*Specific blood substances: serum glucose, potassium, sodium, prothrombin time (PT), SGOT/SGPT (serum glutamic-oxaloacetic transaminase, glutamic-pyruvic transaminase), serum uric acid, blood urea nitrogen (BUN), bilirubin. The possible effects of the drugs on laboratory tests are noted as follows: *blank spaces*, no reported effect; *(+)*, possible increase; *(−)*, possible decrease.

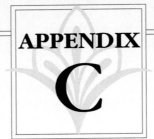
Food-Drug Interactions

Drug category/medication	Foods to avoid	Reason
ANTIBIOTICS		
erythromycin, penicillins*	Meals, acidic fruit juices, citrus fruits, or acidic beverages, such as cola drinks	The antibiotics are acid labile (reduced absorption). Take medication 1 hour before meals or apart from acidic foods or 2 hours after meals.
tetracyclines	Calcium-containing foods: milk, ice cream, yogurt, cheeses, and others	Calcium may complex with tetracycline, resulting in reduced absorption of the antibiotic. Most tetracyclines, with the exception of doxycycline and minocycline, should be administered 1 hour before or 2 hours after meals.
ANTICOAGULANTS		
warfarin (Coumadin), dicumarol, heparin	Beef liver and green leafy vegetables contain vitamin K (spinach, cabbage, brussel sprouts)	Vitamin K can counteract therapeutic action of anticoagulants. A normal, balanced diet will not interfere with this medication. Fad or extreme diets with foods high in vitamin K can affect anticoagulant activity.
MAO INHIBITORS		
isocarboxazid (Marplan), phenelzine (Nardil), tranylcypromine (Parnate)	Foods with high tyramine content, such as aged cheese, (brie, cheddar, processed American, camembert, and others), aged meat, sour cream, yogurt, pickled herring, chicken liver, canned figs, raisins, bananas, avocados, soy sauce, yeast extract, meat tenderizers, alcoholic beverages such as beer and wine (chianti, sherry, or hearty red wines), sausages, chocolate, anchovies	Concurrent use may result in severe headache, nosebleed, chest pain, eyes sensitive to light, or severe hypertension which may result in a hypertensive crisis.

*Erythromycin base (E-Mycin, Ery-Tab, E-Mycin Eryc) or stearates (Erypar, Erythrocin Stearate, Ethril, Wyamycin S) are best absorbed in the fasting state. Erythromycin ethylsuccinate (E.E.S.), estolate (Ilosone), and enteric-coated erythromycin may be given before or with meals. Penicillin, such as penicillin G, ampicillin, cloxacillin, cyclacillin, dicloxacillin, nafcillin, and oxacillin may have decreased absorption if given with food or acidic-type products.

Patient Teaching Tips for Medication Administration

GENERAL INFORMATION FOR HOME CARE

1. To hasten transport and action of oral solid medications, advise client to take water (1 to 2 ounces) before taking solid dosage forms. Whenever possible, a full glass of water should be taken with the ordered medications (Kikendall, 1983).
2. Advise client/family members not to transfer medication to other containers nor to allow others to take their medications.
3. Be sure medication orders are clearly written and understood by all. Include medication, concentration, dosage, time interval, and purpose for written orders.
4. Clearly print any specific medication instructions given for the care of this client.

GENERAL DRUG INFORMATION FOR THE NURSE

1. Antacids, milk of magnesia, Metamucil (and other bulk-forming laxatives) and antidiarrheal agents, unless specifically ordered for concurrent drug administration by the physician, should always be spaced 1 to 2 hours apart from all medications. (Concurrent drug administration may result in a reduction in drug absorption.)
2. Metamucil (and other bulk-forming laxatives) should be mixed in a glass of water or juice immediately before administration. It is recommended that a full glass of fluid follow the previous glass, if not contraindicated by disease process. (Reduced fluid intake can lead to G-I blockade/impaction.)
3. Antacid tablets — instruct client to chew tablets thoroughly and take with a glass of water. (Reduced fluid intake can lead to G-I blockade.)
4. Iron products (Fer-in-sol, Mol Iron, and others) — advise client and/or family not to administer with antacids, eggs, milk or milk products, or fiber cereal. (Concurrent administration may reduce iron absorption.)

Time to Draw Blood Levels for Specific Medications

Serum drug levels are used to aid the physician (1) in determining dosage adjustments for drugs that have a narrow range between therapeutic effect and toxicity, thus ensuring drug efficacy and decreasing the potential for toxicity, and (2) to providing information to help evaluate a suspected toxicity or noncompliance.

Blood samples are usually drawn according to the pharmacokinetics of the individual drug. For example, to obtain a steady state (SS) serum level, the blood sample should be drawn at approximately 5 half-lives after therapy was instituted. For theophylline and phenytoin (Dilantin), the time to withdraw blood would be just before a dose, after at least 2 days of drug therapy.

Gentamicin (Garamycin) has a relatively short half-life; therefore peak and trough levels are usually ordered to ensure adequate therapy. The peak serum level (P) is usually obtained 15 to 30 minutes after an intravenous dose or 1 hour after an intramuscular dose. The trough (T) serum level should be drawn 15 minutes before the next scheduled dose. Trough serum levels are used to predict the risk of adverse reactions; a rising trough level or levels above 2 μg/ml have been associated with increased toxicity.

Therapeutic Ranges of Serum Drug Concentrations

Drug	Serum concentration		Time for blood sampling (hours after last dose)*
	Ther (µg/ml)	Tr (µg/ml)	
ANTIBIOTICS			
amikacin (Amikin)	15-25	5	See previous discussion on gentamicin
gentamicin (Garamycin)	4-10	2	See previous discussion on gentamicin
netilmicin (Netromycin)	6-10	4	See previous discussion on gentamicin
tobramycin (Nebcin)	4-10	2	See previous discussion on gentamicin
ANTICONVULSANTS			
carbamazepine (Tegretol)	4-12		SS 1-2 wk. Before next dose (Tr).
phenobarbital	15-40		SS 10-30 days Before next dose (Tr).
phenytoin (Dilantin)	10-20		SS 1-2 wk. Oral (Tr). before next dose; IV, 2-4 hr after loading dose.
primidone (Mysoline)	5-12		SS 2-3 days for primidone; phenobarbital as above. Before next dose (Tr.)
valproic acid (Depakene, Depakote)	50-100		SS 1-2 days. Before next dose (Tr).
CARDIOVASCULAR DRUGS			
digoxin (Lanoxin)	0.9-2 ng/ml		SS 1 wk. Before next dose (Tr). At least 6 hr after last dose to allow for drug distribution in the body.
lidocaine (Xylocaine)	1.5-5		SS 6-12 hr. Anytime during IV infusion.
procainamide (Pronestyl)	4-10		SS 12-24 hr. Before next dose (Tr.)
quinidine (various drugs)	2.3-5		SS 1.5 days. Before next dose (Tr.)
RESPIRATORY DRUGS			
theophylline (various drugs)	asthma 10-20		SS 1-2 days in adults, up to 1 week in neonates. IV infusion, anytime; oral, before next dose (Tr).

*SS, Time to reach drug steady state. The SS time is noted first, then the suggested appropriate time of blood sampling for the specific drug.

Appendix Bibliography

Carey, KW, and Goldberg, KE, eds: Clinical pocket manual: medications and I.V.s, Springhouse, Pa, 1987, Nursing 87 Books.

Elenbaas, RM: When to monitor blood drug levels, Hosp Ther 11(7):27-39, 1986.

Hahn, NH, and Nissen, JC: Compatibility of pre-op medications mixed in a syringe, Parenterals 6(2):7, 1988.

Knoben, JE, and Anderson, PO: Handbook of clinical drug data, ed 5, Hamilton, Ill 1983, Drug Intelligence Publications, Inc.

Powers, DE, and Moore, AO: Food medication interactions, ed 5, Phoenix, 1986. Food-Medication Interactions.

Riemer, WE: The laboratory manual, Miami, Fla, 1982, Baptist Hospital of Miami, Inc.

Trissel, LA: ASHP handbook on injectable drugs, Bethesda, Md, 1986, American Society of Hospital Pharmacists, Inc.

United States Pharmacopeial Convention: Drug information for the health care provider, vols IA, IB, and II, ed 8, Rockville, Md, The Convention.

Wallach, J: Interpretation of diagnostic tests, ed 4, Boston, Little, Brown & Co.

Zwiebel, N: Brand-generic comparison handbook, Rockford, Ill, 1984, UDL Laboratories, Inc.

Index

Pyrroleacetic acid derivatives, 992-993

Q

QRS complex, 445, 445i
Quaalude♣; *see* methaqualone
Quarzan; *see* clidinium
Quelicin; *see* succinylcholine
Questran; *see* cholestyramine
Quick Pep; *see* caffeine
quinacrine HCl
   action and pharmacokinetics of, 952, 979
   alopecia induced by, 1044
   contact dermatitis caused by, 1046
   dosage and administration of, 952-953, 979
   fixed eruptions caused by, 1045
   for helminthiasis, 974t
   interaction of
      with other agents, 952
      with primaquine phosphate, 955
   lichenoid reactions caused by, 1044
   morbilliform reactions caused by, 1044
   nursing considerations for, 953, 979-980
   side effects/adverse reactions of, 952t, 979
Quinaglute; *see* quinidine gluconate
Quinamm; *see* quinine sulfate
quinethazone
   dosage and administration of, 587t
   photosensitivity caused by, 1047
Quinidex; *see* quinidine sulfate
quinidine, 465, 475
   adverse reactions to, in anesthetized client, 224
   classification and comparative electrophysiologic
      properties of, 466t
   diarrhea caused by, 708
   fixed eruptions caused by, 1045
   interaction of
      with acetazolamide, 289, 583, 731
      with carbonic anhydrase inhibitors, 731
      with dichlorphenamide, 731
      with diltiazem, 517
      with direct-acting cholinergic drugs, 373
      with group I-A antidysrhythmics, 467
      with methazolamide, 731
      with oral anticoagulants, 547t
      with rifampin, 965
   intoxication from, urine pH and, 75
   lichenoid reactions caused by, 1044
   ototoxic effects of, 751t
   pharmacokinetics of, 468t
   photosensitivity caused by, 1047
   purpura caused by, 1044
   resting membrane potential and, 467i
   side effects/adverse reactions of, 469t
quinidine gluconate
   dosage and administration of, 473
   interactions of, 473
   nursing considerations for, 473-475
   properties of, 472-473
quinidine polygalacturonate
   dosage and administration of, 473
   interactions of, 473
   nursing considerations for, 473-475
   properties of, 472-473
quinidine salts, dosage and administration of, 474t
quinidine sulfate
   dosage and administration of, 473
   interactions of, 473
   nursing considerations for, 473-475
   properties of, 472-473
Quinidine syncope, 475
quinine
   abuse of, 146
   alkalinity of, 47

quinine—cont'd
   contact dermatitis caused by, 1046
   fixed eruptions caused by, 1045
   as heroin adulterant, 151t
   ocular side effects of, 737t
   photosensitivity caused by, 1047
   signs and symptoms of abuse of, 152, 153
quinine sulfate
   action and pharmacokinetics of, 951
   dosage and administration of, 951
   interactions of, 951
   nursing considerations for, 951-952
   side effects/adverse reactions of, 952t
Quinite; *see* quinine sulfate
Quinolones, 929-930
   side effects/adverse reactions of, 918t
Quinora; *see* quinidine sulfate
Quotane; *see* dimethisoquin

R

Rabies immune globulin, dosage and nursing considerations for, 1029t
Rabies vaccine
   administration and nursing considerations for,
      1025t
   during pregnancy, 1020t
racepinephrine inhalation solution
   dosage and administration of, 632-633
   interactions of, 632
   properties and pharmacokinetics of, 632
Rad, defined, 1144
Radiation, ionizing, 1144
Radioactive agents
   dosage and administration of, 1146-1147
   indications for, 1144-1145
   mechanism of action of, 1142, 1144
   nursing considerations for, 1147
   pharmacokinetics of, 1146
radioactive iodine; *see* sodium iodide I 131
Radioactive tracers, diagnostic tests using, 1142t
Radioimmunoassay tests, drugs causing false-positive results in, 148
radioiodinated I 125 fibrinogen, diagnostic tests using, 1143t
Radionuclides, 1142
Radiopaque agents
   action and pharmacokinetics of, 1139
   diagnostic tests using, 1140i
   dosage and administration of, 1141
   interactions of, 1141
   nursing considerations for, 1141-1142
   side effects/adverse reactions of, 1140-1141
Radiostol; *see* ergocalciferol
Radiostol Forte; *see* ergocalciferol
ranitidine
   interaction of, with ketoconazole, 939
   for peptic ulcer
      dosage and administration of, 693t-694t
      interactions of, 691-692
      nursing considerations for, 692
      pharmacokinetics of, 691t
      properties of, 691
      side effects/adverse reactions of, 692t
RAS; *see* Reticular activating system
Rash, drug overdoses causing, 152
Rauwolfia alkaloids
   for hypertension, pharmacokinetics of, 488t
   interactions of, with monoamine oxidase (MAO)
      inhibitors, 332
   sexual function and, 849t
Receptor antagonists, H₁; *see* H₁ receptor antagonists

Receptors, 308
   adrenergic, 367
      sensitivities of, 387
   alpha, 367
   alpha adrenergic, 387
   beta, 367
      classes of, 417
   beta adrenergic, 387
   in bronchial smooth muscle, 621
   defined, 53
   dopaminergic, 367
   estrogen; *see* Estrogen receptors
   hormones and, 757
   muscarinic; *see* Muscarinic receptors
   opioid; *see* Opioid receptors
   presynaptic adrenergic, 387
   progesterone; *see* Progesterone receptors
   relationship of, to drugs, 53
Rectum, drug absorption by, 47
Red blood cells; *see* Erythrocytes
red petrolatum as sunscreen, 1050
Redoxon; *see* ascorbic acid
Redoxon♣; *see* ascorbic acid
Reentry phenomenon, 465i
   ectopic beats and, 464
Reflex act
   processes of, 357-358
   sensory input, CNS connection, and motor output
      of, 358t
Reflex arc
   defined, 357
   sensory input, CNS connection, and motor output
      of, 358t
Reflex control system, 357-358
Reflexes, monosynaptic and polysynaptic, blockade
   of, by benzodiazepines, 246
Reflux esophagitis, 671
Refractoriness, 444
Refractory period
   digitalis glycosides and, 454
   effective, 444
Refractory responses, 308
Regibon♣; *see* diethylpropion
Regitine; *see* phentolamine HCl
Reglan; *see* metoclopramide
Regonol; *see* pyridostigmine bromide
Rela; *see* carisoprodol
Relaxation techniques
   in pain management, 196
   as substitution for drug therapy, 133-134
Relefact TRH; *see* protirelin
Rem, defined, 1144
Renal damage, drug-caused, 58
Renal disease
   end-stage, 612
   pharmacologic therapy for, nurse's role in, 613-
      615
Renal failure
   acute, causes of, 611
   chronic
      causes of, 611-612
      special needs of client with, 612
   drug modifications in, 612-613
   signs and symptoms of, 612
Renal function, measurement of, 612
Renal insufficiency
   dosing methods for client with, 613
   dosing recommendations in, 614t
   signs and symptoms of, 612
Renal system, drugs for dysfunction of, 611-615
RenAmin, components of, 1115
Renese; *see* polythiazide

ALSO AVAILABLE!

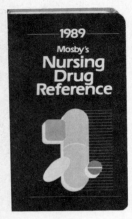

MOSBY'S 1989 NURSING DRUG REFERENCE
by Linda Skidmore-Roth, R.N., M.S.N., N.P.
(5757-1)

MOSBY'S 1989 NURSING DRUG REFERENCE is a practical, A-to-Z drug handbook that helps you administer the most frequently prescribed drugs with confidence. Organized alphabetically for quick clinical reference, the text details information on over 1,000 generic drugs, including 4,000 trade names. Thoroughly revised and updated, this new edition contains over 30 drugs recently approved by the FDA.

- Each drug monograph contains generic name, U.S. and Canadian trade names, pronunciation, functional and chemical classifications, action, use, dosages and routes, side/adverse reactions, contraindications, precautions, pharmacokinetics, interactions/incompatibilities, nursing considerations, and where appropriate, toxicity and treatment of overdose.
- Shows common side effects in *italics* and life-threatening adverse reactions in ***bold italics*** for quick differentiation.
- Highlights nursing considerations in a separate color that allows for instant retrieval of essential clinical information.
- Includes chemical classifications to help you understand how drugs within the same chemical class are related.
- Includes several helpful appendixes: drug incompatibility table, FDA pregnancy categories, nomogram, abbreviations, formulas for drug calculations, and a controlled substances schedule.

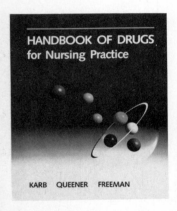

HANDBOOK OF DRUGS FOR NURSING PRACTICE
by Virginia Burke Karb, R.N., M.S.N.; Sherry F. Queener, Ph.D.; and Julia B. Freeman, Ph.D.
(2608-0)

HANDBOOK OF DRUGS FOR NURSING PRACTICE groups more than 1,000 commonly administered drugs by class, to highlight the similarities and dissimilarities of related drugs. A feature unique to this handbook, nursing considerations are grouped into three categories: those related to side effects and toxicities; those related to drug administration; and those related to patient and family education. This practical handbook includes information specific to special patient populations — pregnant, pediatric, and elderly clients — for each drug listed.

- Provides helpful summary tables on related drugs in the same family to aid you in comparing drug similarities and dissimilarities.
- Groups nursing considerations into a consistent, clinical framework, giving you a reliable source for specific concerns for special patient populations.
- Includes FDA pregnancy categories.
- NEW! Integrates side effects with specific nursing actions throughout the reference to demonstrate cause and effect relationships that you can readily apply in the clinical setting.

These references are ideal for every nursing student and practitioner that administers drugs. To order, ask your bookstore manager or call toll-free 800-221-7700, ext. 15A. We look forward to hearing from you.

FACTORS ALTERING DRUG RESPONSES AND SUMMARY OF NURSING CONSIDERATIONS

Factor and pertinent description	Nursing considerations
AGE Infants—immature systems Children—smaller doses needed Elderly—depressed hepatic and renal systems	Modify dosages. Children have a different physiologic profile and body mass distribution. Thus, dose per kilogram is individualized. It could be more or less than in an adult. Elderly clients may also have concomitant physical conditions that alter drug effects; altered excretion mechanism, too, may require less drug or different scheduling of medication.
BODY MASS The greater the volume of distribution, the lower the concentration of drug in the body compartments Calculation: average adult dose based on drug quantity that will produce a particular effect in 50% of population between the ages of 18 and 65 and weighing about 150 pounds (70 kg)	Adjust dosage in proportion to body mass. For children, dosage frequently is determined on the basis of amount of drug per kilogram of body weight or body surface area.
SEX Women smaller than men; definite differences during pregnancy and in relative proportions of fat and water; drugs vary by water or fat solubility	Allow for size differential and whether a drug is water or lipid soluble. Avoid drugs during pregnancy unless an absolute necessity exists.
ENVIRONMENTAL MILIEU Mood and behavior modified by (1) drug itself, (2) personality of the user, (3) environment of the user, and (4) interaction of these three factors; other factors: sensory—deprivation or overload; physical environment—cold vs heat, oxygen deprivation (altitude)	Be aware of the physical situation of the client with regard to heat and cold, interactions with other individuals, drug effects, and how the client generally reacts to situations.
TIME OF ADMINISTRATION Food—presence or absence Biologic rhythms—sleep-wake cycle, drug-metabolizing enzyme rhythms, corticosteroid secretion rhythm, blood pressure rhythms, circadian (24-hour) cycle in absorption and urinary excretion; also rhythm of drug receptor susceptibility	Give irritating drugs when there is food in the client's stomach. Make every effort to understand the client's normal and abnormal rhythms, and seek possible relationships between the client's biologic rhythms and reactions to drug therapy. Administer drugs at same time of day. Altered body cycles (shift workers) may result in altered response to a drug.
PATHOLOGIC STATE Presence and severity of pathologic state—pain intensifies need for opiates; anxiety produces resistance to large doses of tranquilizing drugs; presence of circulatory, hepatic, and/or renal dysfunctions interferes with physiologic processes of drug action	Take into account any pain, disease, or altered metabolic state of the client and adjust dosage accordingly.
GENETIC FACTORS Genetically determined abnormal susceptibility to a chemical, or "idiosyncratic response"	Be aware that any client may show an idiosyncratic response. Always monitor closely, especially when beginning therapy, for abnormal susceptibility. Be aware of common drug idiosyncrasies.
PSYCHOLOGIC FACTORS Symbolic investment in drugs and faith in their efficacy Placebo effect Hostility toward or mistrust of medicine or health personnel	Be aware of the attitude and the impression the nurse creates at the time of drug administration, and use them to enhance the drug's effects.